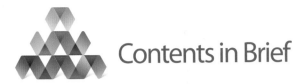 Contents in Brief

 W9-ABN-225

# Critical Care Nursing
## A Holistic Approach

**Patricia Gonce Morton, RN, PhD, ACNP-BC, FAAN**
Dean and Professor
Louis H. Peery Presidential Endowed Chair
University of Utah College of Nursing
Salt Lake City, Utah

**Dorrie K. Fontaine, RN, PhD, FAAN**
Sadie Heath Cabaniss Professor of Nursing and Dean
University of Virginia School of Nursing
Charlottesville, Virginia

*ELEVENTH EDITION*

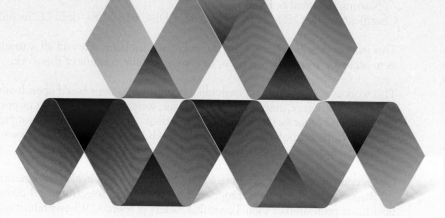

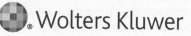

Philadelphia • Baltimore • New York • London
Buenos Aires • Hong Kong • Sydney • Tokyo

*Senior Acquisitions Editor:* Kelley Squazzo
*Senior Development Editor:* Helen Kogut
*Freelance Editor:* Rosanne Hallowell/Beverly Tscheschlog
*Editorial Assistant:* Leo Gray
*Production Project Manager:* Marian Bellus
*Design Coordinator:* Teresa Mallon
*Illustration Coordinator:* Jennifer Clements
*Manufacturing Coordinator:* Karin Duffield
*Marketing Manager:* Katie Schlesinger
*Prepress Vendor:* S4Carlisle Publishing Services

11th edition

**Library of Congress Cataloging-in-Publication Data**

Names: Morton, Patricia Gonce, 1952–editor. | Fontaine, Dorrie K., editor.
Title: Critical care nursing: a holistic approach / [edited by] Patricia
   Gonce Morton, PhD, RN, ACNP-BC, FAAN, Dean and Professor, Louis H. Peery
   Presidential Endowed Chair, University of Utah College of Nursing, Salt
   Lake City, Utah, Dorrie K. Fontaine, PhD, RN, FAAN, Sadie Heath Cabaniss
   Professor of Nursing and Dean, University of Virginia School of Nursing,
   Charlottesville, VA.
Description: 11th edition. | Philadelphia: Wolters Kluwer Health, [2018] |
   Includes bibliographical references and index.
Identifiers: LCCN 2016049219 | ISBN 9781496315625 (hardback)
Subjects: LCSH: Intensive care nursing. | Holistic nursing. | BISAC: MEDICAL
   / Nursing / Critical & Intensive Care.
Classification: LCC RT120.I5 C744 2018 | DDC 616.02/8—dc23 LC record available at https://lccn.loc.gov/2016049219

CCS1216

*To all critical care nurses. Thanks for all you do for critically ill patients and families. Your expertise and compassionate caring transform the lives of those you serve.*

*To our husbands John and Barry. Thanks for your never-ending support, love, and encouragement.*

Trish and Dorrie

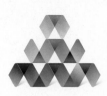# Contributors to the Eleventh Edition

**K. Brooke Anderson, RN, BSN, ACNP-BC**
R Adams Cowley Shock Trauma Center
University of Maryland Medical Center
Baltimore, Maryland

**Sara Angle, RN**
Clinical Nurse Educator of Surgical ICU
University of Utah Hospital
Salt Lake City, Utah

**Nathaniel M. Apatov, PhD, MSN, MHS, CRNA**
Associate Professor
Old Dominion University
Virginia Beach, Virginia

**Carla A. Aresco, CRNP**
Senior Clinical Program Manager
R Adams Cowley Shock Trauma Center
University of Maryland Medical Center
Baltimore, Maryland

**Elyse Atkielski, RN, BSN**
Dialysis Nurse
The University of Arizona Medical Center
Tucson, Arizona

**Mona N. Bahouth, MD, MSN**
Johns Hopkins Hospital
Baltimore, Maryland

**Micah Baker, RN, BSN, NPDS**
Staff Development Educator
University of Utah Hospital and Clinics
Salt Lake City, Utah

**Kara C. Barquist, RN, BSN, CCRN**
Interim Nurse Manager
University of Iowa Hospitals and Clinics
Iowa City, Iowa

**Kathryn S. Bizek, MSN, ACNS-BC, CCRN**
Nurse Practitioner, Cardiology
VA Ann Arbor Healthcare System
Ann Arbor, Michigan

**Nancy Blake, RN, PhD, CCRN, NEA-BC, FAAN**
Director, PCS Critical Care Services
Associate Adjunct Professor UCLA
Children's Hospital Los Angeles
Los Angeles, California

**Shawn Brast, RN, MSN, CCRN, NREMT-P**
Team Educator, Critical Care Transport Nurse
Johns Hopkins Lifeline
The Johns Hopkins Hospital
Baltimore, Maryland

**Sharee Brinton, RN, BSN, CCRN**
Clinical Nurse Educator
University of Utah Hospital
Salt Lake City, Utah

**Tacia Bullard, RN, MSN**
Assistant Nurse Manager, Cardiovascular Intensive Care Unit
University of Iowa Hospitals and Clinics
Iowa City, Iowa

**Ameera Chakravarthy, MS, ACNP-BC, FNP-BC**
Clinical Instructor
University of Maryland School of Nursing
Baltimore, Maryland

**Garrett K. Chan, PhD, APRN, BC-PCM, CEN**
Director of Advanced Practice, Stanford Health Care
Clinical Associate Professor, Stanford School of Medicine
Stanford, California

**Dennis J. Cheek, RN, PhD, FAHA**
Abell-Hanger Professor of Gerontological Nursing
Texas Christian University
Harris College of Nursing and Health Sciences
Fort Worth, Texas

**Vicki J. Coombs, PhD, RN, FAHA, CES**
Chief Nursing Administrator, Keiser University
Ft. Lauderdale, Florida
Senior Vice President, Spectrum Clinical Research, Inc.
Towson, Maryland

**Christine M. Couchman, RN, MS, BSN**
Clinical Education Specialist
AHA Training Center Coordinator
University of Maryland Medical Center
Baltimore, Maryland

**Joan M. Davenport, RN, PhD**
Assistant Professor, Vice Chair
Department of Organizational Systems and Adult Health
University of Maryland School of Nursing
Baltimore, Maryland

**Meghan E. DelMastro, RN, BSN, CWOCN**
Certified Wound, Ostomy and Continence Nurse Specialist
University of Utah Hospital and Clinics and The Huntsman
 Cancer Hospital and Institute
Salt Lake City, Utah

Tamara Ekker, RN, MS
Clinical Instructor
University of Utah College of Nursing
Salt Lake City, Utah

Nicholas Fawcett, RN, BSN
Registered Nurse
University of Utah Hospital
Salt Lake City, Utah

Nancy Kern Feeley, RN, MS, CRNP
Nephrology Adult Nurse Practitioner
Divisions of Nephrology, Johns Hopkins University School
    of Medicine
Baltimore, Maryland

Joshua A. Ferguson, RN, MS, ACNP, ANP-BC
Nurse Practitioner Pulmonary Critical Care
Intermountain Healthcare
Murray, Utah

Dorrie K. Fontaine, RN, PhD, FAAN
Sadie Heath Cabaniss Professor of Nursing and Dean
University of Virginia School of Nursing
Charlottesville, Virginia

Brittany Garey, RN, BSN
Registered Nurse
University of Utah Hospital
Salt Lake City, Utah

Stephanie Gire, RN, MSN, ACCN
Clinical Nurse Educator
University of Utah Hospital
Salt Lake City, Utah

Christine Grady, RN, PhD
Chief, Department of Bioethics
Clinical Center
National Institutes of Health
Bethesda, Maryland

Debby Greenlaw, MS, CCRN, ACNPC, ACHPN
Director of Palliative Care, Acute Care Nurse
    Practitioner
Providence Hospitals
Columbia, South Carolina

Thomasine D. Guberski, PhD, CRNP
Director, Health Program—Nursing
Institute of Human Virology
University of Maryland School of Medicine
Baltimore, Maryland

Janis Gunnel, BS, RN, CCRN
RN-Nurse Educator
Huntsman Cancer Hospital
Salt Lake City, Utah

John C. Hagan, RN, MS, CCRN, ACNP-BC
Acute Care Nurse Practitioner
University of Maryland Medical Center
Baltimore, Maryland

Beth Hammer, MSN, RN, ANP-BC
Program Manager for Nursing Excellence/Nurse Practitioner
Clement J. Zablocki VA Medical Center
Milwaukee, Wisconsin

Jan M. Headley, RN, BS
Principal
Consultants in Acute and Critical Care
Yankee Hill, California

Janie Heath, PhD, APRN-BC, FAAN
Dean and Warwick Endowed Professor of Nursing
University of Kentucky College of Nursing
Lexington, Kentucky

Genell Hilton, PhD, CRNP
Nurse Practitioner, Traima Service
San Francisco City and County
San Francisco, California

Janice J. Hoffman, PhD, RN, ANEF
Associate Dean of Academic Affairs
University of Missouri, Sinclair School of Nursing
Columbia, Missouri

Dorene M. Holcombe, RN, MS, ACNP, CCRN
Nephrology Acute Care Nurse Practitioner
Division of Nephrology, Johns Hopkins University School
    of Medicine
Baltimore, Maryland

Karen L. Johnson, PhD, RN
Research Director, Nursing
Banner Health
Phoenix, Arizona

Karen L. Johnson, PhD, RN
Research Director, Nursing
Banner Health
Phoenix, Arizona

Dennis W. Jones, RN, DNP, NREMT-P
Safety & Quality Officer, Lifeline Critical Care Transport Team
The Johns Hopkins Hospital
Baltimore, Maryland

Roberta Kaplow, APRN-CCNS, PhD, AOCNS, CCRN
Clinical Nurse Specialist
Emory University Hospital
Atlanta, Georgia

Jane Faith Kapustin, PhD, CRNP, BC-ADM, FAANP,
FAAN
Clinical Science Liaison, Diabetes, Medical Affairs
AstraZeneca Pharmaceuticals
Columbia, Maryland

Elizabeth Kozub, RN, MS, CCNS, CCRN, CNRN
Clinical Nurse Specialist, Neurosciences
Abbott Northwestern Hospital
Minneapolis, Minnesota

Megan Cecere Lynn, RN, PhD, FNE-A
Clinical Practice Coordinator
University of Maryland Medical Center
Baltimore, Maryland

Rebecca E. MacIntyre, MSN, RN, ACNP-BC
Neurocritical Care Nurse Practitioner
Christiana Hospital
Newark, Delaware

Cathleen R. Maiolatesi, RN, MS
Program Coordinator, Informatics Advanced Practice Nurse High
   Risk Obstetrics
The Johns Hopkins Hospital
Baltimore, Maryland

Esmeralda Liu Matthews, MS, RN, ACNP-BC
Acute Care Nurse Practitioner, Cardiac Surgical Telemetry Unit
University of Maryland Medical Center
Baltimore, Maryland

E. Jane McCarthy, PhD, CRNA, FAAN
Professor
Brooks College of Health, University of North Florida
Jacksonville, Florida

Patricia C. McMullen, PhD, JD, CRNP, FAANP, FAAN
Dean and Ordinary Professor
School of Nursing
The Catholic University of America
Washington, District of Columbia

Sandra A. Mitchell, PhD, CRNP, AOCN
Research Scientist
National Cancer Institute
Rockville, Maryland

Patricia A. Moloney-Harmon, RN, MS, CCNS, FAAN
Clinical Nurse Specialist, Children's Services
Sinai Hospital of Baltimore
Baltimore, Maryland

Patricia Gonce Morton, RN, PhD, ACNP-BC, FAAN
Dean and Professor
Louis H. Peery Presidential Endowed Chair
University of Utah College of Nursing
Salt Lake City, Utah

Donna M. Mower-Wade, RN, ACNS-BC, CNRN
Lead Neurological-Critical Care APN
Christiana Care Health System
Newark, Delaware

Colleen Krebs Norton, RN, PhD, CCRN
Associate Professor and Director, BSN and CNL Program
Georgetown University
School of Nursing and Health Studies
Washington, District of Columbia

Nayna C. Philipsen, RN, JD, PhD, CFE, FACCE
Professor and Director of Affiliations
Coppin State University
Baltimore, Maryland

Leigh Bastable Poitevent, RN, FNP-BC
Nurse Practitioner
Minuteclinic
Cambridge, Massachusetts

Kim Reck, RN, DNP, CRNP
Clinical Program Manager for Cardiology, Interventional
   Radiology, and Pulmonary Medicine
University of Maryland Medical System
Baltimore, Maryland

Michael V. Relf, PhD, RN, AACRN, ACNS-BC, CNE,
FAAN
Associate Professor
Associate Dean for Global and Community Affairs
Duke University School of Nursing
Durham, North Carolina

Barbara Resnick, PhD, CRNP, FAAN, FAANP
Professor and Sonya Ziporkin Gershowitz Chair in Gerontology
University of Maryland School of Nursing
Baltimore, Maryland

Sarah Jane Mooney Rorick, RN, BSN, BA
Clinical Nurse
University of Utah Hospital
Salt Lake City, Utah

Sarah R. Rosenberger, RN, MS, CRNP, CCNS
Adult Emergency Department
The Johns Hopkins Hospital
Baltimore, Maryland

Valerie K. Sabol, PhD, AGACNP-BC, ANEF, FAANP
Professor & Division Chair, Healthcare in Adult Populations
Duke University School of Nursing
Adult-Gerontology Acute Care Nurse Practitioner
Department of Medicine, Division of Endocrinology,
   Metabolism and Nutrition
Duke University Medical Center

Eric Schuetz, BS Pharm, CSPI
Poison Specialist
Maryland Poison Center
Baltimore, Maryland

Julie Schuetz, MS, CRNP
Lead Nurse Practitioner, Medical Oncology
University of Maryland St Joseph Medical Center
Towson, Maryland

Brenda K. Shelton, DNP, RN, APRN-CNS, CCRN,
AOCN
Clinical Nurse Specialist
Sidney Kimmel Comprehensive Cancer Center at
   Johns Hopkins
Baltimore, Maryland

Jo Ann Hoffman Sikora, MS, CRNP
Senior Clinical Program Manager, Cardiac Surgery Advanced
    Practice
University of Maryland Medical System
Baltimore, Maryland

Kara A. Snyder, RN, MS, CCRN, CCNS
Clinical Nurse Specialist, Surgical Trauma Critical Care
The University of Arizona Medical Center
Tucson, Arizona

Mandy L. Snyder, RN, MSN, ACNP-BC
Acute Care Nurse Practitioner
Intermountain Heart Institute Cardiology
Murray, Utah

Lisa M. Spannbauer, MSN, APNP
Electrophysiology/Cardiology Nurse Practitioner
Clement J. Zablocki Milwaukee VA Medical Center
Milwaukee, Wisconsin

Kathleen Stevenson, RN, BSN
Consultant
Saugus, California

Louis R. Stout, RN, MS
Chief Nurse
62nd Medical Brigade
Joint Base Lewis-McChord, Washington

Paul A. Thurman, RN, MS, ACNPC, CCNS, CCRN
Clinical Nurse Specialist
R Adams Cowley Shock Trauma Center
University of Maryland Medical Center
Baltimore, Maryland

Kathleen Turner, RN, DNP
Assistant Professor
Duke University School of Nursing
Durham, North Carolina

Connie M. Ulrich, RN, PhD, FAAN
Professor of Nursing and Bioethics
University of Pennsylvania School of Nursing
Philadelphia, Pennsylvania

Kathryn T. Von Rueden, RN, MS, ACNS-BC, FCCM
Associate Professor
University of Maryland School of Nursing
Clinical Nurse Specialist
R Adams Cowley Shock Trauma Center
University of Maryland Medical Center
Baltimore, Maryland

Carol R. Wade, RN, MS, CRNP
Senior Nurse Practitioner
University of Maryland Medical System
Baltimore, Maryland

Cheryl A. Walsh, RN, MS
Registered Nurse, Informatics
Veterans Health Administration
Salt Lake City, Utah

Denise E. Ward, RN, DNP, ACNP-BC, FNP-BC
Assistant Professor (Clinical)
Specialty Director, Adult-Gerontology Acute Care Nurse
    Practitioner Program
University of Utah College of Nursing
Salt Lake City, Utah

Robert H. Welton, RN, MSN, MDE
Retired, Director, Office of Clinical Practice & Professional
    Development
University of Maryland Medical Center-Midtown Campus
Baltimore, Maryland

Erin Tilson Wice, RN, BSN
Clinical Course Coordinator
Neurological Critical Care Unit
University of Utah Hospital
Salt Lake City, Utah

Clareen Wiencek, RN, PhD, ACNP, ACHPN
Director of Advanced Practice
University of Virginia School of Nursing
Charlottesville, Virginia
AACN President, 2016–2017

Tracey L. Wilson, RN, MS, CRNP
Acute Care Nurse Practitioner
Medical Intensive Care Unit
University of Maryland Medical Center
Baltimore, Maryland

Amy M. Winkelman, RN, MSN, ACNP-BC
Neurosurgery Nurse Practitioner
San Francisco General Hospital and Trauma Center
San Francisco, California

Janet A. Wulf, RN, MS, CHPN
Clinical Instructor
University of Maryland School of Nursing
Baltimore, Maryland

Allison Steele York, BSN, MSN, CRNP
Nurse Practitioner, Gastrointestinal Medicine
Veterans Administration, Maryland Health Care System
Baltimore, Maryland

Elizabeth K. Zink, RN, MS, CCNS, CNRN
Clinical Nurse Specialist
Neurosciences Critical Care Unit
The Johns Hopkins Hospital
Baltimore, Maryland

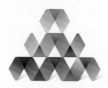 Contributors to the Tenth Edition

Susan E. Anderson, RN, MS
Senior Quality Assurance Specialist
U.S. Army Graduate Program in Anesthesia Nursing
Fort Sam Houston, Texas

Nathaniel M. Apatov, PhD, MSN, MHS, CRNA
Program Director, Nurse Anesthesia Program
Old Dominion University
Norfolk, Virginia

Sue Apple, RN, PhD
Retired
Formerly Assistant Professor
Georgetown University
Washington, District of Columbia

Richard Arbour, RN, MSN, CCRN, CNRN, CCNS, FAAN
Critical Care Nurse Specialist
Albert Einstein Medical Center
Philadelphia, Pennsylvania

Carla A. Aresco, RN, MS, CRNP
Nurse Practitioner, Shock Trauma
R Adams Cowley Shock Trauma Center
University of Maryland Medical Center
Baltimore, Maryland

Mona N. Bahouth, MSN, CRNP
Nurse Practitioner
Baltimore, Maryland

Kathryn S. Bizek, MSN, ACNS-BC, CCRN
Nurse Practitioner, Cardiology
VA Ann Arbor Healthcare System
Ann Arbor, Michigan

Nancy Blake, RN, PhD, MN, CCRN, NEA-BC, FAAN
Director, PCS Critical Care Services
Associate Adjunct Professor UCLA
Children's Hospital Los Angeles
Los Angeles, California

Kay Blum, PhD, CRNP
Nurse Practitioner and Coordinator
Cardiac Risk Reduction Center
Southern Maryland Hospital Center
Clinton, Maryland

Garrett K. Chan, PhD, APRN, BC-PCM, CEN
Director of Advanced Practice, Stanford Health Care
Clinical Associate Professor, Stanford School of Medicine
Stanford, California

Donna Charlebois, RN, MSN, ACNP-CS
Acute Care Nurse Practitioner
Interventional Cardiology
University of Virginia Health System
Charlottesville, Virginia

Dennis J. Cheek, RN, PhD, FAHA
Abell-Hanger Professor of Gerontological Nursing
Harris College of Nursing and Health Sciences, Texas Christian University
Fort Worth, Texas

Mary Ciechanowski, RN, MSN, ACNS-BC, CCRN
Stroke Program Advanced Practice Nurse
Christiana Care Health Systems
Newark, Delaware

JoAnn Coleman, RN, DNP, ACNP, ANP, AOCN
Acute Care Nurse Practitioner
Gastrointestinal Surgical Oncology
The Johns Hopkins Hospital
Baltimore, Maryland

Vicki J. Coombs, RN, PhD, FAHA
Senior Vice President
Spectrum Clinical Research Incorporated
Towson, Maryland

Kelley Caldwell Crusius, RN, CCRN
Staff Nurse
University Medical Center
Tucson, Arizona

Joan M. Davenport, RN, PhD
Assistant Professor, Vice Chair
Department of Organizational Systems and Adult Health
University of Maryland School of Nursing
Baltimore, Maryland

Marla J. De Jong, RN, PhD, CCNS, Col
Dean
United States Air Force School of Aerospace Medicine
Wright-Patterson Air Force Base, Ohio

Emily Smith Des Champs, RN, MS, CCRN
Clinical Nurse Specialist, Neurology
University Medical Center
Tucson, Arizona

Nancy Kern Feeley, RN, MS, CRNP, CNN
Nephrology Adult Nurse Practitioner
Division of Nephrology, Johns Hopkins University School of Medicine
Baltimore, Maryland

Charles Fisher, RN, MSN, CCRN, ACNP-BC
Acute Care Nurse Practitioner
Medical Intensive Care Unit
University of Virginia Health System
Charlottesville, Virginia

Dorrie K. Fontaine, RN, PhD, FAAN
Sadie Heath Cabaniss Professor of Nursing and Dean
University of Virginia School of Nursing
Charlottesville, Virginia

Conrad Gordon, RN, MS, ACNP
Assistant Professor
Department of Organizational Systems and Adult
    Health
University of Maryland School of Nursing
Baltimore, Maryland

Christine Grady, RN, PhD
Chief, Department of Bioethics
Clinical Center
National Institutes of Health
Bethesda, Maryland

Debby Greenlaw, MS, CCRN, ACNPC, ACHPN
Director of Palliative Care, Acute Care Nurse
    Practitioner
Providence Hospitals
Columbia, South Carolina

Thomasine D. Guberski, PhD, CRNP
Director, Health Program—Nursing
Institute of Human Virology
University of Maryland School of Medicine
Baltimore, Maryland

Kimberli Haas, RN, BSN
Staff Nurse II
University Medical Center
Tucson, Arizona

John C. Hagen, MS, CCRN, CRNP-AC
Acute Care Nurse Practitioner
University of Maryland Medical Center
Baltimore, Maryland

Jillian Hamel, MS, ACNP-BC, CCNS, CCRN
Nurse Practitioner
University of Maryland Medical Center
Baltimore, Maryland

Kathy A. Hausman, RNC, PhD
Assistant Professor
University of Maryland School of Nursing
Baltimore, Maryland

Jan M. Headley, RN, BS
Director, Clinical Marketing and Professional Education
Edwards Lifesciences LLC
Irvine, California

Janie Heath, PhD, APRN-BC, FAAN
Dean and Warwick Professor of Nursing
University of Kentucky College of Nursing
Lexington, Kentucky

Genell Hilton, PhD, CRNP
Nurse Practitioner, Trauma Services
San Francisco General Hospital
San Francisco, California
Adjunct Faculty
Santa Rosa Junior College
Santa Rosa, California

Janice J. Hoffman, PhD, RN, ANEF
Associate Dean of Academic Affairs
University of Missouri, Sinclair School of Nursing
Columbia, MO

Dorene M. Holcombe, RN, MS, ACNP, CCRN
Nephrology Acute Care Nurse Practitioner
Johns Hopkins University School of Medicine
Baltimore, Maryland

Elizabeth Holderness, RN, MS, ACNP-BC
Nurse Practitioner, Cardiac Surgery
University of Maryland Medical Center
Baltimore, Maryland

Christina Hurlock-Chorostecki, PhD(c), APN
Nurse Practitioner
St. Joseph Health Care, London
London, Ontario, Canada

Karen L. Johnson, RN, PhD
Director of Nursing, Research, and Evidence-Based Practice
University of Maryland Medical Center
Associate Professor
University of Maryland School of Nursing
Baltimore, Maryland

Lisa M. Johnson, RN, MS, ACNP-BC, CCRN
Major, U.S. Army Nurse Corps
Nurse Manager, Burn Intensive Care Unit
U.S. Army Medical Department
Sam Houston, Texas

Dennis W. Jones, RN, DNP, CFRN
Critical Care Flight/Transport Nurse
The Johns Hopkins Hospital
Baltimore, Maryland

Kimmith M. Jones, RN, DNP, CCNS
Advanced Practice Nurse in Critical Care
Sinai Hospital of Baltimore
Baltimore, Maryland

Roberta Kaplow, APRN-CCNS, PhD, AOCNS, CCRN
Clinical Nurse Specialist
Emory University Hospital
Atlanta, Georgia

Jane Faith Kapustin, PhD, CRNP, BC-ADM, FAANP, FAAN
Associate Professor
Assistant Dean for Masters and Doctor of Nursing Practice
   Programs
University of Maryland School of Nursing
Adult Nurse Practitioner, Joslin Diabetes Center
University of Maryland Medical Center
Baltimore, Maryland

Elizabeth Kozub, RN, MS, CCNS, CCRN, CNRN
Nurse Clinician III
Sharp Memorial Hospital
San Diego, California

Sun-Ah Lee, RN, MS, CRNP
Nurse Practitioner
University of Maryland Medical System
Baltimore, Maryland

Barbara Leeper, RN, MN, CNS, M-S, CCRN, FAHA
Clinical Nurse Specialist, Cardiovascular Services
Baylor University Medical Center
Dallas, Texas

Tara Leslie, RN, BSN
RN Extender
St. Joseph Cardiology Associates
Lexington, Kentucky

Susan Luchka, RN, MSN, CCRN, ET
Director of Clinical Education
Memorial Hospital
York, Pennsylvania

Christine N. Lynch, RN, MS, ACNP, CCRN
Acute Care Flight Nurse Practitioner
Cleveland Clinic, Critical Care Transport
Cleveland, Ohio

Megan Cecere Lynn, RN, MS, MBA, FNE-A
Clinical Instructor
University of Maryland School of Nursing
Baltimore, Maryland

Cathleen R. Maiolatesi, RN, MS
Advanced Practice Nurse
The Johns Hopkins Hospital
Baltimore, Maryland

E. Jane McCarthy, PhD, CRNA, FAAN
Visiting Professor
University of Maryland School of Nursing
Baltimore, Maryland

Sandra W. McLeskey, RN, PhD
Professor
University of Maryland School of Nursing
Baltimore, Maryland

Patricia C. McMullen, PhD, JD, CRNP, FAANP, FAAN
Dean and Ordinary Professor
School of Nursing
The Catholic University of America
Washington, District of Columbia

Paul K. Merrel, RN, MSN, CCNS
Advanced Practice Nurse 2—CNS, Adult Critical Care
University of Virginia Health System
Charlottesville, Virginia

Sandra A. Mitchell, PhD, CRNP, AOCN
Nurse Scientist
National Institute of Health Clinical Center
Bethesda, Maryland

Patricia A. Moloney-Harmon, RN, MS, CCNS, FAAN
Advanced Practice Nurse
Children's Services
Sinai Hospital of Baltimore
Baltimore, Maryland

Patricia Gonce Morton, RN, PhD, ACNP-BC, FAAN
Dean and Professor
Louis H. Peery Presidential Endowed Chair
University of Utah College of Nursing
Salt Lake City, Utah

Donna Mower-Wade, RN, MS, CNRN, ACNS-BC
Trauma Clinical Nurse Specialist
Christiana Care Health System
Newark, Delaware

Nancy Munro, RN, MN, CCRN, ACNP
Acute Care Nurse Practitioner
Critical Care Medicine Department
National Institutes of Health
Bethesda, Maryland

Angela C. Muzzy, RN, MSN, CCRN, CNS
Clinical Nurse Specialist, Cardiovascular Intensive Care Unit
University Medical Center
Tucson, Arizona

Colleen Krebs Norton, RN, PhD, CCRN
Associate Professor and Director, BSN and CNL Program
School of Nursing and Health Studies
Georgetown University
Washington, District of Columbia

Dulce Obias-Manno, RN, MHSA, CCDS, CEPS, FHRS
Nurse Coordinator, Cardiac Arrhythmia Device Clinic
Washington Hospital Center
Washington, District of Columbia

Mary O. Palazzo, RN, MS, FACHE
Senior Director of Transition Planning
Mercy Medical Center
Baltimore, Maryland

Archana D. Patel, MS, CRNP
Acute Care Nurse Practitioner, Thoracic Surgery
University of Maryland Medical Center
Baltimore, Maryland

Nayna C. Philipsen, RN, JD, PhD, CFE, FACCE
Professor and Director of Affiliations
Coppin State University
Baltimore, Maryland

Clifford C. Pyne, RN, MS, ACNP
Nurse Practitioner—General Cardiology
Buffalo Cardiology and Pulmonary Associates
Williamsville, New York

Kim Reck, RN, MS, CRNP
Adult Nurse Practitioner
Clinical Program Manager, CRNP
Division of Cardiology
University of Maryland Medical Center
Baltimore, Maryland

Michael V. Relf, RN, PhD, CNE, ACNS-BC, AACRN, FAAN
Associate Professor
Associate Dean for Global and Community Health Affairs
Duke University School of Nursing
Durham, North Carolina

Kenneth J. Rempher, RN, PhD, MBA, CENP
Associate Chief Nursing Officer
University of Iowa Hospitals and Clinics
Iowa City, Iowa

Cynthia L. Renn, RN, PhD
Assistant Professor
University of Maryland School of Nursing
Baltimore, Maryland

Barbara Resnick, PhD, CRNP, FAAN, FAANP
Professor and Sonya Ziporkin Gershowitz Chair in Gerontology
University of Maryland School of Nursing
Baltimore, Maryland

Valerie K. Sabol, PhD, ACNP-BC, GNP-BC
Associate Professor, Specialty Director
Acute Care Nurse Practitioner and Critical Care Clinical Nurse
   Specialist Program
Duke University School of Nursing
Durham, North Carolina

Eric Schuetz, BS Pharm, CSPI
Specialist in Poison Information
Maryland Poison Center
Baltimore, Maryland

Julie Schuetz, MS, CRNP
Nurse Practitioner
Department of Hematologic Malignancies
The Sidney Kimmel Comprehensive Cancer Center
Johns Hopkins Medicine
Baltimore, Maryland

Brenda K. Shelton, RN, MS, CCRN, AOCN
Critical Care Clinical Nurse Specialist
The Sidney Kimmel Comprehensive Cancer Center at Johns
   Hopkins
Baltimore, Maryland

Jo Ann Hoffman Sikora, RN, MS, CRNP
Nurse Practitioner, Cardiac Surgery
University of Maryland Medical Center
Baltimore, Maryland

Kara Adams Snyder, RN, MS, CCRN, CCNS
Clinical Nurse Specialist
Surgical Trauma Critical Care
University Medical Center
Tucson, Arizona

Debbi S. Spencer, RN, MS
Chief Nurse, Joint Trauma System
U.S. Army Institute of Surgical Research
Fort Sam Houston, Texas

Allison G. Steele, RN, MSN, CRNP
Nurse Practitioner
Division of Gastroenterology and Hepatology
University Physicians Inc.
Baltimore, Maryland

Louis R. Stout, RN, MS
Lieutenant Colonel, United States Army Nurse Corps
United States Army Medical Department
Fort Lewis, Washington

Paul A. Thurman, RN, MS, ACNPC, CCNS, CCRN, CNRN
Clinical Nurse Specialist
R Adams Cowley Shock Trauma Center
University of Maryland Medical Center
Baltimore, Maryland

Sidenia S. Tribble, RN, MSN, ACNP-BC, CCRN
Acute Care Nurse Practitioner
Augusta Health
Fisherville, Virginia

Kathleen Turner, RN, DNP
Assistant Professor
Duke University School of Nursing
Durham, North Carolina

Connie M. Ulrich, RN, PhD, FAAN
Professor of Nursing and Bioethics
University of Pennsylvania School of Nursing
Philadelphia, Pennsylvania

Jeffrey S. Upperman, MD
Associate Professor of Surgery
Director, Trauma Program
Children's Hospital Los Angeles
Keck School of Medicine
University of Southern California
Los Angeles, California

**Mary van Soeren, RN, PhD**
Director
Canadian Health Care Innovation
Guelph, Ontario, Canada

**Kathryn T. Von Rueden, RN, MS, ACNS-BC, FCCM**
Associate Professor
University of Maryland School of Nursing
Clinical Nurse Specialist
R Adams Cowley Shock Trauma Center
University of Maryland Medical Center
Baltimore, Maryland

**Amanda S. Walther, MS, CRNP**
Nurse Practitioner
Department of Cardiology
University of Maryland Medical Center
Baltimore, Maryland

**Tracey L. Wilson, MS, CRNP**
Acute Care Nurse Practitioner
Medical Intensive Care Unit
University of Maryland Medical Center
Baltimore, Maryland

**Janet A. Wulf, RN, MS, CNL, CHPN**
Staff Nurse
Union Memorial Hospital
Baltimore, Maryland

**Karen L. Yarbrough, MS, CRNP**
Acute Care Nurse Practitioner
Director, Stroke Program
University of Maryland Medical Center
Baltimore, Maryland

**Elizabeth K. Zink, RN, MS, CCRN, CCNS, CNRN**
Clinical Nurse Specialist
Neurosciences Critical Care Unit
The Johns Hopkins Hospital
Baltimore, Maryland

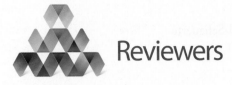

# Reviewers

**Nezam Al-Nsair, PhD, BSN, MSN**
Director of Nursing, Chair of the Department of Nursing,
    and Associate Professor of Nursing
University of Mount Union
Alliance, Ohio

**Roxie Barnes, MSN, RN, CCRN**
Clinical Assistant Professor
Indiana University
Bloomington, Indiana

**Mali M. Bartges, DNP, RN, CNE, CCRN**
Professor
Northampton Community College
Bethlehem, Pennsylvania

**Lyndele Bernard, RN, MSN**
Professor
Anne Arundel Community College
Arnold, Maryland

**Catherine Berry, MSN, BSN, CNE, CCRN**
Clinical Assistant Professor Emerita
University of Wisconsin-Eau Claire
Eau Claire, Wisconsin

**Joy Borrero, BS, MS, ANP**
Academic Chair/Associate Professor of Nursing
Suffolk County Community College
Brentwood, New York

**Destiny Brady, MSN, RN, CCRN**
Instructor
Saint Anselm College
Manchester, New Hampshire

**Audrey Charchenko, MSN, MMA, BSN**
Assistant Professor of Nursing
Dickinson State University
Dickinson, North Dakota

**Audrey Cornell, PhD, MSN, RN, CNE**
Clinical Associate Professor
Western Kentucky University
Bowling Green, Kentucky

**Ann Crawford, PhD, MSN, BSN, RN**
Professor
University of Mary Hardin-Baylor
Belton, Texas

**JoAnn Daugherty, PhD, RN, CNL**
Lecturer
California State University San Marcos
San Marcos, California

**Tammie Davis, BSN, MSN**
Clinical Associate Professor
Walsh University Byers School of Nursing
North Canton, Ohio

**Denise Dawkins, DNP, MSN, RN, CNL**
Simulation and Skills Labs Director and Lecturer
California State University
Bakersfield, California

**Carol Diehl, MSN, MSED, RN**
Simulation Coordinator
The Reading Hospital School of Health
    Sciences
Reading, Pennsylvania

**Judy Donnelly**
Lancaster County Career & Technology Center
Willow Street, Pennsylvania

**Tina Dorsey, RN, MSN**
Instructor
Chipola College
Marianna, Florida

**Deborah Drummonds, RN, MN, CCRN, CCN**
Assistant Professor
Abraham Baldwin Agricultural College
Tifton, Georgia

**Mary Louanne Friend, RN, PhD**
Assistant Professor
Capstone College of Nursing
Tuscaloosa, Alabama

**Linda Gambill, BSN, MSN/Ed**
Clinical Simulation Center
Southwest Virginia Community College
Cedar Bluff, Virginia

**Virginia Hackett, RN, PhD**
Assistant Professor
Barry University College of Nursing and Health
    Sciences
Miami Shores, Florida

**Cam Hamilton, PhD, MSN, BSN**
Assistant Professor
Auburn University at Montgomery
Montgomery, Alabama

**Julie Isaacson**
Professor
Arkansas State University
Jonesboro, Arkansas

Verena Johnson, MSN, RN, CNE
Associate Professor
Amarillo College
Amarillo, Texas

Robin Kappler, MSN, RN
Assistant Professor
Bryan College of Health Sciences
Lincoln, Nebraska

Tonia Kennedy, EdD, MSN, RN, CCRN
Associate Professor
Liberty University
Lynchburg, Virginia

Stephen Krau, PhD, RN, CNE
Associate Professor of Nursing
Vanderbilt School of Nursing
Nashville, Tennessee

Patricia Lea, DNP, MSEd, RN, CCRN
Associate Professor
Baccalaureate Program Director—Senior Level
University of Texas Medical Branch School of
    Nursing
Galveston, Texas

Stephen Lomax, MSN, MBA, RN
Assistant Professor
Austin Peay State University
Clarksville, Tennessee

Naomi Lungstrom, FNP, MN, BSN
Clinical Assistant Professor
Washington State University College of Nursing
Spokane, Washington

Susan Malkemes, PhD
Associate Professor, Chair
Wilkes University
Wilkes-Barre, Pennsylvania

Annette Mattea, DNP, MSN, RN, APN/CCNS
Assistant Professor, Nursing
University of St. Francis
Joliet, Illinois

Catherine McCoy-Hill, RN, MSN, CNS, ANP-C
Assistant Professor
Azusa Pacific University
Azusa, California

Carrie Morgan, DNP
Retired
Western Kentucky University
Bowling Green, Kentucky

Betty Nash, MSN
Associate Professor
Bluefield State College
Bluefield, West Virginia

Crystal O'Connell-Schauerte
Program Coordinator
Algonquin College
Ottawa, Ontario

Kristin O'Neail
Lourdes University
Sylvania, Ohio

Jeanne Marie Papa, BSN, MSN, MBE
Instructor
Neumann University
Aston, Pennsylvania

Carol Penrosa, MSN, RN
Nursing Faculty
Southeast Community College
Lincoln, Nebraska

Sherily Pereira
University of Puerto Rico School of Nursing
San Juan, Puerto Rico

Debra Peterson, PhD, MSN, RN, CMSRN, CNE
Professor
University of St. Francis
Joliet, Illinois

Donna Polverini, MS
Associate Professor of Nursing
American International College
Springfield, Massachusetts

Joyce Pompey, RNC, DNP
Assistant Professor
The University of South Carolina
Aiken, South Carolina

Carrie Pucino, DED, RN, CCRN
Assistant Professor of Nursing
York College of Pennsylvania
York, Pennsylvania

Deanna Reising, PhD, RN, ACNS-BC, ANEF
Associate Professor
Indiana University
Indianapolis, Indiana

Kim Resanovich, MSN, RN-BC
Lecturer
Ohio University
Athens, Ohio

Karen Roberts, MSN
Associate Professor
Marian University
Fond du Lac, Wisconsin

Martha K. Roper
Nursing Faculty
Wallace State Community College
Hanceville, Alabama

Susan Rouse, RN, PhD
Assistant Professor
Indiana University Northwest
Gary, Indiana

Mary Runde, RN, BScN, MScN, APN, CNCC
Professor
Durham College
Sault Ste. Marie, Michigan

Alice Santiago
Interamerican University of Puerto Rico
Puerto Rico

Deborah Jane Schwytzer, MSN, BSN, BS, DNP
Associate Professor
University of Cincinnati College of Nursing
Cincinnati, Ohio

Pamela Sealover, MSN
Associate Director of Nursing
Ohio University Zanesville
Zanesville, Ohio

Tonya Sellars, MSN, RN
Instructor
Armstrong State University
Savannah, Georgia

Joanne Serembus, EdD, RN, CCRN, CNE
Associate Clinical Professor
Drexel University
Philadelphia, Pennsylvania

Margaret Sherer, RN, MS, CEN, CNE
Faculty Department Chair
Portland Community College
Portland, Oregon

Brenda Sloan, MA, RN
Assistant Professor
Indiana Wesleyan University
Marion, Indiana

Jacqueline J. Stewart, PhD
Associate Professor
Wilkes University
Wilkes-Barre, Pennsylvania

Betsy Swinny, MSN, RN, CCRN
Professional Nursing Faculty
Baptist Health System, School of Health Professions
San Antonio, Texas

Annie Thomas, RN, PhD
Assistant Professor
Loyola University Chicago
Chicago, Illinois

Charlene Thomas, RN, PhD
Assistant Professor
Aurora University
Aurora, Illinois

Yvonne Tolson-Myers, CNP
Trinity Health System
Steubenville, Ohio

Kim Kilpatrick Uddo, DNP
Professor
Delgado Community College, Charity School of Nursing
New Orleans, Louisiana

Tammy Vant Hul, RN, MSN, ACNP
Associate Professor
Riverside City Community College
Riverside, California

Barbara Voshall, DNP
Professor of Nursing
Graceland University
Independence, Missouri

Judy Walloch, RN, EdD
Part Time Clinical Instructor
Graham Hospital School of Nursing
Canton, Illinois

Linda Warren, EdD, RN, MSN, CCRN
Assistant Professor
Western Connecticut State University
Danbury, Connecticut

Marline Whigham, MSN
Assistant Professor
College of Nursing, Nova Southeastern University
Miami, Florida

Rachel Wilburn, RN, MSN, CNS
Assistant Professor
McNeese State University
Lake Charles, Louisiana

Phyllis Wille, MSN, FNP-C, CNE
Instructor
Danville Area Community College
Danville, Illinois

Michael L. Williams, PhD, RN, CCRN, CNE
Director, Associate Professor
Eastern Michigan University
Ypsilanti, Michigan

Sharon Wing, PhDc, BSN, MSN
Associate Professor
Cleveland State University School of Nursing
Cleveland, Ohio

Karen Wood, RN, DNSc, CCRN, CNL
Associate Professor
Saint Xavier University
Chicago, Illinois

Shirley Woolf, MSN
Clinical Assistant Professor
Indiana University
Indianapolis, Indiana

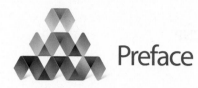

# Preface

The practice of critical care nursing has changed dramatically since its inception in the 1960s. Critical care nurses, more than ever before, must possess an extensive body of knowledge in order to provide competent and holistic care to critically ill patients and their families. Critically ill patients are no longer found just in intensive care units. Instead, they are cared for in the emergency department, in progressive care units, in postanesthesia care units, and in the home. Today, critically ill patients are liable to be older and sicker than ever before, thus demanding extensive knowledge to meet their complex needs. Advances in nursing, medicine, and technology; the rapidly changing healthcare climate; and the shortage of nursing staff and faculty are other factors that have come together to effect great changes in the practice of critical care nursing.

Some of the requisite knowledge for the practice of critical care nursing can be attained through formal education and textbooks, like this one. The rest can only be gained through experience. It is our goal, with this 11th edition of *Critical Care Nursing: A Holistic Approach*, to assist readers on their journey by providing a comprehensive, up-to-date resource and reference.

As in past editions, this 11th edition promotes excellence in critical care nursing. Presenting theory and principles within the context of practical application helps the reader to gain competence and confidence in caring for critically ill patients and their families. As always, the patient as the center of the healthcare team's efforts is emphasized throughout. In the highly specialized and complicated technical environment of critical care, knowing how to deliver holistic care and demonstrating caring behaviors are just as important as knowing how to operate complex equipment and perform difficult procedures.

New to this 11th edition, the reader will find a continued emphasis on evidence-based practice, and an even more streamlined text that focuses on the key knowledge and practices that all nurses need to care for critically ill patients.

## An Overview

*Critical Care Nursing: A Holistic Approach*, 11th edition, consists of 13 parts. The following is a brief overview of those parts and the information they contain.

### Part 1: The Concept of Holism Applied to Critical Care Nursing Practice

The six chapters that make up Part 1 introduce the student to the concept of holistic care, as it applies in critical care practice. In Chapter 1, the student is introduced to critical care nursing practice. Chapters 2 and 3 review the psychosocial effects of critical illness on the patient and the family, respectively. These chapters also describe the effect of the critical care environment on the patient and review actions the nurse can take to help reduce environment-induced stress and promote healing. Chapter 4 emphasizes the role of patient and family education in critical care. Chapter 5 focuses on strategies for relieving pain and promoting comfort. We conclude the part with Chapter 6, which concentrates on end-of-life and palliative care.

### Part 2: Professional Practice Issues in Critical Care

This part consists of three chapters that are of concern to the nursing profession. In Chapters 7 and 8, ethical and legal issues are explored. Chapter 9 describes characteristics of critical care nurses, delineates aspects of nursing professionalism, and defines critical attributes of nursing excellence.

### Part 3: Special Populations in Critical Care

The four chapters in this part focus on the special needs of certain groups of people who are critically ill. Chapters 10, 11, and 12 focus on the pediatric patient, the pregnant patient, and the elderly patient, respectively. Chapter 13 describes the role of the nurse in caring for the patient who is recovering from anesthesia.

### Part 4: Special Situations in Critical Care

This section opens with a chapter that focuses on the care of the patient who is being transported within or between facilities as well as the role of the rapid response team. The second chapter in this section describes the role of the critical care nurse in disaster management.

### Part 5: Cardiovascular System

This part, the first of eight organ system–based parts, focuses on the care of the patient with a cardiovascular disorder. Each organ system–based part begins with a chapter that reviews the anatomy and physiology of the organ system under discussion (e.g., Chapter 16). The part then continues with a chapter on patient assessment (e.g., Chapter 17), general patient management (e.g., Chapter 18), and common disorders (e.g., Chapter 19). In Part 5, heart failure and acute myocardial infarction are each given their own chapters (Chapters 20 and 21, respectively). The unit concludes with a discussion of the most recent developments in cardiac surgery (Chapter 22). Throughout the unit, the latest diagnostic tests, the newest medications for treating cardiovascular disorders, and updates on technologies (such as the left ventricular assist device, the implantable cardioverter defibrillator, and the cardiac pacemaker) are discussed.

### Part 6: Respiratory System

In this part, current assessment technologies (such as end-tidal carbon dioxide monitoring) and the newest modes of ventilation for patients in respiratory failure are discussed. Evidence-based treatment strategies for respiratory disorders such as pneumonia, pleural effusion, and chronic obstructive pulmonary disease are described. Chapter 27 is devoted to the latest developments in the assessment and management of the patient with acute respiratory distress syndrome (ARDS).

### Part 7: Renal System

In this edition of the text, Part 7 includes a more in-depth discussion of the assessment and management of fluids, electrolytes, and acid–base balance. Updates on laboratory and diagnostic tests are included. The newest dialysis technologies and the latest drugs are discussed in Chapter 30. Chapter 31 focuses on common renal disorders, including recent developments in the care of the patient with acute kidney injury and chronic kidney disease.

### Part 8: Nervous System

This part offers updates on neurologic diagnostic studies and the newest approaches to treating the patient with increased intracranial pressure. The latest drugs for treating neurologic disorders and the most recent developments in neurosurgery are addressed. Separate chapters are devoted to care of the patient with a head injury and spinal cord injury.

### Part 9: Gastrointestinal System

In Part 9, the latest diagnostic tests for evaluating patients with gastrointestinal disorders are discussed. The management of patients with gastrointestinal disorders has been updated to include the newest drugs, the latest developments in the use of enteral and parenteral nutrition, and recent trends in the treatment of common disorders such as liver failure and hepatitis.

### Part 10: Endocrine System

In this edition, Part 10 includes an assessment chapter covering multiple components of the endocrine system. The content is organized by the major gland, and for each gland addressed in the chapter, the reader is given information on the history, laboratory tests, and diagnostic tests. The most current information on the treatment of endocrine disorders, especially glycemic control and diabetic emergencies, is included in Chapter 44.

### Part 11: Hematologic and Immune Systems

This part continues to be a unique feature that is not included in many critical care texts. The numerous recent developments in organ and hematopoietic stem cell transplant are described in Chapter 47. Chapter 48 addresses up-to-date information on the assessment and management of critically ill patients with HIV/AIDS as well as those with oncologic emergencies. The latest trends in the treatment of patients with hematologic disorders such as disseminated intravascular coagulation are included in Chapter 49.

### Part 12: Integumentary System

This part includes three chapters not covered in other critical care texts: the anatomy and physiology of the integumentary system, assessment of the integumentary system, and management of integumentary disorders, respectively. Evidence-based assessment and management of wounds are addressed.

In addition, care of the critically ill burn patient is covered in Chapter 53.

### Part 13: Multisystem Dysfunction

In Chapter 54, hypoperfusion states such as shock, systemic inflammatory response syndrome (SIRS), and multiple organ dysfunction syndrome (MODS) are discussed. The latest understanding of the pathophysiologic process is described, as well as how this knowledge guides the selection of the most recent interventions. Chapter 55 reviews care of the trauma patient, including the latest trends in the management of these complex patients. Chapter 56 reviews care of the patient with a drug overdose or poisoning, a problem that is becoming more common in the critical care setting.

## Features

The features of the 11th edition of *Critical Care Nursing: A Holistic Approach* have been designed to assist readers with practice as well as learning.

### Practice-Oriented Features

- **Considerations for the Older Patient boxes** highlight the special needs of this patient population that constitutes the largest numbers of critically ill patients.
- **Health History boxes** summarize key areas that should be covered and relevant information that may be revealed during the health history.
- **Teaching Guides** help the nurse to prepare patients and family members for procedures, assist patients and family members with understanding the illness they are dealing with, and explain postprocedure or postoperative activities.

### Pedagogical Features

**Learning Objectives,** at the beginning of each chapter, help focus the reader's attention on important topics.

**Clinical Applicability Challenges,** at the conclusion of each chapter, consists of three to five **short-answer questions** or a **case study** followed by three to five short-answer questions.

## New to This Edition

- **New case study/short-answer questions** in every chapter guide the reader from knowledge to application. Discussion points for these questions are available on thePoint.
- **Updated Evidence-Based Practice Highlights** help the reader to understand the importance of research-based practice and include excerpts from the latest AACN practice alerts as well as from recently published research.
- **New Spotlight on Genetics boxes** appear in selected chapters and include important genetic information and summaries of selected genetic disorders. These disorders may be the result of random genetic mutations, genetic mutations caused by environmental influences, or inherited mutated genes.
- **QSEN** Because the Quality and Safety Education for Nurses (QSEN) competencies have become such an important part of every nursing curriculum, a new QSEN icon has

been added to pertinent features to highlight this essential content related to the core competencies.

- **Patient Safety boxes** alert readers to risk factors, signs and symptoms, side effects, and complications that the critical care nurse must anticipate and continuously monitor to maintain patient safety.
- **Collaborative Care Guides** describe how the health-care team works together to manage a patient's illness and minimize complications. The information incorporates nursing diagnoses and emphasizes outcomes and interventions based on teamwork and collaboration.
- **Evidence-Based Practice Highlights** help the reader to understand the importance of research-based practice.

## Student and Instructor Resources

A wide variety of resources that support the student and instructor are available online on thePoint.

### Student Resources

Students who purchase this book have access to all of these additional resources via thePoint website:

- References
- Selected Readings
- Chapter NCLEX-Style Review Questions and Answers with accompanying rationales
- Journal articles
- Internet resources
- Spanish–English audio glossary
- Concepts in Action animations
- Watch and Learn video clips
- Practice and Learn activities

- Clinical Simulation Case Studies and Tutorial
- Dosage calculation quizzes
- Learning objectives
- Nursing professional roles and responsibilities
- Heart and breath sounds
- Discussion points for the case study/short-answer questions in the text

### Instructor Resources

In addition to all of the student assets, instructors who adopt this text also have access to a special instructor's resource section on thePoint. The following are included on the website:

- Test generator, featuring over a thousand questions
- Image bank, containing over 300 illustrations
- PowerPoint presentations and accompanying guided lecture notes for each chapter
- Syllabi
- Strategies for effective teaching

It is with great pleasure that we introduce these resources—the textbook and the accompanying interactive resource package—to you. One of our primary goals in creating these resources has been to promote excellence in critical care nursing practice so that nurses can help patients and families cope with the consequences of critical illness. It is our intent that these resources will provide aspiring and currently practicing critical care nurses the tools to make their optimal contribution to the care of critically ill patients and their families and to the nursing profession. We hope that we have succeeded in that goal, and we welcome feedback from our readers.

Patricia Gonce Morton
Dorrie K. Fontaine

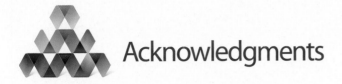

# Acknowledgments

This project required the help and cooperation of many people. First, we want to thank our many colleagues who contributed to the text, either by authoring a chapter or by sharing their expertise as a reviewer. Our publisher, Wolters Kluwer, through all editions of this book remains committed to producing the best text possible. We especially want to thank Helen Kogut, Senior Development Editor, for her superb work and guidance, commitment to excellence, and words of positive encouragement as she cheered us on to the finish line with this project.

We also wish to express our thanks to Jordan Ciulla who assisted with all the additional selected readings. His hours of work were an enormous help to us.

In addition, we wish to thank Dr. Dennis Cheek, a nationally known expert in genetics, for creating the genetics feature, *Spotlight on Genetics*, that appears throughout the text.

And finally, we wish to express a word of thanks to our families and nursing colleagues who endured the time we took to complete this project.

Trish and Dorrie

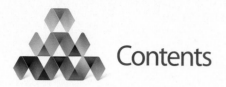

# Contents

# The Concept of Holism Applied to Critical Care Nursing Practice

## 1

## Critical Care Nursing Practice: Promoting Excellence Through Caring, Collaboration, and Evidence

ROBERTA KAPLOW, KATHLEEN TURNER, AND MICHAEL V. RELF

### LEARNING OBJECTIVES

*Based on the content in this chapter, the reader should be able to:*

1. Describe the value of certification in critical care nursing.
2. Describe the value of evidence-based practice in caring for critically ill patients.
3. Discuss the value of collaborative practice in critical care.
4. List the underlying premises of the Synergy Model to promote positive patient outcomes.
5. Discuss methods to mitigate alarm fatigue.
6. Discuss future issues facing critical care nursing practice.

As the health care delivery system continues to evolve and transform, so too does the discipline of nursing and the specialty of critical care nursing. Today, the care of critically ill patients occurs not only in the traditional setting of the hospital intensive care unit but also on the progressive care unit, on medical and surgical clinical units, in the subacute facility, in long-term care, in the community, and even in the patient's home. As a consequence of recent health care reform legislation, coupled with an aging population and application of genomics in personalized medicine, critical care nursing practice as we know it today will continue to evolve.

Since the first critical care unit opened in the late 1960s, significant technological, procedural, and pharmacological advances have occurred, accompanied by a knowledge explosion in critical care nursing and medicine. Consequently, critical care nurses, progressive care nurses, and home health nurses of the 21st century are routinely caring for the complex, critically ill patients who just a few decades ago would not have survived a critical illness. As a result, nurses are increasingly being challenged to integrate sophisticated technologies and interventions and to implement care based on contemporary evidence while simultaneously caring for the whole person by addressing the psychosocial challenges and ethical conflicts associated with critical illness. At the same time, nurses are expected to deliver care not only to the patient but also to the patient's family, as defined by the patient, and not in professional isolation but in collaboration with the interdisciplinary team.

In response to the ever-changing health care delivery system, critical care nurses are championing the needs of the patient and the family, integrating evidence to improve standards of care, striving to maintain patient safety, engaging in interdisciplinary collaboration, and developing healthy work environments (HWEs)—all in the pursuit of quality clinical outcomes. During the past several decades, critical care nurses have experienced firsthand what nurse scientists have consistently demonstrated: critical illness is not only a physiological alteration but also a psychosocial and spiritual process as well as a threat to individuals and their families. Through specialty certification by the American Association of Critical-Care Nurses (AACN), nurses voluntarily demonstrate their knowledge of critical care nursing. Furthermore, as health care becomes increasingly technical, the need for humanization is increasingly essential. Compatible with the need for "humanized" health care is the need to provide effective evidence-based interventions instead of those steeped in tradition or based on intuition.

This chapter describes select aspects of the critical care environment. These include the value of certification, evidence-based practice (EBP), quality and safety, healthy environments, and the AACN Synergy Model for Patient Care. Each of these, when implemented, helps promote optimal outcomes for acute and critically ill patients and their families. This chapter also describes etiologic factors and detrimental effects of alarm fatigue, as well as some suggestions to help mitigate this phenomenon.

## Value of Certification

"Certification is a process by which a nongovernmental agency validates, based on predetermined standards, an individual nurse's knowledge for practice in a defined functional or clinical area of nursing."[1] A white paper, *Safeguarding the Patient and the Profession*, published by the AACN, demonstrated the value of specialty certification.[2] Certification promotes continuing excellence in the critical care nursing profession, helping nurses achieve and maintain an up-to-date knowledge base essential in the practice of critical care nursing.[2–4] In addition, it validates nurses' knowledge to patients and families, employers, and themselves.

## Value to the Patient and Family

As a consequence of medical errors, adverse outcomes, and complicated regulations governing reimbursement, many consumers are wary of today's health care delivery system. Certification provides patients and families with validation that the nurses caring for them have demonstrated experience and knowledge that exceeds that which is assessed in entry-level licensure examinations.[2] Nurses who have had their knowledge validated through a certification examination make decisions with greater confidence.[3] A decreased likelihood of death has also been suggested to be related to patients being cared for by certified nurses.[5–7] Although "failure to rescue" a patient in trouble cannot always be avoided, experienced and knowledgeable nurses are able to recognize signs and symptoms earlier and respond accordingly. In addition, certified nurses have demonstrated commitment to continual learning. This attribute is needed to care for patients with complex, multisystem problems requiring aggressive intervention and advanced technologies.

## Value to Employers and Nurses

Certification allows the employer to know that the nurses working for them have the knowledge and expertise to promote optimal patient outcomes. Nurses who become certified have demonstrated their commitment to quality since they have taken the time to become certified in a specialty area of practice. Evidence across studies demonstrates that certified nurses have higher perceptions of workplace empowerment and do not intend to leave the profession.[3,4,8] In a review of the literature examining the perceived effects of specialty nurse certification, both communication and collaboration are essential to quality patient outcomes. Additionally, evidence indicates that certified nurses intend to remain employed in an area where they can apply their knowledge. It has been suggested that health care organizations that support and recognize the value of certification experience decreased turnover rates and higher nurse retention rates.[3,4]

As health care organizations apply to achieve Magnet designation by the American Nurses Credentialing Center (ANCC), certification is one of the many important factors considered.[7,9] Certification is also a means for hospitals to distinguish themselves from competitors.[2] In addition, hospital administrators must demonstrate to The Joint Commission that nurses are competent to provide care: Certification is a clear demonstration of knowledge competency.[2]

Certification provides nurses with a sense of professional pride and achievement.[1] A survey by the American Board of Nursing Specialties revealed that most nurses who sat for certification examinations did so for personal fulfillment and commitment to excellence in practice.[3] Certified nurses demonstrate to their employers that they are taking responsibility for their own professional development, which may give them a competitive edge when seeking promotion or new career opportunities.

Research has identified that certified nurses perceive higher empowerment, recognize the intrinsic value of certification, experience enhanced collaboration with other members of the interdisciplinary team, and perceive knowledge being enhanced and validated through certification.[4,8]

## EBP in Critical Care Nursing

EBP is "applying the best available research results (evidence) when making decisions about health care. Health care professionals who perform EBP use research evidence along with clinical expertise and patient preferences."[10] EBP is essential to help optimize patient outcomes in today's dynamic health care environment. In the United States, the Institute of Medicine (IOM), the ANCC, and The Joint Commission acknowledge EBP as a crucial step in improving health care quality.[11] Although knowledge about effective nursing interventions continues to increase, practice lags behind the available evidence. Practice based on intuition or information that does not have a scientific basis is not in the best interest of patients and families and should be discouraged when care decisions are being made.

EBP is often confused with conducting research. Research is conducted to generate new knowledge. Through translation of new knowledge, EBP takes what is known and uses it to guide patient care to achieve the best possible outcomes.[10] In the translation of knowledge into clinical practice, it is essential for the critical care nurse to consider the strength or level of the evidence.

- Much of health care and nursing practice has little or no evidence or research to support it. Consequently, other sources of evidence must be considered.
- Different research designs have limitations that affect generalizability of findings to populations other than those studied.[11]
- Nurses and other health care professionals must critically examine the evidence that they use in their clinical reasoning, but should not restrict their definition of what constitutes evidence to only what can be measured in a randomized controlled trial (RCT).

Therefore, it is essential for critical care nurses to familiarize themselves with the levels of evidence in order to evaluate the evidence or research and determine the applicability to their patients.[12]

The AACN was one of the first nursing organizations to develop a rating system for evidence. In 2008, a work group was charged by the AACN board of directors to review the evidence-leveling system and to align the AACN hierarchy with other health care organizations.

## Levels of Evidence

In EBP, the lowest levels of evidence include the opinions of authorities or expert committees. This level of evidence would result from clinical practice committees and professional organizations that may convene to discuss guidelines when higher levels of evidence are not available. The next level of evidence is a single descriptive, qualitative, or physiologic study. Continuing up the evidence hierarchy is the systematic review of descriptive, qualitative, or physiologic studies. A systematic review refers to rigorous and systematic synthesis of findings from several studies in a focused area of inquiry. Proceeding in the hierarchy, a single correlational or observational study provides the next level of evidence. To guide clinical practice, these quantitative studies lend themselves to precise measurement allowing for examination of relationships. The next level is the systematic review of correlational or observational studies, examining relationships and evaluating cause and effect. Moving toward the stronger levels of evidence is a single RCT and nonrandomized control trial (quasi-experimental). The highest level of evidence is the systematic review of RCTs, also referred to as a meta-analysis. A meta-analysis is a statistical approach to combine the data derived from a systematic review; therefore, every meta-analysis should be based on an underlying systematic review, but not every systematic review leads to a meta-analysis. For studies using qualitative methods, a meta-synthesis is analogous to a meta-analysis.[13]

Using postoperative delirium as an example, a critical care nurse would identify much literature on postoperative delirium, yielding editorials from experts, descriptive studies, single RCTs, and meta-analyses. Since meta-analyses, the highest level of evidence, exist for postoperative delirium, critical care nurses can revise protocols and implement interventions based on evidence to prevent this condition.[14] To improve quality of care and to protect patient safety during critical illness, critical care nurses must be able to systematically gather, review, synthesize, and evaluate the evidence to guide practice changes and promote quality clinical outcomes. For example, rather than just using the clinical practice guidelines available at the National Guidelines Clearinghouse (www.guideline.gov), the critical care nurse needs to perform a meta-analysis or systemic review of the available evidence in order to determine best practice.

## Barriers to Implementation

Despite the value of EBP, it unfortunately takes an average of 17 years to translate research findings into clinical practice.[15] Barriers to implementation include lack of knowledge of the research process, limited access to literature, lack of skill to critique research, limited interest in scientific inquiry, limited power to change practice, time factors, lack of organizational support and commitment (including resources), volume of research being published, and availability of mentors.[16]

An organization's culture, climate, or environment has significant impact on the nurses' autonomy to change nursing practice and the ability to adapt to change.[17] Critical care nurses are often adept and skillful in direct patient care, but when care is not based on evidence, it is difficult to optimize outcomes, use resources efficiently, and protect patient safety. Thus, it is essential for critical care nurses to have the required knowledge, skills, and abilities for locating and evaluating relevant evidence and translating the evidence into practice.

## Strategies to Promote Implementation

Several strategies have been proposed to help enhance the incorporation of evidence into clinical practice, including the use of protocols, clinical pathways, algorithms, and educational interventions. Increasing critical care nurses' awareness of available resources and educating and mentoring them to implement EBP activities are essential. Similar to building a house, an organization committed to EBP must first establish EBP as a foundation of everyday practice and create a culture of clinical inquiry and commitment to lifelong learning.

Several resources are available for critical care nurses to facilitate adoption of an EBP culture. Superb databases include PubMed, CINAHL, and MEDLINE. The Cochrane Collaboration, a website containing high-quality, independent evidence to inform health care decision making and obtain evidence-based information, is available via the worldwide web. In addition, professional nursing organizations have research-based practice recommendations frequently available via their websites. For example, AACN's Practice Alerts section is available to members as well as to the public. Other EBP resources include the websites and publications from the Agency for Healthcare Research and Quality (www.ahrq.gov), Centers for Disease Control and Prevention (www.cdc.gov), Institute for Healthcare Improvement (www.ihi.org), IOM (www.iom.edu), National Guidelines Clearinghouse (www.guidelines.gov), National Institute for Health and Clinical Excellence (NICE) in the United Kingdom (www.nice.org.uk), U.S. National Library of Medicine (www.nlm.nih.gov), and American Nurses Association (www.nursingworld.org) as well as the Society of Critical Care Medicine (www.sccm.org). Table 1-1 summarizes perceived barriers to the implementation of EBP and outlines strategies for those perceived barriers.

## Healthy Work Environments

The current nursing shortage calls for major change in the workplace. An HWE can lead to positive patient outcomes. In addition, nurses gravitate to facilities that have optimal work conditions. Conversely, unhealthy work environments play a role in health care errors, result in ineffective care, waste scarce resources, leading to increased costs associated with health care, and contribute to moral distress and adverse outcomes.

AACN affirms that the best way to address the nursing shortage is to focus on HWEs. After conducting an extensive literature search, AACN developed the HWE initiative based on data indicating that harmful health care working environments exist nationwide, and that these environments result in medical errors, poor health care delivery,

**TABLE 1-1** Barriers and Recommended Strategies to Optimize Evidence-Based Practice in Critical Care

| Perceived Barriers to EBP | Strategies to Overcome Perceived Barriers |
| --- | --- |
| **Time** | |
| • No time to read and evaluate research or implement EBP<br>• Heavy workload/lack of time | • Schedule time for review and discussion of evidence in the form of EBP committees<br>• Nurses need time away from clinical bedside responsibilities for EBP activities |
| **Knowledge** | |
| • Unaware of research<br>• Literature not compiled in one place<br>• Not capable of evaluating quality of research<br>• Misconceptions about evidence-based practice<br>• Lack of ability to understand research<br>• Poor understanding of statistics<br>• Inadequate understanding of jargon used in research articles | • Invest, as a student, in the process of searching and evaluating the evidence<br>• Be a change agent in the facility, mentoring nurses who are less familiar with the process<br>• Commit to lifelong learning |
| **Resources and Mentoring** | |
| • Lack of evidence<br>• Isolated from knowledgeable colleagues<br>• Lack of computers, computer skills, library access, search skills<br>• Difficulty understanding research<br>• Lack of access to resources | • Administration must recognize and commit to EBP, putting systems in place to support the clinical nurses in their role with EBP<br>• Managers need to recognize the ability of clinical nurses, provide the necessary resources, and document the effectiveness of initiatives<br>• Implementation of an evidence-based champion<br>• Designated work groups |
| **Culture** | |
| • No authority to change practice<br>• Other staff and disciplines not supportive<br>• Research not generalizable to setting<br>• Lack of value of research in practice<br>• Lack of administrative support<br>• Difficulty changing behavior<br>• Organizational culture rewarding routine, task-based practice<br>• Lack of nursing autonomy | • A research-based needs assessment to provide an evidence-based foundation for organizational strategic planning<br>• Performance appraisals and clinical ladder reviews require examples of EBP<br>• Educational activities that help clinicians critically review the literature<br>• Clinical resources available 24 h a day<br>• Streamlined processes for practice<br>• Incorporating the doctor of nursing practice role as leader of this process<br>• Progress reported to a central source and shared among clinical areas and facilities<br>• Mentors and champions at the bedside<br>• Utilize clinical nurse specialists who may have a better understanding of research and EBP |

Data from Brown CE, Wickline MA, Ecoff L, et al: Nursing practice, knowledge, attitudes and perceived barriers to evidence based practice at an academic medical center. J Adv Nurs 65(2):371–381, 2009; Majid S, Foo S, Luyt B, et al: Adopting evidence-based practice in clinical decision making: Nurses' perceptions, knowledge and barriers. J Med Libr Assoc 99(3):229–236, 2011; Ross J: Information literacy for evidence-based practice in perianesthesia nurses: Readiness for evidence based practice. J Perianesth Nurs 25(2):64–70, 2010; Schulman CS: Strategies for starting a successful evidence based practice program. Adv Crit Care 19(3):301–311, 2008; and Wallis L: Barriers to implementing evidence-based practice remain high for U.S. nurses. Am J Nurs 112(12):15, 2012.

and dissatisfaction among health care providers. The HWE initiative focuses on barriers to employee and patient safety and identifies six essential standards, which encompass the aspects that are most important as nurses strive to provide optimal care.[18] Box 1-1 lists these six standards, including the critical elements inherent in each.

## Standard 1: Skilled Communication

Miscommunication is identified as a cause of many sentinel events in health care; skilled communication is essential to prevent these errors from occurring. A large majority of sentinel events reported to The Joint Commission from 2004 through the fourth quarter of 2010 were related to communication issues.[19]

The AACN partnered with VitalSmarts, L.C., to conduct a study of conversations that do not occur in hospitals, to the detriment of patient safety and provider well-being. The "Silence Kills" study used focus groups, interviews, workplace observations, and surveys of nurses, physicians, and administrators in urban, rural, and suburban hospitals nationwide.[20] Overwhelming data indicated that poor communication and ineffective collaboration were prevalent among health care provider interactions. In this report, 53% of nurses related concern about a peer nurse's competence, but only 12% spoke with this peer about their concerns.[20] Similarly, 34% of nurses were concerned about a physician's competence, but only 12% spoke with this peer to discuss concerns. In both situations, failure to communicate skillfully and professionally can be linked to poor patient care and clinical outcomes.

The "Silence Kills" study included the following example of a situation where poor communication can adversely affect patient outcome: A group of nurses considered a nurse colleague to be absentminded and negligent. They reported that, unknown to this nurse, they rechecked her work, performed safety checks and vital signs after the nurse had just done so, and performed other "work-arounds" rather than speak with her about it. This went on for over a

---

**BOX 1-1** **Essential Elements of a Healthy Work Environment**

**Standard 1: Critical Elements of Skilled Communication**
*Nurses must be as proficient in communication skills as they are in clinical skills.*
- The health care organization provides team members with support for and access to education programs that develop critical communication skills including self-awareness, inquiry/dialogue, conflict management, negotiation, advocacy, and listening.
- Skilled communicators focus on finding solutions and achieving desirable outcomes.
- Skilled communicators seek to protect and advance collaborative relationships among colleagues.
- Skilled communicators invite and hear all relevant perspectives.
- Skilled communicators call on goodwill and mutual respect to build consensus and arrive at common understanding.
- Skilled communicators demonstrate congruence between words and actions, holding others accountable for doing the same.
- The health care organization establishes zero-tolerance policies and enforces them to address and eliminate abuse and disrespectful behavior in the workplace.
- The health care organization establishes formal structures and processes that ensure effective information sharing among patients, families, and the health care team.
- Skilled communicators have access to appropriate communication technologies and are proficient in their use.
- The health care organization establishes systems that require individuals and teams to formally evaluate the impact of communication on clinical, financial, and work environment outcomes.
- The health care organization includes communication as a criterion in its formal performance appraisal system, and team members demonstrate skilled communication to qualify for professional advancement.

**Standard 2: Critical Elements of True Collaboration**
*Nurses must be relentless in pursuing and fostering true collaboration.*
- The health care organization provides team members with support for and access to education programs that develop collaboration skills.
- The health care organization creates, uses, and evaluates processes that define each team member's accountability for collaboration and how unwillingness to collaborate will be addressed.
- The health care organization creates, uses, and evaluates operational structures that ensure the decision-making authority of nurses is acknowledged and incorporated as the norm.
- The health care organization ensures unrestricted access to structured forums, such as ethics committees, and makes available the time needed to resolve disputes among all critical participants, including patients, families, and the health care team.
- Every team member embraces true collaboration as an ongoing process and invests in its development to ensure a sustained culture of collaboration.
- Every team member contributes to the achievement of common goals by giving power and respect to each person's voice, integrating individual differences, resolving competing interests, and safeguarding the essential contribution each must make in order to achieve optimal outcomes.
- Every team member acts with a high level of personal integrity.
- Team members master skilled communication, an essential element of true collaboration.

- Each team member demonstrates competence appropriate to his or her role and responsibilities.
- Nurse managers and medical directors are equal partners in modeling and fostering true collaboration.

**Standard 3: Critical Elements of Effective Decision Making**
*Nurses must be valued and committed partners in making policy, directing and evaluating clinical care, and leading organizational operations.*
- The health care organization provides team members with support for and access to ongoing education and development programs focusing on strategies that ensure collaborative decision making. Program content includes mutual goal setting, negotiation, facilitation, conflict management, systems thinking, and performance improvement.
- The health care organization clearly articulates organizational values, and team members incorporate these values when making decisions.
- The health care organization has operational structures in place that ensure the perspectives of patients, and their families are incorporated into every decision affecting patient care.
- Individual team members share accountability for effective decision making by acquiring necessary skills, mastering relevant content, assessing situations accurately, sharing fact-based information, communicating professional opinions clearly, and inquiring actively.
- The health care organization establishes systems, such as structured forums involving all departments and health care disciplines, to facilitate data-driven decisions.
- The health care organization establishes deliberate decision-making processes that ensure respect for the rights of every individual, incorporate all key perspectives, and designate clear accountability.
- The health care organization has fair and effective processes in place at all levels to objectively evaluate the results of decisions, including delayed decisions and indecision.

**Standard 4: Critical Elements of Appropriate Staffing**
*Staffing must ensure the effective match between patient needs and nurse competencies.*
- The health care organization has staffing policies in place that are solidly grounded in ethical principles and support the professional obligation of nurses to provide high-quality care.
- Nurses participate in all organizational phases of the staffing process from education and planning—including matching nurses' competencies with patients' assessed needs—through evaluation.
- The health care organization has formal processes in place to evaluate the effect of staffing decisions on patient and system outcomes. This evaluation includes analysis of when patient needs and nurse competencies are mismatched and how often contingency plans are implemented.
- The health care organization has a system in place that facilitates team members' use of staffing and outcomes data to develop more effective staffing models.
- The health care organization provides support services at every level of activity to ensure nurses can optimally focus on the priorities and requirements of patient and family care.
- The health care organization adopts technologies that increase the effectiveness of nursing care delivery. Nurses are engaged in the selection, adaptation, and evaluation of these technologies.

*(continued)*

---

**BOX 1-1** | **Essential Elements of a Healthy Work Environment (Continued)**

**Standard 5: Critical Elements of Meaningful Recognition**
*Nurses must be recognized and must recognize others for the value each brings to the work of the organization.*

- The health care organization has a comprehensive system in place that includes formal processes and structured forums that ensure a sustainable focus on recognizing all team members for their contributions and the value they bring to the work of the organization.
- The health care organization establishes a systematic process for all team members to learn about the institution's recognition system and how to participate by recognizing the contributions of colleagues and the value they bring to the organization.
- The health care organization's recognition system reaches from the bedside to the board table, ensuring individuals receive recognition consistent with their personal definition of meaning, fulfillment, development, and advancement at every stage of their professional career.
- The health care organization's recognition system includes processes that validate that recognition is meaningful to those being acknowledged.
- Team members understand that everyone is responsible for playing an active role in the organization's recognition program and meaningfully recognizing contributions.
- The health care organization regularly and comprehensively evaluates its recognition system, ensuring effective programs that help to move the organization toward a sustainable culture of excellence that values meaningful recognition.

**Standard 6: Critical Elements of Authentic Leadership**
*Nurse leaders must fully embrace the imperative of an HWE, authentically live it, and engage others in its achievement.*

- The health care organization provides support for and access to educational programs to ensure that nurse leaders develop and enhance knowledge and abilities in skilled communication, effective decision making, true collaboration, meaningful recognition, and ensuring resources to achieve appropriate staffing.
- Nurse leaders demonstrate an understanding of the requirements and dynamics at the point of care and within this context successfully translate the vision of an HWE.
- Nurse leaders excel at generating visible enthusiasm for achieving the standards that create and sustain HWEs.
- Nurse leaders lead the design of systems necessary to effectively implement and sustain standards for HWEs.
- The health care organization ensures that nurse leaders are appropriately positioned in their pivotal role in creating and sustaining HWEs. This includes participation in key decision-making forums, access to essential information, and the authority to make necessary decisions.
- The health care organization facilitates the efforts of nurse leaders to create and sustain an HWE by providing the necessary time and financial and human resources.
- The health care organization provides a formal co-mentoring program for all nurse leaders. Nurse leaders actively engage in the co-mentoring program.
- Nurse leaders role-model skilled communication, true collaboration, effective decision making, meaningful recognition, and authentic leadership.
- The health care organization includes the leadership contribution to creating and sustaining an HWE as a criterion in each nurse leader's performance appraisal. Nurse leaders must demonstrate sustained leadership in creating and sustaining an HWE to achieve professional advancement.
- Nurse leaders and team members mutually and objectively evaluate the impact of leadership processes and decisions on the organization's progress toward creating and sustaining an HWE.

From American Association of Critical-Care Nurses: AACN standards for establishing and sustaining healthy work environments: A journey to excellence. Aliso Viejo, CA: American Association of Critical Care-Nurses, 2005. Retrieved January 29, 2015, from http://www.aacn.org/WD/HWE/Docs/HWEStandards.pdf.

---

year. Physicians had also avoided confronting the situation and had compensated for the nurse in question. The data suggest that physicians are as unlikely as nurses to confront an incompetent peer or other health care provider. In fact, 88% of physicians reported working with people who had persistently poor clinical judgment that caused deleterious complications.[20]

Seventy-seven percent of nurses were concerned about the disrespect they experience in the health care environment. They reported being treated discourteously or abusively in at least 25% of their interactions. This study found a significant correlation between the frequency of being mistreated and the intent to resign from the job. The study concluded that health care providers repeatedly observe errors and dangerous levels of incompetence, yet they do not speak up; rather, they consider leaving their respective units because of their concerns.[20]

## Standard 2: True Collaboration

True collaboration occurs when "the unique knowledge and abilities of every professional are respected to achieve safe quality care for patients. Without the synchronous, ongoing collaborative work of health care professionals from multiple disciplines, patient and family needs cannot be optimally satisfied within the complexities of today's healthcare system."[18]

Many studies have been conducted regarding nurse–physician collaboration. Ninety percent of all AACN members have reported that collaboration with physicians and administrators is among the most important elements in creating an HWE.[18] A collaborative work environment is equally essential for establishing a safe work environment.[21] A number of outcomes have been linked to positive nurse–physician collaborative relationships. Recently reported outcomes include decreased morbidity and mortality rates, fewer errors, and decreased costs of care, as well as increased nurse retention and increased nurse job satisfaction.[22] Despite studies supporting the outcomes of nurse–physician collaboration, data continue to regularly reveal significant differences in perception of collaboration between these two groups.[22]

In the fall of 2011, following collaboration with the IOM, the Robert Wood Johnson Foundation (RWJF) assembled nurse and physician leaders from their professional organizations to outline an interdisciplinary consensus document. Following an initial negative reaction by some medical professional organizations, the Center for Applied Research, which led the consensus-building process, organized a meeting in early 2012. Results from this later meeting included a new understanding and respect between nurses and physicians and agreement that "the patient must be at the center of interprofessional collaboration, although challenges remain in implementing that focus." Physicians agreed that a team-based approach was "great as long as I'm the leader." There were identified differences in approaches to patient care between nurses and physicians and agreement that further understanding of these differences was required.[23]

In one study of collaboration between nurses and physicians, frequently and infrequently used behaviors were evaluated. Collaborative behaviors that were most frequently reported by the 114 nurses who participated were related to sharing patient information. The collaborative behaviors that were reported by the 33 physicians were relationships between the physicians and nurses. The most infrequent collaborative behaviors reported by both groups were related to decision-making processes regarding patient care or cure.[24]

Despite the reported benefits of collaboration, it is not practiced often.[23] A number of barriers exist that preclude collaboration in health care organizations. In addition to the lack of an agreed-upon definition for collaboration, other barriers have historically included professional cultures, immaturity of nurses and physicians, coupling of unassertive nurse behavior and aggressive physician behavior, the challenges of human relationships and personalities, hierarchical barriers, power imbalances, decision-making processes in organizations, hierarchical structure of health care organizations, nurses' perceived power differences, territorial boundaries, different perceptions of what patients need, which lead to different goals being set for patients, and role socialization.[24]

## Standard 3: Effective Decision Making

Clinical decision making is an essential component of nursing responsibilities in relation to quality patient outcomes. In clinical practice, where true collaboration does not exist and the elements of an HWE are not embraced, it is difficult for nurses, who are accountable for a scope of practice, to fully participate in decisions that affect quality and safe, effective care. The HWE standards reveal that only a small percentage of physicians acknowledge nurses as part of the decision-making team.[18]

Today's health care climate is ever changing.[25] As severity of patient illness increases, so does nurses' responsibility for patient outcomes. Nurses caring for high acuity and critically ill patients are confronted with a plethora of challenging and complex situations. These situations require that nurses make a multitude of decisions each day. Effective decision making and high levels of critical thinking are central to optimizing quality patient outcomes. Dorgham and Al Mahmoud[25] describe two types of decisions with regard to nursing practice: patient care decisions, which impact direct care, and condition of work decisions, which impact patient groups and the work environment. The complex course of action of making choices regarding patient care is the core of effective decision making.[26]

A greater amount of clinical experience correlates with improved decision making. This is evidenced by the percentage of errors made by novice nurses.[27] Errors that have been reported were related to critical thinking and experience. Therefore, it is suggested that enhancing clinical decision making may be one way to mitigate nursing errors.[28]

Effective clinical decision making is essential to the delivery of quality care. Factors reported to affect nurses' clinical decision making include clinical experience, competent education, relationship with instructors, values, beliefs, stress, and cognitive abilities.[28] To promote quality patient outcomes, nurses must use the nursing process, apply critical thinking, and draw on knowledge and experience to make salient clinical decisions promptly.

## Standard 4: Appropriate Staffing

For appropriate staffing, one must consider the knowledge, skills, and abilities—collectively referred to as competencies— of staff assigned in relation to the individualized, holistic needs of the patient and family. When the needs of patients and families are matched with the competencies of the assigned nurse, optimal outcomes may be achieved.

In a landmark study, Aiken et al[29] documented an increased risk for patient mortality when the nurse-to-patient ratio increased in the medical–surgical setting. In this study, when the nurse-to-patient ratio was 1:8, the patient's risk for death was 31% higher than when the nurse-to-patient ratio was 1:4 or lower. After the fourth patient, each surgical patient added to a nurse's assignment resulted in a 7% increase in chance of patient death within 30 days of hospital admission and a 7% increase in failure to rescue. Later data corroborate improved quality metrics with lower nurse-to-patient ratios in adult patients and fewer hospital readmissions in pediatric patients with lower nurse-to-patient ratios.[30]

Researchers found significant relationships between lower nurse staffing and adverse patient outcomes. These outcomes included postoperative sepsis, pneumonia, deep vein thrombosis, pressure ulcers, and mortality.[31,32] In its report, the IOM acknowledged the relationship between nurse staffing and quality of care. Nurse staffing levels and knowledge and skill level have an impact on patient outcomes and safety.

## Standard 5: Meaningful Recognition

HWEs as well as programs that effectively recognize nurses and nursing contribution to quality, safe patient care are important to retain high-performing nurses, to engage them actively in enhancing patient satisfaction, to use scarce nursing resources appropriately, and to enhance nursing accomplishment.

Nurse recognition can have a significant effect on job satisfaction. Because of generational, gender, and cultural differences in today's nursing workforce, nurses find workplace satisfaction through a variety of mechanisms and frequently desire more out of a job than just a salary. Staff recognition has been identified as one of the simplest, most cost-effective approaches to retain experienced staff, and is essential to maintain nurse morale.[33,34]

There seems to be universal agreement that to retain nursing staff during a critical shortage, in addition to monetary rewards when possible, expression of appreciation by recognition for excellent performance is part of the strategy.[33] Nurses in one study rated recognition from patients, families, and other nurses to be of greater value than recognition from nursing leaders and physicians. In a follow-up study, nurses continued to value recognition from patients and families most (48.9%). This was followed by recognition from other registered nurses (27%), administration (8.5%), immediate supervisor (7.7%), physicians (4.6%), and other coworkers (3.3%).[35]

Meaningful recognition is associated with increased self-esteem. This can enhance job performance, improve communication with patients, families, and colleagues, and improve patient safety.[34] Meaningful recognition has been found to be associated with a number of positive outcomes, such as job satisfaction, commitment to an organization and career, collaboration, perceived organizational support, feeling valued, job embeddedness, and work group cohesion.[36–38] This will likely translate into retention. Absence of meaningful recognition is associated with absenteeism, staff turnover, stress, burnout, and decreased quality of care. Therefore, in addition to appropriate staffing, effective decision making, and true collaboration, critical care nurses, like all nurses, value meaningful recognition, which in turn improves job satisfaction and morale while reducing turnover and improving quality patient outcomes.[34]

## Standard 6: Authentic Leadership

Nurses are attracted to health care systems that promote an HWE. Nursing leaders, from unit manager to chief nurse executive, as well as nursing peers are essential to creating and sustaining a healthy environment in today's dynamic health care climate.[18] It has been demonstrated that positive nursing leadership is linked to quality patient outcomes.[39] This has been corroborated by The Joint Commission, which asserts that leadership is essential to obtain high-quality, safe health care, and that ineffective leadership is a contributing factor when sentinel events occur.[19] Attributes of an authentic leader include good communication skills, integrity, inspiring others, working as part of the team, asking for and giving 100%, and establishing a vision.[39]

## The Synergy Model

The Synergy Model developed by the AACN has served as the foundation for certified practice since the late 1990s.[40,41] The model describes nursing practice on the basis of patients' characteristics. The underlying premises of the Synergy Model are that (1) patients' characteristics are of concern to nurses; (2) nurses' competencies are important to patients; (3) patients' characteristics drive nurses' competencies; and (4) when patients' characteristics and nurses' competencies match and synergize, outcomes for the patient are optimal.[40,41] The Synergy Model has also been described as a framework that can be used as a basis for work to be done by facilities seeking Magnet designation.[41]

Eight patient characteristics and eight nurse competencies that constitute nursing practice form the basis of the model (Fig. 1-1; Boxes 1-2 and 1-3). The patient characteristics range in intensity and are expressed as level 1, 3, or 5. The level can change from 1 minute to the next. Like the patient characteristics, the nurse competencies exist on a continuum and are expressed as level 1, 3, or 5. The level can vary based on level of expertise in a given clinical situation.

The Synergy Model is also used to determine outcomes. Outcomes are evaluated based on those derived from the patient, nurse, and health care system. Patient-derived outcomes may include functional change, trust, satisfaction,

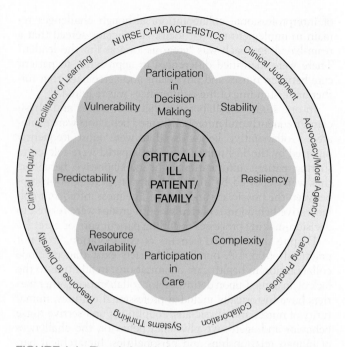

**FIGURE 1-1**   The relationship between the patient/family and the nurse in the Synergy Model.

comfort, and quality of life. Nurse-derived outcomes may include physiological changes, absence of complications, and extent to which treatment objectives are attained. Health care system–derived outcomes may include recidivism (a negative outcome), costs (savings or overrun), and resource utilization (under- or overutilization or optimal utilization).

Since its development, the Synergy Model has been used in a variety of clinical settings as a basis for nursing clinical advancement, determining staffing ratios, preceptorship, safe critical care patient transport, building a nursing productivity measure, and guiding practice of rapid response teams, and as a foundation for advanced practice nursing.[41,42]

## Alarm Fatigue

The amount of medical equipment with alarms has grown exponentially.[43] Alarms are integrated into infusion pumps, mechanical ventilation, beds (indicating that a patient may be attempting to get up without assistance), sequential compression devices, feeding pumps, cardiac monitors, and pulse oximeters, to name a few.

The purpose of alarms on medical devices is to notify care providers of either a change in a patient's physiologic status or that a predetermined threshold for a variable has been exceeded.[44] While hundreds or thousands of alarms may sound on a patient each day,[44] as few as 1% necessitate a nursing intervention.[44,45] "Alarm fatigue" occurs when the nurse is surrounded by harsh noise from too many alarms, including false alarms—also termed "nuisance alarms," meaning that there was not a valid triggering event[43]—that did not require intervention. Nuisance alarms distract the health care provider from patient care. The high incidence of nuisance alarms has been well documented in the literature over the past two decades.[44]

**The Synergy Model: Characteristics of Patients, Clinical Units, and Systems of Concern to Nurses**

- **Resiliency**—the capacity to return to a restorative level of functioning using compensatory/coping mechanisms; the ability to bounce back quickly after an insult
  *Level 1: Minimally resilient.* Unable to mount a response; failure of compensatory/coping mechanisms; minimal reserves; brittle
  *Level 3: Moderately resilient.* Able to mount a moderate response; able to initiate some degree of compensation; moderate reserves
  *Level 5: Highly resilient.* Able to mount and maintain a response; intact compensatory/coping mechanisms; strong reserves; endurance

- **Vulnerability**—susceptibility to actual or potential stressors that may adversely affect patient outcomes
  *Level 1: Highly vulnerable.* Susceptible; unprotected, fragile
  *Level 3: Moderately vulnerable.* Somewhat susceptible; somewhat protected
  *Level 5: Minimally vulnerable.* Safe; out of the woods; protected, not fragile

- **Stability**—the ability to maintain a steady-state equilibrium
  *Level 1: Minimally stable.* Labile; unstable; unresponsive to therapies; high risk of death
  *Level 3: Moderately stable.* Able to maintain steady state for limited period of time; some responsiveness to therapies
  *Level 5: Highly stable.* Constant; responsive to therapies; low risk of death

- **Complexity**—the intricate entanglement of two or more systems (eg, body, family, therapies)
  *Level 1: Highly complex.* Intricate; complex patient/family dynamics; ambiguous/vague; atypical presentation
  *Level 3: Moderately complex.* Moderately involved patient/family dynamics
  *Level 5: Minimally complex.* Straightforward; routine patient/family dynamics; simple/clear cut; typical presentation

- **Resource Availability**—extent of resources (eg, technical, fiscal, personal, psychological, and social) the patient/family/community bring to the situation
  *Level 1: Few resources.* Necessary knowledge and skills not available; necessary financial support not available; minimal

personal/psychological supportive resources; few social systems resources
  *Level 3: Moderate resources.* Limited knowledge and skills available; limited financial support available; limited personal/psychological supportive resources; limited social systems resources
  *Level 5: Many resources.* Extensive knowledge and skills available and accessible; financial resources readily available; strong personal/psychological supportive resources; strong social systems resources

- **Participation in Care**—extent to which patient/family engages in aspects of care
  *Level 1: No participation.* Patient and family unable or unwilling to participate in care
  *Level 3: Moderate participation.* Patient and family need assistance in care
  *Level 5: Full participation.* Patient and family fully able to participate in care

- **Participation in Decision Making**—extent to which patient/family engages in decision making
  *Level 1: No participation.* Patient and family have no capacity for decision making; requires surrogacy
  *Level 3: Moderate participation.* Patient and family have limited capacity; seek input/advice from others in decision making
  *Level 5: Full participation.* Patient and family have capacity and make decisions

- **Predictability**—a characteristic that allows one to expect a certain course of events or course of illness
  *Level 1: Not predictable.* Uncertain; uncommon patient population/illness; unusual or unexpected course; does not follow critical pathway, or no critical pathway developed
  *Level 3: Moderately predictable.* Wavering; occasionally noted patient population/illness
  *Level 5: Highly predictable.* Certain; common patient population/illness; usual and expected course; follows critical pathway

From the American Association of Critical-Care Nurses Certification Corporation. Retrieved January 29, 2015, from http://www.aacn.org/wd/certifications/content/synmodel.pcms?menu=certification#Patient.

**The Synergy Model: Nurse Competencies of Concern to Patients, Clinical Units, and Systems**

- **Clinical Judgment**—clinical reasoning, which includes clinical decision making, critical thinking, and a global grasp of the situation, coupled with nursing skills acquired through a process of integrating formal and informal experiential knowledge and evidence-based guidelines
  *Level 1:* Collects basic-level data; follows algorithms, decision trees, and protocols with all populations and is uncomfortable deviating from them; matches formal knowledge with clinical events to make decisions; questions the limits of one's ability to make clinical decisions and delegates the decision making to other clinicians; includes extraneous detail
  *Level 3:* Collects and interprets complex patient data; makes clinical judgments based on an immediate grasp of the whole picture for common or routine patient populations; recognizes patterns and trends that may predict the direction of illness; recognizes limits and seeks appropriate help; focuses on key elements of case, while sorting out extraneous details
  *Level 5:* Synthesizes and interprets multiple, sometimes conflicting, sources of data; makes judgment based on an

immediate grasp of the whole picture, unless working with new patient populations; uses past experiences to anticipate problems; helps patient and family see the "big picture"; recognizes the limits of clinical judgment and seeks multidisciplinary collaboration and consultation with comfort; recognizes and responds to the dynamic situation

- **Advocacy and Moral Agency**—working on another's behalf and representing the concerns of the patient/family and nursing staff; serving as a moral agent in identifying and helping to resolve ethical and clinical concerns within and outside the clinical setting
  *Level 1:* Works on behalf of patient; self-assesses personal values; aware of ethical conflicts/issues that may surface in clinical setting; makes ethical/moral decisions based on rules; represents patient when patient cannot represent self; aware of patients' rights
  *Level 3:* Works on behalf of patient and family; considers patient values and incorporates in care, even when differing from personal values; supports colleagues in ethical and clinical issues; moral decision making can deviate from rules;

*(continued)*

demonstrates give and take with patient's family, allowing them to speak/represent themselves when possible; aware of patient and family rights

*Level 5:* Works on behalf of patient, family, and community; advocates from patient/family perspective, whether similar to or different from personal values; advocates ethical conflict and issues from patient/family perspective; suspends rules—patient and family drive moral decision making; empowers the patient and family to speak for/represent themselves; achieves mutuality within patient/professional relationships

- **Caring Practices**—nursing activities that create a compassionate, supportive, and therapeutic environment for patients and staff, with the aim of promoting comfort and healing and preventing unnecessary suffering. Includes, but is not limited to, vigilance, engagement, and responsiveness of caregivers, including family and health care personnel

*Level 1:* Focuses on the usual and customary needs of the patient; no anticipation of future needs; bases care on standards and protocols; maintains a safe physical environment; acknowledges death as a potential outcome

*Level 3:* Responds to subtle patient and family changes; engages with the patient as a unique patient in a compassionate manner; recognizes and tailors caring practices to the individuality of patient and family; domesticates the patient's and family's environment; recognizes that death may be an acceptable outcome

*Level 5:* Has astute awareness and anticipates patient and family changes and needs; is fully engaged with and sensing how to stand alongside the patient, family, and community; caring practices follow the patient and family lead; anticipates hazards and avoids them, and promotes safety throughout patient's and family's transitions along the health care continuum; orchestrates the process that ensures patient's/family's comfort and concerns surrounding issues of death and dying are met

- **Collaboration**—working with others (eg, patients, families, health care providers) in a way that promotes/encourages each person's contributions toward achieving optimal/realistic patient/family goals. Involves intradisciplinary and interdisciplinary work with colleagues and community

*Level 1:* Willing to be taught, coached, and/or mentored; participates in team meetings and discussions regarding patient care and/or practice issues; open to various team members' contributions

*Level 3:* Seeks opportunities to be taught, coached, and/or mentored; elicits others' advice and perspectives; initiates and participates in team meetings and discussions regarding patient care and/or practice issues; recognizes and suggests various team members' participation

*Level 5:* Seeks opportunities to teach, coach, and mentor and to be taught, coached, and mentored; facilitates active involvement and complementary contributions of others in team meetings and discussions regarding patient care and/or practice issues; involves/recruits diverse resources when appropriate to optimize patient outcomes

- **Systems Thinking**—body of knowledge and tools that allow the nurse to manage whatever environmental and system resources exist for the patient/family and staff, within or across health care and non–health care systems

*Level 1:* Uses a limited array of strategies; limited outlook—sees the pieces or components; does not recognize negotiation as an alternative; sees patient and family within the isolated environment of the unit; sees self as key resource

*Level 3:* Develops strategies based on needs and strengths of patient/family; able to make connections within components; sees opportunity to negotiate but may not have strategies; developing a view of the patient/family transition process; recognizes how to obtain resources beyond self

*Level 5:* Develops, integrates, and applies a variety of strategies that are driven by the needs and strengths of the patient/family; global or holistic outlook—sees the whole rather than the pieces; knows when and how to negotiate and navigate through the system on behalf of patients and families; anticipates needs of patients and families as they move through the health care system; utilizes untapped and alternative resources as necessary

- **Response to Diversity**—the sensitivity to recognize, appreciate, and incorporate differences into the provision of care. Differences may include, but are not limited to, cultural differences, spiritual beliefs, gender, race, ethnicity, lifestyle, socioeconomic status, age, and values.

*Level 1:* Assesses cultural diversity; provides care based on own belief system; learns the culture of the health care environment

*Level 3:* Inquires about cultural differences and considers their impact on care; accommodates personal and professional differences in the plan of care; helps patient/family understand the culture of the health care system

*Level 5:* Responds to, anticipates, and integrates cultural differences into patient/family care; appreciates and incorporates differences, including alternative therapies, into care; tailors health care culture, to the extent possible, to meet the diverse needs and strengths of the patient/family

- **Facilitation of Learning**—the ability to facilitate learning for patients/families, nursing staff, other members of the health care team, and community. Includes both formal and informal facilitation of learning

*Level 1:* Follows planned educational programs; sees patient/family education as a separate task from delivery of care; provides data without seeking to assess patient's readiness or understanding; has limited knowledge of the totality of the educational needs; focuses on a nurse's perspective; sees the patient as a passive recipient

*Level 3:* Adapts planned educational programs; begins to recognize and integrate different ways of teaching into delivery of care; incorporates patient's understanding into practice; sees the overlapping of educational plans from different health care providers' perspectives; begins to see the patient as having input into goals; begins to see individualism

*Level 5:* Creatively modifies or develops patient/family education programs; integrates patient/family education throughout delivery of care; evaluates patient's understanding by observing behavior changes related to learning; is able to collaborate and incorporate all health care providers' and educational plans into the patient/family educational program; sets patient-driven goals for education; sees patient/family as having choices and consequences that are negotiated in relation to education

- **Clinical Inquiry (Innovator/Evaluator)**—the ongoing process of questioning and evaluating practice and providing informed practice. Creating practice changes through research utilization and experiential learning

*Level 1:* Follows standards and guidelines; implements clinical changes and research-based practices developed by others; recognizes the need for further learning to improve patient care; recognizes obvious changing patient situation (eg, deterioration, crisis); needs and seeks help to identify patient problem

---

**BOX 1-3** **The Synergy Model: Nurse Competencies of Concern to Patients, Clinical Units, and Systems (*Continued*)**

*Level 3:* Questions appropriateness of policies and guidelines; questions current practice; seeks advice, resources, or information to improve patient care; begins to compare and contrast possible alternatives

*Level 5:* Improves, deviates from, or individualizes standards and guidelines for particular patient situations or populations;

questions and/or evaluates current practice based on patients' responses, review of the literature, research, and education/learning; acquires knowledge and skills needed to address questions arising in practice and improve patient care. (The domains of clinical judgment and clinical inquiry converge at the expert level; they cannot be separated.)

From the American Association of Critical-Care Nurses Certification Corporation. Retrieved January 29, 2015, from http://www.aacn.org/wd/certifications/content/synmodel.pcms?menu=certification#Patient.

---

Alarm fatigue may result in apathy toward alarms, limits being changed, alarms being turned down, deactivation of alarms, individuals becoming insensitive to the alarms, failure to respond to alarms, ignoring the alarms, or alarms not being heard.[43,45–47] Alarm fatigue has been implicated in numerous patient deaths.[43,47–49] As a result, alarm fatigue has been identified as the top technology hazard for the past 4 years.[43,45,47,50–52] There are 98 alarm-related events recorded in The Joint Commission sentinel event database from January 2009 to June 2012; 80 of these events led to patient death, 13 patients had permanent loss of function, and 5 had increased length of hospital stay.[53]

In 2003, The Joint Commission added alarm safety to the National Patient Safety Goals (NPSG). Part of this mandate requires alarms to be set appropriately so that health care providers can be notified of changes in a patient's status or of equipment malfunction. Subsequently, as a result of 23 reported deaths or injuries involving patients on mechanical ventilation, clinical alarms were changed from an NPSG to an Environment of Care standard in 2005.[54] In October 2011, a clinical alarms summit was assembled by the Association for the Advancement of Medical Instrumentation (AAMI), the U.S. Food and Drug Administration (FDA), The Joint Commission, and the American College of Clinical Engineering to address this issue.[43,44]

Alarms are now designed with varying levels of intensity to help distinguish those situations requiring an immediate response from those that do not. Improvements are being made in clinical settings to mitigate nuisance alarms and alarm fatigue. Some interventions include changing alarm delays, workflow changes, daily electrode changes, and individualizing alarms based on a patient's status.[43,45,47,53,54]

## Future Challenges in Critical Care Nursing

Because health care, nursing, and the world are dynamic, critical care nursing must continue to evolve. As the United States becomes increasingly diverse, nursing must increase its ability to deliver evidence-based care that is culturally congruent and relevant. The growing US Hispanic population makes it increasingly essential for health care systems to have a multilingual, culturally diverse workforce. This requires not only the need to recruit and retain diverse professionals but also the need to expand the skill set of today's already experienced critical care nurses.[55–57]

As new and emerging infectious diseases present, critical care nurses must be prepared to identify, manage, and treat unknown threats. Similarly, Hurricane Katrina clearly demonstrated the impact that natural disasters have on a nation, health outcomes, and the nursing workforce. Furthermore, in the era after September 11, critical care units must be prepared to handle any actual or potential bioterrorism threat.

Finally, as critical care continues to evolve and becomes increasingly technologically sophisticated, critical care nurses must continue to expand their repertoire of skills and evidence-based interventions to address not only the physiological needs but also the psychosocial, spiritual, ethical, and advocacy needs of patients and families. With implementation of advances in technology, the critical care unit will continue to require caring, competent, and knowledgeable nurses who can foster collaboration, navigate complex delivery and reimbursement systems, and facilitate patient and family learning while responding to vulnerable diverse communities with complex needs.[58] These exciting challenges await critical care nurses—challenges that they will overcome with commitment, dedication, and grace!

## Clinical Applicability Challenges

### SHORT ANSWER QUESTIONS

1. Describe a situation in your workplace when nurses experienced alarm fatigue. What were the underlying issues and sequelae?
2. Describe a time when nurses overcame system barriers and implemented a practice change based on evidence.
3. Describe a clinical situation that exemplifies high levels of competence with the nurse competency advocacy and moral agency from the AACN Synergy Model for Patient Care.

---

**WANT TO KNOW MORE?**

A wide variety of resources to enhance your learning and understanding of this chapter are available on thePoint.

You will find:

- References
- Selected readings
- NCLEX-style review questions
- Internet resources
- And more!

# 2

# The Patient's Experience With Critical Illness

### DORRIE FONTAINE AND KATHRYN S. BIZEK

## LEARNING OBJECTIVES

*Based on the content in this chapter, the reader should be able to:*

1. Explore relationships among stress, response to illness, and anxiety.
2. Examine the role of the nurse in controlling environmental stressors to promote healing and limit posttraumatic stress disorder.
3. Compare and contrast techniques that the patient and family can learn in an effort to manage stress and anxiety.
4. Describe strategies to promote sleep and early mobilization in critically ill patients.
5. Develop nursing interventions that foster the ability of patients to draw strength from their personal spirituality.
6. Discuss alternatives to the use of physical restraint in the intensive care unit.

The patient's experience in an intensive care unit (ICU) has lasting meaning for the patient and his or her family members and significant others. Although actual painful memories may be blurred by drugs and the mind's need to forget, attitudes that are highly charged with feelings about the nature of the experience survive. These attitudes shape the person's beliefs about nurses, physicians, health care, and the vulnerability of life itself.

This chapter describes specific measures that nurses use to support patients in managing the stressors associated with critical illness and injury. It is the caring presence and emotional support given by the nurse that will be remembered and valued.

## Perception of Critical Illness

Admission to an ICU may signify a threat to the life and well-being of the patient who is admitted. Critical care nurses perceive the unit as a place where fragile lives are vigilantly scrutinized, cared for, and preserved. However, patients and their families often perceive admission to critical care as a sign of impending death, based on their own past experiences or the experiences of others. Understanding what critical care means to patients may help nurses care for their patients. However, effective communication with critically ill patients is often challenging and frustrating.[1-3] Barriers to communication may relate to the patients' physiologic status; the existence of endotracheal tubes, which inhibit verbal communication; medications; and other conditions that alter cognitive function.

About 30% to 100% of former ICU patients could recall part or all of their stay in the ICU.[4] Although many of the patients recalled feelings that were negative, they also recalled neutral and positive experiences. Negative experiences were related to fear, anxiety, sleep disturbance, cognitive impairment, and pain or discomfort. Positive experiences were related to feelings of being safe and secure. Often, these positive feelings were attributed to the care provided by nurses. The need to feel safe and the need for information were predominant themes in other research studies.[2,5-7] Nurses' technical competence and effective interpersonal skills were cited by patients as promoting their sense of security and trust.

## Stress

Stress exists when an organism is faced with any stimulus that causes disequilibrium between psychological and physiologic functioning. Patients admitted to the ICU are subject to multiple physical, psychological, and environmental stressors. Stimulation of the body's stress response involves activation of the hypothalamic–pituitary–adrenal axis. The resultant increase in catecholamine, glucocorticoid, and mineralocorticoid levels leads to a cascade of physiologic responses.[8]

### Acute Stress Response

Critical injury or illness can initiate the first phase of the stress response. This phase is characterized by the body's efforts to survive and involves the stimulation of the sympathetic nervous system and activation of multiple neuroendocrine responses. This "ebb phase" results in increased heart rate and contractility, vasoconstriction, and increase in blood pressure. Blood flow is redirected to vital organs. Pain sensations are temporarily attenuated. Body temperature and nutrient consumption fall. A sensation of thirst may be prominent. Other physiologic effects include increase in minute ventilation and respiratory rate, hyperglycemia, insulin resistance, and coagulopathies. This initial phase is deeply catabolic as protein stores are mobilized to respond to the threat and begin to repair the injury. If this phase is prolonged, it can result in impaired oxygen and nutrients delivery to tissues secondary to alterations in microcirculatory blood flow. Table 2-1 summarizes the effects of hormones released in response to major stress.[9-19]

The second phase of the stress response, or the "flow phase," is a hyperdynamic state that occurs as the body

| TABLE 2-1 | Major Stress-Related Hormones and Effects | |
|---|---|---|
| **Stress Hormones** | **Source** | **Major Effects** |
| Adrenocorticotropic hormone | Anterior pituitary | Stimulates adrenal cortex to release cortisol |
| Catecholamines | Adrenal medulla and the sympathetic nervous system | Increases overall strength, blood flow to vital organs, glyconeogenesis |
| Epinephrine | | Increases myocardial contractility (inotropic effect), heart rate (chronotropic effect), venous return to the heart, and cardiac output |
| Norepinephrine | | Constricts smooth muscle in all blood vessels, increases blood pressure, dilates pupils, inhibits gastrointestinal activity |
| Cortisol | Adrenal cortex (following stimulation by adrenocorticotropic hormone from the anterior pituitary) | Gluconeogenesis; hyperglycemia; decreases protein synthesis, immunoglobulin synthesis, number of lymphocytes, and leukocytes (at inflammatory site); promotes muscle and lymphoid tissue catabolism; delays healing; suppresses cell-mediated immune response |
| Antidiuretic hormone | Posterior pituitary | Increases water retention |
| Aldosterone | Adrenal cortex | Increases sodium and water retention |
| Growth hormone (somatotropin) | Anterior pituitary | Increases immune function; levels are increased during stress |
| Prolactin | Anterior pituitary | β-Cell activation and differentiation; levels are reduced during stress |
| Testosterone | Testis | Regulates male secondary characteristics; levels are decreased during chronic stress |
| Endorphins | Anterior pituitary | Endogenous opiates, elevated during stress, downregulate pathways to the stress response |
| Enkephalins | Adrenal medulla | Endogenous opiates, elevated during stress, downregulate pathways to the stress response |

From Lusk B, Lash AA: The stress response, psychoneuroimmunology, and stress among ICU patients. Dimens Crit Care Nurs 24(1):25–31, 2005, with permission.

compensates for the oxygen deprivation. This phase is also characterized by multiple hormonal influences. Pain and discomfort are now prominent. Movement is minimized to conserve metabolic costs. Prolonged activation of the stress response can lead to immunosuppression, hypoperfusion, tissue hypoxia, and eventual death. Treatment is directed at eliminating the stressors and providing supportive care in the form of nutrition, oxygenation, pain management, anxiety control, and specific measures related to the cause of illness or injury.[16,20–22]

## Environmental Stressors in the Intensive Care Unit

The ICU is a stressful environment for patients and caregivers. Walk into any ICU and you will find blinking monitors, ventilators, intravenous (IV) pumps, noise from equipment and the many practitioners talking at the bedside, bright lights, and a hurried pace in a crowded space. Multiple sophisticated technologies are commonplace. The specialty of critical care nursing developed in response to this setting, where the most acutely ill and injured receive concentrated nursing care to enhance survival.

In the early ICUs of the 1950s, nurses were confronted daily with pain, suffering, and death while caring for patients in a confined, though open, space.[23] In older hospitals, these ICUs were often a few beds, carved out of existing wards, which brought the sickest patients together in one area. The most distinctive feature of the first ICUs was this concentration of nursing care; this is where the specialty of intensive care nursing was born. As the design of ICUs evolved over the decades, care needs for the patient and family also evolved. The concept of the healing environment emerged—that is, the idea that the hospital environment can make a difference in how quickly the patient recovers.[24]

Key design features of ICUs from the 1950s through the present reflects the notion of close observation and rapid intervention.[25] Meeting patient needs through continuous monitoring is the hallmark of all critical care. However, close monitoring has led to patient complaints of noise, lighting with no day–night distinction, and frequent interruptions of sleep and rest. Intensive care beds were often so close to each other that patients could hear everything happening to the critically ill patient in the next bed. Lack of privacy and fears related to overheard procedures and conversations in the unit created undue anxiety and the potential for physiologic instability in vulnerable patients.

The evolution of ICUs has demonstrated increasing use of the precepts of patient- and family-focused care.[26] Early units typically had no space for family to visit, and visits were not encouraged. Emphasis today is on how the design of the ICU can best meet the needs of the patient and family as a unit, despite the important life-sustaining technology. Signs that welcome family and visitors to the ICU often suggest the philosophy of the hospital and the culture of the unit. The more welcoming the ICU is to visitors, the more likely the environment is to offer a healing culture of care and support. Does the sign on the door read "Stop, Do Not Enter" or "Welcome to the ICU"?

Patients are more likely to experience a positive outcome in an environment that incorporates natural light, elements of nature, soothing colors, meaningful and varied stimuli, peaceful sounds, and pleasant views.[27] In fact, research demonstrates less pain medication is needed and a faster recovery may occur when careful attention is given to providing a soothing environment. Hospitals that combine creative design elements with an emphasis on patient- and family-focused care are the leaders in creating healing spaces for recovery.

## Noise

Despite third-generation unit design and architecture, the problems of noise and bright lighting have remained a challenge. Beds surrounded by noisy machines and equipment are intimidating to patients, family, and novice nurses in critical care. Noise is an environmental hazard that creates discomfort in a patient. Consequences of noisy environments include disrupted sleep, impaired wound healing, and activation of the sympathetic nervous system. Moderate noise levels may produce vasoconstriction. Hyperarousal related to noise can occur over many days to even weeks for patients with prolonged ICU stays.

Patient complaints include listening to banging noises, alarms going off at all times, water sounds (such as the bubbling of chest tubes), and doors opening and closing. Sources of noise include equipment, alarms, telephones, televisions, ventilators, and staff conversations. Health care providers are often unaware of the loudness of their conversations and the irritation they may create for patients. Nurses should perform an objective assessment of the environment for noise.

Noise is measured in decibels using a logarithmic scale. An increase of 10 decibels makes a sound seem twice as loud. Sleep occurs best below 35 decibels. The Environmental Protection Agency recommends unit noise be less than 45 decibels during the day and 35 decibels at night. Numerous studies measuring noise levels in the ICU consistently demonstrate elevations as high as 80 to 90 decibels. Background noise is often above 50 decibels day and night.[28] New technology can be an additional source of noise, although some manufacturers attempt to provide equipment that lowers the total unit volume of sound.

Decades of studies consistently point to noise as a key aspect of the ICU environment. Noise was measured in two ICUs using a sound meter placed at the head of a patient's bed.[29] More than 50% of the noise in the environment was attributed to human behavior, with a mean sound level of 84 decibels in the medical ICU. Television and talking were two of the most frequent disruptive sounds for patients. Another study investigated the perceptions of 203 patients who filled out a questionnaire on discharge from the ICU and found that noise from talking and alarms was the most disruptive to sleep.[30] Sound peaks greater than 80 decibels are common in ICUs and are directly related to arousals from sleep.[31] Although noise is not the only culprit in limiting sleep in the ICU, it remains an important one.[32]

In recent years, alarm fatigue has been recognized as detrimental to nurse well-being as well as patient safety. Between 72% and 99% of clinical alarms may be false,[33] leading to "alarm fatigue"—that is, nurses become desensitized to alarms because of the high percentage of alarms that are false. Strategies to consider in the case of cardiac alarms include changing electrocardiogram electrodes every day, better skin preparation, education, and making the alarm parameters individualized to decrease the number of false alarms. Studies are underway to uncover the deficiencies of current alarm systems in order to implement better computer algorithms.[34]

## Lights and Color

Light is a powerful *zeitgeber*, or environmental synchronizer, that assists in entraining sleep by promoting the normal circadian cycle of sleep and wakefulness. Many critical care settings could benefit from more natural lighting and lights that are lowered during normal sleep times. In addition to natural lighting, providing a soothing view for the patient to look on instead of the ceiling or a hospital curtain may foster recovery. A classic study found that when a patient had a view of natural scenery and the outdoors, as opposed to viewing a brick wall, less pain medication was used and the hospital stay was shorter.[35] Other studies have demonstrated that impaired cognition occurs more often in windowless units than in those with windows.

In the hospital setting, artificial light is provided by fluorescent bulbs and tubes. If unshielded, this harsh light leads to visual fatigue and headaches. Glare reflected off environmental surfaces such as glass, shiny metal, mirrors, and enameled or polished finishes is troublesome to patients, especially elderly patients. Bright lights may be left on for many hours in ICUs, even when no direct patient care is being performed. Lack of control over artificial lighting is a source of frustration to critical care patients.

Interruptions in normal light–dark patterns can disrupt normal physiologic processes. For example, artificial light exposure for as little as 20 minutes during a normal sleep cycle caused a drop in melatonin levels.[36] In addition, constant lighting and high-intensity light can lead to a complete disruption of the normal melatonin concentration rhythm. Melatonin secreted at night synchronizes the sleep–wake and dark–light cycles.[37] Patients with sepsis in an ICU are likely to have disrupted melatonin secretion not linked to the normal circadian pattern.[38] However, therapy with exogenous melatonin is not a clear recommendation to increase sleep duration in critically ill patients at this time.[39]

The ideal ICU environment has windows with natural views, soothing artwork, and calm colors. The nurse and other health care providers have access to work and computer stations with glass soundproof partitions that permit proximity to the patient for easy observation while shielding the patient from noise. Equipment is selected for its low noise level. Stress created by unnecessary noise and light is diminished for the good of the patients, families, and staff. This vision may already be a reality in some institutions. For example, muted colors of beige, blue, and green were used to design a holistic nursing unit in a Minnesota hospital.[40] Art on the walls depicts many different cultures and the peacefulness of nature. The goal of a more peaceful, healing ICU environment is possible to attain.

## Anxiety

Anxiety is an emotional state of apprehension in response to a real or perceived threat. Typically, the threat is associated with motor tension, increased sympathetic activity, and hypervigilance.

### Causes of Anxiety

Any stressor that threatens a person's sense of wholeness, containment, security, and control can cause anxiety. Illness and injury are such stressors. Other common causes of anxiety include feelings of increased vulnerability and decreased security, which occurs when patients admitted to ICUs perceive a loss of control, a sense of isolation, and fear of death or loss of functionality. Anxiety, pain, and fear can initiate or perpetuate the stress response. Left untreated or undertreated, anxiety can contribute to the morbidity and mortality of critically ill patients.

Anxiety occurs when people experience the following:

- Threat of helplessness
- Loss of control
- Sense of loss of function and self-esteem
- Failure of former defenses
- Sense of isolation
- Fear of dying

### Assessment of Anxiety

Assessment of anxiety is challenging in the critical care population because of the severity of illness, barriers to communication, and altered cognitive states. However, most critical care nurses believe that assessment of anxiety is important. Multiple-item, self-report scales of anxiety may be used, but they have specific drawbacks in critical care areas, especially for patients receiving mechanical ventilation, because of communication barriers. According to many critical care nurses, the top five physiologic and behavioral indicators of anxiety are agitated behavior, increased blood pressure, increased heart rate, verbalization of anxiety, and restlessness. Monitoring of these patient parameters is useful, but there is still a need for a reliable and comprehensive anxiety assessment tool.[11,17] Use of a visual analog scale to assess anxiety with selected patients can be useful.[41]

## Delirium

Delirium may be an unintended consequence of a patient's ICU experience that can lead to a prolonged stay and higher mortality. Often undetected, delirium is increasingly recognized as a factor in morbidity and mortality that can affect up to 80% of patients. The American Association of Critical Care Nurses practice alert on delirium assessment and management recommends tools such as the Confusion Assessment Method for the ICU (CAM-ICU) developed by Ely et al.[42] Early mobility and limiting sedation are the current best practices for delirium prevention and treatment. The ABCDE bundle includes multiple evidence-based practices to support patients; it consists of spontaneous **A**wakening and **B**reathing trial coordination,

Careful sedation choice, **D**elirium assessment, and **E**arly progressive mobility and exercise.[42] Family engagement and empowerment is advocated through adding an **F** to this bundle and highlighting the essential role of families in the healing process.[43]

## Nursing Interventions

In caring for the critically ill patient, the nurse helps the patient manage a multitude of stressors. Stress management includes not only physical and environmental stressors but also psychological stressors. This complex and labor-intensive process requires advanced assessment skills, adept manipulation of a variety of highly technological treatment strategies, and creativity in care and compassion.[44-47]

### Creating a Healing Environment

Florence Nightingale, the founder of modern nursing, often wrote about the nurse's role in creating an environment that would allow healing to occur. She emphasized holism in nursing—that is, caring for the whole person. In today's technological age, critical care nurses are challenged to create an environment of healing. These environments must allow critically ill patients to have their psychological as well as physical needs met. Manipulating the milieu may involve timing interventions to allow adequate sleep and rest, providing pain-relieving medication, playing music, and teaching relaxation and mindfulness approaches such as breathing exercises. The physical environment of the ICU can be altered to create a more healing and restful environment.

### Promoting Rest and Sleep

#### Sleep Assessment

Promotion of sleep and rest for critically ill patients begins with an understanding of sleep, the major environmental disruptions, and a sleep assessment.

Sleep involves two very distinct types of brain activity: rapid eye movement (REM) sleep and non-REM sleep. The sleep stages are described in Box 2-1. Healthy adults progress through sleep stages in a specific order, from a light stage to a deeper stage, in 90-minute cycles. REM sleep increases later in the normal nighttime sleep patterns of most people, with morning naps containing primarily REM sleep. Specific sleep stages have a circadian rhythm and are controlled by brainstem mechanisms.[48]

Although sleep patterns are individual, most patients can tell when they feel rested and have had a "good night's sleep." Unfortunately, this is a rare occurrence in the hospital. Sleep, once thought to be a quiescent state, actually involves physiologic activation while the brain and body rejuvenate themselves. Sleep is often appreciated only when it has been "lost" and is typically taken for granted by health care providers, who often do not make sleep a priority for patients. Often in the ICU, sleep is severely fragmented and nonconsolidated,[49] with those receiving mechanical ventilation experiencing some of the most severe sleep disruption.[39]

---

**BOX 2-1**    **Stages and Characteristics of Sleep**

| | |
|---|---|
| Stage 1 | Transitional stage between wakefulness and sleep |
| | Relaxed state where person is somewhat aware of surroundings |
| | Involuntary muscle jerking that may awaken the person |
| | Normally lasts only minutes |
| | Easily aroused |
| | Constitutes only about 5% of total sleep |
| Stage 2 | Beginning of sleep |
| | Arousal occurs with relative ease |
| | Constitutes 50% to 55% of sleep |
| Stage 3 | Depth of sleep increased and arousal increasingly difficult |
| | Constitutes about 10% of sleep |
| Stage 4 | Greatest depth of sleep (*delta sleep*) |
| | Arousal from sleep difficult |
| | Physiological changes in the body—slow brain waves on electroencephalogram, decreased pulse and respiratory rates, decreased blood pressure, relaxed muscles, slow metabolism, and low body temperature |
| | Constitutes about 10% of sleep |
| Stage REM | Sleep with vivid dreaming (rapid eye movement [REM]) |
| | REM, fluctuating heart and respiratory rates, fluctuating blood pressure |
| | Skeletal muscle tone lost |
| | Most difficult to arouse |
| | Duration of REM sleep increased with each cycle and averages 20 minutes |
| | Constitutes about 20% to 25% of sleep |

Adapted from Taylor C, Lillis C, LeMone P, et al: Fundamentals of Nursing: The Art and Science of Nursing Care, 8th ed. Philadelphia, PA: Lippincott Williams & Wilkins, 2015.

---

Sleep deprivation in patients in ICUs can have cumulative effects and can lead to altered cognition, confusion, impaired wound healing, and the inability to wean from the ventilator because of muscle fatigue and carbon dioxide retention. For over four decades, researchers have noted that patients in ICUs have frequent awakenings, little to no REM sleep, shorter total sleep time than at home, and perceived poor quality of sleep.[32,50,51] Drugs can interrupt sleep in critically ill patients.[52] In addition, care interventions, such as unnecessary baths between the hours of 2:00 and 5:00 AM, can disturb the sleep of critically ill patients on a routine basis.[53] A poor sleep pattern is characteristic of all age groups in the ICU, from elderly to pediatric patients.[54] The impact of sleep disruption on the clinical outcome of ICU patients is not fully known. However, patients often report that sleep disruption is one of the most unpleasant aspects of their illness.

The patient's own report of sleep quality is the best measure of sleep adequacy, although this is inherently difficult when the patient is receiving mechanical ventilation. As with pain assessment, only the person affected can make the assessment: "I slept well" or "I didn't sleep at all." Monitoring brain waves by polysomnography is the gold standard for measuring patient sleep but is not feasible as a standard measure in the ICU.[52] If self-report of sleep is unobtainable, systematic observation of patients by nurses has been shown to be somewhat valid and reliable.[55] A visual analog scale is recommended for select patients at high risk for sleep disruption owing to extended stay in the ICU.[56] Wrist actigraphy is used as a research tool to continuously monitor activity and rest but may overestimate sleep in sedentary and elderly people.[52]

### Promoting Sleep

Despite four decades of research into reasons why patients do not sleep in the ICU, little has been done to facilitate what patients often rate as their number one priority after pain relief: sleep. Box 2-2 outlines strategies that are most often recommended to promote sleep. The challenging environment dictates that the nurse first is sensitive to the patient's needs and attuned to the environment and then has the tools and resources to implement sleep promotion.

A time-honored idea for promoting sleep is the 5-minute backrub. The concept of using back massage to ease patients to sleep seems intuitive; however, until recently, it had never been systematically studied. In a study of 69 patients in an ICU, a 5-minute slow back massage (or *effleurage*) was demonstrated to increase patient sleep by 1 hour as compared with a control group.[57] It should be noted that an effective backrub does not consist of the application of cold lotion and a quick one-handed massage while holding the patient on his or her side with the other hand, but rather a soothing, slow-stroke massage, in which the nurse first becomes centered and truly present with the patient.

The role of the nurse as a gatekeeper to protect patient sleep time will be more difficult to fulfill as patient–nurse ratios escalate, but it must remain a priority. According to the 2013 clinical practice guidelines for sedatives and analgesics

---

**BOX 2-2**    **Nursing Interventions**

For Promoting Sleep
- Provide large clocks and calendars.
- Block sleep times.
- Provide a quiet time during the day shift.
- Have the patient use earplugs and eye masks.
- Assess sleep time and quality of sleep by asking the patient when possible.
- Provide opportunity for music therapy.
- Provide a 5-minute backrub before sleep.
- Consider using white noise or ocean sounds.
- Eliminate pain.
- Position patient for comfort with pillows.
- Stop the practice of bathing patients in the middle of the night for the convenience of the nursing staff.
- Titrate environmental stimuli: turn down lights, turn down alarms, and decrease noise from television and talking.
- Evaluate the need for nursing care interruptions.
- At bedtime, provide information to lower anxiety. Do a review of the day and remind patient of progress made toward recovery, then add what to expect for the next day.
- Institute "PM Care" back to basics, brushing teeth, and washing face before "bedtime."
- Allow family to be with the patient and provide open visiting.
- Use relaxation techniques, mindfulness meditation, and guided imagery.
- Ensure patient privacy: close door or pull curtains.
- Post sign at designated times: "Patient Sleeping."

in the critically ill adult developed by a multidisciplinary team of physicians, pharmacists, and nurses, sleep promotion should include optimization of the patient's environment through the use of strategies to control light and noise, to cluster patient care activities, and to decrease stimuli at night in order to protect the sleep cycle.[58] One intervention is to implement a sleep protocol that institutionalizes the importance of sleep,[59] blocks sleep times, and truly controls the environment. In several studies, it was shown that having a "quiet time" helped improve the opportunity for sleep.[60,61] Earplugs and eye masks can be considered,[62] as well as staff behavior modification programs for limiting noise.[63] Another innovation in sleep promotion that decreased noise and promoted sleep involved moving all routine chest radiographs from 3:00 am to 10:00 pm.[64] Although this increased the workload of the radiology department on the evening shift, patient and nurse satisfaction rose dramatically.

All health care providers need to be aware of the importance of restorative sleep and its impact on a patient's well-being and work toward a "sleep-friendly ICU."[65] Sleep of the health care provider is also an important aspect of the healing dyad in the ICU. Nurses who work nights are routinely sleep deprived; they may have young children to care for at home or school to attend when the next day begins. The growing interest in patient safety makes the work patterns of nurses, including 12-hour shifts and overtime, a focus of study.[66] Nurses' vigilance to patient needs is threatened with longer work hours, and the risk for error is increased. Antidotes for working at night include scheduling of shifts to phase-advance the sleep cycle (ie, going from days to evenings to nights), eating healthy snacks, using bright lights during a shift away from patient rooms, and obtaining regular exercise.[66] Compassionate caring includes the nurse caring for himself or herself in order to better meet the demands of patients, families, and colleagues. Prioritizing clinician well-being is increasingly viewed as one of the best ways to enhance patient safety and quality outcomes.[67]

## Fostering Trust

Almost every nurse in critical care can relate stories of special bonds that formed with individual patients and families. They can describe special situations where a trusting relationship developed and they made a difference in the patient's recovery or even dignified death. In contrast, research has shown that when patients mistrust their caregivers, they are more anxious and more vigilant of staff behaviors and lack the feeling of safety and security. The goals, then, are to display a confident, caring attitude, demonstrate technical competence, and develop effective communication techniques that will foster the development of a trusting relationship. Communication can be especially difficult with mechanically ventilated and intubated patients. Use of nonverbal signals, writing pads, or commercial communication boards can help make communication of basic needs easier.[68]

## Providing Information

Aside from the need to feel safe, critically ill patients identify the need for information as a high priority.[47,69,70] This "need to know" involves all aspects of care. Patients need to know what is happening at the moment. They also need to know what will happen to them, how they are doing, and what they can expect. Many patients also need frequent explanations of what happened to them. These explanations reorient them, sort out sequences of events, and help them distinguish real events from dreams or hallucinations. Anxiety can be greatly relieved with simple explanations. Consider the patient, for example, who is being weaned from the ventilator who just needs reassurance that if he did not breathe, the machine would do it for him.

Families, too, have identified the need for information as a high priority. This is followed closely by the need to have hope. Most families identify physicians as the primary source of information. It is important for nurses to be mindful of patient confidentiality issues when speaking to family members. Nurses should have the patient's permission before giving confidential medical information to family members. If that is not possible because of the patient's condition, a family spokesperson should be identified as the person who may receive confidential information, and this should be recorded in the patient's medical record.

## Allowing Control

Nursing measures that reinforce a sense of control help increase the patient's autonomy and reduce the overpowering sense of a loss of control. The nurse can help the patient exert more control over his or her environment in the following ways:

- Providing order and predictability in routines
- Using anticipatory guidance
- Allowing the patient to make choices whenever possible
- Involving the patient in decision making
- Providing information and explanation for procedures

Providing order and predictability allows the patient to anticipate and prepare for what is to follow. Perhaps it creates only an illusion of control, but anticipatory guidance keeps the patient from being caught off guard and allows the mustering of coping mechanisms. Allowing small choices when the patient is willing and ready increases the patient's feeling of control over the environment. Would the patient prefer to lie on his or her right or left side? In which arm should the IV line be placed? What height is preferred for the head of the bed? Does the patient want to cough now or in 20 minutes after pain medication? Any decisions that afford the patient a certain amount of control and predictability are important. These small choices may also help the patient accept lack of control during procedures that involve little choice.

## Encouraging Early Mobilization

Efforts to prevent delirium and PTSD increasingly point to encouraging early mobilization for patients. Getting patients up and moving in spite of being attached to the ventilator, drains, monitors, and other equipment has demonstrated benefits of improved healing, positive mood, and shorter lengths of stay. Nursing coordination of the team to make early mobilization possible is a priority.[71]

## "Presencing" and Reassurance

Presence, or just "being there," can in itself be a meaningful strategy for alleviating distress and anxiety in the critically ill patient. *Presencing* is the therapeutic use of self, adopting a caring attitude, and paying attention to a person's needs. Presence implies more than just physical presence. It means giving one's full attention to the person, focusing on the person, and practicing active listening. When a nurse uses presence, the focus is not on a task or outside thoughts. Energy and attention are directed at the patient and his or her needs or feelings. This means the nurse makes a conscious effort to use all of his or her capacity, including eyes, voice, energy, and touch, in a more intentionally healing way. Reassurance can be provided to the patient in the form of presencing and caring touch. Reassurance can also be verbal. Verbal reassurance can be effective for patients if it provides realistic encouragement or clarifies misconceptions. However, verbal reassurance is not valuable if it prevents a patient from expressing his or her emotions or stifles the need for further dialogue. Reassurance is intended to reduce fear and anxiety and evoke a calmer, more passive response. It is best directed at patients who are expressing unrealistic or exaggerated fears.

## Cognitive Techniques

Techniques that have evolved from cognitive theories of learning may help anxious patients and their families. They can be initiated by the patient and do not depend on complex insight or understanding of one's own psychological makeup. They can also be used to reduce anxiety in a way that avoids probing into the patient's personal life. Furthermore, the patient's friends and family members can be taught these techniques to help them and the patient reduce tension.

### Internal Dialogue

Highly anxious people are most likely giving themselves messages that increase or perpetuate their anxiety. These messages are conveyed in one's continuously running "self-talk" or internal dialogue. For example, the patient in the ICU may be silently saying to himself, "I can't stand it in here. I've got to get out." Another unexpressed thought might be, "I can't handle this pain." By asking the patient to share aloud what is going on in this internal dialogue, the nurse can bring to awareness the messages that are distracting the patient from rest and relaxation and suggest substitute messages to the patient. It is important to ask the patient to substitute rather than delete messages because the internal dialogue is continuously operating and will not turn off, even if the patient wills it to do so. Therefore, asking the patient to substitute constructive, reassuring comments is more likely to help the patient significantly reduce his or her tension level. Comments such as, "I'll handle this pain just 1 minute at a time" or "I've been in tough spots before, and I am capable of making it through this one!" automatically reduce anxiety and help the patient shape coping behaviors accordingly. Any message that enhances the patient's confidence, sense of control, and hope and puts him or her in a positive, active role, rather than the passive role of victim, increases the patient's sense of coping and well-being.

The nurse helps the patient develop self-dialogue messages that increase the following:

- Confidence
- Sense of control
- Ability to cope
- Optimism
- Hope

### External Dialogue

A similar method can be applied to the patient's external conversation with other people. By simply requiring patients to speak accurately about themselves to others, the same goals can be accomplished. For example, patients who exclaim, "I can't do anything for myself!" should be asked to identify the things that they are able to do, such as lifting their own bodies, turning to one side, making a nurse feel good with a rewarding smile, or helping the family understand what is happening. Even the smallest movement in the weakest of patients should be acknowledged and claimed by the patient. This technique is useful in helping patients correct their own misconceptions of themselves and the way others see them. This reduces patients' sense of helplessness and therefore their anxiety.

### Cognitive Reappraisal

The cognitive reappraisal technique asks the patient to identify a particular stressor and then modify his or her response to that stressor. In other words, the patient reframes his or her perception of the stressor in a more positive light so that the stimulus is no longer viewed as threatening. The patient is given permission to take personal control of responses to the stimulus. This technique may be combined with guided imagery and relaxation training.

## Guided Imagery and Relaxation Training

Guided imagery, meditation, and relaxation training are useful techniques that can be taught to the patient to help reduce tension.[72] The nurse can use the concept of mindfulness or meditation to guide patients to achieve a sense of calm. Guided imagery also can be used to help reduce unpleasant feelings of depression, anxiety, and hostility. Patients who must relearn life-sustaining tasks, such as walking and feeding themselves, can use imagery to prepare mentally to meet the challenge successfully. In these instances, patients should be taught to visualize themselves moving through the task and successfully completing it. If this method seems trivial or silly to the patients, they can be reminded that this method demands concentration and skill and is commonly used by athletes to improve their performance and to prepare themselves mentally before an important event. Guided imagery is a way of purposefully diverting or focusing the patients' thoughts and has been shown to empower patients, improving their satisfaction and well-being.[73,74]

The nurse can also use techniques that induce deep muscle relaxation to help the patient decrease anxiety. Deep muscle relaxation may reduce or eliminate the use of tranquilizing and sedating drugs. In progressive relaxation, the patient is first directed to find as comfortable a position as possible and then to take several deep breaths and let them out slowly. Next, the patient is asked to clench a fist or curl toes as tightly as possible, to hold the position for a few seconds, and then to let go while focusing on the sensations of the releasing muscles. The patient should practice this technique, beginning with the toes and moving upward through other parts of the body—the feet, calves, thighs, abdomen, chest, and so on. This procedure is done slowly while the patient gives nonverbal signals (eg, lifting a finger) to indicate when each new muscle mass has reached a state of relaxation. Extra time and attention should be given to the back, shoulders, neck, scalp, and forehead because many people experience physical tension in these areas.

Once a state of relaxation is achieved, the nurse can suggest that the patient fantasize or sleep as deeply as he or she chooses. The patient must be allowed to select and control the depth of relaxation and sleep, especially if the fear of death is prominent in his or her mind. A moderately dark room and a soft voice facilitate relaxation. Asking the patient to relax is frequently nonproductive compared with directing him or her to release a muscle mass actively, let go of tension, or imagine tension draining through the body and sinking deeply into the mattress. Again, the patient is assisted to take an active rather than passive role by the nurse's careful use of language. In addition, a number of commercially available recordings can be used to assist in guided imagery and relaxation.

## Deep Breathing

When acutely anxious, the patient's breathing patterns may change, and the patient may hold his or her breath. This could be physically and psychologically detrimental. Teaching diaphragmatic breathing, also called abdominal breathing, to the patient may be useful as both a distraction and a coping mechanism. Diaphragmatic breathing can be taught easily and quickly to the preoperative patient or to a patient experiencing acute fear or anxiety. The patient may be asked to place a hand on the abdomen, inhale deeply through the nose, hold briefly, and exhale through pursed lips. The goal is to have the patient push out his or her own hand to demonstrate the deep breath. The nurse may demonstrate the technique and perform it along with the patient until the patient is comfortable with the technique and is in control. The mechanically ventilated patient may be able to modify this technique by concentrating on breathing and on pushing out the hand. However, a mechanically ventilated patient experiencing severe agitation may not be able to respond to this technique.

## Music Therapy

Music therapy has been used in the critical care environment as a strategy to reduce anxiety, provide distraction, and promote relaxation, rest, and sleep.[75–78] The patient receives a choice of specially recorded audiotapes and a set of headphones. Usually, music sessions are 20 to 90 minutes long, once or twice daily. Music selections may vary by individual taste, but the most commonly used selections have a tempo of 60 to 70 beats; a simple, direct musical rhythm; and a low-pitched sound with primarily a string composition. Most patients prefer music that is familiar to them. Many ICUs maintain a CD library with a variety of genres to satisfy patient choices. Patients or family members are also encouraged to bring in their own MP3 players with the patient's favorite music selections already programmed. This intervention has proved effective for relaxing mechanically ventilated patients. Some hospitals have used loudspeakers to play music overhead in their ICUs, emergency rooms, and postanesthesia units to promote a healing environment.

## Humor

A good belly laugh produces positive physiologic and psychological effects. Laughter can increase the level of endorphins, the body's natural pain relievers, which are released into the bloodstream. Laughter can relieve tension and anxiety and relax muscles. Humor is a universal emotion that can help patients cope with stressful experiences. The use of humor by nurses in critical care, which can be spontaneous or planned, can help reduce procedural anxiety or provide distraction. Once again, the humor must be compatible with the context in which it is offered and with the person's cultural perspective. Many nurses report using humor cautiously after they have established a rapport with the individual. Nurses also report that they are able to take cues from the patient and visitors regarding the appropriate use of humor. Patients have reported that nurses who have a good sense of humor are more approachable and easier to talk with. Humor that is lighthearted, witty, and, of course, timed just right, is the most well received by adults.

Humor therapy has been used successfully in a variety of treatment settings, including pediatrics, surgery, oncology, and palliative care. In an effort to incorporate the positive effects of humor into health care settings, some institutions have developed humor resource rooms or mobile humor carts. These provide patients with a variety of lighthearted reading materials, videotapes, and audiotapes. Also included on the cart may be games, puzzles, and magic tricks. Some nurses have created their own portable therapeutic humor kits, comic strips, jokes, or humorous stories to which their patients can relate.

Use of humor by patients may help them reframe their anxiety and channel their energy toward feeling better. Some patients link humor with spirituality, noting that humor helped them cope better with serious illness and develop a closer relationship with God. In addition, appropriate use of humor can relieve stress among critical care nurses who work in complex, challenging environments with significant economic pressures.

## Massage, Aromatherapy, and Therapeutic Touch

Massage is the purposeful stroking and kneading of muscles with the goal of providing comfort and promoting relaxation.[79–82] Nurses have traditionally used effleurage for backrubs for patient comfort. Effleurage uses slow, rhythmic strokes from distal to proximal areas of long muscles such as the back or extremities. Consistent, firm, yet flexible, hand pressure is applied with all parts of the hand to conform to body contours. Lotion may be used to decrease friction and add moisture. Massage has been effective at reducing anxiety and promoting relaxation.

Patient selection is an important consideration when electing massage as a therapeutic intervention. Patients who are hemodynamically unstable, for example, would not be appropriate candidates. In addition, nurses require additional training in massage therapy to effectively incorporate more advanced massage techniques such as pétrissage or pressure points into plans of care for critically ill patients.

Massage can be combined with aromatherapy, in which massage is carried out with scented oils or lotions. Some scents have been associated with specific beneficial effects.

For example, lavender oil and other floral scents are said to be relaxing, citrus oils to be positive mood enhancers, and peppermint oils to be promoters of mental stimulation. Aromatherapy can also be accomplished with use of scented bath water or unlit scented candles placed in the room.

Therapeutic touch is a set of techniques in which the practitioner's hands move over a patient in a systematic way to rebalance the patient's energy fields. An important component of therapeutic touch is compassionate intent on the part of the healer. Therapeutic touch as a complementary therapy has been used successfully in acute care settings to decrease anxiety and promote a sense of well-being. It is a foundational technique of healing touch. Healing touch involves a number of full-body and localized techniques to balance energy fields and promote healing. Implementation of healing touch therapy involves a formal educational program for healers, and its potential benefits are under active investigation.

## Animal-Assisted Therapy

The human–animal bond has been well documented. Pet ownership has been linked to higher levels of self-esteem and physical health. Pet therapy (or, more broadly, animal-assisted therapy) has had measurable benefits for schoolchildren and residents of nursing homes. More recently, this concept has been introduced to the acute and critical care settings with positive results. Some hospitals have developed guidelines for pet visitation—for example, a patient's leashed pet may be brought to the hospital to visit with the patient. This type of program has been well received by patients and staff; however, it does require coordination between staff and family members. Pets must be in good health, have up-to-date vaccinations, and be well behaved in unfamiliar environments. The handler must be familiar with the pet and agree to follow hospital guidelines regarding time limits (generally 20 to 30 minutes per visit). A private patient room or visiting room is required. It is recommended that pets be leashed and wear a "shirt," which reduces shedding and identifies the pet. In some hospitals, a formal program exists in which volunteer owner–dog teams visit patients in the hospital on a variety of units. In addition, one hospital reported patients' delight in having fish aquariums placed in their rooms while they were awaiting heart transplantation.

## Fostering Spirituality and Healing

Caring in nursing includes recognition and support of the spiritual nature of human beings. Spirituality refers to the realm of invisible and intangible factors that influence our thoughts and behaviors. This includes religious beliefs and extends beyond them. When people sense power and influence outside of time and physical existence, they are said to be experiencing the metaphysical aspects of spirituality.

Spirituality, which includes one's system of beliefs and values, can be defined as the means or manner by which people seek meaning in their lives and experience transcendence or connectedness to that which is beyond the self.[83–85] Intuition and knowledge from unknown sources and origins of unconditional love and belonging typically are viewed as spiritual power. A sense of universal connection, personal empowerment, and reverence for life are also aspects of spirituality; these elements also may be viewed as benefits of spirituality.

Spirituality includes the following:

- Religion
- Beliefs and values
- Intuition
- Knowledge from the unknown
- Unconditional love
- A sense of belonging
- A sense of connection with the universe
- Reverence for life
- Personal empowerment

Critical care patients and their families frequently find strength in prayer, which is used by people of many faiths. Research on prayer and health has demonstrated prayer to be a powerful tool to help patients cope with difficult situations, chronic illnesses, and impending death.

Nursing goals related to spirituality include the recognition and promotion of patients' spiritual sources of strength. By allowing and supporting patients to share their beliefs about the universe without disagreement, nurses help patients recognize and draw on their own sources of spiritual courage. Recognition of the unique spiritual nature of each patient is thought to assist personal empowerment and healing.

Nurses who find their own spiritual values in religion must acknowledge and respect that nonreligious people may also be spiritual and experience spirituality as a life force. Regardless of personal views, the nurse is obligated to assess patients' spiritual belief systems and assist them to recognize and draw on the values and beliefs already in existence for them.

Critical illness may deepen or challenge existing spirituality. Patients have reported deeper faith after coping with critical illness. During these times, it may be useful for the nurse or family to call on a spiritual or religious leader, hospital chaplain, or pastoral care representative to help the patient make meaningful use of the critical illness experience. Patients may also gain support from members of their congregation or family. It is important for nurses to assess and recognize the spiritual nature of their patients, to allow time for spiritual and religious practices, and to make referrals when needed. Referrals may be made to the hospital chaplain or to a clergy person of the patient's choice.

## Restraints in Critical Care

Restraints in critical care include any drug or device that is used to restrict the patient's mobility and normal access to his or her body. Physical restraints may include limb restraints, mittens with ties, vests or waist restraints, geriatric chairs, and side rails. Side rails are considered a restraint if used to limit the ability of the patient to get out of bed rather than to help him or her sit or stand up.

## Chemical Restraint

Chemical restraints refer to pharmacologic agents that are given to patients as discipline or to limit disruptive behavior. Medications that have been used for behavior control include, but are not limited to, psychotropic drugs such as haloperidol, sedative agents such as benzodiazepines (eg, lorazepam, midazolam), and the anticholinergic antihistamine diphenhydramine. This definition does not apply to medications that are given to treat a medical condition. The use of sedative, analgesic, and anxiolytic medications is an important adjunct in the care of the critically ill patient.

Care must be taken to provide adequate comfort for patients experiencing life-threatening illnesses and a variety of noxious interventions. It is desirable to use the least amount of medication that is feasible to achieve the goals of patient care because all medications have potential side effects and adverse reactions. Patients must be continually assessed for adequacy of comfort. Behaviors that seem to indicate pain may actually indicate a change in the patient's physiologic status. Agitation, for example, may be a sign of hypoxemia. Caution must be exercised when using as-needed (prn) medications to reduce pain and promote comfort. Without consistency in assessment, goal setting, and administration, prn dosing may inadvertently lead to overmedication or undermedication in the critically ill patient. In addition, these medications can have rebound effects if abruptly withdrawn. Weaning a patient from analgesic or sedative medication may be as important as weaning a patient from a mechanical ventilator. Many ICUs incorporate assessment tools for patient comfort on their daily flow sheets.

## Physical Restraints

Historically, physical restraints have been used for patients in critical care to prevent potentially serious disruptions in patient care through accidental dislodgment of endotracheal tubes or lifesaving IV lines and other invasive therapies. Other reasons that have been cited for use of restraints include fall prevention, behavior management, and avoidance of liability lawsuits resulting from patient injury. However, research related to restraint use, especially in elderly patients, has demonstrated that these reasons, although well intentioned, are seldom valid.[86–90] Patients who are restrained have been shown to have more serious injuries secondary to falls as they "fight" the device that limits their freedom. In addition, there are reportedly a greater number of lawsuits related to improper restraint use than to injuries sustained when restraints were not used. Critically ill, intubated patients have been known to self-extubate despite the use of soft wrist restraints.

The forced immobilization that results from restraining a patient can prolong a patient's hospitalization by contributing to skin alterations, loss of muscle tone, impaired circulation, nerve damage, and pneumonia. Restraints have been implicated in accelerating patients' levels of agitation, resulting in injuries such as fractures or strangulation.

Standards on physical restraint use are published and monitored by The Joint Commission and the Centers for Medicare and Medicaid Services. A summary of these standards is given in Box 2-3. These standards may be viewed on the websites of the respective agencies. Many hospitals have revised their policies, procedures, and documentation of the use of restraints to comply with the most recent revision of these standards. Clinical practice guidelines have been published by the Society of Critical Care Medicine.

---

**BOX 2-3** | **Summary of Care Standards Regarding Physical Restraints**

**Initiating Restraints**
- Restraints require the order of a licensed independent practitioner who must personally see and evaluate the patient within specified time periods.
- Restraints are used only as an emergency measure or after treatment alternatives have failed. (Treatment alternatives and patient responses are documented.)
- Restraints are instituted by staff members who are trained and competent to use restraints safely. (A comprehensive training and monitoring program must be in place.)
- Restraint orders must be time limited. (A patient must not be placed in a restraint for longer than 24 hours, with reassessment and documentation of continued need for restraint at more frequent intervals.)
- Patients and families are informed about the reason/rationale for the use of the restraint.

**Monitoring Patients in Restraints**
- The patient's rights, dignity, and well-being are to be protected.
- The patient will be assessed every 15 minutes by trained and competent staff.
- The assessment and documentation must include evaluation of adequate nutrition, hydration, hygiene, elimination, vital signs, circulation, range of motion, injury due to the restraint, physical and psychological comfort, and readiness for discontinuance of the restraint.

---

## Alternatives to Restraints

What, then, is the well-meaning nurse to do when a patient is experiencing confusion or delirium and is pulling at his or her lifesaving devices and tubes? Remember that physical restraint is the last resort, to be used only when the patient is a danger to self or others and when other methods have failed. Restraints may actually potentiate the dangerous behavior. The nurse should attempt to identify what the patient is feeling or experiencing. What is the meaning behind the behavior? Is the patient cold? Does the patient itch? Is the patient in pain? Does the patient know where he or she is and why he or she is there? Sometimes addressing the patient's needs or concerns and reorienting the patient is all that is needed to calm him or her. Other interventions may include modifying the patient's environment, providing diversionary activities, allowing the patient more control or choices, and promoting adequate sleep and rest (Box 2-4). Some hospitals have instituted restraint protocols and decision trees to help nurses with assessment and care of patients in restraints.

## Posttraumatic Stress Disorder/Post–Intensive Care Syndrome

New evidence suggests that as many as 25% of survivors of critical illness experience posttraumatic stress disorder (PTSD) symptoms. PTSD has been identified as common in mechanically ventilated patients post-ICU.[91] Other factors that may contribute to the syndrome of PTSD include larger doses of sedation, agitation, and reports of scary memories from their ICU stay.[92] Existing psychological problems may

**BOX 2-4** **Alternatives to Physical Restraints**

Modifications to Patient Environment
- Keep the bed in the lowest position.
- Minimize the use of side rails to what is needed for positioning.
- Optimize room lighting.
- Activate bed and chair exit alarms where available.
- Remove unnecessary furniture or equipment.
- Ensure that the bed wheels are locked.
- Position the call light within easy reach.

Modifications to Therapy
- Frequently assess the need for treatments and discontinue lines and catheters at earliest opportunity.
- Toilet patients frequently.
- Disguise treatments, if possible (eg, keep intravenous [IV] solution bags behind patient's field of vision, apply loose stockinette or long-sleeved gown over IV sites).
- Meet physical and comfort needs (eg, skin care, pain management, positioning wedges, hypoxemia management).
- When possible, guide the patient's hand through exploration of the device or tube and explain the purpose, route, and alarms of the device or tube.
- Mobilize the patient as much as possible (eg, consider physical therapy consult, need for cane or walker, reclining chairs, or bedside commode).

Involvement of the Patient and Family in Care
- Allow patient choices and control when possible.
- Family members or volunteers can provide company and diversionary activities.
- Consider solitary diversionary activities (eg, music, videos or television, books on tape).
- Ensure that the patient has needed glasses and hearing aids.

Therapeutic Use of Self
- Use calm, reassuring tones.
- Introduce yourself and let the patient know he or she is safe.
- Find acceptable means of communicating with intubated or nonverbal patients.
- Reorient patients frequently by explaining treatments, devices, care plans, activities, and unfamiliar sounds, noises, or alarms.

also be a factor. Researchers are looking into using ICU diaries as a promising therapeutic tool to prevent PTSD in ICU survivors. Post–intensive care syndrome (PICS) is becoming increasingly diagnosed and is broader than PTSD.[93] A constellation of physical, cognitive, and mental health problems comprise this syndrome that is seen in up to 50% of ICU survivors as well as family members. The Society of Critical Care Medicine has instructional videos that assist in understanding and treatment.[94]

## Clinical Applicability Challenges

**SHORT ANSWER QUESTIONS**

1. What nonpharmacologic interventions are included in best practices for sleep promotion in the ICU patient, based on the 2013 Society of Critical Care Pain, Agitation and Delirium Guidelines?
2. PTSD is considered increasingly common in ICU survivors. How should the nurse intervene to prevent this syndrome?
3. Sandy is a 34-year-old multiple-trauma patient who has three small children at home. She has been in the ICU for 5 days and is slowly improving postsepsis and post–acute respiratory distress syndrome (ARDS). What interventions are most important for Sandy's recovery?

*WANT TO KNOW MORE?*

A wide variety of resources to enhance your learning and understanding of this chapter are available on thePoint.

You will find:

- References
- Selected readings
- NCLEX-style review questions
- Internet resources
- And more!

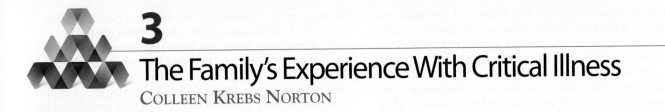

# 3

# The Family's Experience With Critical Illness

COLLEEN KREBS NORTON

## LEARNING OBJECTIVES

*Based on the content in this chapter, the reader should be able to:*

1. Comprehend the impact of a critical illness and the critical care environment on the family.
2. Identify various methods to assess the needs of individual family members.
3. Demonstrate nursing behaviors that help families cope with crisis.
4. Discuss palliative care issues in the critical care environment that have an impact on the family.
5. Define the components and application of the Critical Care Family Needs Inventory and the Critical Care Family Assistance Program.
6. Outline items to include in a plan of care that reflect the needs of the family.
7. Describe the role of the interprofessional team in the care of the critically ill patient and associated family.

Why did he die with a hole in his chest?…

Final moments.

Last breath….

If only she'd come then,

or we had thought to ask.

Her heart, an empty vessel of mourning

would ache, but the tortured anguish

of the unanswered question

never needed to be.[1]

This poem, a personal reflection that a family member shared with her nurse, demonstrates the suffering and torment she experienced when exposed to a critical illness in someone she loved. A critical illness is an unplanned, significant, and often life-altering experience that affects each family member in some way. Nurses who strive to deliver consistent, quality critical care need to recognize the importance of assessing and caring for patients and their families. The interaction between the family, the nurse, and the patient in the critical care environment, and the needs that result from this interaction, remain a challenge and responsibility of the contemporary critical care nurse.

What is meant by the word *family*? The *Oxford English Dictionary* defines family as "a group of persons consisting of the parents and their children whether actually living together or not; in a wider sense, the unity formed by those who are nearly connected by blood and affinity."[2] The Institute for Patient- and Family-Centered Care refers to family as "two or more persons who are related in any way—biologically, legally, or emotionally." In the patient- and family-centered approach, this definition, as well as the amount of involvement in decision making, should be determined by the patient if competent to do so. For the purpose of this chapter, family is defined as any people who share routine day-to-day or intimate living with the critically ill patient.[3] Additionally, anyone who is a significant part of the patient's normal lifestyle and routine is considered a family member. The term *family* describes the people whose social balance and well-being are altered by the patient's entrance into the arena of critical illness or injury. A philosophy that acknowledges that patients are part of a larger entity is essential to provide the best possible care to the patient and family.[4]

This chapter addresses the family in crisis, stressors in the critical care environment, family assessment, coping mechanisms, and the nursing process. The use of the Critical Care Family Needs Inventory (CCFNI) and the benefits of the Critical Care Family Assistance Program (CCFAP), family presence during resuscitation in the intensive care unit, and palliative care are also discussed. The role of the interdisciplinary team in the care of the critically ill patient and family is presented.

## Stress, Critical Illness, and the Impact on the Family

A critical illness is a sudden, unexpected, and often life-threatening occurrence for both the patient and the family that threatens the steady state of internal equilibrium usually maintained in the family unit. It can be an acute illness or trauma, an acute exacerbation of a chronic illness, or an acute episode of a previously unknown problem. A family member's entrance as a participant in the life–death sick role of a loved one threatens the well-being of the family and can trigger a stress response in both the patient and the family. Family members of patients in the critical care unit (CCU) may experience stress, disorganization, and helplessness, which may ultimately result in difficulty in mobilizing appropriate coping resources, thus leading to anxiety. Anxiety often includes both physiologic and behavioral factors. Physiologic aspects can include a rapid heartbeat, dry mouth, and diaphoresis. Behavioral signs can include an inability to act, inability to express oneself, and difficulty dealing with life events.[5]

When a family enters this unplanned situation with its unexpected outcomes, family members are often forced into the role of decision makers. The balance of strengths and limitations within the family, including the degree of cohesion within the family and conflict resolution strategies, often determines how stress is confronted.[6] The astute critical care nurse recognizes that the fear and anxiety demonstrated by the patient and family is an expected consequence of activation of the stress response, a somewhat protective, adaptive mechanism initiated by the neuroendocrine system in response to stressors. The stress response of family members varies.

## Stress Syndrome

Studied initially by Selye in 1956,[7] *stress* has been defined as a specific syndrome that was nonspecifically induced. Selye also discussed the role of stressors, the stimuli that produce tension and that could contribute to disequilibrium. Stressors can be physiologic (eg, traumatic, biochemical, environmental) and psychological (eg, emotional, vocational, social, cultural). The critical care environment is rich in both physiologic and psychosocial stressors that threaten the state of well-being of the patient and family.

In response to a stressor, the fight-or-flight mechanism is activated, releasing the catecholamines norepinephrine and epinephrine through the sympathetic nervous system. These hormones are responsible for the increased heart rate, increased blood pressure, and vasoconstriction that make up the physiologic response to the *alarm stage*, the initial stage of the general adaptation to stress syndrome described by Selye. The alarm stage is followed by the *stage of resistance*, which attempts to maintain the body's resistance to stress. According to Selye's theory, all people move through the first two stages many times and become adapted to the stressors encountered during ordinary life. If the person is unsuccessful at adaptation, or if the stressor is too great or prolonged, alarm and resistance are followed by the *stage of exhaustion*, which can lead to death, the result of a wearing down of the human body. The work of Selye made it possible to integrate into the nursing assessment the role that stress plays in the life of those to whom critical care is delivered. Science continues to make advances today in the study of the connection between stress and illness.

Caring practices, including the creation of a compassionate, supportive, and therapeutic environment in which the nurse has an acute awareness of the patient's and family's changing needs, are an expectation of the critical care nurse.[8] The critical care nurse is expected to help the patient's family resolve the crisis response and facilitate adaptive coping. Family members expect nurses to intervene and meet their needs, and they have high expectations for family-centered care.[9]

After the initial fear and anxiety over the critical illness and possible death of the family member, other family issues become evident, including shifts in responsibilities and role performance, unfamiliarity with the routines of the CCU, and a lack of knowledge concerning the course and outcome of the disease. These issues can develop and persist over the duration of the patient's stay in the CCU.

The patient's previous contributions to the family unit now become the responsibilities of other family members. Financial issues are often a major concern, and routine daily activities become difficult to manage. The patient is often the wage earner. Chores that had been the patient's responsibility, such as balancing a checkbook, participating in a car pool, or preparing meals, can have significant consequences if left undone. The social role that the patient plays in the family is absent during the critical illness. Comforter, organizer, mediator, lover, friend, and disciplinarian are examples of important roles in family functioning that may be, under normal circumstances, fulfilled by the patient. When that role function is unfulfilled, havoc and grief may ensue.

The circumstances surrounding the nature of the patient's illness can also be a stressor for the family. With a sudden, unexpected event, such as a blunt trauma or an acute myocardial infarction, family routines can be brought to a halt in a matter of minutes. Having little or no time to prepare for such an event, the family is overwhelmed with a massive amount of unmanageable stress and can be thrown into crisis. The hospital CCU, in most instances an unknown entity, becomes the center of the family's life. When allowed to visit in the CCU, the family observes sophisticated, intimidating equipment that causes additional fear. Such stress often can manifest itself as anger toward the caregiver. The caregiver, absorbed with the physical care of the patient, frequently has limited or inadequate time to respond to family members' emotional needs; family members may have unrealistic goals, and expectations of the health care staff.[10]

In other instances, the critical event is an acute exacerbation of a chronic but life-threatening illness. Such an episode brings with it a different set of stressors, reminding the family of difficult and painful times in the past when they have faced similar circumstances. Prolonged critical illness can present emotional difficulties for the family, which may increase the likelihood of crisis. Quality-of-life issues such as prolonged mechanical ventilation may occur and should be approached with empathy and understanding.

## Coping Mechanisms

Coping mechanisms can be defined as a person's response to a change in the environment; they can be healthy or unhealthy. The critical care nurse, as caregiver to both the patient and family, should be aware of the use of coping mechanisms by the family as a means of maintaining equilibrium. A sense of fear, panic, shock, or disbelief is sometimes followed by irrational acts, demanding behavior, withdrawal, perseveration, or fainting. The family attempts to obtain some sense of control over the situation, often demonstrated by refusing to leave the bedside or, alternatively, by minimizing the severity of the illness through denial. Reactions to crisis are difficult to categorize because they depend on the different coping styles, personalities, and stress management techniques of the family. The nurse must be able to interpret the feeling that a person in crisis is experiencing, particularly when that person cannot identify the problem or the feeling to himself or herself or to others. The following are five generalizations about crisis:

- Whether people emerge stronger or weaker as a result of a crisis is based not so much on their character as on the quality of help they receive during a crisis state.
- People are more open to suggestions and help during a crisis.

- With the onset of a crisis, old memories of past crises may be evoked. If maladaptive behavior was used to deal with previous situations, the same type of behavior may be repeated in the face of a new crisis. If adaptive behavior was used, the impact of the crisis may be lessened.
- The primary way to survive a crisis is to be aware of it.
- Dealing with a crisis demands patience, understanding, and time.

## The Family and the Nursing Process

### Nursing Assessment

In 2010, the Institute of Medicine (IOM)[11] recommended that health care delivery systems become patient centered rather than disease or clinician centered, and that an assessment be made of the patient's preferences and beliefs. In the CCU, this translates into an increase in family involvement. Nursing assessment by the critical care nurse involves primarily, but not exclusively, an appraisal of the patient. It also includes an assessment of the members of the family.[12] Accurately assessing the needs of the critically ill patient's family allows for nursing interventions to reduce the family's stress and strengthen family members' ability to interact positively; it increases family satisfaction with care and promotes trust and confidence.[13]

Patient- and family-centered care is an "approach to the planning, delivery, and evaluation of health care that is grounded in mutually beneficial partnerships among health care providers, patients, and families."[14] Initially introduced and modeled in both the pediatric and maternity setting, family-centered care is described as an expansion of total patient care, and includes the family in the planning and implementation phases of care in the critical care setting. The patient and the family are now viewed as the unit of care.[15] Family-centered care is advocated by both The Joint Commission as well as the American Association of Critical-Care Nurses (AACN) Standards for Acute and Critical Care Nursing.[16]

The nursing assessment serves as a database and identifies strengths and concerns on which care of the patient and family can be based. It includes not only physiologic data but also psychological, social, environmental, cultural, economic, and spiritual information. It involves an assessment and validation of verbal and nonverbal behavior and requires clinical expertise. A thorough nursing assessment guides the formulation of nursing diagnoses. The AACN Standards emphasize and support the importance of an assessment of the family and the continual involvement of the family in implementing the plan of care and participating, to the extent they are able, in decision making about the nursing care.[17]

An important part of the family assessment is a history of the family. Whom does the patient include in the description of his or her family? Although all patients belong to a family, the family might not include or be restricted to blood relatives. Who are the people most disturbed about the patient's illness? Is there a formal or informal leader identified by the group? This becomes important when communicating with the family in decision making, as well as in legal matters, such as obtaining consent and withdrawing life support. What is the coping style of the family? Does the family have a history

of dealing with a critical illness? What are the relationships between the members of the family? How close is the family? Do the family members identify any unresolved issues? The family history can aid the nurse in interpreting how the family is coping with stress, how their coping mechanisms will affect the patient, and how they are adapting to the patient's illness. Family assessment should include recognition of the families' values and respecting diversity.

Numerous assessment tools are available to aid the nurse in determining the needs and problems the family faces. One of the initial assessment tools was developed by Molter in 1979.[17] This method includes a 45-item needs assessment tool, which became an instrument to describe the needs of critical care family members. Leske modified the tool used by Molter by adding an open-ended item and calling it the CCFNI.[18] The CCFNI has been used widely during the past two decades to identify the needs of family members in the CCU.[18–20] The CCFNI, after analysis, was found to contain five distinct subscales: support, comfort, information, proximity, and assurance.[1] Lee and Lau found the need for assurance as the highest category among family members of critical care patients 24 to 72 hours after the patient's admission.[19] The family remains the most important social context to assess and consider when determining interventions to influence patient outcomes in a positive way.[14]

Nursing research conducted using these assessment tools reveals consistency in relation to which areas are important to be addressed with family members. These areas include but are not limited to:

1. family satisfaction with care given;
2. explanations that the family can understand;
3. the need for close proximity to the patient;
4. honest information about the patient's condition;
5. an understanding of why things are done;
6. delivery of care by staff members who are courteous and show interest in how the family is doing; and
7. assurance that someone will notify the family of any changes.

The tools also suggest assessing how comfortable the family is in the waiting room, and inquiring about what could be made better for them. Identified needs included physical needs (eg, having comfortable furniture, having the waiting room near the patient, and having a bathroom nearby) as well as emotional needs, such as a place to be alone in the hospital and the opportunity to discuss negative feelings. In addition, families of critically ill patients have other needs that should be addressed frequently, including the following:[15]

- to feel that there is hope;
- to feel that hospital personnel care about the patient;
- to know the prognosis;
- to receive information about the patient at least once a day;
- to see the patient frequently.

In summary, recent research has shown that the top needs of families of critically ill patients are the need for information, the need for support from hospital staff, and the need for hope.[21]

Although the needs perceived by the family may differ from those perceived by the nurse, strong communication

---

**BOX 3-1**   **Examples of Nursing Diagnoses**

**For the Family with Critical Illness or Injury**

- Anticipatory grieving
- Anxiety
- Caregiver role strain
- Comfort, impaired
- Communication, readiness for
- Confusion, acute
- Coping, defensive

- Coping, disabled family
- Coping, ineffective

- Decisional conflict

- Denial, ineffective
- Family process: dysfunctional
- Fatigue
- Fear

- Grieving
- Hopelessness
- Insomnia
- Knowledge deficit
- Loneliness, risk for

- Neglect, self
- Power, readiness for enhanced
- Powerlessness
- Resilience, risk for compromised
- Role performance, ineffective
- Sleep pattern disturbed
- Social interaction, impaired
- Stress overload
- Spiritual distress

---

skills as well as an atmosphere of concern and caring help the nurse gather the subjective and objective assessment data and formulate the appropriate nursing diagnoses for the family. Having questions answered in an honest fashion, being provided with understandable expectations, feeling the patient's dignity was respected, and feeling the patient is treated as a person and not as a case are all areas of strength in current practice.[22] Examples of nursing diagnoses appropriate to the family members of a critically ill patient are listed in Box 3-1. These diagnoses guide both the nurse and the family in establishing mutual goals.

## Nursing Interventions

The critical care nurse's time with the family is often limited because of the crucial physiological and psychosocial needs of the patient. Therefore, it is important to make every interaction with the family as useful and therapeutic as possible. A high-quality nursing staff that demonstrates professional behavior and competence is central to family satisfaction with care. Compassion and respect, which include treating the patient and family with kindness and listening to special requests, are also listed as important by patients and families.[23] Nursing interventions should address cognitive, affective, and behavioral domains and should be designed to help the family:

- learn from the crisis experience and move toward adaptation;
- regain a state of equilibrium;
- experience the normal (but painful) feelings associated with the crisis, to avoid delayed depression and allow for future emotional growth.[24]

Family meetings are considered an important component in the practice of family-centered care. Recommendations include a family meeting within 12 to 24 hours of admission to the CCU, and repeated as dictated by the patient and interprofessional team. Second, it is recommended that caregivers receive training in communication, appropriate communication behaviors, and conflict management.

Treatment goal updates to the interprofessional team are also recommended to maintain consistent messages to the family.[25] The patient–family dyad establishes the family not as a visitor but rather as a participant in care. Following the IOM recommendations:[11]

- Patients and families are kept informed and actively involved in medical decision making and self-management.
- Patient care is coordinated and integrated across the group of health care providers.
- Health care delivery systems provide for the physical comfort and emotional support of patients and family members.
- Health care providers have a clear understanding of the patient's concept of illness and their cultural beliefs.

Conducting family meetings is just one of several ideas to improve the family's experience. The use of family visiting kits has also been explored; these kits include activities that can be performed at the bedside (eg, hand massage), directions on personal care activities (eg, applying lip balm around an endotracheal tube), cognitive recovery tools (eg, dominoes, playing cards), and personal care items for the families themselves (eg, toiletries, a log for questions).[26] Suggestions for nursing interventions with the family in crisis are outlined in Box 3-2. Considerations for the older patient are presented in Box 3-3.

---

**BOX 3-2**   **Nursing Interventions**

**For Care of the Family in Crisis**

- Guide the family in defining the current problem.
- Help the family identify its strengths and sources of support.
- Prepare the family for the critical care environment, especially regarding equipment and purposes of the equipment.
- Speak openly to the patient and the family about the critical illness.
- Be realistic and honest about the situation, taking care not to give false reassurance.
- Convey feelings of hope and confidence in the family's ability to deal with the situation.
- Try to perceive the feelings that the crisis evokes in the family.
- Help the family identify and focus on feelings.
- Assist the family to determine the goals and steps to take in facing the crisis.
- Provide opportunities for the patient and the family to make choices and avoid powerlessness and hopelessness.
- Assist the family in finding ways to communicate with the patient.
- Encourage the family to help with the care of the patient.
- Discuss all issues as they relate to the patient's uniqueness; avoid generalizations.
- Help the family to set short-term goals so that progress and positive changes can be seen.
- Ensure that the family receives information about all significant changes in the patient's condition.
- Advocate for the adjustment of visiting hours to accommodate the needs of the family as permitted by the situation in the unit.
- Determine whether there is space available in the hospital near the unit where the family can be alone and have privacy.
- Recognize the patient's and family's spirituality, and suggest the assistance of a spiritual advisor if there is a need.

---

**BOX 3-3**    *CONSIDERATIONS for the Older Patient*

**Providing Care for the Critically Ill Older Patient**

- Respect the dignity, intelligence, privacy, and maturity of the patient at all times.
- Maintain the patient's right to make decisions as long as possible.
- Avoid paternalism in patient care.
- Integrate the physiological and cognitive changes of aging with the assessment and care of the patient.
- Allow the family to share in the care of their family member.
- Provide active participation and a sense of control for the patient and family.
- Make sure that the patient remains the focus of care and that interventions are performed for the good of the patient.
- Assess the impact that medical and nursing interventions have on quality of life and sense of well-being.
- Determine family burdens resulting from the critical illness.

## Visitation Advocacy

Open visiting hours are another method for enhancing family-centered care. Visiting hour policies should be evaluated periodically. Research demonstrates that novel approaches to visitation, such as allowing children who are accompanied by an adult to visit a relative in the CCU and the use of animal-assisted therapy in the CCU, can have positive effects on the patient, including increased feelings of happiness and calmness and reduced feelings of loneliness.[27]

Visiting hours in CCUs have been restricted for many years, with the rationale that rest, quiet, and an undisturbed environment were therapeutic nursing interventions. Families often interpreted these restrictions as denying access to their loved ones. As early as 1978, Dracup and Breu[28] reported that satisfying the needs of the families of patients was improved by relaxing a policy of restricted visiting hours and initiating set communication with patients' spouses. It is strongly suggested that visiting hours for the critically ill be used as simple guidelines, and that they be relaxed and specific to the needs of the patient, with knowledge of the responsibilities of the nurse as well as the climate on the unit at the time the visit is requested.

Restricting visiting hours is sometimes seen as a way to maintain control over families. However, patients have a need to receive comfort and support, and families appreciate a caregiving supportive role. It is not the duration of the visit, but rather the flexibility of the visit and how appropriate it is for the patient, that is important.[29] Unrestricted visiting policies in CCUs have been linked to a decrease in septic complications; a decrease in the amount of cardiovascular complications, specifically shock and pulmonary edema; and an improvement in the physiologic presentation of blood pressure, heart rate, and intracranial pressure.[30] See Evidence-Based Practice Highlight 3-1.

When choosing a less-restrictive visitation policy, the physical layout of the unit must be considered. Smaller units may be less appropriate for unrestricted visiting hours with unlimited visitors. However, the focus should be on what proves to be best for the patient, not for the nurse. The effectiveness of changes in visiting hours must also be evaluated. Additional nursing research is needed to determine the current trends in visiting, as well as the outcomes of changes in visiting hours on the needs of patients and families.

---

**QSEN**

### EVIDENCE-BASED PRACTICE HIGHLIGHT 3-1
### Family Visitation in the Adult ICU

**Expected Practice**

- Facilitate unrestricted access of hospitalized patients to a chosen support person (eg, family member, friend, or trusted individual) who is integral to the provision of emotional and social support 24 hours a day, according to patient preference, unless the support person infringes on the rights of others and their safety, or it is medically or therapeutically contraindicated.[1] (Level D)
- Ensure that the facility/unit has an approved written practice document (ie, policy, procedure, or standard of care) for allowing the patient's designated support person—who may or may not be the patient's surrogate decision maker or legally authorized representative—to be at the bedside during the course of the patient's stay, according to the patient's wishes.[1-6] (Level D)
- Evaluate policies to ensure that they prohibit discrimination based on age, race, ethnicity, religion, culture, language, physical or mental disability, socioeconomic status, sex, sexual orientation, and/or gender identity or expression.[1-6] (Level D)
- Ensure that there is an approved written practice document (ie, policy, procedure, or standard of care) for limiting visitors whose presence infringes on the rights of others and their safety or are medically or therapeutically contraindicated to support staff in negotiating visiting privileges.[6] (Level D)

**AACN Levels of Evidence**

**Level A** Meta-analysis of quantitative studies or metasynthesis of qualitative studies with results that consistently support a specific action, intervention, or treatment (including systematic review of randomized controlled trials)

**Level B** Well-designed, controlled studies with results that consistently support a specific action, intervention, or treatment

**Level C** Qualitative studies, descriptive or correlational studies, integrative reviews, systematic reviews, or randomized controlled trials with inconsistent results

**Level D** Peer-reviewed professional and organizational standards with the support of clinical study recommendations

**Level E** Multiple case reports, theory-based evidence from expert opinions, or peer-reviewed professional organizational standards without clinical studies to support recommendations

**Level M** Manufacturer's recommendations only

Excerpted from American Association of Critical-Care Nurses Practice Alert. Available online at http://aacn.org.

---

The names, roles, and responsibilities of all members of the interprofessional health care team should be identified for both the patient and family. Additionally, the nurse must prepare family members for the initial visit to the CCU because it can be an overwhelming environment. The functions of monitors, intravenous drips, ventilators, and other technologies, as well as the meaning of alarms, should always be explained before and during the family visits to avoid causing anxiety and the potential for the technology to become a barrier between nurse, patient, and family. The nurse, by example, can demonstrate the value of communication and touch to the family. Encouraging family members to provide direct care to the patient, if they are interested, can help decrease anxiety and provide the family with some control. Direct care activities for the family to perform may include brushing teeth, combing hair, helping with a meal, and providing skin care.

Allowing children to visit a CCU may require special arrangements on the part of the staff. Visits should include short, simple explanations to the child concerning the patient's condition. Answering the child's questions in developmental terms that he or she can understand helps reduce possible fears. The person who is escorting the child into the CCU should be aware that invasive monitoring and other equipment might upset a youngster. If a visit from the child is not possible, arrangements can be made for videoconferencing or telephone visit.

Family presence during invasive procedures and resuscitation should be discussed. Positive and compelling evidence has emerged in the research about the benefits of family presence in the emergency department (ED), indicating that family presence in adult CCUs should continue to be investigated. Terminal weaning, support of an organ donor, and planned invasive procedures seem suitable situations for the family to be present, although differences exist between the CCU and the ED in terms of appropriateness. Support was found for family presence among physicians, physician assistants, and nurses.[31,32] Families believe it is their right to be present, but nurse perceptions continue to vary widely. However, there are still differences between what is recommended in the nursing literature and what is actually practiced related to witnessed resuscitation. Interventions to increase positive attitudes and practices by ICU nurses during witnessed resuscitation should be encouraged.[14]

## Use of the Nurse–Family Relationship

Initiating nursing interventions and establishing a meaningful relationship with the family tend to be easier during crisis than at other times. People in crisis are highly receptive to an interested, caring, and empathetic helper. When first meeting the patient's family, the nurse must demonstrate the desire and ability to help. Help that is specific to the family's needs at that time demonstrates the nurse's interest in their comfort and well-being. The nurse will need to determine who in the family is to be notified of the patient's status, and validate that person's contact information; determining who will be the family representative can be an overwhelming decision for the family. Assisting the family to determine immediate priorities is essential in the early phase of crisis intervention. The existence of an advance directive, a living will, and a health care power of attorney should be determined. In the absence of these documents, support and methods to obtain them should be given to the family.

With this type of timely involvement, the family will begin to trust and depend on the nurse's judgment. This process then allows family members to believe the nurse when the nurse conveys feelings of hope and confidence in the family's ability to cope with whatever is ahead. It is important to avoid giving false reassurance; rather, the reality of the situation should be expressed in a kind, supportive fashion.

## Problem Solving With the Family

As the relationship between the nurse and the family develops, the nurse begins to understand the dynamics of the problem facing the family. Problem solving with the family takes into consideration items such as:

- the meaning the family has attached to the event;
- other crises with which the family may be coping;
- the adaptive and maladaptive coping behaviors previously used in time of stress;
- the normal support systems of the family, which might include friends, neighbors, clergy, and colleagues.

Using the information collected and recorded in the assessment base enables the nurse to help the family deal with stress. Interventions include defining the problem, identifying support, focusing on feelings, and identifying steps.

### Defining the Problem

A vital part of the problem-solving process is to help the family clearly state the immediate problem. Often people are overwhelmed and immobilized by the anxiety or panic caused by acute stress. Being able to state the problem and acknowledge the difficulty or threat it poses reduces the family's anxiety by helping family members realize that they have achieved some sort of understanding of what is happening. Defining the problem is a way of delimiting its parameters. Simply asking the family members their understanding of the problem and the greatest concern for them at this time helps in problem definition. In addition, the family's response helps the nurse to clarify his or her understanding of what the family needs.

Defining and redefining problems can and should occur many times before the problem is solved. Stating the problem clearly helps the family assign priorities and direct needed actions. Goal-directed activities help decrease anxiety.

### Identifying Support

Under high levels of stress, some people may become reluctant to involve their usual resources. Asking family members to identify the person to whom they usually turn when they are upset, and encouraging them to seek assistance from that person now, helps direct the family back to the normal mechanisms for handling stressful issues. Few families are truly without resources; rather, they only have failed to recognize and call on them.

Defining and redefining the problem may also help put the problem in a different light. The process of helping the family view a problem from a different perspective is called *reframing*.

The nurse can also help the family call on its own inherent strengths. What is it as a family that they do best? How have they handled stress before? Encouraging the family members to capitalize on their strengths as a family unit is both helpful and therapeutic.

### Focusing on Feelings

A problem-solving technique emphasizing choices and alternatives helps the family achieve a sense of control over part of their lives. Helping the family focus on feelings is extremely important to avoid delayed grief and protracted depression in the future. The reflection of feelings or active listening is necessary throughout the duration of the crisis. Valuing the expression of feelings may help the family avoid the use of unhealthy coping mechanisms, such as alcohol or excessive sleep. Adaptation takes time.

During the difficult days of the critical illness, the family may become dependent on the judgment of professionals. The family may have some difficulty identifying the appropriate areas in which to accept the judgments of others. It is important that the nurse acknowledges the family's feelings and recognizes the complexity of the problem, while emphasizing the responsibility each member of the family has for his or her feelings, actions, and decisions. Encouraging family members to focus on things they can change helps to give them a sense of control. For example, if the patient is experiencing pain, the family can be encouraged to advocate for the patient by requesting that the nurse evaluate the patient's pain control.

### Identifying Steps

Once the problem has been defined and the family begins goal-directed activities, the nurse may help further by asking the family members to identify the steps they must take. Such anticipatory guidance may help reduce the family's anxiety. However, the nurse must recognize moments when direction is vital to health and safety. It is often necessary to advise families, for example, to return home to rest. This can be explained by stating that by maintaining their own health, family members will, at a later date, be as helpful to the patient as possible. To make each interaction more meaningful and therapeutic, the nurse should focus on the crisis situation and avoid involvement in long-term chronic problems.

### Interprofessional Management

The health care providers who most often meet the needs of family members are generally thought to be nurses and physicians. Communication with families is not the responsibility of a single profession, and it is an essential component of care. Few researchers have examined interventions aimed at improving communication between the entire health care team and the family.[33] Interprofessional collaboration occurs "when multiple health care workers from different professional backgrounds work together with patients, families, carers, and communities to deliver the highest quality of care."[34] Communication is essential to successful interprofessional collaboration, and also contributes to patient safety and positive patient outcomes.

In some cases, nurse-coached hospital volunteer programs have proved effective in providing family support.[35] An example would be an in-service program taught by nurses and followed by the assignment of a nurse mentor to the volunteer. Some families benefit by a referral to a mental health clinical specialist, a social worker, a psychologist, or a chaplain. Other interdisciplinary teams can include pharmacists, family care specialists, and therapists. It may be appropriate for the nurse to set up the first meeting with the consultant, with follow-up meetings coordinated between the family and the consultant. Many CCUs have such resources on a 24-hour on-call basis to ensure prompt interventions. An objective professional with experience in critical illness and its impact on the family can be an excellent resource. Family members of former patients have also been used as a method of sharing experiences and providing information to assist with the critical care experience.[34]

An additional method for improving family-centered care in critical care is the Patient and Family Advisory Council (PFAC).[36] An advisory council composed not just of nurses and other health care providers but also of past patients and family members represents the needs of family members. Driven by the consumer movement, this concept has at its core respect and dignity, information sharing, participation, and collaboration. PFACs have the potential to provide new insights leading to improved family care. The opportunity exists for the advanced practice nurse to spend more time as a resource to enhance good communication with patients and their families as well as to serve as a teacher and a mentor to other nurses.[37]

## Palliative Care Issues in Critical Care

According to the World Health Organization, palliative care is an "approach that improves the quality of life of patients and their families facing the problem associated with life-threatening illness, through the prevention and relief of suffering by means of early identification and impeccable assessment and treatment of pain and other problems, physical, psychosocial, and spiritual."[38] Important components of palliative care are the inclusion of the family in decision making and the provision of patient care. Families are faced with complex palliative care decisions that must be made in the unfamiliar environment of the CCU. Developing CCU nurses' "mastery of communication skills using palliative care principles is gaining momentum as an effective strategy."[37] Nurses' personal issues and practices, such as previous experiences with the death of their own family members, have the potential to either enhance or threaten assessment and intervention.

Caring for a patient's family at any point during the dying process encompasses three major areas: access, information and support, and involvement in caregiving activities. Family members of dying loved ones should be allowed more liberal access in both visiting hours and number of visitors allowed. Ensuring that a family can be with their critically ill loved one will be a source of comfort. Access to information has been identified as a crucial component in the family's coping, and support in the form of the nurse's caring behaviors is influential in shaping the critical care experience for both the patient and family. Honesty and truth-telling are important skills in this emotionally charged time. Finally, family involvement in caregiving, in tasks as simple as being physically present as well as those as complex as assisting with postmortem care, may help families work through their grief. Facilitation of family involvement is a practical nursing intervention. See Chapter 6 for further discussion of end-of-life and palliative care issues in the critical care setting.

## The Critical Care Family Assistance Program

Numerous research studies during the past 20 years have focused on the environmental and social issues of anxious families awaiting the outcome of a family member's stay in the CCU; these studies demonstrate that attending to the needs of family members cannot be ignored.[38] Additionally, a crucial initiative of the AACN focuses on establishing respectful, healing, and humane nursing care environments. As a result of collaboration between the Chest Foundation and Eli Lilly and Company Foundation, the first CCFAP was developed as an example of a renewed awakening to the concepts of family-centered care. The objectives of the CCFAP

---

**BOX 3-4**   **Components of the Critical Care Family Assistance Program (CCFAP)**

**Communication**
*Example*: "ICU Navigators," weekly group family sessions that provide information about equipment, medical procedures, and assertiveness skills

**Environmental Changes**
*Examples*: Expanding the waiting area, brightening the look of the room, acquiring new and more comfortable furniture

**Educational Materials**
*Example*: Publications that are up-to-date and written in non-technical language

**Information Kiosk**
*Examples*: Electronic messaging system, Internet access, CCFAP family satisfaction surveys

**Hospitality Programs**
*Examples*: Hotel discounts, meals for families

**Other Services**
*Examples*: Music therapy, pet therapy

---

are driven by the following two factors: a growing evidence that family support positively impacts the recovery rates of ICU patients and high levels of dissatisfaction reported by the families of patients in CCUs. Initial analysis at the third-year mark of utilization of the program demonstrated a provision of high-quality care and above-average communication. Families reported increased satisfaction with decision making, safety and security, and an understanding of the treatment the patient was receiving.[38] Commonly noted gaps in supporting the families of patients included the following:

- discrepancies in the viewpoint among health care workers with regard to the sharing of information;
- the need of the family to involve more family members in decision making; and
- a lack of resources and services offered during this time of crisis.

Because of shortened lengths of stay and nursing shortages, family members are increasingly more active participants in the care of their loved ones. Family-centered care focuses on better integration of the family into the care-planning process. Engaging family members early and encouraging them to work in partnership with the nursing staff can make a difference. Box 3-4 lists the components of the CCFAP model. It is hoped that with expanded use of this model, the quality of critical care delivered will increase, whereas cost of critical care delivery will decrease.

## Cultural Issues Related to Critical Illness

Nursing interventions for the critically ill patient include recognition and appreciation of the cultural uniqueness of each person. In today's diverse society, culture affects the nursing care of patients in many ways, from pain control and visitation expectations to care of the body after death. Critical care nurses must recognize the uniqueness of each person in this diverse, multicultural population and realize the ways in which that uniqueness affects the care of the patient and the needs of the family.

Health care providers in Western medicine often address a critical illness as a disease process and focus on the physical symptoms, the pathology of organ function, or injury to a body part. The patient and family, having a different cultural perspective, may view the illness in a more psychophysiological manner, focusing on the physical, psychological, personal, and cultural ramifications of the illness. In other cultures, the patient's critical illness may be viewed as a curse or disharmony in the universe. Culture is an important influence on the patient's attitudes about approach to suffering and beliefs about life-prolonging treatments, palliative care, and advanced directives and health care proxies.[35]

Cultural competence is a reflection of one's attitudes, knowledge base, acquired skills, and behavior. Although it is unrealistic to expect that the nurse should know the customs and beliefs of all critically ill patients he or she cares for, it is not unreasonable to expect some degree of cultural competence. Institute for Patient-and-Family Centered Care make the following suggestions:[36]

- Be aware of one's own ethnocentrism.
- Assess the family's beliefs about illness and treatment.
- Consistently convey respect.
- Request that the family and patient act as guides for cultural preferences.
- Ask for the patient's personal preference.
- Respect cultural differences regarding personal space and touch.
- Note appropriate complementary and alternative medical practices, and allow their use if possible.
- Incorporate the patient's cultural healing practices into the plan of care.
- Be sensitive to the need for a translator.

Cultural characteristics, such as language, values, behavioral norms, diet, and attitudes toward disease prevention, death and dying, and management of illness, vary from culture to culture. Critical illness may be viewed by the family from a religious or spiritual perspective. Flower writes about five aspects of cultural competence: cultural awareness, cultural knowledge, cultural skill, cultural encounter, and cultural desire (Box 3-5).

Astuteness and sensitivity on the part of the critical care nurse helps ensure a health care system that supports cultural beliefs in response to wellness and response to illness including complementary and alternative health practices.

---

**BOX 3-5**   **Model for Cultural Competence**

**Cultural Awareness:** Perform self-examination and in-depth exploration of cultural background.
**Cultural Knowledge:** Seek and obtain an information base on different cultures.
**Cultural Skill:** Collect relevant data that permit a culture-specific physical assessment.
**Cultural Encounter:** Directly engage in cross-cultural interaction with patients.
**Cultural desire:** Be motivated to become culturally aware and seek cultural encounters.

Adapted from Flowers D: Culturally competent nursing care: A challenge for the 21st century. Crit Care Nurse 24(4):48–52, 2004.

# Clinical Applicability Challenges

## SHORT-ANSWER QUESTIONS

1. Mrs. J. is a 40-year-old Caucasian critically ill patient with multiple trauma status post–motor vehicle crash who has been admitted to the critical care unit with head trauma and on mechanical ventilation. She is not expected to survive her injuries. Mrs. J.'s husband, her two children ages 16 and 20, and her parents have just arrived to see her for the first time. Formulate a plan of care that reflects sensitivity to the issues that will assist the patient's family in dealing with the probable death of their loved one.

2. Mr. E., 73 years old, is admitted to the critical care unit following resuscitation in the ED. He has a long-standing history of cardiac disease. Mr. E. collapsed at home after what has been interpreted as a life-threatening rhythm disturbance. Although he received cardiopulmonary resuscitation, he was unconscious for 10 minutes before the rescue team arrived. His older daughters are arguing over the maintenance of ventilatory support. Mr. E. does not respond to any stimuli and is not generating any spontaneous breaths. Discuss how you would help his daughters at this difficult time.

3. Mr. and Mrs. P. are the parents of a 9-year-old critically ill, newly diagnosed type 1 insulin-dependent diabetic child in the critical care unit. They are Indian and speak very little English. Describe the nonverbal criteria the nurse would use to assess the parents' degree of stress and anxiety. How can the nurse be certain that the cultural needs of the family are met while the child is a patient on the unit? How can the nurse assess the readiness to learn in the parents?

---

**WANT TO KNOW MORE?**

A wide variety of resources to enhance your learning and understanding of this chapter are available on thePoint.

You will find:
- References
- Selected readings
- NCLEX-style review questions
- Internet resources
- And more!

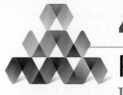

# 4

# Patient and Family Education in Critical Care

LEIGH BASTABLE POITEVENT

## LEARNING OBJECTIVES

*Based on the content in this chapter, the reader will be able to:*

1. Differentiate between the concepts of education, teaching, and learning.
2. Identify the three domains of learning.
3. Recognize the six principles of adult learning.
4. Describe the barriers to teaching and learning that are unique to the critical care environment.
5. Assess learning in the critical care environment.
6. Evaluate learning outcomes of critically ill patients and their families based on appropriate teaching strategies.

Patient and family education is a fundamental nursing competency.[1] In the critical care setting, it can be a challenge to meet the educational needs of patients and families or significant others (hereinafter referred to as family) because of the life-threatening nature of critical illness and limited time for teaching. The critical care nurse must deal with not only the physical aspects of acute or chronic illness (eg, pain, fatigue, delirium) but also the emotional effects (eg, anxiety, fear, confusion) while trying to teach difficult concepts in an environment that can be overwhelming and poorly suited for learning.[2] However, studies show that early and adequate patient education decreases hospital lengths of stay, lessens risks for acute and chronic complications, and reduces hospital readmission rates.[3]

Health care is no longer solely defined in terms of sound clinical decision making. Today, it also encompasses prudent use of resources and financial accountability. The passage of The Affordable Care Act (ACA) in March 2010 has been deemed the broadest health care reform legislation in the US history. The overall goals of this legislation are to reframe the financial and health insurance relationship between Americans and the US health care system.[4] The ACA reform shifts the payment structure for hospitals and health care providers from a traditional fee-for-service model to an incentive model.[5] Reimbursement for care is now based on hospital performance against several clinical outcome measures. Quality outcomes are monitored for conditions such as myocardial infarction, congestive heart failure, pneumonia, surgical site and nosocomial infections, screening and intervention for tobacco and alcohol abuse, and patient satisfaction.[6] Additionally, many of the quality indicators that are being tracked include patient and family education components. Reforms to the health care infrastructure necessitate clear evidence through documentation of nurses' involvement in patient and family instruction and of quantifying outcomes based on the delivery of nursing care and patient education.[5]

Today, it is not unusual for a patient to be transferred to a step-down unit or directly discharged to home from an intensive care unit (ICU), placing an even greater responsibility for self-care on the patient and family. The ICU nurse not only manages the physical instabilities and emotional needs of the patient with a critical illness, but also prepares the patient and family for the likelihood of early discharge from the hospital.

Use of the ICU has increased over the past 20 years and is expected to expand in the future as medical technology improves, the older adult population grows, and more people survive critical illnesses.[7] At the same time, hospitals are facing an ongoing shortage of experienced nurses. ICUs that were once reserved for expert registered nurses (RNs) are now training grounds for the newly graduated nurse.[8] The novice RN is preoccupied with prioritizing care and managing the myriad equipment used to support the critically ill patient while also working to apply his or her knowledge of the pathophysiology of multisystem illness. The new nurse may be overwhelmed by these responsibilities and thus find it difficult to appropriately address the educational needs of the patient and family. In addition, the highly variable nursing shift patterns likely disrupt continuity of care and are not ideal for fostering nurse–patient relationships or for creating continuity for teaching and learning.

These are just a few examples of the realities of the current health care landscape that may pose obstacles to patient education in the ICU. The purpose of this chapter is to assist nursing students and staff nurses in acquiring the skills and tools needed to meet the challenges of patient and family education in the presence of critical illness. ICU nurses who comprehend the standards of education, the principles of teaching and learning, the process of adult education, the barriers to teaching and obstacles to learning, the strategies for effective educational interventions, and the process of evaluating teaching and learning are better prepared to address the informational needs of patients and families. Nurses grounded in these skills have the potential to positively influence quality of care and health-related outcomes of their patients.

## Standards of Patient and Family Education

The emphasis on patient and family education stems from the patient care standards put forth by The Joint Commission

(TJC).[9,10] Hospitals voluntarily participate in TJC surveys to ensure that the patient care provided meets or exceeds the criteria set forth in the standards for high-quality patient care. Some examples of TJC standards related to patient and family education are as follows:

- The hospital provides, coordinates, and evaluates patient education and training based on each patient's needs and abilities.
- Education provided is appropriate to the patient's condition and clearly addresses the patient's identified learning needs.
- Communication between patients and providers requires written documentation of all health teaching with patients and families. It is not acceptable for practitioners to text orders for patients to the hospital because the senders cannot be verified.
- The hospital performs a learning needs assessment, which includes cultural and religious beliefs, emotional barriers, health literacy level, desire and motivation to learn, physical or cognitive limitations, and barriers to communication.[10]

The goal of these educational standards is to guide hospitals to create an environment in which both the patient and family and the health care team members are responsible for teaching and learning. The medical record should reflect an interdisciplinary approach to patient education throughout the hospital stay. TJC's recommended educational topics are detailed in Box 4-1.[10] An initial assessment of learning needs and the teaching plan should indicate the learning topics and how they relate to the patient's health issues. Evaluation should document the patient's current response to treatment and whether home health care or community resources are necessary to support the safe transition of the patient from the hospital to home. The medical record should reflect evidence of coordination of these services before discharge.

ICU nurses routinely teach patients and families, but often the patient education record is left blank because "there isn't enough time to teach." Nurses must remember that much of patient and family teaching is informal and may not be obviously recognized as a teaching encounter. Nurses are taught to explain each procedure, medication, intervention, and diagnostic test to the patient beforehand. For example, nurses who take the time to explain their actions, such as hanging an IV antibiotic, measuring urine output, changing a dressing, or monitoring vital signs, are taking advantage of each opportunity to teach. Yet, many nurses do not recognize this action as patient education, and they often do not document it in the teaching record.[11] Nonetheless, these types of informal instructions meet TJC's standards for patient education. If ICU nurses would remember to document informal teaching sessions, the patient's educational records would be filled with teaching entries.

## Education, Teaching, and Learning

Often the terms *education* and *teaching* are used interchangeably, but there is a difference between these two concepts. *Education* is defined as a systematic process that is scientifically based to promote changes in the knowledge, behavior, and attitudes of people, groups, or communities.[11] More specifically, *patient education* is a process of assisting people to learn health-related behaviors with the goal of achieving optimal health and self-care. *Teaching* is one part of the education process and is defined as an informal or formal deliberate act with the goal of producing learning.[11] *Learning* is defined as an internal individual behavior change due to acquisition of knowledge, skills, and attitudes that can be observed or measured. The process of teaching and learning should be a partnership between health care providers and patients and families.[11]

## Three Domains of Learning

Three categories of human behavior—the cognitive, affective, and psychomotor domains—must be considered when developing an education plan for teaching and learning. The ICU nurse must keep these three domains in mind while assessing learning needs and developing teaching plans.

The *cognitive domain (knowledge)* involves the development of a mental skill set that provides a basis for behavior. In this "thinking" domain, knowledge expands, and teaching and learning material is organized from simple to complex.[12] Learning is enhanced when information builds on previous knowledge; therefore, basic ideas should be introduced before attempting to teach more difficult material. As an example, cognitive learning occurs when a family member learns to assess wound healing. The ICU nurse provides basic information about the healing process and the appearance of a healthy incision. Once the family member understands how a healed wound should look, the nurse can explain the signs and symptoms of infection and when to notify the health care team. Once prepared, the family member should be able to apply the learned principles to provide appropriate home care for the patient.

The *affective domain (attitudes)* permeates all spheres of learning because it encompasses the patient's emotions, values, beliefs, motivations, and feelings.[12] When formulating a teaching plan, the nurse should take a nonthreatening approach to assessing what the patient and family consider important to learn. Listening to the patient and family and respecting their individual and cultural attributes provide the opportunity for the ICU nurse to establish a trusting relationship. Establishing rapport with clients is key to increasing their motivation to learn. An example of addressing the affective domain is smoking cessation classes that take place

---

**BOX 4-1** **The Joint Commission's Recommended Topics for Patient and Family Education**

- Explanation of the plan of care
- Basic health practices and safety
- Safe and effective use of medications
- Nutrition interventions
- Pain management
- Safe and effective use of medical equipment
- Techniques that help the patient reach maximum independence
- Fall reduction strategies

Data from The Joint Commission: Advancing Effective Communication, Cultural Competence, and Patient- and Family-Centered Care: A Roadmap for Hospitals. Oakbrook Terrace, IL: The Joint Commission, 2010. Retrieved from: http://www.jointcommission.org/assets/1/6/ARoadmapforHospitalsfinalversion727.pdf; and The Joint Commission: 2015 Comprehensive Accreditation Manual for Hospitals (CAMH). Joint Commission Resources. Oakbrook Terrace, IL: The Joint Commission, 2014.

in an interactive group setting. In this situation, the teacher demonstrates behaviors that the learner wants to imitate and provides positive feedback to the participants to encourage them to stop smoking. If learning experiences are satisfying and patients and family members associate positive feelings with these experiences, then behavioral changes are likely to result.

The *psychomotor domain (skills)* involves gross and fine motor skills that are performed in an ordered sequence of movement and that must be practiced for learning to occur. The learner must have an intact neuromuscular system that is capable of performing the skill and the ability to form a mental image when watching a demonstration. The nurse may use written, step-by-step instructions as a reference guide when demonstrating the skill and should allow the patient to ask questions. For instance, learning to inject insulin is an example of psychomotor learning. It takes practice for the patient or family member to become proficient at performing this task. The thought of learning a new skill is intimidating to many adults; therefore, it is important that the nurse provides praise and encouragement with each teaching session.[12]

## Adult Learning Principles

The fundamental principles of adult learning are grounded in developmental psychology and education theory. Adults must be ready to learn and know why it is important to learn something new. Orientation to learning for adults is "life centered" and thus should be taught with a focus on current problem resolution. Motivation to learn is also a key principle of adult learning and arises from internal pressures such as self-esteem and the desire for quality of life.

The contemporary father of adult learning, Malcolm Knowles, expounded upon the *andragogy model*. This model emerged from research studies that identified some of the unique characteristics of the adult learner.[13] According to this model, adult education is "learner centered" rather than "teacher centered." This model of learning can be used as a framework for education of adult patients and their family members as well as health care staff education.[14] The andragogy model has six core principles related to the science of teaching an adult learner:

1. *The need to know.* Adults need to understand why they need to learn something before they are willing to commit the energy and time to learn it. To raise the learner's level of awareness of their needs, the facilitator should use real or simulated experiences to help the learner discover gaps in their knowledge.
2. *The learner's self-concept.* Adults are self-directed and responsible for their own decision making. Therefore, educators need to create learning situations that give adults options and independence.
3. *The learner's life experience.* Life experiences define and shape adult beliefs, values, and attitudes. Adult education methods emphasize experiential techniques such as case method, simulation, and problem-solving exercises. In addition, adults learn well from their peers, making group learning an effective teaching method.
4. *Readiness to learn.* Adults are ready to learn the things they need to know. The information should be relevant and applicable to real-life situations.
5. *Orientation to learning.* Adults are motivated to learn if the information will help them to perform useful tasks or to deal with problems in their lives.
6. *Motivation to learn.* Adults are more motivated by internal forces such as improved quality of life, increased job satisfaction, and heightened self-esteem. External factors such as job promotion or increased salary are less likely to sustain learning.[13]

An example of how the ICU nurse might use adult learning principles in the practice setting is presented in the case scenario outlined in Box 4-2.

## The Process of Adult Education

Patient and family education requires more than just providing an educational brochure or turning on an instructional videotape; it is an ongoing, interactive process based on a therapeutic relationship. The most important strategy for effective patient and family teaching is to begin with an assessment of learning needs and readiness to learn. Developing a plan, implementing the plan, and evaluating the teaching all follow the assessment phase.[1,11] The education process provides a framework for the ICU nurse to use for patient education. Figure 4-1 portrays how the education process parallels the nursing process.

The mnemonic ASSURE can be applied by ICU nurses to help organize and carry out the education process:

**A:** Analyze the learner.
**S:** State the objectives.
**S:** Select the instructional methods and materials.
**U:** Use the instructional methods/materials.
**R:** Require learner performance.
**E:** Evaluate the teaching plan and revise as necessary.[11]

Just as ICU nurses apply clinical judgment to recognize and treat hemodynamic instability, they are also expected to diagnose and intervene to meet the learning needs of patients and their family members. Each teaching and learning session enhances the knowledge of the patient and family, and offers the nurse a chance to evaluate the success or failure of what he or she has taught based on the learning outcomes that have been achieved.

## Assessing Learning Needs in a Time of Crisis

A learning need is defined as a gap between what the learner knows and what the learner needs to know.[15] Learning needs, especially in the ICU environment, can rapidly change. In the critical care setting, it is preferable to use an informal and open-ended dialogue between the nurse and the patient and family.

The first step in the assessment process is to get to know the patient and family. Taking a few minutes to learn the family members' names and their relationship to the patient signifies respect and begins to build a therapeutic and trusting relationship. Start by assessing the patient and family's current knowledge and understanding of the patient's condition.[1] Asking for feedback on what has been learned to date is helpful in developing a care plan.[3] Use of open-ended questions—for example, "What is your understanding of your

---

**BOX 4-2**   Case 1: Patient and Family in Crisis

Johaun is a 54-year-old man who sustained a traumatic motor vehicle accident during his morning commute to work. He was airlifted to a nearby hospital. Upon arrival in the ER he was awake, alert, and oriented, with lacerations to the face and torso. He rated the pain in his chest as 5 on a scale of 1 to 10. X-ray in the ER revealed two closed rib fractures.

Shortly after admission to the ICU, his respiratory status began to decompensate and he reported worsening chest pain, now rated as 7/10, which he described as constant, sharp, and radiating to his back. Further workup revealed a dissecting aortic aneurysm. He was immediately taken to the operating room for emergent surgical repair of this life-threatening condition. The surgery was successful and he was transferred back to the ICU with bilateral chest tubes and intubation.

Johaun's wife Charvel anxiously waited in the ICU and had not yet seen Johaun since the accident occurred earlier that morning. She was in shock about all that had occurred in such a short period of time. Johaun had left for work like any other normal day and now he was lifeless and unrecognizable in front of her in a hospital bed.

Manny, the critical care nurse caring for Johaun, greeted Charvel and began to speak to her in a calm, clear manner. He recognized her obvious look of concern and acknowledged her anxiety and fear for Johaun's life. Manny began to explain

Johaun's condition, his frightful appearance, and the purpose of all the equipment. Meanwhile as the nurse was providing education to Charvel, he also began to speak gently to Johaun and leaned down to him explaining, "My name is Manny and I am the nurse caring for you. You are in the hospital. You have a tube in your throat to help you breathe. This tube is only temporary. Our goal is to keep you comfortable. Your wife, Charvel, is here at your bedside and you are making good progress."

Manny encouraged Charvel to speak to Johaun in short phrases that offered support and reassurance. Charvel reached over and held Johaun's hand and began to speak to her husband saying, "I am here with you and you are doing well, I love you so much. Everyone in the hospital is taking really good care of you." Manny explained the ICU surroundings and encouraged Charvel to reorient her husband frequently to the situation, date, and time of day. Manny offered Charvel general information on the visitation hours and also offered resources for support, such as chaplain services and social work. In addition, he mentioned that he would be available to answer any questions she may have until shift change at 7 PM, when Tamera, the night shift nurse, would take over Johaun's care. He then offered her some time alone with her husband.

*See Clinical Applicability Challenges at the end of this chapter for questions related to this case.*

---

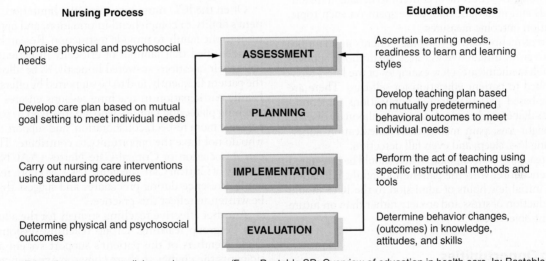

**Nursing Process**

Appraise physical and psychosocial needs → **ASSESSMENT**

Develop care plan based on mutual goal setting to meet individual needs → **PLANNING**

Carry out nursing care interventions using standard procedures → **IMPLEMENTATION**

Determine physical and psychosocial outcomes → **EVALUATION**

**Education Process**

**ASSESSMENT** → Ascertain learning needs, readiness to learn and learning styles

**PLANNING** → Develop teaching plan based on mutually predetermined behavioral outcomes to meet individual needs

**IMPLEMENTATION** → Perform the act of teaching using specific instructional methods and tools

**EVALUATION** → Determine behavior changes, (outcomes) in knowledge, attitudes, and skills

**FIGURE 4-1**   Education process parallels nursing process. (From Bastable SB: Overview of education in health care. In: Bastable SB, Alt MF: Nurse as Educator: Principles of Teaching and Learning for Nursing Practice, 4th ed. Burlington, MA: Jones & Bartlett Learning, 2014, p 14)

---

mother's condition?" or "What did the nurse practitioner tell you about the surgery?"—helps identify actual learning needs and gives the nurse a starting point for teaching. Also, assessing age, cognitive abilities, goals of treatment, motivation, and physical and psychosocial well-being are key to effective teaching.[1]

Assessment is a dynamic and ongoing process that provides the foundation for teaching and reflects principles of patient-centered care.[1] Assessment engages the patient in learning and provides the ICU nurse with many opportunities to assist patients and families to cope with the stress and anxiety associated with critical illness while meeting their learning needs. It also entails knowing when the patient or

family is unable to learn. For example, a patient who is experiencing pain is not able to focus well on learning a new skill, like insulin administration; adequate pain control is necessary before learning can take place. Setting unrealistic educational goals hinders learning and frustrates both the nurse and the learner.

The ICU nurse must be very sensitive to the heightened anxiety that accompanies an admission to the ICU. A high level of anxiety markedly reduces a person's ability to perform, concentrate, and retain information. However, a moderate level of anxiety acts as a motivator and creates readiness to learn; this is considered the best situation to take advantage of teaching opportunities.[15]

## Assessing Learning Needs for End-of-Life Care

The critical care setting is a common site for delivery of end-of-life (EOL) care. The main goals expressed by patients in the EOL stage are relief of pain, a sense of control, open discussions with the health care team and the family, dedicated time to be with loved ones, and limiting the burdens of loved ones. Thus, it is recommended that palliative care specialists and concepts associated with palliative care be embedded into ICU treatment plans, thereby facilitating open discussions with the health care team and the patient and family about prognosis.[16] During EOL care, effective delivery of information to family members has a positive impact on their satisfaction with care.[17] Refer to Chapter 6 for specifics about EOL issues in critical care.

## Effective Teaching Strategies

Once the ICU nurse has completed and summarized the assessment of patient and family learning needs, he or she can begin to develop a teaching plan. Standardized patient teaching plans contain information that is essential for most patients, but they are flexible enough to accommodate individual needs. Teaching plans include an overall goal, specific behavioral objectives, outline of content to be taught, teaching methods and materials, time to be spent on each topic, and evaluation outcome measures.

The role of technology in teaching patients and families continues to grow. Interactive websites, smartphone applications, and telemedicine are a few examples of the latest technology applied to patient education for self-care. There are smartphone-based patient-oriented applications for conditions such as diabetes, chronic obstructive pulmonary disease, asthma, weight loss, pain management, medication adherence, hearing loss, sleep, and even fall detection.[18]

Patient teaching is an ongoing task; it should be integrated into every encounter with the patient and family. Education during the initial few hours of admission to the ICU should focus on reduction of stress and anxiety rather than on future management objectives.[14]

## Learning Opportunities

Life-threatening illness, which thrusts patients into a vulnerable state, often stimulates patients to change unhealthy behavior patterns that may have contributed to their situation. Therein arises a "teachable moment" when patients are inspired to learn how to take control of their lives by altering their former habits.[6] Smoking cessation, dietary restrictions, and activity limitations are the types of lifestyle changes that patients frequently struggle to achieve and maintain.

Other opportunities to learn often arise in the course of routine patient care.[6] For example, while performing skin assessment the nurse often conducts a brief teaching session on postoperative incision care. This review can include the signs and symptoms of infection, proper wound cleansing, and a description of a healthy healing incision. Likewise, teaching pertinent information about the indications or side effects of medications while giving them to the patient is another

way to initiate or reinforce learning. Both of these examples highlight informal teaching and the importance of focusing on a single concept (eg, wound care or medication administration), especially considering the typical limited attention span of a patient who is recovering from a critical illness.[3]

Learning is best accomplished when the message is consistent and the knowledge progresses from simple to more complex concepts. Because of time limitations in the ICU setting, supplemental resources should be given when appropriate to augment verbal instruction; these may include written material or audiovisual resources. All health information (written and online) should be evaluated for quality and readability before dissemination to patients.[1,19]

## The Family Connection

A patient- and family-centered care model, based on the concepts of dignity, respect, participation, and information sharing, has become the emphasis of the US health care system. Optimal care requires collaboration between health care professionals, patients, and the patients' family members. Family support during critical illness is cited as a positive factor in patient survival as well as a contributor to the overall health and well-being of patients. In a research study examining burn survivors, family support reduced the risk of long-term psychosocial issues, such as depression, post-traumatic stress disorder (PTSD), and anxiety.[20]

Often the ICU nurse recognizes the limitations of the patient's ability to comprehend information, and appropriately turns to the family to provide instruction. Research evidence has identified that families of critically ill patients need to have their questions answered honestly, to be allowed to see the patient frequently, and to be supported by offers of hope.[20] Family participation in teaching sessions ensures success of teaching plans, and families who are involved in patient care perceive more respect, collaboration, and support than those who do not have the opportunity to contribute. The American Association of Critical-Care Nurses (AACN) and the Society of Critical Care Medicine (SCCM) both recommend family presence during procedures and suggest that policies be written to reflect this practice.[20]

Another effective teaching strategy for the adult learner may be group learning. Group teaching sessions that include members of the patient's support system allow participants the chance to share common experiences, express concerns about the recovery process, voice fears about potential complications, and provide the opportunity to ask questions.[15]

A strong positive support system has the potential to decrease anxiety levels of patients and their family members. The ICU nurse should acknowledge feelings of fear, uncertainty, and anxiety, and provide the family with emotional support while giving them information and teaching them skills to ensure safe care upon discharge to home. A newly learned skill, such as subcutaneous injection of insulin or a simple dressing change, may require both the patient and a family member to learn and demonstrate the basic steps of the procedure to ensure that adequate learning has occurred before the patient leaves the hospital. It may become apparent that a home health care consultation is indicated for further teaching to reinforce newly learned skills that facilitate a safe transition from the hospital to home.

## Barriers to Teaching and Obstacles to Learning

Factors that affect the ability of the nurse to deliver educational services are considered *barriers to teaching*, whereas factors that negatively impact the ability of the learner to process information are considered *obstacles to learning*.[11]

### Critical Illness and Stress

Typically, the patient and family enter an ICU unexpectedly because of a life-threatening event. The onset of severe illness or sudden accident signals the beginning of a physical and emotional crisis for all involved. Altered metabolic states, pain, sepsis, exposure to sedating medications, organ failure, episodes of hypoxia, delirium, and marked sleep deprivation, to name a few, are common conditions seen in the critically ill patient. Each of these factors can compromise mental acuity and hinder a person's ability to take in new information, learn, and recall facts.[1] In addition, combating a severe illness or injury consumes much of the patient's energy, leaving the patient with a limited capacity to learn.

Critically ill patients experience not only the physical effects related to their altered status but also emotional and spiritual distress. When facing life-threatening situations, patients often express feelings of powerlessness, profound anxiety, and fear of death. The ICU nurse who recognizes a patient's fear and anxiety during an unfamiliar course of illness, treatment, and recovery can support the patient's need for safety, reassurance, and comfort. For example, patients frequently report that the process of ventilator weaning is difficult to endure. Many experience feelings of "air hunger" and heightened anxiety when the ventilator support is reduced and the patient assumes more of the work of breathing. The nurse who provides clear explanations and reassurances during this period can greatly enhance the patient's probability of successful extubation and prevent undue emotional distress. Other examples of nursing interventions involving patient education include preparation of the patient for an invasive procedure or for transition to another level of care.

In the ICU setting, depending on the patient's state of consciousness, the focus of education may be redirected to meet the learning needs of the family members. Family members of patients in the ICU often take on the role of the surrogate decision maker (SDM) as a result of a life-threatening condition that renders the patient incapable of making his or her own health care decisions. As one can imagine, the SDM's responsibilities can lead to increased levels of anxiety, depression, and PTSD.[2] While coping with the crisis of a critically ill patient, family members may demonstrate changes in their sleeping and eating patterns, as well as an increased use of tobacco, over-the-counter medications, alcohol, and prescription drugs. Stress can also manifest in hypervigilant behaviors, such as repetitive questions, frequent telephone calls, and numerous hospital visits. Family members of ICU patients also need to be supported, comforted, informed, given assurance, and allowed proximity to the patient to maintain their desired vigilance. Research reveals that family members of critically ill patients want to know basic information about the care, the unit, the equipment, and what they can do for the patient during their visits, but these factors are often overlooked.[17] Evidence-based studies have resulted in changes to hospital visitation policies. Many ICUs now offer "open visitation," or unrestricted visiting hours. This paradigm shift creates greater opportunity for the ICU nurse to educate the family members and to help them to feel more comfortable when immersed in this stressful environment. The ICU nurse can encourage the family to participate in the basic care of a loved one. Simply getting ice chips, providing mouth care, or combing their loved one's hair may assist families in feeling that they are doing something to help the patient in an otherwise "helpless" situation.

The case study presented in Box 4-3 demonstrates how the interventions of the ICU nurse are used to support the educational and emotional needs of a family in crisis. This brief case example illustrates the unpredictability of illness and just how quickly a crisis can develop. In this scenario, the bedside nurse initiates family education through an informal discussion of the patient's status and the care that is being delivered. The initial interaction with family is fundamental to reduce stress and for the care delivery team and the family

---

### BOX 4-3 Case 2: A Patient Who Is Motivated to Learn

Sonal is an 18-year-old college student. At age 14 she was diagnosed with Type 1 diabetes. Recently she was found unconscious by her roommate and was admitted to the ICU suffering from her first episode of diabetic ketoacidosis with a blood sugar of 556. Sonal had been consistent about taking her insulin in the past, but this semester she has not been regularly checking her blood sugar or urine, frequently eating fast food, enduring stress from her heavy course schedule, and not taking her insulin like she should.

By day 3 in the ICU her condition had been corrected with insulin, fluids, and electrolyte replacement, and she was doing much better. Sonal explained to Maria, the ICU nurse, that this hospitalization was a huge "wake up call" and has expressed a desire to learn more about diabetes self-management now that she is away at school and facing new lifestyle challenges. Sonal expresses aspirations to pursue her bachelor's degree in education, which includes a teaching internship abroad in a few semesters. She recognizes that to achieve this goal she must first maintain her health by keeping her blood sugar under control.

Maria takes advantage of Sonal's motivation to learn and submits a referral to the diabetes educator and the nutritionist for counseling, and also provides contact information for a diabetes support group. Maria also provides Sonal with adequate readability level patient education material on dietary guidance for type 1 diabetics. Further, Sonal mentions that she has seen advertisements for insulin pumps and would like to find out if she would be a candidate. Maria asks her, "What other things do you think you can do to better control your blood sugar?" Sonal responds that she plans to pack healthy, low-carbohydrate lunches for class, and to briskly walk 15 minutes to class instead of taking the bus.

Because of this life-threatening event, Sonal has vowed to regain control of her disease and be responsible for self-management. Maria capitalized on Sonal's new motivation by helping her set important and realistic lifestyle changes prior to discharge.

*See Clinical Applicability Challenges at the end of this chapter for questions related to this case.*

to establish frequent and open communication about the patient's situation. In the course of talking with the patient's wife, the nurse is continually assessing her learning needs and developing an understanding of her coping mechanisms. By allowing the family to spend time with the patient at the bedside, the nurse supports the wife's need to keep watch over her loved one. Moreover, consistent and accurate information about the patient enables the family to deal with the crisis phase of illness. Research has demonstrated that up-to-date information is the highest priority for family members who are coping with critical illness.[2]

Rather than overwhelm patients and families with detailed knowledge and pathophysiology, nurses should teach the "need to know" basic information first in a manner that reflects their readiness or capacity to learn.[1] The adage "you don't need to know how an engine works to drive a car" can be applied to various illness states managed in the critical care setting.[19] For example, a newly diagnosed diabetic patient should first be taught basic education about the types of diabetes, general concepts of glucose and insulin, types of food that need to be in balance, and prevention of complications from diabetes. Education should focus on what the person can do to get better, how to stay that way, and the resources that are available. The nurse should avoid instilling fear, as this emotion decreases a person's ability to learn. Also, the nurse should remember to allow time for the patient and family to comment and ask questions. This will allow the patient and family to remain in control of their learning, as well as providing cues as to what they have actually learned and what they think is most important to learn.[3]

## Prolonged Illness and Stress

Frequently, the period of critical illness extends well beyond the initial crisis phase and creates additional burdens for the patient and family. The critically ill patient may experience an unpredictable course, and recovery can be tedious. Families are forced to balance their home and work schedules with time spent at the hospital, which can be stressful and evoke feelings of guilt. Having a critically ill family member disrupts daily routines, can require long travel distances, and can have an economic impact when the patient is the breadwinner or when family members take time off from work. It can trigger conflict within the family unit, and can impose physical and mental fatigue.[2] Substantial caregiver burden is experienced by many SDMs and has been reported to continue for as long as 1 to 2 years after the ICU survivor's illness.[7] Health care providers' schedules are often unpredictable and do not always mesh well with family visits, which further underscores the vital role that the ICU nurse plays as the primary link to the family.

As a patient and family advocate, the nurse must provide accurate information and share the plan of care with the family. Including families in hands-on patient care, goal setting, daily rounds, and interdisciplinary meetings can be effective strategies to enhance family support in the ICU setting.[2] To reduce stress and improve communication with families, open-ended questions should be asked to allow the family members to express in their own words their understanding of the patient situation and the current plan of care. This allows the health care team to clarify misunderstandings and

to provide additional opportunity for consensus building. Patient conferences offer a therapeutic method of shared decision making between the health care team and the patient's family. The following are effective communication and relationship strategies that have been found to ease family members' stress and increase confidence in their role as SDMs:

- Perceived transparency of information conveyed between health care providers and the SDM
- Inclusivity
- Availability of providers to answer questions
- Clarity of information
- Patience
- Responsiveness and empathy toward SDM concerns
- Extended social support network of friends and family
- Communication with nurses
- Knowledge of patient's wishes related to treatment preferences or advanced directives
- Faith and spirituality.[2]

As the patient's condition improves, the ICU nurse begins to prepare the patient and family for eventual discharge from the ICU. This milestone in recovery that will lead to a step down in care from the ICU environment can create a feeling of uneasiness in patients and families. Moving from a more secure ICU environment to one that is unfamiliar can result in "transfer anxiety."[21] A family member once stated that the discharge/transfer experience was like "going from a five-star to a one-star hotel and you really need a halfway house."[22]

Well-written and thoughtful discharge summaries are a valuable part of the rehabilitation process, as they can reduce "transition stress," optimize recovery, and provide patients with an opportunity to begin to understand all that they have been through in the ICU.[23,24] However, time constraints, competing priorities, and lack of motivation of the health care team have been identified as barriers to writing effective ICU discharge summaries.[6] Well-written discharge summaries personalize information, actively involve the patient and family in identifying self-care needs, and offer an avenue for reflection, all of which motivate both the patient and family and the staff to meet predetermined goals. The best time to begin to present discharge information is 24 to 48 hours prior to discharge from the ICU.[24]

Research has found that ICU patients receiving well-written discharge summaries with self-directed exercises and patient diaries of their experiences, in addition to routine follow-up care upon discharge, have improved physical functioning and quality of life at 6 months postdischarge.[7] Also, patient discharge summaries have been found to help nurses in the step-down units better understand a patient's experiences, relieving some of the nurses' anxiety when taking over the care of an ICU patient.[23] Furthermore, the ICU nurse can provide anticipatory guidance by spending time educating the patient and family about the new unit routine, staffing patterns, and visiting hours before making the transfer. This approach helps mitigate some of the negative feelings and anxiety associated with the change in environment.[2] Overall, well-written information and personalized discharge summaries, combined with effective verbal communication about discharge, likely increases psychosocial well-being for family members and physical recovery for patients.[24]

## Environmental Stress

Ringing telephones, chiming call lights and pagers, overhead announcements, equipment alarms, staff conversations, banging automatic doors, and pneumatic tubes are just a few examples of the sounds that fill the typical ICU. Also, structural factors such as limited space to visit, restricted visiting hours, rules on age and number of visitors, and constricted waiting room areas contribute to stress and family discomfort in the ICU environment.[2] Patients and families are not accustomed to the constant sounds and lack of privacy in an ICU, and yet, as difficult as it may be, nurses ask patients and families to learn in this distracting environment.

Simple measures can help to reduce environmental stress and enhance the success of learning. The mere act of closing the door to the patient's room can reduce the background noise sufficiently. Placing a comfortable chair at the bedside can enhance the learner's attention span. Reducing the alarm volumes and muting or turning off the television while the nurse is talking with the patient or family helps minimize the number of interruptions or distractions, and may improve the learner's ability to focus on a teaching session.[25]

Health care providers must be mindful of their surroundings when discussing confidential details of a patient's case. Ensuring privacy while sensitive or confidential information is being exchanged can markedly reduce the anxiety of a patient or family member. This regard for patient confidentiality also applies to teaching rounds that are held in the halls and at the bedside in the ICU.

## Cultural and Language Differences

As the demographics of the US population changes, the patients and families whom nurses care for in hospital settings are becoming increasingly diverse. Currently, Asians and Hispanics are the two largest immigrant groups in our country. The U.S. Census Bureau projections estimate that by 2060 minority groups will constitute over 57% of the US population.[25] Therefore, cultural awareness and sensitivity need to be the hallmark of nurse communication now and in the future.[17]

Cultural competence in health care is defined as having the knowledge, abilities, and skills to deliver care congruent with the patient's beliefs and practices.[26] Culture influences a patient's beliefs about health and illness, treatment options, relationships within families and between health care providers, privacy needs, and dietary preferences.[1]

Galanti describes an effective method of questioning patients to ascertain information that is culturally sensitive by using the *Four Cs of Culture*:

1. *Call*. Attempt to identify the problem by asking the patient, "What do you call your problem?"
2. *Cause*. Explore the patient's belief surrounding the origin of the illness by asking, "What do you believe has caused your problem?"
3. *Cope*. Figure out how the patient has been managing the problem by asking, "What have you or other health care providers done to treat this problem?"

4. *Concern*. "What concerns do you have about your condition or the recommended treatment?"

The Four Cs of Culture is an open-ended method of seeking information that can also be used when speaking with family members.[27]

Successful education of culturally diverse patients and families requires more than just basic knowledge about ethnic groups. ICU nurses must recognize their own individual biases and examine their personal beliefs about health and nursing care. Many of our health beliefs are based on ethical principles and values of Western medicine, such as patient autonomy, self-determination, justice, "do no harm," truth telling, independence, privacy, clock time, physical fitness, and beauty.[26,27] The imposition of these Euro-American values on other cultures impedes communication between the nurse and patient and hinders the education process.[28] Racial and ethnic health disparities also exist in the critical care setting; evidence suggests that minority patients receive lower-quality EOL care than whites, and nonwhite patients are less likely to have documentation of advance directives.[29] Although ICU nurses may not have the time to complete a thorough cultural assessment, several key pieces of information should be obtained, as outlined in Box 4-4.

Language barriers also pose a major obstacle to patient and family education, especially in the stressful and complex ICU environment. Although it is convenient for health care providers to rely on a family member or friend to serve as the interpreter of verbal messages or the translator of written materials, it may be difficult for the family member or friend to understand the complex medical terminology or keep personal bias from entering the context of the conversation. In some cultures, the oldest male makes the health care decisions; if a child is asked to interpret medical information, it disrupts the social order of the family and can lead to conflict. Therefore, every effort should be made to provide a professional interpreter for the non–English-speaking patient and family to communicate sensitive, important health care information. During the assessment, questions should be directed to the patient, not to the interpreter.[26] Written instructions also should be translated and reviewed in the presence of a professional translator so that any questions can be immediately addressed. Culturally competent health care organizations must provide language assistance and make

---

**BOX 4-4** | **Key Pieces of Information to Obtain as Part of the Cultural Assessment**

- Does the patient live in an ethnic community?
- When medical decisions are made, who should be consulted before making the decision?
- Primary and secondary languages (speaking and reading ability)
- Religious practices
- Health and illness beliefs and practices
- Family expectations to remain with a hospitalized family member
- Communication practices (verbal and nonverbal)
- How decisions are made in the context of the patient and family

Adapted from Galanti GA: Caring for Patients from Different Cultures, 5th ed. Philadelphia, PA: University of Pennsylvania Press, 2014.

readily available printed instructions in several languages for use by patients and their families.[26]

## Low Health Literacy

Effective communication is the foundation of high-quality patient-centered health care.[30] The Institute of Medicine's (IOM's) report "Health Literacy: A Prescription to End Confusion" states that more than 50% of adult Americans struggle to understand and follow the health information instructions they are provided. In a study conducted at various public hospitals, roughly 42% of patients misinterpreted directions to "take medication on an empty stomach."[31,32]

The term *literacy* refers to the ability to read and write, whereas the term *health literacy* indicates skills to navigate and act on instructions given in the health care setting.[19,30] *Healthy People 2010* and the IOM define health literacy as the "degree to which individuals have the capacity to obtain, process, and understand basic health information and services needed to make appropriate health decisions."[33] In recent years the concept of *e-health literacy* has emerged. *E-health literacy* is defined as the "ability to seek, find, understand, and appraise health information from electronic sources and apply the knowledge gained to address a health problem."[19,32] Ashton and Oermann[1] found that 81% of US adults use the Internet, and among those, 72% have searched online for health-related information.

More than two thirds (about 66%) of people soon to be insured under the ACA will come from vulnerable populations most affected by low health literacy.[30] Vulnerable populations are identified as adults over age 64, racial or ethnic minorities, and those with income at or below the poverty level. This population is also at risk for having complicated physical and mental health needs requiring proficient health literacy skills.[30] Low heath literacy has been associated with less use of preventive health services, lower rates of medication adherence, worse clinical outcomes, an increased use of emergency services, greater racial and ethnic disparities in health care, and higher medical costs for patients and the health care system. In addition, poor health literacy has been identified as an independent predictor of admission to the hospital, hospital readmission within 30 days of discharge, and higher rates of mortality. Thus, low health literacy is a significant problem that can be difficult to identify, not only because patients often mask their lack of literacy skills, but also because no standardized health literacy screening guidelines currently exist.[17,30,33]

The average reading grade level for most Americans is the 8th grade level, with one out of five people (20%) reading below the 5th grade level. A vast majority of patient education materials published by national professional organizations are written at the 9th grade level or higher, which is not suitable for understanding by most patients.[34] For example, a 10th grade reading level is needed to understand directions on an aspirin bottle.[19] To compound the problem, shame is the most common emotion associated with low health literacy, and this poses additional barriers to accessing health information. In fact, patients who have difficulty reading often have not told spouses, children, and health care providers for fear of being negatively judged.[19] Also, nurses should not assume that attainment of a particular educational grade level accurately reflects a person's reading grade level.[34] Numerous studies have shown that many people read two to four grades below their reported level of education.[19] TJC supports the practice of effective communication between health care professionals and patients by mandating that written patient education materials are prepared at an appropriate reading level, with pictures and simple wording that address issues relevant and appropriate for family members.[9]

Patients and families in the ICU are often overwhelmed and anxious by the gravity of their situation. During such times of crisis, patients and families are expected to process and use complex information to make health decisions. Because ICU nurses are familiar with the fast-paced ICU environment, they can easily overestimate the ability of patients and families to comprehend their overall situation. In fact, patients retain only about 50% of the information they receive while in the hospital, and in the critical care setting the percentage is even less. Too often, patients and families will say "yes" when asked if they understand health communication because they are overwhelmed, when in reality they do not understand.[17]

In the ICU setting, abstract concepts and complex problems can be scary and difficult to comprehend for people with low health literacy skills. Rather than ask family members to leave when care needs to be done, the ICU nurse should include the family and patient, if able and alert, to be involved in the care to begin to build knowledge of self-care skills. To effectively educate the patient and family about what is happening, nurses should take time to establish rapport and listen uninterrupted, and provide them with appropriate education materials. Without sufficient knowledge, patients and families will not be able to succeed with self-care requirements as they transition through the health care setting.

Several strategies have been shown to improve written and oral communication for patients with low health literacy skills. Verbal sharing of information remains the most trusted form of communicating with patients and families, but many health care professionals rely solely on providing written materials for patient education.[30] Since patients typically remember less than half of what is discussed, limiting the amount of information presented at one time can improve learning recall.[30] Provide only the "need to know" information, and be sure to repeat information that is essential. Avoid medical terminology and complex explanations of pathophysiology. Speak in short sentences (less than 15 words), using words with fewer than 3 syllables. Solicit information from patients using open-ended questions. For example, rather than asking a "yes/no" question such as "Do you understand?" ask, "What questions do you have for me?" to engage the patient in discussion. Be interactive by presenting education topics using multiple modalities (oral, written, video, and pictures). Visual communication is the best form of communication for patient understanding and knowledge retention; it has been shown to improve comprehension of information by 27% as compared with information presented without visuals.[30]

An education strategy called the "teach-back" method is a well-established, effective way of assessing patient comprehension of orally presented material, yet it is used less than 40% of the time by health care providers when educating patients.[19,30] It requires the health care provider to ask a patient to repeat, in his or her own words, the information that was just presented.[34] The three main goals of "teach-back" are as follows:

1. To confirm that a patient or family member has understood what is being said
2. To correct misconceptions
3. To open dialogue between the patient and family and the health care provider.[17]

The teach-back method not only improves information retention but also exposes gaps in knowledge.[1] Although this method may seem to take extra time and effort, the teach-back interactive communication style has been proven, especially in the hectic ICU environment, to build nurse–patient and nurse–family trust and improve communication, and to actually save time in the long run.

Written material can reinforce and support key messages that have been conveyed verbally. If written material is used, however, it is important to take time to review the handout with the patient and family for the purpose of highlighting key points.[32] All written materials provided in the health care environment should be written at a simplified level (fifth to sixth grade or below) and augmented with illustrations to improve comprehension, as noted earlier.[19]

When evaluating appropriateness of printed education materials (PEMs), nurses should ask themselves, "Is the purpose of the handout clear?" Fairly simple modifications to format and layout, language, and graphics can greatly improve the readability of PEMs. For example, bolding and underlining are encouraged. The use of 12- or 14-point font and high-contrasting colors, with important "need-to-know" information up front, followed by headings and subheadings as well as bullet points and lists, makes information more readable.[19] In 2010, the Agency for Healthcare Research and Quality (AHRQ) released the *Health Literacy Universal Precautions Toolkit*, which encourages health care providers to treat all patients as though they have low health literacy by applying "universal precautions" to deliver clear and plain language to ensure effective health care communication to everyone.[32,30]

The elderly (patients 65 years and older) are the largest consumers of health care, including ICU admissions, yet this cohort has the lowest health literacy skills.[34] Guidelines for developing PEMs that are appropriate for use with older adult patients are presented in Box 4-5.

Low health literacy has been called the "silent epidemic," with millions of Americans lacking skills needed to navigate health care systems successfully, especially complex settings like the ICU, resulting in multiple adverse health-related outcomes.[17] Recognition of low health literacy skills is lacking among nurses, physicians, and other health professionals, as is awareness of practices designed to address low health literacy. Negative attitudes exist as well among health professionals about patients with low health literacy.[26]

The Department of Health and Human Services report entitled *National Action Plan to Improve Health Literacy*, also known as the NAP, has urged all health care providers to be aware of health literacy, understand how to assess it, and develop interventions to address it in their practice setting.[19,30] The AACN places ICU nurses in the role of patient advocate; to truly embrace this role, nurses must continue to be responsive to all health information needs of their patients

---

**BOX 4-5**  *CONSIDERATIONS for the Older Patient*

**Guidelines for PEMs**

- Font should be 12 points or larger
- Serif type is preferred over sans-serif type
- Avoid script or stylized types
- Use boldface headings
- Avoid using all uppercase letters for body type
- Use specific language and avoid generalizations
- Use "calls to action" to highlight important points
- Use four to five lines of text broken up with white space
- Avoid paper with a glossy finish because the glare makes reading difficult. Use matte-finish paper instead
- Enhance legibility by using black ink printed on white or off-white paper
- Avoid printing over a designed or customized background

From Bastable SB, Myers GM, Poitevent LB: Health literacy. In: Bastable SB (ed): Nurse as Educator: Principles of Teaching and Learning for Nursing Practice, 4th ed. Burlington, MA: Jones & Bartlett Learning, 2014, pp 229–283.

---

and families and facilitate effective communication.[17] It can be fairly simple to modify health communication by applying the techniques suggested within this section—techniques designed to improve patient and family relationships with health care providers, to create workable management plans, to share decision making, and to help understand care, all of which lead to adherence and improved outcomes.[35] Overall, nurses can empower patients by showing respect, and they can create patient-centered, comfortable, and shame-free environments that allow patients and family members to ask for help or to convey that they do not understand something.[17] The overarching goals of our health care system to provide patient- and family-centered care and medical home models cannot be achieved without paying attention to the problem of low health literacy.

## Sensory Deficits

The Americans with Disabilities Act prohibits discrimination against people with disabilities, including those who are blind, deaf, or hearing impaired.[36] Under the law, people with disabilities must be able to communicate with hospital staff, and the medical facility must be ready to meet that requirement.[36] To ensure that deaf or hearing-impaired patients and families can communicate effectively, an oral interpreter should be used in the ICU setting for the discussion of treatment options; informed consent for procedures, blood administration, or surgery; and discharge instructions.

Intubated patients frequently experience frustration, anxiety, and exhaustion because they lack the ability to communicate a need or thought.[17] The health care team must learn strategies to allow the ventilated patient, when able, to communicate decisions, wishes, and the plan of care. The ICU nurse can alleviate anxiety by asking simple yes/no questions rather than open-ended questions and by giving directions in a calm, confident, and reassuring manner—for example, "if you are having pain, squeeze my hand." Grossbach and coauthors provide six strategies to facilitate communication with ventilator-dependent patients:

1. *Establish a trusting and friendly environment for communication.* Ensure you are visible to the patient, maintain eye contact when speaking, use adequate lighting, limit excess noise, ensure that the call bell is within reach, and allow adequate time for patient responses.

2. *Assess functional skills that affect communication.* Identify visual and auditory acuity, dominant handedness, and muscle strength. If the patient wears glasses or hearing aids, ensure these are in place and functioning.

3. *Anticipate needs.* Ask questions about basic care needs, be consistent with communication methods, and ensure other staff are aware of patient-specific techniques.

4. *Facilitate lip reading.* Position the bedside light to illuminate the lips. Avoid interruptions when communicating via this mode. Speak normally, avoiding overly exaggerated speech.

5. *Use alternative communication methods and devices.* Use gestures, head nods, writing, picture boards, or computer assistive devices to communicate with the health care team and family members. Consider consultations with a speech and language pathologist.

6. *Educate the patient and family.* To encourage consistent use of communication methods, share with the family (in oral and written form) the communication strategies established specifically for the patient.[37]

## Evaluating the Teaching and Learning Process

Evaluation includes a review of the learning objectives established in the teaching plan to determine achievement of outcomes. Evaluation provides evidence about patient accomplishments and skill acquisition. Evaluation can be done through the "teach-back" method to help identify gaps in knowledge that indicate where further teaching may be required.[1,21] Questioning the learner provides the teacher with immediate feedback to validate the level at which the learner has grasped the information. Also, questions by the learner indicate where gaps in learning may still exist.

Direct observation of the performance of newly learned skills or procedures should also be part of evaluation. Because adults do not want to appear awkward or clumsy when performing a task, it is important to have a relaxed, positive learning environment whereby the teacher establishes a good rapport with the patient or family member before asking them to return-demonstrate a new task or skill.

Often the success or failure of patient and family education influences the discharge plans. Patients who are unable to perform new tasks need supervision and further practice to learn required skills. Therefore, adequate evaluation of the learning process is an essential component of the health care continuum. If the teaching plan is ineffective or the learner's

---

> **BOX 4-6**   **Components of Teaching Documentation**
>
> - Participants (Who was taught?)
> - Date and time (When was it taught?)
> - Patient status (What was the patient's condition at the time?)
> - Content (What was taught?)
> - Teaching methods and materials (How was the patient taught?)
> - Evaluation of learning (How well was the information absorbed?)
> - Follow-up and learning evaluation (If teaching was incomplete, what was the reason? What additional education needs does the patient have?)
>
> Bastable SB: Chapter 10: Behavioral objectives. In: Bastable SB (ed): Nurse as Educator: Principles of Teaching and Learning for Nursing Practice, 4th ed. Burlington, MA: Jones & Bartlett Learning, 2014, pp 424–468.

needs change, it should be altered. Each nursing intervention should document the content, method, and media used for teaching and the extent of what was learned by the patient or family member. In addition, the patient's barriers to learning should be addressed, and the nursing interventions should be aimed at meeting those personal needs. In the ICU, families are often included in the teaching plans because of the limited learning ability of the patient.

The details of teaching documentation are outlined in Box 4-6.

## Summary

The past decade has seen a tremendous increase in understanding of critical illness, the needs of the critically ill, and the long-term effects of critical illness on patients and families. Effective communication and information help minimize patient and family anxiety as well as prevent adverse outcomes in the critical care setting.[38] The ICU is an environment that is overwhelming to most patients and families. Care can become fragmented between multiple providers, and the complex needs, terminology, and equipment can be unfamiliar and frightening.[2] First, by finding out through assessment what the patient and family "need to know," the nurse can capture their attention and begin to lower anxiety. Then, by devoting time and attention to educating ICU patients and their families using evidence-based information and appropriate patient education tools, the nurse not only supports patient empowerment and self-care, but also improves outcomes for patients and families.[34,38] The impact that a nurse educator can have on patients and families can be summarized well by a quote from John C. Maxwell: "People don't care how much you know until they know how much you care." Once patients and their families feel supported, the nurse has paved the way to educate them for self-care.

# Clinical Applicability Challenges

## CASE STUDY QUESTIONS

**Case 1**

*Please refer to Box 4-2 on page 35 to answer these questions.*

1. Discuss the teaching and learning strategies used by Manny, the critical care nurse, to effectively manage the initial shock felt by Johaun's wife Charvel.
2. What learning needs do you anticipate for Charvel during this time of crisis?
3. As Johaun's condition improves, how else can the ICU health care team assist Johaun and Charvel in dealing with the long-term effects of the crisis?

**Case 2**

*Please refer to Box 4-3 on page 37 to answer these questions.*

1. What would be an appropriate initial approach for the ICU nurse, Maria, to take when working with Sonal to help her manage her Type 1 diabetes?
2. What principles from Malcolm Knowles' andragogical model did the ICU nurse employ to assist Sonal, who is now considered to be a young adult learner, with self-management of her diabetes?
3. What techniques could Maria use to assess and evaluate Sonal's learning?

## WANT TO KNOW MORE?

A wide variety of resources to enhance your learning and understanding of this chapter are available on thePoint.

You will find:

- References
- Selected readings
- NCLEX-style review questions
- Internet resources
- And more!

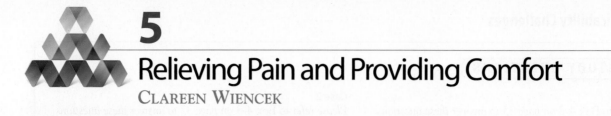

# 5

# Relieving Pain and Providing Comfort

CLAREEN WIENCEK

## LEARNING OBJECTIVES

*Based on the content in this chapter, the reader should be able to:*

1. Differentiate between acute and chronic pain
2. Identify factors that exacerbate the experience of pain in the critically ill
3. Prepare patients for the common sources of procedural pain in intensive care
4. Compare and contrast tolerance, physical dependence, and addiction

5. Discuss clinical practice guidelines for the management of pain, agitation, and delirium in intensive care unit patients
6. Identify appropriate analgesics for high-risk critically ill patients
7. Describe nonpharmacologic interventions for alleviating pain and anxiety

Pain is one of the greatest stressors and most common symptoms in critically ill patients.[1,2] In addition to being a coexisting symptom of critical illness, patients experience increased levels of pain during many critical care interventions and routine procedures.[3,4]

Even though pain management has become a national priority in recent years, pain continues to be misunderstood, poorly assessed, and undertreated in intensive care units (ICUs) and many other health care settings.[1,2] Uncontrolled pain triggers physical and emotional stress responses, inhibits healing, increases the risk of other complications, and increases the length of ICU stay. Critical care nurses need a clear understanding of concepts related to pain assessment and management. Because optimal pain and comfort management in the critically ill requires an integrated approach by the interdisciplinary team, the critical care nurse performs a critical role as the member of the team who is most consistently at the bedside, assessing and relieving patients' pain.

Chapter 5 provides an overview of key concepts related to managing acute pain and comfort in the critically ill adult patient. For an overview of the physiologic processing of pain, refer to Chapter 32.

## Pain Defined

Pain is a complex, subjective phenomenon. It is a protective mechanism, causing one either to withdraw from or to avoid the source of pain and seek assistance or treatment. The International Association for the Study of Pain defined pain as "an unpleasant sensory and emotional experience associated with actual or potential tissue damage or described in terms of such damage."[5] McCaffery provides an operational definition of pain that considers the subjectiveness and individuality of the pain experience. This definition is based on the premise that the individual experiencing the pain is the true authority: "Pain is whatever the experiencing person says it is, existing whenever he or she says it does."[6]

Not all pain is the same. The various types of pain are categorized based on the duration (acute or chronic) and source (somatic, visceral, or nerve) of the pain. It is essential that the types of pain a patient is experiencing be properly identified so that the most efficacious management strategies can be implemented.

The type of pain that most ICU patients experience is classified as *acute pain*. Acute pain is a physiologic response to an identifiable cause, is generally time-limited, and typically responds well to opioid and nonopioid therapies. For example, the pain experienced during endotracheal suctioning or a dressing change is expected to end when the treatment is completed. Similarly, pain at an incision or area of injury is expected to cease once healing has occurred. Often, patients in the critical care setting will experience pain from more than one source. For example, a postoperative patient will likely have somatic pain stemming from the site of the incision, visceral pain from organs that were manipulated, and possibly nerve pain from nerves that were cut or damaged during the surgical procedure.

In contrast, *chronic pain* is caused by physiologic mechanisms that are less well understood. Chronic pain differs from acute pain in terms of etiology, adaptive mechanisms, and expected duration. Chronic pain extends past the usual course of an acute illness or injury for an indefinite period of time, usually exceeding 3 to 6 months, and serves no adaptive purpose. It is difficult to treat, responds poorly to routine pain management strategies, and adversely affects the quality of life for the individual.[7,8] It is essential for the critical care nurse to be aware that, in addition to acute pain associated with the critical illness or injury, ICU patients will frequently have a concomitant chronic pain condition that must be properly managed as well.

## Pain in the Critically Ill

Acute critical illness, regardless of the etiology, is painful. Consider the most common illnesses or injuries treated in the ICU: sepsis, myocardial infarction, cardiothoracic surgery and neurosurgery, multiple trauma, and extensive burns. All of these conditions can be associated with moderate to severe pain, and most critically ill patients will likely experience pain during their ICU course.[1]

Beyond the acute ICU phase, patients with the syndrome of chronic critical illness are likely to experience a combination of acute pain (due to a new illness, injury, or procedure) and chronic pain that is often associated with additional symptoms, such as respiratory distress, fatigue, and cognitive impairment.[9] The syndrome of chronic critical illness is associated with post–intensive care syndrome (PICS), based on decades of research into the long-term consequences of critical illness.[10,11] Evidence now refutes the previously held belief that critically ill patients were unable to remember their painful experiences because of the acute nature of the illness or injury. Recent research demonstrates that up to 82% of ICU patients do remember painful experiences, and that 17% to 38% still remembered severe pain episodes 6 months after discharge from the ICU.[1] In addition, studies have shown that inadequately managed pain has significant short- and long-term consequences, including sleep deprivation, persistent recall of painful episodes, posttraumatic stress disorder symptoms, higher prevalence of chronic pain, and lower quality of life.[10] PICS is addressed in more detail in the section, Pain Management in Specific Populations.

In addition to the patient's illness-, injury-, or procedure-induced pain, the critical care nurse must also be cognizant of the many factors inherent to an ICU admission and the ICU environment that will increase the patient's pain experience (Box 5-1). Each of these factors alone will exert a significant negative effect on the patient's pain; when experienced in combination, they act synergistically to further increase pain. For example, pain and anxiety act in a cyclical fashion to exacerbate each other.

---

| BOX 5-1 | Factors Contributing to Pain and Discomfort in the Critically Ill |

**Physical**
- Symptoms of critical illness (eg, angina, ischemia, dyspnea)
- Wounds: Posttrauma, postoperative, postprocedural, or penetrating tubes and catheters
- Sleep disturbance and deprivation
- Immobility; inability to move to a comfortable position due to tubes, monitors, restraints
- Temperature extremes associated with critical illness and the environment (fever, hypothermia)

**Psychosocial**
- Anxiety and depression
- Impaired communication; inability to report and describe pain
- Fear of pain, disability, or death
- Separation from family and significant others
- Boredom or lack of pleasant distractions
- Sleep deprivation, delirium, or altered sensorium

**Intensive Care Unit Environment or Routine**
- Continuous noise from equipment and staff
- Continuous or unnatural patterns of light
- Awakening and physical manipulation every 1 to 2 hours for vital signs or positioning
- Continuous or frequent invasive, painful procedures
- Competing priorities in care (unstable vital signs, bleeding, dysrhythmias, poor ventilation) may take precedence over pain management

## Procedural Pain

Procedural pain is commonly experienced by critically ill patients.[1,2] Efforts to provide pain relief and comfort measures are complicated by the fact that critical care nurses must continuously perform procedures and treatments that are inherently painful. Procedures like chest tube insertion and removal, endotracheal suctioning, and wound debridement are obviously painful. Less obvious are the simple procedures, such as turning and positioning, that can also cause considerable pain for critically ill patients.

The landmark, multisite Thunder Project I and II reported patients' responses to six procedures frequently performed on critically ill patients: position changes, tracheal suctioning, deep line removal, deep breathing and coughing exercises, dressing changes, and drain removal. Turning and dressing changes were found to be the most painful.[3,4] Additional research shows that less than 25% of patients receive analgesia prior to procedures.[1] Critical care nurses must advocate for adequate preemptive pain management, especially related to common ICU procedures.

Before performing procedures known to be associated with pain, patients should be premedicated, and the procedure should be performed only after the medication has taken effect. During procedures, intravenous (IV) opioids, such as morphine or fentanyl, are usually used for analgesia. The nurse needs to know that onset of action for IV morphine occurs within 5 to 10 minutes, and IV fentanyl within 1 to 2 minutes.[1,2] The patient's response must be monitored during the procedure, with additional doses given as needed. Anxiolytic medications, such as midazolam or propofol, can be given to relieve anxiety during the procedure; however, these agents should *only* be used *as adjuncts*, because they provide sedation and no analgesia. In addition to providing preemptive analgesia and anxiolytic medications, the nurse should educate the patients about the procedure to help him or her prepare for anticipated pain and discomfort. The nurse can also use diversionary interventions, such as imagery, distraction, and family support, as part of the pain management plan.

## Consequences of Pain

Pain produces many harmful effects that have a negative impact on the function of all body systems, inhibit wound healing, and slow recovery from critical illness.[1,10] These effects can extend beyond the ICU phase, contributing to the development of PICS.[10]

The autonomic nervous system responds to pain by causing vasoconstriction and increased heart rate and contractility. Additionally, pulse, blood pressure, and cardiac output all increase, leading to concomitant increases in myocardial workload and oxygen use, both of which can cause or exacerbate myocardial ischemia in an already compromised critically ill person. Patients in pain are also hesitant to move, cough, or breathe deeply because the associated movements increase pain. This decrease in movement manifests as pain-induced respiratory alterations that include splinting, decreased respiratory effort, and reduced pulmonary volume and flow. These pain-induced respiratory alterations can then lead to pulmonary complications, such as atelectasis and pneumonia. In the gastrointestinal system, undertreated pain can cause decreased gastric emptying and intestinal motility, which can result in impaired function and ileus.

Unrelieved pain also negatively affects the musculoskeletal system by causing muscle contractions, spasms, and rigidity, and by suppressing immune function, which predisposes the patient to pneumonia, wound infections, and sepsis.

The negative effects of uncontrolled pain on the course of a critical illness are clear. It is vital for the critical care nurse to understand that the impact of uncontrolled pain during a critical illness can extend beyond the time of recovery from the critical illness. The benefits of effective pain relief are summarized in Table 5-1.

## Barriers to Effective Pain Control

Pain continues to be undertreated in many settings, even though the negative consequences of uncontrolled pain and the benefits of pain relief have been well documented.[1,7,12,13] Often, optimizing pain relief may be perceived to conflict with other clinical goals, such as hemodynamic stability, ventilator weaning, neurologic assessment, or discharge planning. Additionally, comfort goals may compete with

regulatory pressures to use evidence-based bundles or checklists that measure quality outcomes, such as the prevalence of catheter associated urinary tract infections or central line associated blood stream infections.[1,2] Critical care teams may be overly concerned that analgesic administration may cause hemodynamic and respiratory compromise, oversedation, or drug addiction.[1,2]

The fear of addiction is one of the greatest concerns and impediments associated with analgesia and pain control. This fear causes anxiety for patients and their families as well as for health care providers. Critical care nurses must have a clear understanding of the differences between, and implications of, addiction, tolerance, and dependence. Patients who require long-term analgesic medication for pain control often develop tolerance or physical dependence. However, these scenarios should not be confused with addiction, which is characterized by behaviors, such as impaired control, compulsive use, and continued use despite serious negative physical or social consequences.[2,12,13] Table 5-2 provides clarification of the concepts of tolerance, physical dependence, and addiction.

Patients with a history of opioid addiction and tolerance provide a unique challenge to nurses trying to manage pain when these patients present with a critical illness. This particular patient population may require much larger doses of pain medication to produce an adequate level of pain control than a patient not addicted to opioids. Research shows that patients with opioid addiction may require 30% to 50% more opioid pain medication than they were taking preoperatively. Continuous epidural delivery and patient-controlled analgesia (PCA) are often beneficial in these patients. Opioid withdrawal is another significant concern when caring for an opioid-addicted patient. The onset of withdrawal can occur between 6 and 48 hours after the last dose, depending on the drug.[14] Symptoms of withdrawal may include flu-like symptoms (nausea, vomiting, diarrhea, headaches, muscle and joint pain, fever), tachycardia, dilated pupils, runny nose, lacrimation, piloerection (hair standing on end), yawning, restlessness, sweating, irritability, anxiety, and hypertension. Although opioid withdrawal does not tend to be fatal, underlying medical conditions (hypertension or recent myocardial infarction) may increase the patient's risk for death.[15] Important to note is that withdrawal can also occur in patients

### TABLE 5-1  Benefits of Effective Pain Relief

| System | Benefit |
|---|---|
| Cardiovascular | Decreased pulse rate, blood pressure, and myocardial workload |
| Respiratory | Enhanced respiration, oxygenation, ability to perform deep breathing and coughing exercises, and decreased incidence of pulmonary complications |
| Neurologic | Decreased anxiety and mental confusion, enhanced sleep |
| Gastrointestinal/ Nutritional | Enhanced gastric emptying, promotion of positive nitrogen balance, increased appetite |
| Musculoskeletal | Earlier ambulation, reducing complications of immobility |
| Economic | Decreased length of stay, decreased costs, enhanced patient satisfaction with care |

### TABLE 5-2  Tolerance, Physical Dependence, and Addiction

| Condition | Definition | Implication |
|---|---|---|
| Tolerance | A state of adaptation in which exposure to a drug induces changes that result in a diminution of one or more of the drug's effects over time | Increase dose by 50% and assess effect. Tolerance to side effects, such as respiratory depression, will increase as the dose requirement increases. |
| Physical dependence | A state of adaptation that is manifested by a drug class–specific withdrawal syndrome that can be produced by abrupt cessation, rapid dose reduction, decreasing blood level of the drug, and/or administration of an antagonist | Gradually taper opioid dosage to discontinuation to avoid withdrawal symptoms. |
| Addiction | A primary, chronic, neurobiologic disease, with genetic, psychosocial, and environmental factors influencing its development and manifestations. It is characterized by behaviors that include one or more of the following: impaired control over drug use, compulsive use, continued use despite harm, and craving. | Rarely seen in critical care patients, unless patient is admitted for drug overdose or other sequelae of illicit drug use |

Definitions from American Pain Society: Definitions related to the use of opioids for the treatment of pain. Retrieved January 15, 2016, from http://american painsociety.org/uploads/education/section_1.pdf.

who do not have a history of opioid drug abuse, but who have been treated for an extended period of time with opioids to control pain. In this patient population, it is vital to taper the use of the opioid and avoid an abrupt stoppage of the drug.

Pain treatment should not be restricted in patients with a history of opioid abuse; rather, it should be more aggressive. The period of critical illness in these patients is not the appropriate time for drug rehabilitation attempts, and the symptoms associated with opioid withdrawal can exacerbate conditions related to the critical illness. The critical care team must focus on providing all necessary measures to allow a full recovery from the illness, which can then be followed by a proper referral for drug-dependence rehabilitation.

## Resources to Promote Effective Pain Control

In recent decades, government agencies, professional organizations, health care institutions, and pain management experts have focused attention on improving pain management

across the United States. The most relevant and extensive set of guidelines, with robust synthesis of current evidence and direct applicability to the critically ill, is the 2013 Clinical Practice Guidelines for the Management of Pain, Agitation, and Delirium (PAD) in Adult Patients in the Intensive Care Unit.[1] These guidelines, developed by an interdisciplinary panel and published in 2013 by the American College of Critical Care Medicine, make evidence-based recommendations using an integrated and interdisciplinary approach to the management of pain. A summary of these recommendations is found in Table 5-3.

The past decade has also seen a significant growth in palliative care; in 2015, 90% of hospitals with more than 300 beds reported having palliative care teams.[16]

## Clinical Practice Guidelines

The concept of clinical practice guidelines was introduced in the early 1990s by the Agency for Healthcare Research and

---

**TABLE 5-3** Clinical Practice Guidelines for the Management of Pain, Agitations, and Delirium in Adult Patients in the Intensive Care Unit

| Statements and Recommendations Related to Pain Management | Rationale |
|---|---|
| **Pain Assessment** | |
| 1. Pain should be routinely monitored in all adult ICU patients.<br>2. The BPS and the CPOT show the most reliability and validity in adult ICU patients who are unable to self-report and have intact motor function.<br>3. Vital signs should not be used alone to assess pain in ICU patients. | • Adult ICU patients routinely experience pain at rest and due to routine procedures.<br>• Routine assessment is associated with better patient outcomes, including lower ICU length of stay, lower use of analgesics, and shorter duration of mechanical ventilation.<br>• Regular use of the BPS or CPOT leads to improved clinical outcomes in ICU patients.<br>• The CPOT and BPS can be implemented after short training sessions.<br>• Changes or trends in vital signs have shown to be unreliable predictors of pain in ICU patients.<br>• Vital signs do not correlate with either patient's self-report of pain or behavioral pain scores.<br>• Vital signs can be used as cues to perform more in-depth pain assessment. |
| **Pain Management** | |
| 1. Preemptive analgesia and/or nonpharmacologic interventions should be administered prior to chest tube removal.<br>2. Preemptive analgesia and/or nonpharmacologic interventions may be needed prior to routine ICU procedures.<br>3. IV opioids should be the first-line drug class of choice to treat nonneuropathic pain in ICU patients.<br>4. All IV opioids are equally effective when titrated to similar end points.<br>5. Use nonopioid analgesics to decrease the amount of opioids administered and/or to reduce opioid related side effects.<br>6. Recommend that the use of enterally administered gabapentin or carbamazepine, in addition to IV opioids, be considered for neuropathic pain.<br>7. Consider thoracic epidural anesthesia/analgesia in patients undergoing abdominal aortic surgery.<br>8. No recommendations exist for thoracic epidural analgesia in patients undergoing thoracic or nonvascular abdominal procedures or regional analgesia in medical ICU patients. | • Studies show that benefits of preemptive analgesia prior to chest tube removal outweigh any negative effects.<br>• Studies show that patients are able to recall painful procedures and episodes after discharge from the ICU.<br>• All IV opioids appear to exhibit similar analgesic efficacy and are associated with similar clinical outcomes.<br>• High quality evidence shows that thoracic epidural anesthesia or analgesia provides superior pain relief for patients undergoing abdominal aortic surgery.<br>• There is no evidence to support the use of neuraxial/regional analgesia in medical ICU patients.<br>• Epidural analgesia to patients with rib fractures improved pain control. |

From Barr J, Fraser GL, Puntillo K, et al: Clinical practice guidelines for the management of pain, agitation, and delirium in adult patients in the intensive care unit. Crit Care Med 41(1):263–306, 2013.

Quality (AHRQ). These guidelines were intended to serve as nationwide standards of care for specific clinical problems. Acute pain management was the topic of the first guideline, and now there are over 2,500 practice guidelines on the National Guideline Clearinghouse, a web-based site sponsored by the American Medical Association and the American Association of Health Plans that evolved from AHRQ's early efforts.[17] Via these various mechanisms, pain management guidelines have been disseminated throughout the United States and have served as a catalyst for several improvements in pain management. These guidelines are also used as legal documents representing the national standard of care for pain management in medical liability. Finally, the reader should make note of the strength of evidence behind the recommendations when referring to clinical practice guidelines.

## Palliative Care

As noted, the past decade has seen an explosive growth in palliative care programs. Palliative care is a multidisciplinary approach to improving the quality of life in persons with serious or life-limiting illnesses based on open communication, patient and family centered goals, and multidimensional pain and symptom management. Palliative care can be offered simultaneously with lifesaving and curative measures in the ICU to all patients, regardless of diagnosis or prognosis. Multiple studies have demonstrated the benefits of integrating palliative care in the ICU, and palliative care is now considered an essential component of high-quality critical care. Some clinicians call for nurses to play a leading role in that integration.[18–22] Critical care teams should incorporate goal-directed palliative interventions to optimize pain management and comfort in the critically ill. Clinical practice guidelines for quality palliative care are available for clinicians, and consumer-focused resources, such as Get Palliative Care, are accessible for consumers.[23,24]

## Internet Resources

The Internet is an important source of information and resources for pain management. Table 5-4 lists websites containing pain management information that may be useful to critical care nurses, teams, patients, and families.

## Pain Assessment

The failure of staff to routinely assess pain and pain relief is one of the most common reasons for unrelieved pain in hospitalized patients.[1] Assessment should be done systematically and at regular intervals using multiple sources of data, including the patient's self-report; observation of behavioral cues, vital signs and other physiologic parameters; and proxy report.

Self-report is considered the gold standard in pain assessment. For patients able to self-report, a numeric rating scale, in which the patient rates the pain on a scale of 1 to 10, with 10 being severe pain, is most commonly used (Fig. 5-1). Pain should be reassessed at an appropriate interval after pain medications or other interventions have been administered. Unfortunately, the absence of physical signs or behaviors is often incorrectly interpreted as the absence of pain; thus, the patient may suffer unnecessarily. The critical care nurse must make every effort to elicit a self-report from the patient to perform an effective pain assessment. Behavioral observation and changes in physiologic parameters can be helpful but should be considered along with the patient's self-report.

Many critically ill patients are unable to report their pain; in this situation, the nurse and team must use validated nonverbal scales and multiple sources of data. Factors that affect self-report in the critically ill include severity of illness, intubation and mechanical ventilation, altered neurologic status, and pharmacologic effects. Vital signs should be used as cues for more in-depth assessment but not as the primary source of data.[1]

In those instances when the patient cannot self-report due to sedation or cognitive impairment, an objective tool for assessing the noncommunicative patient should be used. The Behavioral Pain Scale (BPS) and the Critical-Care Pain Observation Tool (CPOT) have the strongest validity and reliability for monitoring pain in critically ill patients unable to self-report with intact motor function (Tables 5-5 and 5-6).[1,25] The patient's pain must be assessed at regular intervals to determine the effectiveness of therapy, the presence of side effects, the need for dose adjustment, or the need for supplemental doses to offset procedural pain.[1]

Pain assessment is an ongoing process; assessment after pain management interventions and prior to procedures is essential.

**TABLE 5-4** Internet Resources on Pain Management

| Website | Resources Provided |
| --- | --- |
| American Chronic Pain Association www.theacpa.org | Offers information and support for people with chronic pain |
| American Pain Foundation www.painfoundation.org | Resource center for people with pain, their families, friends, care givers, the media, legislators, and the general public |
| American Society for Pain Management Nursing www.aspmn.org | Information about society membership, conferences, resources, guidelines, and position statements |
| City of Hope Pain/Palliative Care Resource Center http://prc.coh.org | Resources to assist others in improving pain management and end-of-life care; a source for assessment tools, patient education materials, quality assurance materials, end-of-life resources, and research instruments |
| National Guideline Clearinghouse www.guidelines.gov | Multiple evidence-based clinical practice guidelines for pain and various other clinical problems; sponsored by the Agency for Healthcare Research and Quality |
| Center to Advance Palliative Care www.capc.org | National data about prevalence of palliative care programs and delivery; educational and quality improvement resources; consumer information |
| American Pain Society http://americanpainsociety.org | Educational resources to promote optimal pain management and practice standards |

### TABLE 5-5   Behavioral Pain Scale

| Item | Description | Score* |
|---|---|---|
| Facial expression | Relaxed | 1 |
| | Partially tightened (eg, brow lowering) | 2 |
| | Fully tightened (eg, eyelid closing) | 3 |
| | Grimacing | 4 |
| Upper limb movements | No movement | 1 |
| | Partially bent | 2 |
| | Fully bent with finger flexion | 3 |
| | Permanently retracted | 4 |
| Compliance with mechanical ventilation | Tolerating movement | 1 |
| | Coughing but tolerating ventilation for most of the time | 2 |
| | Fighting ventilator | 3 |
| | Unable to control ventilation | 4 |

*Score ranges from 3 (no pain) to 12 (maximum pain).
Stites, M. Observational pain scales in critically ill adults. *Crit Care Nurs.* June 2013;Vol.33:68-78:Table 3.

After pharmacologic therapy, pain reassessment should correspond to the time of onset or peak effect of the drug administered and the time the analgesic effect is expected to dissipate. Response to therapy is best measured as a change from the patient's baseline pain level. Occasionally, there may be discrepancies between the patient's self-report and behavioral and physiologic manifestations. For example, one patient may report pain as 2 out of 10, while being tachycardic, diaphoretic, and splinting with respirations. Another patient may give a self-report of 8 out of 10 while smiling. These discrepancies can be due to the use of diversionary activities, coping skills, beliefs about pain, cultural background, fears of becoming addicted, or fears of being bothersome to the nursing staff. When these situations occur, they should be discussed with the patient. Any misconceptions or knowledge deficits should be addressed and the pain treated according to the patient's self-report.

## Patient Self-Report

Because pain is a subjective experience, the patient's self-report is considered to be the gold standard in pain assessment. A numeric pain scale should be used, as mentioned above (Fig. 5-1). In addition, family members and care givers can be used as proxies for the patient self-report in situations, such as critical illness, where significant communication barriers can be present.[2] A self-report or proxy assessment of pain should be obtained not only when the patient is resting, but also during routine activities and procedures such as coughing, deep breathing, and turning.

Critical care nurses are frequently more attuned to objective indicators of pain than to the patient's self-report. If the patient can communicate, the ICU nurse must accept the patient's description of pain as valid. In the conscious and coherent patient, behavioral cues or physiologic indicators should *never* take precedence over the patient's self-report of pain. Behavioral and physiologic manifestations of pain are extremely variable and may be minimal or absent, despite the presence of significant pain.

During the pain assessment, the nurse should elicit a specific verbal description of the quality of the patient's pain, such as burning, crushing, stabbing, dull, or sharp, whenever possible. The location, duration, and exacerbating and alleviating measures should also be established in the assessment process. Often, this descriptive information helps to determine the cause of the pain and the best treatment strategies to employ. All of the information gathered during the pain assessment must be clearly documented in the patient record with a quotation from the patient's self-reported description included.

Pictures or word boards can also facilitate communication about the patient's pain. The board should include questions, such as "Do you have pain?" "Where is the pain located?" "How bad is your pain?" and "What helps your pain?" Developing a simple system of eye movements ("blink once for

### TABLE 5-6   Critical-Care Pain Observation Tool

| Indicator | Description | Score | |
|---|---|---|---|
| Facial expression | No muscular tension observed | Relaxed, neutral | 0 |
| | Presence of frowning, brow lowering, orbit tightening, and levator contraction | Tense | 1 |
| | All of the above facial movements plus eyelid tightly closed | Grimacing | 2 |
| Body movements | Does not move at all (does not necessarily mean absence of pain) | Absences of movements | 0 |
| | Slow, cautious movements, touching or rubbing the pain site, seeking attention through movements | Protection | 1 |
| | Pulling tube, attempting to sit up, moving limbs/thrashing, not following commands, striking at staff, trying to climb out of bed | Restlessness | 2 |
| Muscle tension (evaluation by passive flexion and extension of upper extremities) | No resistance to passive movements | Relaxed | 0 |
| | Resistance to passive movements | Tense, rigid | 1 |
| | Strong resistance to passive movements, inability to complete them | Very tense or rigid | 2 |
| Compliance with the ventilator (intubated patients) | Alarms not activated, easy ventilation | Tolerating ventilator or movement | 0 |
| | Alarms stop spontaneously | Coughing but tolerating | 1 |
| | Asynchrony: blocking ventilation, alarms frequently activated | Fighting ventilator | 2 |
| OR Vocalization (extubated patients) | Talking in normal tone or no sound | Talking in normal tone or no sound | 0 |
| | Sighing, moaning | Sighing, moaning | 1 |
| | Crying out, sobbing | Crying out, sobbing | 2 |
| Total, range | | | 0–8 |

Stites, M. Observational pain scales in critically ill adults. *Crit Care Nurs.* June 2013;Vol.33:68-78:Table 4.

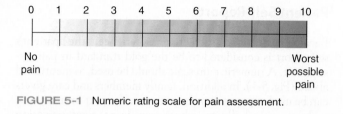

FIGURE 5-1   Numeric rating scale for pain assessment.

yes and twice for no") or finger movements can be effective for the patient who cannot speak or move his or her hands.

If the patient is unable to use any of the above methods to verbalize or indicate that he or she is in pain, the nurse will have a dilemma when attempting the pain assessment and planning the subsequent treatment. In this situation, it is appropriate to observe for the behavioral cues or physiologic indicators discussed in the next section. However, the absence of physiologic indicators or behavioral cues should *never* be interpreted as absence of pain. If the procedure, surgery, or condition is believed to be associated with pain, the presence of pain should be assumed and the patient should be treated appropriately.[1]

## Observation

Nonverbal behaviors, such as guarding, withdrawal, and avoidance of movement, protect the patient from painful stimuli. Attempts by the patient to seek relief, such as touching or rubbing the affected area and changing positions, are palliative behaviors. Crying, moaning, or screaming are affective behaviors and reflect an emotional response to pain. Facial expressions, such as frowning, grimacing, clenching of the teeth, tight closure of the eyes, and tears, can indicate pain. If one or more of these behaviors are present in the nonverbal/noncommunicative patient, it should be assumed that the patient has pain and the proper treatment should be administered.

Patients who are alert and oriented but who are unable to speak may use eye or facial expressions or movement of hands or legs to communicate their pain. Restlessness, agitation, and muscular bracing may be indicators of pain in the nonverbal patient. Since nonverbal cues can be difficult to interpret as indicators of pain, input from family members or other care givers is often helpful in interpreting specific behavioral manifestations of pain based on their knowledge of the patient's behavior before hospitalization.

## Physiologic Parameters

Critical care nurses are skilled in assessing the patient's physical status in terms of changes in blood pressure, heart rate, or respirations. Therefore, the observation of the physiologic effects of pain will assist in pain assessment. Unfortunately, the physiologic response to pain is highly individualized. Vital signs, such as heart rate, blood pressure, and respirations, may increase or decrease in the presence of pain.[1] Therefore, vital signs and physiologic data should be used by the nurse as cues for further assessment and not as the sole source of data from which to determine intervention.[1] The potential for physiologic changes can also be masked by medications that are administered to manage the critical illness—for example, medications that slow the heart rate or decrease blood pressure. When physiologic changes do occur in critically ill patients, it can be difficult to attribute these physiologic changes specifically to pain rather than other causes.

## Pain Intervention

The nurse plays a key role in providing pain relief. While pharmacologic intervention is the most commonly used strategy, nursing management of pain also includes physical, cognitive, and behavioral measures.

## Pharmacologic Interventions

Opioids administered by the IV route should be the first-line drug class of choice for critically ill patients with all types of pain except neuropathic.[1] For neuropathic pain, patients should receive IV opioids and enteral gabapentin or carbamazepine. All available opioids in IV form are equally effective when used in equianalgesic doses.[1]

In general, the ideal method of analgesia should allow adequate serum drug levels to be achieved and maintained. Therefore, analgesic medications should be administered on a regular schedule around the clock and not on an "as needed" (PRN) basis. The efficacy of analgesia depends on the presence of an adequate and consistent serum drug level. The traditional PRN analgesic order is a major barrier to effective pain control in all patient populations. The PRN order suggests that the nurse should administer a dose of analgesic only when the patient requests it and only after a certain time interval has elapsed since the previous dose. Invariably, a delay occurs between the time of the request and the time of administration. The PRN order poses another problem when the patient is asleep. As serum drug levels decrease, the patient is suddenly awakened by severe pain, and a greater amount of the drug is needed to achieve relief. PRN analgesic medication doses should be reserved for breakthrough pain, for when the patient has recovered from the critical illness or is predominantly pain free, or when continuous analgesia is no longer required.

### Nonopioid Analgesics

Though opioids are considered to be the most evidence-based pharmacologic intervention for pain in the critically ill patient, other types of nonopioid or adjuvant agents may be added to the pain regimen. Nonsteroidal anti-inflammatory drugs (NSAIDs), IV acetaminophen, anticonvulsants, antidepressants, and local and regional anesthesia can be used for selected populations as adjunctive medications to optimize the patient's response and overall comfort. Nonopioid analgesics should be considered by the critical care team to decrease the amount of opioid required and the potential for opioid-induced side effects, or to treat concomitant symptoms such as anxiety or depression.[1] NSAIDs decrease pain by inhibiting the synthesis of inflammatory mediators (prostaglandin, histamine, and bradykinin) at the site of injury and effectively relieve pain without causing sedation, respiratory depression, or problems with bowel or bladder function. Many NSAIDs are supplied in oral forms only, which may not be appropriate for some critically ill patients. Ketorolac

(Toradol) is available in parenteral form, but it can cause renal impairment if administration exceeds 5 days; therefore, it must be used with caution in patients with renal insufficiency or those receiving dialysis. Indomethacin (Indocin) is available in suppository form and can be combined with opioids to provide effective pain relief.[2]

When administering NSAIDs as a complement to opioid medications, it is important to consider the potentially harmful side effects. Prostaglandins help protect the gastric mucosa, are active in the aggregation of platelets, and are involved in the autoregulatory response of the vasculature in the kidneys. The inhibition of prostaglandins by NSAIDs can lead to impaired platelet aggregation, renal dysfunction, and gastric irritation, resulting in increased bleeding risk, sodium and water retention, increased creatinine, and gastric ulceration. NSAIDs can also put a patient at higher risks for bronchospasms. Because of these potential risks, NSAIDs should be used with extreme caution in any critically ill patient with renal dysfunction, cardiac failure, coagulation problems, or respiratory failure.[1,15]

Acetaminophen is commonly used in critical care. IV acetaminophen (Ofirmev) has recently been approved for use in the United States in conjunction with opioids for postoperative pain in surgical ICU patients.[1] When it is combined with opioids, it produces a greater effect than opioids alone. In addition to mild analgesia, acetaminophen is an effective antipyretic; however, it does have the potential to cause hepatic damage. Dosages should be limited to a maximum of 2,400 mg/d in patients who have a history of, or high potential for, liver impairment.

Nonopioid analgesics that are commonly used in critical care and their recommended doses are listed in Table 5-7.

## Opioid Analgesics

Opioids are the pharmacologic cornerstone of pain management in the critically ill.[1] They provide pain relief by binding to various receptor sites in the central and peripheral nervous systems, thus changing the perception of pain. Since all opioids are effective in the critically ill, opioids are selected based on individual patient needs and tolerance, formulary availability, and the potential for adverse effects. Commonly used opioids are compared in Table 5-8.

**DOSING GUIDELINES.** *Equianalgesia* means approximately equal analgesia. This term is used when changing a patients' regimen from one opioid to another. Morphine, 10 mg parenteral, is generally considered the gold standard dose for comparison. Dosing guidelines for opioid analgesics are presented in Table 5-8. Opioid dosage varies depending on the individual patient, the method of administration, and the pharmacokinetics of the drug. Adequate pain relief will occur once a minimum serum level of the opioid has been achieved. Each patient's optimal serum level will be different, and this level can change as pain intensity changes. Therefore, the dosing and titration of opioids must be individualized, and the patient's response and any undesirable effects, such as respiratory depression or oversedation, must be closely assessed. If the patient has previously received an opioid, doses should be adjusted above the previous required dose to achieve an optimal effect. Factors such as age, individual pain tolerance, coexisting disease(s), type of surgical procedure, and the concomitant use of sedatives warrant consideration as well. Older patients are often more sensitive to the effects of opioids; therefore, decreasing the initial opioid dose and slow titration are recommended for older patients.

**METHODS OF ADMINISTRATION.** Opioids can be administered by the oral, sublingual, parenteral, rectal, buccal, subcutaneous, transdermal, topical, or nebulized routes. However, the parenteral route is most commonly used in the ICU setting.[26]

**Oral Administration.** Oral administration is simple, noninvasive, and inexpensive and provides effective analgesia. The oral route is the preferred route for patients with cancer and chronic nonmalignant pain. The oral route is used infrequently in the ICU setting because many patients are unable to take anything by mouth. Serum drug levels obtained after oral administration of opioids are variable and difficult to titrate. In addition, the transformation of oral opioids by the liver causes a significant decrease in serum levels.

**Rectal Administration.** Morphine and hydromorphone are available in a rectal form. This provides an alternative for patients who cannot take anything by mouth. Unfortunately, this route has many of the same disadvantages as oral

**TABLE 5-7** Nonopioid Analgesic Drugs

| Drug | Adult Dose | Usual Pediatric Dose | Comments |
|---|---|---|---|
| Acetaminophen | 325–650 mg every 4–6 h | 10–15 mg/kg every 4–6 h | Available in liquid form<br>Lacks anti-inflammatory action<br>Doses exceeding 4,000 mg/d increase the risk of hepatic toxicity. |
| Aspirin | 325–650 mg every 4–6 h | 10–15 mg/kg every 4–6 h | Can cause gastrointestinal or postoperative bleeding |
| Celecoxib (Celebrex) | 100–400 mg twice a day | | Less adverse effects than other nonsteroidal anti-inflammatory drugs<br>Considerably more expensive |
| Ibuprofen (Motrin) | 200–400 mg every 4–6 h | 4–10 mg/kg every 6–8 h | Available in liquid form |
| Indomethacin (Indocin) | 25–50 mg every 8–12 h | | Available in rectal and IV forms<br>High incidence of side effects |
| Ketorolac (Toradol) | 30–60 mg IM initially, then: 30 mg IV every 6 h or 30 mg IM every 6 h<br>10 mg PO every 4–6 h | | Available in parenteral form<br>Limit use to 5 d<br>Contraindicated with renal insufficiency |
| Naproxen (Naprosyn) | 500 mg initially then 250 mg every 6–8 h | 5 mg/kg every 12 h | Available in liquid form |

All doses are oral, unless noted otherwise.

**TABLE 5-8** Opioid Analgesic Drugs

| Drug | Equianalgesic Dose (mg) | | Onset of Action | Comments |
| | Oral | IM/IV | | |
|---|---|---|---|---|
| Morphine | 30 | 10 | 5–10 min IV route<br>30 min oral dose, usually given every 3–4 h | Gold standard for comparing opioids<br>Not recommended with hemodynamic instability or hepatic/renal insufficiency |
| Fentanyl | N/A | 0.1 | Onset 1–2 min IV | Drug of choice for rapid onset of analgesia<br>Preferred in patients with hepatic or renal insufficiency<br>With transdermal form, 12–24 h delay to peak effect |
| Hydromorphone (Dilaudid) | 7.5 | 1.5 | Onset of IV dose 5–10 min | More potent and slightly shorter duration than morphine<br>Rectal form available |
| Methadone (Dolophine) | 2.5–10 | 2.5–10 IV/IM | 10–15 min oral dose | Long half-life, unpredictable steady state<br>Accumulates with repetitive dosing, causing excessive sedation<br>Consult pain or palliative specialists because of highly variable and complex metabolism in individual patients |
| Oxycodone (OxyContin) | 20 | N/A | 30 min oral dose | Dosing must be individualized because of high variability in pharmacokinetics. |

administration, including variability in dosing requirements, delays to peak effect, and unstable serum drug levels.

**Transdermal Administration.** Fentanyl is available as a transdermal patch. This form is used primarily to control stable, chronic cancer pain because it takes 12 to 16 hours to see substantial therapeutic effects and up to 48 hours to achieve stable serum concentrations. If used for acute pain, such as postoperative pain, high serum concentrations may remain after the pain has subsided, putting the patient at risk for respiratory depression. Therefore, transdermal fentanyl is not recommended for acute postoperative pain.[2,26,27]

The nurse must exercise caution when administering fentanyl by a transdermal patch. Gloves should be worn when handling the patch to avoid accidental exposure to the drug. The site where the patch will be applied should be chosen carefully. The skin must be intact. Any open areas in the skin (eg, abrasions, rashes, wounds) could cause the drug to be absorbed more rapidly than anticipated, leading to increased serum concentrations and a possible overdose. Avoid using lotion in the area where the patch will be applied; the lotion can act as a barrier and reduce or prevent the absorption of the drug, thus decreasing the serum concentration and the analgesic effect. When the fentanyl patch is changed, the old patch must be disposed of properly to avoid accidental exposure to the drug or illicit use of the discarded patch.

**Intramuscular Injection.** Intramuscular (IM) injections should not be used to provide acute pain relief for the critically ill patient for several reasons:

- IM injections are painful.
- IM drug absorption is extremely variable in critically ill patients because of alterations in cardiac output and tissue perfusion.
- Anticipated discomfort associated with the injection increases the patient's anxiety.
- Repeated IM injections can cause muscle and soft-tissue fibrosis.

**Intravenous Injection.** IV administration is usually the preferred route for opioid therapy, especially when the patient requires short-term acute pain relief—for example, during procedures such as chest tube removal, diagnostic tests, suctioning, or wound care. IV opioids have the most rapid onset and are easy to administer. With morphine, the time to peak effect is 15 to 30 minutes; for fentanyl, peak effect is achieved within 1 to 5 minutes. However, the duration of analgesia is shorter with intermittent IV injections, and this can cause serum drug levels to fluctuate.

Continuous IV administration has many benefits for critically ill patients, especially those who have difficulty communicating their pain because of an altered level of consciousness or an endotracheal tube. Continuous IV infusions are easily initiated and maintain consistent serum drug levels. For continuous IV opioid infusions, fentanyl and morphine are commonly used because of their short elimination half-life. Before starting a continuous IV infusion, an initial IV loading dose is given to achieve an optimal serum level. Appropriate dosing and titration must be individualized; this can be difficult, because many critically ill patients have hepatic or renal dysfunctions that result in decreased metabolism of the opioid. A disadvantage of continuous IV infusions is that pain occurring during painful procedures may not be managed unless additional IV bolus injections are given.

PCA is an effective method of pain relief for the critically ill patient who is conscious, able to participate in PCA therapy, and exhibiting no signs of delirium. The PCA method of opioid administration produces good quality analgesia, stable drug concentrations, less sedation, less opioid consumption, and fewer adverse effects.[2,26] Effective use of PCA is based on the assumption that the patient is the best person to evaluate and manage his or her pain. With PCA, the patient self-administers small, frequent IV analgesic doses using a programmable infusion device. The PCA device limits the opioid dose within a specific time period, thus minimizing the risk of oversedation and respiratory depression. If the patient is physically or cognitively unable to use "conventional" PCA, continued usage of PCA therapy must be reevaluated. Clinician-administered doses can be delivered, but nurses should check their hospital policy regarding the use of clinician or family-assisted PCA dosing.

**Subcutaneous Administration.** In some situations, venous access may be limited or impossible to obtain. When this occurs, continuous subcutaneous infusion and subcutaneous PCA may be used, though absorption is slower than via the IV route. Typically, volume should not exceed 1 mL in intermittent injections and 3 mL in continuous infusions.[2,26]

**Spinal Administration.** Spinal opioids can provide superior pain management for many patients. Spinal opioids selectively block opioid receptors, while leaving sensation, motor, and sympathetic nervous system function intact. This results in fewer opioid-related side effects than oral, IM, or IV routes of administration. Analgesia from spinal opioids has a longer duration than other routes, and significantly less opioid is needed to achieve effective pain relief. Opioids such as fentanyl or morphine can be given as a single injection in the epidural or intrathecal space, as intermittent injections, or as continuous infusions through an epidural catheter or epidural PCA.

Epidural analgesia is noted for providing effective pain relief and improved postoperative pulmonary function. This method is especially beneficial for critically ill patients after thoracic, upper abdominal, or peripheral vascular surgery, patients with rib fractures or orthopedic trauma, and postoperative patients with a history of obesity or pulmonary disease. With epidural analgesia, opioids are administered through a catheter inserted in the spinal canal between the dura mater and vertebral arch. Opioids diffuse across the dura and subarachnoid space and bind with opioid receptor sites.

Intermittent injections may be given before, during, or after surgical procedures. For more sustained pain relief, continuous epidural infusions are recommended. For patient-controlled epidural analgesia, the same parameters are used as with IV PCA, except that smaller opioid doses are used. Contraindications to epidural analgesia include systemic infection/sepsis, bleeding disorders, and increased intracranial pressure.

Preservative-free morphine and fentanyl are most commonly used for epidural analgesia, because preservatives can be neurotoxic and may cause severe spinal cord injury. Morphine is more water soluble than fentanyl and thus is more likely to accumulate in the cerebrospinal fluid and systemic circulation; with increased accumulation, side effects are more likely. Fentanyl diffuses more quickly to the opioid receptors and causes fewer opioid-related side effects.

The most serious adverse effect of epidural analgesia is respiratory depression. Although the incidence of serious respiratory depression is extremely low with epidural analgesia, respiratory assessments should be performed hourly during the first 24 hours of therapy and every 4 hours thereafter.

Because epidural analgesia is more invasive than the other drug delivery methods discussed, the patient must be closely monitored for signs of local or systemic infections. The insertion site is covered with a sterile dressing, and the catheter is taped securely. To avoid accidental injection of preservative-containing medications, the epidural catheter, infusion tubing, and pump should be clearly marked.

With intrathecal analgesia, the opioid is injected into the subarachnoid space, located between the spinal cord and dura mater. Intrathecal opioids are significantly more potent than those given epidurally; therefore, less medication is needed to provide effective analgesia. The intrathecal method is usually used to deliver a one-time dose of analgesic, such as before surgery, and is infrequently used as a continuous infusion because of the risk of central nervous system infection.

With epidural or intrathecal analgesia, a local anesthetic, such as bupivacaine (Marcaine), can be added to the continuous opioid infusion. Local anesthetics block pain by preventing nerve cell depolarization. They act synergistically with intraspinal opioid and have a dose-sparing effect. Less opioid is needed to provide effective analgesia, and the incidence of opioid-related side effects is decreased. This combination is more commonly administered via the epidural route.

**OPIOID EFFECTS.** Opioids cause undesirable side effects, such as constipation, urinary retention, sedation, respiratory depression, and nausea. These side effects represent a major drawback to their use but can be managed for optimal comfort. Opioid-related side effects are best managed in the following ways:

- *Decreasing the opioid dose:* This is the most effective strategy because it is directed at the *cause* of the side effect. Side effects are usually seen with excessively high serum levels of the drug.
- *Rotating the opioid:* Adverse side effects of a particular drug that are unacceptable to the patient are common reasons to rotate or switch the opioid—for example, switching from morphine to hydromorphone (Dilaudid). Equianalgesic tables should be consulted to calculate the therapeutic dose, including a reduction in the dose of the new drug because of incomplete cross-tolerance at the opioid receptor sites.[27]
- *Avoiding PRN dosing:* When opioids are administered on a PRN basis, fluctuating serum drug levels occur, causing a greater tendency toward sedation and respiratory depression. Around-the-clock administration of analgesics is recommended.
- *Adding an NSAID to the pain management plan:* Using an NSAID in addition to an opioid can decrease the amount of opioid needed while still provide effective pain relief, thus decreasing opioid-related side effects.

Medications can be given to minimize or alleviate some side effects (eg, laxatives for constipation, antihistamines for pruritus, and antiemetics for nausea). However, medications commonly prescribed to treat the opioid-related adverse effects can actually cause other adverse effects. For example, promethazine, a commonly prescribed antiemetic, can cause hypotension, restlessness, tremors, and extrapyramidal effects in the older patient.

Respiratory depression, a life-threatening complication of opioid administration, is often a concern for nurses and physicians. Though the evidence varies, the incidence of opioid-induced respiratory depression is estimated to be 1.1% or less in patients receiving general opioid therapy and between 0.19% and 5.2% in patients receiving PCA therapy.[28] The critical care nurse plays a key role in assessing and monitoring all patients, especially those with known risk factors, for these adverse events.

Opioid-induced respiratory depression is defined as a respiratory rate of less than 8 to 10 per minute, with associated shallow or ineffective respirations, decreasing $SpO_2$ levels, or elevated end-tidal $CO_2$ levels.[28] Risk factors for opioid-induced respiratory depression include age over 55 years, obesity (body mass index greater than 30 $kg/m^2$), obstructive sleep apnea, prolonged surgery that lasted more than 2 hours, the first 24 hours of opioid therapy, frequent or large changes in opioid dosing, history of snoring or apneic periods, smoking history greater than 20 packs/year, and pre-existing pulmonary or cardiac disease such as chronic obstructive pulmonary disease or heart failure. Specifically, the nurse should be aware that the opioid-naïve patient and any patient in the first 24 hours of opioid therapy are at the highest risk of opioid-induced advancing sedation and respiratory depression. Typically, sedation precedes respiratory depression.[28]

Owing to the critical importance of close monitoring and systematic assessment to prevent the life threatening events of sedation and respiratory arrest, and because of the critical role of the bedside nurse, the American Society for Pain Management Nursing (ASPMN) issued expert guidelines in 2011 for monitoring for opioid-induced sedation and respiratory depression. Box 5-2 presents the recommendations from ASPMN.

### Opioid Antagonists

If serious respiratory depression does occur, naloxone (Narcan), a pure opioid antagonist that reverses the effects of opioids, can be administered. The dose of naloxone is titrated to effect—which means reversing the oversedation and respiratory depression, not reversing analgesia. This usually occurs within 1 to 2 minutes. After giving naloxone, the nurse needs to continue observing the patient closely for oversedation and respiratory depression because the half-life of naloxone (1.5 to 2 hours) is shorter than that of most opioids.

---

| BOX 5-2 | **American Society for Pain Management Nursing (ASPMN) 2011 Recommendations for Monitoring for Opioid-Induced Sedation and Respiratory Depression** |

- The frequency and nature of monitoring should be individualized to the patient. Nurses should identify patients at high risk for opioid-induced respiratory depression.
- Monitoring guidelines should be followed according to hospital policy.
- Serial assessment should be performed using validated sedation scales.
- Transfers of patients should be avoided during peak effect times of opioid medications.
- Respiratory rate should be counted for a full minute when patients are on opioid therapy.
- Patients with signs of respiratory depression should be aroused immediately and instructed to perform deep breathing.
- Technologically supported monitoring, such as continuous pulse oximetry and capnography ($ETCO_2$), can be effective for high-risk patients.

Data from Jarzyna D, Jungquist CR, Pasero C, et al: American Society for Pain Management Nursing guidelines on monitoring for opioid-induced sedation and respiratory depression. Pain Manag Nurs 12(3):118–145, 2011. Retrieved from http://www.aspmn.org/documents/Guidelineson MonitoringforOpioid-InducedSedationandRespiratoryDepression.pdf.

Naloxone should be diluted (0.4 mg in 10 mL of saline solution) and given IV, very slowly. Giving the drug too quickly or giving too much can precipitate severe pain, withdrawal symptoms, tachycardia, dysrhythmias, and cardiac arrest. Patients who have been receiving opioids for more than a week are particularly at risk.

### Sedatives and Anxiolytics

Acute pain is often accompanied by anxiety and agitation, both of which occur frequently in the critically ill and can increase the patient's perception of pain.[1] Several decades of research have led to different approaches to sedation in order to produce optimal outcomes in the critically ill. We now know that maintaining light levels of sedation (the patient is arousable and able to follow simple commands) is preferred over deep sedation (patient is unresponsive to painful stimuli), and is strongly associated with shorter length of ICU stay and shorter duration of mechanical ventilation.[1] The 2013 Clinical Practice Guidelines for the Management of Pain, Agitation, and Delirium in Adult Patients in the Intensive Care Unit recommends that patients be assessed using the Richmond Agitation-Sedation Scale (RASS) or the Sedation-Agitation Scale (SAS), the most valid and reliable tools for measuring quality and depth of sedation in adult critically ill patients.

Benzodiazepines, propofol, and dexmedetomidine are the most commonly used sedative and anxiolytic agents in the ICU setting. Use of nonbenzodiazepine agents such as propofol or dexmedetomidine are preferred in patients on mechanical ventilation.[1,29] Table 5-9 provides a comparison of sedatives commonly used in critical care according to the 2013 Clinical Practice Guidelines for Management of Pain, Agitation, and Delirium.[1]

**BENZODIAZEPINES.** Benzodiazepines, such as midazolam (Versed), diazepam (Valium), and lorazepam (Ativan), can control anxiety and muscle spasms, and produce amnesia for uncomfortable procedures. In the ICU, benzodiazepines may be given IV as an intermittent bolus or by continuous infusion, and titrated according to the patient's response. Because these medications have no analgesic effect (except for controlling pain caused by muscle spasm), an analgesic must be administered concomitantly to relieve pain. If an opioid and benzodiazepine are used together, the doses of both medications should usually be reduced because of their synergistic effects. The patient should also be closely monitored for oversedation and respiratory depression.

Midazolam is recommended for conscious sedation and short-term relief of anxiety because of its rapid onset (1 to 5 minutes with IV administration) and its short half-life (1 to 12 hours). Another advantage is its retrograde amnesia effect, which is particularly beneficial during procedures. The duration of effect of midazolam can be longer in older or obese patients and those with liver disease.[1]

A major advantage of benzodiazepines is that they are reversible agents. If respiratory depression occurs from benzodiazepine administration, IV flumazenil (Romazicon) can be administered. A major disadvantage of benzodiazepines is the strong correlation with delirium, formerly referred to as ICU psychosis. Benzodiazepines should be limited or avoided in order to reduce the high risk of delirium in the ICU population.[1] Two methods of sedation are currently recommended

**TABLE 5-9** Comparison of Sedatives Commonly Used in Critical Care

| Drug | Recommended Use | Onset After IV Loading Dose (IV) | Adverse Effects |
|---|---|---|---|
| Diazepam (Valium) | For rapid sedation of acutely agitated patients | 2–5 min | Respiratory depression<br>Hypotension<br>Phlebitis |
| Lorazepam (Ativan) | For long-term sedation of most patients via intermittent or continuous infusion | 15–20 min | Respiratory depression<br>Hypotension<br>Acidosis/renal failure with high doses |
| Midazolam (Versed) | For conscious sedation and rapid sedation of acutely agitated patients<br>For short-term use only | 2–5 min | Respiratory depression<br>Hypotension<br>Prolonged wakening and delayed weaning from ventilator if used long term |
| Propofol | Preferred sedative when rapid awakening is important<br>Preferred for patients on mechanical ventilation | 1–2 min | Pain on injection<br>Elevated triglycerides<br>Respiratory depression<br>Hypotension<br>Pancreatitis<br>Allergic reactions |
| Dexmedetomidine | Short-term sedation<br>Preferred for patients at risk of delirium and on mechanical ventilation | 5–10 min | Bradycardia<br>Hypotension<br>Loss of airway reflexes |

for critically ill patients: daily sedation interruption or maintenance of light levels of sedation. Evidence supports that both are safe and proven to improve outcomes for critically ill patients requiring sedation. As more research is needed to determine if one approach is superior to the other, ICU teams must continue to choose management techniques that are individualized to the patient.[1,30]

**PROPOFOL.** Propofol (Diprivan) is a rapid-acting sedative/hypnotic agent that has no analgesic properties and minimal amnesic effects. With appropriate airway and ventilatory management, propofol can be an ideal agent for patients requiring sedation during painful procedures. Because of its ultrashort half-life and high rate of elimination, it is reversible simply by discontinuing the infusion: patients will awaken within a few minutes. Propofol can also be used as a continuous infusion for mechanically ventilated patients who require deep, prolonged sedation.

Because propofol is only slightly water soluble, it is formulated in a white, oil-based emulsion containing soybean oil, egg lecithin, and glycerol. It is contraindicated, therefore, in patients allergic to eggs or soy products. Propofol contains no preservatives. Each ampule or vial must be used as a "single-dose" product vial and should be discarded within 6 to 12 hours after breaking the sterile seal to minimize the risk of systemic infections. Adverse effects commonly associated with propofol include respiratory depression, hypotension, elevated triglycerides, and pain and stinging at the injection site.

**DEXMEDETOMIDINE.** Dexmedetomidine is a selective alpha-receptor agonist with sedative, sympatholytic, and analgesic/opioid-sparing properties. The pattern of sedation differs from other agents; patients are more easily arousable and the risk of respiratory depression is less. Onset of action is 15 minutes after the IV infusion is started, with peak sedation in 1 hour. Though dexmedetomidine is approved in the United States for short-term sedation only (less than 24 hours) at a maximal dose of 0.7 µg/kg/h, there are some studies that show efficacy of treatment longer than 24 hours.[1] The most common side effects that should be monitored by

the critical care nurse are hypotension and bradycardia, especially if IV loading doses are administered.

## Nonpharmacologic Comfort Measures

The critical care nurse can lead the team in incorporating nonpharmacologic interventions as adjuncts to promote optimal pain relief and general comfort for the critically ill patient. Though pharmacologic interventions are often the most utilized, usually owing to predictable effects, a growing body of evidence supports the use of nonpharmacologic interventions to provide better pain control with less use of opioid analgesics, decreased incidence of anxiety, and increased patient satisfaction.[31-37] In addition, nonpharmacologic interventions are usually low cost, easy to provide, and safe, and include therapies that are already part of the critical care nurse's practice.[2] Environmental modification, sleep hygiene, early mobility, complementary therapies such as music, pet and massage therapy, and therapeutic touch, among others, should be considered as part of the comprehensive approach to optimal pain and comfort management in the ICU population.

### Environmental Modification

In the ICU, the most basic and logical nonpharmacologic intervention is environmental modification. The excessive noise and light in ICUs can disrupt sleep and increase anxiety and agitation, in turn contributing to pain and discomfort. Sources of noise include multiple alarms, equipment, telephones, ventilators, and staff conversations.

The critical care nurse has the primary role in modifying the environment in which care of the patient and family is delivered. As evidence has grown in the past decades about the detrimental effects of the ICU environment on comfort and other outcome measures, especially on sleep quality, nurse-initiated interventions are now common. Nurse initiated environmental modifications include but are not limited to noise control, turning down lights to allow for sleep hygiene, temperature control per patient's comfort, allowing privacy, and the use of music or aromatherapy, if tolerated by the patient and family.

### Sleep Hygiene

Sleep disruption is a significant barrier to comfort and a source of stress for patients in the ICU that can negatively impact both recovery and survival.[1,31] The severity of illness has also been shown to be associated with sleep disturbances. The negative consequences of poor sleep quantity and quality include delirium, poor quality of life, diminished physical and cognitive function, mood instability, and amplification of other symptoms such as increasing pain intensity.[1,31] Studies suggest that almost 40% of ICU patients report difficulty falling asleep and 61% report a greater need for sleep.[31] Current guidelines recommend that sleep hygiene be promoted by controlling light and noise and by clustering patient care activities rather than using sleep agents.[1] It is generally recommended that all sleep-disrupting medications, such as sedatives and analgesics, be discontinued as soon as possible, because these agents alter sleep patterns and normal sleep physiology.[31]

### Early Mobility

Historically, early and daily physical activity, such as getting out of bed or walking, was considered too risky for the average ICU patient owing to hemodynamic instability or technology dependence. However, strong evidence now exists to support the benefits, safety, and feasibility of early mobility for critically ill patients, and expert guidelines outline early mobility strategies.[1,32]

Specific approaches to early mobilization of patients in neurologic, general, step-down, and hematology–oncology units have been reported.[38–40] For patients on mechanical ventilators, early mobility has been shown to decrease days of mechanical ventilation and ICU and hospital length of stay.[1,41] In addition, nurse-driven quality improvement projects have shown the benefits of early mobility in a variety of ICU settings.[42]

### Complementary and Alternative Therapies

A wide variety of complementary and alternative therapies exist as nonpharmacologic alternatives to the management of pain and other distressing symptoms in the critically ill. The critical care nurse can offer music therapy, pet therapy, art therapy, healing touch or massage, aromatherapy, and other therapies. The positive effects of music therapy on a wide variety of acutely and chronically ill patient populations have been repeatedly demonstrated, especially on the reduction or relief of pain.[34–37] Many hospitals now employ specialists in integrative medicine and art, music, and pet therapy. The nurse and ICU team can consult members of the interdisciplinary team to provide a multidimensional approach to pain relief and comfort.

### Relaxation Techniques

Relaxation can be described as a state of calmness or peacefulness. Relaxation exercises involve repetitive focus on a word, phrase, prayer, or muscular activity and a conscious effort to reject other intruding thoughts. Most relaxation methods require a quiet environment, a comfortable position, a passive

---

| **BOX 5-3**   *TEACHING GUIDE*   *Instructions for the Quieting Reflex* |
| :--- |
| 1. Inhale using an easy, natural breath. |
| 2. Think "alert mind, calm body." |
| 3. Smile inwardly (with your internal facial muscles). |
| 4. As you exhale, allow your jaw, tongue, and shoulders to go loose. |
| 5. Allow a feeling of warmth and looseness to go down through your body and out through your toes. |

attitude, and concentration. Though these conditions can be challenging to achieve in the ICU environment, the nurse is encouraged to include relaxation and breathing or quieting exercises in the care of patients with pain and comfort challenges.

Breathing exercises, which have been used with much success in childbirth, can also be used successfully in the critically ill patient. The quieting reflex is a breathing and relaxation technique that reduces stress and can easily be taught to the conscious and coherent patient (Box 5-3). The nurse encourages the patient to perform the quieting reflex frequently during the day. This relaxation technique can be done in only 6 seconds, and it calms the sympathetic nervous system and gives the patient a sense of control over stress and anxiety.

### Touch

Historically, one of the greatest contributions nurses have made is the comfort and caring of presence and touch. These contributions still have an important place in today's highly technical ICUs. Nurses may feel that touching is too simple to be effective; however, few medical advances can replace the benefits of warm and caring touch. The need for touch is thought to intensify during times of high stress and cannot be totally met by other forms of communication. Nurses, when using touch, are usually trying to convey understanding, support, warmth, concern, and closeness to the patient. Touching not only contributes to the patient's sense of well-being but also promotes physical recovery from disease. It has a positive effect on perceptual and cognitive abilities and can influence physiologic parameters, such as respiration and blood flow. Touch represents a positive therapeutic element of human interaction.

The effects of touch in the clinical environment are far-reaching. Touch has played a major part in promoting and maintaining reality orientation in patients prone to confusion about time, place, and personal identification. Nursing touch may be most helpful in situations in which people are experiencing fear, anxiety, depression, or isolation. It may also be beneficial for patients who have a need for encouragement or nurturing, who have difficulty verbalizing needs, or who are disoriented, unresponsive, or terminally ill.

### Patient Education

To effectively educate the patient and family about the pain management plan, the critical care nurse must be a fully contributing member of the interdisciplinary team that develops the plan. Full participation by the patient and family, when appropriate, is essential. Any information given should be reinforced periodically during the course of therapy, and the patient should be encouraged to verbalize any questions or concerns. Plans for pain management should be discussed with patients when they are most able to understand—for example, prior to surgery rather than during the recovery period. Emphasis is on prevention or proactive management of pain before it becomes severe.

Patients and families need to know that most pain can be relieved, and that unrelieved pain may have serious consequences on physical and psychological well-being and may interfere with recovery. The nurse helps patients and families understand that pain management is an important part of their care and that the health care team will respond quickly to reports of pain. Patients should also be given instructions about nonpharmacologic interventions and traditional methods to minimize pain. Splinting the incisional area with a pillow while coughing or ambulating is a traditional pain-relief measure.

The potential for drug addiction or overdosage is often a major concern for the patient and family. These issues should be addressed and clarified because they create a barrier to effective pain relief. The patient also needs a clear understanding of any specialized pain management technology, such as PCA or epidural analgesia.

## Pain Management in Specific Populations

Some critically ill populations present unique pain management challenges; these populations include the elderly patient, the patient at risk for PICS, and the patient at the end of life. Special considerations for the elderly patient are noted in Box 5-4.[43]

## Post–Intensive Care Syndrome

Comprehensive management of the critically ill patient by the interdisciplinary team must extend beyond the ICU doors. More than 80% of the 4 million patients admitted to ICUs each year in the United States survive the critical illness but are at risk of developing PICS.[32] PICS is the term used to describe new or worsening impairments in the physical, cognitive, or mental health status of survivors of critical illness that persist beyond the acute hospitalization. It is estimated that disabling weakness and associated impairments occur in up to 50% of survivors of sepsis, multiple organ failure, and prolonged mechanical ventilation.[32] Growing data show that 20% to 30% of ICU survivors experience cognitive impairment, anxiety, depression, posttraumatic stress disorder, or inability to perform activities of daily living.[32,44,45]

The critical care nurse and the team must include specific interventions for the patient in the ICU to minimize the negative long-term consequences of critical illness. Though more research is needed, the current state of evidence suggests that effective pain management, sleep regulation, and early mobility are key interventions that hold promise to minimize the negative outcomes related to PICS.[32,44,45]

## The Patient at End-of-Life

Death is common in the ICU: it is reported that one in five Americans die in the ICU or via an ICU-related episode annually.[2] There are significant barriers to optimal end-of-life care in the ICU setting, including poor communication between the patient and family and the care team, unrealistic expectations of ICU care and resuscitation, prognostic uncertainty, ethical conflicts over end-of-life decision-making, the lack of advance care planning, and the high prevalence of surrogate decision makers.[2]

Just as the ICU episode is a stressful experience for patients and families, the shift in goals to end-of-life is a particularly sensitive and challenging phase. Thus, each critical care nurse must develop knowledge and skills in communication and in providing pain and comfort management for patients at end-of-life and their families. Nurses and other team members are expected to provide primary palliative care that includes effective pain and symptom management, and to consult palliative care teams for secondary palliative care in complex situations.[18,22] Proactive integration of palliative care principles or consult teams has shown to positively benefit patient outcomes in a variety of ICU settings.[20,21]

Critical care nurses play the central role in providing a good death for patients and a positive memory for families of dying ICU patients. They accomplish this through environmental modification, informed use of pharmacologic and nonpharmacologic therapies to relieve pain, and skilled communication. General guidelines when caring for the patient at end-of-life are as follows:

- Patient–family meetings should be held as frequently as needed to clarify the goals at end-of-life. Ideally, a patient–family meeting should be held within 5 days of ICU admission for all patients.[2]
- The goal of comfort and relief from suffering should take priority over hemodynamic stability, mechanical ventilation parameters, or mental status unless the patient or surrogate decision maker has stated other priorities.
- Analgesics should be administered in the amount necessary to provide relief from pain and distressing symptoms without concern about actual total dose.
- All routes for opioid administration can be used at end-of-life.

---

**BOX 5-4**  *CONSIDERATIONS for the Older Patient in Pain*

- Painful chronic diseases often compound the acute pain of critical illness in older patients.
- Arthritis, the most common cause of chronic pain in older patients, often affects the back, hips, knees, and shoulders, increasing the patient's pain when being turned, particularly in the ICU.
- Some older patients can experience acutely painful conditions, such as myocardial infarction or appendicitis, without feeling pain.
- Older patients often use words such as "aches" or "tenderness" rather than "pain."
- Family care givers can help assess pain in older patients who have cognitive or language impairments.
- Older patients are particularly sensitive to opioids; higher peak concentrations and longer duration of actions are achieved in older adults.
- Meperidine (Demerol), pentazocine (Talwin), propoxyphene (Darvon), and methadone should not be used to treat pain in older adults.
- Some older patients often have an increased need for meaningful touch during episodes of crisis.

Data from Derby S, Tickoo R, Saldivar R: Elderly patients. In: Ferrell BR, Coyle N, Paice JA (eds): Oxford Textbook of Palliative Nursing, 4th ed. New York: Oxford University Press, 2015.

- Although all opioids are equally effective at equianalgesic doses, fentanyl and hydromorphone are preferred agents for patients with renal or hepatic failure because of short half-life and metabolic qualities.
- There is no universally accepted method of withdrawal of life-sustaining technologies. Currently, there are two methods used to withdraw the ventilator: immediate extubation and terminal weaning. The nurse and team must anticipate the patient's need for pharmacologic therapy before and during the process of withdrawal. Refer to unit or hospital policies.[2]

- The needs of the family of the dying ICU patient should be assessed early, and interdisciplinary team members used as needed to meet these needs. ICU family members typically need access, updates, and information, assurance that their loved one will not suffer, and, for some, involvement in caregiving activities.[2]

The critical care nurse should take a leading role in providing end-of-life care focused on the patient and family and based on clinical expertise, compassion, and empathy.

## Clinical Applicability Challenges

---

**CASE STUDY**

Mr. B, a 53-year-old male has been hospitalized for 1 week on a progressive care unit. He was recently diagnosed with metastatic malignant melanoma and presents with severe pain and weakness in his lower extremities, ptosis of the right eye, fluctuating mental status, incontinence, and dependence in all ADLs. Magnetic resonance imaging (MRI) scans show extensive intracranial and extracranial metastatic disease and T8–T12 vertebral body compression and epidural neoplasm. He is married with three children. His pain regimen is:

  PCA hydromorphone 0.6 demand dose with 6 minute lockout; no basal rate
  Morphine sustained release 90 mg po q12 hours
  Oxycodone 10 mg po q4 hour prn for severe pain

Mr. B's most recent pain assessment is: 10/10 sharp numbing pain in his back, burning pain in both legs; cannot move his legs secondary to pain, worse with movement. Due to his fluctuating mental status, his wife is acting as his surrogate decision maker. She states that his goal is to spend as much time with his children as possible and therefore prefers active treatment for his metastatic disease, aggressive interventions including admission to the ICU, and that his resuscitation status be full code. Overnight, the patient has a change in mental status and hypotensive episode and is transferred to the Medical ICU. All opioid therapy is discontinued and the patient is placed on vasopressors for suspected sepsis.

1. What are possible explanations for Mr. B's change in mental status?
2. Discuss alternatives to discontinuing Mr. B's pain regimen.
3. What nonpharmacologic interventions could the nurse include in Mr. B's care to alleviate pain and increase comfort?

---

**WANT TO KNOW MORE?**

A wide variety of resources to enhance your learning and understanding of this chapter are available on thePoint.

You will find:

- References
- Selected readings
- NCLEX-style review questions
- Internet resources
- And more!

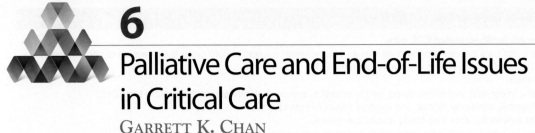

# 6

# Palliative Care and End-of-Life Issues in Critical Care

GARRETT K. CHAN

**LEARNING OBJECTIVES**

*Based on the content in this chapter, the reader should be able to:*

1. List at least three end-of-life issues related to critical care nursing.
2. List at least three components of palliative care.
3. Describe how palliative care can be integrated into curative or disease-modifying care.
4. Identify at least three symptoms commonly experienced at the end of life.
5. Recognize the importance of flexible visiting hours for a patient at the end of life.
6. Describe activities by the nurse in preparing for and coordinating a family conference.
7. Identify strategies for self-care of the nurse.

About 2 million people die in the United States every year. Although some people die in peace and comfort, others die in severe distress and suffering. Over the past decade, nurses in the acute care setting have been increasingly concerned about how people die. Thoughts about critical care have slowly shifted; clinicians now recognize that death may be inevitable and that the use of technology to prevent death is limited. Critical care nurses are well positioned to help patients and families during this difficult transitional period. "Being with" patients and families in addition to "doing things to" them enables critical care nurses to provide the holistic care that is central to nursing.[1]

## The Need for Quality End-of-Life Care

In the early 20th century, the average life expectancy was 50 years. Common causes of death included infection, accidents, and childhood diseases.[2] Few life-extending measures were available, and death occurred after hardly any interventions. The focus was on caring for the dying person by family members, who witnessed the death.

However, in the middle to late 20th century, medical interventions such as antibiotics, cardiopulmonary resuscitation (CPR), mechanical ventilation, dialysis, intra-aortic balloon pumps, and pulmonary artery catheters were discovered and routinely used to combat morbidity and mortality. These technologies, combined with other public health initiatives such as improved sanitation, carried the promise of treating the causes of death and therefore extending life. By the year 2000, the average life expectancy had been extended to 77 years.

Critical care nurses became focused on these life-extending procedures, and critical care units were developed to house seriously ill patients in one area of a hospital and closely monitor their response to curative, lifesaving, and aggressive treatments.[3] Increasingly, people died in the hospital setting surrounded by health care practitioners rather than

their families. Over the course of the years of technological advancement, nurses increasingly viewed patients in terms of disease processes or technologies. The perception of the patient lying in the bed as a person who experienced physical, emotional, psychological, social, and spiritual suffering was lost.[4]

Over the past decade, evidence has shown that skillful communication, family-centered care, and shared decision making among the patient, family, and interdisciplinary team can lead to healthy work environments for the staff as well as decreased moral distress and mitigation of traumatic stress experienced by the patient and all persons involved in the care of the patient.[5-7] It is important to recognize that people approach death in a variety of ways. Therefore, instituting these caring practices from the moment the patient reaches the critical care environment is vital to providing good care. While palliative and end-of-life (EOL) care education is important, there has been a paucity of prelicensure and continuing education programs addressing these topics.[8,9] The End-of-Life Nursing Education Consortium–Critical Care (ELNEC-CC) project was designed specifically to educate nurses about palliative and EOL care in critical care settings.[10]

## Understanding Human Death

Over the past decade, there has been an increase in understanding the human experience of dying in the acute care setting. In 1995, the *Study to Understand Prognoses and Preferences for Outcomes and Risks of Treatment* (SUPPORT) was published.[11] This study, conducted in five major academic medical centers across the United States, involved more than 9,000 seriously ill patients. The goal was to improve EOL decision making and reduce the frequency of mechanically supported, painful, and prolonged death. Despite use of an intervention designed to communicate preferences among providers, patients, and families, the wishes of patients and

**BOX 6-1** Recommendations to Improve End-of-Life Care

**1. Delivery of person-centered, family-oriented EOL care**

Government health insurers and care delivery programs as well as private health insurers should cover the provision of comprehensive care for individuals with advanced serious illness who are nearing the EOL.

Comprehensive care should:

- be seamless, high-quality, integrated, patient-centered, family-oriented, and consistently accessible around the clock;
- consider the evolving physical, emotional, social, and spiritual needs of individuals;
- approaching the EOL, as well as those of their family and/or caregivers;
- be competently delivered by professionals with appropriate expertise and training;
- include coordinated, efficient, and interoperable information transfer across all providers and all settings; and
- be consistent with individuals' values, goals, and informed preferences.

Health care delivery organizations should take the following steps to provide comprehensive care:

- All people with advanced serious illness should have access to skilled palliative care or, when appropriate, hospice care in all settings where they receive care (including health care facilities, the home, and the community).
- Palliative care should encompass access to an interdisciplinary palliative care team, including board-certified hospice and palliative medicine physicians, nurses, social workers, and chaplains, together with other health professionals as needed (including geriatricians). Depending on local resources, access to this team may be on site, via virtual consultation, or by transfer to a setting with these resources and this expertise.
- The full range of care that is delivered should be characterized by transparency and accountability through public reporting of aggregate quality and cost measures for all aspects of the health care system related to EOL care. The committee believes that informed individual choices should be honored, including the right to decline medical or social services.

**2. Clinician–patient communication and advanced care planning**

Professional societies and other organizations that establish quality standards should develop standards for clinician–patient communication and advance care planning that are measurable, actionable, and evidence based. These standards should change as needed to reflect the evolving population and health system needs and be consistent with emerging evidence, methods, and technologies. Payers and health care delivery organizations should adopt these standards and their supporting processes, and integrate them into assessments, care plans, and the reporting of health care quality.

Payers should tie such standards to reimbursement, and professional societies should adopt policies that facilitate tying the standards to reimbursement, licensing, and credentialing to encourage:

- all individuals, including children with the capacity to do so, to have the opportunity to participate actively in their health care decision making throughout their lives and as they approach death, and receive medical and related social services consistent with their values, goals, and informed preferences;
- clinicians to initiate high-quality conversations about advance care planning, integrate the results of these conversations into the ongoing care plans of patients, and communicate with other clinicians as requested by the patient; and
- clinicians to continue to revisit advance care planning discussions with their patients because individuals' preferences and circumstances may change over time.

**3. Professional education and development**

Educational institutions, credentialing bodies, accrediting boards, state regulatory agencies, and health care delivery organizations should establish the appropriate training, certification, and/or licensure requirements to strengthen the palliative care knowledge and skills of all clinicians who care for individuals with advanced serious illness who are nearing the EOL.

Specifically:

- all clinicians across disciplines and specialties who care for people with advanced serious illness should be competent in basic palliative care, including communication skills, interprofessional collaboration, and symptom management;
- educational institutions and professional societies should provide training in palliative care domains throughout the professional's career;
- accrediting organizations, such as the Accreditation Council on Graduate Medical Education, should require palliative care education and clinical experience in programs for all specialties responsible for managing advanced serious illness (including primary care clinicians);
- certifying bodies, such as the medical, nursing, and social work specialty boards, and health systems should require knowledge, skills, and competency in palliative care;
- state regulatory agencies should include education and training in palliative care in licensure requirements for physicians, nurses, chaplains, social workers, and others who provide health care to those nearing the EOL;
- entities that certify specialty-level health care providers should create pathways to certification that increase the number of health care professionals who pursue specialty-level palliative care training; and
- entities such as health care delivery organizations, academic medical centers, and teaching hospitals that sponsor specialty-level training positions should commit institutional resources to increasing the number of available training positions for specialty-level palliative care.

**4. Policies and payment systems to support high-quality EOL care**

Federal, state, and private insurance and health care delivery programs should integrate the financing of medical and social services to support the provision of quality care consistent with the values, goals, and informed preferences of people with advanced serious illness nearing the EOL. To the extent that additional legislation is necessary to implement this recommendation, the administration should seek and Congress should enact such legislation. In addition, the federal government should require public reporting on quality measures, outcomes, and costs regarding care near the EOL (eg, in the last year of life) for programs it funds or administers (eg, Medicare, Medicaid, the Department of Veterans Affairs). The federal government should encourage all other payment and health care delivery systems to do the same.

Specifically, actions should:

- provide financial incentives for:
  - medical and social support services that decrease the need for emergency room and acute care services,
  - coordination of care across settings and providers (from hospital to ambulatory settings as well as home and community), and
  - improved shared decision making and advance care planning that reduces the utilization of unnecessary medical services and those not consistent with a patient's goals for care;
- require the use of interoperable electronic health records that incorporate advance care planning to improve communication of individuals' wishes across time, settings, and providers, documenting (1) the designation of a surrogate/decision maker, (2) patient values and beliefs and goals for care, (3) the presence of an advance directive, and (4) the presence of medical orders for life-sustaining treatment for appropriate populations; and
- encourage states to develop and implement a Physician Orders for Life-Sustaining Treatment (POLST) paradigm program in accordance with nationally standardized core requirements.

**5. Public education and engagement**

Civic leaders, public health and other governmental agencies, community-based organizations, faith-based organizations, consumer groups, health care delivery organizations, payers, employers, and professional societies should engage their constituents and provide fact-based information about care of people with advanced serious illness to encourage advance care planning and informed choice based on the needs and values of individuals.

Specifically, these organizations and groups should:

- use appropriate media and other channels to reach their audiences, including underserved populations;
- provide evidence-based information about care options and informed decision making regarding treatment and care;
- encourage meaningful dialogue among individuals and their families and caregivers, clergy, and clinicians about values, care goals, and preferences related to advanced serious illness; and
- dispel misinformation that may impede informed decision making and public support for health system and policy reform regarding care near the EOL.

Adapted from Pizzo PA, Walker DM: Dying in America: Improving Quality and Honoring Individual Preferences Near The End of Life. Washington, DC: Institute of Medicine, 2014

families were often overlooked, and aggressive treatment was common. Physicians were not aware that their patients preferred to avoid CPR. In addition, nearly 40% of patients who died spent at least 10 days in an intensive care unit (ICU), and 50% of family members of conscious patients reported that the patients were in moderate to severe pain at least half the time.

After publication of the SUPPORT study, the Institute of Medicine (IOM) released two reports, Approaching Death: Improving Care at the End of Life[12] and When Children Die: Improving Palliative and End-of-Life Care for Children and their Families.[13] The IOM conducted another study released in 2014, Dying in America: Improving Quality and Honoring Individual Preferences Near the End of Life.[14] This group of experts listed five recommendations to improve EOL care (Box 6-1). These recommendations are important for critical care nurses because it is estimated that about 20% of deaths in the United States occur while patients are using ICU services.[15] Critical care nurses play an important role in recognizing opportunities for interventions that support patients, families, and staff members during this difficult transition in life. Although technology, urgency, uncertainty, and conflict are common in critical care practice, these characteristics may inhibit or fragment a coordinated effort that aims to provide good EOL and palliative care.[1]

## Palliative Care

The introduction of palliative care principles into critical care can provide a framework to address EOL issues or life-threatening situations. Palliative care originated from hospice care, which was designed to improve the quality of death and dying for patients and their families by addressing aspects of care that are unrelated to disease-specific treatments, cure, or rehabilitation.[16] According to the World Health Organization[17] and the IOM,[12] palliative care from an interdisciplinary perspective includes the following core principles: symptom management; advanced care planning; family-centered care; emotional, psychological, social, and spiritual care; facilitating communication; awareness of ethical issues; and caring for the care giver. These principles should be addressed and incorporated into the total care of the patient, even when disease-modifying or curative therapies are used. In critical care nursing, it is vital that these core palliative care principles are incorporated in the daily plan of care of patients using an interdisciplinary approach.[18–20] Figure 6-1 illustrates how palliative care can be incorporated throughout the patient's illness.

Palliative care services in critical care have demonstrated an improvement in symptom management, family support, reduction in length of hospital stay, increased discharges to home with hospice referrals, and reduced costs.[18,21,22] The American Association of Critical-Care Nurses (AACN) has developed protocols for critical care practice in palliative and EOL care.[23] These protocols provide a good overview of core issues and clinical recommendations for critical care nurses. Resources to assist nurses in addressing issues surrounding the EOL phase are given in Table 6-1.

A particular therapeutic intervention may be either curative or palliative depending on its intent. For example, a packed red blood cell transfusion may be curative in a patient with an acute hemorrhage or palliative in a patient with chronic anemia and severe fatigue following chemotherapy. Whether an intervention attempts to cure or to palliate determines whether it is curative or palliative. Additional examples of treatments that can be either curative or palliative are surgeries that resect the bowel to remove a tumor that is causing an intestinal obstruction or administering furosemide in a patient who has severe pulmonary edema. If the treatment relieves the patient's suffering, then it is considered palliative.

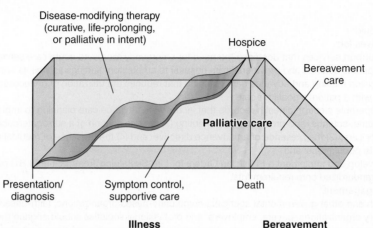

**FIGURE 6-1**    The continuum of care. (Adapted from Emanuel L, von Gunten C, Ferris F, et al: The Education in Palliative and End-of-Life Care [EPEC] Curriculum: The EPEC Project. Chicago, IL: EPEC, 2003)

Central to developing any relationship is the establishment of trust. For the critical care nurse to deliver high-quality palliative care, the nurse must take steps to foster a trusting relationship. For example, the nurse can demonstrate concern and assess the patient's and family's physical, emotional, psychosocial, and spiritual well-being.[24,25] Critical care nurses can build rapport and strengthen therapeutic relationships by holding the patient and family members in high esteem, being approachable, and being affable.[24] Nurses can also demonstrate professionalism by showing respect for the patient and family, demonstrating a professional demeanor, and providing evidence that they are collaborating with other health care providers (eg, oncology, pulmonology, or surgery providers), and by remaining calm and confident.[24,25]

## Symptom Management

In critical care, patients experience a wide range of symptoms from their diseases as well as from the therapies that are used to treat those diseases. Common symptoms at the end of life include pain, dyspnea, anxiety and agitation, depression, delirium, and nausea and vomiting. The nurse assesses for the presence and severity of each of these symptoms. It is important that the nurse also assesses for the underlying causes of the symptoms—an essential step in symptom management. Interventions appropriate for the symptoms and an evaluation of those interventions are crucial in providing good palliative care.

## Pain

Pain is the most prevalent symptom in critical care units and is distressing to patients and families.[11] Diseases, procedures, and interventions such as turning, suctioning, and wound care can be sources of painful stimuli.[26,27] Assessing for the presence of pain and intervening to prevent or treat it using pharmacological and nonpharmacological interventions should be incorporated into every patient's care plan. Dose escalation to treat severe pain is an appropriate treatment modality in the hands of skilled clinicians provided there are accurate pain assessments.[26] Including a bowel regimen to prevent constipation is crucial in the management of pain. Chapter 5 describes in detail the assessment of pain and nursing interventions that can be used to treat it.

## Dyspnea

It is estimated that dyspnea is present in 21% to 90% of all patients with a life-threatening illness.[28] Causes of dyspnea can include the underlying disease pathology (eg, chronic obstructive pulmonary disease, pulmonary embolism, pleural effusion); anxiety; or family, spiritual, or social issues. Investigation for the source of the dyspnea directs the nurse to the appropriate intervention. Accurate and frequent assessment of dyspnea will also alert the nurse to the presence and severity of this distressing symptom.[29] Instruments that can accurately assess dyspnea include the Modified Borg Scale[30] for

| TABLE 6-1 | End-of-Life Care Resources |
| --- | --- |
| **Organization** | **Website** |
| American Association of Critical-Care Nurses (AACN) | http://www.aacn.org |
| Association of Organ Procurement Organizations (AOPO) | http://www.aopo.org |
| Center to Advance Palliative Care (CAPC) | http://www.capc.org |
| City of Hope Pain & Palliative Care Resource Center | http://prc.coh.org/ |
| Education in Palliative and End-of-Life Care (EPEC) | http://www.epec.net |
| Emergency Nurses Association (ENA) | http://www.ena.org |
| End-of-Life Nursing Education Consortium (ELNEC) | http://www.aacn.nche.edu/elnec |
| Hospice and Palliative Nurses Association (HPNA) | http://www.hpna.org |
| National Consensus Project for Quality Palliative Care (NCP) | http://www.nationalconsensusproject.org |
| National Hospice and Palliative Care Organization (NHPCO) | http://www.nhpco.org |
| Nursing Leadership Academy on End-of-Life Care | http://www.palliativecarenursing.net |

patients who can verbally respond and the Respiratory Distress Observation Scale (RDOS)[31] for patients who cannot verbally respond. Common interventions used for dyspnea include oxygen, opioids, and anxiolytics.[29] Nonpharmacological interventions such as pursed-lip breathing, relaxation strategies, reducing the room temperature (but not chilling the patient), reducing the number of people in the room at one time, keeping an unobstructed line of sight between the patient and the outside environment, and using a fan to blow gently across the face (not directly into mucous membranes) have all been found to be effective in decreasing dyspnea.[29,32]

## Anxiety and Agitation

Patients and families who face life-threatening illnesses commonly experience anxiety.[32] Anxiety can be related to any number of physical, emotional, psychological, social, practical, and spiritual issues. Assessment of anxiety can be complex, and an interdisciplinary approach, including nursing, social services, psychology, and chaplaincy, may be needed to evaluate the patient accurately and treat the anxiety properly. Nonpharmacological interventions may include counseling, taking care of practical matters (eg, arranging for the care of a pet), and arranging for spiritual concerns to be addressed (eg, arranging for a visit from a clergy member). If medication is needed, short- or long-acting benzodiazepines and atypical antidepressants may be helpful. Additional interventions for anxiety are discussed in Chapter 2.

## Depression

When confronted with a serious illness, many patients experience intense sadness and anxiety accompanied by depressive symptoms such as anhedonia (loss of pleasure); loss of self-esteem; pervasive despair; thoughts of suicide; or feelings of helplessness, hopelessness, or worthlessness.[32] These are natural feelings and are usually present for only a short time. It is a myth that depression is "normal" at the end of life. If these feelings of depression persist, appropriate treatment needs to be initiated using a multidimensional approach, such as supportive psychotherapy, cognitive–behavioral therapy, and antidepressants.

## Delirium

Delirium is an acute change in awareness or cognitive status that may manifest as agitation, withdrawal, or confusion. "Confusion" is an all-inclusive term that refers to inappropriate behavior, disorientation, or hallucinations. Terminal delirium is common in patients near death and may manifest as day–night reversal.[32] Management of delirium during the EOL phase is focused more on symptom control and relief of the distress of the patient and family than on the diagnosis and treatment of the underlying cause of the delirium. Benzodiazepines or neuroleptics (eg, haloperidol) are helpful in managing this symptom.

## Nausea and Vomiting

Nausea is very common in patients with advanced disease. Nausea can be acute, delayed, or anticipatory. It can be exhausting, debilitating, and frustrating for the patient and the family. The pathophysiology of nausea and vomiting is complex and can vary based on the underlying etiology. Causes of nausea and vomiting may include physiological factors such as gastrointestinal causes (eg, intestinal obstruction, constipation, pancreatitis); metabolic causes (eg, hypercalcemia, uremia); central nervous system causes (eg, increased intracranial pressure); emotional factors; treatment-related factors (eg, chemotherapy); and vestibular disturbances.

A careful assessment and investigation of the source of nausea and vomiting is important in determining the appropriate treatment course. Drug classes that are commonly used to treat nausea and vomiting are serotonin (5-hydroxytryptamine) receptor agonists (eg, ondansetron), anticholinergics (eg, hyoscine hydrobromide), antihistamines (eg, dimenhydrinate), phenothiazines (eg, prochlorperazine), steroids (eg, dexamethasone), prokinetic agents (eg, metoclopramide), butyrophenones (eg, haloperidol), and benzodiazepines (eg, lorazepam). A nasogastric tube may be used to decompress the stomach to prevent vomiting, but it may cause discomfort. To relieve persistent nausea and vomiting, surgery to resect an intestinal obstruction may be appropriate. If a patient has an unresectable intestinal obstruction, a draining percutaneous endoscopic gastrostomy tube may also be placed. Lastly, patients should be positioned to avoid any aspiration of emesis.

## Palliative or EOL Sedation

Palliative sedation, also known as EOL or terminal sedation, may be considered when all interventions have failed to control the symptoms. Palliative sedation is used when the patient (1) is experiencing unbearable and unmanageable pain or other symptoms, and (2) is approaching the last hours or days of his or her life.[32] The goal of EOL sedation is to produce a level of obtundation sufficient to relieve suffering without hastening death.[32] Before palliative sedation is considered, specialists in pain or palliative care are consulted, and it is verified that all therapies have been attempted without success. In addition, other disciplines such as social services, chaplaincy services, and psychology should be consulted to investigate other potential causes of suffering before resorting to palliative sedation.

## Advanced Care Planning

Advanced care planning involves deciding how a patient would like to be treated in the event that he or she becomes unable to make decisions or communicate his or her wishes regarding care.[6] Advanced care planning involves more than just advance directives—it also involves issues such as determining health care proxies as well as trying to discover from the patient or the health care proxy the preferences for the goals of care during the EOL phase.

The critical care nurse communicates with the patient's primary care provider, who may have a long-standing relationship with the patient and know the patient's preferences regarding EOL treatment. The primary care provider may have had conversations with the patient on this subject. It is important to note that some patients want aggressive treatment despite a poor prognosis, whereas other patients want to forego any aggressive treatment despite the treatment's probable success. Patients are allowed, by federal law, to refuse treatment.

## Advance Directives

Advance directives are written or oral instructions about future medical care that are to be followed in the event that the person loses the capacity to make decisions.[33] Types of advance directives include living wills and health care proxies (durable powers of attorney for health care). Each state regulates the use of advance directives differently. Advance directives are not "set in stone"; they can be revised, orally or in writing, at any time.

A health care proxy is a person who has been designated to make decisions in the event that the patient cannot make decisions for himself or herself. The designation of a person as a health care proxy must be in written form and should always be up to date. The proxy should know the preferences of the patient and be able to communicate and adhere to those preferences. He or she should not confuse his or her own wishes and desires with those of the patient. Health care proxies are also known as "surrogate decision makers" (SDMs) or "health care agents."

## "Do Not Resuscitate" and "Do Not Attempt Resuscitation" Orders

The standard of care for patients who suffer a cardiac or respiratory arrest is to initiate CPR. "Do not resuscitate" (DNR) or "do not attempt resuscitation" (DNAR) orders are orders placed by a physician, most often with the consent of the patient or the health care proxy, to alert other care givers that if the patient has a cardiac or pulmonary arrest, no attempts to restore cardiac or pulmonary function should occur.[12,34]

Although resuscitation efforts should not be initiated for a patient with a DNR or DNAR order, the patient should continue to receive appropriate care. In one study of critically ill cancer patients in a surgical ICU, researchers noted that the patients with a DNR or DNAR order received less medical care than other patients.[35] However, supportive nursing care remained unchanged. It is important to recognize that DNR and DNAR are not intended to give the impression that nurses should give inappropriate care.[36]

## Family-Centered Care

Family-centered care is a cornerstone of critical and palliative care. In palliative care, the patient is recognized as being part of a larger social network. Serious illness and death affect not only the patient but also the family. The Society of Critical Care Medicine published clinical practice guidelines[7] delineating recommendations to support families during critical illness. These recommendations include endorsement of a shared decision-making model, early and repeated care conferencing to reduce family stress and improve consistency in communication, honoring culturally appropriate requests for truth-telling and informed refusal, spiritual support, staff education and debriefing to minimize the impact of family interactions on staff health, family presence at both rounds and resuscitation, open flexible visitation, way-finding and

family friendly signage, and family support before, during, and after a death.

When the patient can communicate, according to Stannard,[37] the ideal definition of family is whoever the patient defines as his or her family. When a patient is unable to communicate, the practical definition of family is anyone who shares a history and a future with the patient. The legal definition of family is based on blood relations and is purposefully narrow and limiting to clearly distinguish who may have authority over the patient should the patient lose decision-making capacity.

## Family Presence During Resuscitation

In a critical review of the literature, Halm[38] noted that research has found that families have a right to be present during resuscitation; in addition, families report that being present during resuscitation was helpful during the bereavement process. Family members who were present during resuscitations did not experience more anxiety, depression, grief, intrusive imagery, or avoidance behavior as compared with family members who did not witness resuscitations. In addition, there is no evidence to substantiate that the presence of family members invites litigation.

However, research studies do report that many health care providers are uncomfortable with family presence. Nurses who have less experience with resuscitation report more discomfort with family presence than nurses who have more such experience. In addition, the staff surveyed expressed concern that family members may take time and attention away from the patient. The AACN recommends that hospitals have policies and procedures about how family presence during resuscitation is to be handled in their institutions.[39] It has been suggested that a successful family presence program depends on having a dedicated staff member attend to the family witnessing the resuscitative efforts. See Evidence-Based Practice Highlight 6-1.

## Visitation

To the greatest extent possible, families should be free to visit a patient who is near death, to allow for coping during this period. Family members may communicate with and touch the patient, which may reassure both the patient and the family. During this period of closure, cultural or spiritual ceremonies may also take place. Staff who have developed a relationship with the family should continue to work with the patient and family to the greatest extent possible. The extended visiting hours provide a continuity of care that is invaluable to families and helps cultivate a trusting relationship to reassure families that the nurses are working for the benefit of the patient.

It is important to be aware of the dynamics of each individual family. For example, if there is tension among certain family members, a visiting schedule may need to be established to allow family members to see the patient without crossing paths. In addition, the nurse should be alert to any signs from the patient that a particular family member is unwelcome. The patient may exhibit signs of agitation when that person is in the room. The nurse acts as an advocate to uphold the patient's wishes. Visitation advocacy as it relates to families and the critical care environment is discussed in more detail in Chapter 3.

## EVIDENCE-BASED PRACTICE HIGHLIGHT 6-1
### Family Presence During Resuscitation and Invasive Procedures

**Expected Practice**

- Family members[1] of all patients undergoing resuscitation and invasive procedures should be given the option of presence at the bedside. (Level B)
- All patient care units should have an approved written practice document (ie, policy, procedure, or standard of care) for presenting the option of family presence during resuscitation and bedside invasive procedures. (Level D)

**AACN Levels of Evidence**

**Level A** Meta-analysis of quantitative studies or metasynthesis of qualitative studies with results that consistently support a specific action, intervention, or treatment (including systematic review of randomized controlled trials)

**Level B** Well-designed, controlled studies with results that consistently support a specific action, intervention, or treatment

**Level C** Qualitative studies, descriptive or correlational studies, integrative reviews, systematic reviews, or randomized controlled trials with inconsistent results

**Level D** Peer-reviewed professional and organizational standards with the support of clinical study recommendations

**Level E** Multiple case reports, theory-based evidence from expert opinions, or peer-reviewed professional orgastandards without clinical studies to support recommendations

**Level M** Manufacturer's recommendations only

Excerpted from American Association of Critical-Care Nurses Practice Alert. Available at: http://aacn.org.

[1]*Family members are those individuals who are relatives or significant others with whom the patient shares an established relationship.*

## Family Conferences

The family conference is a mechanism for sharing information in an organized way among clinicians and family members. During the family conference, the health care team (1) provides information about the condition of the patient and the patient's prognosis and (2) reviews recommendations from the primary and consult services. Family conferences also serve as a forum for exploring future care preferences with the family—how family members may wish to participate in determining the goals of care for the patient.[40] Cultural or religious beliefs may influence how these conversations develop and how the family reacts to the information.

Careful planning should occur before the family conference as family conferences can be very stressful to all participants. Curtis et al[40] describe the nurse's role before and after the family conference (Box 6-2). Box 6-3 describes how to facilitate a family conference. Encouraging the family to be active participants during the family conference increases their level of satisfaction and improves the quality of communication among providers and families.[41] Early and proactive multidisciplinary meetings help reduce confusing or conflicting messages and improve emotional and spiritual support to the family.[42]

## Bereavement Care

The death of a patient can affect the family members and the staff in different ways. Previous coping skills, cultural and spiritual beliefs, and the circumstances surrounding the death influence the grief experience. A multidisciplinary

### BOX 6-2  The Nurse's Role Before and After the Family Conference

**Before the Conference**

- Explain to the family about the patient's medical equipment and therapies.
- Tell the family what to expect during their conference with the health care team members.
- Talk with the family about their spiritual or religious needs, and take actions to address the unmet spiritual or religious needs.
- Talk with the family about specific cultural needs and take actions to address unmet cultural needs.
- Talk with the family about what the patient valued in life.
- Talk with the family about the patient's illness and treatment.
- Talk with the family about their feelings.
- Reminisce with the family about the patient.
- Tell the family it is all right to talk to and touch their loved one.
- Discuss with the family what the patient might have wanted if he/she were able to participate in the treatment decision-making process.
- Locate a private place or room for the family to talk among themselves.

**After the Conference**

- Talk with the family about how the conference went.
- Talk with any other health care team members who were present at the conference about how the conference went.
- Ask the family if they had any questions following the conference.
- Talk with the family about their feelings.
- Talk with the family about any disagreement among the family concerning the plan of care.
- Talk with the family about changes in the patient's plan of care as a result of the conference.
- Support the decisions the family made during the conference.
- Assure the family that the patient will be kept comfortable.
- Tell the family it is all right to talk to and touch their loved one.
- Locate a private place or room for the family to talk among themselves.

From Curtis JR, Patrick DL, Shannon SE, et al: The family conference as a focus to improve communication about end-of-life care in the intensive care unit: Opportunities for improvement. Crit Care Med 29(2 Suppl):N26–N33, 2001

### BOX 6-3  Facilitating a Family Conference

**Preparing for an ICU Family Conference About EOL Care**

- Review previous knowledge of the patient and/or family.
- Review previous knowledge of the family's attitudes and reactions.
- Review your knowledge of the disease—prognosis, treatment options.
- Examine your own personal feelings, attitudes, biases, and grieving.
- Plan the specifics of location and setting: a quiet, private place.
- Discuss with the family in advance about who will be present.

**Holding an ICU Family Conference About EOL Care**

- Introduce everyone present.
- If appropriate, set the tone in a nonthreatening way: "This is a conversation we have with all families. . . ."
- Discuss the goals of the specific conference.
- Find out what the family understands.
- Review what has happened and what is happening to the patient.

(continued)

---

**BOX 6-3**   **Facilitating a Family Conference** (*continued*)

- Discuss prognosis frankly in a way that is meaningful to the family.
- Acknowledge uncertainty in the prognosis.
- Review the principle of substituted judgment: "What would the patient want?"
- Support the family's decision.
- Do not discourage all hope; consider redirecting hope toward a comfortable death with dignity if appropriate.
- Avoid temptation to give too much medical detail.
- Make it clear that withholding life-sustaining treatment is not withholding caring.
- Make explicit what care will be provided including symptom management, where the care will be delivered, and the family's access to the patient.
- If life-sustaining treatments will be withheld or withdrawn, discuss what the patient's death might be like.
- Use repetition to show that you understand what the patient or family is saying.
- Acknowledge strong emotions and use reflection to encourage patients or families to talk about these emotions.
- Tolerate silence.

**Finishing an ICU Family Conference About EOL Care**
- Achieve common understanding of the disease and treatment issues
- Make a recommendation about treatment.
- Ask if there are any questions.
- Ensure basic follow-up plan, and make sure the family knows how to reach you for questions.

From Curtis JR, Patrick DL, Shannon SE, et al: The family conference as a focus to improve communication about end-of-life care in the intensive care unit: Opportunities for improvement. Crit Care Med 29(2 Suppl):N26–N33, 2001

---

**BOX 6-4**   **Spiritual Assessment**

F    Faith, belief, meaning
"Do you consider yourself spiritual or religious?" or "Do you have spiritual beliefs that help you cope with stress?" If the patient responds "no," the nurse might ask "What gives your life meaning?"

I    Importance and influence
"What importance does your faith or belief have in your life? Have your beliefs influenced you in how you handle stress? Do you have specific beliefs that might influence your health care decisions?"

C    Community
"Are you a part of a spiritual or religious community? Is this of support to you and how? Is there a core group of people you really love or who are important to you?" Communities such as churches, temples, and mosques can serve as strong support systems for some patients.

A    Address/action in care
"How should the health care provider address these issues in your health care?" Referral to chaplains, clergy, and other spiritual care providers.

From Puchalski CM: Spirituality and the care of patients at the end-of-life: An essential component of care. Omega (Westport) 56(1):33–46, 2007

---

team consisting of other nurses, social workers, chaplains, physicians, and volunteers can assist family members and staff with managing their grief. Critical care nurses should be familiar with the bereavement information and support services available within their institutions for both family members and themselves. Bereavement support includes providing family members with information regarding what to do after the death and who can be contacted at the hospital if questions arise.

Critical care staff should do everything possible to allow the family sufficient time to go through their leave-taking rituals by creating sacred spaces to recognize the loss of a loved one.[25,43] Bed shortages can make this difficult. However, not allowing family members the chance to say goodbye can complicate the grieving process. Survivors have reported that they remember unsatisfactory interactions with staff for a very long time. Sensitivity must be exercised during this potentially traumatic period.

## Emotional, Psychological, Social, and Spiritual Care

Patients nearing the end of their lives may experience emotional, psychological, social, and spiritual crises. Critical care nurses play a vital role in helping patients identify these concerns. An interdisciplinary team can attend to these potential feelings of loss, isolation, fear, and existential distress. At times, these crises can manifest as physical symptoms, such as pain, dyspnea, and fatigue. To assist patients at the end of life, assessment and interventions by social services, chaplaincy, psychologists, and volunteers are encouraged. One way to conduct a spiritual assessment is by using the FICA tool (Box 6-4).[44]

## Facilitating Communication

Communication among the health care team, the patient, and family is the most important aspect of caregiving in critical care, especially at the end of life. Through good communication, all people involved in the patient's care have a better understanding of how to care for the patient and family through this hospitalization. In addition, good communication facilitates a healing environment that supports the physical and psychosocial needs of the patient, family, and providers. Three significant communication issues that surface frequently in EOL care include establishing treatment goals and priorities, ensuring interdisciplinary communication, and delivering bad news. Critical care nurses can build trusting relationships by providing factual information about the ICU environment, treatments, and the patient's health status. The nurse serves as an informational guide and helps interpret information and findings during the critical care process to help the family understand and cope.[24]

### Assessing Patient and Family Learning Needs

Roughly 40% of adult deaths in the United States occur in the hospital, and more than 25% of those deaths occur in the ICU. Thus, the critical care setting is a common site for delivery of EOL care.[45-47] A good death, as defined by the IOM, is "one that is free from avoidable distress and suffering for patients, families, and caregivers; in general accord with patients and families wishes; and reasonably consistent with clinical, cultural, and ethical standards."[46] Unfortunately, the harsh and sterile ICU atmosphere is far from a natural environment for patients at their life's end. The main goals expressed by patients in the EOL stage are relief of pain, a sense of control, open discussions with the health care team and their family, dedicated time to be with loved ones, and limiting the burdens of loved ones. Thus, it is recommended that palliative care specialists and concepts associated with palliative care be embedded into ICU treatment plans, thereby facilitating open discussions with the health care team and the patient and family about prognosis.[46] During EOL care, effective delivery of information to family members has a positive impact on their satisfaction with care.[47]

Despite efforts to promote the completion of advanced directives (ADs), only 5% to 11% of ICU patients have an AD.[48] Completion of ADs, such as living wills and health care proxies (durable power of attorney for health care decision making), promotes patient autonomy related to quality of life and EOL wishes. Health care providers may find it difficult to broach the topic of EOL choices with critically ill patients and their family members. Instead, focusing the discussion on quality of life, such as important aspects that make life worth living, may help initiate the discussion and assist the health care team to honor a patient's specific wishes.[48]

Because many critically ill patients are unable to fully participate in decision making, health care providers must turn to SDMs to make choices surrounding EOL. Because a majority of ICU patients do not have advance directives in place outlining their desires for what should and should not be done at the end of their lives, the role of the SDM becomes even more complicated and stressful.[49] Ideally, the SDM and health care team will come to a shared decision surrounding withdrawal or continuation of care if an AD has not been completed.

Health care providers can do the following to support SDM decisions at the EOL:

- Build trust by communicating frequently with the SDM.
- Regularly educate the SDM about prognosis and inform him or her about the patient's condition.
- Provide the SDM with adequate time to make decisions.
- Involve other family members in supporting the SDM.
- Help the SDM reflect on the patient's values to assist with decision making.[49]

Appropriate nursing considerations for EOL care are as follows:

- Allow for privacy and create a comfortable space for the patient and family.
- Allow family to express emotions during the process of death.
- When possible, remove technology devices to eliminate artificial noises.
- Create a dignified and uncluttered environment in the room.
- Allow time for family to be alone with the patient after death occurs.[50]

## Establishing Treatment Goals and Priorities

Establishing treatment goals and priorities is essential to facilitating decision making with regard to care. The way in which options are presented can influence the decisions the

patient and family make. For example, if a nurse asks the family, "Do you want the health care team to do everything for your loved one," it sets the family up for a "yes" answer. In the family's mind, the opposite of "everything" is "nothing"; therefore, if the family answers "no" to the question, they may feel as if they are abandoning their loved one. In addition, it is important that nurses avoid ambiguous language and clearly define terms to ensure a shared knowledge. For example, the critical care nurse's understanding of "everything" commonly means intubation, CPR, defibrillation, and other aggressive procedures, whereas the family's understanding of "everything" may include only those interventions that might be helpful and calling a spiritual leader. Across the lifespan (ie, in neonatal, pediatric, adult, and geriatric settings), nurses can support family decision making by involving the family in the decision-making process, remaining unbiased in the face of decision making, avoiding personal opinions, and accepting the decisions that the family members make.[24,51,52]

Emanuel et al[32] suggest a seven-step approach to help negotiate goals for patient care:

1. Create the proper setting. Sit down, ensure privacy, and allow adequate time.
2. Determine what the patient and family know. Clarify the current situation and the context in which decisions about goals of care should be made. For example, if the family thinks that the renal failure is transient, yet the nurses believe the kidneys are beyond recovery, the determination of goals of care must be delayed until everyone has agreed about the clinical situation.
3. Explore what the patient and family are expecting or hoping. For example, ask the family what they hope will happen during this last hospitalization, or what outcomes they think will be attained while the patient is in the ICU. Understanding these hopes and expectations will assist in tailoring communication and reorienting families to what is or might be possible. Focus on what you will do to achieve the family's expectations and hopes. As appropriate, identify those things that you cannot do, perhaps because they will not help achieve the goals or because they are not possible.
4. Suggest realistic goals. To assist with decision making, share your knowledge about the patient's illness, its natural course, the experience of patients in similar circumstances, and the effects that contemporary health care may have. After sharing this information, suggest realistic goals (eg, comfort, peace, closure, loving care, withdrawal of interventions) and how they can be achieved. Work through unreasonable or unrealistic expectations.
5. Respond empathetically to the emotions that may arise.
6. Make a plan and follow through with it.
7. Review and revise the goals and treatments as appropriate.

## Ensuring Interdisciplinary Communication

A clear and unified communication process is important to minimize confusion and distress among patients, families, and the health care team.[53] Critical care nurses should explore their understandings and beliefs about prognosis, goals, and the plan of care and share these understandings with other health care providers to develop a unified message before discussing these issues with the family. An interdisciplinary approach in which all health care workers are giving the same information consistently is ideal. Consensus among providers is an important step in deciding how treatment choices are presented.[53] Providing conflicting information creates confusion for everyone involved and may lead families to request nonbeneficial interventions. Being asked to provide care that is not helpful for the patient can create moral distress in nurses. Other disciplines such as social services, chaplaincy, and the bioethics committee can assist in clarifying issues and values among patients, families, and providers.

## Delivering Bad or Serious News

Despite the best efforts of the health care team, patients may not respond positively to interventions. Keeping an honest and open line of communication is essential to preserve the trust of the patient and family. For this reason, it is important that critical care nurses practice strategies for delivering bad news. Such news can range from reporting that an antibiotic is not reducing an infection or a vasopressor medication is not maintaining an acceptable blood pressure, to telling a family member that a patient has died. Because nurses are at the bedside 24 hours a day, communicating with the family early on that a patient is not doing well may help avoid a "surprise" announcement that the patient has died. Critical care nurses must remember that family members are not health care professionals. The health care system requires that patients and their proxy decision makers be active in making decisions about health care treatment. However, at times the health care team may try to place the responsibility of making a crucial decision, such as withdrawing mechanical ventilation, on the family; because of fear of legal action, clinicians may try to abdicate responsibility for the decision. A better approach would be to help the family understand the benefits and drawbacks of continuing mechanical ventilation, thus setting the stage for making the decision jointly. Even if family members are health care professionals, they are family members first and health care professionals second, and they may make decisions based more on their relationship with their loved one than on sound medical or nursing knowledge.

Simple strategies for communicating bad news may include phrases such as the following:

- "The blood pressure is worrisome given the amount of medication that we are giving your sister. We have reached the limit of how much we can safely give, and her blood pressure is not responding."
- "The ventilator alarm keeps ringing. It is letting me know that your father's lungs are becoming more resistant to mechanical ventilation. This is not a good sign."
- "I have noticed that your mother's kidneys have not been working well for the past couple of days. We have been trying to reverse her disease. However, now it seems that her heart and lungs are having difficulty as well."

Phrasing bad news in this way clearly indicates that the patient is not doing well but that the health care team is doing its best to help the patient. If discussions regarding withholding or withdrawing life-sustaining measures become

necessary, the family may be more receptive because they see what the nurses are seeing.

Notifying family members that the patient has died is a special case of delivering bad news. The manner that the nurse uses to deliver the bad news has a significant impact on how the family members remember the last moments of the patient's life. An excellent resource to help nurses learn more about how to communicate bad news to families is the book by Dr. Kenneth Iserson, *Grave Words: Notifying Survivors About Sudden, Unexpected Deaths*.[54] This book recommends that nurses divide death notification into four stages: prepare, inform, support, and afterwards.

1. In the preparation stage, the nurse gathers all the facts surrounding the death of the patient in order to answer any questions that might come up. Family members try to make sense of the death by requesting information.
2. In the inform stage, the nurse uses the person's name instead of "the patient" or "the deceased."
3. In the support stage, the nurse is available to the family members to answer any questions.
4. In the afterwards stage, the nurse provides information for the family, such as the names of funeral homes, medical examiner or coroner's office information, and whom to contact at the hospital if the family has any questions.

How to discuss these issues with the family and many more interventions are found in Dr. Iserson's book. Using clear, unambiguous language is important when delivering the bad news. Supporting the family members after the notification is essential. Becoming comfortable with the wording of the message (eg, by practicing phrases before they are needed) allows the nurse to focus on the family and their reaction to the message, instead of the message itself and how that message is delivered.

## Ethical Issues

Ethical issues affect how nurses work and provide care in the critical care environment. Ethical and legal issues are discussed in general terms in this chapter and in Chapter 8. Four ethical issues with special significance when talking about EOL care are the principle of double effect, moral distress, the withdrawal of life-sustaining technology, and organ and tissue donation.

### Principle of Double Effect

The principle of double effect is an ethical principle that distinguishes between consequences a person intends and consequences that are unintended but foreseen; this principle may be applicable in various situations where an action has two effects, one good and one bad.[55] The principle of double effect is most commonly applied to the administration of pain medications to patients who are dying. Opioids are used to relieve pain and other symptoms of suffering (ie, the good effect). However, opioids also may cause respiratory and cardiovascular depression that may, if left untreated, lead to death (ie, the bad effect). If the primary intention is to relieve pain and suffering with the recognition that the patient may die, it is morally and legally permissible to administer the opioid. If the primary intention is to cause death, it is not morally or legally permissible to administer the opioid.

The Center to Advance Palliative Care (CAPC) provides Fast Facts on their website, which are quick step-by-step instructions about how to deal with a variety of EOL issues (see Table 6-1).

## Moral Distress

Moral distress occurs when nurses cannot turn moral choices into moral action.[56,57] This distress occurs when the nurse knows the proper course of action to take, but institutional or interpersonal constraints make it nearly impossible to do so.[56] For example, nurses tend to recognize when therapies are no longer beneficial or helpful to a patient sooner than family members. For families, it is difficult to realize that therapies may no longer be helpful. Moral distress can arise when the family's understanding about the utility of therapy differs from that of the nurse.

The AACN has identified moral distress as a key issue affecting the work environment. To produce a more healthy occupational environment, the AACN has developed a resource for nurses to use to address this issue.[58] This resource, *The Four A's to Moral Distress*, provides a framework for nurses to address their moral distress and find avenues for its resolution. The four A's— **A**sk, **A**ffirm, **A**ssess, and **A**ct—facilitate change, thus creating a healthier nursing environment. Copies of this resource are available to AACN members or by contacting the AACN office (see Table 6-1). In addition, hospital bioethics or ethics committees are available to staff to help work through situations in which moral distress is a factor.

## Withholding or Withdrawing Life-Sustaining Measures

When it becomes clear to both the nurse and family that additional treatment will not be beneficial, the decision may be made to withdraw life-support methods. Mechanical ventilation is one intervention that is often withdrawn in such circumstances. Other life-sustaining measures that may be stopped include implantable cardiac defibrillators or pacemakers and hemodialysis.

When the decision is made to withdraw a therapy, special considerations are taken to reduce the suffering of the patient and to minimize the exhibition of distress to the family members. In the case of withdrawing mechanical ventilation, the decision is first made jointly with the family. In the case of extubation, opioids and sedatives are administered to the patient to reduce the pain and discomfort. In addition, the alarms to both the ventilator and the cardiac monitor are silenced to focus the family on the patient rather than the technology. Campbell[59] has published recommendations to successfully withdraw a mechanical ventilator. Additionally, many of the Fast Facts on the CAPC website relate to withdrawal of therapies, including mechanical ventilation and tube feeding (see Table 6-1).

## Organ and Tissue Donation

Organs and tissues can be procured after cardiac death or brain death. Federal law (Public Law 99-5-9; section 9318), Medicare, and the Joint Commission (formerly the Joint Commission on Accreditation of Healthcare Organizations) all require that (1) hospitals have written protocols regarding organ and tissue donation and (2) these institutions give the surviving family members the chance to authorize donation of their family member's tissues and organs.[60] When organ or tissue procurement is an issue, it is important that all family members are given the information they need to make a decision with which they are comfortable and that their grief is respected. In some cases, family members have initiated the conversation with their health care providers independently.

The local organ procurement organization (OPO) can provide additional resources. To find the OPO in your area, see Table 6-1.

## Caring for the Nurse

Some deaths can affect the nurse significantly. The death of a child, the death of a friend or colleague, mass casualties, or a particularly horrific, traumatic death can have a profound effect on the nurse. Nurses must explore ways to support each other in such situations, rather than dismissing the impact the death has on a colleague. According to Badger,[61] some self-care strategies for coping with a significant death include asking to be relieved from care responsibilities and taking a break; discussing the experience with a colleague, a friend, or a nurse leader; taking a moment to reflect on one's feelings after the event; focusing on what was done right; and following basic health principles, such as physical exercise, meditation, humor, music, eating properly, and obtaining adequate rest.

Working in a critical care unit is demanding physically, intellectually, and emotionally. Dealing with death on a consistent basis can take its toll on the nurse's well-being.[61] In the critical care setting, nurses caring for a patient who died may delay attending to their own grief because the demands of the unit and the needs of the family members may take precedence. It is important to be vigilant in recognizing signs and symptoms of unexpressed grief, burnout, and posttraumatic stress. Symptoms may include an increase in the number of sick days; indecision; difficulty with problem solving; isolation or withdrawal; behavioral outbursts; denial and shock; fixation on a single detail; immobilization; a feeling of extreme serenity; emotional numbing responses, such as withdrawal, pessimism, or a diminished capacity for experiencing pleasure; and intrusive responses, such as unwanted or unpleasant recollections or flashbacks.[61] To maintain emotional health, it is important to seek assistance in dealing with these issues. Nurse leaders and human resources representatives can provide resources to assist with the stresses of working in critical care.

## Clinical Applicability Challenges

### CASE STUDY

You are caring for Mr. J., a 42-year-old man who suffered a massive myocardial infarction. From the emergency department, he was admitted to the cardiac catheterization laboratory (CCL). He had occlusions in the left anterior descending artery and the left circumflex coronary artery that were opened via angioplasty and stent. In the CCL, the patient had persistent hypotension of systolic blood pressures in the 70s, cardiac index of 1.2, and pulmonary edema suggestive of cardiogenic shock. Dobutamine and an intra-aortic balloon pump were initiated in the CCL, and the patient was transferred to the ICU.

On hospital day 7, the patient's blood pressure, cardiac index, and mentation have not improved, and the interdisciplinary team has scheduled a family conference.

The patient continues to decline, and on hospital day 10 the family decides to withdraw the intra-aortic balloon pump and dobutamine. It is 6:30 PM, and Mr. J.'s wife wants to go home to take a shower and eat dinner and come back at 9:00 PM, which is past the posted visiting hours. In addition, the change of shift will occur at 7:00 PM, and you will transfer care to the oncoming nurse.

1. A foundational aspect of providing good palliative care is to develop a trusting relationship. How can critical care nurses establish and maintain a trusting relationship with families?

2. Palliative care includes the physical, psychological, emotional, social, and spiritual suffering dimensions for both the patient and the family. What are common concerns or manifestations of suffering in critical care settings in each of these dimensions?

3. Dealing with critical illness and end of life can be emotional not only for the patient and family but also for the staff. How can critical care nurses assess their colleagues for burnout, and how can they support each other?

### WANT TO KNOW MORE?

A wide variety of resources to enhance your learning and understanding of this chapter are available on thePoint.

You will find:

- References
- Selected readings
- NCLEX-style review questions
- Internet resources
- And more!

# PART 2

# Professional Practice Issues in Critical Care

## 7

# Ethical Issues in Critical Care Nursing

CONNIE M. ULRICH AND CHRISTINE GRADY

**LEARNING OBJECTIVES**

*Based on the content in this chapter, the reader should be able to:*

1. Explain the way ethics assists nurses and other clinicians in resolving moral problems.
2. Name and describe ethical principles applicable to clinical ethics.
3. Describe steps in the process of ethical decision making.
4. Identify resources available to nurses to help resolve ethical dilemmas.
5. Discuss an example of an ethical issue confronted by critical care nurses in practice and how applying ethical principles may help to resolve it.

Practicing critical care nurses face daunting ethical challenges. Nurses who work in intensive care and step-down units, operating rooms, emergency rooms, and other fast-paced, highly specialized settings must be able to recognize ethical issues they face in the daily care of patients and be prepared to address them in collaboration with patients, families, colleagues, administrators, and relevant others. Because of the precarious condition of critically ill patients, difficult ethical issues often arise that may cause conflicts among health care team members surrounding the benefits and burdens of treatment. How do nurses alleviate suffering when the patient or family want to continue aggressive measures? How do nurses and other health care team members openly discuss end-of-life issues when these discussions are often perceived as giving up hope? How do nurses provide beneficent care in the context of finite resources? How can nurses feel good about the choices that are made in critical practice environments, reflecting their professional goals for optimal care? This chapter provides a foundational overview of nursing ethics, the application of ethical principles, and ethical reasoning skills in critical care to enable nurses to confidently advocate for their patients' best interests.

## What is Ethics?

*Ethics* is the study of morality or standards of conduct and critical reflection and evaluation of moral choices.[1] Nurses help critically ill patients and their families make moral choices every day in intensive care environments. These choices range from the initiation of treatment following critical injury to the withdrawal of medical procedures at the end of life. Moral choices are not easy; there is often disagreement among stakeholders about what is best in a given situation. The intensity and complexity of patient care require all nurses to have an ethical foundation to help them address these difficult moral choices.

Nurses often struggle with ethical issues because they are strong patient advocates who develop intimate human relationships when caring for critically ill patients. Issues are especially challenging when there is limited consensus about what the ethically right or wrong approach may be in any given situation. For example, what "ought" the nurse do if a family member asks that the patient with a poor prognosis not be told about a cancer diagnosis? Should the truth *always* be told in these types of situations? Ulrich et al[2] noted that an ethical problem can occur in any clinical or research situation when there are salient questions about the "rightness" or "wrongness" of particular aspects of the care and treatment of patients. Applying ethical principles and considerations helps nurses articulate sound reasons for ethical positions, clarify ethical principles that might be in conflict, and address the issues they encounter.

## Ethical Principles

Ethical principles serve as general guidelines in health care decision making. Principles such as autonomy, beneficence, nonmaleficence, veracity, fidelity, and justice can guide conduct and ethical reasoning. These principles are not, however, absolute and can conflict with one another. Understanding and applying these principles can help critical care nurses determine an ethically appropriate course of care for their patients.

## Autonomy

Autonomy is the right to self-determination or the right to make decisions about one's own body or actions free from interference or coercion from others.[1] It is a central value in the Western world and reflects personal values, goals, and convictions for self-governance.

Critical care nurses are known for their advocacy roles and their willingness to speak up for their patients. In fact, the patient population that they care for seems to require advocacy. Critical care patients range from those who are ventilator dependent for long periods of time to patients whose families must make immediate decisions pertaining to end-of-life care. It is not unusual for nurses to be "caught in the middle" as they struggle to promote patients' autonomous decision making, including ensuring that patients give their informed consent and have opportunities to plan advance directives.[3] In a study investigating the everyday ethical issues that nurses face, nurses (including those in acute care settings) reported frequently encountering issues associated with protecting patients' rights and informed consent to treatment procedures.[2]

Informed consent respects autonomy by providing patients and families with the pertinent information they need to make an ethically sound decision. In essence, "respect for autonomy obligates professionals in health care and research involving human subjects to disclose information, to probe for and ensure understanding and voluntariness, and to foster adequate decision-making."[1] Conflict may occur when health care professionals' views about care in a patient's best interests do not match the patient's autonomous wishes. Critical care nurses can use the Nursing Interventions Classification (NIC) system for guidance when developing activities to facilitate autonomous decision making in the critical care setting (Box 7-1).[4]

## Beneficence

Nurses are ethically, legally, and professionally obligated to avoid harm and promote benefit for their patients. The American Nurses Association (ANA)[5] notes that nurses' primary commitment is to the "health, welfare, and safety of the client"; this includes acts of caring and compassion as well as protection from harm. The ethical principle of beneficence is the *sine qua non* for the nursing profession, guiding all nurses in their daily interactions and activities with patients. Beneficence presupposes that any harms patients are exposed to are justified by potential benefits. Beauchamp and Childress[1] outline three obligations of beneficence: preventing harm to others, promoting and acting for the good of others, and eliminating untoward or harmful circumstances.

In the critical care setting, beneficence often conflicts with other ethical principles, including that of autonomy. Sometimes patients and their families may be more comfortable deferring treatment decisions to their health care provider, especially because the crisis and chaotic nature of intensive care may make it difficult to make decisions. In other instances, the critical care nurse and physician may need to act on behalf of a patient who is neurologically or cognitively impaired. With limited or no knowledge of the patient's autonomous wishes, the nurse acts to promote the patient's best medical interests. Intentionally acting on

---

**BOX 7-1** **Nursing Interventions Classification**

**Decision-Making Support**

**Definition**

Providing information and support for a patient who is making a decision regarding health care.

**Activities**

- Determine whether there are differences between the patient's view of his or her own condition and the view of health care providers.
- Assist patient to clarify values and expectations that may assist in making critical life choices.
- Inform patient of alternative views or solutions in a clear and supportive manner.
- Help patient identify the advantages and disadvantages of each alternative.
- Establish communication with patient early in admission.
- Facilitate patient's articulation of goals for care.
- Obtain informed consent, when appropriate.
- Facilitate collaborative decision making.
- Be familiar with institution's policies and procedures.
- Respect patient's right to receive or not to receive information.
- Provide information requested by patient.
- Help patient explain decision to others, as needed.
- Serve as a liaison between patient and family.
- Serve as a liaison between patient and other health care providers.
- Use interactive computer software or Web-based decision aides as an adjunct to professional support.
- Refer to legal aid, as appropriate.
- Refer to support groups, as appropriate.

From Bulechek GM, Butcher HK, Dochterman JA, et al (eds): Nursing Interventions Classification (NIC), 6th ed. St. Louis, MO: Mosby, 2013, p 139.

---

behalf of another without the other's explicit consent may be considered paternalistic. "Paternalism is commonly framed in terms of the conflict between the primary obligation of physicians, nurses, and other provider-practitioners to abide by the principle of beneficence in their practice and the assertion of the rights of persons who are receiving services to make autonomous decisions about their lives."[6] Paternalism can be acceptable in the critical care setting when there are benefits to the patient that justify the paternalistic action. A common example is helping the patient turn, breathe deeply, cough, and ambulate following an extensive surgical procedure when the patient is in pain, is sleep deprived, or wants to be left alone.

## Nonmaleficence

The ethical principle of nonmaleficence obligates us to avoid causing undue pain and suffering or harm to another. This principle is often discussed along with the principle of beneficence because the two are intricately linked. Nonmaleficence is a *prima facie* duty for the nurse, meaning that it is morally binding unless other conflicting moral obligations outweigh its primacy.[1,7] Nonmaleficence obligates nurses to avoid unnecessary physical or bodily harm as well as psychological or emotional distress; in some cases, harm can be caused by a breach of professional standards of care. Nurses are constantly balancing the benefits and harms of decisions, treatments, and procedures for critically ill patients to make sure harms are justified by the benefits. Indeed, medications meant to improve a patient's condition, including steroids, morphine, amphotericin B, heparin, and others, may have serious adverse effects. Nurses must constantly apply the principle of nonmaleficence in critical care where the quality of life of patients is an important consideration.

## Veracity

Nurses remain the most trusted professional groups in the United States,[8] and veracity or truth-telling is foundational to the nurse–patient relationship. The ANA Code for Nurses states: "Truth-telling and the process of reaching informed choice underlie the exercise of self-determination, which is basic to respect for persons. . ... Clients have the moral right to determine what will be done with their own person; to be given accurate information, and all the information necessary for making informed judgments."[5]

Much current research suggests that patients want to be told the truth about their diagnosis, including full disclosure of potential risks and benefits of specific treatments and alternatives, in order to make informed decisions related to their care.[9-11] Sometimes information can be presented in ways that are misleading or biased, even though accurate; this can create conflict and uneasiness. Truth-telling in the clinical setting preserves autonomy and trust and maintains sound communication patterns with patients.

## Fidelity

Fidelity in the context of nursing care is the duty to be faithful to one's patients by keeping promises and fulfilling contracts and commitments. It is the moral covenant between individuals in a relationship.[1] Nurses are involved in many aspects of patients' immediate care: physical, emotional, spiritual, and psychological. For this reason, they often develop close relationships with patients and their families, and are called upon to be forthright and to keep their promises to inform, update, and communicate unforeseen circumstances that might occur. However, there are times when keeping promises can be problematic, as in the following situation:

> A patient previously asked the nurse and the team to keep the fact that he is HIV-positive a secret. He has been afraid to tell his wife and asked the team not to tell her. He is now ventilator dependent, suffering from sudden onset bacterial pneumonia.

Should the nurse agree to keep the patient's secret and withhold the information from the patient's wife until he can work through his emotions and the best way to discuss the issue? Does the nurse have obligations to the patient's wife, because she is at risk of infection, and because she will now become the patient's caregiver? How should the nurse handle the situation after the patient is weaned from the ventilator?

*Confidentiality* is an aspect of fidelity that is an essential component of trusting relationships. Patients have the right to know who has access to their personal health care information, and assurance that it will be kept confidential and that there are safeguards in place for privacy, security, and authorized access.[12] A commitment to maintain confidentiality in patient–provider relationships is part of every professional health care code of ethics. But confidentiality is not absolute, and in certain circumstances can be overridden, such as when there is imminent danger to the patient or a third party. Additionally, disclosure is required for public health reporting purposes related to certain infectious diseases or abusive situations.[13]

## Justice

Justice, an important ethical principle in critical care settings and in health care, is often discussed in terms of distributive justice, or how one allocates scarce or finite resources. Recent national health care debates have brought to light ethical concerns associated with escalating costs of US health care, the quality of care that is provided, and the cost-effectiveness and cost–benefit analysis of current standard therapies. The Patient Protection and Affordable Care Act[14] (more commonly known as ACA, or "Obamacare"), signed into law by President Obama in 2010, was an important legislative achievement to redress US health care access, equity, and equality concerns. Many more Americans now have health insurance since the passage of the ACA.[15] The ACA addressed ethical concerns such as access to primary care providers and health insurance coverage for preexisting illnesses and other conditions but raised new concerns related to its successful implementation. Individuals who previously did not have health care insurance will enter the health care system with varying conditions, and in some instances, with multiple comorbidities. This has the potential to increase the volume of patients who are admitted to critical care units as well as add to the complexity of needed care.

Questions of distributive justice arise on a daily basis in intensive care and emergency settings because of the need to prioritize care. ICU care is expensive; about one of five Americans die annually in ICUs, with the elderly accounting for up to half of all ICU admissions.[16] Distributive justice is concerned not only with the appropriate allocation of technology and aggressive measures, but also with the unit- and nursing-based resources needed to provide that care.

Staffing is an ethical concern and an indicator of distributive justice because it directly affects the beneficent care of patients. Understaffing has emerged as a major concern in the care of critically ill patients. Aiken et al[17] reported an association between nurse staffing levels and patient mortality in relation to "failure to rescue" (mortality following complications) in adult surgical patients cared for in Pennsylvania hospitals. In this research, nurses were important for surveillance and safety measures within hospitals, with higher patient-to-nurse ratios negatively affecting outcomes of care. More recent research by Kelly et al[18] did not find an association between staffing, nurse experience, and patient mortality in critical care units. These researchers did show, however, that a positive work environment and the proportion of critical care nurses with bachelor's degrees were significantly related to lower patient mortality.

Staffing inadequacies are also a major source of ethics-related stress that ultimately affects job satisfaction and retention of nurses.[19] Organizational ethical climate is also key to addressing the ethical concerns of critical care nurses. Feeling respected and valued, believing in the mission of the institution in which one works, and resolving tensions that might arise in the course of caring for patients are important to all critical care nurses. In fact, Ulrich et al[19] reported that a positive ethical climate was significantly associated with job satisfaction and retention of nurses and other providers. Critical care nurse managers and staff nurses are constantly allocating resources as they weigh the patient care needs required on their units, the number of admissions and available beds, and the ability of staff to meet those needs. Staffing shortages sometimes require utilizing personnel who are not readily familiar with a particular unit or hospital, including novice nurses or those designated as "float" or contract staff. Critical care unit–based orientation and other special training sessions are imperative to address standards of practice, policies, procedures, and additional technological aspects of caring for critically injured patients.

## Ethics as a Foundation for Nursing Practice

Nursing is guided by historical precepts and ethical norms that form the basis of nursing's contract with society. This fiduciary relationship is based on trust. In fact, nurses are consistently ranked highly in public polls on issues of trust and ethical standards. Nursing's primary commitment is to the patient and to ensure the delivery of safe, quality care; however, there is also a collective moral responsibility to serve the good of society. All professional groups define themselves by their body of scholarly knowledge, degree of self-regulation, and the professional code of ethics that underlie their beliefs, practices, and norms.[20,21]

Understanding the ethical and philosophical foundations of the nursing profession can help maintain focus on the profession's values, duties, and obligations to patient care within a society with changing demographics (ie, a chronically ill and aging society) and rising health care costs. Ongoing evaluations of the professional standards of nursing and, specifically, critical care nursing are necessary as the profession continues to evolve and develop new knowledge that will address advancing technology and its use in the care of the critically ill.

## Nursing Code of Ethics

The ANA *Code of Ethics for Nurses*, first adopted in 1950, has gone through several revisions to reflect the ethical, professional, and societal concerns of the day.[22] The most recent *Code of Ethics for Nurses With Interpretive Statements* (2015)[5] embodies the moral values of the profession. It represents not only expectations for ethical conduct in clinical practice but also the duty of the nurse to protect his or her own integrity. The Code symbolizes collective agreement among its members for societal good and serves as a guideline for nurses to follow in ethical decision making related to patient, family, and community care. Every profession, including nursing, is bound to a code of ethics that represents the moral basis for its professional standards of practice and helps to ensure the public's trust in their care.

## Ethical Issues

An ethical issue or problem can occur in clinical situations where there are concerns about what might be "morally right or wrong" in the care of critically ill patients and their families. There are many ethical issues in critical care, including,

but not limited to, end-of-life treatment decisions, futility, truth-telling, harvesting and allocating organs for transplantation, do not resuscitate (DNR) decisions, informed consent, clinical research with critically ill patients, assisted suicide, the use of aggressive measures, conflict among colleagues, and resource allocation. Ulrich et al[2] reported that these everyday ethical issues occur frequently and often reflect providers' concerns about protecting their patients' rights.

Although nurses interact daily with patients and their families, some evidence suggests they are hesitant to speak up about the ethical issues they encounter for fear of retaliation.[23] Sulmasy et al[24] stress that nurses can be included in sensitive conversations (eg, DNR) because they are both confident and capable. They are in a key position to listen, explain, and comfort patients and address unmet needs. Health care organizations should develop policies and procedures that provide support to nurses to seek consultation for ethical concerns. Ethics education, in professional training and continuing education, is also essential, as is interdisciplinary teamwork, because the complex needs of intensive care patients require all members of the health care team to be part of the discussion.

## Withholding and Withdrawing Treatment

Determining when to withhold or withdraw treatment for critically ill or injured patients can be stressful for all involved. This is true not only for families who surrender hope for continued survival, but also for health care providers who have been caring for a patient. Withholding care may be at the request of the patient or family, and is sometimes a consideration for patients deemed critically or irreversibly ill for whom there is no foreseeable recovery regardless of the treatment offered. Withdrawing life-supportive treatments (eg, ventilator and respiratory support, nutrition, and hydration) once they have been started is also sometimes ethically appropriate, but can create psychological distress for physicians and nurses. Ethical and legal advice is often sought, and professional guidelines (eg, Society of Critical Care Medicine) and in-house hospital and ethics committee policies and procedures can assist both physicians and nurses with these determinations. Brock[25] notes that "any set of circumstances that would morally justify not starting life-sustaining treatment would justify stopping it as well."

Open communication is imperative in critical care because "the majority of deaths in the intensive care setting involve withholding or withdrawing multiple life-sustaining therapies."[26] Families are often confronted with the difficult task of deciphering medical information about the prognosis of their loved ones. Some patients and their families prefer a shared decision-making model in which decisions are made with clinicians; others prefer recommendations from the physician.[27] Critical care nurses can help prepare families for difficult discussions about withdrawing or withholding life-supportive treatments by facilitating care conferences to address patients' health status as well as cultural, spiritual, and value-based needs. When a patient cannot speak for himself, nurses can help talk with families about their loved one's wishes and present timely information about the patient's plan of care with up-to-date, clear, and honest expectations about the situation at hand. Sadly, in a large

European and Israeli study that examined intensive care physicians' and nurses' perceptions of the appropriateness of care in intensive care units, 31.7% of nurses reported not being present during end-of-life family discussions.[28]

## Medical Futility

Medical futility is frequently discussed in critical care situations. When the health care team believes an intervention has no prospect of helping the patient, they may describe the intervention as futile. This can create conflict and turmoil if family members hold out hope of recovery and seek to pursue all aggressive measures. Medical futility includes both a qualitative value judgment and a quantitative aspect.[29] Schneiderman et al[29] note that "when physicians conclude (either through personal experience, experiences shared with colleagues, or consideration of reported empirical data) that in the last 100 cases, a medical treatment has been useless, they should regard that treatment as futile." Furthermore, the Hastings Center remarks that physicians have no obligation to comply with a patient's or surrogate's request for treatment if that treatment will provide no physiologic benefit.[30] Critical care nurses, who work with patients and their families day after day, are not immune to distress in such situations. Questions about futility are often accompanied by conflict among stakeholders and necessitate careful deliberation and communication, and sometimes consultation, about the plan of action.

## Moral Distress

Moral distress has become a frequent topic of discussion in the literature and remains a common concern among health care providers, including nurses and physicians. This phenomenon was originally defined by Jameton[31] as the distress that one feels when one knows the ethically correct action to take but is precluded from doing so for a variety of reasons. Constraints can be individual, societal, or organizational. Patient demands, limited resources, authoritative structures, and other circumstances within the workplace can make nurses feel powerless. Bell and Breslin[32] add that acting against one's personal and professional values creates moral distress. Physical and emotional symptoms, such as anger, anxiety, frustration, powerlessness, and fatigue, are common outcomes associated with moral distress. Additionally, studies have shown that moral distress is linked to nurses' intent to leave their positions.[19,33]

Moral distress is prevalent in intensive care environments because aggressive treatments may be offered to patients and their families without clear benefit. This perception of "futility" is disturbing to many nurses, in particular, as they encounter ethical tensions between continuing aggressive treatments and initiating conversations on end-of-life care options. Piers et al[28] reported that both physicians and nurses in ICUs (27.1%) perceived that inappropriate care was given to at least one patient during the day in which they were surveyed.

Strategies to minimize moral distress and create a healthy workplace have been outlined by the American Association of Critical Care Nurses (AACN)[34] and include the four As: Ask, Affirm, Assess, and Act. Ulrich and Hamric[35] also urge nurses to foster an open communication plan with other health care team members, seek ethics consultation services as needed, uphold a zero tolerance policy for retaliation if members speak out, and continually assess and dialogue about the needs of complex patients.

## Ethical Decision Making: The Case Method Approach

Several models exist to assist clinicians in the ethical decision-making process. A pragmatic case method approach is useful because it allows all health care team members to focus on a specific clinical case, address the ethical issues that may be morally problematic, and develop a plan of action. Steps in the case method of ethical decision making, similar to those in the nursing process, are listed in Box 7-2.

### Step 1: Assessing the Problem

Assessment is an initial task of any medical or nursing clinician, and this applies to the ethical decision-making process as well. Identifying the ethical problem is the most critical part of the assessment. One needs to understand the patient's medical condition or problem, as well as the prognosis, potential sequelae, and treatment goals, and any additional contextual factors that may influence the ethical decision-making process, including family and organizational systems. It is always important to gather sociodemographic information, such as age, gender, education, setting of care, and other factors (eg, religion, culture, language), which might influence decisions or communication.

Assessment questions that might be helpful include the following: Is the patient legally competent and capable of making a decision associated with his or her care? What are the patient's and family's preferences? Are there advance directives that outline the patient's wishes for treatment? Are there competing interests that need further discussion such as conflict amongst family members, and/or conflict between the patient, family members, and clinicians? Are institutional factors contributing to the ethical problems presented by the clinical case? The usual goals in the critical care setting, for example, trend toward aggressive treatment rather than palliation or support.

### Step 2: Defining the Issues

Explicating and ranking the relevant ethical issues or moral considerations associated with a particular case is the second step in the ethical decision-making process. Clinicians can use relevant literature, institutional policies, professional groups, commissions, their past clinical experiences,

---

**BOX 7-2** **Steps in Ethical Decision Making**

1. Assess the problem.
2. Define the ethical issues.
3. Delineate the goals, make decisions, and implement a plan of action.
4. Evaluate the process and modify actions as needed.

Adapted from Spencer E: A case method for consideration of moral problems. In: Fletcher JC, Spencer EM, Lombardo PA (eds): Fletcher's Introduction to Clinical Ethics, 3rd ed. Hagerstown, MD: University Publishing Group, 2005.

or other resources to seek out information on cases that pose similar ethical challenges. This can help illuminate how to resolve the specific problem and identify the morally acceptable options available to the clinician.

## Step 3: Goal Setting, Decision Making, and Implementing

Step 3 focuses on goal setting, decision making, and implementation. During this step, all personnel involved in the decision-making process are encouraged to clarify their own values and moral convictions so that the needs of the patient can be discussed forthrightly. Spencer[36] notes that "moral problem-solving and planning for the care of the patient go hand in hand." Weighing the benefits and burdens of each option, as well as examining the ethical principles and underlying theories in regard to the case at hand, can assist clinicians in making a decision. Sometimes, ethics consultations, referral to an ethics committee, or other types of assistance are needed to provide an impartial outside voice and to facilitate open dialogue among clinicians or family members when discussions appear to be at an impasse.

## Step 4: Evaluating and Modifying Actions

Evaluation of an ethical decision allows all parties to reflect on the decision at hand and address any missed opportunities. Some questions to consider include the following: Was the ethical problem adequately addressed? Were the goals of treatment met? If not, why? Were all parties satisfied with the outcome? Is there an alternative option that could be used if there is a need to rethink the plan of care? What factors contributed to a positive resolution of the case? What factors led to a less than desirable outcome? What have I (we) learned from this process? What, if any, educational changes can be made in the clinical environment to resolve similar ethical challenges in the future?

## Strategies for Promoting Ethical Decision Making

The highly charged environment in which critical care nurses work calls for strategies to assist them with the increasing demands they encounter. Two strategies for developing an environment that is supportive of ethical concerns are briefly discussed here: institutional ethics committees (IECs) and ethics rounds and conferences.

## Institutional Ethics Committees

Many health care facilities have IECs to help resolve ethical conflicts in patient care as well as address ethics-related questions that might arise in clinical practice.[37-40] Ethics committees usually involve a diverse group of individuals, including physicians, nurses, social workers, pastoral care counselors, legal counsel, administrators, and community members. IECs provide ethics consultation and can assist practitioners by providing an external voice on contentious ethical issues that may seem irresolvable and facilitate education for all members of the health care team. These ethical issues can include concerns about research with seriously ill patients in intensive care settings, surrogate decision making for patients at end of life, professional or patient-family-related conflicts in treatment goals and preferences, and pain or symptom management strategies.

Recommendations by the IEC can be either binding or nonbinding, depending on the individual committee. However, an IEC can offer support to practitioners, patients, and families and improve their satisfaction with the delivery of care. Some institutions provide an ethics consultation service as a subset of the IEC or an independent consultant. Nurses have full authority to ask for an ethics consultation; they are critical members of interdisciplinary teams working toward the beneficent care of critically ill patients, helping these patients and families achieve desirable goals in critical care settings.

## Ethics Rounds and Conferences

Ethics rounds may be an important and useful aspect of patient care, as they provide an opportunity to discuss a particular patient's health care needs in depth and identify clinical, social, or ethical problems early in the course of care. Importantly, ethics rounds allow providers to express their views on issues of concern as well as clarify the most salient values and preferences at stake. This can include questions on DNR status, palliative care versus curative care, advance directives, conflicts associated with family systems, disagreements among health care providers about future goals of care, organ donation, cultural and religious differences, and many others.

Nurses can make ethics rounds a regular part of their unit's activities and focus on a specific case that raised ethical concerns or was particularly distressing for the staff. Interdisciplinary ethics rounds also provide an opportunity to build trusting work relationships with multidisciplinary care providers and develop a team approach to addressing value conflicts that arise in the unit. An individual patient ethics conference can be useful in resolving complex cases and opening a dialogue with patients, families, and the nursing staff or a multidisciplinary group.

## Clinical Applicability Challenges

### CASE STUDY

Mr. B, age 88 years, was admitted to the Postanesthesia Care Unit (PACU) following surgery for an unresectable malignant gastrointestinal tumor. Mr. B was still sedated and intubated, and nurses decided to let him wake up on his own, not being sure how he would clear the anesthesia. Mr. B's two sons arrived at his bedside and were quite emotional and teary-eyed with worry for their father, holding his hands and stroking his arms.

Mr. B began awakening and, after a few minutes, he started thrashing about and accidentally extubated himself. He then said to his sons at the bedside: "You two are so stupid—I told you I didn't want this." For the rest of the night, Mr. B. would not cooperate with his primary nurse on any aspects of his care. He would not answer questions the PACU nurse asked while attempting to make sure he was alert and oriented, and not somnolent from retaining $CO_2$ after pulling out his endotracheal tube. Mr. B would

see his primary nurse across the 23 bed unit and shut his eyes to avoid her, so all the efforts of the PACU nurse to care for Mr. B fell short.

1. What strategies might the nurse use to work with Mr. B, given his apparent anger over his situation in the PACU?
2. What factors might have a bearing on the plan of care for Mr. B, based on his nonresectable tumor?
3. How would you determine the best course of action for this patient's plan of care, and what resources would you call on to help you?

#### Acknowledgment

Thanks to Kimberly Mooney-Doyle, PhD, RN, for her assistance on clinical applicability challenges with critically ill patients.

### WANT TO KNOW MORE?

A wide variety of resources to enhance your learning and understanding of this chapter are available on thePoint.

You will find:

- References
- Selected readings
- NCLEX-style review questions
- Internet resources
- And more!

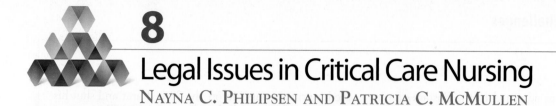

# 8

# Legal Issues in Critical Care Nursing

NAYNA C. PHILIPSEN AND PATRICIA C. MCMULLEN

**LEARNING OBJECTIVES**

*Based on the content in this chapter, the reader should be able to:*

1. Describe major areas of the law that affect critical care nursing practice.
2. Define the four elements of malpractice (professional negligence).
3. Delineate allegations commonly made against critical care nurses.
4. Explain types of vicarious liability.
5. Apply knowledge of informed consent and advance directives to critical care patient situations.

Because society in the United States seems to be more litigious than ever, legal issues involving critical care are of increasing concern. Contemporary research indicates that approximately 210,000 deaths occur each year as a result of preventable harm in hospitals.[1]

This chapter begins with an overview of the major areas of law of governmental organizations and major areas of law that impact the practice of nursing. Next, the legal principles of negligence, vicarious liability, and patient autonomy are reviewed, with pertinent critical care case examples. The chapter then proceeds to identify and address selected current legal issues that are most applicable to the practice of critical care nursing.

## Overview of Governmental Organization and Major Areas of the Law

The US Constitution provides the basic principles and guiding policy for all law in the land. Three branches of government were established to create a "balance of powers" to minimize the risk of abuse of the law by those in power. The structure of each state government is similar to the federal structure. The *legislative branch*, composed of representatives of the people, creates and modifies *statutes*. The *executive branch* is headed by the president or a state governor, and consists of federal and state agencies that write and enforce *regulations* that give the people *notice* of what they need to do to comply with the statutes. The *judicial branch* consists of the federal and state court systems, which interpret statutes and regulations and examine constitutionality when disputes arise. The courts generate *case law*, which becomes *precedent or common law*, providing guidance for future interpretation of the law.

A legal dispute is first heard by a *trial court*, which examines the evidence and makes a decision based on the facts of the case. Some disputes then go on up to higher courts, called *appeals courts*. These courts make decisions about alleged legal and procedural mistakes by the judges or lawyers in the trial courts. They do not retry the initial dispute.

Three types of law affect the practice of critical care nurses. These are administrative law, criminal law, and civil law.

## Administrative Law

Administrative law includes state and federal statutes, their accompanying regulations, and the regulatory agencies that enforce those laws. Nurses deal with state agencies and state laws and regulations when they apply for a nursing license to enter the profession. Every state legislature has enacted a Nurse Practice Act (NPA). The NPA defines the practice of nursing, requires nursing licensure, establishes standards for nursing schools, and delegates enforcement powers to a state agency, usually the State Board of Nursing. This agency develops regulations that give notice to the public and to nurses of how the NPA will be interpreted and implemented in that state. The Boards of Nursing work together to develop common standards and address common challenges through the National Council of State Boards of Nursing, Inc. (NCSBN), where their representatives conduct research, pool resources, and publish model practice acts and position statements. The NCSBN is also responsible for the development and integrity of the national licensure examination known as the NCLEX.

Practicing nurses are expected to know the provisions of the NPA and any regulations dealing with the practice of nursing in every state where they practice. If a nurse is unfamiliar with the NPA, it is important that he or she contact the State Board of Nursing to obtain access to and review this act. State boards of nursing increasingly place their NPA and regulations on a Web site. The NCSBN Web site, www.ncsbn.org, provides links to the Web sites of all of the boards of nursing, as well as other useful information related to legal aspects of nursing licensure and practice.

Why do state governments regulate nursing practice? The United States Constitution charges the states with protecting the health, safety, and well-being of their citizens. For nurses, this begins with nursing licensure, a process in which the new nurse applicant must show that he or she can enter practice as a safe practitioner by completing an approved nursing education program, passing a national examination (the NCLEX), and demonstrating good moral character. While public protection during initial licensure is proactive, assurance of continuing competency after licensure is often reactive. As long as they continue to pay their renewal fees, nurses may be required to practice a certain number of hours per year or attend approved continuing education seminars, but they typically do not have to return to nursing school or face reexamination to renew a license. Instead, the boards identify loss of competency by responding to complaints.

Complaints, whether to the Board of Nursing or to the courts in the form of a lawsuit, are a special concern of critical care nurses. Because their patients are not as stable as patients in most other areas of health care, they are at high risk for an undesired outcome. These complaints can come from many sources, such as patients, their families, other health care workers, or the nurse's employer. Even a revengeful ex-spouse of a nurse can allege any of the violations listed in the NPA.

For example, if a patient feels that he or she has received incompetent or unethical nursing care, he or she may contact the State Board of Nursing and file a complaint against the nurse or nurses involved in the care. The state board then determines whether the complaint, if true, would violate the NPA and possibly result in limits on or loss of the nurse's license to practice. If so, the board conducts an investigation to determine whether the claim has merit.

Under the Fifth Amendment of the US Constitution, all citizens are afforded the right to *due process* before the state or federal government can take any property. Case law indicates that a nurse's license is a form of property because it helps a person earn a living. Therefore, due process rights are attached to a nursing license. This means that the State Board of Nursing must meet certain procedural requirements before it can discipline a nurse by taking away or placing conditions or limitations on his or her nursing license. First, the nurse is entitled to *notice* that someone has filed a claim against his or her license. The nurse is also entitled to a *hearing* that follows the procedures outlined in the NPA, in order to answer and defend alleged violations.

In most states, the final defense against charges on a nurse's license takes the form of a hearing before the State Board of Nursing, whose members typically include nurses. To be sure that the hearing is fair, the nurse should attend the hearing and should arrange to have representation at the hearing by an attorney whose practice includes nursing licensure. The American Association of Nurse Attorneys (TAANA) is an excellent source of attorneys with this special expertise. At a hearing, the board members listen to the case against the nurse's license, which is presented by an attorney or other representative for the state. Witnesses who have knowledge of facts surrounding the complaint will testify and introduce evidence. These witnesses may include board staff members who investigated the complaint or who acquired the related medical records and other documents, the person who filed the complaint, any witnesses to the incident, and people who supervised the nurse. Then the nurse, either directly or through legal counsel, can question the board's witnesses and can introduce evidence or testimony to refute the allegations in the complaint. Based on the presentations by the state and

by the nurse, the State Board of Nursing makes a determination as to whether the nurse violated the NPA and what, if any, discipline is warranted to protect the public. Typically, the decision of the State Board of Nursing is final, and unless there were violations of the nurse's due process rights, a court will uphold the state board's findings if either side appeals.

Although the nurse's right of due process cannot be abridged, state boards of nursing have the right to *immediately* suspend a nurse's license for acts that the Board deems so dangerous to the public welfare that the complaint, if true, would constitute an emergency. When the state immediately suspends a license, the nurse must stop any nursing practice immediately. The NPA provides the nurse with the right to an accelerated hearing, within a short period of time from the date of the suspension.

### HIPAA

A federal agency that has a major impact on nursing practice is the U.S. Department of Health and Human Services (HHS), which generates regulations and enforces federal statutes such as the Health Insurance Portability and Accountability Act (HIPAA), Medicare, and Medicaid, including the rules for reimbursement to providers and health care institutions. Critical care nurses are familiar with HIPAA, a statute enacted by Congress in response to concerns about the security of electronic health records. The Title II HIPAA Privacy Rule in particular has raised the awareness of critical care nurses about their need to verify who can have access to patient information before sharing it. HIPAA made it clear that patients have a great deal of control over their health information, and in many circumstances the right to decide with whom the nurse can share that information. HIPAA also provides guidelines for communicating this right to the patient. The exceptions to HIPAA privacy rules include sharing information in the record needed for care with other care givers, information needed for billing payers, information that is de-identified (personal and all possibly identifying information are removed), and information needed for the general welfare, such as public health data and the regulation of health care facilities and professionals, including HIPAA enforcement. HIPAA's security rules also impact nursing practice. As the use of electronic health records increases, nurses must comply with regulations designed to protect electronic information, including the use of passwords and biometric identification and the location of computer screens to protect them from unauthorized eyes. Violation of relevant federal regulations and standards can have serious consequences, including the loss of federal reimbursement for care.

### Employment Law

Workplace statutes and their supporting regulations form another area of administrative law that clearly impacts nursing practice. A full discussion of this topic is beyond the scope of this chapter, but critical care nurses should be aware that a number of statutes affect their practice, their conditions of employment, their right to a safe workplace, and the responsibilities of health care supervisors and employers. Each statute is enforced by the federal or state government agency that is also responsible for drafting and revising such regulations. For example, the Fair Labor Standards Act,

P.B., a Certified Registered Nurse Anesthetist who was going through a traumatic divorce, expressed suicidal thoughts to co-workers at the hospital where she worked. On at least one occasion, she cried and had difficulty performing a routine task. Her supervisors then placed her on sick leave. They required her to meet certain requirements, including a psychiatric evaluation and communication of the results, before she could return to work. When P.B. met the requirements, she was reinstated.

P.B. sued the hospital, claiming that this action was not work-related, but was discrimination against her solely because her employer regarded her as disabled, in violation of the Americans with Disabilities Act (ADA). The court found that P.B.'s behavior would cause a "reasonable person" to question whether she could do her job. The action taken by the hospital was therefore a job-related necessity, and not a violation of the ADA.

*Barnum v. The Ohio State University Medical Center, et al: 2016 U.S. App LEXIS 2957; 2016 FED App. 0106N (6th Cir.).

**BOX 8-2** **Five Legal Responsibilities of the Registered Nurse**

- Performs only those functions for which he or she has been prepared by education and experience
- Performs those functions competently
- Delegates responsibility only to personnel whose competence has been evaluated and found acceptable
- Takes appropriate measures as indicated by observations of the patient
- Is familiar with policies of the employing agency

the Occupational Health and Safety Act, and the Family Medical Leave Act are enforced by the U.S. Department of Labor. The U.S. Equal Employment Opportunity Commission enforces Title VII of the Civil Rights Act of 1964 with Amendments, including the Lilly Ledbetter Fair Pay Act of 2009. The National Labor Relations Board is a federal agency formed to enforce the National Labor Relations Act. A number of federal agencies share responsibility for enforcing the Americans with Disabilities Act (ADA), including the Office of Civil Rights of HHS and the U.S. Department of Justice. Box 8-1 presents the case of a nurse who sued her employer for violating the ADA.

## Criminal Law

Criminal law is public law. It encompasses cases in which the local, state, or federal government has filed a lawsuit against an individual alleging that he or she has committed a wrongful and illegal act against society. In criminal cases, the victim has the role of witness for the state. If the nurse is the victim of the charged crime, he or she is a witness. If the state files charges against the nurse for committing a crime, the nurse is the defendant. Criminal cases involving nurses have included intentional assault and battery, fraud, theft, negligent homicide, and murder. If a nurse intended harm to a patient through substandard treatment, the nurse may be charged by the state under criminal law, in addition to any civil case for malpractice damages filed by the patient. In general, criminal cases are unusual in nursing situations. Nurses caring for trauma patients whose injuries may have resulted from criminal acts sometimes find themselves involved in a criminal case as a witness to the injury. In some states, they may be required to report certain injuries to criminal law enforcement authorities. An example of a criminal case is presented in Box 8-5 later in this chapter.

## Civil Law

Civil law is private law, and deals with conflicts among individuals. Civil law includes tort law, contract law, and the concepts of vicarious liability and product liability. Torts include trespass, assault, battery, and negligence.

## Nursing Negligence in Critical Care

The fundamental legal responsibility of the registered nurse in critical care settings does not differ from that of the registered nurse in any work setting. The registered nurse adheres to five principles for the protection of the patient and the practitioner (Box 8-2). The most common lawsuits against nurses and their employers are based on *negligence by a professional*, which is called *malpractice*.

A nursing malpractice case can begin when a patient experiences bad bedside manner or an undesired outcome related to nursing care. If a significant financial loss can be attributed to that outcome, the distressed patient might file a lawsuit against the nurse in a civil court, alleging nursing malpractice. The nurse then becomes the defendant in a civil malpractice case. This experience is a great burden for any nurse, even in the best of times. First, the nurse should contact his or her malpractice insurance carrier and obtain legal counsel who has expertise in nursing malpractice. The nurse may soon be involved with the next step of the civil lawsuit, called *discovery*. This can involve requests for documents, preparing written answers to written questions called "interrogatories," and, most stressful of all, a deposition, which is oral testimony given under oath and recorded by a court reporter, but out of court. In the best case, the plaintiff patient's attorney will advise dropping the case after hearing the nurse's testimony, but in the worst case this testimony will be used later to challenge the nurse's credibility during the next major phase of the lawsuit, the *trial*. During trial, witnesses will testify for both sides and introduce evidence for cross-examination in the courtroom. To prove a malpractice case, the complaining patient must prove all of the required "elements" of malpractice: duty, breach of duty, damages, and causation.

### Duty

A duty is a legal relationship between two or more parties. In most nursing cases, duty arises out of an implied contractual relationship between the patient and the health care facility. The patient, the insurer, or both agree to pay for any health care services the patient receives. In return, the health care facility agrees to supply "reasonable care." One way the duty of an individual nurse to the patient may be confirmed is by the appearance of the nurse's name in the patient's record. A nurse has a legal duty to provide reasonable care to all of his or her patients. This means that the nurse must provide care that complies with the established *standard of care* for a reasonable nurse under the circumstances present at the time of the incident.

Arguing the standard of care is the core of many malpractice cases. In a typical malpractice lawsuit, this is done by both sides hiring expert witnesses, sometimes called "dueling experts," to introduce evidence arguing for their different versions of the standard of care. The following factors can be used to determine the standard of care for a critical care nurse:

- Testimony from experts in critical care, which may include a critical care nurse who is working as an expert witness
- The employing institution's procedure and protocol manuals
- Nursing job descriptions
- Nursing research, textbooks, professional journals, medication books
- Professional organization standards and guidelines (eg, Advanced Cardiac Life Support [ACLS] and Certified Critical Care Registered Nurse [CCRN] standards)
- Laws and regulations governing professionals and institutions
- Standards of private accrediting bodies
- Equipment manufacturers' instructions

### Breach of Duty

What was the standard of care? What would a reasonable critical care nurse have done under the circumstances? After the plaintiff patient establishes duty, the patient must show that the nurse breached (violated) that duty—that is, the nurse was negligent. The critical care nurse who fails to meet the standard of care has breached (violated) his or her duty to the patient.

Negligence may be either "ordinary" or "gross." Ordinary negligence implies professional carelessness. Gross negligence suggests that the nurse willfully and consciously ignored a known risk for harm to the patient. Most cases involve ordinary negligence, but gross negligence can be found if, for example, the nurse ignored sound nursing advice or harmed a patient while under the influence of drugs or alcohol.

### Causation

Malpractice law requires a causal relationship between the critical care nurse's breach of the standard of care and the injury to the patient. To prove malpractice, the plaintiff patient has to show that injury or harm occurred as a result of the nurse's action or inaction; that is, the injury would not have occurred without the conduct in question. The plaintiff must also show that the injury was reasonably anticipated. For example, if a critical care nurse administered digoxin to a cardiac patient who had a pulse of 30 beats/min and the patient suffered a cardiac arrest, the court would likely find that the critical care nurse caused the patient's arrest; that is, the wrongful administration of the digoxin was the "proximate cause" of the arrest. However, if the patient had a pulse of 70 beats/min when the digoxin was administered, and the patient suffered a totally unanticipated seizure, it is probable that the nurse's action would not be found to be careless such as to be the cause of the seizure. In this case, the nurse would normally be exonerated, because seizures are not an expected complication of digoxin administration.

### Damages

The intent of malpractice negligence law is to make the injured party "whole." The law attempts to return the plaintiff as close as possible to a position that he or she would have been in had the nurse's conduct not caused this injury. Unfortunately, injuries sustained usually cannot be undone. Therefore, most court awards attempt to give the injured plaintiff an award of monetary "damages" that will compensate the plaintiff for his or her injuries. Monetary damages are grouped under the broad headings of economic and noneconomic damages.

Economic damages relate to those damages that can be calculated within a degree of certainty. Medical costs and lost wages are the two major types of economic damages. Noneconomic damages are more difficult to calculate. These damages include pain and suffering and loss of consortium (eg, relations, ability to perform household tasks) that occurred as a result of the malpractice. Many state and federal governments place monetary limits on the amount a patient can recover for pain and suffering, regardless of the amount that may be awarded by a jury.

The spouse and minor children of a patient may also be able to recover economic and noneconomic damages that they suffer as a consequence of injuries to the patient. When a minor child is the plaintiff, it is not unusual for the parents to file for noneconomic losses due to the loss of society and affection of their child. On the economic side, a parent can sue for his or her own lost wages due to a need to care for the child.

Many types of malpractice complaints are lodged against critical care nurses. The cases presented in Boxes 8-3, 8-4, and 8-5 illustrate reasons why nurses are named in malpractice suits.

In 1999 the Institute of Medicine (IOM) released a study, *To Err is Human: Building a Safer Health System*,[2] which raised awareness of medical errors, including serious medication errors, which occur in 5% to 10% of patients admitted to hospitals. Experts agreed that the most common cause of error is the system itself, not the individual practitioners in the system. This report triggered the formation of the National

---

**BOX 8-3** **Case Study: Failure to Comply with Reasonable Standards of Care\***

J.W., a patient with multiple risk factors, was admitted to the hospital for a second surgery to treat an abscess on his buttock 10 days after his first surgery. His surgeon ordered that sequential compression devices be placed on J.W.'s legs after surgery, but the nurses failed to carry out the order. J.W. developed deep venous thrombosis (DVT), ultimately resulting in the below-knee amputation of both legs.

At trial, a jury found that the nurses had breached the standard of care when they failed to carry out the surgeon's order. However, expert testimony conflicted regarding whether this negligence caused the DVT, or whether it was established after the first surgery and before this second surgery. The jury concluded that the negligence by nurses more than likely caused the DVT. J.W. was awarded $650,000 in damages, and the verdict was upheld on appeal.

\*Providence Hospital, Inc., Appellant/Cross Appellee v. John Willis, Appellee/ Cross-Appellant. Nos. 13-CV-920 & 13-CV-921. 103 A.3d 533; 2014 D.C. App. LEXIS 511.

**Case Study: Improper Medication Administration\***

N.D. was a 24-year-old woman who had been born with velo-cardiofacial syndrome, a heart anomaly. As she grew, N.D. developed severe pulmonary hypertension, and now was receiving hospice care. Nevertheless, she reportedly was taking classes at a community college and was preparing to go on a vacation when she elected to go to the hospital for an outpatient paracentesis, a palliative procedure. During the procedure, a doctor noticed that N.D. had cellulitis, so she decided to stay overnight for IV antibiotic treatment. Her mother said that she gave the nurse a container full of N.D.'s medications, with accurate dosages on them.

The admission nurse incorrectly recorded N.D.'s dose of Vasotec from an earlier medical record. All of the doctors and nurses subsequently involved in her care failed to notice this error and continued to prescribe and administer a double dose of Vasotec, in spite of falling blood pressure, which can be a side effect of Vasotec, and acute kidney failure, which caused her death days later.

N.D.'s estate sued three of the doctors and two of the nurses. At trial, experts opined that the doctors and nurses deviated from the standard of care by doubling N.D.'s medication, not properly checking it, not noticing or correcting the error, not withdrawing the Vasotec when her blood pressure fell and her kidneys failed, and incorrectly transcribing the family's statements about N.D.'s prescriptions. One expert noted that the number-one reason that people die in hospitals when they should not die is because of medication errors.

The jury determined that N.D. died because of her heart disease. Since the medication error was not the cause of her death, N.D.'s family received no damages. This decision was upheld on appeal.

*Virginia Dickerson, as Lawful Heir of Nicole Dickerson, Appellant v. Saint Luke's South Hospital, Inc., et al, Appellees. No. 110,513. 51 Kan. Ap. 2d 337; 346 P.3d 1100; 2015 Kan. App. LEXIS 25.

**Case Study: Criminal Liability in Critical Care\***

C.C. was a registered nurse who had been disciplined and terminated from six hospitals in different states. When he applied for new positions, former employers did not disclose the reasons for his termination, nor did they report him to the Board of Nursing. C.C. was arrested after investigation of an unexpected death in the seventh hospital revealed the presence of a lethal dose of digoxin in the patient. Because it was the second unexplained overdose in 2 weeks, the hospital initiated further investigation, which eventually revealed that C.C. had killed at least 40 patients over a 16-year period by injecting them with lethal doses of medications, including pancuronium bromide (Pavulon) and insulin. He may have killed as many as 400 patients.

C.C. stated that he killed patients to relieve suffering. He was charged under the state criminal code with murder, and received six life sentences.

*Sackman B: When the ICU becomes a crime scene. Crit Care Nurs Q 38(1): 30–35, 2015.

Patient Safety Foundation by the American Medical Association, and the creation of a nonpunitive sentinel events reporting system by the Joint Commission for the Accreditation of Healthcare Organizations (JCAHO), now known as the Joint Commission. Remaining controversies include what type of errors should be reported, and whether individual practitioners should be disciplined for this type of

error. In the case of gross negligence, the nurse is likely to be found liable for a medication error, regardless of the answers to these questions.

## Vicarious Liability

Vicarious liability means to hold someone (a person or institution) responsible for the actions of another. Critical care nurses sometimes find themselves in situations where various types of vicarious liability apply, including respondeat superior, corporate liability, negligent supervision, and the rule of personal liability.

### Respondeat Superior

The doctrine of respondeat superior is translated as "let the master answer for the sins of the servant." Under this legal theory, hospitals are held liable for the negligence of their employees. Respondeat superior is a legal doctrine based on public policy that notes that because a hospital profits from the patients seeking care, the hospital should pay for some of the damages caused by hospital personnel if negligence occurs. This doctrine applies only when hospital employees act within the scope of their employment.

Respondeat superior does not apply in situations involving temporary agency personnel, because they are usually employees of the agency, not of the hospital. Nor does it typically apply to physicians, because they are usually not employed by the hospital. This doctrine would not apply to nurses who are employed by a hospital but who are accused of malpractice for work outside of their hospital employment.

Because hospitals may be held liable for nursing activities conducted by their employees, they carry professional liability insurance that is intended to cover the cost of defending individuals named in a malpractice case. However, many nurses also carry their own malpractice insurance, to cover off-the-job nursing activities and to cover the cost of choosing their own independent counsel where multiple parties from their institution are sued, because they are likely to have conflicting interests.

### Corporate Liability

Corporate liability is vicarious liability that occurs when a hospital is found liable for its own unreasonable conduct. For example, if it is found that a unit is chronically understaffed and a patient suffers an injury as a result of short staffing, the hospital can be held accountable. It is reasonable to expect any hospital that has an ICU or an emergency department to take precautionary measures to ensure adequate staffing or that beds or admissions are reduced.

Corporate liability may also occur within "floating" situations. A nurse working in a critical care setting must be competent to make immediate nursing judgments and to act on those decisions. If the nurse does not possess the knowledge and skills required of a critical care nurse, he or she should not be attempting to render critical care. A nurse who is not well versed in critical care should notify the charge nurse or nursing supervisor of this fact. The nurse needs to clearly state which nursing care activities he or she can and cannot implement. The supervisor and charge nurse must then

## BOX 8-6 Commonly Asked Questions When Rotating to an Unfamiliar Unit

1. *If I am asked to go to another unit, must I go?*
Usually, you will be required to go to the other unit. If you refuse, you can be disciplined under the theory that you are breaching your employment contract or that you are failing to abide by the policies and procedures of the hospital. Some nursing units negotiate with hospitals to ensure that only specially trained nurses rotate to specialty units.

2. *If I rotate to an unfamiliar unit, what types of nursing responsibilities must I assume?*
You will be expected to carry out only those nursing activities that you are competent to perform. In some instances, this will be the performance of basic nursing care activities, such as blood pressures, and uncomplicated treatments. If you are unfamiliar with the types of medications used on the unit, you should not be administering them until you are thoroughly familiar with them. Consider the medication cards the student completes in nursing school. They were assigned because a reasonable, prudent nurse does not give medications without knowledge of their pharmacology, dosage, method of administration, side effects, and interactions with other medications. The same reasoning applies for any other type of critical care monitoring.

3. *What should I do if I feel unprepared when I get to the unit?*
Suggest that you assist the unit with basic nursing care requirements and that specialized activities (eg, invasive monitoring, cardiac monitoring, or the administration of unfamiliar drugs) be performed by staff members who are adequately prepared. Do not feel incompetent because you are not familiar with all aspects of nursing care. After all, when is the last time you saw the neurologist go to labor and delivery and perform a cesarean birth?

4. *What if the charge nurse orders me to do something I am not able to do safely?*
You are obligated to say you are unqualified and request that another nurse carry out the task. The charge nurse also needs to remember that she could be held liable for negligent supervision if she orders you to do an unsafe activity and a patient injury results.

## BOX 8-7 Case Study: Rule of Personal Liability and Independent Nursing Judgment*

R.K., a 35-year-old man, was struck in the back of the head by a softball while running to home plate and fell face down, briefly losing consciousness. He was transported to a hospital emergency department by ambulance. There a CT scan showed a left parietal acute epidural hematoma with depressed skull fracture. The nurses assessed R.K. at 3½ hours and again 5 hours after admission, noting that he was stable. One hour later a nurse notified the surgeon that R.K.'s condition was deteriorating, with unequal pupils and possible seizures. He was intubated and physicians requested that R.K. be transferred. When he could not be transported by air, doctors proceeded with emergency surgery to evacuate the hematoma.

R.K. sued the hospital, doctors, and nurses for negligence. The hospital responded that it was not responsible for the physicians because they were independent contractors, not hospital employees. A board certified and practicing emergency medicine physician testified, as the hospital's expert witness, that the nurses met the standard of care.

R.K.'s expert was a physician who did not work in acute care. The court determined that his expert witness was not qualified by training and experience to testify about the specialty of emergency care. This meant that R.K. gave the court no basis to support his claims of negligence, and he lost his lawsuit.

*Kunkel, et al. v. Universal Health Services of Rancho Springs, Inc. E0532776 2012 Cal. App. Unpub. LEXIS 3649.

delegate the remaining nursing duties to staff members with adequate education, training, and experience. Box 8-6 addresses issues of concern to the floating nurse.

### Negligent Supervision

Negligent supervision is vicarious liability claimed when a supervisor fails to reasonably supervise people under his or her direction. For example, if a nurse rotates to an unfamiliar unit and informs the charge nurse that he or she has never worked in critical care, it would be unreasonable for the charge nurse to ask the floating nurse to perform invasive monitoring. If the charge nurse did assign such responsibilities to the floater and a patient injury resulted, the charge nurse could be held accountable to the patient for negligent supervision.

### "Captain of the Ship" Doctrine vs. Rule of Personal Liability

At one time, the physician was viewed as the "captain of the ship" in relation to the nurse. Therefore, the nurse was expected to follow any order from the physician. This doctrine has largely been replaced by a legal concept known as

the *rule of personal liability*. As a result, nurses are responsible for making sound decisions by virtue of their own specialized education, training, and experience. A critical care nurse today who is unsure about whether a physician's order is safe or appropriate should not follow it as a matter of course, but should seek clarification from the physician or, if needed, from the nursing supervisor. Box 8-7 presents a case study related to the rule of personal liability.

### The Questionable Medical Order

The questionable medical order is a difficult situation for nurses, who frequently feel that their employment may be threatened if they do not follow the order of a physician. However, an order that is patently wrong can harm the patient if it is followed. A secondary consequence can be liability for the physician, the nurse, and the hospital (as the employer) if the patient suffers harm as a direct result of the order. Both ethics and professional preservation (where can a critical care nurse work without a license?) argue the wisdom of refusing to obey orders in some situations.

A policy statement should exist in procedures or by directive that indicates the manner of resolving the issue of the "questionable" medical order. This is important for all medical orders, but particularly for those given for critically ill patients where unusual doses of medications are frequently ordered. The nurse who questions an order should express his or her specific reasons for concern to the physician who wrote the order. This initial approach frequently results either in an explanation of the order and a medical justification for the order in the patient's medical record, or in an alteration of the order based on additional information from the nurse. If this approach is unsuccessful, many hospitals require that the attending physician or the nursing supervisor be notified. Others have a policy that the chief of the service must be consulted about questionable orders. If these options are unavailable or are unsuccessful, a critical care nurse or any other nurse can refuse to give a medication, and should if patient harm is the expected result.

## Establishment of Protocols

If the critical care nurse is required to perform medical acts and is not under the direct and immediate supervision of the delegating physician, the activities must be based on established protocols. These protocols should be created by the medical and nursing departments and should be reviewed for compliance with the state's NPA. Protocols must be reviewed frequently so health care professionals can make sure that they reflect current medical and nursing regulations and standards of care. In the event of a malpractice suit, the critical care protocols and procedures can be introduced as evidence to help establish the applicable standard of care. Although it is important that protocols provide direction, excessive detail restricts the critical care nurse's flexibility when selecting a proper course of action and is more likely to be different from actual practice, increasing the liability risk of the nurses and the institution.

## Liability for Defective Medical Equipment

A medical device, defined as virtually anything used in patient care that is not a drug, includes intricate pieces of equipment (eg, intra-aortic balloon pumps, endotracheal tubes, pacemakers, defibrillators), along with less complicated ones, such as bedpans, suture materials, and tampons. Before 1976, medical devices were unregulated; since 1976, the U.S. Food and Drug Administration (FDA) within HHS has regulated medical devices sold in the United States. The Safe Medical Devices Act of 1990 requires user facilities, which include hospitals and ambulatory surgery facilities, but not physician offices, to report to the manufacturer medical device malfunctions that result in serious illness, injury, or death to a patient. They are also required to report to the FDA malfunctions that result in a patient's death. A serious illness or injury includes not only a life-threatening injury or illness but also an injury that requires "immediate medical or surgical intervention to preclude permanent impairment of a body function or permanent damage to a body structure."[3] Therefore, the rupture of an intra-aortic balloon pump that requires that the balloon-dependent patient immediately be transported to the operating room for removal and replacement of the device is a reportable event. Nursing and other staff must now participate in reporting device malfunctions, including those associated with user error, to a designated hospital department. Personnel in that area are usually responsible for determining which malfunctions engender an obligation to report and to whom they should be reported.

In 2009 the Secretary of HHS directed the FDA commissioner to issue regulations for class III devices, those with the greatest risk to harm patients, to ensure that they are approved through the most stringent premarket review process.[4] There is a duty not to use equipment that is patently defective. If the equipment suddenly ceases to do what it was intended to do, makes unusual noises, or has a history

---

**BOX 8-8** **Case Study: Defective Equipment and Negligence***

P.B. had severe heart failure and underwent HeartMate II Left Ventricular Assistive Device (LVAD) placement surgery. The nurse gave postoperative instructions to P.B. and his wife on the alarms the LVAD could emit, stating that intermittent alarms were not life threatening, but continuous alarms were.

One month post-LVAD surgery, Thoratec Corporation, the manufacturer of the HeartMate II, issued a warning notice that the device "may require a reoperation to replace the pump." PB was not informed about the warning notice.

Mrs. B. testified that the night before her husband died, they "heard a lot [of] little beep[s], light beep[s]" and that they checked all of the machine's systems, which seemed to be working properly. In the morning the same alarms appeared and they changed Mr. B.'s "controller." With the change of controller, they heard a noise coming from the controller and nothing was being displayed on the power base to indicate a problem. They called the nurse and requested she call them back. A few hours following their call, the nurse called them back and Mrs. B. placed the telephone up to the equipment in order for the nurse to hear the beeps. During the call, P.B. complained of dizziness, and the nurse instructed Mrs. B. to keep her husband on battery power while she ascertained the nature of the problem. She assured them not to worry unless they heard a loud beep, which would mean Mrs. B. should take her husband to the hospital. The nurse said she would call the manufacturer for additional information.

Shortly after Mrs. B. spoke with the nurse, the LVAD sounded a loud beep and a red light was displayed. Despite a prompt 911 call by Mrs. B., her husband died. Mrs. B. filed suit against the LVAD manufacturer and the U.S. government as the employer of the nurse and cardiac surgeon, alleging they were negligent in failing to alert the family about the problems with the LVAD.

The court found that the nurse and surgeon were both liable for malpractice because they failed to reasonably inform Mr. and Mrs. B. about the device's difficulties. The government moved to dismiss the case because Mrs. B. had not secured the testimony of an expert witness to establish a breach of the standard of care. However, the court applied the state law's "common knowledge exception" to the expert witness requirement, and upheld judgment in favor of P.B.'s wife. The estate also settled a parallel case against the LVAD manufacturer.

*Bush v. United States of America. No. 14-30896. 802 F.3d 680; 2015 U.S. App. LEXIS 16594.

---

of malfunction and has not been repaired, the hospital could be liable for damage caused by it. Likewise, the nurses could be liable if they know or should know of these problems and use the equipment anyway. The case presented in Box 8-8 involved liability for defective equipment.

## Patient Decision-Making Autonomy

Laws protecting patient autonomy require that patients receive enough information to make an informed, intelligent decision to accept or reject a proposed treatment. This is called *informed consent*. It can be especially challenging for nurses caring for patients who are critically ill. Obtaining informed consent from the patient, or from the family or designated proxy in the case of a patient who is not competent, is the responsibility of the caregiver who is ordering the care, usually a physician. The nurse is frequently asked to witness the signing of the consent form. In these cases, the nurse is merely attesting that the signature on the consent form is that of the patient or the patient's surrogate decision maker. When the nurse actually witnesses a physician's explanation concerning the nature of the proposed treatment, the risks and benefits of the treatment, alternative treatments, and potential consequences if the patient or surrogate decides to do nothing, the nurse may place a note in the nurse's notes or designated part of the patient's record stating, "consent procedure witnessed." This information may be vital in the rare case in which the patient or family alleges that the caregiver failed to provide informed consent.

## Advance Directives: Living Wills and Powers of Attorney

*Advance directives* are legal documents that preserve a patient's right to determine his or her care by permitting the patient to make decisions about health care ahead of time, in case the patient becomes incompetent to make decisions later. Incompetence can occur due to illness, age, or trauma, or by court determination. If a patient is deemed incompetent, the nurse must identify the patient's surrogate decision maker and contact the surrogate to make health care decisions on the patient's behalf.

If the patient's surrogate is not designated in writing, state law identifies the appropriate family members to make decisions. The surrogate should refer to the patient's advance directives and any other known wishes for guidance. This situation can become complex, especially when the surrogate decision maker disagrees with the advice of the physician or other caregiver, with the wishes stated by the patient in an advance directive or otherwise, or with another surrogate, which can occur in a situation where the patient's children, parents, or siblings share this responsibility. While the nurse should not implement procedures that he or she identifies as unethical, neither nurses nor physicians can substitute their judgment for the patient's right to make the decision about accepting or rejecting available procedures.

A *living will* is a written directive from a competent patient to family and health care team members concerning the patient's wishes in the event the he or she is unable to express these wishes in the future. A living will only applies to the limited situations that it describes, which may not include the particular decision that must be made. A living will becomes effective only if the patient is both terminally ill, or permanently comatose and incompetent to communicate his wishes. Consequently, when the patient is critically ill or temporarily unable to make health care decisions, the living will may not be operative.

To provide broader coverage, patients must prepare a *durable power of attorney for health care*, a legal document that allows the patient to appoint a surrogate decision maker while he or she is still competent. The surrogate, also known as a health care agent or proxy, allows a trusted friend or relative to make treatment and health care decisions in the event that the patient is not able to do so.

Savvy patients will prepare both a living will and the durable power of attorney for health care. This ensures that the decision maker's decisions will be as close as possible to what the patient wants. Many advance directives give the health care agent specific instructions concerning health matters.

For example, the advance directive may provide instructions concerning artificial nutrition and hydration, or it may outline specific treatments, such as a "no code" status under specified circumstances.

In response to a federal statute referred to as the Patient Self-Determination Act of 1991,[5] all 50 states have statutes that allow patients to execute living wills, durable powers of attorney for health care, and advance directives. However, each state may place unique requirements on the drafting of these documents. Some states require that the directive be notarized. Other states mandate that a state-appointed ombudsman outlines the pros and cons associated with the advance directive counsel the patient. Witness requirements also vary from state to state. Consequently, it is important to know the laws concerning advance directives that apply in your state. An excellent starting point is the web page of the National Hospice and Palliative Care Organization (caringinfo.org), where you can download advance directives and instructions from each state. The Web site of the American Association of Retired Persons (aarp.org) provides lay people and health care providers with up-to-date information about advance planning for health care as well.

In most states, it is likely that a recent living will would be taken as evidence of what the patient would have wanted had he or she been competent when the decision was presented. Although there have not been any cases concerning a written living will, there have been several involving patients who had expressed wishes orally about life-sustaining measures.

## Issues That Involve Life-Support Measures

Several basic issues regarding refusal and termination of treatment can involve the critical care nurse. Do not resuscitate (DNR) orders, refusal of treatment for religious reasons, advance directives, and withdrawal of life support all fall into this category.

## Do Not Resuscitate Orders

Cardiopulmonary resuscitation (CPR) success rates for those receiving in-hospital care are variable and are affected by patient environment and resuscitative factors.[6] However, CPR is not appropriate for all patients who experience a cardiac arrest, because it is highly invasive and may constitute a "positive violation of an individual's right to die with dignity." Furthermore, CPR may not be indicated when the illness is terminal and irreversible and when the patient can gain no benefit.

Prestigious authorities (eg, the President's Commission for the Study of Ethical Problems in Medicine and Biomedical and Behavioral Research; hereafter "the President's Commission") have recommended that hospitals have an explicit policy on the practice of writing and implementing DNR orders.[7] Most hospitals and medical societies, and some states, have published DNR policies.[8]

Whether to resuscitate any patient is a decision that is made with the attending physician, the patient, and the family, although critical care nurses and other nurses often have substantial input into the decision. However, in general, the consent of a competent patient or the patient surrogate is required when a DNR decision is made and the order is written.

Once the DNR decision has been made, the order should be written, signed, and dated by the responsible physician. It should be reviewed periodically; hospital policies may require review every 24 to 72 hours. The more informal methods of designating patients with whom CPR is not to be undertaken can lead to uncertainty and inappropriate responses if an arrest occurs. If an arrest occurs in an emergency department or in another situation in which a formal DNR decision has not been made and written, the presumption of the medical and nursing staffs should be in favor of intervention, and a code should be called. A "slow code" (in which the nurse takes excessive time to call or the health care team takes its time responding) is never permissible. Either CPR is indicated, or it is not.

Courts sometimes become involved in DNR decisions and provide legal guidance through case law. In 2004, a California court ruled that a physician may lawfully write a DNR order for a minor patient for whom there is no lifesaving or life-prolonging treatment. This case involved a DNR order for Christian, an 11-year-old boy with cystic fibrosis who developed the flu and then pneumonia after his parents had rejected the flu shot for him. A nurse testified that she was present during the discussion between the doctor and the parents, and that both parents agreed to the DNR order "in view of (Christian's) chronic irreversible condition."[9] Box 8-9 presents another case in which the courts became involved, where there was a dispute between the hospital and the family related to a patient's care.

It is estimated that the majority of Americans do not have an advance directive.[10] An advance directive can facilitate difficult decisions. It is also important for patients to speak with their families and their attending physician, nurse practitioner, or designated provider concerning end-of-life decisions.

## Right to Refuse Treatment for Religious Reasons

Some courts are unwilling to rule against the religious-based decisions of a patient to refuse treatment, but they are most likely to do so if the welfare of a dependent child is at stake.

---

**BOX 8-9** | **Case Study: Discontinuation of Ventilator Support\***

H.M. had no living will. Her husband, C.M., stated that she had asked him to make decisions regarding life support if she were ever not able to. She also had told him that she wanted to continue life support and remain alive.

Following surgery on her wrist, H.M. developed an infection and was placed on a ventilator. Staff repeatedly asked C.M. about removing H.M.'s ventilator. C.M. refused, and instructed them to never "pull the plug."

After about 3 months the ventilator was removed, and H.M. died. Her husband filed a lawsuit against the hospital, based on the premise that the hospital had "ignored the wishes" of H.M. The claims against the hospital included medical malpractice, H.M.'s pain and suffering, wrongful death, C.M.'s loss of consortium, and intentional infliction of emotional distress on C.M. and his children. The hospital asked the courts to give summary judgment in its favor. The court agreed to do that on most of the allegations, but the malpractice claim remained, and was to be tried before a jury. This case is still in review, and the final outcome is not available.

*Marsala, et al. v. Yale-New Haven Hospital, Inc. AANCV12601861, AANCV126011711. 2015 Conn. Super. LEXIS 588.

---

For example, in one case, the Connecticut Supreme Court found that a hospital could not "thrust unwanted medical care on a patient who. . . competently and clearly denied that care." Critical care nurses need to consult the hospital's risk management department or legal counsel in such situations to ensure proper handling of these types of legal issues.[11] There are exceptions to the informed consent requirements. For example, an emergency situation in which time and circumstances create critical barriers does not require informed consent before initial procedures are implemented. A patient can also waive the right to informed consent by stating that he or she does not want information about a proposed treatment or procedure. Box 8-10 illustrates a case involving a Jehovah's Witness patient related to blood transfusion.

---

**BOX 8-10** | **Case Study: Lifesaving Transfusion for a Jehovah's Witness\***

G.R., a 55-year-old woman of Jehovah's Witness faith with end-stage renal disease, received a kidney transplant and was discharged after 2 days. She returned to the hospital about a week later complaining of abdominal pain. A CT-guided needle biopsy confirmed antibody-mediated vascular rejection, and she began plasmapheresis treatment, also known to affect coagulation parameters and clotting factors.

The next day G.R.'s hemoglobin and hematocrit levels were low, and an abdominal CT scan confirmed a large mass. She was taken to the operating room, where the transplanted kidney was removed because her bleeding and refusal of blood precluded its survival. Her husband confirmed her rejection of a blood transfusion because of her religious faith, even to save her life. The operation was completed and G.R. was taken to recovery. She died the next day.

G.R.'s husband sued the hospital and physicians for negligence and medical malpractice, alleging breaches of the standard of care, including treatments and failure to make an earlier diagnosis of internal bleeding. He argued that the doctors caused G.R.'s predicament, requiring her to make the decision about blood transfusions. Experts for both sides agreed that G.R. would have lived if she had accepted a blood transfusion, meaning that, under an objective standard, it was unreasonable for her to refuse the life-saving treatment.

The court held that the Free Exercise and Establishment Clauses of the First Amendment of the Constitution did not permit a jury to subjectively decide whether G.R.'s religious-based decision to prohibit transfusion was reasonable, because that required the jury to decide whether her religion was reasonable. Instead, the jury could only determine whether the refusal was objectively reasonable.

A concurring opinion pointed out that that this conclusion reflects the guarantee of every person's right to freely exercise religious beliefs of his or her choice. In this case, G.R. and her family made a choice to forgo the blood transfusion that would have saved her life. Choices have consequences. "However unfortunate the nature of that consequence, it does not provide a basis for shifting responsibility for the consequence of that choice to others. . ... The choice was hers, and hers alone, to make, and with that choice came the consequences that naturally flowed from it, irrespective of the righteousness of the reasons for which she made the choice." Because no evidence supported the claim that the hospital or the physicians were responsible for G.R.'s death, summary judgment was upheld on appeal, and the claims against the hospital and the health care team were dismissed.

*Rozier v. Grnager, et al, No. 309528 303 Mich. App. 587; 844 N.W.2d 485; 2015 Mich. App. LEXIS 39.

## Landmark Legal Cases on Withdrawal of Treatment

What constitutes life support, when these measures must be used, and when they may be terminated are issues that have been raised in many court cases. However, the law in these areas is still developing and will continue to do so as each state creates its own guidelines and as technology continues to introduce new possibilities.

In the matter of *Schiavo v. Schiavo*,[12] the United States was drawn into a legal and emotional battle over the issue of the right to die and, barring advance directives, who may speak for an unconscious patient. Theresa (Terri) Schiavo was in a vegetative state for 13 years. In 2003, Ms. Schiavo's husband, Michael, petitioned to cease his wife's feeding and hydration over the objections of her parents and brother. In response, Terri's parents, Robert and Mary Schindler, led a battle before the Florida State Courts, the U.S. Courts of Appeal, the Florida State Legislature and Executive Branch, the U.S. Congress, the White House, and, eventually, the U.S. Supreme Court.[13] Aside from the legal activities, the parties to the action also presented Terri's circumstances and future before the court of public opinion.

Although it is unusual for this type of case to be heard in the U.S. Supreme Court, lower court involvement in this type of situation is not unusual. When a disabled person is unable to understand and coherently speak on his or her own behalf, the law requires that health care providers first obtain the patient's personal advance directives. Courts have repeatedly struggled over who should make decisions about the disabled patient's care when there is no advance directive and relatives cannot agree on the appropriate plan of care for the patient, such as occurred in the Schiavo case.

Initially the Schiavo case was representative of a typical guardianship action. The petitioner (husband Michael Schiavo) petitioned the court to act on behalf of the alleged disabled patient (his wife, Terri). Notice of the proposed order to name Mr. Schiavo as Terri's guardian was given to all interested persons, including her parents, Mr. and Mrs. Schindler.[12] In addition, courts may appoint a temporary *guardian ad litem*, charged with the duty to represent the interests of the alleged disabled. The temporary guardian ad litem, usually an attorney, is an independent, disinterested party whose responsibilities are to review the medical records, interview all medical providers, interview the petitioner (ie, Mr. Schiavo) and any interested persons, and, most importantly, interview the alleged disabled as to his or her mental and physical capacity. The temporary guardian ad litem reports independently to the court on his or her findings of the status of the alleged disabled.

In the Schiavo case, a custodial hearing was held allowing the petitioner, witnesses, and any other interested persons to testify as to (1) the competency of the alleged disabled, (2) whether the alleged disabled would be best served with a guardianship, and (3) who would be best to act as *permanent* guardian ad litem. In deciding these issues, the courts place great weight on the findings of the temporary guardian ad litem.

Michael Schiavo prevailed in maintaining his position as permanent guardian ad litem of Terri[13] and her tube feeding was discontinued. As a result of this and other cases, families throughout the nation became more aware that they might be faced with the awful possibility of being pitted emotionally, legally, and monetarily against each other when advance directives are not executed.

Nurses, particularly those working in critical care areas, are frequently confronted with patients who are incompetent to understand the nature of their care. Nurses are instrumental in educating patients, families, friends, and society about the importance of understanding and executing advance directives. From an attorney's perspective, the consensus is, "Pay me a little now to prepare a valid advance directive, or pay me dearly when we need to litigate guardianship and end-of-life issues."

Given the regularity with which life-support decisions must be made in health care facilities, it is remarkable that it was not until 1976 that the first case, *In re Quinlan*, focused national attention on the "right to die" controversy.

The cases concern competent minors and adults who have a disease or condition that would eventually be terminal. States have not been consistent in their decisions, even when the situations are arguably similar. For example, the New Jersey court in the case of Karen Ann Quinlan, a 21-year-old woman in a persistent vegetative state, held that the decision about treatment is in the hands of the patient's guardian in consultation with the hospital ethics committee.[14] The President's Commission stated (p. 6) that judicial review of these decisions should be reserved for occasions when "adjudication is clearly required by state law or when concerned parties have disagreements that they cannot resolve over matters of substantial import."[15]

Box 8-11 presents the case of Nancy Cruzan related to withdrawal of a feeding tube. Although the Cruzan case is still applicable law, the way in which this landmark case has been interpreted and implemented has been extremely variable at state court levels. This case received much publicity, but it did not change the law in any state except Missouri. Most states continue to permit surrogate decision making by relatives and

---

**BOX 8-11** | **Case Study: Right to Restrict Food and Fluids**

Nancy Cruzan, a young woman who suffered anoxic brain damage in an automobile accident, remained in a persistent vegetative state in Missouri and was fed by gastrostomy. After rehabilitation was unsuccessful, Ms. Cruzan's parents (as coguardians) requested withdrawal of the feeding tube. When the employees of the residential rehabilitation center where Ms. Cruzan was receiving care refused to withdraw the feedings, her parents sought judicial review of their request. After testimony, the trial court approved the parents' request.

On appeal, the Missouri Supreme Court reversed the lower court. First, it held that Missouri law does not permit surrogate decision making in decisions of this importance. For a person to exercise the right to terminate artificial feeding in Missouri, that person must have previously expressed his or her wishes, either orally or in writing. Evidence of those wishes had to meet a relatively high evidentiary standard, a standard that the court held had been met in the lower court proceeding.

This case was appealed to the U.S. Supreme Court, and in 1990, it was affirmed on constitutional grounds.* After the decision was issued, the Cruzans returned to the Missouri lower court and presented further evidence (through additional witnesses) about what their daughter had expressed while competent. The lower court found that they had presented clear and convincing evidence and affirmed the rights of the coguardians to authorize withdrawal of the feeding tube.

*Cruzan v. Director, Missouri Department of Health, et al, III L Ed2d 224, 110 S Ct 2841, 1990.

require a lower evidentiary standard than that required in Missouri. Also note that, unlike the Schiavo case described previously, family members were all in agreement that Ms. Cruzan's artificial nutrition and hydration should be discontinued.

The right to consent to treatment is meaningless without the right to refuse treatment before or after it is initiated. In recent years, as health care providers have become more comfortable recommending rejection or termination of treatment in selected cases, they have met resistance from some families who wish to continue treatment no matter what the chance of success. Although no law or legal principle requires that extraordinary, but clearly futile, treatment be provided, it is probably also true that health care providers have little legal recourse against families who refuse to withdraw life support—that is, unless the patient has left written indications of his or her wishes before incompetence. This may change as society reexamines the allocation of limited resources in health care.

In most states, problems of terminating treatment need not be resolved in court. This is not an easy decision, but decisions regarding treatment or nontreatment that meet accepted medical standards and with which the patient concurs are made virtually every day in health care settings such as critical care. Hospital ethics committees typically play a crucial role in such circumstances.

A distinction should be made between termination of treatment and termination of care. Ending treatment is not the same as giving up. Patients who are not being "treated" for their terminal condition require competent and sensitive nursing and medical care. Palliative care provides pain relief and symptom management, and a better quality of life for those nearing the end of life and their families. The duty to provide good nursing care does not end with the decision to move from treatment for cure to providing comfort care and (ideally) timely referral to hospice.

## Brain Death

In 1968, an ad hoc committee at Harvard Medical School established the Harvard criteria for determining brain death, or irreversible coma. In 1981, the President's Commission for the Study of Ethical Problems in Medicine and Biomedical and Behavioral Research published *Defining Death*. The Commission recommended a uniform statute defining death, to address "general physiological standards rather than medical criteria and tests, which will change with advances in biomedical knowledge and refinements in technique."[16] All states have laws addressing the definition of death in the state. Some states adopted the Harvard criteria by statute, whereas other states enacted legislation that defines brain death in broader, less restrictive terms. Some states use brain

death as the sole criterion; other states rely on a number of factors, such as response to pain and cessation of cardiac function. It is important that the nurse know the legal definition of death in any state where he or she is practicing, although such a determination typically rests with the patient's attending physician and may require the concurrence of other consulting physicians.

A patient who is brain-dead is legally dead, and there is no legal duty to continue to treat him or her. It is not necessary to obtain court approval to discontinue life support on a patient who is brain-dead. Furthermore, although it can be desirable to obtain family permission to discontinue treatment of a brain-dead patient, it is not a legal requirement. Before terminating life support, physicians and nurses should determine whether the patient is an organ donor.

## Organ Donation

Every state in the United States has a law based on the Uniform Anatomical Gift Act. The statutes establish the legality of organ donation by people and their families, and set procedures for making and accepting the gift of an organ. Every state also has some provision to enable people to consent to organ donation using a designated place on a driver's license. More recently, many states have enacted "required request" laws. These laws attempt to increase the supply of organs for transplantation by requiring hospital personnel to ask patients' families about an organ gift at the time of the patient's death.

## Clinical Applicability Challenges

### SHORT ANSWER QUESTIONS

1. Nurse Jacqui's patient was admitted with a history of seizures and was found later out of his bed and on the floor. The patient's guardians sued for malpractice, alleging failure to keep the bedrails up and failure to monitor. How can Jacqui defend against these charges?

2. Nurse Jacqui's patient was diagnosed with disseminated intravascular coagulation. His doctor ordered that he was not to be administered heparin, but another order included IV heparin flush q 12 hours, and Jacqui administered the heparin. What is Jacqui's status in this situation?

3. Nurse Jacqui believes her colleague has been taking pain medication and diverting it to personal use or selling it instead of administering it to the patients for whom it was ordered. How should she respond?

4. Nurse Jacqui's patient was just admitted to the Emergency Department and is unable to communicate, has no one else with him, and delay in treatment would likely result in serious harm to the patient. How should Jacqui respond?

### WANT TO KNOW MORE?

A wide variety of resources to enhance your learning and understanding of this chapter are available on thePoint.

You will find:

- References
- Selected readings
- NCLEX-style review questions
- Internet resources
- And more!

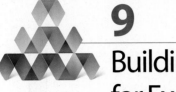

# 9

# Building a Professional Practice Model for Excellence in Critical Care Nursing

JANIE HEATH

## LEARNING OBJECTIVES

*Based on the content in this chapter, the reader should be able to:*

1. Discuss nursing professionalism and nursing excellence.

2. Recognize characteristics of professional development.

3. Explore personal and professional attributes to build a professional practice model of critical care nursing excellence.

In today's fast-paced critical care environment, nurses respond to the needs of patients and families who have entered a chaotic and frightening world of illness, trauma, and pain. Often, finding the time for professional growth can be challenging. Building a professional practice of excellence requires a "passion" to profoundly affect the lives of patients and families. At the same time, it requires advancing the critical care nursing profession through evidence-based practice, best practice models of care, or both. This chapter discusses how a professional practice for excellence in critical care nursing can be built with the attributes of values, vision, mastery, passion, action, and balance as the framework.

## Defining the Critical Care Nurse

Like their patients and patients' families, critical care nurses are an exceptional and diverse group of people. "Knowledgeable," "highly skilled," and "caring" are a few of the professional attributes that can be applied to critical care nurses. However, the term *nursing professionalism* may bring to mind different images, especially to health care consumers who have seen nurses portrayed in television series such as *ER*, *House*, and *Nurse Jackie*. Fortunately, the face of nursing is changing, with more nurses filling local, state, and national seats of legislation and organizational boards. The image has clearly changed since the days when Kalisch and Kalisch[1] first reported that "90% of the public thought nurses were nice ladies who help doctors" to the public seeing or experiencing the high level of intellectual, interpersonal, ethical, and clinical skill abilities of nurses.

Critical care nurses know all too well that responding to lethal dysrhythmias, administering blood products, and weaning patients from ventilators is more about having a specialized body of knowledge, competent skills, and clinical experience in holistic nursing than about just "helping doctors." For both the novice and the experienced critical care nurse, the journey of nursing professionalism and nursing excellence goes beyond the bedside skills required to take care of the sickest and most vulnerable patients and families. Critical care nursing started being recognized as a specialty when the first intensive care units (ICUs) emerged in the

1950s, yet Buresh and Gordon[2] have found increasing evidence of a large communication gap between the profession and the greater public. To sustain recognition as a respected and valued profession, critical care nurses must boldly speak up to define who they are and what they do.

The annual demographic membership survey conducted by the American Association of Critical-Care Nurses (AACN),[3] the world's largest specialty nursing organization, provides a starting point for defining who critical care nurses are. Since 1969, the AACN has been serving the needs of more than 500,000 nurses who care for critically ill patients and their families. The majority of the AACN's approximately 100,000 members (43%) are younger than 40 years of age and have a bachelor of science in nursing (58%) (Fig. 9-1A), and 26% have been in critical care practice for more than 21 years (Fig. 9-1B).[3] Although membership continues to be predominantly female (86%), the number of men in critical care nursing (14%) is increasing.[3] The largest ethnic background represented was Caucasian (75%), followed by Asian (12%), African American (5%), Hispanic (4%), and Pacific Islander (1%).[3] Of interest, the AACN membership data are consistent with the average findings of today's 3 million registered nurses (RNs) reported in the initial findings from the 2012 National Sample Survey of Registered Nurses.[4]

These data reflect trends and issues that have policy and advocacy implications, helping to drive decision making that affects critical care nursing practice, patients and families, and health care systems. Currently, the majority of AACN members (17%) work in ICU settings; 14% work in progressive care settings; 11% in combined ICU and coronary care unit (CCU) settings; 9% in cardiovascular–surgical ICU settings; 9% in combined medical ICU and medical–surgical ICU; 4% in surgical ICU; and 4% in pediatric ICU. The remaining top categories make up less than 4% of the total and include the emergency department, recovery room/post–anesthesia care unit, trauma unit, and neuro/neurosurgical ICU (Fig. 9-2A).[3] The vast majority of the AACN members surveyed (58%) have positions providing direct care as staff nurses (Fig. 9-2B). The AACN membership data are consistent with the average findings of Kirchhoff and Dahl's[5] national survey of facilities and units that provide critical care. Their study revealed that

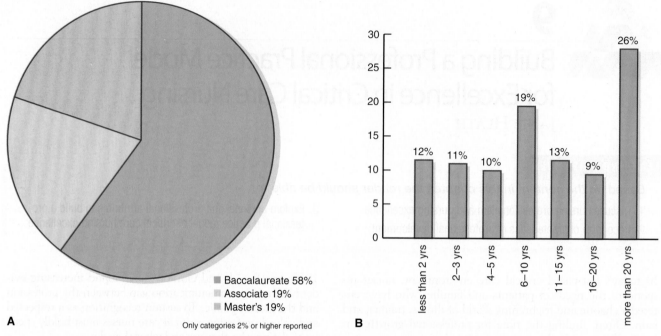

**A** Only categories 2% or higher reported

■ Baccalaureate 58%
■ Associate 19%
■ Master's 19%

**B**

**FIGURE 9-1** Mastery of the profession. **A:** The nursing degrees earned by critical care nurses. **B:** Years of experience in critical care nursing. (From American Association of Critical-Care Nurses: 2014 Demographics. Retrieved July 10, 2015, from http://www.aacn.org.)

74% of the facilities participating in the study were nongovernment, not-for-profit organizations with a mean of 217 operating beds and 13,000 admissions per year.[5]

## Defining Nursing Professionalism

The struggle to define nursing professionalism expands beyond critical care environments. There continues to be ongoing dialogue about whether nursing is a true profession. For more than two decades, Kelly has emphasized that the status of nursing as a profession is important because it reflects the value society places on the work of nurses.[6] However, some think that because entry into nursing practice does not require a baccalaureate degree, it is, at best, an emerging profession that requires new models of nursing education.[7] Widespread efforts are underway to optimize opportunities for higher education in nursing to meet the landmark 2010 Institute of Medicine recommendation for 80% of the nursing workforce to be educated at the baccalaureate level by 2020.[8,9] Accelerated online RN-to-BSN programs, clinical nurse leader programs, and Doctor of Nursing Practice programs are preparing nurses to lead change and advance health, but controversy remains about whether progress to meet full-fledged professional status is possible with current models of nursing education.[10]

One of the first definitions of professionalism came from Flexner,[11] who wrote the classic Flexner Report in the early 1900s to reform medical education. Flexner defines professionalism as a process by which an occupation achieves professional status. Although other professions have developed their own criteria, Flexner's work remains the benchmark and foundation for many. In 1981, Kelly was the first to expand his work for the nursing profession by providing a theoretical framework from which professional nursing characteristics are defined today[6] (Box 9-1).

One legendary nurse leader, Margretta Styles, argued that the professionalism of nursing can only be achieved through the "professionhood" of its members.[7] Like Kelly, Styles believes there must be a sense of social significance, commitment to professional performance, and appreciation of collegiality and collectivity.[7] However, as Styles approached the end of her nursing career, she proposed a new term to describe the work of nurses: *professionalist*.[7] In her words, "professionalists strive to build a solid foundation for their calling—an ethical, academic, political, and socioeconomic foundation to serve as the underpinning for a strong profession to evolve and serve" (p 89).[7]

Researchers have studied professionalism among critical care nurses as well. In 1994, Holl[12] investigated such critical care nursing characteristics as professional beliefs, decision making, level of education, membership in professional nursing organizations, and certification. Holl[12] found that nurses who continue their education and belong to professional organizations are more likely than others to be independent thinkers and to participate in creative problem solving. In a similar study, Heath et al[13] found that there was a high level of "passion about nursing and promoting the profession," and that self-motivation was the leading influential factor for fostering individual professional development among critical care nurses. Other professional development characteristics evaluated included participation in employing agency committees, community service, and recognition of peers.[13] Several of the professional characteristics initially identified by Kelly and studied by others[14,15] are identified in this chapter as hallmarks of excellence for critical care nursing practice.

## Defining Nursing Excellence

The term *excellence* can be difficult to define, similar to the expression *best practice*. No single definition captures the

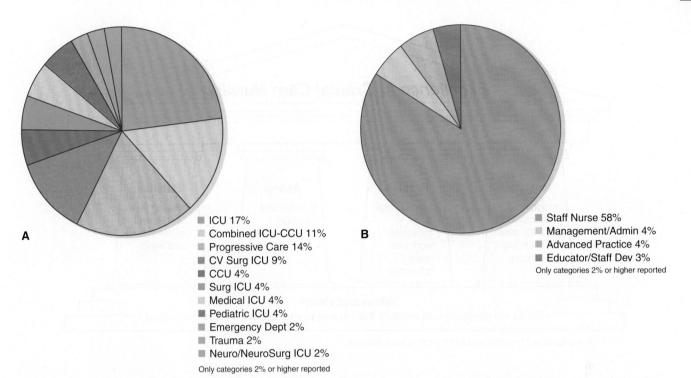

FIGURE 9-2   Who are critical care nurses? **A:** Practice settings for critical care nurses. **B:** The positions held by critical care nurses. (From American Association of Critical-Care Nurses: 2014 Demographics. Retrieved July 10, 2015, from http://www.aacn.org.)

**A:**
- ICU 17%
- Combined ICU-CCU 11%
- Progressive Care 14%
- CV Surg ICU 9%
- CCU 4%
- Surg ICU 4%
- Medical ICU 4%
- Pediatric ICU 4%
- Emergency Dept 2%
- Trauma 2%
- Neuro/NeuroSurg ICU 2%

Only categories 2% or higher reported

**B:**
- Staff Nurse 58%
- Management/Admin 4%
- Advanced Practice 4%
- Educator/Staff Dev 3%

Only categories 2% or higher reported

---

**BOX 9-1**   **Kelly's Characteristics of a Profession**

- The services provided are vital to humanity and the welfare of society.
- There is a special body of knowledge that is continually enlarged through research.
- The services provided involve intellectual activities where accountability is a strong feature.
- Practitioners are educated in institutions of higher learning.
- Practitioners are motivated by service, and work is an important component of their lives.
- There is a code of ethics to guide the decisions and conduct of practitioners.
- There is an association that encourages and supports standards of practice.

Data from Kelly L: Dimensions of Professional Nursing. New York, NY: Macmillan, 1981; and Joel L: Kelly's Dimensions of Professional Nursing, 10th ed. New York, NY: McGraw-Hill, 2011.

---

essence of excellence for everyone. For some, excellence can be defined as a "sixth sense"—for example, the way a critical care nurse sees a patient going "bad" before laboratory values or hemodynamic numbers are known may be evidence of excellence. Excellence may also be demonstrated by the way a critical care nurse hears an $S_3$ or $S_4$ heart sound before a patient becomes symptomatic, or the way a critical care nurse "feels" the pain of a postoperative patient on neuromuscular blockade without analgesics.

Weston et al[16] define nursing excellence as a dynamic process that is continually redefined and reinforced. They further describe excellence as an ongoing comparison with a standard that one continuously tries to improve.[10] Six attributes of advanced-practice nursing excellence have been identified by Weston et al[16] as values, vision, mastery, passion, action, and balance. These attributes have been

adopted and modified for this chapter to propose a professional practice model for critical care nursing (Fig. 9-3). The foundation for this model consists of strong values and a vision. The supporting structures of the model are composed of mastery, passion, action, and balance. The top of the model captures the essence of the structure: critical care nursing excellence. Each structure of the professional practice model has defining characteristics that are instrumental for ongoing self-reflection, which is necessary to develop and commit to excellence in critical care nursing.

## Values

True excellence is seen when professionals reflect their core values. The values of one's profession, the values of one's employing organization, and one's own personal values are the behaviors that guide professional practice for excellence. The unique contributions that critical care nurses bring to the bedside are often a reflection of an inner core value of caring. It is this deep and personal connection to caring that brings many into the nursing profession. The word *nursing* is derived from the Latin word *nutrire*, which means "to nourish." The term *nurturing* describes an ability to care for, sustain, and provide for another. Critical care nurses are privileged to care for individuals who face life-threatening conditions during the most vulnerable and private times of their lives. It is through this value of altruism (the desire to help others) that critical care nurses have the ability to creatively bridge high-tech and high-touch with everyday practice.

The everyday busyness of critical care nursing is labor intensive, but taking the time to share joyful, painful, and tearful experiences with complex patients and families is the core of the critical care nursing experience. The art of nursing, rather than the science of nursing, is probably the dominant

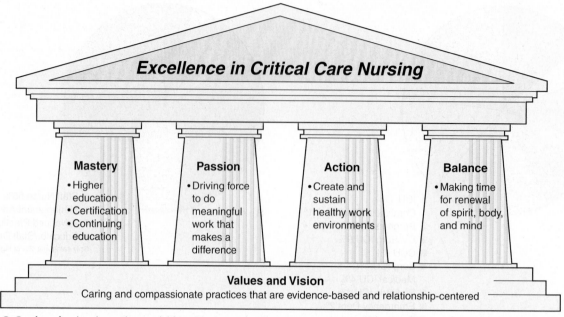

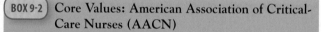

**FIGURE 9-3**   A professional practice model for critical care nursing.

image of nursing for the public. For 12 years in a row, Gallup polls have reported that the public rates nursing as the most honest and ethical profession.[17] In their book *From Silence to Voice*, Buresh and Gordon[2] reported that the Gallup poll results about nurses reflect a paradox. These non-nurse authors discuss how the public holds nurses in the highest regard, even though the public has limited information about the science involved in nursing practice.[2]

The power inherent in the nursing profession is evident when nurses articulate the core values of their profession—not only caring but also evidence-based practice, advocacy, accountability, autonomy, and collaboration. Many believe that nurses have been silent for too long, and that the days of "It is just my job" or "I am just a nurse" need to come to an end.[2,18,19] AACN's presidential themes, such as "Stand Tall," "Together, Stronger, Bolder," "Dare To," "Step Forward," and "Focus the Flame," help empower nurses to make their voices heard for their patients, families, and profession.[20] Strong personal and professional core values at AACN (Box 9-2) inspired a nine-person panel to develop the AACN Healthy Work Environment Standards to help address work environments that tolerate ineffective interpersonal relationships that result in medical errors, ineffective delivery of care, and conflict and stress among health professionals.[19] Creating and sustaining healthy work environments ensure safe patient care and set a path toward the AACN core value to "commit to quality and excellence."[21] Box 9-3 presents a Case Study related to this core value.

## Vision

A clear vision, based on core values, is essential to building a professional practice model of critical care nursing excellence. It requires envisioning the future's possibilities and then taking the challenge of making the vision a reality, as reflected in the Case Study in Box 9-4. Over a decade ago, the AACN made a strategic decision to promote the creation of

**BOX 9-2**   Core Values: American Association of Critical-Care Nurses (AACN)

- **Ethical accountability and integrity** in relationships, organization decisions, and stewardship of resources.
- **Leadership to enable individuals to make their optimal contribution** through lifelong learning, critical thinking, and inquiry.
- **Excellence and innovation** at every level of the organization to advance the profession.
- **Collaboration** to ensure quality patient- and family-focused care.

From American Association of Critical-Care Nurses: Core values. Retrieved July 10, 2015, from http://www.aacn.org/wd/aacninfo/content/mission-vision-values-ethics.pcms?menu=aboutus, with permission.

healthy work environments that embrace a culture of excellence when taking care of acute and critically ill patients.[19] Based on the escalating evidence from the Institute of Medicine and the Joint Commission about unhealthy work environments and how they contribute to medical errors, the AACN had a vision to propose solutions to improve patient safety.[25-27] Through a partnership with VitalSmarts, a national study was conducted to evaluate communication and collaboration challenges among hospital providers of care. The findings of the study indicated a need to develop standards addressing six essential areas: skilled communication, true collaboration, effective decision making, appropriate staffing, meaningful recognition, and authentic leadership.[19]

As risk takers and agents for change, today's critical care nurses are making history by embracing the AACN Healthy Work Environment Standards. Winston Churchill once said, "The pessimist sees difficulty in every opportunity and the optimist sees the opportunity in every difficulty."[22] It is challenging to create and sustain work environments of excellence, especially when there are concerns about nurse-to-patient ratios, mandatory overtime, unionization, and nursing recruitment and retention. It is also difficult to

**BOX 9-3** Case Study

*"Our lives begin to end the day we become silent about things that matter."—Martin Luther King Jr.*[22]

**Reflection on "Values" for Critical Care Nursing Excellence**
"A group of nurses, participating in a focus group for the AACN–VitalSmarts Silence Kills Study, describe a peer as careless and inattentive. Instead of confronting her, they double check her work—sometimes running into patient rooms to retake a blood pressure or redo a safety check. They have 'worked around' this nurse's weaknesses for over a year. The nurses resent her but never talk to her about their concerns, nor do any of the physicians who also avoid her and compensate for her" (p 2).[18] Further data reveal that out of 1,700 health care providers and administrators throughout US hospitals, 84% of physicians and 62% of nurses and other clinical care providers have seen co-workers taking shortcuts that could be dangerous to patients.[22] McCauley summed the significance of the study well by stating, "This research (Silence Kills) validates what our 100,000 constituents have communicated to us as the number one barrier hindering optimal care for patients. Too often, improving workplace communications is seen as a 'soft' issue—the truth is, we must build environments that support and demand greater candor among staff if we are to make a demonstrable impact on patient safety."[23]

Self-reflection
- Do you value communication about competence and accountability?
- Do you value having a healthy work environment where skilled communication protects patients and fosters collaborative relationships?
- What are your values to foster care nursing excellence and make a difference in the lives of the acute and critically ill?

provide critical care nurses with the tools, resources, and support they need to meet patient and family needs effectively and at the same time enhance their own professional growth, learning, and satisfaction. Nursing has a long tradition of taking "bumpy" roads to make a vision reality. No matter how many times nurses fall down and get bruised on the way to reach a vision, they maintain their resilience by having the courage to listen, learn, and act for themselves, their patients, and their professional practice.

## Mastery

Studer,[28] author of *Hardwiring Excellence,* believes that excellence in health care occurs when "employees feel valued, physicians feel their patients are getting great care, and patients feel the service and quality they receive are extraordinary" (p 45). Studer[28] further believes that creating and sustaining a culture of excellence requires the willingness to take individual ownership of problems and opportunities—in other words, to be an owner, not a renter of an organization. To value lifelong learning and to have a vision for personal mastery is essential to building a professional practice model for critical care nursing excellence (see Fig. 9-3).

There are many pathways for personal mastery. Weston et al[16] believe that seeking feedback and peer review for self-improvement is one of the most effective pathways for building mastery. Other pathways for personal mastery include seeking a degree in higher education, making a commitment to ongoing continuing education, and demonstrating competence through certification. The rewards of mastery often go beyond these pathways. Mastery combines expert professional skills with leadership and interpersonal and organizational proficiency, and often leads to the most coveted role of all: the role of mentoring.

The importance of demonstrating personal mastery of knowledge and skills can also be seen in the mounting

**BOX 9.4** Case Study

*"There is no power greater than a community discovering what it cares about."—Margaret Wheatley*[22]

**Reflection on "Vision" for Critical Care Nursing Excellence**
Excerpt from Teri Lynn Kiss, RN, MSN, APRN-BC, 2014–2015 AACN President Speech: "Focus the Flame"
    Remember the excitement of passing boards? Writing RN after my name lit the flame of my dream to make a genuine difference in people's lives. Then one night I was caring for an older postoperative patient who didn't have a good outcome because, plain and simple, I didn't know all I needed to be an effective nurse. I could blame it on the patient's age, multiple comorbidities, even the surgery itself. But in my heart and mind I knew I didn't have the right knowledge, skills, and abilities. I still feel the pain that almost extinguished my flame. Almost, because the experience generated a new lifelong goal—focusing my flame on becoming the best nurse I could be.
    I believe words create worlds, and the following words represent the world I want to help create: "AACN is dedicated to creating a healthcare system driven by the needs of patients and families, where acute and critical care nurses make their optimal contributions." Creating a world requires a huge inner source of energy. It requires fire. Each of us has an internal flame driving our desire for excellence when we make our optimal contribution.

Focus our internal flame, and we prepare ourselves for the future....Think of F-I-R-E as an acronym, and it identifies the aptitude we need to develop to meet tomorrow's demands.

**F**  stands for fearlessness. Fearless people recognize fear, then confront it with brave and smart decisions.
**I**  stands for inquiry. Asking what if and why helps us see beyond where we are by uncovering a trail of new possibilities.
**R**  stands for resilience—the ability to adapt, overcome, and bounce back, which grows from anticipating disruptions and healing after we've been aggrieved.
**E**  stands for engagement. Shifting emphasis from my task to our task, we develop deeper communication and a sense of shared ownership across organizational silos.[24]

Self-reflection
- Do you have a vision to apply the "FIRE aptitude skills" (Fearlessness, Inquiry, Resilience, and Engagement) to advance professional growth and engagement in the work environment?
- Do you have a vision to have a bold voice for a culture in which people hold themselves and others accountable to professional standards and collaborative relationships?
- What is your vision to foster nursing excellence and make a difference in the lives of the acute and critically ill?

evidence about how poor communication and lack of collaboration among health care professionals contribute to medical errors and staff turnover.[18,25,26] The Case Study in Box 9-5 presents a nurse's reflections on this topic. The Silence Kills Study revealed that 88% of physicians and 48% of nurses and other providers work with people who show poor clinical judgment, and unfortunately, fewer than 10% of them confront their colleagues about their concerns.[18] Avoiding crucial conversations about observed incompetent or inappropriate practices, such as violation of infection standards or verbal abuse, impairs patient safety and impedes quality care. It is essential that critical care nurses achieve the personal mastery of knowledge and skills that promotes high-quality health care delivery and patient safety.

To emphasize the importance of validating clinical competency, a landmark white paper documents the benefits that specialty certification brings to the public, employers, and nurses.[28] The document, *Safeguarding the Patient and the Profession: The Value of Critical Care Nurse Certification*, raises awareness about the responsibility nurses have to honor and validate the public's trust for patient safety. The AACN believes that certification validates competency of knowledge, skills, and experience for quality patient care.[25] Consumers of nursing services must be able to recognize the contributions critical care nurses make to ensure high-quality and competent care to patients and families.

---

**BOX 9-5** **Case Study**

*"Education is our passport to the future, for tomorrow belongs to the person who prepares for today."* —Malcolm X[22]

**Reflection on "Mastery" for Critical Care Nursing Excellence**
"At 3:30 AM in a busy ICU, a nurse prepares to give insulin to a patient with an elevated blood glucose level. The sliding scale doses of insulin on the medication sheet are unclear, and the physician's order sheet is difficult to read. From past experience, the nurse knows how late night calls to this physician often result in verbal outbursts and demeaning slurs, no matter how valid the inquiry. Needing to act but not wanting another harassing encounter with the physician, she makes a judgment of the appropriate dose and administers the insulin. Two hours later, she finds the patient completely unresponsive. To treat the critically low blood glucose level, she administers concentrated injections of glucose and calls for additional emergency help. Despite all attempts to restore the patient's brain to consciousness, he never awakens and his brain never functions normally again" (p 10).[19]

Barden summarized this scenario well by stating, "Nurses must be as proficient at handling personal communication as they are in clinical skills. A culture of safety and excellence requires that individual nurses and healthcare organizations make it a priority to develop communication skills that are on par with expert clinical skills."[23]

Self-reflection
• What mastery of knowledge and skills have you achieved to stop verbally abusive behavior in the workplace?
• What mastery of knowledge and skills have you achieved to seek solutions that preserve a nurse's personal integrity and ensure a patient's safety?
• What are you mastering to foster nursing excellence and make a difference in the lives of the acute and critically ill?

---

The Chief Clinical Officer for AACN, Connie Barden, believes that there should only be two types of critical care nurses at the bedside: (1) those who are certified, and (2) those who are in the process of becoming certified.[29] Certification is a process of achieving the highest recognition of excellence. It is more than "another initial"[30]; it is a mark of excellence that can be referred to as "the Good Housekeeping Seal of Approval." Credentials on name badges, such as CCRN (critical care registered nurse), PCCN (progressive care certified nurse), or CCNS (clinical nurse specialist in acute and critical care), make personal mastery visible to the consumer and ensure public protection.

Since 1975, the AACN Certification Corporation has promoted and enhanced mastery of patient health and safety by certifying and recertifying nurses in the care of acute and critically ill patients.[31] The first national study on certification revealed more than 410,000 nurses were certified in 134 specialties by 67 different certifying bodies granting the use of at least 95 different credentials.[32] Currently, there are more than 87,000 certified critical care nurses with the credentials of CCRN, CCRN-E (e-ICU nurses), PCCN, CCNS, ACCNS (acute and critical care CNS), CMC (cardiac medicine certification), CSC (cardiac surgery certification), ACNPC (acute care nurse practitioner), and ACNP-AG (acute care NP adult gerontology).[31]

Achieving a culture of excellence requires meaningful recognition of achievements such as mastery of certification.[19] Cary[33] reported four avenues through which certification status can be recognized: public acknowledgment, financial compensation, career advancement, and retention. In addition, findings revealed that there is a perception, especially among newly certified nurses, that certification gives autonomy, enhances collaboration with other health care providers, allows control over practice, and results in higher patient satisfaction ratings.[33]

A growing body of knowledge related to the value of specialty certification in critical care is being developed to determine the effect of certified nursing practice. Most recently, Kendall-Gallagher et al[32] conducted a secondary analysis of over 1.2 million discharged patients and found that a 10% increase in certified baccalaureate-prepared staff nurses decreased the odds of adjusted inpatient 30-day mortality and failure to rescue. Fitzpatrick et al[34] found that AACN-certified nurses with higher empowerment scores were less likely to leave their current position, and Krapohl et al[35] found similar positive associations with empowerment among 866 nurses. In addition, Kirchhoff and Dahl[5] found that 42% of CCUs provided public acknowledgment of certification and that 25% provided financial compensation with a certification bonus, whereas Ulrich et al[36] reported less support for an initial certification bonus and slightly higher support for certification recognition among critical care nurses.

## Passion

Just as a link is seen between values, vision, and mastery, passion is the essential thread to link together all the professional practice attributes for critical care nursing excellence (see Fig. 9-3). Passion involves enthusiastically striving for what is best for ourselves and those we serve. In *You Are the Leader You've Been Waiting For*, Klein described how to enjoy high performance and high fulfillment at work by being passionate about your calling or purpose.[37] He stated, "When your values, gifts, and calling operate in unison your work has a sense of inner congruence and outer effectiveness. You are clear about who you are and enjoy the ways in which you bring your gifts to life through your work" (p 119).[37] Similarly, others believe passion fuels results so that there is a "flywheel" effect, building in momentum with every step, action, decision, and turn.[37,38]

Weston et al[16] stated that "passion involves ardently striving for the best, even when repeated efforts seem tedious or appear exceedingly strenuous" (p 310). The truly passionate critical care nurse is not satisfied with providing less than the highest quality care possible to patients and families. Achieving this goal often requires going beyond an 8- or 12-hour shift. Acts of passion for critical care nursing excellence can be seen in bringing the latest research findings to the bedside, revising unit policy and procedure books with the most up-to-date procedures, and teaching coworkers the most effective therapies to produce the best outcomes for patients and families. Acts of passion for critical care nursing excellence can be seen when people take ownership to become engaged and transform work environments so that they are respectful, healing, and humane. The Case Study in Box 9-6 presents a flight nurse's personal experience that renewed her passion for nursing.

Passion can be felt in critical care nursing not only at the bedside but throughout the profession. Nursing leaders in critical care are partnering with interdisciplinary groups and talking to legislators to improve patient safety issues such as the workforce shortage, computerized physician and provider order entry, intensivist models of practice, evidence-based practice, and appropriate staffing. Being passionate about something requires time, energy, and commitment. The journey to excellence for healthy work environments started in 2001 for AACN because leadership was passionate about its mission of providing the highest quality resources to maximize nurses' contribution to caring and improving the health care of critically ill patients and their families.[17]

In *Good to Great*, Collins[38] describes why some organizations make the leap and sustain the leap from being a good organization to a great organization. He challenges people and organizations to pick up their rocks and look at the "ugly squiggly things" underneath them, rather than putting the rocks back down and covering them up. Using resources from AACN, critical care nurses are picking up their rocks and addressing the "ugly squiggly things" in their workplace environments that impede quality patient care. Acts of passion for healthy work environments are taking place as the AACN standards for skilled communication, true collaboration, effective decision making, appropriate staffing, meaningful recognition, and authentic leadership are established.[19]

## Action

Nightingale[41] once said, "One's feelings waste themselves in words, they ought all to be distilled into action which brings results" (p 44). In other words, part of professionalism in critical care nursing is "to walk the talk" for excellence. As values, vision, mastery, and passion for critical care nursing excellence build, the attribute of action (see Fig. 9-3) becomes another essential pillar for the framework, and one that resonates well for tangible results in critical care. The Case Study in Box 9-7 presents one example of nursing action for excellence.

Recognizing that so many vulnerable patients' lives are at risk and the invaluable contributions that nurses make, the AACN leadership decided it was time to act deliberately and definitively. In 2003, AACN launched the Beacon Award for Critical Care Excellence, an award specifically designed to recognize the leading critical care units in the United States.[37] Currently, 323 critical care units have been recognized for demonstrating high-quality standards, exceptional care of patients, families, and healthy work environments. Of those units, 88 have gold recognition, 191 have silver recognition, and 44 have bronze recognition.[43]

When the Beacon Award was first launched, a *beacon* was defined as "a source of light, an inspiration, or signal of

---

**BOX 9-6** | **Case Study**

*"Perpetual optimism is a force multiplier."—General Colin Powell, U.S. Army, retired, and former Secretary of State[22]*

Reflection on "Passion" for Critical Care Nursing Excellence Excerpt from The American Nurse Project by Caroline Jones: "They Understand How Hard It Is to Feel Helpless"

My father was in a motorcycle accident four years ago. He lived in rural Iowa, and he was very badly injured. Another flight team went out to get him, but he didn't survive, and that shook my whole foundation. When I came back to work, everything seemed more personal to me. I used to not want to know the name of the patient or make it personal in any way when we picked someone up in the helicopter. I thought it made it easier to pick them up and then drop them off if I didn't make any emotional connection. But after my dad died, I started making it a point to talk to the families before we took off. I take 2 minutes to say, "My name is Venus, and I'm going to be flying your loved one to Omaha. Can I get your phone number? When we get there, I'll call you and let you know how it went." I make sure they come into the helicopter to give their loved one a kiss good-bye or say

whatever they want to say to him or her. I realized that one thing that killed me was not knowing what was going on with my dad during the process. I don't think this gesture is a waste of time anymore.[39]

*Venus Anderson, BSN, CFRN, Nebraska Medical Center/Lifenet in the Heartland, Omaha, Nebraska. In addition to working in a pediatric ICU at Children's Hospital in Omaha, Venus Anderson is a member of a select group of about 5,000 flight nurses currently working in the United States.*

Self-reflection
• Do you have a passion to understand how hard it is to feel helpless, and to influence the care of patients and families by putting their care first regardless of the challenges?
• Do you have a passion to follow or lead evidence-based initiatives such as *AACN Practice Alerts for Family Presence for Visitation in the Adult ICU*?[40]
• What are you passionate about in order to foster nursing excellence and make a difference in the lives of the acute and critically ill?

**BOX 9-7** Case Study

*"We are what we repeatedly do. Excellence then is not an act but a habit."—Aristotle*[22]

**Reflection on "Action" for Critical Care Nursing Excellence**
Excerpt from Kathryn E. Roberts, RN, MSN, CNS, CCRN, CCNS, 2012–2013 AACN President Speech: "Dare To"

History is not made without daring. And creating a preferred future doesn't just happen; it takes vision followed by courageous action....If we act boldly, this will be the time people look back on and see that nurses were the driving force behind positive change. They'll see that nurses dared to take on the problems that threatened to render our health care system more dangerous than it is healing for our patients....

For example, one nurse dared to end the bullying behavior of some colleagues that had escalated due to a very divisive issue the unit was facing. After seeing how the conflict was damaging relationships and their work environment, she initiated what she described as one of the most crucial conversations of her life. She wrote, "I began the conversation with how I loved our unit and thought that we had something very special. I said that I was sure none of us wanted to ruin what we had. I talked. They listened. They talked and I listened. When the conversation was over, we all hugged to acknowledge the mutual respect and new understanding among us. We repaired our unhealthy environment. We have since received the Beacon Gold Award."[42]

*Self-reflection*
- What action have you dared to take on to improve your workplace environment or personal self?
- What scares or excites you enough to take action?
- When was the last time you dared to foster nursing excellence and make a difference in the lives of the acute and critically ill?

---

guidance" with the belief that "every critical care unit could be a Beacon unit."[43] Since that time, the 42-item Beacon application has been modified to a new application with 38 items, and any hospital unit that has high acuity and critically ill patients and meets evidence-based standards of excellence and patient safety is now eligible to apply. Although the new application includes three levels (bronze, silver, and gold) for units to chart their journey and receive a 3-year designation, the Beacon application continues to address innovation, excellence, or both in six categories: recruitment and retention; education, training, and mentoring; evidence-based practice and research; patient outcomes; creating and promoting healing environments; and leadership and organizational ethics. In addition, the Beacon Award provides a mechanism for individual and collective critical care units to measure progress against evidence-based initiatives and national criteria for performance, learn and refine their processes and systems, and be recognized for their achievements.[43] What bolder action or stronger message can be conveyed to the public and the patients whom critical care nurses serve than to validate excellence in practice?

Seeking opportunities and partnerships to further extend action to ensure optimal health outcomes for individuals experiencing an acute and life-threatening illness requires a relentless and fearless voice by critical care nurses. These nurses have been using their innate gift of inquiry for decades to tackle patient care issues. Nightingale is perhaps nursing's most famous leader who first used research to change practice.[40] Even though she lacked the theoretical bases that we have today, she had a core set of values, a vision, the mastery, and a passion to improve England's hospital care in the mid-19th century. Today, critical care nurses are witnessing once-revered "sacred cows" being eliminated from practice. Examples include the use of dye in enteral feeding, restricting family presence during cardiopulmonary resuscitation, and restricting visitation hours in ICUs: nursing research demonstrated that all of these practices should be eliminated.

Even though new models of nursing education are evolving, it does not take a doctorate-prepared critical care nurse to raise questions and put a plan in place for collecting, analyzing, and reporting patient and family outcomes. Outcome-based practice is the responsibility of all nurses, whether one is actually doing the research, disseminating the research to the bedside, or reporting the research findings. In addition, it is important for all nurses to celebrate and showcase high-quality nursing outcomes, no matter what nursing specialty provided the body of knowledge. Focusing on quality indicators and performance improvement in acute and critical care settings as daily practice is a bold and powerful action for improving patient care.

Practice alerts from AACN are another example of nursing actions for excellence. AACN practice alerts consist of efforts to prevent and minimize infection, reduce complications from critical illness, promote patient safety, and establish best practices. First launched in 2004, the AACN practice alerts are succinct dynamic directives that are well supported with current authoritative evidence to ensure best practice. There are more than a dozen practice alerts that bridge the gap between practice and research, provide guidance, standardize care, and identify and inform new trends and provide information about them.[42] Examples of recent practice alerts include assessing pain in the critically ill adult, alarm management, and verification of feeding tube placement.[40] Promoting the science of nursing by adopting the AACN practice alerts informs the public that critical care nurses have the knowledge and understanding necessary to protect the welfare of patients and their families.

## Balance

Balance is the final component of the professional practice model for critical care nursing excellence illustrated in Figure 9-3. Balance can bring renewal to the spirit and allow for more moments of "full presence," which often breaks down in our busy professional and personal lives. Taking the time to care for one's self is essential to keep the body and mind in balance. Otherwise, it can be difficult to maintain a clear perspective. Today, nurses are increasingly blurring the lines between home and work, and between work and leisure. The lines of communication are continuously open because of the proliferation of electronic devices and communication options such as pagers, cell phones, text messaging, e-mail, and voicemail. It is important to say "no" to being "supernurse" and "supermom" or "superdad" and find the time to take care of oneself. Nurses do not do their patients, their families, or

**BOX 9-8**   Case Study

*"Balance isn't either/or, it's AND." (Steven Covey)*[22]

Reflection on "Balance" for Critical Care Nursing Excellence
Excerpts from Critical Care Nurse: "The Pause" by Jonathan Bartels BSN, RN

A... young woman is wheeled into the trauma bay. She'd been crossing a busy intersection at night....Smears of blood streak her face like war paint, and her arms are bent at unnatural angles. Her body lies exposed, her clothing in snipped tatters about her small frame.... These are the final moments of her life, but no one knows that yet...there is no blood pressure, then no pulse, and the monitor chirps asystole. The tension escalates as compressions begin....Drugs and fluids are rapidly infused. We expertly move in a choreographed dance dedicated to saving lives.... We try to bring her life back for 45 minutes before we realize it's too late, and the code is called.

On this day...I remember defeat and exhaustion, but also...a kind of vacancy, a space where the pull of emotion gets tamped down by time, fatigue, and grief, leaving an empty numbness in its place.... I watch my colleagues throw off their gloves and stride out of the room, leaving the naked, lifeless body on the table. Not a glance back, just a step back out into the world of the emergency department where patients stream in like locusts.

It isn't heartless: it's force-fed anguish. There is no time for a breath, or thought or tears. A death that gives us pause as

humans leaves us as clinicians with no time to pause. Maybe, I think, that's the problem....

Her death wasn't our first, and it would not be the last, but I remember it because it did mark the end of the old way and the beginning of the new—our pause.... After a death in the emergency department, I would stand, ask that no one leave, and invite my peers to bear witness with me, to be together and present in a singular moment of grief and loss...to remember that the person who had died loved and was loved, to understand that the person's passing deserved recognition, and to acknowledge that our own efforts, too, were worthy of honor.

Forty-five seconds, maybe a minute, a minute and a half. For us, pausing has made all the difference...in its own way, breathes life back into what can feel like an airless, emotionless room where we work.[44]

Self-reflection

• When was the last time you rose above the high-tech, fast-paced, and emotionally charged patient care environment to allow a few moments of stillness and reflection?
• When was the last time you took care of yourself, mentally and physically, to have the energy and resiliency to foster nursing excellence and make a difference in the lives of the acute and critically ill?

---

themselves any good if they consistently place the needs of others above their own needs. Critical care nurses listen to patients and families at all hours of the day and night. They must also have time to listen to their own minds and hearts and those who love them most. The Case Study in Box 9-8 presents a reflection on balance for the critical care nurse.

In *You Are the Leader You've Been Waiting For*, Klein stresses the importance of letting go. He believes letting go of the old can make space for something new. He believes that during a time of transformation one should not act but be still.[37] This is particularly true for critical care nurses, as the intense pressures of managing the care of complex patients in chaotic environments for long hours at one stretch can take a toll on health and welfare. Whether it is sitting quietly and listening to music, reading, or exercising, the minds and hearts of nurses need time to renew and be recharged for the next day of taking care of critically ill patients and their families. When nurses are balanced, it is easier not to give in to the cynicism and frustration that abound in the workplace or home. To be truly engaged and energized requires nurturing oneself first and then empowering others to do the same. Look around your unit today and ask yourself some questions. Who are the critical care nurses who reach out to others the most? Who are the critical care nurses who smile the most? Who are the critical care nurses who say "thank you" and give compliments the most? You may find that your answer is with nurses who have discovered how to make balance a priority in their professional and personal lives.

## Conclusion

In today's fast-paced critical care environment, finding the time for professional growth can be challenging yet rewarding (Box 9-9). Building a professional practice of excellence

**BOX 9-9**   Closing Thoughts on Critical Care Nursing Excellence

REMEMBER... Ready or not, someday it will all come to an end.
There will be no more sunrises, no shift work, no change of report.
All the things you valued, whether treasured or forgotten, will pass to someone else.
It will not matter what you owned or what you were owed.
Your challenges, frustrations, and disappointments will finally disappear.
So too your hopes, ambitions, and plans.
What will matter is not your success, but your significance.
What will matter is not what you learned, but what you taught.
What will matter is every act of integrity, compassion, courage,
or sacrifice that enriched, empowered, or encouraged others
to emulate your example of critical care nursing excellence.
Living a life that matters doesn't happen by accident.
It's not a matter of circumstance but of choice.
Live your contribution and choose to live a life that matters.
Become engaged and transform your practice for critical care nursing excellence.

Modified from Josephson M: What will matter. Retrieved July 10, 2015, from http://charactercounts.org/pdf/WhatWillMatter.pdf.

requires a passion to profoundly affect the lives of those who trust critical care nurses most: complex, unstable, and vulnerable patients and their families. At the same time, it requires advancing the critical care nursing profession through a healthy work environment that is patient centered, collaborative, interdisciplinary, and evidence based. The desire for and commitment to critical care nursing excellence requires self-reflection about the values, vision, mastery, passion, action, and balance in one's practice. Critically ill patients and their families expect and deserve nothing but the best care.

Building a professional practice model of excellence can give critical care nurses the confidence to use their bold voice and presence to make significant contributions to improving the delivery of care to the patients and families who have entered a chaotic and frightening world of illness, trauma, and pain. In the fast-paced critical care environments of today, finding the time for professional growth is challenging but, as evidence demonstrates, essential. For the profession of critical care nursing to advance, nurses must acquire the necessary clinical experience and competencies to provide best practice models of care for critically ill patients and their families. Whether it is participating on a patient safety hospital committee or recruiting younger people to critical care nursing, endless opportunities exist for building a professional practice of excellence. The days of landmark studies reporting that nursing is a silent and unknown profession[45,46] will soon come to an end as more bold and committed voices are heard about excellence in critical care nursing practice.

## Clinical Applicability Challenges

### SHORT ANSWER QUESTIONS

1. How can nurses collaborate effectively with integrated health care teams to bring the distinct gifts and diversity of perspectives to optimize the care provided for acute and chronically ill patients, families, and health care systems?

2. How can nurses relentlessly continue to advance their professional development and fill their knowledge and skill gaps to help ensure that patient safety is never compromised?

3. Why would a health care organization require a potential new hire critical care nurse to have, or commit to earning, a baccalaureate degree in nursing and specialty certification?

### WANT TO KNOW MORE?

A wide variety of resources to enhance your learning and understanding of this chapter are available on thePoint.

You will find:

- References
- Selected readings
- NCLEX-style review questions
- Internet resources
- And more!

# PART 3

# Special Populations in Critical Care

## 10

# The Critically Ill Pediatric Patient

PATRICIA A. MOLONEY-HARMON

### LEARNING OBJECTIVES

*Based on the content in this chapter, the reader should be able to:*

1. Analyze anatomical and physiologic differences in the infant and child that necessitate the modification of physical assessment parameters and intervention techniques.

2. Describe special considerations in ventilatory management and medication administration for the critically ill child.

3. Evaluate pain assessment tools that can be used for the critically ill child.

4. Examine important aspects of interaction with the critically ill child and family that will enhance interventions.

Many critical care clinicians feel ill equipped to care for children seen in adult intensive care units (ICUs), emergency departments (EDs), procedural suites, and recovery rooms. To facilitate smooth and optimal care of the critically ill child, it is wise to adopt a framework for the modification of the adult critical care practice to include the pediatric patient. A comprehensive framework is beyond the scope of this chapter, but readers are referred to the PEDS framework, discussed in more detail elsewhere.[1] This chapter highlights prominent anatomical and physiologic differences and related implications, equipment selection, recognition of the decompensating child, and unique challenges in caring for the pediatric patient in a critical care environment.

## Prominent Anatomical and Physiologic Differences and Implications

### Vital Signs

Infants and young children have an age-appropriate, but higher, heart rate and respiratory rate than do adults. The higher heart and respiratory rates assist in meeting the need for a higher cardiac output, despite a smaller stroke volume and a higher basal metabolic rate. Blood pressure in children is lower than that of adults. Vital signs (Table 10-1), although important parameters, should not be evaluated in isolation but rather in a trending fashion.

Tachycardia is a nonspecific response to a variety of entities, such as anxiety, fever, shock, and hypoxemia. Although the child is predisposed to bradycardia, tolerance is poor. Persistent bradycardia produces significant changes in perfusion because cardiac output is heart rate dependent. Bradycardia

is most often caused by hypoxemia, but any vagal stimuli, such as suctioning, nasogastric tube insertion, and defecation, may precipitate an event.

As for respiratory rate, an infant or child increases his or her respiratory rate to compensate for an increased oxygen demand. Tachypnea is often the first sign of respiratory distress. A slow respiratory rate in a sick child often indicates impending respiratory arrest. Associated conditions, such as fever and seizure activity, which further increase the metabolic rate, also increase oxygen requirements. These conditions can cause rapid deterioration in an already compromised child.

Unlike that of the adult, the child's blood pressure is the last parameter to fall in the face of shock. Children can compensate for up to a 25% blood loss before the systolic blood pressure falls. A normal blood pressure should never discourage interventions for the child showing signs of circulatory failure. The pulse pressure is often a more reliable indicator for assessing the adequacy of perfusion. Hypertension is uncommon unless the child has renal disease.

| TABLE 10-1 | Pediatric Vital Signs | | |
|---|---|---|---|
| Age | Heart Rate (beats/min) | Respirations (breaths/min) | Systolic Blood Pressure (mm Hg) |
| Newborn | 100–160 | 30–60 | 50–70 |
| 1–6 wk | 100–160 | 30–60 | 70–95 |
| 6 mo | 90–120 | 25–40 | 80–100 |
| 1 y | 90–120 | 20–30 | 80–100 |
| 3 y | 80–120 | 20–30 | 80–110 |
| 6 y | 70–110 | 18–25 | 80–110 |
| 10 y | 60–90 | 15–20 | 90–120 |
| 14 y | 60–90 | 15–20 | 90–130 |

## Neurologic System

Brain growth occurs at a rapid rate during the first few years of life. Because brain growth is rapid during this time, measurement of head circumference is important in the child until 2 years of age. The circumference of the child's head is related to intracranial volume and estimates the rate of brain growth.

The child's cranial sutures are not completely fused until 18 to 24 months of age. The posterior fontanelle closes by 3 months of age, and the anterior fontanelle closes by 9 to 18 months of age. The fontanelles provide a useful assessment tool in the infant. The characteristics of the fontanelles can be used to assess hydration status or the presence of increased intracranial pressure (ICP). Bulging fontanelles may indicate increased ICP or fluid overload. Sunken fontanelles may be seen with fluid deficit.

Like adults, infants and children have protective reflexes (eg, the cough and gag reflexes). There are also several newborn reflexes (ie, the Moro, rooting, grasp, and Babinski reflexes), which differ from adult reflexes. For example, the Babinski reflex is present until 9 to 12 months of age or until the child starts walking. A positive Babinski reflex response (fanning of the toes and dorsiflexion of the big toe when the lateral aspect of the sole of the foot is stroked) is expected in an infant, yet is considered an abnormal finding in an older child or adult. In-depth discussion of these reflexes is beyond the scope of this chapter; the reader is referred to a developmental anatomy text for further information.

An infant's or child's mental status is assessed the same way as an adult's, by noting the level of consciousness, interaction with the environment, and appropriateness of behavior for age. Level of consciousness is assessed by noting whether the child is arousable and oriented. This can be done by observing for spontaneous arousability or by providing verbal, tactile, or noxious stimuli. Even though the assessment is the same, the assessment techniques must be age appropriate. Specific techniques are provided in the section in this chapter on interaction. An important difference to note when interacting with the child is paradoxical irritability (ie, the inability of the child to be calmed with normal comfort measures, such as cuddling). Paradoxical irritability, when present with meningeal irritability, nuchal rigidity, and positive Brudzinski and Kernig signs, may indicate meningitis.

Infants and young children are at high risk for ineffective thermoregulation, resulting in physiologic instability from a variety of maturational and environmental factors. Closely monitoring body temperature and providing a temperature-controlled environment help to manage temperature regulation. The temperature is measured at regular intervals, and external factors affecting body temperature should be controlled.

## Cardiovascular System

Decreased perfusion to the skin is an early and reliable sign of shock. Because a child's skin is thinner than an adult's, skin characteristics change easily and rapidly with changes in perfusion. Skin color, texture, and temperature and capillary refill are of great significance during assessment of the child. Before assessing the skin, it is important to note the room temperature because some findings may be a normal response to the environment (such as mottling in a drafty operating room). Mottling in a bundled infant or warm environment is the reason for further investigation. The nurse assesses skin temperature and the line of demarcation between extremity coolness and body warmth. Coolness or the progression of coolness toward the trunk may be a sign of diminishing perfusion.

Peripheral cyanosis is normal in newborns but abnormal in young children and adults. Central cyanosis (circumoral) is always abnormal. Capillary refill time is normally recorded in seconds rather than as "brisk, normal, or slow" and normally is no longer than 2 seconds. Estimated blood volume varies with age; despite a higher volume per kilogram of body weight in children, the overall total circulating volume is small. A small amount of blood loss can be significant in a child.

## Respiratory System

The infant's or child's large head (in proportion to body size); weak, underdeveloped neck muscles; and lack of cartilaginous support to the airway lead to an easily compressible or obstructed airway. The nurse must avoid overextending or overflexing the neck because the airways are easily collapsible. Head and neck position alone can facilitate a patent airway. Ideal positioning for the decompensating child is in a neutral ("sniffing") position; this can be accomplished by placing a small roll horizontally behind the shoulders (Fig. 10-1).

Infants, until 6 months of age, are obligate nose-breathers, and so any obstruction of nasal passages can produce significant airway compromise and respiratory distress. Secretions, edema, inflammation, poorly taped nasogastric tubes, or occluded nasal cannulas can cause obstructed nasal passages in an infant. The infant's and young child's airways are smaller both in diameter and in length, thus requiring smaller artificial airways. Airway compromise can be caused by the slightest amount of inflammation or edema of the natural airway, or from a mucus plug in either the natural or artificial airway. The narrowest part of the child's airway (until approximately 8 years of age) is at the level of the cricoid ring, as opposed to the glottic opening in the adult.

The young child's thin, compliant chest wall allows for easy assessment of air entry, which is assessed by observing the rise and fall of the child's chest with adequate ventilatory efforts. Unequal chest movement may indicate the development

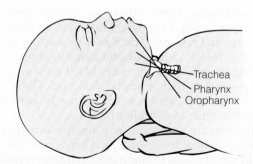

Trachea
Pharynx
Oropharynx

**FIGURE 10-1**   The neutral ("sniffing") position can improve airflow in a decompensating child by aligning the oropharynx, pharynx, and trachea with the mouth.

of a pneumothorax or atelectasis, but may also indicate endotracheal tube obstruction or displacement into the right mainstem bronchus. The child's flexible rib cage and poorly developed intercostal muscles offer little stability to the chest wall; therefore, suprasternal, sternal, intercostal, and subcostal retractions may be seen during respiratory distress. The presence and location of retractions should be noted. Accessory muscles are also poorly developed, and so an infant or child may use the abdominal muscles to assist with breathing. This gives the appearance of "seesaw" breathing, a paradoxical movement of the chest and abdomen. Seesaw breathing becomes more exaggerated with respiratory distress. As in the adult, the major muscle of respiration is the diaphragm. However, the child is more diaphragm dependent.

Because of the thin chest wall, breath sounds are more audible than in the adult. In addition, obstructed airways often produce sounds that are easily heard during assessment. The nurse listens for expiratory grunting, inspiratory and expiratory stridor, and wheezing. Expiratory grunting is a sound produced in an attempt to increase physiologic positive end-expiratory pressure to prevent small airways and alveoli from collapsing. The infant's and child's thin chest wall may allow breath sounds to be heard over an area of pathology when sounds are actually being referred from another area of the lung. The nurse listens for changes in the breath sounds as well as for their presence or absence.

## Gastrointestinal System

Children normally have a protuberant abdomen; however, there are numerous causes of abnormal abdominal distention. A nasogastric or orogastric tube should be inserted early rather than later in a critically ill child to minimize the risk for distention. Abdominal distention can interfere with respiratory excursion and may even cause respiratory arrest. Active removal of air with a syringe may be necessary if distention is not relieved by putting the tube to straight drainage. In addition, the abdominal girth is measured every shift or more often if there is a concern about abdominal distention.

Stomach capacity varies with the age of the child. A newborn's stomach capacity is 90 mL, a 1-month-old's is 150 mL, and a 12-month-old's is 360 mL; in comparison, an adult's stomach capacity is 2,000 to 3,000 mL. Because stomach capacity is smaller, care is taken when formula and other fluids are instilled into the abdomen. Bolus feedings are of an appropriate amount, consistent with the child's stomach capacity.

The infant and young child have a gastric emptying time of 2.5 to 3 hours, which increases to 3 to 6 hours in the older child. An appropriate amount of time to allow for absorption of formula is taken into account when measuring residuals. If the child is receiving chest physiotherapy, the amount of time between therapy and feeding is considered, or the gastric contents are checked to avoid problems with reflux and aspiration.

## Renal System

Infants have less ability to concentrate urine and therefore have a normal urine output of 2 mL/kg/h. For children and adolescents, normal urine output is 1 and 0.5 mL/kg/h, respectively. Because of the infant's limited ability to concentrate urine, a low specific gravity does not necessarily mean that the infant is adequately hydrated. The immaturity of the child's kidney means that the child may not process fluid as efficiently as the adult and is less able to handle sudden large amounts of fluid, leading to fluid overload.

Infants and young children have a larger body surface area in relation to body weight. Maintenance fluid requirements are determined on the basis of body weight (Table 10-2). Children have a higher percentage of total body water, most of which is composed of extracellular fluid (ECF), as compared with adults. The ECF makes up 50% of the body weight in infants but 20% in adults. In addition, children have a higher insensible water loss because of a higher basal metabolic rate, higher respiratory rate, and larger body surface area. The child's higher percentage of total-body water and higher insensible water loss increase the risk for dehydration. Sudden weight loss or gain may indicate fluid imbalance. Children should be weighed daily at the same time using the same scale.

Signs of dehydration include dry mucous membranes, decreased urine output, increased urine concentration, sunken fontanelles and eyes, and poor skin turgor (Table 10-3). The severity of dehydration varies with the degree of dehydration and the child's fluid and electrolyte status. Circulatory compromise accompanies severe dehydration. Treating a child's dehydration in an adult ICU requires pediatric consultation. Fluid overload is manifested by bulging fontanelles, taut skin, edema (usually periorbital and sacral), hepatomegaly, and other signs of congestive heart failure.

## Endocrine System

Infants and young children have smaller glycogen stores and increased glucose demand because of their larger brain-to-body size ratio. The smaller stores and increased demand predispose infants and young children to the development of hypoglycemia. Blood glucose levels are closely monitored, especially when the infant or child is not permitted to have anything by mouth and numerous adjustments are being made to nutritional support.

## Immune System

Immunologic differences in infants and small children may predispose them to infection. The skin of newborns

| TABLE 10-2 | Calculation of Maintenance Fluid | |
|---|---|---|
| Body Weight (kg) | Fluid Requirements per Day | Fluid Requirements per Hour |
| Less than 10 | 100 mL/kg | 4 mL/kg |
| 10–20 | 1,000 mL + 50 mL/kg for each kg above 10 | 2 mL/kg for each kg above 10 |
| More than 20 | 1,500 mL + 20 mL/kg for each kg above 20 | 1 mL/kg for each kg above 20 |

From Roberts KE: Fluid and electrolyte regulation. In: Curley MAQ, Moloney-Harmon PA (eds): Critical Care Nursing of Infants and Children, 2nd ed. Philadelphia, PA: WB Saunders Co, 2001, pp 369–392, with permission of Elsevier Science.

**TABLE 10-3**   Clinical Assessment of Severity of Dehydration

| Patient | Mild Dehydration | Moderate Dehydration | Severe Dehydration |
|---|---|---|---|
| Infant (%) | 5 | 10 | 15 |
| Adolescent (%) | 3 | 6 | 9 |
| Infants and young children | Thirsty, alert, restless | Thirsty, restless, or lethargic but irritable to touch or drowsy | Drowsy, limp, cold, sweaty, cyanotic extremities, may be comatose |
| Older children and adults | Thirsty, alert, restless | Thirsty, alert, postural hypotension | Usually conscious, apprehensive, cold, sweaty, cyanotic extremities, wrinkled skin of fingers and toes, muscle cramps |
| **Signs and Symptoms** | | | |
| Tachycardia | Absent | Present | Present |
| Palpable pulses | Present | Present (weak) | Decreased |
| Blood pressure | Normal | Orthostatic hypotension | Hypotension |
| Cutaneous perfusion | Normal | Normal | Reduced and mottled |
| Skin turgor | Normal | Slight reduction | Reduced |
| Fontanelle | Normal | Sunken | Very sunken |
| Eyes | Normal | Slightly depressed | Sunken |
| Tears | Present | Present or Absent | Absent |
| Mucous membranes | Moist | Dry | Very dry |
| Respirations | Normal | Deep, may be rapid | Deep and rapid |
| Urine output | Normal | Oliguria | Anuria and severe oliguria |
| Estimated fluid deficit (mL/kg) | 30–50 | 60–90 | ≥100 |

Data from World Health Organization. Table adapted from Greenbaum LA: Fluids and electrolytes. In: Kliegman RM, Jenson HB, Marcdante KJ, et al (eds): Nelson Essential of Pediatrics, 7th ed. St. Louis, MO: Saunders, 2015, Table 33-5, p 109, with permission from Elsevier Science.

is thinner; therefore, it provides less of a barrier to outside pathogens. Because infants and young children have fewer stored neutrophils, they are less able to repeatedly replenish white blood cells in the face of an overwhelming infection. The complement levels are lower, which affects the chemotactic activity of phagocytes and the opsonization of bacteria. There is also a relative deficiency of immunoglobulins, making infants and young children more susceptible to infections caused by viruses, *Candida* species, and acute inflammatory bacteria. In addition, infants may not demonstrate fever and leukocytosis in response to an infection. It is important to observe for subtle signs, such as changes in feeding behaviors, altered glucose metabolism, and hypothermia.

## Integumentary System

Expected differences in the skin, hair, nails, and glands depend on the age of the child. Infants and children without exposure to the sun or wind are expected to have smooth-textured skin without coarse adult terminal hair. Infants up to about 14 days of age may be covered with lanugo, a fine, silky-textured hair. Infants have less developed hypodermal fat and, as a result, are at risk for hypothermia. The sweat glands do not begin to function until 1 month of age and are not fully functional until adolescence.

In the young child, the most noticeable skin variation may be that of bruising as the child increases activity and play becomes more aggressive. It is very important to attend to bruising seen in the child because it may be associated with abusive situations. The nurse notes the location and color changes of bruising indicating the stage of healing. Bruising is more common and not unexpected on the lower legs and

the face. Bruising on the upper arms, buttocks, and abdomen occurs less often and may indicate abuse.

In the adolescent, the sweat glands and sebaceous glands become fully functional. The adolescent may be expected to experience body odor, increasing axillary perspiration, and acne. The development of axillary and pubic hair is expected related to the increasing levels of circulating androgen levels in both male and female adolescents.

# Selected Pediatric Challenges

## Ventilatory Issues

The most common cause of cardiopulmonary arrest in children is respiratory in nature. This fact mandates that respiratory distress and failure be recognized early, and that airway management interventions be immediate (Table 10-4). Signs of respiratory decompensation include diminished level of consciousness, tachypnea, minimal or no chest movement with respiratory effort, evidence of labored respirations with retractions, seesaw breathing, minimal or no air exchange noted on auscultation, and the presence of nasal flaring, grunting, stridor, or wheezing.

The initial intervention for respiratory decompensation is positioning the child to open the airway. If the child does not respond to position alone, manual ventilation with 100% oxygen using a bag-mask device is initiated. There are several sizes of pediatric manual resuscitation bags; the correct size is determined by noting the child's tidal volume and deciding whether the bag is capable of delivering 1.5 times the child's tidal volume. Even though a pressure manometer may assist

**TABLE 10-4** Quick Examination of a Healthy versus Decompensating Child

| Assessment | Healthy Child | Decompensating Child |
|---|---|---|
| **Airway** | | |
| Patency | Child requires no interventions; child verbalizes and is able to swallow, cough, gag | Child self-positions and requires interventions, such as head positioning, suctioning, adjunct airways. Unmaintainable airway requires intubation |
| **Breathing** | | |
| Respiratory rate | Breathing is within age-appropriate limits | Breathing is tachypneic or bradypneic compared with age-appropriate limits and conditions* *Note:* Warning parameter: more than 60 breaths/min |
| Chest movement (presence) | Chest rises and falls equally and simultaneously with abdomen with each breath | Child has minimal or no chest movement with respiratory effort |
| Chest movement (quality) | Child has silent and effortless respirations | Child shows evidence of labored respirations with retractions. Asynchronous movement (seesaw) is observed between chest and abdomen with respiratory efforts |
| Air movement (presence) | Air exchange is heard bilaterally in all lobes | Despite movement of the chest, minimal or no air exchange is noted on auscultation |
| Air movement (quality) | Breath sounds are of normal intensity and duration | Nasal flaring, grunting, stridor, and/or wheezing are noted |
| **Circulation** | | |
| Heart rate (presence) | Apical beat is present and within age-appropriate limit* | Heart rate is absent; bradycardia or tachycardia occurs as compared with age-appropriate limits* *Note:* Warning parameters: Infant: <80 beats/min Child <5 y: more than 180 beats/min Child older than 5 y: more than 150 beats/min |
| Heart rate (quality) | Heart rate is regular with normal sinus rhythm | Heart rate is irregular, slow, or very rapid; common dysrhythmias include supraventricular tachycardia, bradyarrhythmias, and asystole |
| Skin | Extremities are warm, pink with capillary refill 2 s or less; peripheral pulses are present bilaterally with normal intensity | Child has pallor, cyanosis, or mottled skin color and cool-to-cold extremities. Capillary refill time is 2 s or more; peripheral pulses are weak or absent; central pulses are weak |
| Cerebral perfusion | Child is alert to surroundings, recognizes parents or significant others, is responsive to fear and pain, and has normal muscle tone | Child is irritable, lethargic, obtunded, or comatose; has minimal or no reaction to pain; and/or has loose muscle tone (floppy) |
| Blood pressure | Blood pressure is within age-appropriate limits | Blood pressure falls from age-appropriate limits,* a late sign of decompensation *Note:* A fall of 10 mm Hg systolic pressure is significant. Lower systolic blood pressure limit: Infant 1 mo or less, 60 mm Hg Infant 1 y or less, 70 mm Hg Child, 70 mm Hg + (2 × age in years) |

*All vital signs are interpreted within the context of age, clinical condition, and other external factors, such as the presence of fever.
Adapted from McCormick CM: Nursing care of the child in the adult intensive care unit (ICU). In: Stillwell S (ed): Mosby's Critical Care Nursing Reference, 4th ed. St. Louis, MO: Mosby, Inc., 2006, p 653, with permission from Mosby, Inc.

in minimizing pressure, the true indicator of delivery of an adequate tidal volume is a clinical one. The adequate amount of tidal volume delivered during a manual resuscitation breath is the amount that causes rise and fall of the child's chest.

If bag-mask ventilation is not successful in restoring the child's ventilatory status, endotracheal intubation is required. Numerous sizes of endotracheal tubes are available for infants and children. To estimate the correct size of endotracheal tube, the size of the child's little finger or the following formula can be used:

$$\text{Internal diameter} = (16 + \text{age in years}) / 4$$

A cuffed tube can be used safely in the in-hospital setting.[2] For cuffed endotracheal tubes, the formula used to estimate the internal diameter is as follows:

$$\text{Internal diameter} = (16 + \text{age in years}) / 4 + 3$$

Because these are both estimations of endotracheal tube size, tubes one-half size smaller and larger should be available for immediate use. Table 10-5 provides information regarding endotracheal tube sizes and other equipment issues.

Monitoring the patient during intubation is critical to assess for desaturation or bradycardia. Once the child is

| TABLE 10-5 | Recommended Resuscitation Equipment for Infants and Children | | | | | | |
|---|---|---|---|---|---|---|---|
| | **Child's Weight** | | | | | | |
| Equipment | 4–8 kg (8.8–17.6 lb) | 8–11 kg (17.6–24.2 lb) | 11–14 kg (24.2–30.8 lb) | 14–18 kg (30.8–39.6 lb) | 18–24 kg (39.6–52.8 lb) | 24–32 kg (52.8–70.4 lb) | 32+ kg (70.4 + lb) |
| Oxygen mask | Newborn | Pediatric | Pediatric | Pediatric | Pediatric | Adult | Adult |
| Oral airway | Infant | Small child | Child | Child | Child | Small adult | Small adult |
| Resuscitation bag | Infant | Child | Child | Child | Child | Adult | Adult |
| Laryngoscope blade | 0–1 straight | 1 straight | 2 straight or curved | 2 straight or curved | 2 straight or curved | 2–3 straight or curved | 3 straight or curved |
| Endotracheal tube (mm) | 2.5 preterm; 3.0–3.5 term infant | 4.0 uncuffed | 4.5 uncuffed | 5.0 uncuffed | 5.5 uncuffed | 6.0 cuffed | 6.5 cuffed |
| Endotracheal tube (cm at the tip) | 10–10.5 | 11–12 | 12.5–13.5 | 14–15 | 15.5–16.5 | 17–18 | 18.5–19.5 |
| Stylet | Small | Small | Small | Small | Large | Large | Large |
| Suction catheter | 6–8 | 8 | 8–10 | 10 | 10 | 10–12 | 12–14 |
| Nasogastric tube (F) | 5–8 | 8–10 | 10 | 10–12 | 12–14 | 14–18 | 18 |
| Urinary catheter | 5–8 | 8–10 | 10 | 10–12 | 10–12 | 12 | 12 |
| Chest tube (F) | 10–12 | 16–20 | 20–24 | 20–24 | 24–32 | 28–32 | 32–40 |
| Blood pressure cuff | Newborn or infant | Infant or child | Child | Child | Child | Child or adult | Adult |
| IV catheter (G) | 22–24 | 22–24 | 20–22 | 18–22 | 18–20 | 18–20 | 16–20 |
| Butterfly catheter | 23–25 | 23–25 | 21–23 | 21–23 | 21–23 | 20–22 | 18–21 |
| Vascular catheter | 3.0 F 5–12 cm | 3.0–4.09 F 5–12 cm | 3.0–4.0 F 5–12 cm | 4.0–5.0 F 5–25 cm | 4.0–5.0 F 5–25 cm | 4.0–5.0 F 5–25 cm | 5.0–8.0 F 5–30 cm |
| Guide wire (mm) | 0.46 | 0.46–0.53 | 0.53–0.89 | 0.53–0.89 | 0.53–0.89 | 0.53–0.89 | 0.89 |

Data from Hazinski M: PALS Provider Manual. Dallas, TX: American Heart Association, 2002; Slota M: AACN Core Curriculum for Pediatric Critical Care Nursing. Philadelphia, PA: WB Saunders, 2006. From the AACN Pediatric Critical Care Pocket Reference Card. © 1998 American Association of Critical Care Nurses (AACN). Adapted with permission of the publisher. Reprinted from Dimens Crit Care Nurs 20(1):23, 2001, with permission.

intubated, observation of chest movement and auscultation of the lungs help determine correct placement. A radiograph is used to confirm proper placement. When placement is confirmed, the tube is securely taped to avoid accidental displacement. In addition, soft restraints should be used to prevent the child from removing the tube. Adequate sedation and analgesia are provided to increase the child's comfort and manage anxiety during intubation.

## Medication Administration

Because a child may differ in weight significantly from the average child in the associated age group, medications are prescribed on a microgram, milligram, or milliequivalent per kilogram of body weight basis rather than on a standard dose according to age. Confirming the weight (in kilograms) that is being used to determine drug dosages is important. This same weight should be used during the child's entire hospitalization unless there is a significant change in the child's weight. Because pediatric dosages may be unfamiliar to the adult clinician, precalculated emergency drug sheets are helpful. The emergency drug sheet should include the recommended resuscitation medication dosages, medication concentration, and final medication dose and volume the individual child is to receive. The recommended dosages should reflect the American Heart Association's Pediatric Advanced Life Support standards.

An important recommendation for medication administration in the pediatric patient is the single-dose system. The single-dose system involves preparing one syringe to contain only the prescribed medication dose. The syringe should be properly labeled with the drug name and dose. The nurse administers the entire volume of the syringe to ensure that the prescribed dose has been given. The single-dose system prevents overmedication or undermedication of the child.

Medication errors have received increased attention since the publication of the 2000 Institute of Medicine report, "To Err Is Human." The most common reason for harm to pediatric patients, medication errors result in a higher risk for death.[3] The prescribing phase is associated with the most errors (dosing errors), and the administration phase results in the second most errors.[4] Nurses are the last potential barrier between an occurrence and an adverse outcome; they are most likely to intercept the error. Preventing medication errors is especially important in children because there is a much smaller margin for error in this patient population. Risk reduction strategies, such as ensuring staff competency and computerized physician order entry, should be in place as best practice. All providers must use vigilance in ordering and administering medications to a pediatric patient.[5]

## Pain Management

Because of the nature of the environment and associated procedures, the critically ill child is at high risk for pain. The first step in assessing pain in children is to understand the child's response to, and communication of, pain. This is based on a variety of factors, including the child's developmental level, past and present experience with pain, cultural aspects, personality, parental presence, and age, as well as the nature of the illness or injury.[6] For instance, critically ill children may be in severe pain but may be unable to communicate because of sedation, paralytic agents, mechanical ventilation, or coma.

Pain assessment is multidimensional. Synthesis of a variety of parameters provides information that can be used to make a decision about the level of the child's pain and the most appropriate intervention. Assessment of pain by nurses is influenced by factors such as educational level, skills, experience, personal beliefs, and different strategies adopted for assessment.[6] Infants and young children cannot communicate verbally, which makes pain assessment challenging. This inability to communicate is also an issue in the sedated or chemically paralyzed child. This requires that the nurse assesses pain using different cues, which include physiologic and behavioral changes.[7]

Physiologic parameters used in pain assessment include heart rate, respiratory rate, blood pressure, and oxygen saturation. Other parameters described by Anand and Carr[8] include sweating, increased muscle tone, and skin color changes. These parameters return to normal as physiologic adaptation occurs. This adaptation can actually occur within minutes, and the nurse must realize that the child may still be in pain. The physical signs are not necessarily specific for pain but may be the only parameter available to the nurse caring for the critically ill child.

Behavioral responses may be helpful for pain assessment, especially in the child who cannot communicate. The next section on interaction with children and families discusses the continuum of responses related to pain and comfort.

Another dimension of pain assessment is self-report. Many of the available tools for assessing pain, however, require children to interact or use their hands, and thus they are not usually helpful in the critical care setting. Examples of self-report tools include the numerical rating scale (see Chapter 5, Fig. 5-1), the FACES scale (Fig. 10-2 A), and the color scale. If the child is unable or unwilling to give a report, the parent's report of pain is often helpful. Multidimensional scales, such as the COMFORT scale, Modified Motor Activity Assessment scale, and FLACC (face, legs, activity, cry, consolability) scale (Fig. 10-2B), are helpful because they combine dimensions of behavioral and physiologic distress and do not require interaction or use of the hands.

Multidimensional pain management interventions are used whenever possible, including nonpharmacologic and pharmacologic approaches. However, pharmacologic intervention is never withheld when it is appropriate. Opioids are usually the first-line drugs for pain management in the critically ill child. A variety of pharmacologic drugs are available, and the choice of medication depends on the child's response and the practitioner's preference. Nursing responsibilities include assessing the child's need for the drug, administering the appropriate dose, and monitoring the child's response. Sedation and analgesia are part of the daily management of the critically ill child. However, inherent in the use of these drugs is the risk of adverse responses. The nurse is responsible

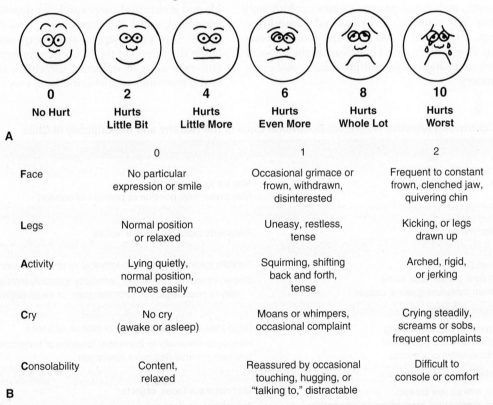

FIGURE 10-2 Tools for assessing pain in children. **A:** The FACES scale. This scale may be used in children 3 years and older. Explain that FACE 0 is a very happy face because there is no pain. FACE 2 hurts just a little bit. FACE 4 hurts a little bit more. FACE 6 hurts even more. FACE 8 hurts a whole lot. FACE 10 hurts very much; the pain can make you cry. Ask the child to choose the face that best describes the pain he or she is feeling. **B:** The FLACC (face, legs, activity, cry, consolability) scale. This scale can be used with children younger than 3 years. To use the FLACC scale, assess the child in each category, assigning a score between 0 and 2. Total the score, and then evaluate the total using the 0 to 10 pain scale parameters. (**A** © 1983 Wong-Baker FACES Foundation, HYPERLINK "http://www.WongBakerFACES.org" www .WongBakerFACES.org. Used with permission. Originally published in *Whaley & Wong's Nursing Care of Infants and Children.* © Elsevier Inc. **B** from Merkel SI, Voepel-Lewis T: The FLACC: A behavioral scale for scoring post-operative pain in young children. Pediatr Nurs 23(3): 293–297, 1997. © 2002, The Regents of the University of Michigan.)

for vigilant monitoring and for implementing changes on the basis of the child's response and recommendations by the multidisciplinary team.[9]

Other methods of pain control include intravenous patient-controlled analgesia (PCA) and epidural analgesia. PCA helps the child maintain a steady state of pain relief and also gives the child some control over pain. Epidural analgesia is also helpful for a variety of children. Epidural narcotics provide selective analgesia but do have associated side effects, including respiratory depression, nausea and vomiting, pruritus, and urinary retention.

Nurses may consider the use of nonpharmacologic methods, such as distraction, relaxation, massage, and hypnosis, in conjunction with pharmacologic methods. The method must be age appropriate, and parental presence is considered. Whatever methods are used, a critical determinant of their effectiveness is the child's response.

## Interaction with Children and Families

Interacting with children demands familiarity with their developmental capabilities and psychosocial needs. Categorization of children into groups according to physical and cognitive age can assist the nurse in predicting the child's expected social, cognitive, and physical capabilities. Developmental and psychosocial assessment is beyond the scope of this chapter; therefore, the reader should consult an appropriate growth and development reference. Although each age group has common developmental capabilities, tasks, and fears, it is helpful to recognize the common fears of all children despite their age. These fears include loss of control, threat of separation, painful procedures, and communicated anxiety.

Unlike the adult patient, the young child does not consciously screen most behavior and spoken words. The young child subconsciously communicates behaviorally through verbal, nonverbal (body language, behaviors), and abstract (play, drawing, storytelling) cues. Although the child's behavior is more natural in a familiar environment, the cues available to the clinician can suggest how a child is feeling or perceiving an event or the presence of a person. In general, the child's behavior is more activity oriented and more emotional than that of adults. These qualities of a child's behavior should be expected as the norm of average, healthy children and may be used as parameters against which to contrast the behavior of the critically ill child (Table 10-6).

Behavioral responses are particularly helpful during the assessment of pain or comfort. The infant or child may display body movement that spans the entire activity continuum from minimal movement, such as rigidity and guarding, to high activity, such as thrashing and kicking. Assessing various behavioral responses (eg, gestures, posture, movement, facial expression) and examining the congruency between these responses are particularly helpful.

Interaction with pediatric patients and their families is also facilitated by the appreciation of the child's significant others. The philosophy of family-centered care is essential to the optimal care of the pediatric patient. Although there are several components of family-centered care, the salient concept is to value, recognize, and support the family in the care of its child. The family is the constant in the child's life and is ultimately responsible for responding to the child's emotional, social, developmental, physical, and health care needs. Appropriate support and incorporation of parents may buffer the threats of the ICU environment to the child. Parents may assist or influence the child's cognitive appraisal of the environment, personnel, and events. The child often

---

**TABLE 10-6** Contrasting Affective Nonverbal Behavioral Cues of the Healthy and the Critically Ill Child

| Healthy | Critically Ill |
|---|---|
| **Posture** | |
| Moves, flexes | May be loose, flaccid |
| | May prefer fetal position or position of comfort |
| **Gestures** | |
| Turns to familiar voices | Responds slowly to familiar voices |
| **Movement** | |
| Moves purposefully | Exhibits minimal movement, lethargy, or unresponsiveness |
| Moves toward new, pleasurable items | Shows increased movement, irritability (possibly indicating cardiopulmo- |
| Moves away from threatening items, people | nary or neurologic compromise, pain, or sleep deprivation) |
| **Reactions/Coping Style** | |
| Responds to parents coming, leaving | Responds minimally to parent presence, absence |
| Responds to environment, equipment | Responds minimally to presence, absence of transitional objects |
| Cries and fights invasive procedures | Displays minimal defensive responses |
| **Facial Expressions** | |
| Looks at faces, makes eye contact | May not track faces, objects |
| Changes facial expressions in response to interactions | Avoids eye contact or has minimal response to interactions |
| Responds negatively to face wash | Minimally changes facial expression during face wash |
| Blinks in response to stimuli | Has increase, decrease in blinking |
| Widens eyes with fear | Avoids eye contact |
| Is fascinated with own mouth | Avoids, dislikes mouth stimulation |
| Holds mouth "ready for action" | Drools or displays loose mouth musculature |
| | Displays intermittent, weak suck on pacifier |

From McCormick CM: Nursing care of the child in the adult intensive care unit (ICU). In: Stillwell S (ed): Mosby's Critical Care Nursing Reference, 4th ed. St. Louis, MO: Mosby, Inc., 2006, p 638, with permission from Mosby, Inc.

uses the reactions of the parent as a barometer in interpreting events in ways ranging from threatening to beneficial.[10]

The tone and manner in which the clinician approaches the bedside of a pediatric patient and his or her family are important. Anxious feelings of the parents or health care team members may be communicated to the child; thus, interventions to relieve the anxiety of parents and fellow health care team members have a direct impact on the child's well-being. Interventions may include assisting parents and staff in anticipating the child's responses to therapy and illness and guiding parents and staff in therapeutic communication techniques.

Parents depend on nurses to humanize the critical care experience for their child. A recent study examined parents' perceptions of nurses' caring practices in the pediatric ICU. Parents reported that nurses used behaviors that demonstrated affection, caring, watching, and protecting. Parents stated that the most desirable nursing behaviors were those that complemented the parental role, which preserved family integrity during a time of crisis.[11] Clinical practice guidelines that support the parents of children in pediatric ICUs facilitate family involvement.[12]

## Clinical Applicability Challenges

<hr>

**( CASE STUDY )**

J. is a 4-year-old, 15-kg (33-lb) girl who presents to the ED with a history of flu-like symptoms for several days. In the ED, her vital signs are as follows: heart rate, 160 beats/min; respiratory rate, 46 breaths/min; blood pressure, 98/52 mm Hg; axillary temperature, 38.5°C; and oxygen saturation, 92%. She is very agitated and crying. Blood and urine cultures are ordered, and a chest x-ray and lumbar puncture are done. She is given the initial diagnosis of fever of unknown origin, possibly related to sepsis. She is then admitted to the pediatric intensive care unit (PICU). In the PICU, her heart rate is 160 and her pulses are full and bounding. Her blood pressure is 96/62 with a widened pulse pressure. Her capillary refill time is 1 second, and peripheral edema is present. Her respiratory rate is 48, and her skin is warm and dry. The symptoms that are occurring are related to the release of mediators due to infection and inflammation. The symptoms indicate vasodilatation, increased capillary permeability, and atypical distribution of blood flow. The child's respiratory rate is high for her age, although tachypnea is to be expected for her clinical condition. She has a fever and is anxious, which may also account for the tachypnea. The anxiety, agitation, and increased work of breathing increase the oxygen demand. The warning parameters at this stage include tachypnea, tachycardia, normal or high blood pressure, bounding pulses, and warm, flushed skin, indicating a child with increased oxygen demands who is at risk for cardiovascular collapse.

Initial management priorities include administering oxygen and fluids while assessing the child's response. In addition, antibiotics are started, an antipyretic is administered, and inotropic agents are considered. After these interventions, her vital signs are as follows: heart rate, 144 beats/min; respiratory rate, 40 breaths/min; blood

pressure, 110/64 mm Hg; and oxygen saturation, 98% on 40% oxygen by face mask.

One hour later, J's level of consciousness, hemodynamic status, and respiratory status begin to decline. Vital signs are as follows: heart rate, 170 beats/min; respiratory rate, 48 breaths/min; blood pressure, palpable only; mottling of the lower extremities, capillary refill greater than 4 seconds, weak peripheral pulses, and oxygen saturation, 86. She is extremely lethargic and is not responding to her parents. Her temperature is 38.6°C (101.5°F). She is demonstrating increased respiratory effort, and her blood gas results indicate metabolic acidosis and respiratory alkalosis. She is intubated and placed on mechanical ventilation. J. is demonstrating signs of uncompensated septic shock. Warning parameters include a change in her level of consciousness, tachycardia, altered peripheral perfusion, delayed capillary refill, and weak or absent peripheral pulses. Management priorities at this time include continuation of interventions started earlier and starting inotropic agents to support her blood pressure.

Treatment is directed toward ensuring hemodynamic stability and oxygenation of vital tissues. Medications include antibiotics and inotropic agents. Mechanical ventilation is also provided until J. shows improvement, as demonstrated by arterial blood gas values, vital signs, and clinical condition. Managing J.'s temperature will help to minimize the mismatch between oxygen delivery and consumption.

1. J. is demonstrating signs of uncompensated septic shock. Describe the signs that indicate septic shock in this child.
2. Discuss the management priorities for J. related to her septic shock.

Describe assessment parameters to determine J.'s response to intervention.

<hr>

**WANT TO KNOW MORE?**

A wide variety of resources to enhance your learning and understanding of this chapter are available on the Point.

You will find:
- References
- Selected readings
- NCLEX-style review questions
- Internet resources
- And more!

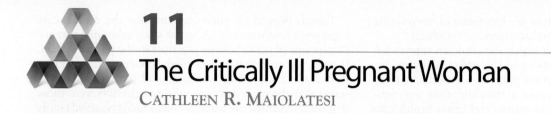

# 11

# The Critically Ill Pregnant Woman

CATHLEEN R. MAIOLATESI

Most women experience a normal pregnancy. However, a small percentage of women experience life-threatening complications that may result from the pregnancy itself or that develop as a result of a preexisting (comorbid) condition. Such critically ill pregnant women provide a unique challenge to nurses. The physical assessment of these patients includes the interaction between the maternal host and the fetus. Critical care nurses are not expected to have the knowledge and skills associated with fetal heart rate monitoring, and perinatal nurses may not possess the knowledge and skills required for patients needing ventilator support or hemodynamic monitoring. When a critically ill pregnant woman is in the intensive care unit (ICU), it is important that a collaborative approach be used to provide care.[1]

The general principles of diagnosis and management of the critically ill pregnant woman are similar to those used for other ICU patients. However, critical care nurses caring for pregnant patients must understand the physiological changes that occur as the body adapts to pregnancy to distinguish normal from abnormal responses, in order to decrease morbidity and mortality.[2] Table 11-1 outlines these changes.

## Physiological Changes in Pregnancy

### Cardiovascular Changes

Normal cardiovascular changes that occur during pregnancy affect pulse, blood pressure, cardiac output, and blood volume (see Table 11-1). Maternal blood volume increases 40% to 50% above baseline values. This increase, which consists mostly of plasma, begins in the first trimester and continues throughout pregnancy. The increase is necessary to provide adequate blood flow to the uterus, fetus, and changing maternal tissues and to accommodate blood loss at birth. Red blood cell volume increases by 20% and is disproportionate to the plasma increase, resulting in maternal physiological anemia. Heart rate increases 10 to 15 beats/min as early as 7 weeks of gestation and returns to the prepregnancy level

by 6 weeks postpartum.[2] Changes in blood volume and heart rate lead to an increase in cardiac output of 30% to 50% (6 to 7 L/min) during pregnancy.[2] Cardiac output increases slightly more intrapartum as a result of the shunting of blood from the placental–fetal unit. Immediately after birth, a larger increase in cardiac output (59% to 80%) occurs when the empty uterus contracts and shunts approximately 1,000 mL of blood back into the systemic circulation[2] (Table 11-2). A woman loses approximately 500 mL of blood during a vaginal birth and approximately 1,000 mL of blood during a cesarean birth. This is usually well tolerated.

Development of the uteroplacental unit provides a low-resistance network for the expanded blood volume, which reduces cardiac afterload.[3] The pulmonary vascular resistance, or right afterload, also decreases in response to increased blood volume and vasodilation. Under hormonal influence, smooth muscles and vascular beds relax, lowering systemic vascular resistance (SVR). Blood pressure decreases during the first and second trimesters and returns to prepregnancy levels by the third trimester. The nurse should keep in mind that the pregnant woman's position has a greater effect on blood pressure then it would if she were not pregnant. Supine hypotension occurs when the mother remains in a flat position. Therefore, when measuring blood pressure, the side-lying position is recommended, but if the patient must be supine, the uterus should be displaced by tilting it away from the inferior vena cava. This can be accomplished by using a wedge under the hip.

### Respiratory Changes

Respiratory changes as noted in Table 11-1 occur to accommodate the enlarged uterus and the increased oxygen demands of the mother and fetus. Structural changes include the upward shift of the diaphragm, which decreases functional residual capacity, and rib cage volume displacement, which increases tidal volume by 30% to 35%.[3] Airway mucosal changes include hyperemia, hypersecretion, increased friability, and edema. These changes are significant when

**TABLE 11-1    Physiological Changes in Pregnancy**

|  | Change | Pregnancy Levels |
|---|---|---|
| **Cardiovascular Changes** | | |
| Blood volume | Increases 40%–50% | 1,260–1,625 mL |
| Red blood cells | Increases 20% | 250–450 mL |
| Blood pressure | | |
|    Systolic | Decreases 5–12 mm Hg | |
|    Diastolic | Decreases 10–20 mm Hg | |
| Cardiac output | Increases 30%–50% | 6–7 L/min |
| Heart rate | Increases 10%–30% | Increased by 15–20 beats/min |
| Systemic vascular resistance | Decreases 20%–30% | $1,210 \pm 266$ dyn s/cm$^{-5}$ |
| Pulmonary vascular resistance | Decreases 34% | $78 \pm 22$ dyn s/cm$^{-5}$ |
| Colloid osmotic pressure | Decreases 10%–14% | Less than $22.4 \pm 0.5$ |
| **Respiratory Changes** | | |
| Functional residual capacity | Decreases 10%–21% | 1,343–1,530 |
| Tidal volume | Increases 30%–35% | 600 mL |
| **Renal Changes** | | |
| Renal blood flow | Increases 25%–50% | 1,500–1,750 mL/min |
| Glomerular filtration rate | Increases 50% | 140–170 mL/min |
| Creatinine clearance | Increases 50% | 100–150 mL/min |

**TABLE 11-2    Cardiac Output Changes in Pregnancy and Labor and Delivery**

| Stage of Pregnancy, Labor, or Delivery | Cardiac Output |
|---|---|
| By 8 wk of gestation | 22%–30% increase |
| By 20 wk of gestation | 50% increase |
| Repositioned from supine to left lateral decubitus | 21% increase |
| Early first stage of labor (dilated less than 3 cm) | 13%–17% increase |
| Late first stage of labor (dilated 4–7 cm) | 23% increase |
| Second stage of labor (dilated more than 8 cm) | 34% increase |
| During each contraction | 11%–15% increase |
| Immediately after delivery (10 min) | 59%–80% increase (dependent on type of anesthesia) |
| Within 1 h of delivery | 49% increase |

inserting nasogastric tubes or nasotracheal tubes because of the risk for epistaxis. Respiratory rate remains unchanged, although some women experience tachypnea or shortness of breath at some time during their pregnancy. The exact cause of dyspnea is unknown, but it may be related to hyperventilation, increased oxygen consumption, or decreased partial pressure of arterial carbon dioxide ($PaCO_2$).

Oxygen consumption increases by 20% to 33% during pregnancy and may increase by 300% during labor.[2] This results in an increased partial pressure of arterial oxygen ($PaO_2$) to 104 to 108 mm Hg. $PaCO_2$ decreases to 27 to 32 mm Hg and allows for the increased diffusion of carbon dioxide from the fetus to the mother.[3] Renal excretion of bicarbonate causes a slight increase in maternal pH, which is usually insignificant.

## Renal Changes

Changes in renal function, also outlined in Table 11-1, accommodate the increase in metabolic and circulatory requirements of pregnancy. Renal blood flow increases by 30% (in some incidences up to 75%) and glomerular filtration rate (GFR) by 50%.[4] These increases allow elevations in the clearance of many substances, such as creatinine and urea, and are reflected in lower serum levels.

## Gastrointestinal and Metabolic Changes

Gastrointestinal changes in pregnancy occur as a result of the growing uterus. Displacement of the esophageal sphincter into the thoracic cavity allows stomach contents to enter the esophagus passively. The pregnant woman is prone to passive regurgitation and aspiration, especially when under general anesthesia or any time she may be unconscious.[4] Hormonal influences cause delayed gastric emptying and increased gastric acid secretion in the third trimester. Smooth muscle relaxation contributes to nausea, heartburn, and constipation. Pregnancy creates a diabetogenic state because the body becomes increasingly resistant to insulin, and hyperinsulinemia occurs. Hepatic and maternal fasting blood glucose levels decrease owing to the constant transfer of glucose to the fetus.

## Hematological Changes

Hematocrit laboratory values decrease because of the hemodilution effect of increased plasma volume. Normal hematocrit values are 32% to 40% during pregnancy.[3] The white blood cell count is elevated from the normal range of 5,000–10,000/mm$^3$ to 6,000–16,000/mm$^3$.[4] There is an increase in clotting factors VII through X and a decrease in factors XI and XIII, which inhibit coagulation. Fibrinogen increases to 300 to 600 mg/dL. Bleeding and clotting times and platelet counts remain the same in pregnancy. A pregnant patient is in a state of hypercoagulability. This state is developed as a defense against postdelivery hemorrhage.[4]

## Fetal and Placental Development Considerations

Clinicians must carefully balance the effects and risks of all treatment decisions on the pregnant woman and her fetus. Maternal circulation and nutrition and exposure to teratogens influence embryonic and fetal development.

There are three stages in fetal development: preembryonic (first 14 days), embryonic (day 15 through 8 weeks), and fetal (8 through 40 weeks and delivery). During the embryonic stage, vital organs such as the heart and brain are in development. It is during this stage that the fetus is most vulnerable to teratogens (Fig. 11-1). Certain medications used in treating the critically ill pregnant woman may cross the placenta and have teratogenic effects on the fetus. For this reason, the clinician must consider the risks and benefits of medication therapy during pregnancy. In 2007, the U.S. Food and Drug Administration revised the five risk categories for labeling drug use in pregnancy (Table 11-3).

The placenta is the organ responsible for the metabolic exchange of oxygen, nutrition, and waste removal between the pregnant woman and the fetus. In early pregnancy, the placenta produces four hormones necessary to maintain the pregnancy. The hormone human chorionic gonadotropin—the basis for pregnancy tests—preserves the function of the corpus luteum. Another hormone, human placental lactogen, stimulates maternal metabolism to supply needed nutrients for fetal growth. This hormone is responsible for the increase in insulin resistance associated with pregnancy. The hormones progesterone and estrogen are eventually produced by the placenta and are responsible for uterine growth and uteroplacental blood flow.

Placental function depends on maternal blood flow. Diseases and conditions that cause vasoconstriction, such as hypertension, cocaine use, or smoking, can diminish blood flow to the placenta and fetus. Even excessive maternal exercise can shunt blood away from the placenta and fetus.

## Critical Care Conditions in Pregnancy

During pregnancy, normal physiological changes occur to provide for growth of the fetus and prepare the mother for birth. Medical or obstetrical complications may alter this adaptation and shift an uncomplicated pregnancy into a critical situation. ICU admissions become necessary in 0.04% to 4.54% of pregnancies, with the majority of indications being hemodynamic instability, obstetrical hemorrhage, and respiratory failure.[5] The most common obstetrical complications requiring ICU admission are severe preeclampsia (sometimes accompanied by HELLP [hemolysis, elevated liver enzymes, and low platelets] syndrome), disseminated intravascular coagulation (DIC), amniotic fluid embolus, acute respiratory distress syndrome (ARDS), and trauma.

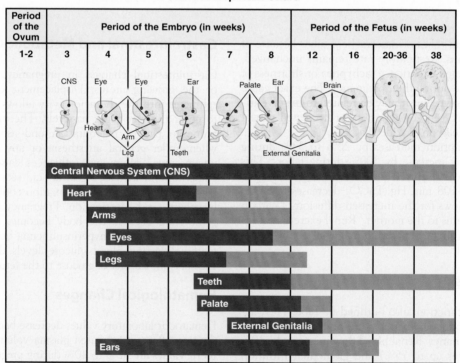

**Fetal Development Chart**

FIGURE 11-1  Critical periods of development. *Dark blue* denotes highly sensitive periods. (Adapted from the National Organization on Fetal Alcohol Syndrome.)

| TABLE 11-3 | FDA Rating System for Teratogenic Effects of Drugs | |
|---|---|
| **Category** | **Description** |
| A | Fetal risk not revealed in controlled studies in humans |
| B | Fetal risk not confirmed in studies in humans but has been shown in some studies in animals |
| C | Fetal risk revealed in studies in animals but not established or not studied in humans, may use if benefit outweighs risk to fetus |
| D | Fetal risk shown in humans, use only if benefits outweigh risk to fetus |
| X | Contraindicated, benefit does not outweigh risk |

Data from http://www.drugs.com/pregnancy-categories.html.

## Severe Preeclampsia

Hypertensive disorders of pregnancy occur in approximately 3% to 10% of all pregnancies and accounts for the majority of obstetric morbidity and mortality.[6,7] They are the third leading cause of maternal death in the United States. Terms used to describe the different types of hypertension that may occur in pregnancy are listed in Box 11-1.

Preeclampsia is a hypertensive disorder occurring in 5% to 7% of pregnancies.[8] The etiology of preeclampsia is unknown; however, predisposing risk factors include nulliparity, multiple gestation, diabetes, age younger than 18 years or older than 35 years and chronic hypertension. Preeclamptic symptoms include hypertension, edema, and proteinuria.

Hypertension in pregnancy is defined as a blood pressure of greater than 140/90 mm Hg.[8] In the past, increases of 30 mm Hg systolically or 15 mm Hg diastolically were used to diagnose hypertension in pregnancy. These criteria have become unreliable and should no longer be used. If the prepregnancy blood pressure is unknown, a blood pressure measurement of 140/90 mm Hg obtained twice at intervals of 6 hours apart in the same position and using the same arm is appropriate to diagnose this complication. In severe preeclampsia, the systolic blood pressure is greater than 160 mm Hg, and the diastolic blood pressure is greater than 110 mm Hg.[7]

<table>
<tr><td>

**BOX 11-1   Clinical Terminology: Hypertensive Disorders During Pregnancy**

- *Preeclampsia:* A pregnancy-specific syndrome observed after the 20th week of pregnancy with systolic blood pressure of greater than or equal to 140 mm Hg or diastolic blood pressure of greater than or equal to 90 mm Hg, accompanied by significant proteinuria. In women with preeclampsia, blood pressure usually returns to baseline within days to weeks after delivery.
- *Eclampsia:* The occurrence, in a woman with preeclampsia, of seizures that cannot be attributed to other causes. Convulsions usually occur after midpregnancy and may occur postpartum.
- *Gestational hypertension:* A blood pressure elevation detected for the first time after midpregnancy, distinguished from preeclampsia by the absence of proteinuria.
- *Chronic hypertension:* Elevated blood pressure in the mother that predated the pregnancy. It can also be diagnosed in retrospect when preeclampsia or gestational hypertension fails to normalize after delivery.

</td></tr>
</table>

From National Institutes of Health, National Heart Lung and Blood Institute: Report of the Working Group on Research on Hypertension During Pregnancy, April 2001.

Edema may be generalized but is more pronounced in the hands and face.

Proteinuria is diagnosed by protein concentrations of 1 g or greater in a 24-hour urine specimen. Target end-organ damage symptoms may also occur, and include oliguria, thrombocytopenia, impaired liver function, epigastric pain, cerebral and visual disturbances, and possibly pulmonary edema.[7] Oliguria is defined as a urine output less than 30 mL/h or less than 500 mL/24 h. Symptoms of visual and cerebral disturbances may include blurred vision and headaches. Liver involvement may be manifested by epigastric pain and impaired liver function tests.

### Physiological Principles

Severe preeclampsia is associated with vascular endothelial damage caused by arteriolar vasospasms and vasoconstriction.[9] Arterial circulation is disrupted by alternating areas of constriction and dilation. Damage to the endothelium results in leakage of plasma into the extravascular space and allows platelet aggregation to occur. Colloidal osmotic pressure decreases as protein enters the extravascular space, and the woman is at risk for hypovolemia and altered tissue perfusion and oxygenation. Physiologic changes in the maternal cardiovascular system, such as increased plasma volume, cardiac output, heart rate, and capillary permeability, and a decrease in colloid osmotic pressure, are exaggerated in preeclampsia and predispose the women to develop pulmonary edema.[9] Symptoms of pulmonary edema include coughing, dyspnea, chest pain, tachycardia, cyanosis, and pink, frothy sputum.

Arterial vasospasm and endothelial damage also decrease perfusion to the kidneys. The decreased kidney perfusion results in a decreased GFR and leads to oliguria. Oliguria may not be an indication of hypovolemia, and should not be treated with diuretics. Glomerular capillary endothelial damage permits protein to leak across the capillary membrane and into the urine, resulting in proteinuria, increased blood urea nitrogen, and increased serum creatinine. If vasospasm and hypercoagulability are long lasting, ischemia occurs in the glomeruli. Complete recovery of renal function usually occurs after delivery.[10]

The liver is also affected by multisystem vasospasm and endothelial damage. Decreased perfusion to the liver can cause ischemia and necrosis. The liver may become edematous as a result of inflammatory infiltrates and obstructed blood flow.[11] Liver damage is reflected in elevated liver function study results, such as serum aspartate aminotransferase, lactate dehydrogenase, and serum alanine aminotransferase.[11]

Neurological sequelae may include seizures, cerebral edema, and cerebral hemorrhage. Symptoms associated with neurological progression are headaches, blurred vision, hyperreflexia and clonus, and changes in the level of consciousness. Increased intracranial pressure and decreased perfusion can lead to hypoxia, coma, and death.[11]

### Management

The only cure for severe preeclampsia is delivery of the fetus. The decision to deliver the fetus versus continuing expectant management (ie, to maintain the pregnancy and monitor changes) is individualized.[9]

Usually these patients require invasive hemodynamic monitoring, frequent blood pressure measurements, strict intake and output monitoring, laboratory report monitoring, aggressive anticonvulsant and antihypertensive drug therapy, and, if undelivered, fetal surveillance. Management is focused on preventing seizures and respiratory complications, controlling hypertension, monitoring cardiovascular status, and maintaining fluid status. If the woman does not deliver, fetal monitoring is necessary. Critical care and obstetrical staff must collaborate to provide close fetal observation. It is important that they consider the fetus to be another patient.

Hemodynamic monitoring permits accurate assessments of cardiac output and fluid volume status. Normal hemodynamic values in pregnancy are listed in Table 11-4.[12] Elevated pulmonary artery occlusion pressure (PAOP) and pulmonary artery pressure (PAP) values may indicate hypervolemia, thereby placing the woman at risk for cardiogenic pulmonary edema. (See Chapter 17 for a more detailed discussion of hemodynamic monitoring.) Interventions to reduce preload include restricting intravenous (IV) fluids, repositioning the patient on her side, and administering diuretics when fluid overload or pulmonary edema is present. Decreased central venous pressure, PAP, and PAOP values indicate hypovolemia, and the patient may need a fluid challenge.

Drug therapy is directed at preventing seizures and hypertensive crises. IV magnesium sulfate is the drug of choice for severe preeclampsia to prevent maternal seizures (Box 11-2). Magnesium sulfate blocks the reuptake of acetylcholine at the nerve end synapses and relaxes smooth muscles. Side effects include drowsiness, flushing, diaphoresis, hyporeflexia, hypocalcemia, and respiratory paralysis.[9] A therapeutic serum level of 4 to 7 mg/dL is maintained through a continuous infusion of 1 to 3 g/h. Serum levels higher than 15 mg/dL may result in respiratory arrest.

Hydralazine hydrochloride (Apresoline) is the antihypertensive agent most commonly used during pregnancy when a hypertensive crisis occurs. It causes arterial vasodilation and decreases mean arterial pressure and SVR. Hydralazine increases cardiac output, heart rate, and renal blood flow. Doses

---

**BOX 11-2** **Magnesium Sulfate Administration**

*Dose concentration*: 20 g in 500 mL normal saline solution or D$_5$W = 2 g/50 mL
*Loading dose*: 4 to 6 g intravenous bolus over 10 to 20 minutes
*Maintenance dose*: 2 to 3 g/h by intravenous infusion

are commonly given in 5- to 10-mg boluses intravenously every 20 minutes until a satisfactory reduction in blood pressure is achieved.[13] Other antihypertensive agents used may include nifedipine (Procardia) and labetalol hydrochloride (Normodyne). These drugs may be used when hydralazine therapy fails, or they may be chosen because they have fewer maternal and fetal side effects.[13]

### Nursing Interventions

The nurse must assess the patient for increased risk of seizures by evaluating neurological symptoms. To reduce the risk of seizures, the nurse can decrease light and sound stimulation to the patient. Treatments and interventions are coordinated to optimize rest periods. If seizures occur, the nurse protects the patient from injury, ensures a patent airway, provides adequate oxygenation, and evaluates possible aspiration. After stabilizing the patient, the nurse quickly assesses uterine and fetal activities. In most instances, immediate delivery of the fetus is indicated.

If the patient is receiving magnesium sulfate therapy, the nurse continuously assesses for symptoms of magnesium toxicity, such as respiratory depression and hyporeflexia. Magnesium is excreted in the urine, and prolonged oliguria allows magnesium to accumulate to toxic blood levels.

If the patient has delivered, magnesium sulfate therapy should be continued for 24 hours. The nurse must assess uterine bleeding. The uterus should be firm after delivery; if it is not firm, uterine massage and oxytocin therapy are needed. Box 11-3 summarizes some of the key nursing interventions for patients with severe preeclampsia.

## HELLP Syndrome

HELLP syndrome accompanies severe preeclampsia and eclampsia in approximately 8% to 24% of diagnosed cases. Maternal mortality rates may be as high as 30%.[14] It is often considered a variation of severe preeclampsia. Women in whom HELLP syndrome develops are usually older than 27 years, Caucasian, and multiparous. Patients with HELLP syndrome are at an increased risk for developing complications such as renal failure, pulmonary edema, DIC, placental

---

**TABLE 11-4** Hemodynamic Values in Nonpregnant and Pregnant Women

| | Nonpregnant | Pregnant |
|---|---|---|
| Central venous pressure (mm Hg) | 5–10 | 1.1–6.1 |
| Pulmonary artery pressure | | |
| Systolic (mm Hg) | 20–30 | 18–30 |
| Diastolic (mm Hg) | 8–15 | 6–10 |
| Mean (mm Hg) | 10–20 | 11–15 |
| Pulmonary artery occlusion pressure (mm Hg) | 6–12 | 5.7–9.3 |
| Cardiac output (L/min) | 4.3–6.0 | 5.2–7.2 |

Risk for Disrupted Maternal–Fetal Dyad Related to Severe Preeclampsia

Strict Bed Rest in Left Lateral Tilt
- Explain rationale and expected benefits.
- Encourage family and friends to visit and provide activities that may prevent boredom.
- Explain seizure precautions.

Medications
- Explain the action of drugs such as magnesium sulfate and antihypertensive drugs.
- Explain the frequency of laboratory tests, vital sign assessment, and urinary output measurement.

Fetal Surveillance
- Explain external fetal monitoring and tests used to monitor fetal well-being, such as the nonstress test, the biophysical profile, Doppler flow studies, and fetal pulse oximetry.
- Explain the rationale used to determine adequate uteroplacental function.

Delivery
- Prepare the patient for the possibility of cesarean delivery.
- Explain the rationale for the need to deliver.
- Explain neonatal intensive care unit (NICU) if unable to physically take the patient on a unit tour.
- Arrange for a discussion with a neonatologist if the infant is premature or expected to be admitted to NICU.

abruption, ARDS, and liver hematoma and rupture. Signs and symptoms of HELLP syndrome may be similar to those of severe preeclampsia, and include epigastric pain, nausea, malaise, and right upper quadrant tenderness. Laboratory results reveal decreased platelets (less than 100,000/mm$^3$) and elevated liver enzymes.

## Physiological Principles

Hemolysis occurs when red blood cells pass through vasospastic vessels, producing burr cells or schistocytes.[11] Liver enzyme levels become elevated as liver damage occurs resulting from ischemia secondary to vasospasm. Prolonged vasospasm can lead to hepatic necrosis. Platelets are consumed because of the aggregation at endothelial damage sites.

## Management

As with severe preeclampsia, delivery is the treatment of choice for HELLP syndrome; however, the timing of delivery remains controversial. Most clinicians recommend expectant management occur no longer than 48 hours after the diagnosis of HELLP is established.[15] If delivery does not occur, management includes bed rest, frequent blood pressure assessments, frequent laboratory evaluation of liver function and coagulation status, and intensive fetal surveillance.[15] The patient is managed in the same manner as in severe preeclampsia, with magnesium sulfate and antihypertensive agents given as needed. Blood products may be given to correct coagulation abnormalities.

HELLP syndrome may mimic other disease entities; differential diagnosis must be made to rule out autoimmune thrombocytopenic purpura, chronic renal disease, pyelonephritis, cholecystitis, gastroenteritis, hepatitis, pancreatitis, thrombotic thrombocytopenic purpura, hemolytic–uremic syndrome, and acute fatty liver disease of pregnancy.[11]

Monitoring changes in vital signs, bleeding, pain, and laboratory values is necessary when caring for patients with HELLP syndrome. Fetal surveillance is important, and should include assessments for fetal heart rate and signs and symptoms of placental abruption. Nurses must be aware of the complications that can occur in patients with HELLP syndrome. Signs of worsening pain, vascular collapse, or shock may indicate liver hematoma or rupture. Accurate monitoring of intake and output must be maintained to assess renal status.

## Disseminated Intravascular Coagulation

Several conditions predispose a pregnant woman to DIC because of changes in the coagulation and fibrinolytic systems. These conditions include preeclampsia, abruptio placentae, amniotic fluid embolus, fetal death, and sepsis.[16] Although the incidence of sepsis has decreased because of antibiotic therapy, it is responsible for 3% to 8% of the maternal deaths in the United States.[17] Sepsis during pregnancy is a result of bacterial invasion of the uterine cavity.

Immunosuppression is a normal consequence of pregnancy and thought to occur so that the fetus is not rejected by the maternal immune system. This alteration increases the woman's susceptibility to infection and decreases the body's ability to fight infection. Septic shock may develop in a few days or several hours. Manifestations of septic shock include tachycardia, tachypnea, temperature instability, increased cardiac output, and decreased peripheral resistance.

Abruptio placentae is the premature separation of the placenta from the uterine wall, and is one of the most common causes of DIC. Blood collects between the uterus and placenta, causing consumption of clotting factors. The placental unit contains high concentrations of thromboplastin. When the placenta prematurely separates, thromboplastin continues to be released systemically, activating the clotting and fibrinolytic systems throughout the body. Parallel to the activation of the fibrinolytic system, the hemostatic system initiates clot formation at the site of the separation.[18] Clinical signs of abruption include acute abdominal pain, uterine tenderness, premature contractions, and vaginal bleeding. Abruptions may be subtle, and blood may not be visible.

Intrauterine fetal death can also lead to DIC. Tissue thromboplastin is released from the dead fetus into the maternal circulation, activating the procoagulant system. Coagulopathy is gradual and consistent with chronic, low-grade DIC.

## Management

Management of patients with DIC includes identifying the underlying condition and initiating appropriate therapy, evaluating and monitoring the coagulation system to restore hemostasis, and preventing further hemorrhage and thrombosis. Management of DIC caused by sepsis includes prompt delivery of the fetus and IV administration of broad-spectrum antibiotics. For abruptio placentae, prompt delivery of the fetus is necessary to control further bleeding.

Nursing care is aimed at preventing further bleeding, monitoring coagulation studies, and assessing the patient for multisystem involvement, altered tissue perfusion, and fluid volume deficits.[18] Nursing care includes monitoring respiratory status, administering IV fluids to prevent hypovolemia, assessing hemodynamic values, and administering and evaluating antibiotics, blood replacement products, and antipyretics. (See Chapter 49 for a more detailed discussion of DIC.)

## Amniotic Fluid Embolism

Amniotic fluid embolism (AFE), although rare, is responsible for approximately 10% of maternal deaths in the United States.[19] AFE occurs when amniotic fluid gains entry into the maternal circulation. This entry may occur during cesarean birth or uterine rupture, or through small tears in the endocervical veins during a vaginal delivery. Once amniotic fluid enters the maternal circulation, it is rapidly transported to the pulmonary vasculature, resulting in pulmonary emboli. The pulmonary response to AFE is vasospasm, which produces transient pulmonary hypertension and profound hypoxia. The maternal system becomes hemodynamically compromised, similar to anaphylactic shock, with elevated PAP and left ventricular failure.[19] Predisposing factors that may lead to AFE include preeclampsia, multiple gestation, polyhydramnios (excess amniotic fluid), low insertion of placenta, post-term pregnancy, hypertonic contractions during labor, abruptio placentae, uterine rupture, maternal seizures, and umbilical cord prolapse. Clinical manifestations of AFE include sudden onset of dyspnea, cyanosis, and hypotension, followed by cardiopulmonary arrest.

### Management

Management of AFE is directed at maintaining left ventricular output and an adequate airway.[19] Interventions include intubation and ventilation with 100% oxygen, IV administration of vasopressors and crystalloid fluids, basic cardiac life support (BLS), administration of blood products, and pulmonary artery catheterization. In extreme cases, extracorporeal membrane oxygenation (ECMO) may be used to provide adequate oxygenation and ventilatory support during treatment of the AFE. Potential sequelae include acute pulmonary edema, respiratory distress, DIC, hemorrhage, and multisystem failure.

The nurse must react quickly when AFE is suspected. Following the basic CAB (compressions, airway, breathing), the nurse can prioritize interventions needed in this stressful situation. If the patient is not intubated, oxygen must be administered using a face mask, and oxygen saturation assessed using a pulse oximeter. The nurse can anticipate that after intubation, a resuscitation bag or mechanical ventilation will be needed. To maximize venous return, the woman should be positioned on her side or a wedge placed under her hip. A large-bore IV line is needed to administer IV fluids and blood products and to correct hypotension. Assessment focuses on the cardiovascular, pulmonary, hematological, and neurological systems.

## Acute Respiratory Distress Syndrome

ARDS is characterized by progressive respiratory distress, severe hypoxemia, low lung compliance, noncardiogenic pulmonary edema, and diffuse infiltrates on chest radiography.[20] Precipitating factors of ARDS associated with pregnancy include abruptio placentae, severe preeclampsia, pyelonephritis, DIC, sepsis, AFE, aspiration, systemic infections, and fetal death in utero. Maternal hypoxemia can lead to spontaneous labor and fetal hypoxia, acidosis, and death; therefore, it should be aggressively managed. Perfusion to vital organs, including the fetus, must be maintained to reduce morbidity and mortality. Adequate fetal oxygenation requires a maternal arterial oxygen saturation ($SaO_2$) of at least 95%.

### Management

Pregnant women with ARDS require cardiovascular support and mechanical ventilation using positive end-expiratory pressure. Hemodynamic monitoring is essential for evaluating changes associated with ARDS, such as central hypovolemia and noncardiogenic pulmonary edema. Ventilator settings include a low tidal volume setting with a plateau pressure less than 30 cm $H_2O$ and a maximum respiratory rate of 32 to 35 breaths per minute.[20]

Nursing care of pregnant women with ARDS is primarily supportive. Interventions are directed at optimizing oxygen transport to tissues and restoring pulmonary capillary integrity. A complete respiratory assessment is made, including evaluation of $SaO_2$ using pulse oximetry; observation of respiratory rate, character, and effort; and auscultation of lungs. The symptoms of noncardiogenic pulmonary edema are similar to those of cardiogenic pulmonary edema (ie, tachypnea, tachycardia, rales, shortness of breath); however, the nurse should be aware that a decrease in PAOP and PAP (from the obstetrical normal; see Table 11-4) may indicate noncardiogenic pulmonary edema. Noncardiogenic pulmonary edema in obstetrical patients can be caused by aspiration of gastric contents, sepsis, blood transfusion reactions, DIC, and AFE. Nursing interventions to improve uteroplacental blood flow include positioning the patient on her side and maintaining adequate fluid volumes.[2]

Nursing care of women who are mechanically ventilated includes psychosocial support to help relieve anxiety, fear, and separation from family. Nurses can facilitate communication between the patient and family and keep them informed about maternal and fetal conditions. In extreme cases of ARDS in the postpartum period, ECMO may be used to provide adequate oxygenation and ventilatory support.

## Trauma

Accidental injuries complicate 1 in 12 pregnancies and are associated with spontaneous abortion, preterm labor, abruptio placentae, and fetal death. Trauma is the leading cause of nonobstetrical maternal death.[21] Common types of trauma include blunt trauma from motor vehicle crashes (51%), falls, and domestic violence (22%) and penetrating trauma from stab wounds or gunshots (4%).[22] Fetal survival depends on maternal survival, so immediate care and stabilization of the pregnant woman are essential.

Hemodynamic instability may not be initially apparent because of the normal physiological cardiovascular changes during pregnancy. A pregnant woman can lose up to 2,000 mL of blood before becoming hemodynamically unstable.[2]

## Management

Management consists of immediate stabilization and care. Immediate stabilization of all trauma patients consists of applying the ABCs of resuscitation: establishment of airway, breathing, and circulation. First an airway is established, and oxygen is provided at a rate of 10 to 12 L/min to produce a $PaO_2$ level of 60 mm Hg or higher. This $PaO_2$ level is necessary for optimal fetal oxygenation. A nasogastric tube should be inserted to avoid aspiration.

If BLS is necessary, the anatomical and physiological changes in pregnancy must be considered to maximize efforts. The uterus compresses major abdominal vessels and displaces abdominal contents, which decreases chest compliance. Placing a wedge under the woman's right hip displaces the uterus and decompresses the vessels (Fig. 11-2). This intervention can increase cardiac output up to 30%.[2] Standard advanced cardiac life support procedures are used, including defibrillation and most standard drugs. The administration of vasopressors should be avoided, however, because the vasoconstrictive action can impair uteroplacental perfusion.[20] Medical antishock trousers and pneumatic antishock garment equipment are rarely used; however, if they are employed, the abdominal compartment should not be inflated.[21]

IV access using large-bore catheters is needed, and aggressive IV infusions are used to increase stroke volume and maintain cardiac output. If hemorrhage occurs, bleeding must be controlled. A decrease in arterial blood pressure may not be an indication of hypovolemia because of low resistance in the uteroplacental system. A 30% to 35% loss can occur with severe consequence to the fetus before hypotension is noted. Fluid replacement therapy must be administered at a higher rate.[21]

Once the pregnant woman has been stabilized, her neurological status is assessed. After this assessment, a fetal assessment, including determination of life, is made. The fetal heart rate can be auscultated using a fetoscope, stethoscope, fetal Doppler, or ultrasonography. Additional assessments can be made on arrival at the hospital or trauma center. These assessments include electrocardiography, a complete physical examination, and laboratory tests, such as arterial blood gases (Table 11-5), complete blood count, platelet count, electrolytes, blood type, and crossmatch. Assessments should include parameters such as the onset of regular contractions (indicating labor may have begun), vaginal bleeding,

**TABLE 11-5 Arterial Blood Gas Values in Nonpregnant and Pregnant Women**

| | Nonpregnant | Pregnant |
|---|---|---|
| $PaO_2$ (mm Hg) | 80–100 | 87–106 |
| $PaCO_2$ (mm Hg) | 36–44 | 27–32 |
| pH | 7.35–7.45 | 7.40–7.47 |
| $HCO_3^-$ (mEq/L) | 24–30 | 18–21 |

and leakage of fluid from the vagina (indicating ruptured membranes).

## Cardiovascular Disease in Pregnancy

An increase in the number of maternal deaths has occurred since 2008 in the United States due to cardiovascular disease. Common causes include cardiomyopathy, chronic hypertension, metabolic syndrome, regurgitant lesions, and obesity.[23] Pregnancy adds a burden to the maternal cardiovascular system because of the increase of circulating fluid needed for the fetus and the hematologic changes that reduce the risk of bleeding at delivery but increase the risk for thrombosis.

Women who are pregnant and who have a WHO risk classification of III or IV should be counseled about their increased risk of morbidity and mortality. The patient will need cardiac consultations during her prenatal period as well as during her labor and delivery. To manage the severest cardiac pregnancies, it may be necessary to monitor and deliver the patient in the cardiac ICU.

## Providing Emotional Support

Emotional support is very important to all critically ill pregnant women and their families. If the woman labors in the ICU, her coach or significant other should be allowed to remain at the bedside. When she gives birth, breastfeeding and bonding can be encouraged when feasible. The mother needs access to her newborn and family during this time. If the newborn is not able to be at the bedside, the staff should provide frequent updates about the newborn. Creating a flexible and individualized atmosphere for a new family is a challenge in the ICU. The importance of coordinating obstetrical and critical care cannot be overemphasized. Box 11-4 lists nursing

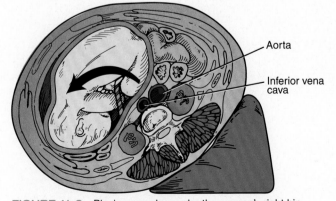

**FIGURE 11-2** Placing a wedge under the woman's right hip decompresses the major abdominal vessels, maximizing the cardiopulmonary resuscitation effort.

Aorta

Inferior vena cava

**BOX 11-4 Nursing Interventions**

Anxiety Related to Poor/Uncertain Pregnancy Outcome
- Shift orientation from the health care team to family-centered care.
- Incorporate cultural beliefs into the environment. Maintain family rituals when possible.
- Understand the role of the pregnant woman and her family members and assist them with their tasks to optimize family function.
- Provide names of family support groups.
- Provide information and education to family members.
- Encourage the family when they are coping well.
- Validate the family's emotions.
- Encourage use of breast pump, if mother chooses breastfeeding to feed infant.

interventions to promote well-being and address anxiety in a high-risk pregnancy.

If the fetus dies as a result of maternal complications, grief support may be needed. The nurse may collaborate with the labor and delivery staff (who may have grief training), psychiatric liaison nurses, social workers, psychologists, psychiatrists, and clergy to offer emotional support to a grieving mother and family.

## Clinical Applicability Challenges

---

### CASE STUDY

K.B. is a 36-year-old G1 P0 with risk factors that include advanced maternal age and a body mass index of 35 kg/m². At 37 weeks' gestation she was driving and had a motor vehicle accident. She was hit on the driver's side of the vehicle; she was wearing her seatbelt and no other persons were in the car with her. Initially K.B. expressed that she felt fine except for a slight pain in her abdomen where she thinks she may have hit the steering wheel. Her vital signs are BP 110/60, pulse 92, respirations 18. She is taken to the nearest emergency room by ambulance where the obstetric team is called to see her. An IV is initiated with D₅RL, her vital signs continue to be monitored, the fetal heart is assessed, and she is placed on a fetal monitor. The team assesses that K.B. is having contractions on the monitor and the fetal heart rate is 152 bpm. Her color is pink, skin warm and dry, there is no evidence of vaginal bleeding, her vital signs remain within normal limits (WNL), her pain is rated 3, and her pulse oximetry is 95%. There is no evidence of any other injuries, so the team decides to observe her further on the Labor & Delivery (L&D) unit.

K.B. arrives on L&D, and immediately complains of increasing pain in her abdomen. Her vital signs are 90/50, pulse 108, respirations 26. The fetal heart rate is 188 and her abdomen becomes hard and rigid to touch. There is no evidence of blood from the vagina. The obstetrics (OB) team decides to take K.B. to the operating room (OR) for an emergency C-section. Once in the OR, the fetal heart rate drops to 60 bpm, K.B.'s BP is 80/40, and the team begins the operative procedure. Once the abdomen and the uterus are opened, the team visualizes a large accumulation of blood. They quickly deliver and hand the infant to the pediatric team. The placenta was completely detached from the uterine wall and a large blood clot was observed. The remainder of the operation is completed, and K.B. is recovered and sent to the floor.

On the second postoperative day, K.B. complains of shortness of breath. Her blood pressure is 90/50, pulse 108, and respirations are 28. Her pulse oximetry is 90%, and her PaO₂/FiO₂ ratio is 112 mm Hg. She has a tomography scan that rules out a pulmonary embolism, but a chest x-ray reveals atelectasis. She is diagnosed with ARDS and transferred to the ICU. In the ICU she is placed on CPAP and monitored. Her vital signs return to 110/62, pulse 82, and respirations 18, but K.B. is anxious and keeps asking about her baby. She is transferred back to the postpartum unit, where she is reunited with her family and is discharged on day 5.

1. What signs and symptoms led to the diagnosis of abruption placenta?
2. What are the risk factors that may contribute to a patient developing ARDS?
3. How can the ICU staff provide a family-centered environment for a postpartum patient?

---

### WANT TO KNOW MORE?

A wide variety of resources to enhance your learning and understanding of this chapter are available on thePoint.

You will find:

- References
- Selected readings
- NCLEX-style review questions
- Internet resources
- And more!

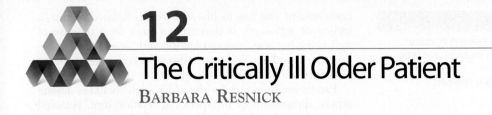

# 12

# The Critically Ill Older Patient

BARBARA RESNICK

**LEARNING OBJECTIVES**

*Based on the content in this chapter, the reader should be able to:*

1. Explain general physical changes that occur as a result of the normal aging process.
2. Describe the developmental tasks of the older person.
3. Discuss specific conditions that affect the major body systems of the older person.
4. Explain cognitive changes that may occur in the older patient.
5. Compare and contrast delirium and dementia in the older patient.
6. Describe assessment indicators of potential abuse or neglect of the older person.
7. Describe why the principle *start low, go slow* is important for the older patient in regard to the absorption, distribution, metabolism, and excretion of medications.

America is growing older. Between 2002 and 2030, the older population is anticipated to more than double, increasing to 71.5 from 35.6 million (Fig. 12-1). Almost 1 in 5 people will be 65 years old or older,[1] and more people will seek medical care for chronic disease, the leading cause of disability among older adults. When older adults have acute exacerbations of their diseases, they often require hospitalization in an intensive care unit (ICU).

As a result, critical care nurses need to understand the many physiologic changes that occur normally with aging. These alterations are progressive and usually are not apparent or pathological. However, these age-related changes put the critically ill older adult at increased risk for complications. Preventive nursing care, focused on avoiding potential problems, is necessary.

Death in older men from heart disease has dropped precipitously, while death from cerebrovascular disease has declined somewhat, but death from cancer overall has not changed much. The pattern for women is very similar. Life expectancy at age 65 continues to increase for both men and women, and the gender gap is narrowing. It is anticipated that the obesity epidemic we now face may alter longevity among current adults. In a recent study, for example, obesity reduced U.S. life expectancy at age 50 years by 1.54 years (95% confidence interval [CI] = 1.37, 1.93) for women and by 1.85 years (95% CI = 1.62, 2.10) for men.[2] Similarly, the number of patients with type 2 diabetes, which is known to be associated with premature death, is increasing rapidly.[3] Life expectancy in the United States has essentially stabilized and continues to be approximately 79 years of age.[4]

## Normal Psychobiologic Characteristics of Aging

### Biologic Issues

Intrinsic aging refers to characteristics and processes that occur universally with all older adults. Changes resulting from the aging process must be distinguished from extrinsic aging, which results from a particular disease process, disuse, or environmental factors, such as ultraviolet radiation. Normal aging is defined as the sum of intrinsic aging, extrinsic aging, and idiosyncratic or individual genetic factors.[5,6]

In most physiologic systems, the normal aging processes do not result in significant impairment or dysfunction in the absence of disease and under resting conditions. It is only in response to stress that an age-related reduction in physiologic reserves causes a loss of homeostatic balance. Examples of intrinsic age changes include reduced resistance to stress, poor tolerance of temperature extremes, reduced sensory perceptions, and greater fluctuations in blood pH. Aging, in one organ or the entire body, may be premature or delayed in relation to actual chronologic age. The effect of aging on cellular tissues is asymmetrical. For example, the changes resulting from aging in relation to the brain, bone, cardiovascular, and lung tissues may be fairly obvious, whereas changes affecting

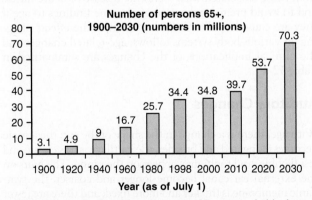

**FIGURE 12-1** Profile of Americans age 65 years and older based on data from the United States Bureau of the Census. Data from the year 1900 to present were used to predict the number of Americans age 65 years and older in the year 2030. (From U.S. Department of Health and Human Services, Administration for Community Living, Administration on Aging: A Profile of Older Americans: 2013. Washington, DC: USDHHS, ACL, AOA, 2013, p 3. Retrieved from http://www.aoa.acl.gov/Aging_Statistics/Profile/2013/docs/2013_Profile.pdf)

- The amount of connective and collagen tissue is increased.
- Cellular elements in the nervous system, muscles, and other vital organs disappear.
- The number of normally functioning cells is reduced.
- The amount of fat is increased.
- Oxygen use is decreased.
- During rest, the amount of blood pumped is decreased.
- Less air is expired by the lungs.
- Excretion of hormones is decreased.
- Sensory and perceptual activity is decreased.
- Absorption of lipids, proteins, and carbohydrates is decreased.
- Presbyesophagus occurs.
- The arterial lumen thickens.

the liver, pancreas, gastrointestinal tract, and muscle tissues are less obvious. Several organic changes that result from aging are listed in Box 12-1.

## Psychosocial Issues

In addition to physical signs of aging, nurses caring for acutely ill older patients must be aware of the older person's normal developmental tasks and the specific dreams or wishes of a particular senior. Developmental tasks of older people are listed in Box 12-2.

The need for support and meaningful relationships continues throughout life. Support can be described as a feeling of belonging or a belief that one is an active participant in the surrounding world. The feeling of mutuality with others in the environment lends strength and helps decrease the sense of isolation. Support by family, friends, and the community can provide an older patient with a greater sense of stability and security.

Self-worth and perceived well-being are feelings that usually coincide in older adults. The perception of well-being arises from the satisfaction of meeting an acceptable proportion of one's life goals. It can be described as an inner

**BOX 12-2** Developmental Tasks of the Older Person

- Deciding where and how to live for his or her remaining years
- Preserving supportive, intimate, and satisfying relationships with spouse, family, and friends
- Maintaining an adequate and satisfying home environment relative to health and economic status
- Providing sufficient income
- Maintaining a maximum level of health
- Attaining comprehensive health and dental care
- Maintaining personal hygiene
- Maintaining communication and adequate contact with family and friends
- Maintaining social, civic, and political involvement
- Initiating new interests (in addition to former activities) that increase status
- Recognizing and feeling that he or she is needed
- Discovering the meaning in life after retirement and when confronted with illness of self or spouse and death of spouse and other loved ones; adjusting to death of loved ones
- Developing a significant philosophy of life and discovering comfort in a philosophy or religion

contentment one has in life as a whole. Related to this, a feeling of self-worth is derived not only from a sense of well-being but also from satisfaction with one's image or acceptance by others. Self-worth also reflects the quality of interactions with family and friends.

Family environment for the older adult includes, among others, dimensions of interpersonal relationships, personal growth, integrity of the family unit, and adaptation to stress. As family members age, all these areas of concern intensify because of changes in roles of family members, alterations in the family power structure, and changes in financial and decision-making dynamics. Acute illness increases the urgency for effective cooperation among all family members as the traditional family structure is suddenly challenged.

When older patients are admitted to intensive care, issues of family cohesion and adaptability often surface. Frequently, families face immediate changes in roles, with adult children and grandchildren assuming the roles of caretakers and nurturers for the older family members. The family must suddenly adjust to dramatically different demands. Frequent visits to the hospital, communication with nurses, physicians, and social workers, and efforts to support and communicate with the patient become primary tasks. Amid these activities, family members (particularly those who have been given power of attorney) find themselves being pressed for decisions about immediate and long-term care. The expanding use of the Medical or Physician Orders for Life-Sustaining Treatment (MOLST, POLST) as part of the health record has greatly helped families during this difficult time.[7]

## Physical Challenges

Chronic changes in one organ system may be associated with changes in other systems. Moreover, there is individual variation in age-related changes. Therefore, each person must be evaluated on the basis of the age-related changes actually present rather than on those that are "normal" for a particular age.

It is equally important to distinguish age-related changes from those associated with a chronic disease or acute illness and to avoid prematurely attributing some findings to age if they are caused by illness. A discussion of the effects of aging on various body systems follows; age-related changes and the clinical implications of the changes are summarized in Table 12-1.

## Auditory Changes

With age, there is a change in the shape of the ear: the auricle becomes elongated and broader, the cartilage is less elastic and less flexible, and tophi may appear on the pinna. The hairs on the external ear canal become longer and coarser, the tympanic membrane is thicker and more fixed, and there are fewer cerumen glands (leading to thicker, drier cerumen). In the cochlea, hair cells, neuron-supporting cells, ganglion cells, and fibers are decreased, causing decreased hearing and balance.

An estimated 7 million people older than 65 years have significant hearing loss, and continuation of current trends indicates that more than 11 million people will have this problem by 2020.[8,9] The aging process affects hearing in two critical ways: reduction in threshold sensitivity (the

**TABLE 12-1    Summary of Age-Related Changes, Clinical Implications, and Key Nursing Interventions**

| Age-Related Changes | Clinical Implications | Key Nursing Interventions |
|---|---|---|
| **Cardiovascular** | | |
| • Atrophy of muscle fibers that line the endocardium<br>• Atherosclerosis of vessels<br>• Increased systolic blood pressure<br>• Decreased compliance of the left ventricle<br>• Decreased number of pacemaker cells<br>• Decreased sensitivity of baroreceptors | • Increased blood pressure<br>• Increased emphasis on atrial contraction with an $S_4$ heard<br>• Increased dysrhythmias<br>• Increased risk for hypotension with position change<br>• Valsalva maneuver may cause a drop in blood pressure<br>• Decreased exercise tolerance | • To prevent falls related to positional hypotension, make sure the person changes position slowly and waits before ambulating |
| **Neurologic** | | |
| • Decreased number of neurons and increase in size and number of neuroglial cells<br>• Decline in nerves and nerve fibers<br>• Atrophy of the brain and increase in cranial dead space<br>• Thickened leptomeninges in spinal cord | • Increased risk for neurologic problems: CVA, parkinsonism<br>• Slower conduction of fibers across the synapses<br>• Modest decline in short-term memory<br>• Alterations in gait pattern: wide based, shorter stepped, and flexed forward<br>• Increased risk for hemorrhage before symptoms are apparent | • To compensate for the decline in short-term memory, provide more time to complete memory-associated tasks |
| **Respiratory** | | |
| • Decreased lung tissue elasticity<br>• Thoracic wall calcification<br>• Cilia atrophy<br>• Decreased respiratory muscle strength<br>• Decreased partial pressure of arterial oxygen ($PaO_2$) | • Decreased efficiency of ventilatory exchange<br>• Increased susceptibility to infection and atelectasis<br>• Increased risk for aspiration<br>• Decreased ventilatory response to hypoxia and hypercapnia<br>• Increased sensitivity to narcotics | • To prevent infection and atelectasis, encourage deep breathing and coughing |
| **Integumentary** | | |
| • Loss of dermal and epidermal thickness<br>• Flattening of papillae<br>• Atrophy of sweat glands<br>• Decreased vascularity<br>• Collagen cross-linking<br>• Elastin regression<br>• Loss of subcutaneous fat<br>• Decreased melanocytes<br>• Decline in fibroblast proliferation | • Thinning of skin and increased susceptibility to tearing<br>• Dryness and pruritus<br>• Decreased sweating and ability to regulate body heat<br>• Increased wrinkling and laxity of skin<br>• Loss of fatty pads protecting bone and resulting in pain<br>• Increased need for protection from the sun<br>• Increased time for wound healing | • To prevent damage to fragile skin, avoid shearing forces<br>• To counteract dryness, immerse skin in water daily and apply emollients<br>• To minimize pain, pad thinned areas with additional layers (eg, extra socks for feet)<br>• Encourage sunscreen use |
| **Gastrointestinal** | | |
| • Decreased liver size<br>• Less efficient cholesterol stabilization and absorption<br>• Fibrosis and atrophy of salivary glands<br>• Decreased muscle tone in bowel<br>• Atrophy of and decrease in number of taste buds<br>• Slowing in esophageal emptying<br>• Decreased hydrochloric acid secretion<br>• Decreased gastric acid secretion<br>• Atrophy of the mucosal lining<br>• Decreased absorption of calcium | • Change in intake due to decreased appetite<br>• Discomfort after eating related to slowed passage of food<br>• Decreased absorption of calcium and iron<br>• Alteration of drug effectiveness<br>• Increased risk for constipation, esophageal spasm, and diverticular disease | • Encourage small, frequent meals to avoid discomfort and improve intake<br>• Encourage fluids and fiber to improve bowel function |

*(continued)*

**TABLE 12-1** Summary of Age-Related Changes, Clinical Implications, and Key Nursing Interventions (*continued*)

| Age-Related Changes | Clinical Implications | Key Nursing Interventions |
|---|---|---|
| **Urinary** | | |
| • Reduced renal mass<br>• Loss of glomeruli<br>• Decline in number of functioning nephrons<br>• Changes in small vessel walls<br>• Decreased bladder muscle tone | • Decreased GFR<br>• Decreased sodium-conserving ability<br>• Decreased creatinine clearance<br>• Increased BUN<br>• Decreased renal blood flow<br>• Altered drug clearance<br>• Decreased ability to dilute urine<br>• Decreased bladder capacity and increased residual urine<br>• Increased urgency | • To prevent complications from medical therapy, monitor drug clearance and alter dosing as necessary<br>• Monitor for UTI |
| **Reproductive** | | |
| • Atrophy and fibrosis of cervical and uterine walls<br>• Decreased vaginal elasticity and lubrication<br>• Decreased hormones and reduced oocytes<br>• Decreased seminiferous tubules<br>• Proliferation of stromal and glandular tissue<br>• Involution of mammary gland tissue | • Vaginal dryness and burning and pain with intercourse<br>• Decreased seminal fluid volume and force of ejaculation<br>• Reduced elevation of the testes<br>• Prostatic hypertrophy<br>• Connective breast tissue is replaced by adipose tissue, making breast examinations easier | • To compensate for vaginal dryness or pain, encourage the use of lubricating creams, estrogen cream, or both<br>• Monitor for urinary retention in men |
| **Musculoskeletal** | | |
| • Decreased muscle mass<br>• Decreased myosin adenosine triphosphatase activity<br>• Deterioration and drying of joint cartilage<br>• Decreased bone mass and osteoblastic activity | • Decreased muscle strength<br>• Decreased bone density<br>• Joint pain and stiffness<br>• Loss of height<br>• Increased risk for fracture<br>• Alterations in gait and posture | • Encourage resistive exercises to reverse a decline in muscle strength<br>• Encourage exercise and intake of calcium and vitamin D<br>• Encourage activity and exercise |
| **Sensory** | | |
| *Vision*<br>• Decreased rod and cone function<br>• Pigment accumulation<br>• Decreased speed of eye movements<br>• Increased intraocular pressure<br>• Ciliary muscle atrophy<br>• Increased lens size and yellowing of the lens<br>• Decreased tear secretion | • Decreased visual acuity, visual fields, and light/dark adaptation<br>• Increased sensitivity to glare<br>• Increased incidence of glaucoma<br>• Distorted depth perception with increased falls<br>• Less able to differentiate blues, greens, and violets<br>• Increased eye dryness and irritation | • Provide materials with large print<br>• Make sure there is adequate lighting without glare<br>• Use contrasting colors for print material |
| *Hearing*<br>• Loss of auditory neurons<br>• Loss of hearing from high to low frequency<br>• Increased cerumen<br>• Angiosclerosis of ear | • Decreased hearing acuity and isolation (specifically, decreased ability to hear consonants)<br>• Difficulty hearing, especially when there is background noise or when speech is rapid<br>• Cerumen impaction may cause hearing loss | • Make sure to face the person; use touch and visual cues to facilitate communication<br>• Evaluate for cerumen impaction, and remove cerumen as necessary |
| *Smell*<br>• Decreased number of olfactory nerve fibers | • Inability to smell noxious odors<br>• Decreased food intake | • Present odors the patient can smell. The ability to smell fruity odors, for example, is retained. Also use spices in foods to augment the sense of taste |
| *Taste*<br>• Altered ability to taste sweet and salty foods; bitter and sour tastes remain | | • Use alternative seasonings |
| *Touch*<br>• Decreased sensation | • Safety risk with regard to recognizing dangers in the environment: hot water, fire, small objects on floor that may result in tripping | • Avoid a cluttered environment |

| TABLE 12-1 | Summary of Age-Related Changes, Clinical Implications, and Key Nursing Interventions (*continued*) | |
|---|---|---|
| **Age-Related Changes** | **Clinical Implications** | **Key Nursing Interventions** |
| **Endocrine** | | |
| • Decreased testosterone, GH, insulin, adrenal androgens, aldosterone, and thyroid hormone<br>• Decreased thermoregulation<br>• Decreased febrile response<br>• Increased nodularity and fibrosis of thyroid<br>• Decreased basal metabolic rate | • Decreased ability to tolerate stressors such as surgery<br>• Decreased sweating and shivering and temperature regulation<br>• Lower baseline temperature; infection may not cause an elevation in temperature<br>• Decreased insulin response, glucose tolerance<br>• Decreased sensitivity of renal tubules to ADH<br>• Weight gain<br>• Increased incidence of thyroid disease | • Monitor the temperature of the room<br>• Provide adequate clothing and blankets to keep the patient warm<br>• Closely monitor blood glucose levels of patients with diabetes |
| **Immune** | | |
| • Decline in both T-cell and B-cell function<br>• The decreased numbers of B cells secreting immunoglobulin G<br>• The thymus gland involutes, and there is a decrease in thymic hormone levels<br>• The number of autoantibodies increases | • Poor immune response and risk for infection | • Encourage exercise, as there is some evidence that exercise helps to boost the immune system<br>• Encourage meticulous use of universal precautions and infection control techniques |

minimum sound level of a pure tone that an average ear with normal hearing can hear with no other sound present) and reduction in the ability to understand speech. The ability to hear sounds that occur between 8,000 and 20,000 Hz is not detectable with a routine hearing test. Therefore, hearing loss because of aging or other factors is not documented clinically until frequencies are at or below 8,000 Hz.

Presbycusis is a sensorineural hearing loss and is the most common form of hearing loss in older adults. Presbycusis is characterized by a gradual, progressive, bilateral, symmetrical, high-frequency sensorineural (perceptive) hearing loss with poor speech discrimination. Thirteen percent of people 65 years of age and older, if tested, would show signs of presbycusis.[10] Sensorineural hearing loss is due to degeneration or changes in the neural receptors in the cochlea, cranial nerve VIII (the acoustic nerve), and central nervous system. Treatment may vary dramatically from simple removal of impacted earwax to surgical removal of an auditory nerve tumor.

Conductive hearing loss is due to the blockage of sound transmission from the external ear through the tympanic membrane and small bones in the middle ear. Like presbycusis, conductive hearing loss is commonly found in older adults, and it is not unusual for older people to have both sensorineural and conductive hearing loss.

### Findings on Physical Examination and Management

The ear canal of the older adult should be evaluated at regular intervals (every few months) because of the tendency to have thicker, drier cerumen, which can occlude the canal and affect hearing. The older patient may retain the ability to hear pure tones, but if these pure tones are grouped to form words, the ability to understand and perceive these sounds as intelligible speech may be lost. This loss is known as impairment of discrimination ability. The patient has increased

difficulty hearing high-frequency stimuli-sibilant sounds (-f-, -s-, -th-, -ch-, and -sh-). Noisy environments further hamper the ability to hear certain sounds. Therefore, the person may respond inappropriately to questions, withdraw, or frequently ask for the speaker to repeat what is said. Eliminating background noise, speaking lower and louder, and using multiple means of getting information across (eg, verbal as well as written formats) can facilitate communication. People with impaired discrimination may also have problems with balance during transfers and ambulation, and they experience frequent falls. Activity and exercise interventions should be implemented as soon as possible to strengthen muscles and bones and improve balance.

## Visual Changes

Like all other body systems, the eye is affected by aging. Structural and functional changes occur slowly and gradually. Visual perception depends on the integration of various neurosensory systems and structures that age at different rates.

Normal visual changes associated with aging may include a loss of elasticity in the eyelids and subsequent wrinkling, ptosis (upper eyelid drooping), and "pouches" resulting from changes in the tissues beneath the eyelid skin and the subsequent formation and accumulation of fatty tissue. The conjunctiva may develop a yellowish or discolored membrane or become thickened as a result of environmental hazards, such as dust and exposure to drying and irritating pollutants. Arcus senilis, which is a white or gray ring around the limbus (junction of the cornea and sclera), may be related to a high blood level of fatty substances accumulated with advancing age. Although there is a decrease in the amount of lacrimation with age, overflow of tears may occur because of impaired drainage of the ductal system.

The iris loses its ability to accommodate rapidly to light and dark and develops an increased need for light. With age, the pupil becomes smaller and fixed. The lens becomes inflexible with less complete accommodation for near and far vision. The vitreous humor behind the lens may pull on the retina, producing holes or tears and predisposing the older person to retinal detachment. The ciliary muscle becomes stiff, which contributes to the problems of accommodating to distances. By the age of 60 years, presbyopia (the inability to shift focus from far to near) may develop—possibly because the older, aging lens, which is less flexible, cannot easily change shape through the action of the focusing muscle to which it is attached.

A cataract is a clouding of the normally clear and transparent lens of the eye. When a cataract interferes with the transmission of light to the retina, some loss in visual acuity may result. The older patient may complain of increased sensitivity to glare, a blurring of vision, halo images, cloudiness, decreased visual acuity, and decreased contrast sensitivity. Risk factors for cataract formation include diabetes mellitus, heredity, ultraviolet-B radiation exposure, smoking, corticosteroid drugs, alcohol use, and insufficient ingestion of antioxidant vitamins. The visual changes can progress to complete loss of vision. Cataracts account for one sixth of all cases of visual impairment in the United States, and most often occur in people older than 50 years.

Glaucoma is one of the major causes of blindness and is especially prevalent in the older adult. Glaucoma is due to increased intraocular pressure that may result in compression of the optic disc of the eye and damage to cranial nerve II (the optic nerve). This causes loss of peripheral vision and visual acuity. Risk factors for glaucoma include African American race, a family history of glaucoma, ocular hypertension, advanced age, myopia, retinal vascular disturbance, corticosteroid drug use, diabetes mellitus, and vascular crisis (elevation in blood pressure). Age-related changes in the canal of Schlemm, infection, injury, swollen cataracts, and tumors are also etiologic factors for glaucoma. Glaucoma is classified on the basis of whether the angle of the anterior chamber is open or narrow and whether the glaucoma is primary or secondary. Primary, open-angle glaucoma is the most common type found in older adults and is generally caused from corticosteroid-induced pressure increases in the eye. This type progresses slowly. Primary, angle-closure glaucoma, commonly caused by a swollen cataract, is less common and is characterized by a sudden and marked increase in intraocular pressure with accompanying redness and pain in the eye, headache, nausea or vomiting, corneal edema, and decreased vision. Secondary glaucoma is characterized by an anatomical or functional blockage of the outflow channels. Early diagnosis of glaucoma is important because the earlier that treatment is started, the easier it is to control the disease.

Retinal degeneration, or macular degeneration, is the third major source of visual disability in the older adult. Macular degeneration is a pigmentary change of the macular area of the retina caused by small hemorrhages. People see a gray shadow in the center of the visual area but can see well at the outer border. This condition rarely results in total blindness; however, visual loss can progress to legal blindness. Early symptoms include a slight blurring of vision, followed by a blind spot. Compensation techniques include wearing sunglasses or visors, looking to the side, and using magnifiers.

Diabetic retinopathy is the leading cause of blindness in the United States. It is caused by the deterioration of the blood vessels nourishing the retina at the back of the eye. Microaneurysms and small hemorrhages in the eye may leak fluid or blood and cause swelling of the retina. If this leaking blood or fluid damages or scars the retina, the image sent to the brain becomes blurred, and the condition eventually can progress to blindness.

### Findings on Physical Examination and Management

The older adult is likely to have smaller pupils, decreased visual acuity, difficulty with depth perception, decreased peripheral vision, and dry eyes. Ectropion and entropion are commonly noted with age. Ectropion is eversion of the eyelid (usually the lower lid), resulting in exposure of the lid, thickening and keratinization, and chronic irritation. When cataracts are present, there is opacity of the lens, and the red reflex may be absent during funduscopic examination. The older adult with cataracts presents with dimming of his or her vision and complains that everything appears clouded. People who have glaucoma present with complaints of blurred vision, halos around lights, or decreased peripheral vision. Older adults with macular degeneration present with a gradual decline in vision, particularly central vision, without a change in peripheral vision.

Good lighting, avoiding glare, and using contrasting colors (eg, black letters on white paper) and large print can facilitate vision. Selected nursing interventions for people with impaired vision are listed in Box 12-3.

## Other Sensory Changes

Although hearing and vision changes are the most researched sensory changes occurring in older people, there also may be declines in other senses. The number of taste buds is reported to decrease with age, in conjunction with a decline in the ability to taste substances. Sweet and salty substances are less detectable as one ages; therefore, many older adults complain that food tastes bitter or sour. There is very little information on smell sensation, but it is thought that a decrease in the sense of smell can result from atrophy of the olfactory organ and increased hair in the nostrils.[11] The loss of taste and smell affects the older person's ability to identify food and make odor discriminations.

The threshold of touch varies with the part of the body stimulated. There is a loss of tactile sensation as one ages,

---

**BOX 12-3** | **Nursing Interventions**

For Visually Impaired Patients
- Identify yourself on approach.
- Approach blind patients from the front.
- Assess impact of failing vision and patient's ability to adapt during hospitalization and after discharge.
- Assess stress level because increased stress can necessitate higher dosages of eye medication for patients with glaucoma.
- Be alert to side effects that other medications may have on the eyes (ie, medications containing antihistamines, caffeine, and atropine-like substances).
- Provide eye lubrications when eyes are dry.
- Instill all prescribed medications.

although this varies individually. Older adults may not feel the effects of lying too long in one position. A key nursing intervention is to vary the positions of the immobile older patient. The older adult also has decreased kinesthetic sense, which is the person's awareness of his or her body in space. Decreased kinesthetic sense results in postural instability and difficulty reacting to bodily changes in space.

### Findings on Physical Examination and Management

With age, the lips tend to become thin and pale, and the tissue of the oral mucosa is thinner, paler, and less elastic. Small yellow sebaceous glands may be seen in the buccal mucosa. The dorsum and margins of the tongue may have decreased number and size of papillae and may be coated with a thin white film, and there are changes in the gums and salivary glands. To facilitate taste and improve oral intake, the nurse provides frequent mouth care (before meals), offers foods in a pleasant setting using liberal seasonings to stimulate taste, and encourages the use of interventions, such as sugar-free candies, to stimulate salivation.

Older adults with decreased sensation may present with complaints of increased difficulty performing fine motor activities such as buttoning clothes or picking up objects. They may also have pressure sores and decreased balance. Frequent position changes are essential and should be instituted every 30 minutes.

## Sleep Changes

It is estimated that sleep disturbances occur in more than half of those older than 65 years.[12] An important aspect of the critical care nurse's assessment is to determine whether sleep problems are the result of normal aging, sleep disorders, or sleep disturbances due to the acute care environment.

Although some age-related changes in sleep patterns are the normal consequences of aging, the prevalence and potential for severe sleep disorders call for increased clinical awareness and evaluation. Such complaints as habitual snoring, frequent awakening, nocturnal sweating, and awakening with anxiety may be signs of a genuine sleep disorder.

The loss of neurons in the brain may be responsible for the normal age changes in the sleep cycle. These include a longer time to fall sleep, increased time in lighter stages of sleep (stages 1 and 2), decreased time in deeper stages of sleep (stages 3 and 4), and increased and shorter repetitions of the sleep cycle. The amount of sleep needed for each person does not change with age. However, there is an increased tendency for older adults to sleep less at night, to be somnolent late in the day or early evening, and to awaken early in the morning. This has been referred to as the advanced sleep phase syndrome.[13] Older adults also have shortened sleep latency, resulting in daytime napping. Daytime napping further compounds the problem because it reduces the need for nighttime sleep. Common complaints (eg, anxiety, waking up due to choking, headaches, sweating at night, nocturia, and snoring) are not normal age-related changes and should be assessed more thoroughly.

The most prevalent and most serious age-related sleep disorder is sleep apnea. There is evidence of an association between sleep apnea and circulatory disorders, including hypertension, stroke, and angina pectoris. There also may be a link between sleep apnea and reduced life expectancy. The prevalence of disordered breathing in the older patient is high. Moreover, there may be an association among habitual snoring, stroke, and angina pectoris in older men.[13]

### Findings on Physical Examination and Management

Older adults with sleep disorders present with an inability to fall asleep, an inability to stay asleep, or both. They may exhibit daytime napping, and fall asleep during activities. Conversely, there may be evidence of sleep deprivation with altered mental status being the major presenting sign. Loud snoring with multiple apnea–hypopnea events is indicative of sleep apnea. These people may have daytime hypersomnolence, fatigue, irritability, and decreased cognitive function because of impaired nighttime sleep patterns. Normal aging, chronic illness, and drug therapy increase the older person's susceptibility to insomnia.

Sleep disturbances in hospitalized older adults are multifactorial and related to illness, medications, change in routines, and a sleep-disruptive environment. Moreover, adherence to useful behavioral intervention in the acute care setting is particularly challenging. Sleep medications are commonly used and initiated during the hospitalization. When used, benzodiazepine receptor agonists should be prescribed in small dosages. Sedating antihistamines such as diphenhydramine should not be used as a sleep aid owing to associated anticholinergic adverse events (eg, delirium, urinary retention, constipation).

Care should be taken in dispensing sedative-hypnotics for people with risk factors for sleep apnea. Nursing interventions include encouraging older patients with disordered breathing to sleep on their sides and to lose weight if obese. Other interventions include giving supplemental oxygen if hypoxemia, caused by chronic lung disease or hypoventilation, is present.

## Skin Changes

Although a variety of cutaneous changes have been associated with age, some of these changes are due to normal or intrinsic age factors, whereas others are due to chronic solar exposure.[8] Photoaging is the combined effect of repeated sun exposure and intrinsic aging on the skin, and it is the cause of what is generally associated with the clinical (and histologic) changes that are consistent with "aging."

The combined skin changes in older adults result in a tendency toward quicker breakdown in the skin barrier and slower recovery of skin integrity. Common interventions to maintain skin integrity are shown in Box 12-4.

---

**BOX 12-4  Nursing Interventions**

For Maintaining Skin Integrity in the Older Adult
- Avoid shearing forces when turning the patient.
- Turn the patient frequently.
- Keep the patient appropriately covered for warmth.
- Bathe the patient daily, preferably with total immersion in water 32.2°C to 40.5°C (90°F to 105°F).
- Apply oil-based emollient to the patient's skin after bathing.
- Monitor responses from transdermal medications.
- Monitor wounds closely for healing and signs and symptoms of infection.

## Findings on Physical Examination and Management

The skin of older adults tends to sag, especially on the hands and forearms, and causes underlying tissue injury. The person may appear pale and may not be able to correctly perceive surface temperature (eg, how hot water is). The hair becomes gray and is coarser, and the nails may break and become more brittle. Additional hairs develop on the eyebrows and in the nose and ears. Wound healing is prolonged, and there is increased risk for contact dermatitis due to increased skin sensitivity. Xerosis, or dry skin, is a common problem for the older adult and is the most common cause of pruritus in this group. The treatment of dry skin focuses primarily on applying emollients to the skin immediately after bathing and avoiding excessive bathing with very hot water.

Skin lesions are more common in the older adult. Any change in a skin growth or any lesion that does not heal in a reasonable time should be suspect for malignancy. Malignant lesions tend to occur in sun-exposed areas but may also be present in other areas.

## Cardiovascular Changes

A number of cardiovascular changes occur with aging (see Table 12-1). These age-related changes, overt and occult cardiovascular disease, and reduced physical activity all affect cardiovascular function in elderly people. Aging changes in the heart have an impact on afterload, preload, contractility, diastolic function, and the cardiovascular response to exercise. Afterload is the resistance to the ejection of blood by the left ventricle and is composed of (1) peripheral vascular resistance and (2) characteristic aortic impedance. With age, the large elastic arteries become dilated, with a reduction in compliance. Progressive thickening of the aortic media and intima is associated with aortic enlargement. There is an age-associated increase in arterial stiffness resulting from changes in the arterial media.

With aging, there is an increase in systolic blood pressure and a widened pulse pressure. A slight reduction in diastolic blood pressure occurs after the sixth decade.[14] The increase in systolic blood pressure is due to an interaction of many factors, with age being only one of them.

Posterior left ventricular wall thickness increases (ie, left ventricular hypertrophy develops) with age, and this is mediated by an increase in systolic blood pressure.[14] This hypertrophy is due to volume, not the number of cardiac myocytes. Fibroblasts undergo hyperplasia, and collagen is deposited in the myocardial interstitium. Increased afterload causes an increase in left ventricular systolic stress and the addition of sarcomeres. These changes result in an increased left ventricular wall thickness with a normal or decreased left ventricular chamber size and an increased relative wall thickness.

Preload is the filling volume of the left ventricle and is determined by numerous factors that influence blood return to the heart. Resting preload does not change with age,[15] although left ventricular early diastolic filling is reduced with age. With age, left ventricular stiffness is increased, left ventricular compliance is decreased, left ventricular wall thickness is increased, left ventricular relaxation is impaired, and left ventricular diastolic filling is decreased. An age-related increase in systolic blood pressure also impairs left ventricular early diastolic filling, leading to hypotension if preload is reduced. Despite this age-related reduction, preload is maintained because left atrial contraction becomes more vigorous and thereby increases late diastolic filling of the left ventricle.[15]

An age-related increase in left atrial size from increased wall stress counteracts the effects of decreased left ventricular compliance with aging. Left atrial contraction can contribute up to 50% of left ventricular filling in a poorly compliant left ventricle. Consequently, in older adults, development of atrial fibrillation may cause a marked reduction in cardiac output because of the loss of left atrial contribution to left ventricular late diastolic filling.

The intrinsic ability of the heart to generate force does not change with age, although the duration of contraction and relaxation is prolonged in older adults. There is no reduction of resting left ventricular ejection fraction or circumferential fiber shortening in healthy older adults.

Aging is associated with prolongation of isovolumic relaxation time, a reduction in early diastolic filling of the left ventricle, and augmentation of the late diastolic filling of the left ventricle.[15] Also with aging, there is a slowing of the rate at which calcium enters the sarcoplasmic reticulum after myocardial excitation, and a subsequent decrease in relaxation of the left ventricle.[16] Reduced oxidative phosphorylation and cumulative mitochondrial peroxidation occurring with aging may also impair left ventricular diastolic function.

The maximum amount of oxygen uptake ($VO_2$ max) decreases with age, although the degree to which oxygen uptake decreases is affected by physical conditioning, subclinical coronary artery disease (CAD), smoking, and body weight. With exercise, older adults have a decrease in heart rate, cardiac index, and left ventricular ejection fraction and increases in the left ventricular end-diastolic and end-systolic volume indices.[16]

## Findings on Physical Examination and Management

In the absence of vascular disease, age-related cardiovascular changes should not interfere with normal tissue perfusion. In the older patient, however, the likelihood of atherosclerosis increases. The narrowing of vessels, coupled with their decrease in compliance, may produce tissue ischemia, which contributes to tissue injury and pressure ulcer formation in older patients on bed rest.

The increased vascular stiffness of aging causes the upstroke of the arterial pulse to appear brisker than usual, potentially masking the slowly rising carotid pulse of aortic stenosis. Older adults commonly present with an early-peaking basal systolic murmur of aortic stenosis, typically accompanied by an $S_4$ sound at the cardiac apex as evidence of reduced ventricular compliance. These people report and demonstrate a limited ability to tolerate physical activity. Older patients may also have a greater amount of pooling in the lower extremities because of decreased muscle mass and poor venous return. If the patient is placed on bed rest, this fluid pool is redistributed and may cause an overload in the cardiovascular system. The nurse must be alert for vascular overload and congestive heart failure.

Another factor to consider is the shifting of fluids when a patient arises after having been on bed rest. The sudden shift in fluid to the lower extremities and the lowered fluid volume that results from bed rest can produce extreme lightheadedness. This is further complicated by a decrease in baroreceptor sensitivity with age. A slow progression of head elevation and dangling the legs before moving the patient to sitting or standing are necessary to prevent syncope and possible injury from falling.

Although chest pressure is the classic symptom of angina in older adults, there is an increased incidence of silent ischemia in this age group. If angina or a myocardial infarction is suspected, a comprehensive history, vital signs, and electrocardiogram (ECG) should be obtained, and a laboratory workup (including cardiac enzymes) should be ordered. If at all possible, it is important to obtain a prior ECG for comparison.

About half of all older adults have abnormalities on the resting ECG, most commonly PR- and QT-interval prolongation, intraventricular conduction abnormalities, reduction in QRS voltage, and a leftward shift of the frontal plane QRS axis. Elderly men more frequently have major ECG abnormalities than do elderly women, and these abnormalities increase with age.[17]

## Respiratory Changes

It is particularly difficult to distinguish age-related changes in the structure and function of the lungs from those changes caused by disease, because the lungs are continually exposed to environmental stressors. However, some commonly identified lung changes with physiologic aging include dilation of alveoli, enlargement of airspaces, decreases in exchange surface area, and loss of supporting tissue for peripheral airways. These changes result in decreased static elastic recoil of the lung and increased residual volume and functional residual capacity.

There is a tendency for older adults to have relative inefficiency in control and monitoring of ventilation. This is especially true with regard to responses to both hypoxia and hypercapnia at rest. Elderly people tend to have increased ventilatory response to exercise-induced carbon dioxide production.[18] The VO$_2$max declines with age owing to a decrease in the diffusing capacity and alveolar capillary volume, along with ventilation–perfusion mismatch. Mucociliary clearance is reduced with age, although there is some evidence to suggest that the cough reflex is unaffected by aging.[19] Older adults tend to have more-frequent and severe bacterial, viral, and fungal infections, but this is due to pathologic processes commonly seen in older people, changes in other body systems, and some of the functional and structural changes identified.

Despite lung changes with aging, the respiratory system remains capable of maintaining adequate gas exchange at rest and during exertion throughout the life span. Aging does tend to result in diminished reserve of the respiratory system in cases of acute disease. Specifically, decreased sensitivity of respiratory centers to hypoxia or hypercapnia results in a diminished ventilatory response in cases of heart failure, infection, or aggravated airway obstruction. Moreover, decreased perception of bronchoconstriction and diminished physical activity may result in less awareness of the disease and delayed diagnosis.[20]

### Findings on Physical Examination and Management

Older adults commonly present with barrel chest (an increased anteroposterior diameter), which has a significant impact on appearance as well as chest wall compliance (particularly in patients who are supine), and may result in lung sounds being more distant and less discernible. It may be helpful to use a pediatric diaphragm to listen for breath sounds in older adults with prominent ribs. This allows for a more firm application of the stethoscope between the interspaces.

Dyspnea is a common complaint; the causes may be cardiac, pulmonary, metabolic, mechanical, or hematologic, or it may be due to deconditioning. Increased lung sounds are also common with age and may be due to deconditioning and age-related fibrotic changes rather than acute disease, such as congestive heart failure. When evaluating the older adult, it is particularly important to match clinical signs and symptoms of disease with objective diagnostic findings, such as chest radiography and laboratory testing.

Pulmonary infections are more common with age because of the changes described previously. However, expectorated tissue specimens in older adults are often unreliable because of pharyngeal colonization. To prevent infection, careful attention to nutrition, especially to sufficient calories, protein, and fluid intake, is needed. Moreover, frequent position changes assist in clearing secretions and aid ventilation and perfusion of the lungs.

## Renal Changes

Age-associated kidney changes can be categorized as anatomical or functional. Anatomical changes include the loss of renal glomeruli, decreased kidney size, renal tubular changes, and renal vascular changes. There are also functional kidney changes, as described in Box 12-5.

The total number of glomeruli decreases by 30% to 40% by the eighth decade. The loss of glomeruli, in conjunction with decreased kidney perfusion, results in a decreased glomerular filtration rate (GFR). However, one longitudinal study revealed that not all people exhibit a decline in GFR.[21] Changes are likely due to a combination of lifestyle factors and associated chronic illness. The decrease in filtration may result in decreased clearance of substances normally excreted. An increase in blood urea nitrogen (BUN) or creatinine may indicate the extent to which the GFR is diminished. However, creatinine levels from muscle breakdown may be less than in younger patients and could mask an elevated creatinine level. Creatinine clearance is a more accurate measure

---

**BOX 12-5**    Age-Associated Functional Kidney Changes

- Decreased GFR
- Decreased mean creatinine clearance rate
- Increased mean creatinine concentrations
- Decreased blood flow through the kidneys
- Decreased tubular transport capacity
- Decreased functional nephrons
- Decreased concentrating ability
- Decreased diluting ability
- Decreased plasma renin activity
- Impaired sodium conservation

of renal function in the older patient. Corrected GFRs can easily be calculated for older adults using the Modification of Diet in Renal Disease formula:

$$mL/min/1.73\ m^2 = 175 \times (SCr)^{-1.154} \times (age)^{-0.203}$$
$$\times\ 0.742\ (if\ female)$$
$$\times\ 1.210\ (if\ black)$$

where SCr equals serum creatinine (see also Chapter 31, Box 31-3).

GFR calculators are available to assist with the calculations at http://kidney.org or http://nephron.com/cgi-bin/MDRD.cgi. Evaluation of renal function is extremely important if the patient is receiving drugs normally excreted by the kidney. Table 12-2 provides an overview of normal laboratory values, including renal function, and how these change with age.

With age, there is also a decrease in renal blood flow, decreased tubular function, and decreased ability to concentrate urine. Basal renin is diminished by 30% to 50% in older adults. Renin alterations and other renal changes diminish the capability of the older adult to maintain sodium and water balance, especially in the presence of stress. There may also be a lessened response to antidiuretic hormone, which can result in a decreased ability to concentrate urine. This decreased ability may lead to problems of fluid–electrolyte balance as sodium, potassium, and water are lost. Loss of hydrogen ions may also make the acid–base balance more difficult to maintain.

## Findings on Physical Examination and Management

Older adults tend to have decreased sensations of thirst and consequently drink less fluid. This change leaves them vulnerable to dehydration, especially when medications with diuretic actions are administered. To prevent renal damage, care must be taken to ensure that the hospitalized older patient has adequate fluid intake by oral, enteral, or parenteral routes. Fluid balance may also be precarious because disease states such as diabetes can produce diuresis. Furthermore, potassium and sodium levels may already be low when the patient arrives in the unit. Care must be taken to ensure that electrolyte balance remains stable or is restored. Confusion, dysrhythmias, coma, and death can occur quickly in the older patient with altered electrolyte balance.

As bladder muscle tone is lost, incomplete emptying with retention can foster the development of urinary tract infections (UTIs) that can ascend and become renal infections.

**TABLE 12-2** **Normal Laboratory Values and Age-Related Changes**

| Laboratory Test | Normal Values | Age-Related Changes |
|---|---|---|
| **Urinalysis** | | |
| Protein | 0–5 mg/100 mL | Rises slightly |
| Glucose | 0–15 mg/100 mL | Glycosuria appears after high plasma levels and is very unreliable |
| Specific gravity | 1.005–1.020 | Lower maximum of 1.016–1.022 |
| Sedimentation rate | Men 0–20 mm/h | Increases with age; no clinical significance |
| | Women 0–30 mm/h | |
| Iron | 50–60 mcg/dL | Slight decrease |
| Iron binding | 230–410 mcg/dL | Decrease |
| Hemoglobin | Men 13–18 g/100 mL | No normal decline with age |
| | Women 12–16 g/100 mL | |
| Hematocrit | Men 45%–52% | No normal decline with age |
| | Women 37%–48% | |
| Leukocytes | 4,300–10,800/mm³ | No normal decline with age |
| Lymphocytes | 500–2,400 T cells/mm³ | Both T- and B-cell levels decrease |
| | 50–200 B cells/mm³ | |
| Platelets | 150,000–350,000/mm³ | No change with age |
| Albumin | 3.5–5.0 g/100 mL | Declines because of a decrease in liver size and enzymes |
| Globulin | 2.3–3.5 g/100 mL | Slight increase |
| Serum protein | 6.0–8.4 g/100 mL | No change with age |
| BUN | Men 10–25 mg/100 mL | Can increase with age |
| | Women 8–20 mg/100 mL | |
| Creatinine | 0.6–1.5 mg/100 mL | Increases, although this is related to lean body mass |
| Creatinine clearance | 104–124 mL/min | Decreases by 10% per decade after age 40 y |
| Glucose | <200 mg/dL fasting | Slight increase in glucose tolerance of 10 mg/dL per decade after age 30 y |
| Triglycerides | 40–150 mg/100 mL | 20–200 mg/100 mL |
| Cholesterol | 120–220 mg/100 mL | Increases with age, more so in women than in men |
| Thyroxine (T₄) | 4.5–13.5 mcg/100 mL | No change |
| Triiodothyronine (T₃) | 90–220 ng/100 mL | Decreases 25% |
| Thyroid-stimulating hormone | 0.5–5.0 mcg/mL | No significant change with age |
| Alkaline phosphatase | 13–39 IU/L | Increases by 8–10 IU/L, although elevations >20% are likely due to disease |
| Prostate-specific antigen | 4 ng/mL | No change with age, although elevated levels may be seen in non-malignant disease |
| Uric acid | Men 44–76 mg/L | Slight increase with age |
| | Women 23–66 mg/L | |

| TABLE 12-3 | Causes of Incontinence |
|---|---|

**Drug Side Effects**

*Diuretics*: Urgency
*Caffeine and alcohol*: Diuretic effect and irritation
*Sedatives*: Inhibition of micturition, functional changes
*Anticholinergics*: Constipation causing obstruction
*Calcium-channel blockers*: Constipation causing obstruction, smooth muscle relaxation
*Nonsteroidal anti-inflammatory drugs*: Blockage of prostaglandin receptors causing decreased force of contraction

**Physiologic Changes**

*Hypoxemia*: Depressed function of brain
*Delirium*: Depressed function of brain
*Hyperglycemia*: Diuretic effect of glycosuria
*Hypercalcemia*: Diuretic effect of hypercalciuria
*Functional impairment*: Inability to get to the toilet in time

**Bladder Inflammation**

Infection: Uninhibited bladder contractions
Atrophic vaginitis: Uninhibited bladder contractions

---

**QSEN**

### EVIDENCE-BASED PRACTICE HIGHLIGHT 12-1
### Catheter-Associated Urinary Tract Infections

**Expected Practice**

- Prior to placement of any indwelling urinary catheter, assess patient for accepted indications and alternatives. (Level C)
- Adhere to aseptic technique for placement, manipulation, and maintenance of indwelling urinary catheters. (Level E)
- Document all instances of indwelling urinary catheters, including insertion date, indication, and removal date. (Level C)
- Promptly discontinue indwelling urinary catheters as soon as indications expire. (Level C)

**AACN Levels of Evidence**

**Level A** Meta-analysis of quantitative studies or metasynthesis of qualitative studies with results that consistently support a specific action, intervention, or treatment (including systematic review of randomized controlled trials)
**Level B** Well-designed, controlled studies with results that consistently support a specific action, intervention, or treatment
**Level C** Qualitative studies, descriptive or correlational studies, integrative reviews, systematic reviews, or randomized controlled trials with inconsistent results
**Level D** Peer-reviewed professional and organizational standards with the support of clinical study recommendations
**Level E** Multiple case reports, theory-based evidence from expert opinions, or peer-reviewed professional orgastandards without clinical studies to support recommendations
**Level M** Manufacturer's recommendations only

Excerpted from American Association of Critical-Care Nurses Practice Alert. Available online at http://aacn.org.

---

Hypertrophy of the prostate gland also places older men at risk for UTI because the enlarged gland interrupts urine flow. Loss of muscle tone, retention with overdistention, and loss of sphincter control lead to incontinence in the older man or woman. For older patients, this loss of control is embarrassing and disconcerting.

If any type of incontinence or retention develops in an older patient during the stay in the ICU, the nurse should perform a comprehensive evaluation to determine the underlying cause of the urinary problem. Specifically, consideration should be given to drugs, particularly anticholinergic drugs, metabolic and neurologic problems, and bladder inflammation as potential causes (Table 12-3). If an indwelling (Foley) catheter is necessary during acute illness, it should be removed as soon as the primary reason for inserting it (eg, hourly urine measurements) has passed. Early removal may prevent deterioration of bladder function and UTI. See Evidence-Based Practice Highlight 12-1 for information about how to prevent catheter-associated UTIs.

## Gastrointestinal Changes

The gastrointestinal system undergoes many age-related changes (see Table 12-1). The mechanical and chemical processes of digestion that begin in the mouth may be impaired because of loss of teeth, poor hygiene, and a decrease in salivary secretions. Many older adults experience diminished senses of taste and smell, which may lead to decreased food intake.[22]

Data are insufficient to make assumptions about changes in absorption in the large and small bowel. Some evidence indicates that absorption is somewhat impaired. Given that the eating patterns of older adults may not include all food groups, deficiencies may arise from lack of intake rather than malabsorption.

The decreased motility of the large bowel is probably not sufficient to produce constipation in the active adult. However, older adults on bed rest, those who have decreased intake of food and fluids, and those exposed to multiple medications may experience constipation and fecal impaction. Dependence on or misuse of laxatives must be assessed when the history is taken, because this may further exacerbate the constipation and management of bowel function.

### Findings on Physical Examination and Management

Examination of the mouth in an older adult commonly reveals a wearing of dental enamel and gum recession, thereby exposing more of the teeth and increasing the likelihood of decay. Oral care is critical, given the associated risk for pneumonia with poor oral care. The oral mucous membranes also tend to be very dry in the older adult, making eating more difficult. Swallowing disorders are common and can be due to functional abnormality of the oral, pharyngeal, or esophageal stage of swallowing.

Older adults commonly report constipation, and stool may be palpable in the large bowel. In addition to an abdominal examination, a rectal examination must be performed to determine the consistency of stool and the anal tone, and to establish an appropriate treatment plan. Heartburn (which may present as chest pain) is also a common complaint, and is often associated with epigastric tenderness. Aortic aneurysms are more common in older adults and present as a pulsatile mass in the abdomen.

Acute abdominal pain in this population is a particularly challenging complaint; causes include diverticulitis, bowel obstruction, appendicitis, pancreatic disease, infarction, and cancer. Even more challenging is identifying older adults with acute abdominal problems who present without pain or any other significant signs and symptoms (eg, fever, anorexia). Careful evaluation of the abdomen in older adults is essential to monitor for acute changes.

Nursing interventions for gastrointestinal changes begin with a careful history. Eating habits, including time and frequency of food intake, food preferences, usual intake, food intolerances, and taste and smell changes must be assessed. Use of laxatives, enemas, and vitamin supplementation also should be explored. Evaluation of the teeth and gums helps to establish how well food can be handled mechanically.

When planning care, the nurse must consider that bed rest slows peristalsis and aggravates any preexisting condition related to motility. Adequate fluid intake, bulk in the diet, use of natural laxatives (eg, prune juice, warm liquids), and as much active or passive exercise as the condition of the patient allows may help maintain a normal pattern of bowel movements. Laxatives may need to be included in the regimen once constipation does occur.

Hospitalized patients of any age can become rapidly malnourished secondary to the stress of acute illness, an increased demand for energy, and lack of nourishment. Therefore, it is important to look for indicators of nutritional risk, such as a history of recent weight loss, a diet lacking in protein and calories, an albumin level less than 3.5 g/dL, and a lymphocyte count less than 1,500/mm.[23] The older patient who enters the hospital already mildly to moderately malnourished and who has a poor intake of protein and calories may quickly become severely malnourished. This malnourished state can markedly compromise the immune response and increase the incidence and severity of infection. Therefore, it is crucial to see that critically ill older patients maintain adequate nutritional intake.

## Musculoskeletal Changes

An estimated 43 million Americans (one in every seven persons) have some form of diagnosed arthritis or other rheumatic condition; this number is expected to rise to 60 million during the next 20 years. Arthritis affects people of all ages, although it is more prevalent among older adults and women. The disease causes pain, stiffness, and tenderness around the joints and typically affects the hands, feet, knees and hips. Symptoms can range from mild to severe. While arthritis rarely kills, it is a chronic disease that causes significant disability and reduces quality of life. Arthritis is not a normal age change, although it does contribute to mobility problems.

Mobility is also often limited among hospitalized older adults, resulting in a decrease in muscle protein synthesis, strength, and lower extremity and whole body mass. Muscle mass may be lost also because of a reduction in the number and size of muscle fibers or an increase in connective tissues. These changes result in less muscle tension and decreased strength of the contraction. The decrease of lean muscle mass and the loss of elasticity contribute to lost flexibility and increased stiffness.

Musculoskeletal function is dictated largely by the size of the muscle mass that is contracting, and to a lesser extent by changes in surrounding connective tissue in the joint, and neural recruitment, conduction velocities, and fatigue. Sedentary people lose large amounts of muscle mass over time. Unfortunately, muscle mass cannot be maintained into old age with habitual aerobic activities in either normal or athletic adults.[24] Only loading of muscle with weight-lifting exercise has been shown to reverse loss of muscle mass and strength in

older adults.[24,25] There is also a decrease in oxidative and glycolytic enzyme capacity with age, a decrease in total number of muscle fibers, selective atrophy of type 2 (fast-twitch) fibers, and shortening of tendons and ligaments with decreased tissue elasticity. Bone changes, as evidenced by osteoporosis, present with decreased height, kyphosis, and scoliosis.

Sarcopenia is a common aging syndrome and is defined as the age-associated loss of skeletal muscle mass and function. The causes of sarcopenia are multifactorial and can include disuse, altered endocrine function, chronic diseases, inflammation, insulin resistance, and nutritional deficiencies. Although cachexia may be a component of sarcopenia, the two conditions are not the same. The diagnosis of sarcopenia should particularly be considered in all older patients who are hospitalized.

### Findings on Physical Examination and Management

Older adults with osteoporosis may have spontaneous fractures that can occur simply from moving in bed. In general, older adults have a decrease in overall muscle strength and an increased tendency to have muscle cramping. Crepitus and pain with range of motion of the joints are common, particularly in the weight-bearing joints (eg, the knee). Changes in gait and posture are common, and older adults tend to have a stooped posture with a slow, shuffling gait. Patients with sarcopenia often cannot independently rise from a chair, and often have a slow gait speed and low muscle mass.

Forced fasting of the critically ill hospitalized patient may further accelerate muscle loss through catabolism and gluconeogenesis. The added burden of bed rest in the older patient leads to a rapid loss of mobility, strength, and energy as well as sarcopenia. Maintaining nutrition, changing position frequently, active and passive exercise, participating in all personal care, and getting out of bed as much as permitted by condition are essential to preserving strength, energy, and bone mass. If the patient is comatose or has suffered loss of function, proper positioning and splinting can help prevent permanent deformity.

## Endocrine Changes

The equilibrium concentrations of the principal hormones are not necessarily altered with age; however, for older adults, there may be a change in how hormonal equilibrium is achieved. Therefore, with advancing age, some alterations in hormone production, metabolism, and action occur. Subtle changes are noted in pituitary dynamics, adrenal gland physiology, and thyroid function; however, the changes in glucose homeostasis, reproductive function, and calcium metabolism are more apparent.[26,27]

The anterior pituitary gland shows unchanged output of stimulating hormones, although the peripheral levels of target hormones decrease. For example, circulating levels of daytime and nighttime thyroid-stimulating hormone and growth hormone (GH) are greatly diminished in old age.[27] In contrast, prolactin and melatonin are decreased only at night. Age-related decreases in hormonal levels are associated with a decrease in the amplitude but not the frequency of secretory pulses.

The decline in GH with age is believed to be associated with the decrease in lean body mass, increase in body fat (especially in the visceral and abdominal compartment), adverse changes in lipoproteins, and reduction in aerobic capacity commonly noted in older adults. Research is ongoing to determine whether replacement of GH in healthy older adults can reverse these changes.[28]

Normal aging is associated with insulin resistance and reduced β-cell function, but it is not known whether changes in proinsulin and the proinsulin/immunoreactive insulin ratio is also related to reduced β-cell function.[26] Glucose tolerance decreases with age. An increase in blood glucose to 200 mg/dL occurs in about half of people older than 70 years.[26] Interpretation of this glucose intolerance requires the use of age-adjusted parameters to avoid the inappropriate diagnosis and treatment of diabetes mellitus. Evaluating glycosylated hemoglobin (HbA$_{1c}$) or glycosylated albumin may help establish the presence or absence of diabetes mellitus in the older patient with elevated blood glucose levels. Because the renal threshold for reabsorption of glucose increases with age, higher degrees of hyperglycemia must be present before glucose spills into the urine. Therefore, monitoring for hyperglycemia with urine testing should be avoided.

Throughout life, the adrenal cortex shows significant morphogenic and steroidogenic changes. This decline is believed to aggravate some age-related diseases.[29] The thyroid gland also undergoes changes and decreases in size with aging. There may be an age-related reduction in the ability of aged tissues to increase receptor numbers in response to a reduction in hormone levels.[27]

### Findings on Physical Examination and Management

The reduction in thyroid hormone levels with increasing age is correlated with many physiologic and pathologic sequelae: changes in cholesterol metabolism, heart rate, cardiac output, strength of cardiac contraction, and alterations in basal metabolic rate and thermoregulation. The symptoms of thyroid disease, such as apathy, weakness, and weight loss, may not be as pronounced in older adults as they are in younger people. Moreover, these symptoms are often attributed to old age rather than to hyperthyroidism or hypothyroidism. The older patient with hyperthyroidism is likely to present with atrial tachycardia, is more likely to be anorexic than hyperphagic, and usually does not experience heat intolerance. The hypothyroid older adult may present with increased susceptibility to hypothermia if exposed to cold, a change in cognitive status, fatigue, dizziness, and a tendency to fall. Being aware of the atypical presentation of thyroid disease in older adults leads the critical care nurse to recognize endocrine imbalance. Once identified, the imbalance can easily be corrected by replacing thyroid hormone or changing the dosage of thyroid replacement.

Diabetes mellitus is often initially diagnosed during times of stress, such as acute illness, trauma, or surgery. The end-organ damage of diabetes mellitus is a factor in stroke, myocardial infarction, decreased renal function, and peripheral vascular disease. Long-standing non-insulin-dependent diabetes may be diagnosed only when the patient presents with a stroke or acute myocardial infarction. Therefore, it is important to differentiate the impaired glucose tolerance of aging, a transient rise in glucose related to acute illness, and the disease process of diabetes.

Recognition of the underlying diabetes and possible end-organ damage may alter the course of the acute illness. For example, knowing that the incidence of congestive heart failure after myocardial infarction is higher in diabetic than in nondiabetic patients, the nurse can be alert for early signs of fluid retention.

Older people with diabetes are, for the most part, not insulin dependent. Therefore, even if they have extremely high blood glucose levels, they are rarely ketoacidotic. In fact, the coma of this age group is usually hyperglycemic, hyperosmolar, and nonketotic (HHNK). Managing this state requires a delicate balance of hydration and rapid reduction of blood glucose without massive brain edema and death. The critical care nurse must be aware that HHNK coma can be triggered by acute illness or surgery. Common problems found in older adults with diabetes, and nursing interventions to prevent these problems, are shown in Box 12-6. It should be particularly recognized that the most prevalent sign of either hypoglycemia or hyperglycemia among older people with diabetes is a change in cognitive status.

## Immunologic Changes

With age, there is a decline in immune function. Specifically, there is a decline in both T-cell and B-cell function, with a dramatic effect on cell-mediated immunity. With aging, the thymus gland involutes; there is a decrease in thymic hormone levels, and the number of autoantibodies increases.[30] Lastly, with age there is a decrease in the production of immunoglobulin E, the antibody associated with allergic responses; thus, these responses decrease in older individuals.

### Findings on Physical Examination and Management

The usual symptoms of infection such as chills, fever, leukocytosis, and tachycardia may be absent or blunted in the

---

**BOX 12-6**  **Nursing Interventions**

**For Preventing Problems in the Older Adult With Diabetes**

**Skin Alterations**
- Monitor for decreased circulation and skin breakdown.
- Provide foot care to maintain skin integrity. Bathe the feet daily and apply emollient.

**Hyperglycemia**
- Maintain a controlled diet.
- Monitor blood glucose levels.
- Monitor for urinary frequency.
- Monitor for hyponatremia.
- Monitor for dry mouth.
- Monitor for changes in cognition.

**Hypoglycemia**
- Monitor for acute changes in cognition.

**Hydration Status**
- Monitor hydration.
- Encourage the intake of 2,000 mL of fluid daily.

**End-Organ Disease**
- Monitor kidney function.
- Monitor for visual changes (eg, blurred or decreased vision).

older adult. Instead, this age group may present with an acute change in cognition, function, or behavior. Delirium, for example, may be the only sign or symptom of a UTI in an older adult. The most common areas of infection in older adults are the lungs, urinary tract, and skin; when subtle changes are noted in an older patient, consideration should be given to each of these areas.

## Psychological Challenges

### Cognitive Changes

Cognition refers to the process of obtaining, storing, retrieving, and using information. The neuroanatomical and neurophysiologic underpinnings of cognitive change are unclear. Studies[5] have shown that younger people have larger ventricular volumes and smaller gray and white matter volumes compared with older people. There is also greater prefrontal cortex activity in younger adults as compared with older adults in the dorsolateral area during memory retrieval. These changes are believed to account for the changes in working memory and executive abilities[5] associated with normal aging. Crystallized intelligence, or the skills and abilities that are lifelong (eg, bathing and dressing), tend to remain stable with age, but there is some decline in fluid intelligence, which is the learning of new information and which involves problem solving and reasoning. For example, there is some decline in perceptual motor skills, concept formation, complex memory tasks, and quick-decision tasks.[5] However, age itself is not the criterion for making decisions about a patient's cognitive functions. Each person's abilities must be judged individually rather than against a norm. Moreover, interventions such as exercise (aerobic and resistive) can improve executive control processes in older adults, particularly older women.[31,32]

Cognitive function should be assessed and described on admission and monitored routinely over time, and whenever the patient's condition changes. While assessing cognitive functions during the patient's stay in intensive care, it is important to remember that physiologic deficits, some medications, and internal and external stress, such as environmental stressors, affect cognitive skills. In older adults, acute physical changes frequently initially present as changes in cognitive status. For example, an older adult with pneumonia may not have symptoms such as fever or cough but rather may present with changes in cognitive status.

The Mini-Cog,[33] which is available for free use, provides the practitioner with a consistent assessment tool to compare responses and monitor results over time. When completing the Mini-Cog, the patient who is unable to recall any of the three words is categorized as "probably demented," whereas the patient who can recall all three words is categorized as "probably not demented." The patient who can recall one or two words is categorized on the basis of the clock drawing test: the patient who draws a clock that is in any way abnormal is considered "probably demented," whereas if the clock is normally constructed the patient is considered "probably not demented." The main drawback to the use of a questionnaire is that some critically ill patients may not be able to hear, see, talk, or write well enough to respond to the questions. In addition, longer, more sensitive tools may be more fatiguing for the critically ill older patient.

Several common syndromes cause cognitive impairment, including dementia, delirium, and depression (discussed later). Dementia is based on impairment of memory plus at least one of the following: a personality change or impairment in abstract thinking, judgment, or higher cortical functions. Delirium is the abrupt onset of clouding of consciousness and is a medical emergency. Table 12-4 identifies factors used to differentiate dementia and delirium. Reversible causes of dementia and delirium are listed in Box 12-7. Tools to evaluate memory

**TABLE 12-4** Summary of Differences Between Dementia, Depression, and Delirium

| | Dementia | | Delirium | Depression |
|---|---|---|---|---|
| | **Alzheimer Disease (AD)** | **Vascular (Multi-Infarct) Dementia** | | |
| **Etiology** | Familial (genetic [chromosomes 14, 19, 21]) Sporadic | Cardiovascular (CV) disease Cerebrovascular disease Hypertension | Drug toxicity and interactions; acute disease; trauma; chronic disease exacerbation Fluid and electrolyte disorder | Biologic, psychological, and social factors |
| **Risk factors** | Advanced age; genetics | Preexisting CV disease | Preexisting cognitive impairment | Family history |
| **Occurrence** | 50%–60% of dementias | 20% of dementias | 6%–56% of hospitalized older people | 2%–32% of older individuals who experience cognitive problems actually have pseudodementia |
| **Onset** | Slow | Often abrupt Follows a stroke or transient ischemic attack | Rapid, acute onset A harbinger of acute medical illness | May be slow or abrupt if it is in response to a life event |
| **Age of onset (y)** | Early-onset AD: 30s–65 Late-onset AD: 65+ Most commonly 85+ | Most commonly 50–70 y | Any age, but predominantly in older persons | Any age, but particularly high in older adults |
| **Gender** | Males and females equally | Predominantly males | Males and females equally | |

**TABLE 12-4**   Summary of Differences Between Dementia, Depression, and Delirium (*continued*)

| | Dementia | | Delirium | Depression |
|---|---|---|---|---|
| | **Alzheimer Disease (AD)** | **Vascular (Multi-Infarct) Dementia** | | |
| **Course** | Chronic, irreversible; progressive, regular, downhill | Chronic, irreversible Fluctuating, stepwise progression | Acute onset Hypoalert–hypoactive Hyperalert–hyperactive mixed hypo–hyper | Chronic, although is treatable and may resolve over time |
| **Duration Symptom progress** | 2–20 y Onset insidious *Early*—mild and subtle *Middle and late*—intensified progression to death (infection or malnutrition) | Variable; years Depends on location of infarct and success of treatment; death due to underlying CV disease | Lasts 1 d to 1 mo Symptoms are fully reversible with adequate treatment; can progress to chronicity or death if underlying condition is ignored | Variable Symptoms are reversible with appropriate treatment; can become chronic |
| **Mood Speech/ language** | Early depression (30%) Speech remains intact until late in disease *Early*—mild anomia (cannot name objects); deficits progress until speech lacks meaning; echoes and repeats words and sounds; mutism | Labile: mood swings May have speech deficit/ aphasia depending on location of lesion | Variable Fluctuating; often cannot concentrate long enough to speak May be somnolent | Depressed Normal |
| **Physical signs** | *Early*—no motor deficits *Middle*—apraxia (70%) (cannot perform purposeful movement) *Late*—dysarthria (impaired speech) *End stage*—loss of all voluntary activities; positive neurologic signs | According to location of lesion: focal neurologic signs, seizures Commonly exhibits motor deficits | Signs and symptoms of underlying disease | No clinical signs aside from depressed mood and decreased affect; may express somatization or overinterpretation and obsession with minor symptoms |
| **Orientation** | Becomes lost in familiar places (topographic disorientation) Has difficulty drawing three-dimensional objects (visual and spatial disorientation) Disorientation to time, place, and person—with disease progression | | May fluctuate between lucidity and complete disorientation to time, place, and person | Normal |
| **Memory** | Impaired memory, especially the ability to remember recent events and newly learned facts; may demonstrate difficulty with word finding and problem solving | | Impaired recent and remote memory; may fluctuate, however, and seem better at some times than others | Intact, but may be unwilling to fully participate in cognitive screening |
| **Personality** | Apathy, indifference, irritability *Early disease*—social behavior intact; hides cognitive deficits; may be paranoid *Advanced disease*—disengages from activity and relationships; suspicious; paranoid delusions caused by memory loss; aggressive; catastrophic reactions | | Fluctuating; cannot focus attention to engage in conversations and respond to questions; may have delusions or hallucinations; paranoid behavior may be present | Depressed affect; may have a change in personality, with less willingness to engage in social activities if once social |
| **Functional status, activities of daily living** | Poor judgment in everyday activities; has progressive decline in ability to handle money, use telephone, function in home and workplace | | Impaired due to difficulty concentrating on activities | Intact, but may be unwilling to engage in activities |
| **Attention span** | Distractible; short attention span | | Highly impaired; cannot maintain or shift attention | Decreased due to apathy |
| **Psychomotor activity** | May be normal or may exhibit wandering, hyperactivity, pacing, restlessness, or agitation, or may be apathetic | | Variable; alternates between high agitation, hyperactivity, restlessness, and lethargy | May be decreased due to apathy or may be hyperactive |
| **Sleep–wake cycle** | Often impaired; wandering and agitation at nighttime; loss of day/night orientation | | Disturbed and may change hourly | May have early morning insomnia and hypersomnia during the day |

---

| BOX 12-7 | Reversible Causes of Dementia and Delirium |
| --- | --- |

**D**rugs
**E**motional illness (including depression)
**M**etabolic/endocrine disorders
**E**ye/ear/environment
**N**utritional/neurologic disorders
**T**umors/trauma
**I**nfection
**A**lcoholism/anemia/atherosclerosis

and differentiate dementia and delirium are available at http://www.geronurseonline.org. See Evidence-Based Practice Highlight 12-2 for the assessment and management of delirium.

## Learning

Older adults may take longer to respond to and assimilate new material. They may also be hesitant to take on new tasks. Motivation continues to be an important aspect of learning new material. If the material is irrelevant or meaningless, motivation is decreased, which is often interpreted as an inability to learn. The person's sensory and cognitive abilities need to be taken into account when teaching older patients. It may be necessary to present information in small segments using varied stimuli, including touching, seeing, hearing, and (if vision permits) writing. If movements are slow, allow time for the completion of motor tasks, such as manipulating equipment or carrying out exercises.

---

### QSEN

## EVIDENCE-BASED PRACTICE HIGHLIGHT 12-2
### Delirium Assessment and Management

**Expected Practice**

- Implement delirium assessment for all critically ill patients using validated tools such as the Confusion Assessment Method for the ICU (CAM-ICU) or Intensive Care Delirium Screening Checklist (ICDSC) (Level B)
- Create strategies to decrease delirium risk factors, including early exercise (Level B)
- Be cautious with benzodiazepine use, giving only what is needed (Level C)
- Consider whether to adopt a core bundle like the ABCDE bundle (Level E)

**Management of ICU Delirium**

- **No drug has been approved by the FDA to treat delirium**. In fact, the FDA has issued an alert that atypical antipsychotic medications are associated with mortality risk among older patients, and another analysis has reported that haloperidol had an even higher mortality risk in non-ICU older patients than atypical antipsychotics.
- Clinical practice guidelines traditionally recommended antipsychotics as the medication class of choice for delirium, yet very little evidence exists to support this internationally adopted treatment. Currently, there are only two placebo-controlled pilot studies involving antipsychotics and delirium treatment in the ICU. The "Modifying the Incidence of Delirium (MIND)" study compared haloperidol, ziprasidone, and placebo and reported no differences in regard to delirium resolution or any other outcomes or safety concerns in the three treatment groups.[34] Another study compared quetiapine to placebo in patients already determined to be delirious who had an as-needed haloperidol order and found that the patients who received quetiapine experienced a faster resolution of delirium, less delirium, less agitation, and more somnolence. These two studies are the first steps in understanding the best pharmacologic treatment; however, larger trials are needed to confirm these findings in order to systematically direct the choice for delirium treatment.
- All patients receiving antipsychotics (haloperidol or any of the atypical antipsychotics) should be routinely and systematically monitored for side effects, especially QT prolongation. Rivastigmine, a cholinesterase inhibitor, has not been shown to be superior to placebo for the treatment of ICU delirium. A large European trial was stopped prematurely because of increased mortality in the rivastigmine group.
- The Society of Critical Care Medicine suggests identification of causes as the first step in delirium management. The following THINK pneumonic may be helpful in determining the cause when delirium is found to be present in ICU patients:
- Toxic situations
  - CHF, shock, dehydration
  - Deliriogenic meds (tight titration of sedatives)
  - New organ failure (eg, liver, kidney)

- Hypoxemia
- Infection/sepsis (nosocomial)
- Immobilization
- Nonpharmacologic interventions (Are these being neglected?)
  - Hearing aids, glasses, sleep protocols, music, noise control, ambulation, K+ or electrolyte problems

**Putting It All Together: ABCDE Bundle**

Several recent reviews have described the idea of implementing a core model of care combining multiple evidence-based practice strategies subsequently incorporated into routine daily care for the purpose of improving overall patient outcomes and allowing a systematic reduction in the modifiable risk factors for delirium.[35–37] The ABCDE bundle includes spontaneous awakening and breathing trial coordination, careful sedation choice, delirium monitoring, and early progressive mobility and exercise. The intent of combining and coordinating these individual strategies is to "(1) improve collaboration among clinical team members, (2) standardize care processes, and (3) break the cycle of oversedation and prolonged ventilation, which appear causative to delirium and weakness."[35] The ABCDE bundle is a helpful paradigm for critical care nurses to consider when focusing on implementing strategies to improve patient care and reduce the impact of modifiable delirium risk factors.

- Awakening and Breathing Trial Coordination (the Wake Up and Breathe Protocol)
- Choice of Sedative
- Delirium Detection
- Early Progressive Mobility and Exercise

**AACN Levels of Evidence**

**Level A** Meta-analysis of quantitative studies or metasynthesis of qualitative studies with results that consistently support a specific action, intervention, or treatment
**Level B** Well-designed, controlled studies with results that consistently support a specific action, intervention, or treatment
**Level C** Qualitative studies, descriptive or correlational studies, integrative reviews, systematic reviews, or randomized controlled trials with inconsistent results
**Level D** Peer-reviewed professional organizational standards with clinical studies to support recommendations
**Level E** Multiple case reports, theory-based evidence from expert opinions, or peer-reviewed professional organizational standards without clinical studies to support recommendations
**Level M** Manufacturer's recommendations only

Excerpted from American Association of Critical-Care Nurses Practice Alert. Available online at http://aacn.org.

## Memory

The older person's memory decline involves short-term memory rather than long-term and remote memory. Recall of memory from the past is least impaired by age. Remote memory recall (items learned many years ago) can be a positive therapeutic strategy for older patients. Reminiscence is an adaptive mechanism that helps the nurse learn about the patient and increases the patient's feelings of self-worth and competence.

## Depression

There are three types of depression disorders:[38] major depression, dysthymia, and bipolar disorder.

- **Major depression** involves at least five symptoms of depression (Box 12-8) for a 2-week period. Such an episode is disabling and will interfere with the ability to work, study, eat, and sleep. Major depressive episodes may occur once or twice in a lifetime, or they may recur frequently. They may also take place spontaneously, during or after the death of a loved one, a romantic breakup, a medical illness, or other life event.
- **Dysthymia, or minor depression,** is a less-severe, long-term, chronic form of depression. It involves the same symptoms as major depression, mainly low energy, poor appetite or overeating, and insomnia or oversleeping. It can manifest as stress, irritability, and mild anhedonia, which is the inability to derive pleasure from most activities. These individuals have at least one symptom of depression over a 2-week period. People with dysthymia might be thought of as always seeing the glass as half empty.
- **Bipolar disorder,** once called manic depression, is characterized by a mood cycle that shifts from severe highs (mania) or mild highs (hypomania) to severe lows (depression).

The symptoms of depression in the older adult can be masked by normal age-related changes or disease states. For example, difficulty sleeping, early morning awakening, and lethargy are common physical complaints of the normal aging person. Alternatively, depression in the older adult may more commonly present with pseudohypochondriasis, preoccupation with past life events, and changes in cognitive ability. In some patients, the dominant emotional mood may not be sadness but anger, anxiety, or irritability.

Causes of depression are multifaceted and include multiple losses associated with aging, underlying illness, and drugs.

---

**QSEN** BOX 12-8  *PATIENT SAFETY*

### Symptoms of Depression
- Depressed mood
- Decreased interest in activities
- Weight changes
- Sleep changes
- Psychomotor changes
- Fatigue
- Feelings of worthlessness or guilt
- Decreased concentration
- Suicidal ideation

---

**BOX 12-9**  **Drug Groups That May Cause Depression in the Older Person**

Analgesics/anti-inflammatory drugs
Anticonvulsants
Antihistamines
Antihypertensives
Antimicrobials
Antiparkinsonian drugs
Hormones
Immunosuppressive drugs
Tranquilizers

---

Box 12-9 lists drug groups that may cause depression. Screening tools such as the Geriatric Depression Scale[30] are useful to identify people who are depressed. Once depression is identified, appropriate interventions, including drug therapy, behavioral modification, and counseling, can be initiated.

The nurse must also be aware of cardiovascular side effects of antidepressants. The tricyclic antidepressive drugs are less commonly used owing to the risk of side effects. For example, tricyclic antidepressants can result in ST-segment and T-wave changes, although these are not necessarily indicative of myocardial damage. Ventricular dysrhythmias and disturbances in cardiac conduction are potential serious side effects, and may result in the drug being reduced or discontinued. Anticholinergic effects, especially in patients with Alzheimer disease, benign prostatic hypertrophy, or CAD, may also be seen. The selective serotonin reuptake inhibitors are much more commonly used now to treat depression. Side effects to monitor include changes related to sleep, appetite, personality or behavior, and blood pressure readings.

Untreated depression may result in suicide, which is a serious problem among older adults. Of all suicides committed in this country annually, 25% involve people older than age 65. White men older than age 85 are at particular risk.[39] Because of their many losses and changes, older adults may view suicide as a means of fulfilling a fantasy of "reunion" with a dead spouse or significant other. The nurse must monitor signs and symptoms of depression, explore the causes of depression, facilitate treatment, and watch for suicide attempts or warnings.

## Abuse of the Older Person

Mistreatment of older people is a problem that affects more than 4% of the older adults in the United States.[40] Abuse of older adults occurs in homes and institutions and takes many forms. Abuse may be blatant or subtle; it may be physical, psychological, or material (eg, financial). Abuse may involve neglect (by others or by self), exploitation, or abandonment. The abused older person is often physically or mentally frail and unable to report the abusive situation. Abuse can also happen to emotionally and intellectually stable older people who are unable to stop the abuse or report it because of their financial or emotional dependence on the abuser. They may also be afraid of being abandoned.

Abuse can occur because of lack of knowledge about the older person's basic needs, a lack of resources to help, or a desire to protect an inheritance. Those responsible for the abuse may or may not live with the older person. Caregivers

**Signs and Symptoms of Elder Abuse**
- Lack of compliance with management of health problems
- Unexplained injuries, such as fractures, bruises, lacerations
- Burns
- Poor personal hygiene
- Sexually transmitted disease
- Altered mood
- Depression
- Failure to thrive (underhydration/impaired nutritional status)
- Impaired skin integrity/fungal rashes

**BOX 12-11** Alcohol Abuse Screening Tools for Older Adults

**Short Michigan Alcoholism Screening Test—Geriatric Version (SMAST-G)**
Blow FC, Brower KJ, Schulenberg JE, et al: The Michigan Alcoholism Screening Test—Geriatric Version (MAST-G): A new elderly-specific screening instrument. Alcohol Clin Exp Res 16:372, 1992.
*Access:* http://consultgerirn.org/uploads/File/trythis/try_this_17.pdf

**CAGE Questionnaire**
Ewing J: Detecting alcoholism: The CAGE Questionnaire. JAMA 252(14):1905–1907, 1984.
*Access:* http://www.integration.samhsa.gov/clinical-practice/sbirt/CAGE_questionaire.pdf

**Michigan Alcoholism Screening Test—Geriatric Version (MAST-G)**
Blow FC, Brower KJ, Schulenberg JE, et al: The Michigan Alcoholism Screening Test—Geriatric Version (MAST-G): A new elderly-specific screening instrument. Alcohol Clin Exp Res 16:372, 1992.
*Access:* http://www.ssc.wisc.edu/wlsresearch/pilot/P01-R01_info/aging_mind/Aging_AppB5_MAST-G.pdf

**Alcohol Use Disorders Identification Test (AUDIT)**
Saunders JB, Aasland OG: WHO Collaborative Project on the Identification and Treatment of Persons with Harmful Alcohol Consumption. Report on Phase I: Development of a Screening Instrument. Geneva: World Health Organization, 1987.
*Access:* http://www.ncbi.nlm.nih.gov/books/NBK64829/#A45987

who are extremely stressed may become abusive. In some situations, the abused older adult is the caretaker.

The nurse must be alert to the signs and symptoms of elder abuse as outlined in Box 12-10. Any suggestion by the patient or family that things are not well at home must be pursued. A statement such as "My son hasn't been here yet. He sometimes forgets his commitments" should open the door for further conversation. It might uncover a mother who is worried about her son's drinking and perhaps about the way he treats her when he has been drinking. Attempts should be made to compare the history given by the patient with that given by the family. Inconsistencies need to be explored. Likewise, it is helpful to ask caretakers if they are able to give the care they feel is needed. Indications from a caretaker that the patient is "getting to be a handful" may be a clue to mismanaged care or a caretaker in need of support and assistance. In either situation, the nurse can provide information and support and refer the patient and caregiver to a social worker or mental health nurse for further assistance. All health care workers, including nurses, must know their responsibility under state law for reporting abuse of the older patient.

## Substance Abuse

The percentage of older adults who abuse alcohol, prescription drugs, and illicit drugs has doubled recently and is expected to increase with the aging of the baby boomers. It is estimated that over half of older adults consume alcohol; 25% consume more than a single drink a day,[41] with a standard drink being equal to 14.0 grams (0.6 ounces) of pure alcohol, 12 ounces of beer, or 5 ounces of wine.[42] Approximately 15% of men and 12% of women are high-risk drinkers, based on information provided by the National Institute on Alcohol Abuse and Alcoholism.[43] Problem drinking in older adults occurs for similar reasons as in younger adults. However, smaller amounts of alcohol create larger problems for older people, and they may be more susceptible to alcohol-induced disease. Differences in metabolism of alcohol in older people, the smaller volume of body water, and the decrease in lean body tissue may increase the propensity to alcoholism or alcohol problems. In addition, older adults are high consumers of psychotropic drugs and are at risk for drug–alcohol interactions.

Nursing interventions include screening the older adult for alcohol use. The CAGE questionnaire[44] is probably the most commonly used screening tool, although the geriatric

version of the Michigan Alcoholism Screening Test (Geriatric MAST, or MAST-G) was developed for older adults and therefore may be a better screening option.[45] Box 12-11 includes links to alcohol abuse screening tools for older adults. When alcohol abuse is suspected, the immediate goals are to stabilize physiologic and psychological responses to alcohol withdrawal and determine the impact of alcohol abuse on whatever other diagnoses have resulted in the need for critical care. As soon as possible, the nurse should refer the patient to a social worker, psychiatric liaison nurse, or alcohol counselor.

Aside from alcohol, the most commonly used substances are opiates, cocaine, and marijuana. It is important to assess patients for their all care interactions.

## Challenges in Medication Use

The rule for giving therapeutic medications to the older patient is *start low, go slow*. In other words, be patient. Changes related to aging can have a great impact on drug response. Changes in renal function, gastrointestinal secretions and motility, and cell receptor sites and concurrent disease states can alter the absorption, distribution, and excretion of drugs. These changes are summarized in Table 12-5.

Before admission to the ICU, older patients may have been taking many different medications, including over-the-counter (OTC) medications such as vitamins, tonics, herbals (eg, Saint John's wort, glucosamine), laxatives, antacids, and pain relievers. They may also have a history of

**TABLE 12-5**    Altered Drug Responses in Older People

| Physical and Physiologic Age-Related Changes | Pharmacologic Impact | Examples |
|---|---|---|
| **Absorption** | | |
| Reduced hydrochloric acid and pepsin; increased pH (less acid) and alteration in enzyme-secreting cells | Rate of drug absorption possibly delayed and decreased | Calcium and iron |
| Possible reduced gastrointestinal motility; unchanged gastric emptying | Extent of drug absorption generally not affected | |
| **Distribution** | | |
| Decreased albumin sites | The importance that decreased albumin may have on protein binding of drugs and the freeing of drugs may be balanced by the effect albumin has on the clearance of those drugs | Acidic drugs (eg, warfarin, salicylic acid, diazepam) bind to albumin and may be reduced <br><br> Water-soluble drugs (eg, digoxin, ethanol, gentamicin) tend to have smaller volumes of distribution and higher serum levels |
| Reduced cardiac output | Decreased perfusion of many bodily organs (eg, decreased renal plasma flow) | May result in a decreased impact of diuretics, such as furosemide |
| Increased percentage of body fat and decreased lean muscle mass | Because the proportion of body fat increases with age, there is an increased ability to store fat-soluble medications, and thus increased drug accumulation, prolonged storage, and delayed excretion | Water-soluble drugs (eg, digoxin, ethanol, gentamicin) have a higher serum level in older adults <br><br> Fat-soluble medications (eg, diazepam, antipsychotics, morphine) have greater volume distribution unless they are distributed in muscle tissue, in which case volume will be reduced |
| **Metabolism** | | |
| Decreased cardiac output and decreased perfusion of the liver | A reduction in first-pass metabolism <br> Decreased metabolism and delay of breakdown of medications, resulting in prolonged duration of action, accumulation, and drug toxicity | The effect of all medications metabolized by the liver and drugs undergoing first-pass metabolism (propranolol and labetalol) may be increased; the effect of drugs that are activated in the liver (enalapril) will be reduced |
| **Excretion** | | |
| Decreased renal blood flow, particularly GFR; decreased liver blood flow and extraction of drug from the blood into the liver | Decreased rates of elimination and subsequent increased duration of action; risk of drug accumulation, toxicity, and overdosage | Medications with prolonged duration of action (eg, aminoglycoside antibiotics, digoxin, lithium) |

heavy alcohol intake. Any of these drugs can cause problems if combined with medications administered in the hospital.

The nurse needs to elicit a careful history of drug use from the patient and family. The family can be asked to bring in all medications the patient has been using; these include OTC medications and herbal remedies. Although alcohol use may be a sensitive topic, establishing the pattern of use can be essential in preventing untoward drug interactions and anticipating problems with liver damage or withdrawal.

Special considerations concerning administration of drugs to the older patient include knowing the drugs the patient has been taking; assessing renal, hepatic, endocrine, and digestive systems; and evaluating lean body mass. Impaired body systems may affect the absorption, metabolism, and excretion of drugs. Additional considerations are listed in Box 12-12. A decrease in lean body mass and an increase in total body fat may alter the distribution of the drug in the body. The nurse should also be aware of drugs that should be avoided when working with older adults; these are provided in the recent update of the Beers Criteria.[46]

## Drug Absorption

Drug absorption is affected by the following age-related changes: decreased gastric acid, decreased gastrointestinal

**BOX 12-12**   Considerations for Medication Use in Older People

- Drug dosage guidelines are usually based on studies in younger people, and recommended adult dosage guidelines may not be appropriate for older patients.
- Older people may be taking numerous prescription drugs and may self-medicate with borrowed, old, and OTC drugs.
- The effects of alcohol use must be considered.
- The potential for drug interactions and adverse reactions is increased because of the effects of aging on drug absorption, distribution, metabolism, and excretion.
- Drug toxicities are different from those in younger people. Fewer symptoms may be identified, and they may develop more slowly but be more pronounced once they occur.
- Behavioral side effects are more common in older people because the blood–brain barrier becomes less effective. When there is an acute change in mental status, medication should always be considered as the cause.

motility, decreased gastric blood flow, changes in gastrointestinal villi, and decreased blood flow and body temperature in the rectum. The increased pH of gastric secretions and delayed stomach emptying time can alter the degradation, and thus the absorption, of drugs. Drugs that are not stable in an acid medium can be severely reduced in bioavailability if they remain in the stomach for long periods. Drugs that are designed to be acted on in the small intestine may be affected by the higher pH of the aging stomach. A coated, pH-sensitive medication, such as erythromycin, may lose its coating in the stomach and be degraded before reaching the absorption sites in the small intestine. Coated gastric irritants may lose their coatings and cause bleeding or nausea and vomiting.

Some drugs are eliminated from the body before they enter the systemic circulation by a process called *first-pass metabolism*. In general, the enzymes responsible for this first-pass effect are decreased in the elderly so that bioavailability of drugs with high hepatic extraction may be increased with age. These drugs require dosage reduction in older adults.

## Drug Distribution

Distribution of drugs in the body can be affected by a decrease in lean body mass, an increase in total body fat, or a decrease in total body fluid, all of which may accompany aging. Drugs that bind to muscle (eg, digoxin) become more bioavailable as lean body mass diminishes, increasing the risk for toxicity. Fat-soluble drugs (eg, flurazepam [Dalmane], chlorpromazine [Thorazine], phenobarbital) can be deposited in fat and result in cumulative effects of oversedation. In patients with a volume deficit, drugs that are water soluble (eg, gentamicin [Garamycin]) may have a higher concentration and may reach toxic levels rapidly.

## Drug Metabolism

The liver is the major organ for biotransformation and detoxification of medications. Drug-metabolizing reactions are classified as phase I reactions, which involve adding or unmasking a polar chemical group to increase water solubility, and phase II or conjugation reactions, which involve linking the drug to another molecule such as glucose, acetate, or sulfate. In older adults, phase I metabolism is often impaired, whereas phase II metabolism is usually unaffected. In the older patient, there may be some decrease in the metabolism of drugs requiring hepatic enzymes for transformation. This results in an increased plasma level and prolonged half-life of the drug. The benzodiazepines (eg, diazepam [Valium], flurazepam), for example, have a half-life increase from 20 to 90 hours in the older patient. Hepatic oxidation of these drugs can further be affected by alcohol-induced changes in the liver. There may be a decrease in drug metabolism with occasional alcohol use. In chronic alcohol use, however, drug metabolism is increased, and excretion is accelerated.

## Drug Excretion

The kidney is the primary excretory organ for clearing drugs. Drugs that are excreted unchanged (eg, digoxin, cimetidine, antibiotics) or have renally excreted active metabolites require dosage reduction in the older adult to avoid accumulation and toxicity. Serum creatinine alone is not a good determinant of renal function in older people. A creatinine clearance study reflects a more accurate estimation for drug clearance.

## Clinical Applicability Challenges

### CASE STUDY

Mr. B., an 88-year-old white man, is admitted to the acute care unit with an acute change in cognition and behavior and increased blood pressure. Mr. B lives in an assisted living facility and is normally independent with bathing and dressing, and has always been very well groomed and appropriate in terms of social behavior. At the time of admission, Mr. B did not have any acute symptoms indicative of infection. There was no prior history of illness provided by the assisted living facility, and it was noted in his transfer records that, aside from remaining in the apartment more than usual, he had been at his baseline over the past week. His past medical history includes degenerative joint disease, mild cognitive impairment with 3/3 recall but some difficulty with problem solving and changes consistent with frontal lobe impairment, hypertension, depression, insomnia, deep vein thrombosis ×2 with the last episode occurring in the previous year, and a history of psoriasis. His physical function at baseline was independent with a walker. Functionally he was limited mostly by significant back, hip, and knee pain due to degenerative joint disease. Current medications included acetaminophen (Tylenol) 1,000 mg PO three times per day PRN for pain; amlodipine besylate 5 mg PO daily; duloxetine (Cymbalta) 40 mg PO daily; warfarin for long-term deep vein thrombosis

prophylaxis; and melatonin 3–10 mg PO at hs for sleep. He does not smoke but does have two drinks a day consistent with a lifelong adult habit of regular alcohol intake—what he reports was his "attitude adjustment" time with his wife throughout their marriage.

On admission, Mr. B. was restless, agitated, and hypervigilant. He kept watching the doorway and telling the staff that there was a male teenager trying to get into his room who wanted to get his wallet. He could not focus on questioning, and kept returning to his focus on the door and monitoring for someone or something. On physical examination, he was afebrile with a temperature of 98.6°F and pulse oximetry score of 95% on room air at rest; blood pressure was 210/110 and heart rate was 120 bpm and regular. Bilaterally he had 1+ edema to below his knees. He had normal vesicular breath sounds in both lung bases and no rales, rhonchi, or wheezes. His respiratory rate was 12, although it increased when he became agitated. Blood samples were drawn for laboratory testing; results included white blood cell 8.0, hemoglobin 13.4, hematocrit 41.0, platelet count 236.0, MCV 105, creatinine 1.17, BUN 21, calcium 9.3, glucose 120 (nonfasting), sodium 134, potassium 3.9, and chloride 109; carbon dioxide was normal at 19; estimated GFR was greater than 60, ALT was 49,

## CASE STUDY CONTINUED

and other liver functions were all within normal limits. His blood alcohol level was 8. Mr. B.'s chest radiograph showed a normal heart size and no evidence of pulmonary disease. The electrocardiogram showed a sinus tachycardia. He was admitted for tachycardia, hypertension, alcohol abuse, and delirium, and treatment included cardiac monitoring, an increase in the amlodipine to 10 mg daily, and a dose of furosemide at 40 mg and then daily at 20 mg. Lorazepam 1 mg PO bid was initiated to manage alcohol withdrawal and his hypervigilant delirium. Consideration was given to starting a neuroleptic for his hallucinations, but the team decided to monitor the delirium before initiating further treatment.

1. What is your immediate concern related to Mr. B.'s medical management and cardiac status?

2. How do you answer Mr. B.'s daughter's questions about the laboratory work?
3. How would you explain to Mr. B.'s daughter why he is suddenly so "crazy"?
4. What nursing care interventions are essential to help Mr. B. recover from this current episode and prevent recurrent episodes of delirium- and alcohol-associated problems?
5. What nursing care interventions are appropriate related to Mr. B.'s associated comorbidities?
6. What nursing care interventions would you implement related to fall prevention and other possible injuries?

How would you manage Mr. B.'s hypervigilant delirium?

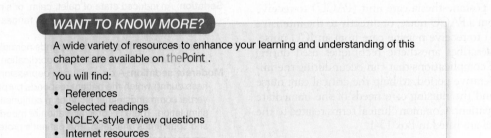

### WANT TO KNOW MORE?

A wide variety of resources to enhance your learning and understanding of this chapter are available on thePoint.

You will find:

- References
- Selected readings
- NCLEX-style review questions
- Internet resources
- And more!

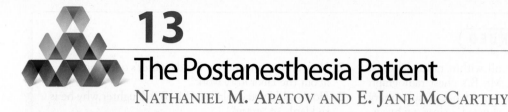

# 13

## The Postanesthesia Patient

NATHANIEL M. APATOV AND E. JANE MCCARTHY

### LEARNING OBJECTIVES

*Based on the content in this chapter, the reader should be able to:*

1. List anesthetic techniques used for surgery and interventional procedures.
2. Describe assessment strategies and nursing interventions for the patient recovering from anesthesia.
3. Explain common complications encountered during the immediate postanesthetic period and the necessary nursing interventions.
4. Compare and contrast moderate IV sedation and general anesthesia.

The time immediately after surgery is the most crucial period in the patient's recovery from anesthesia. The patient is taken to the postanesthesia care unit (PACU) to receive nursing care from a PACU nurse, or directly to the intensive care unit (ICU) to receive nursing care from an ICU nurse. This chapter describes anesthetic techniques used during surgery and the complications that can occur during the immediate postoperative period, to help the critical care nurse better understand the nursing care needs of the immediate postanesthetic patient. Common clinical terms related to the use of anesthesia are listed in Box 13-1.

## Preoperative Anesthesia Patient Assessment

The anesthesia provider interviews and examines the patient before surgery. From this preanesthetic examination and discussions with the patient and surgeon, the anesthesia provider decides which anesthetic technique to use. This decision is based on the patient's age, anesthetic history, and medical history, and the operation to be performed. The anesthesia provider's options range from conscious sedation with the use of regional or IV agents to general anesthesia with the use of IV or inhalational anesthetic agents. Whenever possible, the patient and family are part of the decision-making process. Anesthetic options are illustrated in Table 13-1 and Figure 13-1.

## Postanesthesia Report to PACU or ICU Nurse

What happens in the operating room (OR) affects the patient's immediate postoperative care and overall recovery. To convey what has occurred during surgery, the anesthesia provider gives a detailed report to the nurse who is assuming immediate postoperative care of the patient. Information given in the report is listed in Box 13-2. The anesthesia provider reports on intraoperative hemodynamic parameters, anesthetic technique, surgical procedure, urine output, blood loss, and fluid replacement. While receiving the report from

### BOX 13-1 | Clinical Terminology

**Sedation:** An induced state of quiet, calm, or sleep by means of a medication. The degree of sedation ranges from anxiolysis to anesthesia.

**Minimal sedation:** The patient responds normally to verbal stimuli. Impairment to cognition and coordination may exist.

**Moderate sedation:** A drug-induced depression of consciousness during which the patient responds purposefully to verbal commands either alone or in conjunction with tactile stimulation. There is some alteration of mood, drowsiness, and sometimes analgesia. The patient's protective reflexes remain intact.

**Deep sedation:** A drug-induced depression of consciousness during which the patient cannot be easily aroused but responds purposefully after repeated or painful stimulation. Spontaneous ventilation and the ability to maintain a patent airway may be impaired. The patient may require assistance in maintaining a patent airway.

**General anesthesia:** A drug-induced loss of consciousness during which a patient cannot be aroused, even by painful stimulation. The ability to independently maintain ventilatory function may be impaired. The patient may require assistance in maintaining a patent airway and positive-pressure ventilation may be required. Cardiovascular function may be depressed.

**MAC:** Monitored anesthesia care A specific anesthesia service in which an anesthesia provider has been requested to participate in the care of a patient undergoing a therapeutic or diagnostic procedure. It does not describe the depth of sedation.

**Regional anesthesia:** Regional anesthesia is achieved by placing local anesthetics close to appropriate nerves to achieve a conduction block that provides analgesia and numbness.

**Spinal anesthesia:** A local anesthetic is injected into the lumbar intrathecal space. The anesthetic blocks conduction in spinal nerve roots and dorsal ganglia. Anesthesia and analgesia usually occur below the level of injection.

**Epidural anesthesia:** A local anesthetic is injected via a catheter into the epidural space. The effects are similar to spinal analgesia.

**Peripheral nerve block:** A local anesthetic is injected at a specific nerve site to achieve a defined area of anesthesia.

**TABLE 13-1** Anesthetic Options for Surgical and Interventional Procedures

| Conscious State | Sedated State | Unconscious State |
|---|---|---|
| **Modalities** | | |
| Conscious sedation | MAC | Regional anesthesia |
| MAC | Local anesthesia | General anesthesia |
| Local anesthesia | Regional anesthesia | |
| Regional anesthesia | | |
| **Medications** | | |
| Local anesthetics | Local anesthetics | Local anesthetics |
| IV medications | IV medications | IV medications |
| | | Inhalation anesthetics |
| | | Muscle relaxants |
| **Effect on Patient** | | |
| Patient cooperative | May follow commands | Unconscious |
| Follows commands | Usually maintains protective reflexes | Diminished or loss of protective reflexes |
| Maintains protective reflexes | | Alterations in cardiopulmonary dynamics |

the anesthesia provider, the nurse simultaneously assesses the patient and develops a nursing plan of care. Initial assessment parameters reported to the anesthesia provider by the nurse are the patient's blood pressure, pulse rate, respiratory rate, temperature, oxyhemoglobin saturation ($SaO_2$), and level of consciousness.

In the PACU or ICU, vital signs are monitored every 15 minutes, or more often if the patient's condition warrants. Box 13-3 provides collaborative care guidelines for the postanesthesia patient. The American Society of Peri Anesthesia Nurses, endorsed by the American Association of Nurse Anesthetists (AANA) and the American Society of Anesthesiologists (ASA), recommends that assessment data be collected and documented on the patient's postoperative record.[1] In addition, while assessing the patient and taking vital signs, the nurse uses the "stir-up" regimen, which involves encouraging the patient to deep-breathe, cough, and move as allowed by the surgical procedure or intervention. The nurse also assesses pain levels and implements appropriate interventions to assist the patient in participating in the "stir-up" regimen. This regimen also allows the nurse to identify changes in the patient's cognitive function.

## Complications in the Postanesthesia Patient

The nurse must be able to assess and treat common complications in the postanesthesia patient. Postanesthesia patient care focuses primarily on cardiopulmonary assessment and management.

**GENERAL**

*Inhalation*
Desflurane
Isoflurane
Nitrous oxide
Sevoflurane
*Muscle Relaxants*
*Depolarizing*
Succinylcholine
*Nondepolarizing*
Atracurium
Cisatracurium
Pancuronium
Rocuronium
Vecuronium

**INTRAVENOUS**

*Barbiturates*
Methohexital
Thiopental
*Benzodiazepines*
Diazepam
Lorazepam
Midazolam
*Benzodiazepine Antagonist*
Flumazenil
*Nonbarbiturate*
Dexmedetomidine
Etomidate
Ketamine
Propofol
*Narcotics*
Alfentanil
Fentanyl
Hydromorphone
Meperidine
Morphine
Remifentanil
Sufentanil
*Narcotic Antagonist*
Naloxone
**NSAID
Ketorolac tromethamine
*Narcotic Agonists/ Antagonists*
Buprenorphine
Butorphanol
Dezocine
Pentazocine
Nalbuphine

**LOCAL ANESTHESIA**

*Amides*
Bupivacaine
*EMLA
Etidocaine
Lidocaine
Mepivacaine
Prilocaine
Ropivacaine
*Esters*
Chloroprocaine
Cocaine
Procaine
Tetracaine

* EMLA, Eutectic mixture local anesthetics
** NSAID, Nonsteroidal anti-inflammatory drugs

FIGURE 13-1   Medication choices for anesthetic options.

**BOX 13-2** Anesthesia Provider-to-Nurse Report: Information to Convey

Name of patient
Surgical procedure
Type of anesthetic (agents and reversal agents used)
Estimated blood loss
Fluid and blood replacement
Intraoperative blood pressure and heart rate range
Intraoperative complications
Preoperative patient history
Language barrier

*Note:* The anesthesia provider should not leave the patient until the nurse is satisfied with the patient's immediate postoperative condition.

**QSEN BOX 13-3** *COLLABORATIVE CARE GUIDE for the Postanesthesia Patient*

| Outcomes | Interventions |
|---|---|
| **Impaired Gas Exchange** | |
| Adequate respiration after extubation<br>SaO$_2$ returns to the preoperative value without supplemental O$_2$<br>Airway maintained with intact protective reflexes<br>No evidence of aspiration | • Monitor respiratory rate and breathing pattern every 15 minutes and PRN<br>• Assess weaning parameters before extubation<br>• Monitor end-tidal CO$_2$ and pulse oximetry of mechanically ventilated patients<br>• Encourage patient to cough and deep-breathe<br>• Elevate head of bed if not contraindicated<br>• Use jaw thrust, head tilt, or oral, oropharyngeal, or nasopharyngeal airway to maintain airway<br>• Stimulate patient every few minutes (eg, call name, touch)<br>• Administer antiemetic as indicated<br>• Position patient on side; suction and maintain airway if patient is vomiting |
| **Decreased Cardiac and Peripheral Tissue Perfusion**<br>**Ineffective Thermoregulation: Risk for Imbalanced Body Temperature**<br>**Hyperthermia** | |
| Heart rate and blood pressure returned to preoperative values within 1 to 2 hours after anesthesia<br>Body temperature within normal limits<br>No evidence of malignant hyperthermia | • Monitor vital signs every 15 minutes and PRN<br>• Assess pulse quality and regularity<br>• Monitor for dysrhythmias<br>• Monitor for hypotension related to bleeding<br>• Monitor for hypotension related to warming and vasodilation<br>• Administer IV solution and blood products as ordered<br>• Anticipate hypothermia; have warming devices readily available<br>• Measure temperature on admission and PRN until normal<br>• Warm patient at 1°C to 2°C/h<br>• Monitor for malignant hyperthermia and immediately notify anesthesia provider of temperature increase of 0.5°C<br>• Administer dantrolene and initiate cooling measures<br>• Assist with malignant hyperthermia protocol |
| **Risk for Imbalanced Fluid Volume** | |
| Patient has stable blood pressure and heart rate<br>Urine output will be 0.5 to 2 mL/kg/h<br>No evidence of hypervolemia or hypovolemia | • Maintain patient IV<br>• Monitor intake and output<br>• Assess skin and mucous membranes for signs of hypovolemia<br>• Measure specific gravity if indicated<br>• Assess for signs of hypervolemia (eg, pulmonary crackles, neck vein distention)<br>• Measure serum electrolytes if indicated |
| **Risk for Acute Confusion**<br>**Risk for Activity Intolerance** | |
| Patient will arouse easily and respond appropriately to commands<br>Patient will move all extremities purposefully and with normal strength | • Assess level of consciousness every 15 minutes and PRN<br>• Monitor motor and sensory function to assess reversal of neuromuscular blockade<br>• Assess level of regional block, epidural, or spinal anesthesia |
| **Impaired Skin Integrity** | |
| Skin will remain intact | • Assess skin immediately postoperatively for pressure areas and burns |
| **Imbalanced Nutrition**<br>**Electrolyte Imbalance** | |
| Nutritional intake will be reestablished without nausea or vomiting | • Resume enteral feeding with return of bowel sounds<br>• Begin oral fluids with return of protective airway reflexes |
| **Impaired Comfort** | |
| Pain will be <4 on numeric pain scale or visual analog | • Assess location, type, and severity of pain<br>• Administer opioids as indicated<br>• Monitor response to analgesics<br>• Institute nonpharmacological pain relief strategies and comfort measures<br>• Evaluate patient-controlled analgesia IV or epidural as postoperative pain management option |
| **Ineffective Coping** | |
| Personal support systems will be used to reduce anxiety | • Encourage significant other visits in early postoperative phase<br>• Validate patient's significant other's understanding of surgery and illness<br>• Initiate referrals to social services, clergy, and so forth |

*COLLABORATIVE CARE GUIDE for the Postanesthesia Patient (contiued)*

| Outcomes | Interventions |
| --- | --- |
| **Teaching/Discharge Planning** | |
| Discharge from postanesthesia care phase will occur within 1 to 2 hours | • Orient patient frequently |
| | • Explain procedures and pain management treatment plan |
| Exercises to prevent postoperative pulmonary complications will be demonstrated | • Teach coughing, deep breathing, and incentive spirometer use |
| | • Teach early mobilization |
| Patient or significant other will state understanding of surgical procedure and outcome of surgery | • Teach pain control strategies |
| | • Provide information regarding the procedure, and discuss probable outcomes |

## Hypoxemia

Hypoxemia characterized by an $SaO_2$ of less than 90% or a partial pressure of arterial oxygen ($PaO_2$) of less than 60 mm Hg is life threatening. General anesthetic drugs can cause hypoxemia in the immediate postoperative period as a result of hypoventilation or ventilation–perfusion mismatch.[2] Signs and symptoms of hypoxemia include tachycardia, cardiac dysrhythmias, dyspnea, tachypnea, disorientation, agitation, and cyanosis. Cyanosis is a late symptom of hypoxemia. Hypoxemia and hypoventilation may also occur postoperatively following general anesthesia, intraoperative opioids, or the use of a spinal, epidural, or other regional anesthetics that have blocked the spinal nerves innervating the muscles of respiration, weakening the respiratory effort.[3]

When nitrous oxide is used for general anesthesia, 100% oxygen is administered in the OR for 3 to 4 minutes at the discontinuance of this anesthetic. These patients are transported receiving oxygen to prevent diffusion hypoxia in the PACU. Patients who receive a general anesthetic or sedation receive supplemental oxygen in the immediate postoperative period because general anesthesia and sedation cause a compromise in respiratory function. Patients in the immediate postoperative period are routinely monitored for adequate oxygenation by using the pulse oximeter, a noninvasive device that continuously monitors $SaO_2$. This device has been used in the OR since the 1980s and more recently in the PACU, resulting in a significant decrease in anesthesia and postanesthesia respiratory mishaps.[4]

Reversal agents are used intraoperatively to antagonize the effects of muscle relaxants, sedatives, and opioids. The effects of muscle relaxants, sedatives, and opioids may last longer than the reversal agent, resulting in hypoventilation and hypoxemia even though a reversal agent has been administered. For this reason, it is important to know the onset and duration of action of drugs used to reverse the effects of the sedative, muscle relaxant, or opioid. This knowledge allows for appropriate assessment and intervention when a change in the patient's condition occurs.

## Hypoventilation

Hypoventilation leading to hypercarbia ($PaCO_2 > 45$ mm Hg) may result from any of the following:

• Inadequate respiratory drive secondary to the effects of residual anesthesia, such as opioids, sedatives, and general anesthesia inhalational agents
• Inadequate functioning of respiratory muscles, causing inadequate tidal volume due to residual neuromuscular blockade;

• Chronic pulmonary disease, such as chronic obstructive pulmonary disease, which may require postoperative ventilatory support
• Laryngospasm or upper airway obstruction resulting from residual general anesthesia (Box 13-4).

The nurse institutes the "stir-up" regimen in the immediate postoperative phase to stimulate the patient, especially if opioids or sedatives were used during surgery. The nurse considers the length of time since reversal agents were administered to antagonize neuromuscular blockade. The patient may not be fully reversed and may exhibit signs of residual neuromuscular blockade, as evidenced by the inability to maintain a head lift for 5 seconds. Moreover, inappropriate use of chest and abdominal wall muscles will result in air hunger, anxiety, and tachycardia. Neuromuscular blocking agents are summarized in Box 13-5. The respiratory effect of neuromuscular nondepolarizing drugs is prolonged with hypothermia. Other conditions that increase the effects of nondepolarizing muscle relaxants are listed in Box 13-6.

**BOX 13-4** | **Managing Laryngospasm and Airway Obstruction**

**Laryngospasm**
Laryngospasm is often caused by blood, mucus, or other oral secretions irritating the vocal cords. Suctioning of the oropharynx before extubation helps to prevent laryngospasm. Laryngospasm is treated with positive-pressure ventilation using 100% $FiO_2$ via a bag-valve mask with a tight seal. If this does not break the spasm, a small dose of depolarizing muscle relaxant (succinylcholine) may be given IV.

**Upper Airway Obstruction**
Upper airway obstruction must be identified and treated promptly and effectively. Airway obstruction may range from minimal to complete. Signs of obstruction include
• paradoxical breathing
• stridor
• lack of, or change in, breath sounds
• hypoxemia
• change in level of consciousness.
Treatment to relieve obstruction must be provided in a systematic fashion.
1. Tilt head/lift chin.
2. Thrust jaw.
3. Call for assistance.
4. Insert an oropharyngeal or nasopharyngeal airway. (An oropharyngeal airway may not be tolerated by the partially anesthetized patient.)
5. Apply positive-pressure ventilation.
6. Perform endotracheal intubation if necessary.

**BOX 13-5** | **Neuromuscular Blocking Agents**

**Muscle Relaxants**

- Muscle relaxant drugs used in anesthesia paralyze patients but provide no sedation or analgesia.
- Muscle relaxants facilitate endotracheal intubation, relax muscles for surgical procedures, terminate laryngospasm, eliminate chest wall rigidity, and provide for ease of mechanical ventilation if indicated.
- Depolarizing and nondepolarizing muscle relaxants are used in anesthesia and work at the myoneural junction by blocking nicotinic acetylcholine receptors.

**Depolarizing Agent (Succinylcholine)**

- Succinylcholine combines with acetylcholine receptors at the neuromuscular junction and mimics the action of acetylcholine.
- Onset of action is 1 to 2 minutes and duration of action is 4 to 6 minutes.
- The enzyme pseudocholinesterase breaks down succinylcholine from plasma, so in conditions involving a decrease in pseudocholinesterase, the length of action of succinylcholine increases, keeping patients paralyzed for longer periods.
- Decreased pseudocholinesterase enzyme may be seen in pregnancy, liver disease, malnutrition states, severe anemia, cancer, and with other pharmacological agents, such as quinidine, phospholine eye drops, and propranolol.

**Nondepolarizing Agents**

- Nondepolarizing agents (atracurium, cisatracurium, pipecuronium, vecuronium, pancuronium, doxacurium, rocuronium) compete with acetylcholine at the neuromuscular junction for muscle membrane receptors.
- Onset of action is within 2 to 3 minutes, depending on dose.
- Duration of action ranges from 20 minutes to 2 hours, depending on the drug and dosage.
- Muscle relaxant reversal agents' (neostigmine, edrophonium, sugammadex) duration of action may be shorter than the duration of action of muscle relaxants, resulting in respiratory muscle weakness and respiratory insufficiency. Anticholinesterases cause muscarinic side effects including bradycardia and increased salivary secretions. These side effects are counteracted with the administration of an anticholinergic drug (atropine, glycopyrrolate) in conjunction with the anticholinesterase.

**BOX 13-6** | **Conditions and Drugs That Increase the Effects of Nondepolarizing Muscle Relaxants**

Local anesthetics
General anesthetics
Antibiotics: aminoglycosides, polypeptides, polymyxin
Antiarrhythmics: quinidine, procainamide
Furosemide (Lasix)
Acid–base status: respiratory acidosis, metabolic alkalosis
Electrolyte imbalance: hypokalemia, hypocalcemia, dehydration, magnesium administration
Hypothermia

## Hypotension

The most common cardiovascular complication seen in the postoperative period is hypotension due to decreased blood volume resulting from preoperative fasting and intraoperative blood loss. Intervention is indicated if the pressure decreases

**QSEN** | **BOX 13-7** | *PATIENT SAFETY*

**Factors That May Cause Postoperative Hypotension**

**Drug and Conditional Factors**
Epidural or spinal anesthetic blockade
Inhalation anesthetic agents
Hypovolemia
Hypothermia
Myocardial depression
Sepsis
Transfusion reaction
Increased intrathoracic pressure from mechanical ventilation
Dysrhythmias (supraventricular tachycardia)
Myocardial infarction
Congestive heart failure
Bradycardia
Bladder/abdominal distention

**Technical Factors**
Blood pressure cuff size and position
Tight abdominal dressing
Transducer balance and calibration
Stethoscope position

by more than 30% of the baseline blood pressure.[5] Risk factors for postanesthesia hypotension are listed in Box 13-7.

General and regional anesthetics also decrease blood pressure. Spinal and epidural regional anesthetic techniques cause vasodilation and decrease blood pressure as a result of the sympathetic blockade. Opioids cause histamine release and vasodilation, resulting in lowered blood pressure. Droperidol and chlorpromazine hydrochloride produce sympathetic blockade and hypotension. Propofol and anesthetic inhalational agents, such as isoflurane, sevoflurane, and desflurane, cause myocardial depression. Often, postoperative orthostatic hypotension is due to hypovolemia and decreased venous return to the heart because of inadequate intraoperative volume replacement, blood loss, loss of fluid into the interstitial space, and diuretics. The patient is evaluated for orthostatic hypotension by measuring blood pressure and heart rate in the supine position and in a position with the head of the bed raised 60 degrees, if not contraindicated by the surgical procedure or the patient's status. With orthostatic hypotension, there will be a significant decrease in blood pressure with the head of the bed raised. Cardiac dysrhythmias, such as supraventricular tachycardia and marked bradycardia, can cause a decrease in cardiac output, leading to hypotension. Other causes of postoperative hypotension include sepsis, pulmonary embolism, and transfusion reaction.

Deliberate, controlled hypotensive intraoperative anesthetic techniques are used during some surgical procedures, such as neurosurgery, shoulder arthroscopy, and maxillofacial surgery. This hypotensive technique minimizes blood loss, decreases intraoperative blood transfusions, decreases oozing, and minimizes hematoma formation. These patients must be monitored closely postoperatively until blood pressure returns to normal.

Treatment of immediate postoperative hypotension depends on the underlying cause. A priority is to ensure adequate oxygenation and ventilation of the patient while the blood pressure is addressed. IV fluids, blood products, plasma expanders, crystalloids, and vasopressor drugs are administered to increase blood pressure caused by intraoperative blood loss. Passive leg raising may be used to increase perfusion to the brain during the hypotensive episode. The nurse inspects wound dressings, drains, and surgical sites for postoperative bleeding. If there is significant postoperative bleeding, the surgeon must be notified and the patient may have to return to the OR.

When assessing and treating a patient with hypotension, the nurse must also rule out the possibility of a technical problem rather than physiological problems. Is the blood pressure cuff the correct size, and is it positioned correctly? Is the stethoscope positioned correctly? Is the patient's position a factor? If an arterial line is present, is the transducer correctly calibrated? Troubleshooting for device errors occurs simultaneously with patient assessment.

## Hypothermia

Heat loss during surgery is due to reduced basal metabolism and depression of the hypothalamic thermoregulatory center caused by inhalational anesthetic agents. Vasodilation also occurs with regional anesthesia because of the sympathetic nervous system blockade, resulting in heat loss and hypothermia. Other intraoperative causes of hypothermia include heat loss through radiation, convection, and conduction because of prolonged skin exposure, saturated surgical drapes, cold ORs, antiseptic prepping solutions, cold irrigation solutions, and cold IV fluids. Geriatric patients are at greater risk for hypothermia because of alterations in their hypothalamic function and decreased body fat. Neonates are at increased risk for hypothermia because of their immature thermoregulatory center and their high body surface-to-volume ratio. Hats, warm blankets, forced air warming devices, and IV fluid warmers are used perioperatively to prevent hypothermia.

Patients admitted to the PACU with hypothermia have prolonged postoperative recovery time and higher incidence of postoperative complications such as wound infection.[6] Rewarming of the postoperative patient is done immediately, using heated blankets, warm IV fluids, and warming devices such as the forced air warmer.

## Postoperative Nausea and Vomiting

Postoperative nausea and vomiting (PONV) is one of the more common problems in the PACU and is a frequent cause of postoperative hospital admission for outpatient surgical patients.[7] Although not life threatening, PONV leaves the patient with a lasting unpleasant memory, may increase the length of stay in the hospital, and may have an impact on future surgical and anesthetic decisions. Frequent causes include opioids, increased gastric secretions, spinal anesthesia, and surgical procedures involving manipulation of eye muscles, abdominal muscles, or genitourinary muscles. Laparoscopic techniques and surgical breast procedures are also associated with an increase in PONV. Risk factors for PONV in adults include female sex, prior history of motion sickness or PONV, nonsmokers, and younger age.

Vomiting is regulated by the vomiting center located in the medulla, which receives stimuli from the gastrointestinal tract, the chemoreceptor trigger zone, the labyrinthine apparatus (motion sickness), and cortical and visual input. Stimuli that can cause vomiting are gastric distention, opioids, anesthetic drugs, hypoxemia, postoperative pain, and hypotension. Antiemetic drugs given to treat PONV in the immediate postoperative period may have a synergistic effect on opioids, and decreasing the dose of narcotic is indicated. Patients at high risk for PONV are treated using a multimodal pharmacologic approach beginning in the preoperative period.

Not only is the anesthetized patient prone to vomiting, but because of the unprotected reflexes, there is a greater chance of regurgitation and pulmonary aspiration. Proper positioning of anesthetized or sedated patient is essential. The ideal position is on the side with the head and neck extended. If the surgical procedure precludes turning the patient on the side or the patient is unable to comply, then the patient must not be left unattended until consciousness and protective airway reflexes are regained. A Yankauer suction device attached to wall suction should be immediately available.[8]

## Postoperative Pain

Postoperative surgical pain is caused by several factors including the surgical incision, tissue manipulation, and the anesthetic technique used intraoperatively. Adequate pain relief is important during the postoperative period because it allows the patient to cough, deep-breathe, and ambulate sooner, thus reducing the incidence of postoperative complications such as atelectasis. The patient for whom the anesthetic was an inhalation agent without opioids or local anesthetics may have more pain than a patient who received intraoperative opioids or a regional anesthetic. Patients who have been given opioids during surgery and who then receive naloxone, an opioid antagonist, at the end of surgery may experience severe pain because the opioid antagonist reversed the analgesic effects of any prior opioid drugs. Because these patients may experience hypoventilation again, the nurse must wait 15 to 45 minutes after the administration of naloxone before giving another opioid-based analgesic drug.

Box 13-8 lists factors that influence the patient's response to pain. Types and methods of administration of analgesic drugs commonly used for the immediate postoperative patient are discussed below.

### IV Opioid Drugs

IV titration of opioids such as morphine, fentanyl, or hydromorphone in the immediate postoperative period offers the fastest and most effective pain relief. Because the patient's basal metabolic rate decreases during surgery and the patient may be hypothermic, the uptake of intramuscular medication is often difficult to predict.

---

**BOX 13-8** | **Factors Influencing Pain**

**Surgical procedure:** Site and nature of the operation
**Anxiety level:** Fear of surgery, disfigurement, death, loss of control, previous experiences
**Patient expectations:** Effectiveness of preoperative teaching, adequately prepared for outcome
**Pain tolerance:** Prior use of medications, including analgesics, individual differences
**Anesthesia technique:** Analgesics used during the intraoperative period, use of naloxone

## Toradol

Toradol (ketorolac tromethamine) may be administered during surgery and has been found effective in treating immediate mild to moderate postoperative pain. Toradol is a nonsteroidal anti-inflammatory drug that exhibits analgesic, anti-inflammatory, and antipyretic activity. Peak analgesia occurs in 45 to 60 minutes after intramuscular or IV injection, and the analgesic effect lasts 6 to 8 hours. This drug is given in doses up to 30 mg and is not used for more than 5 days postoperatively. The drug is contraindicated in patients with active peptic ulcers, recent gastrointestinal bleeding, or renal insufficiency.

## IV Acetaminophen

IV acetaminophen is a non-opioid centrally acting analgesic that has been available in Europe for several years and is now approved for use in the United States. It is the only non-opioid that does not have a "black-box" label from the Food and Drug Administration (FDA) and is approved for use in adults and in children. The drug does not increase the incidence of nausea and vomiting, does not depress respirations, and does not increase the risk of postoperative bleeding. The drug may be administered for mild to moderate pain before, during, or after surgery.

## Patient-Controlled Analgesia

The use of patient-controlled analgesia (PCA) in the PACU allows the patient to administer his or her own analgesic intravenously using a PCA device. Clinical studies show that patients report less pain when they are able to control the administration of opioids for their pain.[9] PCA may also be used to inject analgesic drugs into the epidural space. Both modalities are effective ways for patients to control their own analgesic needs.

## Epidural Opioid Drugs

Epidural opioid analgesia is effective in treating acute postoperative pain.[10] Patients who receive epidural opioids are less sedated, are able to ambulate sooner, and have improved respiratory function. Preservative-free epidural opioids are administered as a bolus injection at the end of surgery or by a continuous epidural infusion through an epidural catheter and infusion pump postoperatively. To ensure patient safety during epidural opioid infusion, the infusion sets have no injection ports, and the infusing pump, infusion bag, and infusion tubing are clearly labeled with the word *epidural*. The reason for these safeguards is that accidental infusion of other drugs with preservatives could cause neural damage, resulting in paralysis or death. The duration of analgesia varies with the opioid administered. Opioids frequently used for epidural administration are preservative-free morphine (duration of action 2 to 24 hours), hydromorphone (duration of action 10 to 14 hours), and fentanyl (duration of action 4 to 6 hours).

## Epidural Local Anesthetic Drugs

Dilute local anesthetic solutions of lidocaine, ropivacaine, bupivacaine, or etidocaine are given epidurally for postoperative pain either with opioids or alone. The combination of local anesthetics and opioids has been used to optimize analgesia and minimize the side effects of local anesthetics and

> **BOX 13-9**　**Side Effects of Epidural Analgesia and Possible Remedies**
>
> **Urinary Retention**
> - Catheterize as needed.
>
> **Postural Hypotension**
> - Give fluid (volume) replacement.
> - Administer ephedrine 5 to 10 mg or phenylephrine 50 to 100 mcg IV as ordered.
>
> **Pruritus (Itching of Face, Head, and Neck)**
> - Treat with diphenhydramine (Benadryl) 25 mg PO, IM, IV.
> - Treat with naloxone (Narcan) 0.1 mg IV.
> - Treat with propofol 10 mg IV.
>
> **Nausea and Vomiting**
> - Administer scopolamine patch.
> - Administer a 5-hydroxytryptamine type 3 antagonist.
> - Administer dexamethasone 0.1 mg/kg.
>
> **Respiratory Depression**
> - Administer naloxone 0.1 mg up to a maximum of 0.4 mg IV.
> - Monitor for 30 minutes after naloxone administration because opioid half-life may be longer.

opioids by using minimal doses for both. Nurses are responsible for recognizing and treating the side effects of patients who are receiving epidural analgesia (Box 13-9).

## Hypertension

Hypertension occurs with perioperative pain, hypoxemia, and hypercarbia because of the endogenous catecholamine release. Ketamine, a nonbarbiturate anesthetic and analgesic drug, stimulates the sympathetic nervous system and may cause tachycardia and hypertension. Naloxone, if given too rapidly, may cause hypertension leading to pulmonary edema or cerebral hemorrhage. Other causes of hypertension include anxiety, urinary bladder distention, fluid overload, a narrow blood pressure cuff, and withholding antihypertensive drugs before surgery. Unless instructed otherwise, patients should take their antihypertensive drugs on the day of surgery. Hypertensive patients require reassurance and close observation. Mild to moderate hypertension in the immediate postoperative period is usually treated with IV vasoactive drugs such as hydralazine (Apresoline) and labetalol (Trandate). Hypertensive crises do occur in the immediate postoperative period, and continuous IV infusions of nicardipine, sodium nitroprusside, or nitroglycerin are used to keep the blood pressure in a safe range. When hypertension accompanies emergent delirium, IV sedatives may be required. If the patient is hypertensive because of anxiety and verbal reassurance is ineffective, benzodiazepines, such as midazolam (Versed), may be necessary. If the hypertension results from fluid overload during surgery, the patient may require urinary catheterization and diuretics, such as furosemide (Lasix).

## Cardiac Dysrhythmias

The cardiac dysrhythmias frequently seen in the postoperative period are those induced by anesthetic agents, as detailed in Table 13-2. (Chapter 17 provides more detailed

**TABLE 13-2 Cardiac Dysrhythmias Associated With Anesthetics**

| Anesthetic Agent | Dysrhythmia |
|---|---|
| Local anesthesia with epinephrine | Tachycardia |
| Spinal and epidural | Bradycardia secondary to vagal response |
| Barbiturates | |
| Sodium pentothal | Bradycardia, AV dissociation, occasional PVCs |
| Nonbarbiturate etomidate | Sinus tachycardia |
| Morphine sulfate | Transient brachycardia |
| Meperidine hydrochloride | Transient tachycardia |
| Fentanyl | Bradycardia |
| Opioid antagonist | |
| Naloxone | PVCs, ventricular tachycardia, occasional ventricular fibrillation |
| Ketamine | Tachycardia |
| Isoflurane | Tachycardia |
| Sevoflurane, desflurane | AV dissociation, tachycardia |
| Muscle relaxants | |
| Succinylcholine | Sinus bradycardia, junctional rhythms, PVCs. Patients with burns, trauma, paraplegia or quadriplegia prone to ST-segment depression, peaked T waves, widening QRS complex leading to ventricular tachycardia, ventricular fibrillation, or asystole |
| Pipecuronium bromide | Atrial fibrillation, ventricular extrasystole |
| Pancuronium | Tachycardia and nodal rhythms |
| Anticholinesterases | Bradycardia, slowed AV conduction, PVCs |
| Anticholinergics | Tachycardia |

AV, atrioventricular; PVC, premature ventricular contraction.

information on cardiac dysrhythmias.) The most common causes of cardiac dysrhythmias in the immediate postoperative period are hypoventilation, electrolyte imbalances, hypoxemia, hypovolemia, fluid overload, hypothermia, and pain (Box 13-10).

## Postoperative Emergence Delirium

Emergence delirium (ED) or emergence agitation is seen on emergence from general anesthesia and consists of combative behaviors, such as waking up in a violent manner, thrashing, and pulling out IVs or monitors. ED has been reported more frequently in the pediatric population and in military service members who have returned from combat having sustained a traumatic brain injury or post-traumatic stress (PTS). Total IV anesthesia seems to help minimize this postoperative complication.[11] If a patient appears to be experiencing ED and is acutely anxious or has flashbacks, the presence of a trusted family member or friend in the PACU may help alleviate these symptoms.[12] Reducing environmental stimuli has also been found to be useful in resolving ED, and intraoperative sympatholytic drugs have been

used to prevent ED.[13] Ketamine has been used to reduce the risk of ED in the PTS patient.[14]

ED has also been observed in the pediatric surgical patient population, especially following the use of sevoflurane or desflurane inhalational anesthetic agents, which have a short duration and fast emergence. Intraoperative analgesics may decrease the incidence of ED, suggesting that pain during impaired consciousness may contribute to this phenomenon.[15] Clonidine and dexamethasone have also been used to prevent ED in the pediatric surgical patient population.[16]

## Malignant Hyperthermia

Malignant hyperthermia (MH) is an autosomal-dominant pharmacogenetic disorder of skeletal muscle characterized by a hypermetabolic response to an anesthetic triggering agent, resulting in skeletal muscle damage, hyperthermia, and death if untreated (see Spotlight on Genetics 13-1). Most MH episodes occur in the OR during general anesthesia and less frequently in the immediate postoperative period. MH is triggered in susceptible individuals by halogenated inhalational anesthetic agents and the muscle relaxant succinylcholine. Nitrous oxide, local anesthetics, opioids, propofol, and the nondepolarizing muscle relaxants do not trigger MH episodes.

MH is more prevalent in people with muscular abnormalities, such as muscular dystrophy. The incidence of MH has been estimated to be as low as 1 in 250,000 patients receiving anesthetics to as high as 1 in 4,200 patients receiving anesthetics using triggering agents. MH was first observed in the 1960s with the introduction of inhalational anesthetic agents, and had a mortality of 80%. Today, with the use of intraoperative monitoring of end-tidal $CO_2$ (ETCO$_2$), SaO$_2$, and the drug sodium dantrolene, the mortality has decreased to 5%. When the MH-susceptible skeletal muscle is exposed to an MH triggering agent, intracellular calcium is released at an abnormally high rate, resulting in excessive muscle contraction,

**BOX 13-10 Causative Factors for Dysrhythmias**

**Hypoxemia:** Sinus bradycardia, sinus tachycardia, premature ventricular contractions (PVCs), supraventricular tachycardia

**Hypoventilation/hypercarbia:** Sinus tachycardia, PVCs, sinus bradycardia

**Hypovolemia:** Sinus tachycardia

**Fluid overload:** PVCs, supraventricular tachycardia, premature atrial contractions, atrial fibrillation/flutter

**Hyperthermia:** Sinus tachycardia, PVCs

**Hypothermia:** Sinus bradycardia, atrial fibrillation, atrioventricular nodal blocks

**Pain:** Sinus tachycardia, PVCs

Malignant hyperthermia susceptibility (MHS):

- Is a rare reaction that occurs with the use of volatile inhalation agents such as isoflurane, enflurane, sevoflurane, and desflurane.
- Is due to the genetic mutation of the *RYR1* gene, which codes for the ryanodine receptor, which regulates calcium release or genetic mutation of the *CACNA1S* genes, which codes for a calcium-channel, voltage-dependent, L-type, alpha 1S subunit, which regulates calcium entry.
- The mutation of the *RYR1* or *CACNA1S* gene, in the presence of the inhalation agent, affects the skeletal muscle, leading to the sustained release of calcium from the sarcoplasmic reticulum causing the hypermetabolic state to occur in the skeletal muscle.
- Can now be identified via genetic testing of those patients and/or family members who have experienced complications during or immediately after surgery.

Genetic Home Reference—http://ghr.nlm.nih.gov—Accessed August 10, 2015

Fiszer D, Shaw MA, Fisher NA, et al: Next-generation sequencing of RYR1 and CACNA1S in malignant hyperthermia and exertional heat illness. Anesthesiology 122(5):1033–1046, 2015.

increased metabolism, high oxygen consumption, high $CO_2$ production, and heat production. This leads to generalized muscle rigidity including masseter muscle rigidity, increased $ETCO_2$, acidosis, hypoxemia, tachycardia, and myoglobinuria. Temperature elevation is a late sign of MH and is preceded by an elevation of $ETCO_2$ and cardiac dysrhythmias.

MH is treated by discontinuation of the anesthetic triggering agent, 100% inspired oxygen, hyperventilation, correction of acid–base imbalances, and cooling measures such as a cooling blanket and cool IV fluids. Dantrolene sodium, 2.5 mg/kg IV, is given and is repeated up to 10 mg/kg as necessary to control MH signs and symptoms. Dantrolene sodium is reconstituted with preservative-free sterile water; this is a labor-intensive process because of the difficulty in reconstituting with an aqueous solution. Most ORs and PACUs have an MH kit that includes 36 vials of dantrolene or 3 vials of the newer drug Ryanodex, which is easier to reconstitute and more concentrated (Box 13-11).

**BOX 13-11** **Contents of Malignant Hyperthermia Kit**

- Methylprednisolone
- Furosemide
- Sodium bicarbonate
- Dextrose (50%)
- Sterile water
- Insulin
- Mannitol
- Refrigerated IV fluids
- Dantrolene sodium or Ryanodex
- New oxygen tubing and delivery devices
- Foley catheter tray
- Nasogastric tubes
- Blood specimen tubes
- Arterial blood gas kits
- MHAUS guidelines and contact information booklet

Recrudescence, or return of the signs and symptoms of MH, can occur in the PACU hours after resolution of the initial event.[12] For that reason, after an episode of MH, the patient is observed in the ICU for 24 hours after the temperature has returned to normal. Dantrolene sodium is administered 1 mg/kg every 6 hours as needed. Monitoring is maintained during this time, including temperature monitoring. Upon discharge, patients are referred to the Malignant Hyperthermia Association of the United States (MHAUS) for support and continued education about this disorder.[17,18]

## Moderate IV Sedation Administered by Registered Nurse Versus Monitored Anesthesia Care

Moderate sedation using midazolam (Versed) and small doses of opioids IV provides a drug-induced depression of consciousness, with the patient able to respond to verbal commands, either alone or associated with light tactile stimulation. No interventions are required to maintain airway patency or spontaneous ventilation. In addition, cardiovascular function is maintained. A patient who has been given moderate sedation has the ability to maintain a patent airway, retain protective airway reflexes, and respond to verbal commands. If these three conditions are not met, the patient is not receiving moderate sedation. The advantage of moderate sedation is that it allows the patient to respond to verbal commands and physical stimulation. Moderate sedation is used for ambulatory surgical and for therapeutic and diagnostic procedures. The regimen usually consists of a narcotic, a sedative, and a local anesthetic.[19]

The goal of moderate sedation is to decrease patient anxiety associated with the surgical procedure or intervention using the least amount of drug necessary. Moderate sedation enhances patient cooperation, maintains stable vital signs, elevates the pain threshold, provides amnesia, and allows for rapid postoperative recovery.[20]

Propofol is used for sedation for surgical procedures and interventional procedures such as endoscopies because of its short onset time and fast recovery time. A disadvantage of propofol is the risk of rapid loss of consciousness and apnea resulting in cardiopulmonary compromise. In a clinical study by Schilling et al,[8] propofol was found to cause a greater incidence of decline in $SaO_2$ and blood pressure as compared with midazolam in patients requiring moderate sedation. Because propofol is an IV general anesthetic, those administering propofol must be trained in the administration of general anesthesia and airway management.[21]

Several entities regulate standards for the administration of moderate sedation, including state boards of nursing, the Joint Commission, and health care facilities. The registered nurse (RN) who is administering the sedation and managing the care of patients receiving moderate sedation must be able to:

- recognize cardiac dysrhythmias;
- demonstrate knowledge of anatomy, physiology, pharmacology, and complications related to moderate sedation and sedative drugs;
- assess patient care requirements during moderate sedation and recovery, including physiological measurements

**TABLE 13-3** Comparison of Moderate Sedation and Monitored Anesthesia Care

| Characteristics | Moderate Sedation | MAC |
|---|---|---|
| Responsiveness | Purposeful response to repeated or painful verbal or tactile stimulation | May have purposeful response after stimulation |
| Airway | No intervention required | Intervention may be required |
| Spontaneous ventilation | Adequate | May be inadequate |
| Cardiovascular function | Usually maintained | Usually maintained |

of respiratory rate and effort, oxyhemoglobin saturation, blood pressure, heart rate and rhythm, and patient's level of consciousness;

- understand the principles of oxygen delivery and respiratory and cardiovascular physiology, and demonstrate the ability to use oxygen delivery and monitoring devices;
- anticipate and recognize complications of moderate sedation related to the sedative drugs administered;
- assess, diagnose, and intervene in undesired outcomes of moderate sedation in compliance with orders (including standard orders) or institutional protocols;
- demonstrate skills in airway management; and
- demonstrate knowledge of the legal responsibilities of administering IV moderate sedation and monitoring patients receiving IV moderate sedation, including the RN's liability for any untoward reactions or life-threatening complications.

Monitored anesthesia care (MAC) is a service in which an anesthesia provider has been requested to provide anesthesia care for a patient undergoing a therapeutic or diagnostic procedure usually requiring sedation. The difference between moderate sedation and MAC is that the anesthesia provider is present to recognize and treat the patient who becomes anesthetized following IV sedation and who develops apnea or an obstructed airway. Sedative drugs, including propofol and fentanyl, are given by the anesthesia provider and local anesthetics are injected into the surgical site by the surgeon. Postoperative care of the patient who has received moderate sedation or MAC is similar, although the patient who has received MAC may require more intervention in the postanesthesia phase.

Table 13-3 provides a comparison of moderate sedation and MAC.

## Clinical Applicability Challenges

**CASE STUDY**

Mr. R., age 49, is scheduled for elective repair of his torn right anterior cruciate ligament. He has suffered with this injury for 10 years and has decided that he cannot tolerate the pain any longer. A review of systems includes history of morbid obesity, obstructive sleep apnea, and well-controlled hypertension. Mr. R. has been kept NPO since midnight. He has not had any food, liquids, or medication since the previous evening.

Mr. R. agrees to general anesthesia, but does not allow the nurse anesthetist to place a peripheral nerve block because he is "afraid of needles." The anesthesia goes well and the patient is brought to the recovery room following the procedure. In recovery, the anesthetist reports the following information to the PACU nurse:

- Patient 5 ft, 7 inches tall, weight 106 kg
- Hemoglobin 15 g/100 mL; hematocrit 44%
- Medications include lisinopril, ibuprofen
- No known drug allergies
- OR time 2 hour, 15 minutes
- General endotracheal anesthesia

- Heart rate 70s, systolic blood pressure 120 to 80 mm Hg, diastolic blood pressure 55 to 75 mm Hg intraoperatively
- Estimated blood loss of 250 mL
- Total crystalloid administered: 2,750 mL of lactated Ringer's solution
- Urine output of 0.55 mL/kg/h.

The patient's initial blood pressure in PACU is 190/110 and the patient is complaining that he has pain, which is characterized as being 7 on a 0-to-10 verbal pain scale. Other data include heart rate of 125 beats/min, respiratory rate of 10 breaths/min, and facial grimacing. The PACU nurse suggests trying IV acetaminophen to treat his pain.

1. Is the elevation in Mr. R.'s blood pressure related to postoperative surgical pain, or could it be something else?
2. Mr. R. was told not to take his morning medications. Is that adding to his elevated blood pressure?
3. Mr R.'s heart rate is elevated. What are possible contributing factors?

**WANT TO KNOW MORE?**

A wide variety of resources to enhance your learning and understanding of this chapter are available on thePoint.

You will find:

- References
- Selected readings
- NCLEX-style review questions
- Internet resources
- And more!

# PART 4

# Special Situations in Critical Care

## 14

# Rapid Response Teams and Transport of the Critically Ill Patient

DENNIS W. JONES AND SHAWN R. BRAST

**LEARNING OBJECTIVES**

*Based on the content in this chapter, the reader should be able to:*

1. Explain the indications for calling a rapid response team (RRT) and the key functions of the team.

2. Contrast the benefits and limitations of an RRT.

3. Describe the indications for interfacility transport of the critically ill patient.

4. Compare and contrast the advantages and disadvantages of air versus ground transport.

5. Discuss the specific planning considerations and implications for care in air transport.

6. Explain the Emergency Medical Transfer & Labor Act (EMTALA) requirements for an appropriate interhospital transfer.

7. Describe the indications and key factors necessary for an effective interfacility transfer plan.

8. Analyze the role of the registered nurse in the five phases of the interfacility transport of the critically ill patient.

9. Outline the best practice approach for team communication and training for an intrahospital transport team.

10. Identify the primary considerations in the use of transport equipment during an intrahospital transport.

## Rapid Response Teams

Patients being cared for in hospitals today are older and sicker and have more comorbidities.[1,2] A rapid response team (RRT) or a medical emergency team (MET) is a resource that can be used to reach hospitalized patients at the first sign of hemodynamic instability. Use of the RRT or MET could prevent deterioration into cardiopulmonary arrest and improve patient outcomes. Outside the United States, MET is considered to be a physician-led team, whereas an RRT is frequently a nurse-led team.[3] Within the United States, a team used for the purpose for rapid evaluation prior to cardiopulmonary arrest is typically called an RRT regardless of whether it is initially led by a physician or a nurse. Critical functions of the RRT are listed in Box 14-1.

---

**BOX 14-1** | **Critical Functions Performed by a Rapid Response Team**

- Rapidly assesses a critically ill patient
- Stabilizes the patient using an RRT protocol or provider-directed medical care
- Rapidly collects patient data (eg, vital signs, radiographic and laboratory data)
- Facilitates consultation with health care specialties to redirect a plan of care
- Provides education and support to nursing staff initiating RRT call
- Assists with triage decisions to the appropriate care area
- Assists with transfer to a higher level of care, if needed

Data from Doty S, Anderson C, Dichter J, et al: Health Care Protocol: Rapid Response Team, 4th ed. Bloomington, MN: Institute for Clinical Systems Improvement, 2011.

In-hospital mortality for patients admitted to an acute care hospital ranges between 2% and 4%.[4] Patients who experience an in-hospital cardiopulmonary arrest have an 80% mortality rate.[5] Nearly one third to one half of patients admitted to the intensive care unit (ICU) in a tertiary care hospital are admitted after an RRT evaluation.[2]

## Benefits of RRTs

The RRT system is based on two major components: early recognition of the deteriorating patient and prompt notification of clinical staff trained in advanced resuscitation. These two major components have supported the implementation of an RRT in both community and tertiary hospitals. RRTs can bring critical care expertise to the bedside of adult patients who are clinically deteriorating outside of an intensive care or emergency department. Having critical care resources brought to the bedside in 5 to 10 minutes has resulted in a reduced number of in-hospital cardiopulmonary arrests in the adult population.[5]

Secondary benefits for RRTs include positive staff perceptions related to teamwork and empowerment of nursing staff.[6] In addition, critically ill patient assignments can be rapidly redistributed to balance nursing workload during a crisis.[6] Last, an RRT with a formalized process for upgrading patient care can improve patient flow for higher-acuity patients.[6]

Six hours is the median time that patients demonstrate physical signs of deterioration before cardiopulmonary arrest.[5] One in five adult patients admitted to the ICU after receiving care from an RRT will have a diagnosis of sepsis, which can have several subtle early warning signs.[2] Frequently, the physical signs of clinical deterioration can be missed or delayed in nonmonitored patient care areas because of the limitations of periodic nursing assessments.[5] Patient triggers for notifying an RRT can be found in Box 14-2.[7] The Medical Emergency Response Intervention and Therapy Trial (MERIT Trial) identified that nursing staff used the "staff member with a significant concern" criteria 35 times more often than the objective criteria.[5] This finding indicates that

---

**BOX 14-2** | **Patient Triggers for a Rapid Response Team**

- Staff member with a significant concern about the patient's condition
- Altered mental status
- Heart rate greater than 140 bpm or less than 40 bpm
- Respiratory rate greater than 22 breaths/min or less than 8 breaths/min
- Systolic blood pressure greater than 180 mm Hg or less than 90 mm Hg
- Oxygen saturation lower than 90% despite supplemental oxygen
- Urine output less than 50 mL over 4 hours
- Chest pain unrelieved with nitroglycerin
- Threatened loss of an airway
- Seizure
- Uncontrolled pain

Adapted from Agency for Healthcare Research and Quality Patient Safety Network (AHRQ PSNet), U.S. Department of Health & Human Services: Patient Safety Primers: Rapid Response Systems. Updated December, 2014. Retrieved June, 2015, from http://psnet.ahrq.gov/primer.aspx?primerID=4.

---

there are challenges in identifying objective indicators in evolving clinical condition in real time and conveying that in a timely and meaningful way to other clinical providers. Approximately 40% to 50% of patients suffering an in-hospital cardiopulmonary arrest had mental status changes or respiratory distress in the hours preceding the event.[8]

## Limitations of RRTs

There have been seven systematic reviews on the effectiveness or implementation of RRTs.[5] The most recent data fail to demonstrate conclusive positive effects of using an RRT on reducing readmissions to the ICU, shortening ICU length of stay, and reducing in-hospital mortality of patients discharged from the ICU.[9] The use of RRTs may even create a greater number of ICU admissions for patients presenting with a borderline illness severity.[10] It is proposed that "staff member with a significant concern" criteria may contribute to this patient population. As a result, patients inappropriately upgraded to an ICU level of care may negatively impact patient throughput and divert staff for variable periods of time from higher-acuity patients in an ICU.[10] This situation could create delays for other patients attempting to access the ICU through an emergency department admission.

Additional reasons for RRTs failing to demonstrate positive effects on patient outcomes include staff knowledge of activation criteria, inconsistent team leadership, poor interprofessional teamwork and communication, and the perceived attitudes by staff about activation of the RRT.[9] Other potential challenges in demonstrating the benefit to RRTs include wide variations in the use of an intensivist as the team leader as opposed to a hospitalist, lack of standardized resuscitation equipment, and lack of protocols to support resuscitative interventions.[9] There are additional criticisms from physicians that the use of RRTs may result in lack of continuity in care owing to the primary care team not being directly involved during the change in a patient's clinical condition.[6] Commonly, less senior physicians are not involved in higher-acuity patient care, potentially creating a missed learning opportunity for junior medical staff.[6] This perception is frequently shared by newer nursing staff working on step-down units who miss the opportunity to participate in high-acuity clinical care when an RRT takes over.

## Strategies for Future Improvement of RRTs

Improving RRT utilization is a recurring theme in published peer-reviewed journal articles on this topic. The predominant strategies to improve the effectiveness of RRTs focus on teamwork training and ways to improve RRT triggers. Secondary benefits of using RRTs in select patient populations are also examined.

Studies demonstrating promising results include those in which staff are trained using interprofessional simulation. The use of simulation for resuscitative training has been shown to improve participant knowledge, product skill, skill time, patient outcomes, interprofessional teamwork, and communication between professionals.[11] Communication techniques developed by the Agency for Healthcare Research and Quality (AHRQ), presented as the Team Strategies and Tools to Enhance Performance and Patient Safety (TeamSTEPPS) program, are demonstrating favorable results

**SBAR Communication Tool**

**SBAR** is an acronym for Situation, Background, Assessment, and Recommendation. Communication tools such as the SBAR provide the RRT leader with a template for gathering pertinent information, facilitating communication with the physician, and facilitating triage decision making.

| | |
|---|---|
| **Situation** | State your name and unit |
| | State the name of the patient you are calling about |
| | State the problem for which the team was consulted |
| **Background** | State the admission diagnosis and the date of admission |
| | State the pertinent medical history |
| | Provide a brief synopsis of the patient's hospital course |
| | State the code status of the patient |
| **Assessment** | Most recent vital signs |
| | BP: _____; pulse: _____; respirations: _____; temp: _____ |
| | Any change from prior assessments: |
| |    Mental status |
| |    Quality of respirations |
| |    Pulse rate/rhythm change |
| |    Pain |
| |    Skin color |
| |    Neurologic changes |
| |    Nausea and vomiting, output |
| **Recommendation** | State your triage recommendations |
| |    For example: |
| |    Transfer to coronary care unit |
| |    Have the physician come see the patient at this time |
| |    Arrange for specialist to see the patient now |
| |    Arrange for tests (eg, chest x-ray, arterial blood gas, ECG, complete blood cell count) |

Adapted from Duncan KD: Nurse-led medical emergency teams: A recipe for success in community hospitals. In: DeVita MA, Hillman K, Bellomo R (eds): Medical Emergency Teams: Implementation and Outcome Measurement. New York, NY: Springer, 2006, pp 122–133.

across medical disciplines.[12,13] One key example of a Team-STEPPS tool is Situation, Background, Assessment, Recommendation (SBAR), which is used for communicating a patient's condition to another health care provider during an emergency, by phone or in person (Box 14-3). Resuscitation team members using TeamSTEPPS tools have demonstrated enhanced perceptions and attitudes toward teamwork, and targeted training has been shown to improve team performance and patient safety.

The process of identifying a deteriorating patient presents numerous obstacles and challenges. Three possible approaches to maximize patient benefit are auto-dispatching of RRT resources, early warning scoring systems, and family-initiated RRT.

The first family-activated RRT was piloted at North Carolina Children's Hospital in 2007.[3] Favorable feedback by families has been reported, but a clear positive effect in adult or pediatric patient outcomes has not been demonstrated.

Early warning scoring systems are being developed to improve objective identification of a deteriorating patient.

Published scoring systems have not been validated and require the use of a tool during the assessment of a deteriorating patient.[4] When compared to simplified criteria that rely on mental status and respiratory distress, a calculated tool may not be clinically practical.[8] A potential improvement in identifying patients requiring RRT is through the use of continuous monitoring and direct dispatching.[5] The concern with this approach is alarm fatigue due to the inherent false alarms. Technology at this point remains heavily dependent on clinical interpretation, however; better patient identification could occur if continuous monitoring were employed on lower-acuity hospital wards.

A novel benefit of an RRT is to assist in end-of-life care. It is estimated that up to one third of patients receiving care by an RRT will have an end-of-life issue, possibly as a result of poor end-of-life provisions or failure in recognizing the symptoms of a dying patient.[14] When compared with traditional code teams, an RRT can better assist in potentially preventing aggressive therapies that are unlikely to improve patient outcomes or patient comfort. An RRT can also potentially assist patients and families in adopting consensus on limiting life-sustaining treatment.[14]

A great deal of future research will be required to identify the value of RRTs in improving patient safety and outcomes for patients. Challenges in team configuration, protocols, teamwork, and communication are the most obvious issues. Deliberate efforts to address these challenges should provide additional opportunities to substantiate the value of RRTs in the treatment of the critically ill patient.

## Interfacility Transport

Critically ill patients often must be transported between health care facilities. To ensure safe and expeditious transport, it is important to consider both the method of transport and the people involved in the transport process.

Typically, transport is indicated when the patient's need for complex diagnostic procedures or sophisticated medical and nursing expertise exceeds what can be provided at a facility. Family requests may also initiate a patient transport. For example, a family may want their family member transferred to a hospital closer to home. Outcomes of evolving health care reform also have increased the demands for interfacility transport of critically ill patients. Third-party payers may require patients to be transported to a facility that is a member of their network. In addition, many hospitals vie for patients and have developed their own transport teams to provide a flow of patients to their particular facility.

Whatever the reason for transporting a patient, a risk–benefit analysis of the transport should always be performed. Risks for the patient range from physical safety to physiologic compromise to emotional distress.[15] When the benefits for the patient exceed the risks, an interfacility transport is warranted. Figure 14-1 provides an algorithm for interfacility transfer.

The American College of Emergency Physicians (ACEP) has outlined physician responsibilities for interfacility transfer:

- The sending physician performs the patient assessment and determines the appropriate level of care during transfer.

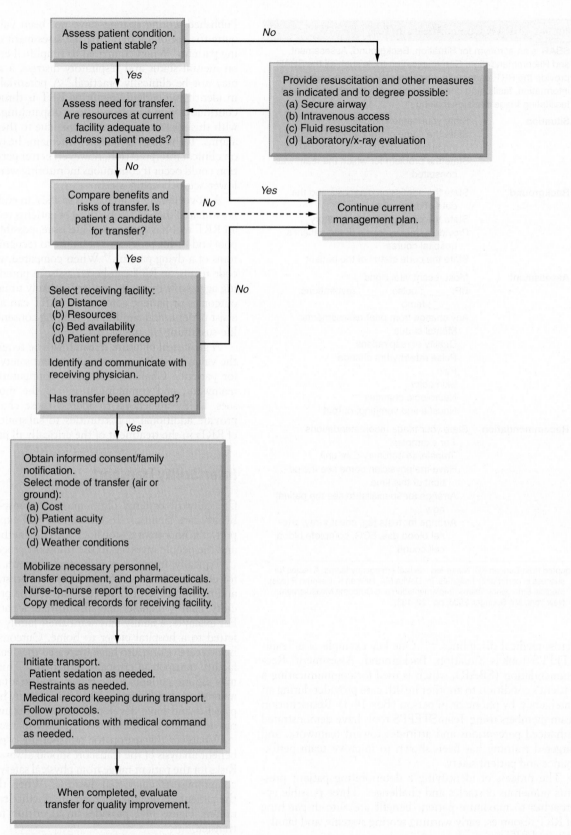

FIGURE 14-1   Interfacility transfer algorithm. (From Warren J, Fromm RE, Orr RA, et al: Guidelines for the inter- and intrahospital transport of critically ill patients. Crit Care Med 32(1):256–262, 2004.)

- The receiving physician ensures that his or her facility is capable of providing necessary patient services to care for the patient.

The medical director of the critical care transportation agency provides medical direction during transport as well as all medical oversight of the transportation operation, which includes, but is not limited to, determining minimal team composition and equipment requirements, education, and practice.[16]

## Modes of Interfacility Transport

Once the decision has been made to transport, the method of transport must be determined. The two primary methods of interfacility transport are ground and air. Ground transport includes ambulances and mobile ICUs. Air transport occurs by either a rotary-wing vehicle (helicopter) or a fixed-wing vehicle (airplane).

When selecting the mode of transport, the following factors must be considered:[17]

- Distance
- The safety of the transport environment
- Patient "out of hospital" time
- The patient's condition and the potential for complications
- The patient's need for critical or time-sensitive intervention (eg, rescue angioplasty)
- Traffic conditions
- Weather conditions

In addition, the advantages and disadvantages of ground versus air transport must be considered. Table 14-1 summarizes the advantages and disadvantages of ground versus air transport.

### Air Transport

Table 14-2 summarizes the special considerations for air transport. It is important for the nurse who may be caring for a patient to have a basic understanding of these considerations to aid in patient preparation prior to flight team arrival and to promote a smooth transfer of care upon the team's arrival.

During air transport, the patient environment differs greatly from the in-hospital setting. Because the patient will be at a higher altitude, where the barometric pressure is reduced, the possibility of hypoxia increases. However, the flight team will assess the patient before departure to determine how much oxygen the patient will need during the transport, based on the patient's clinical condition and the flight plan.

Any air-filled cavity in the patient's body, such as the stomach or lungs, as well as containers (air splint, glass intravenous bottle), can be affected physiologically by changes in barometric pressure. The degree to which any deleterious effects to the patient may occur during transport depends on the type of aircraft and altitude flown. The flight team screens the patient carefully and takes preventive measures to ensure a safe and uneventful transport.

Other environmental factors affecting the patient during transport include changes in temperature and humidity as well as the presence of noise and vibration. The mode of transport will dictate the degree to which each of these factors occurs—that is, whether the vehicle is a fixed-wing or rotary-wing aircraft—and the type of aircraft. The flight crew takes the necessary steps to either prevent or decrease the effects of each of these factors on the patient.

If the critically ill patient is conscious and aware of the need for air transport, the sending nurse screens the patient for fear or anxiety related to flying and a history of motion sickness while in a moving vehicle. Medical consultation is indicated when any of these factors exist, since treatment with an anxiolytic or antiemetic medication could aid in preventing clinical problems during the flight. Again, the flight crew screens the patient for these factors during the preflight assessment.

## Transfer Guidelines and Legal Implications

To facilitate the appropriate transfer of patients, ACEP has developed guidelines. These principles of appropriate patient transfer are listed in Box 14-4.

Legislation provides guidelines, regulations, and penalties for patient transfer. One such law, the Consolidated Omnibus Reconciliation Act (COBRA) of 1985, contains provisions addressing the transfer of patients from hospital to hospital. The purpose of the legislation is to prevent inappropriate transfers of patients who seek emergency department care. In 1986, Congress enacted the Emergency Medical Treatment & Labor Act (EMTALA) to ensure public access to emergency services regardless of ability to pay; this legislation has

**TABLE 14-1** Advantages and Disadvantages of Ground Versus Air Transport

| Mode of Transport | Advantages | Disadvantages |
|---|---|---|
| Ground | Adequate work space for personnel and equipment | Longer transport time |
| | Sensitive monitoring equipment may work better | Unfavorable road conditions may make transport uncomfortable for patient |
| | No weight restrictions | |
| | Adequate lighting | Interventions difficult to perform in a moving vehicle |
| | Able to travel in most types of weather | Ambulance unavailable for other calls in the community |
| Air | May shorten "out of hospital" time | Weather conditions restrict availability of the vehicle |
| | Crew generally composed of advanced-level care providers | Potentially more costly |
| | | Limited space (helicopters) |
| | Improved communication capability | Weight limitations |
| | Ground emergency medical services remain available in the community | Physiologic impact on patient and crew |
| | | Psychological impact on patient (eg, fear of flying) |

From Holleran R: Prehospital Nursing: A Collaborative Approach. St. Louis, MO: CV Mosby, 1994.

**TABLE 14-2** Special Considerations for Air Transport

| Stressors | Effect | Nursing Interventions |
|---|---|---|
| Altitude change | Hypoxia is due to the following:<br>Decrease in the partial pressure of oxygen<br>Decrease in the diffusion gradient for oxygen molecules to cross the alveolar membrane<br>Decrease in oxygen availability | Provide supplemental oxygen<br>Use pulse oximeter and end-tidal $CO_2$ monitor |
| Barometric pressure (atmospheric pressure) change | With increasing altitude, the barometric pressure decreases and gases expand<br>Expansion of gases affects eardrums, sinuses, gastrointestinal tract, pleural spaces, and hollow organs<br>Expansion of gases affects air splints, pressure bags or cuffs, balloon cuffs on endotracheal tubes, intravenous fluid bags and bottles, pneumatic antishock garments | Insert a nasogastric tube to decompress the stomach<br>If possible, fill cuffs with water or saline solution rather than air<br>Monitor equipment and decompress with higher altitudes<br>Vent glass bottles and wrap to protect against breakage<br>Apply pressure cuffs to intravenous solution bags |
| Thermal change | As altitude increases, temperature decreases<br>Oxygen demand increases as the body tries to maintain warmth | Use blankets to keep the patient warm |
| Humidity change | As air is cooled, it loses moisture<br>Mucous membranes dry | Humidify supplemental oxygen<br>Provide adequate fluid intake |
| Gravitational change | Gravitational change affects acceleration and deceleration forces<br>Transient increase in venous return occurs for patients positioned with head at the back of the aircraft<br>Potential exists for motion sickness | Use a head-forward position for patients with fluid overload or increased intracranial pressure<br>To minimize motion sickness, provide oxygen, cool cloth to face, cool air to face<br>Administer medications, such as transdermal scopolamine patches and promethazine |
| Noise | It is difficult to monitor blood pressure, breath sounds, endotracheal tube air leak | Explain sounds to patient<br>Monitor blood pressure by Doppler device<br>Provide continuous airway assessment<br>Wear headsets or ear plugs |
| Vibration | Vibration may distort readings on equipment<br>Equipment may loosen or move | Secure all equipment<br>Check equipment function frequently |

From Harrahill M: Interfacility transfer. In: Kitt S, Selfridge-Thomas J, Proehl J, et al (eds): Emergency Nursing: A Physiologic and Clinical Perspective, 2nd ed. Philadelphia, PA: WB Saunders, 1995, pp 12–18.

**BOX 14.4** **Appropriate Interfacility Patient Transfer**

- The optimal health and well-being of the patient should be the principal goal of patient transfer.
- Emergency physicians, advance practice providers, and facility personnel should abide by applicable laws regarding patient transfer. All patients should be provided a medical screening examination (MSE) and stabilizing treatment within the capacity of the facility before transfer. If a competent patient requests transfer before the completion of the MSE and stabilizing treatment, these services should be offered to the patient and informed refusal documented.
- The transferring facility is responsible for informing the patient or responsible party of the risks and the benefits of transfer and documenting these. Before transfer, patient consent should be obtained and documented whenever possible.
- The medical facility's policies and procedures and/or medical staff bylaws should identify the individuals responsible for and qualified to perform MSEs. The policies and procedures or bylaws must define who is responsible for accepting and transferring patients on behalf of the hospital. The examining physician at the transferring hospital will use his or her best judgment regarding the condition of the patient when determining the timing of transfer, mode of transportation, level of care provided during transfer, and the destination of the patient.
- The mode of transportation used for transfers should be at the discretion of the treating provider and based on the individual clinical situation, available options, needed equipment, and patient preference. Options for transport include but are not limited to ambulance, air transport, and private vehicle. Regardless of the method of transfer, intravenous access may remain in place if deemed appropriate by the referring provider.
- Payment for transport should not be retrospectively denied by insurance companies.
- Agreement to accept the patient in transfer should be obtained from a physician or responsible individual at the receiving hospital in advance of transfer. When a patient requires a higher level of care other than that provided or available at the transferring facility, a receiving facility with the capability and capacity to provide a higher level of care may not refuse any request for transfer.
- All pertinent records and copies of imaging studies should accompany the patient to the receiving facility or be electronically transferred as soon as is practical.
- When transfer of patients is part of a regional plan to provide optimal care at a specialized medical facility, written transfer protocols and interfacility agreements should be in place.

Data from American College of Emergency Physicians: Appropriate Interfacility Patient Transfer. Clinical & Practice Management, Policy Statements, revised January, 2016. Available at: https://www.acep.org/content.aspx?id=29114

become known as the "antidumping law." The Centers for Medicare and Medicaid Services (CMS) impose regulations on Medicare-participating hospitals that offer emergency services.

Provisions of the COBRA legislation prevent any patient from being denied an initial screening in an emergency department, transferred to another hospital, or discharged without receiving care:

1. Hospitals must provide screening examinations for every person who comes to the emergency department and requests care.
2. If the patient has an emergency medical condition, the hospital must provide stabilizing treatment or transfer the patient to another medical facility. The physician must document that the medical benefits outweigh the risks of the transfer.
3. The receiving medical facility agrees to accept the patient and provide appropriate medical treatment. The receiving medical facility must have adequate space and qualified personnel to care for the patient.
4. The transfer is conducted by qualified personnel, and appropriate equipment needed to provide care during the transfer is available.[18]

If a patient is not stabilized, conditions may nevertheless be appropriate for transfer in the following circumstances:

1. The risks of remaining at the initial facility are outweighed by the benefits of transfer.
2. The patient or family requests the transfer.
3. A physician is not present at the initial facility but a qualified medical person certifies that the benefits outweigh the risks.
4. The transfer occurs with appropriate equipment and qualified personnel.

Additional information about EMTALA can be found at https://www.cms.gov/Regulations-and-Guidance/Legislation/EMTALA/.

Figure 14-2 presents the requirements for evaluating a patient's suitability for transfer, as outlined by EMTALA. In addition, the Air and Surface Transport Nurses Association (ASTNA, formerly known as the National Flight Nurses Association, or NFNA) developed nursing standards for transport of the critically ill patient by rotary-wing transport.[18]

## Phases of Interfacility Transport

Five phases of transport have been identified: notification and acceptance by the receiving facility; preparation of the patient by the transport team; the actual transport; turnover of the patient to the receiving hospital; and continuous quality improvement monitoring after transport. Each phase is described in detail as it applies to the transport.

### Phase 1: Notification of and Acceptance by the Receiving Facility

The first phase of transport requires contacting the receiving facility and confirming that it is willing to accept the patient and to provide an accepting physician and an appropriate patient care unit to receive the patient. Additionally, the mode of transport is determined at this time. Communication is a key element in this phase of the process. All personnel (sending, transporting, and receiving) must have the necessary information to make the appropriate transport decision. Standards of care or protocols are necessary for the transport process to be carried out in an organized way. A transfer checklist is helpful to ensure that no steps in the transfer process are missed. In addition, an awareness of the policies and procedures of the transporting agencies is needed for a smooth transport process.[18]

The identification of a responsible physician is essential so that a medical provider is available for consultation while en route and on arrival. ACEP has described medical direction for interfacility transfers as a shared responsibility. The transferring physician ensures that the transport team is composed of professionals appropriate to the needs of the patient and that an appropriate vehicle and equipment are used for transport.[18] If the local emergency medical system is not providing medical direction en route, then the responsible physician must be identified as being part of the hospital-based or private ambulance program.

The Commission of Air Medical Transport Services, which is the certifying body for the air medical industry, maintains the staffing standard on critical care transports; either a registered nurse (RN) or a licensed physician must be present as the primary care provider.[19] Transport teams should have standard orders or protocols if they are unable to contact a physician during transport. The transport flight team has practice protocols that guide their practice; however, they may also receive medical direction from the medical director of the transport program.

Once the specific transporting agency is determined, an overview of the patient's condition and specific clinical needs is communicated. Necessary information includes the patient's name, age, diagnosis, reason for transfer, vital signs, intravenous and special monitoring devices, continuous infusion medications, airway and oxygenation or ventilation status, and special equipment needs (eg, intra-aortic balloon pump). This information assists in determining the composition of the transport team as well as the equipment and medications needed. The American Association of Critical-Care Nurses (AACN), the American College of Critical Care Medicine, and the Society of Critical Care Medicine (SCCM) offer guidelines for accompanying personnel for interfacility transfers (Box 14-5).[15]

Interhospital critical care transport is a highly specialized nursing practice area that requires specific knowledge and skills. Before agreeing to accompany a patient during interhospital transport, nurses who have not received training or who are inexperienced in this practice area must be aware of practice standards or regulations governing nursing practice in this situation, such as those promulgated by a state board of nursing.

The AACN and the SCCM have developed a transfer curriculum and competencies for accompanying staff that may assist in identification of issues related to the role of the nurse in the field.[15] Current regulations require that the patient or a legally authorized representative give informed consent for the transport. If consent cannot be obtained, documentation

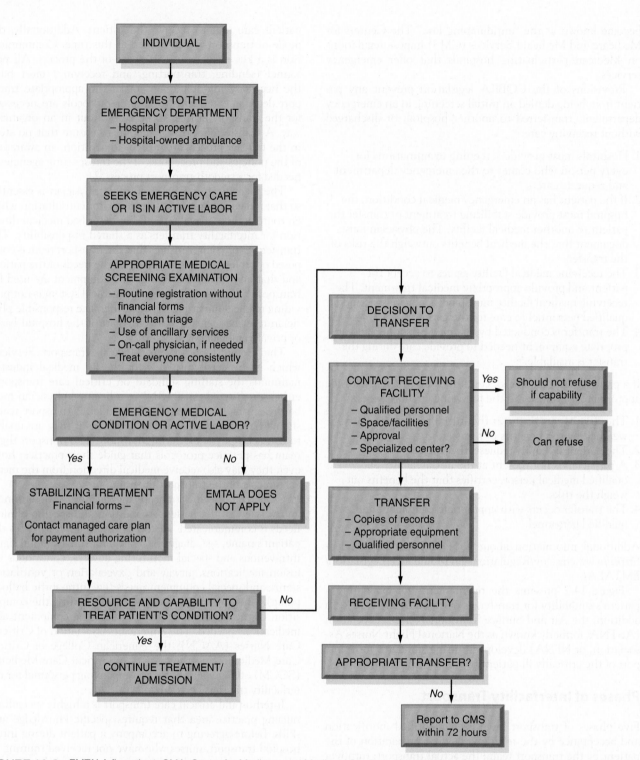

**FIGURE 14-2** EMTALA flow chart. CMA, Center for Medicare and Medicaid Services. (Adapted from Lee NG: Legal Concepts and Issues in Emergency Care. Philadelphia, PA: WB Saunders, 2001, p 140, with permission.)

of the indications for the transport and the reason consent was not obtained must appear in the medical record.[15]

### Phase 2: Preparation of the Patient by the Transport Team

Phase 2 begins upon arrival of the transport team. A thorough patient report is provided to the arriving team; it should include chief complaint, allergies, medical history, reason for transport, patient's age, vital signs, and treatments already provided and their outcomes. Copies of the chart and all radiographs are sent with the patient. To avoid duplication of efforts, the sending and transporting nurses decide who will provide a patient report to the receiving hospital. If the transport is arranged by the sending nurse, the transport nurse updates the receiving nurse as needed.

The transport team performs an assessment of the patient and compares its findings to the previous assessment and

BOX 14.5 | Guidelines for Accompanying Personnel for Interfacility Transfer

- A minimum of two people in addition to the vehicle operator should accompany the patient.
- At least one of the accompanying personnel should be a registered nurse, physician, or advanced emergency medical technician.
- When a physician does not accompany the patient, there should be a mechanism available to communicate with the physician any changes in the patient status and obtain additional orders. If an accompanying physician is not possible, advanced authorization by standing orders to perform acute life-saving interventions must be established.

From Commission on Accreditation of Medical Transport Systems (CAMTS): 10th Edition Accreditation Standards for Medical Transport Systems. Anderson, SC: CAMTS, 2015, pp 9–23. Available at: http://www.camts.org/.

plan of care. If interventions are indicated prior to transport, the transport team and the referral facility personnel determine who assumes responsibility for the interventions. It is important that all stabilization procedures (eg, endotracheal intubation) are completed before departure from the referring facility to ensure the procedures are completed successfully. Completion of these procedures in the less-controlled transport environment increases the risk of error related to unpredictable lighting, movement, and vibration. Although resuscitation and stabilization are initiated at the referral hospital, full stabilization may not be achieved until the patient arrives at the receiving hospital.

The psychosocial preparation of the patient and family for transport is an important step before transport begins. The sending nurse ensures that the patient and family understand all facets of the transport process, including the reason, transport mode, time of transport, and transport destination. Information about the family is also communicated at this time, and includes identification of a family spokesperson and the family's plan for getting to the receiving hospital. If the transport team is unable to meet with the family, the sending nurse supplies information about how to contact the family. The transport team, particularly the flight team, in order to allay any further anxiety related to flying, explains all procedures, safety precautions, and the need for preflight medications (eg, antiemetics) to the patient and family before departure.

Physical preparation of the patient is the next important step to ensure a safe transport. The ABCs of care (airway, breathing, and circulation) are the top priority. Adequate oxygenation and ventilation are ensured before transport begins. As noted earlier, procedures deemed necessary, such as intubation, are performed prior to departure. Most intubated patients are sedated to prevent them from dislodging the endotracheal tube and to decrease fear and discomfort during transport. Furthermore, a nasogastric tube may be inserted to prevent aspiration of stomach contents into the airway. Because auscultation of breath sounds is difficult en route, end-tidal carbon dioxide levels and oxygen saturation are used to monitor respiratory status. Supplemental oxygen is almost universally administered during transport to maintain adequate oxygenation.

The patient's circulatory and hemodynamic statuses are stabilized before transport. Any bleeding is controlled, and adequate intravenous access is established and well secured. For a patient with an unstable volume status, several large-bore intravenous lines are indicated. If the patient is already on intravenous drips, the transport team transfers the drips over to its own equipment and will remix drips as needed. The patient's circulatory status is continuously assessed through blood pressure and cardiac monitoring during the entire transport process. Cardiac arrest medications and a defibrillator should be easily accessible.

Patients with actual or potential spinal injuries should have immobilization devices in place prior to transport. The transport team may request that the staff of the sending facility facilitate this before the arrival of the transport team. A patient with a skeletal long-bone fracture must have the fractured limb immobilized before departure to prevent pain and further complications.

Pain control during transport is also addressed through transport orders or medical protocols. The best agents for pain management are those with a rapid onset, short duration, and ease of administration and storage.

## Phase 3: The Transport Process

Phase 3 is the actual transport of the patient. The time spent in careful planning of the transport and stabilization of the patient eases the transport process. The transport vehicle must contain the essential equipment needed for transporting a critically ill patient. Box 14-6 lists the minimal necessary equipment.[17]

The ABCs of care continue to be the primary focus of the transport team. Box 14-7 lists the minimum and recommended standards for monitoring the critically ill patient during the transport. Each member of the transport team must have a clear understanding of their role in the continuous assessment, planning, and intervention that takes place when caring for the patient. Throughout the transport, the team also provides explanations and reassures the patient,

BOX 14-6 | Minimally Essential Equipment Necessary for Transport

Airway and ventilatory management equipment:
- Resuscitation bag and mask of proper size and fit for the patient
- Oral airways, laryngoscopes, and endotracheal tubes of proper size for the patient
- Oxygen source with a quantity sufficient to meet the patient's anticipated consumption with at least 1-hour reserve in addition
- Suction apparatus and catheters

Cardiac monitor/defibrillator/transcutaneous pacemaker
Blood pressure cuff and stethoscope
Materials for intravenous therapy and devices for regulation of infusion
Drugs:
- For advanced cardiac resuscitation
- For the management of acute physiologic derangements
- For special needs of the patient

Spinal immobilization devices
Communication equipment

From Commission on Accreditation of Medical Transport Systems (CAMTS): 10th Edition Accreditation Standards for Medical Transport Systems. Anderson, SC: CAMTS, 2015, pp 35–40. Available at: http://www.camts.org/.

because transport can be very stressful. The transport team is responsible for documenting all facets of care provided during transport as well as the patient's response to the care.

Before arriving at the receiving facility, if able, the transport nurse calls either a full or updated report to the RN on the receiving unit. This report includes an estimated time of arrival at the receiving facility. The nurse also communicates any special needs, changes in patient status, and unchanged but pertinent findings. In some situations, a flight nurse may not be able to provide a patient update; therefore, an updated bedside report is provided on arrival.

### Phase 4: Turnover of the Patient to the Receiving Facility

Phase 4 of transport involves handing over the patient to the receiving unit staff at the receiving facility. Backup plans on how to handle an acutely deteriorating patient in transit between the transport vehicle and the ICU should also be identified. This plan may include stopping at the emergency department to stabilize the patient; it is essential for the emergency department staff to be aware of this possibility. Once the patient arrives safely in the receiving unit, the transport team and the receiving staff determine when the receiving staff will take over the responsibility for the patient's care. A final verbal update and all medical documents and patient belongings are given to the receiving staff. The written report of the transport is also completed.

### Phase 5: Post-transport Continuous Quality Improvement Monitoring

The final phase of transport is very important and involves continuous quality improvement monitoring. Ideally, the referring facility, the transport team, and the receiving facility are involved in the review process. The first phase of the quality improvement monitoring involves evaluation of the current transport, including any quality indicators developed by the transporting agency. These indicators may include appropriateness of the transfer, accompanying personnel, timeliness of the transfer, patient outcome, management of complications, and transfer outcome. The second phase entails the ongoing review of the transport system. Such reviews focus on system functioning. Indicators may include

complications, deaths in transport, and deaths after transport.[15] The multidisciplinary continuous quality improvement monitoring team scrutinizes the collected data for patterns and trends, identifies solutions to patient care problems, initiates corrective action, and communicates such action to all involved in the transport process. Through a quality improvement plan, the transport process is improved and results in optimal care of the critically ill patient during the transport process.[15]

## Intrahospital Transport

The movement of patients out of the ICU to diagnostic procedure areas for optimizing a plan of care constitutes an intrahospital or intrafacility transport.[20] Patients being transported from the operating room to an ICU or patients being transported from the ICU to a step-down patient care area are excluded from the definition.[21] Much of the current peer-reviewed literature studying this patient population is focused on the potential risks associated with the transport of critically ill patients requiring diagnostic procedures. The reported rate of adverse events during an intrahospital transport ranges from 5.9% to 70%.[22]

The patient care team should consider how the potential information from the diagnostic test would affect a patient's plan of care. Can the required diagnostic tests be completed at the patient's bedside without losing diagnostic quality in the exam? If the answer is no, the patient must be screened carefully for the appropriateness in the timing of diagnostic tests, team configuration, and transport equipment.

## Adverse Events During Intrahospital Transport

In the pretransport assessment, appropriateness of a patient transport is determined in order to avoid adverse events during transport. Although there is no consensus on the definition of adverse events during transport, adverse events can be related to insufficient patient stabilization prior to transport, competency of the team when managing care during the transport, and equipment issues.[22]

Patients requiring an intrahospital transport are vulnerable to acute changes in their clinical condition, and transport may further exacerbate their deterioration.[22] No consensus has been reached about how long to delay transport after treatment modifications. This decision tends to be a clinical decision made by a patient's clinical care team. A well-developed pretransport checklist can help reduce a patient's adverse event risk (Box 14-8).

## Team Composition for an Intrahospital Transport

Standard team configuration for an intrahospital transport consists of a physician or advanced practice clinician, a critical care nurse, and a respiratory therapist.[22] Few hospitals that are using specialized teams without a physician or advanced practice clinician have demonstrated low adverse event rates, but the financial investment may be cost-prohibitive for many institutions.[22] In 2009, the AHRQ identified that there is insufficient data to set a standard for

BOX 14-8 **Pre-intrahospital Transport Assessment Checklist**

- Can the diagnostic test be performed at bedside without losing diagnostic quality?
  - If yes, complete test at bedside.
- Coordinated procedure time
- Procedure consents and screening forms
- Preprocedure lab work reviewed:
  - Blood urea nitrogen/creatinine for patients receiving intravenous contrast
  - Glucose for patients receiving a positron emission tomography scan that requires glucose-bound radioactive tracer
  - Arterial blood gas or oxygen saturation and end-tidal carbon dioxide concentration in expired air for a patient with a compromised airway
- Patient's weight and height evaluated for procedural area diagnostic tables
- Will the patient's bed fit through doorways and elevators that will be encountered during patient movement?
  - Are there any other obstacles between the unit location and the procedure area?
  - Is there a need for additional resources to move the patient once in the procedure area (eg, human, or mechanical lifts, slide boards)?
- Is the patient hemodynamically stable?
  - Have there been modifications in treatment within the last hour?
    - Initiation or titration of a vasoactive medication?
    - Initiation or titration of a sedative or analgesic agent?
- Can the patient lay flat?
  - Consider pretransport supine trial to evaluate for oxygen desaturation in patients with:
    - Respiratory distress
    - Noninvasively ventilated patients are at high risk for aspiration if positioned less than 45 degrees.
- Has the patient taken anything by mouth or received gastric tube feedings within the last hour?
- Consider removal of nonessential equipment:
  - Maintenance IV fluids
  - Compression stockings

team composition for the transport of critically ill patients without a physician, but recommended further research in utilizing a critical care nurse team as a pilot study in the care of pediatric patients during an intrahospital transport.[23]

A best practice in team preparation for intrahospital transports is team training. As mentioned previously, the AHRQ has developed TeamSTEPPS as a structured approach to managing team dynamics, team communication, and strategies to improve patient safety.[24] A key TeamSTEPPS component that can benefit health care team members is the "brief, huddle, debrief" tool, which is a structured communication strategy that is easily implemented and evidence based. By briefing prior to intrahospital transports, calling for a huddle during a transport (if required), and debriefing post-transport, team members maximize the opportunity to improve communication, team performance, and patient safety.

Team composition and skill sets can directly affect patients' adverse event risk during an intrahospital transport.[11,22,23] Skills required to safely transport a patient during an intrahospital transport can best be acquired through simulation. Resuscitation of a patient and the transportation of

a patient have several overlapping skill sets and challenges. The use of simulation for resuscitation training resulted in positive learner outcomes that far exceeded other teaching modalities. In the same way, adverse events during an intrahospital transport may be mitigated with the use of team training and simulation.

## Equipment Considerations During an Intrahospital Transports

Equipment-related incidents have been shown to account for more than 25% of adverse events during an intrahospital transport.[22] Lack of staff experience with the equipment used during a transport is a key factor in equipment failure. A conventional approach that has been used in intrahospital transport involves augmenting the team with a less-experienced physician or advanced practice clinician who has not had the opportunity to become familiar with the transport equipment, and to rely on the patient's primary nurse for technical assistance and troubleshooting. However, if all team members are not familiar with the transport equipment, a single team member may become task-saturated and not have the benefit of additional resources when troubleshooting of equipment is required.

How equipment is used and set up can have a dramatic impact on patient safety. Deciding what equipment will accompany an intrahospital transport should be based on the resources that are readily available in and around procedure areas, and the scope of practice of the transport team members. Carrying large amounts of equipment in a transport box when equipment can be easily obtained from nearby crash carts or supply areas can result in equipment waste. In addition, staff members must regularly check transport equipment and then be able to carry it during the transport phase.

Accidental dislodgement of intravenous lines (IV), drainage catheters (Foley catheters, chest tubes, or wound drains), and airway adjuncts (endotracheal tubes or supraglottic devices) is relatively infrequent, but can have devastating consequences to a patient.[22] In considering patient safety during transport, equipment without clear value during the transport should be removed from the patient. This may include maintenance intravenous fluids, warming/cooling blankets, additional pillows, or compression stocking devices. A patient's physician or advanced practice clinician should be involved in the decision of necessary equipment. The greater the number of items attached to a patient, the greater the risk in dislodging a critical piece of equipment and patient injury.

Using a standardized approach in keeping IV lines separated from a patient's ventilator tubing and monitor cables will reduce the incidence of accidental dislodgements and lessen the readmission time once the patient returns to the critical care unit. Accidental dislodgements and extubations remain a high-volume risk during lateral transfers onto procedural tables; a high level of situational awareness and procedure area familiarity is needed to support patient safety. Knowing where to stage equipment (eg, IV poles, ventilators) in procedure areas to allow for procedural table movement improves patient care and reduces potential adverse events.

Equipment issues that frequently arise during intrahospital transports include transport equipment battery charge and the duration of portable oxygen tanks. Battery charge of critical equipment like IV pumps, portable ventilators, ventricular assist devices, and intra-aortic balloon pumps should be checked pretransport and routinely checked during a transport, and equipment should be plugged in when feasible. Oxygen consumption can be predicted by using the patient's ventilator minute volume or oxygen device liter flow. The value can then be used in an oxygen tank duration calculation. Applications to perform this calculation are readily available for commercial smartphones and from numerous websites. However, it is not uncommon for this estimation to be only as accurate as a point-in-time estimate in ventilated patients; it should not be relied upon during transport because of varying minute volumes.

Planning during the briefing stage of a transport can identify "what if" scenarios and how to locate additional resources or equipment that is not carried or readily available. Planning and thoughtfully positioning equipment on a patient's bed or arranging for equipment to be carried by the transport team will further support a quick transport and improve staff performance during an adverse clinical event.

All staff members involved in an intrahospital transport should be knowledgeable about how transport equipment and beds or stretchers operate. This includes troubleshooting of devices and alarms and common device failures. Each team member should be familiar with the route to a procedure area and any obstacles or "choke points," such as elevators that may delay transport, in the event of equipment battery failure or oxygen device failure.

The final consideration in planning a safe patient transport is the "what if" plan: whom you call and how you call for more resources. This plan should be discussed before each and every transport. Items like a second cell phone should be available in case emergency resources need to be contacted. Contact numbers for emergency resources and attending-level physicians should be on hand, with access familiar to all team members.

## Clinical Applicability Challenges

---

### CASE STUDY

Ms. R., a 55-year-old white woman, was admitted to the medical surgical floor from the emergency department with fever of unknown origin and acute myeloid leukemia. Cultures were drawn and antibiotics were started in the emergency department. The previous nurse reported the patient was resting comfortably at shift change. During rounds immediately after shift change, Ms. R. is found to be unresponsive with a BP of 88/60; HR 150, weak and regular; RR 35; and $SaO_2$ 88%. The primary nurse calls for a RRT. Upon arrival of the RRT, the bedside nurse relays her assessment of Ms. R. to the team leader.

1. What indicated that Ms. R. required a RRT?
2. How would the primary nurse structure his or her report to the RRT team leader?
3. Which clinical changes are most indicative that Ms. R. is at risk for a life-threatening event?
   - Change in mental status
   - Respiratory distress

---

### WANT TO KNOW MORE?

A wide variety of resources to enhance your learning and understanding of this chapter are available on thePoint.

You will find:

- References
- Selected readings
- NCLEX-style review questions
- Internet resources
- And more!

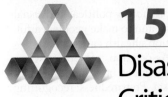

# 15

# Disaster Management: Implications for the Critical Care Nurse

Nancy Blake and Kathleen Stevenson

**LEARNING OBJECTIVES**

*Based on the content in this chapter, the reader should be able to:*

1. Describe the nurse's role in mass casualty incidents.
2. Explain the nurse's role in triage.
3. Describe strategies for surge management.
4. Describe how an explosive attack can occur and how to treat patients who have experienced an explosive attack.
5. Describe how a radiologic attack can occur and how to treat patients who have experienced a radiologic attack.
6. Discuss how a chemical attack can occur and how to treat patients who have experienced a chemical attack.
7. Describe how a biologic attack can occur and how to treat patients who have experienced a biologic attack.

Communities rely on hospitals in times of disaster. After recent disasters and terrorist attacks in the United States exposed weaknesses in emergency planning, lawmakers passed legislation for federal funding for hospital-based disaster preparedness planning and resources. The 1995 Oklahoma City bombing and the 2001 attacks on the World Trade Center and the Pentagon alerted the nation to the major terrorist threats that exist around the world; if hundreds or thousands of survivors suddenly needed emergency treatment, hospitals could easily be overwhelmed. In 2005, the catastrophic hurricane Katrina surprised and shocked many hospital administrators and health care workers, revealing the potential vulnerability of the nation's health care system. The devastating earthquake in Haiti in 2010 and the earthquake and tsunami in Japan in 2011 demonstrated that, in the event of widespread destruction, there may be numerous patients with traumatic injuries needing hospitalization and care in intensive care units (ICUs). The 2013 Boston Marathon bombings demonstrated that one or two are capable of doing great harm despite heightened emergency planning and preparation. More recent active shooter incidents have pushed the emergency providers, including police, firefighters, and hospitals, to care for patients and families with little to no time to prepare.

The Institute of Medicine convened a group of experts in 2009 to develop guidance that health officials could use to establish and implement standards of care in disasters. In 2012, the committee released a report that defined "crisis standards of care" (CSC) as a state of being that is a significant change in health care operations and level of care that is delivered in a public health emergency.[1]

## Fundamentals of Disaster Science

Critical care nurses should participate in their facility's disaster planning process. The critical care nurse's role is crucial in all phases of the disaster planning and response cycle.

When disaster strikes, the job of critical care nurses depends on the impact of the disaster on the facility's structures, its surrounding environment, and the available staffing. For instance, if the hospital's electricity is out and the generators do not work, important equipment in the ICU, such as ventilators and monitors, will not function; in this circumstance, the role of critical care nurses may be to evacuate patients from the ICU. This may also be the case when structures are unstable and resources are scarce. At these critical times, critical care nurses will prioritize evacuation based on available resources and patient condition.

After the initial crisis, resources may be scarce, and vital medications may be unavailable and thus need to be rationed; in this situation, critical care nurses must work closely with physicians and pharmacists to determine alternative methods of care or medications. Under austere conditions, critical care nurses caring for the sickest patients face a daunting task. These nurses need to consider CSC, and work with the health care team when faced with futile care decisions.

During the recovery phases, critical care nurses are a crucial resource in leading and participating in the transitional delivery of care in their facilities. In September 2011, a Pediatric and Emergency Mass Critical Care Task Force published guidelines for triage and treatment, supplies and equipment, neonatal and pediatric regionalized systems, education, community preparedness, legal considerations, family-centered care, ethical issues, and the reality of pediatric and mass critical care in the developing world.[2]

In catastrophic disaster situations, such as Haiti after the earthquake and Japan after the earthquake and tsunami, in which entire communities were devastated, the level of care for the community depends on the equipment, supplies, and facilities on hand. Health care staff may be disaster victims themselves and thus not available to care for patients. Victims of the disaster may present to a hospital that is badly damaged, looking for care despite the devastation the hospital has been subjected to. If all buildings have been destroyed, physicians and nurses must care for patients in alternative care sites, such as tents or shelters. In this situation, the goal becomes providing the highest care possible with limited resources and equipment. Wall oxygen and suction may not be available; portable oxygen tanks become a vital resource. Nurses may need to attach a syringe to a suction catheter to provide manual suction. Portable or disposable handheld short-term ventilators may be all that is available.

One must not forget the psychological and social distress that health care workers experience in major disasters. In cases of severe disruption, psychosocial resources are needed to assist the critical care nurses, because many critically ill patients may die.

As a valued health resource during a disaster response, critical care nurses dictate how and when patients move in the facility for internal evacuation and surge capacity (see Triage, on page 165). Nurses perform best with adequate training, preparation, and practice; therefore, as this chapter discusses, plans must delineate the appropriate deployment of nurses during a disaster and the resources needed for them to be successful.

## Response to Mass Casualty Incidents

By definition, a mass casualty incident (MCI) is characterized by large numbers of patients needing medical treatment that exceeds the capabilities of local emergency and health care personnel. Examples of MCIs include chemical, biologic, radiologic, nuclear, explosive events, and more recently active shooter events. To be integrated into the community's plan for emergency preparedness during an MCI, nurses must have a basic level of skills and education to appropriately respond and protect themselves and others. Critical care nurses may be among the first responders to large MCIs, because public health teams and the emergency medical system (EMS) may be overwhelmed. However, every nurse must have sufficient knowledge and skill to understand the potential for an MCI, identify when such an incident may have occurred, and protect himself or herself while caring for victims.

The trauma and public health system in the United States is continuously improving its ability to respond, at the local, state, and federal level, to MCIs and critically ill patients who have suffered multiple traumas. During an MCI, nurses must perform the primary and secondary surveys as with any other trauma patient. They must know how to recognize their own roles and limitations, as well as where to seek additional information and resources. A group initially known as the International Nursing Coalition for Mass Casualty Education (INCMCE) has developed basic competencies for entry-level registered nurses related to MCIs (Box 15-1). This group is now known as the Nursing Emergency Preparedness Education Coalition.[3] In addition to these guidelines, there are numerous other resources that can be found on the Disaster Information Research Center at http://sis.nlm.nih.gov/dimrc/professionalcompetencies.html.

## Response to Terrorism

Terrorism is the unlawful use of force or violence against persons or property to intimidate civilians or coerce government or a civilian population while promoting political and social objectives.[4] Ultimately, terrorists aim to make people fearful. Terrorism can overwhelm a nation's health care system.

In 2002, the American Association of Critical-Care Nurses (AACN) released a Statement of Commitment to Mass Casualty and Bioterrorism Preparedness recognizing that critical care nurses will be called on to respond to disaster and mass casualty situations. This statement includes the following:

> Bioterrorism and the potential of mass casualties is a significant public health threat facing the United States. The nation's capacity to respond to this threat depends in part on the ability of the health care professionals and public health officials to rapidly and effectively detect, manage, and communicate during an event resulting in mass casualties.[5]

The AACN works closely with the Red Cross to help support critical care nurses during times of disaster.

In August 2003, a report to the Congressional Committee from the US General Accounting Office (GAO) on hospital preparedness for a bioterrorist incident was published. Some of the GAO's findings were alarming. Although most urban hospitals across the country reported that they participated in basic planning and coordination of activities for bioterrorism response, they did not have the medical equipment, especially ventilators, to handle the number of people who would likely require care following a bioterrorist incident. Most hospitals stated that they lacked the necessary resources to handle a large influx of patients.[6] Because many facilities would not be prepared to handle an attack, even fewer would be able to handle a large influx of critically ill patients who needed critical care. The GAO report also recounted many projected scenarios surrounding a possible influenza pandemic, suggesting that the United States would be severely short of ventilators and trained staff to care for patients on ventilators. There has not been a report of this type done to evaluate hospital preparedness nationally in over 10 years.

In 2004, a working group in Pittsburgh, Pennsylvania, made recommendations to hospital and clinical leaders regarding the delivery of critical care services in the wake of a bioterrorist attack resulting in hundreds or thousands of critically ill patients. In these situations, traditional hospital and clinical care standards in general, and critical care standards in particular, likely could no longer be maintained. The study group came up with no clinical guidelines to deal with these situations. However, it did develop the following six planning assumptions regarding the current critical care medicine response for bioterrorism:

1. Future bioterrorist attacks may be covert and could result in hundreds, thousands, or more critically ill victims.
2. Critical care will play a key role in decreasing morbidity and mortality rates after a bioterrorist attack.
3. Mass critical care cannot be provided without substantial planning and new approaches to providing critical care.
4. A hospital has limited ability to divert or transfer patients to other hospitals in the aftermath of a bioterrorist attack.

**BOX 15-1** **Competencies for Entry-Level Registered Nurses Related to Mass Casualty Incidents**

## Core Competencies

### I. Critical Thinking

1. Use an ethical and nationally approved framework to support decision making and prioritizing needed in disaster situations.
2. Use clinical judgment and decision-making skills in assessing the potential for appropriate, timely individual care during a MCI.
3. Use clinical judgment and decision-making skills in assessing the potential for appropriate, individual ongoing care after an MCI.
4. Describe at the predisaster, emergency, and postdisaster phases the essential nursing care for
   a. individuals,
   b. families,
   c. special groups (eg, children, elderly, and pregnant women), and
   d. communities.
5. Describe accepted triage principles specific to MCIs, for example, the START or Simple Triage and Rapid Treatment System.

### II. Assessment

**A. General**

1. Assess the safety issues for self, the response team, and victims in any given response situation in collaboration with the incident response team.
2. Identify possible indicators of a mass exposure (ie, clustering of individuals with the same symptoms).
3. Describe general signs and symptoms of exposure to selected chemical, biologic, radiologic, nuclear, and explosive (CBRNE) agents.
4. Demonstrate the ability to access up-to-date information regarding selected nuclear, biologic, chemical, explosive, and incendiary agents.
5. Describe the essential elements included in an MCI scene assessment.
6. Identify special groups of patients that are uniquely vulnerable during an MCI (eg, very young, aged, and immunosuppressed).

**B. Specific**

1. Conduct a focused health history to assess potential exposure to CBRNE agents.
2. Perform an age-appropriate health assessment including
   a. airway and respiratory assessment;
   b. cardiovascular assessment, including vital signs and monitoring for signs of shock;
   c. integumentary assessment, particularly a wound, burn, and rash assessment, and pain assessment;
   d. injury assessment from head to toe;
   e. gastrointestinal assessment, including stool specimen collection and basic neurologic assessment;
   f. musculoskeletal assessment; and
   g. mental status, spiritual, and emotional assessment.
3. Assess the immediate psychological response of the individual, family, or community following an MCI.
4. Assess the long-term psychological response of the individual, family, or community following an MCI.
5. Identify resources available to address the psychological impact (eg, Critical Incident Stress Debriefing [CISD] teams, counselors, Psychiatric/Mental Health Nurse Practitioners [P/MHNPs]).
6. Describe the psychological impact on responders and health care providers.

### III. Technical Skills

1. Demonstrate the safe administration of medications, particularly vasoactive and analgesic agents, via oral, subcutaneous, intramuscular, and intravenous administration routes.
2. Demonstrate the safe administration of immunizations, including smallpox vaccination.
3. Demonstrate knowledge of appropriate nursing interventions for adverse effects from medications administered.
4. Demonstrate basic therapeutic interventions including
   a. basic first aid skills,
   b. oxygen administration and ventilation techniques,
   c. urinary catheter insertion,
   d. nasogastric tube insertion,
   e. lavage technique (ie, eye and wound), and
   f. initial wound care.
5. Assess the need for and initiate the appropriate CBRNE isolation and decontamination procedures available, ensuring that all parties understand the need.
6. Demonstrate knowledge and skill related to personal protection and safety, including the use of PPE, for
   a. level B protection,
   b. level C protection, and
   c. respiratory protection.
7. Describe how nursing skills may have to be adapted while wearing PPE.
8. Implement fluid and nutrition therapy, taking into account the nature of injuries and/or agents exposed to and monitoring hydration and fluid balance accordingly.
9. Assess and prepare the injured for transport, if required, including provisions for care and monitoring during transport.
10. Demonstrate the ability to maintain patient safety during transport through splinting, immobilization, monitoring, and therapeutic interventions.

### IV. Communication

1. Describe the ICS during an MCI.
2. Identify your role, if possible, within the ICS.
3. Locate and describe the emergency response plan for the place of employment and its role in community, state, and regional plans.
4. Identify one's own role in the emergency response plan for the place of employment.
5. Discuss security and confidentiality during an MCI.
6. Demonstrate appropriate emergency documentation of assessments, interventions, nursing actions, and outcomes during and after an MCI.
7. Identify appropriate resources for referring requests from patients, media, or others for information regarding MCIs.
8. Describe principles of risk communication to groups and individuals affected by exposure during an MCI.
9. Identify reactions to fear, panic, and stress that victims, families, and responders may exhibit during a disaster situation.
10. Describe appropriate coping strategies to manage self and others.

## Core Knowledge

### I. Health Promotion, Risk Reduction, and Disease Prevention

1. Identify possible threats and their potential impact on the general public, EMS, and the health care community.
2. Describe community health issues related to CBRNE events, specifically limiting exposure to selected agents, contamination of water, air, and food supplies, and shelter and protection of displaced persons.

*(continued)*

**BOX 15-1**   **Competencies for Entry-Level Registered Nurses Related to Mass Casualty Incidents** (*continued*)

II. Health Care Systems and Policy
1. Define and distinguish the terms *disaster* and *MCI* in relation to other major incidents or emergency situations.
2. Define relevant terminology, including
   a. CBRNE,
   b. WMD,
   c. triage,
   d. ICS,
   e. personal protective equipment,
   f. scene assessment, and
   g. comprehensive emergency management.
3. Describe the four phases of emergency management: preparedness, response, recovery, and mitigation.
4. Describe the local emergency response system for disasters.
5. Describe the interaction between local, state, and federal emergency response systems.
6. Describe the legal authority of public health agencies to take action to protect the community from threats, including isolation, quarantine, and required reporting and documentation.
7. Discuss principles related to an MCI site as a crime scene (eg, maintaining integrity of evidence and chain of custody).
8. Recognize the impact MCIs may have on access to resources and identify how to access additional resources (eg, pharmaceuticals and medical supplies).

III. Illness and Disease Management
1. Discuss the differences and similarities between an intentional biologic attack and that of a natural disease outbreak.
2. Assess, using an interdisciplinary approach, the short-term and long-term effects of physical and psychological symptoms related to disease and treatment secondary to MCIs.

IV. Information and Health Care Technologies
1. Demonstrate use of emergency communication equipment that you will be required to use in an MCI response.
2. Discuss the principles of containment and decontamination.
3. Describe procedures for decontamination of self, others, and equipment for selected CBRNE agents.

V. Ethics
1. Identify and discuss ethical issues related to CBRNE events:
   a. Rights and responsibilities of health care providers in MCIs, for example, refusing to go to work or report for duty, and refusal of vaccines
   b. Need to protect the public versus an individual's right for autonomy, for example, right to leave the scene after contamination

c. Right of the individual to refuse care, informed consent
   d. Allocation of limited resources
   e. Confidentiality of information related to individuals and national security
   f. Use of public health authority to restrict individual activities, require reporting from health professionals, and collaborate with law enforcement
2. Describe the ethical, legal, psychological, and cultural considerations when dealing with the dying and/or the handling and storage of human remains in an MCI.
3. Identify and discuss legal and regulatory issues related to
   a. abandonment of patients,
   b. response to an MCI and one's position of employment, and
   c. various roles and responsibilities assumed by volunteer efforts.

VI. Human Diversity
1. Discuss the cultural, spiritual, and social issues that may affect an individual's response to an MCI.
2. Discuss the diversity of emotional, psychosocial, and sociocultural responses to terrorism or the threat of terrorism on one's self and others.

Professional Role Development
1. Describe these nursing roles in MCIs:
   a. Researcher
   b. Investigator/epidemiologist
   c. EMT or first responder
   d. Direct care provider, generalist nurse
   e. Direct care provider, advanced practice nurse
   f. Director/coordinator of care in hospital/nurse administrator or emergency department nurse manager
   g. On-site coordinator of care/incident commander
   h. On-site director of care management
   i. Information provider or educator, particularly the role of the generalist nurse
   j. Mental health counselor
   k. Member of planning response team
2. Identify the most appropriate or most likely health care role for oneself during an MCI.
3. Identify the limits to one's own knowledge, skills, abilities, and authority related to MCIs.
4. Describe essential equipment for responding to an MCI, for example, stethoscope, registered nurse license to deter imposters, packaged snack, change of clothing, bottles of water.
5. Recognize the importance of maintaining one's expertise and knowledge in this area of practice and of participating in regular emergency response drills.
6. Participate in regular emergency response drills in the community or place of employment.

From Nursing Emergency Preparedness Education Coalition (formerly International Nursing Coalition for Mass Casualty Education). July 2003. Retrieved from http://www.aacn.nche.edu/leading-initiatives/education-resources/INCMCECompetencies.pdf.

5. Currently deployable medical teams of the federal government have a limited role in increasing a hospital's immediate ability to provide critical care to large numbers of victims of a bioterrorist attack.
6. Hospitals may need to depend on nonfederal sources or reserves of medications and equipment necessary to provide critical care for the first 48 hours following discovery of a bioterrorist attack.[7]

## Role of Hospital Emergency Incident Command System

Hospitals respond to MCIs using the Hospital Incident Command System (HICS). HICS is an incident management system based on the Incident Command System (ICS) that assists hospitals in improving their emergency management planning as well as response and recovery capabilities for unplanned and planned events. HICS is consistent with ICS and the National Incident Management System principles, which allow for multiagency response to events. The Hospital Incident Management Team organizational chart is shown in Figure 15-1. Critical care nurses need to be aware of how they specifically fit into their hospital disaster plan; they may be called on to take on a major role in the HICS organizational system.

## Triage

Triage is a system for rationing resources in response to an overwhelming medical emergency event. Effective triage is one of the first procedures that the critical care nurse uses in responding to a disaster. Patients are quickly categorized into minimal, delayed, immediate, and expectant or deceased categories (Box 15-2). Triage is a fluid process that needs to be monitored throughout the event; patients' condition may change, or resources may become more or less available to care for patients, necessitating a recategorizing of patients.

In addition to triage occurring outside the facility, health care workers should also perform triage inside the facility and ensure that salvageable patients are appropriately categorized. As patients are triaged, personnel should send them to the area where they will receive the appropriate level of care for their triage category. The latter form of triage requires policy, education, and practice for desirable results.

An emerging concept in triage is surge management—a health care system's ability to expand quickly above and beyond normal services to meet an increased demand for medical care in the event of large-scale health emergencies. The goal of surge management is "to maintain operations and increase capacity in order to preserve the life and safety of the patients and ensure appropriate healthcare delivery to the community." Nursing responsibility and patient care ratios will adjust during a disaster event, with surge capacity depending on nurses caring for more patients. Strategies used to manage surge capacity include managing space, staff, and materials. The goal of management of space is to increase the ability to maintain operations or take on additional patients. This may be accomplished through discharge or transfer of patients, use of patient care space that is not currently occupied, or expansion into approved alternate surge areas. The goal of the management of staff is to increase the ability to maintain staffing levels or expand the workforce. This may be accomplished through staff taking on additional patients to care for, use of staff in alternate roles, or enhancing staff through return of staff members who are not currently working. The goal of management of materials is to ensure adequate supplies and equipment. This may be accomplished through delivery of additional items from vendors through prearranged agreements, redistribution of supplies on site, conservation methods, and, in extreme cases, rationing of supplies or materials.

Nurses serve as a focal point for assessing patients for movement and assembling the necessary materials for continuing the care of these patients at the new site. It is important to periodically practice the movement of patients for internal evacuation.

## Terrorist Attacks

Terrorist attacks can take many forms, including explosion/blast, nuclear or radiologic, chemical, and biologic attacks.

## Explosions and Blast Attacks

Explosives and bombs are the weapons of choice for terrorists; ingredients and instructions are readily available to the person determined to cause harm. Victims of an explosive event typically require evaluation by hospital personnel. Since these victims are being received from a crime scene, nurses caring for such patients need to be familiar with preservation of evidence if at all possible. Although some injured victims do not need hospital admission, more severely injured victims will need critical care. After the Boston Marathon bombing, 264 victims sought treatment.

Explosive injuries can result from primary, secondary, or tertiary blast effects. Primary blast injuries are the result of sudden changes in atmospheric pressure caused by an explosion. Examples of primary blast injuries are as follows:

- Ear injuries, such as perforated eardrums
- Pulmonary injuries, including hemorrhagic contusion and hemopneumothorax
- Gastrointestinal hemorrhage, bowel perforation, or bowel rupture.

Secondary blast injury occurs when victims are struck by flying objects and debris. Tertiary blast injuries occur when the victim's body is hurled through the air and strikes other objects.

### Response to Attack

The response to this type of attack is similar to that for any other traumatic injury. Where there are multiple victims, there should be a triage setup and with victims sorted on the basis of their injuries. A thorough evaluation of each victim needs to be done for blast injuries that are not visible but nevertheless life threatening.

## Nuclear or Radiologic Attacks

The medical consequences of a nuclear or radiologic attack or accident depend on the nuclear or radiation source. Radiation accidents or attacks can occur as the result of problems with nuclear reactors, as well as from industrial sources and medical sources. It is important that clinicians understand how a radiologic attack can occur and how to treat patients. A radiologic or nuclear attack can occur in one of five ways:

1. *Simple radiologic device* (SRD): An SRD is a device designed to spread radioactive material without the use of explosives, thereby exposing many people to various levels of radiation. This type of attack could be accomplished by placing a container of radioactive material in a public area or by spreading radioactive materials through the air in a powder or aerosolized form, exposing people who come in contact with it.
2. *Radiologic dispersal device* (RDD): An RDD, or "dirty bomb," is a device formed by combining an explosive agent with radioactive materials. Radioactive materials

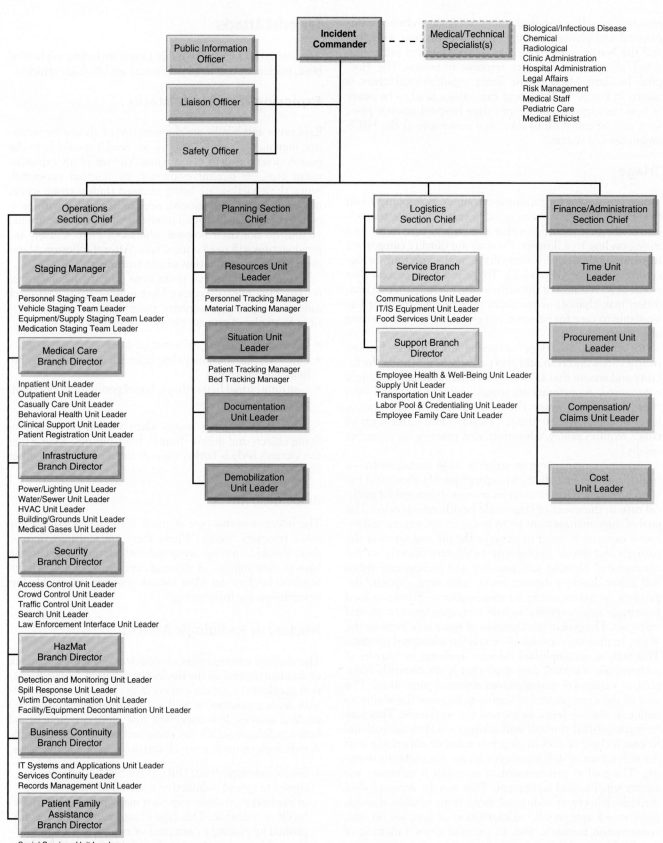

Public Information Officer

Liaison Officer

Safety Officer

Incident Commander

Medical/Technical Specialist(s)

Biological/Infectious Disease
Chemical
Radiological
Clinic Administration
Hospital Administration
Legal Affairs
Risk Management
Medical Staff
Pediatric Care
Medical Ethicist

**Operations Section Chief**

Staging Manager

Personnel Staging Team Leader
Vehicle Staging Team Leader
Equipment/Supply Staging Team Leader
Medication Staging Team Leader

Medical Care Branch Director

Inpatient Unit Leader
Outpatient Unit Leader
Casualy Care Unit Leader
Behavioral Health Unit Leader
Clinical Support Unit Leader
Patient Registration Unit Leader

Infrastructure Branch Director

Power/Lighting Unit Leader
Water/Sewer Unit Leader
HVAC Unit Leader
Building/Grounds Unit Leader
Medical Gases Unit Leader

Security Branch Director

Access Control Unit Leader
Crowd Control Unit Leader
Traffic Control Unit Leader
Search Unit Leader
Law Enforcement Interface Unit Leader

HazMat Branch Director

Detection and Monitoring Unit Leader
Spill Response Unit Leader
Victim Decontamination Unit Leader
Facility/Equipment Decontamination Unit Leader

Business Continuity Branch Director

IT Systems and Applications Unit Leader
Services Continuity Leader
Records Management Unit Leader

Patient Family Assistance Branch Director

Social Services Unit Leader
Family Reunification Unit Leader

**Planning Section Chief**

Resources Unit Leader

Personnel Tracking Manager
Material Tracking Manager

Situation Unit Leader

Patient Tracking Manager
Bed Tracking Manager

Documentation Unit Leader

Demobilization Unit Leader

**Logistics Section Chief**

Service Branch Director

Communications Unit Leader
IT/IS Equipment Unit Leader
Food Services Unit Leader

Support Branch Director

Employee Health & Well-Being Unit Leader
Supply Unit Leader
Transportation Unit Leader
Labor Pool & Credentialing Unit Leader
Employee Family Care Unit Leader

**Finance/Administration Section Chief**

Time Unit Leader

Procurement Unit Leader

Compensation/ Claims Unit Leader

Cost Unit Leader

FIGURE 15-1  Hospital Incident Management Team organizational chart. (From Hospital Incident Command System Guidebook, 5th ed, p 45. Retrieved from http://hicscenter.org/Shared%20Documents/HICS_Guidebook_2014_7.pdf.)

**BOX 15-2** | **START: Triage Categories**

In disaster situations, the Simple Triage and Rapid Treatment (START) system offers a quick and efficient way to prioritize victims' treatment needs based on respiratory, perfusion, and mental status observations. Categories include

- **Minor:** Victims who can get up and walk are determined to be in less need and care may be delayed for up to 3 hours.
- **Delayed:** Victims who are breathing and have adequate circulation, and who can follow simple commands, such as "open your eyes; close your eyes" may be considered for care that can be delayed up to 1 hour.
- **Immediate:** Victims who are unresponsive and cannot follow simple commands.
- **Deceased:** Victims whose breathing, perfusion, and mental status are absent and/or unresponsive to stimuli may be considered deceased, and therefore, not in need of urgent care.

Source: Community Emergency Response Team Unit, LAFD Disaster Preparedness Section. Retrieved from www.cert-la.com.

are common to laboratories, medical centers, and industry, and relatively small amounts of radioactive material can be found to be contained inside common household items. Strict guidelines exist for the handling of these materials, and they are safe when the source is not tampered with. The possibility of obtaining the material through tampering, gathering from multiple sources, or illegal access to disposal collection points exists. The initial explosion of an RDD kills or injures those closest to the bomb, and the radioactive material remains to expose and contaminate survivors and possibly emergency responders.

3. *Nuclear reactor sabotage:* This likelihood of this type of incident is low because of sophisticated shielding, but it could occur with an attack on a nuclear reactor.
4. *Improvised nuclear device* (IND): An IND is any device designed to cause a nuclear detonation. It is not easy to make such a weapon detonate correctly. This type of incident is actually an RDD. Although an IND is unlikely because of the necessary engineering sophistication, a stolen device would generate high levels of radiation.
5. *Nuclear weapon:* This method of exposure could occur if a weapon were stolen. As with nuclear reactor sabotage,

the likelihood of this type of exposure is low, but it could happen.[8]

There are two categories of radiation incidents: (1) *external exposure* is irradiation from a source distant or in close proximity to the body. External irradiation can be subdivided into *whole-body exposure* and *local exposure*. (2) *Contamination* is unwanted radioactive material in or on the body.[8]

### Response to Attack

The response to a nuclear or radiologic exposure is based on the type of incident. Most external exposures result in irradiation of the victim. Once the person is removed from the source of radiation, the irradiation ceases. A person exposed to external radiation does not become radioactive and poses no hazard to people nearby.

Contamination incidents require an entirely different approach to dealing with the victim. Caregivers and support personnel must be careful not to spread the contamination to uncontaminated parts of the victim's body, to themselves, or to the surrounding area. Internal contamination can result from inhalation, ingestion, direct absorption through the skin, or penetration of radioactive materials through open wounds. Serious or significant medical condition treatment should always take precedence over radiologic assessment or patient decontamination.

After radiation exposure, individuals may develop acute radiation syndrome (ARS). Strong, healthy people are often resistant to minimal exposure. The factors that determine whether ARS occurs include exposure to high-dose radiation (minimum 100 cGy) and rate of radiation with whole-body exposure and penetrating-type radiation. There are several stages of radiation exposure, as detailed in Table 15-1.

### Management

Treatment priorities after a radiologic attack are as follows:

1. Treat and stabilize life-threatening injuries. It is essential to stabilize the patient and treat life-threatening injuries first. Once that is done, a health care provider with radiologic health training should perform a radiologic assessment. Use a Geiger counter for radiologic

**TABLE 15-1** | **Phases of Effects of Radiation Exposure**

| Phase | Time of Occurrence | Signs and Symptoms |
|---|---|---|
| Prodromal phase (presenting symptoms) | 48–72 h after exposure | Nausea, vomiting, loss of appetite, diarrhea, fatigue<br>High-dose radiation: fever, respiratory distress, increased excitability |
| Latent phase (a symptom-free period) | After resolution of prodromal phase; can last up to 3 wk<br>With high-dose radiation, latent period is shorter | Decreasing lymphocytes, leukocytes, thrombocytes, red blood cells |
| Illness phase | After latent period phase | Infection, fluid and electrolyte imbalance, bleeding, diarrhea, shock, and altered level of consciousness |
| Recovery phase Or | After illness phase | Can take weeks to months for full recovery |
| Death | After illness phase | Increased intracranial pressure is a sign of impending death |

From Smeltzer SC, Bare BG, Hinkle JL, et al (eds): Brunner & Suddarth's Textbook of Medical-Surgical Nursing, 12th ed. Philadelphia, PA: Lippincott Williams & Wilkins, 2010, p 2007.

From Pediatric Preparedness for Disaster and Terrorism: A Natural Consensus Conference. National Center for Disaster Preparedness Mailman School of Public Health, Columbus University, March 2007.

**TABLE 15-2** Potassium Iodide (KI) Administration

| Patient | KI Dose (mg) |
| --- | --- |
| Adults | 130 |
| Women who are breastfeeding | 130 |
| Children 3–18 y | 65 |
| Infants and children 1 mo to 3 y | 32 |
| Newborns to 1 mo | 16 |

measurements. Nurses will need to be working together with the radiation safety officer to treat the patients' injuries.

2. Prevent and minimize internal contamination. Time is critical to prevent radioactive uptake. Administration of potassium iodide within 2 hours of contamination prevents radioiodine from accumulating in the thyroid gland (Table 15-2). It is important for the nurse to work with the pharmacy to make sure there is an adequate supply of the drugs in the hospital.
3. Assess internal contamination and decontamination. (This information is covered in the section on Chemical Attacks.) Contaminated patients who are not seriously injured should be decontaminated before treatment.
4. Contain contamination and decontamination. Nurses should be trained to the organization's decontamination procedures.
5. Minimize external contamination to medical personnel. Staff should wear personal protective clothing. Respirators are necessary if the patient is highly contaminated.
6. Assess local radiation injuries/burns and flush them if contaminated.
7. Follow up on patients with significant whole-body irradiation or internal contamination.
8. Counsel patient and family about the potential for long-term risks and effects. Nurses should make sure that the appropriate professionals are working together to care for the patients in the future.[9]

## Chemical Attacks

Chemical warfare agents are hazardous chemicals designed to irritate, incapacitate, injure, or kill.[10] Although several of these agents have been used during wartime, many of the most recent uses have been in terrorist attacks. For example, the sarin gas attacks in the Tokyo subway in Japan in 1995 resulted in few deaths but caused an overwhelming influx of contaminated patients to medical facilities. More recently, the United Nations confirmed the use of chemical weapons in the Syrian Civil War in 2013.

Combinations of chemical attacks with explosions and blast attacks are sometimes called "dirty bombs." To have chemical contamination associated with explosions, the victims need to be in close proximity to the explosion or blast attack.

Chemical agents pose a genuine threat for many reasons. First, they are readily accessible; for example, tear gas is sold in stores. Second, they are easy to find and easy to transport without being considered unusual; for example, transporting of pesticides is not out of the ordinary, and transport of many nerve agents occurs on a daily basis by truck or rail. By the time a chemical attack is completed, the terrorist or criminal can be gone.

Toxic chemicals can be absorbed through the eyes, skin, or airways, or a combination of these routes. Table 15-3 and the text below summarize the common types of chemical agents, their mechanisms of action, signs and symptoms of exposure, and treatment for exposure.

### Types of Chemical Agents

**NERVE AGENTS.** Nerve agents are the most toxic of all weaponized military agents. Examples of these agents are tabun, sarin, soman, and VX. Nerve agents inhibit cholinesterase, and they can cause sudden loss of consciousness, seizures, apnea, and death. Diagnosis is usually made on the basis of clinical signs and symptoms.

**TABLE 15-3** Common Chemical Agents and Antidotes

| Agent | Action | Signs and Symptoms | Decontamination and Treatment |
| --- | --- | --- | --- |
| **Nerve agents:** sarin, soman, organophosphates | Inhibition of cholinesterase | Increased secretions, gastrointestinal motility, diarrhea, bronchospasm | Soap and water<br>Supportive care<br>Benzodiazepine<br>Pralidoxime<br>Atropine |
| **Blood agent:** cyanide | Inhibition of aerobic metabolism | Inhalation—tachypnea, tachycardia, coma, seizures; can progress to respiratory arrest, respiratory failure, cardiac arrest, and death | Sodium nitrate<br>Sodium thiocyanate<br>Amyl nitrate<br>Hydroxocobalamin |
| **Vesicant agents:** lewisite, sulfur mustard, nitrogen mustard, phosgene | Blistering agents | Superficial to partial-thickness burn with vesicles that coalesce | Soap and water<br>Blot; do not rub dry |
| **Pulmonary agents:** phosgene, chlorine, ammonia | Separation of alveoli from capillary bed | Pulmonary edema, bronchospasm | Airway management<br>Ventilatory support<br>Bronchoscopy |
| **Skin and eye irritants:** mace (CN), tear gas (CS) | Local reaction to skin and eyes; may cause respiratory difficulties | Tearing of the eyes; burning of the skin; possible respiratory difficulty | Irrigate eyes—water only<br>Soap and water to skin |

From Slota M (ed): Core Curriculum for Pediatric Critical Care Nursing. St. Louis, MO: Elsevier, 2006; and Smeltzer SC, Bare BG, Hinkle JL, et al (eds): Brunner & Suddarth's Textbook of Medical-Surgical Nursing, 12th ed. Philadelphia, PA: Lippincott Williams & Wilkins, 2010, p 2203.

**VESICANTS.** Vesicants cause blistering. The most commonly used vesicants are sulfur mustard and lewisite. These agents injure the eyes, skin, airways, and some internal organs. Vesicants may be commonly used as a mass casualty weapon because they are potent and difficult to detect, have delayed effect, produce prolonged disability, are stable in storage, can be transported easily, and are inexpensive to produce. They remain active in an area for up to 1 week. Some may have an odor of mustard or garlic.

**CYANIDE.** Cyanide is a widely used chemical in the United States. Terrorists use cyanide in confined spaces, such as subway cars, shopping centers, convention centers, and small buildings. Shortly after inhaling cyanide, victims may become anxious and hyperventilate. Inhalation of cyanide can cause convulsions, asystole, and death. Antidotes must be administered immediately.

**PULMONARY INTOXICANTS.** Pulmonary intoxicants cause severe life-threatening lung injury after inhalation. The effects are generally delayed for several hours. Examples are phosgene, perfluoroisobutene, ammonia, and chlorine. In 1984, an industrial accident—not a terrorist attack—involving a pulmonary intoxicant occurred at the Union Carbide plant in Bhopal, India. The released chemicals, including methyl isocyanate, caused great morbidity and death. To this day, this industrial accident remains one of the worst to occur in India.

Pulmonary intoxicants are irritating to the eyes and respiratory tract. These agents can cause severe pulmonary edema of a noncardiac nature. The pathophysiology involves a permeability defect in the alveolar capillary membrane, and there may be a clinical latency period following exposure.

**RIOT CONTROL AGENTS.** Riot control agents, which have an immediate effect, irritate the eyes, nose, mouth, skin, and respiratory tract. They stimulate tear production by the lacrimal glands. The effect lasts about 30 minutes. Examples of these agents, which are routinely used by police, are chloroacetophenone (CN; Mace), oleoresin capsicum (pepper spray), and chlorobenzylidenemalononitrile (CS; tear gas).[10]

### Management

In the event of chemical exposure, decontamination is necessary. Staff need to be trained to decontaminate patients appropriately and should have access to appropriate personal protective equipment (PPE). With most chemical agents, only a splash-resistant gown, much like that used every day in hospitals, and an N95 mask used for respiratory isolation in hospitals are necessary. Some of the more potent chemicals also require a self-contained breathing apparatus and a chemical-resistant suit. People who use these specialty suits and breathing devices should receive training in putting on the suit and have a respiratory evaluation annually.

The Joint Commission requires hospitals to have decontamination protocols and procedures in place. A decontamination shelter can be a room designated at the entrance to the emergency department with appropriate drainage and shower capability, a designated decontamination mobile trailer, or simple capabilities such as a pool or other containment device with hoses. The decontamination shelter should

1. have a water connection with adjustable water temperature
2. have the ability to collect and contain large quantities of water
3. have something to mix with the water to remove the various chemical agents (Most chemical agents respond to soap and water.)
4. have adequate lighting
5. have some connection to electricity, whether through the hospital or a generator
6. have heater capability to maintain comfortable ambient temperature
7. have a conveyor system for nonambulatory patients
8. allow for patient privacy
9. have room for about two or three personnel (These personnel are preferably not health care providers because all clinical staff will be needed to provide medical care.)
10. have sufficient room for families. (It may be necessary to decontaminate parents as well as children. Parents can also help decontaminate their children.)[11]

Decontamination of children involves some special considerations. Because children may not understand what is happening, they may be uncooperative or even combative. Size may be an issue: children are lower to the ground, which means that they may have been exposed to more of the contaminant. Children have a large surface-to-volume ratio, which places them at higher risk for absorption and exposure to the contaminant. In addition, because even a small dose may be lethal in a child, children need to be decontaminated as quickly as possible. Children are also at a higher risk for cold stress from a rapid drop in temperature, or fever from exposure to very warm temperatures; it is necessary to get them into a neutral thermal environment and out of extreme heat or cold. Finally, whenever possible, it helps to keep the family unit together so that the parents can keep the smaller children safe. If the parents are not present, appropriate arrangements must be made for supervision.

## Biologic Attacks

A biologic attack, referred to as bioterrorism, is the deliberate release of microorganisms (bacteria, viruses, fungi, or microbial toxins) into a community to produce death, disease, or poisoning.[10] Humans, animals, and plants may be affected. Many bioterrorist agents are readily accessible. For example, anthrax is naturally occurring and can be found on some farms, and terrorists can pick it up and haul it away without being noticed. Because they are relatively inexpensive to produce and disseminate, biologic weapons are often called the "poor man's bomb." A bioterrorist attack is a real threat, as evidenced by the anthrax attacks of 2001 in the United States: letters with anthrax spores arrived by post at some media and legislative offices, closing down many post offices and federal buildings for long periods. The attacks resulted in 22 cases of anthrax, 5 deaths, and a nation on high alert.

Smallpox, a viral disease, is a strong bioterrorism threat because it has a high morbidity in an otherwise healthy population. Figure 15-2 shows the smallpox rash. In 1980, the World Health Organization (WHO) declared smallpox eradicated.[10] However, samples of the virus are still available in laboratories for research. These samples could be deadly if

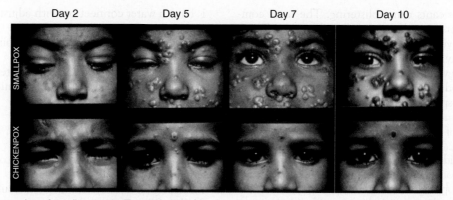

Day 2          Day 5          Day 7          Day 10

**FIGURE 15-2** Progression of smallpox rash. (From World Health Organization: WHO slide set on the diagnosis of smallpox. 2001. Reproduced by permission of the World Health Organization.)

they fell into the wrong hands and used in an attack. In 2003, a smallpox vaccine became available for health care workers, but the US Food and Drug Administration recalled it, and few people received the vaccine because of issues related to the exclusion criteria and the occurrence of some cardiac problems after administration of the vaccine.

The plague has a negative historical connotation because people still remember references to biblical plagues and the "Black Death," a deadly pandemic caused by bubonic plague in the 14th century. Animals such as squirrels and other rodents that live on farmland and in city parks and campgrounds still carry the bacteria that cause plague. Humans bitten by infected animals can become ill.

Botulism still occurs today in developed countries. A person can contract the disease from eating food that has been infected with the botulism toxin. Treatment is available. Children who develop infantile botulism can take an antidote, commonly known as "Baby Big"—botulism immune globulin intravenous (human)—if the disease is diagnosed early and verified by a laboratory approved by the Centers for Disease Control and Prevention (CDC). At the time of diagnosis, the local health department provides the hospital the necessary dosage. The main issue is that the botulism is not always diagnosed promptly enough.

One of the more common viral hemorrhagic fevers is caused by the Ebola virus, which is found more commonly in Third World countries. The virus is spread through direct contact with a sick person's blood or body fluid, objects contaminated with infected body fluids, and infected animals. In 2014, a deadly natural outbreak of Ebola occurred in West Africa, killing over 11,000 people. This outbreak garnered worldwide attention when, for the first time in history, cases were cared for on US soil. This recent Ebola outbreak validated the importance of careful attention to infection control standards and use of PPE by health care workers to prevent contracting or spread of the disease. Ebola treatment guidelines are constantly being updated; the most recent guidelines can be found on the CDC website (http://www.cdc.gov/). Critical care nurses should know where to find these guidelines, and hospitals that have been identified as treatment centers or assessment centers should be practicing the response procedures.

### Management

Biologic agents result in specific signs and symptoms, and every nurse should know the basics of caring for affected patients. In 1999, the Association of Professionals in Infection Control developed a template, the *Bioterrorism Readiness Plan: A Template for Healthcare Facilities*, for hospitals to follow when dealing with bioterrorism.[11] In 2002, this group made some minor modifications to this plan.

## Natural Disasters

A natural disaster is a result of the combination of a natural event (eg, earthquake, extreme heat, flood, hurricane, landslide, tornado, tsunami, volcanic eruption, wildfire, winter storm) and human involvement. By definition, a natural disaster does not occur without human involvement; therefore, an earthquake that destroys an uninhabited island is technically not a natural disaster. In a natural disaster, an unprepared or ill-prepared population is vulnerable; therefore, a lack of preparation amplifies the unfortunate outcomes.

Hospitals and other health care facilities play a unique role in the community during a natural disaster. These facilities already contain an unhealthy, weak population, and yet are expected to receive casualties resulting from disasters. Therefore, hospital personnel and administrators must actively prepare for any event that threatens the structure, function, and recovery of their organization, and practice the appropriate responses to a hazardous event.

Some experts consider pandemic influenza a potential natural disaster. Currently, the health care and corporate industries are working together to address the problem, and new vaccines and antiviral agents have been developed. Nurses are critical to the disaster response because they have direct patient care roles and will be present if an unforeseen event arises.

The H1N1 influenza virus (swine flu) outbreak in 2009 increased the census in hospitals and ICUs across the country. Cases spread quickly, especially in the younger population (25 years and younger).[12] The most common symptoms were fever, cough, and sore throat. A small percentage of patients required hospitalization, and many patients who ended up in the critical care units were put on extracorporeal membrane oxygenation, as pulmonary bypass, to treat respiratory failure. A small percentage of the patients treated in the critical care units died. Within 3 months of the first identified H1N1 case, the WHO raised the H1N1 outbreak to a level of pandemic because there were community-level outbreaks in at least one country other than where it was first identified. The H1N1 outbreak mobilized hospitals and government agencies to identify the issues and plan strategies to protect the public in this global emergency. Excellent resources are available for H1N1 and are noted on the CDC and the WHO websites. The Association of Infection Control Practitioners (APIC) also developed a reference document for infection prevention in alternate care sites; it can be found on their website, www.apic.org.

## Psychological Effects of Terrorism and Natural Disasters

It is natural to be fearful during and after a major disaster, whether or not it is a terrorist incident. People exhibit various responses to stress and stressful events such as a terrorist attack or a major natural disaster. The responses include fear, grief, and deep sadness. People may complain that they feel "sick to their stomach" and have no appetite. Their sleep patterns and conduct in daily activities may change. Several weeks to months may pass before they feel normal and stable again. In severe cases, the psychological stress remains months after the event.

Multiple factors affect how people respond to a major disaster. The perception of numerous losses generally has a negative impact and may be related inversely to disaster recovery. Research has found that when there are large numbers of deaths and high levels of symptoms, the presence of long-term psychiatric disorders may be quite high.[13] People affected by a major disaster should undergo screening for post-traumatic stress disorder (PTSD). PTSD is an intense emotional and physical response to thoughts and reminders of the event, which lasts for many weeks or months after the traumatic event. Victims of PTSD may complain of nightmares, flashbacks, and severe emotional and physical reactions to thoughts of the event. Los Angeles County has adopted a triage model of PsySTART information and resiliency plan to triage those who need further psychiatric or mental health care.[14]

In addition to assessing disaster victims for PTSD, nurses should assess whether their peers are able to function in times of high stress. Major disasters may overwhelm health care workers, rendering them unable to care for others. If a coworker is exhibiting symptoms of stress, a nurse should inform his or her supervisor so that further assessments can be made as to whether the coworker is fit for duty.

## Clinical Applicability Challenges

---

**CASE STUDY**

An earthquake of magnitude 9.0 has hit a remote town in Northern California. Buildings have been destroyed, and police and fire resources are searching for victims. Numerous casualties have been identified, and ambulances are beginning to deliver patients with crushing injuries to the hospital. Because of the remote location and the fact that the roads have been destroyed, patients cannot be transferred to other hospitals at this point in time. The hospital is initiating the hospital disaster procedures and preparing to receive disaster victims.

1. What are the first priorities for the critical care nurses?
2. The critical care nurses are expecting to receive 10 critically ill victims; there is no other transport facility available at this time. What are the next steps for the critical care nurses?
3. The power is cutting in and out, and the generator is not working consistently. What should the critical care nurses do if the power is not working?

---

**WANT TO KNOW MORE?**

A wide variety of resources to enhance your learning and understanding of this chapter are available on thePoint.

You will find:

- References
- Selected readings
- NCLEX-style review questions
- Internet resources
- And more!

# PART 5

# Cardiovascular System

# 16

# Anatomy and Physiology of the Cardiovascular System

PATRICIA GONCE MORTON

## LEARNING OBJECTIVES

*Based on the content in this chapter, the reader should be able to:*

1. Briefly describe the characteristics of cardiac muscle cells.
2. Differentiate the electrical events from the mechanical events in the heart.
3. Explain depolarization and repolarization.
4. Describe the normal conduction system of the heart.
5. Explain the formula for calculating cardiac output.
6. Compare and contrast the role of the parasympathetic and sympathetic nervous systems in the regulation of heart rate.
7. Explain the three factors involved in the regulation of stroke volume.
8. Describe the coronary artery blood source for the cardiac chambers and conduction system.
9. Discuss the influence of blood volume and blood pressure on peripheral circulation.

During the 70 years in the life of the average person, the heart will pump approximately 70 times per minute, 24 hours a day, and 365 days a year. The heart pumps about 5 quarts of blood a minute, 75 gallons an hour, and 1,800 gallons in a day.[1] Although the work accomplished by this organ is out of proportion to its size, for most people, the heart functions normally throughout the life span. The pumping action of the heart moves blood, a vital substance, throughout the body, supplying oxygen and nutrients to cells, and removing waste. Without this action, cells die. For people in whom cardiac problems develop, the results may be dramatic and the outcome drastic. This chapter reviews the principles of cardiovascular anatomy and physiology.

## Cardiac Microstructure

Microscopically, cardiac muscle contains visible stripes, or striations, similar to those found in skeletal muscle (Fig. 16-1). The ultrastructural pattern also resembles that of striated muscle. The cells branch and connect freely and form a three-dimensional, complex network. The elongated nuclei, like those of smooth muscle, are found deep in the interior of the cells and not next to the cell membrane as they are in striated muscle.

Cardiac muscle (myocardial) cells are endowed with extraordinary characteristics, most of which belong to the cell membrane or sarcolemma. To pump effectively, the heart muscle must begin contraction as a single unit. To contract myocardial cells simultaneously, cell membranes must depolarize at the same time. The heart does this, without using much neural tissue, by rapidly conducting impulses from cell to cell through intercalated disks. At each end of every myocardial cell, adjacent cell membranes are folded elaborately and attached strongly. These areas comprise the intercalated disks, where depolarization is conducted extremely rapidly from one cell to the next (see Fig. 16-1).

Another extraordinary characteristic of myocardial cells, seen mainly in cell membranes, is automaticity. Selected groups of cardiac cells are capable of initiating rhythmic action potentials, and thus waves of contraction, without any outside humoral or nervous intervention. Automaticity and other terms used to describe cardiac tissue functions are listed in Box 16-1.

Within each cardiac cell lie thousands of contractile elements, the overlapping actin and myosin filaments. Many cross-bridges extend like rows of oars from the surface of the thicker myosin filaments. During diastole, these bridges are unattached to other filaments. The arrangement of actin and myosin filaments gives cardiac muscle its banded or striated

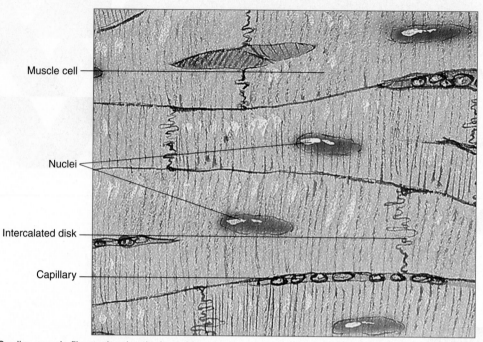

**FIGURE 16-1** Cardiac muscle fibers, showing the branching structure and intercalated disks. (From Anatomical Chart Company: Atlas of Human Anatomy. Springhouse, PA: Springhouse, 2001, p 167.)

---

**BOX 16-1** | Terms Used to Describe Cardiac Tissue Function

**Automaticity:** The ability of specialized cells in the heart known as pacemaker cells to spontaneously generate an action potential, thus causing depolarization

**Conductivity:** The ability of cardiac cells to conduct action potentials, thus transmitting the electrical signal from one cell to another

**Contractility:** The ability of cardiac muscle to shorten in response to depolarization

**Excitability:** The ability of cardiac tissue to respond to a stimulus and generate an action potential

**Rhythmicity:** The ability of cardiac cells to spontaneously generate an action potential at a regular rate

---

appearance. One grouping of actin and myosin filaments is called a *sarcomere*.

## Mechanical Events of Contraction

When an action potential causes depolarization of the sarcoplasmic reticulum, calcium ions move from the sarcoplasmic reticulum into the myocardial cell cytoplasm and bind to troponin molecules on actin filaments. Rapid, successive uncoupling of cross-bridges and their reattachment to new actin-binding sites lead to rapid and dramatic shortening of the sarcomere. This shortening is the essence of myocardial contraction (systole). Contraction ceases when the calcium ions return to their storage sites on the sarcoplasmic reticulum, thereby causing the binding sites on the actin filaments to be covered again.

Contraction requires calcium and energy. The presence of adequate ATP stores and the movement of calcium provide the essential link between the electrical events of depolarization and the mechanical events of contraction in the heart.

## Electrical Events of Depolarization

Membranes of all the cells in the human body are charged, that is, they are polarized and therefore have electrical potentials. The charges are separated at the membrane. In humans, all cell membranes, regardless of type, are positively charged at rest, with more positively charged particles at the outer surface of the cell membrane than at the inner surface. Figure 16-2A illustrates this "resting stage."

In the depolarized state, the cell membrane is negatively charged, with more negatively charged particles at the outer surface of the cell membrane than at the inner surface. Figure 16-2B illustrates this "depolarized stage." *Excitability* is the term used to describe the ability of a cell to depolarize in response to a given stimulus.

Cardiac muscle membranes are polarized, and the electrical potential can be measured, as it can in any of the cells in the human body. The potential results from the difference between intracellular and extracellular concentrations of electrolytes.

In the resting myocardial cell, there are more potassium ions inside than outside the cell and more sodium and unbound calcium ions outside than inside the cell. All three of these cations (positively charged ions) may diffuse through pores, or channels, in the cell membrane. If each ion freely obeyed the law of diffusion, however, potassium would diffuse out of the cell, whereas sodium and calcium would diffuse into it. Very soon there would be equal concentrations of each ion between the intracellular and extracellular fluids, and no resting potential would exist. It is through selective regulation of the concentrations of these ions on either side of the membrane that the resting membrane potential is maintained. Several factors contribute to this regulation. The first factor is the presence of sodium–potassium "pumps" in the cell membrane. These pumps move sodium out of the

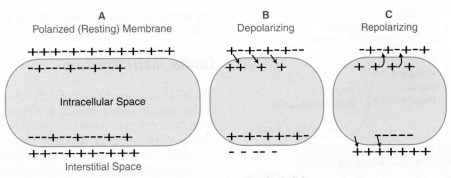

**FIGURE 16-2** Electrical events at rest (diastolic) and preceding contraction (systolic).

cell and potassium into the cell, with both movements occurring against the concentration gradients for each of these ions. The second factor is the active movement of calcium out of the cell against the concentration gradient in response to the passive diffusion of sodium into the cell. The third factor is the regulation of membrane channels, whereby calcium ions can enter the resting myocardial cell. The fourth factor is the presence of intracellular anions (negatively charged particles) that are too large to exit from the cell.

## Physiologic Basis of the Resting Potential

The cardiac cell contains large anions that cannot exit the cell. These anions attract sodium and potassium cations, which diffuse through membrane channels into the cell. The anions would attract the calcium cation also, except that the membrane channels for the entry of this ion are closed when the cell is at rest. The potassium ions remain within the cell, but the sodium ions are pumped out of the cell almost as fast as they can enter by the sodium–potassium pumps located in the cell membrane. While forcing sodium out of the cell, these pumps actively transport potassium ions into the cell against their concentration gradients. This increase in intracellular potassium still is insufficient to offset all the intracellular anions. Thus, the inside of the myocardial cell remains negative with respect to the outside—as long as the pumps are operative. As a result, the resting potential is approximately –80 mV. For each molecule of an ion pumped from the cell, one molecule of ATP is required to provide the energy necessary to effect the chemical bond between ion and carrier. Maintaining a resting potential thus requires energy. Factors that maintain resting membrane potential of myocardial cells are listed in Box 16-2.

## Physiologic Basis of the Action Potential

When a stimulus is applied to the polarized cell membrane, the membrane that ordinarily is only slightly permeable to sodium permits sodium ions to diffuse rapidly into the cell. This rapid diffusion occurs because of inactivation of the sodium active transport enzymes (pumps). The result is a reversal of net charges. The outer surface is now more negative than positive, and the membrane is said to be depolarized (see Fig. 16-2B).

When the sodium influx changes the polarity from –80 mV to approximately –35 mV, the electrical change opens the previously closed "calcium channels" in the myocardial cell membrane. Once open, these channels permit the influx of calcium. The entry of this cation, together with the continued entry of sodium, is responsible for the remainder of the depolarization, which continues until the polarity of the extracellular side equals approximately +30 mV. Such a maximal depolarization inactivates sodium–potassium pumps in nearby membranes. This can cause depolarization in these areas. When the original depolarization becomes self-propagating in this way, it is termed an *action potential*. In a myocardial cell, an action potential triggers the release of intracellular calcium from its storage sites on the sarcoplasmic reticulum. This release plus the calcium influx across the sarcolemma elevates intracellular calcium levels, thereby initiating muscular contraction, as previously described.[1]

If the depolarization remains below a certain critical (threshold) point, it dies out without having opened any calcium channel or inactivated any adjacent sodium–potassium pumps. Because it does not become self-propagating and remains localized, such a depolarization is termed a *local depolarization*.

During depolarization, the elevated intracellular sodium concentration frees potassium ions to diffuse out of the cell in accordance with their concentration gradient. Just as this potassium efflux gains some momentum, however, the sodium–potassium pumps automatically reactivate (they can be inactivated only temporarily). Once reactivated, the pumps begin to restore the original resting potential, a process termed *repolarization* (see Fig. 16-2C). During the initial phase of repolarization, the efflux of potassium and sodium ions exceeds their influx, but as the intracellular sodium ions are removed from the cell, potassium ions remain as the major cation to be electrostatically held within the cell by the intracellular anions. This halts the potassium efflux. The remainder of repolarization consists of pump activity that increases intracellular potassium and decreases intracellular

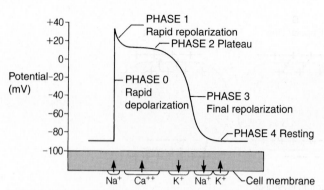

FIGURE 16-3  Cardiac action potential. Phase 0 is the rapid depolarization phase. During this phase, the fast sodium channels in the cell membranes are stimulated to open, resulting in the rapid influx of sodium. Contraction of the myocardium follows depolarization. Phase 1 is the rapid repolarization phase and occurs at the peak of the action potential. This phase indicates the inactivation of the fast sodium channels with an abrupt decrease in sodium permeability. Phase 2 represents the plateau of the action potential. During this phase, potassium permeability is low, allowing the membrane to remain depolarized throughout phase 2. The influx of calcium that occurs during the plateau phase is much slower than that of sodium and lasts for a longer time. Phase 3 is the final repolarization phase and begins with the downslope of the action potential curve. During this phase, the influx of calcium and sodium ends, and there is a rapid outward movement of potassium. By the end of phase 3, sodium and potassium return to their normal resting state. Phase 4 is the resting membrane potential and corresponds to diastole. During this phase, the sodium–potassium pump is activated, resulting in the active transport of sodium out of the cell, and potassium is moved back into the cell. The *arrows* below the diagram indicate the approximate time and direction of movement of each ion influencing membrane potential. The phase of calcium moving out of the cell is not well defined but is thought to occur during phase 4.

sodium; thus, the resting potential is reestablished. The electrical events at the start of repolarization also reclose the calcium entry channels, thereby halting calcium influx. Intracellular calcium levels are reduced when the diffusion of sodium into the cell causes a movement of calcium out of the cell against the latter's concentration gradient.[1] The phases of the action potential are shown in Figure 16-3.

## Cardiac Macrostructure

The heart is about the size of a clenched fist. The right side of the heart is almost entirely in front of the left side of the heart, and the right ventricle occupies most of the anterior cardiac surface (Fig. 16-4). Only a small portion of the left ventricle is in the frontal plane of the heart. The left ventricle forms the left lateral margin of the heart with a tapered inferior tip that is often termed the *cardiac apex*.[2]

The heart is made up of four layers: the endocardium, the myocardium, the epicardium, and the pericardium. The inner layer, known as the *endocardium*, consists of endothelial tissue that lines the inner surface of the heart and the cardiac valves. The middle layer, known as the *myocardium*, is composed of muscle fibers that enable the heart to pump. The outer layer, known as the *epicardium*, is tightly adherent to the heart and the base of the great vessels. A thin, fibrous, double-layered sac, known as the *pericardium*, surrounds the heart. This structure has two parts: an outer layer called the *parietal pericardium* and the inner layer called the *visceral pericardium*. Between these two layers is a small amount of pericardial fluid (30 to 50 mL) that serves as a lubricant between the two layers.[1]

The heart consists of four chambers: right and left atria, and right and left ventricles. The atria are smaller, thinner-walled, low-pressure chambers. Approximately 30% of blood flow to the ventricles is the result of atrial contraction, also known as *atrial kick*. The remaining 70% of blood that reaches the ventricles is the result of pressure differences between the atria and the ventricles. The ventricles are larger, higher-pressure chambers with thicker walls than the atria. The walls of the left ventricle are thicker than the right ventricle because the left ventricle must generate a large amount of force to eject blood into the aorta. Deoxygenated

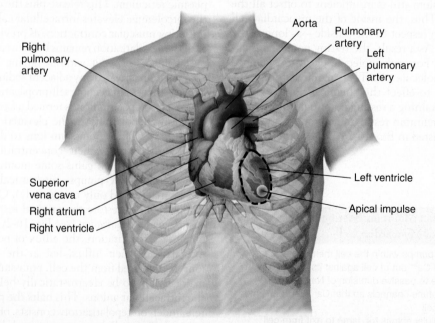

FIGURE 16-4  Structure of the heart. (From Bickley LS: Guide to Physical Examination and History Taking, 10th ed. Philadelphia, PA: Lippincott Williams & Wilkins, 2009, p 324.)

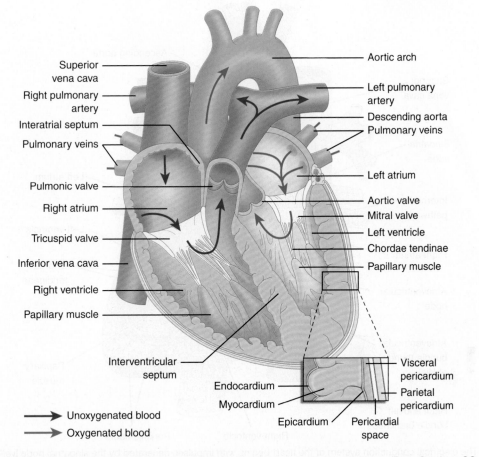

**FIGURE 16-5** Structure of the heart. *Arrows* show course of blood flow through the heart chambers. (From Smeltzer SC, Bare BG, Hinkle JL, et al: Textbook of Medical–Surgical Nursing, 13th ed. Philadelphia, PA: Lippincott Williams & Wilkins, 2014, p 656.)

blood enters the right atrium from the superior and inferior venae cavae. The blood passes through the tricuspid valve into the right ventricle, which then pumps the blood through the pulmonic valve into the pulmonary circulation. After gas exchange in the lungs, oxygenated blood returns to the left atrium, passes through the mitral valve, enters the left ventricle, passes through the aortic valve, and finally enters the aorta (Fig. 16-5).

The cardiac valves are composed of fibrous tissue and allow blood to flow in one direction. The valves open and close as a result of blood flow and pressure differences. The tricuspid and mitral valves are known as the *atrioventricular (AV) valves* because they are located between the atria and the ventricles. The chordae tendineae and the papillary muscles attach to the AV valves and help maintain closure and prevent eversion of the valve leaflets during ventricular contraction so that blood does not move into the atria. The pulmonic and aortic valves are known as the *semilunar valves* because each has three leaflets shaped like half-moons.

## Cardiac Conduction

To pump effectively, large portions of cardiac muscle must receive an action potential nearly simultaneously. Special cells that conduct action potentials extremely rapidly are arranged in pathways through the heart. All these cells have automaticity (see Box 16-2).

The heart chambers and specialized tissues are diagrammed in Figure 16-6. The sinoatrial (SA) node is located between the opening of the inferior and superior venae cavae in the right atrial wall. The cells of the SA node have the property of automaticity. Because the SA node normally discharges faster than any other heart cell with automaticity (60 to 100 beats/min), this specialized tissue acts as a normal cardiac pacemaker. Atrial action potentials travel through atrial cells by intercalated disks, although some specialized conductive tissue in the atria has been discovered.

In the lower right portion of the interatrial septum is the AV node, also known as the AV junction. This tissue conducts, yet delays, the atrial action potential before it travels to the ventricles. Action potentials reach the AV node at different times. The AV node slows conduction of these action potentials until all potentials have exited the atria and entered the AV node. After this slight delay, the AV node passes the action potential all at once to the ventricular conduction tissue, allowing for nearly simultaneous contraction of all ventricular cells. This AV node delay also allows time for the atria to eject fully their load of blood into the ventricles in preparation for ventricular systole.

From the AV node, the impulse travels down the bundle of His in the interventricular septum into either a right or left bundle branch and then through one of many Purkinje fibers to the ventricular myocardial tissue itself. An action potential can traverse this conducting tissue three to seven

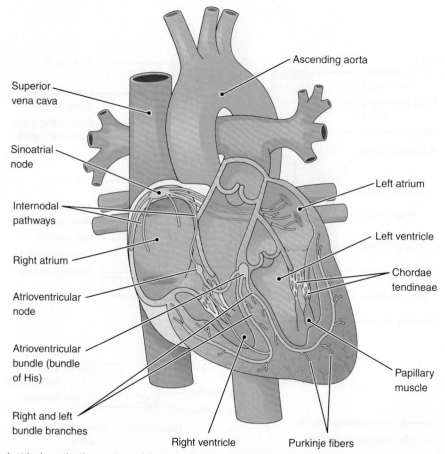

FIGURE 16-6   The electrical conduction system of the heart begins with impulses generated by the sinoatrial node (*yellow*) and circuited continuously over the heart. (From Weber J, Kelley K: Health Assessment in Nursing, 5th ed. Philadelphia, PA: Lippincott Williams & Wilkins, 2014, p 418.)

times more rapidly than it can travel through the ventricular myocardium. Thus, the bundle branches and Purkinje fibers enable a near-simultaneous contraction of all portions of the ventricle, thereby allowing a maximal unified pump action to occur.[1]

## Electrocardiograms

Conduction of an action potential through the heart can be shown by an electrocardiogram (ECG; Fig. 16-7). Because ECGs are extensively covered in Chapter 17, discussion here is brief. An ECG does not show mechanical events of the heart, but in the normal heart, coupling of electrical and mechanical events can be assumed (see Chapter 17).

In Figure 16-7, point 1 shows early ventricular diastole, when the atria and ventricles are at rest. Blood from the large veins is passively filling both atria. As the atria fill, the pressure in the atria exceeds the pressure in the ventricles, and the AV valves open in response to the pressure gradient. The blood from the atria now passively fills the ventricles.

At point 2, the beginning of late ventricular diastole, both ventricles remain relaxed and are about three-fourths full. The SA node fires spontaneously (due to automaticity), and both atria depolarize, generating a P wave. The atria contract, and blood is actively moved from the atria into the ventricles: this "atrial kick" supplies approximately 20% to 30% of the ventricular blood volume.

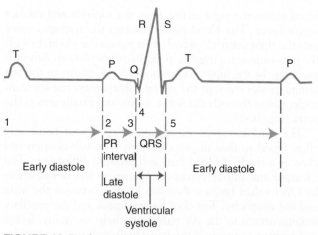

FIGURE 16-7   Comparison of electrical and mechanical events during one cardiac cycle, using a normal electrocardiogram tracing.

At point 3, late in the PR interval, the action potential begun in the SA node is being delayed and "collected" in the AV node and travels to the bundle of His. The atria and ventricles are at rest.

At point 4, the action potential moves to the septum, which depolarizes and leads to the Q wave. Septal depolarization is rapidly followed by action potential movement down the right and left bundles into the Purkinje fibers to all cardiac muscle cells. These electrical events are seen as the RS wave on the ECG and are followed rapidly by mechanical contraction of both ventricles. The AV valves close, and the aortic and pulmonic valves open.

At point 5, the heart returns to early ventricular diastole, and the ventricles repolarize. This repolarization shows as a large, wide T wave. The aortic and pulmonic valves close about midway through repolarization.[1]

## Rhythmicity and Pacing

Automaticity is an inherent property of myocardial conduction cells and occurs as a result of a spontaneous and rhythmic inactivation of the sodium pumps. Under abnormal conditions, cardiac muscle cells also gain automaticity and can produce their own rhythmic series of action potentials and thus their own stimulus for contraction. Coordination of automaticity is important for rhythmic cardiac contraction and is achieved through the varying rates of automaticity found in different cardiac tissues.

The SA node discharges normally in an adult at a resting rate of 60 to 100 times per minute. The remainder of the conduction system and ventricles has progressively slower rates of firing. The AV node discharges at a rate of 40 to 60 times per minute. The conduction tissues in the ventricles fire about 20 to 40 times per minute. The group of cells with the fastest rate of automaticity paces the heart. Normally, this is the SA node.

If the SA node should fail to fire, a pacemaker site lower in the heart should take control because of the automaticity of cardiac tissue. This new pacemaker site is usually the AV node; however, the heart rate (HR) will most likely be slower. If conduction from the SA node is blocked (unable to pass through the AV node), the fastest pacemaker tissue on both sides of this interruption will govern their respective areas, and the ECG may show independent atrial and ventricular rhythms. Atrial systole is not needed for the ventricle to fill with blood because most ventricular filling is passive and occurs in early diastole. The clinically important rhythm is that of the ventricles; they are the chambers that supply the lungs and the rest of the body with blood. Their systolic rate helps determine true perfusion. The slower the rate, the less able are the ventricles to meet the perfusion needs of the body during exercise or activities of daily living. A very rapid ventricular rhythm also compromises perfusion needs because the shorter the diastole, the less time for filling of the chambers. Decreased ventricular filling reduces cardiac output (CO).

## Cardiac Output

A traditional measure of cardiac function, CO is the amount of blood, in liters, ejected from the left ventricle each minute. CO is the product of HR and stroke volume (SV), which is the volume of blood ejected per ventricular contraction:

$$CO = HR \text{ (beats / min)} \times SV \text{ (L/beat)}$$

Normal CO for an adult ranges from 4 to 8 L/min. The output can be altered to meet changing bodily demands for tissue perfusion, but the CO equation does not account for differences in body size. An output of 5 L/min may be adequate for a 50-kg man but insufficient for a 120-kg man. Because perfusion is a function of body size, a more accurate measure

of cardiac function is cardiac index (CI), which represents the amount of blood, in liters, ejected each minute from the left ventricle (or CO) per square meter of body surface area. CI typically averages $3.0 \pm 0.2$ L/min and ranges from 2.8 to 4.2 L/min/m²:

$$CI = CO \text{ (L/min) / body surface area (m}^2)$$

## Regulation of Heart Rate

Although the heart has the ability to beat independently of any extrinsic influence, cardiac rate is under autonomic and adrenal catecholamine influence. Parasympathetic and sympathetic fibers innervate the SA and AV nodes. In addition, some sympathetic fibers terminate in myocardial tissues.

Parasympathetic stimulation releases acetylcholine near the nodal cells and decreases the rate of depolarization, thereby slowing cardiac rate. Sympathetic stimulation increases HR (Table 16-1). The adrenal medulla also releases norepinephrine and epinephrine into the bloodstream. These circulating catecholamines act on the heart in the same way as sympathetic stimulation.

Two reflexes adjust HR to blood pressure: the aortic reflex and the Bainbridge reflex. In the aortic reflex (Fig. 16-8A), a rise in arterial blood pressure stimulates aortic and carotid sinus baroreceptors to fire sensory impulses to the cardioregulatory center in the medulla. The result is an increase in parasympathetic stimulation or a decrease in sympathetic stimulation to the heart. Thus, a rise in arterial blood pressure reflexively causes a slowing of cardiac rate. The decrease in HR results in a decrease in output, which can decrease arterial blood pressure. Conversely, a fall in arterial blood pressure, such as in shock, reflexively increases HR. This aortic reflex is an ongoing regulatory mechanism for homeostasis of arterial blood pressure.

The Bainbridge reflex (see Fig. 16-8B) uses receptors in the venae cavae. An increase in venous return stimulates these receptors, which then fire sensory impulses that travel to the cardioregulatory center. These reflexively cause a decrease in parasympathetic cardiac stimulation and an increase in sympathetic cardiac stimulation, thereby increasing cardiac rate. A fall in venous return causes a decrease in HR. Thus, the Bainbridge reflex adjusts cardiac rate to handle venous return.

## Regulation of Stroke Volume

Stroke volume is the amount of blood ejected by the left ventricle during systole. Normal values range from 60 to 100 mL/beat. Three factors are involved: preload, afterload (or wall tension), and inherent inotropic myocardial contractility.

### Preload

Preload is the amount of stretch placed on a cardiac muscle fiber just before systole. Usually, the amount of stretch in any chamber is proportional to the volume of blood the chamber contains at the end of diastole, before systole. However, in some situations, the chamber can hold a large amount of volume with little change in pressure.

The concept of preload is related to the Frank–Starling law of the heart, which states that the force of myocardial contraction is determined by the length of the muscle cell

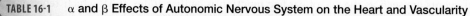

**TABLE 16-1**    α and β Effects of Autonomic Nervous System on the Heart and Vascularity

| Effector Organ | Cholinergic Impulses Response | Noradrenergic Impulses Receptor Type | Noradrenergic Impulses Response |
|---|---|---|---|
| **Heart** | | | |
| Sinoatrial (SA) node | Decrease in HR; vagal arrest | β₁ | Increase in HR |
| Atria | Decrease in contractility and (usually) increase in conduction velocity | β₁ | Increase in contractility and conduction velocity |
| Atrioventricular (AV) node and conduction system | Decrease in conduction velocity; AV block | β₁ | Increase in conduction velocity |
| Ventricles | — | β₁ | Increase in contractility and conduction velocity |
| **Arterioles** | | | |
| Coronary, skeletal muscle, pulmonary, abdominal viscera, renal | Dilation | α β₂ | Constriction Dilation |
| Skin and mucosa, cerebral, salivary glands | — | α | Constriction |
| **Systemic Veins** | | | |
| | — | α β₂ | Constriction Dilation |

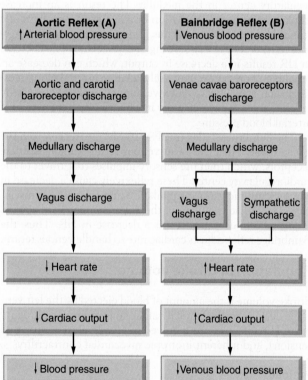

FIGURE 16-8    Effects of aortic reflex (**A**) and Bainbridge reflex (**B**) on heart rate (HR).

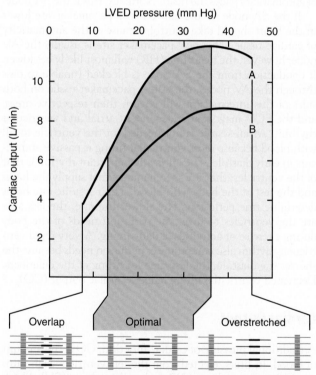

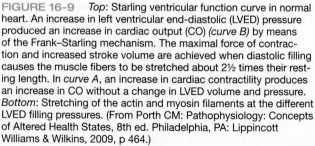

FIGURE 16-9    *Top*: Starling ventricular function curve in normal heart. An increase in left ventricular end-diastolic (LVED) pressure produced an increase in cardiac output (CO) *(curve B)* by means of the Frank–Starling mechanism. The maximal force of contraction and increased stroke volume are achieved when diastolic filling causes the muscle fibers to be stretched about 2½ times their resting length. In *curve A*, an increase in cardiac contractility produces an increase in CO without a change in LVED volume and pressure. *Bottom*: Stretching of the actin and myosin filaments at the different LVED filling pressures. (From Porth CM: Pathophysiology: Concepts of Altered Health States, 8th ed. Philadelphia, PA: Lippincott Williams & Wilkins, 2009, p 464.)

fibers (Fig. 16-9). Within a certain range, increasing myofibril stretch increases the force of systole. Beyond optimal fibril length, it is hypothesized that too few actin–myosin binding sites overlap to provide an adequate contraction. Below optimal shortening, there is little room for filaments to slide, and cell walls limit further sliding. Also, actin filaments may have begun to overlap, decreasing the number of binding sites available to myosin fibers.

When the force of systole decreases, the chamber pumps poorly and does not empty properly. Excessive blood is left in the chamber at the end of systole. During diastole, when the chamber fills, this extra blood causes overfilling of the chamber and increases stretch. The next systole will be even weaker, as preload increases during every diastole.

Because preload is affected by the volume at the end of diastole, it is often equated with end-diastolic volume or pressure. Thus, left ventricular preload is represented by left ventricular end-diastolic pressure.

An example of rapid and normal adjustments to changes in preload occurs during the Valsalva maneuver. The first part of the Valsalva occurs when one holds one's breath and bears down, such as during defecation or heavy lifting. Bearing down increases intra-abdominal and intrathoracic pressures, decreasing venous return to the right atrium and ventricle. Right heart preload decreases. Bearing down also stimulates the vagus nerve, and the HR slows.

On exhalation, during the second part of the Valsalva maneuver, intrathoracic pressures decrease rapidly, allowing a sudden increase in venous return. Right atrial and ventricular preloads increase dramatically, stretch increases, and the right ventricular SV increases. Atrial stretch receptors also signal the medulla and lead to sympathetic nervous discharge. HR increases.

### Afterload

Afterload is the force or pressure against which a cardiac chamber must eject blood during systole. The most critical factor determining afterload is vascular resistance, in the systemic or pulmonic vessels. Afterload is often equated with systemic vascular resistance or pulmonary vascular resistance.

Afterload affects SV by increasing or decreasing the ease of emptying a ventricle during systole. A decrease in systemic vascular resistance, through vasodilation, presents the left ventricle with relatively large, open, relaxed arteries into which it can pump. Because it is easier to pump, the left ventricle empties easily, which increases SV.

If systemic vascular resistance increases, for example through catecholamine-induced constriction of arteries, it takes a great deal more force for the left ventricle to pump into such a tightened vasculature. SV decreases.

### Contractility

Inotropic capabilities and cardiac workload refer to contractile forces. Cardiac muscle forces change in response to neural stimuli and circulating levels of catecholamines. It is thought that through cyclic adenosine monophosphate mechanisms, cardiac cells change intracellular levels of calcium and ATP. These changes lead to increased inotropic actions, although the mechanisms remain unknown.

However, increased inotropic action increases the oxygen consumption of heart cells. This increased consumption is also called *increased workload* and *increased oxygen demand*.

CO depends on HR and SV. Regardless of the initial cause of increased SV (increased preload, increased afterload, or increased inotropic force), an increase in SV increases workload. Similarly, an increased HR, no matter what the cause, increases oxygen demand.

## Coronary Circulation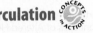

Blood supply to the myocardium is derived from the two main coronary arteries, the left and the right (Fig. 16-10). The left main coronary artery has two major branches known as the left anterior descending (LAD) and the left circumflex (LCA) artery. The LAD passes down the anterior wall of the left ventricle toward the apex of the myocardium. The LAD supplies blood flow to the anterior two-thirds of the ventricular septum, the anterior left ventricle, the apex, and most of the bundle branches (Table 16-2).

The LCA, the other branch of the left main coronary artery, sits in the groove between the left atrium and the left ventricle and wraps around the posterior wall of the heart. The LCA supplies blood flow to the left atrium, the lateral wall of the left ventricle, and the posterior wall of the left ventricle. In about 10% of the population, the LCA is the source of blood flow to the posterior descending coronary artery; when this pattern of flow occurs, the patient is referred to as left dominant.

The right coronary artery (RCA) branches toward the right atrium; the anterior, lateral, and posterior regions of the right ventricle; and the posterior ventricular septum. The RCA provides blood flow to the right atrium, the right ventricle, and the inferior wall of the left ventricle. In about 90% of the population, the RCA is the source of blood flow to the

| **TABLE 16-2** | Coronary Artery Blood Supply for Cardiac Muscle and Conducting System | |
|---|---|---|
| **Coronary Artery** | **Cardiac Muscle Supplied** | **Conducting Tissue Supplied** |
| **Left Main Coronary Artery** | | |
| Left anterior descending | Anterior ventricular septum | Bundle branches |
| | Anterior left ventricle | |
| | The apex | |
| Left circumflex | Left atrium | SA node in 45% of hearts |
| | Left ventricular lateral wall | AV node in 10% of hearts |
| | Left ventricular posterior wall | |
| **Right Coronary Artery** | | |
| | Right atrium | SA node in 55% of hearts |
| | Right ventricle | AV node in 90% of hearts |
| | Posterior ventricular septum | |
| | Inferior wall of left ventricle | |

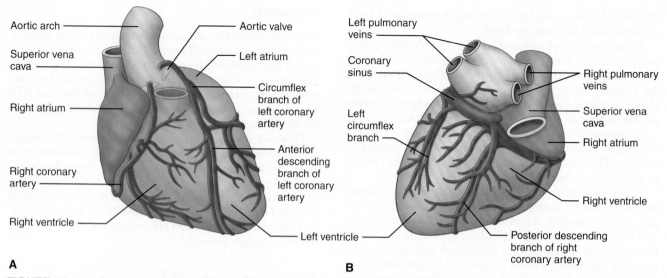

**FIGURE 16-10** Coronary arteries and some of the coronary sinus veins. A is the anterior view and B is the posterior view. (Adapted from Porth CM: Pathophysiology: Concepts of Altered Health States, 8th ed. Philadelphia, PA: Lippincott Williams & Wilkins, 2009, p 547.)

posterior descending coronary artery, a pattern of flow known as right dominant.

The coronary arteries initially supply the epicardial layer of the heart and then pass deeper into the heart muscle to provide blood flow to the endocardium. As a result of this flow pattern, poor coronary blood flow initially deprives the subendocardial area of oxygenated blood. If the interruption to flow continues, the effects of decreased oxygenation expand throughout the thickness of the wall of the heart to the subepicardial surface.

Because the coronary arteries derive from the aorta (above the aortic valve) and lie between myocardial fibers, blood flow through the coronary arteries occurs when the aortic valve is closed during ventricular diastole, not systole. Therefore, anything that decreases the diastolic time (eg, tachycardia) decreases coronary perfusion.

## Peripheral Circulation

The biologic significance of the cardiovascular system is tissue perfusion. Such perfusion supplies the body's cells with oxygen and nutrients while carrying away metabolic wastes, including carbon dioxide. Tissue perfusion is directly proportional to the rate of blood flow, which depends on several factors. One factor is the difference between the mean arterial blood pressure and the right atrial pressure (usually represented by the central venous pressure [CVP]). The greater this difference, the faster the flow rate (all else being unchanged). Conversely, if arterial pressure falls or venous pressure rises, flow rate, and thus tissue perfusion, will be decreased.

Another factor affecting flow rate is vascular resistance. The relationship between vascular resistance and blood flow has two general applications. The first describes the flow rate through vessels of differing diameters (eg, arteries, capillaries). The second concerns the ongoing regulation of blood flow by means of adjustments in arteriole diameters (ie, constriction, dilation). Arteriole constriction reduces the radius, thereby increasing the resistance and decreasing the flow rate. Conversely, arteriole dilation increases the flow rate.

The other two factors that can affect the flow rate normally are held constant. They are the sum of all vessel lengths and

blood viscosity. Because these factors do not normally change significantly, they are usually omitted from flow rate considerations. However, their relationships are obvious. The greater the length of the vessel, the more the resistance and thus the slower the flow rate. Also, the more viscous the blood, the slower the rate of its flow. Blood viscosity is determined by the proportion of solvent (water) to solute and other particles, including blood cells and platelets. The less water and more particles that exist, the more viscous is the blood. The complete equation that describes all four factors is as follows:

$$\text{Flow rate} = \frac{(\text{mean arterial pressure} - \text{central venous pressure})}{(\text{resistance} \times \text{viscosity} \times \text{vessel length})}$$

Because blood volume and pressure have such an important influence on tissue perfusion, the factors that alter and regulate them are examined.

## Blood Volume

Urinary output and fluid input are the major normal mechanisms for regulating volume. If output is greater or fluid input is less, the volume is less—if all else is held constant. Factors that alter the volume of urine excreted every 24 hours include those that alter the glomerular filtration rate and the tubular reabsorption of water, with or without electrolytes. (For a more detailed explanation of these factors see Chapter 42, specifically the discussion of normal endocrine physiology that considers the antidiuretic hormone.) Pathologic conditions that promote any type of fluid loss (eg, burns, severe diarrhea, osmotic diuresis) or a shift of water from the vascular to the interstitial compartment have the potential to reduce blood volume.

## Blood Pressure

Because the difference between arterial and venous pressures is the driving force for blood circulation and tissue perfusion, factors that influence CVP are examined first, followed by the factors that regulate arterial blood pressure. CVP is, strictly speaking, the pressure of blood in the venae cavae just before its entry into the right atrium. CVP can be increased by an increase in blood volume (eg, intravenous fluid overload) or a decrease in the pumping ability of the heart (eg, cardiac failure). Because the pulsatile effects of the cardiac cycle are removed by capillary networks, venous pressure is recorded as an average, or mean, and reported in millimeters of mercury (mm Hg).

Arterial blood pressure is the pressure of blood in the arteries and arterioles. It is a pulsatile pressure due to the cardiac cycle, and systolic (peak) and diastolic (trough) numbers are reported in millimeters of mercury. Average or mean arterial blood pressure can be clinically useful as an indicator of average perfusion pressures.

Arterial blood pressure is regulated by the vasomotor tone of the arteries and arterioles, the amount of blood entering the arteries per systole (ie, CO), and blood volume itself. The greater the volume or output, the greater the blood pressure, and vice versa, if vasomotor tone were held constant. The normal regulation of vasomotor tone involves neural and hormonal mechanisms.

Neural regulation is mediated by the vasomotor center of the medulla oblongata. This center consists of vasopressor and depressor subdivisions. The vasomotor center receives neural input from baroreceptors in the carotid sinuses and aorta, atrial diastolic stretch receptors, the limbic system and hypothalamus, the midbrain, and pulmonary stretch receptors. In addition, the center is directly responsive to local hypoxia or hypercapnia. Neural outputs from the vasopressor center result in increased sympathetic stimulation to arterial smooth muscle cells. This increase in sympathetic stimulation results in arterial constriction and an increase in arterial blood pressure. Stimulation of the depressor area decreases such sympathetic stimulation.

Rapid adjustments in arterial blood pressure are effected primarily by the baroreceptor reflexes. An increase in the pressure on these receptors (directly by elevated blood pressure or manual compression and indirectly by increased blood volume) reflexively stimulates the depressor area. This stimulation of the depressor area results in decreased sympathetic stimulation to major arteries and the aorta, which causes a decrease in arterial blood pressure. The decreased baroreceptor stimulation caused by a fall in arterial blood pressure reflexively stimulates the pressor area and results in increased sympathetic stimulation to arterial muscles, causing a rise in arterial blood pressure. Thus, homeostasis of arterial pressure is maintained.

In orthostatic hypotension, the baroreceptor reflex is sluggish. Because arterial pressure is not elevated rapidly enough, the postural change results in a temporary decrease in brain perfusion that leads, in extreme cases, to syncope.

Other factors may alter arterial blood pressure reflexively by their influences on the vasomotor center. Nerve fibers from the limbic system and hypothalamus are believed to mediate emotionally produced alterations in blood pressure. An example of this is fainting, caused by neurally mediated vasodilation in response to the sight of blood or very bad (or good) news. Neural inputs from the midbrain and possibly from ascending spinothalamic fibers in the medulla result in the elevation in arterial pressure that initially accompanies severe pain and in the later decrease in arterial pressure that occurs when severe pain is prolonged. Lung inflation stimulates pulmonary stretch receptors. Their input to the vasomotor center reflexively decreases arterial pressure. Hypercapnia and, to a lesser extent, hypoxia of vasomotor neurons stimulate the pressor area, reflexively causing an increase in arterial pressure. Such stimuli obviously are not part of a normal daily regulatory mechanism but can operate as a normal compensatory mechanism in certain pathologic situations. Elevated intracranial pressure can promote medullary hypercapnia and hypoxia. The increase in arterial pressure reflexively produced by these stimuli (Cushing's reflex) increases medullary perfusion, which can ameliorate the medullary hypoxia, hypercapnia, or both. Hormonal regulation of arterial blood pressure is effected by adrenal medullary catecholamines and the renin–angiotensin system. In the former, adrenal medullary catecholamines mimic the action of sympathetic fibers innervating the muscle layer of arteries (tunica media), causing arterial constriction and elevating arterial pressure. The renin–angiotensin system is discussed in Chapter 28. Briefly, a decreased glomerular filtration rate, which can result, for example, from a decrease in blood volume or renal perfusion, stimulates the secretion of renin from the juxtaglomerular apparatus. This stimulation of renin leads to the production of angiotensin II, which acts directly on the tunica media to promote vasoconstriction. Thus, renin elevates arterial pressure, which increases renal perfusion and glomerular filtration.

Finally, arterial blood pressure can be influenced by alterations in the level of unbound calcium in tunica media cells. Such levels are influenced by factors that open or close calcium channels in the membranes of these muscle cells. Drugs that block calcium channels ("calcium blockers") inhibit the entry of calcium into cells. Such decreased calcium influx can lower intracellular calcium levels sufficiently to decrease muscle contractility, including contractility of the heart, thereby promoting a degree of vasodilation and lowering the arterial pressure.

## Clinical Applicability Challenges

### SHORT ANSWER QUESTIONS

1. Mr. W. was diagnosed with aortic stenosis and will be having surgery to replace the valve. Mr. W. asks you where is the aortic valve located and what does it do?

2. Mrs. K. has been diagnosed with 90% occlusion of her RCA. Describe which anatomical walls of the heart are affected. Explain which parts of her cardiac conducting system may be affected by the occlusion.

3. Ms. M. is taking a drug that has side effects of stimulating the sympathetic nervous system. What are the implications for her HR?

### WANT TO KNOW MORE?

A wide variety of resources to enhance your learning and understanding of this chapter are available on thePoint.

You will find:

- References
- Selected readings
- NCLEX-style review questions
- Internet resources
- And more!

# 17

# Patient Assessment: Cardiovascular System

PATRICIA GONCE MORTON, KIM RECK, AND JAN M. HEADLEY

## LEARNING OBJECTIVES

*Based on the content in this chapter, the reader should be able to:*

1. Explain the components of the cardiovascular history and physical examination.
2. Discuss the mechanisms responsible for the production of the first, second, third, and fourth heart sounds and their timing in the cardiac cycle.
3. Explain the attributes of heart murmurs.
4. Describe components of hematologic studies, coagulation studies, blood chemistries, and serum lipid studies.
5. Describe current techniques used for diagnostic purposes in cardiology and the nursing implications.
6. Describe potential complications of cardiac diagnostic procedures.
7. Explain the major features of an electrocardiogram (ECG) monitoring system and steps to troubleshoot the system.
8. Describe the components of the ECG tracing and their meaning.
9. Explain the steps used to interpret a rhythm strip.
10. Describe the causes, clinical significance, and management for each of the dysrhythmias discussed.
11. Describe the parameters of a normal 12-lead ECG and the determination of electrical axis.
12. Explain the causes, clinical significance, and treatment of bundle branch blocks, atrial enlargement, and ventricular enlargement.
13. Describe the ECG changes associated with serum potassium and calcium abnormalities.
14. Describe the system components required to monitor hemodynamic pressures.
15. Analyze the characteristics of normal systemic arterial, right atrial, right ventricular, pulmonary artery, and pulmonary artery occlusion pressure waveforms.
16. State nursing interventions that ensure accuracy of pressure readings.
17. Discuss the major complications that can occur with an indwelling arterial, central venous, and pulmonary artery catheter.
18. Describe methods for measuring cardiac output and for obtaining hemodynamic data through minimally invasive and noninvasive methods.
19. Evaluate the factors influencing oxygen delivery and consumption.
20. Use $SvO_2$ or $ScvO_2$ monitoring to assess oxygen delivery and consumption.

The application of complex technology to the assessment and management of cardiovascular and cardiopulmonary conditions has increased greatly in the past several decades. Use of advanced and complex technologies is an integral part of the care of critically ill patients. Nevertheless, the value of a comprehensive cardiovascular assessment should never be underestimated.

## CARDIAC HISTORY AND PHYSICAL EXAMINATION

The cardiovascular nursing assessment and health history provide physiologic and psychosocial information that guides the physical assessment, the selection of diagnostic tests, and the choice of treatment options. During the history, the nurse asks about the patient's chief complaint and the history of the present illness, including a complete analysis of each sign and symptom. Next, the nurse asks about the patient's past health history, family history, and personal and social history. The history concludes with a review of systems that provides additional clues to the patient's health status.

The information gathered during the history gives the nurse insight into risk factors and behaviors that promote or jeopardize cardiovascular health. The nurse uses this information to guide health teaching. During the process of taking a thorough history and performing a physical examination, the nurse has an opportunity to establish rapport with the patient and to evaluate the patient's general physical and emotional status.

## History

### Chief Complaint and History of Present Illness

The nurse begins the history by investigating the patient's chief complaint, asking the patient to describe the problem or reason for seeking health care in his or her own words. The nurse then asks for more information about the present illness, using the NOPQRST format and the questions presented in Box 17-1. Answers to these questions are essential to understanding the patient's perception of the problem. To gain a better understanding of the current illness, the nurse also asks the patient about any associated symptoms, including chest pain, nausea or vomiting, dyspnea, edema of feet or ankles, palpitations, syncope or dizziness, cough and hemoptysis, nocturia, cyanosis, and extremity pain or paresthesias.

**Assessment Parameters: Questions to Ask in a Symptom Assessment**

**N  Normal:** Describe your normal baseline. What was it like before this symptom developed?

**O  Onset:** When did the symptom start? What day? What time? Did it start suddenly or gradually?

**P  Precipitating and palliative factors:** What brought on the symptom? What seems to trigger it—factors such as stress, position change, or exertion? What were you doing when you first noticed the symptom? What makes the symptom worse? What measures have helped relieve the symptom? What have you tried so far? What measures did not relieve the symptom?

**Q  Quality and quantity:** How does it feel? How would you describe it? How much are you experiencing now? Is it more or less than you experienced at any other time?

**R  Region and radiation:** Where does the symptom occur? Can you show me? In the case of pain, does it travel anywhere such as down your arm or in your back?

**S  Severity:** On a scale of 0 to 10, with 0 being the absence of pain and 10 being the worst ever experienced, rate your symptom. How bad is the symptom at its worst? Does it force you to stop your activity and sit down, lie down, or slow down? Is the symptom getting better or worse, or staying about the same?

**T  Time:** How long does the symptom last? How often do you get the symptom? Does it occur in association with anything, such as before, during, or after meals?

## Chest Pain

Chest pain is one of the most common symptoms of patients with cardiovascular disease (CVD). Therefore, it is an essential component of the assessment interview. Chest pain is often a disturbing or even frightening experience for a patient, so the patient may be hesitant to initiate a discussion of chest pain. The questions listed in Box 17-1 are particularly useful when assessing chest pain because the answers help determine whether the pain is cardiac in origin.

Because cardiac pain (angina pectoris) is the result of an imbalance between oxygen supply and oxygen demand, it usually develops over time. Typically, anginal pain does not start at maximal intensity. Because not all chest pain is cardiac in origin, it is necessary to carefully reporting the characteristics of the pain and the behaviors (or lack thereof) that precede the onset of pain. The nurse asks the patient about his or her normal baseline status before the symptoms developed. It is also important to ask about the onset of the symptoms to determine the date and time of the start of symptoms and whether the onset was sudden or gradual. Symptoms that may accompany chest pain caused by heart disease include nausea and vomiting.

Chest pain caused by coronary artery disease (CAD) is often precipitated by physical or emotional exertion, a meal, or being out in the cold. Palliative measures to relieve anginal pain may include rest or sublingual nitrates; these measures usually do not relieve the pain of a myocardial infarction (MI). The quality of cardiac chest pain is often described as heaviness, tightness, squeezing, or a choking sensation. If the pain is reported as superficial, knifelike, or throbbing, it is not likely to be anginal. Cardiac chest pain is usually located in the substernal region and often radiates to the neck, left arm (LA), back, or jaw. Although the pain is often referred to other areas, anginal pain is visceral in origin, and most complaints include a reference to a "deep, inside" pain. When the patient is asked to point to the painful area, the painful area is about the size of a hand or clenched fist. It is unusual for true anginal pain to be localized to an area smaller than a fingertip. Using a scale of 0 to 10, with 10 being the worst pain the patient has ever experienced and 0 being the absence of pain, the patient is asked to rate the severity of the pain. When asked about time, the patient with cardiac chest pain reports the pain lasting anywhere from 30 seconds to hours.

Pain may be secondary to cardiovascular problems that are unrelated to a primary coronary insufficiency. Therefore, when obtaining the patient's history, the nurse must consider other causes. For example, if the patient reports the pain is made worse by lying down, moving, or deep breathing, it may be caused by pericarditis. If the pain is retrosternal and accompanied by sudden shortness of breath and peripheral cyanosis, it may be caused by a pulmonary embolism.

## Dyspnea

Dyspnea occurs in patients with both pulmonary and cardiac abnormalities. In patients with cardiac disease, it is the result of inefficient pumping of the left ventricle, which causes a congestion of blood flow in the lungs. During history taking, dyspnea is differentiated from the usual breathlessness that follows a sudden burst of physical activity (eg, running up four flights of stairs, sprinting across a parking lot). Dyspnea is a subjective complaint of true difficulty in breathing, not just shortness of breath. The nurse determines whether the breathing difficulty occurs only with exertion or also at rest. If dyspnea is present when the patient lies flat but is relieved by sitting or standing, it is orthopnea. If dyspnea is characterized by breathing difficulties starting after approximately 1 to 2 hours of sleep and relieved by sitting upright or getting out of bed, it is paroxysmal nocturnal dyspnea.

## Edema of the Feet and Ankles

Heart failure is one of many possible causes of swollen feet and ankles. With heart failure, the heart is unable to mobilize fluid appropriately. Because gravity promotes the movement of fluids from intravascular to extravascular spaces, the edema becomes worse as the day progresses and usually improves at night after lying down to sleep. Patients or families may report that shoes do not fit anymore, socks that used to be loose are now too tight, and the indentations from sock bands take more time than usual to disappear. The nurse inquires about the timing of edema development (eg, immediately after lowering the extremities, only at the end of the day, only after a significant salt intake) and duration (eg, relieved with temporary elevation of the legs or with constant elevation).

## Palpitations and Syncope or Dizziness

Palpitations refer to the awareness of irregular or rapid heartbeats. Patients may report the "skipping" of beats, a rushing of the heart, or a loud "thudding." The nurse asks about onset and duration of the palpitations, associated symptoms, and any precipitating events that the patient or family can remember. Because a cardiac dysrhythmia may compromise blood flow to the brain, the nurse asks about symptoms of dizziness, fainting, or syncope that accompany the palpitations.

## Cough and Hemoptysis

Abnormalities such as heart failure, pulmonary embolus, or mitral stenosis may cause a cough or hemoptysis. Side effects of medications such as angiotensin-converting enzyme (ACE) inhibitors may also include a cough. The nurse asks the patient about the presence of a cough and inquires about the quality (wet or dry) and frequency of the cough (chronic or occasional, only when lying down or after exercise). If the cough produces expectorant, the nurse inquires about its color, odor, consistency, and amount perceived by the patient. If the patient reports spitting up blood (hemoptysis), the nurse asks if the substance spit up was streaked with blood, frothy bloody sputum, or frank blood (bright or dark).

## Nocturia

Kidneys that are inadequately perfused by an unhealthy heart during the day may finally receive sufficient flow during rest at night to increase their output. The nurse asks about the number of times the patient urinates during the night. If the patient takes a diuretic, the nurse also evaluates frequency of urination in relation to the time of day the diuretic is taken.

## Cyanosis

Cyanosis is a reflection of the reduced oxygenation and circulatory status of the patient. Central cyanosis is generally distributed and best found by examining the mucous membranes for discoloration and duskiness, and reflects reduced oxygen concentration. Peripheral cyanosis is localized in the extremities and protrusions (hands, feet, nose, ears, and lips) and reflects impaired circulation.

## Extremity Pain or Paresthesias

Extremity pain occurs when the blood supply to exercising muscles is inadequate; this type of pain is known as claudication. Usually, the cause of claudication is significant atherosclerotic obstruction to the lower extremities. The limb is asymptomatic at rest unless the obstruction is severe. Blood supply to the legs is inadequate to meet metabolic demands during exercise, and ischemic pain results. The patient describes a cramping, "charley horse" ache, or weakness in the foot, calf, thigh, or buttocks that improves with rest. The patient is asked to describe the severity of the pain and how much exertion is required to produce the pain.

## Past Health History

When assessing the patient's past health history, the nurse inquires about childhood illnesses and other previous illnesses, as well as past surgeries, previous diagnostic tests and interventions, medication use, allergies, and transfusions (Box 17-2). The nurse also asks about risk factors for CVD (Box 17-3).[1,2]

---

**BOX 17-2**   *HEALTH HISTORY for Cardiovascular Assessment*

**Chief Complaint**
- Patient's description of the problem

**History of the Present Illness**
- Complete analysis of the following signs and symptoms (using the NOPQRST format; see Box 17-1)
- Chest pain
- Nausea and/or vomiting
- Dyspnea
- Edema
- Palpitations
- Syncope/dizziness
- Cough and hemoptysis
- Nocturia
- Cyanosis
- Extremity pain or paresthesias

**Past Health History**
- Relevant childhood illnesses and immunizations: rheumatic fever, murmurs, congenital anomalies, streptococcal infections
- Past acute and chronic medical problems including treatments and hospitalizations: heart failure, hypertension, CAD, MI, hyperlipidemia, valve disease, cardiac dysrhythmias, diabetes mellitus, endocarditis, thrombophlebitis, deep venous thrombosis, peripheral vascular disease, chest injury, pneumonia, pulmonary embolism, thyroid disease, tuberculosis
- Risk factors: age, heredity, gender, race, tobacco use, elevated cholesterol, hypertension, physical inactivity, obesity, diabetes mellitus (see Box 17-3)
- Past surgeries: coronary artery bypass grafting, valvular surgery, peripheral vascular surgeries
- Past diagnostic tests and interventions: ECG, echocardiogram, stress test, electrophysiology studies, myocardial imaging studies, thrombolytic therapy, cardiac catheterization, percutaneous transluminal cardiac angioplasty, stent placement, atherectomy, pacemaker or ICD implantation, valvuloplasty
- Medications, including prescription drugs, over-the-counter drugs, vitamins, herbs, and supplements: ACE inhibitors, anticoagulants, antihypertensives, antiplatelets, antiarrhythmics, angiotensin II receptor blockers (ARBss), β-blockers, calcium-channel blockers, antihyperlipidemics, diuretics, electrolyte replacements, nitrates, inotropes, hormone replacement therapies, oral contraceptives
- Allergies and reactions to medications, foods, contrast dye, latex or other materials
- Transfusions, including type and date

**Family History**
- Health status or cause of death of parents and siblings: CAD, hypertension, diabetes mellitus, sudden cardiac death, stroke, peripheral vascular disease, lipid disorders

**Personal and Social History**
- Tobacco, alcohol, and substance use
- Family composition
- Occupation and work environment
- Living environment
- Diet: restrictions, supplements, caffeine intake
- Sleep patterns: number of pillows used
- Exercise and leisure activities
- Cultural, spiritual, and/or religious beliefs
- Coping patterns and social support systems
- Sexual activity: use of agents for erectile dysfunction

**Review of Other Systems**
- HEENT: retinal problems, visual changes, headaches, carotid artery disease
- Respiratory: shortness of breath, dyspnea, cough, lung disease, recurrent infections, pneumonia, tuberculosis
- Gastrointestinal: nausea, vomiting, weight loss, change in bowel habits
- Genitourinary: incontinence, erectile dysfunction
- Musculoskeletal: pain, weakness, varicose veins, change in sensation, peripheral edema
- Neurologic: transient ischemic attacks, stroke, change in level of consciousness, changes in sensations
- Endocrine: thyroid disease, diabetes mellitus

**BOX 17-3** **Risk Factors for Cardiovascular Disease**

## Major Uncontrollable Risk Factors

- **Age:** There is an increased incidence of all types of atherosclerotic disease with aging. More than 83% of people who die from CAD are age 65 or older. Women at older ages who have an MI are more than likely as men to die of it within a few weeks.
- **Heredity (including race):** The tendency for development of atherosclerosis seems to run in families. The risk is thought to be a combination of environmental and genetic influences. Even when other risk factors are controlled, the chance for development of CAD increases when there is a familial tendency. African Americans have more severe hypertension than Caucasians and a higher risk of heart disease. The risk of heart disease is higher in Mexican Americans, American Indians, native Hawaiians, and some Asian Americans. This risk is partly due to higher rates of obesity.
- **Gender:** Men have a greater risk for development of CAD than women at earlier ages. After menopause, women's death rate from MI increases but is not as great as men's.

## Major Risk Factors That Can Be Modified, Treated, or Controlled

- **Tobacco smoking:** A smoker's risk for developing heart disease is much higher than the risk of nonsmokers. For smokers with coronary heart disease, cigarette smoking is a powerful independent risk factor for sudden cardiac death. Cigarette smoking, combined with other risk factors, greatly increases the risk of coronary heart disease. Exposure to smoke from others increases the risk of coronary heart disease for nonsmokers.
- **High blood cholesterol levels:** The risk for coronary heart disease increases as the blood cholesterol level rises. When other risk factors are present, this risk increases even more.
- **Hypertension:** Known as the "silent killer," hypertension is a risk factor with no specific symptoms and no early warning signs. Men have a greater risk for hypertension than women until the age of 55 years. The risk for development of hypertension is about the same for men and women between the ages of 55 and 75 years. After the age of 75 years, hypertension is

more likely to develop in women than in men. African Americans are more likely to have hypertension than whites. Hypertension increases the risk for stroke, MI, kidney failure, and heart failure.

- **Physical inactivity:** A lack of physical exercise is a risk factor for CAD. Moderate to vigorous regular exercise plays a significant role in preventing heart disease and blood vessel disease. Even moderate-intensity exercise is beneficial if performed regularly and long term. Physical activity also plays a role in controlling cholesterol, diabetes, obesity, and hypertension.
- **Obesity:** People who have excess body fat, especially at the waist, are more likely to develop heart disease and stroke even if they have no other risk factors. Excess weight raises blood pressure, blood cholesterol, and blood triglyceride levels. Excess weight lowers high-density lipids and makes diabetes more likely to develop.
- **Diabetes mellitus:** Even when blood glucose levels are under control, diabetes greatly increases the risk for heart disease and stroke. If blood glucose is not well controlled, the risk is even greater. Most people with diabetes die of some form of heart or blood vessel disease. Many people with diabetes also have high blood pressure, increasing their risk even more.

## Other Contributing Factors

- **Stress:** A person's response to stress may be a contributing factor to heart disease. Stress in a person's life, his or her health behaviors, and socioeconomic status may all contribute to established risk factors. For example, individuals under stress may overeat, smoke, and not exercise.
- **Excessive alcohol intake:** Drinking too much alcohol can raise blood pressure, cause heart failure, lead to stroke, contribute to high triglycerides and obesity, and produce dysrhythmias. The risk for heart disease in individuals who drink moderate amounts of alcohol (an average of one drink for women and two drinks for men per day) is lower than in those who do not drink alcohol.
- **Diet and Nutrition:** Diet is one of the best means to prevent CVD. Food also can affect other controllable risk factors such as cholesterol, blood pressure, diabetes, and obesity.

## Family History

The nurse asks about the age and health, or age and cause of death, of immediate family members, including parents, grandparents, siblings, children, and grandchildren. The nurse inquires about cardiovascular problems, such as CAD, hypertension, diabetes mellitus, sudden cardiac death, stroke, peripheral vascular disease, and lipid disorders (see Box 17-2).

## Personal and Social History

Although the physical symptoms provide many clues about the origin and extent of cardiac disease, the personal and social history provided additional information about the patient's health status. An understanding of the topics listed in Box 17-2 contributes to the nurse's knowledge of the patient as a person and guides interaction with the patient and family as well as patient education.

## Review of Other Systems

The health history concludes with a review of relevant systems. This information gives the nurse a better understanding

of the patient's total health status, and it also helps the nurse determine the impact of CVD on the functioning of other body systems (see Box 17-2).

## Physical Examination

Cardiac assessment requires examination of all aspects of the individual, using the standard steps of inspection, palpation, percussion, and auscultation. A thorough and careful examination helps the nurse detect subtle abnormalities as well as obvious ones.

## Inspection

### General Appearance

Inspection begins as soon as the patient and nurse interact. General appearance and presentation of the patient are key elements of the initial inspection. Critical examination reveals a first impression of age, nutritional status, self-care ability, alertness, and overall physical health. It is necessary to note the ability of the patient to move and speak with or without distress. Consider the patient's posture, gait, and musculoskeletal coordination.

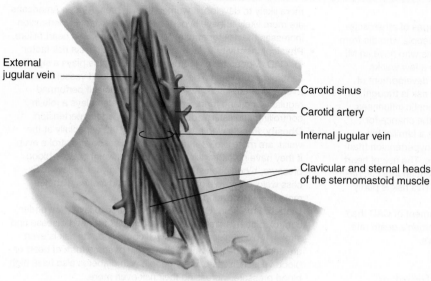

External jugular vein

Carotid sinus

Carotid artery

Internal jugular vein

Clavicular and sternal heads of the sternomastoid muscle

**FIGURE 17-1**   Internal jugular veins. (From Bickley L: Bates' Guide to Physical Examination and Health History, 10th ed. Philadelphia, PA: Lippincott Williams & Wilkins, 2009, p 237.)

## Jugular Venous Distention

Pressure in the jugular veins reflects right atrial pressure (RAP) and provides the nurse with an indication of heart hemodynamics and cardiac function. The height of the level of blood in the right internal jugular vein is an indication of RAP because there are no valves or obstructions between the vein and the right atrium.

The internal jugular veins are not directly visible because they lie deep to the sternomastoid muscles in the neck (Fig. 17-1). The goals of the examination are to determine the highest point of visible pulsation in the internal jugular veins, to note the level of head elevation, and to measure this point of visible pulsation as the vertical distance above the sternal angle. The patient is positioned supine in the bed with the head of the bed elevated 30, 45, 60, and 90 degrees. The patient is examined at each elevation with the head slightly turned away from the examiner. The nurse uses tangential light to observe for the highest point of visible pulsation.[3,4]

Next, the angle of Louis is located by palpating where the clavicle joins the sternum (suprasternal notch). The examining finger is slid down the sternum until a bony prominence is felt; this prominence is known as the angle of Louis. A vertical ruler is placed on the angle of Louis; another ruler is placed horizontally at the level of the pulsation. The intersection of the horizontal ruler with the vertical ruler is noted, and the intersection point on the vertical ruler is read (Fig. 17-2).

Normal jugular venous pulsation should not exceed 3 cm above the angle of Louis. A level more than 3 cm indicates an abnormally high volume in the venous system. Possible causes include right-sided heart failure, obstruction of the superior vena cava, pericardial effusion, and other cardiac or thoracic diseases. An increase in the jugular venous pressure of more than 1 cm while pressure is applied to the abdomen for 60 seconds (hepatojugular or abdominojugular test) indicates the inability of the heart to accommodate the increased venous return.

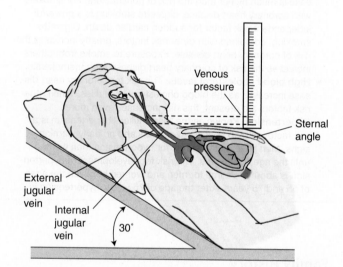

Venous pressure

Sternal angle

External jugular vein

Internal jugular vein

30°

**FIGURE 17-2**   Assessment of jugular venous pressure. Place the patient supine in bed and gradually raise the head of the bed to 30, 45, 60, and 90 degrees. Using tangential lighting, note the highest level of venous pulsation. Measure the vertical distance between this point and the sternal angle. Record this distance in centimeters and the angle of the head of the bed.

## Chest

The chest is inspected for signs of trauma or injury, symmetry, chest contour, and any visible pulsations. The inspection may reveal the location of the point of maximal impulse (PMI). In most patients, the apical pulse is the PMI; however, in some pathologic conditions, these may be two distinct areas on the chest.[3] Thrusts (abnormally strong precordial pulsations) are noted. Any depression (sternum excavatum) or bulging of the precordium is recorded.

## Extremities

The extremities are examined for lesions, ulcerations, unhealed sores, and varicose veins. Distribution of hair on the extremities also is noted. A lack of normal hair distribution on the extremities may indicate diminished arterial blood flow to the area.

### Skin

Skin is evaluated for moistness or dryness, color, elasticity, edema, thickness, lesions, ulcerations, and vascular changes. Nail beds are examined for cyanosis and clubbing, which may indicate chronic cardiac or pulmonary abnormalities. (For a further discussion of nail assessment, see Chapter 51). General differences in color and temperature between body parts may provide perfusion clues.

## Palpation

### Pulses

Cardiovascular assessment continues with palpation. Using the pads of the fingers, the nurse palpates the carotid, brachial, radial, femoral, popliteal, posterior tibial, and dorsalis pedis pulses. The peripheral pulses are compared bilaterally to determine rate, rhythm, strength, and symmetry. The 0-to-4 scale described in Box 17-4 is used to rate the strength of the pulse. The carotid pulses should never be assessed simultaneously because this can obstruct flow to the brain.

Pulses can also be described according to their characteristics. For example, pulsus alternans is a pulse that alternates in strength with every other beat; it is often found in patients with left ventricular failure. Pulsus paradoxus is a pulse that disappears during inspiration but returns during expiration.

To determine whether the condition is pathologic, the sphygmomanometer is deflated until the pulse is heard only during expiration and the corresponding pressure noted. As the cuff continues to deflate, the point at which the pulse is heard throughout the inspiratory and expiratory cycle is noted. The second systolic pressure reading is subtracted from the first; if the difference is greater than 10 mm Hg during normal respirations, it is considered pathologic. During the assessment of pulses, the nurse compares the warmth and size of the palpated areas to monitor perfusion.

### Precordium

The chest wall is palpated to assess for the PMI, thrills, and abnormal pulsations. Palpation starts with locating the PMI, which in most patients is the point at which the apical pulse is most readily felt. Using light pressure, the nurse first uses the palmar surface of the hand to feel for pulsations and then uses the pads of the finger to palpate the apical pulse (Fig. 17-3). The nurse palpates the PMI, noting its location, diameter, amplitude, and duration. Usually, the PMI is located in the midclavicular line at about the fourth or fifth intercostal space. If the pulse is difficult to palpate, it may be necessary to ask the patient to turn on the left side (left lateral decubitus position).

Next, the nurse palpates the lower left sternal border area, the upper left sternal border area, the sternoclavicular area, the right upper sternal border area, the lower right sternal border area, and finally the epigastric area. During palpation of these areas, the nurse feels for a thrill, which is a palpable vibration. A thrill usually represents a disruption in blood flow related to a defect in one of the semilunar valves.

## Percussion

With the advent of radiologic means of evaluating cardiac size, percussion is not a significant contributor to cardiac assessment. However, a gross determination of heart size can be made by percussing for the dullness that reflects the cardiac borders.

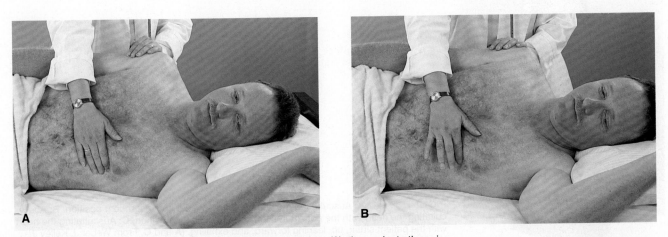

**FIGURE 17-3** Locate the apical impulse with the palmar surface (**A**), then palpate the apical pulse with the fingerpad (**B**). (From Weber J, Kelley J: Health Assessment in Nursing, 4th ed. Philadelphia, PA: Lippincott Williams & Wilkins, 2010, p 367.)

## Auscultation

Data obtained by careful and thorough auscultation of the heart are essential in planning and evaluating care of the critically ill patient. In this section, the following topics are discussed: the basic principles underlying cardiac auscultation; the factors responsible for the production of normal heart sounds; and the pathophysiologic conditions responsible for the production of extra sounds, murmurs, and friction rubs.

To facilitate accurate auscultation, the patient should be relaxed and comfortable in a quiet, warm environment with adequate lighting. The patient is placed in a recumbent position with the trunk elevated 30 to 45 degrees. To help hear abnormal sounds, the patient may be asked to roll partly onto the left side (left lateral decubitus position). This position helps bring the left ventricle closer to the chest wall. The patient also may be asked to sit up, lean forward, and exhale.

In this position, it may be easier to hear murmurs caused by aortic regurgitation (Fig. 17-4).

A good-quality stethoscope is essential. The head of the stethoscope should be equipped with both a diaphragm and a bell on a valve system that allows the clinician to switch easily between the two components. The diaphragm is used to hear high-frequency sounds, such as the first and second heart sounds ($S_1$, $S_2$), friction rubs, systolic murmurs, and diastolic insufficiency murmurs. The diaphragm should be placed firmly on the chest wall to create a tight seal. Low-frequency sounds, such as the third and fourth heart sounds ($S_3$, $S_4$) and the diastolic murmurs of mitral and tricuspid stenosis, are best heard with the stethoscope bell, which should be placed lightly on the chest wall only to seal the edges.

The precordium is auscultated systematically (see Fig. 17-5). Some authorities suggest the use of anatomical names for the auscultation areas (eg, aortic and pulmonic),

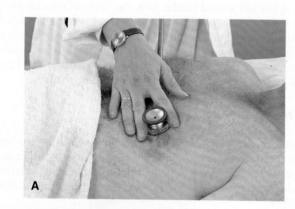

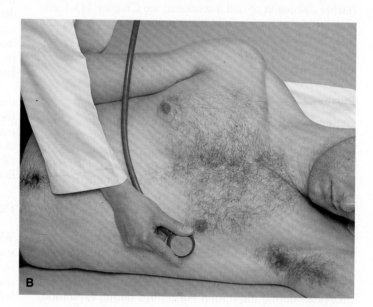

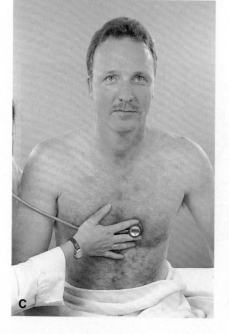

FIGURE 17-4    **A:** Auscultating the heart with the patient in a recumbent position. **B:** Auscultating the heart with the patient in a left lateral decubitus position. **C:** Auscultating the heart with the patient sitting up, leaning forward, and exhaling. (**A** and **C**, From Weber J, Kelley J: Health Assessment in Nursing, 4th ed. Philadelphia, PA: Lippincott Williams & Wilkins, 2010, pp 368–369. **B**, From Bickley L: Bates' Guide to Physical Examination and Health History, 10th ed. Philadelphia, PA: Lippincott Williams & Wilkins, 2009, p 363.)

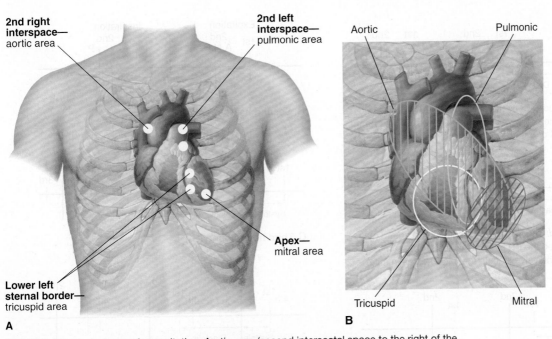

**2nd right interspace—**
aortic area

**2nd left interspace—**
pulmonic area

Aortic

Pulmonic

**Apex—**
mitral area

**Lower left sternal border—**
tricuspid area

Tricuspid

Mitral

**A**

**B**

FIGURE 17-5  **A:** Areas of auscultation. Aortic area (second intercostal space to the right of the sternum). Pulmonic area (second intercostal space to the left of the sternum). Tricuspid area (fifth intercostal space to the left of the sternum). Mitral or apical area (fifth intercostal space, midclavicular line). **B:** Heart sounds and murmurs that originate in the four valves range widely. Use anatomical location rather than valve area to describe where murmurs and sounds are best heard. (**A** From Bickley L: Bates' Guide to Physical Examination and Health History, 10th ed. Philadelphia, PA: Lippincott Williams & Wilkins, 2009, p 362. **B** Redrawn from Leatham: Introduction to the Examination of the Cardiovascular System, 2nd ed. Oxford, Oxford University Press, 1980.)

whereas others discourage the use of such labels because murmurs of more than one origin can be heard in a given area.[3,4] Instead, some suggest the use of anatomical landmarks such as intercostal spaces and relationship to the sternal border.[3,4]

The nurse begins the examination by listening with the stethoscope diaphragm in the right second intercostal space along the sternum. This area is sometimes called the aortic area and is the place where $S_2$ is loudest. Next, the nurse places the stethoscope in the left second intercostal space along the sternum, which is known as the pulmonic listening area, and from there moves the stethoscope down the left sternal border between the second and fifth spaces, one intercostal space at a time. The lower left sternal border area is sometimes referred to as the tricuspid area. Finally, the nurse moves the stethoscope to the mitral area or apex of the heart, where $S_1$ is the loudest. This pattern is then repeated with the stethoscope bell.

In each area auscultated, the nurse identifies $S_1$, noting the intensity of the sound, respiratory variation, and splitting. $S_2$ should then be identified and the same characteristics assessed. After $S_1$ and $S_2$ are identified, the presence of extra sounds is noted—first in systole, then in diastole. Finally, each area is auscultated for murmurs and friction rubs.

### First Heart Sound (S₁)

$S_1$ is timed with the closure of the mitral and tricuspid valves at the beginning of ventricular systole (Fig. 17-6A). Because mitral valve closure is responsible for most of the sound produced, $S_1$ is heard best in the mitral or apical area. The

upstroke of the carotid pulse correlates with $S_1$ and can be used to help distinguish $S_1$ from $S_2$.

The intensity (loudness) of $S_1$ varies with the position of the atrioventricular (AV) valve leaflets at the beginning of ventricular systole and the structure of the leaflets (thickened or normal). A loud $S_1$ is produced when the valve leaflets are wide open at the onset of ventricular systole and corresponds to a short PR interval on the surface electrocardiogram (ECG) tracing. A lengthening of the PR interval produces a soft $S_1$ because the leaflets have had time to float partially closed before ventricular systole. Mitral stenosis also increases the intensity of $S_1$ due to a thickening of the valvular structures.

In general, $S_1$ is heard as a single sound. However, if right ventricular systole is delayed, $S_1$ may be split into its two component sounds. The most common cause of this splitting is delay in the conduction of impulses through the right bundle branch; the splitting correlates with a right bundle branch block (RBBB) pattern on the ECG. Splitting of $S_1$ is heard best over the tricuspid area.

### Second Heart Sound (S₂)

$S_2$ is produced by the vibrations initiated by the closure of the aortic and pulmonic semilunar valves and is heard best at the base of the heart (Fig. 17-6B). (The term "base of the heart" is a clinical term that refers to the superior aspect of the heart at right and left second intercostal spaces next to the sternum.) This sound represents the beginning of ventricular diastole.

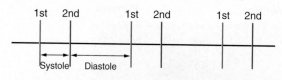

*Normal:* $S_1$ is produced by the closure of the AV valves and correlates with the beginning of ventricular systole. It is heard best in the apical or mitral area.

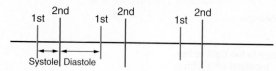

*Loud First Sound:* The intensity of the first heart sound may be increased when the PR interval is shortened, as in tachycardia, or when the valve leaflets are thickened as in mital stenosis.

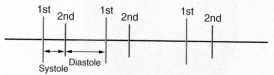

*Soft First Sound:* A soft $S_1$ is heard when the PR interval is prolonged.

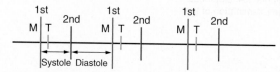

*Split First Sound:* A split $S_1$ is heard when right ventricular emptying is delayed. The mitral valve closes before the tricuspid valve and "splits" the sound into its two components.

**A. First heart sound ($S_1$)**

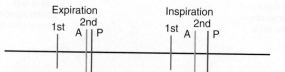

**B. Second heart sound ($S_2$)**

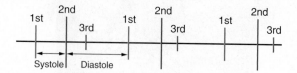

**C. Third heart sound ($S_3$)**

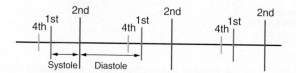

**D. Fourth heart sound ($S_4$)**

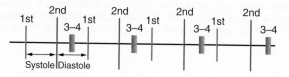

**E. Summation gallop**

**FIGURE 17-6** **A:** First heart sound. **B:** Second heart sound. The second heart sound is produced by the closure of the semilunar valves (aortic and pulmonary). During inspiration, there is an increase in venous return to the right side of the heart, which causes a delay in the emptying of the right ventricle and the closure of the pulmonic valve. This allows the two components of the second heart sound to separate or split during inspiration. **C:** Third heart sound. An $S_3$ or ventricular gallop is heard in early diastole, shortly after the second heart sound. The presence of a pathologic $S_3$ may be indicative of heart failure. **D:** Fourth heart sound. An $S_4$ is a late diastolic sound that occurs just before $S_1$. It is a low-frequency sound heard best with the bell of the stethoscope. **E:** Summation gallop. With rapid heart rates, $S_3$ and $S_4$ may become audible as a single, very loud sound that occurs in middiastole. This sound is a summation gallop.

Like $S_1$, $S_2$ consists of two separate components. The first component of $S_2$ is aortic valve closure; the second component is pulmonic valve closure. With inspiration, systole of the right ventricle is slightly prolonged because of increased filling of the right ventricle; this causes the pulmonic valve to close later than the aortic valve and $S_2$ to become "split" into its two components. This normal finding, termed physiologic splitting, is heard best on inspiration with the stethoscope placed in the second intercostal space to the left of the sternum.

The intensity of $S_2$ may be increased in the presence of aortic or pulmonic valvular stenosis or with an increase in the diastolic pressure forcing the semilunar valves to close, as occurs in pulmonary or systemic hypertension.

### Third Heart Sound ($S_3$)

An $S_3$ may be physiologic or pathologic (Fig. 17-6C). A physiologic $S_3$ is a normal finding in children and healthy young adults; it usually disappears after 25 to 35 years of age. An $S_3$ in an older adult with heart disease signifies ventricular failure.

An $S_3$ is a low-frequency sound that occurs during the early, rapid-filling phase of ventricular diastole. A noncompliant or failing ventricle cannot distend to accept this rapid inflow of blood; this causes turbulent flow, resulting in the vibration of the AV valvular structures or the ventricles themselves, producing a low-frequency sound. An $S_3$ associated with left ventricular failure is heard best at the apex with the stethoscope bell. The sound may be accentuated by turning the patient slightly to the left side. A right ventricular $S_3$ is heard best at the xiphoid or lower left sternal border and varies in intensity with respiration, becoming louder on inspiration.

## Fourth Heart Sound ($S_4$)

An $S_4$ or atrial gallop is a low-frequency sound heard late in diastole just before $S_1$ (Fig. 17-6D). It is rarely heard in healthy patients. The sound is produced by atrial contraction forcing blood into a noncompliant ventricle that, by virtue of its noncompliance, has an increased resistance to filling. Systemic hypertension, MI, angina, cardiomyopathy, and aortic stenosis all may produce a decrease in left ventricular compliance and an $S_4$. A left ventricular $S_4$ is auscultated at the apex with the bell of the stethoscope. Conditions affecting right ventricular compliance, such as pulmonary hypertension or pulmonic stenosis, may produce a right ventricular $S_4$ heard best at the lower left sternal border; it increases in intensity during inspiration.

## Summation Gallop

With rapid heart rates, as ventricular diastole shortens, if $S_3$ and $S_4$ are both present, they may fuse together and become audible as a single diastolic sound. This is called a summation gallop (Fig. 17-6E). This sound is loudest at the apex and is heard best with the stethoscope bell while the patient lies turned slightly to the left side.

## Heart Murmurs

Murmurs are sounds produced either by the forward flow of blood through a narrowed or constricted valve into a dilated vessel or chamber or by the backward flow of blood through an incompetent valve or septal defect.

Murmur classification is based on several attributes (Box 17-5). Timing in the cardiac cycle is an important attribute that refers to the presence of the murmur during either systole or diastole. Systolic murmurs occur between $S_1$ and $S_2$; diastolic murmurs occur after $S_2$ and before the onset of the following $S_1$. Location of maximum intensity refers to the anatomical location on the anterior chest where the sound of the murmur is heard the loudest. Anatomical landmarks are used to describe the radiation of the sound. The pitch of the sound helps further differentiate the type of murmur. The shape of the murmur refers to any changes in intensity over time. The intensity or loudness of a murmur is described using a grading system from 1 to 6. The quality of the sound produced is described as blowing, harsh, rumbling, vibratory, or musical. The effect of ventilation or a change in body position on the murmur is another important attribute.

**SYSTOLIC MURMURS.** As previously described, $S_1$ is produced by mitral and tricuspid valve closure and signifies the onset of ventricular systole. Murmurs occurring after $S_1$ and before $S_2$ are therefore classified as systolic murmurs.

During ventricular systole, the aortic and pulmonic valves are open. If either of these valves is stenotic or narrowed, a sound classified as a midsystolic ejection murmur is heard. Because the AV valves close before blood is ejected through the aortic and pulmonic valves, there is a delay between $S_1$ and the beginning of the murmur. The murmurs associated

---

**BOX 17-5** | **Attributes of Heart Murmurs**

**Timing:** A systolic murmur is heard between $S_1$ and $S_2$. A diastolic murmur is heard between $S_2$ and $S_1$.
*Systolic murmurs* are classified into three groups:
*Midsystolic* murmur begins after $S_1$ and stops before $S_2$.
*Pansystolic (holosystolic)* murmur starts with $S_1$ and stops with $S_2$ without a gap between the murmur and the heart sound.
*Late systolic* murmur starts in mid to late systole and continues up to $S_2$.
*Diastolic murmurs* are also divided into three categories:
*Early diastolic* murmur starts right after $S_2$ and fades before the next $S_1$.
*Middiastolic* murmur starts a short time after $S_2$ and fades away or merges into a late diastolic murmur.
*Late diastolic* murmur starts late in diastole and continues up to $S_1$.
**Location of maximal intensity:** The anatomical location where the murmur is heard best. The location is identified based on intercostal space and its relation to the sternum, the apex, the midclavicular line, or one of the axillary lines.
**Radiation or transmission from the point of maximal intensity:** The nurse notes the site farthest from the location of the greatest intensity at which the sound is still heard. The farthest site is identified using anatomical landmarks as described previously.
**Pitch:** The terms *high, medium,* and *low* are used to describe the pitch of the murmur.
**Shape:** The shape of a murmur is determined by its intensity over time. A *crescendo murmur* grows louder. A *decrescendo murmur* grows softer. A *crescendo–decrescendo murmur* first rises in intensity, then falls. A *plateau murmur* has the same intensity throughout.
**Intensity:** A grading system is used to describe the intensity of the murmur.
Grade 1: barely audible in a quiet room, very faint; may not be heard in all positions.
Grade 2: quiet, but clearly audible.
Grade 3: moderately loud.
Grade 4: loud with palpable thrill.
Grade 5: very loud with an easily palpable thrill; may be heard when the stethoscope is partly off the chest.
Grade 6: very loud with an easily palpable thrill; may be heard with stethoscope entirely off the chest.
**Quality:** The terms such as *harsh, rumbling, vibratory, blowing,* and *musical* are used to describe the quality of the sound.
**Ventilation and position:** Note if the murmur is affected by inspiration, expiration, or a change in body position.

---

with aortic stenosis and pulmonic stenosis are described as crescendo–decrescendo or diamond shaped (Table 17-1), meaning that the sound increases and then decreases in intensity. The quality of these murmurs is harsh, and they are of medium pitch. The murmur caused by aortic stenosis is heard best in the aortic area and may radiate into the neck. The murmur of pulmonic stenosis is heard best over the pulmonic area. In severe pulmonic stenosis, $S_2$ may be widely split.

Systolic regurgitant murmurs are caused by the backward flow of blood from an area of higher pressure to an area of lower pressure. Mitral or tricuspid valvular insufficiency or a defect in the ventricular septum produces systolic regurgitant murmurs, which are harsh and blowing in quality. The sound is described as holosystolic, meaning that the murmur begins immediately after $S_1$ and continues throughout systole up to $S_2$ (see Table 17-1).

# TABLE 17-1   Common Systolic and Diastolic Murmurs

| Type | Possible Causes | Where to Auscultate | Radiation | Pitch | Shape | Quality | Ventilation and Position |
|------|-----------------|---------------------|-----------|-------|-------|---------|--------------------------|
| **Systolic Murmurs** | | | | | | | |
| Aortic stenosis | Calcification, rheumatic fever, congenital malformation of valve cusps, degenerative process | Aortic area, right second intercostal space | Neck, upper back, right carotid, down the left sternal border to the apex | Medium | Crescendo-decrescendo May be diminished $S_1$ $S_2$ | Harsh, may be musical at the apex | Heard best with the patient sitting and leaning forward, loudest during expiration |
| Pulmonic stenosis | Congenital malformation | Pulmonic area, second and third left intercostal spaces | Left side of neck, toward left shoulder | Medium | Crescendo-decrescendo $S_1$ $S_2$ | Often harsh | Loudest during inspiration |
| Mitral regurgitation | Chronic rheumatic fever, acute bacterial endocarditis, myocardial ischemia or infarction, calcification, dilation of valvular apparatus secondary to dilated left ventricle (eg, heart failure), mitral valve prolapse | Mitral area, apex | Left axilla, less often to the left sternal border | Medium to high | Plateau Diminished $S_1$ $S_2$ | Blowing, harsh | Heard best with patient in the left lateral decubitus position, does not become louder with inspiration |
| Tricuspid regurgitation | Right ventricular failure, dilation of valvular apparatus secondary to dilated right ventricle, bacterial endocarditis (rare) | Tricuspid area, lower left sternal border | Right sternal border, to the xiphoid area, and perhaps to the left midclavicular line, but not to the axilla | Medium | Plateau Diminished $S_1$ $S_2$ | Blowing, harsh | May increase slightly with inspiration |
| **Diastolic Murmurs** | | | | | | | |
| Aortic regurgitation | Bacterial endocarditis, trauma, rheumatic fever, congenital malformation | Aortic area, right second intercostal space | Sternal border, apex | High | Decrescendo $S_1$ $S_2$ | Blowing | Heard best with the patient sitting, leaning forward, with breath held after exhalation |
| Mitral stenosis | Rheumatic fever, congenital malformation (rare) | Mitral area, apex | Usually none | Low | Decrescendo-crescendo Loud $S_1$ $S_2$ | Rumbling | Best heard with the patient in a left lateral position Mild exercise and listening during exhalation also make the murmur easier to hear |

Mitral insufficiency produces a murmur, heard most easily in the apical area with radiation to the left axilla. The type of murmur associated with tricuspid regurgitation is heard loudest at the left sternal border and increases in intensity during inspiration (see Table 17-1). Both types of regurgitant murmurs are often accompanied by a diminished $S_1$.

**DIASTOLIC MURMURS.** Diastolic murmurs occur after $S_2$ and before the next $S_1$. During diastole, the aortic and pulmonic valves are closed while the mitral and tricuspid valves are open to allow filling of the ventricles.

Aortic or pulmonic valvular insufficiency produces a blowing diastolic murmur that begins immediately after $S_2$ and decreases in intensity as regurgitant flow decreases through diastole. These murmurs are described as early diastolic decrescendo murmurs (see Table 17-1).

The murmur associated with aortic regurgitation is heard best in the aortic area and may radiate along the sternal border to the apex. Pulmonic valve regurgitation produces a murmur that is loudest in the pulmonic area.

Stenosis or narrowing of the mitral or tricuspid valve also produces a diastolic murmur. The AV valves open in mid-diastole shortly after the aortic and pulmonic valves close, causing a delay between $S_2$ and the start of the murmur of mitral and tricuspid stenosis. This murmur decreases in intensity from its onset and then increases again as ventricular filling increases because of atrial contraction; this is termed decrescendo–crescendo (see Table 17-1).

The murmur associated with mitral stenosis is heard best at the apex with the patient turned slightly to the left side. Tricuspid stenosis produces a murmur that increases in intensity with inspiration and is loudest in the fifth intercostal space along the left sternal border.

### Friction Rubs

A pericardial friction rub can be heard when the pericardial surfaces are inflamed. This high-pitched, scratchy sound is produced by these inflamed layers rubbing together. A rub may be heard anywhere over the pericardium with the diaphragm of the stethoscope. The rub may be accentuated by having the patient lean forward and exhale. A pericardial friction rub, unlike a pleural friction rub, does not vary in intensity with respiration.

## CARDIAC LABORATORY STUDIES

Knowledge of the purpose and significance of laboratory values in relation to the diagnosis and prognosis of CVD can enhance the quality of nursing care available to patients. Laboratory studies include both routine serum analysis and special studies, such as serum and cardiac enzymes.

## Routine Laboratory Studies

Appropriate assessment of normal and compromised cardiac function is essential to ensure accurate evaluation and correct diagnosis of the patient experiencing symptoms consistent with a cardiovascular disorder or CAD. Nurses can more appropriately plan the care of the patient and initiate interventions if they have an understanding of these laboratory tests and recognize their implications. Valuable information

may be obtained by assessing levels of hematologic components, coagulation factors, electrolytes, and phospholipids. Determination of these laboratory studies may vary with institutional techniques and equipment used. Normal and abnormal assay ranges have been universally established, and a brief listing of frequently ordered laboratory studies with their normal values can be found in Table 17-2. A more extensive explanation of the effects of abnormal laboratory determinations is provided elsewhere in this text.

## Hematologic Studies

Accurate assessment of the patient with a possible cardiac disorder merits review of hematologic function. It is important for the critical care nurse to understand the role of blood cells in cardiac function and their contribution to the maintenance of healthy tissue. Blood is the transport medium for nutrients, such as oxygen and glucose, as well as electrolytes, plasma proteins, hormones, and medications. It is also the vehicle for removal of the products of metabolism. Changes in blood cell integrity and total cell count may reflect specific disorders of the cardiac system and should be considered an integral part of the laboratory assessment.

Knowledge of normal blood values is vital to understand deviations from normal that can be seen with various cardiac disruptions. It is necessary to review both the red blood cell count, which assesses cellular nutrition, and the white blood cell (WBC) count, which assesses defensive capability against infections, when diagnosing specific insults. Table 17-2 lists the components of these helpful hematologic studies.

## Coagulation Studies

Coagulation studies are also warranted in the laboratory assessment of patients with cardiac disease. Establishment of a baseline for coagulation function provides important information about the patient's ability to form, maintain, and dissolve blood clots. Such information may prove instrumental in patient care decisions. This is especially true in relation to the administration of anticoagulation agents, whether for long-term management, such as warfarin for the management of atrial fibrillation, or for emergency interventions, such as the use of fibrinolytic therapy during an acute MI. Coagulation studies are listed in Table 17-2.

## Blood Chemistries

Mechanisms that ensure homeostatic function at the cellular and tissue level depend on the appropriate production and modulation of intracellular and extracellular electrolytes. It is important that the nurse understand normal electrolyte functions and the unique, perhaps life-threatening, situations that may occur when they are significantly abnormal. A thorough analysis of basic electrolyte chemistries is always appropriate in screening of the patient with cardiac disease, whether in the inpatient or outpatient setting. These studies are almost universally obtained during the initial clinical examination. The blood chemistries most commonly assessed are sodium, potassium, chloride, carbon dioxide, calcium, glucose, magnesium, and phosphorus. Table 17-2 provides the normal assay values for common electrolytes.

| TABLE 17-2 | Normal Reference Ranges for Laboratory Blood Tests | | |
|---|---|---|---|
| **Blood Test** | **Reference Range** | **Blood Test** | **Reference Range** |
| **Hematologic Studies** | | **Blood Chemistries (continued)** | |
| Red blood cell count | | Blood gases | |
| Men | $4.6–6.2 \times 10^6$ | pH | 7.35–7.45 |
| Women | $4.2–5.4 \times 10^6$ | $PaO_2$ | 80–105 mm Hg |
| Hematocrit | | $PaCO_2$ | 35–45 mm Hg |
| Men | 40%–50% | Bicarbonate | 22–29 mEq/L |
| Women | 38%–47% | Base excess, deficit | $0 \pm 2.3$ mEq/L |
| Hemoglobin | | $SaO_2$ | 98% |
| Men | 13.5–18.0 g/100 mL | $Sv–CO_2$ | 75% |
| Women | 12.0–16.0 g/100 mL | Bilirubin | |
| Corpuscle indices | | Total | 0.2–1.3 mg/dL |
| Mean corpuscular volume | 82–98 FL | Direct | 0–20 mg/dL |
| Mean corpuscular hemoglobin | 27–31 pg/cell | Calcium | |
| Mean corpuscular hemoglobin concentration | 32%–36% | Total | 8.9–10.3 mg/dL |
| | | Free (ionized) | 4.6–5.1 mg/dL |
| WBC count | | Creatinine | |
| Total | 4,500–11,000/mm$^3$ | Men | 0.9–1.4 mg/dL |
| Differential (in number of cells/mm$^3$ blood) | | Women | 0.8–1.3 mg/dL |
| Total leukocytes | 5,000–10,000 (100%) | Glucose (fasting) | 65–110 mg/dL |
| Total neutrophils | 3,000–7,000 (60%–70%) | Magnesium | 1.3–2.2 mEq/L |
| Lymphocytes | 1,500–3,000 (20%–30%) | Phosphorus | 2.5–4.5 mg/dL |
| Monocytes | 375–500 (2%–6%) | Phosphatase, alkaline | 35–148 units |
| Eosinophils | 50–400 (1%–4%) | Protein (total) | 6.5–8.5 g/dL |
| Basophils | 0–50 (0.1%) | Urea nitrogen | 8–26 mg/dL |
| Sedimentation rate | 0–30 mm/h | Uric acid | 65–110 mg/dL |
| **Coagulation Studies*** | | Men | 4.0–8.5 mg/dL |
| Platelet count | 250,000–500,000/mm$^3$ | Women | 2.8–7.5 mg/dL |
| Prothrombin time | 12–15 s | **Serum Enzymes*** | |
| Partial thromboplastin time | 60–70 s | CK-MM | 95%–100% |
| Activated partial thromboplastin time | 35–45 s | CK-MB | 0%–5% |
| Activated clotting time | 75–105 s | CK-BB | 0% |
| Fibrinogen level | 160–300 mg/dL | Aspartate aminotransferase | <50 units/L |
| Thrombin time | 11.3–18.5 s | **Myocardial Proteins** | |
| **Blood Chemistries** | | Troponin-I | <0.1 ng/mL |
| Serum electrolytes | | Troponin-T | <0.1 mcg/mL |
| Sodium | 135–145 mEq/L | Myoglobin | |
| Potassium | 3.3–4.9 mEq/L | Men | 20–90 ng/mL |
| Chloride | 97–110 mEq/L | Women | 10–75 ng/mL |
| Carbon dioxide | 22–31 mEq/L | | |

*Examples; regional laboratory techniques, and methods may result in variations.

## Common Electrolytes

Sodium is the most abundant cation in the body. It is essential in the maintenance of acid–base balance and osmolality of extracellular fluids as well as in the transmission of nerve impulses. It plays a pivotal role in fluid balance, and its concentration is primarily regulated by the kidneys. Significant alterations of cellular function are evident when sodium levels are lower than normal (hyponatremia) or greater than normal (hypernatremia).

Potassium is the major intracellular cation. Its role in the evaluation of cardiac patients is important because it is released when cells are damaged. It is essential for maintenance of oncotic pressure, intracellular osmolality, and acid–base balance, as well as for its role in cellular reactions. In addition, potassium is vital to the normal functioning of skeletal, smooth, and cardiac muscle. It is particularly important in the regulation of cardiac rate and force of contraction.

Chloride is another major extracellular cation. Like sodium and potassium, it plays a role in acid–base balance and is an important component in the evaluation of acid–base balance.

The carbon dioxide electrolyte is a reflection of carbon dioxide content (mainly bicarbonate), not carbon dioxide gas. In some settings, carbon dioxide is reported as bicarbonate ($HCO_3^-$).

## Other Blood Chemistries

Calcium, like potassium, is important for cardiac function. It plays a significant role in the initiation and propagation of electrical impulses and in myocardial contractility. It is also important for blood clotting, teeth and bone formation, and intracellular energy production. Ionized calcium (free calcium) is responsible for cardiac and neuromuscular excitability. Calcium is reported as total and free (ionized) values.

Glucose levels are important to monitor with baseline laboratory studies because they reflect the nutritive status of the cell. Alterations in glucose, such as in diabetes mellitus, can provide the clinician with both diagnostic as well as prognostic information.

Magnesium is the second major intracellular cation after potassium. It is important in many metabolic processes and is necessary for the normal functioning of the neuromuscular system. It facilitates enzyme activities that help maintain protein synthesis and metabolism, carbohydrate and lipid metabolism, and nucleic acid synthesis. Alterations in normal magnesium levels are reflected in disruptions in neuromuscular activity, such as in the patient with dysrhythmia.

Phosphorus reflects levels of serum phosphate. It is controlled by the parathyroid gland and regulated in the kidneys. Phosphate is important for normal cellular function and for oxygen delivery. It is reciprocal to calcium. Abnormalities can be seen with alterations in heart rate, alterations in neuromuscular function, and reciprocal changes in serum calcium.

## Serum Lipid Studies

A review of serum lipid levels is a critical part of the information needed by the nurse to assess cardiovascular risk in any given patient. Patients without a history of CAD need lipid analysis for primary prevention (ie, prevention of the development of CAD). Patients with a new or past history of CAD need lipid analysis for secondary prevention to prevent progression of known disease after a cardiac event. Standard elements of a lipid profile are total cholesterol, low-density lipoprotein cholesterol (LDL-C), very low-density lipoprotein cholesterol (VLDL-C), high-density lipoprotein cholesterol (HDL-C), and triglycerides. Treatment of lipids for primary and secondary prevention is based on LDL-C and triglyceride values, as well as age and the presence of relevant comorbidities such as diabetes mellitus.

In 2013, the American Heart Association (AHA) and American College of Cardiology (ACC) updated their guidelines for care of patients with a history of coronary and other atherosclerotic diseases.[5] The ACC/AHA guidelines, along with the National Cholesterol Education Program (NCEP) Adult Treatment Panel (ATP) IV, identified four major "statin benefit groups."[5] Table 17-3 summarizes the recommended treatment for each group. The ACC/AHA's suggested approach to identifying patients in need of cholesterol reduction therapy was controversial, largely because it represented a departure from previous treatment guidelines, which had advocated for treating to specific LDL-C or non-HDL-C target goals. However, after examining available evidence, the ACC/AHA elected to categorize patients based on the presence or absence of arteriosclerotic cardiovascular disease (ASCVD), age, and the presence of diabetes. The patient's tolerance of statin therapy also affected the decision to treat. There was also a new emphasis on lifestyle modification as the foundation for the reduction of ASCVD risk (see Table 17-3). The nurse is ideally positioned to advocate for this element of care.

Cholesterol, a pearly, fatlike substance, is a precursor of bile acids and steroid hormones. Most of the body's cholesterol is synthesized in the liver, but some is absorbed from the diet. The NCEP IV recommends treatment with statins to decrease the probability of CAD in patients with no history of cardiac disease, and to slow the progression of disease in patients with known CAD. Patients with known CAD should be treated with statin therapy if they have no contraindications for the class of drugs.[5]

LDL-C constitutes 60% to 70% of the total cholesterol in the bloodstream. Based on numerous large-scale studies, LDL-C is known to be directly correlated with the development of CAD and subsequent CVD in susceptible individuals. Current guidelines recommend initiation of therapy in individuals without known CAD when LDL-C is greater than 190 mg/dL or when triglycerides are greater than 500 mg/dL. All patients with known CAD should be started on statin therapy as long as no contraindications exist.[5]

Triglyceride originates from VLDL-C. Although VLDL-C is not considered to be atherogenic, elevated levels can be a

| TABLE 17-3 | Statin Benefit Groups and Treatment Recommendations | |
|---|---|---|
| | **Treatment Groups** | **Treatment Recommendations** |
| Group 1: | Individuals with clinical ASCVD (ACS, MI, angina, coronary or other revascularization) | Heart-healthy lifestyle habits<br>Age less than 75 years old, high-intensity statin or moderate-intensity statin if not a candidate for high-intensity statin<br>Age greater than 75 years old, or if not a candidate for high-intensity statin, moderate intensity statin |
| Group 2: | Individuals with primary elevations of LDL-C greater than 70–189 mg/dL | Heart-healthy lifestyle habits<br>High-intensity statin or moderate-intensity statin if not a candidate for high-intensity statin |
| Group 3: | Individuals 40–75 years of age with diabetes with LDL-C 70–189 mg/dL | Heart-healthy lifestyle habits<br>Moderate-intensity statin if 10-year ASCVD risk less than 7.5%<br>High-intensity statin if 10-year ASCVD risk greater than 7.5% |
| Group 4: | Individuals without clinical ASCVD or diabetes who are 40–75 years of age with LDL-C 70–189 mg/dL and an estimated 10-year ASCVD risk of 7.5% or greater | Heart-healthy lifestyle habits<br>Moderate- to high-intensity statin |

Adapted from Stone NJ, Robinson J, Lichtenstein, AH, et al: 2013 ACC/AHA Guideline on the Treatment of Blood Cholesterol to Reduce Atherosclerotic Cardiovascular Risk in Adults: A Report of the American College of Cardiology/American Heart Association Task Force on Practice Guidelines. Circulation published online November 12, 2013.

**TABLE 17-4  Lipid Abnormalities and Associated Mechanisms**

| Lipid Abnormality | Mechanisms |
|---|---|
| Elevated total cholesterol | High dietary intake of saturated fat and cholesterolLDL receptor deficiency or downregulation |
| Elevated LDL cholesterol | LDL receptor deficiency |
| | Apoprotein B-100 genetic defect |
| | High dietary intake of saturated fat and cholesterol |
| Elevated triglycerides | Deficiency in lipoprotein lipase |
| | Obesity, physical inactivity, insulin resistance, glucose intolerance |
| | Excessive alcohol intake |
| Low HDL | Apoprotein A-1 deficiency |
| | Reduced VLDL clearance |
| | Cigarette smoking, physical inactivity |
| | Insulin resistance |
| | Elevated triglycerides |
| | Overweight and obesity |
| | Very high CHO intake (more than 60% total calories), certain drugs (beta-blockers, anabolic steroids, progestational agents) |
| Increased lipoprotein remnants (VLDL is a surrogate marker for lipoprotein remnants when Tg is more than 200 mg/dL) | Defective apolipoprotein E, seen in familial combined hyperlipidemia |
| Lipoprotein(a) | Level is genetically determined |
| Small LDL particles | Particle size is determined by level of Tg; LDL particle is denser and more atherogenic at higher levels of Tg |
| HDL subspecies | Low levels of HDL 2 and 3 may increase CVD risk, genetically determined vs. lifestyle and other lipid levels |
| Apolipoprotein B | May be potential marker for all atherogenic lipoproteins |
| Apolipoprotein A-1 | Increased CVD risk when Apo A-1 is low |
| Combined dyslipidemias (small, dense LDL, high triglycerides, low HDL, elevated LDL and triglycerides) | Defects in VLDL and LDL receptor activities coexisting with environmental influences such as obesity, physical inactivity, diet high in saturated fat, and cigarette smoking |

HDL, high-density lipoprotein; LDL, low-density lipoprotein; Tg, triglycerides; VLDL, very-low-density lipoprotein; CHO, cholesterol.
From Woods SL, Froelicher ESS, Motzer SU, et al: Cardiac Nursing, 6th ed. Philadelphia, PA: Lippincott, Williams & Wilkins, 2009.

marker for a genetic form of cholesterol disorder. The NCEP ATP IV recommends treatment of triglycerides above 500 mg/dL because of the association between hypertriglyceridemia and pancreatitis.[5] Table 17-4 describes lipid abnormalities and associated mechanisms.

## Enzyme Studies

Enzymes are found in all living cells and act as catalysts in biochemical reactions. They are present in low amounts in the serum of healthy people. When cells are injured, enzymes leak from damaged cells, resulting in serum enzyme concentrations greater than the usual low levels.

No single enzyme is specific to the cells of a single organ. Each organ contains a variety of enzymes, and there is considerable overlap among organs in the enzymes they contain. However, the distribution of enzymes in the cells of organs is relatively organ specific. When organ damage occurs, the presence of abnormally high levels of enzymes in the serum, their distribution, and the timing of their appearance and disappearance make the clinical use of serum enzyme studies relevant.

Cardiac enzymes are enzymes found in cardiac tissue. When cardiac injury occurs, as in acute MI, these enzymes are released into the serum, and their concentrations can be measured. Cardiac tissue enzymes are present in other organs as well, so elevation of one or more of these enzymes is not a specific indicator of cardiac injury. However, because cardiac damage does result in above-normal serum concentrations of these enzymes, the quantification of cardiac enzyme levels, along with other diagnostic tests and the clinical presentation of the patient, is routinely used for diagnosing cardiac disease, particularly acute MI.

The challenge is to identify an enzyme or "marker" that correctly identifies cardiac cell death. In essence, a cardiac marker is a surrogate for thrombus formation in the coronary arteries. An ideal marker for cardiac injury should have several important characteristics. It should be easy to measure; be inexpensive; be cardiac specific, with a direct proportional relationship between the extent of myocardial injury and the measured level of the marker (zero blood concentration in the absence of cardiac injury); have rapid serum levels after the onset of injury; and stay in the serum long enough to be measured in patients who delay seeking treatment. No available biomarkers fit these criteria, but troponins, discussed later in this text, have several important features, making them the most useful of the biomarkers at present.

Since 2000, the Multinational Third Global Taskforce, representing the European Society of Cardiology, The American College of Cardiology Foundation, the AHA, and the World Heart Federation, has been tasked with providing a cohesive definition of MI. In their third set of guidelines, published in 2012, they outlined the appropriate use of cardiac enzymes to detect myocardial necrosis. Historically held biomarkers such as myoglobin, CK, and CK-MB are no longer recommended for use. In the Third Universal Definition of Myocardial Infarction, the preferred biomarker of necrosis is the highly sensitive and specific cardiac troponin (cTn).[6]

## Biochemical Markers: Myocardial Proteins

Troponins are cardiac proteins that are released into the circulation after necrosis and rupture of myocardial cells. Three subforms have been identified: cardiac troponin-I (cTnI), troponin-T (cTnT), and troponin-C (cTnC). Both cTnI and cTnT are highly specific to cardiac tissue. Assays for both isoforms have become increasingly sensitive, and very minute elevations of the troponins can be detected. Both cTnI and cTnT have equal sensitivity and specificity in detecting myocardial necrosis. Troponins will be detectable in the blood 2 to 3 hours after myocardial damage occurs, and values will remain elevated for up to 6 days (Box 17-6).

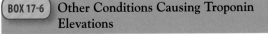

**BOX 17-6** Other Conditions Causing Troponin Elevations

- Sepsis/systemic inflammatory response syndrome
- Hypovolemia
- Supraventricular tachycardia
- Stroke
- Heart failure
- Pulmonary embolism
- Myocarditis
- Pulmonary hypertension
- Myocardial contusion
- Renal failure
- Left ventricular hypertrophy
- Chronic obstructive pulmonary disease

## Neurohumoral Hormones: Brain-Type Natriuretic Peptide

Brain-type natriuretic peptides (BNP) and pro-BNP are neurohormonal hormones released by the heart in response to decompensation. BNP and pro-BNP are sometimes used in evaluating patients with heart failure. BNP and pro-BNP are discussed more thoroughly in Chapter 20.

## CARDIAC DIAGNOSTIC STUDIES

Cardiovascular diagnostic techniques have expanded dramatically in the past few years, especially in the area of noninvasive testing. Understanding the principles on which the procedures are based enables the nurse to answer questions, incorporate diagnostic findings into the patient's plan of care, and provide high-level nursing care. The critical care nurse also can decrease the anxiety of patients and their families by providing an explanation of the procedure.

## Standard 12-Lead Electrocardiogram

The standard ECG records electrical impulses as they travel through the heart. In patients with normal conduction, the first electrical impulse for each cardiac cycle originates in the sinus node and is spread to the rest of the heart through the specialized conduction system—the intra-atrial tracts, AV node, bundle of His, and right and left bundles. As the impulse traverses the conduction system, it penetrates the surrounding myocardium and provides the electrical stimuli for atrial and ventricular contraction. The change in electrical potential in cells of the specialized conduction system as the impulse proceeds is very small and cannot be measured from electrodes outside the body. However, the change in electrical potential of myocardial cells produces an electrical signal that can be recorded from the surface of the body, as is done with an ECG.

Impulses that originate in sites other than the sinus node or impulses that are prevented from traversing the conduction system because of disease or drugs interrupt the normal order of electrical sequences in the myocardium. An ECG may be used to record these abnormal patterns of impulse formation or conduction. A clinician then has a visual record of the abnormal pattern from which to identify the dysrhythmia.

In addition, an abnormal ECG tracing may result from diseased myocardial cells. For example, in patients with left ventricular enlargement, impulses traversing the enlarged muscle mass of the left ventricle produce a larger electrical signal than normal. In contrast, impulses are unable to traverse myocardial cells that are irreversibly damaged, such as in MI, and no electrical signal is present in the infarcted cells of the left ventricle.

### Procedure

The standard 12-lead ECG is so named because the usual electrode placement and recording device permit the electrical signal to be registered from 12 different views. The four limb and six precordial lead wires are attached to the patient as shown in Figure 17-7. For the limb leads, the recording device alternates the combination of electrodes that are active during recording of electrical signals from the heart (Fig. 17-8). This results in six standard views or leads (I, II, III, augmented voltage of the right arm [aVR], augmented voltage of the left arm [aVL], and augmented voltage of the left foot [aVF]) that are recorded in the heart's frontal plane. The six precordial leads ($V_1$, $V_2$, $V_3$, $V_4$, $V_5$, and $V_6$) are arranged across the chest to record electrical activity in the heart's horizontal plane (see Fig. 17-7).[7]

Used routinely in intensive care unit (ICU) patients, ECGs assess dysrhythmias and myocardial ischemia or MI. An ECG is performed easily at the bedside, with the patient ideally placed in the supine position and the electrodes arranged as previously described. In some patients, chest bandages may preclude placement of the precordial leads. It is important that the patient remain still during the ECG recording so that skeletal muscle movement does not result in extraneous noise or artifact in the electrical signal. Additional horizontal plane leads may be recorded by placing electrodes on the right side of the chest to view right ventricular activity or the back of the chest to view left ventricular posterior wall activity (see Fig. 17-7).

In the clinical setting, it is important that the nurse remembers where the positive electrode is located in each of the 12 leads of the ECG. The positive electrode is like a camera and provides a view of the heart from that perspective. In lead I, the positive electrode is on the patient's LA, giving a left lateral view of the heart. In leads II and III, the positive electrode is on the patient's left leg (LL), resulting in an inferior view of the heart. For the augmented leads, the name of the lead corresponds with the placement of the positive electrode. In lead aVR, the view of the heart is poor because the positive electrode is far from the heart on the right arm. In lead aVL, the positive electrode is on the LA, providing a left lateral view of the heart. In lead aVF, the positive electrode is placed on the patient's LL, resulting in an inferior view of the heart. Each of the electrodes placed on the patient's chest is a positive electrode. Therefore, $V_1$ through $V_4$ provide a view of the anteroseptal wall of the heart, and $V_5$ and $V_6$ provide a view of the left lateral wall of the heart. Figure 17-9A and B shows the six limb leads in the frontal plane and the six chest leads in the horizontal plane, and the location of the positive electrode in each. The right-sided chest leads $V_4R$ through $V_6R$ offer the best view of the right ventricle. Leads $V_7$ through $V_9$ give the best view of the posterior wall of the

Supplemental Right Precordial Leads

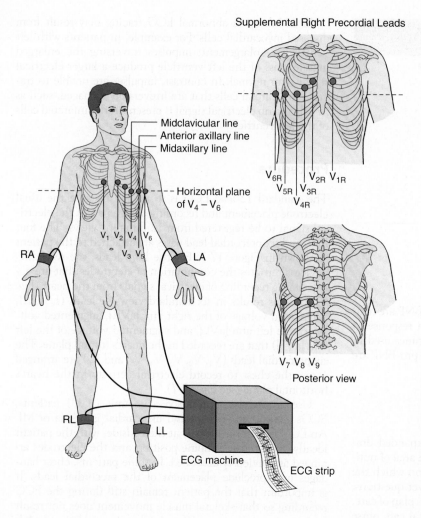

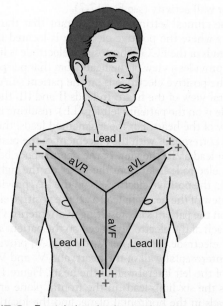

**FIGURE 17-7** ECG electrode placement. The standard left precordial leads are $V_1$, fourth intercostal space, right sternal border; $V_2$, fourth intercostal space, left sternal border; $V_3$, diagonally between $V_2$ and $V_4$; $V_4$, fifth intercostal space, left midclavicular line; $V_5$, same horizontal line as $V_4$, midway between $V_4$ and $V_6$; $V_6$, same horizontal line as $V_4$ and $V_5$, midaxillary line. The right precordial leads, placed across the right side of the chest, are the mirror opposite of the left leads. For the posterior leads, $V_7$ is placed at the left posterior axillary line, $V_8$ is placed at the left midscapular line, and $V_9$ is placed at the left border of the spine. All are placed on the same horizontal line as $V_6$.

heart (see Fig. 17-7). Table 17-5 summarizes the electrocardiographic leads and the corresponding views of the heart.

## Nursing Assessment and Management

Critical care nurses often record an ECG when there is a change in patient status, such as the development of dysrhythmias. Evaluation of a rhythm strip in relation to dysrhythmias is discussed later in this chapter. Often, an ECG is obtained during episodes of chest pain before and after the administration of sublingual nitroglycerin. The ECG provides documentation of ST-segment changes associated with the pain.

Some patients fear being shocked by the ECG recorder. Preparatory instruction for patients should include an explanation of the manner in which the electrical impulses of the heart are recorded and that the patient will feel no sensation during the recording of the ECG.

## Electrophysiologic Studies

## Holter or 24-Hour Monitoring

Holter monitoring involves the use of ECG monitoring to quantify the frequency and complexity of cardiac ectopic

**FIGURE 17-8** Frontal plane leads: standard limb leads, I, II, III, plus augmented leads aVR, aVL, and aVF. This allows an examination of electrical conduction across a variety of planes (eg, LA to LL, RA to left arm).

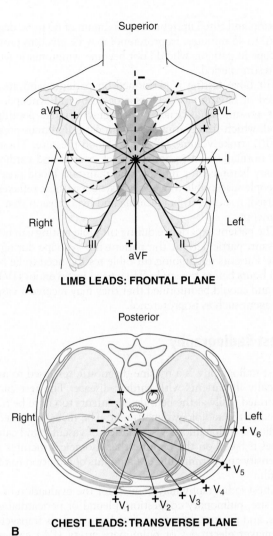

**FIGURE 17-9 A:** Positioning of the positive and negative electrodes for the limb leads in the frontal plane. **B:** Positioning of the positive electrodes on the chest wall giving a horizontal plane view. (From Bickley L: Bates' Guide to Physical Examination and Health History, 10th ed. Philadelphia, PA: Lippincott Williams & Wilkins, 2009, p 331.)

activity that occurs during a patient's usual activities. It is a noninvasive method of assessing for dysrhythmias, response to antiarrhythmic therapy, and development of ECG changes suggestive of ischemia.

Holter monitoring involves placement of anterior chest electrodes that are then connected to a portable recording device, or Holter monitor. The Holter monitor is a small recording device that may be carried in a shirt pocket and is worn

| TABLE 17-5 | Electrocardiographic Leads and Corresponding Views of the Heart |
| --- | --- |
| **Lead** | **View of the Heart** |
| II, III, aVF | Inferior |
| I, aVL, V$_5$, and V$_6$ | Left lateral |
| V$_1$ through V$_4$ | Anteroseptal |
| Right-sided V$_4$ through V$_6$ | Right ventricle |
| V$_7$ through V$_9$ | Posterior |

for about 24 to 48 hours. Holter monitoring is indicated for patients with syncope, near syncope, dizziness, or palpitations. Patients with infrequent symptoms may not benefit from this method of gathering data because Holter monitoring is most useful in patients who are experiencing their dysrhythmias multiple times in a day. Holter monitoring is rarely used in the inpatient setting where telemetry monitoring is also available.

Holter monitoring requires significant patient participation. Patients receive instructions about keeping a diary to record medications, activities, and symptoms during the monitoring period. Usually, patients should maintain normal activities while wearing the monitor and record an entry in the diary at least every 2 hours. An understanding of the physical and emotional stressors, as well as the patient's symptoms, enhances analysis of the recordings. Compliance with record keeping is necessary.

## Event (Continuous Loop) Monitoring

In event (continuous loop) monitoring, the patient wears electrodes and a recording device, but the device does not record continuously. Instead, the patient is required to activate the recorder when a symptom occurs, and recording can go on for the duration of symptoms. The ECG is recorded on a continuous loop tape so that information before, during, and after the event is recorded. Results can be communicated to a monitoring agency by telephone, allowing for rapid analysis and feedback to patient and caregiver. Cardiac event recorders can be worn for up to 1 month.

Cardiac event recorders are most useful for patients who have relatively infrequent episodes of dysrhythmias, who are aware and able to respond to symptoms, and who are willing to wear electrodes and carry the recorder, possibly for as long as a month. As with Holter monitoring, electrode placement on clean, intact skin is crucial. Electrodes must be kept in place for the duration of the study, making immersion bathing impractical. The patient diary, a source of detailed information, requires significant participation on the part of the patient.

## Implantable Loop Monitoring

The implantable loop monitor (ILR) is a device that is implanted subcutaneously and provides continuous ECG monitoring for up to 14 months. ILRs were developed to provide long-term monitoring for patients with presyncope and syncope. The major limitations of the ILR are its requirement for subcutaneous implantation and cost. The use of the device requires familiarity with implantation techniques and programming. The ILR is used for patients in whom less expensive tests, such as Holter monitoring, have failed to provide a diagnosis.

Implantation of the ILR is a surgical procedure that exposes the patient to the risk of infection and bleeding. Patients undergoing ILR implantation must understand the potential risks of the procedure. They need instruction regarding postoperative site care and use of the device.

## Diagnostic Electrophysiology Study

The diagnostic electrophysiology study is a type of heart catheterization during which access to the heart is obtained through the femoral veins, or, for some more complex studies, the upper extremity (brachial, external jugular, or subclavian) veins. Multiple catheters are usually placed in one or more vessels. An arterial line is typically placed to provide continuous blood pressure monitoring during the case.

Diagnostic electrophysiology studies are performed to evaluate a broad spectrum of cardiac dysrhythmias. They can help assess the function of the sinoatrial (SA) node, the AV node, and the His-Purkinje system; determine the characteristics of reentrant dysrhythmias; map the location of dysrhythmogenic foci for potential ablation; and assess the efficacy of antiarrhythmic drugs and devices. The basic electrophysiology protocol involves measurement of baseline conduction intervals; atrial pacing to assess SA node and AV node properties; assessment of the His-Purkinje system conductivity; ventricular pacing to evaluate for retrograde conduction and ventricular dysrhythmia potentials; and drug testing.

Diagnostic electrophysiology studies are very safe. The risks associated with the procedure are similar to those encountered with cardiac catheterization and include hemorrhage, thromboembolism, phlebitis, and infection. Because most diagnostic electrophysiology studies do not require arterial puncture, the risk of serious vascular damage is very low. The risk of death due to the induction of lethal dysrhythmias is close to zero, in part because the procedural setting is uniquely equipped to terminate hemodynamically unstable dysrhythmias.

The following preprocedure preparations are necessary for patients undergoing diagnostic electrophysiology studies:

- The physician or nurse reviews the procedure so that the patient clearly understands its purpose and nature. Appropriate personnel obtain informed consent.
- Because sedation is used, the patient must be NPO for 8 hours before the procedure.
- The ordering physician or nurse practitioner must review patient medications to be sure they are to be administered on the day of the procedure. Antiarrhythmic drugs are typically withdrawn before the procedure.
- Excessive anxiety can increase catecholamine release and affect sympathetic tone, so the nurse should alert the ordering physician or nurse practitioner to signs of anxiety.

Postprocedure, the following nursing care applies:

- The nurse checks the patient's blood pressure and heart and respiratory rates frequently according to the institution's protocols.
- If the diagnostic electrophysiology study failed to induce dysrhythmias, the patient may not require telemetry monitoring. If dysrhythmias were induced, the patient does need continuous telemetry monitoring.
- The nurse monitors venous and arterial access sites for bleeding. This monitoring may include serial complete blood counts to ensure stable hemoglobin and hematocrit counts.

## Tilt Table Testing for Syncope

Tilt table testing, or upright tilt table testing, refers to maintaining the patient in a head-up position for a brief period to provoke syncope, bradycardia, or hypotension. In tilt table testing, the patient is positioned on a tilt table in the supine position and tilted upright to a maximum of 60 to 80 degrees for 20 to 45 minutes. Isoproterenol may be given to provoke syncope in patients who do not become symptomatic within the testing period.

Tilt table testing is performed on patients who are suspected of having vasodepressor or vasovagal syncope. Upright posture is associated with gravitational pooling of blood, which results in a decline in central venous pressure (CVP), stroke volume (SV), and blood pressure. These effects normally lead to activation of arterial and cardiopulmonary baroreceptor reflexes that maintain blood pressure. In people susceptible to vasovagal syncope, these reflexes are reversed, resulting in bradycardia and hypotension that lead to syncope.

The patient experience during tilt table testing can be unpleasant, particularly if the patient has syncope during the study. Patients undergoing tilt table testing need to be NPO for 8 hours before the study. They need intravenous (IV) access and should be informed that they may receive a vasoactive agent such as isoproterenol.

## Chest Radiography

Chest radiography is a routine diagnostic test used to assess critically ill patients with cardiac disease. The test can be performed easily at the bedside in patients too ill to be transported to the radiology department. The image obtained on a radiograph that allows visualization of vascular and cardiac shapes is based on the premise that thoracic structures vary in density and permit different amounts of radiation to reach the film.

Chest radiography may be used for the evaluation of cardiac size, pulmonary congestion, pleural or pericardial effusions, and position of intracardiac lines, such as transvenous pacemaker electrodes or pulmonary artery (PA) catheters. Figure 17-10 shows the structures that can be seen on a normal posteroanterior chest radiograph.

### Procedure

Cardiac size is evaluated best in the radiology department, where the procedure can be standardized with the patient standing and the radiograph taken from posterior and lateral views at a distance of 6 feet. Portable bedside chest radiographs are usually taken only from an anterior view with the patient lying supine or sitting erect and are not standardized.

Patients undergoing radiography of the chest are instructed not to move while the radiograph is being taken. Proper positioning of the radiographic plate behind the patient is important to ensure that thoracic structures are aligned on the film. Care is taken to remove all metal objects, including fasteners on clothing, from the field of view because metal blocks the x-ray beam. Patients are usually asked to take a deep breath and hold it when the radiograph is taken to displace the diaphragm downward; this may be uncomfortable for patients who have undergone recent thoracic surgery.

### Nursing Assessment and Management

The critical care nurse's role in obtaining diagnostic thoracic radiographic films is often limited to the ICU, where portable

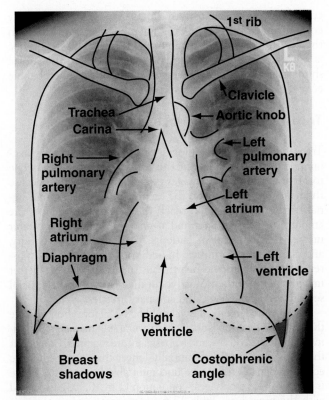

**FIGURE 17-10** Outline of structures visible on normal postero-anterior chest radiograph. (Adapted from Woods SL, Froelicher ESS, Motzer SU, Bridges EJ: Cardiac Nursing, 6th ed. Philadelphia, PA: Lippincott Williams & Wilkins, 2010, p 268.)

radiographs are made. With unstable patients, the nurse must decide when the film can be taken. It is important that IV lines not become tangled or loosened while one is trying to place the radiographic plate in the proper position.

Female patients of childbearing potential should have a lead drape placed over the abdomen to protect the ovaries from any radiation scatter. For the same reason, caregivers and family members should leave the patient's room when the radiograph is taken. When caregivers cannot leave the patient's bedside, a lead apron should be worn.

## Echocardiography

Echocardiography refers to a group of tests that use ultrasound technology to provide information about cardiac structures. Specifically, a transducer emits ultrasound waves and receives a signal from the reflected sound waves; it alternates periods of sound transmission and reception. As the sound waves are emitted and travel through tissues with a homogeneous density, such as when the sound waves move through the left ventricular wall, the signal travels in a straight line. When the density of the structures changes, such as when the waves move from the ventricular wall into the blood-filled left ventricle, the direction of the sound waves changes, and this difference is recorded by the receiver. These density changes are called interfaces, and they form the basis for distinguishing one structure from another. Ultrasound waves do not travel well through bone; thus, bony paths are avoided during the examination.

Echocardiography is most often used to assess ejection fraction, wall motion and thickness, systolic and diastolic ventricular volumes, valvular function and disease, vegetations, intracardiac masses or thrombi, and pericardial fluid. It is a helpful diagnostic tool in the presence of sudden clinical deterioration in acute MI, in which significant complications may be observed or suspected. In addition, it may also be used in evaluating function of all four cardiac valves, including calculation of gradients and orifice size, intracardiac tumors, and aortic dissection. Contrast echocardiography is a technique for improving resolution during echocardiographic studies. Agitated saline solution, injected intravenously, is used to identify intracardiac shunts. In addition, several phospholipid IV contrast agents have been developed to improve visualization of the endocardial border. These agents would be used when visualization of the endocardial border is hindered by body habitus or artifact.

The quality and usefulness of echocardiographic studies depend on the relative age of the technology being used, the skill of the technologist performing the study, the habitus of the patient, and the skill of the study's interpreter. Accuracy may decrease up to 20% in patients who are obese or who have chronic obstructive pulmonary disease or chest wall deformities. These physical features increase the distance the ultrasound waves must travel and thus increase the likelihood of artifact. Transthoracic echocardiography is of limited usefulness in investigating the left atrium and left atrial (LA) appendage because these structures are at the back of the heart.

Echocardiography is performed in a specifically designed laboratory with dim lighting and minimal sound distraction. It can also be performed at the bedside with lighting optimized to enhance the quality of the study. Patients should be able to tolerate lying flat or nearly flat. The technician asks them periodically to change position, and they should be able to turn onto their left side for several minutes at a time. In addition, they should be able to breathe in deeply or hold their breath. They do not need to be fasting.

### M-Mode Echocardiography

Motion mode, or M-mode, echocardiography allows recording of amplitude and of the rate of motion of moving objects with great accuracy. It is often referred to as an "ice pick" view because it uses a single beam of sound that allows a small region of the heart to be visualized at any point in time. The four positions of the transducer depicted in Figure 17-11 are the typical views used during an M-mode echocardiogram. It provides rapid assessment of valvular motion and chamber wall thickness. The transmitter is placed on the anterior chest in an intercostal space or subcostal position to avoid bony structures.

### Two-Dimensional Echocardiography

Two-dimensional (2D) images of cardiac structures can be obtained by using multiple crystals to generate a cross-sectional imaging plane. The ultrasound beam is pie shaped, resulting in a "plane" of reflected echoes. Visually, 2D echocardiography creates a cross-sectional slice of the heart from parasternal, subcostal, apical, and suprasternal positions. This approach is

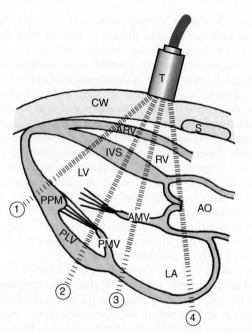

FIGURE 17-11 Echocardiographic views of the heart. A cross-section of the heart shows the structures through which the ultrasonic beam passes as it is directed from the apex (1) toward the base (4) of the heart. AMV, anterior mitral valve; AO, aorta; ARV, anterior right ventricular wall; CW, chest wall; IVS, interventricular septum; LA, left atrium; LV, left ventricle; PLV, posterior left ventricular wall; PMV, posterior mitral valve; PPM, posterior papillary muscle; RV, right ventricular cavity; S, sternum; T, transducer.

useful for evaluating the thickness of the left ventricular wall, left ventricular wall mass, and wall motion abnormalities.

## Three-Dimensional Echocardiography

3D echocardiography allows for the imaging and analysis of cardiac structures as they move in time and space. 3D echocardiography uses the principles of ultrasound imaging with advanced real-time reconstruction capabilities to generate a more authentic representation of the heart. Early in the evolution of 3D echocardiography, the generated images required lengthy postprocedure processing, which meant that immediate results were not available. Current technology allows for real-time images, making this modality a valuable diagnostic and treatment tool.

## Doppler Echocardiography

Doppler echocardiography superimposes Doppler techniques on either M-mode or 2D images. The direction of blood flow can be assessed by measuring echoes reflected from red blood cells as they move away from or toward the transducer. This type of study is particularly useful in patients with valvular disease. Stenotic valves cause turbulence in the forward flow of blood through the heart, and regurgitant valves cause turbulence in blood flowing retrograde through the cardiac chambers. When the direction of flow is color encoded, the study is known as a color Doppler echocardiogram. Audio signals are usually recorded during Doppler studies. Contrast material may also be used in conjunction with M-mode or 2D echocardiography. Although many agents have been used as

contrast material, almost any liquid injected intravenously contains microbubbles. As the microbubbles travel through the heart, they produce multiple echoes. This technique is especially useful in identifying right-to-left intracardiac shunts because of the early appearance of the microbubble echoes on the left atrium or ventricle.

## Transesophageal Echocardiography

Transesophageal echocardiography (TEE) involves the placement of a 2D transducer at the end of a flexible endoscope to obtain high-quality images of cardiac structures. Because the heart rests directly on the esophagus, the ultrasound signal travels millimeters to reach the heart. This reduces the amount of signal artifact and attenuation, yielding a clearer image. TEE is useful in patients with emphysema, obesity, and chest wall deformities. In addition, TEE provides a posterior approach to the heart; thus, it also allows for better imaging of the aorta, PA, valves of the heart, both atria, atrial septum, LA appendage, and coronary arteries.

Patients undergoing TEE should be NPO for 6 hours before the study. IV sedation is given, and several staff members, including technicians, nurses, and a physician, are required throughout the study. TEE takes substantially longer than a transthoracic echocardiogram and can be uncomfortable for patients. There is also a risk for esophageal perforation (1 in 10,000) associated with the procedure. Table 17-6 summarizes nursing considerations for caring for the patient undergoing TEE.

## Bedside Vascular Access Testing

Obtaining vascular access in a critically ill patient frequently represents a challenge. Portable devices have been designed for use at the bedside to locate vascular anatomy in real time, allowing placement of IV lines with great accuracy.

## Intravascular Ultrasound

Intravascular ultrasound (IVUS) uses ultrasound technology to visualize the lumen and wall structure of the coronary arteries. Optical coherence tomography (OCT) is a CT scan–based technology that also provides additional information on the structure of coronary arteries. Both methods are adjuncts to cardiac catheterization and are discussed more fully in that section (see Cardiac Catheterization, Coronary Angiography, and Coronary Intervention).

## Stress Testing

Stress testing is an important tool in the evaluation of the patient with suspected ischemic CVD. Stress testing is used to assess prognosis and to determine functional capacity. Stress testing involves monitoring physiologic parameters, such as blood pressure and ECG, when the heart is in a resting state and again when the heart has been stressed either by exercise or by a pharmacologic agent chosen to simulate exercise. A great deal of more information can be obtained by also looking at images of the heart at rest and with activity. These images can be obtained by a variety of methods, including radioactive tracers and echocardiography. Box 17-7 presents indications and contraindications for stress testing. The

| TABLE 17-6 | Nursing Interventions for the Patient Undergoing Transesophageal Echocardiography (TEE) | |
|---|---|
| **Nursing Action** | **Rationale** |
| **Preprocedure** | |
| 1. Evaluate patient for contraindications | Patients with history of dysphagia or esophageal disease are not candidates for TEE |
| 2. Instruct patient and family about procedure | Some discomfort may occur; patient will receive moderate sedation but will be closely monitored |
| 3. Ensure that documented patient history is adequate and informed consent has been signed | Medication allergies should be noted; procedure requires consent signature |
| 4. Ensure that patient has been NPO for 6 h before procedure | Aspiration precaution is vital |
| 5. Prepare patient for procedure | Remove oral prosthetics, as indicated; have patient void |
| 6. Insert peripheral IV catheter | IV access is required for routine medication administration; emergency vascular access line should be available |
| 7. Place patient on cardiac monitor with blood pressure and pulse oximetry | Patient must be continually monitored during procedure |
| 8. Ensure that emergency resuscitation equipment is nearby, including medications, defibrillator, and suction apparatus | Cardiac arrest precaution |
| **During Procedure** | |
| 1. Monitor cardiac rhythm, blood pressure, pulse oximetry, and airway patency per institutional policy | Continuous observation is required after moderate sedation |
| 2. Assist physician with patient positioning and endoscope placement | Allaying fears enhances patient cooperation<br>Vagal stimulation may occur with a resultant vasovagal reaction; transient tachycardia/bradycardia and blood pressure alterations may appear; patient may experience hypoxia or laryngospasm |
| 3. Monitor for complications | |
| 4. Reassure patient throughout procedure | Allaying fears enhances patient cooperation |
| 5. Document patient response to procedures | Per institutional protocol |
| **Postprocedure** | |
| 1. Assess vital signs at conclusion of procedure; document per institutional policy | Comparison with baseline is necessary to monitor sedation recovery |
| 2. Assist patient to position of comfort or on one side | Position provides comfort and patent airway support<br>Prudent, given aspiration risk |
| 3. Keep patient NPO until gag reflex is assessed | Interventions provide patient opportunity to clear residual secretions and obtain comfort |
| 4. If gag reflex is present, encourage patient to cough; offer lozenges or ice to soothe sore throat; keep NPO per physician order | If patient was sedated during procedure, it is best if family member or another drives patient home |
| 5. If outpatient, instruct patient not to drive for at least 12 h | If symptoms of complications occur, patient should be reevaluated |
| 6. Instruct patient to seek care or contact physician in event of dyspnea, hemoptysis, or severe pain | |

BOX 17-7 **Indications and Contraindications for Stress Testing**

Indications
- Differential diagnosis of chest pain (ie, evaluation of patients with suspected ischemic heart disease)
- Assessment of the level of exercise at which ischemic manifestations occur in a patient with known ischemic heart disease
- Evaluation of therapy for dysrhythmias and angina
- Evaluation of functional disability secondary to organic heart disease (eg, valvular heart disease)
- Risk stratification of the asymptomatic patient with multiple risk factors for ischemic heart disease

Contraindications
- Recent MI (4 to 6 weeks), except when submaximal protocols are used (65% of maximum predicted heart rate or symptom-limited exercise stress testing before hospital discharge)
- Unstable angina or angina at rest
- Rapid ventricular or atrial dysrhythmias
- Advanced AV block, unless chronic
- Uncompensated congestive heart failure
- Acute noncardiac illnesses
- Severe aortic stenosis
- Blood pressure greater than 170/100 mm Hg before the onset of exercise

contraindications largely relate to advanced disease states; stress testing in patients with these conditions could precipitate a catastrophic event.

Fundamentally, stress testing provides information about the heart's response to activity. The heart extracts 70% of the oxygen carried by each unit of blood perfusing the myocardium. Cardiac metabolism is nearly entirely aerobic, meaning that the heart is unable to create energy in anaerobic conditions or when the oxygen supply is insufficient. Therefore, an increase in oxygen demand on the heart requires additional coronary artery blood flow to meet the new metabolic requirements. Narrowing of the coronary arteries can limit the amount of blood delivered to a portion of the myocardium, resulting in ischemia.

## Exercise Stress Testing

Patients must be ambulatory to participate in exercise stress testing. Functional limitations due to orthopedic, neurologic, pulmonary, or peripheral vascular issues can affect the patient's ability to complete the stress test protocol.

### Procedure

In exercise stress testing, the heart rate is monitored continuously while exercise is performed on a treadmill or bicycle.

The patient is exercised to a target heart rate that is 85% of the maximum predicted for that individual. By convention, the maximum predicted heart rate is calculated as 220 beats/min for men (210 beats/min for women) minus the patient's age in years. Attainment of maximum heart rate is a good prognostic sign.

The blood pressure, heart rate and rhythm, ECG, presence or absence of symptoms, and workload performed are monitored. Workload is determined by metabolic equivalents (METs) or by the double product (blood pressure × heart rate). METs are defined as the resting respiratory oxygen uptake for a 70-kg, 40-year-old man, and 1 MET is equivalent to 3.5 mg/min/kg of body weight. Work activities are calculated in terms of METs. Stair climbing, for example, is approximately equivalent to 4 METs. A reasonable workload for most active adults is 10 METs. Although the double product correlates well with the degree of CVD, it is less often used as a measure of workload.

Initial ECG readings are performed before exercise to document a baseline, with continuous 12-lead monitoring used throughout the study. The lead system is the same as used for the standard 12-lead ECG. However, it is necessary to move the limb leads to the torso to prevent arm or leg movement during exercise from interfering with ECG recording. Skin preparation and electrode attachment require careful attention to permit interpretable recordings during maximal exercise. It may be necessary to wrap material or fishnet over the electrodes and cables on the patient's torso to reduce movement artifact. Treadmill stress testing without a concomitant imaging modality is less reliable in females; therefore, exercise stress testing in females is typically paired with radionuclide or echocardiographic imaging. Baseline ECG abnormalities, such as left bundle branch block (LBBB), make analysis of exercise-induced ECG changes more complex.

The treadmill protocol chosen should reflect the patient's physical capacity and the purpose of the test. All treadmill protocols are multistaged, using increments in time, speed, and elevation of the treadmill platform. The protocol is selected based on the condition of the patient and the purpose of the study. For example, the Ellestad protocol uses small increments in workloads of shorter duration, whereas the Bruce protocol uses larger workload increments of longer duration. The Ellestad protocol may be better suited to a patient with less exercise tolerance. The Bruce protocol is among the most popular in use for reasonably functional people; a large body of diagnostic and prognostic data supports its use.

Patients who have not previously undergone exercise testing should be allowed briefly to practice walking on the treadmill or riding the bicycle. Before starting the test, a resting baseline ECG and blood pressure are obtained with the patient in sitting and standing positions. The ECG and heart rate are monitored continuously throughout the test, and blood pressure is monitored every few minutes. The monitoring continues for at least 6 to 10 minutes into recovery, or until symptoms or blood pressure and ECG changes have resolved to document the patient's return to baseline values.

It is mandatory that emergency personnel and equipment be available in areas where exercise testing is performed. Indications of myocardial ischemia during exercise testing are the development of ST-segment depressions, chest pain or the anginal equivalent, or failure to increase blood pressure to 120 mm Hg or the sustained decrease of 10 mm Hg with progressive stages of exercise. The test is terminated for any of the following reasons:

- The target heart rate is reached.
- The patient is unable to continue exercising because of shortness of breath, fatigue, claudication, or severe chest pain.
- There is ECG evidence of complete AV block, ventricular tachycardia (VT), or premature ventricular contractions (PVCs).
- There is ECG evidence of ST-segment changes consistent with ischemia or infarction.
- The patient's systolic blood pressure is greater than 220 mm Hg or diastolic blood pressure is greater than 120 mm Hg during exercise, or the patient's blood pressure drops below baseline at any time during the exercise protocol.

In the absence of ECG evidence of ischemia or the development of life-threatening dysrhythmias, every effort should be made to reach the maximum predicted heart rate to improve the diagnostic accuracy of the test. When the maximum predicted heart rate is not reached, the diagnostic reliability of the study is low. Exercise stress test results are considered reliable only if patients reach the maximum predicted heart rate value (85% of their maximal predicted effort).

### Nursing Assessment and Management

Adequately preparing patients for the stress test maximizes the information obtained from the study. Patients should be NPO for 4 to 6 hours before the test to minimize blood diversion to the gastrointestinal tract, which decreases available coronary blood supply. In particular, they should not drink caffeine-containing beverages because of the effect of caffeine on the heart rate. Beta blockers blunt the heart rate response to exercise and may prevent achievement of the maximum predicted heart rate, so they should be withheld on the day of the test. Digitalis may also be withheld because of its negative chronotropic effects. Badly deconditioned patients, or those with comorbidities that could affect their ability to ambulate, may not be able to complete the required exercise. Appropriate attire, including comfortable walking shoes, is necessary to maximize patient comfort and performance.

The critical care nurse may be responsible for explaining the general format of the exercise test to the patient and family. It is important that patients understand why the test is indicated and what will be expected of them. The nurse reassures patients that someone will observe them closely throughout the test and encourages them to express any concerns before, during, and after the procedure. Patients should also understand that they may have to continue exercising after angina develops but will not be expected to exercise more than is safe.

### Pharmacologic Stress Testing

Pharmacologic stress testing is performed in patients who are unable to bike or walk on a treadmill. Patients referred for stress testing may have limitations that prevent them from performing adequate physical exercise. This has led to the development of alternative methods of simulating the effect of exercise on the heart using adrenergic agents, such as dobutamine, or vasodilators, such as adenosine or dipyridamole. These studies require no activity on the part of the patient. There is continuous monitoring of the ECG, along with frequent blood pressure measurements. In addition, an imaging modality, such as echocardiography, nuclear imaging, positron emission tomography (PET), or magnetic resonance imaging (MRI), is always used.

Pharmacologic agents used include several drugs. Dobutamine increases myocardial oxygen demand by increasing contractility, heart rate, and systemic blood pressure. Because dobutamine has some heart rate–blunting characteristics, supplemental atropine may be required to achieve target heart rate values. With the infusion of dobutamine, coronary blood flow increases up to twofold in normal coronary arteries but less so in arteries with flow-limiting lesions. Vasodilators, such as adenosine and dipyridamole, also cause an increase in coronary blood flow. They simulate the effects of exercise on the heart by producing arteriolar and coronary artery vasodilation. Regadenoson is a selective adenosine agonist that incites coronary vasodilation, producing maximal effects quickly, and maintaining hyperemia for the duration of perfusion imaging. Although information on functional capacity is not obtained during pharmacologic stress testing, it is expected to provide a reasonable equivalent to that gathered during physical exercise.

ECG changes, secondary to the infusion of dobutamine, adenosine, and dipyridamole, have a very low sensitivity for the detection of significant CAD. Therefore, pharmacologic stress testing is always accompanied by an imaging modality to increase the sensitivity of the study.

## Nuclear Imaging with Stress Testing

Noninvasive, rapid, and accurate imaging of cardiac structure and function using radiotracers is a routine part of inpatient assessment of patients with known or suspected CVD. Broadly speaking, this is known as radionuclide cardiac imaging. Single-photon emission computed tomography (SPECT) and positron emission tomography (PET) are both widely available types of radionuclide imaging. SPECT and PET cameras capture the photons emitted by infused radiotracers and provide information on the magnitude and location of the uptake. The images are ECG gated, or collected in synchrony with ongoing ECG monitoring, so that the final data interpretation can be presented in the context of the full cardiac cycle of contraction and relaxation. In SPECT imaging, the final result is also referred to as myocardial perfusion imaging (MPI). PET is discussed at greater length later in this chapter (see Positron Emission Tomography).

Nuclear imaging is combined with exercise or the infusion of a pharmacologic agent in a variety of protocols. Protocols may involve the injection of several radiotracers over several hours, with imaging performed 24 hours later. The purpose of the protocols is to obtain information on the heart at rest and with stress. Protocols vary widely because of patient comorbidities, patient size, and available personnel and equipment.

### Myocardial Perfusion Imaging

MPI uses SPECT technology to look at coronary blood flow, giving information about the location, quantity, and severity of cardiac disease. MPI uses radiopharmaceutical agents that, once injected into the venous bloodstream, accumulate in viable myocardium in proportion to the blood flow to a particular area. After injection of the tracer, the SPECT camera is used to record an image of radioactive counts from the entire myocardium.

During MPI studies, images are obtained of the heart at rest and with stress. Typically, at rest in the normal heart, the radiotracer is spread uniformly throughout the myocardium, and the camera reads counts equally from throughout the myocardium. During exercise, a similar scan is obtained in patients without significant coronary artery stenosis because blood flow increases uniformly to meet myocardial oxygen demands.

However, in patients with significant CAD, the image obtained during exercise is altered. The amount of coronary blood flow is limited in stenotic arteries, and the quantity of tracer in myocardial segments supplied by stenotic arteries is diminished or absent compared with segments supplied by nonstenotic arteries. An area of decreased tracer uptake during exercise compared with at rest is known as a reversible perfusion defect. Reversible perfusion defects are suggestive of impaired blood flow, or ischemia, in a region. In patients with previous infarction, decreased uptake may be present on both the rest and exercise scans in the infarcted segments; this pattern is known as a fixed perfusion defect and usually signifies nonviable myocardium. It is possible for patients to have fixed perfusion defects in some myocardial segments, reversible defects in others, and normal perfusion in the remaining segments.

Because of the many patients who are physically unable to exercise, pharmacologic agents may be used to mimic the heart's response to exercise. Vasodilating agents, such as dipyridamole, adenosine, and dobutamine, administered IV mimic exercise conditions in the heart by dilating nonstenotic coronary arteries. Coronary blood flow is increased preferentially through normal, nonstenosed arteries; this results in relative hypoperfusion in myocardial segments supplied by stenosed coronary arteries. A radiotracer injected during the peak action of the pharmacologic agent produces images similar to those seen with exercise. Currently, only dipyridamole is approved by the U.S. Food and Drug Administration (FDA) for use in perfusion imaging.

**PROTOCOLS.** Three radioactive tracers, thallium-201, technetium (Tc)-99m, and sestamibi, are approved for perfusion imaging. Characteristics of the three agents differ and are responsible for the varying imaging protocols used.

**Thallium Protocol.** The cardiac half-life of thallium is approximately 7.5 hours, meaning that 50% of the tracer is still present in myocardial cells 7.5 hours after it is administered. It also redistributes readily, so thallium in normally perfused areas moves to previously underperfused areas after the myocardial blood flow demands in that territory have decreased. The standard protocol for thallium perfusion studies begins first with the exercise portion; thallium is injected at the peak of exercise, and imaging starts within 5 minutes of injection. The rest portion is obtained 2 to 4 hours later. Because of redistribution, no additional thallium is required. However, in some patients with perfusion defects on both the rest and exercise scans, significant redistribution may not occur, and it is recommended that an additional dose of thallium be administered.

**Sestamibi Protocol.** Perfusion imaging with sestamibi typically begins with the rest scan. Because significant uptake also occurs in the liver, imaging is delayed for approximately 60 minutes. This delay allows sestamibi to be cleared from the liver but not the heart. In addition, a glass of milk or small fatty meal is taken shortly after radiotracer injection to enhance hepatic clearance. A second dose of sestamibi is administered during peak exercise, and the exercise scan is obtained 60 minutes after injection, again allowing time for hepatic clearance. Because sestamibi redistributes very slowly, the image obtained 60 minutes after peak exercise reflects the perfusion conditions at the time of injection. Initially, perfusion studies with sestamibi were performed on two different days, but it is now customary to complete both portions of the study in 1 day. It has been shown that exercise sestamibi myocardial perfusion SPECT can provide incremental prognostic information in patients who have not suffered a previous MI or undergone cardiac catheterization and who are determined to be at low risk.

## NURSING ASSESSMENT AND MANAGEMENT.
All the directions and precautions that pertain to exercise ECG also apply to exercise radionuclide imaging. When pharmacologic agents are used in place of exercise, minor side effects, such as flushing, headache, and nausea, may occur. Serious side effects due to the radiotracer are extremely rare. Medications to counteract serious side effects should be readily available. Some patients who receive sestamibi report a metallic taste several minutes after injection. Patients are often anxious about the radiation involved and the appearance of the equipment. It is important for the nurse to allay these anxieties. Table 17-7 outlines some of the tests that are used to detect the presence of myocardial ischemia.

## Radionuclide Angiocardiography

A radionuclide ventriculogram or multigated acquisition (MUGA) scan is a precise means of calculating both right and left ventricular ejection fraction. The MUGA scan has, for many years, been the gold standard for measuring ejection fraction, but other technologies, such as cardiac MRI, echocardiography, and angiography, can now provide equally useful information. The MUGA scan is performed by labeling the patient's red blood cell pool with a radioactive tracer, usually technetium 99m, and measuring radioactivity with a gamma camera positioned over the chest. The number of counts recorded per unit of time is proportional to the blood volume moving through the cardiac chambers. Information is collected on cardiac wall motion, dilation, and wall thickness.

A *first-pass MUGA scan* is performed specifically when information is required regarding right ventricular function. In this study, the gamma camera is positioned to begin counting before the radioactive tracer is injected. That way, when the venous blood makes its first pass through the right side of the heart, information can be obtained on right ventricular function. Once the tracer completes a circulatory cycle, leading to labeled blood in both the right and left ventricles, right ventricular function is obscured by the left ventricle.

Nurses caring for patients who have undergone radionuclide imaging should be aware of precautions; this information is available through the radiation safety department of their institution. The length of time that any precautions may be necessary is related to the half-life of the radiotracer used. In general, nurses who are pregnant should avoid caring for patients for 24 to 48 hours after the study, and all nurses should wear gloves when handling body fluids during the 24- to 48-hour period.

---

**TABLE 17-7** Diagnostic Tests Used to Detect Myocardial Ischemia

| Procedure | Abnormal Findings | Special Considerations |
|---|---|---|
| Standard 12-lead ECG | Transient ST-segment and T-wave changes in patients with chest pain at rest or of prolonged duration | |
| Holter monitoring | Transient ST-segment and T-wave changes occurring at rest or with activity | Only two ECG leads monitored |
| Stress echocardiogram | Segmental wall motion abnormality associated with echocardiogram obtained during exercise | May be used in patients with ventricular conduction defects<br>Pharmacologic agents may be used in patients who cannot exercise |
| Exercise ECG | Transient ST-segment and T-wave changes occurring with exercise | Cannot be used in patients who are unable to exercise or who have LBBB or paced rhythm<br>Does not provide good information on the location of the CAD |
| Radionuclide perfusion stress study | "Cold spot" image or perfusion defect associated with scan obtained during exercise | May be used in patients with ventricular conduction defects<br>Pharmacologic agents may be used in patients who cannot exercise |
| Online ischemia analysis | Myocardial ischemia dynamic analysis (MIDA)* analyzing eight leads to detect ST-segment levels indicating ischemia and QRS complex changes corresponding to infarct evolution | Noninvasive<br>Hastens clinical decision making<br>Graphic trends monitored online<br>Reocclusion readily identified<br>Helps differentiate chest pain related to ischemia from nonischemic symptoms |

*Data from MIDA CoroNet, Hewlett-Packard, Andover, MA, Product Literature.

## Stress Echocardiography

There are several important advantages to the use of echocardiography as the imaging modality with stress testing. The echocardiogram identifies regional wall motion abnormalities, which are the final result of myocardium that is poorly perfused, secondary to CAD. Echocardiograms can be read immediately, do not involve ionizing radiation, and are more cost effective than nuclear imaging. The disadvantages of stress echocardiography include the difficulty in obtaining quality images secondary to the experience of the technologist and because of the patient's body habitus. Images must be obtained both at rest and at peak exercise for comparison.

Stress echocardiography can be used with exercise stress testing or pharmacologic stress testing. A baseline 2D echocardiogram is performed before exercise is performed or the drug is infused. (For pharmacologic stress testing, dobutamine or dipyridamole is used as the provocative agent.) The imaging is continued through and for 10 minutes after stopping the exercise or drug infusion. The echocardiogram is examined for wall motion abnormalities indicative of poor regional myocardial perfusion. A study is considered positive if, after exercise or drug infusion, new wall motion abnormalities are detected.

## Computed Tomography

Computed tomography (CT) scanning is a noninvasive technique used to evaluate the heart and its surrounding structures. CT scanning involves passing x-ray beams through a patient's body while a detector gathers and records images generated by the beams. Computers reconstruct the images into 2D or 3D images that provide strikingly detailed views of the anatomy (Fig. 17-12). Cardiac CT scanning is used to detect structural diseases of the heart, including congenital anomalies and aneurysms.

Coronary artery calcium (CAC) is an indicator of atherosclerosis that can be assessed by CT. Atherosclerotic plaque evolves though stages where instability and rupture may be followed by calcification. Although arterial calcification

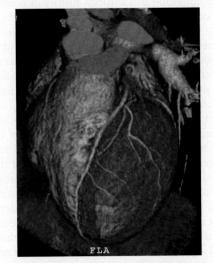

FIGURE 17-12 Multislice CT image of the heart, a 64-slice cardiac computed tomography scan of the heart, frontal plane.

indicates a later stage of vascular disease, its absence does not exclude the presence of noncalcified plaque that is vulnerable to rupture. A CAC score (CACS) of zero, consistent with no detectable CAC, may be falsely reassuring as this measurement does not identify plaque that has yet to be calcified. There is no direct association between the CACS and degree of stenosis of atherosclerotic lesions. In other words, it is possible to have a very high CACS with no flow-limiting intravascular lesions, or a very low CACS with significant flow-limiting intravascular lesions. CACS is most useful in determining a patient's CVD event risk by virtue of its strong association with total coronary atherosclerotic disease burden. The Agatston Score is used to measure the amount of calcium detected during a coronary CT. Scores of less than 10, 11 to 99, 100 to 400, and greater than 400 are used to categorize individuals into groups having minimal, moderate, increased, or extensive amounts of calcification, respectively. Although it has not replaced coronary angiograms as the gold standard of detection and quantification of CAD, the CACS adds independent prognostic information of all-cause mortality when used in conjunction with risk assessment algorithms (such as the Framingham risk score).[8,9]

Coronary computed tomography angiogram (CCTA) is a noninvasive method to visualize the actual lumen of the coronary arteries. CCTA can identify narrowings and stenoses of coronary arteries, whether or not calcium deposits are present. Patients undergoing ECG-gated CCTA may need heart rate modulation. Optimal heart rates are 55 to 60 beats/min and can be safely achieved in most patients with medications, particularly β-blockers. Patients require placement of an IV line for contrast administration. Monitoring for contrast-induced allergic reactions and renal toxicity is also necessary.[10]

## Magnetic Resonance Imaging

MRI allows high-resolution assessment of cardiovascular anatomy, function, blood flow, metabolism, and perfusion. It permits assessment of cardiac structure and function at rest or during exercise or pharmacologic stress testing during the assessment for presence of CAD. Cardiac magnetic resonance imaging (CMRI) has emerged as an alternative to stress nuclear cardiac imaging and stress echocardiography, particularly in patients who are undergoing pharmacologic stress testing.[11,12] MRI is also used in the diagnosis of cardiomyopathy, valvulopathy, congenital heart disease, cardiac masses, intracardiac thrombi, and diseases of the pericardium. Myocardial viability studies can be performed using MRI; thus, viable or ischemic tissue can be distinguished from scarred or infarcted tissue. Centers performing electrophysiology procedures use MRI to map pulmonary veins before an atrial fibrillation pulmonary vein ablation procedure. Atrial septal defects can be characterized before the percutaneous placement of an occlusion device.

Cardiovascular MRI has other advantages. It is useful in patients unable to tolerate iodine-based contrast material because of allergy or renal insufficiency. Gadolinium, the MRI contrast medium, can cause both allergic reactions and nephrotoxicity, but the frequency of both complications appears to be less than that associated with iodinated contrast material. In addition, cardiovascular MRI with a stress testing protocol

| BOX 17-8 | Contraindications to Magnetic Resonance Imaging |
|---|---|

**Absolute**
Cardiac pacemaker
Aneurysm clips
Epicardial pacing wires
Metal prosthetic heart valves
Implanted cardioverter–defibrillator
Implanted infusion pumps
Cochlear implants
Metal intrauterine devices
Metal debris (eg, bullets, shrapnel)

**Relative (Individual Assessment Required)**
Prosthetic joints
Certain foreign objects in body (eg, dental braces)
Nonmetallic prosthetic heart valves
Surgical staples
Coronary stents (if recently deployed)

is being used to provide a comprehensive evaluation of cardiac structure, wall function, valvular function, myocardial perfusion, angiography, and viability. The provocative agent used for MRI stress testing can be adenosine, dobutamine, or dipyridamole.

Obesity may be a contraindication for MRI (or magnetic resonance angiography) because the patient is required to fit into a fixed-sized tunnel within the scanner. The patient must be able to lie flat and remain composed despite confinement and loud noises generated by the scanner. Non–MRI-compatible aneurysm clips, implanted devices (including implanted cardiac defibrillators and pacemakers), and other body metal are all contraindications to MRI scanning. Patients with a history of metalworking may have metal shards in their eyes, making them unsuitable for MRI scanning. Contraindications to MRI are listed in Box 17-8. Although tattoo dye may contain metallic oxides that heat up during MRI, tattoos are not contraindicated in MRI scanning. Breath holding is required to avoid breathing artifacts at intervals during MRI, so cardiac MRI scanning may not be appropriate for patients who are unable to hold their breath. An IV line is required for instilling the contrast medium. Central catheters are not used because of the high pounds per square inch injection pressure used.

## Positron Emission Tomography

PET has significantly contributed to the knowledge of cardiac physiology and metabolism. It detects coronary stenoses (perfusion) and assesses myocardial viability (metabolism). PET scanning is the gold standard for testing myocardial viability.

Rubidium-82 and nitrogen-13–labeled ammonia are tracers used in evaluating regional myocardial blood flow. Fluorodeoxygenase (FDG) and carbon-11–labeled acetate are used for evaluating glucose and fatty acid metabolism, respectively. If perfusion testing with rubidium-82 and nitrogen-13 ammonia demonstrates decreased blood flow, and metabolic testing with FDG and carbon-11 acetate demonstrates absent metabolic activity, then that region of myocardium is considered nonviable. That is, there is a matched decrease in

flow and metabolism. If, on the other hand, the flow appears reduced by the perfusion tracers but the metabolic activity is preserved, that region of myocardium is considered ischemic and viable. This would indicate a mismatch of flow and viability, and it would direct the patient's treatment to an intervention that would restore flow to a viable area of tissue.

The patient should be NPO for 6 hours before the study. Caffeinated beverages should be restricted for 24 hours before the procedure.

PET scanning is also used as a myocardial imaging modality during stress testing. It provides additional prognostic information during evaluations for CAD.[13]

## Cardiac Catheterization, Coronary Angiography, and Coronary Intervention

During cardiac catheterization and related procedures, radiographic contrast is injected into the chambers of the heart and the coronary arteries under fluoroscopic guidance. These studies are commonly performed and are well established as the gold standard for evaluating the coronary artery lumen. Intracoronary lesions may be targets for a variety of interventions, including angioplasty and stenting, or coronary artery bypass. Coronary anomalies and other disease states, including aneurysms and myocardial bridging, can also be seen. Coronary interventions are performed based on the information gained during the diagnostic cardiac catheterization.

The major limitations related to cardiac catheterization involve cost, experience of the operator, level of risk afforded, and ability to determine whether an identified lesion can cause ischemia. The cost of cardiac catheterization, which is in the thousands of dollars, is much greater than for noninvasive modalities. Extensive data indicate that the physician operator must perform at least 75 procedures annually to maintain the skills necessary to perform a safe and interpretable procedure. Although this procedure can locate blockages in the coronary arteries, more information may be required to understand the ischemic potential of a given lesion before an angioplasty is performed.

Patients undergoing cardiac catheterization require careful preprocedure evaluation, including a recent history and physical examination to identify a history of contrast media allergy as well as a recent set of laboratory studies, including a complete blood count, prothrombin and partial thromboplastin time, International Normalized Ratio, and chemistry panel (serum potassium, creatinine, and blood urea nitrogen levels). Women who are premenopausal and could be pregnant must have pregnancy tests performed within 48 hours of the procedure. The patient must also be NPO for at least 8 hours before the procedure; appropriate medications may be taken with a sip of water on the morning of the procedure. Patients need IV line placement, and consideration may be given to insertion of a Foley's catheter if the patient may have difficulty urinating postprocedure. Patients must be able to lie still and almost flat on a procedure table for the duration of the examination. For nursing considerations for the patient undergoing cardiac catheterization, see Box 17-9.

After the procedure, the patient requires careful monitoring of vital signs (blood pressure, heart rate, and respirations with pulse oximetry). The percutaneous entry site of the procedure needs close monitoring for signs of bleeding. When a

**BOX 17-9** **Nursing Interventions**

**For the Patient Undergoing Cardiac Catheterization**

**Preprocedure**
- Explain procedure to patient and family.
- Verify that the patient has taken nothing by mouth for at least 6 hours before the procedure except prescribed medications as advised by the physician.
- Ensure that ordered preoperative laboratory studies have been completed and results are available.
- Verify patient, identify allergy information; alert physician if patient is allergic to radiographic dye, medications, or specific foods.
- Ensure that informed consent has been obtained.
- Establish IV access per institutional protocol or physician order.
- Place patient on cardiac monitoring system with blood pressure and pulse oximetry monitoring.
- Provide supplemental oxygen as ordered/indicated.
- Premedicate patient per physician order.
- Obtain vital signs before transfer to catheterization laboratory.

**During Procedure**
- Continually assess patient vital signs, oxygenation, level of consciousness, and cardiac rhythm per institutional protocol.
- Alert attending physician to significant changes in vital signs, oxygenation, and presence of malignant cardiac dysrhythmias (eg, PVCs, ventricular tachycardia, VF).
- Be prepared to initiate cardiac resuscitation with emergency equipment and medications.

**Postprocedure**
- Ensure that patient vital signs are stable before transfer.
- Check catheterization site dressing for bleeding and integrity.
- Check distal pulse below catheterization site; if femoral site was used, check distal pulse, extremity color, capillary refill, and neurosensory status.
- With transfemoral approach, keep extremity straight and instruct patient not to bend leg or arm.
- With transradial approach ensure that hemostasis band is properly placed and inflated. Follow manufacturer's instructions regarding deflation/removal.
- Maintain IV infusion per physician order or institutional protocol.
- Maintain supplemental oxygenation support as ordered or indicated.
- Encourage oral fluids as ordered.
- Check patient's coagulation status per institutional protocol before sheath removal.
- When femoral artery catheter is removed:
  - Apply direct pressure over invasive site for 20 to 30 minutes to prevent bleeding or apply commercial hemostatic compression device per institutional protocol.
  - Check distal extremity for pulse, color, capillary refill, and sensorium.
  - Remind patient to lie flat for 4 to 6 hours per institutional protocol.
  - Check site dressing every 4 to 6 hours for bleeding and integrity.

transfemoral approach has been used, any bleeding or hematoma formation must be managed to prevent serious vascular complications, including retroperitoneal bleeding IV fluids after the procedure promote elimination of the renal-toxic contrast media and protect the patient from hypotension due to dehydration or increased vagal tone during potentially painful portions of the recovery. Bed rest for several hours after a femoral arteriotomy is mandatory to allow the site to stabilize and

further protect the patient from vascular bleeding complications. A summary of patient teaching for patients undergoing cardiac catheterization can be found in Box 17-10.

Diagnostic cardiac catheterization and coronary angioplasty can also be performed via the radial artery for selected patients. This approach offers the advantage of fewer vascular and bleeding complications, less postprocedure bedrest and increased patient satisfaction.[14]

**BOX 17-10** *TEACHING GUIDE* *Cardiac Catheterization*

**Preprocedure**
- Instruct the patient not to take anything by mouth for at least 6 hours before the procedure, except prescription medications as advised by the physician to reduce the chance of nausea and vomiting during the procedure.
- Tell the patient that an IV line will be placed to allow fluid and medication administration before, during, and after the procedure.
- Tell the patient that preoperative medication will be given before transport to the catheterization laboratory.
- Inform the patient that only a patient gown will be worn during the procedure.
- Advise the patient that the catheterization laboratory is usually cool, and the procedure table is firm and may be uncomfortable after a prolonged time.
- Explain that the patient may be asked to turn the head, hold the breath, or cough during the procedure.
- Advise that some discomfort may be experienced during the procedure but that local anesthesia will be administered to minimize pain.
- Inform the patient that a cardiac monitor will be used for the duration of the procedure and for a few hours after the procedure.

- Tell the patient that lying flat for several hours after the procedure will minimize the chance of bleeding from the catheter site.
- Inform the patient that oral fluids should be consumed as tolerated after the procedure to assist in eliminating the radiographic contrast material.
- Encourage the patient and family to ask questions.

**During Procedure**
- Instruct the patient to inform the physician and team of any chest pain experienced.
- Remind the patient to lie still.
- Reassure the patient and allay anxiety.
- Encourage and answer the patient's questions.

**Postprocedure**
- If a transfemoral approach is used, remind the patient to lie still and keep the extremity straight.
- If a transradial approach is used a wrist band will be placed to prevent bleeding from the radial artery.
- Instruct the patient to verbalize any chest pain or shortness of breath if present.
- Tell the patient when the catheter sheath is due for removal.
- Encourage the patient to take oral fluids as ordered.
- Advise the patient that the physician will review and explain the catheterization findings.

IVUS is an adjunctive technique performed in patients undergoing cardiac catheterization. IVUS uses ultrasound technology to obtain information regarding the lumen and wall structure of the coronary artery. It permits detailed cross-sectional imaging of coronary arteries and allows for a risk assessment of individual lesions. It is frequently performed in conjunction with coronary angiograms to determine lumen measurements and characteristics, including plaque morphology and burden. The information obtained from IVUS can be used to determine the need for coronary angioplasty or stenting. It is also used to evaluate the final outcome from coronary angioplasties with and without stenting.

OCT is a light-based intravascular imaging modality that is similar to IVUS, but images are of better resolution and provided more quickly. OCT is an emerging modality that is still being studied in comparison to the widely utilized IVUS.[15]

The standard method for determining when to use angioplasty to treat an intracoronary lesion is angiography alone. However, determining which lesions cause ischemia can be difficult, and coronary angiography may under- or overestimate a lesion's functional severity. Fractional flow reserve (FFR) is a measurement that is obtained to help determine the ischemic potential of coronary stenoses. FFR is performed in the cardiac catheterization laboratory in conjunction with angiography and is defined as the ratio of maximal blood flow in a stenotic blood vessel compared with normal maximal blood flow. A pressure-sensor guidewire is threaded beyond the lesion in question, and the pressure gradient across the blockage is measured at peak hyperemia, usually induced by intracoronary adenosine infusion. It is calculated as the mean distal coronary pressure divided by the mean aortic pressure during maximum blood flow. FFR in a normal coronary artery is a value of 1. An abnormal value of less than 0.75 indicates a flow-limiting lesion and is associated with ischemia. While not mandatory to perform, FFR-guided interventions have been associated with a reduced rate of primary composite end point of death, MI, and repeat vascularization at 1 year, when compared with standard percutaneous coronary interventions guided by angiography alone.[16]

Coronary interventions that may be necessary include percutaneous transluminal coronary angioplasty (PTCA), which involves the displacement of intracoronary plaque or thrombus for intracoronary blockages of 70% or greater. Intracoronary stents are intraluminal scaffolds placed after PTCA to decrease the reclosure rate of angioplasty sites. In directional coronary atherectomy (DCA), the plaque is removed rather than displaced. DCA is a specialized procedure, used far less frequently than PTCA in most centers. Extraction atherectomy is performed using a transluminal extraction catheter and suction to remove thrombi. A more detailed discussion of coronary interventions can be found in Chapter 18.

## Left Heart Catheterization

Left heart catheterization provides information about the lumen of the aorta, coronary arteries, aortic and mitral valvular competencies, and wall motion of the left ventricle. Many studies also include pressure measurements in the left atrium and left ventricle, with pressure gradients measured across the aortic and mitral valves, as well as over the left ventricular outflow tract.

A diagnostic left heart catheterization is typically performed percutaneously from either the radial or femoral artery. This procedure delineates baseline coronary anatomy, and it can identify abnormalities of the coronary arteries, great vessels, and cardiac chambers. Injection of the coronary vessels with radiographic contrast shows the actual lumen of the vessel and defines plaque, thrombus, and dissections that cause obstruction to blood flow. The left ventricular filling pressure is obtained as an indicator of the fluid status of the patient. A left ventriculogram, which involves rapid filling of the left ventricle with contrast media, provides the left ventricular ejection fraction as well as information regarding wall motion abnormalities and size of the left ventricle. Patients with valvular disease can have additional studies to measure valvular gradients and chamber pressures to allow for mathematical calculations of valve area and flow dynamics.

The risk profile for left heart catheterization is significant because the procedure involves cannulation of an artery and use of contrast media. The risks include bleeding at the percutaneous entry site, dissection of any of the vessels traversed during the procedure, perforation of peripheral or coronary arteries, mechanical irritation of the cardiac tissue, plaque embolization leading to MI or cerebrovascular accident, allergic reactions to the contrast media or any other drug given during the procedure, and renal compromise because of the renal toxic effects of the contrast media.

## Right Heart Catheterization

Right heart catheterization aids in the differentiation of left ventricular failure versus pulmonary disease as a cause of dyspnea. It is performed in patients with a history of dyspnea, valvular heart disease, and intracardiac shunts.

Diagnostic right heart cardiac catheterizations can be performed from the right or left external jugular or the femoral veins. Right heart chamber pressures and information about the pulmonic valve and PA pressures are obtained. More commonly, the procedure may be performed through the inferior jugular vein to the superior vena cava. The goal is to sample oxygen saturations and pressures in the right atrium, right ventricle, pulmonary capillary bed, and PA.

The most common problem during right heart catheterization is dysrhythmia resulting from stimulation of the myocardium. The dysrhythmias are self-limiting and usually do not require treatment. Postprocedure restrictions are minimal because a vein is accessed, and the risk for bleeding is low.

# ELECTROCARDIOGRAPHIC MONITORING

Cardiac monitoring is used in a variety of settings where it is necessary to monitor continuously a patient's heart rate and rhythm or the effects of a therapy.

Although the type of monitor may differ in each setting, all monitoring systems have three basic components: a display system, a monitoring cable, and electrodes. Electrodes are placed on the patient's chest to receive the electrical current from the cardiac muscle tissue. The electrical signal is then carried by the monitoring cable to a screen, where it is magnified and displayed. The display can be obtained both at the patient's bedside and at a central station, along with displays from other patients' monitors.

Today's monitors have expanded capabilities such as the diagnosis of complex dysrhythmias, the detection of myocardial ischemia, and the identification of prolonged QT intervals. These expanded features are made possible through development of computerized dysrhythmia detection algorithms,

ST-segment monitoring software, noise reduction features, multilead monitoring systems, and derived 12-lead ECGs with a minimum number of electrodes.

## Equipment Features

Two types of cardiac monitoring equipment are in use: continuous hard-wire monitoring systems and telemetry monitoring systems.

### Hard-Wire Monitoring Systems

Hard-wire monitors require the patient to be linked directly to the cardiac monitor through the ECG cable. Information is displayed and recorded at the bedside along with simultaneous display and recording at a central station. Because this type of cardiac monitoring limits patient mobility, patients using this system are usually confined to bed rest or are allowed to be up at the bedside only. Hard-wire monitors operate on electricity but are well isolated so that water, blood, and other fluids do not pose an electrical hazard as long as the machine is maintained properly.

### Telemetry Monitoring Systems

In telemetry monitoring, no direct wire connection is needed between the patient and the ECG display device. Electrodes are connected by a short monitoring cable to a small battery-operated transmitter. The ECG is then sent by radio-frequency signals to a receiver that picks up and displays the signal on an oscilloscope, either at the bedside or at a distant central recording station. Batteries are the power source for the transmitter and make it possible to avoid electrical hazards by isolating the monitoring system from potential current leakage and accidental shock. Because the patient is mobile, stable ECG tracings are often more difficult to obtain. Some hard-wire systems have built-in telemetry capability so that patients may be switched easily from one system to another as monitoring needs change.

### Display Systems

Modern electronic technology continues to make sophisticated advances in monitoring equipment, and current display systems incorporate features such as the following:[7]
- Computerized storage capability that permits retrieval of dysrhythmia data
- Automatic chart documentation, in which the ECG recorder is activated by alarms or at preset intervals
- Expanded alarm systems for a variety of parameters
- Multilead or 12-lead ECG display, which facilitates interpretation of complex dysrhythmias
- ST-segment analysis for monitoring ischemic events
- Computer systems that store, analyze, and trend monitored data, allowing the information to be retrieved at any time to aid in diagnosis and to note trends in the patient's status
- Wireless communication devices carried by the nurse that provide data and alarms
- QT-interval monitoring.

## Monitoring Lead Systems

All cardiac monitors use lead systems to record the electrical activity generated by cardiac tissue. Each lead system is composed of a positive or recording electrode, a negative electrode, and a third electrode used as a ground. As the heart depolarizes, the waves of electrical activity move inferiorly because the normal route of depolarization moves from the SA node and atria, downward through the AV node, His-Purkinje system, and ventricles, and to the left because the muscle mass in the left side of the heart is greater than the muscle mass of the right side of the heart. Each lead system views these waves of depolarization from a different location on the chest wall and thus produces P waves and QRS complexes of varying configuration.

The terminology used to describe lead systems can be confusing. The wires attached to the patient's chest are called leads, and the pictures produced by these wires are also called leads. A standard ECG uses 10 lead wires with electrodes at the ends (4 placed on the limbs, and 6 placed on the chest) and produces 12 electrical views of the heart, known as 12 leads.

Cardiac monitoring systems currently on the market vary from a simple three-electrode device to the more common five-electrode system. Other systems less commonly used aim to reduce the number of electrodes while monitoring all 12 leads. The discussion of monitoring in this chapter will focus on the three- and five-lead systems.

The three-electrode system produces limited selections of leads I, II, or III with only a single lead viewed on the screen at one time (single-channel recording). Five-electrode systems allow the possibility of viewing any of the 12 ECG leads and permit the nurse to view two or more leads on the monitor screen simultaneously (multichannel recording).

### Three-Electrode Systems

Monitors that require three electrodes use positive, negative, and ground electrodes that are placed in the right arm (RA), LA, and LL positions on the chest as designated by markings on the monitor cable. When the electrodes are placed appropriately, the standard leads (leads I, II, III) may be obtained by moving the lead selector on the bedside monitor to the lead I, II, or III position (Fig. 17-13). The lead selector automatically

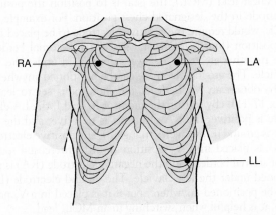

**FIGURE 17-13**  Three-electrode monitoring system. Leads placed in this position allow the nurse to monitor leads I, II, and III. The LL electrode must be placed below the level of the heart.

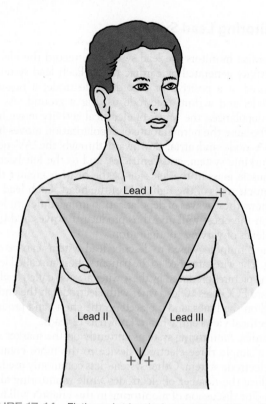

FIGURE 17-14 Einthoven's triangle. Leads I, II, and III are known as the standard leads. When placed together over the chest, they form what is known as Einthoven's triangle. Lead I: LA is positive and RA is negative. Lead II: LL is positive and RA is negative. Lead III: LL is positive and LA is negative.

adjusts which electrode is positive, which electrode is negative, and which electrode is ground to obtain an appropriate tracing. When lead I is selected, the LA is positive, the RA is negative, and the LL is ground. For a lead II configuration, the LL is positive, the RA is negative, and the LA is ground. To obtain a lead III, the LL is positive, the LA is negative, and the RA is ground. The configuration of leads I, II, and III, known as Einthoven's triangle, is illustrated in Figure 17-14.

To obtain a chest lead on the monitor that replicates the chest lead from the 12-lead ECG, a 5-wire system is needed. (See Fig. 17-7 for a review of chest lead placement.) When only three wires are available, a modified version of any of the six chest leads may be obtained. To configure a modified chest lead (MCL), the goal is to position the positive electrode in the designated chest position. For example, an MCL$_1$ would require the positive electrode to be placed in a V$_1$ position (fourth intercostal space, right sternal border). The negative electrode is always positioned under the left clavicle. The ground electrode can be positioned anywhere.

To obtain an MCL$_1$ lead, the monitor is set to lead I (Box 17-11). (By setting the monitor to lead I, the LA electrode is positive, the RA electrode is negative, and the leg wire is ground [Einthoven's triangle].) The positive electrode (LA) is placed in a V$_1$ position (fourth intercostal space, right sternal border), and the negative electrode (RA) is positioned under the left clavicle. The ground electrode (LL) can be positioned anywhere, but if it is placed in a V$_6$ position, it is helpful when switching to an MCL$_6$ lead.

To obtain an MCL$_6$ lead, the goal is to place a positive electrode in a V$_6$ position, a negative electrode under the left clavicle, and a ground wire anywhere. By setting the monitor to

**BOX 17-11** **Three-Electrode System**

To monitor MCL$_1$ using a three-electrode monitor:
1. Select lead I on the monitor.
2. Refer to Einthoven's triangle to remember that LA is positive, RA is negative, and LL is ground for lead I.
3. Place the positive electrode (LA) in a V$_1$ position (fourth intercostal space, right sternal border).
4. Place the negative electrode (RA) under the left clavicle.
5. Place the ground wire (LL) in the V$_6$ position (fifth intercostal space, left midaxillary line).

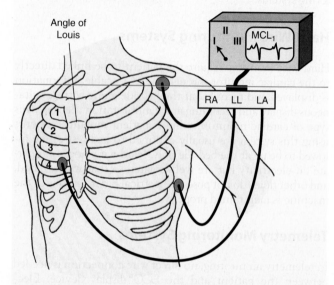

To monitor MCL$_6$ using a three-electrode monitor:
1. Select lead II on the monitor.
2. Refer to Einthoven's triangle to remember that LL is positive, RA is negative, and LA is ground for lead II.
3. Place the positive electrode (LL) in the V$_6$ position (fifth intercostal space, left midaxillary line).
4. Place the negative electrode (RA) under the left clavicle.
5. Place the ground wire (LA) in a V$_1$ position (fourth intercostal space, right sternal border).

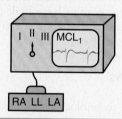

*Note:* The electrodes are in the same position on the chest for the MCL$_1$ lead and the MCL$_6$ lead. To view the two leads, the nurse merely switches the monitor from lead I to lead II.

lead II, the LL electrode is positive, the RA electrode is negative, and the LA electrode is ground (Einthoven's triangle). The positive electrode (LL) is placed in the V$_6$ position and the negative electrode (RA) is placed under the left clavicle. The ground wire can be placed anywhere, but if it is placed in a V$_1$ position, it will be helpful when switching to an MCL$_1$ lead.

By arranging the electrodes as described, the nurse can monitor both MCL$_1$ and MCL$_6$ merely by switching the monitor from a lead I to a lead II without changing the electrode placement on the patient's chest. MCL$_1$ and MCL$_6$ are ideal leads for detecting bundle branch block (BBB) rhythms and for differentiating supraventricular wide-QRS tachycardias from VT.

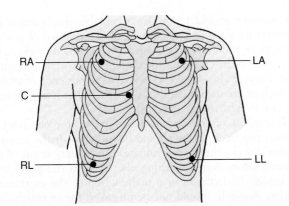

FIGURE 17-15 Five-electrode monitoring system. Using a five-electrode system allows the nurse to monitor any of the 12 leads of the ECG. The chest electrode must be moved to the appropriate chest location when monitoring the precordial leads.

## Five-Electrode Systems

The five-electrode system that increases the monitor's capability beyond the three-electrode system is preferred over the three-electrode system. (The four-electrode monitor requires a right leg electrode that is the ground for all leads described in the three-electrode system.) The five-electrode monitor adds an exploring "chest" electrode that allows one to obtain any one of the six chest leads and the six limb leads. In essence, a five-wire monitor system provides all the capabilities of the 12-lead ECG machine. The only difference is that the five-wire monitor has only one chest electrode, whereas the 12-lead ECG machine has six chest electrodes. Newer cardiac monitors now have all six chest electrodes and allow the nurse to view all 12 leads of the ECG simultaneously on the monitor screen.

To monitor a patient with a five-wire system, the four limb electrodes are positioned on the body according to their designations. The fifth chest electrode is placed on the chest in the designated precordial position. For example, if the nurse wants to monitor $V_1$, the chest electrode is placed in the fourth intercostal space, right sternal border (Fig. 17-15). If the nurse wants to switch to a different chest lead for monitoring, the electrode must be repositioned on the patient's chest. A five-electrode monitor offers the additional advantage of allowing the nurse to view two or more different leads simultaneously on the monitor screen.

## Lead Selection

No single monitoring lead is ideal for every patient. Table 17-8 summarizes the use of various leads and the reasons for their use. Lead II is used commonly because it records clear upright P waves and QRS complexes that are helpful in determining the underlying rhythm. In addition to lead II, leads III, aVF, and $V_1$ or $MCL_1$ show well-formed P waves and are therefore helpful in identifying atrial dysrhythmias. $V_1$ or $MCL_1$ is useful in recognizing RBBB and in differentiating ventricular ectopy from supraventricular rhythms with aberrancy. $V_6$ or $MCL_6$ is helpful in identifying LBBB and is also useful in differentiating ventricular ectopy from supraventricular rhythms with aberrancy. Lead I may be tried in the patient with respiratory disease who has much artifact on the tracing because there is less movement of the positive electrode in this lead than in a lead II or a $V_1$.

As mentioned, there is no one ideal monitoring lead for every patient, and in several situations, multilead recording is desirable. Multilead ECG systems offer multiple views of the heart

| Lead | Rationale for Use |
|---|---|
| II | Produces large, upright visible P waves and QRS complexes for determining underlying rhythm |
| $V_1$ or $MCL_1$ | Helpful for detecting RBBB and to differentiate ventricular ectopy from supraventricular rhythm aberrantly conducted in the ventricles |
| $V_6$ or $MCL_6$ | Helpful lead for detecting LBBB and to differentiate ventricular ectopy from supraventricular rhythm aberrantly conducted in the ventricles |
| III, aVF, $V_1$ | Produce visible P waves; useful in detecting atrial dysrhythmias |
| I | Useful in patients with respiratory distress |
| | Left arm and RA electrodes involved and placements less affected by chest motion compared with other leads |
| II, III, aVF | Helpful in detecting ischemia, injury, and infarction in the inferior wall |
| | Ischemia related to the right coronary artery is best seen in lead III |
| I, aVL, $V_5$, $V_6$ | Helpful in detecting ischemia, injury, and infarction in the lateral wall |
| $V_1$ through $V_4$ | Helpful in detecting ischemia, injury, and infarction in the anterior wall |
| | Ischemia related to the left anterior descending coronary artery or the left circumflex coronary artery is best seen in lead $V_3$ |

**TABLE 17-8   Suggested Monitoring Lead Selection**

because they reflect a tracing from each of the major heart surfaces. One of the major uses of multilead monitoring is in the interpretation of complex cardiac dysrhythmias, especially when differentiating aberrancy from ventricular ectopy and in identifying complex atrial dysrhythmias, uncharacteristic-looking ventricular premature beats, and fascicular blocks. Another use of multilead monitoring is in assessment of myocardial ischemia, injury, and infarction. By continuously viewing one lead from each area of the heart, episodes of anginal pain or silent ischemia can be documented. As soon as possible, these changes should be confirmed by a full 12-lead ECG.

## Procedure

### Electrode Application

Proper skin preparation and application of electrodes are imperative for good ECG monitoring. An adequate tracing should reflect (1) a narrow, stable baseline; (2) absence of distortion or "noise"; (3) sufficient amplitude of the QRS complex to activate the rate meters and alarm systems properly; and (4) identification of P waves.

The type of electrode currently used for ECG monitoring is a disposable silver- or nickel-plated electrode centered in a circle of adhesive paper or foam rubber. Most electrodes are pregelled by the manufacturer. They may have disposable wires attached to the electrodes or nondisposable wires that snap onto the electrodes. Electrodes should be comfortable for the patient. If not properly applied, undue artifact and false alarms may result.

When applying electrodes, the following procedure should be followed:

1. Select a stable site. Avoid bony protuberances, joints, and folds in the skin. Areas in which muscle attaches to bone have the least motion artifact.
2. Shave excessive body hair from the site.

3. Rub the site briskly with a dry gauze pad to remove oils and cellular debris.
4. Remove the paper backing and apply each electrode firmly to the skin by smoothing with the finger in a circular motion. Attach each electrode to its corresponding ECG cable wire. Sometimes it is necessary to tape over the cable wire connection or make a stress loop with the cable wire for extra stability.
5. Change electrodes at least daily, and monitor for skin irritation.

While applying the electrodes, explain the purpose of the procedure to the patient. Reassure the patient that monitor alarm sounds do not necessarily indicate a problem with the patient's heart beat; alarms often occur when an electrode becomes loose or disconnected.

## Monitor Observation

Cardiac monitors are useful only if the information they provide is "observed," either by computers with alarms for programmed parameters or by the human eye, and appropriately acted on by competent, responsible people. Those observing the monitor should know the acceptable dysrhythmia parameters for each patient and should be notified of any interruptions in monitoring, such as those caused by changing electrodes or by changing the patient to a portable monitor. The observer also should be aware of the presence of artifact from chest physical therapy or hiccups so that it may be considered in dysrhythmia diagnosis.

Regardless of the system used for monitor observation, certain practices always should be followed. If the monitor alarms sounds, the nurse evaluates the clinical status of the patient before doing anything else to see if the problem is an actual dysrhythmia or a malfunction of the monitoring system. Asystole should not be mistaken for an unattached ECG wire, nor should a patient inadvertently tapping on an electrode be misread as VT. In addition, monitor alarms always should be in the functioning mode. Only when direct physical care is being given to the patient can the alarm system safely be put on "standby." This ensures that no life-threatening dysrhythmia goes unnoticed. If the change on the monitor is not caused by an artifact or a disconnected wire, a full 12-lead ECG should be recorded to evaluate the rhythm change further. See Evidence-based Practice Highlight 17-1 regarding alarm management.[17]

---

**QSEN**

### EVIDENCE-BASED PRACTICE HIGHLIGHT 17-1
### Alarm Management: Scope and Impact of the Problem

Alarm fatigue develops when a person is exposed to an excessive number of alarms. This situation can result in sensory overload, which may cause the person to become desensitized to the alarms. Consequently, the response to alarms may be delayed, or alarms may be missed altogether.[1] Several strategies for alarm management have been suggested to reduce alarm fatigue and improve patient safety.

#### Expected Practice and Nursing Actions

**Provide proper skin preparation for ECG electrodes. (Level B)**
● Wash the isolated electrode area with soap and water, wipe the electrode area with a rough washcloth or gauze, and/or use the sandpaper on the electrode to roughen a small area of the skin.
● Do not use alcohol for skin preparation; it can dry out the skin.

**Change ECG electrodes daily. (Level E)**
● Change daily or more often if needed.

**Customize alarm parameters and levels on ECG monitors. (Level E)**
● Customize the alarms to meet the needs of individual patients.
● Set customized alarms within 1 hour of assuming care of a patient and as the patient's condition changes.

**Customize delay and threshold settings on oxygen saturation via pulse oximetry (SpO$_2$) monitors. (Level E)**
● Collaborate with an interprofessional team, including biomedical engineering, to determine the best delay and threshold settings.
● Use disposable, adhesive pulse oximetry sensors, and replace the sensors when they no longer adhere properly to the patient's skin.

**Provide initial and ongoing education about devices with alarms. (Level E)**
● Provide education on monitoring systems and alarms, as well as operational effectiveness, to new nurses and all other health-care staff on a periodic basis.
● Budget for ongoing education when purchasing monitoring systems.

**Establish interprofessional teams to address issues related to alarms, such as the development of policies and procedures. (Level E)**
● Determine the default alarms for the equipment being used.
● Evaluate the need to upgrade to next-generation pulse oximetry.
● Consider developing a culture of suspending alarms when nurses perform patient care that may produce false alarms.
● Standardize monitoring practices across clinical environments.

**Monitor only those patients with clinical indications for monitoring. (Level C)**
● Collaborate with an interprofessional team to determine those patients in a population or care unit who should be monitored and what parameters to use.
● Use the AHA's *Practice Standards for ECG Monitoring in Hospital Settings: Executive Summary and Guide for Implementation.*[14]

#### AACN Levels of Evidence

**Level A** Meta-analysis of quantitative studies or metasynthesis of qualitative studies with results that consistently support a specific action, intervention, or treatment (including systematic review of randomized controlled trials)
**Level B** Well-designed, controlled studies with results that consistently support a specific action, intervention, or treatment
**Level C** Qualitative studies, descriptive or correlational studies, integrative reviews, systematic reviews, or randomized controlled trials with inconsistent results
**Level D** Peer-reviewed professional and organizational standards with the support of clinical study recommendations
**Level E** Multiple case reports, theory-based evidence from expert opinions, or peer-reviewed professional orgastandards without clinical studies to support recommendations
**Level M** Manufacturer's recommendations only

Excerpted from American Association of Critical-Care Nurses Practice Alert. The full practice alert is available online at http://aacn.org.

## BOX 17-12 Troubleshooting: ECG Monitor Problem Solving

**Excessive Triggering of Heart Rate Alarms**
- Is the high–low alarm set too close to the patient's heart rate?
- Is the monitor sensitivity level set too high or too low?
- Is the patient cable securely inserted into the monitor receptacle?
- Are the lead wires or connections damaged?
- Has the monitoring lead been properly selected?
- Were the electrodes applied properly?
- Are the R and T waves the same height, causing both waveforms to be sensed?
- Is the baseline unstable, or is there excessive cable or lead wire movement?

**Baseline but No ECG Trace**
- Is the size (gain or sensitivity) control properly adjusted?
- Is an appropriate lead selector being used on the monitor?
- Is the patient cable fully inserted into the ECG receptacle?
- Are the electrode wires fully inserted into the patient cable?
- Are the electrode wires firmly attached to the electrodes?
- Are the electrode wires damaged?
- Is the patient cable damaged?
- Call for service if the trace is still absent.
- Is the battery dead (for telemetry system)?

**Intermittent Trace**
- Is the patient cable fully inserted into the monitor receptacle?
- Are the electrode wires fully inserted into the patient cable?
- Are the electrode wires firmly attached to the electrodes?
- Are the electrode wire connectors loose or worn?
- Have the electrodes been applied properly?
- Are the electrodes properly located and in firm skin contact?
- Is the patient cable damaged?

**Wandering or Irregular Baseline**
- Is there excessive cable movement? This can be reduced by clipping to the patient's clothing.
- Is the power cord on or near the monitor cable?
- Is there excessive movement by the patient? Are there muscle tremors from anxiety or shivering?
- Is site selection correct?
- Were proper skin preparation and application procedures followed?
- Are the electrodes still moist?

**Low-Amplitude Complexes**
- Is size control adjusted properly?
- Were the electrodes applied properly?
- Is there dried gel on the electrodes?
- Change electrode sites. Check 12-lead ECG for lead with highest amplitude, and attempt to simulate that lead.
- If none of the preceding steps remedies the problem, the weak signal may be the patient's normal complex.

**Sixty-Cycle Interference**
- Is the monitor size control set too high?
- Are there nearby electrical devices in use, especially poorly grounded ones?
- Were the electrodes applied properly?
- Is there dried gel on the electrodes?
- Are lead wires or connections damaged?

## Troubleshooting Electrocardiogram Monitor Problems

Several problems may occur in monitoring the ECG, including baseline but no ECG trace, intermittent traces, wandering or irregular baseline, low-amplitude complexes, 60-cycle interference, excessive triggering of heart rate alarms, and skin irritation. Box 17-12 outlines the steps to follow when such problems occur.

## DYSRHYTHMIAS AND THE 12-LEAD ELECTROCARDIOGRAM

Dysrhythmias and abnormalities of the 12-lead ECG commonly encountered in monitored patients can be recognized with a little practice. The types that occur most frequently are discussed in this chapter. Before presenting the individual dysrhythmias and 12-lead ECG abnormalities, the method for evaluating a rhythm strip is addressed.

To understand the causes, clinical significance, and treatment of dysrhythmias, knowledge of the conduction system is essential. Chapter 16 provides a review of the essential elements of the cardiac conducting system.

## Evaluation of a Rhythm Strip

### Electrocardiogram Paper

An ECG tracing is a graphic recording of the heart's electrical activity. The paper consists of horizontal and vertical lines, each 1 mm apart. The horizontal lines denote time measurements. When the paper is run at a sweep speed of 25 mm/s, each small square measured horizontally is equal to 0.04 second, and a large square (five small squares) equals 0.20 second. Height or voltage is measured by counting the lines vertically. Each small square measured vertically is 1 mm, and the large square is 5 mm (Fig. 17-16). Some ECG paper is also

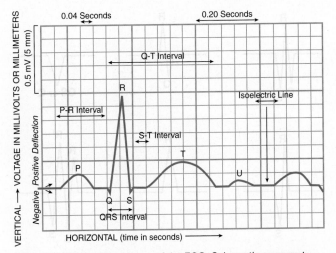

**FIGURE 17-16** Waveforms of the ECG. Schematic representation of the electrical impulse as it traverses the conduction system, resulting in depolarization and repolarization of the myocardium.

marked by vertical slash marks across the top or bottom. The distance between two vertical markings represents 3 seconds. The distance between 6 seconds is used for rate calculation.

## Waveforms and Intervals

During the cardiac cycle, the following waveforms and intervals are produced on the ECG surface tracing (see Fig. 17-16):

- **P wave:** The P wave is a small, usually upright and rounded deflection representing depolarization of the atria. It is normally seen before the QRS complex at a consistent interval.
- **PR interval:** The PR interval represents the time from the onset of atrial depolarization until the onset of ventricular depolarization. Included in the interval is the brief delay of the electrical signal at the AV node that allows time for the blood to move from the atria to the ventricles before the ventricles are depolarized. The interval is measured from the beginning of the P wave to the beginning of the QRS complex. A normal PR interval is 0.12 to 0.20 second.
- **QRS complex:** The QRS complex is a large waveform representing ventricular depolarization. Each component of the waveform has a specific connotation. The initial negative deflection is a Q wave, the initial positive deflection is an R wave, and the negative deflection after the R wave is an S wave. Not all QRS complexes have all three components, even though the complex is commonly called the QRS complex. A normal QRS complex is 0.06 to 0.11 second in width. Figure 17-17 illustrates different kinds of QRS complexes.
- **ST segment:** The ST segment is the portion of the tracing from the end of the QRS complex to the beginning of the T wave. It represents the time from the end of ventricular depolarization to the beginning of ventricular repolarization. Normally, it is isoelectric. An isoelectric ST segment means the ST segment joins the QRS complex at the baseline. ST segments may be elevated or depressed in a variety of conditions. Elevated ST segments could indicate acute myocardial injury. Depressed ST segments may signify acute myocardial injury or myocardial ischemia. For a more detailed discussion of ST-segment abnormalities, see Chapter 21.

- **T wave:** The T wave is the deflection representing ventricular repolarization or recovery. The T wave appears after the QRS complex. The atria also have a repolarization phase. However, there is no visible wave on the ECG to represent atrial repolarization because it occurs at the same time as the QRS complex.
- **U wave:** A U wave is a rarely seen, small, usually positive deflection after the T wave. Its significance is uncertain, but it is typically seen with hypokalemia.
- **QT interval:** The QT interval is the period from the beginning of ventricular depolarization to the end of ventricular repolarization. The QT interval is measured from the beginning of the QRS complex to the end of the T wave. Because the QT interval varies with heart rate, it is necessary to use a table in which QT intervals for various heart rates are listed. Tables are available for this purpose in most texts about dysrhythmias (Table 17-9). If such a table is not available, a corrected QT interval (QTc) can be calculated for comparison with normal values. Normal QTc usually does not exceed 0.42 second for men and 0.43 second for women. A quick method for obtaining a QTc is to use half of the preceding RR interval (described later).

## Calculation of Heart Rate

Although cardiac monitors and ECG strips can be used to calculate heart rate, the calculated rate is merely an estimate of the number of times per minute the heart has been electrically excited. In the normal heart, each excitation should be followed by cardiac contraction. However, in some situations, electrical activity can occur without contraction, resulting in a lack of perfusion. Therefore, the heart rate obtained from the cardiac monitor or ECG strip should never be substituted for the determination of heart rate by palpating the pulse.

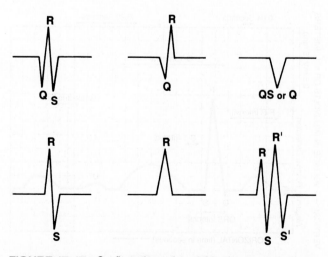

FIGURE 17-17 Configurations of the QRS complex. A Q wave is a negative deflection before an R wave, an R wave is a positive deflection, and an S wave is a negative deflection after an R wave.

| TABLE 17-9 | Approximate Normal Limits for QT Intervals in Seconds | |
|---|---|---|
| **Heart Rate/Minute** | **Men and Children** | **Women** |
| 40 | 0.45–0.49 | 0.46–0.50 |
| 46 | 0.43–0.47 | 0.44–0.48 |
| 50 | 0.41–0.45 | 0.43–0.46 |
| 55 | 0.40–0.44 | 0.41–0.45 |
| 60 | 0.39–0.42 | 0.40–0.43 |
| 67 | 0.37–0.40 | 0.38–0.41 |
| 71 | 0.36–0.40 | 0.37–0.41 |
| 75 | 0.35–0.38 | 0.36–0.39 |
| 80 | 0.34–0.37 | 0.35–0.38 |
| 86 | 0.33–0.36 | 0.34–0.37 |
| 93 | 0.32–0.35 | 0.33–0.36 |
| 100 | 0.31–0.34 | 0.32–0.35 |
| 109 | 0.30–0.33 | 0.31–0.33 |
| 120 | 0.28–0.31 | 0.29–0.32 |
| 133 | 0.27–0.29 | 0.28–0.30 |
| 150 | 0.25–0.28 | 0.26–0.28 |
| 172 | 0.23–0.26 | 0.24–0.26 |

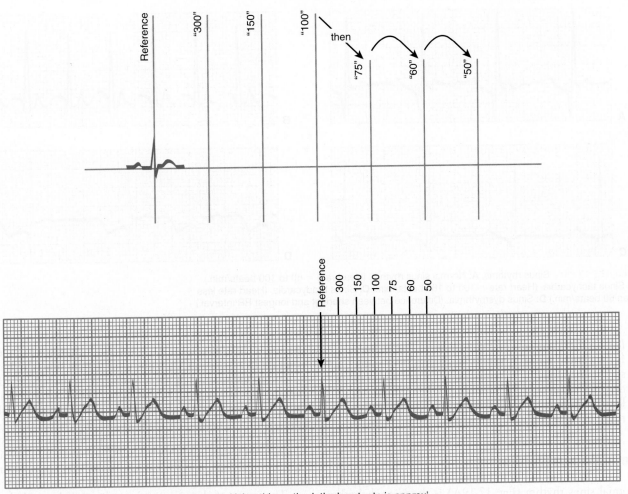

**FIGURE 17-18**   Method for estimating heart rate. Using this method, the heart rate is approximately 85 beats/min.

Both the atrial and the ventricular rates can be estimated by examining the ECG. To determine the ventricular rate, count the number of QRS complexes in a 6-second strip and multiply by 10. To estimate the atrial rate, count the number of P waves in a 6-second strip and multiply by 10. In the normal patient, the atrial and the ventricular rates should be the same. This method of rate calculation provides an estimate of heart rate for regular and irregular rhythms.

Another method of rate calculation can be used if the rhythm is regular. The ventricular heart rate is estimated by dividing 300 by the number of large boxes on the ECG paper between two R waves (the RR interval). The atrial rate is calculated by dividing 300 by the number of large boxes on ECG paper between two P waves (the pulse pressure [PP] interval).

Another quick method for estimating rate involves the use of a series of numbers. To use this method for estimating ventricular rate, the nurse first finds a QRS complex that falls directly on a dark line of the ECG paper. This dark line is the reference point. The next six dark lines of the paper are labeled 300, 150, 100, 75, 60, and 50 (Fig. 17-18). Then, the nurse finds the next QRS complex immediately after the reference point and estimates the ventricular rate using the sequence of numbers. The same method can be used for estimating atrial rate by using the P waves.

## Steps in Assessing a Rhythm Strip

The following analysis represents a systematic approach to assessment of a cardiac rhythm strip. Whether or not this method is used, it is important to take the time to complete each step because many dysrhythmias are not as they first appear.

1. *Determine the atrial and ventricular heart rates.* Are they within normal limits? If not, is there a relationship between the two (ie, one a multiple of the other)?
2. *Examine the rhythm to see if it is regular.* Is there an equal amount of time between each QRS complex (RR interval)? Is there an equal amount of time between each P wave (PP interval)? Are the PP and RR intervals the same?
3. *Look for the P waves.* Are they present? Is there one or more P waves for each QRS complex? Do all P waves have the same configuration?
4. *Measure the PR interval.* Is it normal? Is it the same throughout the strip, or does it vary? If it varies, is there a pattern to the variation?
5. *Evaluate the QRS complex.* Is it normal in width, or is it wide? Are all complexes of the same configuration?
6. *Examine the ST segment.* Is it isoelectric, elevated, or depressed?

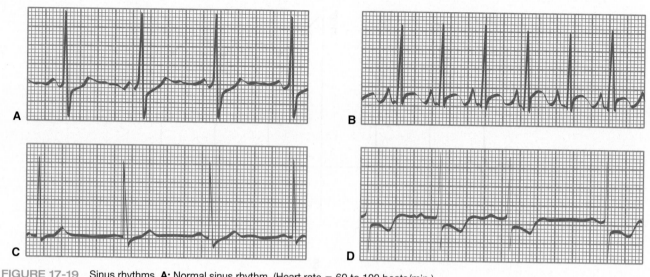

**FIGURE 17-19** Sinus rhythms. **A:** Normal sinus rhythm. (Heart rate = 60 to 100 beats/min.) **B:** Sinus tachycardia. (Heart rate = 100 to 180 beats/min.) **C:** Sinus bradycardia. (Heart rate less than 60 beats/min.) **D:** Sinus dysrhythmia. (Difference between shortest and longest RR interval.)

7. *Identify the rhythm and determine its clinical significance.* Is the patient symptomatic? (Check skin, neurologic status, renal function, coronary circulation, and hemodynamic status or blood pressure.) Is the dysrhythmia life-threatening? What is the clinical context? Is the dysrhythmia new or chronic?

## Normal Sinus Rhythm

Normal sinus rhythm (Fig. 17-19A) is the normal rhythm of the heart. The impulse is initiated at the sinus node in a regular rhythm at a rate of 60 to 100 beats/min. A P wave appears before each QRS complex. The PR interval is within normal limits and of equal duration (0.12 to 0.20 second), and the QRS is narrow (less than 0.12 second) unless an intraventricular conduction defect is present.

## Dysrhythmias Originating at the Sinus Node

Table 17-10 summarizes and compares ECG characteristics of sinus rhythms.

## Sinus Tachycardia

In sinus tachycardia, the sinus node accelerates and initiates an impulse at a rate of 100 times per minute or more (see Fig. 17-19B). The upper limits of sinus tachycardia extend to 160 to 180 beats/min. All other ECG characteristics, except for heart rate, are the same as in normal sinus rhythm.

Sinus tachycardia is usually caused by factors relating to an increase in sympathetic tone. Stress, exercise, and stimulants such as caffeine and nicotine can produce this dysrhythmia. Sinus tachycardia is also associated with such clinical problems as fever, anemia, hyperthyroidism, hypoxemia, heart failure, and shock. Drugs, such as atropine, which blocks vagal tone, and the catecholamines (eg, epinephrine, dopamine) also can produce this rhythm.

The cause of the sinus tachycardia and the underlying state of the myocardium determine the prognosis. Sinus tachycardia alone is not a lethal dysrhythmia but often signals an underlying problem that should be pursued. In addition, the rapid rate of sinus tachycardia increases oxygen demands on the myocardium and decreases the filling time of the ventricles. In people who already have depleted cardiac reserve, ischemia, or heart failure, the persistence of a fast rate may worsen the underlying condition.

Treatment of sinus tachycardia is usually directed at eliminating the underlying cause. Specific measures may include sedation, oxygen administration, digitalis, and diuretics if heart failure is present, or β-blockers if the tachycardia is caused by thyrotoxicosis.

## Sinus Bradycardia

Sinus bradycardia is defined as a rhythm with impulses originating at the sinus node at a rate of less than 60 beats/min

**TABLE 17-10** A Comparison of the Electrocardiographic Characteristics of Sinus Rhythms

|  | Normal Sinus Rhythm | Sinus Tachycardia | Sinus Bradycardia | Sinus Dysrhythmia |
|---|---|---|---|---|
| Rate | 60–100 beats/min | More than 100 beats/min | Less than 60 beats/min | 60–100 beats/min |
| Rhythm | Regular | Regular | Regular | Irregular |
| P waves | Present, one per QRS | Present, one per QRS | Present, one per QRS | Present, one per QRS |
| PR interval | Less than 0.20 s, equal | Less than 0.20 s, equal | Less than 0.20 s, equal | Less than 0.20 s, equal |
| QRS complex | Less than 0.12 s | Less than 0.12 s | Less than 0.12 s | Less than 0.12 s |

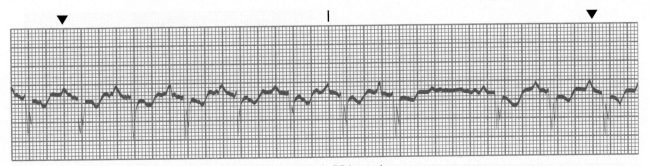

FIGURE 17-20   Sinoatrial block. The pause is a multiple of the basic PP interval.

(see Fig. 17-19C). The rhythm (RR interval) is regular, and all other parameters are normal.

Sinus bradycardia is common among people of all ages and may be normal in highly trained athletes. It is present in both healthy and diseased hearts. It may be associated with sleep, severe pain, inferior wall MI, acute spinal cord injury, and certain drugs (eg, digitalis, β-blockers, verapamil, diltiazem). In people with healthy hearts, slow heart rates are tolerated well. However, in those with severe heart disease, the heart may not be able to compensate for a slow rate by increasing the volume of blood ejected per beat. In this situation, sinus bradycardia leads to a low cardiac output (CO).

No treatment is indicated unless symptoms are present. If the pulse is very slow and the patient is symptomatic, appropriate measures include atropine (to block the vagal effect) or cardiac pacing.

## Sinus Dysrhythmia

Sinus dysrhythmia (formerly sinus arrhythmia) is a disorder of rhythm (see Fig. 17-19D) that is said to be present if the RR intervals on the ECG, from the shortest RR interval to the longest, vary by more than 0.12 second. This dysrhythmia is caused by an irregularity in sinus node discharge, often in association with phases of the respiratory cycle. The sinus node rate gradually increases with inspiration and gradually decreases with expiration.

Sinus dysrhythmia is a normal phenomenon, seen especially in young people in the setting of lower heart rates. It also occurs after enhancement of vagal tone (eg, with digitalis or morphine). Because it is a normal finding, sinus dysrhythmia does not imply the presence of underlying disease. Symptoms are uncommon unless there are long pauses between heart beats, and usually no treatment is required.

## Sinus Arrest and Sinoatrial Block

Sinus arrest is a disorder of impulse formation. The sinus node fails to form a discharge, producing pauses of varying lengths because of the absence of atrial depolarization. The P wave is absent, and the resulting PP interval is not a multiple of the basic PP interval. The pause ends either when an escape pacemaker from the junction or ventricles takes over or when sinus node function returns.

An SA block is often difficult to differentiate from sinus arrest on a surface ECG tracing. In SA block, the sinus node fires, but the impulse is delayed or blocked from exiting the

sinus node. If the block is complete, the duration of the pause is a multiple of the basic PP interval (Fig. 17-20).

Both dysrhythmias may result from disruption of the sinus node by infarction, degenerative fibrotic changes, drugs (digitalis, β-blockers, calcium-channel blockers), or excessive vagal stimulation. These rhythms are usually transient and insignificant unless a lower pacemaker fails to take over to pace the ventricles. Treatment is indicated if the patient is symptomatic. The goal is to increase the ventricular rate, which may require the use of atropine or, in the presence of serious hemodynamic compromise, a pacemaker.

## Sick Sinus Syndrome

Sick sinus syndrome refers to a chronic form of sinus node disease (Fig. 17-21). Patients exhibit severe degrees of sinus node depression, including marked sinus bradycardia, SA block, or sinus arrest. Often, rapid atrial dysrhythmias, such as atrial flutter or fibrillation ("tachycardia–bradycardia syndrome"), coexist and alternate with periods of sinus node depression.

Management of sick sinus syndrome requires control of the rapid atrial dysrhythmias with drug therapy and, in selected cases, control of very slow heart rates, often requiring implantation of a permanent pacemaker.

## Atrial Dysrhythmias

### Premature Atrial Contraction

A premature atrial contraction (PAC) occurs when an ectopic atrial impulse discharges prematurely and, in most cases, is conducted in a normal fashion through the AV conducting system to the ventricles (Fig. 17-22A). On the ECG tracing, the P wave is premature and may even be buried in the preceding T wave; it often differs in configuration from the

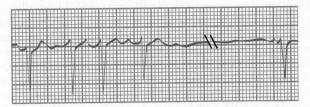

FIGURE 17-21   Sick sinus syndrome. Atrial fibrillation is followed by atrial standstill. A sinus escape beat is seen at the end of the strip.

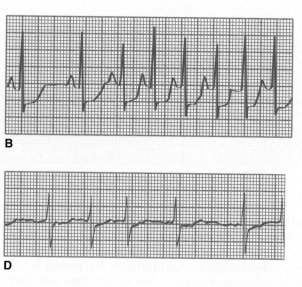

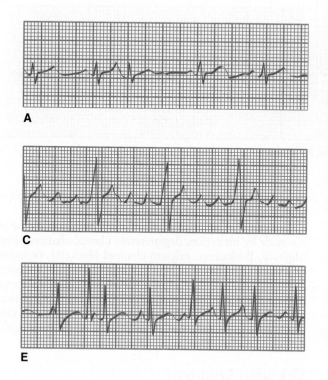

**FIGURE 17-22** **A:** PAC. **B:** PSVT, which begins with a PAC. **C:** Atrial flutter. (Atrial rate = 250 to 350 beats/min. P wave shows characteristic sawtoothed pattern.) **D:** Atrial fibrillation. (Atrial rate = 400 to 600 beats/min with a variable ventricular response. Characteristic atrial fibrillatory waves seen.) **E:** Multifocal atrial tachycardia. (The atrial rate exceeds 100 beats/min with three or more different P-wave morphologies.)

sinus P wave. The QRS complex is usually of normal configuration. However, because of timing, the QRS complex may appear wide and bizarre if conducted with some degree of delay (aberrant PAC) or may not appear at all if the atrial impulse is blocked from being conducted to the ventricles (blocked PAC). A short pause, usually less than "compensatory," is present (see later section on PVC).

People of all ages experience PACs. PACs may occur in healthy people as a result of various stimuli, such as emotions, tobacco, alcohol, and caffeine. PACs also may be associated with rheumatic heart disease, ischemic heart disease, mitral stenosis, heart failure, hypokalemia, hypomagnesemia, medications, and hyperthyroidism. Alternatively, PACs may be a precursor to an atrial tachycardia, atrial fibrillation, or atrial flutter, indicating an increasing atrial irritability. They also may indicate an underlying condition (eg, heart failure). Patients may have the sensation of a "pause" or "skip" in rhythm when PACs are present.

No treatment is necessary in many cases. The patient should be monitored and frequency of premature beats documented. In addition, the patient should be assessed for underlying conditions and treated.

## Paroxysmal Supraventricular Tachycardia

Paroxysmal supraventricular tachycardia (PSVT) describes a rapid atrial rhythm occurring at a rate of 150 to 250 beats/min (Fig. 17-22B). The tachycardia begins abruptly, in most instances with a PAC, and it ends abruptly. P waves may precede the QRS complex but also may be hidden in the QRS complex or precede the T wave at faster rates. (If some of the P waves are not followed by a QRS complex, this is referred to as PSVT with block and is usually caused by digitalis toxicity.) The P waves may be negative in leads II, III, and aVF because of retrograde conduction from the AV node to

the atria. The QRS complex is usually normal unless there is an underlying intraventricular conduction problem. The rhythm is regular, and the paroxysms may last from a few seconds to several hours or even days.

The term PSVT is used to identify rhythms previously called paroxysmal atrial tachycardia and paroxysmal nodal or junctional tachycardia, rhythms similar in all respects except in their sites of origin. PSVT is also known as AV nodal reentrant tachycardia because the mechanism most commonly responsible for this dysrhythmia is a reentrant circuit or chaotic movement at the level of the AV node.

PSVT must be differentiated from other narrow QRS complex (supraventricular) tachycardias. Table 17-11 is a guide to the differential diagnosis. The following points favor the diagnosis of PSVT versus a sinus tachycardia:

- An atrial premature beat often initiates the rhythm.
- The tachycardia begins and terminates abruptly.
- The rate is often faster than a sinus tachycardia and tends to be more regular from minute to minute.
- In response to a vagal maneuver, such as carotid sinus massage, the ectopic tachycardia is either unaffected or reverts to a normal sinus rhythm; however, sinus tachycardia slows slightly in response to increased vagal tone.

Like PACs, PSVTs often occur in adults with normal hearts for the same reasons (eg, emotions, tobacco, alcohol, caffeine). When heart disease is present, such abnormalities as rheumatic heart disease, acute MI, and digitalis toxicity may serve as the background for a PSVT. Often the patient has no underlying heart disease and may experience only palpitations and some lightheadedness, depending on the rate and duration of the PSVT. If the patient has underlying heart disease, dyspnea, angina pectoris, and heart failure may occur as ventricular filling time, and thus CO, is decreased.

**TABLE 17-11** Differential Diagnosis of Narrow QRS Tachycardia

| Type of Supraventricular Tachycardia (SVT) | Onset | Atrial Rate | Ventricular Rate | RR Interval | Response to Carotid Massage |
|---|---|---|---|---|---|
| Sinus tachycardia | Gradual | 100–180 beats/min | Same as sinus rate | Regular | Gradual slowing |
| PSVT | Abrupt | 150–250 beats/min | Usually same as atrial; block seen with digitalis toxicity and AV node disease | Regular, except at onset and termination | May convert to normal sinus rhythm |
| Atrial flutter | Abrupt | 250–350 beats/min | Occurs with 2:1, 3:1, 4:1, or varied ventricular response | Regular or regularly irregular | Abrupt slowing of ventricular response; flutter waves remain |
| Atrial fibrillation | Abrupt | 400–650 beats/min | Depends on ability of AV node to conduct atrial impulse; decreased with drug therapy | Irregularly irregular | Abrupt slowing of ventricular response; fibrillation waves remain |

Vagal stimulation often terminates the PSVT, either through carotid massage or the Valsalva maneuver. If vagal stimulation is unsuccessful, IV adenosine may be given. Cardioversion or overdrive pacing may be required if drug therapy is unsuccessful. Long-term prophylactic therapy may be indicated.[18]

## Atrial Flutter

Atrial flutter is a rapid atrial ectopic rhythm in which the atria fire at rates of 250 to 350 beats/min (Fig. 17-22C). The AV node functions as a "gatekeeper," preventing too many impulses from reaching the ventricle. If the ventricles are stimulated 250 to 350 times per minute, they are unable to respond with effective contractions, and CO is insufficient to sustain life. The AV node may allow only every second, third, or fourth atrial stimulus to proceed to the ventricles, resulting in what is known as a 2:1, 3:1, or 4:1 flutter block.

The rapid and regular atrial rate produces "sawtooth" or "picket-fence" P waves on the ECG. It is usual for a flutter wave to be partially concealed in the QRS complex or T wave. The QRS complex exhibits a normal configuration except when aberrant conduction is present.

When the ventricular rate is rapid, the diagnosis of atrial flutter may be difficult. Vagal maneuvers, such as carotid sinus massage or the administration of adenosine, increase the degree of AV block and allow recognition of flutter waves. Atrial flutter is often seen in the presence of underlying cardiac disease, including CAD, cor pulmonale, and rheumatic heart disease. If atrial flutter occurs in conjunction with a rapid ventricular rate, the ventricular chambers cannot fill adequately, resulting in varying degrees of hemodynamic compromise. Likewise, if atrial flutter is accompanied by a very slow ventricular rate, CO is diminished. The loss of "atrial kick," because atrial contraction is not occurring, is also a concern. The lack of atrial kick can compromise CO. Finally, without atrial contractions, thrombi can form on the walls of the atria. If these thrombi break loose, the result could be pulmonary embolus, cerebral embolus, or MI.

Treatment goals for atrial flutter are to reestablish sinus rhythm or to achieve ventricular rate control. When the ventricular rate is rapid, prompt treatment to control the rate or revert the rhythm to a sinus mechanism is indicated. Drugs may be selected to slow the conduction of the impulses through the AV node or to achieve pharmacologic conversion of the rhythm. If pharmacologic conversion is not successful, electrical cardioversion can be used. Synchronized cardioversion is especially useful in the prompt treatment of atrial flutter. The patient should be NPO before the procedure and receive sedation. (For a more detailed discussion of cardioversion, see Chapter 18.) If the patient has been experiencing atrial flutter for more than about 72 hours, anticoagulation may be needed before pharmacologic or electrical conversion of the rhythm is attempted. Other modes of therapy may be indicated for the long-term management of atrial flutter, such as ablation, pacing, and implantable devices.

## Atrial Fibrillation

Atrial fibrillation, which is a rapid atrial ectopic rhythm, occurring with atrial rates of 350 to 500 beats/min (Fig. 17-22D), is characterized by chaotic atrial activity with the absence of definable P waves. Instead, the P waves appear as small, quivering fibrillatory waves. Like atrial flutter, the ventricular rate and rhythm depend on the ability of the AV junction to function as a gatekeeper. If too many atrial stimuli pass through the AV junction, the ventricular response is rapid. If too few atrial stimuli pass through the AV junction, the ventricular response is slow. The ventricular rhythm is characteristically irregular.

Although atrial fibrillation may occur as a transient dysrhythmia in healthy young people, the presence of chronic atrial fibrillation is usually associated with underlying heart disease. One or both of the following are present in patients with chronic atrial fibrillation: atrial muscle disease or atrial distention together with disease of the sinus node. This rhythm commonly occurs in the setting of heart failure, ischemic or rheumatic heart disease, or pulmonary disease, and after open heart surgery. Atrial fibrillation is also seen in congenital heart disease.

The immediate clinical concern in patients with atrial fibrillation is the rate of the ventricular response. If the ventricular rate is too fast, end-diastolic filling time is decreased, and CO is compromised. If the ventricular rate is too slow, CO may again be decreased. As in atrial flutter, patients with atrial fibrillation have lost AV synchrony and atrial kick, resulting in a compromised CO. Patients are also at risk for the formation of mural thrombi and embolic events, such as stroke, MI, and pulmonary embolus.

The treatment principles for atrial fibrillation are the same as those for atrial flutter. The goal of therapy is to achieve rate control or to convert the rhythm to sinus. If a patient has chronic atrial fibrillation, anticoagulant therapy is added to the drug regimen to prevent an embolic event. Cardioversion is indicated for rhythm control when drug therapy fails or in the setting of hemodynamic compromise. Ablation, pacing, and implantable devices are among the therapeutic options.[19]

## Multifocal Atrial Tachycardia

Multifocal atrial tachycardia is a rapid atrial rhythm with varying P-wave morphology, resulting from the firing of three or more atrial foci (Fig. 17-22E). The atrial rate exceeds 100 beats/min, and the rhythm is usually irregular. The P waves vary in shape because of the multiple foci. The PR intervals may vary also, depending on the proximity of the focus to the AV node. The QRS complexes are normal unless an impulse is conducted with aberrancy.

This rhythm characteristically occurs in patients with severe pulmonary disease. Such patients often exhibit hypoxemia, hypokalemia, alterations in serum pH, or pulmonary hypertension. They usually manifest symptoms associated with the underlying disease rather than with the dysrhythmia itself. Treatment is directed at controlling the underlying pulmonary disease and slowing the ventricular rate if necessary.

## Junctional Dysrhythmias

### Junctional Rhythm

A junctional rhythm, also known as a nodal rhythm, is a rhythm originating in the AV node. When the SA node fails to fire, the AV node usually takes control, but the rate is slower. The rate of a junctional rhythm ranges between 50 and 70 beats/min. The P wave in the dysrhythmia can have one of three possible configurations.

1. The AV node fires, and the wave of depolarization travels backward (retrograde conduction) into the atria. The impulse from the AV node then moves forward into the ventricle. When this sequence occurs, the P wave appears as an inverted wave before a normal QRS complex (Fig. 17-23A).
2. The retrograde conduction into the atria occurs at the same time as the forward conduction into the ventricles. The resulting rhythm strip shows an absent P wave with a normal QRS complex. In reality, the P wave is not absent. Instead, it is buried inside the QRS complex (see Fig. 17-23B).
3. Forward conduction of the ventricles precedes retrograde conduction of the atria. When this sequence occurs, a normal QRS complex is followed by an inverted P wave (see Fig. 17-23C).

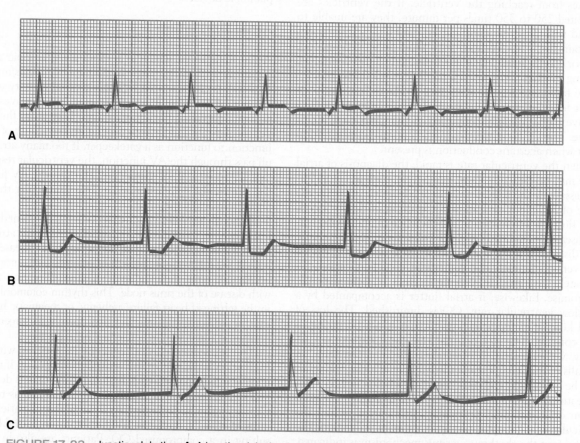

**FIGURE 17-23**    Junctional rhythm. **A:** A junctional rhythm in which the inverted P wave appears before a normal QRS complex. **B:** A junctional rhythm in which the inverted P wave is buried inside the QRS complex. **C:** A junctional rhythm in which the inverted P wave follows the QRS complex.

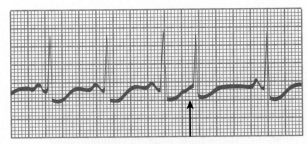

**FIGURE 17-24** Premature junctional contraction.

A junctional rhythm may be the result of hypoxia, hyperkalemia, MI, heart failure, valvular disease, drugs (digoxin, β-blockers, calcium-channel blockers), or any cause of SA node dysfunction. Patients with a junctional rhythm may become symptomatic as a result of the slower rate. Hypotension, decreased CO, and decreased perfusion may occur. The benefit of AV synchrony and atrial kick may be lost when the atria are stimulated with or after ventricular depolarization.

Treatment should be directed at the underlying cause. Symptomatic patients may require immediate treatment. The heart rate can be increased through the use of atropine or cardiac pacing. Interventions are also directed toward improving CO.

## Premature Junctional Contractions

A premature junctional contraction (PJC) is an ectopic impulse from a focus in the AV junction, occurring prematurely, before the next sinus impulse (Fig. 17-24). As in all rhythms originating in the AV junction, the QRS complex is narrow (less than 0.12 second), reflecting normal ventricular conduction. On rare occasions, the QRS complex may be wide if the impulse is conducted aberrantly. The atria are depolarized in a retrograde fashion before, during, or after ventricular excitation, producing inverted P waves that may occur before, during, or after the QRS complex. As with PACs, PJCs may occur in healthy people or in those with underlying heart disease. Ischemia or infarction may activate an ectopic focus in the AV junction, as may stimulants, such as nicotine or caffeine, or pharmacologic agents (eg, digitalis).

Frequent PJCs may indicate increasing irritability and may be a precursor of a junctional rhythm. Although usually asymptomatic, patients may experience a "skipped beat." Treatment for PJCs is not necessary.

## Ventricular Dysrhythmias

### Premature Ventricular Contractions

A PVC is an ectopic beat originating prematurely at the level of the ventricles (Fig. 17-25A). The beat is ventricular in origin and results in no electrical activity in the atria. As a result, no P waves appear. The ventricular depolarization does not travel through the normal rapid ventricular conduction system. Instead, ventricular conduction spreads more slowly through the Purkinje system, resulting in a wide QRS complex with a T wave that is opposite in direction to the QRS complex. A compensatory pause often follows the premature beat as the heart awaits the next stimulus from the

sinus node. The pause is considered fully compensatory if the cycles of the normal and premature beats equal the time of two normal heart cycles.

Ventricular premature beats can be described by their frequency and pattern. They can be rare, occasional, or frequent; optimally, they are described as number of PVCs per minute. If PVCs occur after each sinus beat, ventricular bigeminy is present (see Fig. 17-25B). Ventricular trigeminy is a PVC occurring after two consecutive sinus beats. When PVCs appear in only one form (from one ventricular site), they are referred to as uniformed, as opposed to multiformed, when two or more forms (from more than one ventricular site) of the QRS complex are apparent (see Fig. 17-25C). Two PVCs in a row are a couplet (see Fig. 17-25D), whereas three in a row are a triplet, which is a short run of VT (see Fig. 17-25E).

The most common of all ectopic beats, PVCs can occur with or without heart disease in any age group. They are especially common in people with myocardial disease (ischemia or infarction) or with myocardial irritability (hypokalemia, increased levels of catecholamines, or mechanical irritation with a wire or catheter). The presence of PVCs is a sign of ventricular myocardial irritability and, in some patients, may lead to VT or ventricular fibrillation (VF). The nature of the patient's underlying heart disease, rather than the presence of PVCs as such, determines the treatment and prognosis. Numerous and multiformed PVCs in the presence of serious heart disease worsen the prognosis. PVCs approaching the apex of the preceding T wave (R-on-T phenomenon) are of clinical concern. The T wave represents ventricular repolarization, when the heart should not be stimulated. If stimulation occurs during this vulnerable period, VF and sudden death may result (Fig. 17-26).

Infrequent, isolated PVCs require no treatment. Multiple or consecutive PVCs may be managed with antiarrhythmic agents. In an emergency situation an IV antiarrhythmic drug is selected. Many oral antiarrhythmic agents are available for chronic therapy. If serum potassium is low, potassium replacement may correct the dysrhythmia. If the dysrhythmia is caused by digitalis toxicity, withdrawal of the digitalis may correct it.[20]

## Ventricular Tachycardia

In the previous section, VT was defined as three or more PVCs in a row. VT is recognized by wide, bizarre QRS complexes occurring in a fairly regular rhythm at a rate greater than 100 beats/min (Fig. 17-27A). P waves are not usually seen and, if seen, are not related to the QRS complex. VT may be a short, nonsustained rhythm or longer and sustained.

In adults with normal hearts, VT is rare but is a common complication of MI. Other causes are the same as those described for PVCs. VT is a precursor of VF, and signs and symptoms of hemodynamic compromise (eg, ischemic chest pain, hypotension, pulmonary edema, and unconsciousness) may be seen if the rate is fast and the tachycardia is sustained. Serious dysrhythmia progression depends on the underlying heart disease.

If the patient is hemodynamically stable with the dysrhythmia, lidocaine may be administered intravenously. If the patient becomes unstable, synchronized cardioversion (or in emergency situations, unsynchronized defibrillation)

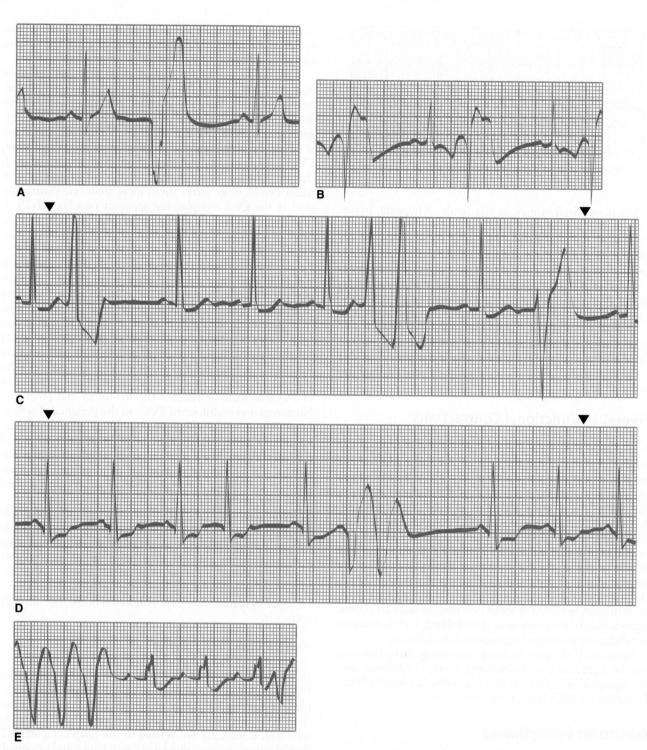

**FIGURE 17-25**   Ventricular dysrhythmias. **A:** PVCs. **B:** Ventricular bigeminy. (Every other beat is a PVC.) **C:** Multiformed PVCs. **D:** Couplet (two PVCs in a row). **E:** Triplet. (Short run of ventricular tachycardia; the first three beats are VT with the rhythm converting to sinus rhythm with first-degree heart block.)

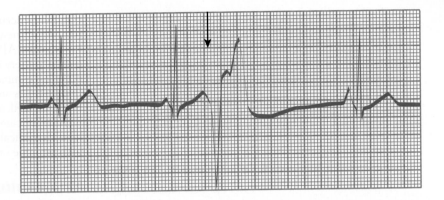

FIGURE 17-26   R-on-T PVC. (From Huff J: ECG Workout, 4th ed. Philadelphia, PA: Lippincott, Williams & Wilkins, 2002, p 195.)

is indicated. Long-term treatment for this dysrhythmia may involve the use of an implantable cardioverter–defibrillator (ICD). See Chapter 18 for a more detailed discussion of ICDs.

## Torsades De Pointes

Torsades de pointes ("twisting of the points") is a specific type of VT (Fig. 17-27B). The term refers to the polarity of the QRS complex, which swings from positive to negative and vice versa. The QRS complex morphology is characterized by large, bizarre, polymorphous, or multiformed QRS complexes of varying amplitude and direction, frequently varying from beat to beat and resembling torsion around an isoelectric line. The rate of the tachycardia is 100 to 180 beats/min but can be as fast as 200 to 300 beats/min. The rhythm is highly unstable; it may terminate in VF or revert to sinus rhythm. This form of VT is most likely to develop in myocardial disease when the underlying QT interval has been prolonged.

Torsades de pointes is favored by conditions that prolong the QT interval. Examples include severe bradycardia; drug therapy, especially with type IA antiarrhythmic agents; and electrolyte disturbances, such as hypokalemia and hypocalcemia. Other factors that can precipitate this dysrhythmia include intrinsic cardiac disease, familial QT-interval prolongation, drug-induced prolongation of the QT interval, hypokalemia, hypomagnesemia, and hypocalcemia. Torsades de pointes may terminate spontaneously and may repeat itself after several seconds or minutes, or it may transform into VF.

Treatment for torsades de pointes consists of shortening the refractory period (and thus the QT interval) of the underlying rhythm. IV magnesium sulfate, magnesium chloride, or isoproterenol is effective in suppression of the dysrhythmia. Overdrive pacing also can be used. Treatment is directed at correcting the underlying problem and may necessitate stopping the offending pharmacologic agent or correcting the electrolyte imbalance. Emergency cardioversion

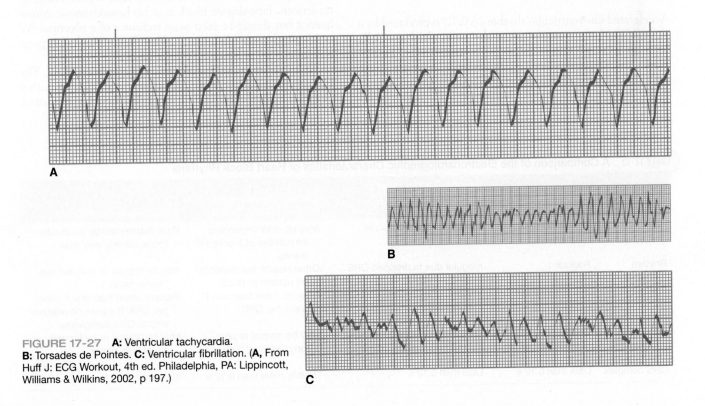

FIGURE 17-27   **A:** Ventricular tachycardia. **B:** Torsades de Pointes. **C:** Ventricular fibrillation. (**A,** From Huff J: ECG Workout, 4th ed. Philadelphia, PA: Lippincott, Williams & Wilkins, 2002, p 197.)

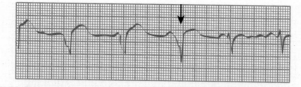

FIGURE 17-28 Accelerated idioventricular rhythm. The first three beats are of ventricular origin. The fourth beat (arrow) represents a fusion beat. The subsequent two beats are of sinus origin.

or defibrillation is indicated if the torsades does not revert spontaneously to sinus rhythm.[21]

## Ventricular Fibrillation

VF is defined as rapid, irregular, and ineffectual depolarizations of the ventricle (Fig. 17-27C). No distinct QRS complexes are seen. Only irregular oscillations of the baseline are apparent; these may be either coarse or fine in appearance.

VF may occur in the following circumstances: myocardial ischemia and infarction, catheter manipulation in the ventricles, electrocution, prolonged QT interval, or as a terminal rhythm in patients with circulatory failure. As in asystole, loss of consciousness occurs within seconds in VF. There is no pulse and no CO. VF is the most common cause of sudden cardiac death and is fatal if resuscitation is not instituted immediately.

If VF occurs, rapid defibrillation is the management of choice (see the discussion of cardiopulmonary resuscitation in Chapter 18). The patient should be supported with cardiopulmonary resuscitation and drugs if there is no response to defibrillation. An ICD may be indicated for long-term management of VF (see Chapter 18 for a discussion of ICDs).

## Accelerated Idioventricular Rhythm

Accelerated idioventricular rhythm (AIVR) is produced by a "speeding up" of ventricular pacemaker cells, which normally have an intrinsic rate of 20 to 40 beats/min (Fig. 17-28). When the idioventricular rate accelerates above the sinus rate, the ventricular pacemaker becomes the primary pacemaker for the heart. AIVR is characterized by wide QRS complexes occurring regularly at a rate of 50 to 100 beats/min. AIVR may last for a few beats or may be sustained.

Typically, AIVR is seen with acute MI, often in the setting of coronary artery reperfusion after thrombolytic therapy. It may occur less commonly as a result of ischemia or digitalis intoxication. Patients are not usually symptomatic. Adequate CO can be maintained, and degeneration into a rapid VT is rare.

In most cases, treatment is not necessary. If a patient is hemodynamically compromised, the sinus rate is increased with atropine or atrial pacing to suppress the AIVR.

## Atrioventricular Blocks

A disturbance in some portion of the AV conduction system causes an AV block. The sinus-initiated beat is delayed or completely blocked from activating the ventricles. The block may occur at the level of the AV node, bundle of His, or the bundle branches because the AV conduction system contains all of these structures. In first- and second-degree AV block, the block is incomplete; some or all of the impulses are eventually conducted to the ventricles. In third-degree or complete heart block, none of the sinus-initiated impulses is conducted. Table 17-12 summarizes and compares heart block rhythms.

## First-Degree Atrioventricular Block

In first-degree block, AV conduction is prolonged and equal in time. All impulses are eventually conducted to the ventricles (Fig. 17-29A). P waves are present and precede each QRS complex in a 1:1 relationship. The PR interval is constant but exceeds the upper limit of 0.20 second in duration.

First-degree heart block occurs in people of all ages and in healthy and diseased hearts. PR prolongation may be caused by drugs, such as digitalis, β-blockers, or calcium-channel blockers; CAD; a variety of infectious diseases; and congenital lesions. First-degree block is of no hemodynamic consequence but should be seen as an indicator of a potential AV conduction system disturbance. First-degree block may progress to second- or third-degree AV block.

No treatment is indicated for first-degree heart block. The PR interval should be monitored closely, watching for further block. The possibility of a drug effect also should be evaluated.

**TABLE 17-12** A Comparison of the Electrocardiographic Characteristics of Heart Block Rhythms

|  | First-Degree Heart Block | Second-Degree Heart Block—Mobitz Type I (Wenckebach) | Second-Degree Heart Block—Mobitz Type II | Third-Degree Heart Block |
|---|---|---|---|---|
| Rate | Usually 60–100 beats/min | Usually 60–100 beats/min | May be slow depending on number of blocked P waves | Rate determined by ventricular focus, usually very slow |
| Rhythm | Regular | Irregular due to dropped QRS | Often regular but depends on pattern of block | May be regular or irregular ventricular focus |
| P waves | Present, one per QRS | Present, one per QRS until QRS is missed | Present, more than one P wave per QRS | Present, more than one P wave per QRS; P waves no relationship to QRS complexes |
| PR interval | Greater than 0.20 s, equal throughout | Progressively gets longer until QRS is missed; pattern repeats | May be normal or prolonged, equal throughout | May be normal or prolonged, unequal throughout |
| QRS complex | Less than 0.12 s | Less than 0.12 s | Usually more than 0.12 s | More than 0.12 s |

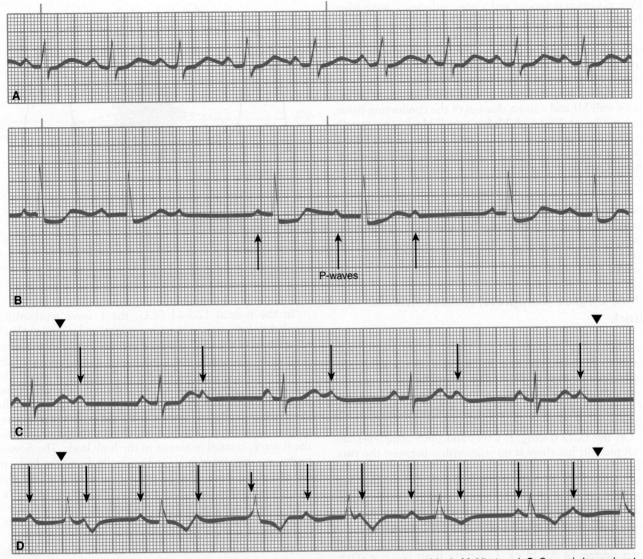

**FIGURE 17-29**   Heart block rhythms. **A:** First-degree heart block. **B:** Second-degree heart block: Mobitz type I. **C:** Second-degree heart block: Mobitz type II. Arrows denote blocked P wave (2:1 block). **D:** Third-degree heart block (complete AV block). Arrows denote P waves. Note the lack of relationship between the atria (P wave) and ventricles (QRS). (**A** and **B**, From Huff J: ECG Workout, 4th ed. Philadelphia, PA: Lippincott, Williams & Wilkins, 2002, pp 150, 156.)

## Second-Degree Atrioventricular Block— Mobitz I (Wenckebach)

Mobitz type I (Wenckebach) block occurs when AV conduction is delayed progressively with each sinus impulse until eventually the impulse is completely blocked from reaching the ventricles. The cycle then repeats itself (see Fig. 17-29B). Of the two types of second-degree block, Mobitz I (Wenckebach) and Mobitz II, Mobitz I occurs more commonly.

On the ECG tracing, P waves are present and related to the QRS complex in a cyclical pattern. The PR interval progressively lengthens with each beat until a QRS complex is not conducted. The QRS complex has the same configuration throughout the underlying rhythm.

A Mobitz type I block is usually associated with block above the bundle of His. Therefore, any drug or disease process that affects the AV node, such as digitalis, myocarditis, or

an inferior wall MI, may produce this type of second-degree block.

Patients with Mobitz type I second-degree AV block are rarely symptomatic because the ventricular rate is usually adequate. Wenckebach block is often temporary, and if it progresses to third-degree block, a junctional pacemaker at a rate of 40 to 60 beats/min usually takes over to pace the ventricles. No treatment is required for this rhythm except to discontinue a drug if it is the offending agent. The patient should be monitored for further progression of block.

## Second-Degree Atrioventricular Block— Mobitz II

Mobitz type II block is described as an intermittent block in the AV conduction, usually in or below the bundle of His. Mobitz type II block is characterized by a fixed PR interval when

AV conduction is present and a nonconducted P wave when the block occurs (see Fig. 17-29C). This block in conduction can occur occasionally or be repetitive with a 2:1, 3:1, or even 4:1 conduction pattern. Because there is no disturbance in the sinus node, the PP interval is regular. Often there is accompanying BBB, so the QRS complex may be wide.

A Mobitz type II pattern is seen in the setting of an anterior wall MI and various diseases of the conducting tissue, such as fibrotic disease. A Mobitz type II block is potentially more dangerous than a Mobitz type I block. Mobitz type II block is often permanent, and it may deteriorate rapidly to third-degree heart block with a slow ventricular response of 20 to 40 beats/min.

Constant monitoring and observation for progression to third-degree heart block are required. Medications, such as atropine, or cardiac pacing may be required if a patient becomes symptomatic or if the block occurs in the setting of an acute anterior wall MI. Permanent pacing is often indicated for long-term management.

### Third-Degree (Complete) Atrioventricular Block

In third-degree or complete heart block, the sinus node continues to fire normally, but the impulses do not reach the ventricles (see Fig. 17-29D). The ventricles are stimulated from escape pacemaker cells either in the junction (at a rate of 40 to 60 beats/min) or in the ventricles (at a rate of 20 to 40 beats/min), depending on the level of the AV block.

On the ECG tracing, P waves and QRS complexes are both present, but there is no relationship between the two. Therefore, complete heart block is considered one form of AV dissociation. The PP and RR intervals are each regular, but the PR interval is variable. If a junctional pacemaker paces the ventricles, the QRS complex is narrow. A pacemaker site lower in the ventricles produces a wide QRS complex.

The causes of complete heart block are the same as for lesser degrees of AV block. Complete heart block is often poorly tolerated. The rate and dependability of the ventricular pacemaker depend on its location. If the escape rhythm is ventricular in origin, the rate is slow, and the pacemaker site is unreliable. The patient may be symptomatic because of a low CO. A pacemaker site high in the bundle of His may provide an adequate rate and is more dependable. The patient may remain asymptomatic if the escape rhythm supports a normal CO.

A temporary pacing wire is usually inserted immediately, and when the patient is stabilized, a permanent pacemaker is implanted.

### The 12-Lead Electrocardiogram

As previously described, the ECG provides 12 electrical views of the heart. The first three electrical views are provided by the standard leads I, II, and III. The next three electrical views are provided by the augmented leads, aVR, aVL, and aVF. The standard and augmented leads are referred to as the limb leads and provide a view from a vertical plane. The remaining six electrical views of the heart, the precordial leads, chest leads, or V leads, $V_1$ through $V_6$, provide a horizontal plane view of the heart (Fig. 17-30).

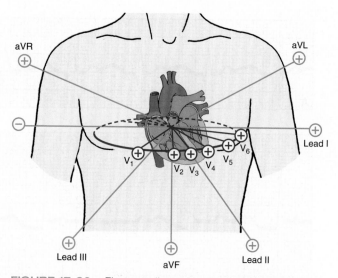

**FIGURE 17-30** Electrocardiographic views of the heart.

In the normal 12-lead ECG, the P wave representing atrial depolarization is usually upright and rounded. Each component of the QRS complex (ventricular depolarization) is analyzed separately. The Q wave, the initial downward deflection of the QRS complex, should be absent or small. The R component is the tallest upright portion of the QRS complex in the limb leads except aVR. In the precordial leads, the R wave begins as a small wave in $V_1$ and gradually progresses to a tall wave by $V_6$. The S wave, the downward stroke after the R wave, is small or absent in the limb leads. The S wave begins as a deep wave in $V_1$ and gradually disappears by $V_6$ in the precordial leads. The ST segment is isoelectric but may be slightly elevated in $V_1$ through $V_3$. The T wave, representing ventricular repolarization, is usually upright, although a variety of configurations can be normal. Table 17-13 summarizes the normal 12-lead ECG.

The 12-lead ECG may be useful in determining the electrical axis of the heart and detecting abnormalities that require more than one electrical view. These abnormalities include BBB; atrial or ventricular enlargement; and patterns of ischemia, injury, or infarction.

### Electrical Axis

Electrical axis refers to the general direction of the wave of excitation as it moves through the heart. In the normal heart, the flow of electrical forces originates in the SA node, spreads throughout atrial tissue, passes through the AV node, and moves throughout the ventricles. This flow of forces is normally downward and to the left, a pattern known as normal axis.

The ventricles make up the largest muscle mass of the heart and therefore make the most significant contribution to the determination of the direction of the flow of forces in the heart. For this reason, the QRS complex is examined when deciding the electrical axis.

A quick way to estimate the axis of the heart is to examine the direction of the QRS complex in leads I and aVF (Fig. 17-31). A QRS complex that is mainly upright in both leads represents a normal axis. A QRS complex that is upright in lead I and downward in lead aVF represents left axis

**TABLE 17-13** The Normal 12-Lead Electrocardiogram

| Lead | P | Q | R | S | S-T | T |
|------|---|---|---|---|-----|---|
| I | Upright | Small, 0.04 s, or none | Dominant | Less than R or none | Isoelectric +1 to −0.5 mm | Upright |
| II | Upright | Small or none | Dominant | Less than R or none | +1 to −0.5 mm | Upright |
| III | Upright Flat Diphasic Inverted | Small or none | None to dominant | None to dominant | +1 to −0.5 mm | Upright Flat Diphasic Inverted |
| aVR | Inverted | Small or large | Small or none | Dominant | +1 to −0.5 mm | Inverted |
| aVL | Upright Flat Diphasic Inverted | Small, none, or large | Small, none, or dominant | Small, none, or dominant | +1 to −0.5 mm | Upright Flat Diphasic Inverted |
| aVF | Upright Flat Diphasic Inverted | Small or none | Small, none, or dominant | None to dominant | +1 to −0.5 mm | Upright |
| $V_1$ | Upright Flat Diphasic | None May be QS | Small | Deep | 0 to +3 mm | Inverted Flat Upright Diphasic |
| $V_2$ | Upright | None | | | 0 to +3 mm | Upright Diphasic Inverted |
| $V_3$ | Upright | Small or none | | | 0 to +3 mm | Upright |
| $V_4$ | Upright | Small or none | | | +1 to −0.5 mm | Upright |
| $V_5$ | Upright | Small | | | +1 to −0.5 mm | Upright |
| $V_6$ | Upright | Small | Tall | Small or none | +1 to −0.5 mm | Upright |

deviation. A QRS complex that is downward in lead I and upright in lead aVF represents right axis deviation. A QRS complex that is downward in leads I and aVF is uncommon and represents indeterminate axis.

The direction of the flow of forces in the heart can change as a result of an anatomical shift of the heart in the chest wall. An anatomical shift may occur in very obese patients or in patients with large abdominal tumors or abdominal ascites. Left axis deviation can be caused by LBBB, left ventricular enlargement, or inferior wall MI. Right axis deviation can be caused by RBBB, right ventricular enlargement, or an anterior wall MI.

Patients with an axis shift are asymptomatic. The only way an axis shift can be detected is through a 12-lead ECG. The axis shift usually represents some underlying abnormality, and treatment is directed at the underlying cause.

## Bundle Branch Block

A BBB develops when there is either a functional or pathologic block in one of the major branches of the intraventricular conduction system. As conduction through one bundle is blocked, the impulse travels along the unaffected bundle and activates one ventricle normally. The impulse is delayed in reaching the other ventricle because it travels outside of the normal conducting fibers. The right and left ventricles are thus depolarized sequentially instead of simultaneously. The abnormal activation produces a wide QRS complex, representing the increased time it takes for ventricular depolarization (Fig. 17-32). The broad QRS complex has two peaks (RSR′), indicating that depolarization of the two ventricles was not simultaneous.

An RBBB and LBBB are diagnosed on the 12-lead ECG but can also be identified on the bedside monitor using a $V_1$ or $MCL_1$ tracing and a $V_6$ or $MCL_6$ tracing (see section on Electrocardiographic Monitoring for description of lead

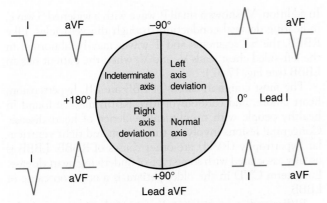

**FIGURE 17-31** Determining electrical axis. To determine the axis of the heart, examine the direction of the QRS complex in leads I and aVF.

| Lead I | Lead aVF | Axis |
|--------|----------|------|
| Negative | Negative | Indeterminate axis |
| Negative | Positive | Right axis deviation |
| Positive | Negative | Left axis deviation |
| Positive | Positive | Normal axis |

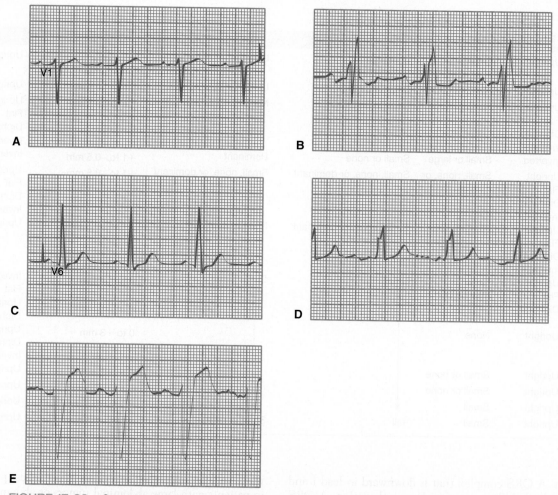

**FIGURE 17-32**   Comparison of right versus LBBB. **A:** A normal V₁ tracing. Note the small narrow R and deep narrow S wave. **B:** V₁ tracing showing the wide QRS complex and double-peaked R wave, indicating a RBBB. **C:** A normal V₆ tracing. Note the tall narrow R wave and absent S wave. **D:** A V₆ tracing showing the wide QRS complex and double-peaked R wave, indicating an LBBB. **E:** A V₁ tracing. Note the small narrow R and deep wide S wave, indicating an LBBB.

selection). To identify the presence of a BBB, the QRS complex duration must be prolonged to 0.12 second or longer, representing the delay in conduction through the ventricles. An RBBB alters the configuration of the QRS complex in the right-sided chest leads, $V_1$ and $V_2$. Normally, these leads have a small, single-peaked R-wave and deep S-wave configuration. With an RBBB, depolarization of the right ventricle is delayed, and the ECG pattern changes. An RBBB is evidenced by an RSR′ configuration in $V_1$. If the initial peak of the QRS complex is smaller than the second peak, the pattern would be described as rSR′. An "r" is used to describe the first, smaller peak, and an "R" is used to describe the second, taller peak. Likewise, if the initial peak of the QRS complex is taller than the second peak, the pattern is described as an RSr′. Whenever ventricular depolarization is abnormal, so is ventricular repolarization. As a result, ST-segment and T-wave abnormalities may be seen in leads $V_1$ and $V_2$ for patients with an RBBB.

An LBBB changes the QRS complex pattern in I aVL, and the left-sided chest leads, $V_5$ and $V_6$. Normally, these leads have a tall, single-peaked R wave and a small or absent S wave. Instead, the double-peaked RSR′ pattern is noted.

In addition, $V_1$ shows a small R wave with a widened S wave, indicating delayed conduction through the ventricles. Like RBBB, the ST segments and T waves may be abnormal in the left-sided chest leads $V_5$ and $V_6$ when the patient has an LBBB (see Fig. 17-32).

The most common causes of BBB are MI, hypertension, heart failure, and cardiomyopathy. RBBB may be found in healthy people with no clinical evidence of heart disease. Congenital lesions involving the septum and right ventricular hypertrophy (RVH) are other causes of RBBB. LBBB is usually associated with some type of underlying heart disease. Long-term CVD in the older patient is a common cause of LBBB.

BBB signifies underlying disease of the intraventricular conduction system. Patients should be monitored for involvement of the other bundles or fascicles or for progression to complete heart block. Progression of block may be very slow or rapid, depending on the underlying cause. A new-onset LBBB in conjunction with an acute MI is associated with a higher mortality rate.

The underlying heart disease determines treatment and prognosis. Patients with an MI and new-onset BBB are

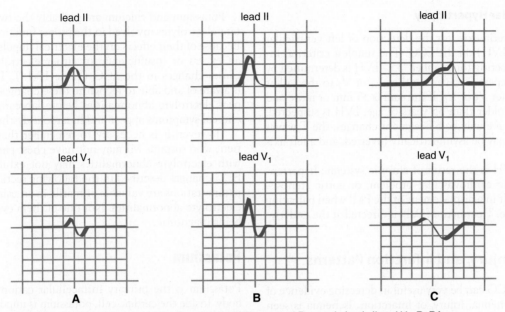

**FIGURE 17-33**  RA versus LA enlargement. **A:** The normal P wave in leads II and V₁. **B:** RA enlargement. Note the increased amplitude of the early, RA component of the P wave in V₁ and the tall, pointed P wave in lead II. **C:** Left atrial enlargement. Note the increased terminal downstroke and duration of the P wave in V₁ and the broad, notched P wave in lead II.

closely monitored for progression to a type of complete heart block. A temporary pacemaker may be inserted.[22]

## Enlargement Patterns

Enlargement of a cardiac chamber may involve hypertrophy of the muscle and/or dilation of the chamber. The most common causes include pumping for a prolonged period against high pressures or pumping for a prolonged period to move blood through narrowed valves. Electrocardiography is not an ideal diagnostic tool for determining the cause of the enlargement. Echocardiography is more helpful in determining if the enlargement is the result of hypertrophy or dilation. The terminology used to describe enlargement patterns on the ECG can be confusing. The term ventricular hypertrophy is commonly used because hypertrophy is the most frequent cause of the enlargement pattern in the ventricles. The general terms atrial abnormality and atrial enlargement are often used rather than the specific terms atrial hypertrophy or atrial dilation because atrial changes on the ECG may result from a variety of causes, including atrial dilation, hypertrophy, or other conditions.[23,24] (See Fig. 17-33A for comparison.)

### Right Atrial Abnormality

When the atria enlarge, changes are seen in the P wave because the P wave represents atrial depolarization. RA abnormality is noted on the ECG by the presence of tall, pointed P waves in leads II, III, and aVF. The P wave in V₁ may show a diphasic wave with an initial upstroke that is larger than the downstroke (Fig. 17-33B).

The right atrium is more likely to enlarge as a result of pressures created by pulmonary causes, such as pulmonary hypertension and chronic obstructive pulmonary disease. For this reason, RA abnormality is often referred to as P pulmonale. RA abnormality is often associated with RVH.

Treatment is directed at the underlying cause. Often, however, the underlying cause may be a chronic condition that cannot be cured.

### Left Atrial Abnormality

Left atrial abnormality is noted on the ECG by the presence of broad, notched P waves in leads I, II, and aVL. The P wave in V₁ may show a diphasic wave with a terminal downstroke that is larger than the initial upstroke (see Fig. 17-33C).

The left atrium is more likely to enlarge because of increased pressures created by trying to pump blood through a stenotic mitral valve. For this reason, LA abnormality is often referred to as P mitrale. When a LA abnormality pattern is noted on the ECG, the patient should be evaluated for the presence of mitral stenosis. An echocardiogram is a helpful diagnostic tool in addition to cardiac auscultation. Treatment is directed at the underlying cause. A valve replacement may be necessary.

### Right Ventricular Hypertrophy

RVH may exist without clear evidence on the ECG because the left ventricle is normally larger than the right and can mask changes in the size of the right ventricle. ECG evidence suggestive of RVH includes RA enlargement and right axis deviation. In addition, the normal QRS complex pattern across the precordial leads is reversed. Normally, R waves are small in V₁ and gradually grow tall by V₆. With RVH, the R wave is tall in V₁ and progresses to small by V₆. Precordial S waves persist rather than gradually disappear.

The presence of RVH is most likely an indicator of a chronic pulmonary condition, most likely chronic obstructive pulmonary disease, pulmonary hypertension, or pulmonic stenosis. RA enlargement is usually seen with an accompanying RVH. Treatment is directed at the underlying pulmonary disease.

### Left Ventricular Hypertrophy

Numerous criteria exist for the detection of left ventricular hypertrophy (LVH) on the ECG. The simplest criterion involves remembering the number "35." LVH is determined by adding the deepest S wave in either $V_1$ or $V_2$ to the tallest R wave in either $V_5$ or $V_6$. If the sum is 35 mm or more and the patient is older than 35 years of age, LVH is suspected. In addition, there may be ST-segment changes, the T waves in $V_5$ and $V_6$ may be asymmetrically inverted, and a left axis shift is likely.

Usually, LVH is the result of chronic systemic hypertension, a chronic cardiovascular problem, or aortic stenosis. LVH may result in a displacement of the PMI when palpating the apical pulse. Treatment of LVH is directed at the underlying condition.

### Ischemia, Injury, and Infarction Patterns

The 12-lead ECG can be very useful in detecting evidence of myocardial ischemia, injury, or infarction. Ischemia is seen on the ECG by ST-segment depressions and T-wave inversions. Acute patterns of injury are noted by ST-segment elevations. The presence of significant Q waves indicates an MI. For a more detailed discussion of patterns of ischemia, injury, and infarction, see Chapter 21.

## EFFECTS OF SERUM ELECTROLYTE ABNORMALITIES ON THE ELECTROCARDIOGRAM

Maintenance of adequate fluid and electrolyte balance assumes high priority in the care of patients in any medical, surgical, or coronary ICU. Patients being treated for renal or CVDs are especially vulnerable to electrolyte imbalances. The cure may well be worse than the disease if electrolyte abnormalities go undetected or ignored because they are frequently caused by the treatment rather than by the disease itself.

Diuresis can very quickly cause major shifts in electrolytes. Certainly, the often insidious drop of serum potassium levels in the patient with cardiac disease, who has been taking digitalis and then starts diuretics, is well known. Diuretics are also used frequently as part of the medical regimen for the control of hypertension. Any addition, deletion, or change in diuretic therapy warrants close monitoring of serum electrolytes. A history of any of these problems should alert the nurse to check the patient's serum electrolytes on an ongoing basis.

Potassium and calcium are probably the two most important electrolytes involved in the proper function of the heart. Because of their effects on the electrical impulse in the heart, an excess or insufficiency of either electrolyte frequently causes changes in the ECG (Table 17-14). The nurse who is aware of and able to recognize these changes may well suspect electrolyte abnormalities before laboratory findings or clinical symptoms appear and hazardous dysrhythmias occur.

However, it is necessary to remember that just as a patient who sustains MI may not have chest pain, the patient with electrolyte abnormalities may not exhibit any of the ECG changes described in the following sections. The ECG manifestations are valuable primarily in arousing suspicion of electrolyte abnormalities. Not one of them even approaches being diagnostic.

## Potassium

Potassium is the primary intracellular cation found in the body. Inside the cardiac cell, potassium is important for repolarization and for maintaining a stable, polarized state.

### Hyperkalemia

The earliest sign of hyperkalemia on the ECG is a change in the T wave. It is usually described as tall, narrow, and "peaked" or "tented" in appearance (Fig. 17-34). As the serum potassium level increases, the P-wave amplitude decreases and the PR interval is prolonged. Atrial asystole occurs, along with a widening of the QRS complex. At high, near-lethal potassium levels, the widened QRS complex merges with the T wave and starts to resemble a sine wave. Various dysrhythmias may occur during this time, with progression to VF and asystole. Clinically, the described changes in T waves begin to appear at serum levels of 6 to 7 mEq/L, and QRS complex widening is seen at serum levels of 8 to 9 mEq/L. Vigorous treatment must be instituted to reverse the condition at this point because sudden death may occur at any time after these levels are reached.

The ECG changes in hyperkalemia also may be associated with other conditions. Tall, peaked T waves may be a normal finding or may occur in the early stages of MI. QRS complex widening may be seen with quinidine and procainamide toxicity.

### Hypokalemia

Hypokalemia is associated with the appearance of U waves. Although the presence of U waves may be normal in many

| TABLE 17-14 | Electrocardiographic Changes Associated With Electrolyte Imbalances | |
|---|---|---|
| Electrolyte Imbalance | ECG Change | Possible Dysrhythmia Associated with the Electrolyte Imbalance |
| Hyperkalemia | Tall, narrow, peaked T waves; flat, wide P waves; widening QRS complex | Sinus bradycardia; SA block; junctional rhythm; idioventricular rhythm; ventricular tachycardia (VT); VF |
| Hypokalemia | Prominent U waves; ST segment depression; T-wave flattening or inversion | Premature ventricular beats; SVT; VT; VF |
| Hypercalcemia | Shortened QT interval | PVCs |
| Hypocalcemia | Lengthened QT interval; T-wave flattening or inversion | VT |

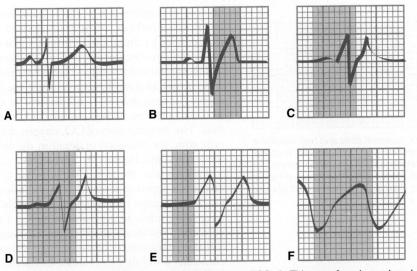

FIGURE 17-34  The effect of hyperkalemia on an ECG. **A:** This waveform is produced when the serum potassium level falls within the normal range—usually considered to be 3.5 to 5 mEq/L. **B:** When the serum potassium level rises above 5.5 mEq/L, the T wave begins to peak (*see highlighted area*). The P wave and QRS complex are normal. **C:** When the potassium level exceeds 6.5 mEq/L, the P wave grows wider, and its amplitude falls. The QRS complex also widens (*see highlighted area*) as intraventricular conduction velocity diminishes. **D:** When the potassium level reaches 10 mEq/L, the P wave becomes almost indiscernible; the QRS complex is slurred and widened (*see highlighted area*). **E:** When the potassium level ranges from 10 to 12 mEq/L, the P wave is undetectable (*see highlighted area*) because the atria are no longer excitable. **F:** When the potassium level exceeds 12 mEq/L, the QRS complex is no longer identifiable. The waves are known as sine waves (*see highlighted area*). Ventricular fibrillation and cardiac arrest follow. (From Springhouse: ECG Interpretation: Clinical Skillbuilders. Springhouse, PA: Springhouse Pub Co, 1990, p 113.)

people, these waves also may be an early sign of hypokalemia (Fig. 17-35). Usually easily recognized (best seen in lead $V_3$), a U wave may encroach on the preceding T wave and go unnoticed. The T wave may look notched or prolonged when it is hiding the U wave, giving the appearance of a prolonged QT interval. With increased potassium depletion, the U wave may become more prominent as the T wave becomes less so. The T wave becomes flattened and may even invert. The ST segment tends to become depressed, somewhat resembling the effects of digitalis on the ECG. Only at very low serum levels is there reasonable correlation between ECG changes and serum potassium concentrations.

The changes seen in hypokalemia are also observed in other conditions. The U wave may be accentuated in association with digitalis, LVH, and bradycardia.

Untreated hypokalemia enhances instability in the myocardial cell. Ventricular premature beats are the most common manifestation of this imbalance, but supraventricular dysrhythmias, conduction problems, and eventually VT and VF may occur. Hypokalemia also increases the sensitivity of the heart to digitalis and its accompanying dysrhythmias, even at normal serum levels. The severity of the dysrhythmias associated with hypokalemia requires early recognition of this problem.

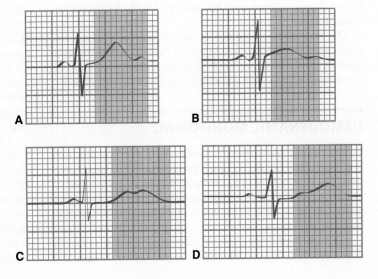

FIGURE 17-35  The effect of hypokalemia on an ECG. **A:** When the potassium level is normal—usually considered to be 3.5 to 5 mEq/L—the T wave is much higher than the U wave (*see highlighted area*). **B:** When the potassium level falls to 3 mEq/L, the T wave and U wave are almost the same height (*see highlighted area*). **C:** When the potassium level falls to 2 mEq/L, the U wave starts rising above the T wave (*see highlighted area*). **D:** As the potassium level reaches 1 mEq/L, the U wave starts to resemble a T wave (*see highlighted area*). The duration of the QT interval remains the same, but it cannot be measured because the two waves are fusing. (From Springhouse: ECG Interpretation: Clinical Skillbuilders. Springhouse, PA: Springhouse Pub Co, 1990, p 114.)

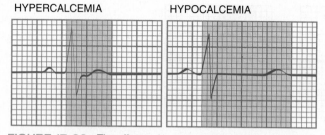

FIGURE 17-36 The effects of hypercalcemia and hypocalcemia on an ECG. Changes in serum calcium levels are reflected in phase 2 of the action potential. Hypercalcemia shortens the QT interval, whereas hypocalcemia lengthens it (*see highlighted areas*). (From Springhouse: ECG Interpretation: Clinical Skillbuilders. Springhouse, PA: Springhouse Pub Co, 1990, p 115.)

## Calcium

Like potassium, calcium is important in normal cardiac function. It is essential for the initiation and propagation of electrical impulses and for myocardial contractility. Abnormal calcium levels are not commonly seen unless they are associated with an underlying disease, and therefore they are not as common as serum potassium abnormalities.

### Hypercalcemia

On an ECG, the major finding associated with hypercalcemia is shortening of the QT interval (Fig. 17-36). Because the QRS complex and T wave are usually unaffected by changes in serum calcium levels, the shortened QT interval is a result of shortening of the ST segment. QT-interval shortening is also seen in patients taking digitalis. In addition, ST-segment depression occasionally occurs, and T-wave inversion may be seen.

### Hypocalcemia

On an ECG, low serum calcium levels prolong the QT interval because of a lengthening of the ST segment (see Fig. 17-36). The T wave itself is not prolonged but may be inverted in some cases. The prolongation of the QT interval in hypocalcemia should not be mistaken for a prolonged QTU interval seen in hypokalemia. In patients with chronic renal failure, hypocalcemia may be associated with decreased potassium levels.

QT interval prolongation also may be seen in cerebral vascular disease and after cardiac arrest. Several antiarrhythmic agents produce prolonged QT intervals and always should be considered when evaluating an ECG for hypocalcemic changes.

## HEMODYNAMIC MONITORING

Hemodynamic monitoring is a means of evaluating intracardiac and intravascular volume, pressures, and cardiac function. The purposes of hemodynamic monitoring are to aid in the diagnosis of various cardiovascular disorders, guide therapies to optimize cardiac function, and evaluate the patient's response to therapy.

Because a primary goal of management of a critically ill patient is to ensure adequate oxygenation of tissues and organs, indications for hemodynamic monitoring include conditions in which CO is insufficient to deliver oxygen to the cells due to alterations in intravascular volume (preload), alterations in vascular resistance (afterload), or alterations in myocardial contractility. Hemodynamic monitoring may be indicated as a mechanism to assess the balance of oxygen supply (oxygen delivery) and demand as evaluated by measurement of oxygen consumption or venous oxygen saturation. The determinants of CO, oxygen delivery, and oxygen utilization are discussed in detail in the later portion of this section and in Chapters 16, 23, and 54.

Patients who are in cardiogenic shock, severe heart failure, severe sepsis or septic shock, multiple system organ dysfunction, or acute respiratory distress syndrome, or those who have had cardiac surgery, are examples of candidates for invasive and minimally invasive hemodynamic monitoring. In addition, noninvasive hemodynamic technology now affords clinicians the ability to evaluate cardiovascular performance in areas outside of the critical care arena and in the outpatient setting.

To incorporate hemodynamic data into the care of the critically ill, the nurse must understand the following:

- Cardiorespiratory anatomy and physiology
- Monitoring system components to measure intracardiac and vascular pressures and CO
- Rationales for interventions directed toward enhancing CO, oxygen delivery, and oxygen utilization potential complications
- Differences between physiologic changes and mechanical or monitoring system problems.

## Pressure Monitoring System

Basic equipment necessary to measure and monitor invasive hemodynamic pressures includes a hollow-tube catheter, a fluid-filled pressure monitoring system composed of flush solution, IV tubing with drip chamber, noncompliant tubing, stopcocks, a flush device, one or more transducers, and a monitor that amplifies and displays the pressures and waveforms (Fig. 17-37). Pressures from the intravascular space or cardiac chambers are transmitted through the catheter and the fluid-filled noncompliant pressure tubing to the pressure transducer, which then converts the physiologic signal from the patient into an electrical one. Transducers are usually disposable and precalibrated, and come packaged with the pressure system. The monitor converts and amplifies the electrical signal generated by the transducer to a pressure tracing and digital value. In general, bedside physiologic monitoring systems have the capability to display several pressure digital readings and waveforms simultaneously. The monitors also include mechanisms to label and color code waveform locations, set or adjust alarms and tracing scale size, and zero the system.

Using a continuous flush solution maintains a patent pressure system. The flush solution is typically normal saline or dextrose and water ($D_5W$) and may be heparinized. The bag of solution is placed in a continuous pressure infusion bag or device to exert approximately 300 mm Hg. This maintains a constant pressure through the restrictor in the flush device and system. A continuous flow of approximately 3 to 5 mL/h prevents backflow of blood through the catheter and tubing, thereby maintaining system patency and accurate

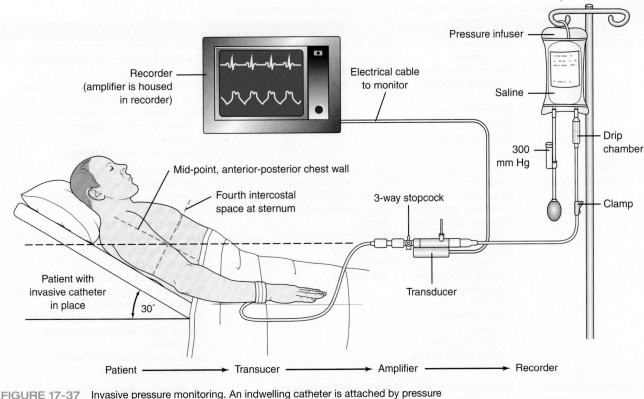

Patient ⟶ Transucer ⟶ Amplifier ⟶ Recorder

**FIGURE 17-37**  Invasive pressure monitoring. An indwelling catheter is attached by pressure tubing to a transducer. The transducer is connected to an amplifier/monitor that visually displays a waveform and systolic, diastolic, and mean pressure values. The system is composed of a flush solution under pressure, a continuous flush device, and a series of stopcocks. Typically, the stopcock closest to the insertion site is used to draw blood samples from the artery, and the stopcock located nearest the transducer is used for zeroing.

transmission of pressures. The system is flushed manually by activating the flush device.

## Optimizing the Pressure Monitoring System

An optimal pressure monitoring system is one that accurately reproduces the physiologic signals transmitted through it. For optimal use of invasive monitoring systems, it is essential to ensure accurate pressure recordings and waveform display. Technical or mechanical factors can produce erroneously high or low pressures and altered waveforms. Before determining whether abnormal pressures are a result of altered physiology or a response to interventions, the nurse assesses the system to determine whether the pressures recorded are accurate. Table 17-15 describes causes of technical factors affecting invasive pressure monitoring and troubleshooting techniques. Any impedance between the patient and transducer, such as air bubbles, blood, or additional stopcocks, can alter the signal and subsequently the pressures and waveforms. Less than 300 mm Hg in the continuous pressure device, soft compliant IV tubing, or additional length of pressure tubing may also distort the signal to the transducer. Stopcocks, used for zeroing the transducer and blood sampling, as well as any other connectors, are kept to a minimum. Luer-Lok–type connections, rather than slip-lock connections, help preserve the integrity of the system.

After assessing the pressure system components to identify any potential mechanical problems, the nurse performs a square-wave test to determine the dynamic response of the system. In addition, the nurse ensures proper leveling of the air–fluid interface and zeroing of the transducer to optimize the system.[25–28]

### Square-Wave Test: Dynamic Response Testing

For a rapid bedside assessment of the dynamic response of the system, a simple evaluation can be obtained by performing a square-wave test and observing the resultant oscillations. Checking the dynamic response of the system determines the natural frequency and damping coefficient. Factors affecting the response of the system include the natural frequency of the system itself, the pressure tubing quality, number of stopcocks, and other components, such as blood sampling systems. The steps required to measure the natural frequency and damping coefficient accurately are complex and time consuming. Other references describe the steps for performing this process.[25,26]

To perform a square-wave test, a flush device that can be activated and released rapidly is required. Activating the flush device opens the internal restrictor and increases the fluid flow through the system. The nurse observes the bedside monitor for the increase in pressure. The waveform sharply rises and "squares off" at the top of the scale. After the flush device is released, the restrictor closes. The nurse observes the waveform as it returns to baseline, counts the number of oscillations, and observes the distance between them.

**TABLE 17-15**   **Troubleshooting Pressure Monitoring Systems and Measurements**

| Problem | Cause | Prevention | Intervention |
|---|---|---|---|
| 1. No waveform | Transducer not open to catheter<br>Settings on bedside monitor incorrect or off<br>Catheter clotted<br>Faulty cable<br>Faulty transducer | Check stopcocks for proper position<br>Use correct setting on bedside monitor<br>Maintain continuous flush<br>Use functioning cables | Check and correct stopcock position<br>Check scale setting and monitor setup<br>Aspirate blood clot<br>Do not fast flush or irrigate with syringe<br>Check function with cable checking device<br>Check function of transducer with mercury, water column, or supplemental pressure device<br>Change transducer if necessary |
| 2. Overdamped waveforms | Improper scale selection<br>Air bubbles in tubing and near transducer<br>Blood clot partially occluding catheter tip<br>Forward migration of catheter<br>Catheter tip occluded by balloon or vessel wall<br>Leak in pressure system<br>Pressure bag not inflated at 300 mm Hg | Flush system by gravity<br>Remove any air bubbles<br>Maintain continuous flush; use heparinized solution according to hospital protocol<br>Tighten all connections and stopcock up on setup<br>Inflate or apply pressure to device to 300 mm Hg | Change to proper scale<br>Flush air from system<br>On initial setup, expel all air from flush solution bag<br>Aspirate clots with syringe<br>Use heparinized solution according to institution policy<br>Reposition patient<br>Check for kinks in catheters<br>Reposition by pulling back catheter while observing waveforms<br>Tighten all connections and stopcocks<br>Change faulty system components if necessary<br>Reinflate bag or activate device<br>Change device if faulty |
| 3. Underdamped waveforms; whip or ringing | Excessive movement of catheter<br>Air bubbles in tubing | Correct catheter placement<br>Use appropriate catheter size for vessel<br>Eliminate excessive length of pressure tubing<br>Check for very rigid pressure tubing | Try different catheter tip position<br>Eliminate excessive tubing<br>Change tubing<br>Eliminate excessive stopcocks |
| 4. False low readings | Leveling or zero reference (transducer) is too high<br>Improper zeroing<br>Overdamped waveforms | Check level periodically. Level air–fluid interface of stopcock nearest the transducer to the phlebostatic axis<br>Check monitor settings. Observe waveforms<br>Perform square-wave test | Relevel transducer air–fluid interface to phlebostatic axis<br>Rezero monitor<br>Optimize length of pressure tubing |
| 5. False high readings | Leveling or zero reference (transducer) is too low<br>Improper zeroing<br>Overdamped waveforms | Check level periodically. Level air–fluid interface of stopcock nearest the transducer to the phlebostatic axis<br>Check monitor settings. Observe waveforms<br>Perform square-wave test | Relevel transducer air–fluid interface to phlebostatic axis<br>Rezero monitor<br>Remove excessive length of pressure tubing |
| 6. Inappropriate pressure waveform | Incorrect catheter position<br>Migration of PAC into mechanical wedge position | Establish optimal position carefully during the insertion process, ensuring use of 1.25–1.5 mL air for proper balloon inflation volume for obtaining a PAOP tracing | Reposition patient<br>Obtain chest x-ray<br>Reposition catheter*<br>Observe waveforms and confirm with initial insertion tracings<br>If right ventricular tracing is observed from PAC distal tip, slowly inflate balloon to allow PAC to "float" into PA<br>If PAOP tracing is observed with balloon deflated, withdraw catheter slightly while observing waveforms<br>Stop withdrawing as soon as a PA tracing is observed |
| 7. Bleed back into pressure tubing or transducer | Loose connections<br>Stopcocks not returned to proper position<br>Pressure bag not at 300 mm Hg | Ensure all connections are tight<br>Return stopcocks to proper positions<br>Maintain 300 mm Hg of pressure | Tighten connections<br>Ensure stopcocks are in correct position<br>Check pressure device |

*Repositioning the PAC is usually done by a physician or advanced practice nurse such as a nurse practitioner and varies with hospital policies.

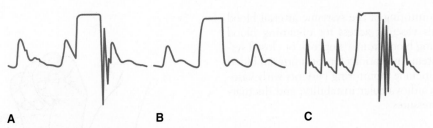

A          B          C

FIGURE 17-38    Steps to perform a square wave test include the following:
1. Activate the snap or pull tab of the flush device.
2. Observe the square wave generated on the bedside monitor.
3. Count the oscillations after the square wave.
4. Observe the distance between the oscillations.
   A. *Optimally damped system*: Activation of the fast flush device generates a sharp vertical up-stroke, horizontal line, and straight vertical downstroke ending with 1.5 to 2 oscillations close together before returning to baseline.
   B. *Overdamped system*: Activation of the fast flush device generates a slurred upstroke and downstroke with less than 1.5 oscillations above or below the baseline. Causes include system leaks, blood clots, or large air bubbles in the tubing or transducer. Systolic pressures read erroneously low, diastolic pressures occasionally read low.
   C. *Underdamped system*: Activation of the fast flush device generates more than 2 to 3 oscillations above and below the baseline. Causes include small air bubbles in the system, very rigid pressure tubing, and additional length of tubing. Systolic pressures read erroneously high, diastolic pressures read erroneously low.
(Courtesy of Edwards Lifesciences LLC.)

In an ideal system, also called optimally damped, the square wave has a straight vertical upstroke from the baseline, a straight horizontal component at the top of the monitor, and more importantly, a straight vertical downstroke back to the baseline with approximately one and one-half to two sharp oscillations. The distance between the oscillations is also close.[25] Figure 17-38 depicts a normal square wave and examples of square waves from nonoptimized hemodynamic monitoring systems. Overdamped systems produce lower than actual systolic pressures and potential loss of dicrotic notch identification. Underdamped systems produce artificially high systolic pressures and artificially low diastolic pressures. By performing a square-wave test, the bedside clinician can quickly assess if the abnormal waveform tracing is a result of the patient's physiology or a less-than-optimal system.[25–28]

### Leveling and Zeroing

After a square-wave test is performed, the system is leveled to an external landmark and then zeroed to atmospheric pressure to ensure accurate pressure monitoring. Typically, the stopcock nearest the transducer is used as the air–fluid interface for leveling and zeroing; however, any stopcock port in the system can be used as long as it is leveled to the phlebostatic axis. The phlebostatic axis is best described as the bisection of the fourth intercostal space and the midpoint of the anterior–posterior chest diameter (see Fig. 17-37); it is often called the zero reference point. Zeroing the transducer is the action of opening the pressure system to atmospheric air and observing a reading of zero on the bedside monitor. With the stopcock turned off to the patient and opened to air, the influence of hydrostatic pressure is negated from the fluid-filled pressure system. Subsequent pressures recorded on the monitor now reflect those generated by the patient, not external forces. Bedside monitor manufacturers vary; however, most have a function key to ensure that the zeroing process has been successful. Newer disposable transducers come from the manufacturer precalibrated and do not require adjustment to an electronic zero. The term "zeroing" is used, however, when referencing to atmospheric pressure.

Once the zero reference point is established, the patient's chest is marked to ensure consistent leveling when other practitioners obtain subsequent pressure readings. With the patient positioned supine, a carpenter-type level or laser-light level device is used to align the air–fluid interface with the phlebostatic axis. Further pressure measurements are taken with the patient in the supine position.

If the alignment of the air–fluid interface changes after initial leveling and zeroing, an inversely related error of approximately 2 mm Hg for every inch misaligned occurs. For example, if the transducer air–fluid interface is raised from initial leveling, the values displayed will be about 2 mm Hg too low, and if lowered from initial leveling, the values recorded will be erroneously too high.

The head of the bed may be elevated as much as 60 degrees, provided that the air–fluid interface is releveled after any changes in patient position. Lateral or side-lying positions may be used if the external landmark is properly identified. Because some patients respond differently to head of bed elevation and side-lying positions, their hemodynamic values should be compared from supine.[25–28]

After the level and zero are verified, the only way to determine whether the pressures displayed on the monitor are accurate is to apply a known value to the transducer with a piece of external tubing and water column. Some transducer manufacturers provide a device that applies a known pressure to the transducer for rapid determination of accurate pressure recordings.

## Arterial Pressure Monitoring

Invasive arterial pressure monitoring uses an intra-arterial catheter connected to the pressure monitoring system. This allows continuous monitoring of the systemic arterial blood pressure and provides vascular access for obtaining blood samples by withdrawing blood from a stopcock or closed system device in the system. Indications for intra-arterial blood pressure monitoring include monitoring patients with vasoactive IV infusions; cardiovascular instability; and fluctuating, unstable blood pressures.

## Arterial Line Insertion

The most common sites for arterial catheter insertions are the radial, brachial, and femoral arteries. Alternative and less frequent sites include the axillary and dorsalis pedis arteries in adults and the temporal and umbilical arteries in neonates. The following factors are considered for selecting the artery for cannulation:

- *Size of the artery in relation to the size of the catheter:* The artery should be large enough to accommodate the catheter without occluding or significantly impeding flow.
- *Accessibility of the site:* The chosen site should be easily accessible and free from contamination by body secretions.
- *Blood flow to the limb distal to the insertion site:* There should be adequate collateral flow in the event that the cannulated artery becomes occluded.

The radial artery, which satisfies these criteria, is the most frequent site for an arterial catheter. It is superficially located and therefore easy to palpate. Cannulation of this artery also usually poses the least limitation on the patient's mobility.

Before a catheter is inserted into the radial artery, the presence of adequate collateral circulation to the hand by the ulnar artery is assessed by performing Allen's test (Fig. 17-39). The Allen's test is performed by having the patient clench his or her fist several times while the nurse is occluding both the radial and ulnar arteries. The patient then extends the hand with the palm side up to show it is blanched. Pressure on the ulnar artery is released, and the hand is observed for return of color. If the hand remains blanched for longer than about 10 seconds, ulnar circulation is considered inadequate, in which case the radial artery should not be cannulated. Use of ultrasound devices for assessing blood flow in place of the Allen's test is becoming more common.[26]

Regardless of the site chosen for arterial catheter placement, the insertion is performed using sterile technique. The pressure monitoring system is assembled and flushed, and the transducer is leveled and zeroed before the catheter is inserted. Once the catheter is in place, it should be secured and the site dressed according to institutional policy.[25–28]

## Arterial Pressure Waveform

The normal arterial waveform should have a rapid upstroke, a clear dicrotic notch, and a definite end-diastole, as shown in Figure 17-40. The mechanical activity of systole and diastole follows the electrical activity of depolarization and repolarization, respectively. The initial sharp upstroke of the waveform results partly from the rapid ejection of blood from the left ventricle into the aorta. On a dual-channel tracing of both the ECG and arterial waveforms, the QRS complex precedes the rapid rise in arterial pressure. The dicrotic notch reflects a slight backflow of blood in the aorta, reflecting

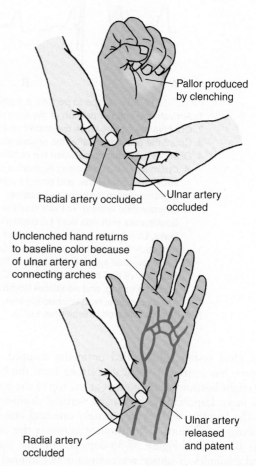

**FIGURE 17-39** Modified Allen's test.

closure of the aortic valve or may be a reflective wave from the periphery.

## Obtaining Arterial Pressures

The value measured at the peak of the waveform is the systolic pressure. A normal arterial systolic pressure is typically 90 to 140 mm Hg. The dicrotic notch typically indicates the end of ventricular systole and the beginning of diastole. As blood flows to the periphery, the pressure in the arterial system decreases. The lowest point of the waveform is the diastolic pressure, which is normally between 60 and 90 mm Hg.

Mean arterial pressure (MAP) is used to evaluate perfusion of vital body organs. Normal MAP is 70 to 105 mm Hg. The MAP calculation incorporates the impact of diastolic time being approximately two times longer than systole during a cardiac cycle. Therefore, MAP = diastolic pressure + 1/3 PP, or

$$\frac{\text{Systolic pressure} + (\text{Diastolic pressure} \times 2)}{3}$$

Most bedside monitors automatically calculate and continuously display the MAP. Manufacturer algorithms to determine MAP may vary; however, most incorporate assessment of the area under the full arterial waveform rather than use a mathematical model.

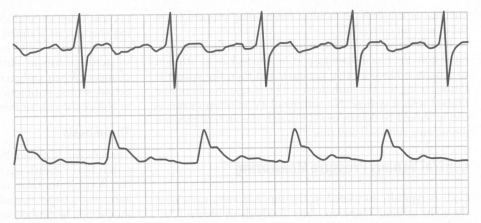

**FIGURE 17-40** Normal relationship of ECG and arterial pressure waveform.

The difference between the systolic and diastolic pressure is the PP. This value more closely reflects the SV from the ventricle. SV is proportional to PP and inversely related to the aortic compliance. Bedside monitors do not automatically display this valuable parameter. Clinicians who want to assess the patient's volume status should include PP in their assessment because it is an indirect reflection of the SV. The range of PP may be as wide as 30 to 100 mm Hg at the far ends of the spectrum. A wide PP occurs typically with elevated systolic pressures resulting from aortic regurgitation and some vascular conditions. A narrow PP may result from hypovolemic states when the diastolic pressure rises.[25–27]

## Complications

### Infection

Proper attention to sterile technique during catheter insertion; care of the insertion site; blood sampling; and maintenance of a sterile, closed monitoring system reduce the risk of infection. The following should be performed according to institution policy: assessment of insertion site for signs of infection; use of sterile technique when changing dressings, tubing, and flush solution; and maintenance of the integrity of the system. Opening the pressure system to air for either zeroing or blood sampling provides opportunity for infection. Applying sterile nonvented or "dead-ender" caps to the stopcock ports helps eliminate contamination. Closed systems for blood sampling help reduce the potential for open stopcock infections and assist with managing potential blood loss.

### Accidental Blood Loss

Accidental blood loss from an arterial catheter can be catastrophic and often can be prevented. All connections in the system should use a Luer–Lok–type connector. The extremity in which the catheter is placed may be immobilized (eg, placing the wrist on an arm board). If some type of patient self-protective device is used, it should not be placed over the insertion site. Easy access to the insertion site and connections is imperative.

### Impaired Circulation to Extremity

Circulation to the extremity in which the arterial line is placed must be monitored frequently. Initial assessment of color, sensation, temperature, and movement of the extremity is made after insertion of the arterial catheter and as frequently as the institution policy states. Any indication of impaired circulation may be an indication for catheter removal and is reported immediately.

## Nursing Considerations

Blood pressures obtained by an intra-arterial catheter and with an optimal pressure monitoring system are most accurate. Comparisons between intra-arterial and cuff pressures may be misleading because the methods of measurement reflect different physiologic events and are therefore not truly comparable. Direct or invasive monitoring measures pressure, and indirect cuff measurements are based on flow. In normotensive patients, intra-arterial pressures are typically higher by about 5 to 10 mm Hg than the pressures obtained using a cuff. Indirect methods tend to overestimate direct measurements in hypotensive patients and underestimate them in hypertensive patients. Variations as wide as 20 to 60 mm Hg occur, depending on specific patient conditions.[26,27]

For interventions when accurate values are important for therapeutic decisions, intra-arterial pressures remain the gold standard. Using a trend value from one source is often more helpful than comparing values obtained between different technologies. Documenting the site of pressure measurements and the type of technique used is key.

Patient safety measures include the proper setting and activation of all alarms on the bedside physiologic monitor. Bedside monitor alarms provide warning that a change has occurred either in the system or in the patient's physiologic status. Alarms are set either around a patient's specific parameter or according to institution policy. Typically, high and low alarms are set for systolic, diastolic, and mean pressures and within 10 to 20 mm Hg of the patient's blood pressure. The alarms must be visible and audible to the caregiver for the specific patient environment. Troubleshooting steps for an alarm are listed in Table 17-15 on page 238.

General steps to ensure accurate pressures from invasive lines include assessing the patient first, then checking the pressure monitoring system, and then inspecting the monitor itself. Assess the insertion site: Is the catheter kinked? Are there any blood clots? Is there any sign of bleeding? Next, evaluate the pressure system: Are any stopcocks turned the wrong way? Is there sufficient pressure in the pressure bag (ie, does the pressure read 300 mm Hg)? Are there any air bubbles? Is the bedside monitor functioning properly? Are the alarms set correctly?

If catheter patency is in question, blood and fluid are aspirated from the blood-drawing port or stopcock in an attempt to remove a blood clot (if present), and then the system is flushed using the fast flush device. The system should not be flushed with a syringe. No additional IV solution or medication should be administered through the arterial pressure monitoring system at any time.[26,27]

## Central Venous Pressure Monitoring

CVP is typically measured in the superior vena cava near the right atrium. There are three methods to obtain CVP readings: via a catheter placed in the jugular or subclavian vein, monitoring the RA lumen of a PA catheter, or by use of a peripherally inserted catheter (PICC). CVP reflects the pressure of blood in the right atrium and provides information about intravascular blood volume, right ventricular end-diastolic pressure (RVEDP), and right ventricular function. To a limited degree in persons with normal pulmonary vasculature and left ventricular function, the CVP indirectly reflects left ventricular end-diastolic pressure (LVEDP) and function because the left and right sides of the heart are linked by the compliant pulmonary vascular bed. Alterations in intravascular volume status or ventricular function are usually associated with abnormally high or low CVP measurements.[25–27]

### Catheter Insertion

The CVP catheter is long and flexible. It is inserted under maximum sterile conditions with a chlorhexidine site preparation. The physician or nurse practitioner uses a sterile field with a full sterile drape, sterile gloves and gown, and a mask and cap. Those assisting the physician also should wear a cap and mask and sterile gloves if near the catheter or insertion site. The best insertion site to minimize infection risk is the subclavian vein.[29] Catheters also can be inserted into an antecubital, jugular, or femoral vein if necessary. It is threaded into position in the vena cava close to the right atrium. Occasionally, the catheter may advance into the right atrium. In this situation, the catheter is withdrawn several centimeters.

The hemodynamic monitoring system components and preparation for CVP monitoring are identical to those described for arterial pressure monitoring. After insertion of the catheter, the pressure tubing is connected to the catheter hub. The CVP waveform and value appear on the bedside monitor.[25–27]

### Complications

#### Infection

Infection may occur within the catheter or around the insertion site. Central venous catheter–associated bloodstream infection is diagnosed and verified by blood cultures. Occasionally after catheter removal, the tip is cut off with sterile scissors and sent to the microbiology laboratory. Signs and symptoms of infection include erythema at the insertion site, fever, or elevated WBC count. Primary measures to prevent infection include routine dressing and IV fluid tubing changes, as outlined by the Centers for Disease Control and Prevention[29] and hospital policy, as well as adherence to sterile technique during catheter insertion and dressing changes. When catheters are left in place for an extended period of time, antibiotic-impregnated catheters may be used to reduce the risk for infection.

#### Thrombosis

Thromboses occasionally form and may vary in size from a thin fibrin sheath over the catheter tip to a large thrombus. A small thrombus may be flushed away without causing harm, but a larger thrombus occluding the catheter and vein should not be flushed into the venous circulation. A large thrombus may be detected by loss of hemodynamic waveform and inability to infuse fluid or withdraw blood from the catheter. The patient may have edema of the arm closest to the catheter site, varying degrees of neck pain (that may radiate), and jugular vein distention. A large thrombus is classified as an emergency because it may impair circulation to a limb. A nurse may attempt to aspirate this clot if hospital policy permits. Frequently, hospitals also have protocols to administer small doses of thrombolytic agents to dissolve the clot. At the very least, the nurse is responsible for reporting suspected catheter occlusion to a physician.

#### Air Embolism

Air embolism occurs as a result of air entering the system and traveling through the vena cava to the right ventricle. Usually, air entry into the catheter is associated with disconnection of the catheter from the IV tubing. Changes in intrathoracic pressure with inspiration and expiration draw air into the catheter and vena cava. Sudden hypotension may be the first indicator of this sometimes lethal problem.

Approximately 10 to 20 mL of air must enter the venous system before the patient becomes symptomatic. Signs of such an emergency may include confusion, lightheadedness, anxiety, and unresponsiveness. The physiologic event is the creation of foam in the ventricle with each heart contraction and loss of SV due to air instead of blood in the ventricle, causing a sudden decrease in CO. Cardiac arrest may occur.

If this problem is suspected, turning the patient on the left side in the Trendelenburg position may allow the air to rise to the wall of the right ventricle and improve blood flow. Oxygen should be started unless contraindicated.

Strategies to prevent disconnections include having Luer–Lok connections on all central line catheters and tubings, careful manipulation of catheter and tubing during dressing changes, and routine monitoring of the connections. There is no substitute for close observation by skilled and educated nursing staff.

### Nursing Considerations

Ensuring the integrity of the monitoring system, obtaining and documenting accurate data, and monitoring trends in CVP are critical to the interpretation and utilization of information to assess a patient's cardiovascular function and response to interventions. Evidence-Based Practice Highlight 17-2 summarizes current evidence related to obtaining accurate measurement of CVP pressure.[28]

and causing blood to "back up" in the right ventricle, right atrium, and vena cava. In extreme cases, the increased intrathoracic pressure associated with mechanical ventilation causes significant right ventricular dysfunction, and the CVP is elevated because of reduced forward blood flow into the pulmonary vasculature, resulting in increased volume and pressure of the blood in the right atrium and vena cava.

Increased CVP is associated with right ventricular failure due to CAD or left ventricular failure. The inability of the right ventricle to pump blood through the pulmonary vasculature because of injured or infarcted myocardium results in increased volume and pressure in the right atrium and vena cava. Left ventricular failure may increase CVP as the pressure of blood volume congests the pulmonary vasculature and impairs flow from the right ventricle, causing right ventricular dilation and subsequent failure. Again, the increased pressure is reflected backward to the right atrium and vena cava. In these instances, interventions are directed toward facilitating forward blood flow by improving ventricular contractility and reducing the intravascular blood volume. A decrease in the CVP is an indication of the effectiveness of therapy.

CVP is always interpreted in conjunction with other clinical observations, such as auscultation of breath sounds, heart and respiratory rate, ECG, neck vein distention, and urine output. For example, increased CVP associated with pulmonary basilar crackles and decreased urine output is often indicative of left ventricular failure. Distended neck veins but clear breath sounds and a high CVP might be caused by increased intrathoracic pressure from mechanical ventilator effects. Patients who are septic may have a low CVP that is associated with fever, elevated WBC count, tachycardia, and tachypnea, whereas patients who are taking vasodilating agents may have a low CVP that is associated with an increased heart rate but none of the other aforementioned clinical signs. A CVP value alone is meaningless, but when used in conjunction with other clinical data, it is a valuable aid in managing and predicting the patient's clinical course.[25–28]

## Pulmonary Artery Pressure Monitoring

The PA catheter provides assessment of right ventricular function, pulmonary vascular status, and, indirectly, left ventricular function. RA, right ventricular (RV), and PA pressures, as well as pulmonary artery occlusion pressure (PAOP), are measured using a PA catheter. PA catheters with a thermistor have the capability of determining CO. The pressures and CO obtained allow the clinician to calculate derived parameters and facilitate diagnosis of cardiovascular and cardiopulmonary dysfunction, determine the therapy needed, and evaluate the effectiveness of the interventions.

## Pulmonary Artery Catheters

Several types of flow-directed, balloon-tipped PA catheters are available in different sizes. The type of catheter used is determined by the parameters to be monitored and additional requirements governed by the patient's condition. The 7.5- or 8-French (F; a measure of catheter size) thermodilution catheter is the size most commonly used (Fig. 17-41). All PA catheters have several external ports or lumen hubs

Normal CVP is less than 8 mm Hg. Low CVP indicates a hypovolemic state often requiring fluid administration. The anticipated response to fluid therapy is an increase in the CVP. Similarly, diuretic therapy reduces intravascular volume, and its administration is expected to be associated with a decrease in the CVP. Vasodilation from sepsis or vasodilating drugs may also lead to a low or decreasing CVP; both create a relative hypovolemia because the intravascular space has become greater relative to the blood volume, which has not changed. Increased CVP may be caused by a number of complex and interrelated factors, each of which requires scrutiny. Two of the more common causes of increased CVP are right ventricular failure and mechanical ventilation. Rarely is intravascular volume overload and hypervolemia alone a cause of increased CVP.

Mechanical ventilation increases intrathoracic pressure, which is transmitted to the pulmonary vasculature, heart, and great vessels. This pressure may directly affect CVP, which may increase as well, because intrathoracic pressure compresses the pulmonary vessels, creating resistance to blood flow from the right side to the left side of the heart

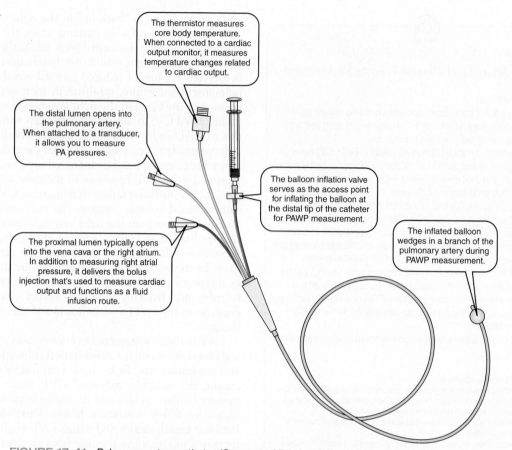

**FIGURE 17-41** Pulmonary artery catheter. (Courtesy of Edwards Lifesciences, LLC.)

corresponding to internal lumens and lumen openings into the right side of the heart and PA. A typical PA catheter has four lumens with external hubs or ports: the proximal hub and lumen, distal hub and lumen, balloon inflation valve and lumen, and thermistor connector and lumen.

The proximal or RA lumen opens into the right atrium; in smaller patients, the location might be in the superior or inferior vena cava, depending on insertion location. The lumen is used for infusion of fluids and is often connected to a transducer to provide RAP measurements and display of the RAP waveform. The RA lumen port is also used as the injectate port for measuring COs.

The distal or PA lumen hub is always attached to a transducer and a continuous flush system. The PA waveform is displayed continuously, as are the PA systolic, diastolic, and mean pressures. The PA port is used for the withdrawal of mixed venous blood, which is necessary for venous oxygen saturation, oxygen extraction, oxygen consumption, and intrapulmonary shunt measurements. Use of the PA distal port for fluid or medication administration is not recommended.

The balloon inflation port and lumen enable inflation of the balloon near the catheter tip with a small volume of air to measure the PA occlusion pressure, known as the PAOP. The balloon capacity of most PA catheters is 1.5 mL, and the balloon should not be inflated with more than this amount of air. Fluid is never inserted into the balloon inflation port.

Near the tip of the PA catheter is a thermistor. A cable to the bedside monitor or to a CO computer connects to the external thermistor port. The thermistor permits measurement of the patient's temperature in the PA (core temperature), and it detects the blood temperature change when solution is injected through the RA port to obtain a CO.

Specialty PA catheters include the previously described components and additional features and lumens. Some of the features include additional lumens in the RA, RV, or both for added infusion. A distal lumen containing fiber-optic filaments allows continuous measurement of mixed venous oxygen saturation ($SvO_2$). The external optic connecting cable is attached to an optics module and then special oximetry monitor. Catheters modified with a thermal filament and combined with a thermal filament connector and special monitor provide and display CO on a continuous basis. Other advanced catheters with advanced monitor algorithms determine RV ejection fraction and additional derived parameters such as end-diastolic volume. Figure 17-42 shows various types of PA catheters.

Specially designed catheters may also be used for temporary pacing. There are PA catheters that house pacing electrodes for both atrial and ventricular pacing as well as PA catheters with lumens in the RA and RV for placing of special probes for pacing.[25-27]

## Pulmonary Artery Catheter Insertion

Before the PA catheter is inserted, all necessary equipment should be assembled and prepared according to institution policies. The flushed pressure monitoring system is placed at

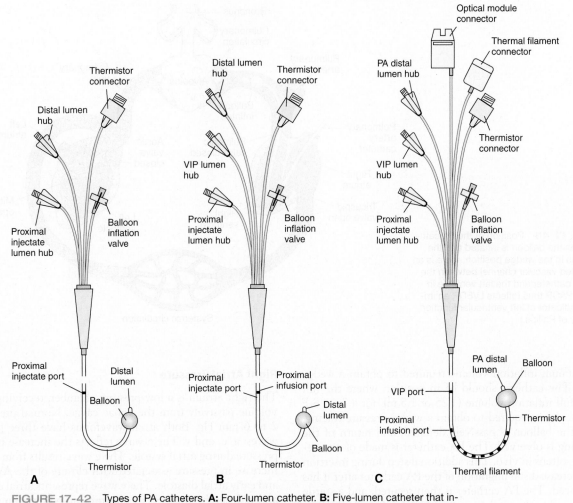

**FIGURE 17-42**   Types of PA catheters. **A:** Four-lumen catheter. **B:** Five-lumen catheter that includes an additional venous infusion port (VIP) into the right atrium. **C:** Seven-lumen catheter that includes a VIP port and two additional lumens for continuous cardiac output (CCO) and thermal filament, and continuous mixed venous oxygen saturation ($SvO_2$) monitoring (optical module connector). An additional option is to combine use of the CCO filament and the thermistor response time to calculate end-diastolic volume monitoring. (Courtesy of Edwards Lifesciences, LLC.)

the zero reference point, leveled, and zeroed. Each lumen of the PA catheter is flushed with sterile solution from the flush system. (Note that fiber-optic $SO_2$-monitoring catheters must be calibrated in the calibration cup housed in the sterile tray package before flushing the PA lumens.) The balloon lumen is inflated with air to ensure proper inflation and to check for leaks; it is then deflated before insertion. The PA port is then connected to the prepared pressure tubing, and the other lumens are connected to either a pressure monitoring system or an IV solution.

Strict sterile technique, including a full sterile drape, is required for the insertion procedure. The clinician performing the procedure wears a cap, mask, gown, and gloves. The nurse assisting wears a cap and mask and, if manipulating the catheter, gloves. The PA catheter is inserted into a large vein through an introducer catheter, which is usually placed by a percutaneous approach. The most common insertion sites are the right internal jugular, right or left subclavian, and femoral veins. Occasionally, the antecubital vein is used; this requires a venous cutdown.

Determination of the catheter tip location is established by monitoring the waveform and pressures on the bedside monitor as the catheter passes through the heart chambers and vessels. Black catheter markings occur every 10 cm, with a heavier black line at the 50- and 100-cm points. Distances are identified from the distal tip (ie, the proximal lumen exits 30 cm from the distal tip). These markings are also used during the insertion procedure to assist with catheter tip placement. When the catheter tip is approximately 15 cm into the introducer, the tip has typically exited the sheath and lies in the vena cava and RA junction. Waveforms on the monitor show respiratory excursions.

At this time, the balloon is inflated with the recommended balloon inflation volume of 1.5 mL air or $CO_2$. The clinician gently but rapidly advances the catheter with the balloon inflated. This helps "float" the catheter into the right atrium, through the tricuspid valve into the right ventricle, across the pulmonic valve into the PA, and eventually into the wedged position (Fig. 17-43). The balloon is allowed to deflate passively after the PA wedge waveform is noted on the monitor and return of the PA waveform is confirmed. The PA catheter is slowly pulled back 1 to 2 cm to reduce or remove any redundant length or loop in the right atrium or right ventricle. The balloon is then reinflated to determine

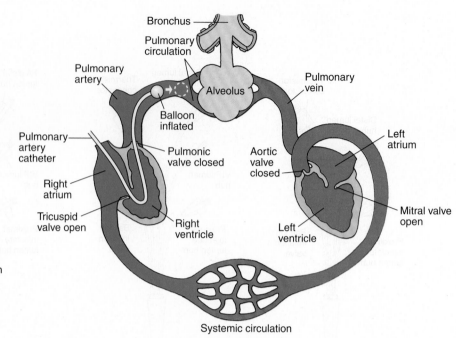

FIGURE 17-43 Position of the PA catheter. When the balloon is inflated and the catheter is in the wedge position, there is an unrestricted vascular channel between the tip of the catheter and the left ventricle in diastole. PAOP thus reflects LVEDP, an important indicator of left ventricular function. (Courtesy of Philips.)

the minimum inflation volume required to obtain a wedge tracing. The catheter should be in position where the full or near-full inflation volume (1.25 or 1.5 mL for a 7- or 8-F PA catheter) is required to obtain a wedge pressure tracing. Again, the balloon is passively deflated, and return of the PA tracing is observed. The PA catheter is made of a material that softens in vivo. This additional step during insertion helps decrease distal migration of the PA catheter after it has been placed. The PA catheter is then secured, and a sterile dressing is placed over the insertion site. Catheter position is also verified with a chest radiograph after the insertion.

Nursing responsibilities during the insertion procedure include ensuring use of sterile technique, monitoring the changes in hemodynamic waveforms, recording the pressures in each chamber of the heart as the catheter is passed through, and monitoring the patient for complications. Ventricular dysrhythmias are the most common complications during PA catheter insertion (see following section on Complications). Therefore, it is advisable to have a lidocaine bolus and defibrillator available for the insertion procedure.[25–27]

## Waveform Interpretation

All hemodynamic pressures and waveforms are generated by pressure changes in the heart during the various phases of the cardiac cycle. Electrical activity (depolarization and repolarization) precedes mechanical activity of systole and diastole. Therefore, interpretation of the hemodynamic waveforms depends on the correlation of mechanical to electrical activities using the ECG. There are three categories of hemodynamic waveforms: atrial, which includes RA, LA, and PA wedge (that indirectly reflects the LA waveform); ventricular, which includes left and right ventricular; and arterial, which includes PA and systemic arterial. The waveforms in each category are similar because they result from the same cardiac events. The measurements are different because the pressures generated in the right side compared with the left side of the heart differ.

### Right Atrial Pressure

The right atrium is a low-pressure chamber, receiving blood volume passively from the venae cavae. Normal pressure is 2 to 6 mm Hg. Both atrial waveforms have three positive waves: a, c, and v. The a wave reflects the increase in atrial pressure during atrial systole. The c wave results from a small increase in pressure associated with closure of the AV valve and early atrial diastole. The v wave represents atrial diastole and reflects the increase in pressure caused by filling of the atrium with blood. It also occurs during ventricular systole. Figure 17-44A shows the RA waveform.

Accurate identification of the a, c, and v waves requires correlation of the waveform with the ECG. On the ECG, the P wave represents atrial depolarization, which causes RA and then LA contraction. Therefore, the a wave occurs after the P wave and usually in the PR interval. The QRS complex represents ventricular depolarization and causes ventricular contraction. Simultaneously, the atria relax and fill with blood. The v wave generated by these events thus falls after the QRS complex and in the T-to-P interval.

Atrial pressure tracings also have two primary negative waves or descents: x and y. The x descent follows the a or c wave if present and represents a decrease in pressure caused by atrial relaxation at the beginning of atrial diastole. The y descent follows the v wave and represents the initial, passive atrial emptying into the ventricle as the AV valve opens.[25–27]

### Right Ventricular Pressure

The RV is a low-pressure chamber. RVEDP is usually 0 to 8 mm Hg. When the tricuspid valve is open, the RAP and the RVEDP are similar. Right ventricular systolic pressure is normally 20 to 30 mm Hg because the RV must generate only enough pressure to open the pulmonic valve and move blood through the low-pressure pulmonary vasculature.

The RV waveform has a distinctive "square root" configuration. Figure 17-44B shows the RV waveform. The initial

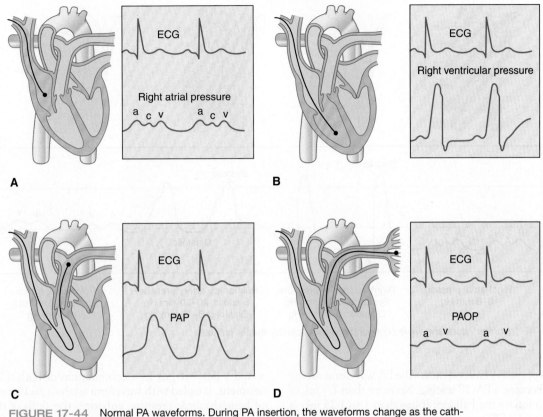

**FIGURE 17-44** Normal PA waveforms. During PA insertion, the waveforms change as the catheter advances through the heart. **A:** When the catheter enters the right atrium (RA), a waveform with three small upright waves appears. The a waves represent the RA systole; the v waves, RA filling. **B:** When the catheter reaches the right ventricle, a waveform with sharp systolic upstrokes and lower diastolic dips appears. **C:** When the catheter "floats" into the PA, a PA pressure (PAP) waveform appears. Note that the upstroke is smoother than on the right ventricle waveform. The dicrotic notch indicates pulmonic valve closure. **D:** When the catheter "floats" into a distal branch of the PA, the balloon wedges where the vessel becomes too narrow for it to pass, and a PAOP waveform, with two small upright waves, appears. The a wave represents LA systole; the v wave, LA filling.

rapid increase in RV pressure represents isovolumetric contraction, which follows the QRS complex of the ECG. The RV pressure continues to increase as the tricuspid and pulmonic valves are closed until the ventricular force generated exceeds the PA pressure. Rapid ejection occurs when the pulmonic valve opens. After ventricular systole, the pulmonic valve closes, and the right ventricular pressure rapidly decreases, creating a diastolic dip. Next in the cardiac cycle, the tricuspid valve opens and the RV passively fills with blood from the RA. Right ventricular diastole occurs within the period from the T wave to the next Q wave on the ECG. The point on the waveform just before the rapid increase in pressure represents RVEDP.[25–27]

### Pulmonary Artery Pressure

The pulmonary vasculature is a relatively compliant low-resistance, low-pressure system in healthy people. Normal PA systolic pressure is 20 to 30 mm Hg. Normal diastolic PA pressure is 8 to 15 mm Hg, with a mean of 10 to 20 mm Hg. Systolic PA pressure and the peak of the PA waveform are generated by RV systolic ejection; therefore, the PA systolic pressure and the RV systolic pressure are the same as long as the pulmonic value is not stenotic. The PA waveform characteristics are similar to the systemic arterial waveform

previously described (see Fig. 17-43). The dicrotic notch in the downward slope of the PA waveform corresponds with pulmonic valve closure at the beginning of RV diastole and is the beginning of the PA diastolic phase. PA diastolic pressure reflects the resistance of the pulmonary vascular bed and, to a limited degree, LVEDP. In normal conditions, with no obstructions or resistance from the PA to the left ventricle, PA diastolic pressure theoretically is an indirect measure of LVEDP because the pulmonary vasculature, left atrium, and open mitral valve allow equalization of pressure from the left ventricle back to the tip of the PA catheter.[25–27]

### Pulmonary Artery Occlusion Pressure

When the PA catheter is properly positioned, the PAOP (also called pulmonary artery wedge pressure) is obtained by inflating the balloon at the catheter tip. The balloon occludes forward flow in the branch of the PA, decreasing the influence of pulmonary vascular resistance (PVR) on the pressure reading, and creates a static column of blood from that portion of the PA through the LA, an open mitral valve during diastole, and the LV. In this way, the PAOP reflects LVEDP. Normal PAOP is 8 to 12 mm Hg. The PAOP more closely measures LA pressure and LVEDP than the PA diastolic pressure.

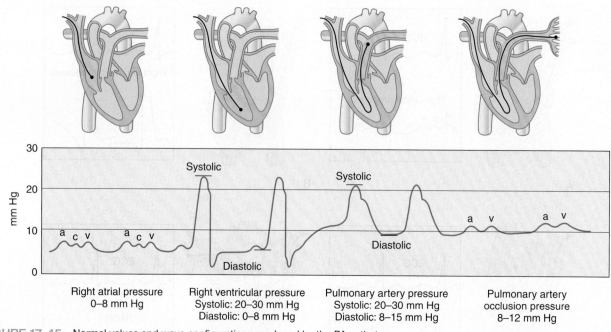

**FIGURE 17-45** Normal values and wave configurations produced by the PA catheter.

Inflation of the PA balloon causes the PA waveform on the monitor to become a PAOP tracing. No more than 1.5 mL of air is used to inflate the balloon. If less than 1 to 1.25 mL of air generates a PAOP tracing, the PA catheter has migrated distally and with the balloon passively deflated, needs to be withdrawn slightly. Depending on institution policies, a physician or advanced practice clinician performs this procedure.

An LA tracing has a, c, and v waves and x and y descents. The electrical and mechanical events of the heart generating these waves are identical to those of the RA waveform. The a wave corresponds to LA contraction and the v wave corresponds to LA filling and LV contraction. With a direct LA line, the c wave is typically visible as in an RA tracing. The c wave is rarely visible on the PAOP tracing because the slight increase in pressure from backward bulging of the mitral valve is difficult to observe.

The ECG may be correlated with the PAOP waveform just as with the RA waveform. The primary difference between the PAOP and the RA waveforms is the slight delay of a and v waves in PAOP relative to the ECG because of the distance from the left side of the heart to transmit pressures to the catheter placed in the right side. The a wave now falls more closely in line with the QRS complex, although it may be within the PR interval. The v wave correlates with the T-to-P interval.[25–27]

Figure 17-45 shows the normal values and waveforms during a PA catheter insertion. Note that the RA pressure is equivalent to the RVEDP, the RV systolic pressure is equivalent to the PA systolic pressure, and the PA diastolic pressure is equivalent to the PAOP. Observe the diastolic value during insertion; it increases when the PA catheter "floats" into the PA, and the systolic pressures from the RV to the PA are similar.

## Physiologic Causes of Abnormal Waveforms

Hemodynamic waveform analysis provides valuable additional information for differential diagnosis. Specific conditions produce abnormalities in the a, c, and v waves, in the x and y descents, or in a combination of both. Clinical assessment, coupled with waveform analysis and interpretation of hemodynamic pressure, enhances the skills of the critical care nurse. Table 17-16 summarizes the causes of abnormal hemodynamic pressures.

Abnormalities of RA waveform include large, elevated a or v waves. Increased resistance to RV filling and impaired atrial emptying cause an elevated a wave. Examples of pathologic causes of large a waves are tricuspid stenosis and RV failure. Elevated v waves are related to regurgitant flow from the ventricle back into the atrium during ventricular contraction. Examples of pathologic causes of large v waves are tricuspid valve insufficiency and RV failure. Elevations in either the a or v wave cause the mean RA pressure to be higher.

Increased PA pressures may be systolic or diastolic or both. Because PA systolic pressure is a reflection of RV systolic pressure, factors that increase RV pressures such as increased PVR, hypervolemia, LV failure, and mechanical ventilation can produce an increased PA systolic pressure. Left ventricular failure, hypervolemia, and increased PVR cause increased PA diastolic pressure. Increased PVR may result from acute respiratory distress syndrome, primary pulmonary hypertension, or pulmonary embolus.

Left ventricular dysfunction and mitral valve disease occur more frequently than RV or tricuspid valve disorders, and therefore abnormal PAOP waveforms are more common than abnormal RA waveforms. Abnormalities of the PAOP waveform are usually large, elevated a or v waves. Increased resistance to LV filling and impaired atrial emptying cause elevated a waves. Examples of pathologic causes of large a waves are mitral stenosis and LV failure. Elevated v waves relate to regurgitation from an incompetent mitral valve, allowing blood to flow from the ventricle back into the atrium during ventricular contraction. In both these valvular diseases, the PAOP does not accurately reflect LVEDP. Left ventricular failure usually causes elevation of both the a and v waves and significantly increases the PAOP because of reduced contractility and forward

**TABLE 17-16** Interpreting Hemodynamic Monitoring Pressures

| Pressure and Description | Normal Values | Causes of Increased Pressure | Causes of Decreased Pressure |
|---|---|---|---|
| **CVP or RAP** | | | |
| The CVP or RAP reflects right ventricular function and end-diastolic pressure | Mean pressure: 2–8 mm Hg | • Right-sided heart failure<br>• Volume overload<br>• Tricuspid valve stenosis or insufficiency<br>• Constrictive pericarditis<br>• Cardiac tamponade<br>• Pulmonary hypertension<br>• Right ventricular infarction | Reduced circulating blood volume |
| **Right Ventricular Pressure** | | | |
| Typically, right ventricular pressure monitored only on initial PA catheter insertion. Right ventricular systolic pressure normally equals PA systolic pressure; RAP reflects RVEDP | Systolic pressure: 20–30 mm Hg<br>Diastolic pressure: 0–8 mm Hg | • Mitral stenosis or insufficiency<br>• Pulmonary disease<br>• Hypoxemia<br>• Constrictive pericarditis<br>• Chronic heart failure<br>• Atrial and ventricular septal defects<br>• Patent ductus arteriosus | Reduced circulating blood volume |
| **Pulmonary Artery Systolic Pressure** | | | |
| Pulmonary artery systolic pressure results from right ventricular systolic pressure and reflects right ventricular function | Systolic pressure: 20–30 mm Hg<br>Mean pressure: 8–15 mm Hg | • Left-sided heart failure<br>• Increased pulmonary blood flow (left or right shunting, as in atrial or ventricular septal defects)<br>• Any condition causing increased pulmonary arteriolar resistance (such as pulmonary hypertension, volume overload, mitral stenosis, or hypoxia) | Reduced circulating blood volume |
| **Pulmonary Artery Diastolic Pressure** | | | |
| Pulmonary artery diastolic pressure is an indirect reflection of LVEDP in a patient without significant PA disease | Diastolic pressure: 8–12 mm Hg | • Any condition causing increased pulmonary arteriolar resistance (such as pulmonary hypertension, volume overload, mitral stenosis, or hypoxia) | Reduced circulating blood volume |
| **Pulmonary Artery Occlusion Pressure (PAOP) or Left Atrial Pressure** | | | |
| PAOP indirectly reflects LA and LVEDPs, unless the patient has obstructions from the tip of the PA catheter to the left ventricle. Changes in PAOP reflect changes in left ventricular filling pressure | Mean pressure: 8–12 mm Hg | • Left-sided heart failure<br>• Mitral stenosis or insufficiency<br>• Pericardial tamponade | Reduced circulating blood volume |
| **PP** | | | |
| PP is the difference between systolic and diastolic arterial pressure. PP can be used to assess the patient's SV. | Normal range: 40–60 mm Hg with a wider range of 30–100 mm Hg | • Increased SV<br>• Decreased vascular resistance<br>• Peripheral vascular disease<br>• Aortic insufficiency | Decreased SV Severe vasodilation in conditions such as late sepsis, various shock states |

Modified from Critical Care Made Incredibly Easy, Philadelphia, PA: Lippincott Williams & Wilkins, 2004, p 170.

blood flow. Elevated PAOP is frequently due to LV dysfunction or hypervolemia. In some cases, such as in acute respiratory distress syndrome or with mechanical ventilator settings that generate extremely high intrathoracic pressure, PAOP is elevated because of noncardiogenic causes. In these cases, the normal PA diastolic pressure/PAOP gradient of 1 to 4 mm Hg widens. A widened pressure gradient is a differential diagnostic sign of pulmonary hypertension or increased PVR.[25–27]

## Complications

Generally, most complications that occur with use of the PA catheter relate to the process of percutaneous central venous access. The other complications such as infection, thrombus, and air embolus are discussed in the earlier section on CVP.

## Pneumothorax

Pneumothorax is a complication from vessel access through the subclavian vein. Anatomical factors can make placement of a PA catheter difficult, particularly if the patient is obese or has torturous subclavian veins. The needle or introducer sheath may pass through the vessel wall and puncture the lung during insertion, causing an apical pneumothorax. Signs and symptoms of a pneumothorax and routine postinsertion chest radiograph are used to diagnose this complication.

## Infection

Systemic infection and sepsis are caused by contamination of the PA catheter, insertion site, or pressure monitoring system. Careful attention to sterile technique during pressure tubing assembly, using the maximum sterile barrier for insertion, and dressing changes helps prevent infection.[29] Protocols for changing the PA catheter and monitoring system should be followed carefully. Diagnosis of PA catheter-related sepsis is based on blood cultures, WBC count, and fever in the absence of other sources of infection.

## Ventricular Dysrhythmias

Ventricular dysrhythmias may occur during the insertion of a PA catheter. As the catheter passes through the right ventricle, it may irritate the endocardium and cause premature ventricular complexes and occasionally ventricular tachycardia. The dysrhythmias typically resolve when the catheter is advanced into the PA. After the PA catheter is in proper position, it may become dislodged if it is not well secured, and the tip may "fall back" into the right ventricle. The patient may experience dysrhythmias, and the hemodynamic pressures and waveform reflect those of the right ventricle. Usually in this situation, because of potential contamination at the insertion site, the catheter is withdrawn or occasionally by inflating the balloon, the catheter may "refloat" into the PA. It is essential to have ready access to emergency drugs and equipment in case the ventricular dysrhythmias persist. Many introducer kits contain sterile sheaths; when placed over the PA catheter, they provide additional protection from contamination.

## Pulmonary Artery Rupture or Perforation

A rare but very serious and potentially fatal complication is rupture or perforation of the PA. Perforation of the PA may occur during insertion, manipulation, or upon subsequent rewedging of the PA catheter. Patients with friable PAs may be at some risk. However, proper advancement of the catheter with the balloon fully inflated with 1.5 mL of air and avoidance of advancing the catheter too far into a small artery minimize the chance of PA perforation. Close observation of the PA waveform as the balloon is inflated and filling the balloon only with the amount of air necessary to obtain a PAOP tracing prevent overdistending a small PA. As previously stated, the catheter should become wedged when inflated with 1.25 to 1.5 mL of air. If less air is required to obtain the PAOP waveform, the catheter has migrated out of proper position.[25,26]

## Nursing Considerations

Nursing care of the patient undergoing PA pressure monitoring is complex. Critical care nurses must be able to interpret waveforms and pressure data as well as be alert to potential complications. It is necessary to ensure accurate readings and minimize operator error. Consistency of leveling and measurement techniques is especially important because small variations in the zero reference point elicit large and erroneous changes in the pressures observed. Table 17-16 outlines problems and troubleshooting strategies associated with hemodynamic pressure monitoring. Evidence-Based Practice Highlight 17-2 summarizes current evidence related to obtaining accurate measurement of PA pressures.

Measurement of all hemodynamic pressures is most accurate when obtained at the end of expiration in the respiratory cycle. In the healthy person, intrathoracic pressure at end expiration is about equal to atmospheric pressure. During the end-expiration period, there is minimal airflow and little variation in pleural pressures that influence cardiac pressures. Thus, end expiration provides a standard reference point for obtaining measurements. Spontaneous breathing causes negative intrathoracic pressure during inspiration, which produces a decline in the waveform. The waveform used for measurement is the last clear wave occurring just before the inspiratory dip. Mechanical ventilation causes increased intrathoracic pressure during inspiration, which produces an inspiratory "push" or rise in the waveform. The end-expiratory wave used for measurement is the last clear wave occurring just before the inspiratory rise (Fig. 17-46).

Closely set alarm parameters alert the nurse to potential physiologic or technical complications. For example, one indication of a pulmonary embolus is an acute increase in PA pressures. Distal migration of the PA catheter may cause the catheter to wedge spontaneously without balloon inflation, and PA pressures may decrease to that of a PAOP. With properly set alarms, conditions such as these are detected.[25,27]

## Determination of Cardiac Output

CO is the volume of blood ejected from the heart per minute, expressed in liters per minute. Normally, CO is 4 to 8 L/min at rest. CO is a function of heart rate and SV. The left ventricle must generate enough pressure in systole to overcome aortic pressure and systemic vascular resistance (SVR) and eject sufficient blood volume to perfuse the organs of the body. The determination of CO and assessment of its determinants are important adjuncts to the care of critically ill patients. Routine evaluation of CO and SV is essential when any CO and SV monitoring technology is used.

Cardiac index relates CO to body size. Normally, the cardiac index is 2.5 to 4 L/min/m$^2$. To obtain an indexed value, the CO is divided by the patient's body surface area (BSA). Standard bedside monitors and CO computers automatically calculate the cardiac index when the patient's height and weight are entered. The BSA is also used to index other valuable hemodynamic parameters (Table 17-17).

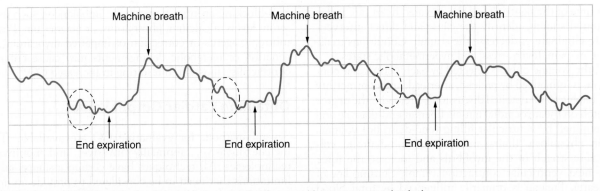

**FIGURE 17-46** PAOP tracing showing respiratory variation from positive pressure mechanical ventilation. Measurement of PAOP is made at the last clear tracing before the inspiratory rise as identified by the open circles.

**TABLE 17-17** Calculation of Cardiac Hemodynamic Parameters

| Parameter | Definition | Formula | Normal Values |
|---|---|---|---|
| CO | The number of liters pumped by the heart per minute | Heart rate × SV | 4–8 L/min |
| Cardiac index (CI) | CO indexed to the patient's BSA | CO/BSA | 2.5–4 L/min/m$^2$ |
| SV | The mL of blood ejected from the ventricle with each contraction | CO/HR × 1,000 | 60–100 mL/beat |
| Stroke volume index (SVI) | SV indexed to the patient's BSA | CI/heart rate | 33–47 mL/beat/m$^2$ |
| MAP | The calculated average arterial pressure over a full cardiac cycle | [Systolic BP + (diastolic BP × 2)]/3 | 70–105 mm Hg |
| RAP | Pressure created by volume of blood in the right heart | Direct measurement | 0–8 mm Hg |
| Left atrial pressure (LAP) | Pressure created by volume of blood in the left heart | Direct measurement | 6–12 mm Hg |
| PAOP | Pressure measured in the PA when the PA catheter's balloon is inflated | Direct measurement | 8–12 mm Hg |
| Right ventricular end-diastolic volume index (RVEDVI) | Amount of volume in the right ventricle at the end of diastole | SVI/RV ejection fraction | 60–100 mL/m$^2$ |
| Left ventricular end-diastolic volume index | Amount of volume in the left ventricle at the end of diastole | SV/LV ejection fraction | 40–80 mL/m$^2$ |
| SVR | Refers to the resistance to blood flow offered by the systemic vasculature | [(MAP–RAP) × 80]/CO | 800–1,200 dyne/s/cm$^{-5}$ |
| Systemic vascular resistance index (SVRI) | SVR indexed to patient's BSA | [(MAP–RAP) × 80]/CI | 1,360–2,200 dyne/s/cm$^{-5}$ |
| PVR | Refers to the resistance to blood flow offered by the pulmonic vasculature | (MPAP–PAOP) × 80/CO | <250 dyne/s/cm$^{-5}$ |
| Pulmonary vascular resistance index (PVRI) | PVR indexed to patient's BSA | (MPAP–PAOP) × 80/CI | <425 dyne/s/cm$^{-5}$ |
| Left ventricular stroke work index (LVSWI) | A measure of work performed by the left ventricle each beat | SVI (MAP–PAOP) × 0.0136 | 40–70 g/m$^2$/beat |
| Right ventricular stroke work index (RVSWI) | A measure of work performed by the right ventricle each beat | SVI (MPAP–RAP) × 0.0136 | 5–10 g/m$^2$/beat |
| SV variation | Variation in SV over a respiratory cycle | SV maximum–SV minimum/ SV mean | <10%–15% |

## Factors That Determine Cardiac Output

CO is determined by heart rate and SV as described in Chapter 16. Alterations in CO are caused by changes in heart rate, preload, afterload, and contractility. Analysis of each of these is essential in directing interventions to address the underlying pathophysiologic process. One strategy to consider is to evaluate CO, then systematically assess the determinants of heart rate, SV with preload first, afterload second, and finally contractility.

An increased or decreased CO provides global information only and needs to be evaluated in light of the components affecting it. Bradycardia due to conduction defects or medications can cause CO to decrease. An increase in heart rate can produce an increase in CO; however, this may be a compensatory physiologic response to emotional or physiologic stress, or to a decreased SV. Tachycardia increases myocardial oxygen demands and may place a compromised patient at risk for myocardial ischemia. Tachycardia also may decrease CO because of shortened diastole and decreased filling time of the ventricles. If the elevated heart rate is due to external stimuli, identify the cause and direct interventions to eliminate or decrease the stimuli. Conditions to assess for are pain, fever, stress, and hypermetabolic states.

SV, the volume of blood ejected by each ventricular contraction, is influenced by preload, afterload, and contractility (see Chapter 16 for detailed discussion). Preload is the degree of stretch on the myocardial muscle fibers at end-diastole and is determined by ventricular filling (end-diastolic) volume. Within physiologic limits, increases in end-diastolic volume cause stretch of the myofibrils and increase the force of the next ventricular contraction (Frank–Starling law of the heart). Preload is primarily influenced by total blood volume. Because the PA catheter measures pressure, not volume, assumptions are made that volume and pressure can be equated. Many factors alter the pressure–volume relationship; therefore, the use of pressures (eg, CVP or PAOP) to evaluate preload must be considered in light of factors that can affect pressures, such as mechanical ventilation or ventricular compliance. A specialized PA catheter is able to provide right ventricular ejection fraction and volumetric data. Indirect assessment of preload uses the RAP or CVP for the right ventricular preload, and the PA diastolic pressure, LA pressure, and PAOP for the left ventricular preload.[25–27]

Decreases in preload can be due to hypovolemia, secondary to blood loss, dehydration, or third spacing of fluids. Preload is also reduced related to massive vasodilation, for example in septic, anaphylactic, or neurogenic shock. Hypovolemia or decreased venous return associated with mechanical ventilation and elevated intrathoracic pressures can cause a decreased preload.

Afterload is often defined as the impedance or resistance to ejection of blood from the ventricles. PVR is a clinical assessment of right ventricular afterload. Left ventricular afterload is clinically evaluated by calculating SVR. PVR and SVR can be indexed to body size using the patient's BSA (see Table 17-17). Primary factors affecting afterload are semilunar valve abnormalities and vascular resistance.

Vasoconstriction causes elevated afterload and has several causes. Increased SVR may be a compensatory response to hypovolemia caused by vasoconstriction to maintain peripheral perfusion in this state. An increase in afterload occurs with some medications, hypothermia, and the compensatory vascular response to cardiogenic shock. This increase in afterload may also be accompanied by a decrease in CO and an increase in myocardial oxygen demand and work. A decrease in afterload due to vasodilation reduces resistance to ejection of blood, thus increasing CO. Vasodilating medications, septic states, and allergic and anaphylactic reactions are all causes of vasodilation and thus increased CO.

Contractility, the third determinant of SV, is an inherent property of the heart. It is not affected by preload or afterload and cannot be directly measured. Indices used to assess contractility include determining SV and calculating the stroke work index for both the left and right ventricles. Myocardial oxygen supply and demand balance, electrolytes, and minerals (eg, calcium) influence myocardial contractility.

Reduction in contractility decreases CO. Examples include insufficient oxygen delivery to the myocardium, causing myocardial ischemia and infarction; medications, such

as β-blocking agents; or metabolic imbalances, such as low serum levels of calcium, phosphorus, or magnesium. Positive inotropic agents or correction of impaired myocardial oxygenation or metabolic derangements may cause enhanced contractility, most often resulting in increased CO.[25–27]

## Obtaining Cardiac Output Values

Several methods for evaluating CO are available. These include invasive, minimally invasive, and noninvasive technologies. All techniques have certain assumptions and limitations that need to be considered to provide an understanding of the indications and applications of each. This section discusses the more common methods of CO monitoring used in the acute and critical care areas.

### Fick's Method for Cardiac Output Determination

The Fick method, originally developed in the 1800s by Adolf Fick, is the historical laboratory gold standard. The Fick method is based on the principle that the uptake or release of a substance by an organ divided by the arterial and venous concentration of that substance is the product of flow or CO. The classic method of determining CO uses oxygen as the substance and the lungs as the organ. For this relationship to be valid, simultaneous samples of arterial and venous blood must be obtained and accurately measured. In addition, inspired and expired oxygen concentration must be measured by indirect calorimetry to determine the oxygen consumption. Other technologies use these principles; however, they use carbon dioxide as the measured substance.

### Indicator-Dilution Methods for Cardiac Output Determination

Stewart proposed the principles of the indicator-dilution method, and Hamilton further refined them. The Stewart–Hamilton equation is based on use of a known indicator as a signal and determination of the dilution rate of that signal over a given period of time. Three indicators in clinical use are dye, thermal, and small doses of lithium. The indicator is injected into the venous system, and a time–concentration curve is generated from a blood sample obtained from the arterial system. Analysis of the curve allows CO calculation.[25–27]

Thermodilution is considered the clinical gold standard for determining CO. Cold or room temperature solution is the indicator and is injected into the RA port of the PAC. A thermistor near the end of the catheter continuously measures the temperature of blood flowing past it. A dilution curve is generated by the change in blood temperature after indicator injection. Based on this curve, CO is calculated by the computer.

Determination of CO through thermodilution is obtained either on an intermittent or continuous basis. Intermittent CO requires the injection of a known amount of "cooler than blood" injectate, and a single CO curve is produced. Specialty catheters house thermal filaments and, with a dedicated thermal cable and computer, emit energy as the indicator. The "warmer than blood" signal is measured at the thermistor, and thermodilution curves are produced on a 30- to 60-second frequency for continuous CO assessment.[25]

## Procedure for Intermittent Thermodilution Cardiac Output Determination

A computation constant, based on the catheter size, volume, and temperature of the injectate, as well as injection method, is set on the computer or programmed into the bedside CO module. Five or ten milliliters of sterile $D_5W$ or normal saline solution is used as the injectate solution and volume. The injectate syringe used should be part of a closed system that remains intact and attached to the RA port by a stopcock (Fig. 17-47). Iced (0°C to 4°C) or room-temperature solution may be used. A temperature difference between the patient's blood temperature and the injectate of at least 10°C improves accuracy. In most conditions, room-temperature injectate with a 10-mL volume provides accurate results. With hypothermia or very low CO states, iced solution and a 10-mL injectate volume provide a greater signal and increased accuracy.

Steps for performing a manual CO determination vary according to bedside monitor or CO computer manufacturer. See specific operations manuals for directions for use. General steps include:

- Ensuring the accurate amount of injectate volume in the syringe
- Injecting the volume in a smooth and rapid manner, in less than 4 seconds
- Waiting approximately 1 minute between injections to allow the catheter thermistor to return to baseline.

When injected, the solution passes a temperature probe in the closed system and flows through the right atrium and right ventricle, past the thermistor at the tip of the PAC. A curve is produced and used for determining the CO. The average of several CO determinations is required to obtain a final measurement. Serial measurements and averaging are necessary because of the number of physiologic variables and the performance of the technical procedure. Three or more consecutive measurements are usually necessary. Measurements included in the averaging process should be within 10% to 15% of the mean, and each one should be associated with a normal CO curve. Abnormal curves are eliminated from the CO averaging process.

### Interpretation of Cardiac Output Curves

Many bedside monitors and CO computers are equipped with a means of visualizing the CO curves. Normal CO curves have a smooth upstroke from the rapid injection followed by a gradual decline (Fig. 17-48). The area under the curve is inversely proportional to the CO. Curves associated with a high CO have a small area under the curve, with a steeper upstroke and more rapid return to baseline, and curves associated with a low CO have a greater area under the curve, with a more sloped upstroke and slower return to baseline.

### Arterial Pressure- and Waveform-Based Cardiac Output Determinations

Various technologies for using the arterial waveform for CO and SV determinations are available. By employing the various methods, SV/CO values can be obtained by invasive arterial lines or noninvasively with modified finger cuff technologies. The basic premise relates to the proportionality relationship of PP to SV and the inverse relationship of PP to aortic compliance. As PP widens, SV increases and aortic compliance

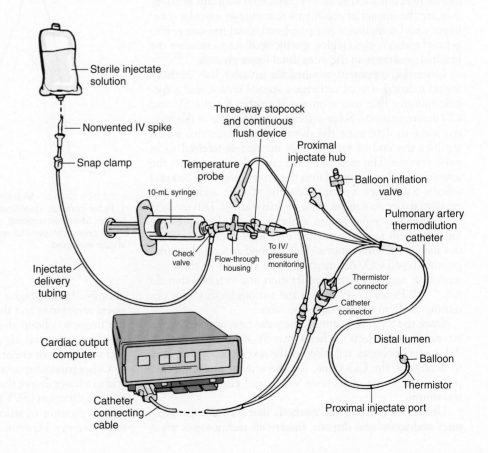

**FIGURE 17-47** A closed room-temperature injectate system for measurement of CO. (Courtesy of Edwards Lifesciences.)

Sterile injectate solution

Nonvented IV spike

Snap clamp

10-mL syringe

Temperature probe

Three-way stopcock and continuous flush device

Proximal injectate hub

Balloon inflation valve

Pulmonary artery thermodilution catheter

Check valve

Flow-through housing

To IV/ pressure monitoring

Injectate delivery tubing

Thermistor connector

Catheter connector

Cardiac output computer

Distal lumen

Balloon

Thermistor

Catheter connecting cable

Proximal injectate port

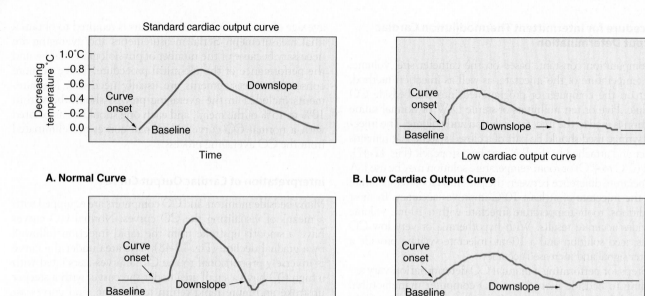

**A. Normal Curve**

Standard cardiac output curve

**B. Low Cardiac Output Curve**

Low cardiac output curve

High cardiac output curve

**C. High Cardiac Output Curve**

Improper injection technique

**D. Irregular Cardiac Output Curve**

FIGURE 17-48 Examples of thermodilution curves observed on a bedside monitor or strip chart recorder. **A:** Normal curve with smooth upstroke and gradual decline to baseline. Note that the temperature change is actually lower than patient baseline temperature; however, the graph is shown in an upright orientation. **B:** Low CO produces a greater area under the curve. The upstroke is normal with a more gradual decline. **C:** A high CO has a smaller area under the curve. The upstroke is more rapid with a faster return to baseline. **D:** Irregular curve shows an erroneously low CO probably due to irregular or uneven emptying of the injectate syringe. (Courtesy of Edwards Lifesciences.)

decreases (becomes more rigid, less elastic). As PP narrows, SV decreases and aortic compliance increase (become less rigid and more elastic). Other factors considered with this relationship are the impact of conditions that change vascular tone: larger vessel compliance and peripheral vessel resistance. Finger cuff technologies employ specific analyses to recreate the brachial pressure from the more distal finger pressure.[25–27,30,31]

General components required for invasive line methods are an existing arterial catheter, a special sensor, and a specific monitor that uses a unique algorithm for the SV and CO determinations. Some systems use the shape of the arterial wave to determine the dicrotic notch location, which signifies the end of systole. This method is referred to as pulse contour. The area under the curve then represents the amount of volume ejected into the arterial vascular bed and reflects SV. Other systems assess the systolic and diastolic pressure to obtain a mean value to arrive at SV. This method is described as pulse power. Another method samples the full waveform for pressures and uses waveform characteristics for CO determinations. This method is termed arterial pressure-based CO. All methods have versions of their systems that require external calibration and versions that do not.[26,30–32] Figure 17-49 depicts the various methods for obtaining SV from the arterial pulse wave.

Once the SV is determined, the pulse rate, assessed by the arterial waves, reflects the heart rate; SV × heart rate = CO. All the technologies, regardless of the specific algorithm used to determine the CO value, use the arterial pressure. This requires obtaining of accurate values and ensuring optimal waveforms.

Unlike the arterial line methods that measure the pressures and waveforms directly, finger cuff technologies use a

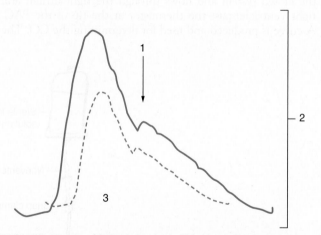

FIGURE 17-49 Methods to obtain SV using arterial pulse wave. 1. Pulse contour: Identification of dicrotic notch required. 2. Pulse power: Mean determined, systolic and diastolic extrapolated. 3. Pulse pressure/flow: Full wave measured for pressure and waveform shape assessed.

photoplethysmographic device in either one or two cuffs to assess waveforms and that also apply a "counter pressure" to the finger to obtain the patient's BP. The finger pressure is then reconstructed algorithmically into a brachial pressure and waveform for enhanced accuracy.[26,32]

Other parameters obtained with an arterial pressure system and to a lesser degree the cuff technologies can include stroke volume variation (SVV), pulse pressure variation (PPV), and systolic pressure variation (SPV). These parameters evaluate the difference between the maximum and minimum values of systolic pressure, PP, or SV during a respiratory cycle. They are called dynamic parameters and are better predictors of fluid responsiveness than static measures such as CVP/RAP in the critically ill. A natural phenomenon occurs during the respiratory cycle in which the arterial pressure falls during inspiration and rises during expiration. The variation is a result of changes in intrathoracic pressure during respiration; a negative pressure during inspiration results in a fall in systolic pressure, and a relatively higher intrathoracic pressure during expiration causes a rise in systolic pressure. The normal variation during a respiratory cycle is 5 to 10 mm Hg. When the difference is greater, the condition is termed *pulsus paradoxus*. Reverse pulsus paradoxus is the same phenomenon that occurs during controlled mechanical ventilation. The mechanics are opposite of spontaneous breathing in that the arterial pressure rises during inspiration and falls during expiration.[25–27,30–33]

Some bedside physiologic monitors have special software that will measure and then display SPV and PPV values. Alternatively, while not as accurate as built-in algorithms or dedicated monitors, these calculations can also be made from the arterial tracings as long as the respiratory variations are noted. However, it must be noted that using the 'eyeball' technique is not as accurate as the actual measurement of the values.[34,35]

**NURSING CONSIDERATIONS.** Patient assessment includes assessing for pulsus paradoxus that occurs during cardiac tamponade, obstructive lung diseases, and hypovolemic states. An SVV greater than 10% to 15% has a high level of sensitivity and specificity for determining the need for fluid and in predicting preload responsiveness. A patient is preload responsive if after a fluid bolus their SV or CO increases by 10% to 15%. Technical considerations for the use of arterial pressure–based technologies include those that affect the accuracy of the arterial waveform. Optimal pressure system maintenance and leveling of the device is required. Limitations to using variation parameters relate to factors that cause changes in intrathoracic pressure and those that affect ventricular filling time. Any cardiac dysrhythmia can affect the overall value because of irregular ventricular responses and therefore the value should be used with caution in those conditions. Intravascular volume resuscitation increases preload, which in turn increases CO.[25–27,30]

With the completely noninvasive finger cuff technologies special attention needs to be paid to finger perfusion due to the cyclic inflation function of the finger cuff. In conditions of severe vasoconstriction, hypoperfusion, edematous fingers, and Reynaud syndrome, the signal may be hampered.[26]

### Bioimpedance- and Bioreactance-Based Cardiac Output Determinations

Two general types of transthoracic noninvasive cardiography technologies are bioimpedance and bioreactance. Both provide noninvasive, continuous, real-time CO and other hemodynamic data using pairs of skin electrode-sensors on the thorax (Fig. 17-50). Electrical stimuli are emitted by the sensors and the amplitude or frequencies from the current are analyzed for changes in impedance (Z) or to the flow (Zo) of an electrical current.[36–38] Bioimpedance cardiography is also known as impedance cardiography, or ICG.

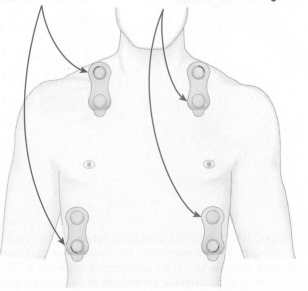

Four sets of paired sensors - two on both sides of the upper thorax and two on both sides below the heart level

Red line denotes the outer sensors where the current is applied. The green inner sensors receive and record the signals.

The electrical field of the blood causes a delay in the signal. The delay is proportional to the volume of blood.

This time delay, called a Phase Shift is recorded and then translated to flow.

**FIGURE 17-50**  Placement of impedance sensors. (Courtesy of Cheetah Medical.)

Both bioreactance and bioimpedance monitors provide traditional hemodynamic determinations such as CO, SV, and SVR if a blood pressure and CVP or RAP are entered into the monitor. If CVP is not entered, the monitors will display total peripheral vascular resistance. Since aortic blood flow causes the most significant change in impedance, these technologies provide more direct indices of left ventricular contractility, which are not available from a PAC. They also provide a baseline impedance, the thoracic fluid content, which reflects all of the fluid in the thorax (interstitial, intravascular, or intracellular). In some instances, when thoracic fluid content is very high, ICG determination of SV and CO may be negatively affected. SV/CO values appear to be less influenced by pleural fluid, pulmonary edema, and chest wall movement in bioreactance technology than in ICG.[36,37]

**NURSING CONSIDERATIONS.** Because bioreactance and ICG are noninvasive technologies, nurses in any inpatient or outpatient setting can initiate this type of hemodynamic monitoring. Thus, the clinical applications are broad. For example, parameters obtained by these methods are used to evaluate patients with heart failure, hypertension, and permanent pacemakers in the emergency department, outpatient clinic, or physician office.

Since electrical impedance is reduced in the presence of fluid, the thoracic fluid content measurement is useful in the differential diagnosis of heart failure or chronic obstructive pulmonary disease as well as in the assessment and management of patients with heart failure who may have pulmonary congestion or pulmonary edema. Adjustment in diuretics, inotropic agents, and vasodilators can be fine-tuned based

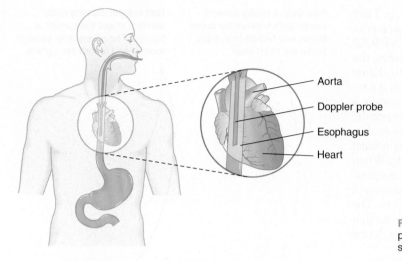

FIGURE 17-51   Location of the esophageal Doppler probe in the esophagus in relation to the heart and descending aorta. (Courtesy of Deltex Medical, Inc.)

on impedance parameters. Similarly, patients with chronic and resistant hypertension can be managed more closely and more aggressively on an outpatient basis using ICG or bioreactance hemodynamic parameters as opposed to using blood pressure alone. Continuous noninvasive CO and hemodynamic parameters are also used to optimize the settings of atrial–ventricular (A-V) sequential cardiac pacemakers to adjust the time for A-V delay to allow appropriate ventricular filling to achieve optimal SV and CO.[36–38]

### Doppler-Based Cardiac Output Determination

Doppler-based technology uses the aortic blood flow velocity waveform to calculate SV and CO. The pulsatile velocity waveform directly reflects left ventricular contractility as well as the patient's intravascular volume status (preload).

The esophageal Doppler monitor (EDM) is a minimally invasive hemodynamic monitoring device that incorporates a Doppler transducer into a nasogastric tube. When placed in the esophagus, EDM monitors the descending aortic blood flow velocity[38] (Fig. 17-51). Continuous CO and SV determinations are calculated in real time relative to changes in blood flow using the Doppler waveform configuration.

USCOM is a noninvasive hemodynamic monitor that determines CO by continuous-wave Doppler ultrasound.(38) Data are obtained using a probe placed on the chest in either the left parasternal position to measure transpulmonary blood flow or the suprasternal notch to measure transaortic blood flow. US-COM does not provide continuous hemodynamic data. Information is obtained intermittently as desired by the clinician.

Both EDM and USCOM provide traditional parameters such as CO, SV, and SVR, if a blood pressure and CVP or RAP is entered into the monitor. Additional parameters derived from the waveform include peak velocity, an indicator of myocardial contractility, and flow time, which reflects systolic ejection time and thus changes in preload.

**NURSING CONSIDERATIONS.** A valuable aspect of Doppler-based technology is use of the waveform shape to determine changes in myocardial contractility and intravascular volume (preload) because the waveform displayed on the monitor reflects the volume and velocity of blood in the aorta. The normal waveform is triangular, consisting of the

beginning of systole, peak systole, and end-systole (Fig. 17-52). As flow from the left ventricle increases, the shape of the waveform changes, becoming a larger, higher, and wider triangle. Conversely, decreased contractility is reflected in a smaller waveform; hypovolemia causes the waveform to become narrower at the base. The baseline shape of the waveform, as well as changes in response to therapy, can significantly contribute to hemodynamic assessment. Thus, Doppler-based data and waveform analysis can guide the clinician in evaluating the patient's need for therapy and responses to fluid administration and titration of vasopressors and inotropes.[38,39]

EDM usually requires the patient to be sedated; therefore, it is most often used in the critical care unit, operating room, postanesthesia care unit, and the emergency department. USCOM is a noninvasive technology; clinicians in any inpatient or outpatient setting can use this type of hemodynamic monitoring. However, training is required and the data obtained depend on proper technique.

## Evaluation of Oxygen Delivery and Demand Balance

One of the primary objectives of hemodynamic monitoring is to use the data in the evaluation of oxygen delivery or transport and the consumption of oxygen by the tissues and organs. Adequate oxygen delivery to the body's organs is essential for maintenance of cell, tissue, and ultimately organ function. Insufficient oxygen delivery and consumption to meet the

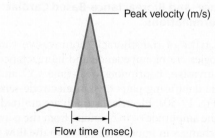

FIGURE 17-52   Esophageal Doppler waveform showing peak velocity and flow time. (Courtesy of Deltex Medical, Inc.)

| TABLE 17-18 | Oxygen Delivery and Utilization Parameters | | |
|---|---|---|---|
| **Parameter** | **Definition** | **Formula** | **Normal Values** |
| Arterial oxygen content ($CaO_2$) | The amount of oxygen carried by hemoglobin in a deciliter of arterial blood | $(Hb \times 1.37 \times SaO_2) + (0.003 \times PaO_2)$ | 20 mL $O_2$/dL |
| Venous oxygen content ($CvO_2$) | The amount of oxygen carried by hemoglobin in a deciliter of venous blood | $(Hb \times 1.37 \times SvO_2) + (0.003 \times PvO_2)$ | 15 mL $O_2$/dL |
| Arterial oxygen delivery index ($DaO_2I$) | The amount of oxygen transported in the blood from the left ventricle through the arteries and capillaries to tissues/organs, in 1 min, indexed to the patient's BSA | $CI \times CaO_2 \times 10$ | 500–600 mL $O_2$/min/m$^2$ |
| Venous oxygen delivery index ($DvO_2I$) | The amount of oxygen in the blood returned to the right ventricle in 1 min, via the veins from tissues/organs, indexed to the patient's BSA | $CI \times CvO_2 \times 10$ | 375–450 mL $O_2$/min/m$^2$ |
| Mixed venous oxygen saturation ($SvO_2$) | The oxygen saturation of venous blood, measured in the PA | Direct measurement | 60%–80% |
| Central venous oxygen saturation ($ScvO_2$) | The oxygen saturation of venous blood, measured in the superior vena cava | Direct measurement | 65%–85% |
| Partial pressure of oxygen, venous blood ($PvO_2$) | Reflects the amount of oxygen dissolved in the plasma of venous blood | Direct measurement | 35–45 mm Hg |
| $O_2$ extraction | Amount of oxygen that is removed (extracted) from hemoglobin for use by cells/tissues/organs | $CaO_2$–$CvO_2$ | 3–5 mL $O_2$/dL |
| Oxygen extraction ratio (OER) | The percent of oxygen delivered that is removed (extracted) from hemoglobin for use by cells/tissues/organs | | 22%–30% |
| Oxygen consumption index ($VO_2I$) | The amount of oxygen used by cells/tissues/organs every minute, indexed to the patient's BSA | $(CaO_2$–$CvO_2) \times CI \times 10$ | 120–170 mL/min/m$^2$ |
| Arterial pH (pHa) | The acidity (pH) of arterial blood | Direct measurement | 7.35–7.45 |
| Base excess/base deficit (BE/BD) | Amount of base required to titrate one liter of arterial blood to a pH of 7.40. Decreases with metabolic acidosis | Direct measurement | −2 to +2 |
| Lactate | A metabolic byproduct of Krebs cycle that increases with anaerobic metabolism | Direct measurement | 0.5–2.2 mmol/L |

cellular requirements for oxygen, or oxygen demand, result in hypoxia and the accumulation of an oxygen deficit. Persistent oxygen deficit causes cell and organ dysfunction and eventually leads to cell death and organ failure.[25] Table 17-18 lists the parameters that are used to evaluate oxygen delivery and demand balance, the formulas, and normal values.

## Determinants of Oxygen Delivery

Arterial oxygen delivery ($DaO_2$) is the amount of oxygen transported to the tissues. $DaO_2$ depends on arterial oxygen content and CO.

### Oxygen Content

Oxygen content is the total amount of oxygen in the blood that is available to the cells. The two primary determinants of oxygen content are hemoglobin and oxygen saturation. Most of the available oxygen in arterial blood (greater than 95%) is reversibly bound to hemoglobin in the form of oxyhemoglobin and is measured by arterial oxygen saturation ($SaO_2$). A very small amount of oxygen (less than 5%) is dissolved in plasma and measured as $PaO_2$. A sufficient amount of hemoglobin is required to ensure adequate oxygen-carrying capacity.

### Cardiac Output

CO is required to deliver oxygenated blood to the cells of the body. $DaO_2$ is assessed by evaluating the adequacy of CO and arterial oxygen content. In nonstressed states, normal $DaO_2$ is 1,000 mL $O_2$/min, or indexed to BSA, 600 mL $O_2$/min/m$^2$.

Increases in the body's oxygen demand associated with injury or illness are initially and primarily met by a compensatory increase in CO. Deficiencies of hemoglobin, arterial saturation, or CO decrease $DaO_2$ to cells and threaten the adequacy of cellular oxygenation.[25,40,41]

## Determinants of Oxygen Consumption

Oxygen consumption ($VO_2$) is the amount of oxygen used by the tissues of the body. The primary determinants of $VO_2$ are the cellular demand for oxygen, the delivery of adequate amounts of oxygen, and the extraction of oxygen from the blood for use by the cells.

### Oxygen Demand

Oxygen demand is the requirement of cells for oxygen and is not directly measurable. Any stress increases the oxygen demand (eg, surgery, infection, mobilization, pain, anxiety). Reduced oxygen demands are associated with lower metabolic rates (eg, hypothermia, sedation, pharmacologic paralysis). Oxygen demands are met through adequate delivery of oxygen and cellular extraction of oxygen.[25,40,41]

### Oxygen Delivery

Cellular use of oxygen depends on an adequate supply of oxygen. This is termed delivery-dependent oxygen consumption (Fig. 17-53). As oxygen delivery increases, oxygen consumption also increases to meet the oxygen demand. When the requirement for oxygen is met, further increases in oxygen

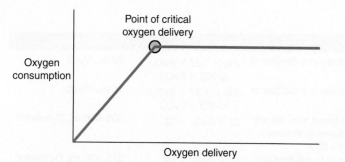

**FIGURE 17-53**  Delivery-dependent oxygen consumption curve reflecting the change in oxygen consumption related to oxygen delivery. At the point of critical oxygen delivery, oxygen delivery is sufficient to meet oxygen demand, and oxygen consumption does not increase further. However, any decrease in oxygen delivery from this point results in a decrease of oxygen consumption due to an inadequate supply of oxygen.

delivery do not increase consumption. The level of critical oxygen delivery is the point at which a decrease in oxygen delivery results in decreased $VO_2$ because of an insufficient oxygen supply.[25,40,41,42]

### Oxygen Extraction

Oxygen extraction ($CaO_2$ - $CvO_2$) is the amount of oxygen removed from the blood for use by the cells. It is measured by comparing the arterial oxygen content to venous oxygen content. Like arterial oxygen content, venous oxygen content ($CvO_2$) is primarily determined by the amount of hemoglobin that is saturated with oxygen. Venous saturation is obtained by withdrawing a mixed venous blood gas sample from the distal port of the PA catheter, or by using an $SvO_2$ or $ScvO_2$ monitoring central venous catheter or PA catheter, as discussed later in this section.

In normal circumstances, provided that oxygen is supplied in adequate amounts, the cells extract the oxygen they need to support tissue and organ function. Increased demand for oxygen results in a compensatory increase in oxygen extraction as more oxygen is "unloaded" from the hemoglobin for cellular use. The decreased amount of oxygen in venous blood means that the $CaO_2$ - $CvO_2$ difference is larger. Conversely, as oxygen demands decrease, less oxygen is required and extracted from the blood, and the $CaO_2$ - $CvO_2$ difference becomes smaller.[25,40,41]

### Oxygen Supply and Demand Imbalance

An imbalance of oxygen supply and demand occurs whenever oxygen delivery is inadequate to meet cellular demand or the cells are unable to extract sufficient quantities of oxygen. Specific threats to the balance of oxygen supply and demand are decreased CO, hemoglobin, or arterial saturation; impaired cellular extraction of oxygen; or oxygen demands that are so great that they cannot be met by increased oxygen delivery or extraction.

### Metabolic Indicators of Oxygen Delivery and Utilization Imbalance

Inadequate oxygen consumption causes an anaerobic state and cellular hypoxia. Cells deprived of oxygen become hypoxic and dysfunctional. Over time, cell damage becomes irreversible and cell death results. Cellular hypoxia is a major

cause of multisystem organ dysfunction and failure. If an oxygen deficit is identified before irreversible cell injury has occurred, it may be reversed by increasing oxygen availability.

Several metabolic parameters can be measured to evaluate cellular hypoxia. When these indicators are used in conjunction with hemodynamic monitoring of oxygen delivery and consumption, therapies may be more specifically directed to achieve a balanced oxygen supply and demand.

Because hypoxia and oxygen debt are associated with anaerobic metabolism, the byproducts of anaerobic metabolism can be used to assess the presence of an oxygen deficit and cellular hypoxia. Lactic acid accumulation causes a metabolic acidosis in a hypoxic state. Therefore, laboratory measurement of lactate levels, serum pH, and base deficit/excess are means to evaluate if oxygen supply is sufficient to meet cell requirements. Serum pH and base deficit/excess are routinely measured and reported with blood gas analysis. Elevated lactate levels (greater than 2.2 mm/L) or metabolic acidosis (pH less than 7.35 with normal $PaCO_2$) correlate with oxygen debt, particularly when the patient has a low or even normal level of $DaO_2$ and $VO_2$. As with all assessment parameters, lactate levels, pH, and base deficit should not be viewed in isolation; they should be evaluated in conjunction with other assessment parameters.[25-27]

### Monitoring of Mixed Venous and Central Venous Oxygen Saturation

Mixed venous oxygen saturation ($SvO_2$) reflects the level of oxyhemoglobin in desaturated blood returning to the right ventricle and PA. Venous oxygen saturation can also be measured in the superior vena cava ($ScvO_2$). $SvO_2$ or $ScvO_2$ can be monitored at the bedside by specialized central venous catheters or PACs containing fiber-optic filaments in one of the lumens ending at the distal end. In addition, specialized PICC catheters can house fiber-optics in which to measure venous oximetry values. The information is updated every few seconds; thus, a continuous $SvO_2$ or $ScvO_2$ reading is obtained.

Both $SvO_2$ and $ScvO_2$ are useful to evaluate the global balance of oxygen supply, oxygen utilization, and oxygen demand. The $SvO_2$ or $ScvO_2$ is significantly lower than arterial saturation because of the extraction of oxygen by the cells and the unloading of oxygen from hemoglobin.

$SvO_2$ or $ScvO_2$ is influenced by the degree of arterial saturation, the quantity of hemoglobin, the CO (the determinants of oxygen delivery), and the amount of oxygen extracted and consumed by the cells. Under normal conditions of oxygen delivery, oxygen consumption, and oxygen demand, approximately 25% of the available oxygen is extracted and used to meet demand. In this situation, the $SvO_2$ or $ScvO_2$ is in the normal range: $SvO_2$ of 60% to 80%, or $ScvO_2$ of 65% to 85%. If oxygen delivery is reduced by a decrease in arterial saturation, hemoglobin, or CO, then more oxygen is extracted from the blood to meet cellular demand. The blood returning to the right side of the heart and PA has had a greater quantity of oxygen removed and is more desaturated, which is reflected by a decrease in $ScvO_2$ or $SvO_2$. Similarly, if oxygen demand increases but oxygen delivery does not increase to meet this requirement, additional oxygen is extracted from the blood and consumed by the cells. Therefore, oxyhemoglobin is reduced in the venous blood, decreasing $SvO_2$ or $ScvO_2$. Persistently low $SvO_2$ or $ScvO_2$ is a warning that cellular hypoxia and an oxygen debt may be

**TABLE 17-19** Causes of Increasing or Decreasing Venous (SvO$_2$/ScvO$_2$) Saturation

| ↓SvO$_2$/ScvO$_2$ | ↑SvO$_2$/ScvO$_2$ |
| --- | --- |
| *Increased oxygen extraction* | *Decreased oxygen extraction* |
| 1. Increased oxygen demand | 1. Decreased oxygen demand |
|     Causes: Stress, pain, anxiety, fever |     Causes: Sedation, pain relief, hypothermia |
| 2. Oxygen delivery insufficient to meet oxygen demand | 2. Increased oxygen delivery |
|     Causes: Decreased CO, Hgb, SaO$_2$ |     Causes: Increased CO, Hgb, SaO$_2$ |
| | 3. Impaired cellular oxygen extraction |
| |     Causes: cytotoxicity, sepsis, cell death |

Hgb, hemoglobin; SaO$_2$, arterial saturation.

developing because of inadequate oxygen delivery or a high oxygen demand not met by the oxygen supply.[40,41]

Three general conditions result in increasing SvO$_2$ or ScvO$_2$:

- An oxygen delivery that is much greater than the oxygen demand; only a small percentage of the delivered oxygen is extracted, causing SvO$_2$ or ScvO$_2$ to increase.
- A low metabolic rate and oxygen demand; the need for oxygen is reduced, and less oxygen is extracted and consumed. SvO$_2$ or ScvO$_2$ reflects the decrease in extraction as greater amounts of oxyhemoglobin are returned to the right side of the heart.
- Pathologic states in which the cells cannot extract oxygen from the blood or in which tissue beds are not well perfused with oxygenated blood; oxygen is not extracted from the blood despite the cellular oxygen demand. The SvO$_2$ or ScvO$_2$, returning to the right side of the heart and PA, is therefore higher because of the decreased oxygen consumption.

Although the SvO$_2$ or ScvO$_2$ may be in the normal range, cells in the body may not use or receive the oxygen they require. In these instances, cells become reliant on anaerobic metabolism because of the reduced cellular oxygen extraction or the shunting of oxygenated blood past tissue beds. Thus, a normal SvO$_2$ or ScvO$_2$ may be misleading when viewed in isolation. Table 17-19 summarizes factors that cause SvO$_2$ or ScvO$_2$ to increase or decrease.[40-42]

Lactate, base deficit and excess, and SvO$_2$ or ScvO$_2$ are measures of global tissue oxygenation status. In shock states, blood is shunted from the splanchnic tissue bed and from the extremities to vital organs. Therefore, assessment of perfusion in these specific tissue beds can be useful in the early detection of reduced oxygen delivery and utilization.

Near-infrared spectroscopy is a noninvasive technology to monitor tissue oxygen saturation (StO$_2$) in muscle. It uses an infrared light emitting and sensing "patch" over the thenar muscle (located at the base of the thumb on the palm of the hand) to measure oxygen saturation in the microcirculation below the sensor (Fig 17-54). As tissue perfusion is reduced, especially when associated with hypovolemia or decreased CO states, StO$_2$ decreases. StO$_2$ values that trend downward and are less than 75% are associated with higher morbidity and mortality. In patients with sepsis and septic shock, StO$_2$ is lower compared with patients who meet SIRS criteria but has not been shown to be superior to ScvO$_2$ in the sepsis population.[43,44]

Gastric tonometry and sublingual CO$_2$ monitoring are methods to evaluate perfusion of specific tissue beds that have early susceptibility to hypoperfusion. In early shock or shock states, compensatory diversion of blood flow from the

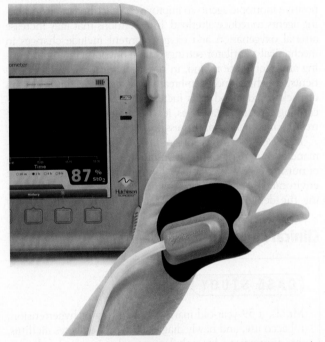

**FIGURE 17-54** Placement of the StO$_2$ sensor over the thenar muscle.

splanchnic bed and digestive tract to vital organs causes the gastric mucosa and upper gastrointestinal tract to be underperfused. Anaerobic metabolism produces increased amounts of CO$_2$ and lactate; thus, measuring the CO$_2$ level or pH of these tissue beds can provide an early indicator of oxygen supply and demand mismatch.

Gastric tonometry uses a nasogastric tube with a gas-permeable balloon near the distal end. CO$_2$ diffuses from the gastric wall into the balloon. Sampling the contents allows measurement of the PCO$_2$ and gastric mucosal pH. Normal gastric mucosal pH is 7.35 to 7.45, and normal gastric mucosal PCO$_2$ is 35 to 45 mm Hg. Decreasing gastric mucosal pH or an increasing gastric PCO$_2$ out of the normal range suggests hypoperfusion and is an indication that oxygen delivery and consumption should be analyzed and optimized. Medications that neutralize gastric pH, such as H-2 blockers, may also affect the gastric tonometer values.

Sublingual capnometry is based on the same physiologic principles as gastric tonometry. Blood flow to the upper digestive tract, including the area under the tongue, is reduced in response to shock or hemorrhage. Sublingual capnometry uses a handheld device similar to a thermometer to measure PCO$_2$ using a sensor that is placed under the tongue. It is important to note that current commercial availability and clinical use of these technologies is limited.[43-45]

## Nursing Considerations

When patients are critically ill, careful evaluation of the adequacy of oxygen delivery, oxygen extraction, and consumption with respect to oxygen demand is paramount. Scrutiny of each determinant of CO (heart rate, preload, afterload, and contractility parameters), oxygen content (arterial saturation and hemoglobin), oxygen consumption ($VO_2$ and $CaO_2 - CvO_2$), and oxygen debt (lactate, pH, base deficit and excess, $SvO_2$ or $ScvO_2$) is important to critical care nursing.

Numerous interventions are used to enhance oxygen delivery. Measures to increase CO include the addition of intravascular volume to increase preload as well as the administration of positive inotropic agents to improve contractility and vasodilating agents to reduce afterload. Interventions that may increase arterial oxygenation and oxygen content include changes in mechanical ventilator settings; chest physiotherapy; positioning and mobilization; and, in nonmechanically ventilated patients, coughing and deep-breathing exercises. Administration of packed red blood cells increases hemoglobin and oxygen-carrying capacity. In all cases, it is necessary to manage both the treatment modalities and assess the patient's response to therapy.

Many of the interventions used to decrease oxygen demand and increase oxygen consumption are important tenets of nursing care. For example, appropriate management of the environment, pain, and anxiety reduces stress, thus decreasing the demand for oxygen. Maintaining normothermia by control of the patient's temperature may decrease oxygen requirements associated with fevers and facilitate impaired perfusion and oxygen consumption associated with hypothermia.

$SvO_2$ or $ScvO_2$ monitoring may be a helpful guide in nursing interventions. For example, endotracheal suctioning may cause a temporary decrease in arterial oxygenation and increase discomfort and anxiety. Monitoring $SvO_2$ or $ScvO_2$ allows the nurse to judge the impact of this activity on the patient's oxygen supply and demand. A decreasing $SvO_2$ or $ScvO_2$ during suctioning is usually caused by increased oxygen demand and decreased arterial oxygenation. Hyperoxygenating and hyperventilating before, during, and after suctioning helps lessen the negative effects on oxygen demand and arterial oxygenation. Before proceeding to another activity such as repositioning, the nurse should monitor the $SvO_2$ or $ScvO_2$ and wait until the value normalizes, thereby avoiding an additional stressor and further increase on oxygen demand.[25,26,40–42]

$ScvO_2$ monitoring has been incorporated into the early, goal-directed management guidelines for patients with sepsis and septic shock.[46] A goal is to maintain an $ScvO_2$ of at least 70% by increasing oxygen delivery. The use of a sepsis bundle and protocol that includes $ScvO_2$ has been associated with improved morbidity and mortality; however, recent RCTs have shown that use of $ScvO_2$ as an end point may not be as significant as reported in earlier papers. Adding dynamic parameters (PPV, SVV, Delta SV) for fluid optimization have been included in the newer guidelines.[47,48]

## Clinical Applicability Challenges

---

**CASE STUDY**

Mr. T., a 59-year-old man with a history of hypertension, tobacco use, and newly diagnosed type 2 diabetes mellitus, was transported by ambulance to the emergency department with complaints of chest burning. The symptoms were precipitated by heavy activity, and were accompanied by dizziness, near syncope, diaphoresis, and nausea. Mr. T. admitted to several less severe episodes in the 2 weeks prior to the ED visit, but decided not to seek medical attention until the third and most severe episode. He called 911 about 15 minutes after his chest burning started, and he arrived in the ED about 45 minutes after his symptoms began.

On arrival to the ED, Mr. T.'s vital signs were BP 100/78 in the RA, 106/80 in the LA. His heart rate was regular and 96 beats per minute, respiratory rate was 22 breaths per minute, and pulse oximeter was 96% on 2 liters per nasal cannula. He was in mild distress, but awake and alert; he admitted to being very frightened by the pain.

He had no chest burning when he arrived because he had received sublingual nitroglycerin in the ambulance, with clearance of all symptoms.

Mr. T.'s telemetry and 12-lead EKG showed a LBBB. Initial troponin I value was 15.9 ng/mL. Mr. T. remained without symptoms. A bedside transthoracic echocardiogram showed concentric LVH, and a remarkable anterior wall motion abnormality. His left ventricular ejection fraction was 35%. No prior medical records were available.

Mr. T. was given an aspirin and placed on a heparin drip and transported to the ICU. You greet him on arrival to the unit. No family is present.

1. The likely diagnosis is MI. What information about the patient's history and presentation supports this diagnosis?
2. What nursing interventions are most critical at the point of Mr. T.'s arrival to the ICU?

---

**WANT TO KNOW MORE?**

A wide variety of resources to enhance your learning and understanding of this chapter are available on thePoint.

You will find:

- References
- Selected readings
- NCLEX-style review questions
- Internet resources
- And more!

# 18

# Patient Management: Cardiovascular System

MANDY L. SNYDER, VICKI J. COOMBS, KARA C. BARQUIST,
TACIA BULLARD, BETH HAMMER, LISA M. SPANNBAUER,
ROBERT H. WELTON, AND CHRISTINE M. COUCHMAN

## LEARNING OBJECTIVES

*Based on the content in this chapter, the reader should be able to:*

1. Compare and contrast commonly used fibrinolytics, anti-coagulants, and platelet inhibitors used to affect thrombosis in the cardiovascular system.
2. Describe the four classes of antiarrhythmic drugs.
3. Discuss the rationale for using inotropic, phosphodiesterase III inhibitor, angiotensin-converting enzyme inhibitor, vasodilator, and antihyperlipidemic drugs for patients with cardiovascular disease.
4. Describe the indications and nursing care for patients undergoing percutaneous coronary interventions (PCIs), including percutaneous transluminal coronary angioplasty and intracoronary stenting.
5. Summarize interventions for complications associated with PCI procedures.
6. Discuss the indications and nursing care for patients undergoing interventions for peripheral arterial disease and percutaneous balloon valvuloplasty for valvular disease.
7. Describe the physiologic effect of intra-aortic balloon pump (IABP) counterpulsation therapy and ventricular circulatory assistance.
8. Explain indications for and contraindications to IABP therapy and ventricular circulatory assistance.
9. Discuss nursing interventions for the patient receiving IABP therapy or ventricular circulatory assistance.
10. Describe the indications, procedure, and nursing management for electrical cardioversion.
11. Explain the indications, procedure, and nursing management for radiofrequency catheter ablation.
12. Describe the indications for a permanent pacemaker.
13. Explain the components, functions, and modes of a pacemaker.
14. Explain the complications of pacing and appropriate interventions.
15. Discuss the nursing management of the patient with a pacemaker.
16. Describe the indications, components, and function for an implantable cardioverter–defibrillator (ICD).
17. Explain the nursing management of a patient with an ICD.
18. Explain the steps of cardiopulmonary resuscitation and the role of each member of the resuscitation team.
19. Discuss the rationale for using targeted temperature management as part of cardiopulmonary arrest management.
20. Describe the pros and cons of having family members present in a cardiopulmonary arrest situation.

Critical care nurses care for many patients with cardiovascular disease. Numerous management options are available for these patients. This chapter discusses pharmacologic therapy, percutaneous coronary interventions and percutaneous valvular interventions, intra-aortic balloon pump counterpulsation and mechanical circulatory support, management of dysrhythmias, and cardiopulmonary resuscitation.

## PHARMACOLOGIC THERAPY

Cardiovascular disease continues to be the leading cause of disease-related death for men and women in the United States. However, recent and remarkable pharmacologic advances have reduced morbidity and mortality related to cardiovascular disease.

Critical care nurses are responsible for administering medications that affect the patient's cardiovascular function. Furthermore, nurses continuously evaluate the effects of these

drugs and use detailed patient assessment data to guide the titration of these drugs.

This section provides a summary of medications used in critical care settings to treat patients with cardiovascular disease. Critical care nurses need to know drug indications, effects, contraindications, dosage, method of administration, and adverse effects. Additionally, many patients require treatment with numerous cardiovascular drugs; therefore, it is important to consider how drugs interact with other drugs.

## Fibrinolytics, Anticoagulants, and Platelet Inhibitors

Atherosclerotic plaque rupture or vascular endothelium damage initiates platelet activation, resulting in platelet aggregation and adhesion. This process initiates the production of thrombin through the activation of the coagulation cascade. Thrombin converts fibrinogen to fibrin, resulting in the formation of a nonsoluble fibrin thrombus. An arterial thrombus may transiently or persistently occlude coronary artery blood flow, causing acute coronary syndrome (ACS). Fibrinolytic, anticoagulant, and platelet inhibitor drugs affect different phases of the thrombotic process and are used to minimize infarct size and prevent future thrombotic events.

For further information about the coagulation process, see Chapter 45. For further information about ACS, see Chapter 21.

## Fibrinolytics

Fibrinolytic agents are indicated for patients with acute ST-segment elevation myocardial infarction (STEMI). These drugs are not effective in patients without ST-segment elevation or nonspecific electrocardiogram (ECG) changes, and should not be administered to these patients.[1,2] Fibrinolytic agents either directly or indirectly convert plasminogen to plasmin, which in turn lyses the thrombus. Early fibrinolytic therapy has been shown to dissolve the thrombus, reestablish coronary blood flow, minimize infarction size, preserve left ventricular (LV) function, and reduce morbidity and mortality.[1] Retavase, streptokinase, tenecteplase, and alteplase are examples of commonly used fibrinolytics.

The decision to administer fibrinolytic therapy is based on the patient's cardiovascular physical assessment data and ECG. Unless contraindicated (contraindications are listed in Box 18-1), fibrinolytics should be given to patients with acute STEMI whose symptoms began within the previous 12 hours and who have ST-segment elevation greater than 0.1 mV in two or more contiguous (adjacent) leads, or who have a new-onset left bundle branch block (BBB).[2] Fibrinolytic therapy produces the greatest reduction in mortality when initiated within the first 4 hours of symptom onset; however, fibrinolytics may be administered up to 12 hours after symptom onset. There is no benefit if there is a delay in presentation of administering fibrinolytics beyond 12 hours after symptom onset. The goal is to administer a fibrinolytic drug within 30 minutes of the patient's arrival in the emergency department. Patients are at risk for recurrent thrombus formation in the coronary artery; therefore, aspirin and heparin are given to most patients who receive fibrinolytic therapy.[2,3]

Reperfusion may be manifested by decreased or resolved ST-segment elevation, abrupt cessation of chest pain, early peak of serum cardiac biomarkers, and reperfusion dysrhythmias, such as premature ventricular contractions, ventricular tachycardia (VT), accelerated idioventricular rhythm, and atrioventricular (AV) blocks. In contrast, reocclusion may be evidenced by recurrent chest pain and ST-segment elevation,

further myocardial ischemia or infarction, lethal dysrhythmias, cardiogenic shock, or death. The most common adverse effects of fibrinolytic therapy are bleeding, intracranial hemorrhage, stroke, and reperfusion dysrhythmias. For more details about the use of fibrinolytic therapy for acute myocardial infarction (AMI), see Chapter 21.

## Anticoagulants

Anticoagulants, such as unfractionated heparin, low-molecular-weight heparins (LMWHs), direct thrombin inhibitors, warfarin (Coumadin), and novel oral anticoagulants limit further fibrin formation and help prevent thromboembolism.[3]

### Unfractionated Heparin

The most commonly used anticoagulant drug for acute cardiovascular conditions, unfractionated heparin is indicated for ACS, venous thromboembolism, percutaneous coronary interventions (PCIs), and patients receiving reteplase or tenecteplase. Heparin prevents clot formation by combining with antithrombin III and inhibiting circulating thrombin. However, unfractionated heparin does not lyse thrombi and is not an optimal anticoagulant because of its narrow therapeutic range, its low bioavailability, the varied anticoagulant response, the requirement for parenteral administration, the need for monitoring the activated partial thromboplastin time (APTT), the risk for bleeding, possible heparin-induced thrombocytopenia (HIT), and hypersensitivity reactions.

The dosage for unfractionated heparin varies according to its indication and administration route. When used with reteplase (Retavase) or tenecteplase (TNKase), the recommended heparin dosage is 60 units/kg intravenous (IV; maximum 4,000 units) bolus given when the fibrinolytic infusion is started, followed by an infusion of 12 units/kg/h (maximum 1,000 units/h) for ST-segment elevation AMI.[1,2] When IV heparin is administered for non–ST-segment elevation myocardial infarction (NSTEMI) and unstable angina, an initial IV bolus of 60 to 70 units/kg (maximum 5,000 units) followed by a 12 to 15 units/kg/h infusion is recommended.[1] The heparin infusion rate is adjusted to maintain an APTT of 50 to 70 seconds for 48 hours.) Protamine sulfate reverses the effects of heparin; however, protamine may cause a life-threatening anaphylactic reaction.

### Low-Molecular-Weight Heparins

LMWHs, such as enoxaparin (Lovenox) and dalteparin (Fragmin), are small fragments derived from unfractionated heparin and are alternatives to heparin for patients with unstable angina, NSTEMI, or deep venous thrombosis.[1,2] These drugs inhibit clot formation by blocking Factor Xa and thrombin. Investigators have shown that enoxaparin is superior to unfractionated heparin for patients with STEMI, unstable angina, and NSTEMI.[1,2] Both enoxaparin and dalteparin are administered subcutaneously every 12 hours based on the patient's weight. Dalteparin is dosed at 120 IU/kg with a maximum of 10,000 international units and enoxaparin is dosed at 1 mg/kg.[1,2]

The advantages of LMWHs are their longer half-life, more predictable anticoagulation effect, greater bioavailability, and cost-effectiveness. In addition, LMWHs are

---

**BOX 18-1** | **Contraindications for Fibrinolytic Therapy**

- Active internal bleeding
- Any history of intracranial hemorrhage
- Ischemic stroke within 3 months
- Intracranial neoplasm, arteriovenous malformation, or aneurysm
- Recent intracranial or intraspinal surgery
- Recent closed-head or facial trauma within 3 months
- Suspected aortic dissection
- Severe uncontrolled hypertension
- Bleeding diathesis

administered subcutaneously twice daily and do not require APTT monitoring.

The most common adverse effects of LMWHs include bleeding, thrombocytopenia, elevated aminotransferase levels, and pain, erythema, ecchymosis, or hematoma at the injection site. Because LMWHs have different molecular weight distribution profiles, activities, and plasma clearance rates, they must not be used interchangeably with each other or unfractionated heparin. LMWH is contraindicated in individuals with morbid obesity because the dose is weight-based and absorption may be unpredictable in obesity. Also, LMWH should not be given to patients with severe renal dysfunction.

## Direct Thrombin Inhibitors

Direct thrombin inhibitors may be administered as alternatives to unfractionated heparin in patients who have a history of heparin-induced thrombocytopenia (HIT). Examples of these drugs include bivalirudin (Angiomax), lepirudin (Refludan), and argatroban (Acova). The medication doses are titrated to maintain optimal anticoagulation and the major risks of using these drugs are bleeding complications.

Bivalirudin (Angiomax), lepirudin (Refludan), and argatroban (Acova) are intravenous direct thrombin inhibitors that may be administered as an alternative to unfractionated heparin in low-risk patients who undergo PCI or patients with HIT.[1,3] The IV bolus dose for bivalirudin and lepirudin are weight based, followed by a continuous infusion for the duration of the PCI procedure. Argatroban is not bolus dosed; it is started at a continuous rate and adjusted to achieve an APTT ratio 1.5 to 3.0 times the baseline level.

An additional bolus dose of bivalirudin may be given in 5 minutes depending on results of the activated clotting time (ACT). The bivalirudin infusion may be continued for 4 hours after the PCI procedure. The lepirudin infusion rate is adjusted to maintain an APTT ratio of 1.5 to 2.5 times the baseline value. As with other anticoagulants, the major adverse effects of these drugs are bleeding complications.[3]

## Warfarin

Warfarin, an oral drug used for chronic anticoagulation therapy, interferes with the synthesis of vitamin K–dependent clotting factors, such as factors II, VII, IX, and X. The most common cardiovascular indications for warfarin include post-AMI anticoagulation for high-risk patients, dilated cardiomyopathy, atrial fibrillation (AF), heart failure (HF), venous thromboembolism, mobile mural thrombus, and presence of a prosthetic heart valve. Studies show that warfarin plus aspirin combination therapy is associated with decreased recurrent AMI, stroke, and revascularization but with increased major bleeding.[4] Thus, oral anticoagulants are not routinely administered after infarction.

Contraindications for warfarin include uncontrolled hypertension; severe hepatic or renal disease; bleeding diathesis; gastrointestinal (GI) or genitourinary (GU) bleeding; cerebral or dissecting aortic aneurysm; recent central nervous system, eye, or other major surgery; recent trauma; pregnancy (first and third trimesters); pericarditis; pericardial effusion; spinal puncture; and recent diagnostic procedures with the potential for uncontrolled bleeding. Patients must be able and willing to adhere to this somewhat complicated therapy.

Warfarin is usually started at 5 mg daily but the initial dose should be decreased for the elderly and patients with liver or renal impairment and HF. The dose is titrated according to the patient's INR.[4] Because warfarin levels do not peak for 3 to 4 days, acute anticoagulant therapy is continued until the INR is at the desired level for the patient's condition, usually between 2.0 to 3.0 for atrial fibrillation and mechanical aortic valves, and 2.5 to 3.5 for a mechanical mitral valve. Once the INR is therapeutic on a stable warfarin dose, less frequent INR monitoring is appropriate. Elevated INR levels predispose the patient to bleeding, warfarin's most common adverse effect.[4] Administration of vitamin K and human prothrombin complex concentrates (Kcentra) can reverse the action of warfarin in situations of life threatening bleeding or the need for emergency surgery.

Patient education is an important part of warfarin therapy. Warfarin interacts with numerous drugs and foods; safe treatment depends on the patient's knowledge of therapy.

## Other Oral Anticoagulants

A new class of anticoagulants, called novel oral anticoagulants, has emerged as an alternative to warfarin therapy. These inhibitors seem to have fewer adverse events related to bleeding. Routine frequent blood testing is not required to monitor the effects. These medications have only been studied in atrial fibrillation and have not been approved by the FDA for thrombus prevention in individuals with mechanical heart valves or valvular atrial fibrillation.[5]

Two recently approved Factor Xa inhibitor agents are rivaroxaban (Xarelto), and apixaban (Eliquis).[5] Dabigatran (Pradaxa) is a direct thrombin inhibitor also used to prevent stroke in nonvalvular atrial fibrillation and falls under the class of novel oral anticoagulants.[5] There are no laboratory tests that can evaluate the effectiveness of the novel oral anticoagulants. If bleeding occurs, laboratory coagulation tests can be used as a qualitative assessment to determine if the medication is contributing to the event. Additionally, there are no reversal agents should severe bleeding occur, though clinical trials are underway to explore novel oral anticoagulant antidotes. Supportive care and control of bleeding are the cornerstones of therapy in this situation.[5]

# Platelet Inhibitors

## Aspirin

Aspirin, the most widely used platelet inhibitor, inhibits thromboxane $A_2$, a platelet agonist, and prevents thrombus formation and arterial vasoconstriction. Aspirin is used to decrease mortality for patients with AMI; to reduce incidence of nonfatal AMI and mortality for patients with stable angina, unstable angina, or previous myocardial infarction (MI); and to prevent graft closure after coronary artery bypass graft (CABG) surgery and coronary artery thrombus after PCI. Aspirin is also indicated to reduce the risk for nonfatal stroke and death in patients with a history of ischemic stroke or transient ischemia resulting from platelet emboli.[1,2,4,6] Aspirin is not indicated for primary prevention of AMI. Patients with a history of aspirin intolerance, GI or GU bleeding, peptic ulcers, severe renal or hepatic insufficiency, or bleeding disorders should not take aspirin.

Common aspirin dosages in the United States range from 81 to 325 mg daily. Depending on the indication, patients may take aspirin for a few weeks or indefinitely. Unless contraindicated, patients with symptoms of ACS should immediately chew 162 to 325 mg of non–enteric-coated aspirin.[2] A 325-mg aspirin suppository is recommended for patients unable to take oral drugs or for patients with severe nausea, vomiting, or upper GI disorders. Aspirin may cause stomach pain, nausea, vomiting, GI bleeding, subdural or intracranial hemorrhage, thrombocytopenia, coagulopathy, and a prolonged prothrombin time (PT).

### P2Y12 Receptor Inhibitors

The adenosine diphosphate receptor antagonists (or P2Y12 receptor inhibitors, as these drugs are also called) prevent platelet activation and platelet aggregation, resulting in an irreversible inhibition of platelet function. Clopidogrel and ticlopidine have been the standard of care, though prasugrel and ticagrelor are newer agents that are now available.

**CLOPIDOGREL.** Clopidogrel (Plavix) is indicated to reduce new AMI, new stroke, and vascular death in patients with ACS (both STEMI and NSTEMI) or atherosclerosis as documented by recent stroke, recent AMI, or established peripheral arterial disease (PAD). The dosage for clopidogrel is 75 mg daily with or without food. A loading dose 600 mg is often used to achieve a rapid onset of action.[2] The effects of clopidogrel begin immediately; steady-state platelet inhibition is achieved after 3 to 7 days of therapy. Once clopidogrel is discontinued, bleeding times and platelet function normalize within 3 to 7 days. Recently, a subgroup of patients has been identified with altered metabolism, which causes a suboptimal clinical response to clopidogrel. The Federal Drug Administration has identified the need for pharmacogenomics testing to identify patients' altered clopidogrel metabolism though routine screening is currently not recommended unless the individual is at high risk for in-stent thrombosis.[2,6]

**PRASUGREL.** Prasugrel (Effient) is started at a loading dose of 60 mg and then 10 mg daily for maintenance. Prasugrel has an increased risk of bleeding especially in individuals with a history of stroke or who are older than 75 years of age.[2]

**TICAGRELOR.** Ticagrelor (Brilinta) is started at a loading dose of 180 mg and then maintenance dose of 90 mg BID. Caution should be used in patients who have altered liver and renal function or who are taking medications that are inhibitors or inducers of the enzyme CYP3A4.[1,2]

**TICLOPIDINE.** Ticlopidine (Ticlid) is used generally for patients who cannot tolerate aspirin. A loading dose of 500 mg can be given with 250 mg twice daily taken with food after that. Maximal platelet aggregation inhibition occurs after 4 to 7 days of therapy. Once ticlopidine is discontinued, bleeding times and platelet function normalize within 2 weeks.

**ADVERSE EFFECTS.** The common major adverse effects of these drugs include bleeding disorders, GI upset, thrombotic thrombocytopenic purpura, and neutropenia. Ticagrelor is also associated with dyspnea. Ticlopidine is associated with rare cases of agranulocytosis and elevated liver aminotransferases. Patients receiving clopidogrel have less GI upset, hemorrhage, and abnormal liver function than patients receiving aspirin. If CABG is planned within 5 days, clopidogrel should be withheld, and even earlier at 7 days for prasugrel.[4]

### GP IIb/IIIa Inhibitors

The three major GP IIb/IIIa inhibitors include abciximab (ReoPro), tirofiban (Aggrastat), and eptifibatide (Integrilin). These drugs inhibit the GP IIb/IIIa receptor, the final common pathway for platelet aggregation, preventing platelet aggregation and thereby inhibiting thrombus formation. These three drugs are all administered with either enoxaparin or unfractionated heparin. Box 18-2 lists the contraindications to GP IIb/IIIa inhibitors. Adverse effects for this class of drugs include bleeding, thrombocytopenia, stroke, and allergic reactions.

Practice guidelines for PCI intervention recommend a GP IIb/IIIa inhibitor for patients with ACS or NSTEMI who undergo PCI.[1,2] Guidelines for managing patients with STEMI recommend abciximab as early as possible before PCI.[2,6]

## Antiarrhythmics

Antiarrhythmic drugs are used to restore the heart to a regular rhythm. Many of these medications have serious side effects, and caution must be used to prevent complications. Antiarrhythmics are classified by their effect on the cardiac action potential, that is, whether they block β-receptors or sodium, potassium, or calcium channels. The action of these drugs is complex; drugs within the same class can work differently, and actions of those in different classes may overlap (Table 18-1). Refer to Chapter 16, Figure 16-3, for a summary regarding the cardiac action potential.

### Class I Antiarrhythmic Drugs

In general, research data do not support the effectiveness of class I antiarrhythmics. The current trend is to treat ventricular dysrhythmias with class II and class III antiarrhythmics, cardioversion, ablative techniques, and implantable cardioverter–defibrillators (ICDs).[7,8]

Class I antiarrhythmics stabilize the cell membrane by blocking the influx of sodium into the cell. Class I drugs are

---

**BOX 18-2** **Contraindications for Glycoprotein IIb/IIIa Inhibitors**

- Internal bleeding
- Bleeding diathesis within 30 days
- Intracranial neoplasm, arteriovenous malformation, or aneurysm
- Stroke within 30 days or any hemorrhagic stroke
- Thrombocytopenia with prior exposure to tirofiban
- Aortic dissection
- Major surgery or severe trauma within the previous month
- Severe hypertension
- Pericarditis (tirofiban)
- Concurrent use of another glycoprotein IIb/IIIa inhibitor
- Dependence on dialysis or serum creatinine 4.0 mg/dL or more (eptifibatide)

CHAPTER 18 Patient Management: Cardiovascular System **265**

| TABLE 18-1 | Classification of Antiarrhythmic Medications | |
|---|---|---|
| **Class** | **Action** | **Medication Examples** |
| IA | Inhibits fast sodium channel, decreases automaticity, depresses phase 0, and prolongs the action potential duration | Quinidine<br>Procainamide<br>Disopyramide |
| IB | Inhibits fast sodium channel, depresses phase 0 slightly, and shortens action potential duration | Lidocaine<br>Mexiletine |
| IC | Inhibits fast sodium channel, depresses phase 0 markedly, slows His-Purkinje conduction profoundly leading to a prolonged QRS duration | Flecainide<br>Moricizine (plus IA and IB effects)<br>Propafenone |
| II | Depresses phase 4 depolarization, blocks sympathetic stimulation of the conduction system | Esmolol<br>Propranolol<br>Sotalol (plus class III effects)<br>Acebutolol |
| III | Blocks potassium channel, prolongs phase 3 repolarization, prolongs action potential duration | Amiodarone<br>Sotalol<br>Ibutilide<br>Dofetilide |
| IV | Inhibits inward calcium channel, depresses phase 4 depolarization, lengthens repolarization in phases 1 and 2 | Verapamil<br>Diltiazem |

further categorized on the basis of the action and effects of the specific medications.

Class IA antiarrhythmics include quinidine (Quinate), procainamide (Pronestyl), and disopyramide (Norpace). These drugs are effective for treating atrial rhythms in the short term but may cause life-threatening dysrhythmias by prolonging the QTc interval. They also interact with other drugs commonly used for cardiovascular disease.

Class IB antiarrhythmics are lidocaine and mexiletine (Mexitil). Lidocaine, a less effective but acceptable alternative to procainamide for ventricular dysrhythmias, is no longer used routinely to prevent ventricular dysrhythmias.

Class IC antiarrhythmics are flecainide (Tambocor) and propafenone (Rythmol). Because these drugs are prodysrhythmic and may increase mortality, they are not commonly prescribed.

## Class II Antiarrhythmic Drugs

β-Adrenergic blockers are class II drugs that interfere with sympathetic nervous system stimulation, contributing to decreased heart rate, prolonged AV node conduction, decreased myocardial contractility, and decreased myocardial oxygen demand. This class of drugs has a broad spectrum of activity and an established safety record, and is currently the best class of antiarrhythmics for general use.[8] This is the only class of medications shown to reduce the incidence of sudden cardiac death following AMI and HF.[1,2]

β-Blockers are categorized as cardioselective (inhibition of $\beta_1$ receptors) or nonselective (inhibition of $\beta_1$ and $\beta_2$ receptors). Examples of cardioselective β-blockers that are used for treating dysrhythmias are esmolol and metoprolol. These medications are available in intravenous form and are used commonly in acute and critical care. Propranolol is also available in an intravenous form, though this drug is nonselective for cardiac tissue effects. These are just a few examples of selective and nonselective β-blockers; others are available in oral forms but may be more common in the outpatient, non–critical care setting.

Inhibition of $\beta_1$ receptors causes decreased heart rate, slowed conduction through the AV node, and depressed cardiac function. Inhibition of $\beta_2$ receptors causes bronchoconstriction, vasoconstriction, and decreased glycogenolysis. Table 16-1 (see Chapter 16) summarizes receptor binding at target organs.

Unless contraindicated, β-blockers should be given indefinitely to all patients with a history of AMI, ACS, or LV dysfunction with or without symptoms of HF.[1,2,9] Other indications include tachydysrhythmias, unstable angina, hypertension, and HF. Acebutolol, esmolol, propranolol, and sotalol are approved to treat dysrhythmias. All β-blockers, except sotalol, are indicated for hypertension.

Metoprolol (Lopressor), atenolol (Tenormin), propranolol, and nadolol (Corgard) are approved for angina, whereas metoprolol and atenolol are indicated as first-line drugs for AMI.[10] The first dose may be given intravenously, and successive doses are usually given orally.

The adverse effects of these medications can exacerbate certain underlying conditions. β-Blockers are contraindicated in patients with severe asthma or bronchospasm, severe chronic obstructive pulmonary disease, cardiogenic shock, severe LV failure, bradycardia (less than 60 beats/min), or second- and third-degree heart block. Cardioselective β-blockers are sometimes used with caution for patients with pulmonary disease. It is important to remember that cardioselective drugs lose their selectivity at higher doses.[1,2] Other adverse effects include hypotension, cold extremities, insomnia, fatigue, decreased libido, and depression. Some patients who experience these adverse effects may respond better to a different β-blocker.[1]

## Class III Antiarrhythmic Drugs

Class III antiarrhythmic drugs include amiodarone (Cordarone), sotalol (Betapace), ibutilide (Corvert), and dofetilide (Tikosyn). It is important to know each drug's unique properties because individual agents contain unique properties not shared by other class III drugs.

Amiodarone is indicated for treating refractory (CPR, defibrillation, and vasopressor therapy) pulseless VT (pVT) and ventricular fibrillation (VF) as well as AF and flutter. The 2015 Advanced Cardiac Life Support (ACLS) algorithms include amiodarone as a first-line option for treating VF, wide-complex tachycardia, and AF.[11] Limitations of amiodarone include its variable onset of action, long half-life, intolerable adverse effects, dangerous drug interactions, and life-threatening complications associated with chronic therapy.[5]

Ibutilide (Corvert) and dofetilide (Tikosyn) are class III drugs that are indicated for the pharmacologic conversion of AF and atrial flutter. Ibutilide inhibits potassium current and enhances sodium current, prolonging repolarization. Dofetilide blocks the rapid potassium current channel, prolonging the action potential duration and refractory period. These drugs may cause a prolonged QT interval and torsades de pointes. Therefore, close monitoring of the QTC is required upon initiation of the medication. These medications have fewer systemic adverse effects than amiodarone and sotalol.[5]

## Class IV Antiarrhythmic Drugs

The class IV calcium channel blocker antiarrhythmics, verapamil (Calan) and diltiazem (Cardizem), decrease automaticity of the sinoatrial (SA) and AV nodes, slow conduction, and prolong the AV nodal refractory period.[5] These agents have negative inotropic and peripheral vasodilation effects. In addition, they have antiplatelet and anti-ischemic effects. Calcium channel blockers are primarily indicated for angina, hypertension, and supraventricular tachycardia (SVT). Verapamil and diltiazem are contraindicated for usual forms of VT, severe sinus bradycardia, sick sinus syndrome, WPW syndrome with AF, digoxin toxicity, hypotension, HF, AV conduction defects, and severe aortic stenosis, and they are not standard therapies for AMI.[9] Calcium antagonists, in general, should be used only in the setting of AMI when β-blockers are contraindicated or maximal dosage has been reached without effect.[1,9]

Adverse effects include hypotension, AV block, bradycardia, headache, dizziness, peripheral edema, nausea, constipation, and flushing.

## Unclassified Antiarrhythmic Drugs

### Adenosine

Adenosine is an antiarrhythmic that effectively converts narrow-complex paroxysmal supraventricular tachycardia (PSVT) to normal sinus rhythm by slowing conduction through the AV node. This agent is effective in terminating dysrhythmias due to reentry involving the SA and AV nodes; however, it does not convert AF, atrial flutter, or VT to sinus rhythm. It is also used to differentiate VT and SVT, treat rare forms of idiopathic VT, and reveal latent preexcitation in patients with suspected WPW syndrome.[11] The dose is 6 mg rapid IV bolus followed by a rapid saline flush. If the 6-mg dose is ineffective, a dose of 12 mg may be administered twice. The half-life of adenosine is less than 10 seconds; therefore, adverse effects are short-lived.

### Magnesium Sulfate

Magnesium sulfate is the drug of choice for treating torsades de pointes. Magnesium is also used for refractory VT and VF,

as well as for life-threatening dysrhythmias from digitalis toxicity. Its mechanism of action is unclear; however, it has calcium channel blocking properties and inhibits sodium and potassium channels. The dose for patients in cardiac arrest is 1 to 2 g diluted in 10 mL of $D_5W$ given by IV push. Adverse effects include hypotension, nausea, depressed reflexes, and flushing.[11]

### Atropine

Atropine, a parasympatholytic agent, is a first-line drug used to treat acute symptomatic bradycardia and slowed conduction at the AV node.[11] Atropine reduces the effects of vagal stimulation, thereby increasing heart rate and improving cardiac function. It is important not to increase the heart rate excessively in patients with ischemic heart disease because this may increase myocardial oxygen consumption and worsen ischemia.[11]

### Digoxin

Digoxin (Lanoxin) is a mild positive inotrope with antidysrhythmic and bradycardic actions. It inhibits the sodium–potassium pump, causing a rise in intracellular sodium. This rise promotes calcium influx and ultimately enhances myocardial contractility. Digoxin also activates the parasympathetic system, decreasing heart rate and increasing AV nodal inhibition. Digoxin is primarily indicated for patients with both HF and chronic AF.[5,12,13] In addition, digoxin may be used to control a rapid ventricular rate associated with non–preexcitation AF or atrial flutter and in combination with verapamil, diltiazem, or β-blockers for patients without HF.[5] Digoxin is not currently used for paroxysmal AF, acute SVTs, or acute LV failure, or as part of inotropic therapy regimens.

The doses and therapeutic blood levels for digoxin are controversial. No longer is it common to administer loading doses.[13] Most patients on digoxin benefit from a low dose, which also reduces the incidence of toxicity.[13] Toxicity is a common occurrence and is frequently associated with serious dysrhythmias. Routine doses are individualized based on the patient's diagnosis, symptoms, underlying disease processes, age, response to therapy, and blood levels. Levels of 0.5 to 0.9 ng/mL are recommended for patients with HF, and levels of 0.8 to 2 ng/mL for those with dysrhythmias.

Signs and symptoms of digitalis toxicity include palpitations, syncope, dysrhythmias, elevated digoxin level, anorexia, vomiting, diarrhea, nausea, fatigue, confusion, insomnia, headache, depression, vertigo, facial pain, and colored or blurred vision. Digitalis levels may be increased by the concurrent use of quinidine, verapamil, amiodarone, captopril, diltiazem, esmolol (Brevibloc), propafenone (Rythmol), indomethacin (Indocin), quinine, or ibuprofen (Motrin).[13] Finally, hypokalemia, hypomagnesemia, and hypothyroidism may predispose patients to digitalis toxicity. Blood serum levels are analyzed if toxicity is suspected.

## Inotropes

Cardiovascular function is regulated by two divisions of the autonomic nervous system: the sympathetic and parasympathetic systems (see Chapter 32). The myocardium and peripheral blood vessels, along with other organ tissues in the body, are innervated by adrenergic sympathetic fibers and

| TABLE 18-2 | Adrenergic Receptors Affecting Cardiovascular Function | |
|---|---|---|
| **Receptor** | **Location** | **Effects of Stimulation** |
| $\beta_1$ | Heart | Positive inotropic (increases contractility) and chronotropic action (increases rate) |
| $\beta_2$ | Bronchial smooth muscle | Bronchodilation |
| | Vascular smooth muscle | Vasodilation |
| | AV node | Positive dromotropic action (increases conduction velocity) |
| $\alpha_1$ | Vascular smooth muscle | Vasoconstriction |
| | Heart | Weak positive inotropic and chronotropic actions |
| $\alpha_2$ | Presynaptic sympathetic nerve endings | Inhibition of norepinephrine release |
| Dopaminergic | Kidney and splanchnic vessels | Renal and splanchnic vessel vasodilation |

respond to stimulation by inotropic agents through antagonistic or agonistic mechanisms. Table 18-2 provides a review of which receptors each inotropic drug stimulates to provide context for this discussion.

Inotropic drugs are used to increase the force of myocardial contraction and cardiac output. Inotropic drugs include sympathomimetics, such as dopamine (Intropin), dobutamine (Dobutrex), epinephrine, isoproterenol (Isuprel), and norepinephrine, and the phosphodiesterase inhibitor milrinone (Primacor). These drugs are commonly given to patients with impaired myocardial contractility or cardiogenic shock. Enhanced ventricular contraction increases stroke volume, cardiac output, blood pressure, and coronary artery perfusion. As the ventricles empty more completely, ventricular filling pressures, preload, and pulmonary congestion are decreased. However, as contractility and heart rate increase, myocardial oxygen demand also increases. Myocardial ischemia can occur if a myocardial oxygen supply–demand mismatch develops. The nurse must closely monitor the patient for evidence of ischemia, angina, and onset of dysrhythmias.

## Dopamine

Dopamine, the most widely used inotropic drug, is administered to patients with conditions that cause hypotension, decreased cardiac output, and oliguria. Dopamine directly stimulates dopaminergic, $\beta$-adrenergic, and $\alpha$-adrenergic receptors and promotes release of norepinephrine from sympathetic nerve terminals. Dopamine is given by continuous IV infusion, and its dose is titrated to achieve the desired effect. Increased myocardial contractility results from dosages of 3 to 10 mcg/kg/min. Higher dosages predominantly cause vasoconstriction and increased blood pressure. Dopamine is usually given through a central line to enhance its distribution and to avoid extravasation, which may cause local vasoconstriction and tissue necrosis. Adverse effects include tachycardia, palpitations, dysrhythmias, angina, headache, nausea, vomiting, and hypertension.[12]

## Dobutamine

Dobutamine acts on $\beta_1$ receptors and increases myocardial contractility. Dobutamine also stimulates the $\beta_2$ receptors as well as the $\alpha_1$ receptors. The result is slight vasodilation.[12,14] Dobutamine is used after cardiac surgery, during some cardiac diagnostic stress procedures, and for patients with HF, shock, or other conditions that cause poor cardiac contractility or a low cardiac output. The dosage for dobutamine is 2 to 20 mcg/kg/min by continuous IV infusion. Adverse effects include tachycardia, dysrhythmias, blood pressure fluctuations, headache, and nausea.[15]

## Epinephrine

Epinephrine stimulates $\alpha_1$, $\beta_1$, and $\beta_2$ receptors and is given for a variety of indications, including cardiac arrest, symptomatic bradycardia, severe hypotension, anaphylaxis, and shock.[11,16] In the intensive care unit (ICU), epinephrine is given by continuous IV infusion through a central line, as an IV bolus, or through an endotracheal tube. Continuous IV dosages of 1 to 2 mcg/min stimulate $\beta_1$ receptors to increase cardiac output by increasing heart rate and myocardial contractility. At higher dosages, epinephrine stimulates $\alpha$ receptors, causing profound vasoconstriction, increased blood pressure and systemic vascular resistance (SVR), and decreased renal and splanchnic perfusion. Epinephrine may cause dysrhythmias, tachycardia, cerebral hemorrhage, pulmonary edema, headache, dizziness, nervousness, myocardial ischemia, and angina.[12]

## Vasopressin

Vasopressin has been used as an alternative to epinephrine for treating shock-refractory VF, asystole, or PEA but has been removed from the 2015 ACLS guideline, because there is no therapeutic benefit to giving vasopressin in lieu of epinephrine.[11] Vasopressin promotes smooth muscle contraction and increases peripheral vascular resistance. The dosage for patients with cardiac arrest is 40 U given by IV push. The drug may also be given as an infusion. Adverse effects include dysrhythmias, myocardial ischemia, angina, MI, tremors, vertigo, sweating, and water intoxication.[11,12,17]

## Isoproterenol

Isoproterenol (Isuprel) stimulates $\beta_1$ and $\beta2$ receptors to increase myocardial contractility, cardiac output, heart rate, and blood pressure. Currently, isoproterenol is used mainly to increase heart rate after cardiac transplantation. Other indications include refractory torsades de pointes, $\beta$-blocker overdose, and symptomatic bradycardia when an external pacemaker is not available. The IV dosage is 0.5 to 10 mcg/min by continuous infusion. Isoproterenol causes a variety of adverse effects, including dysrhythmias, tachycardia, palpitations, myocardial ischemia, hypotension, pulmonary edema, bronchospasm, headache, nausea, vomiting, and sweating.[15]

## Norepinephrine

Norepinephrine (Levophed) primarily affects $\alpha_1$ receptors, causing peripheral vasoconstriction, increased blood pressure, and increased SVR. The increased SVR may actually increase myocardial oxygen demand and work, thus decreasing cardiac output. Norepinephrine is used for patients with cardiogenic shock and significant hypotension accompanied by a low SVR. The dosage is 2 to 12 mcg/min by continuous IV infusion. Adverse effects include tachycardia, bradycardia, dysrhythmias, headache, hypertension, and tissue necrosis from extravasation.[12,18]

## Phosphodiesterase III Inhibitor

The phosphodiesterase III inhibitor milrinone (Primacor) increases contractility, venous vasodilation, and peripheral arterial vasodilation by inhibiting an enzyme that breaks down cyclic adenosine monophosphate. There is a reduction of ventricular filling pressures and a slight reduction of arterial pressure; however, there is minimal effect on the heart rate.

Milrinone is frequently used for the short-term treatment of acute HF. Some patients with HF may be on a milrinone infusion long term at home for palliative care.[13,18] The IV bolus dose of 50 mcg/kg is given over 10 minutes and is followed by a maintenance IV infusion of 0.375 to 0.75 mcg/kg/min. Patients who receive milrinone may experience ventricular dysrhythmias, hypotension, headache, bronchospasm, and thrombocytopenia.[13,15]

## Vasodilators

Vasodilators decrease preload and afterload. Preload is the distending force that stretches the ventricular muscle at the end of filling. The greater the stretch, the better the contraction. However, if the cells are overstretched, contractile force decreases. Afterload is the force against which the heart has to work to eject its contents. If afterload is too low, blood pressure and tissue perfusion may be low. If afterload is too high, the heart has to work harder.

## Nitrates

Patients with myocardial ischemia or infarction may have an increased preload and afterload, which further strains their hearts. Nitrates cause peripheral vasodilation, which in turn decreases venous return to the heart and reduces preload. These drugs promote coronary artery vasodilation, improve collateral blood flow, reduce platelet aggregation, enhance perfusion to ischemic myocardium, and decrease myocardial oxygen demand, thus reducing ischemia, chest pain, and infarct size. Nitrates reduce blood pressure and previously elevated pulmonary vascular resistance, SVR, and central venous and pulmonary artery occlusion wedge pressures. At high doses, nitrates reduce afterload by arterial vasodilator effects.[12,16]

Nitrates are indicated for unstable angina; large anterior AMI; AMI associated with acute and chronic HF, acute pulmonary edema, or hypertension; angina unresponsive to other therapies; and prophylaxis of effort angina. Nitroglycerin has been shown to raise the threshold for VF in the setting of AMI. Contraindications to IV nitrates include, but are not limited to, hypotension, uncorrected hypovolemia, hypertrophic obstructive cardiomyopathy, and pericardial tamponade. When a right ventricular (RV) AMI is suspected, nitrates are used with extreme caution because these patients require an adequate venous return to maintain cardiac output and blood pressure. Patients should not receive nitrates for 24 hours after sildenafil (Viagra), vardenafil (Levitra), or tadalafil (Cialis) use because the resulting drug interactions predispose patients to life-threatening hypotension.[1]

Nitrates are available in a variety of dosage forms. In the ICU, nitrates are often given by the IV, sublingual, or topical routes. An IV nitroglycerin drip is initiated at 5 to 20 mcg/min and increased every 5 to 15 minutes, up to 200 mcg/min, to achieve the desired effects. When used to treat or prevent angina, a 0.3- to 0.6-mg tablet is placed under the patient's tongue and may be repeated twice at 5-minute intervals. The usual dose for nitroglycerin ointment is 1 to 2 inches every 8 hours; however, treatment is often initiated with 0.5 inch and increased gradually to achieve the desired effects.[1]

The adverse effects of nitrates include headache, hypotension, syncope, and tachycardia. Tolerance may develop to the antianginal, hemodynamic, and antiplatelet effects of nitrates, especially with continuous or high-dose therapy; however, dosing regimens that allow for nitrate-free intervals for at least 12 hours may prevent this occurrence.[12]

## Sodium Nitroprusside

Nitroprusside (Nipride) is a potent arterial and venous vasodilator that is used to treat severe LV HF, hypertension after CABG, hypertensive crisis, and dissecting aneurysm. Nitroprusside decreases SVR and increases cardiac output. The usual IV infusion dosage is 0.5 to 10 mcg/kg/min; however, to prevent cyanide toxicity, the maximal dose should not be given for longer than 10 minutes. The dose is titrated to effect; if blood pressure does not respond after 10 minutes, the drug is discontinued. Because nitroprusside is sensitive to light, the infusion bag must be covered with an opaque material to prevent the drug's degradation. Adverse effects include hypotension, myocardial ischemia, nausea, vomiting, abdominal pain, and cyanide toxicity.[12,16]

## Nesiritide

Nesiritide (Natrecor), a recombinant form of human B-type natriuretic peptide, is identical to the hormone produced by the left ventricle in response to volume overload and increased wall stress. A venous and arterial vasodilator, nesiritide reduces preload and afterload and increases cardiac output without increasing heart rate. Nesiritide is indicated for acutely decompensated HF with dyspnea at rest or with minimal activity and is often used with IV diuretics.[12] The bolus dose is 2 mcg/kg/min, followed by an IV infusion of 0.01 to 0.03 mcg/kg/min. Contraindications include cardiogenic or distributive shock, valvular stenosis, constrictive pericarditis, and restrictive or obstructive cardiomyopathy. Adverse effects include hypotension, bradycardia, ventricular dysrhythmias, angina, dizziness, and apnea. Nesiritide should not be infused through heparin-coated catheters or IVs containing furosemide (Lasix), insulin, hydralazine (Apresoline), enalapril (Vasotec), and bumetanide (Bumex).

## Clevidipine

Clevidipine (Cleviprex) is an ultra-short acting nonhydropyridine calcium channel blocker that is used to treat hypertension when rapid results are required or when oral medications are not ideal or desirable therapy.[19] It is clinically useful in situations in which blood pressure control is critical, including cardiac surgery, carotid enterectomy, aneurysm clipping, intracranial tumor resection, and peripheral vascular surgery. Clevidipine is also used to prevent extension of aortic dissection in hypertensive individuals. The advantages of this medication include a rapid onset of action and offset of effect once the IV drip is discontinued with a half-life of approximately 1 minute, though clearance following CABG can be reduced in hypothermic states. Hypotension can develop when β-blockers are administered at the same time.

The dose is started at 1 to 2 mg/h and titrated upwards until BP control is achieved or the maximum dose of 32 mg/h is reached. It is contraindicated in individuals with soy or egg allergies because the drug is formulated in a lipid emulsion that contains both of these substances. Clevidipine does not raise lipid levels but it is contraindicated in individuals who have defective lipid metabolism. Clevidipine also improves dyspnea with BP control in the setting of hypertensive induced heart failure. This drug reduces MAP, SVR, and PVR while increasing stroke volume, cardiac output, and direct coronary vasodilation. There is no reflex tachycardia, though modest increases in heart rate are associated with the use of this medication.

## Angiotensin-Converting Enzyme Inhibitors

Angiotensin-converting enzyme (ACE) inhibitors are indicated to treat HF, hypertension, AMI with or without LV dysfunction or failure, and asymptomatic LV dysfunction. They are also used to decrease morbidity and mortality for patients at high risk for AMI, stroke, or cardiovascular death. Unless contraindicated, patients with a STEMI with anterior infarction, pulmonary congestion, or LV ejection fraction (EF) less than 40% should receive an ACE inhibitor within 24 hours of admission to the hospital.[2]

The ACE inhibitors block the conversion of angiotensin I to the potent vasoconstrictor angiotensin II, reduce aldosterone synthesis, and may promote fibrinolysis.[2,13] As a result, these agents mitigate LV remodeling, increase cardiac output, and decrease sodium retention, blood pressure, central venous pressure, SVR, pulmonary vascular resistance, and pulmonary capillary wedge pressure. Numerous research trials conducted in the late 1980s through the early 2000s showed that ACE inhibitors prevent HF, prevent hospitalization due to HF, and decrease mortality.[13,16]

All ACE inhibitors are contraindicated in pregnancy, angioedema, bilateral renal artery stenosis, and preexisting hypotension. They should be used with caution in patients with renal failure or hyperkalemia. Patients with impaired renal function, hypotension, or concurrent diuretic use should receive a lower dosage. Adverse effects of ACE inhibitors include hypotension, dizziness, angioedema, cough, headache, fatigue, nausea, vomiting, diarrhea, hyperkalemia, and impaired renal function.

## Antihyperlipidemics

Hydroxymethylglutaryl coenzyme-A reductase inhibitors (statins) decrease total and LDL cholesterol, decrease triglycerides, and increase HDL cholesterol by inhibiting the rate-limiting enzyme that promotes cholesterol biosynthesis. Although there are several statin medications available for treatment of chronic hyperlipidemia and primary prevention of atherosclerotic disease, atorvastatin (Lipitor), 80 mg, is the only one recommended for patients with NSTEMI and STEMI. Atorvastatin can reduce low-density lipoprotein (LDL) cholesterol by greater than 50% and reduce the risk of death from coronary heart disease, recurrent MI, stroke, or need for myocardial revascularization procedures.[1,2]

# PERCUTANEOUS CORONARY INTERVENTIONS AND PERCUTANEOUS VALVULAR INTERVENTIONS

## Percutaneous Coronary Interventions

### Historical Background

Although the death rate from cardiovascular diseases (CVD) has declined 31% since 2000, CVD remains the number one cause of death in the United States. According to the American Heart Association,[1] CVD accounts for 1 of every 3 deaths in the United States. These statistics suggest that although the death rates attributable to CVD have declined, the burden of the disease remains high.

The first major advance in the palliative treatment of coronary artery disease (CAD) was the implantation of an aortocoronary saphenous vein bypass graft in 1967. Since that time, the coronary artery bypass grafting procedure (CABG) has been refined and has been the treatment of choice for many patients with CAD. The first percutaneous transluminal coronary angioplasty (PTCA), performed by Andreas Gruentzig in 1977, marked another major innovation in CAD treatment.

Since the late 1970s, techniques to treat CAD have expanded beyond PTCA. Today, the term PCI is used to describe less invasive procedures to treat CAD and includes PTCA, laser angioplasty, atherectomy, and stenting—interventions described in this chapter.

The path to PCI began in 1964, when Dotter and Judkins introduced the concept of mechanically dilating a stenosis in a blood vessel with a technique of inserting a series of progressively larger catheters to treat peripheral vascular disease. After experimenting with this technique, Gruentzig modified the procedure by placing a polyvinyl balloon on the tip of a catheter; the balloon was passed into a narrowed vessel and then inflated. This revised procedure produced a smoother luminal surface with less trauma than the Dotter–Judkins approach and reduced the risk for complications, including vessel rupture, subintimal tearing, and embolism. Gruentzig performed successful dilation of more than 500 peripheral lesions. He subsequently designed a smaller version of the dilation catheter for use within the coronary arterial tree. Gruentzig performed the first human PTCA in 1977.[2]

Improvements in technique and device technology during the past three decades have made PCI the treatment of choice for managing CAD. In 2010, some 492,000 PCIs (75% utilizing drug-eluting stents [DESs]) and 397,000 CABGs were performed in the United States.[1] PTCA is a nonsurgical technique used as an alternative to CABG in treating obstructive CAD. When indicated and if successful, PTCA can alleviate myocardial ischemia, relieve angina pectoris, and prevent myocardial necrosis. PTCA is the hallmark procedure and serves as the basis of almost all other percutaneous intracoronary interventions. During PTCA, a coaxial catheter system is introduced into the coronary arterial tree and advanced into an area of coronary artery stenosis. A balloon attached to the catheter is then inflated, increasing the luminal diameter and improving blood flow through the dilated segment. Several inflations ranging from 30 to 300 seconds may be performed.

## Physiologic Principles

The process that leads to successful dilation is complex and not clearly defined. Angiographic evaluation and animal and human histologic studies indicate that PTCA stretches the vessel wall, leading to fracture of the inelastic atherosclerotic plaque and to tearing or cracking within the intima and media of the vessel. This cracking or slight dissection of the inner lumen of the vessel may be necessary for successful dilation.[2]

## Comparisons Between PCI and CABG

As an alternative treatment for CAD, PCI compares favorably with CABG in terms of risk, success rate, the patient's physical capacity after the procedure, length of hospital stay, and cost.[1]

Mortality rates associated with first-time PCI and CABG are somewhat similar. According to the National Healthcare Cost and Utilization Project Statistics in 2011, the in-hospital death rate for patients undergoing PCI was 1.13% as compared to CABG in-hospital death rates of 1.63%.[1] In the event that a second surgical procedure becomes necessary to alleviate the symptoms of progressive CAD, the mortality and complication rates for the bypass procedure are significantly greater than for a second PCI. The BARI 2D study revealed that at 5 years, rates of survival did not differ significantly between the revascularization group (PCI or CABG, 88.3%) and the group treated with just medical therapy (87.8%, $P = 0.97$). The rates for major cardiovascular events also did not differ significantly among the groups: in the PCI stratum, there was no significant difference in death, myocardial infarction, stroke, or repeat revascularization between the CABG group and the medical-therapy group. In the CABG stratum, the rate of major cardiovascular events was significantly lower (22.4%) than in the medical-therapy group (30.5%). Adverse events and serious adverse events were generally similar among the groups.[3]

Successful PCI, which is defined as a significant reduction of the luminal diameter stenosis without in-hospital death, MI, or CABG, ranges from 80% to 100%, depending on the severity of the patient's angiographic and clinical presentation. Overall, PCI in-hospital mortality is approximately 1.27%, ranging from 0.65% in elective PCI to 4.81% in ST-segment elevation myocardial infarction patients. Multiple preprocedural clinical factors are significantly associated with in-hospital mortality. These include the patient's age, gender, hemodynamic stability, presence of a preprocedural myocardial infarction, presence of congestive heart failure, peripheral arterial disease, serum creatinine level, and presence of left main coronary artery disease. PCI risk calculators can be found in many online formats; an example is on the Zunis Foundation site at http://www.zunis.org/PCI%20Risk%20Calculator2.htm. Angiographic variables (like the location and severity of stenosis) provide only modest incremental information to preprocedural risk assessment.[4]

Restenosis of vessels is a concern for patients after CABG and after PCI. Saphenous vein graft failure after CABG is 10% to 20% in the first year, 20% to 30% in years 1 through 5, and 30% to 45% in years 6 through 10; only 50% remain patent after 10 years.[5] Restenosis or patency data differ greatly between CABG and PCI. Within 6 months after angioplasty, 20% to 30% of lesions recur or re-stenose. Bare metal intracoronary stenting reduces the incidence of restenosis by an additional 5% to 10%. DES placement further reduces the risk for restenosis to approximately 2%.[6-8] Recently, late loss, defined as late restenosis following DES, has been observed. Stent manufacturers are addressing the concern of late loss through DES platform design and a variety of drug coatings applied directly to the stent.

Psychological advantages of PTCA over surgery may argue favorably for the less invasive procedure. The emotional stress of awaiting dilation is less than that of awaiting open-heart surgery. However, this reduction in anxiety is partly offset by the risk for psychological crisis if the angioplasty fails and surgery—especially emergent (immediate) surgery—is needed. The psychological impact of this discouraging situation is significant, but it occurs in a relatively low percentage of cases.

Barring complications with either procedure, PCI requires a hospital stay of 8 to 24 hours, whereas CABG requires a stay of 3 to 5 days. Because the average hospital stay is shorter with PCI, and because it is performed in the cardiac catheterization laboratory with the patient receiving local anesthesia, the average cost of PCI may be substantially lower than that of CABG. However, the following factors can increase the cost of PCI:

- Complications occurring during the procedure that necessitate emergency surgery (eg, coronary perforation, acute closure)
- Lesions that recur, requiring repeat dilation, or bypass surgery
- Lesions that require multiple devices to alleviate the lesion
- Complications associated with the anticoagulation regimen or arterial and venous access
- Long-term anticoagulation or antiplatelet therapy

In general, after a PCI, patients can expect a faster return to work (5 to 7 days) as opposed to patients who have had CABG (6 to 8 weeks). Depression in patients following CABG is common, although reports of quality of life in both groups are similar.[9]

In conclusion, the major advantages of PCI compared with CABG may include reduced mortality and morbidity, shorter convalescence, and lower cost to the patient and third-party payers.

## Diagnostic Tests for Patient Selection: PCI and CABG

Before deciding between PCI and CABG, all objective evidence of coronary insufficiency must be documented. Noninvasive methods of evaluation that may be used before and after PCI include standard treadmill stress testing and thallium stress and redistribution myocardial imaging. These tests allow the physician to discover the areas of ischemia in the myocardium when the patient is subjected to stress (ie, exercise; see Chapter 17 for a discussion of these tests). Nurses must familiarize themselves with the results of thallium stress tests because an understanding of the patient's diagnosis, related symptoms, and indications for PCI promotes informed patient care.

Coronary angiography performed by cardiac catheterization, another method of documenting coronary insufficiency, is performed if the previous tests suggest the presence of CAD. Although this procedure is more invasive than treadmill testing and thallium imaging, it is the gold standard test to pinpoint the location of any stenoses and the degree of involvement of the artery or arteries (see Chapter 17 for a discussion of this test). This procedure yields a 35-mm or digital image of the coronary artery anatomy. The physician can then analyze the areas of narrowing (stenosis) and gain precise information to decide the appropriate treatment (Fig. 18-1).

## Equipment Features

Since the introduction of the PCI procedure, the device technology has been refined and improved, resulting in fewer contraindications, lower rates of mortality, and fewer incidences of emergent bypass surgery. The guiding catheters used to direct and support the advancement of the dilation catheter into the appropriate coronary artery ostium have an outer diameter of 5 to 10 French (Fr). The tips of the guiding catheters have curves that are preshaped for selective access to either the right or left coronary artery.

Balloon dilation systems have evolved since Gruentzig's original design, in which the guidewire tip and catheter shaft were integral. In the early days of PTCA, physicians were limited by catheter performance and could address lesions only in the proximal anatomy. In 1982, Simpson introduced a coaxial "over-the-wire" system, an improvement that has become predominant in current catheter designs. The main innovation is an independently movable guide wire within the balloon dilation catheter. This guide wire can be manipulated to select the correct vessel despite side branches and permits safe advancement of the dilation catheter across the lesion. Currently, the available guide wires measure between 0.010 and 0.018 inch in diameter and thus usually pose little threat of interference with the blood flow through a stenosis.

Coronary balloon dilation catheter shafts range in size from 2.0 to 4.2 Fr, small enough for easy passage through the guiding catheter and for visualization around the catheter during contrast injection. Figure 18-2 shows the contrast injection through the guiding Catheter to verify position. The balloon dilation catheter has one or more radiopaque markers that can be imaged by fluoroscopy, allowing the interventional cardiologist to position the balloon accurately across the lesion. The inflated balloon size ranges from 1.5 to 5 mm wide and from 10 to 40 mm long. The size (inflated diameter) of the balloon to be used for a particular PCI procedure is usually the same as the smallest-diameter segment of the coronary artery proximal or distal to the stenosis (ie, 3-mm vessel, 3-mm balloon). Lesion and balloon length also are approximated.

The interventional cardiologist manually inflates the balloon with a contrast-filled, disposable inflation device that connects to the side arm or balloon lumen of the coronary dilation catheter. The device incorporates a pressure gauge that indicates the amount of pressure exerted against the balloon wall during inflation. Balloon pressure is measured in pounds per square inch (psi) or atmospheres (atm). The average initial inflation is between 60 and 150 psi or 4 to 10 atm and lasts from 30 to 180 seconds. Longer inflations may promote a smoother, more regular vessel wall as assessed by angiography and are used primarily for treating major dissections and abrupt closure. Extended inflations are performed safely with perfusion catheters that simultaneously dilate and perfuse the coronary artery.

A number of factors must be considered when selecting the most appropriate equipment for performing PCI. Technological advances in balloon dilation catheter systems have improved the success and safety associated with PCI and have expanded the clinical and anatomical indications for these procedures. Many interventional cardiologists consider the coaxial "over-the-wire" system a workhorse catheter because it can approach any anatomy well. However, the interventional cardiologist might select a rapid-exchange system to accomplish more easily the dilation of a bifurcation lesion. This type of device incorporates a "rail" system that facilitates the exchange process. A fixed-wire catheter is used to reach and dilate lesions in distal, tortuous anatomy, and its small shaft also makes it an option for the use of two coronary dilation catheters in one guiding catheter when the strategy

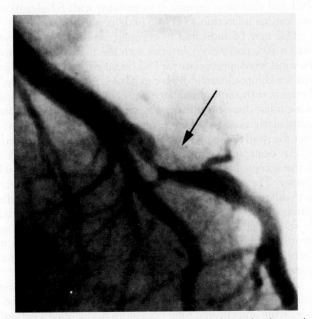

**FIGURE 18-1**   An eccentric stenosis in the left anterior descending artery. The term *eccentric* defines a plaque involving only one side of the intraluminal wall. (Courtesy of John B. Simpson, MD, Palo Alto, CA.)

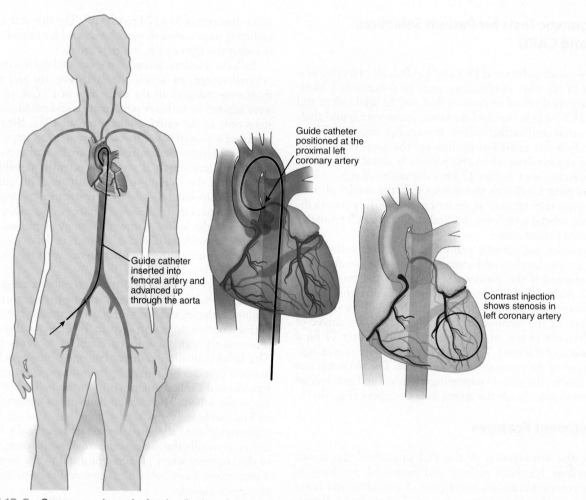

Guide catheter inserted into femoral artery and advanced up through the aorta

Guide catheter positioned at the proximal left coronary artery

Contrast injection shows stenosis in left coronary artery

**FIGURE 18-2** Coronary angiography for visualization of stenosis in left coronary artery.

calls for side-by-side balloons; this is also referred to as a "kissing balloon" technique.

Each PCI intervention also encompasses an inflation strategy. The main elements of an inflation strategy are the duration and pressure of balloon inflation required to open a lesion. Today, balloons that can withstand greater pressure for treating calcific lesions are available.

The outcome of any PCI procedure is greatly affected by[1] the selection of a guiding catheter that provides a platform for the advancement of the dilation system while preserving flow to the coronary artery; and[2] the selection of a balloon dilation system and intracoronary DES that best address the vessel's anatomy and the lesion's location and characteristics.

## Indications for PCI

When choosing to treat with PCI, the physician's purpose is to alleviate angina pectoris unrelieved by medical treatment and to reduce the risk for MI in symptomatic patients and asymptomatic patients with significant stenosis. Indications for PCI have expanded as device technology, techniques, and operator experience have improved. Guidelines for PCI were introduced in 2011 and can be found at the American Heart Association website, www.heart.org.[10] A focused update was published in 2016 that describes guidelines for multivessel

PCI and thrombus aspiration in patients with ST-elevation myocardial infarction (STEMI) undergoing primary PCI.[11]

PCI may be indicated in coronary arteries that have at least a 70% narrowing. Arteries with less narrowing may not be considered appropriate for PCI because they are equally at risk for abrupt closure, which can have serious consequences. Patients with surgical risk factors, such as severe underlying noncardiac diseases, advanced age, and poor LV function, are particularly suited for PCI because successful dilation obviates the need for an operation that would be poorly tolerated.

An example of the wide spectrum of candidacy for PCI is the accepted practice of treating patients with multivessel disease. The common technique for dilating multiple lesions is to dilate the most critical stenosis first. With successful dilation of this "culprit" lesion, remaining lesions are dilated in stages (ie, at different intervals during the procedure or over several days). However, dilation of multiple vessels is technically more demanding and carries a higher risk for complications.

Another expanded indication is the approach to treating the patient with a totally occluded vessel. Early in PCI practice, acute and chronic total occlusions disqualified a patient for the procedure because the stenosis could not be crossed with the guide wire and balloon dilation catheter without causing severe trauma to the artery. Refinement of device technology and the increased physician experience have allowed dilation of total occlusions attempts in appropriate candidates. Total occlusions of short duration (ie, 3 months or less) are easier to cross and dilate successfully than total occlusions of longer duration (chronic total occlusions).

Additional candidates for PCI are those who have undergone CABG in whom symptoms have recurred because of stenosis and graft closure or progression of coronary disease in the native vessels or in vein grafts. For these candidates, successful PCI makes second surgery, with its increased potential for complications, unnecessary. It is thought that the proliferative disease in the graft wall generates fibrous stenosis that is much less dense than most fibrotic tissue in the native vessels, so certain vein graft stenoses respond favorably to percutaneous intervention.

Historically, patients experiencing an AMI as documented by significant ST-segment elevation, increased cardiac enzyme levels, and pain unrelieved by thrombolysis, surgery, or pharmacologic treatment were treated with complete bed rest in a coronary care unit. Today, if thrombus and underlying stenosis are causing the infarction, thrombolytic therapy, PCI, or both offer alternatives. If a blood clot has impeded flow to the distal myocardium and precipitates an ischemic episode, a thrombolytic agent can be administered intravenously or directly into the coronary artery. On successful lysis of the thrombus, dilation of the underlying stenosis often further enhances blood flow to the reperfused myocardium, reducing the risk for rethrombosis or critical narrowing caused by normal or spastic vasomotion superimposed on an organic stenosis.

Primary PCI is a dilation of an infarction-related coronary artery during the acute phase of an AMI without prior administration of a thrombolytic agent. Meyer et al[12] first used PTCA in the AMI setting in 1982. They reported an 81% success rate in PTCA of the infarction-related artery after intracoronary thrombolytic therapy. In 2006, the TRITON TIMI 38 trial[13] reported a PCI with stenting success rate of 95% and a patency rate of 53% 1 year post PCI. Parameters routinely assessed in patients selected to receive primary angioplasty are depicted in Box 18-3.

In the setting of AMI, PCI may benefit patients deemed ineligible for traditional medical therapy. Such patients include those in cardiogenic shock, those believed to be at high risk for bleeding complications (CVA, prolonged cardiopulmonary resuscitation [CPR], bleeding diathesis, severe hypertension, or recent surgery), and those of advanced age (>75 years). Primary PCI does not preclude the use of thrombolytic therapy if residual thrombus is observed. In fact, AMI patients deemed high risk (extensive ST-segment elevation, new-onset left BBB, previous AMI, Killip Class 2 or greater, anterior MI, or EF 35% or less) who receive fibrinolytic therapy at a non-PCI hospital should be transferred as soon as possible to a PCI-capable facility for evaluation and possible intervention. Patients who are not deemed to be at high risk and who receive fibrinolytic therapy at a non-PCI hospital may also be transferred as soon as possible to a PCI-capable facility.[14]

Primary PCI may offer distinct advantages in reducing the length of hospital stay and eliminating the need for additional intervention in many cases. Indications for PCI are summarized in Box 18-4.

In a recent meta-analysis, Stergiopoulos and colleagues reviewed the literature for randomized clinical trials of PCI and medical therapy for stable CAD conducted over the past 40 years. Over a median follow-up of 5 years, mortality, nonfatal MI, unplanned revascularization, and angina were no different between patients treated medically versus those treated with PCI. Thus, medical therapy, as opposed to PCI, may be a viable option for many patients.[15]

Complications of primary PCI include retroperitoneal or vascular hemorrhage, other bleeding requiring transfusion, late restenosis, and early acute reocclusion (subacute thrombosis). These complications occur at approximately the same rate as those experienced in routine elective PCI.

## Contraindications to PCI

There are very few contraindications to PCI. Patients with left main CAD were once not considered candidates for PCI. The obvious drawback of PCI in left main artery disease is

---

**BOX 18-3** | **Parameters Evaluated in Patients Selected to Receive Primary Angioplasty**

Age
Hemodynamic status
- Angiographic anatomy:
- Single-, double-, or triple-vessel disease
- Vessel involvement: left anterior descending artery (LAD), right coronary artery (RCA), left circumflex artery (LCX)
- Lesion location ostial: proximal, mid, or distal disease
- Percent grade stenosis
- Thrombolysis in myocardial infarction flow: 0, I, II, III
Left ventricular (LV) ejection fraction (EF) (%)
Presence of chest pain consistent with acute myocardial infarction (AMI)
Electrocardiogram (ECG) evidence of AMI:
- 1-mm ST-segment elevation in two contiguous leads
- or
- 1-mm ST-segment depression believed to represent reciprocal changes to an area of infarction

---

**BOX 18-4** | **Indications and Contraindications for Percutaneous Coronary Intervention**

Clinical
Symptomatic (angina unrelieved by medical therapy)
Asymptomatic but with severe underlying stenosis
Stable/unstable angina
Acute myocardial infarction
High-risk surgical candidates

Anatomical
Severe stenosis (70% or more)*
Proximal and distal lesions
Single and multivessel disease
Bifurcation lesions
Ostial lesions
Totally occluded vessels
Bypass graft lesions
"Protected" and unprotected left main coronary artery (previous LAD or LCX coronary artery bypass graft)

*Contraindicated in mild stenosis (<70%)

LAD, left anterior descending artery; LCX, left circumflex artery.

the possibility of acute occlusion or spasm of the left main artery during the procedure, which would result in severe LV dysfunction. Patients who have a "protected" left main artery (ie, those who have had previous bypass surgery to the left anterior descending or circumflex arteries with patent grafts present) are often candidates for PCI. One-year clinical outcomes of protected and unprotected left main coronary artery stenting revealed that those who had unprotected left main stenting had increased major adverse cardiac events, and their survival was decreased at 1 year. However, left main stenting should be considered in the absence of other options.[16] For high-risk patients (ie, patients with left main vessel disease, severe LV dysfunction, or dilation of the last remaining patent artery), percutaneous support devices may improve the safety of PCI. These devices include perfusion balloons, intra-aortic balloon counterpulsation, coronary sinus retroperfusion, and cardiopulmonary support.

## Procedure

The PCI procedure is carried out in a sterile fashion, with the use of local anesthesia and either the Judkins (percutaneous femoral) approach or, less often, the Sones (brachial cutdown) approach (Fig. 18-3). With the Judkins approach, the interventional cardiologist cannulates the femoral vein and artery percutaneously by inserting a needle (usually 18-gauge) containing a removable obturator. The obturator is then removed to confirm by the presence of blood flow that the outer needle is within the lumen of the vessel. Once proper placement is established, a guide wire is introduced through the outer cannula into the artery to the level of the diaphragm. The cannula then is removed and replaced by a valved introducer sheath. The sheath provides hemostasis

and support at the puncture site in the groin and reduces potential arterial trauma if multiple catheter exchanges are necessary. The guiding catheter is preloaded with a 0.038-inch J-wire and introduced into the sheath. The 0.038-inch J-wire is advanced over the arch, and the guiding catheter is advanced over the wire. The 0.038-inch J-wire is removed, and the guiding catheter is rotated precisely to the appropriate coronary ostium.

The European Society of Cardiology published a detailed consensus document which recommends that the radial or wrist approach to angioplasty should become the default access method, with the femoral approach to be used as a "bail-out" when radial is not feasible.[17] This is a major change in the techniques utilized worldwide by interventional cardiologists. The use of the radial artery in the wrist (Fig. 18-4) instead of the femoral artery in the groin for catheter access may result in fewer vascular complications for patients and significant cost-savings for the healthcare system. From a patient perspective, radial access offers significantly less discomfort and significantly improved quality of life as compared to femoral access. Patients who have experienced both access routes strongly prefer radial access, primarily because they are able to ambulate immediately after the procedure.

Regardless of the mode of access, coronary angiography is then carried out in both the left anterior oblique (30 degrees) and right anterior oblique (60 degrees) views. These views allow for visualization of the heart along its transverse and longitudinal planes. Opposing views provide a thorough assessment of both the lesion and the anatomical approach. A "freeze frame" of each view is obtained as a road map or guide throughout the procedure. A final lesion assessment is made, confirming lesion severity and vessel diameter for appropriate balloon and stent sizing.

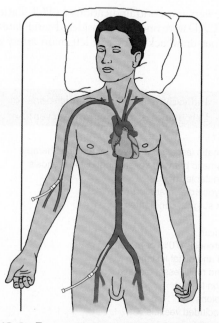

**FIGURE 18-3**  Two approaches to left heart catheterization. The Sones technique uses the brachial artery, and the Judkins technique uses the femoral artery. With either method, the catheter is passed retrograde through the ascending aorta to the left ventricle. (Reprinted with permission of Advanced Cardiovascular Systems [ACS] Inc., Santa Clara, CA.)

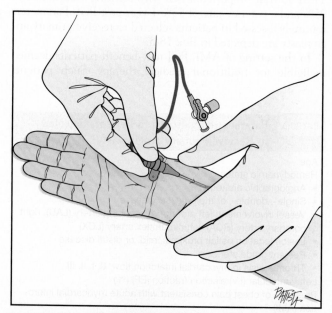

**FIGURE 18-4**  The use of the radial artery in the wrist instead of the femoral artery in the groin for catheter access may result in fewer vascular complications for patients and significant cost savings for the healthcare system. From a patient perspective, radial access offers significantly less discomfort and significantly improved quality of life as compared to femoral access.

If PCI is indicated, the patient may be anticoagulated with 70 to 100 IU/kg of heparin to prevent the formation of clots on or in the catheter system during the procedure. Intracoronary nitroglycerin is kept on the sterile field throughout the procedure and given intermittently as needed for vasospasm and for dilation to facilitate visualization of the culprit coronary artery.

The balloon dilation catheter and intracoronary stent system is introduced into the guiding catheter through a bifurcated adapter that provides access and is a port for contrast injections and aortic pressure measurement. The balloon dilation catheter, stent, and guide wire are advanced to the tip of the guiding catheter while their position is checked by fluoroscopy. The guide wire then is advanced and manipulated to negotiate the branches of the coronary artery. Proper advancement can be confirmed by injecting contrast through the guiding catheter and fluoroscopically visualizing the coronary tree. Once the guide wire is positioned safely beyond the stenosis, the balloon dilation catheter (with or without a stent) can be advanced slowly over the guide wire into the narrowing without risk for injury to the intima.

Exact placement of the dilation balloon and stent in the stenosis is facilitated under fluoroscopy by the radiopaque marker on the balloon and by contrast injections for visualization. Initially, the balloon is inflated at 1 to 2 atm of pressure to confirm its position. Many PTCA balloon catheters expand at both ends and not in the center, where they are pinched by the stenosis (Figs. 18-5). The central indentation usually disappears as the stenosis is dilated. After each inflation, the interventional cardiologist injects a small bolus of contrast medium to assess any changes in coronary blood flow through the stenosis and to assess any increase in luminal diameter. At this time, the need for additional inflations is determined. Complications, such as vessel recoil and abrupt closure, occur most often during this early phase; however, their incidence is low, and redilation can be performed readily at this time. After dilation is complete, the guiding catheter, balloon dilation catheter, and stent delivery platform are removed. Postdilation angiography is performed to define more clearly the results of the PCI procedure.

Reasons for failure to complete a PCI procedure include inability to cross the target lesion with a guidewire or dilation catheter due primarily to chronic total occlusions, inability to dilate the lesion because of rigid lesions or severe dissection, and embolization of friable vein graft material or of thrombus.

Successful dilation of a lesion commonly is defined as a reduction of the luminal diameter stenosis by about 40% or 50%. Clinical success commonly is defined as angiographic success with clinical improvement and without significant in-hospital complications, such as death, MI, or CABG or repeat PCI for abrupt closure.

Angiography after successful PCI demonstrates an immediate increase in the intraluminal diameter of the involved vessel (Fig. 18-6). Clinical improvement of the patient is demonstrated by improved or normalized myocardial perfusion deficits, as shown by comparison of a post-PCI thallium stress image with the pre-PCI stress image. Post-PCI treadmill test results compared with the preprocedure test results reveal increased exercise endurance and a decrease in exercise-induced angina or angina equivalent.

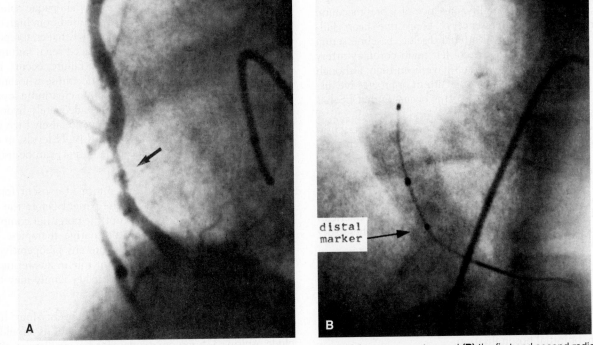

A                                                                  B

FIGURE 18-5   Thirty-five-spot frames showing **(A)** stenosis involving the midright coronary artery and **(B)** the first and second radiopaque markers revealing the position of the dilation balloon across the stenosis, with the distal marker referring to the tip of the catheter beyond the narrowing. (Courtesy of John B. Simpson, MD, Palo Alto, CA.)

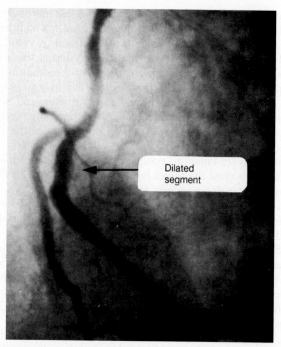

**FIGURE 18-6** Repeat angiography after PTCA of a right coronary artery stenosis showing increased flow and increased diameter of the dilated segment. (Courtesy of John B. Simpson, MD, Palo Alto, CA.)

## Results

Excellent short- and long-term results have been achieved in patients undergoing PCI. The results vary depending on the patient's clinical presentation (stable or unstable angina) and angiographic characteristics, that is, subtotal or total occlusion. Preprocedural clinical factors that have an impact on short-term and long-term results include the patient's age, gender, hemodynamic stability, presence of a preprocedural myocardial infarction, presence of congestive heart failure, existence of peripheral arterial disease, baseline serum creatinine level, and presence of left main coronary artery disease.[4] Long-term survival rates have been high, although repeat PCI may be necessary for recurrent or progressive disease. The frequency with which this occurs with DES has decreased dramatically.

Patients with high-risk clinical or angiographic presentations have lower success rates. However, PCI is often preferable to surgical revascularization because of the latter's increased risk of mortality in older adults or those with depressed LV function. On the other hand, success of a PCI procedure can be defined angiographically, procedurally, or clinically. According to a joint statement by the American College of Cardiology (ACC) and the AHA,[14] these successes are defined as follows:

- *Angiographic success* is defined as a successful PCI procedure: one in which the minimum residual vessel stenosis is less than or equal to 20%.
- *Procedural success* is defined as angiographic success without complications (ie, death, CABG, MI) during the procedure or initial hospitalization.
- *Clinical success* is defined as anatomical and procedural success with relief of the signs of symptoms of myocardial

ischemia. Long-term success requires that the relief of the signs and symptoms persists for more than 6 months after the procedure. Restenosis is the principal cause of failure to achieve long-term success.[16]

## Assessment and Management

### Patient Preparation

When the decision has been made to proceed with any PCI procedure, the patient typically is admitted to the hospital the day of the procedure.

**LABORATORY TESTS.** The nurse monitors all preliminary laboratory tests, including cardiac enzymes, serum electrolytes, coagulation studies (PT and partial thromboplastin time), and serum potassium, creatinine, and blood urea nitrogen (BUN) levels.

Potassium levels must be within normal limits because low levels result in increased sensitivity and excitability of the myocardium and subsequent dysrhythmias. The cardiac muscle also is sensitive and becomes irritable when the flow of oxygen-rich blood decreases, as it does for a controlled period of time during placement and inflation of the dilation balloon and stent across the lesion. The irritability arising from hypokalemia, ischemia, or both can give rise to life-threatening ventricular dysrhythmias.

Elevation in the levels of serum creatinine, BUN, or both may indicate problems in kidney function. Good kidney function is important because during PCI, radiopaque contrast material (which permits fluoroscopic visualization of the coronary anatomy and of catheter placement) is introduced into the bloodstream.[18] This contrast material is a hyperosmotic solution that the kidneys must filter and excrete from the blood. High levels of creatinine and BUN may reflect decreased renal filtration capability and vulnerability of the kidney in processing the extra load of radiopaque solution. Instances of acute renal failure have resulted from high doses of radiopaque contrast agent. A study by Rihal et al reported a 3.3% incidence rate of contrast-induced renal failure following PCI. Contrast-induced renal failure occurs more frequently in patients who are diabetic, those who are dehydrated, and those with higher baseline creatinine levels.[19] The nurse ensures that the patient is adequately hydrated, either orally or with IV solutions, to avoid falsely high electrolyte levels. Trends in creatinine and BUN levels, in conjunction with measurement of urine output, can be used to monitor kidney function.

**INFORMED CONSENT.** The informed consent for the PCI procedure is obtained from the patient before the procedure after a detailed discussion of the potential complications, anticipated benefit, and alternative therapies. This discussion should be conducted before any preoperative sedation. The nurse plays an important role in answering any questions that the patient and his or her family may have regarding the procedure and follow-up care.

**PREOPERATIVE MEDICATIONS.** Twenty-four hours before the procedure, the patient's medications should include aspirin, 325 mg once a day, for its antiplatelet effect. Diabetic patients taking metformin should be advised to discontinue this medication before their procedure because it is

| BOX 18-5 | *TEACHING GUIDE* | *Precautions for Patients Post-Percutaneous Transluminal Coronary Angioplasty* |

The nurse needs to remind the patient to:
- Remain on bed rest for 4 to 6 hours.
- Maintain the involved leg in a straight position (for Judkins technique).

- Avoid an upright position.
- Avoid vigorous use of the abdominal muscles, as in coughing, sneezing, or moving the bowels.

contraindicated with intravascular contrast agents. Anticoagulants, such as warfarin, are often withheld for a number of days before the PCI procedure. Studies show that administration of clopidogrel before and after a PCI decreases adverse events such as acute closure and subacute thrombosis.[20,21]

### SURGICAL STANDBY.

Surgical standby for PCI is controversial at this time. Surgical availability is required, but the degree to which the operating room is held for availability varies according to the patient's risk factors, patient acuity, and hospital policies. Many smaller community hospitals across the United States are performing PCI procedures without in-house surgical standby. These patients are typically low risk and reside near larger academic centers that can accept the patient by immediate transfer if complications arise during the PCI. A comparison of patients treated with PCI at hospitals without on-site cardiac surgery with those treated only with thrombolytic therapy reveals that the former group has better clinical outcomes at 1, 3, and 6 months.[22]

### Nursing Management During PCI

Both before and during the procedure, nurses in the cardiac catheterization laboratory are responsible for understanding all aspects of equipment use in patient care. They should be experienced in ACLS, and knowledgeable about the proper administration of emergency medications and the correct application of emergency equipment, including the defibrillator, the intra-aortic balloon pump (IABP), the ventilator, and the temporary pacemaker. They observe and communicate with the patient intermittently and report any changes in patient status to the physician. The nurse monitors the ECG and arterial pressure, noting significant changes that may accompany the administration of drugs, symptoms of ischemia, or chest pain. The nurse must recognize signs and symptoms of contrast sensitivity, such as urticaria, blushing, anxiety, nausea, and laryngospasm. The nurse should understand the proper assembly and use of all PCI equipment and should be able to troubleshoot any situation that may arise.

The patient's anticoagulation status during the PCI procedure is of utmost importance. Subtherapeutic levels may result in serious complications, including acute closure or thrombotic events. An ACT should be measured in the catheterization laboratory at baseline (before the PTCA), 5 minutes after the heparin bolus (70 to 100 IU/kg and every 30 minutes thereafter for the duration of the procedure). ACT levels of 250 to 300 seconds are desirable after the initial heparin bolus. Subsequent boluses of 2,000 to 5,000 U of heparin may be required to achieve and maintain these ACT levels during the PCI procedure.

Patients at high risk for abrupt closure or with unstable lesions, such as in the setting of AMI, may be administered a platelet GP IIb/IIIa antagonist in addition to aspirin and heparin; this is referred to as a "facilitated PCI." These agents are typically initiated just before or during PCI. Eptifibatide (Integrilin) or tirofiban (Aggrastat) should be administered, in addition to aspirin and either unfractionated heparin or LMWH, to patients with continuing ischemia, an elevated troponin, or other high-risk features in whom an invasive management strategy is not planned.[22]

After the PCI is complete, the nurse instructs the patient in the precautions necessary to prevent bleeding from the puncture site (Box 18-5). The patient is then transferred to a telemetry unit or catheterization recovery area for observation.

### Nursing Management After PCI

The nurse in the catheterization laboratory recovery area, coronary care unit, or telemetry unit plays an important role in observing and assessing the patient's recovery. Post-PCI care is designed to monitor the patient closely for signs and symptoms of myocardial ischemia. The most overt symptom of a possible complication—early recurrence of angina pectoris—requires prompt nursing action.

As soon as possible on receiving the patient from the cardiac catheterization laboratory, the nurse attaches the ECG monitor, which allows a quick initial cardiac assessment and establishes a baseline in case the patient's condition should change suddenly. The nurse assesses the patient's status from head to toe, noting the overall skin color and temperature and carefully observing the level of consciousness. After the patient is transferred to the bed and attached to the monitor, the nurse listens closely to heart and breath sounds. The nurse evaluates the peripheral circulation by noting peripheral skin color and temperature and the presence and quality of dorsalis pedis and posterior tibial pulses.

If the Judkins approach was used, the patient will have an entry port in either the right or the left groin through which sheaths have been placed percutaneously in a vein and artery. If the Sones technique was used, there is an arterial catheter in the brachial area (see Fig. 18-5). A variety of mechanical devices and clamps may be used to facilitate hemostasis after sheath removal. The insertion of collagen plugs or the application of a surgical suture around the opening of the blood vessel is also routinely performed to obtain hemostasis. After sheath removal, the nurse pays careful attention to the area distal to the puncture site, checking pulses frequently and reporting immediately to the physician any changes that may indicate bleeding. Bleeding at the sheath site may result in a major hematoma that can require surgical evacuation or compromise distal blood flow to the lower extremity. To prevent excessive bleeding and to aid hemostasis, the physician may order that a 5-lb sandbag be placed over the puncture site after sheath removal if hemostasis is achieved with manual compression.

The nurse instructs the patient on the importance of keeping the involved leg straight and the head of the bed angled at 45 degrees or less. To prevent clotting in the lumens of the introducing sheaths, an IV infusion is attached to the venous sheath, and a pressurized arterial flush is attached to the arterial line. This arrangement also ensures patency should an immediate return to the cardiac catheterization laboratory be necessary because of a complication. The physician chooses both the type of solution to be infused through the venous sheath and the rate of infusion. His or her decision depends on the patient's fluid volume status.

Radial artery access is in general more comfortable for the patient and carries a lower risk of hematoma, pseudo-aneurysm, and AV fistula formation. Nurses caring for the patient post-PCI should be alert for the loss of the radial pulse. Hand ischemia does not occur if adequate collateral circulation from the ulnar artery could be demonstrated with Allen's test before the procedure.

Although initial post-PCI laboratory blood tests vary by institution, they may include coagulation studies, cardiac enzymes, and serum electrolytes. Elevation of the cardiac enzymes can indicate that a silent MI has occurred (ie, infarction unannounced by chest pain). If a cardiac enzyme laboratory value is abnormal, the nurse notifies the physician immediately because the patient's postoperative care may need to be modified to prevent further injury.

The nurse plays a significant role in observing and assessing angina that recurs soon after a PCI procedure. Any chest pain demands immediate and careful attention because it may indicate either the start of vasospasm or impending subacute thrombosis. The patient may describe angina as a burning, squeezing heaviness or as sharp midsternal pain. Other signs and symptoms of myocardial ischemia include ischemic ECG changes (elevation of the ST segments or T-wave inversion), dysrhythmias, hypotension, and nausea. The nurse notifies the physician immediately of any such change in the patient's condition because it is impossible to tell merely by observation whether the change indicates a transient vasospastic episode, which can be resolved with vasodilation therapy, or an acute occlusion requiring emergent intervention (repeat PCI or CABG).

If vasodilation therapy is indicated, it may be administered as described subsequently unless the patient is hypotensive; in that case, vasodilation is contraindicated. At the first sign of vasospasm, the nurse gives oxygen by mask or nasal cannula. For fast, temporary (and possibly permanent) relief, 0.4 mg of nitroglycerin, 5 mg of isosorbide (Imdur), or 10 mg of nifedipine (Procardia) is administered sublingually. In addition, the IV drip of nitroglycerin should be titrated to maintain a blood pressure adequate to ensure coronary artery perfusion and to alleviate chest pain.

With the onset of the chest pain, a 12-lead ECG reading is recorded to document any acute changes. If the angina resolves and any acute ECG changes caused by medical therapy disappear, it is safe to assume that a transient vasospastic episode occurred; however, if the angina continues and the ECG changes persist, redilation or emergency bypass surgery should be considered.

If the post-PCI course is uncomplicated, the sheaths are removed after 2 to 4 hours and a pressure dressing is applied to the site. A variety of mechanical clamps or hemostasis devices may be used to facilitate hemostasis after sheath removal. The sheaths are often removed before the patient leaves the cardiac catheterization laboratory, and a hemostasis device is used. The patient must continue complete bed rest for 4 to 6 hours after the sheaths are removed. A normal, low-sodium, or low-cholesterol diet may be resumed, depending on the preference of the physician and the needs of the patient.

During the recovery period, the nurse can introduce the patient to the rehabilitation process, emphasizing lifestyle modifications to combat the advance of CAD. Efforts should be made during this instruction to reinforce the importance of aerobic conditioning with regular, moderate exercise. Risk factor and secondary prevention are also discussed, including stress reduction, weight loss, and smoking cessation. See Box 18-5 for instructions for the patient after PCI. Box 18-6 describes implications for the older patient.

After PCI, the patient is asked to take medications that help prevent thrombus formation and maintain maximal dilation at the culprit lesion site. Current guidelines recommend dual antiplatelet therapy (DAPT) that includes aspirin and the platelet $P2Y_{12}$ ADP receptor antagonist clopidogrel after percutaneous coronary intervention (PCI). These recommendations are based on data that indicate DAPT with the $P2Y_{12}$ inhibitors clopidogrel reduces major adverse cardiac events after PCI in stable angina and acute coronary syndrome (ACS) patients when compared with aspirin, or aspirin in combination with warfarin.

Current American College of Cardiology/American Heart Association/Society for Cardiovascular Angiography and Interventions recommendations for the prevention of stent thrombosis after coronary stent implantation state that, at a minimum, patients should be treated with clopidogrel (Plavix), 75 mg, and aspirin, 325 mg, for 1 month after bare-metal stent implantation, 3 months after sirolimus DES implantation, 6 months after paclitaxel DES implantation, and, ideally, up to 12 months if they are not at high risk for bleeding.[10] These recommendations were based on the antiplatelet regimen used in trials that were conducted to obtain US Food and Drug Administration approval (low-risk lesions in low-risk patients) and the anticipated time it takes for the metal stent struts to become adequately endothelialized to reduce the risk of stent thrombosis. However, DESs are now being used in high-risk lesions, and they may be associated

---

**BOX 18-6** **CONSIDERATIONS for the Older Patient**

**Before and After PCI**

- Assess whether the patient will have assistance in the home with meals, cleaning, self-care, and transportation to medical appointments.
- Closely monitor kidney function before and after PCI because elderly patients may be sensitive to small amounts of radio-contrast material.
- Monitor vital signs frequently, including temperature, because elderly patients are prone to excessive body heat loss.
- Assess all preexisting comorbidities: arthritis, peripheral vascular disease, diabetes, and so forth.
- Provide clear, precise, written instructions in preparation for discharge.
- Assess patient's ability to purchase/afford required medications.

with delayed (or absent) endothelialization and late stent thrombosis. In patients taking clopidogrel in whom elective CABG is planned, the drug should be withheld for 5 to 7 days. Often, long-acting nitrates, calcium channel blockers, ACE inhibitors, and lipid-lowering agents are added to the medical regimen.

The nurse may be responsible for explaining to the patient the indications for the specific medications ordered by the physician, including side effects and signs of overdose. The nurse should also answer any questions that the patient may have regarding his or her follow-up care. Box 18-7 summarizes medications currently associated with PCI.

Four to six weeks after the patient's discharge, an exercise treadmill stress test and a thallium imaging study may be performed to test the efficacy of the PCI. Compared with the pre-PCI tests, an increase in exercise capacity and a decrease in or disappearance of exercise-induced chest pain (without ST-segment changes) suggest improved blood flow and normalization of cardiac function in the previously hypoperfused muscle. Treadmill stress testing should be performed annually after PCI.

## Complications

The indications for PCI have expanded to include patients with more severe CAD (ie, total occlusions, multivessel disease, recent or ongoing MI, and poor LV function). The rate of complications associated with PCI has not increased. Major complications that can result in ischemia and possible severe LV dysfunction necessitating emergent CABG include angina unrelieved by maximal administration of nitrates and calcium channel blockers (see Box 18-7), MI, coronary artery spasm, abrupt closure of a dilated segment, coronary artery dissection leading to occlusion, and restenosis.

### Angina, Myocardial Infarction, and Vasospasm

Some degree of angina is anticipated during the PCI procedure owing to the temporary occlusion of the involved vessel during dilation. This angina is handled with intracoronary nitroglycerin or removal of the balloon dilation catheter while the guide wire is left across the lesion. Evidence of persistent chest pain after PCI, reflected in changes in heart

---

| BOX 18-7 | Summary of Medications Most Often Associated With PCI |

Anticoagulants/Antiplatelets

**Aspirin**
*Indications:* Prophylaxis of coronary and cerebral arterial thrombus formation
*Actions:* Blocks platelet aggregation
*Adverse effects:* (Usually well tolerated) nausea, vomiting, diarrhea, headache, and vertigo occasionally

**Heparin (Fractionated)**
*Indications:* Prophylaxis of impending coronary occlusion and prophylaxis of peripheral arterial embolism
*Actions:* Inhibits clotting of blood and formation of fibrin clots; inactivates thrombin, preventing conversion of fibrinogen to fibrin; prevents formation of a stable fibrin clot by inhibiting the activation of fibrin stabilizing factor; inhibits reactions that lead to clotting but does not alter normal components of blood; prolongs clotting time but does not affect bleeding time; does not lyse clots
*Adverse effects:* Uncontrollable bleeding, hypersensitivity

**Low–Molecular-Weight Heparin (Enoxaparin Sodium, Dalteparin Sodium)**
*Indications:* Treatment of unstable angina and myocardial ischemia, complete and non–Q-wave myocardial infarction (MI).
*Action:* Prevents clotting of blood and formation of thrombin.
*Adverse effects:* Thrombocytopenia, hematoma, pain or reaction at the injection site, rash, hemorrhage, fever.

**Glycoprotein IIb/IIIa Antagonists (Abciximab, Eptifibatide, Tirofiban)**
*Indications:* Prevention of clotting and abrupt closure during interventional procedures and prevention of restenosis.
*Action:* Blocks the receptor on the platelet membrane that leads to the final common pathway of platelet aggregation.
*Adverse effects:* Thrombocytopenia, hemorrhage, nausea, hematoma

**Clopidogrel (Plavix)**
*Indications:* Reduction of atherosclerotic events (AMI, stroke, and vascular death) in patients with atherosclerosis documented by a recent stroke or AMI or established peripheral arterial disease
*Action:* Blocks platelet aggregation

*Adverse effects:* Diarrhea, rash, gastrointestinal (GI) disturbances, hemorrhage, neutropenia.

Coronary Vasodilators
**Isosorbide Dinitrate (Isordil, Sorbitrate)**
*Indications:* Prophylaxis of angina
*Actions:* A nitrate that acts as a smooth muscle relaxant; causes coronary vasodilation without increasing myocardial oxygen consumption; secondary to general vasodilation, blood pressure decrease
*Adverse effects:* Cutaneous vasodilation that can cause flushing; headache, transient dizziness, and weakness; excessive hypotension

**Nitroglycerin**
*Indications:* Control of blood pressure and angina pectoris
*Actions:* Potent vasodilator; affects primarily the venous system; selectively dilates large coronary arteries increasing blood flow to ischemic subendocardium
*Adverse effects:* Excessive and prolonged hypotension; headache; tachycardia, palpitations; nausea, vomiting, apprehension; retrosternal discomfort

Calcium Channel Blockers
**Nifedipine (Procardia), Diltiazem (Cardizem)**
*Indications:* Treatment of angina pectoris resulting from coronary artery spasm and fixed vessel disease; hypertension; dysrhythmias
*Actions:* Inhibits calcium ion flux across the cell membrane of the cardiac muscle and vascular smooth muscle without changing serum calcium concentration; decreases afterload through peripheral arterial dilation and
1. Reduces systemic and pulmonary vascular resistance
2. Vasodilates coronary circulation
3. Decreases myocardial oxygen demands and increases myocardial oxygen supply
*Adverse effects:* Contraindicated in patients with sick sinus syndrome; hypertension after IV use; GI distress; headache, vertigo, flushing; peripheral edema, occasional increase in angina, tachycardia
See text for full discussion of antiarrhythmic medications.

rate and blood pressure and elevated ST segments, indicates ischemia predisposing to an insult to the myocardium and requiring immediate intervention. Coronary artery spasm sometimes requires emergent surgical intervention (CABG) when the vasoconstriction, occlusion, or ischemia cannot be reversed by administering nitrates.

## Abrupt Closure of Dilated Segment

Abrupt closure is a serious complication of coronary artery dilation that occurs in approximately 3% of those undergoing angioplasty.[16] An estimated 70% to 80% of abrupt closures occur while the patient is still in the cardiac catheterization laboratory. Approximately one third to one half of those patients whose vessel abruptly closes undergo a successful repeat dilation. Abrupt closure can be caused by coronary artery dissection, coronary artery spasm, and thrombus formation. Treatment options include immediate repeat dilation, emergent CABG surgery, and pharmacologic therapy. To maintain blood flow through the occlusion while the patient is being prepared for emergent CABG surgery, the physician can use a perfusion balloon catheter, which has side holes along its shaft to allow blood to flow through the catheter at the site of occlusion and perfuse the distal myocardium.

## Coronary Artery Dissection

Coronary artery dissection or an intimal tear in the coronary artery can be visualized in the form of intraluminal filling defects or extraluminal extravasation of contrast material. Mild interruptions in the intraluminal wall are an expected result of the splitting and stretching of the intima on inflation of the balloon dilation catheter at the lesion site. However, a dissection may cause a major luminal obstruction associated with coronary artery occlusion, leading to deterioration in blood flow with resultant severe ischemia or MI that requires emergent bypass surgery.

## Stent Thrombosis

As the number of stent implantations increased, so has the incidence of stent thrombosis. The Food and Drug Administration (FDA) met in 2006 and concluded that there appeared to be an issue of late stent thrombosis with DESs, but the magnitude was deemed uncertain, and off-label use of the DES, as with bare metal stents, is associated with increased risk when compared with on-label use. The panel also agreed that, in the future, new DES studies should have longer follow-up, enroll greater numbers of patients, and include stent thrombosis as a study end point. The advisory panel concurred with the joint clinical practice guideline recommendation for 12 months of dual antiplatelet therapy after placement of a DES in patients who are not at high risk of bleeding.[20]

There is some evidence, however, that DESs may be susceptible to an event known as *late stent thrombosis*, which is defined as a blood clot inside the stent that occurs 1 or more years after stent implantation and can be extremely dangerous, even fatal. To prevent subacute thrombosis (SAT), dual anti-platelet therapy (DAPT) is crucial, and patients should be carefully and repeatedly instructed not to stop taking aspirin, Plavix, or Ticlid without consulting their interventional cardiologist. The FDA concluded that more information is

needed, especially in the use of devices in off-label settings. However, when DESs are used as directed, no greater risks of death or heart attack are reported.

The development of devices to remove atherosclerotic plaque (atherectomy catheters) and implantable devices to maintain the opening mechanically (stents) has provided effective adjuncts or alternatives to PTCA for the problem of recurring lesions. Restenosis of de novo lesions after atherectomy is similar in character and prevalence to that in PTCA; however, intracoronary stenting has resulted in a lower restenosis rate in native and vein graft lesions of approximately 10%.

The cause of restenosis is still unclear. It appears to be the result of an excessive healing response to balloon dilation that exposes the subintimal structures of the vessel to circulating blood. These exposed areas are then potential sites for platelet adhesion and aggregation and for thrombus formation. The degree of this "healing" response varies from lesion to lesion and may be influenced by the clinical and angiographic factors associated with restenosis that were discussed previously. Factors associated with increased incidence of restenosis are listed in Box 18-8.

## Other Complications

Other major complications of PCI requiring medical intervention are coronary perforation, which may be treated with a sheathed stent to stop the leak of blood into the pericardium; bradycardia, which requires temporary pacing; VT or VF, which requires immediate defibrillation; and a central nervous system event causing transient or persistent neurologic deficit.

Peripheral vascular complications occurring primarily at the catheter site include arterial thrombosis, excessive bleeding that causes a significant hematoma, pseudoaneurysm, femoral arteriovenous fistula, and arterial laceration. If any of these complications persists or compromises distal blood flow to the involved extremity, surgical intervention may be required.

Table 18-3 summarizes the complications that may result from PCI, including general signs of the complications and possible interventional actions.

Box 18-9 provides a complete outline of care for the patient undergoing PCI.

---

**BOX 18-8** | **Factors Associated With Increased Incidence of Restenosis**

**Clinical Factors**
Severe angina
Noncompliance with antiplatelet regimen
Diabetes
Smoking cigarettes
Substance abuse
Uncontrolled hyperlipidemia

**Angiographic Factors**
Lesion location
Lesion length
Lesion severity before and after PCI
Adjacent arterial diameter
Gaps between overlapping stents

**TABLE 18-3** Complications of PCI: Signs and Symptoms and Possible Interventions

| | General Signs/Symptoms | Possible Interventions |
|---|---|---|
| Angina<br>Myocardial infarctions (MI)<br><br>Abrupt reclosure<br>Dissection/intimal tear | Chest pain or anginal equivalent<br>Dysrhythmias: tachycardia, bradycardia, VT/<br>    fibrillation, ST elevation<br>Marked hypotension<br>Acute ECG changes (ST-segment change) | CABG or repeat PCI<br>Redo PCI<br>Oxygen<br>Medication: vasodilators (nitrates), calcium<br>    channel blockers, analgesics, anticoagu-<br>    lants, vasopressors<br>Intra-aortic balloon pump (IABP) |
| Hypotension<br>Coronary branch occlusion<br>Restenosis | Nausea/vomiting<br>ST-segment elevation<br>Angina pectoris<br>Positive exercise test | Possible repeat PCI<br>Redo PCI<br>Coronary artery bypass graft |
| Marked change in heart rate (bradycardia,<br>    VT, ventricular fibrillation) | Rate below 60 beats/min<br>Rate above 250 beats/min<br>No discernible cardiac rhythm<br>Pallor<br>Loss of consciousness<br>Hypotension | Temporary pacemaker<br>Defibrillation<br>Medications: antiarrhythmics, vasopressors |
| Vascular complication: excessive blood loss | Hypotension<br>Decreased urine output (from hypovolemia)<br>Decreased hemoglobin/hematocrit<br>Pallor<br>Hematoma at puncture site | Possible surgical repair<br>Fluids<br>Transfusion<br>Oxygen<br>Flat in bed |
| Allergic complications | Hypotension, urticaria, nausea/vomiting,<br>    hives, laryngospasm, erythema, shortness<br>    of breath | Medication: antihistamines, steroids,<br>    antiemetics<br>Clear liquids/NPO<br>Oxygen<br>With anaphylaxis: fluids for volume expan-<br>    sion, epinephrine, vasopressors for<br>    hypotension |
| Central nervous system events | Changes in level of consciousness<br>Hemiparesis<br>Hypoventilation/respiratory depression | Oxygen<br>Discontinue/withhold sedatives<br>Medication: narcotic antagonist as a respira-<br>    tory stimulant<br>Computed tomography, magnetic resonance<br>    imaging |

*Miscellaneous complications*: conduction defects, pulmonary embolism, pulmonary edema, coronary air embolism, respiratory arrest, febrile episodes, nausea, minor bleeding.

---

**QSEN BOX 18-9** *COLLABORATIVE CARE GUIDE for the Patient Undergoing PCI*

| Outcomes | Interventions |
|---|---|
| **Impaired Gas Exchange**<br>**Ineffective breathing pattern** | |
| Patient will maintain normal arterial blood gases, or pulse oximeter reading. | • Provide supplemental oxygen per face mask or nasal cannula per hospital post-PCI protocol.<br>• Monitor blood gases/pulse oximeter per protocol.<br>• Auscultate breath sounds when taking vital signs.<br>• Monitor for signs of pulmonary edema or respiratory distress. |
| **Decreased cardiac and tissue perfusion**<br>**Decreased peripheral tissue perfusion**<br>**Risk for bleeding**<br>**Decreased cardiac output** | |
| The patient will have stable vital signs following PCI.<br>There is no evidence of post-PCI myocardial ischemia or infarction due to coronary reocclusion (eg, no ECG changes or angina).<br>There is no evidence of cardiac dysrhythmias after PCI.<br>There is no evidence of bleeding at the puncture site.<br>There is no evidence of arterial occlusion at puncture site. | • Monitor blood pressure, heart rate, respiration rate, arterial puncture site, distal pulses, and distal motor function and sensation:<br>• every 15 minutes × 4, every 30 minutes × 4<br>• every 1 hour × 4, then every 4 hour<br>• Monitor cardiac rhythm in leads specific to myocardium most affected by PCI location.<br>• Administer medications to treat coronary artery spasms (eg, nifedipine and nitroglycerin).<br>• Administer heparin per protocol.<br>• Report type and frequency of dysrhythmias.<br>• Administer antiarrhythmic medication as indicated and ordered. |

*(continued)*

**QSEN BOX 18-9**   *COLLABORATIVE CARE GUIDE for the Patient Undergoing PCI (continued)*

| Outcomes | Interventions |
|---|---|
| | • Temporary transvenous or external pacemaker and defibrillator are readily available.<br>• Monitor site for hematoma as above with vital signs.<br>• Assess for tenderness, ecchymosis, and warmth over puncture site.<br>• Apply direct pressure to puncture site for 15 to 30 minutes after sheath is removed.<br>• Apply sandbag to puncture site if oozing continues, per hospital protocol.<br>• Apply a pressure dressing to puncture site when oozing has stopped.<br>• Monitor activated clotting time, prothrombin time, partial thromboplastin time, and platelets, reporting coagulopathies per protocol.<br>• Monitor involved extremity with vital signs for mottling, coolness, pallor, diminished pulses, numbness, tingling, pain, and so forth. |
| **Ineffective renal perfusion**<br>**Imbalanced fluid volume**<br>**Electrolyte imbalance** | |
| Patient is euvolemic.<br>Renal function is maintained after administration of radiographic IV contrast agent. | • Monitor intake and output.<br>• Obtain type and cross-match, complete blood count, electrolytes prior to PCI.<br>• Maintain IV patency.<br>• Obtain pre-PCI and post-PCI blood urea nitrogen, creatinine, and electrolyte levels.<br>• Closely monitor urine output; report if <30 mL/h.<br>• Monitor urine specific gravity or osmolarity for clearance of IV contrast.<br>• Administer diuretic agents as ordered. |
| **Impaired physical mobility**<br>**Risk for impaired skin integrity** | |
| | • The patient is on bed rest for 4 to 6 hours post-PCI per hospital protocol.<br>• While sheath is in place and while on bed rest, keep head of bed <45 degrees. |
| **Skin Integrity** | |
| Patient's skin will remain intact. | • Assess skin immediately after PCI for pressure areas.<br>• Reposition to relieve pressure from bony prominences, maintaining alignment of extremity involved in procedure.<br>• Consider pressure relief/reduction mattress. |
| **Imbalanced nutrition** | |
| Nutritional intake is reestablished.<br>Patient does not experience nausea or vomiting after PCI. | • Resume oral fluids and diet per protocol.<br>• Monitor swallowing and protective airway reflexes while patient is receiving sedatives or narcotics.<br>• Monitor nausea and vomiting.<br>• Administer antiemetic medication as appropriate. |
| **Impaired comfort** | |
| Patient will not experience anginal pain.<br>Patient will not experience pain from mobility restrictions. | • Instruct patient to verbally report discomfort and pain.<br>• Evaluate severity and location of pain, distinguishing angina from other causes of discomfort.<br>• Administer nitrates or narcotics per order or protocol for angina.<br>• Evaluate patient response to medication.<br>• Reposition patient frequently, keeping involved extremity straight.<br>• Use mattress overlay or egg crate for comfort.<br>• Administer analgesics as appropriate, after distinguishing joint or muscular pain from angina. |
| **Risk for ineffective coping**<br>**Anxiety** | |
| Patient and family state risks associated with PCI.<br>Patient uses personal support systems to reduce anxiety. | • Provide information for informed procedural consent.<br>• Encourage verbalization of questions, concerns, and fears.<br>• Encourage significant other to visit in early postprocedural recovery phase.<br>• Validate patient/significant others' understanding of surgery and illness.<br>• Initiate referrals to social services, clergy, and so forth as necessary. |
| **Teaching/Discharge Planning** | |
| Patient and family are prepared for possibility of emergent repeat PCI or cardiac surgery.<br>Patient cooperates with post-PCI mobility restrictions.<br>Patient states lifestyle changes required to reduce risk for worsening coronary artery disease. | • Preprocedure teaching includes discussion regarding causes for coronary reocclusion or perforation and rationale for surgery or repeat PCI.<br>• Provide preprocedure and postprocedure instruction and rationale for bed rest and limited movement of involved extremity.<br>• Provide verbal and written instruction/information regarding risk factors and pathophysiology, activity, diet, stress reduction, medication administration, and appropriate times/indications to seek medical attention. |

## Other Interventional Cardiology Techniques

The immediate and long-term efficacy of PCI in treating symptomatic patients with single-vessel disease has been well established. In many centers, PTCA also is routinely and successfully used in patients with multivessel disease. The safety and efficacy with which angioplasty has been used have fostered research into treating patients with unstable angina, AMI, and cardiogenic shock.

Technologies have been developed to address the challenges associated with complex PCI. These include laser angioplasty, thrombectomy devices, atherectomy devices, DES, brachytherapy, and distal protection devices.

### Laser Angioplasty

The acronym *LASER* stands for light amplification through stimulated emission of radiation. Through a series of mirrors and lenses, the laser beam is directed into a catheter containing numerous glass fibers. These fibers transmit the light energy through the catheter to the plaque that is to be ablated.[23] The laser is used to ablate plaque or as an adjunct to other PCI procedures to make a pathway in total occlusions to facilitate the passage of a PTCA balloon or stent.

Laser angioplasty is performed much like a standard PCI procedure. The guide catheter is advanced to the ostium of the coronary artery targeted by fluoroscopy. Once the lesion location is ascertained through contrast injection, a guide wire is advanced up and through the lesion. Before the laser is activated, everyone in the room (including the patient) must don protective eyewear. The laser catheter is then advanced through the guide wire and brought into contact with the lesion. Depending on anticipated lesion morphology, energy settings are chosen that will presumably suffice to ablate the plaque. The laser settings include the fluency (millijoules per square millimeter) to be delivered and the repetition rate (pulses per second). The plaque is then vaporized by the laser energy. Several passes down the length of the lesion may be performed. Laser success is determined by fluoroscopy and coronary injections with contrast dye. If there is residual stenosis after use of the laser, adjunctive PCI procedures, including stenting, can be performed to achieve an optimal final result (Fig. 18-7).

Stenotic lesions best suited for laser angioplasty include those that are long and diffuse (longer than 15 to 20 mm), ostial in location, highly calcified, in vein grafts, and totally occluded. Risks associated with laser angioplasty include

perforation of the coronary artery, dissections, and aneurysms. Now considered a "niche" procedure, laser angioplasty is performed less frequently in the percutaneous treatment of cardiovascular disease.

### Atherectomy

Atherectomy is the process of removing atherosclerotic plaque from the coronary artery by cutting or ablating and thus "debulking" the lesion. Atherectomy devices include directional coronary atherectomy (DCA) and rotational ablation (Rotablator).

Potential complications of all atherectomy devices include perforation of the coronary artery, abrupt closure, embolization distal to the lesion site, and MI. The rate of restenosis and other complications is comparable to that with standard balloon angioplasty and less successful than those results achieved with DESs.

### Directional Coronary Atherectomy

The directional coronary atherectomy (DCA) device is a cutting catheter that is inserted over a guidewire into the coronary artery across the stenotic lesion. It is positioned so that the opening for the blade faces the lesion. A low-pressure balloon on the opposite side of the catheter is inflated, thus forcing the atherosclerotic plaque into the opening near the cutting blade. The cutting blade turns at approximately 1,200 revolutions/min (rpm) and is then slowly advanced along the length of the lesion, cutting the plaque and collecting it in the catheter nosecone. The DCA catheter is turned a complete 360 degrees in the artery to shave all sides of the atherosclerotic plaque with repeated passes. The procedure is repeated until the atherosclerotic plaque is sufficiently removed. The catheter, laden with plaque, is then withdrawn from the patient.

### Rotational Ablation Device

The Rotablator device (Boston Scientific, Natick, MA) is a high-speed rotating, abrasive, burr-tipped catheter that ablates the atherosclerotic plaque in the coronary artery. The Rotablator has proved especially effective for complex stenotic lesions that are calcified, tortuous, small in diameter, ostial, or diffuse in character. The device consists of a football-shaped, diamond-studded burr attached to a drive shaft. The Rotablator is advanced over a guide wire to the lesion site. The burr rotates at 160,000 to 190,000 rpm and pulverizes the atherosclerotic plaque into microparticles that are absorbed into the patient's circulatory system. The spinning burr is advanced across the lesion several times to debulk the stenotic lesion. Adjunctive balloon angioplasty may be performed after use of the Rotablator device.

The AngioJet device (Possis) is a thrombectomy system used to extract clot from coronary arteries, saphenous vein grafts, or peripheral arteries. The system consists of three components: (1) the drive unit (Fig. 18-8A); (2) the pump set, which achieves isovolumetric balance between the fluid and thrombus that is removed from the artery and the fluid that is delivered (see Fig. 18-8B); and (3) the catheter, which is disposable and 4- to 6-Fr compatible (see Fig. 18-8C). The AngioJet System has been shown to be safe and effective in removing fresh clot from patients

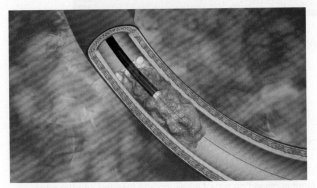
FIGURE 18-7 LASER ablation of a coronary artery stenosis.

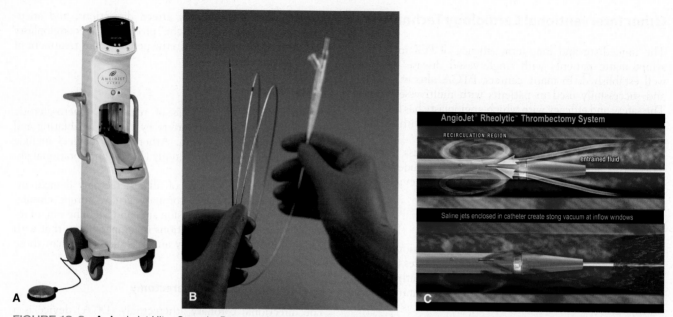

**FIGURE 18-8** **A:** AngioJet Ultra Console. Power and control console for AngioJet Rheolytic Thrombectomy System. **B:** The AngioJet Spiroflex Thrombectomy Catheter is a 4-Fr thrombectomy catheter with a spiral-cut shaft for tracking. **C:** The mechanism of action of the Angio-Jet Thrombectomy Catheter. (Courtesy of Possis Medical Inc., Minneapolis, MN.)

undergoing PCI for AMI[24] and in instances in which there is clot in saphenous vein grafts.[25]

## Stents

Intracoronary stents are hollow stainless steel tubes that act as "scaffolding" in the coronary artery. After predilation with a PTCA balloon catheter, most stents are premounted on a balloon catheter and inserted through the guide catheter along a guide wire to the lesion site. Once placed across the stenotic lesion, the balloon is inflated, and the stent is expanded and left in the coronary artery (Fig. 18-9).

Traditional and older stent designs are bare metal. Because many bare metal stent designs use stainless steel, they are potent thrombogenic prostheses. Stent thrombus is a major short- and long-term complication. Success of the stenting procedure depends on endothelialization of the stent to provide a smooth flow of blood in the coronary artery and through the stent yet controlled to prevent stent thrombosis. Anticoagulation and antiplatelet medication regimens

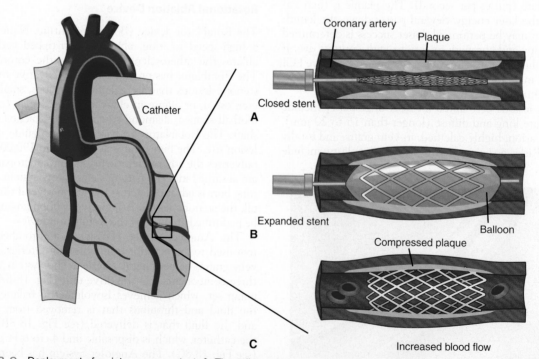

**FIGURE 18-9** Deployment of an intracoronary stent. **A:** The collapsed stent is placed on top of a balloon and inserted into the artery. **B:** The balloon is inflated thus opening the stent. **C:** The balloon is removed and the stent is left in place.

are crucial to successful stenting and long-term prognosis. Stenting has been shown in numerous trials to reduce restenosis rates and improve long-term prognosis. Stents made of newer alloys and compounds are currently undergoing investigation. There are three main components to a DES: (1) the type of stent that carries the drug coating, (2) the method by which the drug is carried (eluted) to the blood vessel wall, and (3) the drug itself. DESs are coated with drugs such as everolimus, paclitaxel, zotarolimus, sirolimus, or rapamycin. It is believed that the gradual release of these drugs into the coronary vasculature at the site of the atherosclerotic plaque inhibits restenosis by limiting smooth muscle cell proliferation and inflammation but allowing reendothelialization to proceed normally. At this time, the FDA-approved DESs include approximately two dozen varieties. An example of a sirolimus-coated stent is known as Cypher (Cordis Corporation; Fig. 18-10). Another stent, known as Endeavor (Medtronic), uses a cobalt chrome Driver stent with a phosphorylcholine coating of zotarolimus. Xience V

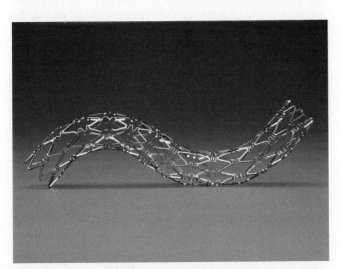

**FIGURE 18-10** Fully expanded Cypher stent. (Used with permission of Cordis Corporation.)

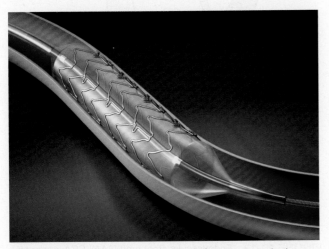

**FIGURE 18-11** Xience V everolimus-eluting coronary stent. (Courtesy of Abbott Vascular. © Abbott Laboratories. All rights reserved.)

(Abbott Vascular; Fig. 18-11) uses an L605 cobalt chromium Multi-Link Vision stent and adds a fluoropolymer multilayer coating with the drug everolimus and the paclitaxel-coated stent called Taxus (Boston Scientific).

The next generation of intracoronary stents includes those that are bioresorbable, such as the Absorb (Abbott Vascular). The first of these bioresorbable stents was approved in July 2016. The Absorb is a DES with a bioresorbable vascular scaffold (BVS) thought to reduce long-term complication rates. Bioresorbable vascular scaffold has many advantages over the metallic stent in the treatment of coronary stenotic lesions. It has added advantages in lesions that are close to the ostium of the culprit vessel, as in the left main coronary artery, right coronary artery, or left internal mammary artery. As the hanging segments of the stent dissolve in approximately 2 years, it reduces difficulty in engaging the vessel for future interventions if needed.

The interventional cardiologist must make several important decisions that lead to a successful stent implantation, including

- correct sizing of the stent length to match the length of the lesion
- correct sizing of the stent diameter to match the thickness of the normal sections of the coronary artery
- accurate and complete deployment of the stent.

Underexpansion of the stent can result in tiny gaps between the stent and arterial wall, which can lead to serious problems such as SAT. Other complications following implantation of bare metal stents or DESs may include bleeding at the access site, stent migration, coronary artery dissection, and abrupt closure.

### Brachytherapy

Intracoronary radiation (brachytherapy) is potentially a potent antiproliferative therapy that is currently being investigated for use with PCI and might therefore provide a means for effective reduction of restenosis. The radiation therapy is emitted in the form of temporarily implanted or inserted radioactive sources, such as seeds, radioactive stents, or radioactive liquid–filled balloons. Radiation works particularly well in inhibiting new growth by attacking the newer, more aggressive neoplastic cells, while often having little effect on normal tissue.[26]

In brachytherapy, endovascular low-dose radiation is applied at the site of balloon dilation or stent implantation by a catheter system. Two types of radiation are used to treat restenosis: gamma and beta emitters. Gamma emitters create a radiation field for a considerable distance away from their source. This requires that the treatment be conducted in a heavily lead-shielded cardiac catheterization laboratory. Gamma-emitter intensity is lower than that of beta emitters, and gamma emitters must be left in place 14 to 45 minutes, depending on the strength of the source used. Beta sources, with a higher intensity of radiation near the source, can be more concentrated, enabling the brachytherapy to last only 3 to 10 minutes. The beta source can be shielded only with approximately 0.5 inch of polymerized methyl methacrylate (Lucite). The FDA currently approves the use of brachytherapy only for in-stent restenosis.

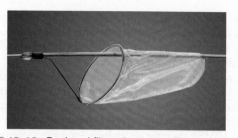

**FIGURE 18-12** Deployed filter wire device. (Photograph courtesy of Boston Scientific Corporation, 2006.)

### Distal Protection Devices

Distal embolization of particulate matter can complicate PCI and peripheral interventional procedures. Tiny microemboli can be showered distally (downstream of the lesion) during revascularization procedures. This can cause end-organ ischemia, AMI, serum cardiac enzyme elevation, stroke, and LV dysfunction. Distal protection devices are designed to reduce or eliminate distal embolization during PCI and peripheral interventions. Distal protection devices are often used during PCI of saphenous vein grafts and during carotid procedures.

To date, the only distal protection devices approved by the FDA are the PercuSurge GuardWire (Medtronic) and the FilterWire (Boston Scientific) (Fig. 18-12). The PercuSurge device consists of a guide wire with a low-pressure occlusive balloon on the distal end. The balloon is inflated to prevent distal embolization, and an aspiration catheter removes the debris from the treated vessel before the balloon is deflated and antegrade flow is restored. The FilterWire device contains a low-profile filter mounted on an angioplasty wire. The filter contains small holes that permit antegrade blood flow while trapping microemboli and thus providing distal protection. Because these distal protection devices are quickly becoming the standard of care for degenerated saphenous veins grafts and carotid stenting, device manufacturers may seek indications for use in ACS interventions and other peripheral procedures in the near future.

## Interventions for Peripheral Arterial Disease

Peripheral arterial disease (PAD) is a condition that affects approximately 8 million Americans, including 12% to 20% of individuals 60 years of age or older.[27] The disease results from the accumulation of plaque in the arteries that constricts normal blood flow and can result in heart attack, stroke, extremity amputation, and death if left untreated. Men and woman are equally affected by PAD; however, Black race/ethnicity is associated with an increased risk. People of Hispanic origin have similar to slightly higher rates of PAD compared to non-Hispanic Whites. Patients with PAD have a 5-year mortality rate of 30%.[27] Refer to Chapter 19 for a discussion of aortic aneurysms and PAD and Chapter 22 for surgical management of carotid disease (endarterectomy). Until recent advances in technology made minimally invasive and percutaneous approaches possible, medical or surgical intervention for these cardiovascular diseases was the only option.

Remote endarterectomy is a minimally invasive endovascular procedure for complete superficial femoral artery revascularization. It provides treatment of lower extremity

arterial disease and serves as an alternative to bypass surgery. The benefits of the remote endarterectomy approach are as follows: (1) it preserves the native vessel; (2) it is less invasive than surgery; (3) there is no limitation on future surgical options; (4) recovery is potentially faster and easier for the patient as compared with bypass procedures; and (5) it has comparable long-term clinical outcomes to surgical endarterectomy.

Percutaneous treatment is an emerging approach in PAD management. Angioplasty, atherectomy, and stenting of the carotid arteries, aorta, renal arteries, iliac and femoral arteries, and upper extremities are routinely performed in many medical institutions. Before undergoing a percutaneous intervention, most patients require magnetic resonance angiography, arterial duplex mapping, or angiography. Percutaneous transluminal angioplasty of the peripheral arteries involves placing a balloon in the blood vessel at the site of the blockage and inflating the balloon to open the blood vessel. Stents can also be inserted into the blocked vessel to serve as scaffolding in opening it. Thrombolytic therapy can also be delivered to the site of the blockages before initiating angioplasty or stenting. Atherectomy, or debulking the peripheral blood vessels, has also been shown to be beneficial in some cases before angioplasty or stenting.

Abdominal aortic aneurysms and thoracic aortic aneurysms can also be treated percutaneously. Endovascular stent grafts are metal-lined fabric tubes that reinforce an aneurysm in a blood vessel. It essentially relines the blood vessel and decreases the incidence of aneurysm rupture. The stent graft seals tightly above and below the aneurysm (Fig. 18-13). The graft is stronger than the weakened aorta and permits blood to pass through without exerting pressure on the aneurysm. Patients are candidates for endovascular stent grafting if aneurysms measure 5 cm wide, the aneurysm and aorta contour are conducible to stent grafting, and the blood vessels are large enough to pass guiding catheters, angioplasty balloons,

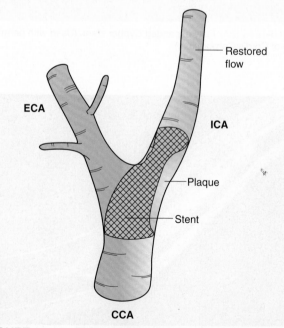

**FIGURE 18-13** Endovascular stent graft (AAA). CCA, common carotid artery; ECA, external carotid artery; ICA, internal carotid artery.

and the stent graft. Potential complications of endovascular stent grafting include endoleaks (leaking of blood around the graft), migration of the stent graft, infection, and restenosis.

Postprocedure care of the patient with PAD is similar to that of patients undergoing PCI of the coronaries. Groin incision observation, extremity assessment, and vital sign measurement are important components of postprocedure care. Patient education and discharge planning should include aggressive management of cardiovascular risk factors, such as smoking cessation, reduction of blood glucose levels, exercise regimens, and lowering of blood pressure and cholesterol level. Antiplatelet therapy is also indicated for the patient undergoing percutaneous treatment of PAD.

With the various tools and technologies available to the interventional cardiologist, as well as improved adjunctive pharmacologic therapy, the future should bring further improvement in the efficacy and predictability of PCI and in the long-term patency of involved atherosclerotic vessels in the coronary system and in the peripheral arterial system.

## Percutaneous Valvular Interventions

### Percutaneous Balloon Valvuloplasty

PBV is a nonsurgical technique for increasing blood flow through stenotic cardiac valves using dilation catheters. This procedure is similar to PCI procedures in that a catheter system is inserted percutaneously and advanced to the region of narrowing using fluoroscopic guidance. A dilation catheter then is inflated to increase the valvular opening and improve blood flow.

#### Historical Background

The first cases of balloon dilation of stenotic cardiac valves were reported in 1979 and 1982, when physicians successfully dilated pulmonary valve stenoses. This technique was considered an effective alternative to open heart surgery, although long-term results could not yet be evaluated. Because surgical commissurotomy was successful in treating mitral valve stenoses and because of the initial success with pulmonary valve dilation, physicians began percutaneous dilation of mitral valves in 1984 to avoid the need for thoracotomy. These procedures improved cardiac function with no serious procedural complications.

The number of PBVs does not approach the volume of PCI procedures. This is due partly to the lesser incidence of valve disease compared with CAD.

Assuming patients have long-term clinical improvement associated with PBV, the advantages compared with surgery are similar to those of PCI versus CABG. PBV is less traumatic, requires no anesthesia, is associated with lower morbidity and a shorter hospital stay, causes no scarring, and is less expensive. Minimally invasive surgical procedures are also available and include mini-thoracotomy approaches.

#### Pathophysiology of Stenotic Valves

Stenotic valves are caused by calcific degeneration, congenital abnormalities, or rheumatic heart disease. Calcific aortic and mitral valve degeneration now appears to be the most frequent causes of valve disease requiring surgical treatment.

Refer to Chapter 22 for a discussion of the pathophysiology and surgical management of specific stenotic valves.

### Diagnostic Tests for PBV and Valve Replacement

Before deciding on the appropriate intervention, the physician evaluates the patient for evidence and severity of valvular stenosis. A variety of noninvasive tests allow the physician to determine the degree of left atrial or LV hypertrophy, pulmonary venous congestion or hypertension, valvular rigidity, and transvalvular gradient. In a 12-lead ECG, the magnitude of the R wave in the left precordial leads reflects the presence of LV hypertrophy associated with AV stenosis. The presence of broad, notched P waves in leads I, II, and aVL reflects left atrial hypertrophy associated with mitral valve stenosis. A chest radiograph illustrates the presence of calcium in or around the valve, LV or atrial hypertrophy, and pulmonary venous congestion or HF. A two-dimensional echocardiogram is used to scan the cardiac valves and chambers. A Doppler ultrasound study allows measurement of the transvalvular gradient, indirect calculation of valve area, and assessment of valvular regurgitation. With this information, the physician is able to (1) estimate the size of the valve orifice, (2) visualize the degree of valve leaflet movement, and (3) determine the extent of LV or atrial hypertrophy.

Right and left heart catheterization is performed if the previous tests indicate valvular disease. Although this procedure is invasive, it is required to determine the pressures within each of the cardiac chambers and to confirm transvalvular gradients. Once the pressures and gradients are obtained, a series of radiographs may be taken by injecting radiopaque contrast medium, either in the aorta to visualize aortic regurgitation or in the left ventricle to visualize mitral regurgitation. This procedure yields a cineangiogram illustrating the function of the cardiac valves and chamber sizes.

After this series of tests, the physician can analyze the valves closely, gaining precise information with which to decide the treatment mode. The nurse should be familiar with the results of these tests because a better understanding of the patient's diagnosis and related symptoms, and thus of the reasons for intervention, promotes better care.

### Equipment Features

Although PBV and PCI catheters are based on similar designs, there are important differences, primarily because of the larger diameters of heart valves compared with coronary arteries. One major difference is the outer diameter of the catheters: PBV catheter shafts range from 7 to 9 Fr, and PBV balloons range from 15 to 25 mm in diameter when inflated. A 10- to 14-Fr introducing sheath may be used at the arterial or venous puncture site to allow for introduction of the valve dilation catheter. A large guide wire, 0.035 to 0.038 inch, is used to provide the added stiffness and support required to introduce the dilatation catheter. PBV dilation catheters have radiopaque markers similar to PCI catheter systems for fluoroscopic imaging.

### Indications for and Contraindications to PBV

The use of PBV initially was limited by the fear of embolization of calcific debris, disruption of the valve ring, acute valvular regurgitation, and valvular restenosis. The incidence of these complications continues to be a concern. Both major and minor complications have been reported in numerous early studies; however, these complications must be assessed in terms of the patient population in which the procedure is performed.

Although surgical valve replacement is an effective treatment for those with aortic valve stenosis and operative mortality rates are low, the operative mortality rate significantly increases in patients with multisystem disease (often, these are older patients). PBV initially has been proved a safe and efficacious alternative for these patients. It also is an effective therapy for children who are high surgical risks because it delays the need for surgery until the child is older and can better tolerate an operation. In addition, the longevity of both mechanical and bioprosthetic valves is approximately 10 to 20 years, so PBV delays or prevents the need for a second operation. Also, the long-term anticoagulation therapy required with mechanical valve prostheses is undesirable in younger patients and pregnant women. PBV also is effective for stabilizing those with poor LV function before surgery; it is contraindicated in patients with moderate to severe valvular regurgitation due to a small but significant risk for increasing valvular insufficiency with the procedure. Box 18-10 summarized the indications and contraindications for PBV.

A complication associated with PBV is excessive bleeding at the puncture site due to the large catheters required to perform dilation. The development of smaller catheters may reduce the incidence of bleeding. As with PCI, PBV catheters are being refined continually to increase procedural safety, time, and efficacy.

## Procedure

The procedure is performed in the cardiac catheterization laboratory and involves many of the same steps as PCI (see earlier section on PCI procedure). Right and left heart catheterization is repeated to evaluate hemodynamic status and to obtain baseline transvalvular gradients. Coronary angiography, when indicated, is repeated to determine whether the patient still meets the criteria for valvuloplasty. Thorough repeat evaluation is necessary because a patient's status can change, precluding treatment with this intervention.

The angiographic catheter is replaced either by an introducing sheath or a dilation catheter. In mitral PBV, a venous

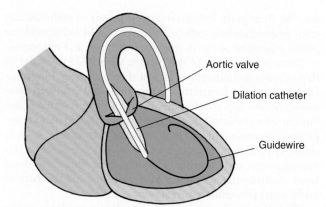

**FIGURE 18-14** Cross-sectional view of heart illustrating guide wire and dilation catheter positions across the aortic valve. The guide wire is curved to prevent ventricular dysrhythmias or puncture.

puncture is made in the right femoral vein. During both aortic and mitral PBV, maintaining patent IV and radial or femoral arterial lines is important to administer medications and draw blood samples.

In aortic PBV, once the sheaths are in place, the patient is anticoagulated with 5,000 to 10,000 U of heparin to prevent clot formation in the catheter system. The dilation catheter and guide wire then are advanced to the root of the ascending aorta. The guide wire is advanced across the stenotic aortic valve, and the dilation catheter is advanced over the guide wire (Fig. 18-14). Exact placement of the dilation catheter is facilitated by fluoroscopy and radiopaque markers on the balloon.

In mitral PBV, a pacing catheter may be positioned through a separate venous sheath at the level of the inferior vena cava or right atrium and placed on standby. The mitral valve then is approached either by way of the femoral artery and aortic valve or, in most cases, through the right heart by perforating the atrial septum to enter the left atrium. Once the mitral valve has been accessed, the patient is anticoagulated with 5,000 to 10,000 U of heparin. The dilation catheter is then advanced over the guide wire through the atrial septal puncture and across the mitral valve (Fig. 18-15). Again, exact

---

**BOX 18-10** | **Indications and Contraindications for PBV**

**Clinical Indications**
High-risk surgical patients (advanced age, severe pulmonary hypertension, renal failure, pulmonary dysfunction, LV dysfunction)
Unstable presurgical patients
Patients not candidates for chronic anticoagulation

**Anatomical Indications**
Moderate to severe valvular narrowing
Moderate to severe valvular calcification
Mild valvular regurgitation

**Anatomical Contraindications**
Inability to access vasculature
Thrombus
Severe valvular regurgitation
History of embolic events

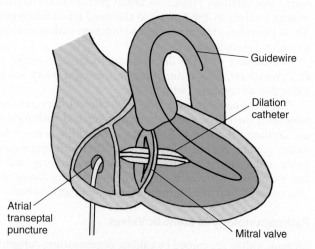

**FIGURE 18-15** Cross-sectional view of heart illustrating guide-wire and dilation catheter placed through an atrial transseptal puncture and across the mitral valve. The guide wire is extended out the aortic valve into the aorta for catheter support.

placement of the dilation catheter in the valve is facilitated by fluoroscopy and radiopaque markers on the balloon.

Average inflation time of the dilation catheter is 15 to 60 seconds in aortic valvuloplasty and 10 to 30 seconds in mitral valvuloplasty. During dilation of either valve, the nurse monitors blood pressure closely because of the imposed decrease in cardiac output. Once the dilation catheter has been deflated, blood pressure should return to normal. During dilation of the mitral valve, there is a temporary increase in the pulmonary artery occlusion pressure (PAOP; formerly known as pulmonary artery wedge pressure [PAWP]). Once the dilation catheter has been deflated, the PAOP should return to baseline. Dysrhythmias, such as VT, VF, or sinus bradycardia, also may occur during dilation.

Once maximal dilation has been obtained, the catheter is removed. Hemodynamic measurements, including transvalvular gradients, are repeated to determine efficacy of the procedure. Repeat angiography is performed to assess for valvular regurgitation. When the procedure is complete, the anticoagulant effects of heparin are reversed to prevent bleeding complications associated with the large puncture site.

### Results

Aortic PBV is associated with a decrease in pressure gradient and end-systolic volume and an increase in aortic valve area, EF, and cardiac output. Although there is an increase in the aortic valve area, it is not as great as with surgical valve replacement. In addition, the restenosis rate associated with PBV is high. Therefore, aortic valvuloplasty is indicated primarily for older and high-risk surgical patients and generally is considered a palliative, not a curative, procedure.

Results of mitral valvuloplasty are more dramatic. There is a more significant increase in valve area and cardiac output and a decrease in valve gradient, PAOP, and mean pulmonary arterial pressure. Three mechanisms have been postulated for improving valvular function due to PBV: (1) fracture of calcific nodules adherent to leaflets (most frequent), (2) separation of fused commissures, and (3) stretching of the annulus and leaflet structure.

### Assessment and Management

**PATIENT PREPARATION.** The patient is admitted to the hospital the day of the PBV procedure. The goal of nursing care is to reduce the cardiac workload, monitor fluid and electrolyte balance, and reduce psychological stress so that the patient remains hemodynamically stable.

In most cases, the patient does not have invasive pressure monitoring lines in place before the procedure. The nurse therefore carefully monitors signs and symptoms of HF: narrowing in the arterial pulse pressure, more frequent increases in heart rate during activity, peripheral edema, presence of a cough, complaints of dyspnea, or rales in lung fields. The nurse also must note any changes in sensorium, color, skin temperature, and pulse volume, and any decrease in urinary output. To monitor fluid and electrolyte balance, the nurse obtains a baseline serum electrolyte level and baseline body weight. In addition, daily fluid intake and output are recorded.

The patient's medications before admission may have included diuretics, digoxin, and anticoagulants. Before the procedure, any anticoagulant medication is discontinued because of the possibility of emergency surgery. Therefore, patients with chronic AF who have the potential for systemic embolization due to thrombus should be monitored closely. The nurse also monitors preliminary laboratory tests and notifies the physician of any abnormalities. (See the section on patient preparation for PTCA for further information on these tests.)

After the patient fully understands the procedure, the physician must obtain an informed consent for PBV, anesthesia, and surgery. Surgical standby usually is provided during PBV due to possible complications requiring emergency valve replacement.

**NURSING ASSESSMENT AND MANAGEMENT DURING PBV.** The nurse continuously monitors pulmonary artery pressure and PAOP and is aware of changes in tracings that may suggest symptoms of HF or pulmonary edema. In the presence of severe hypotension, the nurse should be prepared to start an IV infusion of dopamine or norepinephrine (Levophed). In the case of ventricular dysrhythmias, a lidocaine drip should be available for infusion.

**NURSING ASSESSMENT AND MANAGEMENT AFTER PBV.** The nurse is important in the patient's recovery. The goal of postvalvuloplasty nursing care is to maintain adequate cardiac output, maintain fluid and electrolyte balance, and verify hemostasis at the puncture site. Alterations in cardiac output can be caused by dysrhythmias secondary to valve manipulation, resulting in edema near the bundle of His; left-to-right atrial shunt through the transseptal puncture created during mitral valvuloplasty; cardiac tamponade; alteration in circulating fluid volume; or blood loss. Alteration in fluid and electrolyte balance results from diuretic therapy and contrast medium used during catheterization. Bleeding at the puncture site is secondary to the combined effect of systemic anticoagulation and the large diameter of catheters used.

Because fluids are important in the hemodynamic balance of the patient with valvular disease, the volume of IV fluids is recorded to establish an accurate intake and output. The decreased circulating volume from diuretic medications given before PBV, combined with improved stroke volume after successful PBV, can be reflected as a decrease in cardiac output. Therefore, careful monitoring of central venous pressure, pulmonary artery pressure, PAOP, and blood pressure, in addition to heart rate, urinary output, and electrolyte balance, is essential in the evaluation and assessment of circulating fluid volume and cardiac pumping status.

In addition, the nurse assesses the patient's status from head to toe, noting overall skin color and temperature and carefully observing the level of consciousness and neurologic signs. The nurse also listens closely to heart and breath sounds. Circulation distal to the puncture site is evaluated by noting peripheral skin color and temperature in addition to the presence and quality of the dorsalis pedis and posterior tibial pulses.

Finally, any drainage appearing on the puncture site dressing or tenderness during palpation should be noted to establish a baseline for the possibility of increased pericatheter bleeding. The nurse reports immediately any changes that may indicate excessive bleeding. Bleeding at the sheath site may result in a hematoma requiring surgical evacuation. To prevent excessive bleeding and to aid hemostasis, the physician may order a sandbag or clamp placed over the puncture site.

If the patient has documented CAD, the physician also may request a serum cardiac enzyme panel. Particular attention should be paid to creatine kinase (CK) and CK isoenzymes (see Nursing Management After Percutaneous Coronary Interventions). The nurse should be aware of the signs and symptoms of myocardial ischemia in addition to the appropriate interventions.

The nurse instructs the patient about the importance of keeping the involved leg straight for the first few hours after valvuloplasty.

Post-PBV laboratory evaluation may include PT, hemoglobin and hematocrit, coagulation studies, serum electrolytes, CK, ECG, and chest radiograph. Teaching points for home care for the patient after PCI or PBV are described in Box 18-11.

**COMPLICATIONS.** A common in-hospital complication associated with PBV is bleeding at the arterial puncture site due to the large diameter of the catheters needed to dilate the valve annulus. In addition, in mitral PBV, a common complication is left-to-right shunting secondary to septal dilation, again due to the large diameter of the dilation catheters. Systemic embolization in both mitral and aortic PBV is a potential and significant complication, although its incidence is low. There have been few reports of significant increases in valvular regurgitation. Complications associated with PBV are listed in Box 18-12.

## Transcatheter Aortic Valve Replacement

For people who have been diagnosed with severe symptomatic calcified native aortic valve stenosis and who are at high risk or too sick for open-heart surgery, transcatheter aortic valve replacement (TAVR) may be an alternative. This minimally invasive surgical procedure repairs the valve without removing the old, damaged valve; instead, it wedges a replacement valve into the aortic valve's place. The surgery may be called a transcatheter aortic valve replacement (TAVR) or transcatheter aortic valve implantation (TAVI).

Somewhat similar to a stent placed in an artery, the TAVI approach delivers a fully collapsible replacement valve to the valve site through a catheter (Fig. 18-16). Once the new valve is expanded, it pushes the old valve leaflets out of the way and the tissue in the replacement valve takes over the job of regulating blood flow. This less invasive procedure allows a new valve to be inserted within the patient's native, diseased aortic valve. The TAVR procedure can be performed through two different approaches: transfemoral (through an incision in the leg) or transapical (through an incision in the chest between the ribs).

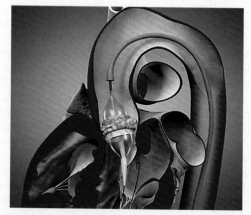

**FIGURE 18-16** Called TAVR or TAVI, this minimally invasive surgical procedure repairs the valve without removing the old, damaged valve. Instead, it wedges a replacement valve into the aortic valve's place. (Courtesy of Edwards Life Science)

# INTRA-AORTIC BALLOON PUMP COUNTERPULSATION AND MECHANICAL CIRCULATORY SUPPORT

## Intra-Aortic Balloon Pump Counterpulsation

IABP counterpulsation is designed to increase coronary artery perfusion pressure and blood flow during the diastolic phase of the cardiac cycle by inflation of a balloon in the thoracic aorta. Deflation of the balloon, just before systolic ejection, decreases the impedance to ejection (afterload) and thus LV work, with subsequent decreased myocardial oxygen consumption. Inflation and deflation counterpulse each heartbeat. With improved blood flow and effective reduction in LV work, the desired results are increased coronary artery perfusion and decreased afterload with subsequent increase in cardiac output. Goals include increasing oxygen supply to the myocardium, decreasing LV work, and improving cardiac output.

The ACC/AHA guidelines for management of AMI consider IABP counterpulsation therapy a class I recommendation for the following conditions: (1) hypotension, defined as systolic blood pressure less than 90 mm Hg, or 30 mm Hg below baseline mean arterial pressure (MAP), in patients with STEMI who do not respond to other interventions; (2) low output state in patients with STEMI; and (3) cardiogenic shock that has not been quickly reversed with pharmacologic agents in patients with STEMI.[1] The ACC/AHA guidelines also regard IABP counterpulsation to be a class I recommendation when used with other medical therapy for patients with STEMI and recurrent ischemic-type chest discomfort with signs of hemodynamic instability, poor LV function, or a large area of myocardium at risk.[1]

## Physiologic Principles

Greater work is required to maintain cardiac output in the failing heart. With this added work requirement, oxygen demand increases. These circumstances may occur at a time when the myocardium already is ischemic and coronary artery perfusion is unable to meet the oxygen demands. As a result, LV performance diminishes even further, resulting in decreased cardiac output. Without interruption of the cycle, cardiogenic shock may be imminent. This cycle can be broken with IABP therapy by increasing aortic root pressure during diastole through inflation of the balloon. With increased aortic root pressure, the perfusion pressure of the coronary arteries is increased (Fig. 18-17).

Effective therapy for the patient in LV failure also involves decreasing myocardial oxygen demand. Four major determinants of myocardial oxygen demand are afterload, preload, contractility, and heart rate. IABP counterpulsation therapy can have an effect on all these factors. It decreases afterload directly and affects the other three determinants indirectly as cardiac function improves.

### Afterload and Preload

The greatest amount of oxygen required during the cardiac cycle is for the development of afterload (see Chapter 16). With greater impedance to ejection, afterload increases,

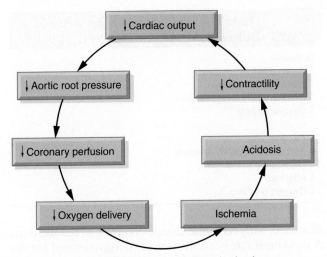

**FIGURE 18-17** Cycle leading to cardiogenic shock.

resulting in increased myocardial oxygen demand. Greater aortic end-diastolic pressures require higher afterload to overcome impedance and ejection. Vascular resistance increases impedance when vessels become vasoconstricted. Vasodilation or lower vascular resistance decreases afterload by decreasing impedance to ejection. Deflation of the balloon in the aorta just before ventricular systole lowers aortic end-diastolic pressure. This decreases impedance to ejection and decreases LV workload. In this way, IABP can effectively decrease the oxygen demand of the heart.

A person in acute LV failure has increased volume in the ventricle at end-diastole (preload; see Chapter 16) as a result of the heart's inability to pump effectively. This excessive increase in preload increases the workload of the heart. IABP therapy helps decrease excessive preload by decreasing impedance to ejection. With decreased impedance, there is more effective forward flow of blood and more efficient emptying of the left ventricle.

### Contractility

Contractility refers to the velocity and vigor of contraction during systole. Although vigorous contractility requires more oxygen, it is a benefit to cardiac function because it ensures good, efficient pumping, which increases cardiac output. In the patient with HF, cardiac contractility is depressed. Contractility is depressed when calcium levels are low, catecholamine levels are low, and ischemia is present with resultant acidosis.

IABP counterpulsation can increase oxygen supply, thereby decreasing ischemia and acidosis. In this way, IABP therapy contributes to improved contractility and better cardiac function (see Fig. 18-17).

### Heart Rate

Heart rate is a major determinant of oxygen demand because the rate determines the number of times per minute the high pressures must be generated during systole. Normally, myocardial perfusion takes place during diastole.

Tension in the muscle retards blood flow, which is why approximately 80% of coronary artery perfusion occurs during diastole. With faster heart rates, diastolic time becomes

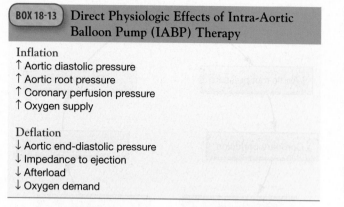

Inflation
↑ Aortic diastolic pressure
↑ Aortic root pressure
↑ Coronary perfusion pressure
↑ Oxygen supply

Deflation
↓ Aortic end-diastolic pressure
↓ Impedance to ejection
↓ Afterload
↓ Oxygen demand

**BOX 18-14** **Indications for IABP Therapy**
- Cardiogenic shock after acute infarction
- LV failure in the postoperative cardiac surgery patient
- Severe unstable angina
- Postinfarction ventricular septal defect or mitral regurgitation
- Short-term bridge to cardiac transplantation

shortened, with very little change occurring in systolic time. A rapid heart rate not only increases oxygen demand but decreases the time available for oxygen delivery. In acute ventricular failure, a person may not be able to maintain cardiac output by increasing the volume of blood pumped with each beat (stroke volume) because contractility is depressed. Cardiac output is a function of both stroke volume and heart rate:

$$\text{Cardiac output} = \text{stroke volume} \times \text{heart rate}$$

If stroke volume cannot be increased, heart rate must increase to maintain cardiac output. This increase is very costly in terms of oxygen demand.

By improving contractility, IABP therapy helps improve myocardial pumping and the ability to increase stroke volume. Decreasing afterload also increases pumping efficiency. With improved myocardial function and cardiac output, the need for compensatory tachycardia diminishes. IABP counterpulsation increases coronary artery perfusion pressure by increasing aortic diastolic pressure during inflation of the balloon, resulting in improved blood flow and oxygen delivery to the myocardium.

The physiologic effects of IABP therapy are summarized in Box 18-13. Proper inflation of the balloon increases oxygen supply, and proper deflation of the balloon decreases oxygen demand. Timing of inflation and deflation is crucial and must coincide with the cardiac cycle.

## Equipment Features

The intra-aortic balloon catheter and the balloon mounted on the end are constructed of a biocompatible polyurethane material. Filling of the balloon is achieved with a pressurized gas that enters through the catheter. Because of its low molecular weight, helium is the pressurized gas of choice. Balloon size should be determined by the patient's physical stature to optimize counterpulsation. With inflation, the addition of the balloon volume into the aorta acutely increases aortic pressure and retrograde blood flow back toward the aortic valve. With deflation, the sudden evacuation of the balloon volume acutely decreases aortic pressure. Catheters have a central lumen with which aortic pressure can be measured from the tip of the balloon.

## Indications for Intra-Aortic Balloon Pump Counterpulsation

Three major applications of IABP therapy are for treatment of cardiogenic shock after MI, low cardiac output following

cardiac surgery, and unstable angina during PCI placement. Other applications of IABP therapy for patients with cardiac pathophysiologic conditions are noted in Box 18-14.

### Cardiogenic Shock

Treatment of cardiogenic shock is complicated, and the mortality rate remains high. Cardiogenic shock develops in approximately 15% of patients with MI.

Initially, patients are treated with various inotropic drugs, vasopressors, and volume. A lack of, or minimal response in, cardiac output, arterial pressure, urine output, and mental status after this therapy indicates a need for assisted circulation with IABP therapy. Once hypotension is present, the self-perpetuating process of injury is in effect. Control of further injury and improvement in survival require early reversal of the shock state.

After IABP therapy is instituted, improvement should be observed within 1 to 2 hours. At this time, steady improvement should be seen in cardiac output, peripheral perfusion, urine output, mental status, and pulmonary congestion. Average peak effect should be achieved within 24 to 48 hours.

### Postoperative Low Cardiac Output

The primary indication for use of IABP therapy in the perioperative cardiac surgery patient is low cardiac output refractory to traditional inotropic support.[2] IABP therapy is also used preoperatively in patients who have sustained mechanical injury resulting from AMI as well as those with refractory angina.

IABP counterpulsation therapy can be used to wean patients from cardiopulmonary bypass (CPB) and to provide postoperative circulatory assistance until LV recovery occurs. In these situations, early recognition of failure is evidenced by the heart's inability to support circulation after CPB. Early recognition and treatment are crucial if LV failure is to be reversed.

In addition to providing circulatory assistance, outcomes in cardiac surgery patients have been positively influenced by IABP through other properties as well. For example, the pulsatile blood flow produced by IABP therapy during CPB has been shown to decrease activation of the systemic inflammatory response.[3] IABP therapy has also been associated with optimized microvascular perfusion, leading to improved patient outcomes in high-risk cardiac surgical procedures requiring prolonged CPB.[3]

### Unstable Angina

IABP counterpulsation therapy may be used during PCI for patients with unstable angina or mechanical problems. In this situation, PCI procedures usually are followed by emergency cardiac surgery. Patients in this category include those with unstable angina, postinfarction angina and postinfarction ventricular septal defects, or mitral regurgitation from papillary muscle injury with resultant cardiac failure. IABP counterpulsation therapy has been used successfully to control the severity of angina in patients in whom previous medical therapy has failed. The use of IABP therapy for patients with cardiac failure after ventricular septal rupture or mitral valve incompetence aids in the promotion of forward blood flow, which decreases shunting through the septal defect and decreases the amount of mitral regurgitation.

## Contraindications to IABP Counterpulsation

There are few contraindications to the use of IABP therapy. A competent aortic valve is necessary if the patient is to benefit from IABP therapy. With aortic insufficiency, balloon inflation would only increase aortic regurgitation and offer little, if any, augmentation of coronary artery perfusion pressure. In fact, the patient's HF could be expected to become worse.

Severe peripheral vascular occlusive disease also is a relative contraindication to the use of IABP therapy. Occlusive disease would make insertion of the catheter difficult and possibly interrupt blood flow to the distal extremity or cause dislodgment of plaque formation along the vessel wall, resulting in potential emboli. In patients who absolutely require IABP therapy, insertion can be achieved through the thoracic aorta, thus bypassing diseased peripheral vessels. Any previous aortofemoral or aortoiliac bypass graft contraindicates femoral artery insertion.

In addition, the presence of an aortic aneurysm is a contraindication to the use of IABP therapy. A pulsating balloon against an aneurysm may predispose the patient to dislodgment of aneurysmal debris with resultant emboli. A more serious complication is rupture of the aneurysm; it is possible for the catheter to perforate the wall of the aneurysm during insertion.

## Procedure

### Insertion

Proper positioning of the balloon is in the thoracic aorta just distal to the left subclavian artery and proximal to the renal arteries (Fig. 18-18). The most commonly used method of catheter placement is percutaneous insertion using a Seldinger technique, although other approaches have been described. The most common alternative is direct insertion into the thoracic aorta. Because this requires a median sternotomy incision, it is restricted to cardiac surgical patients whose chests have been opened for the surgery.

Once in place, the catheter is attached to a machine console that has three basic components: a monitoring system, an electronic trigger mechanism, and a drive system that moves gas in and out of the balloon. Monitoring systems have the capability of displaying the patient's ECG and an arterial waveform showing the effect of balloon inflation–deflation. Consoles also are capable of displaying a balloon waveform that illustrates the inflation and deflation of the balloon itself. The standard trigger mechanism for the balloon pump is the R wave that is sensed from the patient's ECG. This trigger signals the beginning of each cardiac cycle

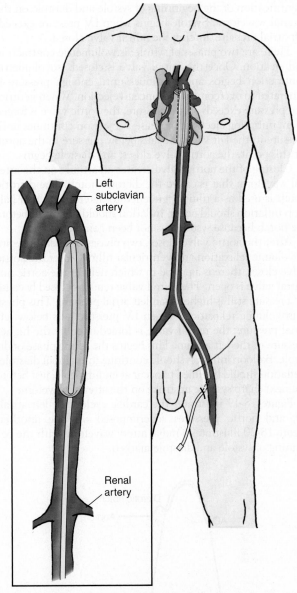

Left subclavian artery

Renal artery

**FIGURE 18-18** Proper position of the balloon catheter; illustrating percutaneous insertion.

for the drive system. Other possible triggers include systolic arterial pressure or pacemaker spikes on the ECG. Adjustment of exact timing is controlled on the machine console. The drive system is the actual mechanism that drives gas into and out of the balloon by alternating pressure and vacuum.

### Timing

Two primary methods of timing can be used with IABP therapy: conventional timing and real timing. Conventional timing uses the arterial waveform as the triggering mechanism to determine both inflation and deflation of the balloon. Real timing uses the same point of reference (the dicrotic notch on the arterial waveform) for balloon inflation but uses the ECG signal as the trigger for balloon deflation. Real timing is discussed briefly after conventional timing.

**CONVENTIONAL TIMING.** The first step to proper timing of the balloon pump using conventional timing is the identification of the beginning of systole and diastole on the arterial waveform. Systole begins when LV pressure exceeds left atrial pressure, forcing the mitral valve closed.

There are two phases of systole: isovolumetric contraction and ejection. Once the mitral valve is closed, isovolumetric contraction begins and continues until enough pressure is generated to overcome impedance to ejection. When ventricular pressure exceeds aortic pressure, the aortic valve is forced open, initiating ejection, or phase 2. Ejection continues until pressure in the left ventricle falls below pressure in the aorta. At this point, the aortic valve closes, and diastole begins.

Closing of the aortic valve creates an artifact on the arterial waveform that is called the dicrotic notch. The dicrotic notch is used as a timing reference to determine when balloon inflation should occur. Inflation should not occur before the notch because systole has not been completed.

After the aortic valve closes, two phases of diastole begin: isovolumic relaxation and ventricular filling. After the aortic valve closes, there is a period in which neither the aortic nor mitral valve is open. The mitral valve remains closed because LV pressure still is higher than left atrial pressure. This phase is isovolumic relaxation. When LV pressure falls below left atrial pressure, the mitral valve is forced open by the higher pressure in the left atrium. This begins the filling phase of diastole. Balloon inflation should continue throughout diastole. Deflation should be timed to occur at end-diastole, just before the next sharp systolic upstroke on the arterial waveform.

Figure 18-19 illustrates the cardiac cycle with left atrial, LV, and aortic pressures superimposed on one another. Figure 18-20 illustrates a radial artery waveform with the beginning of systole and diastole marked.

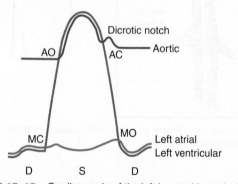

**FIGURE 18-19** Cardiac cycle of the left heart with aortic, left ventricular (LV), and left atrial pressure waveforms. AC, aortic valve closure; AO, aortic valve opening; D, diastole; MC, mitral valve closure; MO, mitral valve opening; S, systole.

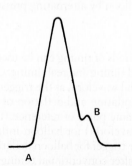

**FIGURE 18-20** Arterial waveform, with *A* representing the point of balloon deflation before the systolic upstroke, and *B* representing balloon inflation at the dicrotic notch, at diastole.

**REAL TIMING.** The main difference between the two timing methods is balloon deflation and the triggering mechanism used. Real timing uses the ECG as the trigger signal for balloon deflation. The QRS complex is recognized as the onset of ventricular systole, and balloon deflation occurs at this time. Triggering off the R wave allows for balloon deflation to occur at the time of systolic ejection and not before (as with conventional timing). This timing mechanism is more effective in patients with irregular heart rhythms because balloon deflation occurs on recognition of the R wave (systolic ejection). It does not need to be approximated by the operator or an algorithm, as in conventional timing. Both a rapid deflation mechanism and a reliable ECG signal are necessary for IABP using real timing to augment blood pressure effectively. Balloon inflation with real timing occurs at the onset of diastole as triggered by the dicrotic notch on an arterial waveform, just as in conventional timing.

Advances in IABP technology have led to the development of automatic timing mechanisms currently available in some IABP models. Automatic timing therapy is possible because of special IABP catheters that have fiber optic pressure sensors in the tip.[2] These pressure sensors, capable of transmitting real-time pressure signals at the speed of light, use Windkessel model algorithms to calculate real-time aortic flow from aortic pressure.[4] This allows the balloon pump to determine the precise time when the aortic valve closes with each contraction of the heart, regardless of the patient's heart rhythm. The closure of the aortic valve signals the onset of diastole, and balloon inflation occurs.

## Interpretation of Results

### Waveform Assessment

Analysis of the arterial pressure waveform and the effectiveness of IABP therapy is an important nursing function. Nurses must be able to recognize and correct problems in balloon pump timing. Figure 18-21 illustrates the five points that are assessed on the waveform.

**STEP 1.** The first step in timing assessment is the ability to recognize the beginnings of systole and diastole on the arterial waveform, as shown in Figure 18-21. Systole begins at point A, where the sharp upstroke begins. Point B marks

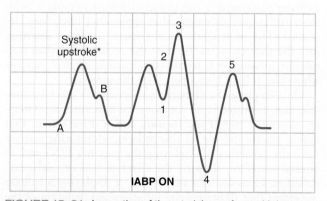

**FIGURE 18-21** Inspection of the arterial waveform with intra-aortic balloon assistance should include observation of (*1*) inflation point, (*2*) inflation slope, (*3*) diastolic peak pressure/diastolic augmentation, (*4*) end-diastolic dip, and (*5*) next systolic peak.

**Criteria for Assessment of Effective IABP Therapy on the Arterial Pressure Waveform**

- Inflation occurs at the dicrotic notch.
- Inflation slope is parallel to the systolic upstroke and is a straight line.
- Diastolic augmentation peak is greater than or equal to the preceding systolic peak.
- An end-diastolic dip in pressure is created with balloon deflation.
- The following systolic peak (assisted systole) is lower than the preceding systole (unassisted systole).

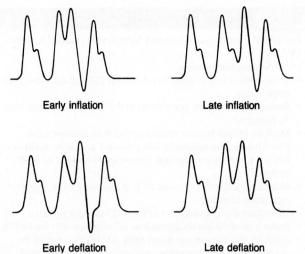

Early inflation            Late inflation

Early deflation            Late deflation

**FIGURE 18-22** Illustration of possible errors occurring with timing.

the dicrotic notch, which represents aortic valve closure. At this point, diastole begins, and the balloon should be inflated. Balloon deflation occurs just before point A, at end-diastole.

Box 18-15 lists five criteria that can be used to measure the effectiveness of IABP therapy on the arterial pressure waveform. To evaluate the waveform effectively, the patient's unassisted pressure tracing must be viewed alongside the assisted pressure tracing. This can be accomplished through adjustment of the console so that the balloon inflates and deflates on every other beat (ie, a 1:2 assist ratio). Most patients tolerate this well for a brief period of time. Machine consoles are capable of freezing the waveform on the console monitor so that it is necessary to assist at a 1:2 ratio only for one screen. Another alternative is to obtain a strip recording of the 1:2 assistance for analysis.

**STEP 2.** After identification of the patient's dicrotic notch, a comparison is made with the assisted tracing to see that inflation occurs at the point of the dicrotic notch. Inflation before the dicrotic notch shortens systole abruptly and increases ventricular volume as ejection is interrupted. Late inflation, past the dicrotic notch, does not raise coronary artery perfusion pressure. The peak-diastolic pressure may not be as high as it would be with proper timing.

**STEP 3.** Next, the slopes of systolic upstroke and diastolic augmentation (also known as diastolic peak pressure) should be compared. The diastolic slope should be sharp and parallel the systolic upstroke, as shown in Figure 18-21. The slope always should be a straight line. The greater the peak in diastolic pressure, the greater the increase in aortic root pressure. For this reason, balloon assistance is adjusted until the highest peak possible is achieved.

**STEP 4.** Deflation should occur just before systole, causing an acute drop in aortic end-diastolic pressure. This quick deflation displaces approximately 40 mL of volume. The result is an end-diastolic dip in pressure that reduces the impedance to the next systolic ejection. The end-diastolic pressure without the balloon assistance should be compared with the end-diastolic pressure with the dip created by balloon deflation. Optimally, a pressure difference of at least 10 mm Hg should be obtained. Better afterload reduction is achieved with the lowest possible end-diastolic dip.

The point of deflation also is crucial. Deflation that is too early allows pressure to rise to normal end-diastolic levels preceding systole. In this situation, there is no decrease in afterload. Deflation that is too late encroaches on the next systole and actually increases afterload because of greater

impedance to ejection from the presence of the still-inflated balloon during systolic ejection. Figure 18-22 demonstrates possible errors in timing.

**STEP 5.** Finally, if afterload has been reduced, the next systolic pressure peak will be lower than the unassisted systolic pressure peak. This implies that the ventricle did not have to generate as great a pressure to overcome impedance to ejection. This may not always be seen because the systolic pressure peak also represents the compliance of the vasculature. If the vasculature is noncompliant due to atherosclerotic disease, the systolic peak may not change very much.

### Balloon Fit

The fit of the balloon to any particular patient's aorta determines how well these criteria are met. Ideally, approximately 80% of the aorta is occluded with balloon inflation. In a dilated aorta, in which less than 80% occlusion occurs, the effect of inflation and deflation is not as dramatic on the waveform. When a patient is hypotensive or hypovolemic, the balloon does not have as pronounced an effect on the waveform because there is less volume displacement as the balloon inflates or deflates.

## Assessment and Management

Patients requiring IABP are managed much like any other critically ill patient in cardiogenic shock or acute LV failure. Nursing assessment and management of these conditions are discussed in Chapter 54. Additional nursing skills and assessment considerations specific to IABP therapy must be included in the care of these patients. These are summarized in Box 18-16.

### Monitoring the Cardiovascular System

Monitoring the cardiovascular system is extremely important in determining the effectiveness of IABP therapy. The basis for this assessment includes vital signs, cardiac output, heart rhythm and regularity, urine output, color, perfusion, and mentation.

---

**BOX 18-16** | **Nursing Interventions**

**For IABP Counterpulsation and Ventricular Assist Devices (VADs)**

**IABP Nursing Interventions**

- Verify correct timing using assist ratio of 1:2 and document settings hourly.
- Reevaluate timing for any change in the heart rate greater than 10 beats/min.
- Maintain proper balloon volume and refill as needed every 2 to 4 hours. Use automatic filling mode if available. Avoid hip flexion, which may impair gas movement in and out of IABP catheter.
- Maintain good arterial waveform and adequate ECG signal for evaluation of timing.
- Transduce aortic arterial line to the IABP per unit protocol.
- Reduce or eliminate situations that will interfere with the IABP's ability to maintain proper assist ratio. Notify physician of the development of tachycardias or irregular rhythms, and treat dysrhythmias with drug therapy or pacing as ordered. Use appropriate trigger (ie, ECG, arterial pressure, pacing).
- Use pacer modes only if the patient is 100% paced.
- Notify physician of significant changes in balloon pressure waveform.

**VAD Nursing Interventions**

- Assess and maintain adequate filling pressures during immediate postoperative phase.
- Monitor and assess heart rate, blood pressure, mean arterial pressure, pump flow, urine output, and neurologic status hourly. Treat changes as ordered.
- Assess and change equipment level for devices that require specific placement of equipment for adequate pump flow.
- Evaluate pump flow and rate of VAD in relation to native heart rate and activity level of patient.
- Manage VAD function and volume status as ordered to maintain adequate device output.

**General Nursing Interventions**

- Monitor and record temperatures every 4 hours and PRN.
- Observe all insertion sites and incisions for signs of infection. Maintain sterile technique with dressing changes.

- Change any dressing that is wet or not intact.
- Change all infusion lines and infusion bags per unit protocol.
- Culture any site with suspicious drainage, redness, or swelling.
- Notify physician of elevation in white blood cell count.
- Treat patient with antibiotics as ordered.
- Auscultate and document breath sounds every 2 to 4 hours.
- Assist patient with pulmonary toilet (ie, coughing, deep breathing, frequent turning). Suction intubated patients as needed.
- Use pulse oximeter to monitor patients with abnormal blood gas levels, excessive secretions, or respiratory difficulty.
- Extubate patient and increase activity level as tolerated—particularly for patients with VADs.
- Document quality of peripheral pulses and neurologic status before IABP or VAD insertion. Assess and document quality of pulses, skin perfusion, and neurologic status per protocol. Evaluate peripheral perfusion with any complaints of leg or foot pain by patient.
- Notify physician of any changes in pulses or neurologic status.
- Maintain anticoagulation as ordered.
- Avoid hip flexion, which might obstruct flow to the affected extremity, by keeping the cannulated leg straight and the bed at angle less than 30 degrees.
- Always maintain balloon motion to avoid thrombus formation on the balloon.
- Assess skin integrity, and document any redness and ulcerations over bony prominences.
- Use sheepskin, foam pads, and specialty beds as needed. Turn patient every 2 hours.
- Ensure that skin remains clean and dry.
- Maintain adequate nutrition by encouraging oral intake or implementing use of parenteral or enteral nutrition when necessary.
- Maintain alarm volumes, monitor noise at lowest level possible, and minimize unnecessary noise in the room.
- Talk with and orient patient to date and time frequently.
- Encourage family visits.
- Explain all procedures and activities to the patient.
- Organize care to allow for periods of uninterrupted sleep. Turn the lights off in room at night if possible.
- Sedate patient if necessary and as tolerated per physician orders.

---

**VITAL SIGNS.** Three important vital signs with respect to IABP therapy are heart rate, MAP, and PAOP. Effective IABP therapy causes a decrease in all three parameters. Acute changes in the MAP may indicate volume depletion. Critically ill patients tolerate little change in their volume status. The PAOP is an important parameter for monitoring volume and provides the clinician with an early indication of volume depletion or overload.

Blood pressure readings require special consideration. Because the balloon inflates during diastole, peak-diastolic pressure may be higher than peak-systolic pressure. Most IABP consoles have monitoring systems capable of distinguishing systole from peak diastole; however, some monitoring equipment can distinguish only peak pressures from low-point pressures. For this reason, a monitor's digital display of systolic pressure actually may represent peak-diastolic pressure. It is advisable to record blood pressure as systolic, peak-diastolic, and end-diastolic, that is, 100/110/60. These pressures can be read from a strip recording of the arterial waveform.

**HEART RHYTHM AND REGULARITY.** Heart rhythm and regularity are important considerations. Early recognition and treatment of dysrhythmias are crucial for effective IABP support. Irregular dysrhythmias may inhibit efficient IABP therapy with some types of consoles because timing is set by the regular R-R interval on the ECG. A safety feature of all balloon pump consoles is automatic deflation of the balloon for premature QRS complexes. If the dysrhythmia persists and timing is ineffective, another alternative might be use of the systolic peak on the arterial waveform as the trigger mechanism for balloon inflation. The primary goal is to treat the dysrhythmia.

**OTHER OBSERVATIONS.** Urine output, color, perfusion, and mentation all are important assessment parameters for determining the adequacy of cardiac output. All should improve in patients responsive to IABP therapy. Any deterioration in these signs also might indicate a fall in cardiac output. Cardiac output measurement is indicated when deterioration is evident, when a major change in volume or pharmacologic therapy has been instituted, and during weaning from IABP support.

The left radial pulse and the cannulated extremity should be frequently assessed. A decrease, absence, or change in character of the left radial pulse may indicate that the balloon has advanced up the aorta and may be partially obstructing or has advanced into the left subclavian artery.

The presence of the balloon catheter in the femoral or iliac artery predisposes the patient to impaired circulation of the involved extremity. The affected extremity needs to be kept relatively immobile. Because flexion of the hip may kink the catheter and impair balloon pumping, it may be helpful to avoid hip flexion. The head of the bed also should not be elevated more than 30 degrees. Hip flexion also contributes to decreased perfusion to the distal extremity. Extremities should be checked hourly for pulses, color, and sensation. Any deterioration in the affected extremity should be reported to the physician. Severe arterial insufficiency necessitates removal of the catheter.

Physicians advocate the use of heparin therapy to prevent possible thrombus formation around the catheter and vascular insufficiency, especially in medical patients. Each physician determines whether the risks of anticoagulation outweigh the benefits for the specific patient. Low-molecular-weight dextran is another possible choice of therapy to prevent thrombus formation. This agent impairs platelet function and prevents triggering of the coagulation cascade. Low-molecular-weight dextran is usually preferred in the cardiac surgical patient for the first 24 hours.

### Monitoring the Pulmonary System

Many patients on IABP therapy require intubation and ventilatory assistance. Some of these patients may have respiratory insufficiency secondary to fluid overload associated with HF. The immobile, intubated patient is always at risk for respiratory infections and the development of atelectasis. Turning the patient is appropriate provided modifications are implemented to keep the extremity cannulated by the balloon catheter straight. Daily chest radiographs are needed to follow pulmonary status and to inspect IV catheter placement. The position of the balloon catheter also can be determined in this manner.

### Monitoring the Renal System

Patients in cardiogenic shock or severe LV failure are at risk for the development of acute renal failure. In the shock state, the kidneys suffer the consequences of hypoperfusion; therefore, urine output and quality should be monitored closely. Serum BUN, creatinine, and creatinine clearance are monitored daily to assess renal function. Creatinine clearance indicates renal dysfunction and possible failure much earlier than elevated serum creatinine. Any acute, dramatic drop in urine output may be an indication that the catheter has slipped down the aorta and is obstructing the renal arteries.

### Weaning

**INDICATIONS FOR WEANING.** Weaning patients from balloon assistance usually can begin 24 to 72 hours after insertion. Some patients require longer periods of support. Weaning can begin when there is evidence of hemodynamic stability that does not require excessive vasopressor support. Ideally, vasopressor support is minimal when weaning begins. After the balloon is removed, it is much easier to increase vasopressor support than to reinsert a balloon catheter for hemodynamic support.

The patient should exhibit signs of adequate cardiac function, demonstrated by good peripheral pulses, adequate urine output, absence of pulmonary edema, and improved mentation. Good coronary artery perfusion is indicated by an absence of ventricular ectopy and no ECG evidence of ischemia or injury.

Complications may require abrupt cessation of IABP. This may or may not result in reinsertion of another balloon catheter. Severe arterial insufficiency, evidenced by a loss of pulses in the distal extremity, pain, and pallor, is definitely an indication to remove the balloon catheter from that particular insertion site. Any balloon that develops a leak also requires removal. The physician may choose to reinsert the balloon catheter in another extremity or to replace the faulty balloon if the patient is hemodynamically unstable. Depending on the philosophy of the institution and physician, a deteriorating, irreversible situation also might be an indication for weaning or discontinuing balloon pump support. Box 18-17 lists major indications for weaning from IABP therapy.

**APPROACHES TO WEANING.** Weaning is commonly achieved by decreasing the assist ratio from 1:1 to 1:2 and so on until the minimal assist ratio is achieved on any particular console. A patient may be assisted at the first decrease for up to 4 to 6 hours. The minimal amount of time should be 30 minutes. During this time, the patient must be assessed for any change in hemodynamic status. An increase in heart rate, a decrease in blood pressure, and a decrease in cardiac output indicate deterioration in hemodynamic status. Weaning should be discontinued temporarily, and therapy should be adjusted before another weaning attempt is made. If the first decrease in assist ratio is tolerated, the assist ratio is decreased to minimum, with 1 to 4

---

**QSEN BOX 18-17** *PATIENT SAFETY*

**Indications for Weaning Patient From IABP**

To ensure patient safety when weaning him or her from IABP, the nurse should be alert for the following:

- Hemodynamic stability
- Cardiac index greater than 2 L/min
- Pulmonary artery occlusion pressure less than 20 mm Hg
- Systolic blood pressure greater than 100 mm Hg
- Minimal requirements for vasopressor support
- Evidence of adequate cardiac function
- Good peripheral pulses
- Adequate urine output
- Absence of pulmonary edema
- Improved mentation
- Evidence of good coronary perfusion
- Absence of ventricular ectopy
- Absence of ischemia on the ECG
- Severe vascular insufficiency
- Deteriorating, irreversible condition

**TABLE 18-4    Injuries Secondary to Balloons**

| Injury | Assessment Findings | Nursing Intervention |
|---|---|---|
| Balloon rupture | Presence of bright red blood or flecks of dried blood in the catheter or helium delivery line<br>Gas alarm sounds<br>Decreased augmentation<br>Signs of embolic event<br>Entrapment (may be the first indication) | Immediate removal of the catheter by the appropriate personnel<br>Before removal:<br>  Turn pump off<br>  Clamp the line<br>  Place the patient on left side in Trendelenburg position |
| Balloon entrapment | Balloon pressure waveform indicates leaks<br>Small amounts of blood in tubing or flecks of dried blood in tubing | Surgical removal is usually indicated<br>Physician may consider pharmacologic dissolution of clot with thrombolytics<br>Physician may consider use of Fogarty embolectomy to remove fresh clot |

hours allowed for each new assist ratio. The patient must be assessed continually for any indications of intolerance to the process. Although less common, weaning can also occur by decreasing balloon volume, which is controlled from the console in many models.

## Complications Specific to IABP Therapy

Patients with IABP counterpulsation need to be monitored for development of poor blood flow to the cannulated extremity, which could lead to compartment syndrome. It may occur within the first 24 hours of support or not until several days after catheter insertion. Compartment syndrome is caused by a rise in the tissue pressure in one of the compartments of the affected lower extremity. Bone, muscle, nerve tissue, and blood vessels all are enclosed by a fibrous membrane called the fascia, and this enclosed space is called a compartment. It is nonyielding, so a rise in volume in the compartment increases the pressure in the compartment. The patient with IABP in whom limb ischemia develops from decreased capillary flow can suffer cellular and capillary damage that leads to increased capillary permeability. The resultant transudation of fluid into the closed compartment space increases tissue pressure to a level that can interfere with capillary blood flow. When this degree of tissue pressure is reached, tissue viability may be threatened. Treatment is directed at improving blood flow. Pressure release by fasciotomy may be needed to prevent tissue death.

Decreased circulating platelets in the first 24 hours of IABP therapy and a minimal decrease in red blood cell count have been reported; however, these problems are not thought to be significant. There is a low incidence of balloon leakage and rupture. These complications may result from balloon inflation against a calcific, atherosclerotic plaque in the aorta. This disruption in the balloon surface may be as small as a pinhole or may be a large tear. The associated danger is gas embolism. In addition, the risk for entrapment is minimal but still exists. Table 18-4 provides additional details about injury secondary to balloons.

Insertion of the catheter in cases of severe atherosclerotic vascular disease may result in arterial perforation or occlusion. Any leak is an indication for immediate balloon removal. Iatrogenic dissection of the aorta is rare but has been reported. Arterial insufficiency is the most common complication of IABP therapy. Arterial insufficiency may be

permanent, or it may be relieved by aortofemoral or ileofemoral bypass grafting. Neuropathy in the catheterized extremity is another reported complication.

## Mechanical Circulatory Support

When there is profound myocardial injury, the augmentation of systemic blood pressure by IABP counterpulsation may not be adequate for patient survival. Use of IABP for circulatory support requires that a patient have a functioning left ventricle because IABP augments cardiac output only by 8% to 10%. Patients with severe, acute LV failure after a MI, after a surgical procedure, or from end-stage HF may need a mechanism for replacing LV function. Circulatory support with a ventricular assist device (VAD) has become a successful treatment for patients with cardiac failure refractory to pharmacologic therapies, revascularization procedures, and IABP counterpulsation. These devices are capable of supporting circulation until the heart recovers or a donor heart is obtained for transplantation.

Interest in the research and development of artificial circulatory support devices has existed since the 1930s. Current research focuses on the use of these devices as a bridge to heart transplantation and as a method of permanent cardiac support for patients with end-stage cardiac disease.

## Physiologic Principles

Patients who are candidates for ventricular assistance suffer from HF resulting from ischemic or myopathic heart disease. Both disease processes lead to a reduction in cardiac output and oxygen delivery. The physiologic response of the body to this low output state is vasoconstriction and increased SVR. Although these compensatory mechanisms are meant to protect and preserve cardiovascular function in the short term, a vicious cycle develops that is characterized by compromised cardiac contractility and a low ventricular EF. Hypotension ensues, leading to hemodynamic instability requiring the use of pharmacologic agents and possibly IABP therapy for cardiovascular support. Should the patient continue to deteriorate despite drug therapy and IABP, a VAD may be necessary for survival. Hemodynamically, these patients usually demonstrate a cardiac index of less than 2 L/min/m$^2$, a PAOP of greater than 20 mm Hg, and a systolic blood pressure of less than 80 mm Hg despite pharmacologic therapies and the use of IABP counterpulsation.

Restoration of adequate blood flow and preservation of end-organ function are the fundamental goals of short- or long-term VAD use. Hemodynamics and perfusion improve as the VAD assumes the workload of the failing ventricle. Ventricular assistance may involve supporting one or both ventricles depending on the extent of myocardial damage and ventricular failure.

LV support usually requires cannulation of the left ventricle with a conduit that leads to the device. The ascending aorta, which receives the output from the device, is also cannulated with a conduit. In certain situations, the left atrium may be cannulated instead of the left ventricle. Circulation in the patient supported by a left ventricular assist device (LVAD) is similar to the normal circulatory process. Venous blood returns to the right heart, passes through the lungs to be oxygenated, and then returns to the left atrium through the pulmonary veins. Blood then passes from the left atrium through the left ventricle and into the LVAD. The LVAD then ejects blood into the ascending aorta during pump systole.

In situations that necessitate biventricular support, two pump units function in synchrony to assume the roles of the native right and left ventricles. One pump supports right heart circulation while the other supports left heart circulation. The addition of RV assistance requires cannulation of the right atrium for inflow to the pump and the pulmonary artery for outflow from the right ventricular assist device (RVAD). During biventricular assistance, blood is diverted from the right atrium to the lungs through the RVAD, bypassing the right ventricle. Circulation continues to the left heart, where the LVAD undertakes support of systemic circulation. Univentricular or biventricular assistance relieves the ventricles of its workload by acting as the primary pump supporting pulmonary circulation or systemic blood pressure. Reducing ventricular workload decreases cardiac oxygen demand.

## Devices

Several VADs are available for use. Certain devices are commercially available, whereas others require special exemption for investigational purposes. Although no universal classification system exists, the devices can be categorized according to four general functional characteristics: the intended duration of support (short term vs. long term), the type of support provided (univentricular vs. biventricular), the actual physical placement of the device (internal vs. external), and the type of blood flow produced (pulsatile vs. nonpulsatile). Short-term support usually refers to assistance for patients expected to recover from episodes of acute LV failure secondary to MI or surgical procedures. Long-term ventricular assistance may be an option for people awaiting heart transplantation, or it may provide an alternative method of permanent cardiac support.

### Nonpulsatile Pumps

Centrifugal and roller pumps are examples of nonpulsatile VADs capable of providing univentricular (to either ventricle) or biventricular support. Centrifugal pumps introduce blood near the center of a rapidly spinning disk that accelerates blood toward the periphery of the disk. They are primarily used for short-term ventricular assistance when myocardial recovery is expected. These devices have been used, infrequently, as bridges to transplantation. Both types are approved by the FDA and are commercially available. Centrifugal and roller pumps are extracorporeal devices designed to support circulation of the patient's blood. Because these devices do not generate pulsatile blood flow, IABP is often used in conjunction with them to create a pulse. Blood is transported from the cannulated chamber to an external pump console that circulates the blood back to the corresponding great vessel by a separate cannula. Should right ventricular failure (RVF) be identified after placement of an LVAD, an RVAD can be added for additional support with these devices.

These devices can be inserted relatively quickly and are adequate methods of deploying short-term circulatory assistance. Methods of cannulation and physical placement of the equipment limit the mobility and activity level of the patient. Patients supported by these VADs are usually sedated and paralyzed. A commonly used centrifugal pump is the Centrimag (Thoratec).

Axial pumps, another type of nonpulsatile pump, use corkscrew-type impellers that propel blood by rapid rotation. These pumps are much more compact than centrifugal pumps and can be used short or long term.[5] In addition, they weigh less than centrifugal pumps, are more compact, and therefore are more comfortable for patients.

Extracorporeal membrane oxygenation (ECMO) or CPB systems are alternative methods of temporary CPR involving circulatory support and oxygenation of the patient's blood. CPB is primarily used for operative situations but has demonstrated effectiveness as a mechanism of support for patients unable to wean from the pump perioperatively or for those requiring cardiopulmonary support refractory to conventional efforts. Circulation of blood between the patient and an external pump is supported by cannulation of the femoral vessels. Venous blood is diverted from central venous circulation; pumped through a membrane oxygenator, where oxygen and carbon dioxide are exchanged; and returned to the arterial circulation through the femoral artery cannula. A heating mechanism in the pump console helps maintain body temperature during circulatory support.

Rapid deployment without the need for surgical intervention and the ability to provide hemodynamic stabilization for a brief period are the major advantages of these resuscitative devices. CPB and ECMO allow time for further assessment and intervention during episodes of acute hemodynamic decompensation. Disadvantages include the need for continuous anticoagulation and the inability to provide extended circulatory support. The presence of occlusive peripheral vascular disease could be a contraindication to use of these devices.

### Pulsatile Pumps

**IMPLANTABLE PULSATILE PUMPS.** Implantable pumps were designed with the intention of providing long-term LV support while allowing the patient a certain amount of physical independence. A few devices have successfully supported a patient for greater than 1 year while awaiting heart transplantation. Many patients with the implantable devices have been physically rehabilitated by participating in regular physical therapy programs and normal activities of daily living while being supported with a VAD. This might better prepare them physically to endure the transplantation process.

Surgical implantation of the VAD necessitates a sternotomy and the use of CPB. Device placement is in an abdominal pocket just below the left diaphragm. Typically, the inflow conduit is tunneled through the diaphragm and anastomosed to the apex of the left ventricle. The outflow conduit is brought around the diaphragm and is anastomosed to the ascending aorta. Drivelines extending from the implanted device are tunneled through the patient's skin and connected to a portable, external power source. This power source may be a portable console or battery pack that is worn by the patient (Fig. 18-23).

Pump units of the implantable VADs are encapsulated in rigid housing and consist of a blood pump sac and single or dual pusher plates (depending on the particular device). Inflow and outflow conduits have valves that support unidirectional blood flow. These devices work on the principle of converting electrical or pneumatic energy to mechanical energy. This mechanical energy activates the pusher plates, causing them to compress the blood sac at the appropriate time. Blood sac compression causes ejection of the blood out of the pump sac and into the ascending aorta through the outflow conduit. These devices have stroke volumes of 70 to 83 mL and can support pump outputs of greater than 10 L/min.

**EXTERNAL PULSATILE PUMPS.** Two commonly used external pulsatile devices are the Thoratec VAD and the Abiomed pump. Both devices have successfully supported patients postcardiotomy and patients bridged to heart transplantation.

The Thoratec VAD is a pneumatically driven device that is positioned externally on the recipient's upper abdomen. Placement of this device requires a sternotomy incision and use of CPB. The structure of the pump drive, the inflow and outflow conduits, and the cannulation techniques of the chambers and great vessels are all similar to that of the implantable devices. A major difference is that the cannulas supporting the blood flow pass through the patient's chest wall to the externally positioned pump. One advantage of this device is the ability to provide univentricular or biventricular support, depending on the extent of HF. Figure 18-24 is an example of biventricular support. Another advantage is that due to its external placement, small patient body size is less of a contraindication when considering the need for ventricular assistance.

Another external VAD, the Abiomed pump, is designed for short-term univentricular or biventricular support. It has been used in patients when myocardial recovery is expected and as a bridge to transplantation. Components consist of cannulas for venous and arterial access, blood pumps to support unidirectional blood flow and systemic circulation, and a pneumatically driven console that provides the power source. Cannulation sites for this device are either atria, the pulmonary artery, and the ascending aorta. Filling of the blood pumps occurs passively by gravity; therefore, the blood pumps must be positioned securely below the level of the heart to promote adequate blood flow into their chambers (Fig. 18-25). A disadvantage of this device is that it significantly impairs patient mobility.

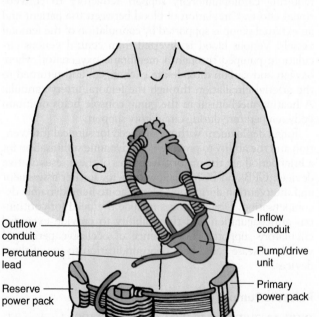

Outflow conduit
Percutaneous lead
Reserve power pack
Compact controller
Inflow conduit
Pump/drive unit
Primary power pack

**FIGURE 18-23** Portable, implantable LV assist device. (Artwork courtesy of the Novacor Division, Baxter Healthcare Corporation, Oakland, CA.)

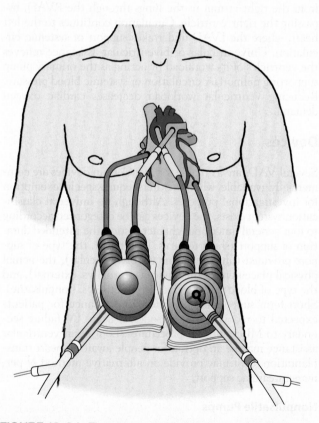

**FIGURE 18-24** Thoratec pneumatic ventricular assist device. External placement with biventricular assist capabilities. (Courtesy of Kathy J. Vaca, RN, Department of Surgery, St. Louis Health Sciences Center, St. Louis, MO.)

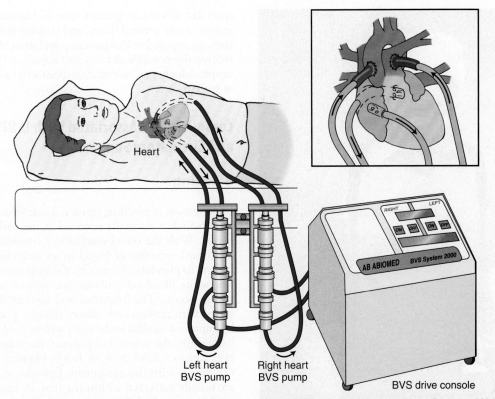

FIGURE 18-25 Abiomed biventricular support system. (Artwork courtesy of ABIOMED Cardiovascular, Inc., Danvers, MA.)

**ADVANCES IN MECHANICAL CIRCULATORY SUPPORT.** There have been many advances in mechanical circulatory support in the last decade. Advances in VAD technology have been introduced through third-generation devices that use rotary pumps to create a centrifugal flow with the help of magnetically levitated propellers. The use of magnetic bearings over traditional blood-coated bearings has positive effects including extended operating life, improved reliability, and decreased blood damage.[6] An example of this type of device is the HVAD (HeartWare).

Another recent advance in mechanical circulatory support has been the introduction of very small pumps that can be incorporated into a transvascular catheter. Major surgical procedures are required for implantation of all other models of VADs, whereas catheter-based LVADs can be placed percutaneously. Several such devices have been developed, including the Tandem Heart LVAD, which is an extracorporeal centrifugal LVAD.

Artificial hearts have been approved in the United States by the FDA for investigational use. Abiomed has developed the first fully implantable replacement heart known as the AbioCor TAH (totally artificial heart). Devices such as the AbioCor are designed for use in patients ineligible to receive a VAD, such as those with both right- and left-sided HF. The AbioCor received Humanitarian Device Exemption from the FDA in September of 2006. In addition, SynCardia Systems has developed the CardioWest device, which is an implantable pneumatic artificial heart. Blood and air in each of the heart's ventricles are separated by a polyurethane sheath and triggered by compressed air from the external console.[6]

Whereas the AbioCor is a self-contained device, the CardioWest device is designed such that patients are connected to a large console by tubes through their chest wall.

**MODES OF OPERATION.** With the exception of the Abiomed device, the pulsatile pumps have several modes of operation. Two primary modes depend on the patient's ECG or the rate of blood flow through the pump during each cardiac cycle. In the ECG trigger mode, the pump initiates blood ejection in conjunction with the patient's QRS complex; the R wave acts as the trigger for pump systole. The second mode is a dynamic mode that allows the pump to respond to the changing heart rate, depending on patient activity level. Pump systole and cardiac output depend on the blood flow sensed by the device, which is programmed to respond to changes in pump filling rate as blood passes from the left ventricle into the blood sac of the pump drive. This ability is particularly important as a patient's level of activity increases during the recovery phase after implantation. A third mode of operation, rarely used clinically, is a fixed-rate mode that functions independently of the native heart.

### Nursing Implications

Historically, VAD recipients have received care in the ICU, usually intubated and sedated. Evolution of the technology and the use of portable devices as bridges to transplantation have changed the mode of care. Now, patients are encouraged to be independent, pursue physical rehabilitation, and engage in normal activities of daily living when possible (Fig. 18-26). Certain patients may even be discharged from the hospital. Nurses have an opportunity to be instrumental in the coordination of patient care and outcome management in this new patient population.

During the immediate postoperative phase, the critical care nurse must be cognizant of the physiologic responses expected and the common postoperative complications

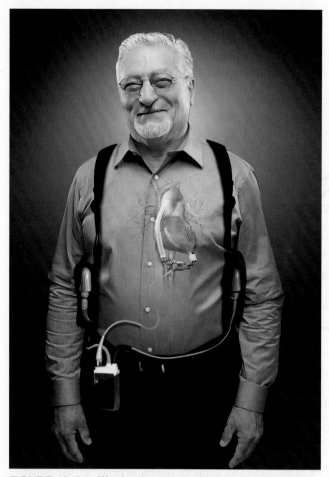

FIGURE 18-26 Wearing the portable LV assist system, a patient is able to enjoy the independence of outdoor activities. Some patients may take day trips or be discharged from the hospital. (Heart-Matell and St. Jude Medical are trademarks of St. Jude Medical, Inc. or its related companies. Reprinted with permission of St. Jude Medical, ©2016. All rights reserved.)

associated with device implantation. The nurse determines whether the equipment is functioning appropriately by monitoring parameters associated with adequate tissue perfusion and improved end-organ function because these are the primary goals of VAD implantation. Hemodynamic instability and the maintenance of adequate filling pressures are critical issues in the immediate postoperative period. Other issues the critical care nurse encounters include, but are not limited to, dysrhythmias, bleeding complications, infections, thromboembolic events, and possible mechanical problems associated with the devices.

As patients are discharged, they and their primary care givers need to be educated about the operation of the equipment and how to troubleshoot malfunctions. A person capable of operating the VAD needs to accompany the patient at all times. Nursing care must facilitate the integration of the patient's lifestyle with the boundaries created by having a VAD implanted for extended support.

An advanced practice nurse is in a pivotal position to assume the role of case manager facilitating the implementation of clinical paths, protocols, and procedures related to patient progress from the acute to chronic phases of rehabilitation. Nursing education facilitated by a clinical nurse specialist is vital to patient care as increasing numbers of nurses on the general floors, and possibly the outpatient setting, are exposed to this patient population. As more patients receive the portable devices and approach the possibility of hospital discharge, case management will be a principal facet of patient care.

## Complications Associated With IABP Therapy and Circulatory Support

### Bleeding

Prolongation of bleeding times is a side effect of exposure to CPB, which is normally reversed in the early postoperative period. With the use of mechanical circulatory support, the continued exposure of blood to an artificial surface causes trauma to platelets. A cascade of events involving the platelets, white blood cells, fibrinolytic system, and complement system occurs. The frequency and severity of bleeding associated with artificial circulatory devices have been reduced by improved surgical techniques and methods of maintaining hemostasis, the reversal of heparin, the infusion of coagulation factors (platelets, fresh frozen plasma), and continued experience with the equipment. Episodes of severe bleeding are usually corrected within the first 24 hours after surgical implantation of a VAD.

Factors associated with increased postoperative bleeding in VAD recipients are preoperative and postoperative use of anticoagulants; coagulopathies secondary to cardiogenic shock, HF, and extended CPB exposure; and the use of multiple cannulation sites. Hemodynamic instability, a reduction in native cardiac output and device output, a risk for ischemia to target organs, and possible cardiac tamponade are all deleterious events associated with uncontrolled bleeding in the patient supported with a VAD. In the patient receiving IABP therapy, bleeding is usually related to use of continuous anticoagulation or the development of coagulopathies. Bleeding commonly occurs at the insertion site of the balloon catheter. In both patient populations, nursing interventions include observing external cannulation sites for oozing, monitoring changes in vital signs (particularly hemodynamic parameters, such as filling pressures for VAD recipients) and laboratory values, and regularly assessing adequate tissue perfusion.

### Thromboembolic Events

Placement of IABP puts a patient at risk for thromboembolic events. At the time of insertion, plaque may become dislodged from the vessel wall, or emboli may break off a thrombus that has formed on the indwelling catheter or balloon. Both situations can impair circulation to distal extremities and other vital organs or cause a stroke. Continuous anticoagulation with a heparin infusion is required during IABP therapy; dextran infusions may also be used.

The development of a thrombus and the migration of emboli have been reported with the use of mechanical circulatory support. Anticoagulation regimens and the prevention of embolic events are unresolved issues in the clinical management of VAD recipients. Currently, anticoagulation therapy is managed differently depending on the device that is inserted. Devices used for short-term support require prophylactic use of low-dose heparin infusions. Similar to IABP, dextran infusions may be used in conjunction with heparin. Patients who are supported with the Novacor, HeartMate, and Thoratec devices and who require long-term support are at greater risk secondary to extended periods of exposure to the device. These patients are usually managed with heparin infusions in the immediate postoperative phase. During the extended support period, the heparin is weaned, and warfarin (Coumadin) therapy is initiated to maintain the PT at an INR median range of 2.0 to 2.5.[7] Antiplatelet agents, such as dipyridamole (Persantine), may be used with warfarin therapy. Obtaining baseline and postimplantation neurologic assessments; monitoring peripheral pulses, especially those distal to cannulation sites; and assessing tissue perfusion are critical to the early recognition and intervention of any embolic event.

## Right Ventricular Failure

RVF is a significant contributor to morbidity and mortality in patients who have undergone LVAD placement. In an effort to detect risk for RVF in patients who are candidates for LVAD placement, researchers at the University of Michigan have developed a preoperative risk assessment instrument.[9] The risk score is calculated using preexisting clinical data and has been scientifically proven to effectively stratify the risk of RVF and death after LVAD implantation.[9]

RVF becomes a problem for patients with LVADs when the pumping capabilities of the device exceed those of the impaired left ventricle, systemic circulation and RV preload increase, subsequently increasing RV workload. RV output is increased in a patient with a healthy right ventricle. However, a patient with underlying RVF may not be able to handle this augmentation in circulatory volume. Evidence of primary RV dysfunction may not become apparent until the right heart is challenged by the cardiac output of the LVAD. When RVF develops after LVAD implantation, vasodilators and IV inotropes, such as prostaglandin E₁, isoproterenol (Isuprel), and epinephrine, are used to reduce pulmonary pressures and improve RV contractility. It may be possible to add an RVAD for additional support if pharmacologic intervention is unsuccessful. Clinical practice has shown that the addition of an RVAD after LVAD placement is a poor prognostic indicator.[9]

## Infection

People requiring mechanical circulatory assistance and IABP therapy are at increased risk for infection secondary to the surgical procedures and the presence of external cannulas, pumps, drivelines, and so forth. Many of these patients suffer from chronic illness that renders them more immunocompromised. Infection may be related to surgical wounds after device insertion, invasive monitoring lines, drain placement, pulmonary status, or nutritional status. Early recognition of signs and symptoms of infection and early intervention can prevent the development of sepsis. Early detection is particularly important because some of these patients await heart transplantation, and an infection could preclude

transplantation. Diligent handwashing, changing or removing invasive lines or drainage tubes when appropriate, adherence to sterile dressing techniques and schedules, and the use of appropriate prophylactic antibiotics are effective barriers to the development of infection. Early extubation and mobilization are goals for patients with the implanted devices. Primary nursing interventions include monitoring invasive sites for signs of infection, encouraging good pulmonary toilet, increasing activity level as tolerated, and promoting adequate nutrition.

## Dysrhythmias

Most patients with cardiomyopathy who require some form of circulatory assistance experience dysrhythmias before insertion of a device. These dysrhythmias often continue after device implantation and may hinder device function, depending on the rhythm. Dysrhythmias should be treated when they occur, and attempts should be made to restore sinus rhythm.

Circulatory assistance with IABP is affected by dysrhythmias. Diastolic augmentation and systolic assistance decrease in the presence of irregular rhythms, such as AF or sinus rhythm with frequent ectopy. These rhythm changes make it difficult to manage the timing of balloon inflation and deflation. Lethal ventricular dysrhythmias need to be treated conventionally because IABP is designed only to augment existing cardiac output.

RV function and the maintenance of adequate pump output are of primary concern in LVAD recipients with lethal ventricular dysrhythmias. These patients may lack sufficient RV function to support cardiac output during ventricular dysrhythmia even though LV function has been assumed by the LVAD. Although LVAD flow and mean blood pressure have been known to decrease by approximately 20%, it has been demonstrated that patients with LVADs do tolerate sustained lethal ventricular dysrhythmias without the need for RVAD support. Symptoms associated with these rhythms and low-flow states are usually weakness and palpitations. Patients receiving biventricular support should be able to maintain adequate device outputs despite the dysrhythmia because left and RV function has been taken over by the VAD. AF is usually tolerated by these patients even though it may have some effect on right heart function. Severe bradycardia and tachydysrhythmia need to be addressed because they will change pump flow and output. Cardiac rhythms require close monitoring for any acute changes.

## Nutritional Deficits

Nutritional status is an important element of any recovery process. Many patients have had end-stage HF and are nutritionally depleted before any surgical intervention, placing them at a higher risk for nutritional deficits during the postoperative phase. Adequate nutrition is necessary for wound healing. Obtaining dietary consultation, encouraging increased oral intake, and providing flexibility with meals will assist these patients in meeting their nutritional goals. Patients who are supported by IABP and VADs and who require intubation and sedation require parenteral or enteral feedings. Those with implanted devices eventually progress to a regular diet but may need smaller, more frequent meals. Experiencing feelings of fullness or early satiety is not uncommon for these patients due to the abdominal placement of the device.

## Psychosocial Factors

Balloon and VAD insertion are usually unplanned, emergent interventions for a deteriorating condition. Abundant monitoring is frightening for both patient and family; therefore, explanations of procedures and surroundings are very important. Family members need to be prepared before visiting their loved one immediately after device insertion. The goal is to alleviate anxiety and to help the patient and family feel more secure in a foreign environment. Honest communication helps family members recognize changes in their loved one's condition and make informed, realistic decisions regarding the patient's care. Putting the family in contact with nonmedical personnel who can objectively provide emotional support is often beneficial. Issues that families and patients struggle with include fear, hopelessness, and death.

Critically ill patients often suffer from disorientation and sleep deprivation. Immobility and unfamiliar noises of the ICU tend to increase stress and anxiety. Mechanisms to help alleviate this stress and anxiety include frequent reorientation by the nursing staff and contact with family members. Better organization of time and procedures also reduces stress because it allows the patient longer periods of uninterrupted rest.

Psychosocial issues and patient education dominate the nursing focus during periods of extended support with a VAD; most of these patients require minimal direct nursing care once stabilized and discharged from the ICU. Increased independence in activities of daily living, continued physical rehabilitation, and patient education are emphasized. All aspects of the rehabilitation phase should include the recipient's family members or identified support person. In addition, feelings of isolation may unfold because investigational device protocols governed by the FDA may restrict the patient's social activity and geographical mobility.

---

## MANAGEMENT OF DYSRHYTHMIAS

## Electrical Cardioversion

Electrical cardioversion is used to convert sustained supraventricular tachycardia (including atrial fibrillation and atrial flutter) or ventricular tachycardia (with a pulse) to sinus rhythm, especially when the arrhythmia causes hemodynamic

**TABLE 18-5** Indications and Energy Requirements for Cardioversion

| Indications | Energy in Joules (J) Monophasic Waveform |
|---|---|
| Monomorphic VT with a pulse | 100–360 |
| Atrial flutter | 50 initially |
| Atrial fibrillation | 200 initially (monophasic) 120–200 (biphasic) |

collapse. It may be used electively for recent-onset dysrhythmias that do not respond to antiarrhythmic drugs. As opposed to defibrillation, which delivers an unsynchronized current to the heart, cardioversion delivers a shock that is synchronized with the heart's activity. By setting the defibrillator to the synchronized mode, the device detects the patient's R wave and delivers the shock during ventricular depolarization. As a result, there is no danger of causing VF, which can occur when a shock is delivered during ventricular repolarization (on the T wave). Indications for synchronized, external cardioversion and recommendations for initial joules (J) used are listed in Table 18-5.[1,2] Precautions and relative contraindications for cardioversion are listed in Table 18-6.

The energy needed to convert monomorphic VT with a pulse may be as low as 100 J initially, followed by 200, 300, or 360 J, as necessary for conversion.[1,2] The energy required for conversion of atrial flutter 50 to 100.[1,2] The energy required to convert AF is greater, starting at 120 to 200 J biphasic or 200 J monophasic.[1,2] After conversion to sinus rhythm, antiarrhythmic therapy may be initiated for rhythm maintenance. Although recommendations are made for the amount of joules needed to convert various rhythms, the actual energy needed may vary depending on the duration of the dysrhythmia, transthoracic impedance, and the waveform morphology of the defibrillator (ie, monophasic vs. biphasic).[2]

## Steps for Cardioversion

1. Explain the procedure to the patient and obtain informed consent.
2. Restrict the patient's food and water for 6 to 8 hours before cardioversion, unless emergency cardioversion is required.
3. If cardioversion of atrial fibrillation or atrial flutter that has been persistent over 48 hours or of unknown duration, ensure that intra-atrial clot has been excluded with either 3 weekly therapeutic INRs, patient compliance of NOACs (Novel Oral Anticoagulants, ie, dabigatran, rivaroxaban, or apixaban) for 3 weeks, or TEE.[3]

**TABLE 18-6** Precautions/Relative Contraindications to Cardioversion

| Condition | Complications |
|---|---|
| Digitalis toxicity | Ventricular irritability, asystole |
| Electrolyte abnormalities (ie hyperkalemia, hypokalemia, hypomagnesemia) | Ventricular irritability/fibrillation |
| AF with slow ventricular response | Postcardioversion bradycardia, asystole |
| AF of unknown duration with inadequate anticoagulation | Thromboembolization |
| Pacemaker dependency | Rise in thresholds with loss of capture |
| Low-amplitude R wave | Synchronization on T wave leading to ventricular fibrillation |

4. If the patient is on chronic digitalis, confirm that digoxin levels are therapeutic. Patients with digitalis toxicity should not undergo elective cardioversion until levels are normalized.

5. Record a 12-lead ECG and vital signs, establish an IV line, monitor blood oxygen saturation levels, and ready all necessary resuscitation equipment.

6. Evaluate potassium and magnesium levels and supplement as needed.

7. Turn on the defibrillator and monitor, and attach the monitoring electrodes to the patient's chest. Avoid placing the electrodes in the area where the defibrillation paddles will be positioned. Some devices permit both monitoring and defibrillation through disposable defibrillation patches.

8. Select a monitoring lead that provides a good ECG pattern with a tall R wave. If monitoring by way of the disposable defibrillator patches, select "paddles" lead.

9. Turn on the synchronizer mode button. The size of the R wave or the monitored lead may need to be adjusted until the synchronization marker appears on each R wave.

10. Sedate the patient, and maintain an adequate airway.

11. Remove paddles from the defibrillator and apply a generous amount of electrode gel to the metal surface. Take care not to smear electrode gel between the two paddles on the chest. Disposable pregelled defibrillator patches may be selected rather than standard paddles.
   a. If hands-free gel patches are used, disconnect the paddles from the defibrillator and connect the terminal pin of the patches to the defibrillator using an adaptor. Place the sternum patch to the right of the sternum, just below the clavicle, and the apex patch below the anterior/axillary margin of the left chest. Apply each patch firmly from the center to the periphery, ensuring that there are no air pockets, which can cause electrical arcing and skin burns.
   b. If using paddles, apply firmly, one just below the right clavicle and the other over the apex of the heart. Make sure paddles or patches are away from electrode wires or from an implanted pacemaker or ICD generator.

12. Set the desired energy level.

13. Press the charge button. A light will flash until paddles are fully charged.

14. Reconfirm the synchronization markers on the R waves on the monitor.

15. Call out "clear" and visually check to make sure no one is touching the patient or the bed.

16. While applying 25 lb of firm pressure on the paddles, push and hold both paddle discharge buttons until the defibrillator discharges. Maintain contact on the chest wall until the machine has delivered the shock. There will be a momentary delay from the pressing of the discharge button to delivery of the shock because of the synchronization with the R wave. Failure to keep the paddles on the chest can result in failure to cardiovert and burns to the chest.

17. Assess the patient's rhythm, airway, and vital signs.

18. Subsequent shocks may need to be delivered. If so, be certain to select the synchronized mode.

19. If the patient's rhythm deteriorates to VF, turn off the synchronizer and immediately defibrillate the patient, starting with 200 J and increasing to 360 J as needed.

20. After cardioversion, observe the patient for changes in rhythm, blood pressure, and respirations. Patients with AF converting with sinus pauses may have underlying tachy–brady syndrome. Be prepared for transcutaneous pacing if needed, or have atropine sulfate readily available. If a patient has a pacemaker, the pacemaker may need to be interrogated or reprogrammed because a temporary rise in capture thresholds may follow cardioversion. Older pacemaker models may revert to a reset or backup mode.

21. Antiarrhythmic agents may need to be initiated to maintain sinus rhythm if patient not already on prior to the cardioversion.

22. Monitor the patient's respiratory status and level of consciousness because sedation was delivered before the procedure. Inspect the chest wall for any signs of burns and treat appropriately.

23. Document the procedure, the outcomes of the procedure, and the patient's status in the medical record.

## Catheter Ablation

Catheter ablation is an invasive procedure used for treating tachydysrhythmias. Prior to consideration of catheter ablation, assessment of the procedural risks and outcomes relevant to the individual patient is recommended. The technique involves percutaneously inserting a catheter into the heart via a vein or artery, and applying radiofrequency or cryoablation. Delivery of the catheter electrode tip to targeted areas responsible for initiating or conducting the dysrhythmia limits the tissue damage.

Clinical use of catheter ablation of cardiac tissue started in the early 1980s with direct current shocks delivered through a catheter attached to a defibrillator. Because this technique was associated with significant risk, safer means to ablate tissue were investigated.

Radiofrequency energy, the primary source of energy used to ablate cardiac tissue, is produced by alternating current (AC) delivered at 500 kHz through the tip of the catheter in unipolar fashion. The circuit is completed through a grounding pad applied on the patient's skin. Resistive heat is created as the energy dissipates around the active electrode, which results in a small localized lesion in cardiac tissue. Tissue temperatures of 50°C or higher lead to irreversible tissue injury. If properly targeted, this localized area of damage can prevent the initiation of the dysrhythmia (the "focus") or interrupt the conduction (the "accessory pathway") of the dysrhythmia. The size of the resulting lesion depends on the electrode temperature, power delivered, and duration of the AC used. When tissue temperature exceeds 100°C, formation of coagulum and char at the electrode tissue interface prevents further energy delivery and adds the risk for steam venting to the endocardial tissue, possibly causing perforation. Electrode cooling (eg, through saline irrigation) reduces the risk for overheating and allows for larger lesion size delivered by higher power. The size, shape, and electrode material of the ablating catheter also influence the resulting lesion.[4]

## Indications for Ablation

Both atrial (AF, atrial flutter, PSVT) and ventricular arrhythmias (VT, PVCs) can be treated with radiofrequency ablation.

Most PSVTs are caused by either atrioventricular nodal reentrant tachycardia (AVNRT) or by atrioventricular reentrant tachycardia (AVRT). PSVT also can be caused by intra-atrial reentrant tachycardia. Recurrent symptomatic or life-threatening ventricular dysrhythmias also may be indications for ablation. Indications for catheter ablation procedures are included in the AHA and Heart Rhythm Society policy statement on catheter ablation.[5]

The most common mechanism for SVT is reentry which occurs when conduction of an impulse through myocardial tissue is initially blocked (or functionally refractory, unresponsive to stimuli) in one direction. The advancing wave front proceeds through an alternate slower route. As the previously refractory pathway recovers, the electrical impulses return through that pathway and then find their way back down to the alternate slower route. As a result, a circuitous reentrant pattern of conduction occurs.

### Atrioventricular Nodal Reentrant Tachycardia

The compact AV node can utilize two functional pathways for conduction—slow and fast—setting the stage for AVNRT. When this phenomenon is observed in the electrophysiology (EP) laboratory, the AV node is described as having dual physiology. AVNRT, the most common type of PSVT, occurs when an AV node with dual physiology is stimulated by a premature atrial contraction. The fast pathway, which is preferentially used in normal sinus rhythm, has not recovered, so the impulse travels down the slow pathway and activates the ventricles. On surface ECG, this initiating rhythm would be viewed as a premature atrial contraction with a long PR interval. The impulse then returns back up to the atria from the ventricles through the fast pathway, which has now recovered excitability, then back down again to the ventricles through the slow pathway, causing the reentrant circuit to perpetuate. Selective ablation of the slow pathway is the preferred method of treating AVNRT. The fast-pathway ablation sites are closer to the compact AV node, and ablation of the fast pathway may be complicated by high-grade AV block.

### Atrioventricular Reentrant Tachycardia

In the normal heart, the AV node and the bundle of His serve as the connection between the atria and the ventricles for the conducting system. AVRT rhythms are characterized by the presence of additional accessory pathways that link conduction between the atria and the ventricles. Conduction through accessory pathways may start from the atria to the ventricles (antegrade conduction), from the ventricles to the atria (retrograde conduction), or in both directions. AVRT rhythms result when circular movement of the impulse occurs because of the ability of the accessory pathways to conduct signals in either direction.

In WPW syndrome, an electrocardiographic pattern associated with PSVT and sometimes associated with Ebstein's anomaly of the tricuspid valve, the person has one or more anomalous conduction accessory pathways linking the atria and the ventricles. Because of these accessory pathways, the person with WPW syndrome is prone to AVRT and AF with rapid ventricular response. When rapidly conducting, these PSVTs may deteriorate into VF. Ablation of the accessory pathways is used to interrupt the rapid limb of the reentrant circuit and eliminate the offending dysrhythmias.

### Atrial Fibrillation or Flutter

Ablation may be indicated for patients with AF or flutter with a rapid ventricular response that has not been controlled by pharmacologic therapy. The AV junction may be ablated, completely disrupting communication from the atria to the ventricles. Successful ablation results in complete heart block with a ventricular rate of 40 to 60 beats/min. A permanent pacemaker is implanted after AV junction ablation to ensure the presence of a reliable rhythm and adequate rate as well as to reduce the risk for bradycardia-dependent torsades de pointes.

In addition, ablation for AF can be performed by creating lines of block around the anatomical triggers (eg, around the orifice of the pulmonary veins), or when the focus is identified, by electrically isolating the foci. The various techniques require special catheters and mapping equipment.[5] However, not all types of AF are amenable to this procedure; the etiology and trigger of the dysrhythmia need to be elucidated before a decision is made to carry out the ablation.

Ablation therapy for primary atrial flutter is indicated in those patients who have reentrant circuits within the right atrium. Ablation lesions are directed at creating a line of block usually along a narrow isthmus between the inferior vena cava and tricuspid annulus to interrupt the circuit.[6] When successful, atrial flutter ablation can provide a permanent cure. Unlike AV node ablation, atrial flutter ablation does not require permanent pacemaker implantation.

### Ventricular Dysrhythmias

The success of ablation for the treatment of VT depends on the cause of the dysrhythmia. Radiofrequency ablation has been effective in patients with VT in structurally normal hearts and in patients with VT due to bundle branch reentry. The technique also has had some limited success in patients with hemodynamically stable, monomorphic VT associated with a healed myocardial scar. However, it is not unusual to have multiple morphologies (forms) of VT in this population, and some unstable morphologies may not be amenable to ablation.

## Procedure

Before an ablation, the patient undergoes an electrophysiologic study (EPS) to evaluate the electrical activity of the heart. The EPS is an invasive test in which catheters are placed in the heart to record intracardiac electrograms (IC-EGM). The test provides information about the sequence of electrical activation of the heart in sinus rhythm and any abnormal sequence of activation during an induced dysrhythmia. An electrical map is inferred from the electrical recordings to help identify the focus of a dysrhythmia or locate an accessory pathway. The map guides the placement of the ablating catheter.

After the catheters are positioned, ECG recordings are made from the surface electrodes on the patient's chest and electrograms (EGMs) from the intracardiac electrodes. Programmed electrical stimulation (PES) is then performed to induce the dysrhythmia so that its mechanism and pathway can be evaluated. Once a diagnosis of the dysrhythmia is confirmed, an ablating catheter is positioned in the targeted area of the heart. Additional catheters are positioned to stimulate atrial and ventricular tissue. The ablation catheter contains multiple electrodes designed to localize the site of the dysrhythmia and to deliver the ablation current. The distal tip of the catheter can be flexed to facilitate access to the tissue and to ensure direct contact. Fluoroscopy and the EGM pattern from the catheter, as well as special mapping equipment and intracardiac ultrasound, help the physician determine the appropriate target area. The clinical ECG of the tachycardia is a useful template of the target dysrhythmia when several morphologies are induced.

When the appropriate site is identified, the radiofrequency current is applied for several seconds until the target tip temperature is achieved. Longer application time is allowed when a cooled or irrigated catheter tip is used. Several lesions may be required to eliminate the abnormal conducting tissue. Successful elimination of the target site is determined by examining the ECG and EGM tracings and confirmed when the dysrhythmia is no longer inducible. When the procedure is finished, the intracardiac catheters and venous or arterial sheaths are removed, and efforts to attain hemostasis at the insertion site are implemented.

## Nursing Management

The nurse plays a vital role in the care of the patient undergoing radiofrequency ablation. In consultation with the electrophysiologist, the nurse provides information to the patient and family about what to expect before, during, and after the procedure. The psychosocial support provided by the nurse may be key in helping the patient and family cope with the uncertainties of dysrhythmia management.

### Preablation

The nurse participates in educating the patient and family about radiofrequency ablation (Box 18-18). During the preablation period, the nurse records a 12-lead ECG, continuously monitors the patient's cardiac rhythm, and treats any dysrhythmias per the physician's orders. Other baseline data obtained include vital signs, breath sounds, fluid status, serum chemistries, PT/INR, and complete blood counts. In some cases, antiarrhythmic drugs may be discontinued 2 to 3 days before the procedure to allow provocation of the dysrhythmia during the procedure. The patient receives nothing by mouth for about 8 hours before the procedure. It is important to verify that a female patient is not pregnant because of x-ray exposure during the test. No activity restrictions are imposed before the procedure.

### During Ablation

The nurse in the EP laboratory is responsible for monitoring the patient throughout the procedure and assisting the physician with necessary interventions. The nurse must be competent in ACLS so that an emergency situation can be handled appropriately.

In the laboratory, the nurse explains each intervention to the patient and helps put the patient at ease. The nurse connects the patient to a cardiac monitor and physiologic recorder and applies a grounding pad for the radiofrequency catheter, defibrillator patches, automatic blood pressure device, and pulse oximeter. Oxygen is provided by nasal cannula. If not already in place, an IV line is inserted. IV conscious sedation is administered to ensure patient comfort. A urinary catheter is inserted if the procedure is anticipated to be lengthy. Both groins and the right subclavian vein sites are shaved and the skin prepared. A sterile field is established and maintained throughout the procedure. A lead apron may be placed under the patient's lower back to block fluoroscopy radiation from penetrating the reproductive system.

Throughout the procedure, the nurse monitors hemodynamic status, activated clotting time (ACT) if heparin is used, sedation level, and patient comfort. Communication with the patient is essential so that the patient is kept informed about the progress of the procedure, and anxiety and fear are minimized. The nurse also warns the patient that a burning sensation may be felt for a brief time during the actual ablation.

### Postablation

Thorough assessment and monitoring of the patient are continued after the ablation procedure. Essential components of

---

**BOX 18-18** | *TEACHING GUIDE* | *Preablation*

Points the patient needs to know before the ablation procedure include the following:
- Purpose of the procedure
- The patient's dysrhythmia and how the procedure will help
- Interventions that will occur before transport to the electrophysiology (EP) laboratory
- The appearance of, equipment, and personnel in the EP laboratory
- The use of IV conscious sedation, including the amnesic/analgesic effect of conscious sedation and possible side effects, such as nausea, vomiting, or hypotension
- Sensations associated with the procedure, such as:
  - Cool sensation from cleansing agents

- Pressure sensation from catheter insertion
- Palpitations, dizziness, or other sensations when dysrhythmia is induced
- possible mild burning sensation during ablation
- Restlessness or back discomfort from lying immobilized
- Anticipated length of the procedure
- Potential for placement of a permanent pacemaker
- Anticipated after effects, such as:
  - Skipped beats or faster than usual resting rate may be felt initially
  - Mild chest discomfort or burning may occur for a few days
  - A "skin effect," a dark outline of the grounding or defibrillation pad, which may persist indefinitely

**TABLE 18-7** Potential Complications of Radiofrequency Ablation and Associated Signs and Symptoms

| Complications | Signs and Symptoms |
|---|---|
| Cardiac perforation/tamponade | Tachycardia, abrupt or gradual fall in BP, dyspnea, pleuritic chest pain |
| Atrioesophageal fistula | May occur 1–4 weeks after ablation. Chest pain, heart burn, dysphagia, hematemesis, unexplained fever/chills |
| Pneumothorax | Dyspnea, decreased oxygen saturation, decreased breath sounds |
| Cerebral embolus | Slurred speech, blurred vision, headache, seizures |
| Pulmonary embolus | Chest pain, dyspnea, tachycardia |
| Femoral pseudoaneurysm or femoral arteriovenous fistula | Hematoma, pain, swelling, bruit, pulsatile mass at groin |
| Pulmonary vein stenosis | Dyspnea, hemoptysis, URI-like symptoms |
| Phrenic nerve injury | Dyspnea, cough, hiccups, elevated hemi-diaphragm |
| Pericarditis | Chest pain |

the assessment include vital signs, cardiac rhythm, catheter insertion sites, peripheral pulses, and level of consciousness. The patient may remain drowsy for several hours and experience nausea and vomiting as a result of the medications. When an arterial site has been used, leg immobilization and bed rest are maintained for about 6 hours. If only venous sites were used, the patient may begin ambulation in about 4 hours. The nurse assesses the patient for any pain or discomfort and provides comfort measures if indicated. Fluid volume status is checked, and when the patient's condition is stable, the urinary catheter is removed.

During the postablation period, the nurse carefully assesses the patient for any evidence of complications. Table 18-7 lists most common potential complications of radiofrequency ablation and associated signs and symptoms.[7]

## Cardiac Pacemakers

Electrical stimulation of the heart was tried experimentally as early as 1819. In 1930, Hyman noted that he could inject the right atrium with a diversity of substances and restore a heartbeat. He devised an "ingenious apparatus" that he labeled an artificial pacemaker, which delivered a rhythmic charge to the heart. In 1952, Zoll demonstrated that patients with Stokes-Adams syndrome could be sustained by the administration of current directly to the chest wall. In 1957, Lillehei affixed electrodes directly to the ventricles during open heart surgery.

From 1958 to 1961, implantable pacemakers became accepted treatment for complete heart block. In the 1970s and 1980s, AV synchrony and "physiologic" pacing became available. At the start of the first decade of the 21st century, clinical trials on right and left ventricular (biventricular) pacing made tremendous progress for symptom management for patients with systolic heart failure.

Technological advances over the past decade have resulted in smaller pacemakers with longer battery life and numerous programmable options for diagnostics and therapies. The goal of individualized, physiologic pacing has been achieved with recent advances.

## Indications for Cardiac Pacing

Cardiac pacing is most commonly indicated for conditions that result in failure of the heart to initiate or conduct an intrinsic electrical impulse at a rate adequate to maintain perfusion. Pacemakers are necessary when arrhythmias or conduction defects compromise the electrical system and the hemodynamic response of the heart. The original pacemakers were designed for antibradycardia. Today's pacemakers also monitor and treat tachyarrhythmias and facilitate electrical remodeling. Further research and advances in technology have allowed the use of pacemakers in heart conditions such as congestive heart failure, long QT syndrome, and neurocardiogenic syncope.[8,9]

Critical care nurses work with members of the health care team to assess potential pacemaker patients who may exhibit arrhythmias, coronary artery disease, AMI, cardiomyopathy or other conditions that alter the conduction of the heart. To assist medical professionals in determining the clinical criteria for pacemaker implantation, a Joint Committee of the ACC, AHA, and Heart Rhythm Society was formed to establish uniform criteria for pacemaker implantation.[8] The committee divided its recommendations for implantation into three classes of indications.

- *Class I:* Implantation recommended; includes conditions for which there is evidence or general agreement that treatment is useful and effective.
- *Class II:* Includes conditions for which there is conflicting evidence or a divergence of opinion about the usefulness or efficacy of a procedure or treatment.
  - Class IIa includes conditions in which treatment is reasonable.
  - Class IIb includes conditions in which treatment may be considered.
- *Class III:* Includes conditions for which there is evidence or general agreement that the procedure or treatment is not useful or effective, and in some cases may be harmful.

The most common indications for pacemaker implantation with recommended pacing modes are summarized in Box 18-19.[8]

## The Pacemaker System

The pacemaker system, consisting of a pulse generator and one to three leads with electrodes, performs two main functions: diagnosis and treatment. The diagnostic function is to sense intrinsic cardiac activity; the treatment function is to emit an electrical impulse that excites endocardial cells and produces a wave of depolarization in the myocardium. Clinical terminology related to pacemakers is listed in Box 18-20.

## BOX 18-19   Indications for Permanent Cardiac Pacing*

### Acquired Atrioventricular (AV) Block in Adults

*Class I:* Third-degree and advanced second-degree AV block at any anatomical level, associated with any one of the following conditions: (1) symptomatic bradycardia; (2) asystole greater than or equal to 3.0 seconds or any escape rate less than 40 beats/min in awake, symptom-free patients; (3) dysrhythmias and other medical conditions that require drugs that result in symptomatic bradycardia; (4) post-AV node ablation; (5) postoperative AV block that is not expected to resolve after cardiac surgery; and (6) neuromuscular diseases with AV block, (7) atrial fibrillation with pause of 5 seconds or greater, and (8) exercise-induced AV block in the absence of myocardial ischemia

*Class IIa:* (1) Asymptomatic third-degree AV block at any anatomical site with average awake ventricular rates of 40 beats/min or faster without cardiomegaly (2) asymptomatic type II second-degree AV block with a narrow QRS; (3) asymptomatic type I second-degree AV block at intra- or infra-His levels found at EPS (4) first- or second-degree AV block with symptoms similar to those of pacemaker syndrome.

*Class IIb:* (1) Neuromuscular diseases, such as myotonic muscular dystrophy, Kearns-Sayre syndrome, Erb's dystrophy (limb-girdle), and muscular atrophy, with any degree of AV block (including first-degree AV block) with or without symptoms. (2) AV block in the setting of drug use when the block is expected to occur even after the drug is withdrawn

*Class III:* Asymptomatic first-degree AV block and type I second-degree AV block, transient AV block

### Chronic Bifascicular Block

*Class I:* (1) Intermittent complete heart block, (2) type II second-degree AV block, and (3) alternating bundle branch block

*Class IIa:* (1) Syncope not demonstrated to be due to AV block when other likely causes have been excluded, specifically VT; (2) prolonged His–ventricular interval on EPS; (3) incidental finding of pacing-induced, nonphysiologic infra-His block at EPS

*Class IIb:* (1) Neuromuscular diseases, such as myotonic muscular dystrophy, Kearns-Sayre syndrome, Erb's dystrophy (limb-girdle), and peroneal muscular atrophy, with any degree of fascicular block with or without symptoms

*Class III:* Fascicular block without AV block or symptoms and asymptomatic fascicular block with first-degree AV block

### AV Block After AMI

*Class I:* (1) Persistent type II second-degree AV block with alternating bundle branch block (BBB) or third-degree AV block (2) transient advanced (second- or third-degree) infranodal AV block and associated BBB; (3) persistent and symptomatic second- or third-degree AV block.

*Class IIb:* (1) Persistent second- or third-degree AV block at the AV node level

*Class III:* Transient AV block

### Sinus Node Dysfunction (SND)

*Class I:* SND (1) with documented symptomatic bradycardia (2) symptomatic chronotropic incompetence (3) Symptomatic bradycardia resulting fromdrug therapy for a medical condition

*Class IIa:* SND (1) with heart rate less than 40 beats/min, (2) syncope of unexplained origin with provoked SND during EPS

*Class IIb:* In minimally symptomatic patients, chronic heart rate less than 40 beats/min while awake.

*Class III:* Asymptomatic SND; SND with symptomatic bradycardia due to nonessential drug therapy; symptoms occur in the absence of bradycardia

### Hypersensitive Carotid Sinus Syndrome and Neurocardiogenic Syncope

*Class I:* Recurrent syncope caused by spontaneous carotid sinus stimulation and asystole of more than 3 seconds induced by minimal carotid sinus pressure.

*Class IIa:* Recurrent syncope without clear, provocative events and a hypersensitive cardioinhibitory response of 3 seconds or longer

*Class IIb:* Significantly symptomatic neurocardiogenic syncope associated with bradycardia documented spontaneously or at head-up tilt

*Class III:* (1) A hyperactive cardioinhibitory response to carotid sinus stimulation in the absence of symptoms or in the presence of vague symptoms such as dizziness, light-headedness, or both and (2) situational vasovagal syncope in which avoidance behavior is effective

### CRT in Patients with Systolic Heart Failure

*Class I:* LVEF ≤ 35%, sinus rhythm, LBBB with QRS duration ≥ 150 ms and NYHA class II, III or ambulatory IV symptoms on optimal medical therapy.

*Class IIa:* (1) LVEF ≤ 35%, sinus rhythm, LBBB with QRS duration 120 to 149 ms and NYHA class II, III, or ambulatory IV symptoms on medical therapy.(2) LVEF ≤35%, sinus rhythm, non-LBBB, QRS ≥ 150 ms, and NYHA class III/ambulatory IV. (3) Atrial fibrillation, LVEF ≤35% on optimal medical therapy if needs ventricular pacing or meets other criteria for CRT, or if AV nodal RFA or pharmacologic rate control resulting in near 100% ventricular pacing. (4) Patients on optimal medical therapy with LVEF ≤ 35% having new or replacement devices and are anticipated to need at least 40% pacing.

*ClassIIb:* (1)Consider if LVEF ≤30%, ischemic etiology of HF, sinus rhythm, LBBB with QRS duration ≥150 ms and NYHA class I symptoms on medical therapy. (2) Consider if LVEF ≤35%, sinus rhythm, non-LBBB, QRS 120 to 149 ms and NYHA class III/ambulatory class IV on optimal medical therpy. (3) LVEF ≤35%, sinus rhythm, non-LBBB, QRS ≥ 150 ms, NYHA class II symptoms.

*Class III:* No Benefit for patients with NYHA class I/II symptoms, non-LBBB, QRS <150 ms. Not indicated if co-morbidities and/or frailty limit survival with good functional capacity to <1 year.

*Box does not include indications for special populations and specific conditions.

Data from Tracy CM, Epstein AE, Darbar D, et al; ACCF/AHA/HRS Focused Update of the 2008 Guidelines for Device-Based Therapy of Cardiac Rhythm Abnormalities: A Report of the American College of Cardiology Foundation/American Heart Association Task Force on Practice Guidelines. Circulation: 126(14):1784–800, 2012; and Gillis AM, Russo AM, Ellenbogen KA, et al: HRS/ACCF expert consensus statement on pacemaker device and mode selection. Heart-Rhythm 2012;9;1344–1365.

### BOX 18-20   Clinical Terminology Related to Pacemakers

**Active fixation lead:** A pacing lead with some design at the lead tip (corkscrew, coil) that allows the tip to be embedded in heart tissue, thus decreasing the likelihood of dislodgment

**Asynchronous pacing:** A pacemaker that fires at a fixed rate regardless of the intrinsic activity of the heart

**Bipolar lead:** A pacing lead containing two electrodes. One electrode is at the tip of the lead and provides stimulation to the heart. A second electrode is several millimeters proximal to the tip and completes the electrical circuit. Both electrodes provide sensing of the intrinsic cardiac activity.

**Capture:** The depolarization of a cardiac chamber in response to a pacing stimulus

**Cardiac Resynchronization Therapy** (CRT): Resynchronizes timing of ventricular depolarization to improve cardiac output in patients with class II, III IV heart failure. Also referred to as "biventricular" pacing.

**Chronotropic incompetence:** Inability of the sinus node to accelerate in response to exercise

**Demand pacing (inhibited pacing):** A pacemaker that withholds its pacing stimulus when sensing an adequate intrinsic heart rate

**Dual-chamber pacing (physiologic pacing):** Pacing in both the atria and the ventricles to artificially restore AV synchrony

**Electromagnetic interference:** Electrical or magnetic energy that can interfere with or disrupt the function of the pulse generator

**Milliamperage (mA):** The unit of measure used for the electrical stimulus (output) generated by the pacemaker

**Multisite pacing:** The ability to stimulate more than one site in a chamber (eg, right ventricle and left ventricle stimulation in biventricular pacing/cardiac resynchronization therapy [CRT])

**Overdrive pacing:** A method to suppress a tachycardia by pacing the heart at a rate faster than the patient's intrinsic rate

**Oversensing:** Inhibition of the pacemaker by events other than those that the pacemaker was intended to sense. These may include tall T waves and EMI.

Pacemaker mediated tachycardia (PMT): Results in ventricle tracking atrial impulses at the upper pacing limit (eg, MTR- max tracking rate). Begins with retrograde conduction to atria. Occurrence limited by programmed safety features, such as post ventricular atrial refractory period.

**Pacing threshold:** The minimal electrical stimulation required to initiate cardiac muscle depolarization consistently (atrial or ventricular).

**Passive fixation lead:** A pacing lead that lodges in the trabeculae of the heart without actually penetrating the cardiac wall

**Rate-responsive (rate-adaptive, rate-modulated) pacing:** A pacemaker that alters pacing rate in response to detected changes in the body's metabolic demand

**Sensing:** The ability of the pacemaker to detect intrinsic cardiac activity and respond appropriately. How the pacemaker responds depends on the programmed mode of pacing.

**Sensing threshold:** The minimal atrial or ventricular intracardiac signal amplitude required to inhibit or trigger a demand pacemaker

**Situational vasovagal syncope:** Syncope associated with bradycardia by vagal stimulation (eg., during coughing, micturition, or severe pain).

**Triggered:** A response to sensing in which the pacemaker fires a stimulus in response to intrinsic cardiac activity. In pacemaker terms, triggered is the opposite of inhibited.

**Undersensing:** Failure of the pacemaker to sense the heart's intrinsic activity. As a result, the pacemaker fires inappropriately.

## Permanent Pacing Systems

**THE PULSE GENERATOR.** The pulse generator for a permanent pacemaker is composed of a lithium iodide battery source and electronic circuits enclosed in a hermetically sealed metal container. The generator weighs 20 to 30 g and is 5 to 7 mm thick; header size determined by number of leads use (Fig. 18-27). The longevity of most permanent pacemakers is about 6 to 12 years, depending on the percentage of pacing the heart requires over time and amount of energy needed to consistently capture. Most permanent pulse generators are inserted in a subcutaneous pocket in the pectoral region below the clavicle (Fig. 18-28). Elderly or thin patients with less subcutaneous tissue may have the device implanted behind the pectoral muscle.

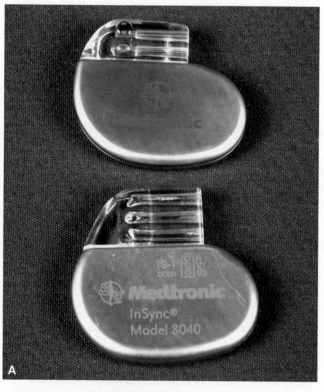

**A**

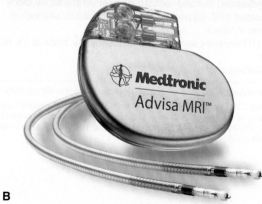

**B**

**FIGURE 18-27** Permanent pulse generators. **A:** Single chamber and atrial-biventricular pulse generators. **B:** Dual chamber pulse generator. (Reproduced with permission of Metronic, Inc., Minneapolis, MN.)

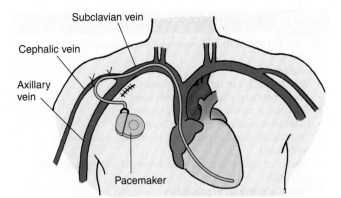

FIGURE 18-28 Transvenous installation of a permanent pacemaker. For dual-chamber pacing, a separate pacing wire would be in the atrium. Left sided implant is most common.

**THE LEAD SYSTEM.** The lead is a wire that provides the communication network between the pulse generator and the heart muscle. One or more electrodes are at the distal end of the lead and provide sensing and pacing of the heart muscle. In a bipolar lead, the negative electrode (cathode) is at the tip, and the positive electrode (anode) is about 1 to 3 cm proximal to the tip (Fig. 18-29). Leadless pacing systems are in development.

The permanent pacemaker lead is typically inserted either through a subclavian vein or a cephalic vein through the chest wall. Alternate insertion sites include epicardial and the external or internal jugular. The lead is then positioned with fluoroscopic guidance and affixed in the right atrial appendage or in the apex of the right ventricle, or in both locations. A third lead may be inserted in a coronary sinus branch to stimulate the left ventricle for biventricular pacing. The leads must provide adequate electrical stimulation, sufficient insulation, and the endurance to withstand pulsatile turbulence.

The permanent pacemaker lead tip can be affixed to the myocardium with a lead fixation mechanism. Over time, fibrotic tissues anchor the tip to the myocardium securing placement and ensuring proper function of the electrode (Fig. 18-30).

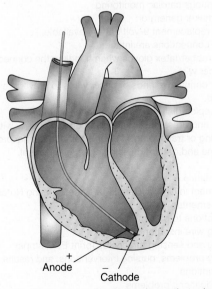

+
Anode

–
Cathode

FIGURE 18-29 Transvenous bipolar pacing catheter in place.

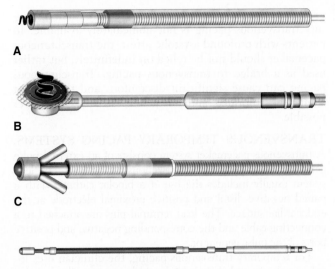

A

B

C

D

FIGURE 18-30 Different pacemaker leads. **A:** Active fixation by a screw. **B:** Epicardial lead. **C:** Passive fixation with barbs. **D:** ICD lead. (Grover F, Mack, MJ. Master techniques in surgery: Cardiac surgery. Wolters Kluwer, 2016 (Fig. 39-2).

**Temporary Pacing Systems**

Temporary pacemaker systems are used in emergency and elective situations. In life-threatening situations, a temporary pacemaker serves as a bridge to permanent pacemaker implantation or until resolution of a reversible cause for symptomatic bradycardia. Electively, temporary pacemakers may be used for overdrive or pace-termination of tachyarrhythmias. Temporary pacing systems can be transcutaneous, transvenous, epicardial, or transthoracic.

**TRANSCUTANEOUS TEMPORARY PACING SYSTEMS.** External transcutaneous pacing involves placing large gelled electrode patches directly on the chest wall. The cathode or negative electrode is applied anteriorly to the left of the sternum, and the anode or positive electrode is applied straight posteriorly on the patient's back and then connected to an external transcutaneous pacemaker (Fig. 18-31).

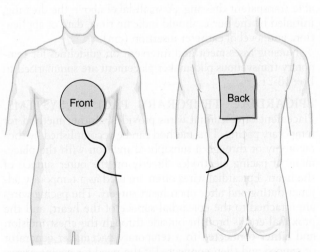

Front

Back

FIGURE 18-31 Transcutaneous pacing. Electrodes are placed on anterior and posterior chest walls and attached to the external pacing unit.

Transcutaneous pacing is used emergently when temporary transvenous pacing is not immediately available. In patients with profound asystolic arrest, the transcutaneous pacemaker should not be relied on indefinitely, but rather used as a bridge to transvenous pacing. Transcutaneous pacing can cause significant discomfort, and the patient should be informed and adequately sedated, whenever possible.

## TRANSVENOUS TEMPORARY PACING SYSTEMS.
A transvenous pacemaker system consists of an external pulse generator and a temporary transvenous pacing lead. The lead system usually includes the use of a bipolar catheter with a paired negative distal and positive proximal electrode at the endocardial surface. The lead terminal pins are attached to a connecting cable and the corresponding negative and positive ports of the pulse generator.

For temporary transvenous pacing, the clinician uses local anesthesia and then introduces the catheter/lead into a superficial vein. The brachial, internal or external jugular, subclavian, and femoral veins may be used. The subclavian and internal jugular sites allow greater lead stability and patient mobility. To maintain sterility at the connection site and terminal tip of the catheter, a sterile protective sleeve is placed over the catheter before insertion and then connected to the end of the sheath after satisfactory position is confirmed. The transvenous lead is threaded through a sheath in the vein, into the vena cava and the right atrium, through the tricuspid valve, and into the right ventricle. The lead tip is placed in contact with the endocardial surface of the RV apex for stability and reliability. For atrial pacing, an atrial bipolar catheter is placed in the right atrial appendage. There are also pulmonary artery balloon flotation catheters with atrial and ventricular pacing ports for dual-chamber pacing. Balloon flotation catheters are useful in the critical care setting because they provide thermodilution and cardiac output determination and do not require fluoroscopy for positioning.

After placement, the leads are affixed at the skin entry site with nonabsorbable suture. The sheath should be sutured and attached to a continuous drip if used for drawing blood or administering drugs. The sheath entry site should be covered with an antiseptic ointment and a self-adhesive, semipermeable transparent dressing. A small label above the dressing, initialed by the nurse, should indicate time, date of application, and level of catheter insertion (cm).

Nursing assessment and intervention guidelines for temporary transvenous pacemaker placement are summarized in Box 18-21.

## EPICARDIAL TEMPORARY PACING SYSTEMS.
Placement of epicardial wires provides another method for temporary pacing. This method can be accomplished by thoracotomy or through a subxiphoid incision with the placement of pacing electrodes directly on the outer surface of the heart. Epicardial wires often are used as a temporary adjunct during and after open heart surgery. The pacing wires are attached to the epicardial surface of the heart, and the proximal end is brought outside through the chest incision and either connected to a temporary pacemaker generator or capped and then connected if the need for pacing arises. The wires are extracted without reopening the incision, even after scar tissue has formed over the tips.

---

### BOX 18-21 Nursing Interventions

**For the Patient With a Temporary Transvenous Pacemaker**

**Assessment**

*During insertion:*
- Vital signs, $O_2$ saturation, peripheral pulses
- Level of sedation/sedative agents used
- Continuous cardiac rhythm monitoring
- Date, time, method, and site of insertion
- Location of wire inserted (atrial, ventricular, atrial and ventricular)
- Measured values: capture (mA) threshold and intrinsic amplitude (mV)
- Patient's tolerance of procedure
- Complications
- 12-lead ECG
- Final settings: mode, rate, output, and sensitivity

*After insertion:*
- Rate setting, mV setting, mA setting, mode of operation (demand, asynchronous) and AV interval (if appropriate), refractory period
- Pacemaker turned off or on
- Rhythm strip, capture and intrinsic, if appropriate; 12-lead ECG
- Status on insertion site, lead insertion level at insertion point (cm) and sutures (if present)
- Chest x-ray performed, results in medical record

*Every change of shift:*
- Pacemaker turned off or on
- Pacemaker secured appropriately to patient
- All connections are secure
- Setting for rate, mA, sensitivity, mode of operation, AV interval, refractory period (if appropriate)
- Rhythm strip (and with any clinical change or intervention)
- Sensing and capture thresholds (compare to baseline)
- Presence/absence of hiccupping or muscle twitching
- Status of insertion site, lead insertion level at insertion point (cm) and sutures (if present)
- Signs of infection (redness, pain, fever, pus)
- Pulse perfusion distal to insertion site (if appropriate)
- Connective ends of pacer wires capped (as appropriate)

**Intervention**
- Continuous cardiac monitoring
- Pacemaker generator:
- Verify replacement 9-volt battery available.
- Verify connections are intact.
- Wear rubber/latex gloves when handling the connective ends of pacer wires.
- Cover connective ends of pacer wires to prevent microshock hazard.
- Label epicardial pacer wires *atrial* or *ventricular*.
- Clean and dress pacer wire insertion site(s) daily with gauze dressing or transparent dressing per institutional protocol. Label time and date of dressing change and initial.

**Documentation**
- Document in Critical Care Flow Sheet/Nursing Notes: Assessments
- Instructions to patient/family
- Pacing wire insertion site care
- Pacing and sensing thresholds (print ECG strips)
- Pacing problems, nursing interventions, and results of interventions
- Complications/problems

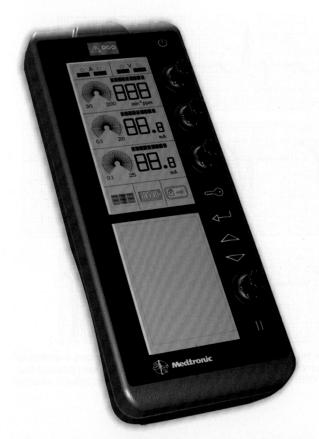

FIGURE 18-32 A dual-chamber temporary pacemaker, model 5392. (Reproduced with permission of Medtronic, Inc., Minneapolis, MN.)

**TRANSTHORACIC TEMPORARY PACING SYSTEMS.** Transthoracic pacing is a temporary pacing method used as a last resort in an emergency situation. This method involves introduction of a pacing needle in the anterior wall of the heart. Transthoracic pacing has limited success rates and a high potential for complications.

**EXTERNAL PULSE GENERATOR.** The temporary pulse generator is an external device powered by a 9-V alkaline or lithium replaceable battery (Fig. 18-32). Often called a temporary pacemaker, the device contains several controls that regulate the current output, rate, sensitivity, and the mode of pacing; for dual-chamber pacing, base and upper rate, AV interval and refractory period settings can be chosen. A dual-chamber pulse generator has separate terminals for the atrial and ventricular inputs. The use of a connecting cable allows the lead tips to tighten into the connector block and a locking mechanism to the pulse generator. Cables should be labeled appropriately near the distal lock (atrial or

ventricular) so as to avoid interchanging the leads when attaching to the atrial or ventricular port of the pulse generator.

## Pacemaker Functioning

When the pacemaker system functions appropriately, it senses and treats the heart rhythm dysfunction. The sensing function is the ability of the pacemaker to detect the heart's intrinsic (underlying) activity, and the sensing amplitude is the largest intrinsic signal that is consistently detected by the pacemaker electrode (eg, the R wave is usually the largest signal sensed by the ventricular lead). At the site of the sensing electrode, the amplitude of the intrinsic depolarization wave is measured in millivolts (mV). The smallest number on the sensor control represents the most sensitive setting, in mV, indicating the smallest signal the pacemaker will sense. If the heart's intrinsic amplitude is smaller than the sensitivity setting, undersensing occurs. This can occur when the electrode has inadequate contact with the heart tissue. The drawback in setting pacemaker sensitivity at its most sensitive setting is that oversensing may occur, such as when the pacemaker senses extraneous signals (eg, T waves) or signals from the other chamber. If oversensing occurs, the pacemaker stimulus may be inhibited (Fig. 18-33).

When intrinsic heart rate is adequate, the pacemaker responds by inhibiting a pacing stimulus. When intrinsic heart rate drops to the programmed minimum rate, the pacemaker delivers a stimulus through the lead. When the pacemaker discharges, an artifact known as a pacing spike appears on the ECG, as shown in Figure 18-34. As a result of this stimulus, the cardiac chamber containing the pacemaker lead is depolarized. *Capture* is the term used to indicate depolarization of the atria or ventricle in response to a pacing stimulus. The minimal amount of voltage required from the pacemaker to initiate consistent capture is known as the pacing threshold. This threshold level is determined by establishing successful pacing at higher energy and then gradually decreasing the energy output of the generator until capture ceases. The pacing threshold is expressed as milliamperage (mA) in the temporary generator and voltage (V) in the permanent pulse generator, within a given pulse width duration. The generator output is then set at two or three times the threshold level to allow for an adequate safety margin.

Many factors affect the pacing threshold, including hypoxia, hyperkalemia, antiarrhythmic drugs, catecholamines, digoxin toxicity, and corticosteroids.

## The Pacemaker Code

A coding system was first developed in 1974 to identify the various modes of pacemaker operation, and since then it has

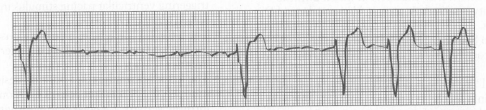

FIGURE 18-33 Failure to pace (discharge) or oversensing with pacing inhibition. In the first half of the strip, the sensing amplifier may have detected electrical noise as an R wave (oversensing) causing pacemaker inhibition.

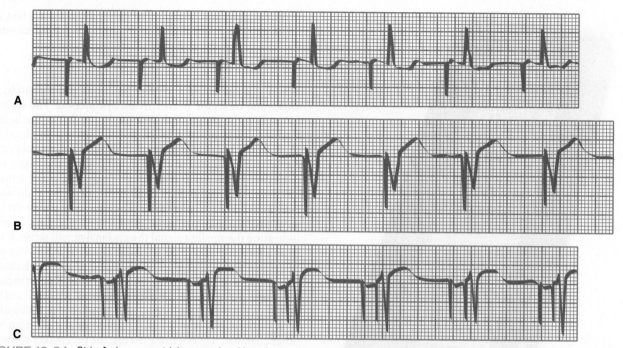

**FIGURE 18-34** Strip **A** shows an atrial pacemaker. Note that each pacing stimulus is followed by a P wave. Strip **B** shows a ventricular pacemaker. Note that each pacing stimulus is followed by a wide QRS complex. Strip **C** shows a dual-chamber pacemaker. Note that the first spike is followed by a P wave and the second spike is followed by a QRS complex. All strips show 1:1 capture. Note: spike is inserted on ECG by monitoring system, not the pacemaker.

**TABLE 18-8    The NBG Pacemaker Code**

| Position: Category | | | | |
| --- | --- | --- | --- | --- |
| **I: Chamber(s) Paced** | **II: Chamber(s) Sensed** | **III: Response to Sensing** | **IV: Rate Modulation** | **V: Multisite Pacing** |
| O = none | O = none | O = none | O = none | O = none |
| A = atrium | A = atrium | T = triggered | R = rate modulation | A = atrium |
| V = ventricle | V = ventricle | I = inhibited | | V = ventricle |
| D = dual (A +V) | D = dual (A + V) | D = dual (T + I) | | D = dual (A + V) |

Adapted from North American Society of Pacing and Electrophysiology/British Pacing and Electrophysiology Group. The revised NASPE/BPEG generic code for antibradycardia, adaptive rate, and multisite pacing. Pacing Clin Electrophysiol 25(2):260–264, 2002.

undergone several revisions. The most recent version of the code was developed in 2002 through the joint efforts of the AHA and Heart Rhythm Society (formerly NASPE) and the British Pacing and Electrophysiology Group (BPEG).[9,10] The NASPE/BPEG Generic (NBG) Pacemaker Code is shown in Table 18-8 and is simply called the NBG pacemaker code.

**I: Chamber(s) Paced.** The first letter in the code describes the chamber or chambers of the heart in which pacing occurs: A, atrium; V, ventricle; and D, dual chamber.

**II: Chamber(s) Sensed.** The second position of the code indicates the chamber or chambers in which intrinsic cardiac activity is sensed: A, atrium; V, ventricle; and D, dual chamber.

**III: Response to Sensing.** The third position of the code denotes the pacemaker's response to sensed intrinsic cardiac activity.

- The letter "I" means that the pacemaker is inhibited from firing in response to a sensed intrinsic event. For example, if the pacemaker is set to a rate of 70, and if the patient's intrinsic rate exceeds 70 beats/min, the pacemaker will not fire. The pacemaker fires only if the patient's intrinsic heart rate drops below the programmed rate. Thus, the pacemaker functions on demand and is known as a demand pacemaker. Because the pacemaker is inhibited by adequate intrinsic heart activity, there is no danger of the pacemaker firing at an inappropriate time that could initiate a dangerous cardiac dysrhythmia, such as VT.

- The letter "T" indicates a pacemaker that triggers pacing stimuli in response to a sensed intrinsic beat. In a patient with complete AV block, a dual-chamber pacemaker is capable of sensing intrinsic atrial activity and triggering ventricular pacing stimulus in response to a sensed atrial event.

- The letter "D" designates a dual response (inhibited pacing output and triggered pacing after sensed event).

- The letter "O" in the third position designates a mode in which the pacemaker does not respond to sensed intrinsic activity. Pacemaker insensitivity to intrinsic activity is known as asynchronous pacing. This can be achieved by setting the sensitivity to the highest number or programming to asynchronous mode (ie, DOO, VOO).

Permanent pacemakers also may be switched temporarily to an asynchronous mode by placement of a large magnet over the pulse generator. This maneuver causes the pacemaker to fire without regard to intrinsic rate (fixed pacing), allowing assessment of firing and capture while the patient's rhythm is overridden by the fixed pacing pulse. This should be used with caution as it could result in R on T, triggering ventricular tachycardia.

**IV: Rate Modulation.** The fourth position of the code describes the presence or absence of rate modulation. The letter "O" denotes no rate modulation, and the letter "R" means that rate modulation is active. This is a feature in which the pacing rate varies in response to a physiologic variable reflecting activity levels. The physiologic variables used are mechanical vibration, acceleration, or minute ventilation. When patients increase their activity, the pacer detects the physiologic response (eg, muscle vibration, increased respiratory rate/thoracic impedance) and increases the pacing rate to meet increased metabolic demands.

**V: Multisite Pacing.** The fifth position of the code describes whether multisite pacing is present: "A" in the atrium, "V" in the ventricle, "D" in both atrium and ventricle, and "O" means that no multisite pacing is present.

In clinical parlance, the absence of a fourth or fifth letter designation signifies no rate modulation and no multisite pacing. The first three positions are required when describing pacemaker mode, although all positions may be indicated for completeness.[9,10]

## Pacing Modes

Knowledge of the pacemaker code helps the critical care nurse determine the type of implanted device, the intended mode of operation, and the actual mode of operation. Modes of operation can be classified as single- and dual-chamber modes.

AAI and VVI are single-chamber modes of operation in the atrium or ventricle. An AAI is a mode of operation for atrial pacemakers. With this mode of operation, there is **a**trial pacing, **a**trial sensing, **i**nhibited response to sensed events, and no rate modulation. Temporary atrial pacemakers most often are set to an AAI mode and are particularly useful in overdrive pacing of atrial dysrhythmias.

DDD mode provides **d**ual-chamber pacing, **d**ual-chamber sensing, **d**ual response to sensed events (inhibited or triggered). Dual-chamber modes allow physiologic pacing, in which atria and ventricles are sequentially sensed or paced. DDDR mode has the additional feature of rate modulation. VDD mode paces only in the ventricle, but this mode senses atrial and ventricular events and has dual response to sensed events. Therefore, an atrial event (P wave) will trigger a ventricular event. If an intrinsic R wave is sensed, ventricular pacing is inhibited. This mode is particularly useful in patients with intact sinus node function but with high-grade AV block.

## Biventricular Pacing (Cardiac Resynchronization)

Device-based therapy guidelines were updated in 2012 to include updated and new recommendations specific to cardiac resynchronization therapy (CRT).[8] CRT, also referred to as biventricular pacing, is achieved by positioning an additional lead in one of the coronary sinus branches to stimulate the left ventricle, restoring ventricular synchrony. Biventricular pacing is primarily used for symptom improvement and treatment of HF in patients with moderate to severe left ventricular dysfunction and bundle branch block. Biventricular pacing corrects intra- and interventricular delay; CRT has been shown to improve functional class and quality of life in select HF populations.[8] It is also approved as initial therapy for patients with CHB who require continuous ventricular pacing, to prevent the development of pacemaker syndrome (Fig. 18-35). Pacemaker syndrome is a possible complication related to loss of atrioventricular synchrony in ventricularly paced patients.[11,12] The pacing codes for biventricular pacing are the same as in traditional pacing (see Table 18-8).

## Pacemaker Malfunction

### Permanent Pacemaker Malfunction

Pacemaker malfunction can be a result of inappropriate programming (pseudomalfunction) or true component malfunction. Although pacemakers are now manufactured to provide more complex capabilities and are generally considered to be more reliable, unanticipated pacemaker malfunction (eg, "advisories") do occur.[11] For this reason, it is important for the patient to know the manufacturer, model, and serial number of his or her pacemaker components (pulse generator and leads) and to ascertain that they have been appropriately registered

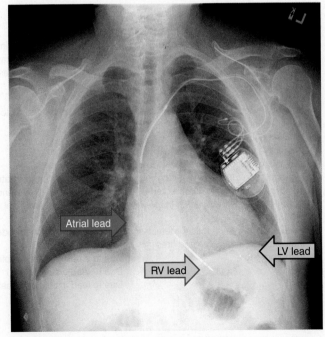

**FIGURE 18-35** Lead placement for atrial biventricular pacing.

with the manufacturer. This information is usually provided to the patient after the implant procedure, and the patient is given an implanted device wallet identification card.

Advisories are issued when devices of a certain lot or model are associated with component or battery failure. Most manufacturers have toll-free telephone numbers that can provide information on advisories. However, it is important that the patient contact his or her physician, who can provide counseling on appropriate interventions for the advisory. At times, simple programming or monitoring may be all that is needed.

## Temporary Pacemaker Malfunction

Temporary pacemaker malfunction should be addressed systematically. First and foremost, immediate action is required to restore pacemaker capture when the patient has no underlying rhythm. These steps are to be followed:

1. Increase pulse generator output (in mA) to the highest setting, asynchronous mode (VOO, DOO).
2. Check patient hemodynamics, simultaneous multiple ECG lead recordings; intervene if appropriate with transcutaneous pacing, atropine sulfate, or isoproterenol.
3. Check all connections.
4. Replace pulse generator or battery; be prepared with transcutaneous pacing backup during replacement.

Proceed with troubleshooting if the patient's condition is stable. Table 18-9 describes troubleshooting strategies for temporary pacemaker malfunction.

## Types of Malfunction

**FAILURE TO DISCHARGE.** If stimulus discharge from the pacemaker causes an artifact, or "spike," to appear on the ECG, failure to discharge may be manifested by absence of

| TABLE 18-9 | Troubleshooting a Temporary Pacemaker | |
|---|---|---|
| **Problem** | **Cause** | **Intervention** |
| **Failure to discharge:** No evidence of pacing stimulus, patient's heart rate below programmed rate | Due to battery depletion or pulse generator failure, output or timing circuit failure Due to loose cable connection | Replace battery or generator. Check all connections for tightness. |
| **Failure to capture:** Pacing stimulus not followed by ECG evidence of depolarization | Due to lead dislodgment Due to broken connector pins or fractured extension connecting cable Due to incompatibility of wire pins with cable or to generator Due to output setting (mA) too low Due to perforation Due to lead fracture without insulation break Due to increase in pacing threshold from medication or metabolic changes | Review chest film, turn patient to left lateral decubitus position until lead can be replaced. Connect wire directly to generator to diagnose cable problem, replace connecting cable. Ascertain a secure fit of the exposed pin to the cable or the generator, adjust connection or replace pulse generator. Check capture thresholds and adjust output to a two- to threefold safety margin. Review 12-lead ECG, report signs of perforation, stabilize hemodynamics. Check intracavitary ECG; if evidence of fracture in one pole, unipolarize lead; if total fracture, replace lead. Check laboratory test results, correct metabolic alterations, review medications and vital signs, increase output. |
| **Oversensing:** Device detects noncardiac electrical events and interprets them as depolarization | Due to oversensitive setting Due to device detecting tall T waves and interpreting them as R waves | Reduce sensitivity (value [in millivolts] should be larger to make pacer less sensitive); if patient is pacer dependent (no intrinsic R wave), program to asynchronous mode until problem is corrected. Increase ventricular refractory period beyond T wave. |
| In dual-chamber pacing, cross-talk is a form of oversensing: The device detects signals from the other chamber and inhibits; in atrial channel, R waves are detected as P waves. | Caused by atrial lead dislodgment | Recheck atrial capture thresholds; if high, dislodgment is probable. |
| In ventricular channel, atrial pacing stimulus afterpotential is detected as an R wave, with V pacing inappropriately inhibited | Due to high output from atrial channel Due to electrical interference, improperly grounded electrical devices | Reduce output from atrial channel, decrease ventricular channel sensitivity (higher millivolt value). Remove nongrounded equipment. |
| **Undersensing:** Device fails to detect intrinsic cardiac activity and fires inappropriately | Due to asynchronous mode setting (VOO, DOO, AOO) Due to small intrinsic amplitude Due to lead dislodgment Due to lead insulation break | Reprogram to synchronous mode (VVI, DDD, AAI). Increase sensitivity (turn sensitivity dial toward lower millivolt value). Recheck capture thresholds; if high, lead probably dislodged and needs repositioning. Check lead with pacing system analyzer, if impedance too low (<200 Ohms), insulation break is likely, and lead needs to be replaced or can be temporarily placed in unipolar configuration |

the spike and unexplained loss of pacing. The cause of this failure may be within the generator itself, either processor or battery failure. Processor failure is not common, but battery failure may occur in permanent pacemakers among patients who are noncompliant with follow-up. This may be evaluated by measuring the output values of the generator through a programmer. When the battery life is significantly low, the generator fails to communicate with the programmer. If the situation is emergent, the physician may insert a temporary transvenous pacemaker to support the patient hemodynamically until the pacemaker generator is replaced.

**FAILURE TO CAPTURE.** Failure of the pacing stimulus to capture the ventricles or atria is noted by the absence of the QRS or P wave immediately after the pacemaker artifact on the ECG (Fig. 18-36). Failure to capture may be caused by elevated threshold, a lead problem (dislodgment lead fracture), or battery depletion. These conditions may create insufficient output delivery to meet the capture threshold. If the patient is pacemaker dependent and becomes symptomatic, BLS and ACLS interventions should be initiated: drug therapy (atropine, isoproterenol), transcutaneous pacing, or CPR may be required until the cause of the problem is found and corrected.

**OVERSENSING.** Oversensing occurs when the pacemaker detects events other than those intended. For example, in VVI pacing, if large T waves are sensed (as R waves) in addition to the R wave, the pacemaker is inhibited, and paces at a slower than programmed rate may be noted. Similarly, electromagnetic interference (EMI) may result in inappropriate sensing and as a result, incorrectly activate the inhibited or triggered mode of a dual-chamber pacemaker. Oversensing may be caused by electrode displacement, inappropriate sensitivity settings, EMI or lead fracture. A partially fractured lead often allows signals to saturate the sensing amplifier, causing oversensing and inhibition of pacing output in demand mode. On the surface ECG, oversensing mimics failure

to discharge because oversensing may cause inhibition of the pacing stimuli; for example, in a DDD pacemaker, a sensed P wave usually triggers a ventricular stimulus after completing the timed P-V interval; however, if the ventricular lead senses an intrinsic signal (eg, oversensing noise), the ventricular stimulus is inhibited. The only way to confirm oversensing is to examine IC-EGM (intracardiac-EGM) through a programmer. If noise is recorded on the IC-EGM, then the problem is due to oversensing.

To correct suspected oversensing in a temporary pacemaker system, the nurse should check the connection between the temporary pacemaker and the lead. Electrical noise from an improperly connected lead could cause oversensing. EMI should be investigated, and the grounding wires of all electrical equipment should be checked. Unipolar leads are particularly prone to EMI because of the broad sensing field from the tip of the lead (negative pole) to the generator (ground). The sensitivity may be decreased by turning the dial toward asynchronous, toward a higher mV value. Oversensing due to partial wire fracture in a temporary transvenous bipolar catheter may also be corrected by converting to a unipolar system.

**UNDERSENSING.** Failure of the pacemaker to sense intrinsic beats is known as undersensing and results in inappropriately placed pacemaker artifacts on the ECG (Fig. 18-37). Undersensing may be a result of lead dislodgment, lead insulation defect, lead wire fracture, or inappropriately programmed sensitivity. Ventricular dysrhythmia caused by the pacemaker firing during the vulnerable phase of the T wave is of concern with undersensing. The most likely cause of sensing failure in the temporary pacemaker is lead displacement.

To correct undersensing problems in the temporary pacemaker, the nurse must first ascertain that the lead is properly connected to the temporary pacer. Undersensing may also be corrected by increasing the sensitivity of the device, which is

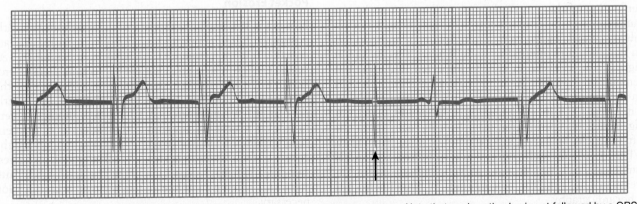

**FIGURE 18-36** Electrocardiogram (ECG) strip showing evidence of failure to capture. Note that pacing stimulus is not followed by a QRS complex.

**FIGURE 18-37** ECG strip showing evidence of undersensing. Failure of the ventricular demand pacemaker to detect the intrinsic rhythm is shown by pacemaker spikes at inappropriate intervals after spontaneous QRS complexes.

done by turning the dial to a lower millivolt value (ie, detect a smaller signal). If problems persist, the physician may need to reposition or replace the lead. In permanent pacemakers, undersensing can sometimes be corrected by reprogramming to a more sensitive setting or by switching bipolar to unipolar sensing mode.

## Pacemaker Complications

Numerous possible complications are associated with cardiac pacemakers. The critical care nurse plays a vital role in the early detection and management of these complications.

### Pneumothorax

Because of the proximity of the subclavian vein to the apex of the lung, insertion of a transvenous lead through the subclavian vein can be complicated by traumatic injury to the lung by the exploring needle, allowing air to escape into the pleural cavity. The symptoms may occur suddenly or may insidiously present up to 48 hours after the procedure. The symptoms include pleuritic pain, hypotension, respiratory distress, or hypoxia. A chest radiograph can reveal the extent of the trauma. When severe, placement of a chest tube is needed for lung reexpansion.

### Ventricular Irritability

Ventricular irritability at the site of the endocardial catheter tip is occasionally encountered in temporary pacing systems during and after initial catheter insertion. The PVC usually appear similar in configuration to the pacemaker complexes (Fig. 18-38). Irritability from the catheter as a foreign body usually disappears after a few hours. Persistent ventricular irritability may indicate lead dislodgment in both temporary and permanent pacing systems.

### Perforation of Ventricular Wall or Septum

Perforation of the ventricular free wall or septum by the transvenous catheter may occur. This may or may not result in cardiac tamponade. Elderly patients and patients on chronic corticosteroid or anticoagulant therapy are at highest risk. Perforation can be suspected if the patient demonstrates a change in precordial lead morphology on cardiac monitoring. RV apical pacing often results in a negative QRS in a V1 lead on a 12-lead ECG recording. Ventricular perforation may result in pacing from the left ventricle, and the QRS becomes positive in polarity. When ventricular wall perforation is suspected, pericardial tamponade, causing a decrease in blood pressure and an increase in sinus rate, can be confirmed by two-dimensional echocardiography.

### Catheter or Lead Dislodgment

Dislodgment of the pacing catheter or lead may occur resulting in oversensing, undersensing, or failure to capture. A chest radiograph usually confirms the findings. Catheter or lead dislodgment usually requires repositioning.

### Infection and Phlebitis or Hematoma Formation

Infection and phlebitis can occur at the temporary pacemaker insertion site, and infection or hematoma may occur at the site of permanent generator implantation. These sites must be inspected for swelling and inflammation and kept dry. Infection in permanent pacemakers needs immediate attention by a physician. In most cases, pacemaker pocket infection requires removal of the entire pacemaker system and replacement at a different site, after systemic antibiotics have been given. In temporary pacing sites, sterile technique must be used to prevent infection when dressings are changed.

### Abdominal Twitching or Hiccups

Abdominal twitching or hiccups occur occasionally as a result of electrode placement against a thin RV wall, resulting in electrical stimulation of the abdominal muscles or diaphragm. In patients with an LV lead for biventricular pacing, abdominal twitching may be due to phrenic nerve stimulation (PNS) by the LV lead in the lateral branch of the coronary sinus vein. PNS is uncomfortable for the patient and can usually be corrected by reprogramming the lead polarity or reducing generator output for that lead.[9,12]

After acute implantation, diaphragmatic stimulation may sometimes be associated with perforation. A drop in the patients' blood pressure and high capture thresholds accompanying diaphragmatic stimulation warrants critical observation and evaluation.

### Pocket Erosion

Erosion at the implantation site occurs rarely in the early postimplantation period and is more often regarded as a late complication of permanent pacemaker implantation. At times, erosion results in significant infection. Pocket erosion may be due to poor skin integrity or pressure of the generator on thinning tissues, particularly in the elderly population. When preerosion is detected, prompt surgery for pocket relocation can protect the patient from a potentially malignant cause of systemic infection and salvage the pacing system. Once a pacemaker pocket erodes, an aggressive infection may occur throughout the lead system into the heart, making complete system removal and relocation necessary.

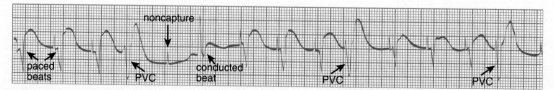

**FIGURE 18-38** Ventricular demand pacemaker with premature ventricular contractions. This strip also shows one noncaptured pacemaker spike followed by an intrinsic beat.

## Nursing Management

Critical care nurses play a key role in caring for patients with a pacemaker. The nurse is responsible for comprehensive assessment of the patient, patient and family education, ECG monitoring, and patient safety. For intervention guidelines for patients with a temporary transvenous pacemaker, see Box 18-21 on page 312.

### Patient Assessment

The critical care nurse may be the first to detect the patient's arrhythmia that necessitates pacing. Knowing the indications for bradycardia related pacing and how to initiate emergent transcutaneous pacing is essential. After a comprehensive assessment and stabilization of the patient, the critical care nurse may need to assist in inserting a transvenous or permanent pacing system.

An important aspect of preimplantation of a pacemaker includes an assessment of the patient's medical and social history. A subclavian approach may be avoided in a person with a history of a collapsed lung or previous lobectomy. A patient with a left arm arterial-venous fistula is best served with a right-sided implant. The patient's social history should be reviewed for activities such as hunting, tennis, golf, and even just preferential arm dexterity. For example, the right pectoral region should not be used in a right-handed tennis player or hunter.

To assess patients with pacemakers accurately, the nurse must understand the pacemaker code to know the type of pacer used and the programmed mode to anticipate appropriate function. The patient's underlying rhythm is assessed so that if the pacemaker fails, the nurse is prepared to treat any life-threatening arrhythmias. A chest radiograph can be used to help determine the type of pacemaker in the absence of the medical record or device wallet card.

A thorough assessment also helps the nurse determine the patient's physiologic response to pacing therapy. Important parameters to assess include pulse rate, underlying cardiac rhythm, blood pressure, activity tolerance, and evidence of dizziness, syncope, dyspnea, palpitations, or edema. The nurse should be attentive to results of chest radiographs, blood tests, and other relevant laboratory tests. If a permanent pacemaker has been implanted, the incision and pocket are examined for swelling, redness, drainage, hematoma, and tenderness.

Psychosocial assessment is another essential component of comprehensive care of the patient with a cardiac pacemaker. Patients' psychosocial responses to the need for cardiac pacing may differ. Some may be relieved to have a device that supports the functioning of their heart, whereas others may be anxious about the technology and express fears of device failure and dying.

### Patient and Family Education

A planned and systematic approach to teaching the patient and family about cardiac pacing is a vital part of nursing care. Teaching a patient about pacemakers begins at the time the decision for pacemaker insertion is made. The nurse can begin by eliciting the patient's previous knowledge of pacemakers and clarifying any misconceptions. If appropriate, clarify the difference between heart block and heart attack. The patient and family should be told why the pacemaker is necessary. The anatomy of the heart is discussed in general terms when explaining the need for pacing and how the pacemaker takes the place of or complements spontaneous rhythm. The insertion procedure and the immediate postinsertion care that can be expected are explained.

Many booklets and media presentations are available to aid the nurse in teaching the pacemaker patient. Visual and written guidelines are helpful for the patient and family to review after discharge from the hospital.

The depth of teaching that is appropriate and the teaching tools used may depend on the patient's age, intellect, attention span, vision, and interest in learning. Initial teaching should be confined to the positive aspects of life with a pacemaker. Knowledge of the function and care of the pacemaker are of no interest until the patient is able to accept it as part of life. Box 18-22 provides a guide for teaching patients and families about living with a pacemaker.

### Electrocardiogram Monitoring

Careful monitoring of the ECG of the patient with a cardiac pacemaker is an essential component of comprehensive patient assessment. The first step in the analysis involves examining the strip for evidence of pacemaker stimulation. This evidence is noted by the presence of pacing spikes on the strip. Unipolar pacing spikes are usually tall and visible, but bipolar pacing spikes may not be visible in certain leads. Each pacing spike should result in capture. If the pacing lead is in the atria, a pacing spike is followed by a P wave. If the pacing lead is in the right ventricle, the spike is followed by a wide QRS complex (Fig. 18-39). A narrower QRS following a pacing spike may be a fusion beat in dual chamber pacing. Biventricular pacing for cardiac resynchronization in HF also results in a narrower QRS (see Fig 18-39A).

The sensing function of the pacemaker is evaluated next. If the pacemaker does not sense intrinsic cardiac activity (undersensing), inappropriate pacemaker spikes may appear throughout the underlying rhythm. An oversensing problem can be detected when the pacemaker senses events other than the intrinsic rhythm and is inappropriately inhibited in that chamber or causes a triggered response in the other chamber.

The third step in evaluating the ECG is to measure various intervals in milliseconds (ms). Each small box on the ECG paper represents 40 ms, and one large box represents 200 ms. The duration of each interval is compared with the programmed setting for that interval.

The first interval, the pacing interval, is the amount of time between two consecutive pacing spikes in the chamber being paced. This interval is used to determine the pacing rate. To calculate the pacing rate, the nurse counts the number of milliseconds between two consecutive atrial spikes or two consecutive ventricular spikes (Fig. 18-40). To convert from milliseconds to beats per minute, the following formula is used: 60,000 ms/min divided by the number of milliseconds between pacing spikes equals the pacing rate.

The next interval to measure is the AV interval, also known as the AV delay. This interval is analogous to the PR interval on the ECG. The AV interval is measured from the beginning of an intrinsic P wave or an atrial pacing spike to

**BOX 18-22** **TEACHING GUIDE** *Living With a Pacemaker*

## Patient Activity

- Start passive and active range-of-motion exercises on the affected arm 48 hours after implantation to avoid "frozen shoulder." For those with new leads implanted, avoid abduction of the affected arm above the shoulder level for 4 to 6 weeks to prevent lead dislodgment.
- Avoid activities that may result in high impact or stress at the implantation site.
- Return to work at the discretion of your physician after discussing the type of work you do and what your job entails.
- Return to whatever degree of sexual activity you prefer.
- Your pacemaker will set off the alarm on metal-detector devices in airports, so avoid going through the detector gates. Show your pacemaker identification card. A manual search may be done or a magnetic wand may be used. Do not allow the wand to linger at the pacemaker site because the magnet in the wand may temporarily put the pacemaker into asynchronous mode. The metal detector or wand will not cause any permanent damage or reprogramming to your pacemaker.

## Signs of Pacemaker Malfunction

- Be alert for symptoms of pacemaker malfunction: those associated with decreased perfusion of the brain, heart, or skeletal muscles. Be particularly mindful of return of symptoms you experienced before pacemaker implantation.
- Report any dizziness, fainting, shortness of breath, undue fatigue, or fluid retention. Fluid retention includes sudden weight gain, "puffy ankles," "tight abdomen" and so forth.
- Take your pulse once daily upon awakening. Report a pulse rate over 5 beats/min slower than that at which pacemaker is set.
- Be aware that your pulse may be somewhat irregular with a demand pacemaker and has some spontaneous beats and paced beats. This does not signify pacemaker malfunction.

## Signs of Infection

- Report any redness, swelling, warmth, drainage, or increase in soreness at the implantation site.
- Report a fever of undetermined source.
- Seek medical attention if infection in other area of the body does not resolve in a reasonable time period.

## Medications

- Antibiotics are usually given within 24 hours of pacemaker implantation. Report any unusual reactions to your physician.
- Medications that were withdrawn before pacemaker implantation may need to be restarted. Check with your physician about such medications as beta blockers, ca channel blocker, digoxin, or blood thinners. Know the name of the medication and the dose, frequency of administration, side effects, and use of each medication.
- If warfarin (Coumadin) therapy is restarted, INR should be rechecked after reinitiation of the medication.

## Considerations for Home Care

- Carry a pacemaker identification card at all times. This card shows the brand and model of your pacemaker, the date of insertion, implanting physician, and manufacturer contact information.
- Wear a medical identification bracelet or necklace stating that you have a pacemaker.
- Adhere to a schedule of follow-up visits with your physician/cardiology team. The follow-up visit will include an interval history and device interrogation. to determine pacemaker and lead performance, battery longevity, frequency of device therapies, and any arrhythmias that may have occurred. Clinics have the capability for obtaining some of this information by telephone ("remote check"), reducing the frequency for clinic visits. Pacemaker should be checked at least once a year in the pacemaker clinic. Remote follow up does not include threshold checks, therefore it is important to follow your team's recommendations for clinic visits. If you have any symptoms similar to those you had before pacemaker insertion, have the pacemaker checked. Be alert for other symptoms of malfunction, such as unexplained dizzy spells, fatigue, or a slow pulse.
- Inform any physician or dentist of the pacemaker and of the medications you are taking.
- Avoid MRI scans, unless you have a specific MRI compatible pacing system.

## Pulse Generator Replacement

- Follow-up is intensified when the pacemaker battery approaches its elective replacement indicator (ERI). Avoid extended absences or vacations without consulting your physician at this time. The generator should be replaced with 6 to 8 weeks of reaching ERI.
- Be aware that when the battery reaches end of life (EOL) it may revert to VVI pacing at 40 bpm.
- The battery cannot be removed from the generator, so the entire generator is replaced when the battery is low (ERI).
- Generator replacement can be done as a same day surgery, as long as the leads are in good condition. Usually only the generator needs to be replaced.

## Considerations for the Older Patient

- Report any changes in skin condition at the pacemaker site. Sudden weight loss or poor nutritional status may predispose elderly patients to pocket erosion.
- Report symptoms, such as fatigue, neck pulsations, and lack of energy. Patients with CHB or high percentage of ventricular pacing over time may develop AV dyssynchrony (pacemaker syndrome).
- If the pacemaker feels like it is "flipping" inside the pocket, report it to your doctor and do not reposition it. When the skin is loose or when the patient "twiddles" with the pacemaker, the leads can become tangled or coiled and may fracture.

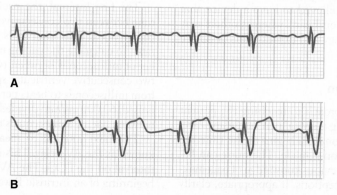

**A**

**B**

**FIGURE 18-39** Pacemaker initiated beats. **A:** The pacemaker artifact is followed by intrinsic QRS complex deflection. **B:** Pacemaker capture (ventricular capture) beats with typical widening of QRS complex.

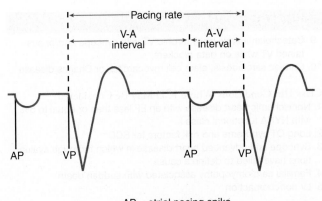

AP = atrial pacing spike
VP = ventricular pacing spike

**FIGURE 18-40** The intervals measured on an ECG strip for a patient with a pacemaker. The pacing interval is the amount of time between two consecutive atrial pacing spikes or two consecutive ventricular pacing spikes. The atrioventricular (AV) interval is measured from the beginning of a P wave or an atrial pacing spike to the beginning of an intrinsic QRS complex or the ventricular pacing spike. The ventriculoatrial (VA) interval is measured from a ventricular pacing or sensed beat to the next atrial pacing spike. The sum of the AV and VA intervals equals the pacing interval.

the beginning of the intrinsic QRS complex or the ventricular pacing spike (see Fig. 18-40).

The third interval to measure is the ventriculoatrial (VA) interval, also called the atrial escape interval. The VA interval is the amount of time from a ventricular paced or sensed event to the next atrial paced stimulus (see Fig. 18-40). The sum of the AV and the VA interval equals the pacing interval.

### Patient Safety

Electrical safety precautions must be observed when the patient has a temporary pacemaker. Electrical equipment in the room is kept at a minimum and must be properly grounded. Electric beds must be properly grounded or remain disconnected from AC. Only battery-operated electric shavers, toothbrushes, or radios are recommended. The nurse should avoid simultaneous contact with the patient and any electrical equipment. The patient's bed must be kept dry at all times. Diathermy and electrocautery equipment should not be used because their output may be sensed by and inhibit the demand pacemaker.

The literature on ensuring electrical safety in temporary pacemaker wires has been sparse; however, manufacturers have been guided by the FDA to increase vigilance over patient safety. Currently manufactured leads have no exposed areas after they are inserted tightly into the connecting cable. The use of rubber gloves to handle temporary pacing lead terminal pins is recommended to help avoid micro shocks. Most manufacturers supply connecting cables with the pulse generator to ensure compatibility. Care should also be taken to ensure that nonsterile cables are not in close proximity with the sterile field during insertion.

The temporary pacing catheter should be taped securely to the patient's skin without direct tension on the catheter. Motion of the extremity nearest the catheter entry site should be minimized, especially if the femoral site has been used.

According to manufacturers of permanent pacemaker generators, very few electrical hazards are associated with the permanent generators. These generators are shielded from external electrical sources and usually are not affected by microwave ovens, small appliances, or small power tools. There have been rare reports of unipolar pacemakers being affected by large electromagnetic fields and radiofrequency signals, such as radio transmitters. The patient should take precautions to avoid large magnetic fields. Patients with pacemakers should use the ear furthest from the device (or an ear piece) when talking on a cell phone, and should avoid carrying the phone in close proximity to the device (ie, less than 6 inches [15 cm]).

## Implantable Cardioverter–Defibrillators

Sudden cardiac arrest, also referred to as sudden cardiac death, continues to be a leading cause of death in the United States.[13] Sudden cardiac death may be caused by the rapid loss of heart pump function due to VF or VT. Rapid VT and fibrillation can be corrected when treated within minutes with defibrillation.

In the late 1960s, Dr. Michel Mirowski and Dr. Morton Mower developed the implantable cardioverter defibrillator (ICD) to treat patients at risk for sudden death due to ventricular dysrhythmia. In 1980, the first device was implanted successfully in a person. The device was found to be safe and effective and, as a result, received FDA approval in 1985. Since its initial use in 1980, the ICD generator and lead technology have undergone many improvements in design and function. With these improvements, as well as with expanded indications and increased understanding of patients at risk, ICD implantation is approved for both primary and secondary prevention of sudden death.[9,14]

### Indications

Uniform criteria for ICD implantation were established by the Joint Committee of the ACC, AHA, and Heart Rhythm Society by class indications.[9] Class I indication recommends implantation. Class II includes conditions for which ICDs may be used, with less than sufficient evidence or divergence of opinion regarding the necessity of insertion. Class III includes conditions for which there is evidence that ICD implantation is unnecessary or may be harmful. Box 18-23 lists the indications for use of ICD therapy.

### The ICD System

The primary purpose of an ICD is to continuously monitor the patient's rhythm, diagnose rhythm changes, and treat life-threatening ventricular arrhythmias. Secondary function is a pacemaker for bradycardia and nonbradycardia indications. Similar to a pacemaker, the ICD consists of a lead system and a pulse generator containing the battery, capacitors, and circuits.

#### The Pulse Generator

Over time, ICD pulse generators have evolved from large, heavy devices implanted in the abdomen to small, lighter-weight devices that are implanted in the pectoral area (Fig. 18-41). The size of the header is determined by the number of leads used. Lithium silver vanadium oxide (Li/SVO) batteries provide the power source for ICDs.

**BOX 18-23** **Indications for Implantable Cardioverter–Defibrillators (ICDs)***

**Class I: Conditions Where ICD Is Effective/Beneficial**

1. Survivors of cardiac arrest due to ventricular fibrillation (VF) or ventricular tachycardia (VT), after evaluation to exclude transient or reversible causes
2. Spontaneous sustained VT associated with structural heart disease
3. Syncope of undetermined origin with induced sustained VT or VF at electrophysiologic study
4. LV dysfunction with EF less than 35% due to prior MI more than 40 days, and NYHA functional class II or III
5. Nonischemic dilated cardiomyopathy (NICM) with an EF less than or equal to 35% and in NYHA functional class II or III

**Class IIa: Conditions Where ICD Is Reasonable**

1. Patients with unexplained syncope, significant LV dysfunction and ND-CM
2. Sustained VT and normal or near normal ventricular function
3. Hypertrophic cardiomyopathy with one or more major risk factors for sudden cardiac death (SCD)
4. Arrhythmogenic right ventricular dysplasia cardiomyopathy with one or more risk factors for SCD
5. Syncope and/or VT while on beta blockers in patients with long QT
6. Nonhospitalized patients awaiting transplantation
7. Brugada syndrome with syncope
8. Brugada syndrome with documented VT that has not resulted in cardiac arrest

9. Catecholaminergic polymorphic VT with syncope and/or sustained VT while on beta blockers
10. Cardiac sarcoidosis, giant cell myocarditis, or Chagas disease

**Class IIb: Conditions Where ICD May Be Considered**

1. Nonischemic heart disease with an EF less than or equal to 5% with NYHA functional class I
2. Long QT syndrome and risk factors for SCD
3. Syncope and advanced heart disease in which thorough evaluations have failed to define a cause
4. Familial cardiomyopathy associated with sudden death
5. LV noncompaction

**Class III: Conditions Where ICD Is Not Useful or May Be Harmful**

1. Conditions that meet Class I, IIa, and IIb but with expected survival less than 1 year
2. Incessant VT or VF
3. Patients with significant psychiatric illnesses that may be aggravated by device implantation or preclude follow-up
4. NYHA Class IV patients with drug-refractory congestive heart failure (HF) and not candidates for cardiac transplantation or CRT-D
5. Syncope of undetermined cause in a patient without inducible VT and without structural heart disease
6. VT or VF amenable to surgical or catheter ablation
7. VT due to reversible cause in the absence of structural heart disease

*Box does not include indications for children, adolescents, and patients with congenital heart disease.

Adapted from Tracy CM, Epstein AE, Darbar D, et al; ACCF/AHA/HRS Focused Update of the 2008 Guidelines for Device-Based Therapy of Cardiac Rhythm Abnormalities: A Report of the American College of Cardiology Foundation/American Heart Association Task Force on Practice Guidelines. Circulation 126(14):1784–800, 2012.

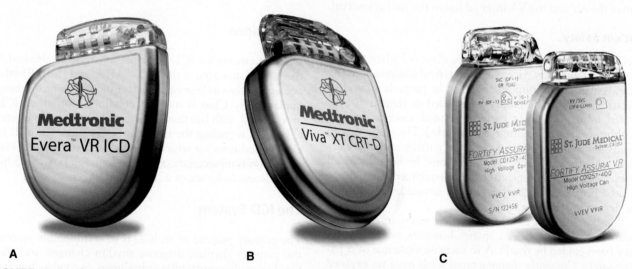

**A** **B** **C**

**FIGURE 18-41** **A:** Medtronic Evera VR single chamber ICD. **B:** Medtronic Viva XT CRT-D atrial-biventricular ICD. **C:** Fortify Assura VR single-chamber ICD. (A and B images courtesy of Medtronic, Inc. C image courtesy of St. Jude Medical, Inc. Fortify Assura and St. Jude Medical are trademarks of St. Jude Medical, Inc. or its related companies. Reprinted with permission of St. Jude Medical, ©2014. All rights reserved.)

Improved circuit design has expanded the capabilities and functions of the ICD.

## The Lead System

Lead systems sense life-threatening ventricular tachyarrhythmias and deliver therapies (rapid pacing or shock) to convert the dysrhythmia. ICD implants use bipolar or tripolar transvenous leads for sensing and defibrillation. The sensing electrodes are bipoles at the tip of the lead. One unipolar coil in the distal portion of the ventricular lead serves as the defibrillation cathode, whereas another coil in the mid-proximal portion or the ICD generator serves as the defibrillation anode, giving rise to the term "active can." With dual-chamber ICDs, an additional bipolar electrode in the right atrium provides atrial sensing and pacing. In biventricular pacing ICDs, a third lead is inserted in the coronary sinus and positioned in a left lateral vein for LV stimulation and resynchronization.

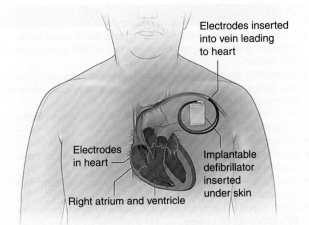

Electrodes inserted into vein leading to heart

Electrodes in heart

Implantable defibrillator inserted under skin

Right atrium and ventricle

**FIGURE 18-42** The ICD mechanical system consists of a generator and a sensing/pacing/defibrillating electrode in the RV. All ICDs also have pacing functions, therefore the system may also include atrial and LV leads. (Courtesy of the National Heart, Lung, and Blood Institute)

Ideally, the ICD generator is implanted in the left pectoral area so that the heart is central to the vector of the defibrillation current (Fig. 18-42). Transvenous pacing and defibrillation leads are implanted similar to permanent pacing leads as previously described. As with initial pacemaker implants, patients can anticipate a 24-hour short stay post-ICD implant.[15]

## ICD Functioning

ICDs function using a tiered therapy approach (Table 18-10). Therapies are programmed based on individual patient needs. Not all patients require all therapies.

The first tier of therapy is antitachycardia pacing (ATP), to treat VT by using rapid pacing intervals that are faster than the detected arrhythmia. ATP is delivered in bursts, ramp pacing or a combination of both. ATP is painless and is delivered quicker than a shock. If ATP is not successful, the second tier of therapy, synchronized cardioversion, is used. The joules for cardioversion can be programmed anywhere from 1 to 36 J, with the highest output dependent on device specifications. To minimize patient discomfort and expedite therapy, ATP is attempted during shock charging. If cardioversion is not successful, the third tier of therapy, defibrillation, is used. The energy delivered for defibrillation can be programmed to a maximum of 43 J, depending on the model and capacity of a device.

The number of defibrillation attempts varies among devices; six attempts in each tier is the maximum. If the patient is successfully converted to a life-compatible rhythm, but the rate is slow, demand pacing is initiated. Bradycardia pacing is programmed in all ICDs. Type and duration of pacing (eg, VVI, DDD, or biventricular) depends upon patient needs.

ICDs have many programmable features that allow the physician to tailor the device to the patient's needs. It is important to remember that an ICD function first as a defibrillator and second as a pacemaker. Bradycardia pacing therapies, including biventricular pacing, are available in most ICDs. Pacing codes for ICDs are the same as in pacemakers (see Table 18-8). An atrial sensing lead allows more specific SVT discrimination algorithms. To improve discrimination of tachyarrhythmias, the device allows programming of discrimination algorithms—for example, withholding VT therapy when PSVT is confirmed. Some devices also have separate tiers of therapy for atrial tachycardia and AF or flutter.

All ICDs are "noncommitted," that is, therapy is aborted if the tachycardia terminates, even while the ICD is charging. This prevents patients with nonsustained VT from suffering the discomfort of an inappropriate shock. Event retrieval involves successive R-wave analysis or EGM recordings of the tachyarrhythmia and therapy. Recordings include arrhythmia before and after the therapy, allowing the physician to analyze the problematic rhythm. These data are correlated to the patient's symptoms to help further diagnose the arrhythmia and appropriate device function.

As with pacemakers, ICDs can be monitored remotely to minimize office visits and assure appropriate device function. Remote transmissions are sent via traditional phone land lines, or using a cell adaptor with the remote transmitter. Many devices are wireless and communicate with the transmitter at routine intervals without the patient needing to interact with the technology. The data are sent to a secure database; cardiology team members then download the information for review and inclusion in the patient's medical record. Information from transmissions include battery voltage, lead impedance, tachyarrhythmia detections and therapies, and percent of pacing.

## Nursing Management

The critical care nurse plays a key role in the pre- and post-implantation management of patients with an ICD. Patient teaching is one of the most important tasks of the critical care nurse. Topics for discussion are included in the Box 18-24. Patients and families need to understand why an ICD is indicated, the purpose of an ICD, the basic parts of the ICD system, how the ICD functions, and what to do if a shock occurs. Once the physician has determined the type of system to be used, the nurse reinforces the physician's explanation

**TABLE 18-10 Implantable Cardioverter–Defibrillator: Tiered Therapy**

| Type of Therapy* | Mode/Energy Level | Condition(s) |
| --- | --- | --- |
| Antibradycardia pacing/Biventricular pacing | VVI/DDD/VDD | Bradycardia CHF |
| Antitachycardia pacing (ATP) | Burst/ramp ATP | AT†/VT (120–200 bpm) |
| Cardioversion‡ | 10–36 J | VT (180–230 bpm) |
| Defibrillation | 30–36 J | VF (>230 bpm) |

*Therapy and detection intervals (rate of tachycardia detected) are programmable.
†AT therapies limited to certain models.
‡ATP while charging, if successful diverts defibrillation shock.
CHF, congestive heart failure; AT, atrial tachycardia; VT, ventricular tachycardia; VF, ventricular fibrillation.

**BOX 18-24** *TEACHING GUIDE* *Implantable Cardioverter–Defibrillator*

When teaching patients receiving an ICD, be sure to include the following points:

- The purpose of an ICD and why it is indicated
- Components of an ICD
- How the ICD works
- How a shock feels
- How the ICD will be implanted
- The expected length of hospitalization
- Activities of daily living that can be tolerated postimplantation
- Rate cutoff and therapies programmed in the ICD, including pacing parameters
- Plans for follow-up care and when to call the doctor
- Importance of carrying an ICD identification card and/or wearing medical identification devices, such as a bracelet or necklace
- Need for carrying a list of current medications and dosages

- Safety precautions (avoid electromagnetic fields, using tools with strong vibrations, no MRI unless has an MRI compatible ICD system)
- Importance of keeping emergency phone numbers readily available and what to do after receiving a shock, especially when not feeling completely recovered
- Importance of calling the physician immediately if you receive more than one shock or several in succession
- What the patient and family should do if a shock occurs
- Information the family, significant others, coworkers, and traveling companions should know about the ICD
- Precautions to be taken when traveling by air and informing airline security personnel of the ICD
- Encouraging of family members to take a cardiopulmonary resuscitation (CPR) course
- Benefits of support groups

of how the device will be implanted and where the leads and pulse generator will be placed. The patient and family should be informed of how the device is programmed and plans for short and long term follow-up care. Many resources for patient education are available from manufacturers of ICDs, including printed materials and videotapes. In addition, the patient and family may find it helpful to meet with a person who has an ICD. This person may be able to alleviate any fears or clarify misconceptions about living with an ICD.[16]

In the immediate postimplantation period, the nurse continuously monitors the patient for the development of any ventricular arrhythmias and intervenes if necessary. If the patient experiences sustained VT and no therapy is delivered, it may be because the rate of the tachycardia is below the programmed rate cutoff (ie, the VT detection rate that triggers device therapies), or because undersensing of the tachyarrhythmias is occurring. Knowledge of the parameters of the ICD and the rate of the patient's arrhythmia is essential for the critical care nurse to assess this situation correctly. A patient with an ICD and who has a sustained, hemodynamically unstable rhythm should not be treated any differently from someone without an ICD. Basic Cardiac Life Support (BCLS) and Advanced Cardiac Life Support (ACLS) should be initiated. External cardioversion can be given in an emergency in the absence of effective therapy from the patient's ICD. Care should be taken not to apply paddles near or above the ICD generator pocket.

The nurse must be aware of the programmed settings and features of the patient's ICD to provide safe and competent care. Device information should be readily available at the bedside and clearly documented in the patient's chart; this includes both pacing and defibrillation therapies. If the device fires, the status of the patient and the patient's rhythm is assessed and documented. If a device fires in the absence of arrhythmias, there is a high probability of R-wave oversensing due to a dislodged or damaged lead, a loose connection at the header, or an oversensitive parameter setting. Immediate intervention by the EP service is necessary to avoid further discomfort to the patient. In the event of inappropriate shocks, VT storm, or emergent surgery in which electrocautery is used, a magnet can be placed over the ICD pocket to inhibit defibrillation therapies. The magnet will not affect

the pacing function of an ICD, nor will it turn the device completely off. Tachyarrhythmia detection and therapies are fully restored when the magnet is removed.[9]

Other immediate postoperative care (wound care, activity instructions) is very similar to that for the patient after pacemaker implantation (see Box 18-22, p. 320). Furthermore, because the operative approach is almost identical to that of a pacemaker, the complications that one might expect from a pacemaker implant can also be encountered after ICD implantation.

After consulting with the implanting physician, the nurse provides discharge instructions about resuming daily activities. Patients are instructed about activity restrictions for the first six weeks post implant while the leads are healing into the myocardium. They are also cautioned against operating equipment that may produce sparks or cause EMI. A complete list of equipment that may interfere with the ICD function is available from the manufacturer. Patient and family teaching points (Box 18-24) should be reviewed with the patient and family with discharge instructions.

Discussion of psychosocial issues regarding living with an ICD also should be part of the discharge preparation. Although the emotional adjustment varies with each patient, many have fears about receiving their first shock. Other potential patient concerns include alterations in body image, return to work, participation in recreational activities, and reaction of family and friends to the device. Patients who are commercial drivers may not be able to return to that type of work. If support groups are available, the patient and family should be encouraged to join.[16]

## CARDIOPULMONARY RESUSCITATION

The acuity of patients in an ICU requires the nurse to be especially vigilant for subtle signs of change in the patient's status. Numerous technologies and monitoring devices assist the nurse in delivering effective interventions, but physical assessment skills must be continually practiced and improved.

In any ICU, there is an increased chance that the patient's condition will deteriorate. The cessation of breathing and circulation is known as cardiopulmonary arrest, also referred

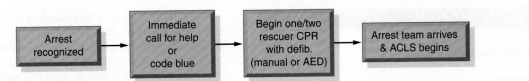

FIGURE 18-43 Sequence of events in CPR.

to as sudden cardiac arrest. When a patient is determined to be in cardiopulmonary arrest, seconds matter: unless definitive action is taken within 4 to 6 minutes, the patient will suffer irreversible brain injury. Prompt intervention is necessary to increase the patient's chances of survival.

Immediate, high quality cardiopulmonary resuscitation (CPR) offers the best chance for neurologically intact patient survival. The American Heart Association (AHA) separates care of adult cardiac arrest patients into three tiers: Basic Life Support (BLS), Advanced Cardiac Life Support (ACLS), and post–cardiac arrest care. Although the abbreviations BLS and CPR are often used interchangeably, BLS also includes emergency care interventions for choking and rescue breathing, and use of an automated external defibrillator (AED) as well as CPR. Rescue breathing alone is administered when a patient has a detectable pulse but is apneic. Figure 18-43 shows the sequence of events in CPR.

Evidence-based recommendations from the AHA identify several critical areas to improve cardiac arrest patient outcomes:[1–3]

- Focus on CPR quality.
- Defibrillate shockable rhythms as soon as possible.
- Minimizing interruption in cardiac compressions.
- Avoid excessive ventilations.
- Incorporate post event de-briefing.
- Measure outcomes, practice, and improve.

These areas are discussed in relation to the role of the nurse during a cardiopulmonary arrest. High-quality CPR (summarized in Box 18-25) is the foundation on which successful BLS and ACLS are based, and it is discussed in several parts of this chapter. The ACLS Pulseless Arrest Algorithm and the ACLS Post Cardiac Arrest Care algorithm are discussed briefly, as well as family presence at an arrest.

ACLS is an advanced set of intra- and postarrest interventions best addressed in its entirety by taking an ACLS Provider course. ACLS guidelines and information about ACLS courses are available at the AHA website, http://www.onlineaha.org/courses. Although transcutaneous pacing is no longer part of the Pulseless Arrest Algorithm, it is discussed as a potential prearrest intervention.

## Causes of Cardiopulmonary Arrest

Box 18-26 outlines some of the causes of cardiopulmonary arrest. This list is not all inclusive; there may be many additional causes of cardiopulmonary arrest. The use of numerous monitoring devices in an ICU, such as continuous electrocardiography, pulse oximetry, wave form capnography, intravascular pressure tracings, and ventilator volume and pressure alarms may allow the nurse to detect changes

---

**BOX 18-25   Components of High-Quality CPR**

Circulation
- Determine unresponsiveness and absence of breathing and pulse
- Place backboard under patient's chest
- Start compressions within 10 seconds of finding no breathing or pulse
- Push Hard and Fast while:
  - Compressing chest at rate of at least 100 to 120/min
  - Compressing chest to a depth at least 2 inches but no more than 2.4 inches
  - Allowing full chest recoil after each compression
  - Minimizing interruptions in compressions to less than 10 seconds
  - Rotating staff doing compressions every 2 minutes
- Palpate pulses (carotid or femoral) to determine effectiveness of compressions

Airway
- Open patients airway using head tilt–chin lift maneuver (jaw thrust for patients with or suspected to have cervical spine injuries
- Place oropharyngeal airway (if possible)
- Provide suction as necessary

Breathing
- Ventilate effectively using a barrier device (face mask or BVM)
  - Maintain seal around patient's mouth and nose
  - Observe for chest rise and fall
- Avoid excessive ventilations
  - 2 ventilations with each 30 compressions or
  - One ventilation every 6 seconds (10 breaths a minute) with an advanced airway
- Use End Tidal $CO_2$ and Pulse Oximetry to determine resuscitation efficacy

Defibrillation
- Defibrillate as soon as possible when a shockable rhythm is detected

Adapted from AHA Adult BLS for HCP algorithm 10/2015.

---

in a patient's status and take definitive actions to prevent a cardiac arrest. But even in the best of circumstances, cardiac arrest can occur without warning, and requires rapid detection and resuscitation. Once cardiac arrest has occurred, determination of the cause of the arrest is secondary to rapid intervention. Once interventions to restore life have been initiated, the cause of the arrest can then be searched for, and any specific interventions designed to correct the underlying cause can be added to the ACLS measures. Treatable causes (commonly referred to as the Hs & Ts) are outlined in the AHA's Adult Cardiac Pulseless Arrest Algorithm.

**Causes of Cardiopulmonary Arrest**

Cardiac Causes
- Myocardial infarction
- Heart failure
- Dysrhythmia
- Coronary artery spasms
- Cardiac tamponade

Pulmonary Causes
- Respiratory failure secondary to respiratory depression
- Airway obstruction
- Impaired gas exchange, such as in acute respiratory distress syndrome
- Impaired ventilation, such as pneumothorax
- Pulmonary embolus

Electrolyte Imbalances
- Hyperkalemia
- Hypomagnesemia
- Hypercalcemia/hypocalcemia

Procedural Causes
- Pulmonary artery catheterization
- Cardiac catheterization
- Surgery

Miscellaneous
- Drug toxicity and drug side effects
- Trauma—myocardial contusion or aortic tear

## Assessment and Management of the Patient in Cardiopulmonary Arrest

Before resuscitative measures are implemented in a cardiopulmonary arrest, the patient must undergo an initial assessment. A myriad of technological monitoring devices are used in the ICU, but it is the everyday physical assessment skills used by nurses that are most accurate in determining a patient's status. The nurse needs to ensure that the alarm parameters of the bedside monitors are set accurately for each patient. The default settings are not always appropriate—remember to treat the patient, not the monitor! Figure 18-44 illustrates the proper sequence for BLS in adults.

Assessment and treatment of the cardiac arrest patient should be done simultaneously, rather than sequentially. After assessing unresponsiveness and calling for help, presence of breathing and pulse can be evaluated at the same time; this decreased the assessment time from 20 seconds to 10 seconds, allowing the rescuer(s) to begin chest compressions more quickly. In healthcare settings where there are trained rescuers, team resuscitation allows multiple people to carryout different action simultaneously—for example, one rescuer calls for help, another does chest compressions, a third rescuer provides ventilations, and another rescuer attaches and operates the defibrillator.[4]

## Positioning the Patient

The patient should be placed supine on a firm, flat surface. This position enables the rescuer to open the airway and assess for the presence and effectiveness of any spontaneous breathing. If the patient is in a standard hospital bed, a back board is placed under his or her torso when help arrives. If the patient is breathing effectively and there is no evidence of trauma, the patient should be placed flat with the head of the bed elevated. Caution must be used when moving patients with suspected or actual spinal cord injuries. One rescuer should ensure that the patient's head remains in a neutral position.

## Determining Responsiveness

The first step in assessment is the determination of responsiveness. If the patient is sedated, comatose, or mechanically ventilated, assessment of responsiveness may not be possible. Unresponsiveness is defined as no response when the patient is shaken and spoken to loudly (eg, "Are you ok?").

After determining responsiveness, the nurse should observe the patient's chest for breathing while simultaneously palpating the carotid pulse. Breathing can only occur if there is blood flow to the respiratory centers in the brainstem. The patient who is breathing is not in cardiac arrest. (*Remember:* This does not apply if the patient is on a ventilator.) Unresponsiveness associated with lack of breathing is considered a cardinal sign of cardiac arrest.

This initial assessment should take no more than 10 seconds. If the patient is unresponsive, not breathing, and has no detectable carotid pulse, the nurse should call for help and request a Code Blue. Once help has been requested, CPR should be started as soon as a backboard can be placed under the patient. CPR always starts with chest compressions. When the "code" is called, the nurse who has the patient acts as the interim team leader until the Code Blue team arrives. When additional staff (responding to the call for help) arrive, they should be assigned appropriate roles using a team approach. Box 18-27 lists the suggested roles and responsibilities of code team members.

## Performing Chest Compressions

### One-Rescuer CPR

BLS typically begins with one rescuer, who assesses the patient for unresponsiveness and breathing, then calls for help. CPR begins with chest compressions, and requires the patient be supine on a hard surface. Many hospital beds now have a CPR mode, which quickly flattens the bed; however, a back board is essential. Chest compressions initially provide blood flow to the brain and vital organs by compressing the heart between the sternum and the spine; without a backboard, it is not possible to get the sternal movement needed to circulate blood.

Maintaining high-quality CPR is vital to the potential recovery of the patient. It should be noted that ventilations are no longer considered the most important initial intervention. Numerous studies compiled by the International Liaison Committee on Resuscitation (ILCOR) have shown that apneic patients have enough oxygen bound to hemoglobin to allow for adequate oxygen delivery during the first few minutes of a cardiac arrest.[5] Early initiation of chest compressions improves survival rates by providing a flow of blood that is already adequately oxygenated.

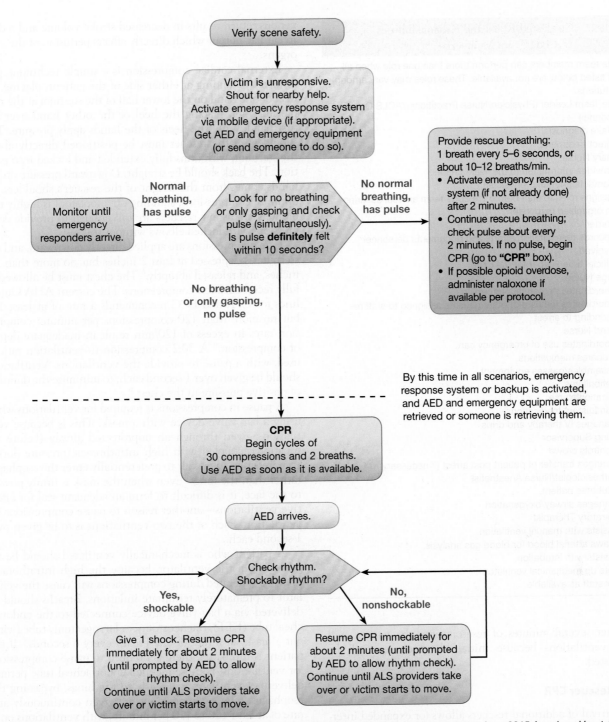

Verify scene safety.

Victim is unresponsive.
Shout for nearby help.
Activate emergency response system
via mobile device (if appropriate).
Get AED and emergency equipment
(or send someone to do so).

Provide rescue breathing:
1 breath every 5–6 seconds, or
about 10–12 breaths/min.
• Activate emergency response
  system (if not already done)
  after 2 minutes.
• Continue rescue breathing;
  check pulse about every
  2 minutes. If no pulse, begin
  CPR (go to **"CPR"** box).
• If possible opioid overdose,
  administer naloxone if
  available per protocol.

Normal
breathing,
has pulse

Monitor until
emergency
responders arrive.

Look for no breathing
or only gasping and check
pulse (simultaneously).
Is pulse **definitely** felt
within 10 seconds?

No normal
breathing,
has pulse

No breathing
or only gasping,
no pulse

By this time in all scenarios, emergency
response system or backup is activated,
and AED and emergency equipment are
retrieved or someone is retrieving them.

**CPR**
Begin cycles of
30 compressions and 2 breaths.
Use AED as soon as it is available.

AED arrives.

Check rhythm.
Shockable rhythm?

Yes,
shockable

No,
nonshockable

Give 1 shock. Resume CPR
immediately for about 2 minutes
(until prompted by AED to allow
rhythm check).
Continue until ALS providers take
over or victim starts to move.

Resume CPR immediately for
about 2 minutes (until prompted
by AED to allow rhythm check).
Continue until ALS providers take
over or victim starts to move.

**FIGURE 18-44** BLS Healthcare Provider Adult Cardiac Arrest-2015 Update. (Reprinted with permission from 2015 American Heart Association Guidelines Update for CPR and ECC. Circulation 123[suppl 2]:S313–S589, 2015. © 2015, American Heart Association, Inc.)

Once 30 compressions have been completed, the airway is assessed and breaths initiated: this is the compression, airway, breathing (C-A-B) sequence. With emphasis placed on the vital activity of chest compressions, less time is lost in establishing an airway (see Box 18-25). For adults, the recommended compression-to-ventilation ratio is 30:2. Ventilations should be deferred until the arrival of a barrier device such as a bag-valve-mask (BVM) or a face mask. The use of mouth-to-mouth ventilations is discouraged.

Compression-only CPR is preferable to mouth-to-mouth contact with a patient whose infectious status is unknown. With universal precautions, all patients are considered infectious. Unless a face mask designed for use by a single rescuer is immediately available, use of a BVM should wait until a second rescuer arrives. A BVM can only be properly used by a rescuer positioned at the patient's head; this position allows the rescuer to adequately seal the mask and anticipate breath delivery.

BOX 18-27 **Suggested Roles and Responsibilities of Code Team Members**

Code team members can perform more than one role when all staff listed below are not available. These roles may vary among institutions.

Code Team Leader (Physician/Nurse Practitioner/ACLS Qualified Personnel)
- Make diagnosis.
- Direct treatment.

Primary Nurse
- Provides information to the Team Leader.
- Contacts attending physician.
- Assigns roles to staff before the code team arrives, assuring an organized response.

Recorder
- Records resuscitation efforts and documents personnel involved.
- Official time keeper for the code.

Charge Nurse
- Coordinates personnel performing CPR.
- Coordinates the care of other patients assigned to staff responding to arrest.

Second Nurse
- Coordinates use of emergency cart.
- Prepares medications.
- Assembles/passes equipment.
- Defibrillates.

Medication Nurse
- Administers medications.
- Manages IV therapy and drips

Nursing Supervisor
- Controls crowd.
- Arranges transfer of patient post arrest (if necessary).

Anesthesiologist/Nurse Anesthetist
- Intubates patient.
- Manages airway/oxygenation.

Respiratory Therapist
- Assists with manual ventilation.
- Draws arterial blood for blood gas analysis.
- Assists with intubation.
- Sets up mechanical ventilator.

Other staff as available

After several minutes of resuscitation, the patient will need ventilations because initial blood oxygen will be exhausted.

## Two Rescuer CPR

The arrival of additional rescuers allows for expanded interventions, including ventilations, defibrillation, and resuscitation documentation. The second rescuer to arrive should relieve the first rescuer by taking over chest compressions. When a second rescuer takes over chest compressions, the first rescuer or additional available staff can open the airway and be ready to deliver breaths via a BVM at the appropriate time in the cycle of 30 compressions to 2 ventilations.

Rescuers doing chest compressions must be rotated every 2 minutes (or after every 5 cycles of 30:2). Rescuer fatigue is a key element in the failure of resuscitation and one that is often overlooked. When rescuers begin to tire, they begin to lean on the chest, not allowing for full recoil (reexpansion) of the chest. When the chest is depressed, intrathoracic pressure is increased, decreasing venous return. This decreased

venous return results in decreased stroke volume and a drop in cardiac output which directly affects perfusion of the vital organs.

External cardiac compression is a simple technique performed by standing at either side of the patient, placing the heel of one hand on the lower half of the sternum at the nipple line, and placing the heel of the other hand over the first hand. Only the heels of the hands apply pressure. The shoulders of the rescuer must be positioned directly above the sternum, with arms fully extended and locked into position. The back should be straight. Downward pressure on the hands comes from the weight of the rescuer's shoulders. To optimize compressions, standing on a footstool is highly recommended, as few rescuers are tall enough to provide compressions with locked elbows without this aid.

Firm compressions are applied directly downward, and the sternum is depressed *at least* 2 inches but no more than 2.4 inches, and released abruptly.[6] The chest must be allowed to fully recoil between compressions. The current AHA Guidelines for CPR and ECC recommends a rate of at least 100 but no more than 120 compressions per minute; compression rates in excess of 120/min result in inadequate depths of compression.[6] A 30:2 compression-to-ventilation ratio is used, with a pause to provide the ventilations. Ventilations should be given over 1 second each, to minimize the duration of positive pressure in the chest.[6]

A pause in compressions is required for ventilations when using a bag valve device with a mask. This is because ventilations given through an unprotected airway (before intubation), coupled with high intrathoracic pressure during compressions, allows air to preferentially enter the esophagus rather than the lungs. Even when the mask is firmly pressed to the face, it is difficult to form an adequate seal for effective ventilations—another reason to pause compressions for ventilation. Each of the two ventilations is to be given over 1 second each.

A patient who is mechanically ventilated should be removed from the ventilator, because the high intrathoracic pressure generated during compressions will cause the ventilator to prematurely terminate inflations. Breaths should be delivered via a bag-valve device connected to the endotracheal tube (ETT), tracheostomy, or laryngectomy tube (without a mask) at a rate of one breath every 6 seconds.[6] If the patient is intubated, there is no need to pause compressions for ventilations, because a cuffed endotracheal tube permits delivery of ventilations directly to the lungs, bypassing the esophagus. Chest compressions are given continuously at a rate of at least 100 to 110 per minute, with ventilations once every 6 seconds.[6] To be effective, these techniques must be learned correctly, practiced frequently, and applied skillfully.

When additional help arrives, one person delivers breaths using a BVM, while another performs chest compressions. A third person can begin to prepare for defibrillation. Circulation checks (using carotid or femoral pulses only) should be performed by any additional rescuers without interrupting CPR.

## Airway

Healthcare providers should assess the patency of the patient's airway. No air exchange detected at the mouth or nose may reflect an obstructed airway or apnea. With the

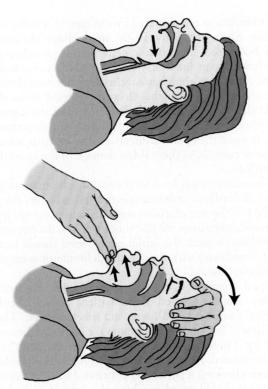

**FIGURE 18-45**  Opening the airway with the head tilt-chin maneuver.

patient supine, the airway is opened using the head tilt–chin lift method: the head is tilted back, and the chin is raised to stretch the airway and advance the tongue in preparation for ventilation The fingertips must be kept on the mandible and away from the submental soft tissues to avoid pushing the tongue against the hard palate (Fig. 18-45).

When caring for patients with confirmed or suspected cervical spine injuries, the jaw thrust method is used (Fig. 18-46). It is most important that the patient's head and neck not be

moved to ensure that no damage (or no further damage) is done to the cervical spine and spinal cord. Keeping the head in a neutral position, the rescuer places a hand on each side of the patient's head behind the temporomandibular joint, gently pushing the jaw forward; this will open the airway to allow for ventilation. Use of an oropharyngeal airway will also ensure that the tongue is not blocking the posterior pharynx. If spontaneous respirations have not returned once a patent airway has been established, then the patient must be ventilated.

## Breathing

If a BVM is connected to oxygen, the rescuer can deliver oxygen as well as ventilate. The BVM is connected to a source of high-flow oxygen (15 L/min), and the face mask is placed over the patient's mouth and nose. When connected to an oxygen source, a BVM can deliver close to 100% oxygen. If the patient has an endotracheal tube or tracheostomy tube, the BVM may be connected to these airways using a universal connector.

Use of a BVM by one person requires the use of the E-C hand clamp technique, with the rescuer positioned at patient's head. The mask is placed on the face of the patient with the narrow end over the nose, and the wide end positioned just below the lower lip. Using the thumb and forefinger of the hand holding the mask (forming a "C"), the rescuer presses directly down on the mask. Using the other three fingers of the same hand (forming an "E"), the rescuer then grasps the bony part of the mandible, pulling the angle of the jaw up and back. This technique allows the rescuer to both position and seal the mask, while at the same time opening the airway.

Once the mask is sealed to the patient's face, the bag is squeezed to deliver ventilations. When using a bag-valve without the mask, the universal connector must be firmly attached to the artificial airway; this allows the rescuer to deliver breaths using one or both hands to squeeze the bag-valve device. Ventilate only until visible chest rise is seen. Measurement of end-tidal $CO_2$ ($ETCO_2$) can be used to confirm proper airway placement and the efficacy of ventilations, and serve as a marker of cardiac output. (See Chapter 25 for additional information on endotracheal intubation.) Pulse oximetry is used to measure oxygenation.

Caution must be used to avoid hyperinflation of the lungs when an advanced airway (supraglottal airway or endotracheal tube) is not in place, because excessive airway pressure will open the esophagus and cause gastric inflation, possibly causing regurgitation and subsequent aspiration. Once an advanced airway has been placed, and position of the airway confirmed, compressions are given continuously at a rate of at least 100/min, but no more than 120/min. Ventilations are given once every 6 seconds, asynchronous with the compressions. Hyperventilation must be avoided, because this increases intrathoracic pressure and decreases venous return, leading to decreased cardiac output.

## Defibrillation

All patients should be connected to a cardiac monitor during a cardiopulmonary arrest. Once BLS has been initiated, additional interventions will be necessary. The delivery of an

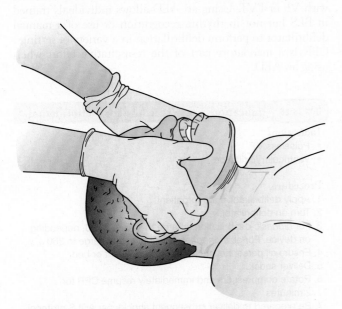

**FIGURE 18-46**  The jaw thrust maneuver without head extension is used if cervical spine trauma is suspected.

electrical impulse by an internal or external defibrillator depolarizes the myocardium and may terminate ventricular fibrillation (VF) or pulseless ventricular tachycardia (PVT). If the myocardium is well oxygenated and has an adequate supply of energy stores, the sinoatrial (SA) node may resume firing after defibrillation resulting in a return to normal sinus rhythm.

If indicated, defibrillation should be attempted as soon as a manual defibrillator or automated external defibrillator (AED) is available. Most defibrillators use multifunctional electrode patches to both monitor and administer electrical therapy. Although paddles are still available, they are seldom used, because their positioning requires additional "hands off" time, which depletes myocardial oxygen and energy stores. The most common placement of the electrode patches (paddles) is the anterior-lateral position: one patch on the upper right chest below the clavicle and the second patch on the left side of the chest in the mid axillary line. This placement puts the heart directly in the current pathway.

Early defibrillation (ie, when oxygen and energy are still present) is most effective when delivered within 3 to 5 minutes of cardiac arrest.[7] To perform rhythm analysis, CPR may need to be interrupted. If the patient is in either VF or PVT, the defibrillator is charged and a shock is administered, followed immediately by 2 minutes of CPR. During compressions, any hands-off time is considered "no flow" time. (*No flow* refers to lack of blood flow when compressions are interrupted.) Research has shown that even with the best CPR, during compressions it is only possible to achieve about 30% of the victim's normal cardiac output. When compressions are interrupted, 10 to 15 compressions are required to resume adequate blood flow. If the heart is not well perfused, the response to defibrillation (shock) is decreased. The longer the pause, the less likely defibrillation will be successful. The quality of CPR prior to defibrillation directly affects clinical outcomes, in that longer preshock pauses and shallow chest compressions are associated with increased defibrillation failure (Fig. 18-47).[6,8]

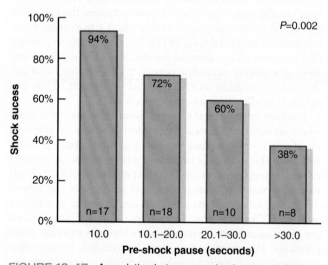

**FIGURE 18-47** Association between preshock pause and shock success. Cases are grouped by preshock pause in 10 s intervals. Note that longer preshock pauses are significantly associated with a smaller probability of shock success. (From Edelson DP, Abella BS, Kramer-Johansen J, et al: Effects of compression depth and preshock pauses predict defibrillation failure during cardiac arrest. Resuscitation 71(2):137–145, 2006, doi:10.1016/j.resuscitation. 2006.04.008. Reprinted with permission.)

Defibrillators are classified by the type of waveform they deliver. Since the early 1970s, monophasic defibrillators have been used. Monophasic defibrillators provide a shock that flows in one direction from one paddle or electrode pad to the other. Newer biphasic technology has been developed that changes the way the electrical current flows during defibrillation. Biphasic defibrillators deliver the current in two phases: the current initially flows in one direction, and then flows in the opposite direction. The biphasic wave uses less peak current, so there is less damage to the heart during defibrillation.

The initial energy level for the first shock when using a biphasic defibrillator is device-specific and may vary from 120 to 200 J. If the manufacturer suggested initial energy level is unknown, administer the first shock at 200 J. If a monophasic defibrillator is used, the initial energy level should be set at 360 J. Familiarity with the specific defibrillator is important for effective use.

Upon completion of five cycles of CPR, the patient's rhythm is again assessed. If the patient is in a "shockable rhythm" (see Fig. 18-48), a second shock is given. The energy (joule) level may be maintained or increased. Immediate CPR for 2 minutes follows the second shock, and the process is repeated. After a shock, CPR is resumed immediately, without checking a pulse, and continued for 2 minutes. All personnel should avoid touching the patient or bed when the shock is delivered. Pulses are only checked if a perfusing rhythm (ie, normal sinus rhythm, bradycardia, tachycardia) is detected after 2 minutes of CPR. If the rhythm remains unchanged (VF or PVT), then there is no pulse check before the next defibrillation. Rhythm checks are done upon completion of compressions.

Box 18-28 outlines the indications and procedure for defibrillation.

## Automatic/Automated External Defibrillator (AED)

Research shows that the sooner a patient in VF is defibrillated, the greater the chance for survival.[7] The development of AEDs has improved the survival of individuals presenting with VF or PVT. Using an AED allows individuals trained in BLS but not in rhythm recognition or use of a manual defibrillator to perform defibrillation in a variety of settings. CPR is a mandatory part of the resuscitative effort when using an AED.

---

**BOX 18-28** Indications and Procedure for Defibrillation

**Indications**
- Pulseless VT
- Ventricular fibrillation

**Procedure**
1. Apply defibrillator pads to patient.
2. Turn on defibrillator.
3. For *biphasic* defibrillation, charge to 120 to 200 J, depending on device. For all *monophasic* defibrillation charge to 360 J.
4. Ensure all personnel are not touching patient or bed.
5. Deliver shock.
6. Rotate compressors and immediately resume CPR for 2 minutes
7. Be prepared to deliver subsequent shocks per ACLS protocol.

AEDs consist of a defibrillator configured with a computer. AEDs are programmed to follow the ACLS guidelines on energy levels and time between periods of rhythm assessment in effect at the time of their manufacture.

Nurses should know the distinction between automatic and automated AEDs. Automatic AEDs charge and independently deliver a shock when indicated, and automated AEDs require action on the part of the user to deliver the shock. Like manual defibrillators, familiarity with the device is important to its safe and effective use. Stand-alone AEDs are available in most hospitals in common areas, allowing for a much shorter time to defibrillation when a patient experiences a "shockable" cardiac arrest.[3] In an ICU setting, the AED function can be a feature of the monitor defibrillator.

### Once the Code Team Arrives

Once the code team arrives, ACLS interventions can be added to BLS efforts, following the adult cardiac pulseless arrest algorithm (Fig. 18-48).

The pulseless arrest algorithm is divided into two branches depending on the patient's rhythm. VF and PVT are "shockable rhythms," while pulseless electrical activity (PEA) and asystole are not. Medications such as epinephrine and amiodarone are an integral part of ACLS interventions. For the patient with PEA or asystole, high-quality CPR while searching for a treatable cause is necessary. According to the American Heart Association, it may be reasonable to administer epinephrine as soon as feasible after the onset of a cardiac arrest from a "nonshockable" rhythm.[9] The classical reversible (treatable) causes are referred to as the "Hs and Ts"; they are listed at the bottom of the sidebar in Figure 18-48. Treatment of the specific cause, coupled with high-quality CPR and early defibrillation (where indicated), is the best path to return of spontaneous circulation (ROSC).

### Resuscitation Team Members

When a cardiopulmonary arrest ("code" or Code Blue) is called, various members of the emergency response team are notified. Each institution has its own policies regarding who responds. In many teaching hospitals, residents, medical students, and other staff may respond. Most institutions now have rapid response teams to care for deteriorating patients in prearrest situations; these teams may also respond to cases of cardiopulmonary arrest (see Chapter 14.)

### Equipment

The equipment used in resuscitative efforts is kept in a central location in what is commonly referred to as the "crash cart." Most hospitals have rolling carts in easy-to-access locations throughout the hospital. These carts are stocked in a standard way so that all hospital personnel are familiar with the contents and layout of the equipment. The carts must be inventoried daily to ensure their contents are complete and available in the event of a cardiopulmonary arrest. Once the cart has been opened, it must be reinventoried and restocked as soon as possible.

There are usually multiple drawers locked with a breakaway lock to ensure that all equipment remains in place and undisturbed unless needed for an emergency situation. The drawers are labeled to assist personnel in locating specific equipment. Intubation equipment may or may not be stored separately from the rest of the cart, because intubation may be the only measure required under some circumstances.

Table 18-11 lists the contents of a typical crash cart and the rationale for the use of the equipment and medications found inside the cart. Crash cart contents may vary among institutions.

## Medications

Numerous drugs are used during and immediately after a cardiopulmonary arrest. These drugs should be readily available in the crash cart and include antiarrhythmic agents, inotropes, vasoconstrictors, and electrolyte replacements. Table 18-12 lists some of these medications and the indications for their use.

Once the patient is resuscitated and achieves return of spontaneous circulation (ROSC), the next phase of care is governed by the AHA's post–cardiac arrest care algorithm (Fig. 18-49, p.334). During cardiac arrest, blood flow to the brain is compromised. After ROSC, the resumption of perfusion may lead to the production of oxygen free radicals and other toxic metabolites.

## Targeted Temperature Management

Targeted temperature management (TTM), as one of several treatments post-ROSC, is indicated when the resuscitated patient is unresponsive, indicating neurologic compromise. The cerebral metabolic rate for oxygen, or $CMRO_2$, is reduced when the body temperature is reduced. Apoptosis (programmed cell death) and the production of free radicals are reduced in a hypothermic state. Some studies have reported improved survival and functional recovery with induced hypothermia.[10]

Many institutions are now implementing TTM protocols. Common among these protocols is the systematic lowering of a patient's core temperature to 32°C to 36°C.[9] This cooling can be accomplished by various methods, including ice packs, cooling blankets, and endovascular cooling devices. Special rectal probes or bladder catheters are used to monitor the cooling process. The patient remains in this hypothermic state at least 24 hours.[10] Passive rewarming is then allowed to occur over the next 8 to 12 hours; actively or rapidly rewarming patients is not recommended.[10]

Care of the patient post-ROSC can be intense, especially if TTM is chosen as a treatment modality. In addition to the monitoring of cardiac rhythm and MAP, potassium levels and blood glucose must also be tracked. Periodic evaluation of arterial gases and ventilator settings is required for mechanically ventilated patients. The nurse must ensure that medications, such as sedatives, neuromuscular blockade medications, and analgesics, are administered in accordance with established protocols. Nursing care includes monitoring of the patients skin and soft tissues for cold thermic injuries that can be caused by the various cooling devices; because these potential injuries are not usually seen in the ICU setting, special vigilance is required. Physical care is otherwise

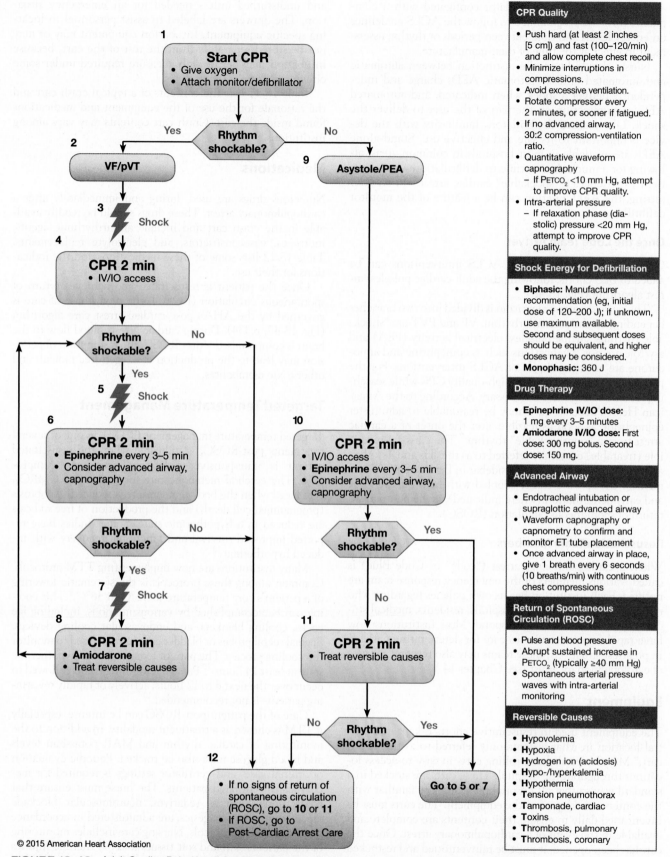

**CPR Quality**

- Push hard (at least 2 inches [5 cm]) and fast (100–120/min) and allow complete chest recoil.
- Minimize interruptions in compressions.
- Avoid excessive ventilation.
- Rotate compressor every 2 minutes, or sooner if fatigued.
- If no advanced airway, 30:2 compression-ventilation ratio.
- Quantitative waveform capnography
  - If PETCO$_2$ <10 mm Hg, attempt to improve CPR quality.
- Intra-arterial pressure
  - If relaxation phase (diastolic) pressure <20 mm Hg, attempt to improve CPR quality.

**Shock Energy for Defibrillation**

- **Biphasic:** Manufacturer recommendation (eg, initial dose of 120–200 J); if unknown, use maximum available. Second and subsequent doses should be equivalent, and higher doses may be considered.
- **Monophasic:** 360 J

**Drug Therapy**

- **Epinephrine IV/IO dose:** 1 mg every 3–5 minutes
- **Amiodarone IV/IO dose:** First dose: 300 mg bolus. Second dose: 150 mg.

**Advanced Airway**

- Endotracheal intubation or supraglottic advanced airway
- Waveform capnography or capnometry to confirm and monitor ET tube placement
- Once advanced airway in place, give 1 breath every 6 seconds (10 breaths/min) with continuous chest compressions

**Return of Spontaneous Circulation (ROSC)**

- Pulse and blood pressure
- Abrupt sustained increase in PETCO$_2$ (typically ≥40 mm Hg)
- Spontaneous arterial pressure waves with intra-arterial monitoring

**Reversible Causes**

- **H**ypovolemia
- **H**ypoxia
- **H**ydrogen ion (acidosis)
- **H**ypo-/hyperkalemia
- **H**ypothermia
- **T**ension pneumothorax
- **T**amponade, cardiac
- **T**oxins
- **T**hrombosis, pulmonary
- **T**hrombosis, coronary

© 2015 American Heart Association

**FIGURE 18-48** Adult Cardiac Pulseless Arrest Algorithm. (Reprinted with permission from 2015 American Heart Association Guidelines Update for CPR and ECC. Circulation 123[suppl 2]:S313–S589, 2015. © 2015, American Heart Association, Inc.)

**TABLE 18-11  Resuscitation Equipment Cart**

| Equipment | Rationale |
|---|---|
| Intubation equipment (usually a separate locked container):<br>• Laryngoscope<br>• Curved and straight blades<br>• Endotracheal tubes<br>• Syringes<br>Laryngeal Mask Airway (LMA)<br>Oropharyngeal airways<br>Nasopharyngeal airways<br>Suction catheters | • Provides adequate, patent airway, thus ensuring oxygenation of the lungs during resuscitation<br>• Allows for patient to be placed on mechanical ventilation<br>• Reduces chances for gastric distention, aspiration, or vomiting<br>• Permits suctioning<br>• Allows for the administration of oxygen in high concentrations<br>• Provides route for certain medications (NAVEL)* |
| Oxygen source (separate tank)<br>Bag-valve-mask device<br>Suction machine (preferably battery powered)<br>Suctioning tubing & catheters | • Ensures that oxygen is available if wall oxygen unavailable<br>• Provides seal over patient's mouth and nose; reduces risk to rescuer<br>• Ensures suctioning available if wall suction unavailable<br>• Clears oropharyngeal (nasopharyngeal) airway before intubation |
| IV fluids and tubing<br>Nitroglycerin tubing<br>Medications (ACLS drugs as a minimum) | • Volume replacement and treatment of hypotension<br>• Prevents precipitation of IV nitroglycerin<br>• Amiodarone<br>• Lidocaine<br>• Atropine<br>• Epinephrine<br>• Sodium bicarbonate<br>• Calcium chloride<br>• $D_{50}$<br>• Premixed dopamine infusion |
| Drip chart (attached to outside of cart) | • Allows for rapid titration of ACLS/Critical Care drugs during and after resuscitation without having to perform complex calculations |
| Blood tubes | • Allows for the rapid drawing and sending of blood for analysis Tube color will be institution specific |
| Arterial blood gas kits<br>Peripheral IV supplies<br>Prefilled flush syringes (normal saline solution)<br>Needles<br>Decompression (cardiac) needles<br>Clipboard with paper and pen; code sheets<br>Pressure bags<br>Gloves (nonlatex, sterile, and nonsterile) | • Allows for rapid drawing and sending of arterial blood gases<br>• Ensures access for fluid and IV drug administration<br>• Allows for faster flushing of IV lines<br>• Allows for drawing up of medications<br>• Used in cardiac tamponade<br>• Used to document the arrest<br>• Used for rapid infusion of fluid boluses<br>• Provides protection for rescuers<br>• Provides sterile gloves for invasive/sterile procedures |
| Portable defibrillator/monitor with the following modes:<br>• Defibrillation<br>• Synchronized cardioversion<br>• Transcutaneous pacing | • Used in defibrillation, cardioversion, and temporary transcutaneous pacing |

**TABLE 18-12  Medications Used to Treat a Patient in Cardiopulmonary Arrest**

| Drug | Class | Uses |
|---|---|---|
| Adenosine | Antiarrhythmic | SVT, AF |
| Amiodarone | Antiarrhythmic | VT, SVT, AF, VF |
| Atropine | Anticholinergic | Bradycardia, PEA |
| Calcium chloride | Electrolyte | Hyperkalemia, hypocalcemia, calcium channel blocker toxicity |
| Dobutamine | Inotrope; β₁ agonist | Decreased cardiac output |
| Dopamine | Inotrope; β₁ agonist | Hypotension<br>Symptomatic Bradycardia |
| Epinephrine | Catecholamine | VF |
| Lidocaine | Antiarrhythmic | VT, VF |
| Magnesium sulfate | Electrolyte | Torsades de pointes |
| Nitroglycerin | Coronary vasodilator | MI, angina |
| Procainamide | Antiarrhythmic | VT, VF |
| Sodium bicarbonate | Alkalinizer | Acidosis |
| Verapamil | Calcium channel blocker | SVT |

The preferred alternate route for medication administration, if IV is not available, is intraosseous (IO). NAVEL is a mnemonic for drugs that may be administered by endotracheal tube: naloxone, atropine, diazepam, epinephrine, lidocaine. The typical dose of drugs administered via the endotracheal tube is 2 to 2½ times the intravenous dose diluted in 5–10 mL. of normal saline or sterile water

AF, atrial fibrillation; NS, normal saline; PEA, pulseless electrical activity; SVT, supraventricular tachycardia; VF, ventricular fibrillation; VT, ventricular tachycardia.

## Adult Immediate Post–Cardiac Arrest Care Algorithm—2015 Update

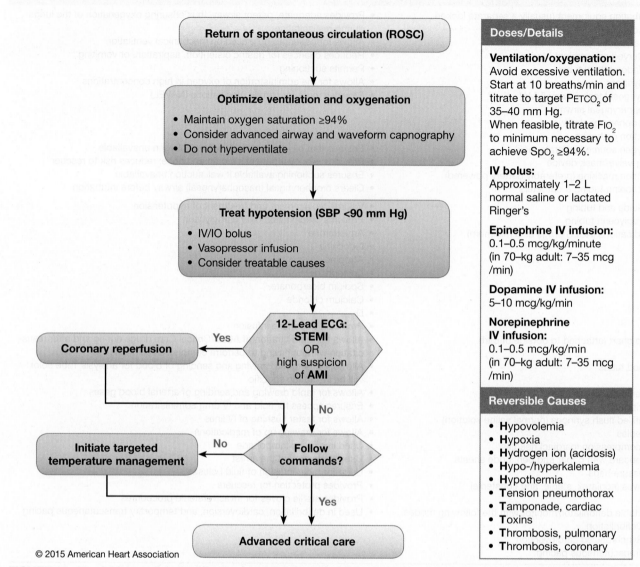

**Return of spontaneous circulation (ROSC)**

**Optimize ventilation and oxygenation**
- Maintain oxygen saturation ≥94%
- Consider advanced airway and waveform capnography
- Do not hyperventilate

**Treat hypotension (SBP <90 mm Hg)**
- IV/IO bolus
- Vasopressor infusion
- Consider treatable causes

**12-Lead ECG: STEMI OR high suspicion of AMI**

Yes → **Coronary reperfusion**

No ↓

**Follow commands?**

No → **Initiate targeted temperature management**

Yes ↓

**Advanced critical care**

© 2015 American Heart Association

**Doses/Details**

**Ventilation/oxygenation:**
Avoid excessive ventilation. Start at 10 breaths/min and titrate to target $P_{ETCO_2}$ of 35–40 mm Hg. When feasible, titrate $F_{IO_2}$ to minimum necessary to achieve $SpO_2$ ≥94%.

**IV bolus:**
Approximately 1–2 L normal saline or lactated Ringer's

**Epinephrine IV infusion:**
0.1–0.5 mcg/kg/minute (in 70-kg adult: 7–35 mcg/min)

**Dopamine IV infusion:**
5–10 mcg/kg/min

**Norepinephrine IV infusion:**
0.1–0.5 mcg/kg/min (in 70-kg adult: 7–35 mcg/min)

**Reversible Causes**
- **H**ypovolemia
- **H**ypoxia
- **H**ydrogen ion (acidosis)
- **H**ypo-/hyperkalemia
- **H**ypothermia
- **T**ension pneumothorax
- **T**amponade, cardiac
- **T**oxins
- **T**hrombosis, pulmonary
- **T**hrombosis, coronary

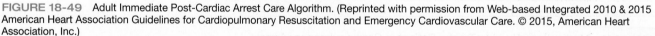

**FIGURE 18-49** Adult Immediate Post-Cardiac Arrest Care Algorithm. (Reprinted with permission from Web-based Integrated 2010 & 2015 American Heart Association Guidelines for Cardiopulmonary Resuscitation and Emergency Cardiovascular Care. © 2015, American Heart Association, Inc.)

no different from that of any other unconscious completely dependent patient.

TTM research continues on optimal temperature, means of cooling, and method of rewarming. Investigative studies are now being conducted as to the efficacy of therapeutic hypothermia in cases of cerebral vascular accidents. One of the major controversies surrounding therapeutic hypothermia is the patient's quality of life following rewarming, as well as the long-term costs if the patient recovers, but with resulting neurologic deficit. If a patient has been cooled, prognosis should not be predicted for at least 72 hours after rewarming, and possibly longer if sedation or paralysis was part of the therapeutic regimen. Actively preventing fever in comatose patients after rewarming is highly recommended, because fevers can lead to increased neurologic damage.[11]

## Family Presence in a Cardiac Arrest Situation

One aspect of the treatment of cardiopulmonary arrest that has gained attention in recent years is the issue of family presence during a code. Nurses and other health care providers have voiced strong opinions for both sides of the issue since its emergence in 1987. Many staff believe that family presence during CPR detracts from their clinical performance and hinders their efforts, and other staff are concerned about the families' emotional and physical well-being during and after a code. Despite the controversies about benefits and harms, major international guidelines for CPR state that available evidence supports family-witnessed resuscitation, and this practice is considered reasonable and generally useful.[12]

Healthcare institutions have become more flexible and accommodating of families. Many emergency departments and ICUs now have protocols in place regarding the presence of families and loved ones at the bedside while resuscitation efforts are taking place. Every effort must be made to have a knowledgeable person explain to the family what measures are being implemented and the rationale. Many family members express a desire to be with the patient during CPR for various reasons, including reassurance that all resuscitative efforts were attempted, the opportunity to say goodbye at the moment of death, and reassurance that the death was as painless as possible.

When discussing advanced directives with patients and their families, the techniques of resuscitation are often described. In the event of a cardiac arrest situation, some family members have seen these measures taking place and make the decision to terminate resuscitation. When the family sees a team of health care professionals working against time to save a patient, the family often expresses the realization and appreciation that the staff strives to deliver excellent and compassionate care.

The prevailing movement in health care to allow the family greater access to their loved one in times of illness will continue to support the practice of family presence during CPR. Institution-specific protocols for family presence during CPR should support providers' ability to give the highest-quality care while also allowing family members appropriate access to their loved ones.[12] Additionally, rules must be in place to escort family members from the room if the rescuers cannot perform resuscitative measures effectively with the family members present.

Box 18-29 outlines cardiopulmonary resuscitation considerations for the older patient.

## Debriefing

Current guidelines suggest that timely and focused debriefing after any cardiopulmonary arrest response can increases survival outcomes.[13] After the code, the responding staff often scatter, and the opportunity for evaluation and learning is lost. Debriefing should occur as soon as possible, and include what went well, what can be improved, and whether there were any safety, procedural, or equipment issues.[2]

Debriefing should not be used as a forum for pointing fingers and assigning blame. Instead, it is an opportunity for all staff involved to improve their performance in preparation for future events. It is best if all members of the team can be debriefed together, because this promotes more effective teamwork; however, this approach is not always possible. Nursing staff should hold their own nursing debriefing

session if it is not possible to debrief with the rest of the code team.[2,13]

## Transcutaneous Pacing

Some bradycardias are at high risk for deterioration into ventricular shutdown. TCP is considered the first line of therapy for second-degree Mobitz Type II block, or a third-degree (complete) heart block. Most defibrillators include a pacer mode. The multipurpose (combination) electrode pads used with the device allow the user to monitor the patient, and to administer electrical therapy including defibrillation, synchronized cardioversion, and TCP. TCP is a continuous therapy, and requires the use of a 3-lead ECG cable in addition to the combo pads to detect the patient's underlying heart rhythm. TCP may be used as a "bridge" (temporary measure) until either a transvenous or permanent pacemaker can be placed. Refer to Box 18-30 for the indications and procedure for transcutaneous pacing.

Before initiating TCP, the nurse must ensure that a conscious patient understands the plan for TCP, and must enlist their cooperation. Although the pain involved in TCP is minimal, it is annoying to the patient. The nursing care plan should include sedation and analgesia during TCP. Electrode (pad) placement is different in TCP than in defibrillation (see Box 18-30). The anterior–posterior pad placement puts the heart directly in the path of the current and allows the use of minimal energy (milliamps). Refer to Figure 18-31 for the proper placement of the electrodes.

The nurse is responsible for placing the pacing electrode pads, and should cut any chest hair with scissors. Shaving the chest is to be avoided because it can lead to skin abrasions and

---

**BOX 18-29**    *CONSIDERATIONS for the Older Patient*

**Cardiopulmonary Resuscitation**

- Assess for fractured sternum after CPR. Continue with CPR even if fracture occurs.
- Keep in mind the effect of medications due to delayed clearance and altered metabolic response
- Be certain the health care team implements the patient's desire for *do not resuscitate* or *do not intubate* orders.
- Consider family presence during code.
- Keep in mind the effect of medications due to delayed clearance and altered metabolic response.

---

**BOX 18-30**    **Indications and Procedure for Transcutaneous Pacing**

**Indications**
- Second-degree heart block Mobitz Type II
- Complete (third-degree) heart block

**Procedure**
1. Explain procedure to patient.
2. Clip excess hair from chest. Ensure skin is dry.
3. Attach the multipurpose electrode pads to the patient
   - Apply anterior electrode to chest at the fourth intercostal space to the left of the sternum.
   - Apply posterior electrode to patient's back in the area of the left scapula
4. Connect the 3-lead EKG cable to the patient
5. Turn on pacer function
6. Set pacemaker heart rate then pacer output (in milliamps).
7. Assess for effectiveness of pacing:
   - Observe for pacemaker spike with subsequent capture (pacer spike followed by a wide waveform indicates electrical capture).
   - Assess increase in heart rate to match rate generated by pacer (mechanical capture).
   - Assess blood pressure.
   - Check level of consciousness.
   - Print a rhythm strip demonstrating electrical capture and document in medical record
   - Observe for patient anxiety and/or pain and treat accordingly.

bleeding, which decreases electrode pad adherence and can lead to pain during electrical stimulation. When initiating TCP, first the rate is set, then the electrical level. Electrical "capture" is identified when the QRS waveform shows a pacer "spike" before every wide QRS complex. Upon electrical capture, effective pacing is confirmed by checking mechanical capture. The nurse checks the patient's pulse to confirm that it has increased to match the rate set on the pacer. The radial pulse is the preferred site for confirmation of mechanical capture. The carotid pulse is not used, because muscle twitching may lead the nurse to think a pulse is present when it is absent. A positive response to TCP is indicated by a rise in blood pressure. Blood pressure should be taken using the right arm to avoid interference from the pacemaker. Adjustment to rate or energy may be necessary to improve outcomes.

Transcutaneous pacing requires diligent monitoring by the nurse. A loss of capture can occur if the electrodes fail to keep good contact with the skin. Inappropriate pacing may occur if the pacemaker cannot detect the heart's intrinsic rhythm. In either case, the nurse must recognize the problem and reposition the patient or the electrodes to ensure efficacious transcutaneous pacing.

## Clinical Applicability Challenges

### CASE STUDY

Mr. M. is a 78-year-old man with a past medical history significant for coronary artery disease (MI, CABG 8 years ago), HTN, and atrial fibrillation. He is admitted today with symptoms of increased fatigue over the past 2 months, dyspnea on exertion, and intermittent rapid heart rates with dizziness.

1. In your initial assessment of Mr. M., what additional objective information do you need to guide interventions?

2. If Mr. M. requires temporary transvenous pacing, what indicators on the ECG will you be monitoring to assure proper pacemaker function? What is your response to common temporary pacemaker malfunctions?

3. Based on Mr. M.'s ECG and echocardiogram, what are some key teaching points if he needs an implanted pacemaker or ICD? What would be unique about a biventricular pacing device?

### WANT TO KNOW MORE?

A wide variety of resources to enhance your learning and understanding of this chapter are available on thePoint.

You will find:

- References
- Selected readings
- NCLEX-style review questions
- Internet resources
- And more!

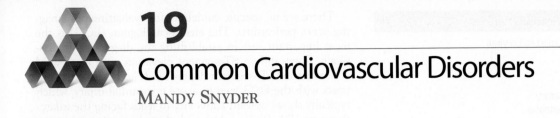

# 19
# Common Cardiovascular Disorders
MANDY SNYDER

**LEARNING OBJECTIVES**

*Based on the content in this chapter, the reader should be able to:*

1. Differentiate between pericarditis and ischemic causes of chest pain.
2. Explain the long-term effects of endocarditis on the heart valves.
3. Discuss key differences in the clinical management of dilated and hypertrophic cardiomyopathy.
4. Describe key differences in clinical presentation between arterial and venous peripheral vascular disease.
5. Compare and contrast the clinical findings of chronic aortic aneurysm with those of acute aortic dissection.
6. Describe the complications of hypertensive crisis when the blood pressure goes untreated for prolonged periods.

This chapter reviews several common cardiovascular disorders, including pericarditis, myocarditis, endocarditis, cardiomyopathies, peripheral vascular disease, aortic diseases, and hypertensive crisis.

## Infection and Inflammation of the Heart

Infectious and inflammatory diseases of the heart have multiple etiologies, making diagnosis and treatment a clinical challenge. Patients may present with acute pain mimicking myocardial infarction (MI) or may seek medical attention because of fatigue and vague flu-like symptoms that fail to resolve over a period of weeks. Because of the permanent damage these diseases can cause to structures of the heart, patients often face serious long-term cardiac disability.

### Pericarditis

The pericardium surrounds the external surface of the heart and the roots of the great vessels. It is composed of two layers: an outer tough fibrous pericardium and an inner serous layer.[1] The serous pericardium has two layers: the parietal and the visceral. The parietal layer lines the internal surface of the fibrous membrane. The parietal pericardium extends to the great vessels, where it then folds over on itself to form the inner visceral layer, also known as the epicardium (Fig. 19-1). Between 10 and 50 mL of clear serous fluid lies between these layers and acts as a lubricant. The pericardium helps restrain the heart and isolate it from infections in the surrounding structures.[1]

Pericarditis is inflammation of the pericardium. Acute pericarditis is pericarditis that lasts no longer than 1 or 2 weeks.[1] Inflammation often involves the adjoining diaphragm. The etiology of pericarditis varies; it can be a primary disease or occur secondarily as the result of another disorder, such as acute MI or renal failure.[1] In almost 90% of patients diagnosed with acute pericarditis, the disease is idiopathic (ie, the exact cause is unknown).[1,2,5] Causes of pericarditis are listed in Box 19-1. Dressler syndrome refers to the development of pericarditis, malaise, fever, and elevated white blood cell count appearing

weeks to months after a MI. This syndrome is believed to be the result of an autoimmune reaction that occurs after the infarction.[1] Infectious pericarditis remains a problem in the immunocompromised patient.[1]

Repeated episodes of pericarditis can lead to the formation of adhesions between the layers of the pericardium or between the pericardium and adjacent structures, resulting in constrictive pericarditis.[1] In constrictive pericarditis, the primary problem is failure of the heart to fill during diastole because of its inability to expand. Unless the diseased pericardium is removed surgically, diastolic filling continues to be impaired, eventually leading to a decrease in cardiac output and systemic signs of heart failure. Even with successful surgical removal of the diseased pericardium, the long-term survival rate for patients with constrictive pericarditis is poor.[1]

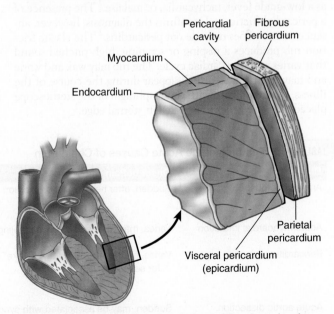

**FIGURE 19-1** Layers of the heart, showing the visceral pericardium, pericardial cavity, parietal pericardium, fibrous pericardium, myocardium, and endocardium. (From Porth CM: Pathophysiology, Concepts of Altered Health States, 8th ed. Philadelphia, PA: Lippincott Williams & Wilkins, 2009, p 459.)

- Idiopathic (usually presumed to be viral)
- Infectious
- Bacterial
- Tuberculosis
- Autoimmune or inflammatory
- Systemic lupus erythematosus
- Drugs
- Vaccinations
- Neoplasms
- Radiation therapy
- Following device implantation, such as an implantable defibrillator
- Acute myocardial infarction
- Trauma to the chest wall or myocardium, including cardiopulmonary surgery
- Chronic renal failure requiring dialysis

Data from Dudzinski DM, Mak GS, Hung JW: Pericardial diseases. Curr Probl Cardiol 37(3):75–118, 2012; and LeWinter MM: Acute pericarditis. N Engl J Med 4(371):2410–2416, 2014.

## Assessment

Important clues to the diagnosis of pericarditis can be obtained from the history and physical examination. The primary symptom in acute pericarditis is chest pain.[2] The pain tends to be pleuritic in nature and classically is made worse by breathing deeply or lying supine. Because of pain from breathing, patients frequently complain of dyspnea. Relief is often obtained by sitting up, leaning forward, and taking shallow breaths. The chest pain of pericarditis may be difficult to distinguish from ischemic chest pain.[1,2] Characteristic features of the acute causes of chest pain are summarized in Table 19-1.[2] One clue in the differentiation is that ischemic chest pain is not relieved by a change in the patient's position.

There may also be general symptoms of an infection, such as a low-grade fever, tachycardia, or malaise.[2] The presence of a pericardial friction rub confirms the diagnosis; however, absence of a rub does not rule out pericarditis.[2] The classic friction rub produces a rasping or scraping, high-pitched sound that varies with the cardiac cycle. The rub may wax and wane and may even transiently disappear during the course of the illness. It is best heard with the diaphragm of the stethoscope placed over the lower to middle left sternal edge.[1]

There are no specific guidelines for evaluating or managing acute pericarditis. The electrocardiogram (ECG) is the most important test in establishing the diagnosis.[1] It classically shows diffuse ST-segment elevation with an upward concavity and PR-segment depression (Fig. 19-2). This contrasts with the ECG seen in acute myocardial injury, which typically shows upward convexity in leads facing the infarction zone (Fig. 19-3).[1,2] Although the echocardiogram is usually normal in acute pericarditis, it is indicated in patients with suspected pericardial disease.[1,2]

Laboratory tests include complete blood count, cardiac enzyme levels (which may be elevated if the inflammation extends to the myocardium), C-reactive protein (CRP), erythrocyte sedimentation rate (ESR), rheumatoid factors, and antinuclear antibody titers.[1,2] Blood cultures may be indicated if there is evidence of infection.[2] Viral studies may be obtained if the rest of the diagnostic workup is negative.[1,2]

### Management

Treatment goals for the patient with pericarditis are relief of symptoms, elimination of any possible causative agents, and monitoring for complications, such as constrictive pericarditis or pericardial effusions that could lead to cardiac tamponade.[1,2] Symptom relief includes the use of nonsteroidal anti-inflammatory drugs (NSAIDs), such as aspirin or ibuprofen.[2] Colchicine has been shown to successfully reduce the recurrence of pericarditis. Steroids may be indicated in refractory cases of autoimmune pericarditis in which infectious causes have been excluded.[2] Anticoagulants should be avoided in the patient recovering from MI, though aspirin is given for recovery and prevention of acute myocardial infarction.[2] Most episodes of pericarditis abate over 2 to 6 weeks. Rarely do patients experience recurrent episodes.[1]

## Myocarditis

Myocarditis is an inflammation of the myocardium.[2–4] Primary myocarditis is believed to be related to an acute viral infection or an autoimmune response to the infection. Secondary myocarditis is inflammation related to a specific organism. Potential causes of both types, which can occur in any age group, are listed in Box 19-2. The prevalence is unknown because the clinical presentation is so varied and

**TABLE 19-1**  Features of the Acute Causes of Chest Pain

| Diagnosis | Onset of Pain | Quality of Pain | Relieved by |
|---|---|---|---|
| Angina pectoris | Sudden, after heavy meal or exertion | Crushing Squeezing Choking | Rest, nitrates |
| Acute myocardial infarction | Varies, may be associated with feeling of doom | Similar to angina, but more severe | No relief with rest |
| Pericarditis | Varies, may be preceded by "flu-like" symptoms for several days to weeks | Pleuritic Sharp, stabbing | Sitting up Shallow breathing NSAIDs |
| Acute aortic dissection | Sudden, may be associated with syncope Intense from the onset | Ripping Tearing Worst pain in patient's life | No relief |

NSAIDs, nonsteroidal anti-inflammatory drugs.
Data from Dudzinski DM, Mak GS, Hung JW: Pericardial diseases. Curr Probl Cardiol 37(3):75–118, 2012; and LeWinter MM: Acute pericarditis. N Engl J Med 4(371):2410–2416, 2014.

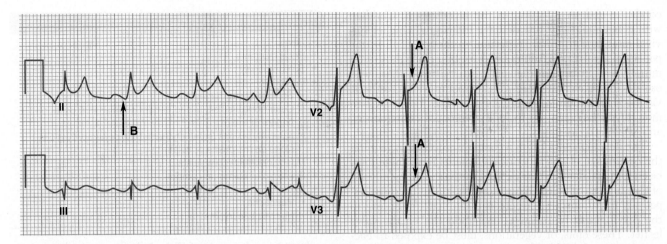

FIGURE 19-2  The 12-lead electrocardiogram in acute pericarditis. Note the diffuse upward concavity ST changes (**A**) and the PR-segment depression (**B**).

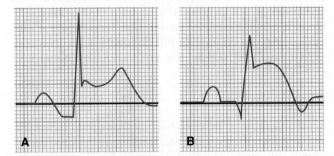

FIGURE 19-3  ST-segment changes seen in (**A**) acute pericarditis and (**B**) myocardial infarction.

### BOX 19-2  Potential Causes of Myocarditis

**Viruses**
- Coxsackie virus
- Adenovirus
- Human immunodeficiency virus
- Influenza virus

**Bacteria**
- *Clostridium* species
- *Corynebacterium diphtheriae*
- Streptococci
- Spirochetes (Lyme disease)

**Fungi**
- *Aspergillus* species
- *Candida* species

**Toxins**
- Tricyclic antidepressants
- Phenothiazines

often subacute.[4] Myocarditis can be a devastating illness that evolves into a chronic, progressive disease with a poor prognosis. The disorder may result in dysrhythmias, congestive heart failure, or death.[3] It is also recognized as a cause of sudden death in young athletes.

### Assessment

The clinical presentation of myocarditis is variable. With viral myocarditis, there is typically a delay before the onset of cardiac symptoms such as congestive heart failure or dysrhythmias.[3] The presence of symptoms, such as fatigue, dyspnea, palpitations, and precordial discomfort, accompanied by a slight rise in serum enzyme levels and nonspecific ST-T wave changes on the ECG suggests a diagnosis of myocarditis. Definitive diagnosis requires a positive endomyocardial biopsy.[3] However, lack of a positive biopsy does not rule out myocarditis. Current research focuses on finding a more reliable and safe method of diagnosing this complex disease.

### Management

Management of myocarditis depends on the etiology and clinical presentation; however, treatment is largely supportive.[3] Although myocarditis evokes a severe inflammatory response, treatment with corticosteroids or immunosuppressive agents has not been effective in changing the clinical course.[4] In some patients, episodes of myocarditis resolve without further sequelae. In other patients, a subacute disease develops with persistent laboratory findings of inflammation (eg, an increased white blood cell count or an elevated sedimentation rate). Athletes with myocarditis should withdraw from competitive sports for a period of at least 6 months following the onset of disease. Return to training and competition depends on normalization of cardiac function and absence of any significant clinical findings, such as dysrhythmias.[1]

Many of the skills required by the nurse to care for the patient with myocarditis are similar to those needed in the care of the patient with heart failure. In addition, the nurse must be prepared to help the patient and family deal with the unexpected reality of a potentially lethal disease that often has no cure and may require heart transplantation or mechanical circulatory support.[4]

### Endocarditis

Endocarditis is an infection of the endocardial surface of the heart, including the valves, caused by bacterial, viral, or fungal agents.[5,6] Infectious endocarditis (IE) is a serious illness associated with considerable morbidity and mortality. The incidence of IE varies with the specific population under study, but overall, the incidence appears to be increasing.[5] Predisposing risk factors for endocarditis are a prior cardiac condition and an infection in the bloodstream. Children with congenital heart disease have increasingly higher survival rates, and this may contribute to the rise of IE in the pediatric population.[7] Adults at risk for IE include those with mitral valve prolapse or rheumatic heart disease, those who use illicit intravenous drugs, and patients with prosthetic valves or long-term indwelling devices (Box 19-3).[6,7] Common infectious organisms include streptococci, enterococci, and *Staphylococcus aureus*.

The development of IE is a complex process that requires the occurrence of several critical elements First, there must be endothelial damage that exposes the basement membrane of the valve to turbulent blood flow. Next, this exposure, especially in patients in a hypercoagulable state, must lead to the development of a platelet and fibrin clot on the valve leaflet. These clots, or vegetations, must be exposed to bacteria by way of the bloodstream, such as occurs after dental manipulations or urologic procedures. Finally, bacterial proliferation must take place. Bacteria proliferate on these vegetations for two reasons: (1) the turbulent blood flow across the valves helps concentrate the numbers of bacteria near the vegetation, and (2) the vegetation itself covers the bacteria with layers of platelets and fibrin, protecting the bacterial colony from the body's natural defense mechanisms. The infected vegetation interferes with normal valve function and eventually damages the valve structure. These incompetent valves eventually lead to severe heart failure. Particles from the infected vegetation or severely damaged valve can break loose and cause peripheral emboli.[6,8]

### Assessment

Symptoms of endocarditis usually occur within 2 weeks of the precipitating event and are related to four underlying processes: bacteremia or fungemia, valvulitis, immunologic response, and peripheral emboli (Box 19-4). Nonspecific complaints, such as general malaise, anorexia, fatigue, weight loss, and night sweats, are common. Because symptoms are nonspecific, a careful history focusing on risk factors for IE and a physical examination are needed when endocarditis is suspected. Fever and a new or changed heart murmur are present in almost all patients.[8] Also, 20% of patients have a presenting symptom of stroke from septic emboli from infected heart valves in endocarditis.[6,8]

---

**BOX 19-3** **Risk Factors for Endocarditis**

Native Valve Endocarditis
- Mitral valve prolapse
- Congenital heart disease
- Rheumatic heart disease
- Degenerative valve disease (such as aortic stenosis)
- Age greater than 60 years
- Intravenous drug abuse

Prosthetic Valve Endocarditis
Early (Within 60 Days of Surgery)
- Nosocomial infections
- Indwelling catheters
- Endotracheal tubes

Late (After 60 Days)
- Dental, genitourinary, or gastrointestinal manipulations

---

**BOX 19-4** **Clinical Features of Endocarditis**
- Fever
- Heart murmurs
- Splenomegaly
- Petechiae
  - Splinter hemorrhages
  - Osler nodes (small, raised, tender nodules that occur on the fingers or toes)
  - Janeway lesions (small erythematous or hemorrhagic lesions on the palms or soles)
- Musculoskeletal complaints
- Systemic or pulmonary emboli
- Neurologic manifestations
  - Headache
  - Mycotic aneurysms

---

Definitive diagnosis of IE includes persistent bacteremia caused by typical IE pathogens and evidence of myocardial involvement, such as echocardiographic visualization of a vegetation or new or worsening murmur (Duke criteria).[8,9] Blood is usually drawn for two to three separate sets of cultures, depending on severity and chronicity of the infection; meticulous blood culture site preparation is necessary to avoid contamination.[8,9]

### Management

Rapid diagnosis of IE, initiation of appropriate treatment, and early identification of complications are the keys to good patient outcomes.[5] Antibiotic therapy is based on culture results and the clinical setting (ie, native valve vs. prosthetic valve IE). Recommended antibiotic therapies have been revised to account for a dramatic increase in drug resistance among common IE organisms.[5] Treatment should not be delayed while waiting for identification of the specific organism but should begin as soon as blood culture specimens are drawn. Immediate surgical intervention is indicated in the presence of native or prosthetic valve dysfunction or dehiscence, severe congestive heart failure secondary to valve dysfunction, and uncontrolled infections.

Cure of IE is difficult and requires complete eradication of the bacterial colony from the vegetation. This usually involves a prolonged course of antibiotic therapy.[8]

## Cardiomyopathies

The cardiomyopathies are diseases of the heart muscle that cause cardiac dysfunction resulting in heart failure, dysrhythmias, or sudden death.[10] The cardiomyopathies have been separated into distinct categories: dilated, hypertrophic, restrictive, arrhythmogenic right ventricular cardiomyopathy, and unclassified.[10] This section focuses on the most common types of primary cardiomyopathies in Western countries: dilated and hypertrophic cardiomyopathies (Table 19-2). See Spotlight on Genetics 19-1 for information about familial restrictive cardiomyopathy.

Exactly how cardiomyopathy develops is not completely understood. Current theories under investigation suggest that ischemic, immune, mechanical, and neurohormonal effects on the pericardium, myocardium, and endothelium lead to remodeling and structural changes that result in functional changes. Structural changes at the cellular

**TABLE 19-2  Primary Cardiomyopathies**

| Cardiomyopathy | Pathology | Clinical Manifestations | Management |
|---|---|---|---|
| Dilated cardiomyopathy (DCM) | Systolic dysfunction<br>Chamber dilation with normal left ventricular wall thickness | • Congestive heart failure<br>• Fatigue, weakness<br>• Dysrhythmias<br>• Systemic or pulmonary | • Identify and eliminate potential causes such as alcohol<br>• Symptomatic treatment<br>• Manage heart failure, dysrhythmias<br>• Biventricular pacing or implantable cardioverter defibrillator (ICD) in selected patients<br>• Genetic testing<br>• Family screening to identify asymptomatic members with DCM |
| Hypertrophic cardiomyopathy (HCM) | Diastolic dysfunction<br>Marked hypertrophy of left ventricle, occasionally also of right ventricle, and usually (but not always) disproportionate hypertrophy of septum | • Dyspnea<br>• Angina<br>• Fatigue<br>• Syncope<br>• Palpitations<br>• Dysrhythmias<br>• Congestive heart failure<br>• Sudden death | • Symptomatic treatment<br>• Medications<br>• ICD<br>• Septal wall ablation or surgery in select patients<br>• Volume reduction surgery<br>• Genetic testing<br>• Family screening to identify asymptomatic members with HCM |

Labels in DCM image: Increased atrial chamber size; Increased ventricular chamber size; Decreased muscle size

Labels in HCM image: Thickened interventricular septum; Left ventricular hypertrophy

Images adapted from the Anatomical Chart Company: Atlas of Pathophysiology. Springhouse, PA: Springhouse, 2010, p 45.

---

**SPOTLIGHT ON GENETICS 19-1**

**FAMILIAL RESTRICTIVE CARDIOMYOPATHY**

• The least common of the cardiomyopathies, the heart muscle is stiff and cannot fully relax after each contraction.
• Is caused by mutations in the *TNNI3* gene, which helps regulate contraction and relaxation of the heart muscle.
• *TNNI3* gene mutations associated with familial restrictive cardiomyopathy result in the production of a defective troponin I-cardiac isoform protein. The altered protein disrupts the function of the troponin protein complex and does not allow the heart muscle to fully relax.
• Genetic testing for the *TNNI3* gene–related familial restrictive cardiomyopathy is available.

Data from Genetic Home Reference. Retrieved August 10, 2015, from http://ghr.nlm.nih.gov; Grupper A, Park SJ, Pereira NL, et al: Role of ventricular assist therapy for patients with heart failure and restrictive physiology: Improving outcomes for a lethal disease. J Heart Lung Transplant 34(8):1042–1049, 2015; and Teekakirikul P, Kelly MA, Rehm HL, et al: Inherited cardiomyopathies: Molecular genetics in the post genomic era. J Mol Diagn 15(2): 158–170, 2013.

level include replacement of contractile and elastic muscle cells with fibrotic elements, which leads to stiffness of the ventricles and smooth muscle layers in the arteries. In hypertrophic cardiomyopathy (HCM), the heart muscle becomes thickened, with increased mass and poor relaxation. In dilated cardiomyopathy (DCM), the ventricular muscle thins, the ventricular chamber dilates and changes from a normally elliptical shape to a less efficient spherical shape, reducing contractility and impairing emptying. Stiffening of arteries seen in aging, atherosclerosis, and arteriosclerosis decreases stroke volume and exacerbates

the ventricular wall stress by overfilling the ventricle. The heart attempts to maintain cardiac output in the face of a decreased stroke volume by increasing heart rate, which decreases relaxation time and impairs filling. This endless spiral of dysfunction is manifested by the progressive nature of heart failure.

The resulting decrease in cardiac output leads to activation of the renin–angiotensin–aldosterone system and the release of catecholamines. As previously described, these neurohormones were meant to respond to temporary decreases in blood pressure, such as hemorrhage. However, blood pressure is chronically decreased in cardiomyopathy, leading to prolonged exposure to compensatory neurohormonal mechanisms.

The persistence of these neurohormones is hypothesized to be the mechanism by which the ventricle remodels from an elliptical shape to spherical, further decreasing its pumping efficiency. The realignment of the muscle fibers has been attributed to long-term exposure to aldosterone. Furthermore, long-term exposure to catecholamines leads to downregulation of β-adrenergic receptors and contributes to decreased contractility. Consequently, this prolonged exposure further exacerbates the problems with decreased cardiac output instead of permanently correcting the issue.

## Dilated Cardiomyopathy

DCM is characterized by increased myocardial cavity size in the presence of normal or reduced left ventricular wall thickness and impaired systolic function.[4,10] The heart gradually assumes a globular shape accompanied by ventricular chamber dilation.[4] A decrease in contractility may occur for many reasons, including ischemia, alcohol abuse, endocrine disorders, pregnancy, viral infections, muscular dystrophy, and valvular disease. The result of the decrease in contractility (ejection fraction less than 40%) is an increase in end-systolic volume. Over time, the ventricle dilates to accommodate the increased intraventricular volumes (preload). The increased preload in a normal heart would lead to an increase in stroke volume, but in the dilated heart, the increased volume leads to a decreasing stroke volume. As ventricular dilation progresses, mitral and tricuspid insufficiency develop as the valve leaflets are stretched and separated. Dysrhythmias, such as ventricular tachycardia, as well as conduction defects commonly occur.

DCM is the third most common cause of heart failure, the most common cause of heart failure in the young, and the most frequent cause of heart transplantation.[10] It occurs most frequently in middle-aged men, and 30% to 50% of cases are familial.[10] In most cases, the specific cause is unknown, or considered idiopathic. The etiology of DCM is various, including familial and genetic factors, viral infections (ie, past episodes of viral myocarditis), immunologic defects, and exposure to toxins.[4] Many researchers believe that alcohol is the most prevalent toxic cause of DCM.[4] DCM can be further divided into two types: ischemic and nonischemic.

## Ischemic Cardiomyopathy

Ischemic cardiomyopathy is the result of oxygen levels that are inadequate to meet the metabolic demands of the myocardial cells. It occurs when there is obstruction in the coronary arteries and may be acute or chronic. Oxygen is essential to the function of cells. It is necessary for the metabolism of nutritional substrates and the formation of adenosine triphosphate (ATP), which powers all intracellular processes. When oxygen is inadequate, ATP becomes insufficient, and the calcium, sodium, and potassium pumps on cell membranes and within the cells fail, leading to interruptions in both the mechanical and electrical function of the cells. The net result is a decrease in contractility and dysrhythmia. If oxygen is restored to the muscle cells, function returns and the dysrhythmia disappears.

If the ischemia is severe or persists, the muscle tissue dies, causing an MI. Dead muscle cannot regenerate and is replaced with scar tissue. The larger the scar, the greater the dysfunction. The decrease in muscle mass leads to decreased energy for pumping blood and therefore decreased cardiac output. The goal in treating unstable angina and acute MI is preservation of muscle mass to prevent systolic dysfunction.

If an MI is small, the damage may be insufficient to cause heart failure because there is still enough muscle to meet the body's demands for oxygen at rest and with exercise.[11] The ejection fraction may still be within the normal range, although it may be decreased somewhat because of the myocardial damage. However, repeated damage from subsequent infarctions or persistent ischemia in other areas of the heart muscle may exhaust the reserve function. "Hibernating" myocardium is an area of myocardial cells that are not dead following myocardial infarction (MI), but lack sufficient oxygen and nutrient substrates to contract. Once a patient's condition is stable after an MI, it is important to identify any viable myocardium that may be hibernating because of reversible ischemia. If perfusion can be restored to this viable but underperforming myocardium, ventricular function can be improved.

If an MI is very large, or if critical structures such as the chordae tendineae are involved, the consequences may be life-threatening. Damage or rupture of the chordae may lead to acute, severe mitral regurgitation and profound heart failure. The loss of ventricular pumping function that results from a massive MI or smaller repeated MIs may produce such an acute loss of pump function that all the body's compensatory mechanisms are not effectively able to overcome the deficit in cardiac output.

This condition represents cardiogenic shock, in which cardiac output is severely inadequate and the left ventricle empties poorly (see Chapter 54). Consequently, left ventricular end-diastolic pressure increases, pulmonary artery pressures increase, and pulmonary edema results. End-organ damage caused by inadequate oxygen delivery to the tissue begins to occur depending on the function of the organ. The skin becomes cool, perhaps clammy and pale. The respiratory rate increases to supply as much oxygen as possible to the blood being pumped because the pulmonary edema severely decreases the effective area for gas transport. The pulmonary edema makes the lungs less compliant and reduces the effective tidal volume. Increases in respiratory rate are necessary to maintain minute volume. In addition, the tissues that are not adequately supplied with oxygen begin to produce lactic acid, leading to metabolic acidosis. The short-term compensation for metabolic acidosis is an increase in minute volume, or hyperpnea. The patient complains of feeling short of breath even at rest and may not be able to breathe in any recumbent position.[11]

The hierarchy of protection in times of inadequate perfusion preserves most of the cardiac output for the brain, heart, and kidneys. Autoregulation mechanisms are present in all these organs to preserve pressure gradients and blood flow even when blood pressure and flow are compromised in other areas such as the skin, muscle, and gut. Indications that the brain is inadequately perfused are confusion, disorientation, somnolence, and agitation.[11] Early indications of inadequate renal flow are an increase in blood urea nitrogen (BUN) and creatinine. Early on, the normal 10:1 to 20:1 ratio of BUN to creatinine increases to greater than 20:1; this signals the onset of prerenal azotemia. If perfusion is restored to the kidney at this time, the BUN and creatinine levels return to normal, as does kidney function. If the poor perfusion is profound or prolonged, the kidneys become damaged, and the BUN and creatinine continue to increase, although the ratio returns to normal. This ischemic damage to the kidneys is known as acute tubular necrosis and may be reversible.

If cardiogenic shock persists uncorrected for an extended period, the damage cannot be reversed, and the patient will die. Even if the patient is treated appropriately, further damage may occur in areas where the oxygen demand is lower than that of the brain and kidneys. Prolonged episodes of low cardiac output may lead to ileus, bowel infarction, liver failure, and increased risk for pneumonia and skin breakdown.

Patients who survive the initial episode of acute heart failure may recover completely if an intervention such as angioplasty or coronary artery bypass restores perfusion to the heart muscle and the damage to the remaining muscle is not severe. Chronic heart failure eventually develops in many patients and is characterized by the same symptoms as acute heart failure, but usually at a lower intensity; the body has had time to compensate for the decreased cardiac output. Usually, chronic heart failure does not have the intense limitations associated with acute heart failure. Patients often modify their activity to match the limited reserve of cardiac output available.

## Nonischemic Cardiomyopathy

Nonischemic cardiomyopathy results from several causes. A large number of people have idiopathic DCM: for some as-yet unknown reason, their hearts dilate, remodel, and become ineffective pumps. Others have myocarditis, often due to viral infection of the myocardium, hypothyroidism or hyperthyroidism, valvular disease, human immunodeficiency virus (HIV), or hemochromatosis. In addition, myocarditis may be bacterial or idiopathic. Nonischemic cardiomyopathy may also result from pregnancy, heavy alcohol use, hypertension, and tachycardia. Heart failure that results from hypothyroidism or hyperthyroidism, hemochromatosis, valvular disease, and tachycardia is reversible and disappears when these problems are corrected.

Nonischemic cardiomyopathy, like ischemic cardiomyopathy, may be acute or chronic. Patients with chronic disease are often quite limited in their ability to carry out everyday activities. The mechanism by which the dilation is triggered and progresses is not well understood. DCM, whether ischemic or nonischemic, produces symptoms after all the compensatory mechanisms have been exhausted.

Consequently, unless the onset of symptoms is acute, pathologic changes may be quite advanced before activity is sufficiently limited and the patient seeks medical care. However, myocarditis frequently has an acute onset. The patient feels fine and is free of symptoms before fatigue and dyspnea on exertion, or, occasionally, pulmonary edema, suddenly develop. Dysfunction results from inflammation of the heart muscle. Metabolic function of inflamed muscle cells is impaired; the cells do not contract properly, leading to decreased cardiac output. Severity of the condition ranges from cardiogenic shock to mild limitation of activity. Once the initial acute phase passes, the patient has a low ejection fraction, with varying levels of physical limitation of activity and shortness of breath, or chronic heart failure.

Alcoholism, hypertension, and idiopathic etiologic factors are nonischemic conditions that may lead to DCM over longer periods—months to years as opposed to days to weeks with acute onset. As the ventricle begins to dilate, compensatory mechanisms, including the previously described catecholamines and other neurohormonal factors, begin to work. The proposed mechanism by which the ventricle remodels from the normal, efficient elliptical dimensions to a thin-walled, inefficient spherical shape involves constant exposure of the myocardium to these neurohormones.[11] The natural progression is from dilation without symptoms to compensated heart failure, to uncompensated heart failure, and to refractory heart failure. Patients most often present when their heart failure is no longer compensated and symptoms interfere with normal daily activities. At this point, medication may relieve all or most symptoms. However, the structural changes that occur are progressive, and, even with medication, symptoms worsen over time. Medication can be adjusted to treat the worsening symptoms, but eventually, the medications will

not be enough; cardiac transplantation is required, ventricular assist devices are implanted, or the patient dies. Usually mortality is due to worsening of the cardiac output, leading to system failure or sudden death from ventricular dysrhythmia. Before the stage of refractory heart failure is reached, much can be done to control the patient's symptoms, improve activity tolerance, control the progression of the disease, and improve quality of life.

**ASSESSMENT.** The natural history of DCM is not well defined. Some patients remain asymptomatic or have minimal clinical findings. Symptoms usually develop gradually and are typically related to left ventricular heart failure. The presence of right-sided heart failure is associated with poor prognosis.[12] Laboratory tests include screening for potentially reversible causes, including HIV. The echocardiogram is needed to differentiate the primary abnormality and determine the ejection fraction. Cardiac catheterization may be needed to rule out coronary artery disease or hibernating myocardium with the heart failure symptoms are of an uncertain cause.[11]

**MANAGEMENT.** Treatment goals include identifying and eliminating potential causes of DCM. Patients and their families should be questioned carefully about alcohol consumption because myocardial damage related to ingesting alcohol is reversible if detected early and the patient abstains from further drinking.[4] Clinical management is focused on control of heart failure and other problems such as dysrhythmias or intracoronary thrombus. Biventricular pacing may be helpful in medically refractory patients with severely symptomatic heart failure and a prolonged QRS on the ECG, dilated left ventricle, and poor ejection fraction.[4] Implantable cardioverter defibrillators (ICDs) may also be indicated in select patients to prevent sudden death associated with lethal dysrhythmias.[4] Mechanical circulatory support, heart transplantation, and some medical therapies have been shown to prolong life.[4]

## Hypertrophic Cardiomyopathy

HCM is distinguished by a hypertrophied, nondilated left ventricle.[13] The most characteristic feature of HCM is diastolic dysfunction. The heart can contract but cannot relax and remains abnormally stiff in diastole. In a few patients, septal wall hypertrophy occurs, leading to a left ventricular outflow tract obstruction during systole.[13]

HCM is probably the most frequently occurring cardiomyopathy in the United States. It appears to be a common autosomal dominant genetic malformation; indeed, it is probably the most common genetic cardiovascular disorder, affecting approximately 1 in 500 of the population.[13] Unlike other cardiac conditions, HCM is not secondary to an underlying systemic cause, such as hypertension or aortic valve stenosis.[10]

Sudden death is a catastrophic outcome of HCM, usually from a ventricular dysrhythmia, in asymptomatic or mildly symptomatic people of any age group. In the United States, HCM is a leading cause of sudden death in competitive athletes as well as in people participating in recreational sports.[10,13] The risk for sudden death is constant; mortality is higher in younger patients.[3] Early identification of patients at risk for HCM (and therefore, sudden death) is imperative. However, there is no agreement on the best method to identify people at high risk at this time, and the intensity of screening through genetic testing can be lengthy and costly.[10]

### Assessment

Many patients with HCM are asymptomatic or have only mild complaints though these symptoms can progress to severe heart failure.[10] The condition is often found unexpectedly during investigation of heart murmurs or family screening. The most common symptom is dyspnea, which may be exacerbated with exertion. Presyncope and syncope also frequently occur. Left ventricular hypertrophy (LVH) present on the echocardiogram confirms the diagnosis. Borderline LVH may be a normal finding in competitive athletes.[13]

### Management

The goals of management include controlling symptoms, preventing complications, and reducing the risk for sudden death. Genetic screening and counseling are also indicated.[13] Most symptomatic patients can be medically managed. ICDs are indicated in patients who have survived an episode of sudden death or have documented potentially lethal ventricular dysrhythmias.[13] In patients with symptoms resulting from septal hypertrophy, percutaneous ablation with ethanol or surgery to remove a portion of the septum may be necessary.[13]

Psychosocial concerns are important as patients and families try to cope with this debilitating and potentially fatal illness. They must deal with feelings of uncertainty and loss of control as well as the financial impact of a serious chronic illness.

## Peripheral Vascular Disease

Peripheral vascular disease includes a group of distinct disorders involving the arteries, veins, and lymphatic vessels of the peripheral circulation—the noncardiac diseases that affect the circulation as a whole. This section focuses on peripheral arterial disease (PAD) and venous disease.

## Peripheral Arterial Disease

PAD refers to processes that obstruct the blood supply of the lower or upper extremities.[14,15] Although the incidence of PAD increases steadily with age, the disease is more likely to occur in patients of any age with risk factors for atherosclerosis, such as smoking or diabetes. Other risk factors for PAD include hypertension, lipid disorders, family history, postmenopausal state, and hyperhomocysteinemia.[15,16] With the aging of the US population, management of PAD is a major focus not only of prevention and cure but also of maintenance of quality of life and independence (Box 19-5).[14,15]

Atherosclerosis is the most common cause of PAD. The disease develops in major bifurcations and areas of acute angulations (Fig. 19-4). In people with diabetes, there is greater involvement of the smaller and more distal vessels.[15] Upper extremity involvement is less common than lower extremity involvement.[17]

Thromboangiitis obliterans, or Buerger disease, is a severe, chronic inflammatory disease affecting the intermediate and small arteries of the extremities. It may also involve adjacent veins and nerves. The etiology is unknown, but it is associated with heavy smoking, especially in young people. The chronic

---

**BOX 19-5** | *CONSIDERATIONS for the Older Patient*

**Peripheral Arterial Disease**

- Management of peripheral arterial disease (PAD) in older adults is often more complicated because of the presence of comorbidities, polypharmacy, financial concerns, physical and cognitive limitations, inadequate social support or isolation, and depression and anxiety.
- The incidence of symptomatic PAD increases with age, directly affecting quality of life.
- Conservative management (eg, smoking cessation, walking, foot care) can reduce symptoms and significantly improve quality of life in people of any age.

---

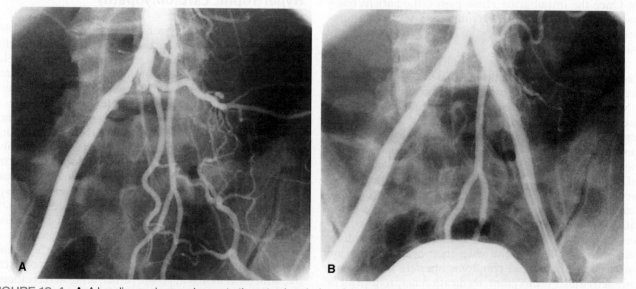

**FIGURE 19-4   A:** A baseline angiogram demonstrating a total occlusion of the left iliac artery. In addition, there is a significant stenosis of the right common iliac artery and occlusion of the internal iliac arteries. **B:** The final result following angioplasty and stenting of the right and left common iliac arteries with Palmaz stents. (Reprinted from Laird JR, Lansky AJ: Percutaneous transluminal angioplasty for the treatment of peripheral vascular disease. In: Apple S, Lindsay J Jr (eds): Principles and Practice of Interventional Cardiology. Philadelphia, PA: Lippincott Williams & Wilkins, 2000, p 196, with permission.)

inflammatory process is often followed by thrombosis, with vascular lesions and fibrous obliteration of the vessel.[18]

## Assessment

Clinical signs of PAD reflect the blood's inability to circulate freely to the extremity. Symptoms depend on the extent of the disease and the presence of collateral circulation. The classic symptom of PAD is intermittent claudication, experienced as a cramping, burning, or aching pain in the legs or buttocks that is relieved with rest.[14,16] Symptoms do not correlate with the extent of the disease. If the PAD is extensive and multilevel, the patient may present with "rest pain," that is, a sensation of burning or numbness in the foot or toes. Patients also experience trophic changes, such as hair loss on the extremities, thickening of the nails, and drying of the skin. Acute arterial obstruction, such as occurs with an embolism, results in the sudden onset of extreme pain and other signs of acute arterial obstruction (Box 19-6).[15]

Practice guidelines should be incorporated in the evaluation of the patient at risk for PAD. This includes a careful vascular examination of the extremities and assessment of all peripheral pulses, including the measurement of segmental pressures in the legs and the ankle/brachial index (ABI). The ABI is the ratio of ankle to brachial systolic blood pressure. A

normal ABI should be 1.0 or greater. The ABI ratio becomes increasingly lower with worsening of the disease (Fig. 19-5).[14]

Treadmill exercise testing can provide an objective measurement of the patient's walking ability as well as an evaluation of possible coronary artery disease. Noninvasive imaging, such as magnetic resonance or computed tomography (CT), may be required to evaluate the extent of disease fully. Angiography is usually limited to revascularization procedures (see Fig. 19-4) or presurgical evaluation.[16]

### BOX 19-6 Clinical Features of Vascular Obstruction

**Acute Arterial Occlusion**
- Pain
- Pulselessness
- Pallor
- Paresthesia
- Paralysis

**Deep Venous Thrombosis**
- Pain when standing
- Inflammation
- Swelling
- Tenderness
- Redness, soreness

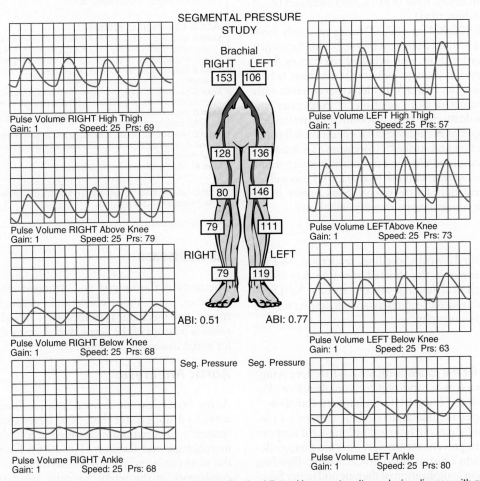

**FIGURE 19-5** Segmental pressures and ankle/brachial indices indicating bilateral lower extremity occlusive disease with more severe involvement of the right lower extremity. There is also a probable significant stenosis of the left subclavian artery, which explains the difference between the right and left brachial pressures. Prs, pressures. (Reprinted from Saucedo JF, Laird JR: Peripheral vascular disease. In: Apple S, Lindsay J Jr (eds): Principles and Practice of Interventional Cardiology. Philadelphia, PA: Lippincott Williams & Wilkins, 2000, p 47, with permission.)

## Management

PAD is associated with an increased risk of atherosclerotic adverse events; the mortality rate is high in symptomatic patients.[14] Therefore, treatment goals include modifying or eliminating risk factors (especially smoking), improving leg symptoms, and maintaining limb viability. Risk factor modification incorporates national guidelines; these include immediate smoking cessation as well as aggressive treatment of hypertension, diabetes, and lipid disorders, with medication, if necessary. Other pharmacologic agents include antiplatelets (aspirin or clopidogrel [Plavix]) to reduce the risk for MI and stroke and cilostazol (Pletal) to increase walking distance. In patients with claudication, exercise improves overall walking ability. Peripheral interventional procedures, such as balloon angioplasty, are successful in restoring circulation in many cases. Surgical bypass may be required when severe or diffuse arterial obstruction is present.[14,16]

## Venous Disease

Superficial thrombophlebitis is a condition in which an injury to the vessel wall causes inflammation and clot formation in the superficial blood vessels.[19] It can lead to the formation of a thrombus, a solid obstruction within the vein that can break loose and form a venous thromboembolism (VTE). Factors that predispose a patient to thrombus formation are vessel wall injury, stasis of blood, and increased blood coagulability (Virchow triad).[20]

An estimated 100,000 to 180,000 cases of death from VTE occur in the United States each year.[20] This incidence increases with age for those with acquired risk factors. Incidences are increased in younger individuals who have inherited thrombophilias (ie, Factor V Leiden) that interact with environmental factors for clot formation.[20,21] Pulmonary embolism has higher death rates than myocardial infarction and is the third most common cardiovascular condition following myocardial infraction and stroke.[20,21] Because VTE is associated with significant morbidity and mortality, it is important for the nurse to be familiar with risk factors for VTE as well as current recommendations for treatment. (See Chapter 26 for more information concerning pulmonary embolism.)

## Assessment

DVT is characterized by pain, swelling, tenderness, and increased temperature over the affected area (see Box 19-6). However, these clinical findings are not specific for DVT. Accurate diagnosis usually requires diagnostic testing such as compression ultrasonography.[22]

## Management

The focus of care for the patient with VTE is to relieve symptoms, increase blood flow, and prevent complications. Patients with DVT are at high risk for pulmonary embolism.[22] Treatment strategies include anticoagulant therapy to prevent the formation of emboli, followed by long-term warfarin (Coumadin) use to prevent recurrence. Specific therapy depends on the patient's history and clinical setting. Bleeding is the most common complication of therapy and major hemorrhage can be fatal in 25% of cases.[22] Patient teaching includes safe administration of home anticoagulants as well as behaviors to decrease the recurrence of DVT. Prevention of VTE is discussed in Evidence-Based Practice Highlight 19-1.

---

**QSEN**

### EVIDENCE-BASED PRACTICE HIGHLIGHT 19-1
### Venous Thromboembolism Prevention

#### Expected Practice

- Assess all patients upon admission to the ICU for risk factors of venous thromboembolism (VTE) and anticipate orders for VTE prophylaxis based on risk assessment. [Level D]
- Review daily—with the physician and during multidisciplinary rounds—each patient's current VTE risk factors including clinical status, necessity for central venous catheter (CVC), current status of VTE prophylaxis, risk for bleeding, and response to treatment. [Level E]
- Maximize patient mobility whenever possible and take measures to reduce the amount of time the patient is immobile because of the effects of treatment (eg, pain, sedation, neuromuscular blockade, mechanical ventilation). [Level E]
- Ensure that mechanical prophylaxis devices are fit properly and in use at all times except when being removed for cleaning and/or inspection of skin. [Level E]
- Implement regimens for venous thromboembolism prophylaxis as ordered.
  - *Moderate-risk patients (medically ill and postoperative patients)*: low-dose unfractionated heparin, low molecular-weight heparin (LMWH), or fondaparinux (Level B)
  - *High-risk patients (major trauma, spinal cord injury, orthopedic surgery)*: LMWH, fondaparinux, or oral vitamin K antagonist (Level B)
  - *Patients at high risk for bleeding*: mechanical prophylaxis, including graduated compression stockings, intermittent pneumatic compression devices, or both (Level B)

#### AACN Levels of Evidence

**Level A** Meta-analysis of quantitative studies or metasynthesis of qualitative studies with results that consistently support a specific action, intervention, or treatment (including systematic review of randomized controlled trials)

**Level B** Well-designed, controlled studies with results that consistently support a specific action, intervention, or treatment

**Level C** Qualitative studies, descriptive or correlational studies, integrative reviews, systematic reviews, or randomized controlled trials with inconsistent results

**Level D** Peer-reviewed professional and organizational standards with the support of clinical study recommendations

**Level E** Multiple case reports, theory-based evidence from expert opinions, or peer-reviewed professional orgastandards without clinical studies to support recommendations

**Level M** Manufacturer's recommendations only

Excerpted from American Association of Critical-Care Nurses Practice Alert. Available online at http://aacn.org.

---

## Aortic Disease

The aorta is the longest and strongest artery in the body. However, over time, congenital, degenerative, hemodynamic, and mechanical factors stress this elastic vessel. The result is dilation of the aortic wall, leaving the patient at risk for aortic dissection or rupture.[23]

## Aortic Aneurysm

Aortic aneurysms are defined as a localized dilation of the aorta to a size greater than 50% larger than its normal diameter.[23] Aneurysms are classified according to their shape, morphology, and location (Fig. 19-6). Fusiform aneurysms, the more common type, are diffuse dilations of the entire circumference of the artery. Saccular aneurysms are localized balloon-shaped outpouchings. Aneurysms may be thoracic or abdominal; rarely, they are both.

True aneurysms involve the entire vessel wall and are classified as fusiform or saccular. False aneurysms are not actually

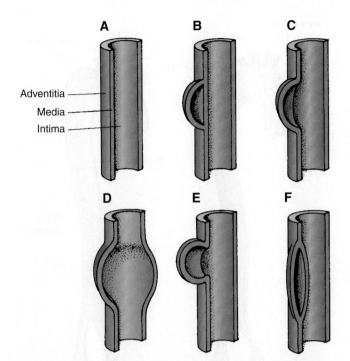

Adventitia
Media
Intima

**FIGURE 19-6** Types of aortic aneurysms. **A:** Normal artery. **B:** False aneurysm—actually a pulsating hematoma. The clot and connective tissue are outside the arterial wall. **C:** True aneurysm. One, two, or all three layers may be involved. **D:** Fusiform aneurysm—symmetric, spindle-shaped expansion of entire circumference of involved vessel. **E:** Saccular aneurysm—a bulbous protrusion of one side of the arterial wall. **F:** Dissecting aneurysm—this usually is a hematoma that splits the layers of the arterial wall.

aneurysms but are formed when blood leaks through the wall of the aorta and is contained by the surrounding tissues (a contained rupture).[22]

## Abdominal Aortic Aneurysm

Abdominal aortic aneurysms (AAAs), which are more common than thoracic aortic aneurysms, occur more frequently in men. Smoking is the leading risk factor for AAAs, followed closely by age, hypertension, lipid disorders, and atherosclerosis.[24] Atherosclerosis is probably a major cause of AAAs, but other factors, such as genetic and environmental influences, almost certainly contribute to their development.[22,24] The major risk from AAAs is rupture, which is associated with a high rate of mortality (up to 90%).[24]

**ASSESSMENT.** Most patients with AAAs are asymptomatic; they are typically identified during health screening for another problem. Abdominal or back pain is the most common complaint. Worsening of symptoms is usually related to expansion or rupture of the aneurysm.

Detection of AAAs by physical examination is difficult, especially in obese patients. The abdomen is examined for the presence of bruits or masses, and peripheral pulses are carefully evaluated. Abdominal ultrasonography is the most practical method of confirming the diagnosis.[25]

**MANAGEMENT.** Management of AAAs includes control of hypertension and elimination of risk factors, such as smoking. The patient should be followed with serial noninvasive tests, such as ultrasonography. Treatment of aneurysms

involves surgical repair, which is usually indicated for AAAs larger than 5.5 cm (Box 19-7).[26]

In addition to surgery, AAAs may be repaired by a minimally invasive approach using an endovascular graft. This approach involves placement of a graft through the femoral artery. The graft is then anchored to the wall of the aorta by means of self-expanding or balloon-expanded stents. Endovascular repair has become the treatment of choice for high-risk patients with AAAs.[26] Periodic monitoring of the graft using surveillance is required to be assured the graft stays anchored, the aneurysm shrinks, and no endoleak has developed.

## Thoracic Aortic Aneurysm

Thoracic aortic aneurysms occur relatively infrequently and are classified by the involved segment of the aorta (root, ascending, arch, or descending). The location is important because the etiology, natural history, and treatment differ for each segment.[22] Most ascending thoracic aortic aneurysms are due to conditions that cause remodeling and cystic medial degeneration. Ascending thoracic aortic aneurysms are also associated with connective tissue disorders, genetic disorders, bicuspid aortic valve, infections, inflammatory diseases, chronic aortic dissection, and trauma.[22]

**ASSESSMENT.** Like most patients with AAAs, most patients with thoracic aortic aneurysms are asymptomatic at the time of diagnosis. Symptoms are related to the size and location of the aneurysm; these include aortic insufficiency and signs of compression of adjacent structures which can lead to symptoms such as hoarseness, dysphagia, dyspnea, heart failure.[22] Rupture or acute dissection of a thoracic aneurysm can be fatal.

**MANAGEMENT.** For most ascending thoracic aortic aneurysms, surgical repair is indicated at a diameter of 5.5 cm or more.[23] These indications vary according to the clinical situation and the existence of comorbidities. Repair of descending thoracic aneurysms is also recommended when the diameter is 5.5 to 6.0 cm or more depending on the risk factors of the patient and the growth rate of the aneurysm.[22,23]

---

**BOX 19-7** **General Indications for Surgical Repair of Aortic Aneurysms**

**Abdominal**
- Diameter 5.5 cm of more (men)
- For women, 4.5 to 5.0 cm (due to greater incidence of rupture)
- Diameter 4.5 to 5.5 cm; clinical setting, patient preference

**Ascending Thoracic**
- Diameter 5.5 cm or more (5 cm in patients with Marfan syndrome)
- Symptoms suggesting expansion or compression of surrounding structures

**Other**
- Rapidly expanding aneurysms (growth rate more than 0.5 cm over a 6-month period)
- Symptomatic aneurysm regardless of size

Data from Rooke TW, Hirsch AT, Misra J, et al: 2011 ACCF/AHA Focused Update of the Guideline for the management of patients with peripheral artery disease (Updating the 2005 Guideline). A report of the American College of Cardiology Foundation/American Heart Association Task Force on Practice Guidelines. Circulation 124:2020–2045, 2011; and Goldfinger JZ, Halperin JL, Marin ML, et al: Thoracic aortic aneurysm and dissection. J Am Coll Cardiol 64(16):1725–1739, 2014.

## Aortic Dissection

Acute aortic dissection, which occurs when the aorta wall tears, is the most common and the most lethal condition involving the aorta. Mortality rates are very high, approaching 1% per hour for ascending aortic dissections.[23,27] Death usually occurs from rupture of the aorta. The incidence is highest in men older than age 60 with a history of hypertension. Other risk factors include connective tissue disorders (ie, Marfan syndrome, Turner syndrome), a preexisting aortic aneurysm, cardiac surgery (aortic valve or coronary bypass), cardiac catheterization, illicit use of stimulants (cocaine, crack, methamphetamine), preexisting vasculitis, strenuous isometric resistance exercises, and trauma.[23,27]

### Pathophysiology

In aortic dissection, the medial layer of the aorta undergoes degeneration due to collagen vascular disorders or genetic diseases, leading to disorganization and loss of medial layer extracellular matrix proteins and loss of vascular smooth muscle and elastic fibers. This remodeling and degeneration weakens the tensile strength of the aortic medial layers, causing wall stress and dissection.[23] Dissection involves a longitudinal separation of the medial layers of the aorta by a column of blood. The dissection begins at a tear in the aortic wall, usually at the proximal end of the dissection. Blood pumped through this tear creates a false channel, or lumen, that rapidly becomes larger than the true aortic lumen. Dissections are typically classified according to location, as illustrated in Figure 19-7.

### Assessment

More than 90% of patients present with sudden, intense chest pain. Frequently, the pain is described as "ripping" or "tearing" and may be accompanied by syncope (see Table 19-1). In most patients, the diagnosis can be determined with a careful history and physical examination. The patient will have a murmur of aortic regurgitation or alteration of the peripheral pulses with a presence of known risk factors, such as hypertension. The chest radiograph may show a widened mediastinum. Cardiac ischemia may be present if the dissection involves the coronary arteries. Cardiac tamponade may be another complication of dissection involving the aortic root.[23] Neurologic deficits may occur if the aortic arch vessels are involved. Dissections involving the renal arteries result in elevated serum creatinine, decreased urine output, and severe hypertension that is difficult to manage. To confirm the diagnosis of acute aortic dissection, transesophageal echocardiography or contrast medium–enhanced CT may be ordered.[22,23,27]

### Management

Survival of the acute phase depends on the location of the dissection, the severity of the complications, and the rapidity with which the diagnosis is confirmed. Clinical management focuses on controlling blood pressure and managing pain. Surgery is the treatment of choice when the dissection involves the ascending aorta.[27,28] Long-term prevention focuses on management of risk factors, which includes blood pressure control, smoking cessation, cholesterol management, avoiding intense isometric exercises, avoiding powerful stimulants, including illicit substances (cocaine, methamphetamine), and controlling stress.[23,28]

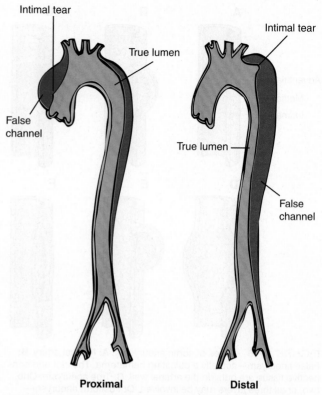

**FIGURE 19-7**    Two major patterns of aortic dissection. Blood pumps through a tear in the wall, creating a false channel or lumen. The false channel rapidly becomes larger than the true lumen.

## Hypertensive Crisis

Hypertension affects approximately 70 million people in the United States and is a major controllable risk factor for the development of cardiovascular diseases.[29] Hypertension is defined as a systolic blood pressure greater than 150 mm Hg in individuals 65 years and older and greater than 140 mm Hg in individuals 18 to 64 years of age, and a diastolic blood pressure greater than 90 mm Hg in all age groups.[30]

Patients with high blood pressure are at risk for experiencing a hypertensive crisis. A hypertensive crisis or emergency is defined as an acute elevation of blood pressure (greater than 180/120 mm Hg) that is associated with acute or imminent target organ damage.[28] This rare but potentially fatal condition strikes about 1% to 2% of hypertensive patients, occurring more frequently in African American men and in elderly patients.

### Pathophysiology

A hypertensive crisis is characterized by a marked rapid increase in blood pressure that initially leads to intense vasoconstriction as the body attempts to protect itself from the elevated pressure. If the blood pressure remains critically high, compensatory vasoconstriction fails, resulting in increased pressure and blood flow throughout the vascular system. In the cerebral circulation, this may quickly lead to hypertensive encephalopathy, as the brain is susceptible to the shear forces of the elevated blood pressure.[28] Hypertensive crisis is associated with a variety of clinical situations (Box 19-8).

BOX 19-8 **Summary of Hypertensive Crisis**

**Causes**
- Acute or chronic renal disease
- Exacerbation of chronic hypertension
- Sudden withdrawal of antihypertensive medications

**Associated Clinical Situations**
- Acute cerebrovascular syndrome
- Acute stroke
- Hypertensive encephalopathy
- Acute cardiovascular syndromes
- Myocardial infarction
- Unstable angina
- Pulmonary edema
- Aortic dissection
- Extensive burns
- Postoperative period
- Pheochromocytoma
- Eclampsia

**Management**
- Intravenous medications with continuous arterial pressure monitoring
- Goal is to reduce mean arterial blood pressure over 1 hour by no more than 25% while avoiding hypoperfusion

## Assessment

Most patients who present with hypertensive crisis are critically ill and in need of immediate treatment. Clinical findings depend on the degree of vascular injury and end organ damage.[28] Signs of encephalopathy include headache, visual disturbances, confusion, nausea, and vomiting. Examination of the retina of the eyes may reveal cotton-wool spots and hemorrhages, indicating damage to retinal nerves and rupture of retinal blood vessels; papilledema is diagnostic of increased intracranial pressure. Chest pain may represent acute coronary syndrome or aortic dissection. Depending on the damage to the kidneys, the patient may present with decreased urine output (oliguria) or azotemia (excess urea in the blood).[28]

## Management

The goal is to reduce the mean blood pressure within 1 hour of starting treatment and to prevent or reverse target organ damage.[28] Several intravenous medications are indicated in treating hypertensive crises; the choice depends on availability and the clinical situation. The selected drug may be a vasodilator, adrenergic blocker, calcium channel blocker, or an angiotensin-converting enzyme inhibitor. Constant monitoring is necessary to avoid lowering the blood pressure too quickly; this is best accomplished with an intra-arterial catheter.

Once the blood pressure has been stabilized, treatment goals depend on the etiology of the crisis. All patients require careful long-term management to control their blood pressure and prevent future episodes.

## Clinical Applicability Challenges

**CASE STUDY**

Mr. P., age 55, is admitted to the coronary ICU with symptoms of shortness of breath with exertion and when lying flat; chest pressure; and extreme fatigue. He has had increased swelling in his feet and abdomen and has been taking an over-the-counter medication for swelling. He has noticed that his heart races with even the mildest exertion and he has to stop and rest after walking very short distances. His symptoms came on gradually over the past 2 weeks and have not been improving. Mr. P. spent the previous night in a recliner because he felt he couldn't breathe when he lay flat.

An echocardiogram shows global left ventricular systolic dysfunction with an ejection fraction of 30% and significant valve disorders. Mr. P. has a history of high blood pressure but stopped taking his medications because of dizziness and impotence. He has not been regularly seen by his primary care provider and thinks he recalls being told at one point that his cholesterol was high. He has worked in construction but has been out of work for 3 months and reports drinking at least a 24-pack of beer daily; he has been a heavy drinker for most of his adult life. He quit smoking cigarettes 2 years ago but uses a vapor cigarette daily. His father died in his 60s from heart failure, alcoholism, and cancer.

Mr. P. is hypoxic with room air saturations of 82%; a chest x-ray shows pulmonary edema and bilateral pleural effusions and a BNP of 2,763. His BUN is elevated at 47 with a serum creatinine of 1.77 with no previous history of kidney disease. His other vital signs on admission include a heart rate of 108 bpm, blood pressure of 159/97 mm Hg, and a respiratory rate of 28 bpm with some mild accessory muscle use. His weight has increased 10 lb over the past week, although his appetite has been decreased.

1. What are Mr. P.'s risk factors for cardiomyopathy?
2. What are the priorities of care for Mr. P.?
3. What are other potential causes of cardiomyopathy for Mr. P.?
4. What are the underlying reasons for Mr. P.'s vital signs and symptoms?

**WANT TO KNOW MORE?**

A wide variety of resources to enhance your learning and understanding of this chapter are available on thePoint.

You will find:

- References
- Selected readings
- NCLEX-style review questions
- Internet resources
- And more!

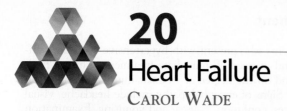

# 20

# Heart Failure

CAROL WADE

**LEARNING OBJECTIVES**

*Based on the content in this chapter, the reader should be able to:*

1. Define heart failure.
2. Describe the classification systems used to define heart failure.
3. Explain the physiologic basis for the clinical manifestations of heart failure.
4. Describe expected clinical assessment findings for patients with heart failure.
5. Explain the standard pharmacologic therapies for chronic heart failure and acute exacerbation of chronic heart failure, and their rationale.
6. Describe the nonpharmacologic therapies for management of heart failure.
7. Define expected outcomes for therapeutic management of patients with heart failure.
8. Formulate a teaching plan for patients and families regarding heart failure.

Approximately 5.1 million Americans 20 years of age and older have heart failure. About 825,000 people receive a new the diagnosis of heart failure each year. Incidence and prevalence statistics indicate that heart failure is a common occurrence in certain patient populations, most notably the elderly and black patient. The incidence of heart failure increases with age, rising from 20 per 1,000 in persons ages 65 to 69 years of age to greater than 80 per 1,000 persons older than 85 years. Heart failure in non-Hispanic black males and females has a prevalence of 4.5% and 3.8%, respectively, while in non-Hispanic white males and females it is 2.5% and 1.8%, respectively. Important risk factors that increase the propensity for heart failure include hypertension, diabetes, metabolic syndrome, and atherosclerotic disease. While the survival rate after a heart failure diagnosis has improved, the death rate remains high: approximately 50% of people diagnosed with heart failure will die in 5 years.[1,2]

Heart failure is the leading cause of hospitalization for the over-65 population. For 2012, the total cost for heart failure was estimated to be 30.7 million dollars, with over half of these costs related to hospitalization. It is projected that by 2030, total costs related to heart failure will increase by 127% to 69.7 billion. An estimated 1,023,000 patients were discharged with heart failure in 2010. Those hospitalized with heart failure have a 1-month all-cause readmission rate of 25%.[1]

Heart failure is a common diagnosis in the intensive care unit (ICU). An acute myocardial infarction (MI) or an acute exacerbation of chronic heart failure is often life threatening. Patients with heart failure are at increased risk for ventricular tachyarrhythmias leading to sudden death. In addition, the physical and emotional burdens of inpatient care are great for patients and their families. Complicating the care of hospitalized heart failure patients is their other comorbidities including chronic kidney disease, hyponatremia, hematologic abnormalities, and chronic obstructive pulmonary disease (COPD).[2]

Management of patients with heart failure requires a collaborative effort on the part of physicians, nurses, pharmacologists, dietitians, and other allied health professionals. The care of patients with heart failure extends across all parts of the health care system. Patients with heart failure may be located in home care, ambulatory care, acute care, critical care, and rehabilitation facilities. As patients take charge of their own disease management, the home serves as a critical location. With the increased emphasis on preventing readmission for heart failure patients, greater attention is being focused on the transition of care from the hospital to the home, and on ensuring that patients have the skills necessary to perform self-care.

## Definition of Heart Failure

Heart failure is a clinical syndrome caused by a structural or functional impairment in the ability of the ventricle to fill or eject blood effectively. The cardinal symptoms of heart failure are fatigue and dyspnea on exertions (DOE); other symptoms include edema, orthopnea, and paroxysmal nocturnal dyspnea (PND). Some patients report profound exercise intolerance owing to fatigue, while other patients complain of symptoms suggestive of volume overload.

The term *heart failure* is used to describe the general clinical syndrome regardless of the type of heart failure or the etiology that produces the symptoms. "Heart failure" is preferred over "congestive heart failure," as not all patients present with symptoms suggestive of fluid retention. Heart failure is caused by a myriad of disorders including diseases of the pericardium, diseases that impact the myocardium such as myocarditis or coronary artery disease (CAD), heart valve abnormalities, and metabolic disturbances.[2] For this reason, it is important to look at the way heart failure is classified, because the pathophysiology and etiology are key to appropriate management.

# Classification of Heart Failure

Heart failure is more difficult to understand when signs and symptoms are common to more than one type of failure, and when types of heart failure are used interchangeably. Several categories are used to describe and classify heart failure. Using these categories to organize information about heart failure and for discussion of any individual patient case makes diagnosis, management, and outcome evaluation clearer.

## Acute Versus Chronic Heart Failure

The terms *acute* and *chronic* describe both the onset of symptoms of heart failure and the intensity of symptoms. Heart failure of acute onset refers to the sudden appearance of symptoms, usually over days or hours. Acute symptoms have progressed to a point at which immediate or emergency intervention is necessary to save the patient's life. Heart failure of chronic onset refers to the development of symptoms over months or years. Chronic symptoms represent the baseline condition, the limitations the patient lives with on a daily basis. If the cause of the acute onset or the acute symptoms is not reversible, then the heart failure may become chronic. For example, a patient who has an acute MI with severe damage to the left ventricle has acute heart failure with pulmonary edema, causing lasting damage to the left ventricle. As a result, the patient has poor contractility (and therefore DOE) after the MI has resolved. The patient's acute onset of heart failure has left him or her with chronic symptoms.

Chronic heart failure does not disappear when the symptoms are controlled or absent. People with heart failure demonstrate various levels of compensation, meaning that they have enough reserve to "compensate" for the loss of function and they appear to be asymptomatic, usually at rest. The lack of symptoms, or compensation, should not be mistaken for absence of disease. Like most chronic conditions, heart failure is characterized by relatively stable periods interrupted by episodes of acute decompensation. Acute decompensation is often life threatening and frequently requires critical care. A common cause of acute decompensation is inadequate treatment for chronic heart failure.

The following discussion focuses on evidence-based care for chronic heart failure and the diagnosis and management of acute decompensated heart failure (ADHF).

## Left-Sided Heart Failure Versus Right-Sided Heart Failure

### Left-Sided Heart Failure

Left-sided heart failure refers to failure of the left ventricle to fill or empty properly. This leads to increased pressures inside the ventricle and congestion in the pulmonary vascular system. Left-sided heart failure may be further classified into systolic and diastolic dysfunction.

**SYSTOLIC DYSFUNCTION (HEART FAILURE WITH REDUCED LEFT VENTRICULAR FUNCTION).** Systolic dysfunction is defined as an ejection fraction (EF) of less than 40% and is caused by a decrease in contractility. Left ventricular function is estimated by EF, or the percentage of the left ventricular end-diastolic volume (LVEDV) that is ejected from the ventricle in one cycle. If the LVEDV is 100 mL and the stroke volume is 60 mL, the EF is 60%. Normal EF is 50% to 70%. With systolic dysfunction, the ventricle does not empty adequately because of poor pumping, and the result is decreased cardiac output (CO).

**DIASTOLIC DYSFUNCTION (HEART FAILURE WITH PRESERVED LEFT VENTRICULAR FUNCTION).** Diastolic dysfunction is less well defined and more difficult to measure. Diastolic dysfunction is caused by impaired relaxation and filling. Left ventricular filling, a complex process that occurs during diastole, is a combination of passive filling and atrial contraction. Pumping is normal or even increased, with an EF as high as 80% at times. If the ventricle is stiff and poorly compliant (due to aging, uncontrolled hypertension, or volume overload), relaxation is slow or incomplete. A reduction in diastolic filling causes a decrease in CO creating worsening symptoms in patients with diastolic dysfunction. Conditions that decrease diastolic filling include tachycardia (due to decreased diastolic filling time) and atrial flutter or fibrillation (due to the loss of atrial kick).

### Right-Sided Heart Failure

Right-sided heart failure refers to failure of the right ventricle to pump adequately. The most common cause of right-sided heart failure is left-sided heart failure, but right-sided heart failure can exist in the presence of a perfectly normal left ventricle, and does not lead to left-sided heart failure. Right-sided heart failure can also result from pulmonary disease (cor pulmonale) and primary pulmonary artery hypertension. Pulmonary embolus is a common cause of acute right-sided heart failure.

## Classification Systems

### New York Heart Association Functional Classification

The New York Heart Association (NYHA) Functional Classification is a measure of how much the symptoms of heart failure limit the activities of patients (Box 20-1). Although EF is used to define left ventricular function, EF is poorly correlated with the patient's functional capacity or prognosis.[3]

### American College of Cardiology/American Heart Association Guidelines

The ACC/AHA Guidelines outline four stages of heart failure that are useful for organizing the prevention, diagnosis, management, and prognosis for patients with heart

---

**BOX 20-1   New York Heart Association Functional Classification of Heart Failure**

**Class I:** No limitation of physical activity. Ordinary physical activity does not cause undue fatigue or dyspnea.

**Class II:** Slight limitation of physical activity. Comfortable at rest, but ordinary physical activity results in fatigue or dyspnea.

**Class III:** Comfortable at rest but minimal activity causes symptoms of heart failure including dyspnea or fatigue.

**Class IV:** Unable to carry on any physical activity without symptoms. Symptoms are present even at rest. If any physical activity is undertaken, symptoms are increased.

failure (Box 20-2).[2] These stages are not meant to replace the NYHA functional classification but rather to augment it. Only stages C and D are applicable to the NYHA functional classification system. See also Evidence-Based Practice Highlight 20-1.

## Factors That Determine Cardiac Output

The underlying result of all types of heart failure is insufficient CO—that is, the volume of blood pumped by the heart in 1 minute is inadequate. Some patients may have a normal CO at rest, but they do not have the reserve function to increase CO to meet the increased demands of exercise, hypoxemia, or anemia. Therefore, it is important to understand the physiologic basis of CO and review the mechanisms of compensation of decreased CO. (See Chapter 16 for a review of cardiovascular physiology.)

### EVIDENCE-BASED PRACTICE HIGHLIGHT 20-1
#### Transition Care for Heart Failure

Heart failure is the leading cause of admission to the hospital in the United States. Up to 25% of all heart failure discharges are readmitted within 30 days, accounting for much of the cost associated with this disease process. The Center for Medicare and Medicaid Services now penalizes hospitals for avoidable all-cause 30-day readmissions when a patient is discharged with a heart failure diagnosis. The National Quality Forum emphasizes the need for effective transition strategies when patients leave the hospital to go home to care for themselves. Multidisciplinary strategies aimed at improving care for the patient with heart failure and ensuring that there is effective communication between providers in the outpatient and inpatient setting have been shown to be effective in reducing readmissions and in decreasing mortality.[2] Additionally, having the patient see a provider within 1 week after discharge and ensuring that this appointment is made before discharge has been shown to effectively prevent a return to the hospital.[4] To safeguard patient understanding of their medications, nursing medication reconciliation at discharge is an important component of transitional care.[5,6] Nursing needs to be involved in research and quality improvement efforts that will prevent readmission to the hospital for heart failure patients.

## Oxygen Demand

The required CO is determined by the body's metabolic demand for oxygen. At rest, the body needs sufficient oxygen to burn calories to support cellular function, as measured by basal metabolic rate. Oxygen delivery to the tissues depends on arterial oxygen content ($CaO_2$) and CO. $CaO_2$, a combination of arterial oxygen saturation ($SaO_2$) and hemoglobin (Hgb), is constant in healthy people. Any factor that increases metabolic demand for oxygen, such as exercise, fever, hyperthyroidism, or trauma, increases CO. If $CaO_2$ is decreased, as it is in hypoxemia or anemia, then CO increases to ensure sufficient oxygen to meet the metabolic demand. Exercise or fever in a patient with anemia puts a tremendous burden on the heart to supply sufficient oxygen to meet the metabolic demands.

A person with a healthy heart has sufficient reserve to meet this increased metabolic demand and increase CO. At best, a patient with myocardial ischemia, cardiomyopathy, valvular disease, dysrhythmia, or lung disease may not be able to meet the metabolic demand for oxygen associated with exercise. At worst, the patient with one or more of these problems may not be able to meet the basal metabolic demand for oxygen and becomes symptomatic, even at rest.

## Mechanical Factors and Heart Rate

CO equals stroke volume multiplied by heart rate. This relationship between stroke volume, heart rate, and CO is critical to understanding why heart failure may be present long before it produces the symptoms that cause patients to seek help.

Preload, afterload, and the contractile force of the left ventricle determine stroke volume (see Chapter 16). These three components are in a constant and dynamic relationship. A decrease in one or more components is compensated by an increase in the others, designed to maintain a constant stroke volume at rest. Catecholamines and other neurohormones contribute to the complex balance that preserves stroke volume over a wide range of supply and demand for oxygen at the tissue level. Relatively minor increases in stroke volume are possible because of neurohormonal regulation of reserve fluid volume stored in the liver and venous system until needed. The largest increase in CO comes not from increased stroke volume but through increases in heart rate. Cardiac reserve is the ability to significantly increase oxygen delivery in response to increased demand. Reserve is meant to meet demand that exceeds that of rest. Patients with heart failure need their reserve just to function at rest. When that reserve is exhausted, they have symptoms even at rest. The increase in catecholamines increases the risk of dysrhythmias such as ventricular tachycardia and sudden death.

### Heart Rate

As stated earlier, CO equals stroke volume multiplied by heart rate; therefore, doubling the heart rate doubles CO without changing stroke volume. The immediate response to a decrease in stroke volume, a decrease in arterial oxygen content, or an increase in metabolic demand is an increase in heart rate. However, at a certain point, increasing the heart rate can actually decrease the stroke volume and, therefore,

CO as well. Because the ventricle fills during diastole, preload becomes compromised at higher heart rates because of the shortened diastolic filling time. A decrease in preload will compromise contractility.

The physiologic role of heart rate in the regulation of CO involves more than just the absolute rate. Cardiac rhythm is important. As previously stated, rapid tachycardia can compromise stroke volume. Any rhythm that does not include a rhythmic atrial contraction, such as atrial fibrillation and flutter, junctional rhythms, ventricular rhythms, and ventricular pacing, can compromise filling and therefore stroke volume and CO. A heart rate that is too slow, such as that which occurs in third-degree atrioventricular (AV) block or sick sinus syndrome, may compromise CO, not by decreasing stroke volume, but by decreasing overall CO.

## Neurohormonal Mechanisms

Metabolic demand for oxygen is the primary factor in the regulation of CO, and the mechanical relationships between loading and contractility provide a means to regulate it. Neurohormones are the messengers that initiate, coordinate, and mediate the complex processes that meet the dynamic need for CO (Fig. 20-1).[7–9]

## Catecholamines

Catecholamines are released from the adrenal medulla as part of the primitive "fight or flight" response to any stressor.

Stressors can be physiologic or psychological. Epinephrine and norepinephrine as well as cortical hormones, such as cortisol and aldosterone, are released.

Epinephrine and norepinephrine are the key catecholamines involved in the regulation of the cardiovascular system. The heart and blood vessels contain α- and β-adrenergic receptors that bind with these hormones to support CO and blood pressure. Norepinephrine has almost exclusively α-adrenergic properties that increase vascular resistance and therefore blood pressure. Epinephrine has both α- and β-adrenergic properties. β-Agonist effects include increased heart rate, increased contractility, and vasodilation. The net effect of epinephrine is increased CO; it increases stroke volume by increasing contractility and decreasing afterload. The increases in heart rate and stroke volume together produce a greater increase in CO than either would alone.[7,9]

### Renin–Angiotensin–Aldosterone System

One of the most important mechanisms of blood pressure control in relation to heart failure is the renin–angiotensin–aldosterone system. Fluids (such as blood) flow down pressure gradients (ie, from higher pressure to lower pressure). Consequently, pressure in the aorta is higher than pressures distal to it, including the arteriolar and capillary levels. Arterial blood pressure is critical to the delivery of blood (and therefore oxygen) to the cells to support cellular function. Several mechanisms maintain normal blood pressure across variable body fluid volumes, in different positions (sitting or standing vs. supine), and with CO demands.

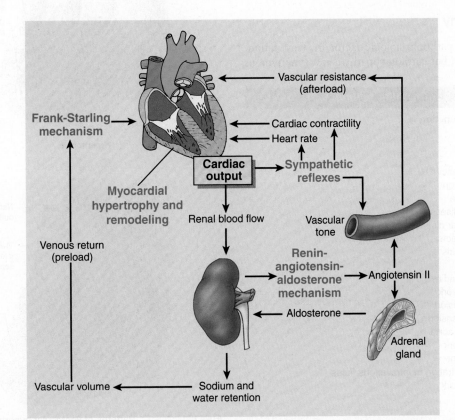

**FIGURE 20-1**  Compensatory mechanisms in heart failure. The Frank–Starling mechanism, sympathetic reflexes, renin–angiotensin–aldosterone mechanism, and myocardial hypertrophy work to maintain CO in the failing heart. (From Porth CM: Pathophysiology: Concepts of Altered Health States, 8th ed. Philadelphia, PA: Lippincott Williams & Wilkins, 2009, p 613.)

Renin is an enzyme produced in the kidney in response to even small decreases in blood pressure. Renin has a direct effect on the kidney, causing increased reabsorption of salt and water. Much of the renin travels to the lung to act enzymatically on angiotensinogen to form angiotensin I. In the presence of angiotensin-converting enzyme (ACE) in the lung, angiotensin I is converted to angiotensin II.

A powerful vasoconstrictor, angiotensin II increases arterial resistance quickly and profoundly, providing immediate support for blood pressure and maintaining perfusion in the short term until a longer-term strategy can be implemented. Although angiotensin II has a much more modest effect on venous resistance, it does increase venous resistance and therefore venous return. Angiotensin II also stimulates the adrenal cortex to release aldosterone. Aldosterone then acts on the kidney to increase salt reabsorption in the distal tubule, and this salt increases water reabsorption in the kidney, resulting in increased circulating volume. Increased circulating volume is the longer-term strategy. The renin–angiotensin–aldosterone system initiates a process that assumes any decrease in blood pressure is a volume loss (eg, hemorrhage), and the long-term strategy is to replace that loss.[7,8]

## Pathophysiology of Heart Failure

Heart failure has many causes (Box 20-3). The physiologic principles discussed in the previous section form the basis for understanding the patient's signs, symptoms, responses, and compensation for the disease process as well as the basis for management strategies.

## Cardiomyopathy

The distinguishing pathophysiologic factor in heart failure is a cardiomyopathy, but cardiomyopathy is not synonymous

---

**BOX 20-3** | **Causes of Heart Failure**

**Impaired Cardiac Function**
Myocardial disease
- Cardiomyopathies
- Myocarditis
- Coronary insufficiency
- Myocardial infarction
Valvular heart disease
- Stenotic valvular disease
- Regurgitant valvular disease
Congenital heart defects
Constrictive pericarditis

**Excess Work Demands**
Increased pressure work
- Systemic hypertension
- Pulmonary hypertension
- Coarctation of the aorta
Increased volume work
- Arteriovenous shunt
- Excessive administration of intravenous fluids
Increase perfusion work
- Thyrotoxicosis
- Anemia

Adapted from Grossman SG, Porth CM: Porth's Pathophysiology: Concepts of Altered Health States, 7th ed. Philadelphia, PA: Wolters Kluwer Health/Lippincott Williams & Wilkins, 2005.

---

with heart failure.[2] Literally, cardiomyopathy is a progressive pathologic process in the heart muscle. Cardiomyopathy may be congenital or acquired. Hypertrophic, nonobstructive cardiomyopathy and dilated cardiomyopathy are the two most common forms. Hypertrophic cardiomyopathy is an increase in muscle mass in the ventricle resulting in a measurable increase in the thickness of the ventricular wall. Hypertrophy is a response to a prolonged increase in resistance (afterload). Dilated cardiomyopathy is an increase in the size of the ventricular chamber without an increase in wall size, and is a response to decreased contractility. For a more detailed discussion of cardiomyopathies, see Chapter 19; see also Figure 20-2.

## Dysrhythmia

Heart failure is commonly associated with dysrhythmias, both atrial and ventricular. The structural and metabolic changes

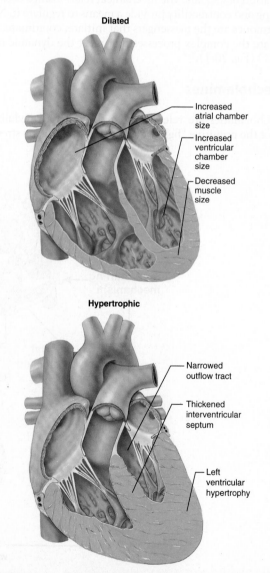

**Dilated**

— Increased atrial chamber size

— Increased ventricular chamber size

— Decreased muscle size

**Hypertrophic**

— Narrowed outflow tract

— Thickened interventricular septum

— Left ventricular hypertrophy

**FIGURE 20-2** Patterns of ventricular hypertrophy and remodeling in dilated and hypertrophic cardiomyopathy. (Anatomical Chart Company: Atlas of Pathophysiology. Springhouse, PA: Springhouse, 2010, p 45.)

that occur in heart failure frequently lead to dysrhythmia, and the dysrhythmia itself may lead to heart failure.

### Atrial Dysrhythmias

Atrial tachycardias may cause heart failure in two ways. First, the shortened diastole leads to decreased filling that may cause or aggravate diastolic dysfunction, resulting in decreased CO and the symptoms of heart failure. When the tachycardia is caused by atrial fibrillation, the loss of atrial kick increases the impact of the atrial dysrhythmia on left ventricular dysfunction.

Patients with heart failure are more likely to develop atrial fibrillation as compared to the general population.[10] The incidence of both atrial fibrillation and heart failure increases with age, increasing the likelihood that patients with heart failure will also have atrial fibrillation at some time. Atrial fibrillation is an independent risk factor for the development of heart failure.[11]

Atrial fibrillation is associated with a functional decline in those with heart failure. Therapy for atrial fibrillation includes the prevention of stroke through the use of anticoagulants. The patient who develops heart failure as a consequence of atrial fibrillation should be converted to sinus rhythm through the use of medication or cardioversion.[2] For the patient who has heart failure and then develops atrial fibrillation, the data suggest there is no benefit to a rhythm control (conversion to sinus rhythm) versus a rate control (controlling the heart rate) strategy.[12] The antiarrhythmics prescribed to treat atrial fibrillation in patients with heart failure are amiodarone, sotalol, and dofetilide. Dofetilide is started when the patient is hospitalized to closely monitor the QT interval for prolongation.[13]

### Ventricular Dysrhythmias

Ventricular dysrhythmias—in particular, premature ventricular beats and nonsustained ventricular tachycardia (NSVT)—are common in patients with dilated cardiomyopathy, whether ischemic or nonischemic. Before the common use of implantable cardioverter–defibrillators (ICDs), sudden death from ventricular dysrhythmia or bradycardia accounted for 30% to 40% of deaths associated with heart failure.[14,15] Since the widespread use of ICDs, the death rate from sudden cardiac death has decreased to 12.7%.[13] The presence of premature ventricular beats or even NSVT has not been shown to reliably predict risk for sudden death for any particular patient. However, the presence of these dysrhythmias does appear to reliably reflect a globally impaired myocardium.

Several mechanisms play a role in the development of ventricular dysrhythmias. The low EF leads to stretch of the myocardial fibers, thus increasing excitability. Excitability is also affected by the presence of increased catecholamines, increased sympathetic tone, and, on occasion, antiarrhythmic drugs. Activation of the renin–angiotensin–aldosterone system contributes to the overall environment that generates dysrhythmia. Ischemia leads to failure of the sodium–potassium pump, and the loss of potassium from the cell increases the risk for premature ventricular beats. Scar tissue from previous infarctions and surgery can stimulate dysrhythmia. Electrolyte shifts involving potassium, calcium, and magnesium are often associated with prolonged or aggressive

diuretic use. Lung disease such as emphysema or chronic bronchitis is often comorbid with heart failure, and the lung disease may lead to hypoxemia, which contributes to the genesis of ventricular dysrhythmias. The traditional sources of ventricular dysrhythmia that occur in patients without heart failure, such as reentry, enhanced automaticity, and delayed after-potentials, may also be involved.

## Acute Decompensated Heart Failure

Chronic disease is characterized by variable periods of relative stability or compensation interrupted by periods of exacerbation or decompensation. Patients with chronic heart failure may live from day to day with no symptoms of heart failure or well-controlled symptoms. However, chronic heart failure may become acutely worse, resulting in an increase in symptoms and limitations associated with left ventricular dysfunction. Management for the hospitalized patient with ADHF is guided by the 2013 American College of Cardiology Foundation/American Heart Association Guideline for the Management of Heart Failure.[2]

Several factors may lead to an exacerbation of ADHF, including but not limited to myocardial ischemia, nonadherence to medial therapy, poorly controlled hypertension, arrhythmias, pulmonary emboli, alcohol or illicit drug use, infections such as pneumonia or endocarditis, and valvular abnormalities. Any factor that increases oxygen demand, and therefore demands for increased CO beyond the ability of the ventricle to function (eg, hypertension, tachycardia, anemia, exercise), causes an exacerbation. Similarly, any factor that depresses the function of the already compromised ventricle leads to exacerbation (eg, alcohol, drugs that exert a negative inotropic effect, such as calcium-channel blockers and β-blockers).[16–18] As the ventricle is called on to work harder, it works less efficiently, and the left ventricular end-diastolic pressure increases, leading to increased pulmonary artery pressures. The increased pulmonary artery pressures, in turn, lead to orthopnea, possibly pulmonary edema, elevated venous pressures, liver congestion, lower-extremity edema, and PND. Patients may also present with lower blood pressures, more rapid heart rates, and prerenal azotemia. Potentially, the acute decompensation is reversible if treated quickly and aggressively.

## Assessment of the Patient With Heart Failure

Heart failure has long been defined by the presence of pulmonary edema characterized by bibasilar rales or crackles. At one time, the absence of crackles ruled out heart failure. However, chronic heart failure is a persistent, not episodic, condition, and it rarely includes pulmonary edema and crackles even in early decompensation. History, physical examination, diagnostic procedures, and hemodynamic evaluation all contribute to diagnosing heart failure, perhaps determining its cause, and evaluating the success of therapy.

### History

The symptoms of heart failure are nonspecific (ie, they are common to many disease processes). The health history is used to put the symptoms into a context that may lead to their interpretation as heart failure and not pulmonary disease, deconditioning, or other conditions that produce shortness of breath, DOE, fatigue, and swelling of the lower extremities. History alone does not confirm the diagnosis, but it helps determine follow-up examinations and diagnostic tests that may be appropriate.

### Onset

The basic question is "When did the symptoms start?" The answer to this question helps categorize the condition as acute or chronic. Most patients indicate an acute onset of 2 weeks or fewer if this is their first visit for their symptoms. If they are asked additional questions about their activity tolerance for the past year or so, patients with chronic heart failure note a gradual slowing of activity to match the amount of energy available or to control symptoms. The recent identification of symptoms indicates that the patient is now aware of them or they have become unbearable. Acuity is important because reversible ischemia is a potentially life-threatening etiology that may present acutely. When identified and treated, chronic heart failure can be avoided, and perhaps a patient's life may be saved.

### Duration

Ask the patient whether the symptoms are persistent and independent of activity or come and go with activity, change of position, food ingestion, or other events. The answer to this question helps differentiate between heart failure and other conditions that can cause the same symptoms. Heart failure symptoms typically worsen with activity and improve with rest. Cough and shortness of breath may increase when lying down and improve with sitting up. Hiatal hernia and gastric reflux may produce shortness of breath, chest pain, and cough but typically occur after eating and more often in the evening. Lung disease or sleep apnea may also cause the shortness of breath that occurs at rest or awakens the patient at night.

### Severity

Severity of symptoms is the basis for establishing functional class (see Box 20-1). Severity of symptoms is also an important standard for evaluating the success of therapy. A major goal of therapy is symptomatic improvement or, if possible, elimination of symptoms. The evaluation of severity requires that patients be asked certain questions about their symptoms (Table 20-1).

### Comorbid Diseases

Many patients with heart failure have comorbid disorders that contribute to or aggravate their heart failure. The most common of these diseases are CAD, hypertension, diabetes mellitus, COPD, and chronic renal insufficiency. Worsening of one or more comorbid diseases may lead to an exacerbation of stable chronic heart failure. In the case of CAD, hypertension, and diabetes, heart failure may be the long-term result of complications of these disease processes. Identification and tight control of these comorbid diseases contribute to the control and treatment of the symptoms of heart failure.

### Medications

It is very important to obtain a complete list of the patient's medications and dosages. The list should include prescription and nonprescription medications. In cases of new-onset

**TABLE 20-1    Assessment of Severity of Heart Failure**

| Symptom | Measure(s) | Questions |
|---|---|---|
| Orthopnea | Number of pillows patient sleeps on regularly | "How many pillows do you sleep on at night? If more than one, is it for comfort or because you cannot breathe with one or two?" |
| DOE | Number of blocks patient can walk without stopping to rest or catch breath<br>Number of flights of stairs patient can climb without stopping to rest or catch breath<br>Number of times patient must rest while doing activities of daily living such as toileting or minor housework | "How many blocks and flights of stairs can you walk without stopping to rest or catch your breath?"<br>"Do you stop because you cannot go further or because you want to avoid getting short of breath?"<br>For patients who are limited by peripheral vascular disease or orthopedic problems: "Do you stop because you cannot breathe or because of pain? Which comes first?" |
| PND | Average number of times per night or week | "After you go to bed, do you ever have to sit up suddenly to catch your breath?"<br>"How much time passes before you can breathe normally?"<br>"Do you need to do anything besides sit up to relieve the shortness of breath?" |
| Dizziness or lightheadedness | Presence or absence (of real concern when symptom occurs when the patient is standing and persists or occurs with activity) | "Do you ever become dizzy or lightheaded?"<br>"What are you doing when this occurs?" |
| Chest pain or pressure* | Presence or absence | "Do you have chest pain or pressure?"<br>"Do you become short of breath with the chest pain or pressure?"<br>"Which comes first, the pain or the shortness of breath?"† |

*Chest pain should be fully investigated to determine whether active ischemia is present. This is especially true in patients who are presenting for the first time for evaluation of symptoms of heart failure. Once ischemia has been ruled out, patients may still have chest pain, and it should be evaluated by using these assessment questions.
†Chest pain that comes after shortness of breath is often caused by the heart failure.

heart failure, prescribed medications may contribute to the severity of symptoms. For example, patients who have been treated with a calcium-channel blocker for hypertension and now present with a decreased EF and heart failure may improve when the medication is changed to one that does not depress myocardial function. Patients taking over-the-counter medications, such as nonsteroidal anti-inflammatory drugs (NSAIDs), may present with worsening heart failure and renal function because of the effect of the NSAIDs on renal blood flow. NSAIDs block the effect of prostaglandins, which the body secretes to maintain renal blood flow in the context of decreased CO. Cold medicines with systemic decongestants can lead to increased blood pressure that precipitates worsening symptoms of heart failure.

## Psychosocial Factors

Noncardiac factors may also affect outcomes in patients with heart failure. Because many affected patients are elderly, they may have problems remembering to fill prescriptions or take medications. Financial hardships may force some patients to choose between buying medication and buying food. Patients may depend on friends or family who may be unreliable for transportation. Housekeeping may be difficult or impossible because of fatigue and shortness of breath. Patients living on the second or third floor of buildings without elevators may become isolated and lonely. A meta-analysis found that 36% of the heart failure patients have depressive symptoms and 20% have a major depressive disorder.[19] Depression and heart failure negatively impact clinical outcomes. In patients with established heart failure, there is an increased risk of hospitalization, and depression is an independent risk factor for cardiac mortality independent of typical risks associated with cardiac disease.[20] Ongoing family dysfunction and family members who depend on the patient for care and financial support (eg, grandchildren, dependent adult children, spouses or partners) add a burden to the patient's management. Illiteracy is still prevalent; even patients who can read may not comprehend medication instructions correctly. Some patients may skip diuretic doses when visiting places where they are uncertain about access to bathroom facilities, and they may not remember to take the diuretic when they return home.

Although many of these factors are significant, they may not be obvious until the patient has visited the same health care facility many times. Screening for depression, early case management, and skillful discharge planning depend on recognizing these problems before they lead to repeated hospitalizations and increased mortality.

## Substance Abuse

Alcohol and drug (eg, cocaine) use may contribute to the development and progression of heart failure. If alcohol use is the cause of cardiomyopathy, abstinence may lead to complete reversal. Patients who have substance abuse problems often forget to buy or take medication. They may be homeless, which increases the likelihood that they will not return to the health care facility for regular follow-up.

## Physical Examination

The physical findings in heart failure differ with acute versus chronic heart failure and with systolic versus diastolic dysfunction. When the physiologic changes of left ventricular dysfunction occur over a long period, the body adapts and compensates. Consequently, many of the findings on physical examination are normal, despite moderate to severe disease. However, when the problem occurs acutely, there is no time for compensation or adaptation, and the symptoms and consequences are severe. Patients who have chronic heart failure from systolic dysfunction and who have abnormal findings have them persistently. Patients with diastolic dysfunction may have abnormal findings only during an exacerbation.

One or more of the following findings characterizes acute decompensation. The patient may be volume overloaded by 5 to 50 pounds over dry weight; dry weight is the patient's weight when he or she is euvolemic. Patient self-monitoring is often geared to maintenance of dry weight. In many cases, maintaining dry weight within 1 to 2 pounds can prevent decompensation. A frequent second finding is renal insufficiency characterized by an increase in both blood urea nitrogen (BUN) and creatinine levels, with a ratio of BUN to creatinine of greater than 20 to 1. The third finding is decreased CO manifested by increased DOE and decreased exercise tolerance in general, often described as "fatigue." Patients may also complain of increased orthopnea, PND, or both.

### General Findings

Patients with acute heart failure or acute decompensation of chronic heart failure appear ill; they are often breathing rapidly, looking anxious, and either sitting up straight or leaning forward and resting their arms on a table or their knees. Patients with stable, chronic heart failure may be quite comfortable but may have evidence of cachexia, muscle wasting, and thin skin.

### Vital Signs

Patients with systolic dysfunction may have quite low, but asymptomatic, blood pressures (systolic, 80 to 99 mm Hg; diastolic, 40 to 49 mm Hg). Heart rates may be rapid (90 beats/min or more), or lower at rest. Patients with diastolic dysfunction may or may not be hypertensive.

Serial weights are very important in following fluid status. Daily weights, when performed properly on a calibrated scale, are more accurate estimates of fluid status than intake and output. Daily weights can be used to evaluate fluid status: 1 L of water weighs 1 kg. Overnight fluctuations in weight are always related to water retention or diuresis.

### Neck

Jugular venous pressure (JVP) is an estimate of right heart filling pressures. When either the total-body fluid volume or the right atrial pressure increases, the JVP increases, and the vein dilates. To estimate JVP, first elevate the patient's head to 45 degrees, then identify the internal jugular vein and measure the height of the pulse from the level of the clavicle in centimeters. Do not use the external jugular vein, which often appears distended and prominent in patients with normal volume and pressure. Normal JVP is no more than 3 cm above the sternal angle.

### Lungs

Determine the respiratory rate and observe the depth of respiration as well as the respiratory rhythm. It is not unusual for patients with severe NYHA class IV heart failure to have a Cheyne–Stokes respiratory pattern.[21] The respiratory symptoms may be chronic in those with class IV, stage D heart failure or may represent an acute exacerbation.

Results of chest auscultation may be completely normal. Because patients with increased pulmonary artery pressures have increased lymph drainage over time, fluid does not collect in the alveoli. Rales or crackles are sounds made by air bubbling through water in the alveoli, and if no water is present, the sounds are not audible. When pressures increase suddenly, water is forced into the alveoli by increased hydrostatic pressure. Consequently, in acute heart failure and acute decompensation, in which pulmonary edema is common, bibasilar crackles occur. Unilateral crackles or nondependent crackles are indicative of a pulmonary process, not heart failure. Pulmonary edema can cause wheezing that may be difficult to distinguish from reactive airway disease, such as asthma.

## Heart

Progressions from left-sided heart failure to left-sided and right-sided heart failure or chronic elevations of pulmonary artery pressure often result in a visible, palpable right ventricular or pulmonary artery pulsation at the left sternal border. The point of maximal impulse may be extremely displaced. In advanced heart failure, the maximal impulse may be inferiorly or laterally displaced in the posterior axillary line and at the fifth or sixth intercostal space.

Cardiac auscultation is an important step in the physical examination of a patient with heart failure. (See Fig. 17-6 for a review of areas of auscultation.) The first ($S_1$) and second ($S_2$) heart sounds are expected. The sudden appearance of a third heart sound ($S_3$) is a warning of impending or worsening heart failure. In chronic heart failure, $S_3$ is a common and chronic finding. A fourth heart sound ($S_4$) is common in patients with long-standing hypertension and is not considered ominous. However, in severe heart failure, all four heart sounds may be heard; this is known as a summation gallop.

When valvular disease is the cause of heart failure, a heart murmur associated with the diseased valve is heard. In patients with dilated cardiomyopathy, a mitral regurgitation murmur is commonly heard. This holosystolic murmur is best heard at the left sternal border or, in patients with very large hearts, at the apex. The mitral valve is usually structurally intact. The dilation of the left ventricle in chronic heart failure dilates the mitral annulus and prevents the close approximation of the valve leaflets. Consequently, blood regurgitates back across the mitral valve into the left atrium with each systole.

When a mitral regurgitation murmur develops acutely, as when there is damage to the papillary muscles that open and close the mitral valve, severe acute heart failure results. The sudden appearance of a mitral regurgitation murmur in a patient with MI is a warning of impending heart failure. The disappearance of this murmur in a patient with severe systolic dysfunction suggests a worsening of the heart failure: the ventricle cannot pump enough to generate the turbulence necessary to make the sound of the murmur.

Tricuspid regurgitation develops in patients with right-sided heart failure alone, and in patients with left-sided heart failure for the same reasons as mitral regurgitation. This murmur is also a holosystolic murmur, and is heard at the right sternal border. It may increase with inspiration. When both mitral regurgitation and tricuspid regurgitation murmurs are present, it may be impossible to distinguish between them.

## Abdomen

Palpate and percuss the abdomen to identify any ascites and the lower liver edge. High right atrial pressures that are translated into high venous pressures characterize right-sided heart failure, and the liver, which becomes a reservoir for the increased venous volume, increases in size (hepatomegaly) when congested. Once the liver becomes engorged, pressure increases in the portal vein and in the capillaries of the intestines. When the lymphatic system can no longer drain sufficient fluid to relieve the pressure, ascites develops. Ascites is the transudation or third spacing of fluid, and sometimes protein, into the abdominal cavity. In the absence of hepatomegaly and ascites, a congested liver may conceal significant fluid. Eliciting hepatojugular reflux may identify this concealed fluid. To assess hepatojugular reflux, observe the internal jugular vein while pressing on the liver. If the height of the pulse increases or the vein engorges, hepatojugular reflux is positive.

## Extremities

Inspect the lower extremities for edema. The edema associated with heart failure is bilateral, dependent, and pitting. Unilateral or nonpitting edema is not related specifically to heart failure, and other causes, such as arterial insufficiency, myxedema, or lymphedema, should be suspected.

In the ambulatory patient, press the skin over the tibia to assess the edema. Pitting here is referred to as pretibial edema. The edema is usually graduated and worse in the ankles than at the calf, and is greater than at the thigh if the edema is present that high. In patients who are confined to bed, the edema is dependent posteriorly, and pretibial edema may be absent even in frank fluid overload. The patient must be assessed for pitting edema on the backs of the legs, the buttocks, and back. Occasionally, an ambulatory patient is so volume overloaded that presacral edema develops. To assess presacral edema and pitting, press the skin over the sacrum against the bone.

There are several schemes for describing the severity of pitting edema. None is superior to another; consistency is the most important factor. It is less important whether a series of pluses on a scale from 0 for no edema to 4+ for severe edema is based on the depth of the pit or the height of the edema on the lower extremity. When in doubt about the scale, a clear description of the depth of the pit and the level of the edema communicates the condition more effectively than a subjective number. A clear description allows for better continuity between clinicians and a better estimate of improvement. See Table 51-6 for the Pitting Edema Scale.

Long-standing venous stasis and the consequent edema produce skin color and texture changes. The skin becomes leathery and discolored, and may be hard to assess. These changes always indicate that the edema is chronic and not acute. Acute increases in the chronic edema may also be hard to assess. Pressing the skin firmly to the side of the tibia

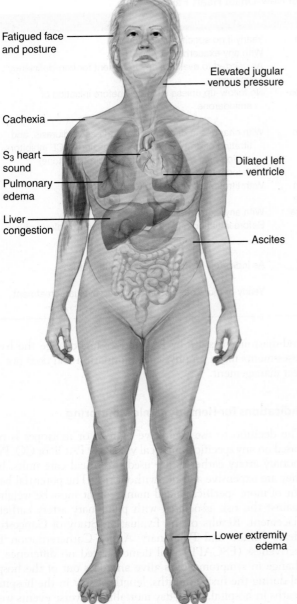

Fatigued face
and posture

Cachexia

S₃ heart
sound

Pulmonary
edema

Liver
congestion

Elevated jugular
venous pressure

Dilated left
ventricle

Ascites

Lower extremity
edema

**FIGURE 20-3**    Physical examination findings for the person with ACC/AHA class D chronic heart failure.

instead of directly over it may be of some help. Figure 20-3 shows the physical assessment findings of a patient with ACC/AHA class D chronic heart failure.

## Laboratory Studies

Laboratory studies are used to rule out some reversible causes of systolic dysfunction and to monitor the effects of management strategies. On initial evaluation of a patient presenting with new-onset heart failure, a battery of baseline laboratory studies is ordered (Table 20-2).

Patients receiving anticoagulation therapy with warfarin are also monitored regularly, using the international normalized ratio to adjust the dose. Before the initiation of amiodarone, thyroid and liver function tests are performed to obtain

baseline values, along with pulmonary function tests that include DLCO (diffusion capacity). These tests are repeated at least yearly and when any complications occur.

Natriuretic peptides (B-type natriuretic peptides, or BNPs, and N-terminal pro BNPs) are naturally occurring substances synthesized and released by the cardiac myocytes when the ventricles are overfilled. As the pulmonary artery occlusion pressure (PAOP) rises and there is more wall stretch on the ventricular wall, a rise in BNP levels occurs. Patients with BNP levels greater than 80 pg/mL show evidence of elevated PAOP, confirming heart failure decompensation as the source of dyspnea.[22–24]

Although the relationship between BNP level and heart failure is clear, the appropriate use of BNP levels in heart failure management is less clear. One important use of BNP levels has been proposed: to distinguish between pulmonary-related and heart failure–related causes of dyspnea in the emergency department.[22] Many patients have both heart failure and lung disease, and the existence of a test that may distinguish between the two conditions as a cause of acute respiratory problems is a real advantage for individualizing and targeting treatment. Serial BNP measurement has been proposed as a marker for the adequacy of treatment in chronic heart failure management and for establishment of the prognosis and severity of chronic heart failure.[25]

## Diagnostic Studies

Diagnostic studies are used to establish baseline values, identify potentially reversible etiologies, evaluate the effectiveness of treatment, and assess changes in condition. Several invasive and noninvasive tests are performed routinely when heart failure is suspected. Some tests are performed initially, when the symptoms of heart failure are first identified; some on a regular basis; and others only if indicated.

### Electrocardiography

The electrocardiogram (ECG) is used to assess heart rate and rhythm; it is also useful in diagnosing dysrhythmias, conduction defects, and MI. In addition, an ECG is often used to identify atrial enlargement and ventricular hypertrophy. However, in such cases, an echocardiogram is more helpful because it can quantify these structural changes.

ECGs are useful in identifying atrial fibrillation and ventricular dysrhythmias common in patients with heart failure. Sudden exacerbation of heart failure symptoms often results from new-onset atrial fibrillation, especially when it is associated with a rapid ventricular response. An ECG can also distinguish frequent premature ventricular beats, which are common in acute and chronic heart failure. Episodes of asymptomatic NSVT often occur in patients who are monitored in ICUs, in telemetry units, or with Holter monitors. These asymptomatic dysrhythmias are usually not treated, and their prognostic importance is unclear. In contrast, symptomatic ventricular tachycardia, even if it is nonsustained, requires evaluation and usually results in placement of an ICD.

Conduction defects are also common in patients with heart failure. A left bundle branch block is the most common conduction defect in patients with systolic dysfunction, and may make interpretation of the ECG very difficult. New

**TABLE 20-2** Laboratory Studies Used in the Baseline Evaluation of New-Onset Heart Failure

| Laboratory Study | Significance | When Performed |
| --- | --- | --- |
| Complete blood count | Used to identify any anemia or infection | Yearly if no specific indication<br>With any exacerbation |
| Iron studies | Anemia workup<br>Used to rule out hemochromatosis | As needed to evaluate any treatment for iron-deficiency anemia |
| Thyroid function tests (thyroid-stimulating hormone and free thyroxine [T4]) | Used to rule out hyperthyroidism or hypothyroidism as a cause of heart failure | No follow-up unless indicated before initiation of amiodarone |
| Electrolytes | Used to assess the effects of diuresis, in particular on potassium level<br>Hyponatremia is common | With changes in diuretic dose, aggressive diuresis, and titration of drugs that affect potassium (ACE inhibitors, angiotensin receptor blockers, spironolactone) |
| BUN and creatinine levels | Used to assess renal function; BUN/creatinine ratio distinguishes between prerenal azotemia and kidney disease | With increased edema or an exacerbation<br>With titration of ACE inhibitors |
| Liver function tests, especially albumin, bilirubin, and alkaline phosphatase (AP) | Bilirubin and AP are often elevated in liver congestion caused by heart failure<br>Low albumin makes peripheral edema more difficult to reduce | With any exacerbation<br>Before initiation of lipid-lowering drugs or amiodarone |
| HIV | Used to rule out HIV/AIDS as etiologic factor | As indicated by history or change in status |
| Lipid panel | Used to assess risk for CAD and nutritional status | Yearly or more often as indicated to evaluate treatment |

anterior ischemia or infarct may be impossible to identify because of this block. Bundle branch blocks and AV blocks require a 12-lead ECG for diagnosis.

ECGs are also useful in diagnosing ischemia, MI, and prior MI that may explain new-onset heart failure. For patients who do not present with typical chest pain (such as those with diabetes mellitus and women), the ECG may show a prior MI that was never diagnosed. New-onset heart failure may be the first indication of MI. An ECG is completed as part of the workup for new-onset heart failure and then repeated as necessary for any new symptoms that may reflect new ischemia or a rhythm change. In addition, ECGs are performed on inpatients who experience chest pain to rule out ischemia as the source of the pain. For further discussion of the 12-lead ECG, see Chapter 21.

Other commonly used diagnostic tests include echocardiogram, echocardiogram with Doppler ultrasonography, transesophageal echocardiogram, radionuclide ventriculogram or multigated acquisition scan, chest radiography, and exercise testing. These diagnostic tests are discussed in more detail in Chapter 17.

## Hemodynamics

The basics of hemodynamic monitoring are discussed in Chapter 17. The application of hemodynamic monitoring in the assessment and management of acute heart failure and acute decompensation of chronic heart failure is discussed here. It may be necessary to obtain more sensitive information about fluid status, cardiac function, and symptom causation to guide evaluation and therapy. For most patients with acute heart failure or acute decompensation of chronic heart failure, the problem is obvious based on history and physical examination. The problem is a combination of decreased CO and increased left ventricular end-diastolic pressure related to volume overload added to poor contractility. Precise quantification of the low CO or the estimation of left ventricular

end-diastolic pressure by PAOP does not change the basic assessments made on physical examination and does not affect management.

### Indications for Hemodynamic Monitoring

The decision to use aggressive diuresis or inotropes is not based on any specific numerical values for PAOP or CO. Pulmonary artery catheters are used in critical care units, but they are expensive and not without risk. The potential benefit of more specific, guided management must be weighed against the risk associated with pulmonary artery catheter placement. Results of the Evaluation Study of Congestive Heart Failure and Pulmonary Artery Catheterization Effectiveness (ESCAPE) trial demonstrated no difference in change in symptoms, days alive and days out of the hospital during the first 6 months, length of stay in the hospital, deaths in hospital, or 30-day mortality. Adverse events were more common with pulmonary artery catheters.[26]

Three types of patients with heart failure may have indications for hemodynamic monitoring in the management of their condition. The first type is the patient who is empirically treated with inotropes and intravenous (IV) diuretics but has not responded appropriately by diuresis and improved symptoms. The second type of patient has both COPD and heart failure; at times, only pulmonary artery pressure measurements can differentiate the source of the current decompensation in such patients. BNP testing in this scenario may rule out heart failure when the result is less than 80 pg/mL, but elevations can be caused by either left-sided heart failure or right-sided heart failure associated with pulmonary embolus or exacerbation of COPD. The third type of patient continues to have congestion associated with peripheral edema or ascites, and has renal function values indicating worsening azotemia. This patient may benefit from a clearer definition of fluid balance; without the aid of a pulmonary artery catheter, it may be impossible to determine fluid status.

In summary, a pulmonary artery catheter is indicated in the following situations:

- The patient does not respond to empirical therapy for heart failure.
- Differentiation between pulmonary and cardiac causes of respiratory distress is necessary.
- Complex fluid status needs to be evaluated.

These categories are not mutually exclusive, and there is much overlap. They are discussed separately here, for clarity.

**INADEQUATE RESPONSE TO EMPIRICAL THERAPY FOR HEART FAILURE.** Respiratory distress, volume overload, and renal insufficiency are common indicators of acute heart failure or acute decompensation of chronic heart failure. Typically, the patient needs inotropic support and IV diuresis to resolve the problem. These therapies are usually started empirically, and the patient's improvement is monitored as a basis for titration of dose. In most patients, improvement follows rapidly, and after 2 to 3 days of therapy, the inotrope is gradually discontinued, and the patient is restarted on oral therapy in preparation for discharge.

**CARDIAC VERSUS PULMONARY CAUSE OF RESPIRATORY DISTRESS.** In the minority of patients who do not respond to empiric therapy, a pulmonary artery catheter may be helpful in identifying any additional factors that have contributed to the persistence of symptoms, especially cardiac and pulmonary causes. It may be particularly difficult to differentiate the cause of worsening DOE, orthopnea, and PND in patients with both pulmonary disease and known heart failure. In COPD and in exacerbations of heart failure, results of history and physical examination are often identical. Pulmonary artery pressures, PAOP, and CO or cardiac index can be very useful in distinguishing COPD from acute heart failure and therefore targeting therapy decisions based on the correct diagnosis. In patients with a predominantly pulmonary cause of their respiratory symptoms, pulmonary artery systolic and diastolic pressures are elevated, but PAOP, CO, and cardiac index are normal. In patients with a primarily cardiac cause, pulmonary artery systolic and diastolic pressures are also elevated, but the PAOP is elevated and the CO or cardiac index is decreased.

**COMPLEX FLUID STATUS.** Patients may respond initially to IV diuresis with or without inotropes. After this initial diuresis, they begin to have decreased urine output associated with increasing BUN and creatinine levels in the presence of persistent peripheral edema. These patients are typically referred to as "intravascularly dry."

The strategy for dealing with this problem is unclear. Insertion of a pulmonary artery catheter may determine whether high pulmonary artery pressures are the cause, and whether those pulmonary artery pressures are elevated because of an elevated left ventricular end-diastolic pressure. The readings can then be evaluated in light of the patient's serum albumin level and any comorbid diseases, such as primary liver failure, sepsis, or vascular insufficiency. Newer hypotheses about the relationship between cardiorenal syndrome and renal venous congestion may better explain this phenomenon. This syndrome involves passive congestion of the kidneys and increased intra-abdominal pressure that further serves to reduce cardiac and renal function.[27,28]

## Pulse Oximetry

Pulse oximetry is a frequently used monitoring device in patients with heart failure. Unfortunately, routine intermittent monitoring is of little value. At best, it gives irrelevant information, and at worst, it enables a false sense of security about the patient's oxygen delivery status (Box 20-4). The results of pulse oximetry should be normal. Decreased oxygen saturation is usually not the result of heart failure unless the patient has severe pulmonary edema.

A low pulse oximetry reading in patients with heart failure and no pulmonary edema suggests that pulmonary disease is complicating the heart failure. Hypoxemia rarely occurs in the absence of comorbid pulmonary disease. Even patients with Cheyne–Stokes respirations associated with an acute decompensation may have blood oxygen saturations greater than 95%. The pulse oximetry reading is only half of the information needed to assess oxygenation accurately. The oxygen saturation is meaningless unless the Hgb level is known as well. Even normal arterial oxygen content in a patient with decreased CO and no reserve may lead to tissue hypoxia. If the arterial oxygen content is decreased, as it is in patients with low Hgb (patients are rarely transfused unless the Hgb is less than 10 g/dL), CO may not be able to increase enough to compensate in the patient with heart failure. Pulse oximetry may be of some value when used continuously in an ICU for patients with acute pulmonary edema. Particularly in patients with ischemic cardiomyopathy and MI, continuous monitoring may alert the nursing staff to impending ischemia or adverse effects of analgesia or conscious sedation.

## Management of Acute Decompensation of Heart Failure

Acute decompensation of heart failure is an acute worsening of chronic heart failure that may occur for many reasons. Left ventricular function may deteriorate; heart failure is a progressive disease. If function deteriorates beyond the patient's ability to compensate, then symptoms worsen. Although heart function may be stable, the development of other problems, such as pneumonia, anemia, dysrhythmia, hypertension, or trauma, may tax the ability of the compromised heart to increase CO to meet the increased metabolic demand. Dietary lapses, medication disruption, or lack of vigilance on the part of the patient regarding progressive water weight gain may all contribute to decompensation. If possible, it is important to identify the cause of a decompensation so that a long-term strategy to control the underlying problem can be implemented. However, in the intervening period, an acute decompensation must be treated aggressively, often to save the life of the patient.

The main concerns for the care of patients with acute decompensation of chronic heart failure are the same as in any patient with any life-threatening condition. They start with the basic priorities: airway, breathing, and circulation. Once these issues are addressed, etiologic factors and long-term strategies can become the focus of care.

**BOX 20-4** **Pulse Oximetry**

Pulse oximetry ($SpO_2$) estimates $SaO_2$ or the percentage of Hgb saturated with oxygen. Oxygen saturation and Hgb are the two major components of arterial oxygen content ($CaO_2$). The dissolved oxygen in the arterial blood ($PaO_2$) contributes only a tiny portion of the arterial oxygen content. Arterial oxygen content multiplied by CO equals tissue oxygen delivery ($DO_2$). If arterial oxygen content is decreased for any reason, CO (mostly heart rate) increases to compensate. This is why patients with anemia or hypoxemia are tachycardic. As long as CO can increase to compensate for a decreased $CaO_2$, tissues have sufficient oxygen to carry out their functions and the patient is asymptomatic. When a patient cannot increase CO, as in heart failure, then even modest decreases in $CaO_2$ produce symptoms and increase the likelihood of an exacerbation or death.

$$(SaO_2 \times Hgb \times 1.34) + (PaO_2 \times 0.0031) = CaO_2$$

$$CaO_2 \times CO \times 10 = DO_2$$

Most nurses would be concerned about a patient with a pulse oximetry reading of 85%, but not one with 98%. The following examples demonstrate that the patient with normal Hgb and a pulse oximetry reading of 85% has more oxygen in the blood and a better oxygen delivery than a person with a 98% saturation and a Hgb of 10. The patients in all these examples have a normal CO at rest but cannot increase CO in response to decreasing arterial oxygen content.

A patient with normal blood gases and a 5-L CO would have a calculated oxygen delivery of 1,000 mL $O_2$/min:

$$(SaO_2 \times Hgb \times 1.34) + (PaO_2 \times 0.0031) = CaO_2$$

$$(0.98 \times 15 \times 1.34) + (90 \times 0.0031) =$$

$$19.7 + 0.3 = 20 \text{ mL } O_2/\text{min}$$

$$CaO_2 \times CO \times 10 = DO_2$$

$$20 \text{ mL } O_2/\text{min} \times 5,000 \text{ mL} \times 10 = 1,000 \text{ mL } O_2/\text{min}$$

Suppose a patient has a low $SaO_2$ and normal Hgb:

$$(SaO_2 \times Hgb \times 1.34) + (PaO_2 \times 0.0031) = CaO_2$$

$$(0.85 \times 15 \times 1.34) + (60 \times 0.0031) =$$

$$17.085 + 0.186 = 17.271 \text{ mL } O_2/\text{min}$$

$$CaO_2 \times CO \times 10 = DO_2$$

$$17.271 \text{ mL } O_2/\text{min} \times 5,000 \text{ mL} \times 10 = 863.55 \text{ mL } O_2/\text{min}$$

Suppose a patient has a normal $SaO_2$ and low Hgb:

$$(SaO_2 \times Hgb \times 1.34) + (PaO_2 \times 0.0031) = CaO_2$$

$$(0.98 \times 10 \times 1.34) + (98 \times 0.0031) =$$

$$13.132 + 0.3 = 13.44 \text{ mL } O_2/\text{min}$$

$$CaO_2 \times CO \times 10 = DO_2$$

$$13.44 \text{ mL } O_2/\text{min} \times 5,000 \text{ mL} \times 10 = 672 \text{ mL } O_2/\text{min}$$

Suppose a patient has low $SaO_2$ and low Hgb:

$$(SaO_2 \times Hgb \times 1.34) + (PaO_2 \times 0.0031) = CaO_2$$

$$(0.85 \times 10 \times 1.34) + (60 \times 0.0031) =$$

$$11.39 + 0.186 = 11.58 \text{ mL } O_2/\text{min}$$

$$CaO_2 \times CO \times 10 = DO_2$$

$$11.58 \text{ mL } O_2/\text{min} \times 5,000 \text{ mL} \times 10 = 579 \text{ mL } O_2/\text{min}$$

## Airway and Breathing

For most patients with acute symptoms of heart failure, airway patency is not a problem. Likewise, oxygenation is not usually compromised unless pulmonary edema is severe or a comorbid pulmonary disease is present. However, when the acute onset of heart failure or the acute exacerbation is accompanied by profound pulmonary edema, such as in MI or flash pulmonary edema, the airway may become compromised. With severe pulmonary edema, surfactant may be washed out of the alveoli, decreasing lung compliance and making ventilation difficult. In patients who also have COPD or restrictive lung disease, the compromise in compliance may make normal minute ventilation difficult if not impossible. An indication that normal minute ventilation is not being maintained is increased partial pressure of arterial carbon dioxide ($PaCO_2$) associated with increased work of breathing and respiratory acidosis. For example, a patient may initially do well but tire as the increased work of ventilating wet lungs is prolonged.

### Supplemental Oxygen and Assisted Ventilation

Treatment for respiratory distress and hypoxia should proceed in a stepwise fashion. First, the patient should be placed in an upright position to support ventilation. Supplemental oxygen should be administered to those patients who appear hypoxic, with the goal of maintaining oxygen saturations greater than 90%. Initial therapy may require a nonrebreather facemask with high-flow oxygen. If respiratory distress, hypoxia, or respiratory acidosis persists, noninvasive positive pressure ventilation (NPPV) may be used provided there are no contraindications to this therapy. This approach to patients with pulmonary edema has been shown to decrease dyspnea, hypercapnia, and acidosis. Those who fail NPPV or who have contraindications to NPPV should be intubated for mechanical ventilation.[29] The usual indications for endotracheal intubation in patients with heart failure are the same as for patients in respiratory distress. Patients who have pulmonary edema and a persistent oxygen saturation level of less than 90% on 100% oxygen or on NPPV should be intubated and supported until they can obtain oxygen on their own. If the increased work of breathing is leading to fatigue of the respiratory muscles, and the $PaCO_2$ is rising in association with a falling pH, intubation is indicated even if the patient is able to breathe unaided. The intubation may not be required for more than 12 to 24 hours, but it may be better to protect the airway than to try to intubate a patient after respiratory arrest. See Chapter 25 for more information about the care of the patient receiving mechanical ventilation.

## Diuresis

Once the airway is protected, attention is directed toward reducing pulmonary edema. In most cases, aggressive IV diuresis is indicated. The presence of bilateral crackles on physical examination is not always an indication of total-body volume excess. Evaluation of crackles, along with peripheral edema, liver congestion or ascites, and renal function, allows for a better assessment of fluid status than evaluation of crackles alone. If the patient has volume overload, IV diuretics are administered to facilitate the rapid excretion of excess fluid, and the patient quickly feels better.

In those who are naive to loop diuretics, aggressive diuresis is usually started with IV furosemide 40 mg, torsemide 10 to 20 mg, or bumetanide 1 mg. In patients treated with oral loop diuretics chronically, the recommended IV dose is equal to or 2.5 times their maintenance dose, adjusted according to their urinary output.[30] An adequate diuretic response is about 1 L of urine within 2 hours of the IV dose. If urine output is less than 1 L, the dose is doubled until a maximum dose is reached (for furosemide, a 400 mg single dose) or until the 1 L urine output goal is met. If the IV loop diuretic is not sufficient to produce this level of diuresis, a thiazide, such as metolazone, may be given orally along with the loop diuretic.[31] The desired weight loss is 1 to 2 kg/d until the patient's dry weight is reached. Initial weight loss may be greater. Careful monitoring of potassium and magnesium is indicated. Hypokalemia and hypomagnesemia may result in the development of dysrhythmias. If the creatinine level begins to rise in response to the diuresis, the ACE inhibitor should be held until after the diuresis is complete.[32]

## Circulation

Once the airway is protected and breathing is adequate to maintain oxygen and carbon dioxide levels, the circulation of blood to perfuse cells and supply oxygen for cellular function becomes the priority. Two indicators are used to determine the adequacy of perfusion. The first indicator is function of organ systems. Inadequate perfusion affects the brain, leading to confusion and change in level of consciousness; the kidneys, leading to increased BUN and creatinine levels; and the gastrointestinal system, leading to ileus and liver failure. The second indicator is metabolic acidosis. If perfusion is severely inadequate or prolonged past the capacity of the body to buffer the lactic acid produced, the level of sodium bicarbonate decreases, as does the pH, producing metabolic acidosis. Metabolic acidosis is a system-wide measure of inadequate oxygen to meet the metabolic demands of tissues.

Hypotension alone is not sufficient to diagnose hypoperfusion in patients with heart failure because many such patients are chronically hypotensive. Hypotension associated with hypoperfusion should be treated in a way that increases flow without increasing afterload. The problem is decreased CO caused by decreased contractility. Whether the patient has acute heart failure associated with cardiogenic shock or acute decompensation of chronic heart failure, the goal of treatment should be to increase CO. Interventions that increase CO include optimizing preload, increasing

contractility, initiating vasodilation, and optimizing heart rate and rhythm.

The normal physiologic response to decreased CO is vasoconstriction and increased afterload. In patients with heart failure, afterload may be increased without a dramatic increase in blood pressure, and it is not safe to assume that a low blood pressure means a decreased afterload. Decreasing afterload increases stroke volume, and even in patients with low blood pressures, the increase in stroke volume and perfusion more than compensates for the low blood pressure.

One system for classifying patient symptoms and severity of congestion was developed by Nohria et al.[33] This 2 × 2 table can be used as a foundation for guiding therapy. Figure 20-4 is a representation of this original work.

## Optimizing Hemodynamics

One way to increase CO is to optimize preload. If a patient is dehydrated or has fluid overload, contractility is compromised. Both the "warm and wet" and "cold and wet" categories benefit from diuresis. The "cold and wet" category may be impossible to diurese without inodilator or mechanical support. The "cold and dry" category usually requires careful rehydration.[33,34]

Decreased preload is usually related to iatrogenic overdiuresis. However, patients who are on stable doses of diuretics may become dehydrated if they become hyperglycemic, or experience vomiting and diarrhea while continuing to take the prescribed diuretic dose. Careful fluid repletion usually corrects this problem and improves CO. The symptomatic hypotension and increased BUN and creatinine that are the hallmarks of decreased preload should quickly return to baseline levels.

More commonly, increased preload or congestion is a problem: patients are total-body volume overloaded. The combination of fluid overload and decreased contractility

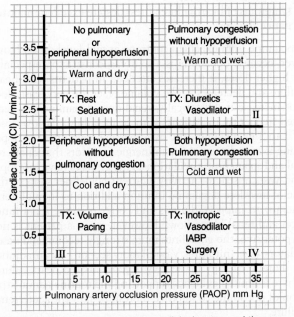

**FIGURE 20-4**  Forrester subsets: clinical states and therapy. IAPV, intra-aortic balloon pumping. (Woods SL, Froelicher S, Motzer SA, et al: Cardiac Nursing, 6th ed. Philadelphia, PA: Lippincott Williams & Wilkins, 2009, p 584.)

leads to cardiopulmonary congestion with increased pulmonary artery pressures and overfilling of the heart. When the heart is overfilled, it becomes stiff and does not empty or fill well. The result is compromised stroke volume and sometimes localized ischemia. The ischemia further worsens contractility. Patients may present with classic angina even if they have no documented CAD. Diuresis with IV loop diuretics often restores the pressure–volume dynamics that optimize stroke volume. For patients who do not respond to diuresis, increasing contractility may decrease preload.

Persistent pulmonary artery pressure elevations lead to jugular venous congestion, liver congestion, ascites, and lower-extremity edema. Newer theories of cardiorenal syndromes suggest that this congestion extends to the renal venous system, raising efferent pressures sufficiently to impair afferent flow and decreasing glomerular filtration rate (GFR). The decreased GFR leads to the increase in BUN, creatinine, and BUN/creatinine ratio, resulting in poor response to diuresis and persistent symptoms despite an adequate CO at rest.[33,34]

### Increasing Contractility

To increase CO, it may be necessary to increase contractility and decrease afterload. Drugs that directly increase contractility are called inotropes. All inotropes increase myocardial oxygen consumption. To be useful in patients with heart failure, there must be greater improvement in oxygen delivery than in oxygen consumption. For this reason, inotropes such as epinephrine and isoproterenol are not used.

The following are indications for using inotropes:

- low CO and high PAOP, especially with symptomatic hypotension
- high PAOP with poor response to diuretics in volume-overloaded patients
- severe right-sided heart failure that is the direct result of left ventricular failure
- symptoms of heart failure at rest despite excellent maintenance therapy.

Dopamine is an excellent inotrope at mid-level doses. However, because dopamine is also a vasoconstrictor, especially at higher doses, it increases afterload in patients with heart failure and decreases stroke volume or, at the very least, does not increase it. Historically, renal-dose dopamine has been used frequently in patients with heart failure. At low doses of 1 to 3 mcg/kg/min, the hypothesized main effect of dopamine is stimulation of dopaminergic receptors that dilate renal and splanchnic circulations. Higher doses have inotropic and vasoconstrictor activity. Current guidelines support the use of low-dose dopamine infusion addition to loop diuretic therapy to improve diuresis and better preserve renal function and renal blood flow.[2] However, when a patient is not hypotensive, the guidelines more strongly recommend vasodilators (see Initiating Vasodilation section) as an adjunct to diuretic therapy for acutely decompensated heart failure. There is limited evidence supporting the routine administration of dopamine to improve diuresis or prevent acute renal failure.[2,35]

Drugs called inodilators are used to stimulate β-adrenergic receptors located in the heart and blood vessels to increase contractility and cause vasodilation.[2] The two inodilators most commonly used in ICUs are dobutamine and milrinone. Although these drugs have different pharmacologic mechanisms, they both increase stimulation of β-adrenergic receptors. Because they stimulate β-adrenergic receptors, they are also chronotropic (ie, they increase heart rate), and they must be used carefully and titrated slowly in patients with tachycardia or ventricular dysrhythmia.

The effect of inotropes and inodilators can be measured when a pulmonary artery catheter is in place. As the drugs are titrated to optimum doses, CO increases and the PAOP decreases. Urine output should increase, and BUN and creatinine levels should return to baseline levels. Any organ function that was compromised because of inadequate perfusion should improve.[34]

Some patients require continued support with inotropes beyond their hospitalization owing to insufficient CO. In these patients, inotropes may be used as a bridge to more definitive advanced heart failure therapies, including cardiac transplantation or mechanical circulatory support. For patients who are not candidates for advanced therapies who have end-stage heart failure, inotropes may be offered to palliate symptoms.

### Initiating Vasodilation

Sometimes an inodilator alone is not sufficient to decrease afterload adequately. In patients with cardiogenic shock and patients who have an exacerbation related to hypertensive emergency, the afterload is the primary limiting factor. Decreasing and controlling the blood pressure or decreasing the workload of the damaged myocardium requires immediate treatment, and vasodilation with parenteral medications is necessary to maintain life or limit end-organ damage. Nitroprusside has the most rapid onset with the shortest half-life of any of these medications. It provides rapid, efficient decrease in blood pressure, and the effect is limited to minutes if the medication is stopped because of an exaggerated response. Nitroprusside must be given as a continuous drip and requires reliable monitoring of blood pressure in a setting where emergency resuscitation is available.

Nesiritide, a BNP, has been approved as a vasodilator for treatment of acute decompensation of chronic heart failure.[35-37] In patients with acute heart failure, the ASCEND-HF trial found using nesiritide decreased the severity of dyspnea more rapidly as compared to the use of diuretics alone; however, there was an increased risk of hypotension. No differences were found with respect to the rate of 30-day readmission, mortality, or renal failure.[37] Caution should be exercised in giving this medication to patients with heart failure with preserved ejection fraction as these patients are more volume sensitive.

For intermittent blood pressure control, IV or oral hydralazine provides vasodilation with a decrease in afterload, without any negative inotropic effects. Sublingual nifedipine should never be used to control blood pressure. IV nitroglycerin is valuable in decreasing preload and in treating angina associated with hypertensive emergency, but it is not a good afterload reducer or antihypertensive.[2]

Intra-aortic balloon counterpulsation has proved very successful in reducing afterload in cardiogenic shock by augmenting perfusion pressure and decreasing the workload of the left ventricle. Intra-aortic balloon counterpulsation is often critical to survival in patients with acute MI who suffer acute left ventricular failure. Intra-aortic balloon counterpulsation is used for a limited time for support of the patient until a revascularization procedure can restore oxygenation and function, or until the stunned myocardium has recovered somewhat (in a patient who cannot be revascularized). For a more detailed discussion of intra-aortic balloon counterpulsation, see Chapter 18.

Improvements in design and increased experience with left ventricular assist devices (LVADs), as well as Food and Drug Administration (FDA) approval and Medicare reimbursement, have led to increased use of these devices in treating intractable heart failure. Where once LVADs were only approved as a bridge to transplant for those patients who were already on a waiting list for transplant, they are now used as destination therapy. That is, for patients who are not eligible for or who do not desire transplant, LVADs are now used to treat heart failure. Continuous-flow pumps with improved durability and battery-operated functions allow the patient to go home, to socialize within the community, and to be an active participant in daily life.[38]

### Optimizing Heart Rate and Rhythm

Heart rate and rhythm must be optimized for adequate CO. If the heart rate is too slow, such as in sick sinus syndrome, second- or third-degree AV block, or sinus bradycardia, stroke volume cannot be increased adequately to compensate, resulting in an exacerbation. A heart rate that is too slow or too fast can compromise filling and, in patients with ischemia, can contribute directly to decreased contractility. A fast rate may be a compensation for a decreased stroke volume and usually responds to increasing stroke volume.

The administration of β-adrenergic inotropes may improve heart rate along with the inotropic effect and greatly improve CO. However, the reason for the bradycardia must be identified and treated if the improvement is to be sustained. In many cases, problems with bradycardia result from ischemic damage to the conduction system. In this situation, a permanent pacemaker resolves the problem. If the bradycardia is the result of active ongoing ischemia, a temporary pacemaker along with treatment of the ischemia is indicated. (For a more detailed discussion of cardiac pacemakers, see Chapter 18.) If the bradycardia is the result of medication, the medication should be withheld or discontinued until the indication for the medication can be reevaluated. In this situation, β-blockers may be withheld for 24 to 36 hours but should not be discontinued suddenly. If the bradycardia is the result of β-blockers, temporary pacing may be required while the drug dosage is titrated down.

Sinus tachycardia is a compensatory mechanism for a decrease in stroke volume. Treatment of the tachycardia without increasing stroke volume leads to worsening end-organ perfusion. Sinus tachycardia usually resolves if the underlying decrease in stroke volume is corrected.

When the tachycardia is caused by atrial flutter or atrial fibrillation with rapid ventricular response, the heart rate is the cause of the problem, and it is necessary to control this directly. If the patient is hemodynamically unstable owing to the heart rhythm, arrangements should be made for urgent cardioversion. Otherwise, mechanical methods such as the Valsalva maneuver or carotid massage may be helpful. If medication is required to slow the rhythm, amiodarone is the least dangerous medication to use in systolic dysfunction. Calcium-channel blockers such as verapamil and diltiazem are powerful negative inotropes and may aggravate the low CO state. In many cases, the tachycardia is associated with ischemia or hypertensive crisis, and treatment of the underlying problem also treats the tachycardia.

After the patient is stabilized and CO has been supported by inodilators or vasodilators, any uncontrolled comorbid diseases that may have triggered or worsened the exacerbation must be treated. Anemia with a Hgb level of less than 10 g/dL has usually been treated with transfusion, although this practice has recently been questioned. Transfusion is more clearly indicated in an anemic individual who is ischemic with diffuse CAD who is not a candidate for PCI and who is symptomatic or unstable, although this remains a decision based more on art than on science.[2] Pneumonia or other infection should be diagnosed and treated with the appropriate antibiotics. Blood glucose levels should be controlled using insulin if necessary.

Effective management of chronic heart failure is a key to the prevention of ADHF. Not all ADHF can be prevented. Even when medical regimens are optimal, patients are excellent at self-care, and providers have frequent and regular contact with patients and their caregivers, events outside of their control can lead to decompensation. There should be a concerted effort to adequately reduce congestion, prescribe guideline-based medication regimens, and educate patients and their caregivers before discharge. It is critical, then, to understand guideline-based management of chronic heart failure.

## Management of Chronic Heart Failure

Heart failure is not a true disease but rather a manifestation of disease. Management is based on the same therapeutic principles that apply to any disease. The cause of disease should be identified and then treated. If an etiologic factor cannot be identified or cannot be treated, then its manifestations should be treated. Often, the cause of heart failure is not identified, and even when it is, it may not be reversible. Reversible causes of heart failure have been discussed previously and are not addressed here. Isolated right-sided heart failure (cor pulmonale) also is not addressed here.

Heart failure due to diastolic dysfunction is a complex and poorly defined entity. Few studies of investigational medications or therapies have included patients with diastolic dysfunction, and consequently, there is little in the way of evidence-based therapy. In general, treatment strategies are directed toward controlling blood pressure, fluid volume, and heart rate and rhythm. There is no consensus as to how this control should be established and maintained.

Chronic heart failure secondary to dilated cardiomyopathy and systolic dysfunction is better defined. This section discusses the current evidence-based guidelines for managing chronic heart failure and acute decompensation. When appropriate, management of acute heart failure is distinguished from management of acute decompensation; the use of IV inotropes, diuresis, and afterload reduction is similar in both conditions.

# Pharmacologic Treatment

The ACC and the AHA have published a consensus of evidence-based guidelines for the pharmacologic management of heart failure.[2] These guidelines present the most current recommendations based on available clinical trials for the medical management of heart failure. For example, heart failure in older patients has particular management implications (Box 20-5).

Table 20-3 lists medications used to treat heart failure.

## Angiotensin-Converting Enzyme Inhibitors

ACE inhibitors are the mainstay of standard therapy for heart failure; they represent one third of the classic three-drug combination used (the other drugs are β-blockers and aldosterone blockers). The Studies of Left Ventricular Dysfunction (SOLVD) and Cooperative North Scandinavian Enalapril Survival Study (CONSENSUS) trials demonstrated improvement in mortality as well as symptom management and exercise tolerance with ACE inhibitors in even the sickest of patients with heart failure.[2,39,40] ACE inhibitors are typically started at low doses and titrated to target doses established in clinical trials. Studies have shown that ACE inhibitors were being underprescribed for appropriate patients, and the Assessment of Treatment With Lisinopril and Survival (ATLAS) trial found that being on the medication alone was not sufficient, and that target doses used in the clinical trials were necessary to achieve the optimum results.[39]

**BOX 20-5** *Considerations for the Older Patient*

**Heart Failure**

Most patients with heart failure are elderly, and many fit the category of "old old." They have a variety of limitations and comorbid diseases that may or may not relate to heart failure, as well as a remarkable resiliency and adaptability not found in younger patients. Therefore, it is critical to evaluate their limitations and strengths on an individual basis. It is important to treat the comorbid diseases aggressively according to patients' wishes and to include them in the planning and treatment decisions at all levels.

It is also critical to assess fall risk, activity level, visual acuity, manual dexterity, cognitive ability, and memory when administering, evaluating, or teaching about any medication. For some older patients, the assistance of a family member or friend is critical to successful medication adherence. Financial considerations are also important because many older patients are on Medicare and have a limited drug plan to pay for expensive medications. Having to choose between medication and food is no choice.

The patient taking ACE inhibitors must be closely monitored for side effects, which include angioedema as a result of allergy to the drug; a persistent, dry, nonproductive cough; hyperkalemia; and hypotension. If patients are unable to tolerate ACE inhibitors, drugs such as hydralazine combined with nitrates or angiotensin II receptor blockers may be considered.

**TABLE 20-3** **Medications Used in the Treatment of Heart Failure**

| Drug | Action |
|---|---|
| **Chronic Heart Failure** | |
| ACE inhibitors | Block renin–angiotensin–aldosterone system, decrease symptoms and mortality |
| Lisinopril | Block conversion of angiotensin I to angiotensin II for afterload reduction |
| Enalapril | |
| Captopril | |
| Hydralazine | Pure vasodilator |
| | Used to decrease afterload |
| Nitrates | Decrease preload |
| Isosorbide dinitrate | Relieve angina |
| Isosorbide mononitrate | Decrease orthopnea |
| Digoxin | Oral inotrope |
| | Blocks neurohormonal bombardment of heart |
| Diuretics | Control fluid volume |
| Spironolactone | Blocks effects of aldosterone and protects potassium |
| β-Blockers | Improve symptoms, increase exercise tolerance, decrease hospitalizations and mortality |
| Metoprolol SR | |
| Carvedilol | |
| Bisoprolol | |
| **Acute Heart Failure and Acute Exacerbation of Chronic Heart Failure** | |
| Inodilators | Increase contractility, decrease afterload, and therefore increase CO |
| Dobutamine | Increased forward flow decreases left ventricular end-diastolic pressure |
| Milrinone | |
| Dopamine | May increase renal perfusion and improve diuresis |
| Nitroprusside | Used for afterload reduction and blood pressure control |
| Nesiritide | Used for afterload reduction |
| Hydralazine | Used for afterload reduction and blood pressure control |

## Digoxin

Cardiac glycosides have been used for centuries in the empirical management of heart failure. In 1993, the Prospective Randomized Study of Ventricular Failure and the Efficacy of Digoxin (PROVED) trial and, more recently, the Randomized Assessment of Digoxin on Inhibitors of Angiotensin-Converting Enzyme (RADIANCE) and Digitalis Investigation Group (DIG) trials provided evidence that digoxin is of value in heart failure treatment. Although none of the studies has shown that digoxin affects mortality, they all have consistently shown that digoxin leads to improvement in symptom management and exercise tolerance as well as decreased hospitalizations for heart failure.[2,41]

Digoxin should be given in daily doses of 0.125 mg. Lower doses are used in patients who have renal insufficiency or who also take amiodarone. Digoxin is safe and has few, if any, adverse effects as long as the blood levels remain less than 2.0 ng/mL. No studies have identified a therapeutic level for digoxin in heart failure or guidelines for interpreting drug levels. The traditional therapeutic levels given in studies of atrial fibrillation may be excessively high; lower levels (ie, 1.0 ng/mL) may be equally beneficial and safer.[2]

## Diuretics

Diuretics have become a mainstay of heart failure management. Edema, a common finding in patients with heart failure, is the result of volume expansion in response to neurohormonally mediated salt and water retention. In certain conditions (eg, ascites, pleural effusions), "third spacing" of fluids is a common result of excess volume and increased hydrostatic pressure. Edema worsens when patients are unwilling or unable to reduce sodium in their diets. Patients who have advanced heart failure are frequently malnourished, and may have low serum albumin levels with a consequent decrease in osmotic gradients to pull fluids back into the circulation. Patients who are symptomatic from volume overload feel dramatically better when diuresis re-establishes their dry weight. Drugs such as ACE inhibitors and β-blockers work best in euvolemic patients.

Loop diuretics, such as furosemide, are standard therapy for diuresis in patients with heart failure.[2] Loop diuretics are threshold drugs, and the threshold varies from patient to patient. This means that the appropriate dosage must be determined by the patient's response. In a patient who requires furosemide in oral doses of 200 mg to maintain dry weight, 100 mg twice daily is not sufficient. Doses in excess of 200 mg daily may be necessary. When patients are receiving oral doses of 240 mg or more, yet continue to have edema or have increased edema, diuretic resistance must be considered. Loop diuretics should not be abandoned; however, a brief course of IV diuretic or the addition of a thiazide, such as metolazone, until the edema is controlled may be required. Alternatively, one may consider a continuous infusion of loop diuretics or rotating loop diuretics (for example, changing to torsemide or bumetanide from furosemide).[2,31,32]

The combination of loop and thiazide diuretics works more efficiently than either type of diuretic alone. However, this drug combination should be reserved for refractory edema, and when the edema resolves, an appropriate dose of loop diuretic should be determined and continued.[32] Finally,

should efforts at diuretic therapy fail or in renal failure the patient may require renal replacement therapy.[2]

As heart failure progresses or when decompensations occur, dose adjustments are necessary. Patients should be taught to weigh themselves daily and record their weights. Increases of 2 pounds or more overnight or of 5 pounds or more in a week are water weight, which can be controlled with additional doses of diuretic (1 L [1.06 quarts] of water weighs 1 kg [2.2 pounds]). Some patients can manage their fluid balance with a sliding-scale diuretic, much like patients with diabetes mellitus manage their blood glucose level with sliding-scale insulin.

## Aldosterone Antagonists

Spironolactone is a weak diuretic with potassium-sparing properties. It is not used specifically for its diuretic activity. The 2013 ACCF/AHA guidelines recommend the addition of aldosterone antagonists to patients with an EF of less than 35% and NYHA class II to IV symptoms. Of concern is the addition of another potassium-sparing drug to the regimen of patients who are already taking an ACE inhibitor, which also spares potassium. These patients must have their potassium level and kidney function evaluated within 1 to 2 weeks after initiation and periodically thereafter. It is essential to educate patients about the possible dangers of elevated potassium levels when using spironolactone or eplerenone. Patients who cannot comply with this monitoring should not be prescribed this therapy.[2]

## β-Blockers

Intuitively, β-blockers, with their negative inotropic properties, ought to be the least likely intervention to benefit patients with systolic dysfunction. For many years, the prevailing standard of care specifically excluded β-blockers for patients with ineffective heart pumps. During the past 40 years, both small studies and large, multicenter, international, randomized, placebo-controlled studies challenged this idea. Multiple studies have demonstrated a significant reduction in mortality with β-blocker use in the heart failure population. Other long-term benefits of β-blockers include improved exercise tolerance, better symptom control, fewer hospitalizations, and improved EF.

Short-term use of β-blockers makes heart failure worse. Consequently, β-blockers should be used as a long-term strategy that is begun only when patients are stable using optimum background therapy with ACE inhibitors, digoxin, and diuretics. β-Blockers should not be started when a patient is in the midst of an decompensation. The specific drug used should be started at a very small dose and gradually increased to the target range. Detailed information about the initiation and titration of β-blockers is beyond the scope of this text but is outlined in detail elsewhere.[2,42–44]

Under no circumstances should β-blockers be stopped suddenly. The rebound tachycardia can be fatal, especially in patients with coronary insufficiency. Patients who come into the hospital because of a decompensation of heart failure who are on β-blockers should continue taking the β-blocker. If a temporal relationship exists between titration of the β-blocker dose and the onset of the exacerbation, the dose should be reduced to the last well-tolerated dose. Patients who are taking β-blockers may receive inotropes without discontinuing the β-blocker and may respond well because of the upregulation of β-adrenergic receptors.

### Calcium-Channel Blockers

First-generation calcium-channel blockers, such as diltiazem, verapamil, and nifedipine, should be avoided in patients with systolic dysfunction. These drugs exert a strong negative inotropic effect without the long-term benefits of β-blockers. Second-generation calcium-channel blockers, such as amlodipine or felodipine, have been used in patients with heart failure because they are vasodilators with minimal negative inotropic effects. They are most commonly used to control blood pressure in patients who are on target doses of ACE inhibitors but who continue to have blood pressure levels that exceed the recommendations of the Eighth Report of the Joint National Committee on Detection, Evaluation, and Treatment of High Blood Pressure (JNC8).[45]

### Nitrates/Hydralazine

Nitrates are venodilators, and their primary effect is to decrease preload. They are used acutely in heart failure to help alleviate the symptoms of orthopnea and DOE.[2,46] Often, when patients lie down, the increased venous return (preload) leads to increased pulmonary artery pressure because the volume is too great for the weakened left ventricle. This sudden increase in preload and pulmonary artery pressure causes the sensation of dyspnea. Sitting up reduces the preload and relieves the symptoms. Nitrates decrease preload and mediate the volume of blood presented to the left ventricle, thus helping to control dyspnea. For this reason, nitrates may be used for patients who do not have angina, specifically for the management of orthopnea and DOE.

Hydralazine combined with nitrates effectively reduces mortality when added to ACE inhibitor and β-blocker therapy in the African American population.[46]

## Nonpharmacologic Treatment

### Role of the Patient

Several nonpharmacologic strategies can be used to manage symptoms and prevent hospitalization of patients with heart failure.[4,47,48] The participation and commitment of the patient is necessary for success.

Sodium restriction is critical. Patients often believe that if they no longer use a salt shaker, they have eliminated all excess salt from their diet, and they may be surprised to learn that canned soup and canned vegetables are extremely high in salt. Education about the natural salt content of foods and the salt that is added as part of food processing is essential. Patients must be taught to read labels and shop for foods that provide optimum nutrition with minimal salt.

Alcohol use should be stopped. As noted previously, alcohol is a powerful cardiac depressant. Many patients have read that a glass of wine or a drink each day decreases the risk for CAD. Although this may be true, the studies were performed in patients who did not have systolic dysfunction. It is important to clarify this fact and explain to the patient the adverse effects of alcohol.

Exercise should be encouraged. Patients with heart failure have limited stamina, and the goal is to increase stamina with low-level exercise over a longer period of time instead of intense exercise for short periods of time. Obviously, some patients with heart failure start at a higher level of functioning and have a better exercise tolerance than patients with advanced heart failure. Exercise for patients with heart failure is not the same as that for development of cardiovascular fitness, and heart rate is not a good indicator of exercise efficacy.

Patients with heart failure should be encouraged to maintain their level of activity. Walking is by far the best exercise. Neither speed nor distance is important. Patients should aim for 15 to 20 minutes each day without stopping to rest or "catch their breath" at whatever pace they are able to manage. Some patients need to take many rests before they begin to exercise, and it may be quite a while before they can exercise for this length of time even at low levels. Weight lifting is not recommended because this activity increases afterload and may worsen symptoms. Medicare recently expanded coverage for cardiac rehabilitation for patients with NYHA class II to IV symptoms and an EF of less than 35% on stable medical therapy for 6 weeks. This is a new option to encourage exercise for those with heart failure.

The most important thing patients can do to stay out of the hospital and control symptoms is to take their medication. The second most important activity is to measure their weight every day. An overnight weight change of more than 3 pounds is due to water weight. If patients take and record their weight every day, modest fluid accumulations of 1 quart or less can be identified. Diuresis can be initiated before patients experience so much fluid overload that hospitalization for IV diuresis is necessary.

Fluid restrictions are punishing, and there is no evidence that water restriction has any value in the absence of significant hyponatremia. Likewise, there is no physiologic basis for decreasing or controlling edema by fluid restriction, or any evidence that restricting fluids is effective.[4] The problem for patients with heart failure is the retention of sodium, which "holds on" to water. Restricting sodium does decrease or control edema, as discussed in the section on diuretics.

### Implantable Cardioverter–Defibrillator

In dilated cardiomyopathy, the incidence of sudden death from ventricular tachycardia or ventricular fibrillation is very high. Asymptomatic ventricular tachycardia is common, but its prognostic impact is unknown. For patients who have syncopal episodes or who survive sudden death, an ICD is usually indicated. An ICD interrupts life-threatening dysrhythmias. If this device fires frequently or symptomatic NSVT occurs, amiodarone may be added to the regimen for rhythm control. See Chapter 18 for more information about the ICD.

### Biventricular Pacing

In the patient with heart failure and intraventricular conduction delays (QRS duration more than 130 milliseconds) that lead to dyssynchronous activation of the left and right ventricles, biventricular pacing or cardiac resynchronization improves CO and therefore symptoms and exercise tolerance.[49] Pacing both ventricles of the spherically dilated heart reproduces the bottom-to-top contraction of a normal ventricle that is lost with myocardial remodeling and bundle branch block.

## Patient Education

Many times, with patient education, severe exacerbations requiring hospitalization can be avoided. If a weight gain of 2 to 3 pounds can be treated with intermittent extra doses of diuretic, then 15- and 20-pound weight gains that require hospitalization will not occur. Helping patients control both their heart failure and their comorbid diseases empowers them and gives them a sense of control that also helps to limit hospitalization. Disease management is an option for patients with multiple comorbidities who find self-care in heart failure to be particularly challenging. There is some evidence that disease management improves quality of life, decreases hospitalizations, and decreases cost of care for patients with heart failure.[50]

Home care provides many opportunities for disease management. As the home care nurse enters the patient's environment, the opportunities for teaching become evident. Even in situations in which the number of visits after a hospital stay are limited, such as with patients covered by Medicare, there are many opportunities for the home care nurse not only to assess but also to intervene.

Discharge planning begins with the first day of hospitalization. A program of education, referral, and follow-up is initiated with the goal of preventing further hospitalization (Box 20-6). Patient teaching alone, however, is not sufficient to enable patients to be effective partners in their care. Carefully planned transitions from hospital to home are linked to decreased hospitalizations for those with heart failure. Clearly, patients must be on target levels of standard medications to reap the benefits supported by clinical studies of heart failure. However, patients must collaborate with health care providers to maximize this benefit (Box 20-7).

---

**BOX 20-6** *TEACHING GUIDE* *Living With Heart Failure*

### Medications

- Take all medications as instructed. If you cannot afford them, please let your provider know so that you can be put in touch with someone to help.
- Do not stop taking medication because you feel better. These are lifetime medications in most instances. Some of the medications will need to be adjusted over time, but your health care provider will discuss the changes with you.
- You may be taking several drugs. These medications do not interfere with each other, and they are given together so that they can work together to do more than any one or two of them can do alone.
- Do not let your medication supply run out because stopping some medications suddenly can cause serious problems.
- Take your medications about the same time every day.
- If you are going out for a few hours and will not have easy access to a bathroom when you need it, hold off on your diuretic until you return home. Do not skip a day's dose of diuretic because this could lead to serious water accumulations and worsening of your heart failure.

### Diet

- Restrict your salt intake by removing the salt shaker from the table and the food preparation area. Do not add salt to any food you are cooking or any food on your plate.
- Avoid foods that have a high salt content naturally or because of the way they are preserved. Foods such as canned soup, canned vegetables, canned meats, foods frozen in sauces, cold cuts, sauerkraut, dill pickles, cheese, and processed foods of any kind are loaded with salt. Seasonings such as garlic and onion salt, Old Bay, and monosodium glutamate are the same as salt. Avoid salt substitutes because they are made with potassium; in combination with the medications you are taking, they can lead to potassium excesses. Avoid fast food such as hamburgers, French fries, fried chicken, and tacos.
- Seasonings such as pepper, Mrs. Dash, onion and garlic powder, herbs, seeds, and spices are acceptable.
- Fresh or frozen vegetables (frozen without sauces), fresh lean meats and poultry, and fish (not fried) are all good choices.

### Daily Weights

- Weigh yourself every day at about the same time and record the value.

- The best time to weigh yourself is in the morning when you first get up and after you go to the bathroom.
- Weigh yourself without clothes if possible.
- Record your weight and the date in a daily diary. Bring this diary with you to the office when you visit your health care provider.
- Call if your weight goes up more than 2 pounds overnight and does not go back to baseline the next day, or if you gain more than 3 pounds in a week.

### Activity

- Stay as active as possible.
- The stronger your skeletal muscles are, the easier it is for your heart.
- Do not use heart rate as a measure of adequacy of exercise effort.
- If you get tired or short of breath, stop and rest, and then try again. The goal is 15 to 20 minutes of continuous activity each day.
- There are no speed or distance goals, and walking at whatever pace you can accomplish is a good choice. Homemaking and gardening are good choices as well. Choose an activity that you enjoy.
- Shortness of breath is uncomfortable but not dangerous. It is an indication that you are nearing the end of your exercise tolerance for this period, but once your breathing normalizes, you can go again. If you stop before you get short of breath out of fear, you will not be able to increase your activity tolerance.
- If you have any questions about how much exercise you can tolerate, discuss it with your health care provider. That person is the best advisor for you because you are well known to him.
- Do not lift weights unless your health care provider has specifically said it is an acceptable activity for you.

### Call Your Health Care Provider If

- Your weight increases or decreases suddenly.
- You begin waking up at night short of breath and need to sit up to breathe.
- You start needing more pillows at night to breathe when you lie down, or you are unable to lie down.
- You become short of breath at rest.
- You cannot walk up stairs that you used to climb regularly because now it makes you too short of breath or tired.
- Your feet and legs start to swell.
- You faint or feel as though you are going to faint.
- You become dizzy and weak when you stand.

**OSEN BOX 20-7**   *COLLABORATIVE CARE GUIDE for the Patient With Acute Decompensation of Chronic Heart Failure*

| Outcomes | Interventions |
|---|---|
| **Decreased cardiac and peripheral tissue perfusion** | |
| There will be adequate oxygen to meet the metabolic demands of the tissue<br>Minimum arterial oxygen content evidenced by:<br>1. Hgb = 10 g/dL or more<br>2. SpO$_2$ = 90% or more | • Consider the transfusion of red blood cells if Hgb is 9.0 g/dL or less<br>• Supplemental oxygen to maintain SpO$_2$ at greater than 90%<br>• Consider intubation and mechanical ventilation if patient develops respiratory acidosis or cannot maintain oxygen saturation on 100% oxygen by mask<br>• Consider primary pulmonary problem as cause of hypoxemia and check brain natriuretic peptide level |
| The patient's symptom of dyspnea will be managed<br>1. Patient denies dyspnea at rest<br>2. Patient reports increased activity before feeling sufficient dyspnea to limit activity<br>3. NYHA class equal to or better than baseline before decompensation | • Elevate head of bed or allow patient to select upright position that best relieves dyspnea<br>• Apply damp washcloth to patient's face<br>• Use a fan or other means to create air movement across the patient's face<br>• Encourage the patient to ambulate as soon and as much as possible once dyspnea at rest is relieved |
| **Decreased CO related to altered preload**<br>**Decreased CO related to contractility**<br>**Decreased CO related to heart rate** | |
| CO will be maximized. Optimum CO evidenced by:<br>1. Cardiac index greater than 2.0<br>2. SvO$_2$ greater than 50%<br>3. Urine output greater than 30 mL/h<br>4. Baseline level of consciousness and orientation | • Optimize preload with diuresis, fluid administration, or vasodilation with agent such as nitroglycerin, nitroprusside, or nesiritide<br>• Increase contractility with inotrope such as milrinone or dobutamine<br>• Decrease afterload with diuresis and vasodilation |
| Hypotension will be asymptomatic, and the patient's blood pressure is at baseline | • Determine the patient's baseline blood pressure; systolic pressure may be less than 90 mm Hg<br>• If blood pressure is less than baseline, assess for orthostatic decreases in blood pressure and increases in heart rate that would suggest dehydration<br>• Continue to give ACE inhibitors and other afterload reducers if hypotension is asymptomatic<br>• If patient is symptomatic on standing, keep on bed rest until orthostasis resolves<br>• If patient is orthostatic, symptomatic, and BUN and creatinine levels are elevated, hold diuretics and consider giving intravenous normal saline solution |
| **Excess Fluid Volume** | |
| Euvolemia will be achieved. Euvolemia evidenced by:<br>1. Absence of peripheral edema<br>2. Absence of ascites<br>3. Documented dry weight<br>4. Baseline BUN and creatinine<br>5. Moist mucous membranes | • Administer loop diuretic sufficient to produce 1 L of urine output within 2 hours of administration<br>• Obtain daily weights<br>• Strive for a weight loss of 1–2 kg/d until dry weight is achieved<br>• Monitor electrolytes at least daily<br>• Replenish potassium, magnesium, and calcium as needed<br>• Measure serum albumin<br>• If inadequate response to loop diuretics, add metolazone or inotropes as above<br>• Report new or worsened rales to physician |
| **Teaching/Discharge Planning** | |
| Refer to Box 20-6 | Refer to Box 20-6 |

# Clinical Applicability Challenges

## CASE STUDY

Mr. S. is a 56-year-old man who had an anterior wall myocardial infarction 5 years ago. His medical history is significant for diabetes type 2, obesity (body mass index of 35), and hypertension. He arrived on the cardiac care unit from the emergency room with three-pillow orthopnea, PND, and lower-extremity edema that has gotten progressively worse over the last week. He denies chest pain or pressure or palpitations.

On examination, his vital signs are as follows: blood pressure 80/50, heart rate 110, respiratory rate 40, pulse oximetry 85%. He is sitting upright and appears to be distressed with intercostal retractions. Jugular venous distention is noted to his mandible. Cardiac examination reveals a point of maximal impulse in the anterior axillary line 6th intercostal space. Auscultation of the heart reveals an irregularly irregular rhythm, S1, S2, S3, and a grade III/VI systolic murmur at the apex. You note bibasilar crackles. The distal pulses are weak and the lower extremities have pitting edema to his knees. Skin is cool and moist.

ECG reveals a sinus tachycardia with frequent premature ventricular contractions (PVCs) and an left bundle branch block (LBBB). There are no ST changes. Labs are as follows:

| | |
|---|---|
| Glucose 186 mg/dL | T bilirubin 2.8 mg/dL |
| Na 124 mg/dL | AST/ALT 163 IU/L/152 IU/L |
| K 5.8 mEq/L | Troponins negative |
| BUN 68 mg/dL | BNP 3,068 pg/mL |
| Creatinine 2.3 mg/dL | EF of 25% |

Home medications include metoprolol XL 50 mg daily, lisinopril 10 mg daily, and atorvastatin 20 mg daily. His wife tells you he works full time as a business consultant and travels extensively. Most of his meals are eaten in a restaurant during the week. He drinks one to two glasses of wine daily and, while he has decreased the amount that he smokes from a full pack to half a pack per day, he has not been able to stop smoking completely since his myocardial infarction.

1. What is your assessment of Mr. S.'s condition, and what are your nursing priorities?
2. You have returned to work 2 days later, and Mr. S. is sitting in chair on room air feeling much improved. His wife is visiting with him and asks how Mr. S. should take care of himself at home. How would you educate Mr. and Mrs. S?
3. The cardiologist would like to place a biventricular ICD in Mr. S. His wife and he do not fully understand why this would be an appropriate option for Mr. S. How would you educate Mr. and Mrs. S. about biventricular ICD placement?

## WANT TO KNOW MORE?

A wide variety of resources to enhance your learning and understanding of this chapter are available on thePoint.

You will find:

- References
- Selected readings
- NCLEX-style review questions
- Internet resources
- And more!

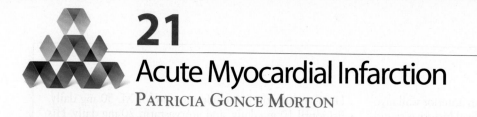

# 21

# Acute Myocardial Infarction

PATRICIA GONCE MORTON

## LEARNING OBJECTIVES

*Based on the content in this chapter, the reader should be able to:*

1. Explain the pathophysiology and risk factors for atherosclerosis.
2. Describe the classification, assessment, and management of patients with angina pectoris.
3. Compare and contrast the pathophysiologic principles and assessment findings of a patient with angina pectoris versus a patient with a myocardial infarction (MI).
4. Discuss the diagnostic tests used for a patient with an MI.
5. Summarize the principles of managing the patient with an MI and the nursing care in the early phase, intensive care phase, and intermediate care phase of management.
6. Describe the complications and nursing care for a patient with an MI.
7. Explain the principles of cardiac rehabilitation and patient education.

Cardiovascular disease is the leading cause of global death, accounting for 17.3 million deaths per year with the figure expected to reach 23.6 million by 2030.[1] Heart disease continues to be the leading cause of death in the United States killing over 375,000 people each year.[1] Heart disease is the number one killer of women and results in more deaths for women than all forms of cancer combined.[1] Approximately 735,000 people in the United States have heart attacks each year, and of that number, about 120,000 die.[1] Heart disease accounts for one in seven deaths in the United States. A person in the United States dies from heart disease about once every 90 seconds.[1]

Although the mortality and morbidity statistics may appear daunting, much progress has been made in the prevention, diagnosis, and management of cardiovascular disease. Since the Framingham Study of risk factors in 1951 and the development of coronary care units in the 1960s, the critical care nurse has played a major role in helping to reduce the mortality associated with heart disease. The critical care nurse uses advanced assessment skills, rapid decision-making, and therapeutic interventions to treat the patient in the acute phase of cardiovascular disease. Patient education and psychological support provided by the nurse have enabled patients and their families to return home and maximize their health status.

## Atherosclerosis

Atherosclerosis is a major cause of cardiovascular disease. The term *atherosclerosis* comes from the Greek words *athere*, meaning "gruel" or "paste," and *sclerosis*, meaning "hardness."

## Pathophysiologic Principles

Atherosclerosis is a complex, insidious process, beginning long before symptoms occur. Although the process is not completely understood, scientific evidence suggests that it begins when the inner, protective layer of the artery (endothelium) is damaged. Three known causes of the damage include elevated levels of cholesterol and triglycerides in the blood, hypertension, and cigarette smoking.

Gradually, as fatty substances, cholesterol, cellular waste products, calcium, and fibrin pass through the vessel, they are deposited in the inner lining of an artery. As a result of the deposition of these materials, a lipid plaque with a fibrous covering, also known as an atheroma, builds up, and blood flow in the artery becomes partially or completely blocked. The injury to the vessel and the resulting accumulation of these substances in the inner lining of the artery cause white blood cells, smooth muscle cells, and platelets to aggregate at the site. As a result, a matrix of collagen and elastic fibers form, and the endothelium becomes much thicker. The core of the fibrous plaque can become necrotic, and hemorrhage and calcification may result. A thrombosis may also form, thus contributing even more to the blockage of the vessel lumen (Fig. 21-1). These fibrous plaques are most often found in the coronary, popliteal, and internal carotid arteries and in the abdominal aorta.

Because of the fibrous plaque, the amount of blood flow through the artery is reduced, resulting in a decreased supply of oxygen to tissues. However, symptoms often do not occur until 75% or more of the blood supply to the area is occluded. The occurrence of symptoms may depend to an extent on the development of collateral circulation. Collateral vessels are small arteries that connect two larger arteries or different segments of the same artery. Under normal conditions, these collateral arteries carry very little of the blood flow. As the larger artery gradually occludes, pressure builds on the proximal side of the occlusion. As a result, flow is redirected through the collateral vessels, which enlarge and dilate over time. Blood is then allowed to flow around an area of blockage through these alternate routes.

Scientific advances have highlighted the role of inflammation in the pathophysiologic process of atherosclerosis. The classic signs and symptoms of inflammation include redness, pain, heat, and swelling. They indicate that the injured tissue is in the process of restoring homeostasis, which includes

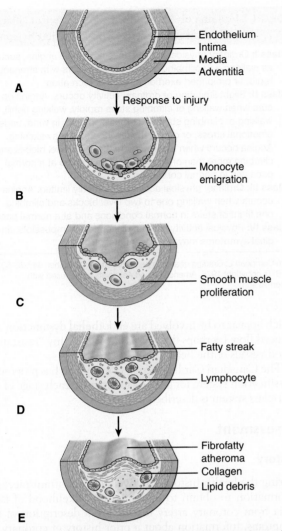

A
- Endothelium
- Intima
- Media
- Adventitia

Response to injury

B
- Monocyte emigration

C
- Smooth muscle proliferation

D
- Fatty streak
- Lymphocyte

E
- Fibrofatty atheroma
- Collagen
- Lipid debris

**FIGURE 21-1 A, B:** Atherosclerosis begins as monocytes and lipids enter the intima of the injured vessel. Smooth muscle cells proliferate within the vessel wall (**C**), contributing to the development of fatty accumulations and atheroma (**D**). As the plaque enlarges, the vessel narrows and blood flow decreases (**E**). The plaque may rupture and a thrombus might form, obstructing blood flow. (From Hinkle JL, Cheever KH: Brunner & Suddarth's Textbook of Medical-Surgical Nursing, 13th ed. Philadelphia, PA: Wolters Kluwer Health/Lippincott Williams & Wilkins, 2014, p 730.)

three phases: vasodilation and increased permeability of the blood vessels, emigration of phagocytes from the blood into the tissue, and tissue repair. This process of restoring homeostasis is meant to be protective, but in the setting of atherosclerosis, the process has been found to be destructive. The atherosclerotic plaque continues to develop, aided by inflammatory molecules, and a fibrous cap forms over the lipid core. As the cap matures, inflammatory substances weaken the cap and cause it to rupture. Once the cap is ruptured, the coagulation cascade is initiated, and a clot is formed, resulting in obstruction of blood flow in the vessel.

## Risk Factors

The cause of atherosclerosis is not clearly known. Through epidemiologic studies, risk factors for the development of atherosclerosis have been identified. These risk factors are usually classified into two groups: major uncontrollable risk

factors and major risk factors that can be modified, treated, or controlled. Major risk factors are those that have been shown through research to increase significantly the risk of cardiovascular disease; they include age, heredity (including race), and gender. Major risk factors that can be modified, treated, or controlled include tobacco smoking, high blood cholesterol levels, hypertension, physical inactivity, obesity, and diabetes mellitus. Other risk factors are known to be associated with an increased risk for cardiovascular disease, but their significance and prevalence are still under investigation. These include stress, excessive use of alcohol, and diet and nutrition. The more risk factors a patient has, the greater the chance of developing coronary heart disease.[2] See Box 17-3 in Chapter 17 for more information on risk factors.

## Acute Coronary Syndrome

The term *acute coronary syndrome* (ACS) is used to describe patients with clinical symptoms compatible with acute myocardial ischemia or infarction that are due to an abrupt reduction in coronary blood flow.[3] This term includes unstable angina and acute myocardial infarction (AMI). Unstable angina refers to unexpected chest pain or discomfort that usually occurs while at rest. Patients with MI are further classified into one of two groups: those with ST-segment elevation MI (STEMI) and those with non–ST-segment elevation MI (NSTEMI).[3] The pathophysiologic origins and clinical presentations of unstable angina and NSTEMI are similar, but differ in severity. An NSTEMI is diagnosed when the ischemia is severe enough to cause myocardial damage and the release of a biomarker indicating myocardial necrosis into the circulation. However, on the electrocardiogram (ECG), ST segments do not elevate. For a patient with unstable angina, biomarkers are not detected in the circulation hours after the initial onset of ischemic pain. Unstable angina can present as rest angina usually lasting more than 20 minutes; new-onset (less than 2 months) severe angina; and a crescendo pattern of occurrence that increases in intensity, duration, frequency, or any combination of these factors. A patient with an STEMI shows the ST changes on the ECG and has detectable biomarkers in the circulation.

## Angina Pectoris

The term *angina* comes from the Latin word meaning "to choke." Angina pectoris is the term used to describe chest pain or discomfort that results from coronary artery disease. The patient may describe the sensation as pressure, fullness, squeezing, heaviness, or pain.

## Pathophysiologic Principles

Angina pectoris is caused by transient, reversible myocardial ischemia precipitated by an imbalance between myocardial oxygen demand and myocardial oxygen supply. In most cases, angina pectoris is the result of a reduced oxygen supply. The most common cause of a reduced supply of oxygen is atherosclerotic narrowing of the coronary arteries. A nonocclusive thrombus develops on a disrupted atherosclerotic plaque, resulting in a reduction in myocardial perfusion. As blood flow to the myocardium decreases, autoregulation of coronary blood flow occurs as a compensatory mechanism. The smooth muscles of the arterioles relax, thus decreasing resistance to blood flow in the arteriolar bed. When this compensatory mechanism can no longer meet the metabolic demands, myocardial ischemia occurs, and the person feels pain.

A less common cause of unstable angina is dynamic obstruction resulting from intense focal spasm of a coronary artery. The spasm is caused by hypercontractility of vascular smooth muscle, endothelial dysfunction, or abnormal constriction of small resistance vessels. As a result of the spasm, perfusion to the myocardium is interrupted, thus reducing the supply of oxygen.

Arterial inflammation may be another cause of decreased oxygen supply that results in unstable angina. The inflammatory process may cause arterial narrowing, plaque destabilization, rupture, and thrombogenesis.

A marked increase in oxygen demand is another cause of unstable angina. Conditions such as fever, tachycardia, and thyrotoxicosis may result in an increased oxygen demand that is unable to be met, especially if the patient has underlying coronary artery disease.

When the balance between oxygen supply and demand is not met, the myocardial tissue's need for oxygen and nutrients continues. The same work of pumping blood must be accomplished with less available energy and oxygen. The tissue that depends on the blood supply becomes ischemic as it functions with less oxygenated blood. Anaerobic metabolism can provide only 6% of the total energy needed. Glucose uptake by the cells is markedly increased as glycogen and adenosine triphosphate stores are depleted. Potassium rapidly moves out of the myocardial cells during ischemia. An acidotic cellular bath develops, further compromising cellular metabolism.

## Classification

Many terms are used clinically to describe angina. *Stable angina* (also known as chronic stable angina, classic angina, or exertional angina) is a term used to describe paroxysmal substernal pain that is usually predictable. The pain occurs with physical exertion or emotional stress and is relieved by rest or nitroglycerin.[4]

*Unstable angina*, also called preinfarction angina or crescendo angina, refers to cardiac chest pain that usually occurs while at rest. The patient with unstable angina has more prolonged and severe chest discomfort than the person with stable angina. Unstable angina is a type of ACS and requires immediate treatment, because the patient is at increased risk for AMI, cardiac dysrhythmias, or cardiac sudden death.[4]

*Variant angina*, also known as Prinzmetal angina or vasospastic angina, is a form of unstable angina. Variant angina usually occurs at rest, most often between midnight and 8:00 AM. It does not usually occur after exertion or emotional stress. Variant angina is the result of coronary artery spasm. Most people who experience variant angina have severe coronary atherosclerosis of at least one major coronary artery, and the spasm occurs very near the area of blockage.[4]

*Microvascular angina*, sometimes referred to as cardiac syndrome X, is angina characterized by chest pain with normal epicardial coronary arteries, the largest vessels on the surface of the heart. The primary cause is unknown, but factors

**BOX 21-1** Grading of Angina Pectoris by the Canadian Cardiovascular Society Classification System

**Class I:** Ordinary physical activity does not cause angina, such as walking and climbing stairs. Angina occurs with strenuous, rapid, or prolonged exertion at work or recreation.
**Class II:** Slight limitation of ordinary activity occurs. Angina occurs when walking or climbing stairs rapidly, walking uphill, walking or climbing stairs after meals, in cold, in wind, under emotional stress, or during the few hours after awakening. Angina occurs when walking more than two level blocks and climbing more than one flight of ordinary stairs at a normal pace and in normal conditions.
**Class III:** Ordinary physical activity is markedly limited. Angina occurs when walking one to two level blocks and climbing one flight of stairs in normal conditions and at a normal pace.
**Class IV:** Physical activity without discomfort is impossible; anginal symptoms may be present at rest.

From Campeau L: Grading of angina pectoris [letter]. Circulation 54:522–523, 1976; copyright 1976, American Heart Association, Inc, used with permission.

which appear to be involved are endothelial dysfunction and reduced flow (perhaps due to spasm) in the tiny "resistance" blood vessels of the heart.[4]

The Canadian Cardiovascular Society also has proposed a classification system for grading for angina. Each stage of the four-class system is described in Box 21-1.

## Assessment

### History

During the health history, the five most important pieces of information to obtain to determine the likelihood of ischemia from coronary artery disease are a description of the symptoms, information about a prior history of coronary artery disease, the patient's sex, the patient's age, and the number of risk factors present.[3]

The nurse uses the NOPQRST method of pain assessment when taking the patient's history. (For a review of the assessment questions, see Box 17-1.) After determining the patient's normal baseline, the nurse asks about the time of onset of the pain. The nurse determines causes (provocative) of the pain and any palliative measures the patient has used to relieve the pain, such as rest or nitroglycerin. The pain of angina is often brought on by exertion or emotion. It may also occur after meals, after exposure to cold, and at rest. Patients with angina often obtain relief from the pain with rest or by taking sublingual nitroglycerin. As the angina becomes more severe (unstable angina), the pain may occur at rest or be caused by less exertion, and is no longer relieved with rest or sublingual nitroglycerin.

The quality of anginal pain is frequently described as deep, poorly localized chest or arm discomfort. Patients often describe heaviness, squeezing, choking, or smothering sensations. When asked about region and radiation of the pain, patients report substernal, left-sided chest, or epigastric pain that may radiate to the left arm, neck, back, or jaw. The severity of the pain is evaluated by asking the patient to rate the pain on a scale of 0 to 10, with 10 being the worst pain they have experienced. Additional information is obtained related to time. The nurse asks how long the pain lasts, how frequently it occurs, and the time of day it occurs. Finally, the nurse asks about associated symptoms, such as dyspnea, nausea, vomiting, and diaphoresis. Box 21-2 summarizes the assessment findings for a patient with myocardial ischemia.

Older patients, and women, who experience angina may have a different presentation because of changes in neuroreceptors. Considerations for the older patient are described in Box 21-3.

## Physical Examination

The physical examination helps determine the cause of the pain, detect comorbid conditions, and assess any hemodynamic consequences of the pain. When taking the vital signs, the nurse should measure the blood pressure in both arms of the patient. During an anginal episode, the patient

---

> **BOX 21-2** | **The NOPQRST Characteristics of Chest Pain Due to Myocardial Ischemia**
>
> **N—Normal**
> - The patient's baseline before the onset of the pain
>
> **O—Onset**
> - The time when the pain/discomfort started
>
> **P—Precipitating and Palliative Factors**
> *Precipitating*
> - Exercise
> - Exercise after a large meal
> - Exertion
> - Walking on a cold or windy day
> - Cold weather
> - Stress or anxiety
> - Anger
> - Fear
>
> *Palliative*
> - Stop exercise
> - Sit down and rest
> - Use sublingual nitroglycerin; pain of myocardial infarction (MI) is often not relieved by sublingual nitroglycerin
>
> **Q—Quality**
> - Heaviness
> - Tightness
> - Squeezing
> - Choking
> - Suffocating
> - Vise-like
>
> **R—Region and Radiation**
> - Substernal with radiation to the back, left arm, neck, or jaw
> - Upper chest
> - Epigastric
> - Left shoulder
> - Intrascapular
>
> **S—Severity**
> - Pain rated on a scale of 0 to 10, with 10 being the worst pain ever experienced, often rated as 5 or above
>
> **T—Time**
> - Pain lasts from 30 seconds to 30 minutes
> - Pain can last longer than 30 minutes for unstable angina or MI

---

> **BOX 21-3** | *CONSIDERATIONS for the Older Patient*
>
> **Acute Coronary Syndrome**
> Coronary artery disease is more common and more severe in the older patient. Older patients often present with special problems because of their numerous comorbidities, such as diminished β-sympathetic response, increased cardiac afterload due to decreased arterial compliance and arterial hypertension, cardiac hypertrophy, and ventricular diastolic dysfunction.
>
> The older patient is more likely to present with atypical symptoms such as dyspnea, confusion, weakness, or fainting rather than with typical substernal chest pain. Because of differences in amount and distribution of subcutaneous fat, the older person may develop anginal symptoms more quickly when exposed to cold. The older person should be taught to dress in warm clothing and to recognize feelings of weakness, shortness of breath, or fainting as possible indicators of angina.

may present with tachycardia and pulsus alternans. Pulsus alternans is a physical finding characterized by a regular alternation of the force of the arterial pulse. During the initial phase of an anginal episode, the patient may be hypertensive or hypotensive. The patient may exhibit pallor with cold, clammy skin. On further examination of the skin, the nurse may detect xanthomas, which are yellow nodules or plaques, especially on the skin. Xanthomas may be indications of hypercholesterolemia. Carotid or femoral bruits may be auscultated, indicating the possible presence of obstructive cardiovascular disease. The nurse may hear a paradoxical split of $S_2$ or auscultate an $S_3$ heart sound; both sounds are indicators of left ventricular failure. An $S_4$ may be heard, which is suggestive of decreased left ventricular compliance. Deficits in peripheral pulses may indicate peripheral vascular disease.

## Diagnostic Tests

A 12-lead ECG is a standard diagnostic test for patients with angina and should be obtained immediately in patients with chest discomfort. During the anginal episode, the ECG may show T-wave inversions and ST-segment depressions in the ECG leads associated with the anatomical region of myocardial ischemia (Fig. 21-2). Transient ST-segment changes (0.05 mV or more) that occur during a symptomatic episode while at rest and that resolve when the patient is asymptomatic are highly suggestive of severe coronary artery disease. Ectopic beats may also be present during an anginal episode. The ECG should be compared with previous ECGs. Between anginal episodes, the ECG may appear normal. Ambulatory ECG monitoring may be used to assist in the diagnosis of angina, especially for patients with angina at rest. The standard 12-lead ECG is a limited diagnostic tool because it does not provide adequate information about the posterior, lateral, and apical walls of the heart. A normal ECG does not exclude the possibility of ACS.[3]

Biochemical cardiac markers are useful in determining both the diagnosis and the prognosis of ACSs. (For a more detailed discussion of cardiac markers, see Chapter 17.) A cardiac-specific troponin (troponin T or troponin I) is the preferred marker to obtain in all patients who present with chest discomfort consistent with ACS. Troponin has replaced creatine kinase-MB (CK-MB) as the preferred biomarker for the diagnosis of myocardial necrosis. Troponin levels usually do not increase until a few hours after the onset

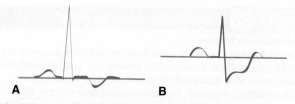

FIGURE 21-2 Inversion of T wave (**A**) and depression of ST segment (**B**). (From Bullock BL: Pathophysiology: Adaptations and Alterations in Function, 4th ed. Philadelphia, PA: Lippincott-Raven, 1996.)

of symptoms.[3] Troponin levels should be obtained at presentation and 3 to 6 hours after symptom onset. If the patient has a negative cardiac marker within 6 hours of the onset of chest discomfort, another blood sample should be drawn in the 6- to 12-hour period after onset of chest discomfort. Troponin levels remain elevated for several days, and therefore may be a useful biomarker for the patient who presents for evaluation several days after the onset of symptoms. Troponin levels are not only useful for the diagnosis of MI, but they also are a reliable tool for therapeutic decision-making.[5] Additional blood tests include chemistry, complete blood count, coagulation studies, and a full lipid profile.

Other diagnostic tests include exercise stress testing, in which the ECG and blood pressure are monitored before, during, and after exercise. The exercise stress test is especially useful in risk stratification of patients. For patients who are unable to exercise, pharmacologic stress testing may be done in which the medication increases myocardial oxygen demand while the patient remains inactive. Intravenous (IV) medications used for pharmacologic stress testing include adenosine, dobutamine, and dipyridamole.

Cardiac imaging studies usually start with chest radiographs, although these have limited value in diagnosing coronary heart disease. Perfusion imaging can be used with exercise or pharmacologic stress testing to detect perfusion defects. Positron emission tomography (PET) may be helpful in differentiating ischemic from infarcted myocardium. Echocardiography is performed to evaluate wall motion abnormalities and thickness, valvular function, and ejection fraction. Magnetic resonance imaging (MRI) and coronary computed tomographic angiography may be used to view structural cardiovascular abnormalities when other diagnostic techniques (eg, the echocardiogram) are inconclusive or ambiguous. (For further discussion of cardiovascular diagnostic tests, see Chapter 17.)

Coronary angiography is an invasive diagnostic test that provides a definitive diagnosis of coronary artery disease. Results from coronary angiography are used to guide the decision whether to manage the patient medically or surgically. (For further discussion of percutaneous coronary interventions, see Chapter 18.)

## Management

The goal of therapy for the patient with angina pectoris is to restore the balance between oxygen supply and oxygen demand. The nurse assesses the patient's vital signs and mental status frequently. The patient is placed on a cardiac monitor for ischemia and dysrhythmia detection. The patient is placed on bed rest until stabilized to minimize oxygen

demands. Supplemental oxygen may be given to unstable patients to increase oxygen supply. A pulse oximeter and arterial blood gases are used to evaluate oxygenation status.

### Pharmacologic Therapy

Pharmacologic therapy is an important component in managing patients with angina pectoris. The severity of symptoms, hemodynamic status of the patient, and medication history guide the drug regimen.

Nitroglycerin is a mainstay of therapy because it is a vasodilator that reduces myocardial oxygen demand by decreasing ventricular preload via vasodilation. Through vasodilation, nitroglycerin improves arterial and collateral flow to ischemic areas. Nitroglycerin is used sublingually or as a spray for acute anginal attacks. If three sublingual tablets (0.4 mg) or spray taken 5 minutes apart (no more than three sprays in 15 minutes) does not relieve the pain of angina, IV nitroglycerin may be started. If signs and symptoms are relieved, there is no need to continue to increase the dose. However, if relief is not obtained, the dose can be increased until a blood pressure response is noted. Once patients have been pain-free and have no other indications of ischemia for 12 to 24 hours, the IV nitroglycerin should be discontinued and replaced with oral or topical nitrates.

Morphine sulfate is indicated for patients whose symptoms are not relieved after three serial sublingual nitroglycerin tablets or whose symptoms recur with adequate anti-ischemic therapy. Morphine is a potent analgesic and anxiolytic with hemodynamic benefits.[3] A dose of 1 to 5 mg IV is recommended to relieve symptoms and maintain comfort. The nurse carefully monitors the patient's respiratory rate and blood pressure, especially if the patient continues to receive IV nitroglycerin.

β-Blockers may be used to decrease myocardial oxygen consumption by reducing myocardial contractility, sinus node rate, and atrioventricular (AV) node conduction velocity. The reduction in myocardial contractility reduces the work of the heart and decreases myocardial oxygen demand. The slowing of the heart rate helps increase the time for diastolic filling, thus improving blood flow to the coronary arteries. β-Blockers are started orally within the first 24 hours for patients with unstable angina and NSTEMI unless contraindicated.[3]

Calcium channel blockers may be beneficial for the patient with unstable angina and NSTEMI. Calcium channel blockers, such as diltiazem or verapamil, decrease myocardial oxygen demand by decreasing afterload, contractility, and heart rate. The nurse carefully monitors the patient for side effects, such as hypotension, worsening heart failure, bradycardia, and AV block. Calcium channel blockers can be administered to treat ischemia-related symptoms in patients unresponsive to or intolerant of nitrates and β-blockers.[3]

The combination of aspirin, an anticoagulant, and an additional antiplatelet drug is recommended for the patient with unstable angina or NSTEMI. Nonenteric coated aspirin should be administered as soon as the diagnosis of unstable angina or NSTEMI is made or suspected, unless contraindicated. A P2Y$_{12}$ inhibitor (either clopidogrel or ticagrelor) in addition to aspirin is used.[3,6] Anticoagulant therapy also is recommended to modify the disease process and its consequences for the patient with unstable angina and NSTEMI.[3]

## Invasive Therapy

Invasive therapy may be indicated for the management of patients with unstable angina. Intra-aortic balloon pump (IABP) support may be used in the critically ill patient to provide increased coronary artery perfusion and to decrease afterload. Percutaneous transluminal coronary angioplasty (PTCA) and stent placement may be used for treating patients with unstable angina. (See Chapter 18 for a more detailed discussion of the IABP, PTCA, and stent placement.) Coronary artery bypass grafting (CABG) is another invasive option for treatment. (See Chapter 22 for a more detailed discussion of cardiac surgery.)

## Risk Factor Modification

Risk factor modification may help prevent an anginal episode or delay the worsening of existing angina. Patients should be encouraged to stop smoking, achieve or maintain optimal weight, and exercise daily. Diet and medications may be prescribed to control hypertension, diabetes, and hyperlipidemia. Patient education, including home care considerations, is essential for patients with angina pectoris. Patient education guidelines and home care considerations are described in Box 21-4.

# Myocardial Infarction

Prolonged ischemia caused by an imbalance between oxygen supply and oxygen demand causes MI. The prolonged ischemia causes irreversible cell damage and muscle death. Although multiple factors can contribute to the imbalance between oxygen supply and oxygen demand, the presence of a coronary artery thrombosis characterizes most MIs. In a classic investigation, DeWood et al[7] demonstrated that 87% of patients studied in the first 4 hours after onset of MI symptoms had a thrombotic occlusion. The incidence of thrombotic occlusion decreases to 65% at 12 to 24 hours.

MI can be determined from several different perspectives, including clinical, electrocardiographic, biochemical, imaging, and pathologic. The European Society of Cardiology, the American College of Cardiology Foundation, the American Heart Association, and the World Heart Federation developed a joint consensus document for the redefinition of MI.[8] Their clinical classification of an AMI is shown in Box 21-5.

## Pathophysiologic Principles

Most patients who sustain an MI have coronary atherosclerosis. The thrombus formation occurs most often at the site of an atherosclerotic lesion, thus obstructing blood flow to the myocardial tissues. Plaque rupture is believed to be the triggering mechanism for the development of the thrombus in most patients with an MI. As mentioned previously, the role of inflammatory processes in the development of atherosclerotic plaque is an area of intense scientific investigation. Cardiovascular risk factors play a role in endothelial damage, resulting in endothelial dysfunction. The dysfunctioning endothelium contributes to the activation of the inflammatory response and the formation of atherosclerotic plaques. When the plaques rupture, a thrombus is formed at the site that can occlude blood flow, thus resulting in an MI. Figure 21-3 shows the atherosclerotic plaque in stable angina and in ACSs.

Irreversible damage to the myocardium can begin as early as 20 to 40 minutes after interruption of blood flow. However, the dynamic process of infarction may not be completed for several hours. Necrosis of tissue appears to occur in a sequential fashion. Reimer and associates demonstrated that cellular death occurs first in the subendocardial layer and spreads like a "wave front" throughout the thickness of the wall of the heart.[9] Using dogs, they showed that the shorter the time between coronary occlusion and coronary reperfusion, the greater the amount of myocardial tissue that could be salvaged. Their classic work indicates that a substantial amount of myocardial tissue can be salvaged if flow is restored within 6 hours after the onset of coronary occlusion. For the clinician, this means time is muscle.

The cellular changes associated with an MI can be followed by the development of infarction extension (new myocardial necrosis), infarction expansion (a disproportionate thinning and dilation of the infarct zone), or ventricular remodeling (a disproportionate thinning and dilation of the ventricle).

---

**BOX 21-4** | *TEACHING GUIDE* | *Angina Pectoris*

**Activity and Exercise**
- Participate in a daily program of exercise that does not precipitate pain.
- Alternate activity with periods of rest and moderate activity level as needed.

**Diet**
- Eat a well-balanced diet with an appropriate caloric intake.
- If obese, participate in a supervised weight-reduction.
- Avoid activity immediately after meals.
- Restrict intake of caffeine because it can increase heart rate.
- Maintain a diet low in fat.

**Smoking**
- Participate in a smoking cessation program. Smoking can increase heart rate, blood pressure, and blood carbon monoxide levels.
- Avoid smoke-filled environments.

**Cold Weather**
- Avoid exposure to cold and windy weather. Exercise indoors when necessary.
- When outdoors, dress in warm clothing and cover mouth and nose with a scarf.
- Use a moderate pace when walking in cold weather.

**Medications**
- Carry sublingual nitroglycerin at all times.
- Keep the pills in a dark-colored glass bottle to protect them from sunlight.
- Do not place cotton in the bottle because the cotton will absorb the active ingredients of the medication.
- If pain occurs, place tablet under the tongue, stop activity, and wait for medication to dissolve. Take another tablet in 3 to 5 minutes if pain does not resolve.
- If pain continues, seek immediate care.
- Be aware of side effects of nitroglycerin, including headache, flushing, and dizziness.

**Universal Classification of Myocardial Infarction**

**Type 1:** Spontaneous myocardial infarction (related to atherosclerotic plaque rupture, ulceration, erosion, or dissection with resulting intraluminal thrombus)

**Type 2:** Myocardial infarction secondary to an ischemic imbalance (where a condition other than CAD contributes to the imbalance between myocardial oxygen supply and/or demand)

**Type 3:** Myocardial infarction resulting in death when biomarker values are unavailable

**Type 4a:** Myocardial infarction related to percutaneous coronary intervention (PCI)

**Type 4b:** Myocardial infarction related to stent thrombosis

**Type 5:** Myocardial infarction related to coronary artery bypass grafting (CABG)

Adapted from Thygesen K, Alpert JS, Jaffe AS, et al; the writing group on behalf of the Joint ESC/ACCF/AHA/WHF Task Force for the Universal Definition of Myocardial Infarction: Third universal definition of myocardial infarction. JACC 60(16):1581–1598, 2012.

### Size of the Infarction

Several factors determine the size of the resulting MI. These factors include the extent, severity, and duration of the ischemic episode; the size of the vessel; the amount of collateral circulation; the status of the intrinsic fibrinolytic system; vascular tone; and the metabolic demands of the myocardium at the time of the event. MIs most often result in damage to the left ventricle, leading to an alteration in left ventricular function. Infarctions can also occur in the right ventricle or in both ventricles.

The term *transmural infarction* is used to imply an infarction process that has resulted in necrosis of the tissue in all the layers of the myocardium. Because the heart functions as a squeezing pump, systolic and diastolic efforts can be significantly altered when a segment of the heart muscle is necrotic and nonfunctional. If the area of the transmural infarction is small, the necrotic wall may be dyskinetic, a term meaning "difficulty in moving." If the damage to the myocardial tissue is more extensive, the myocardial muscle may become akinetic, meaning "without motion."

The normal myocardial muscle contracts with systole and relaxes with diastole. When normal motion is not possible because of infarction, diastolic filling and systolic pumping are altered. As a result, cardiac output is compromised. The larger the area of infarction, the greater is the impact on ventricular function.

### Location of the Infarction

In addition to size, location of the infarction is an important determinant of ventricular function. MIs can be located in the anterior, septal, lateral, posterior, or inferior walls of the left ventricle. MIs also can occur in the right ventricle.

**ANTERIOR LEFT VENTRICLE.** Infarctions of the anterior wall of the left ventricle and the interventricular septum result from occlusion of the left anterior descending (LAD) coronary artery. The LAD coronary artery supplies oxygenated blood to the anterior wall of the left ventricle, the interventricular septum, and the ventricular conducting tissue. (See Chapter 16 for a more detailed discussion of coronary artery anatomy and physiology.)

Anteroseptal wall MIs are the most frequent type of infarction and have the potential for causing a significant amount of left ventricular dysfunction. Patients with an anteroseptal MI are at high risk for heart failure, pulmonary edema, cardiogenic shock, and death because of an inadequate pump. Anteroseptal wall MIs are also associated with increased risk for intraventricular conduction disturbances, such as bundle

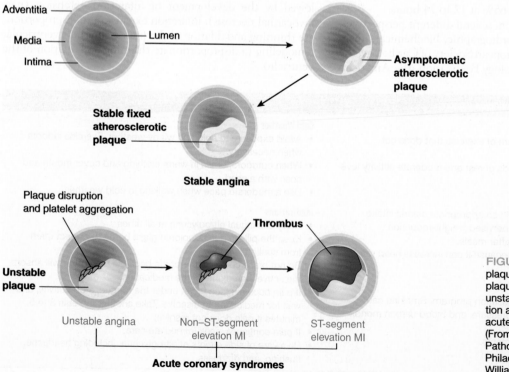

**FIGURE 21-3** Atherosclerotic plaque. Stable fixed atherosclerotic plaque in stable angina and the unstable plaque with plaque disruption and platelet aggregation in the acute coronary syndromes (ACSs). (From Porth CM: Essentials of Pathophysiology, 3rd ed. Philadelphia, PA: Lippincott Williams & Wilkins, 2011, p 453.)

branch blocks and fascicular blocks, which are also known as hemiblocks.

### LATERAL AND POSTERIOR LEFT VENTRICLE.

Infarctions of the lateral and posterior walls of the left ventricle result from occlusion of the left circumflex vessel. In addition to supplying oxygenated blood to the lateral and posterior walls, the left circumflex vessel is the source of blood supply to the sinoatrial (SA) node in about 50% of the population and to the AV node in about 10% of the population. Infarctions of the lateral and posterior walls are less common than infarctions of the anteroseptal wall. Although muscle necrosis occurs with lateral and posterior wall MIs, the impact on left ventricular function is usually less than for patients with anteroseptal MI. Patients with a lateral or posterior wall MI are also at risk for dysrhythmias associated with dysfunction of the SA or AV nodes. Examples include sinus arrest, wandering atrial pacemaker, sinus pause, or junction rhythm.

### INFERIOR LEFT VENTRICLE.

Infarctions of the inferior wall result from occlusion of the right coronary artery. The right coronary artery supplies oxygenated blood to the inferior wall and the right ventricle. In addition, it is the source of blood supply to the SA node in about 50% of the population and the AV node in about 90% of the population. Infarctions of the inferior wall are less common than anteroseptal MIs but occur more frequently than MIs of the lateral or posterior walls. The potential impact on left ventricular function usually is less for a patient with an inferior wall MI than for a patient with an anteroseptal wall infarction. Because the right coronary artery supplies oxygenated blood to much of the conducting tissue, patients are at frequent risk for dysrhythmias related to altered function of the SA and AV nodes.

### RIGHT VENTRICLE.

The right coronary artery provides the blood supply to the inferior wall and the right ventricle. Consequently, right coronary artery disease causing an inferior wall MI is likely to be associated with concomitant right ventricular infarction. Patients may experience significant hemodynamic compromise due to biventricular dysfunction. Dysrhythmias associated with right ventricular infarction involve dysfunction of the SA and AV nodes.

### Type of Infarction

Patients with chest pain may present with or without ST-segment elevations on their ECG. In most patients with ST-segment elevation, a Q wave ultimately develops on the ECG, and the term Q-wave MI is used to describe the type of MI they experience. In a much smaller number of patients who present with ST-segment elevation, a Q wave does not develop, and the term non–Q-wave MI is used to classify these patients. Patients who present without ST-segment elevations are diagnosed with either unstable angina or an NSTEMI (Fig. 21-4).[3] The ST segment is the portion of the ECG tracing from the end of the QRS complex to the beginning of the T wave. Normally, the ST segment is isoelectric, meaning it joins in the QRS complex at the baseline. When the ST segment is elevated, the amount of elevation is measured in millimeters on the ECG paper.

A Q wave is a portion of the QRS complex on the ECG. Specifically, the Q wave is the initial downward deflection of the QRS complex. A Q wave is not present on the normal

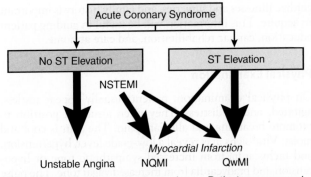

**FIGURE 21-4** Acute coronary syndrome. Patients may present with or without ST-segment elevation on electrocardiography. Most patients with ST-segment elevation (*large arrows*) ultimately develop a Q-wave acute myocardial infarction (QwMI), whereas a minority (*small arrow*) develop a non–Q-wave AMI (NQMI). Most patients who present without ST-segment elevation are experiencing either unstable angina or NSTEMI (non–ST-segment elevation MI). (Adapted from Amsterdam EA, Wenger NK, Brindis RG, et al: 2014 AHA/ACC guidelines for the management of patients with non–ST-elevation acute coronary syndromes: A report of the American College of Cardiology/American Heart Association Task Force on Practice Guidelines. J Am Coll Cardiol 64:e147, 2014.)

ECG. The presence of significant Q waves indicates an MI. (For a review of ECG waveforms, see Chapter 17.)

## Assessment

The nursing assessment of a patient with a probable MI must be organized and thorough. It is best to start with the history because this establishes rapport and provides valuable data. The history is followed by the physical examination and evaluation of diagnostic tests. Based on the data, a management plan is developed initially for the acute phase. Once the patient is stabilized, plans for cardiac rehabilitation are initiated.

### History

The most common presenting complaint of a patient with an MI is the presence of chest discomfort or pain. Other assessment findings are similar to those described in Box 21-2. Like patients with angina, patients with MI describe a heaviness, squeezing, choking, or smothering sensation. Patients often describe the sensation as "someone sitting on my chest." The substernal pain can radiate to the neck, left arm, back, or jaw. Unlike the pain of angina, the pain of an MI is often more prolonged and unrelieved by rest or sublingual nitroglycerin. For a review of the assessment questions, see Box 17-1. Women and the elderly may present differently and often present with a primary complaint of shortness of breath.

Associated findings on history include nausea and vomiting, especially for the patient with an inferior wall MI. These gastrointestinal complaints are believed to be related to the severity of the pain and the resulting vagal stimulation. Patients may initially seek relief of the gastrointestinal symptoms through antacids and other home remedies, thus delaying their decision to go to the hospital. Additional complaints described during the history include diaphoresis, dyspnea, weakness, fatigue, anxiety, restlessness, confusion, shortness of breath, or a sense of impending death.

After the patient is stabilized, a more comprehensive history is obtained. Information about risk factors, previous cardiac illnesses and surgeries, and family history is important to acquire. This information will be useful in guiding patient education, cardiac rehabilitation, and care at home.

## Physical Examination

On physical examination, patients usually appear restless, agitated, and in distress. They often assume a position to promote breathing and alleviate pain. The skin is cool and moist. Vital signs may reveal a low-grade fever, hypertension, and tachycardia from increased sympathetic tone or hypotension and bradycardia from increased vagal tone. The pulse may be irregular and faint.

The cardiovascular examination may reveal additional abnormalities. When the patient is placed in the left lateral decubitus position, abnormalities of the precordial pulsations can be felt. These abnormalities include a lack of a point of maximal impulse or the presence of diffuse contraction. On auscultation, the first heart sound may be diminished as a result of decreased contractility. A fourth heart sound is heard in almost all patients with MI as a result of decreased left ventricular compliance. A third heart sound may be detected due to left ventricular systolic dysfunction. Transient systolic murmurs may be heard because of papillary muscle dysfunction. After about 48 to 72 hours, many patients acquire a pericardial friction rub. Additional findings on physical examination, such as jugular venous distention, may be related to the development of complications, such as heart failure or pulmonary edema. Breathing may be labored and rapid, and fine crackles, coarse crackles, or rhonchi may be heard when auscultating the lungs. These sounds may indicate the presence of heart failure or pulmonary edema.

Patients with right ventricular infarctions may present with jugular venous distention as well as peripheral edema and elevated central venous pressure. Their lungs may be clear because the failing right ventricle has not provided adequate forward flow.

## Diagnostic Tests

**THE ELECTROCARDIOGRAM.** When a coronary artery becomes about 70% occluded and oxygen demand exceeds oxygen supply, myocardial ischemia may result. If the ischemic state is not corrected, injury to the myocardium may occur. Eventually, if adequate blood flow to the myocardium is not restored, an MI may result. Ischemia and injury are reversible processes; however, infarction is not.

An ECG can be used to detect patterns of ischemia, injury, and infarction. When the heart muscle becomes ischemic, injured, or infarcted, depolarization and repolarization of the cardiac cells are altered, causing changes in the QRS complex, ST segment, and T wave in the ECG leads overlying the affected area of the heart. Table 21-1 shows location of the MI, the artery affected, findings from the ECG, and clinical implications.

**Ischemia.** Myocardial ischemia may be a transient finding on ECG, or ischemic patterns may be more prolonged due to the presence of ischemic tissue surrounding a region of infarcted tissue. On the ECG, myocardial ischemia results in T-wave inversion or ST-segment depression in the leads facing the ischemic area. The inverted T wave representative of ischemia is symmetrical, relatively narrow, and somewhat pointed. In contrast, asymmetrical inversion of the T wave usually does not indicate ischemia. Instead, it may signify ventricular hypertrophy or bundle branch block (Fig. 21-5). ST-segment depressions of 1 to 2 mm or more for a duration of 0.08 second may indicate myocardial ischemia. Ischemia also should be suspected when a flat or depressed ST segment makes a sharp angle when joining an upright T wave rather than merging smoothly and imperceptibly with the T wave (Fig. 21-6).

**TABLE 21-1** Location of Myocardial Infarction, Electrocardiographic (ECG) Findings, and Clinical Implications

| Anatomical Location | Coronary Artery | ECG Evidence | Clinical Implications |
|---|---|---|---|
| Anteroseptal wall | Left anterior descending: Supplies blood to the anterior wall of left ventricle, the interventricular septum, and the ventricular conducting tissue | $V_1$ through $V_4$, Q waves and ST-segment elevations | Potential for significant hemodynamic compromise; heart failure, pulmonary edema, cardiogenic shock; intraventricular conduction disturbances |
| Lateral wall | Left circumflex: Supplies blood to the left lateral and left posterior walls and to the sinoatrial (SA) node in 45% of people and atrioventricular (AV) node in 10% of people | I, aVL, $V_5$, and $V_6$, Q waves and ST-segment elevations | Evaluation for posterior wall involvement; some hemodynamic changes; dysrhythmias caused by SA and AV node dysfunction |
| Posterior wall | Left circumflex: Supplies blood to the left lateral and left posterior walls and to the SA node in 45% of people and AV node in 10% of people | $V_1$ and $V_2$, tall upright R waves with ST-segment depression; Q waves and ST-segment elevation in $V_7$ through $V_9$ | Evaluation for lateral wall involvement; some hemodynamic changes; dysrhythmias caused by SA and AV node dysfunction |
| Inferior wall | Right coronary artery: Supplies blood to the inferior wall of the left ventricle, the right ventricle, and the SA node in 55% of people and the AV node in 90% of people | Q waves and ST-segment elevation in II, III, aVF | Evaluation for right ventricular wall involvement; some hemodynamic changes; potential for significant dysrhythmias caused by SA and AV node dysfunction |
| Right ventricular wall | Right coronary artery: Supplies blood to the inferior wall of the left ventricle, the right ventricle, and the SA node in 55% of people and the AV node in 90% of people | Q waves and ST-segment elevations in right precordial chest leads ($RV_1$ through $RV_6$) | Evaluation for inferior wall involvement; some hemodynamic changes; potential for significant dysrhythmias caused by SA and AV node dysfunction |

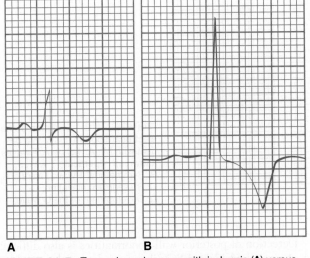

FIGURE 21-5 T-wave inversion seen with ischemia (**A**) versus T-wave inversion seen with left ventricular hypertrophy (**B**).

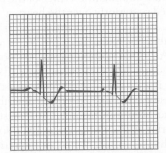

FIGURE 21-6 An ST-segment pattern consistent with myocardial ischemia. Notice how the ST segment forms a sharp angle when joining an upright T wave rather than merging smoothly and imperceptibly with the T wave.

**Injury.** ECG patterns of myocardial injury indicate a state of cellular damage beyond ischemia. Like ischemia, myocardial injury is a reversible process if interventions are instituted rapidly. As described previously, the injury process begins in the subendocardial layer and moves throughout the thickness of the wall of the heart like a wave. If the injury process is not interrupted, it eventually results in a transmural MI.

On ECG, the hallmark of acute myocardial injury is the presence of ST-segment elevations. In the normal ECG, the ST segment should not be elevated more than 1 mm in the standard leads or more than 2 mm in the precordial leads. With an acute injury, the ST segments in the leads facing the injured area are elevated. The elevated ST segments also have a downward concave or coved shape and merge unnoticed with the T wave (Fig. 21-7).

Continuous monitoring of the ST segment is essential for assessing ischemia and injury patterns on the ECG. Ideally, the ST-segment monitoring should be performed using all 12 leads of the ECG. If 12-lead monitoring is unavailable, the nurse monitors the most appropriate leads for ST-segment monitoring based on the patient's needs and risk for ischemia and injury and/or dysrhythmias.

**Infarction.** When myocardial injury persists, MI is the result. The pattern of the ECG indicative of an MI is seen on the ECG in stages and involves changes in the T wave, the ST segment, and the Q wave in the leads overlying the

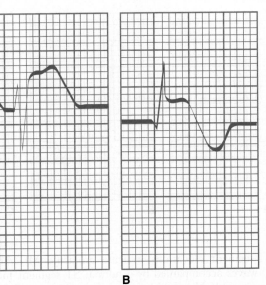

FIGURE 21-7 ST-segment pattern consistent with acute myocardial injury. **A:** ST-segment elevation without T-wave inversion. **B:** ST-segment elevation with T-wave inversion. The elevated ST segments have a downward concave or coved shape and merge unnoticed with the T wave.

infarcted area. Figure 21-8 shows the evolution of the ECG in an MI. During the earliest stage of MI, known as the hyperacute phase, the T waves become tall and narrow. This configuration is referred to as hyperacute or peaked T waves. Within a few hours, these hyperacute T waves invert.

Next, the ST segments elevate, a pattern that usually lasts from several hours to several days. In addition to the ST-segment elevations in the leads of the ECG facing the injured heart, the leads facing away from the injured area may show ST-segment depression. This finding is known as reciprocal ST-segment changes. Reciprocal changes are most likely to be seen at the onset of infarction, but their presence on the ECG does not last long. Reciprocal ST-segment depressions may simply be a mirror image of the ST-segment elevations. Or, reciprocal changes may reflect ischemia due to narrowing of another coronary artery in other areas of the heart.

The last stage in the ECG evolution of an MI is the development of Q waves, the initial downward deflection of the QRS complex. Q waves represent the flow of electrical forces toward the septum. Small, narrow Q waves may be seen in the normal ECG in leads I, II, III, aVR, aVL, $V_5$, and $V_6$. Q waves compatible with an MI are usually 0.04 second or more in width or one fourth to one third the height of the R wave. Q waves indicative of infarction usually develop within several hours of the onset of the infarction, but in some patients, they may not appear until 24 to 48 hours after the infarction.

Within a few days after the MI, the elevated ST segments return to baseline. Persistent elevation of the ST segment may indicate the presence of a ventricular aneurysm. The T waves may remain inverted for several weeks, indicating areas of ischemia near the infarcted region. Eventually, the T waves should return to their upright configuration. The Q waves do not disappear and therefore always provide ECG evidence of a previous MI.

The ECG pattern can be used to distinguish acute MIs from "old" MIs. Abnormal Q waves accompanied by

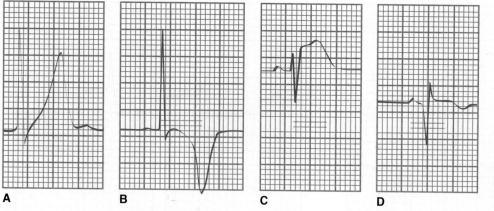

**A** **B** **C** **D**

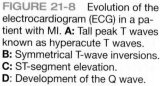

FIGURE 21-8    Evolution of the electrocardiogram (ECG) in a patient with MI. **A:** Tall peak T waves known as hyperacute T waves. **B:** Symmetrical T-wave inversions. **C:** ST-segment elevation. **D:** Development of the Q wave.

ST-segment elevations indicate an acute MI. Abnormal Q waves accompanied by a normal ST segment indicate a previous MI. How long ago the infarction occurred cannot be determined by the ECG. The pattern could signify an infarction that occurred 2 weeks or 20 years before.

The ECG is helpful not only in determining patterns of ischemia, injury, and infarction but also in revealing the anatomical region of the heart where the abnormality has occurred. ECG leads $V_1$ through $V_4$ show the anteroseptal wall of the left ventricle. The inferior wall is seen in leads II, III, and aVF. Leads I, aVL, $V_5$, and $V_6$ reveal the lateral wall of the left ventricle (see Fig. 21-9). The routine 12-lead ECG does not provide an adequate view of the right ventricle or of the posterior wall of the left ventricle. As a result, additional leads are needed to view these anatomical areas. To attain an accurate view of the right ventricle, right-sided chest leads are recorded by placing the six chest electrodes on the right side of the chest using landmarks analogous to those used on the left side (see Fig. 17-7 on page 200). These six right-sided views are examined for patterns of ischemia, injury, and infarction in the same way left-sided chest leads are evaluated.

Detection of posterior wall abnormalities is also difficult on the standard 12-lead ECG because none of the six chest leads provides an adequate view of the posterior wall. To detect posterior wall abnormalities, three of the precordial electrodes are placed posteriorly over the heart, a view known as $V_7$, $V_8$, and $V_9$. $V_7$ is positioned at the posterior axillary line; $V_8$, at the posterior scapular line; and $V_9$, at the left border of the spine. All three posterior leads are positioned along the same horizontal line established by $V_6$ (see Fig. 17-7). The recording is examined for evidence of ischemia, injury, or infarction using the same criteria as described previously. If posterior leads were not recorded, it may still be possible to detect posterior wall abnormalities. To do so, the principle of reciprocal change is used. When an infarction in the posterior wall is suspected, the leads anatomically opposite the posterior wall are examined. These include $V_1$ and $V_2$ because the anterior wall is anatomically opposite the posterior wall. If tall R waves with ST-segment depressions are noted in $V_1$ and $V_2$, the pattern is consistent with a posterior wall MI. Figures 21-10 through 21-13 show the 12-lead ECGs of patients with MIs.

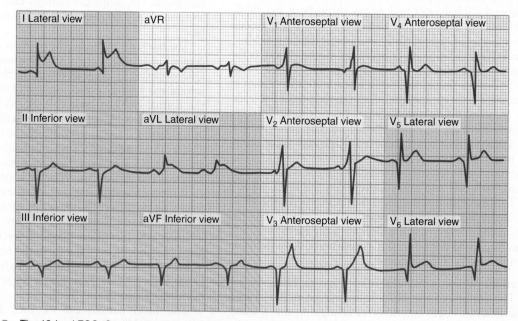

FIGURE 21-9    The 12-lead ECG: Correlation of lead with the view of the heart.

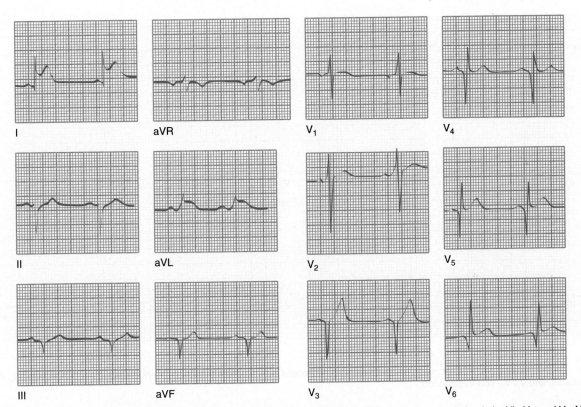

FIGURE 21-10 Twelve-lead ECG showing an acute lateral wall MI. ST-segment elevations can be seen in leads I, aVL, $V_5$, and $V_6$. Note also the deep Q waves in II, III, and aVF and normal ST segments, indicating a previous inferior wall MI.

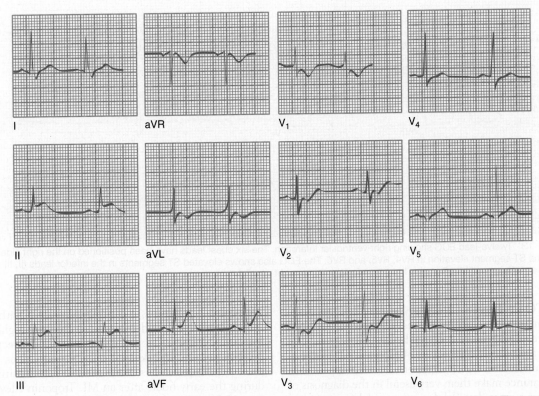

FIGURE 21-11 Twelve-lead ECG showing an acute inferior wall MI. Note the ST-segment elevations in II, III, and aVF. The posterior wall infarction is evidenced by a tall R wave, ST-segment depression, and inverted T wave in $V_1$ and $V_2$.

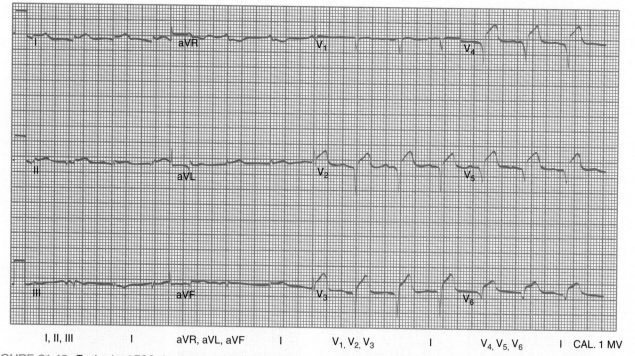

**FIGURE 21-12** Twelve-lead ECG showing an acute anterior and lateral wall MI. Note the ST-segment elevations and Q waves in I, aVL, V₅, and V₆ (lateral), and V₂, V₃, and V₄ (anterior).

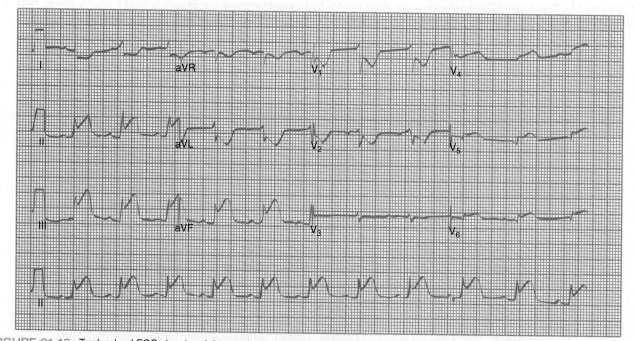

**FIGURE 21-13** Twelve-lead ECG showing right ventricular infarction. The six chest leads have been positioned on the right side of the chest. Note the ST-segment elevation in RV4, RV5, and RV6. The ECG also shows elevated ST segments in the inferior leads (II, III, aVF). Patients with an inferior wall MI often also have an infarction in the right ventricle.

**LABORATORY TESTS.** When myocardial cells are damaged by an infarction, biochemical markers are released into the bloodstream and can be detected by laboratory tests. The presence of abnormally high levels of biochemical markers, their distribution, and the time pattern for their appearance and disappearance make them very useful in the diagnosis of acute MI. For a more detailed discussion of laboratory tests, see Chapter 17.

**Troponin.** Troponin is a contractile protein with two subforms (troponin T and troponin I) that are highly specific for cardiac muscle. Troponin levels are not detected in the healthy person, and skeletal muscle injury does not affect the level. Troponin has been found to be a sensitive marker during the early hours after an MI. Troponin I levels rise in 3 to 12 hours, peak at 24 hours, and remain elevated for 5 to 10 days. Troponin T levels rise in 3 to 12 hours, peak in

12 hours to 2 days, and remain elevated for 5 to 14 days. Because the cardiac troponins are highly sensitive and specific for MI, they are the preferred biomarker for diagnosing this coronary event.[3,5] Other laboratory tests are the same as described previously for the patient with suspected angina and include blood chemistry, complete blood count, coagulation tests, lipid panel, and white blood cell count.

### Other Diagnostic Tests

Patients with an MI should have a chest radiograph. An echocardiogram may be done to detect structural abnormalities, such as valvular problems. Other tests may include radionuclide angiocardiography, MRI, myocardial perfusion imaging, positron emission tomography, or computed tomography (CT) scans. For a more detailed discussion of these diagnostic tests, see Chapter 17.

## Management

### Early Management

When a patient with a possible MI arrives in the ED, the diagnosis and initial management of the patient must be rapid because the benefit of reperfusion therapy is greatest if therapy is initiated quickly. An initial evaluation of the patient should occur ideally within the first 10 minutes after arrival. The patient's history and 12-lead ECG are the primary methods used to determine initially the diagnosis of MI. The ECG is examined for the presence of ST-segment elevations of 1 mm or greater in contiguous leads. This pattern provides evidence of thrombotic coronary arterial occlusion. The patient is placed on a continuous cardiac monitor with ST-segment monitoring capabilities.

If the initial screening suggests an MI, the interventions listed in Box 21-6 are initiated. The nurse checks the vital signs frequently, establishes IV access, and continuously assesses the patient's cardiac rhythm. Blood is drawn to assess troponin levels. Also, hematology, chemistry, and lipid profiles are performed. If indicated, a chest radiograph and echocardiogram are obtained to rule out an aortic dissection and acute pericarditis. During the initial evaluation, the patient and family may be anxious, necessitating brief and clear explanations of the interventions. Reassurance and support are essential components of the nurse's responsibilities.

### PERCUTANEOUS CORONARY INTERVENTION.

Reperfusion therapy should be administered to all eligible patients with STEMI with symptom onset within the prior 12 hours.[10] Primary percutaneous coronary intervention (PCI) is the recommended method of reperfusion when it can be performed in a timely way by experienced physicians.[10] If the patient is brought to a non–PCI-capable hospital, ideally the patient should be transferred immediately to a PCI-capable hospital. If the transfer is not possible in a timely way, fibrinolytic therapy should be administered to patients with a STEMI in the absence of contraindications.[10] The ideal door to drug time for these patients is 30 minutes. Once the patient is stabilized, the patient is evaluated for transfer to a hospital for angiography and revascularization within 3 to 24 hours.

Early reperfusion of myocardial tissue is essential to preserve myocardial function. PCI is an effective intervention to reestablish blood flow to ischemic myocardium.

---

> **BOX 21-6** **Initial Management of the Patient With STEMI**
>
> **Action:** Administer aspirin, 160 to 325 mg chewed.
> **Rationale:** Aspirin is used because it diminishes platelet aggregation. This effect is important because platelets are one of the main components in thrombus formation when a coronary plaque is disrupted. Aspirin has been shown to reduce mortality rates independently in patients with acute myocardial infarction (AMI). Patients diagnosed with an MI should be continued on aspirin indefinitely.
> **Action:** After recording the initial 12-lead electrocardiogram (ECG), place the patient on a cardiac monitor and obtain serial ECGs. Use continuous ST-segment monitoring.
> **Rationale:** The 12-lead ECG is central in the decision pathway for the diagnosis and treatment of the patient. The patient is placed on a continuous cardiac monitor after the 12-lead ECG is recorded to detect dysrhythmias and to monitor ST-segment changes.
> **Action:** Give oxygen by nasal cannula if the oxygen saturation is <90%
> **Rationale:** Hypoxemia often occurs in patients with an MI because of pulmonary edema. If severe pulmonary edema is present and the patient is in respiratory distress, intubation may be necessary. A pulse oximeter is used, and, when time permits, an arterial blood gas may be drawn.
> **Action:** Administer sublingual nitroglycerin (unless the systolic blood pressure is <90 mm Hg or the heart rate is <50 or >100 beats/min). Give 0.4 mg every 5 minutes for a total of three doses.
> **Rationale:** Nitroglycerin helps to promote vasodilation but is relatively ineffective in relieving pain in the early stages of an MI. Intravenous nitroglycerin is recommended for patients with AMI with persistent pain, for control of hypertension, or for management of pulmonary congestion.
> **Action:** Provide adequate analgesia with morphine sulfate.
> **Rationale:** Morphine is the drug of choice to relieve the pain of an MI. The drug is given intravenously in small doses (2 to 4 mg) and can be repeated every 5 minutes until the pain is relieved. Close respiratory and blood pressure monitoring are indicated because morphine can depress respirations and cause hypotension.
> **Action:** Administer β-blocker within the first 24 hours unless contraindicated.
> **Rationale:** β-Blocking agents may diminish myocardial oxygen demand by reducing heart rate, systemic arterial pressure, and myocardial contractility.
> **Action:** Administer an angiotensin-converting enzyme (ACE) inhibitor within the first 24 hours.
> **Rationale:** Angiotensin-converting enzyme (ACE) inhibitors interfere with the formation of the hormone (angiotensin II) that can narrow (constrict) blood vessels. ACE inhibitors help lower blood pressure and reduce the workload on the heart.

Data from O'Gara PT, Kuschner FG, Ascheim DD, et al: 2013 ACCF/AHA guideline for the management of ST-elevation myocardial infarction: A report of the American College of Cardiology Foundation/American Heart Association Task Force on Practice Guidelines. J Am Coll Cardiol 61:e78–e140, 2013.

---

Percutaneous transluminal coronary angioplasty (PTCA), an invasive procedure in which the infarction-related coronary artery is dilated with a balloon catheter, is the type of PCI used. Once the artery is opened by the balloon, a stent may be placed in the artery. (See Chapter 18 for a more detailed discussion of the PTCA procedure.)

A dose of 162 to 325 mg of Aspirin is given to the patient before the primary PCI and the aspirin is continued indefinitely.[10] A loading dose of a $P2Y_{12}$ receptor inhibitor is given as early as possible or at the time of the PCI. Drugs that may be used include: clopidogrel, prasugrel, or ticagrelor. If the patient receives a stent, a $P2Y_{12}$ drug is continued for 1 year.[10] Anticoagulant regimens also are recommended for patients undergoing PCI. Unfractionated heparin is used to maintain therapeutic activated clotting time levels.[10] In selected patients, a GP IIb/IIIa receptor antagonist also may be used. If the PCI is unsuccessful, the patient may be evaluated for coronary artery bypass grafting surgery. Care of the patient undergoing PCI is described in Chapter 18 (see Box 18-9).

**FIBRINOLYTIC THERAPY.** In the absence of contraindications, fibrinolytic therapy is given to the patient with STEMI and onset of ischemic symptoms within the previous 12 hours when it is anticipated that a primary PCI cannot be performed within 120 minutes of the first medical contact.[10] Fibrinolytic therapy also is recommended for patients with STEMI who are unable to receive PCI if there is clinical and/or electrocardiographic evidence of ongoing ischemia within 12 to 24 hours of symptom onset and a large area of myocardium is at risk or hemodynamically unstable.[10]

Fibrinolytic drugs lyse coronary thrombi by converting plasminogen to plasmin. This conversion causes the degradation of fibrin and fibrinogen, resulting in clot lysis. Box 21-7 lists contraindications to fibrinolytic therapy.[10] Fibrinolytic agents used for treating patients with STEMI include streptokinase, alteplase, reteplase, and tenecteplase.[10]

---

**BOX 21-7** **Contraindications and Cautions for Fibrinolysis in ST-Segment Elevation Myocardial Infarction***

**Absolute Contraindications**
- Any prior intracranial hemorrhage
- Known structural cerebral vascular lesion (eg, arteriovenous malformation)
- Known malignant intracranial neoplasm (primary or metastatic)
- Suspected aortic dissection
- Active bleeding or bleeding diathesis (excluding menses)
- Significant closed-head or facial trauma within 3 months
- Intracranial or intraspinal surgery within 2 months
- For streptokinase, prior treatment within the previous 6 months

**Relative Contraindications**
- History of chronic, severe, poorly controlled hypertension
- Significant hypertension on presentation (systolic blood pressure >180 mm Hg or diastolic blood pressure >110 mm Hg)
- History of prior ischemic stroke greater than 3 months
- Dementia
- Known intracranial pathology not covered in contraindications
- Traumatic or prolonged (>10 minutes) CPR
- Major surgery (<3 weeks)
- Recent (within 2 to 4 weeks) internal bleeding
- Noncompressible vascular punctures
- Pregnancy
- Active peptic ulcer
- Oral anticoagulant therapy

*Viewed as advisory for clinical decision-making and may not be all-inclusive or definitive.

From O'Gara PT, Kuschner FG, Ascheim DD, et al: 2013 ACCF/AHA guideline for the management of ST-elevation myocardial infarction: A report of the American College of Cardiology Foundation/American Heart Association Task Force on Practice Guidelines. J Am Coll Cardiol 61:e96, 2013.

---

The goal is to complete the assessment of the patient and the administration of the fibrinolytic drug (if indicated) within 30 minutes of the patient's arrival to the ED. There is a time-dependent reduction in both mortality and morbidity rates during the initial 12 hours after symptom onset.[10]

For the patient receiving fibrinolytic therapy, two to three 18-gauge peripheral IV lines are usually started. One line is for the fibrinolytic agent, and one to two lines are for the administration of other drugs. Subclavian and jugular sites are avoided because they are noncompressible, and blood could be lost into the chest or neck. Some type of blood sampling device is also inserted so that peripheral venous punctures can be avoided.

The patient is closely monitored during and after the infusion of a fibrinolytic agent. The nurse assesses the patient for resolution of chest pain, normalization of elevated ST segments, development of reperfusion dysrhythmias, any allergic reactions, evidence of bleeding, and the onset of hypotension. Commonly seen reperfusion dysrhythmias include an accelerated idioventricular rhythm, ventricular tachycardia, and AV heart block.

Adjunctive antiplatelet therapy with aspirin and clopidogrel are also used with patients undergoing fibrinolytic therapy. Aspirin is continued indefinitely and clopidogrel should be continued for at least 14 days. Anticoagulant therapy also is initiated to improve vessel patency and prevent reocclusion.

Evaluation of complications remains a key nursing intervention. The patient is closely monitored for evidence of reocclusion of the coronary artery. Indicators of reocclusion include chest pain, ST-segment elevation, and hemodynamic instability. Close observation for evidence of bleeding also is essential. The patient is carefully assessed for indications of subcutaneous or mucous membrane bleeding. The nurse also monitors the patient for signs of internal bleeding, including positive results of urine and stool for blood or altered levels of consciousness due to intracranial bleeding.

## Intensive and Intermediate Care Management

The management goal for the patient in the intensive care unit and intermediate care unit continues to be maximizing cardiac output while carefully minimizing cardiac workload. To achieve this goal, the patient frequently has vital signs taken and continues on a cardiac monitor with ST-segment monitoring. The lead selected for monitoring should be based on the infarct location and underlying rhythm. Serial ECGs and serial evaluations of serum cardiac markers of infarction are recorded. Serum hematology and chemistry are monitored.

For the first 12 hours of hospitalization, patients who are hemodynamically stable and free of ischemic-type chest discomfort remain on bed rest with bedside commode privileges. Activity level increases gradually in hemodynamically stable patients. Careful attention is paid to maximal pain relief. Nitroglycerin is not an appropriate substitute for analgesics. A pulse oximeter is used to monitor oxygen saturation continuously and is a good indicator of early hypoxemia. Oxygen is appropriate for patients who are hypoxemic (oxygen saturation less than 90%).

The patient is often not given anything by mouth until pain free. When pain free, the patient is given clear liquids and progressed to a heart-healthy diet as tolerated. Daily weights are recorded, and intake and output are measured to detect fluid retention. Stool softeners are administered so that the patient avoids a Valsalva maneuver. During a Valsalva maneuver, forced expiration against a closed glottis causes sudden and significant changes in systolic blood pressure and heart rate. These changes may influence regional endocardial repolarization and place the patient at risk for ventricular dysrhythmias.

**PHARMACOLOGIC THERAPY.** Prophylactic antidysrhythmics during the first 24 hours of hospitalization are not recommended. However, easy access to atropine, lidocaine, amiodarone, transcutaneous pacing patches, transvenous pacing wires, a defibrillator, and epinephrine is essential for management of dysrhythmias. Daily aspirin is continued on an indefinite basis. Clopidogrel is added to the aspirin regimen for patients with an STEMI and is continued for 14 days.[10] β Blockers and ACE inhibitors are initiated in the first 24 hours unless contraindicated. β Blockers are continued during and after hospitalization. During the first several days after STEMI, it is important to normalize the patient's blood glucose levels. An insulin infusion may be required to achieve this goal. Lipid management therapy is initiated if indicated.

**HEMODYNAMIC MONITORING.** Use of a pulmonary artery catheter for hemodynamic monitoring is indicated in the patient with MI who has severe or progressive heart failure or pulmonary edema, cardiogenic shock, progressive hypotension, or suspected mechanical complications, such as ventricular septal defect, papillary muscle rupture, or pericardial tamponade. The pulmonary artery occlusion pressure (PAOP) is closely followed for assessment of left ventricular filling pressures. A PAOP below 18 mm Hg may indicate volume depletion, whereas a PAOP greater than 18 mm Hg indicates pulmonary congestion or cardiogenic shock. Using the thermodilution technique, frequent measurements of cardiac output and cardiac index can be made to evaluate hemodynamic status further. In some situations, monitoring venous oxygen saturation may also be useful. (For a more detailed discussion of hemodynamic monitoring, see Chapter 17.)

Invasive arterial monitoring is indicated for patients with MI who have severe hypotension or for those receiving vasopressor or vasodilator drugs. The collaborative care guide for the patient with an MI (Box 21-8) provides further information about the care of these patients.

**ADDITIONAL DIAGNOSTIC TESTING.** At times, additional testing may be needed after the patient is stabilized. These include stress testing, echocardiograms, myocardial perfusion imaging, radionuclide angiocardiography, CT

---

**QSEN BOX 21-8** *COLLABORATIVE CARE GUIDE for the Patient With Myocardial Infarction*

| Outcomes | Interventions |
| --- | --- |
| **Ineffective Breathing Pattern** <br> **Impaired Gas Exchange** | |
| Patient has arterial blood gases within normal limits and pulse oximeter value >90%. | Assess respiratory rate, effort, and breath sounds every 2 to 4 hours. Obtain arterial blood gases per order or signs of respiratory distress. Monitor arterial saturation by pulse oximeter. Provide supplemental oxygen by nasal cannula or face mask for oxygen saturation <90%. Provide intubation and mechanical ventilation as necessary. (Refer to Chapter 25, Box 25-15.) |
| There is no evidence of pulmonary edema on chest x-ray and by clear breath sounds. | Obtain chest x-ray per order. Administer diuretics per order. Monitor signs of fluid overload as described below. Weigh patient daily. |
| There is no evidence of atelectasis. | Encourage nonintubated patients to use incentive spirometer, cough, and deep breath every 4 hours and PRN. While on bed rest, turn patient side to side every 2 hours. |
| **Decreased Cardiac Tissue Perfusion** <br> **Risk for Shock** <br> **Decreased Cardiac Output** <br> **Risk for Bleeding** | |
| Vital signs are within normal limits, including MAP >70 mm Hg and cardiac index >2.2 L/min/m². | Monitor HR and BP every 1 to 2 hours and PRN during acute failure phase. Assist with pulmonary artery catheter insertion. Monitor PAP and pulmonary artery occlusion pressure (PAOP), CVP, or right atrial pressure (RAP) every 1 hour and cardiac output, SVR, and PVR every 6 to 12 hours if pulmonary artery catheter is in place. Maintain patent IV access. Administer positive inotropic agents, and reduce afterload with vasodilating agents guided by hemodynamic parameters and physician orders. Evaluate effect of medications on BP, HR, and hemodynamic parameters. Prepare patient for intra-aortic balloon pump assist if necessary. |
| Patient has no evidence of heart failure due to decreased cardiac output. | Restrict volume administration as indicated by PAOP or CVP values. Assess for neck vein distention, pulmonary crackles, S₃ or S₄, peripheral edema, increased preload parameters, elevated wave of CVP, RAP, or PAOP waveform. Monitor 12-lead ECG daily and PRN. |
| Patient has no evidence of further myocardial dysfunction, such as altered ECG or cardiac enzymes. | Monitor cardiac markers, magnesium, phosphorus, calcium, and potassium as ordered. Monitor ECG for changes consistent with evolving MI. Consider obtaining right precordial and posterior chest leads, 12-lead ECG, if inferior wall/right ventricle is involved. Report and treat abnormalities per protocols or orders. |
| Dysrhythmias are controlled. | Provide continuous ECG and ST-segment monitoring in the appropriate leads. Document rhythm strips every shift. Anticipate need for/administer pharmacologic agents to control dysrhythmias. |

*(continued)*

**OSEN** BOX 21-8 *COLLABORATIVE CARE GUIDE for the Patient With Myocardial Infarction (continued)*

| Outcomes | Interventions |
|---|---|
| After PCI or fibrinolytic therapy, patient will have relief of pain; no evidence of bleeding; no evidence of allergic reaction. | Assess, monitor, and treat pain as described below. Monitor signs of reperfusion, such as dysrhythmias, ST-segment return to baseline. Monitor for signs of bleeding, including neurologic, GI, and GU assessment. Monitor PT, aPTT, ACT per protocol. Have anticoagulant antidotes available. Assess for itching, hives, sudden onset of hypotension, or tachycardia. Administer hydrocortisone or diphenhydramine (Benadryl) per protocol. |
| There is no evidence of cardiogenic shock, cardiac valve dysfunction, or ventricular septal defect. | Monitor ECG, heart sounds, hemodynamic parameters, level of consciousness, and breath sounds for changes. Report and treat deleterious changes as indicated. |

**Electrolyte Imbalance**
**Ineffective Renal Perfusion**
**Risk for Imbalanced Fluid Volume**

| | |
|---|---|
| Renal function is maintained as evidenced by urine output >30 mL/h and normal laboratory values. | Monitor intake and output every 1 to 2 hours. Monitor blood urea nitrogen, creatinine, and electrolytes daily and PRN. Take daily weights. Administer fluid volume and diuretics as ordered. |

**Risk for Falls**
**Impaired Physical Mobility**
**Risk for Activity Intolerance**

| | |
|---|---|
| Patient will comply with activity of daily living limitations. | Provide clear explanation of limitations. Provide bed rest with bed side commode privileges first 6 hours. Progress to chair for meals, bathing self, and bathroom privileges. Continually assess patient response to all activities. |
| Patient will not fall or accidentally harm self. | Provide environment to prevent falls, bruising, or injury. Use self-protective devices as indicated and per hospital policy. |

**Impaired Skin Integrity**

| | |
|---|---|
| Patient has no evidence of skin breakdown. | Turn side to side every 2 hours while patient is on bed rest. Evaluate skin for signs of pressure areas when turning. Consider pressure relief/reduction mattress for high-risk patients. Use Braden scale (see Chapter 51, Fig. 51-4) to monitor risk for skin breakdown. |

**Imbalanced Nutrition**
**Electrolyte Imbalance**

| | |
|---|---|
| Caloric and nutrient intake meets metabolic requirements per calculation (eg, basal energy expenditure). | Provide appropriate diet: oral, parenteral, or enteral feeding. Provide clear or full liquids during the first 24 hours. Restrict sodium, fat, cholesterol, fluid, and calories if indicated. Consult dietitian or nutritional support services. |
| Patient has normal laboratory values reflective of nutritional status. | Monitor albumin, prealbumin, transferrin, cholesterol, triglycerides, total protein. |

**Impaired Comfort**

| | |
|---|---|
| Patient has relief of chest pain. | Use visual analog scale to assess pain quantity. |
| There is no evidence of pain, such as increased HR, BP, RR, or agitation during activity or procedures. | Assess quality, duration, and location of pain. Administer IV morphine sulfate, and monitor pain and hemodynamic response. Administer analgesics appropriately for chest pain and assess response. Monitor physiologic response to pain during procedures or after administration of pain medication. Provide a calm, quiet environment. |

**Ineffective Coping**
**Ineffective Health Maintenance**
**Impaired Individual Resilience**

| | |
|---|---|
| Patient demonstrates decreased anxiety by calm demeanor and vital signs during, for example, procedures and discussions. | Assess vital signs during treatments and interactions. Provide explanations and stable reassurance in calm and caring manner. Cautiously administer sedatives and monitor response. |
| Patient/family demonstrates understanding of MI and treatment plan by asking questions and participating in care. | Consult social services and clergy as appropriate. Assess coping mechanism history. Allow free expression of feelings. Encourage patient/family participation in care as soon as feasible. Provide blocks of time for adequate rest and sleep. |

**Teaching/Discharge Planning**

| | |
|---|---|
| Patient reports occurrence of chest pain or discomfort. | Explain importance of reporting all episodes of chest pain. Provide frequent explanations and information to family. |
| Family demonstrates appropriate coping during the critical phase of an acute MI. | Encourage family to ask questions regarding treatment plan, patient response to therapy, prognosis, and so forth. |
| In preparation for discharge to home, patient understands activity levels, dietary restrictions, medication regimen, and what to do if pain recurs. | Make appropriate referrals and consults early during hospitalization. Initiate family education regarding heart-healthy diet, cardiac rehabilitation program, stress-reduction strategies, and management of chest pain after crisis phase has passed. |

---

**BOX 21-9** Complications of Acute Myocardial Infarction Hemodynamic Complications

**Hemodynamic Complications**
- Hypotension
- Pulmonary congestion
- Cardiogenic shock
- Right ventricular infarction
- Recurrent ischemia
- Recurrent infarction

**Myocardial Complications**
- Diastolic dysfunction
- Systolic dysfunction
- Heart failure

**Mechanical Complications**
- Mitral valve regurgitation from papillary muscle rupture
- Left ventricular free wall rupture
- Ventricular septal rupture
- Left ventricular aneurysm

**Pericardial Complications**
- Pericarditis
- Dressler syndrome
- Pericardial effusion

**Thromboembolic Complications**
- Mural thrombosis
- Systemic thromboembolism
- Deep venous thrombosis
- Pulmonary embolism

**Dysrhythmia Complications**
- Ventricular tachycardia
- Ventricular fibrillation
- Supraventricular tachydysrhythmias
- Bradydysrhythmias
- Atrioventricular block (first, second, or third degree)

Data from O'Gara PT, Kuschner FG, Ascheim DD, et al: 2013 ACCF/AHA guideline for the management of ST-elevation myocardial infarction: A report of the American College of Cardiology Foundation/American Heart Association Task Force on Practice Guidelines. J Am Coll Cardiol 61:e78–e140, 2013.

---

scans, MRI, or positron emission tomography. (See Chapter 17 for a discussion of these tests.)

## Complications

The nurse closely monitors the patient with MI for evidence of complications. Numerous complications can occur, and a list of possible complications is provided in Box 21-9. Prompt recognition and management of complications are essential in reducing mortality and morbidity.

### Hemodynamic Complications

Recurrent myocardial ischemia can occur in patients and is often transient. A recurrent MI is another possible complication. If the reinfarction occurs within the first 24 hours, it may be hard to diagnose because the cardiac serum markers have not yet returned to baseline. Early recognition and management are essential for both of these vascular complications. Efforts are made to lower myocardial oxygen demand and to relieve pain. Emergent surgical revascularization may be considered.

Cardiogenic shock is the most serious myocardial complication of MI. It occurs because of the loss of contractile forces in the heart, resulting in left ventricular dysfunction. This loss or contractile forces can result from mechanical complications such as papillary muscle rupture, ventricular septal rupture, free-wall rupture with tamponade, and right ventricular infarction. (For a more detailed discussion of cardiogenic shock, see Chapter 54.)

Clinical manifestations of cardiogenic shock include a rapid, thready pulse; a narrow pulse pressure; dyspnea; tachypnea; inspiratory crackles; distended neck veins; chest pain; cool, moist skin; oliguria; and decreased mentation. Arterial blood gas analysis reveals a decreased $PaO_2$ and respiratory alkalosis. Hemodynamic findings include a systolic blood pressure less than 85 mm Hg, a mean arterial blood pressure less than 65 mm Hg, a cardiac index less than 2.2 L/min/m$^2$, and a PAOP greater than 18 mm Hg. Cardiac enzymes may show an additional rise or a delay in reaching peak values.

The goal of treatment for cardiogenic shock is to minimize myocardial workload and maximize myocardial oxygen delivery. Immediate actions must be taken to improve tissue perfusion and preserve viable myocardium. To improve oxygenation, supplemental oxygen is given to the patient and, if necessary, the patient may be intubated and placed on a mechanical ventilator. Efforts are aimed toward restoring blood pressure. This may require discontinuation of vasodilator drugs and drugs with negative inotropic effects. Inotrope and vasopressor agent use is individualized and guided by invasive hemodynamic monitoring.[10] Treatment may also require the use of an IABP. This invasive device helps improve coronary artery perfusion and decrease left ventricular afterload. A left ventricular assist device may be considered. (For a more detailed discussion of IABP therapy and left ventricular assist devices, see Chapter 18.)

### Mechanical Complications

Mechanical complications most often occur either in the first 24 hours or within the first week.[10] The most catastrophic mechanical complications of MI are intraventricular septal rupture and left ventricular free wall rupture. These clinical situations develop rapidly and result in almost immediate physiologic deterioration.

**VENTRICULAR SEPTAL WALL RUPTURE.** Ventricular septal wall rupture occurs most often within the first 24 hours in patients with STEMI treated with fibrinolytic therapy.[10] The patient presents with a new, loud, systolic murmur associated with heart failure and cardiogenic shock. In addition, the patient has progressive dyspnea, tachycardia, and pulmonary congestion. The patient is supported with fluid administration, inotropic support, vasodilator agents, and IABP counterpulsation until emergency surgery is possible. Often it is impossible to maintain the patient medically until surgical repair occurs.

**LEFT VENTRICULAR FREE WALL RUPTURE.** Left ventricular free wall rupture occurs most frequently in patients with their first MI, anterior infarctions, the elderly, or women. Other risk factors include hypertension during the acute phase of STEMI, lack of antecedent angina or MI, absence of collateral blood flow, Q waves on ECG, use of corticosteroids or nonsteroidal anti-inflammatory drugs, and administration of fibrinolytic therapy more than 14 hours after symptom onset.[10] The patient experiencing free wall rupture presents with recurrent chest pain and ST-T wave changes, with rapid progression to hemodynamic collapse, electromechanical dissociation, and death.[10] This event occurs so suddenly and with such severity that lifesaving efforts are often futile.

**MITRAL REGURGITATION.** Mitral regurgitation after STEMI results from either papillary muscle rupture or postinfarction left ventricular remodeling with displacement of the papillary muscles, leaflet tethering, or annular dilation. Patients with acute severe mitral regurgitation may develop a systolic murmur, pulmonary edema, and/or shock. Temporary stabilization with diuretics and afterload-reducing agents or the IABP may be attempted until emergent surgery is performed.

**PERICARDIAL COMPLICATION.** The incidence of acute pericarditis after STEMI has decreased with the use of reperfusion therapy.[10] The patient reports chest pain that may be confused with ischemic pain. The precordial pain of pericarditis intensifies with deep breathing, coughing, and swallowing, and is positional. The pain is lessened when the patient sits up and leans forward. The patient may have a fever, with a temperature usually less than 101.5°F (38.6°C) that lasts for several days. Often on auscultation, a friction rub can be heard along the left sternal border. Some friction rubs are transient; therefore, the absence of such a rub is not conclusive. Often, the ECG shows concave upward ST-segment elevation on five or more leads. Aspirin is recommended for treatment.

**THROMBOEMBOLIC AND BLEEDING COMPLICATIONS.** Thromboembolisms occur in fewer MI patients than previously because of the routine use of anticoagulants. Those patients with a deep venous thrombosis (DVT) may be predisposed because of the systemic inflammatory response associated with infarction, immobility, venous stasis, and reduced cardiac output. Pulmonary embolism is a risk for patients with DVT. After MI, patients are also at risk for systemic emboli that usually originate in the wall of the left ventricle. These emboli can occlude the cerebral, renal, mesenteric, or iliofemoral artery.

STEMI patients who receive heparin therapy are closely monitored for heparin-induced thrombocytopenia. Bleeding complication is another condition the nurse closely monitors. Hemoglobin and hematocrit levels are assessed regularly and early signs of bleeding must be identified.

**DYSRHYTHMIA COMPLICATIONS.** Cardiac dysrhythmias and conduction disturbances often accompany acute MIs and can be life-threatening. The causes of electrical complications are many and include myocardial ischemia, myocardial necrosis, altered autonomic tone, electrolyte imbalances, acid–base disturbances, and adverse drug effects.

Ventricular dysrhythmias that occur in the prehospital phase cause the majority of sudden cardiac deaths. Ischemic myocardium has a lower fibrillatory threshold, and few ventricular dysrhythmias are considered benign after an infarction. Patients may experience tachydysrhythmias or bradydysrhythmias during the hospital phase of treatment. Supraventricular rhythms may be the result of high left atrial pressures caused by left ventricular failure.

Conduction disturbances after MI can include those caused by SA node, AV node, or ventricular conducting tissue abnormalities. The right coronary artery supplies the SA node in about half of all patients, and the left circumflex coronary artery supplies the SA node in the other half. Because the right coronary artery is also the source of oxygenated blood for the inferior, right posterior, and right ventricular walls, patients with inferior, right posterior, or right ventricular wall MIs are at risk for conduction disturbances resulting from poor SA node functioning. Patients with lateral wall MIs also are at risk for SA nodal conduction disturbances because the left circumflex vessel supplies the lateral wall of the heart.

The right coronary artery also is the source of oxygenated blood for the AV node in about 90% of people. Therefore, patients with inferior, right posterior, or right ventricular wall infarctions due to right coronary artery occlusion are at risk for AV nodal conduction disturbances. First-degree heart block and Mobitz type I (Wenckebach) block may appear, but often are transient. These rhythm disturbances may progress to complete heart block and require pacing therapy.

The LAD coronary artery is the primary source of blood supply to the bundle of His and bundle branches. Therefore, patients with an anterior wall MI caused by an LAD occlusion are at risk for ventricular conduction defects. Conduction defects, such as right bundle branch block, left bundle branch block, anterior fascicular block, posterior fascicular block, bifascicular block, or trifascicular block, may occur.

For patients with MI, the nurse continuously monitors the cardiac rate and rhythm, assesses the apical and peripheral pulses, auscultates the heart, and monitors blood pressure and other indicators of hemodynamics, such as urine output and level of consciousness. The goals of therapy for cardiac dysrhythmias and conduction disturbances are to restore normal rate, rhythm, and AV synchrony and to maintain adequate cardiac output. To achieve these goals, pharmacologic therapy may be indicated. Cardioversion may be used to treat patients with supraventricular dysrhythmias, such as atrial fibrillation or atrial flutter. Transcutaneous pacing may be indicated in an emergent situation for heart block dysrhythmias until a transvenous temporary pacemaker can be initiated. The patient may require permanent pacemaker implantation to maintain an adequate rate and rhythm. Some patients may require an implantable cardioverter–defibrillator to manage ventricular dysrhythmias. (For a more detailed discussion of pacemakers and implanted cardioverter–defibrillators, see Chapter 18.)

### Acute Kidney Injury

Multiple factors place the STEMI patient at risk for acute kidney injury such as age, baseline renal function, medications, and hemodynamic status. Contrast agent-induced nephropathy after angiography is always a risk requiring careful monitoring and optimal hydration.[10]

## Hyperglycemia

Careful glucose control is essential for the patient post-STEMI. The mortality rate associated with hyperglycemia appears to be as high as the mortality rate associated with hypoglycemia. Ideally, the patient's glucose level should be maintained below 180 mg/dL.

## Cardiac Rehabilitation

Preparation for discharge must begin early in the patient's course of hospitalization. Patient and family education is an essential component of the process. A severely compromised, critically ill patient may lack the ability to process and retain new information but usually is motivated to learn after the life-threatening event. Guidelines for patient and family education after an acute MI are described in Table 21-2.

Cardiac rehabilitation is recommended for most patients after MI. Cardiac rehabilitation involves a combination of prescribed exercise, education, and counseling. The goals of cardiac rehabilitation are to limit the adverse physiologic and psychological effects of heart disease, modify risk factors, reduce the risk for sudden death or reinfarction, control cardiac symptoms, stabilize or reverse the atherosclerotic process, and enhance the patient's psychosocial and vocational status. Components of cardiac rehabilitation programs include exercise, smoking cessation, lipid management, weight control, blood pressure control, psychological interventions, and guidance for return to work.

Cardiac rehabilitation programs have been shown to improve the patient's functional capacity and quality of life and to decrease emotional distress, risk for subsequent coronary events, and cardiovascular mortality.[10] However, although the benefits of cardiac rehabilitation are well known, fewer than one third of patients receive information or counseling about cardiac rehabilitation before being discharged from the hospital.

Depression is common among people with coronary heart disease and has been associated with increased risk for adverse outcomes for patients with ACS. Therefore, patients should be assessed for evidence of depression and a treatment plan needs to be developed as part of the rehabilitation process.[11]

Family members of patients with MI should be included in the educational process so that they can learn about heart disease and help the patient achieve the goals of rehabilitation. Family members also should be given the opportunity to learn cardiopulmonary resuscitation because most episodes of cardiac arrest in patients with MI occur within the first 18 months after discharge from the hospital.

**TABLE 21-2   Patient Teaching: Goals After Acute Myocardial Infarction**

| | When Mastery of Content Is To Be Expected: | | |
| --- | --- | --- | --- |
| | **Acute Phase** | **Before ICU Discharge** | **At Hospital Discharge** |
| Pathophysiology of heart disease | Can identify angina, using 0–10 pain scale for reference | Can initiate treatment of angina (rest, nitroglycerin, O$_2$ use) | Knowledgeable about medications, when to seek medical assistance |
| Environment of hospital | Understands procedures | Asks appropriate questions | Knowledgeable about disease process and therapy |
| Lifestyle modifications | Complies with activity limitations Complies with dietary limitations | Can state relationship between activity and cardiac workload Begins light activity States risk factors Selects appropriate meals | Can progress activity as tolerated Placement in cardiac rehabilitation program Can state dietary restrictions |
| Treatment of disease | Accepts medications as ordered | Can identify medications Can identify risk factors | Knowledgeable about medications, dose, timing, action, and side effects Plans for risk factor reduction Begins cardiac rehabilitation program |
| Emotional adaptation | Able to define support system | Begins to communicate about lifestyle changes Becomes involved with resolving emotions related to surviving a critical illness | Involves self and loved ones in plans for lifestyle changes Expresses feelings Participates in group recovery program |

# Clinical Applicability Challenges

### CASE STUDY

Mrs. T., a 74-year-old white woman, drove herself to the emergency department, arriving at 10:30 AM. She complained of substernal chest pain with radiation to her back that began 1 hour ago. The pain is not relieved by rest or one sublingual nitroglycerin. She describes the pain as dull and rates it a 7 on a scale of 10. She feels nauseated but has not vomited. Mrs. T. has a history of hypertension, diabetes, and elevated cholesterol levels. She has no known drug allergies.

On physical examination, Mrs. T. is awake, alert, oriented, and anxious. Her skin is cool and diaphoretic. Blood pressure is 96/52 mm Hg; heart rate, 112 beats/min and regular; respiratory rate, 22 breaths/min; oxygen saturation, 92%; and temperature, 98°F (36.7°C). Cardiac examination reveals $S_1$, $S_2$, and an $S_3$. She has no jugular venous distention. Peripheral pulses are present but thready, and there is 1+ pedal edema bilaterally. Auscultation of the lungs reveals bilateral basilar crackles. She has no evidence of cyanosis or clubbing. Her abdominal examination shows positive bowel sounds in all quadrants. Her abdomen is soft and nontender with no palpable masses.

The nurse immediately records a 12-lead ECG that shows a 4-mm ST-segment elevation in leads II, II, and avF. Blood samples are drawn that reveal an elevated troponin level. Mrs. T. is given an aspirin, and an intravenous (IV) line is started. Her pain is treated with IV morphine sulfate. Mrs. T. is diagnosed with an acute STEMI in the inferior wall and is admitted to the coronary care unit. On day 2 after admission, Mrs. T complains of chest pain that is made worse by deep breathing and is somewhat relieved when she sits up and leans forward. She has a low-grade fever. On physical examination, she displays a pericardial friction rub upon auscultation of her heart.

1. Mrs. T. was diagnosed with an inferior wall myocardial infarction. What coronary artery is most likely occluded and what potential complications are priorities for you to monitor?
2. In addition to the routine 12-lead ECG, what other electrocardiographic monitoring steps should you take and why?
3. What may be the cause of Mrs. T.'s pain on day 2?

### WANT TO KNOW MORE?

A wide variety of resources to enhance your learning and understanding of this chapter are available on thePoint.

You will find:

- References
- Additional selected readings
- NCLEX-style review questions
- Internet resources
- And more!

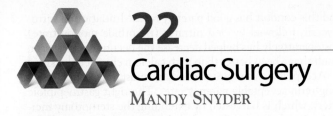

# 22

# Cardiac Surgery

MANDY SNYDER

**LEARNING OBJECTIVES**

*Based on the content in this chapter, the reader should be able to:*

1. Discuss the indications for coronary artery bypass grafting surgery and valvular surgery.
2. Describe the nursing care of the patient before and after coronary artery bypass grafting surgery.
3. Compare and contrast the pathophysiologic implications of stenosis and insufficiency in the mitral and aortic valves.
4. Explain nursing interventions used to prevent complications after cardiac surgery.
5. Discuss the nursing care of the patient before and after carotid endarterectomy.

Despite emphasis on modifying and eliminating risk factors, cardiovascular disease remains a leading cause of disability and death in the United States. Development of new treatments, such as thrombolytic and anticoagulation therapy, balloon angioplasty, and coronary artery stenting, has improved medical management of cardiac disease. These nonsurgical approaches are discussed in Chapter 18. However, surgical intervention remains the treatment of choice in some patient populations with coronary artery disease (CAD) and valvular disease.

## Indications for Cardiac Surgery

### Coronary Artery Diseased

A discussion of the pathophysiology of coronary artery disease (CAD) is found in Chapter 21.

#### Coronary Artery Bypass Graft Surgery

In coronary artery bypass graft (CABG) surgery, native vessels or conduits are "harvested" during the initial phase of surgery and used to reroute or bypass blood flow past diseased areas of the coronary arteries. CABG surgery has become an acceptable treatment for CAD. Compared with medical treatment, CABG surgery has proved effective in relieving angina and improving exercise tolerance, and it prolongs life in patients with left main CAD, three-vessel disease with poor left ventricular function, and two vessel disease with significant stenosis in the proximal left anterior descending.[1–3]

Increased use of percutaneous transluminal coronary angioplasty and stenting has decreased the need for CABG surgery in many cases. Patients selected for such a surgery today are older, have more advanced coronary disease, have more impaired left ventricular function, and, in many cases, have had previous CABG surgery. To decrease the mortality associated with bypass surgery, it is necessary to consider several factors: urgency of operation, age, previous heart surgery, sex, left ventricular ejection fraction, percentage stenosis of the left main coronary artery, and number of major coronary arteries with greater than 70% stenosis.[1]

Desired characteristics for a graft or conduit are (1) diameter similar to the coronary arteries, (2) no disease or vessel wall abnormalities, and (3) adequate length. Commonly used grafts include saphenous vein grafts and internal mammary artery grafts.

**SAPHENOUS VEIN GRAFTS.** Saphenous vein grafts are used to bypass the obstruction in the coronary artery by anastomosing one end of the vein to the aorta (proximal anastomosis) and the other end to the coronary artery just past the obstruction (distal anastomosis) (Fig. 22-1).

Although the saphenous vein can be taken from above or below the knee, a vein from below the knee is generally preferred because of the vessel size. To remove the vein, an incision is made along the inner aspect of the leg. Alternatively, small incisions can be made in the area of the vein, and a flexible fiberoptic scope is inserted to visualize the vessel and remove it. The fiberoptic method of vein removal is

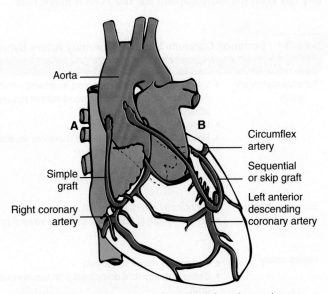

FIGURE 22-1 Aortocoronary bypass grafts using saphenous vein. **A:** Simple graft from aorta to right coronary artery. **B:** Sequential graft from aorta to left anterior descending coronary artery to diagonal or circumflex artery.

associated with improved wound healing and reduced complications involving the incision site.[2]

About 50% of saphenous vein grafts are occluded after 10 years. Three main processes account for saphenous vein failure: thrombosis, fibrointimal hyperplasia, and atherosclerosis. Thrombosis is most common in the first month but may occur as long as 1 year after surgery. Aspirin is the drug recommended for use postoperatively to prevent early saphenous vein graft closure and should be continued indefinitely.[1,2]

**INTERNAL MAMMARY ARTERY GRAFTS.** Compared with saphenous vein grafts, internal mammary artery grafts have superior graft patency rates: 90% were patent 10 years after surgery. In addition, internal mammary artery grafts exhibit less atherosclerosis over time, and they have been associated with lower long-term morbidity and improved long-term survival.[1,2]

The left or right internal mammary artery is used with the proximal end remaining attached to the subclavian artery. The left internal mammary artery (LIMA) is usually used to bypass the left anterior descending coronary artery. The right internal mammary artery (RIMA) is used to bypass to the right coronary artery or the circumflex coronary artery. To isolate the internal mammary artery, the pleural space is entered, the internal mammary artery is dissected free from the chest wall, and the intercostal artery branches are cauterized.

IMA grafts may spasm or atrophy if there is significant residual blood flow in the native coronary artery. Sternal wound infections may develop if both the LIMA and RIMA are used as bypass grafts in diabetic or obese individuals.

**OTHER GRAFTS.** The search for other native vessels to serve as conduits continues as patients return for reoperation. The use of the radial artery has gained popularity; occlusion rates have lowered as harvesting techniques have improved. The radial artery—a thick, muscular artery—is prone to spasm with mechanical stimulation; to prevent spasm, the artery is perfused with a calcium channel blocker solution during surgery and minimally stimulated. After the radial artery has been implanted, spasm has not been a major issue,

and this conduit has good patency rates.[2] Initiation of nitroglycerin followed by oral nitrates (isosorbide mononitrate) postoperatively has helped decrease the occurrence of spasm; results have been better than with calcium channel blockers.[2]

Acceptable alternative conduits must have short- and long-term acceptable patency rates. The right gastroepiploic artery, which is harvested by extending the sternotomy incision toward the umbilicus and dissecting the artery off the greater curvature of the stomach, is used for coronary grafting. Early patency rates of this artery are 90%, but they decrease over time to 60% after 10 years.[1] Homologous (nonnative) conduits using the saphenous vein, umbilical vein, or bovine internal mammary artery have had poor patency rates and are therefore not recommended. A comparison of common conduits used for revascularization is presented in Table 22-1.

### Off-Pump Coronary Artery Bypass Graft Surgery

CABG surgery began as a surgical procedure performed on a beating heart, because the cardiopulmonary bypass machine, which assumes the job of oxygenating the patient's blood and circulating it throughout the body, was not yet available. Once the cardiopulmonary bypass machine was perfected, "beating heart" surgery was used less often. However, intraoperative complications of cardiopulmonary bypass occur with cannula insertion, inducing cardiac standstill, and when weaning from the bypass machine. These complications have led surgeons to reconsider performing CABG surgery "off pump" (OPCABG) in the hope of improving patient outcome.

Patients who have had OPCABG surgery have shorter lengths of stay in the ICU and the hospital as compared with patients who have had on-pump CABG surgery.[1,4] Additionally, patients who have had OPCABG have decreased transfusion needs, less postoperative atrial fibrillation and hemodynamic instability, and fewer inotrope needs, wound infections, and prolonged ventilation times. The stroke rate is similar in patients who undergo OPCABG and those who undergo on-pump CABG, although the timing is

---

**TABLE 22-1  Common Conduits Used for Coronary Artery Bypass Grafting**

| Type of Graft | Advantages | Disadvantages |
|---|---|---|
| Internal mammary artery | • Vascular endothelium adapted to arterial pressure and high flow, resulting in decreased intimal hyperplasia and atherosclerosis<br>• Improved long-term patency<br>• Retains nerve innervation and therefore its ability to adapt diameter to blood flow<br>• No leg incision<br>• Diameter closer to coronary artery | • Dissection off the chest wall takes more time; long dissection time may increase risk for postoperative bleeding<br>• Pleural chest tube needed because pleural space violated<br>• Increased postoperative pain<br>• Use of bilateral internal mammary arteries may increase risk for infection and sternal infection, especially in patients with diabetes |
| Saphenous vein | • Technically easier to harvest<br>• Longer length (if able) may allow for several grafts | • Less long-term patency compared with internal mammary artery graft<br>• Leg incision has tendency toward edema and infection; less common with fiberoptic approach |
| Radial artery | • Technically easier to harvest<br>• Better patency rate compared with saphenous vein graft<br>• Vascular endothelium adapted to arterial pressure and high flow, resulting in decreased intimal hyperplasia and atherosclerosis | • Tendency to spasm, although this can be treated medically<br>• Preoperative assessment of ulnar artery's ability to supply alternative blood flow is important |

immediate after on-pump CAGB and within 48 to 72 hours after OPCABG.[1,4] The explanation for the difference in stroke timing is that systemic inflammatory response syndrome (SIRS, discussed in detail in Chapter 54) causes diffuse microembolic events in patients who undergo OPCABG as a result of the inflammation of the endothelium, which activates the coagulation cascade.

Traditional agents such as heparin, aspirin, clopidogrel (Plavix), and low-molecular-weight heparin are aggressively implemented to prevent platelet activation and suppress activation of the coagulation cascade. Nursing assessment focuses on detecting embolic events in any body system (eg, neurologic changes or electrocardiographic [ECG] ST-segment changes) and monitoring for side effects of anticoagulation, such as gastrointestinal bleeding and heparin-induced thrombocytopenia. A high index of suspicion for evolving patient complications is the key nursing intervention after OPCABG surgery and may improve patient outcomes. While it would seem that OPCABG would provide more benefits than on-pump CABG, there is no advantage of one surgical procedure over the other.[4]

### Minimally Invasive Direct Coronary Artery Bypass Grafting

Minimally invasive direct coronary artery bypass grafting (MIDCABG) uses the less invasive "mini" left and right thoracotomy approaches while performing CABG surgery, on or off bypass. Because the small incision does not allow access to the entire heart surface, only certain types of grafts can be performed using this technique. MIDCABG is most frequently used for grafts to the left anterior descending artery. Depending on where the "mini" incision is placed, grafts to the right coronary artery and the posterior descending artery can also be made using this technique.[1] MIDCABG has not been as successful as anticipated, but the technique is still used depending on the patient situation. An additional consideration with the thoracotomy approach is the increased need for pain medication, which may decrease patient compliance to cough and deep-breathe postoperatively.

## Valvular Disease

Cardiac valves maintain the unidirectional flow of blood in a "forward" direction through the heart chambers and vessels. Disease may cause structural changes to the valves that disrupt their function, resulting in either valvular stenosis or insufficiency (regurgitation). The stenotic valve has a narrowed orifice that creates a partial obstruction to blood flow, resulting in increasing pressure behind the valve and decreasing forward blood flow. The insufficient or regurgitant valve is incompetent or leaky: blood flows backward, increasing the pressure and volume behind the valve. Stenosis and insufficiency (Fig. 22-2) can occur alone or in combination, in the same valve, or in more than one valve. Abnormalities

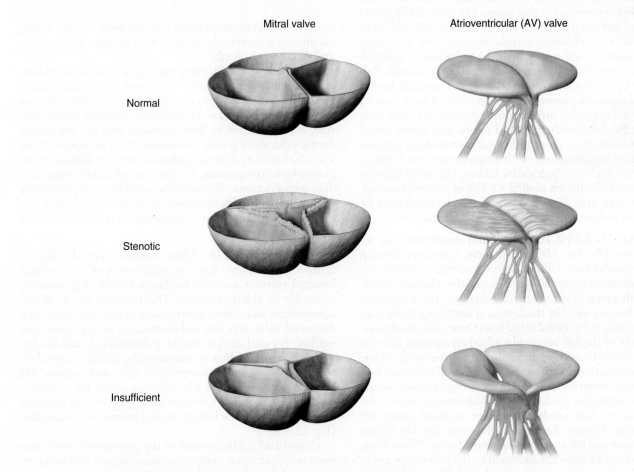

Mitral valve

Atrioventricular (AV) valve

Normal

Stenotic

Insufficient

**FIGURE 22-2**   Normal and diseased heart valves. (From Anatomical Chart Company: Atlas of Pathophysiology. Springhouse, PA: Springhouse, 2010, p 77.)

can affect all four valves, but mitral and aortic abnormalities are more common and produce profound hemodynamic changes.

The diagnosis of valvular disease is suggested by the history, clinical signs and symptoms, physical examination, and auscultation of the characteristic murmur. Diagnosis is confirmed by echocardiography and catheterization of both sides of the heart, at which time the pressure across the valves or valvular gradients are measured.

To determine the gradient across the aortic valve, the left ventricular and aortic root pressures are measured on echocardiogram or during systole with a pressure catheter inserted into the heart during catheterization. A peak gradient of more than 60 mm Hg and an aortic valve area less than 1 cm$^2$ are associated with clinically significant aortic stenosis.[3] Valvular insufficiency is diagnosed by regurgitation of the contrast medium backward through the incompetent valve.

### Pathophysiology

**MITRAL STENOSIS.** Mitral stenosis (Fig. 22-3A) occurs most frequently as a result of rheumatic heart disease. The disease process causes fusion of the commissures and fibrotic contraction of valve leaflets, commissures, and chordae tendineae. A valve area decreased to less than 1.5 cm$^2$ signifies critical mitral stenosis. The decrease restricts blood flow from the left atrium to the left ventricle; as forward flow from the left atrium to the left ventricle decreases, cardiac output falls, creating a decrease in systemic perfusion. Blood backed up behind the stenotic valve causes left atrial dilation and increased left atrial pressure. This pressure is reflected backward into the pulmonary circulation, and with prolonged high pressures, fluid moves from the pulmonary capillaries into the interstitial space and, eventually, the alveoli. Pulmonary hypertension develops, which can eventually lead to left- and right-sided heart failure. A gradient of more than 15 to 20 mm Hg (ie, left atrial diastolic pressure is higher than left ventricular diastolic pressure) means that severe mitral stenosis exists. As a result of this pathophysiology, patients with mitral stenosis present with fatigue, exertional dyspnea, orthopnea, and even pulmonary edema. Left atrial dilation causes atrial fibrillation in 40% to 50% of affected patients. Patients with critical mitral stenosis may be candidates for surgery or balloon valvuloplasty (see also Chapter 18).[3]

**MITRAL INSUFFICIENCY.** Mitral insufficiency or regurgitation (see Fig. 22-3B) can occur acutely or develop over a period of time. Chronic mitral insufficiency may result from rheumatic heart disease, degenerative changes associated with aging, or left ventricular dilation. The basic valve dysfunction is caused by thickening or stretching of the leaflets, resulting in backward blood flow. During ventricular systole, some of the left ventricular blood regurgitates into the atrium rather than being ejected through the aortic valve. This regurgitation decreases the forward cardiac output. Left ventricular hypertrophy occurs in an attempt to improve the cardiac output, but the hypertrophy can actually worsen the regurgitation. Left ventricular volume overload causes left ventricular dilation. Regurgitant flow into the left atrium causes increased left atrial pressure and dilation. This volume overload can be reflected backward to the pulmonary circulation; however, pulmonary and right-sided heart symptoms usually do not develop until late in the disease process. As a

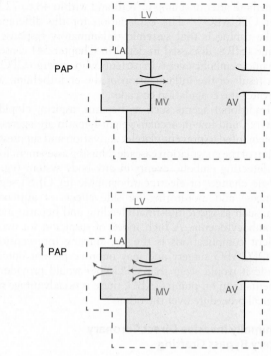

**FIGURE 22-3** Mitral valve dysfunction. **A:** Mitral stenosis. **B:** Mitral insufficiency. AV, aortic valve; LA, left atrium; LV, left ventricle; MV, mitral valve; PAP, pulmonary artery pressure.

result of this pathophysiology, patients with chronic mitral insufficiency commonly present with fatigue, palpitations, and shortness of breath.

Acute mitral insufficiency may result from endocarditis, chest trauma, or myocardial infarction (MI). Endocarditis erodes or perforates the valve leaflets or chordae. Trauma may rupture the chordae. MI may cause papillary muscle rupture, allowing blood to flow backward into the left atrium during ventricular systole. Because of the acute nature of the valve dysfunction, there is inadequate time for dilation or hypertrophy to compensate. In acute mitral insufficiency, cardiac output decreases dramatically, cascading into pulmonary edema and shock. The treatment of choice for hemodynamically significant acute mitral regurgitation is emergent mitral valve replacement.

**AORTIC STENOSIS.** Aortic stenosis may develop as a result of rheumatic fever or calcification of a congenital bicuspid valve; it may also be due to calcific degeneration, especially in elderly patients. The resultant fusion of the commissures and fibrous contractures of the cusps leads to a decreased valve area size and obstruction of left ventricular outflow. Forward cardiac output is diminished, and the left ventricle hypertrophies to maintain the cardiac output. As the stenosis worsens, compensation fails, and volume and pressure overload in the left ventricle causes left ventricular dilation. Increased left ventricular pressures are reflected backward through the left atrium and pulmonary vasculature (Fig. 22-4A).

Diminished cardiac output in the person with aortic stenosis may lead to two major problems: angina and syncope. Extreme left ventricular hypertrophy decreases ventricular cavity volume and filling and increases myocardial oxygen demand at the same time that cardiac output and coronary artery perfusion are decreased. Ischemic myocardium develops, which may lead to angina. Syncope occurs in the late stages of aortic stenosis, when the forward cardiac output cannot increase to meet the body's demands. As a person with severe aortic stenosis exercises, the blood vessels to the skeletal muscles dilate to increase the blood supply. The normal response to this increased demand is increased cardiac output. However, the person with aortic stenosis is unable to respond in such a way. The vasodilation without a concomitant increase in cardiac output results in insufficient cerebral perfusion and syncope. Patients with aortic stenosis also experience exertional dyspnea, orthopnea, and paroxysmal nocturnal dyspnea. Perfusion to all areas of the body decreases as the person experiences decreasing cardiac output. Fatigue becomes more advanced with minimal exertion. Also, renal perfusion becomes compromised, which may result in a decreased urine response to diuretics, and laboratory evaluation of renal function can show increased BUN and creatinine.

**AORTIC INSUFFICIENCY.** Aortic insufficiency, like mitral insufficiency, can occur acutely or develop over a period of time. Chronic aortic insufficiency is commonly caused by rheumatic fever and aneurysm of the ascending aorta. Rheumatic disease results in thickened and retracted valve cusps, whereas aortic aneurysm causes annular dilation. Both conditions prevent the edges of the valve leaflets from approximating, allowing blood to regurgitate backward from the aorta into the left ventricle during ventricular diastole. Cardiac output decreases, and left ventricular volume and pressure increase; left ventricular hypertrophy ensues. Eventually, the increase in left ventricular pressure is reflected backward into the left atrium and pulmonary circulation (see Fig. 22-4B).

Patients with chronic aortic insufficiency present with fatigue, and they have a low diastolic blood pressure and a widened pulse pressure. The pulse may rise rapidly and collapse suddenly (water-hammer or Corrigan pulse) because of the forceful ventricular contraction and subsequent diastolic regurgitation from the aortic root into the left ventricle. Angina may occur, because aortic insufficiency creates an imbalance between left ventricular myocardial oxygen supply and demand: as left ventricular hypertrophy worsens, the oxygen demand increases, but regurgitant flow from the aortic root during diastole decreases coronary artery perfusion.

Acute aortic insufficiency may be caused by blunt chest trauma, ruptured ascending aortic aneurysm, or infective endocarditis. Left-sided heart failure and pulmonary edema develop rapidly in the patient with acute aortic insufficiency because compensatory left ventricular hypertrophy does not have time to develop. In response to the diminished cardiac output, systemic vascular resistance (SVR) increases to maintain the blood pressure. The elevated SVR increases the degree of regurgitation and worsens the situation.

### Surgical Treatment

Surgical intervention for valvular disease consists of either valve reconstruction or valve replacement. The goals of valvular surgery are to relieve symptoms and restore normal hemodynamics. Surgery is indicated before left ventricular function deteriorates significantly and the patient's activity

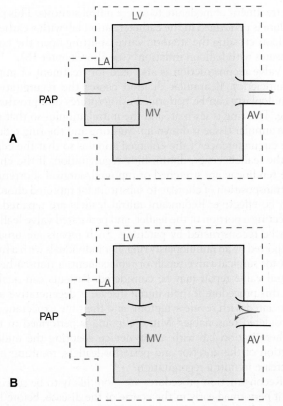

**FIGURE 22-4** Aortic valve dysfunction. **A:** Aortic stenosis. **B:** Aortic insufficiency. AV, aortic valve; LA, left atrium; LV, left ventricle; MV, mitral valve; PAP, pulmonary artery pressure.

becomes severely limited or before severe signs and symptoms, such as angina or syncope from aortic stenosis or pulmonary hypertension from mitral stenosis, develop. Percutaneous balloon valvuloplasty and transcatheter aortic valve replacement (TAVR) are procedures that are indicated primarily for patients considered too high risk for surgery (see Chapter 18). TAVR is performed in a hybrid catheterization lab and operating suite using catheters and valve delivery performed off bypass through the blood vessels or alternate access sites.[5]

**VALVE RECONSTRUCTION.** Continuous transesophageal echocardiography is used to assess the effectiveness of repair during surgery. Most valve reconstruction procedures are performed on the mitral valve. Reconstruction eliminates the need for long-term anticoagulation, decreases the risks for thromboembolism and endocarditis, decreases the need for reoperation, and increases survival rates. However, for aortic valve disorders, most attempts at reconstruction have not been successful because of late insufficiency and restenosis.

A common reconstruction technique for mitral stenosis is surgical commissurotomy. Although not indicated for patients with severe mitral stenosis, commissurotomy may be effective for patients with moderate stenosis with minimal calcification and regurgitation.[5] During commissurotomy, the fused commissures are surgically divided. Calcified tissue is debrided and fused, and shortened chordae are incised. This procedure decreases the degree of stenosis by improving leaflet mobility and increases the mitral valve area. Percutaneous mitral balloon commissurotomy is also recommended for treatment of moderate to severe mitral stenosis. This procedure is performed in the catheterization lab with a catheter balloon crossing the stenotic valve, splitting open the commissures with balloon inflation[5] (see also Chapter 18).

Valve reconstruction is also used for treatment of mitral insufficiency. If annular dilation causes the regurgitation, annuloplasty can be performed using sutures or a prosthetic ring. The ring is sewn around the mitral annulus so that excess annular tissue is drawn up. Suturing and the ring reduce the circumference of the enlarged annulus so that the edges of the leaflets coapt, diminishing regurgitation. If the chordae tendineae are stretched or ruptured, surgical shortening or transposition of chordae to substitute for ruptured chordae can be effective. Redundant mitral leaflets are repaired by resecting a portion of the leaflet, and perforated valve leaflets can be reconstructed by patching. Such repairs are usually supported by an annuloplasty ring. For individuals with a high risk for surgical valve repair or replacement, a transcatheter mitral valve repair may be considered. Patients can qualify for this procedure if their mitral disease is degenerative and associated with severe symptoms and their life expectancy is considered reasonable.[5] Mitral clipping is performed in the catheterization lab with a clip device coapting the middle portion of the anterior and posterior leaflets, resulting in a decrease in mitral regurgitation.

Reconstruction procedures are more likely to be successful if performed early in the course of the disease, before left ventricular function deteriorates and irreparable damage occurs. Anticoagulation is not usually needed after valve repair unless an annuloplasty ring is used. In such cases, anticoagulants are given for only 3 months until the ring is endothelialized. If reconstruction cannot be accomplished, valves are replaced.[5]

**VALVE REPLACEMENT.** Valve replacement surgery is done through a median sternotomy incision; cardiopulmonary bypass and myocardial preservation techniques (discussed in detail later in this chapter) are used. Transcatheter valve replacement options continue to be studied, with ongoing research on expanding this option to individuals with lower and moderate surgical risk profiles.[5]

The mitral valve is approached through the left atrium. Rather than excising the native valve, the chordae and papillary muscles are preserved when the prosthetic valve is sutured in place; this technique helps maintain left ventricular function and ejection fraction. The aortic valve is approached through the ascending aorta; the native aortic valve is excised, the annulus is sized, and the prosthetic valve is sutured to the annulus.

Ideally, a prosthetic valve would be durable, last for a patient's life, and perform exactly like a normal human valve. The valve would have normal hemodynamics with unimpeded, nonturbulent blood flow through a central opening, no transvalvular gradient, and no regurgitation when closed. It would be nonthrombogenic and not damaging to blood components, and acceptable to the patient in terms of noise and the need for anticoagulation. Unfortunately, no artificial valve currently meets these criteria, so research continues.

**Choosing a Valve.** The first valve replacement was performed with a caged ball prosthesis. Many new prosthetic valve designs have evolved. Two major types of prosthetic valves are available: biologic and mechanical. Mechanical valves are made entirely of synthetic materials, whereas biologic valves combine synthetic materials with chemically treated biologic tissues. When choosing an appropriate valve for a patient, it is necessary to compare the advantages and disadvantages of the various valve types. The advantages and disadvantages of prosthetic cardiac valves are listed in Box 22-1.

Patients with a long life expectancy may receive mechanical valves because they are particularly durable. However, the patient's lifestyle and occupation must be taken into consideration, because a mechanical valve may increase the risk of bleeding in the setting of chronic anticoagulation.[5] Biologic valves studied at autopsy have shown structural deterioration beginning as early as 6 years after implantation, and their total useful lifetime is usually considered to be less than 10 years.

**Biologic Valves.** Older patients may receive biologic valves because less calcification and deterioration occur in older people, long-term durability is less important, and the risk of anticoagulation may increase with advancing age. Biologic valves are indicated for patients who are unable to comply with an anticoagulation regimen, for those in whom a long-term anticoagulation regimen is contraindicated, and for women of childbearing age who plan to become pregnant (the anticoagulant warfarin crosses the placental barrier).[5]

**Mechanical Valves.** Mechanical valves include the caged ball, tilting disk, and bileaflet designs. The caged ball valve consists of a plastic or metal ball inside of a metal cage attached to a sewing ring. When pressure behind the valve increases, the ball is forced down into the cage, and blood flows around it. When pressure in front of the valve increases, the ball is forced upward against the sewing ring, preventing regurgitant flow.

Hemodynamically, the ball in the cage produces a central obstruction to blood flow, which can result in a small stenotic pressure gradient, and ventricular outflow may be partially obstructed because of the cage's size and high profile. Because of the thrombogenicity of the plastic and metal and the turbulent flow around the ball and through the cage, blood clots can form on or around the valve. Clotting is also a concern with the tilting disk design.

---

**BOX 22-1** | **Advantages and Disadvantages of Prosthetic Cardiac Valves**

**Mechanical Valves**
- Good long-term durability
- Adequate hemodynamics
- High risk for thromboembolism; necessity for long-term anticoagulation
- Increased risk for anticoagulation related bleeding

**Biologic Valves**
- Limited long-term durability
- Better hemodynamics than mechanical valves (except in small sizes)
- No hemolysis
- Low incidence of thromboembolism; possibly no necessity for anticoagulation
- Decreased bleeding events

The tilting disk and bileaflet tilting disk valves consist of one to two semicircular disks or leaflets hinged to a sewing ring (see Fig. 22-5). When the pressure behind the valve increases, the leaflets open perpendicular to the sewing ring, and blood flows through the central opening with minimal obstruction. When pressure in front of the valve increases, the leaflets return to their flat position against the sewing ring, preventing insufficiency. The tilting disk valves have good hemodynamic characteristics and durability.

**Biologic Prostheses.** Biologic prostheses, or tissue valves, offer another alternative for valve replacement (Fig. 22-6). The porcine heterograft is constructed of an excised pig aortic valve preserved in glutaraldehyde and mounted on a frame attached to a sewing ring. Biologic prostheses provide good hemodynamics, except in smaller sizes, where obstruction to flow can occur and a gradient can develop. Their main advantage is a lower risk for thromboembolism compared with mechanical valves. Because most thromboembolic events occur during the first 3 months after implantation, before the sewing ring is endothelialized, most patients with biologic valves receive anticoagulants during that time only. However, the decision regarding anticoagulation must be based on the patient's condition and other risks for thromboembolism. Patients in chronic atrial fibrillation who undergo mitral valve replacement will frequently receive long-term anticoagulation therapy even with a biologic prosthesis because of stagnant blood flow in the atria, a condition that may lead to clot formation.

## Cardiac Surgery

When caring for patients undergoing cardiac surgery, the unique challenge for the critical care nurse is to integrate theoretical knowledge, assessment skills, and problem-solving ability to provide optimal nursing care and maintain high-quality outcomes while decreasing resource consumption, yet always keeping the patient as the focus.

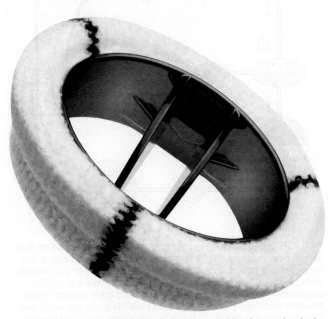

FIGURE 22-5   Open pivot valve is an example of a mechanical valve. (Courtesy of Medtronic, Inc.)

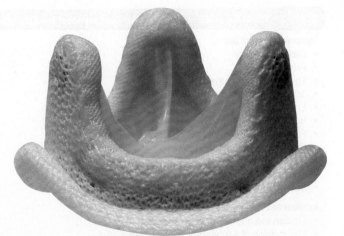

FIGURE 22-6   Hancock II bioprosthetic valve is an example of a biologic valve. (Courtesy of Medtronic, Inc.)

## Preoperative Phase

Preoperative preparation for cardiac surgery includes physiological and psychological components. The physiologic preparation is similar to that for any preoperative patient and includes history, physical examination, chest radiography, and an ECG. The history and physical examination are extremely important; they can provide information about previous neurologic status, current medications, and any other coexisting conditions (eg, diabetes mellitus, pulmonary disease, renal disease). The chest radiograph can give the surgeon general information about aortic calcification, and the ECG provides baseline information about the patient's heart rhythm. Laboratory tests include complete blood count (CBC), electrolytes, prothrombin time (PT), partial thromboplastin time (PTT), blood urea nitrogen (BUN), and creatinine. Pulmonary function tests and arterial blood gas (ABG) analyses may be performed if a patient has underlying pulmonary problems.

Effective preoperative teaching, which reduces anxiety and physiologic responses to stress before and after surgery, is an important aspect of psychological preparation. The surgical procedure and the intraoperative and postoperative experiences are explained. A tour of the ICU helps familiarize the patient and family with the specialized equipment and environment. The sight of a patient who is successfully recovering from cardiac surgery helps instill confidence and allay anxiety. Incorporating family members or significant others in the education process is pivotal in patient care. Specific teaching topics related to the patient's stay in the ICU are listed in Box 22-2.

## Intraoperative Phase

### Surgical Approach

The surgical approach most commonly used for myocardial revascularization and valve surgery is median sternotomy. The sternum is split with a sternal saw from the manubrium to below the xiphoid process, and the ribs are spread to expose the anterior mediastinum and pericardium. If the mediastinal approach is used in a reoperation for CABG surgery,

**Equipment to Point Out**
- Cardiac monitor
- Arterial line
- Thermodilution catheter
- IV lines and IV infusion pumps
- Endotracheal tube and ventilator
- Suctioning
- Foley catheter (increased sensation to urinate)
- Chest tubes (anticipated removal)
- Pacing wires
- Nasogastric tube
- Soft hand restraints

**Incisions and Dressings to Expect**
- Median sternotomy or other incision
- Leg incision (if saphenous vein is used)

**Patient's Immediate Postoperative Appearance**
- Skin yellow from use of Betadine solution in operating room
- Skin pale and cool to touch because of hypothermia during surgery
- Generalized "puffiness," especially noticeable in neck, face, and hands because of third spacing of fluid given during cardiopulmonary bypass

**Awakening From Anesthesia**
- Explain how to communicate when intubated; unable to talk
- Explain when extubation can be anticipated
- Patient recovers in the intensive care unit (ICU); does not go to the postanesthesia care unit (PACU)

- Each patient recovers from anesthesia differently
- Patient may feel certain sensations
- Patient may hear certain noises
- Patient may be aware or able to hear but unable to respond

**Discomfort**
- Amount of discomfort to be expected
- When pain might be expected
- Relief mechanisms
- Positioning/splinting
- Medications
- Patient-controlled analgesia (PCA) and the importance of early administration of pain medication

**Postoperative Respiratory Care**
- Turning
- Use of pillow to splint median sternotomy incision
- Effective coughing and deep breathing after extubation; have patient practice exercises before surgery
- Incentive spirometry
- Early mobilization

**Miscellaneous**
- Postoperative activity progression
- Hospital visiting policy in intensive care area
- Avoiding use of arms to protect stability of sternotomy

---

injury to old bypass grafts or embolization of debris resulting from manipulation of diseased grafts may cause problems.[6] Hybrid stent-bypass grafting procedures may decrease the need for a redo sternotomy and risks of vessel injury and other complications.[2]

Additionally, adhesions along the incision line make redo procedures more technically difficult and alter the stability of the tissue when attempting to close the incision at the end of the surgery. As myocardial revascularization has become increasingly sophisticated, new interventions to minimize the invasive nature of the surgery have been developed. A smaller lateral thoracotomy incision may be used to decrease the risks associated with reentry into the mediastinum. The choice of incision is based on the specific needs of each patient and the experience of the surgeon.

## Cardiopulmonary Bypass

Cardiac surgery as it is known today was made possible by the development and practical application of cardiopulmonary bypass procedure by Gibbon in 1953.[3,7] Because the heart must be still (not beating) and empty during the surgery, a cardiopulmonary bypass machine is used, unless OPCABG surgery is to be performed. The patient's deoxygenated venous blood is brought to the pump either through one cannula placed in the right atrial appendage or by two cannulas, one of which is placed directly in the inferior vena cava and the other directly in the superior vena cava. Another cannula is placed in the ascending aorta to return oxygenated blood to the patient's systemic circulation (Fig. 22-7). Heparin is administered throughout cardiopulmonary bypass to prevent massive extravascular coagulation as the blood circulates through the mechanical parts of the bypass system. During

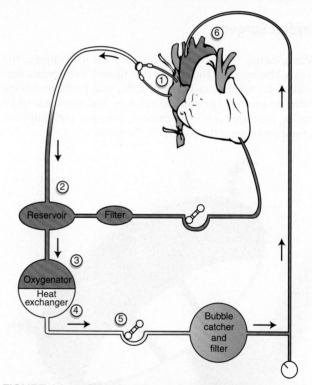

**FIGURE 22-7**   Blood flow through the circuit of the cardiopulmonary bypass machine: (1) Patient's deoxygenated blood enters the bypass circuit from the venous cannulas in the superior and inferior vena cavae. (2) The reservoir holds the blood temporarily. (3) The oxygenator removes carbon dioxide from and adds oxygen to the patient's blood. (4) The heat exchanger initially cools the blood and then rewarms the blood. (5) Roller pumps pump the blood through the circuit and back to the patient. (6) Oxygenated blood is returned to the ascending aorta by way of the aortic cannula.

bypass, the patient's core body temperature is lowered to 28° to 32°C (82.4° to 89.6°F) to decrease metabolism. This reduction in metabolic demands helps protect the major organ systems from possible ischemic injury and the adverse effects of nonpulsatile perfusion during cardiopulmonary bypass.[2,7]

Oxygenated blood is filtered and returned to the patient's ascending aorta through the arterial cannula (see Fig. 22-6). Once extracorporeal circulation is established and systemic hypothermia is achieved, the aorta is cross-clamped just above the coronary arteries, and either crystalloid or blood cardioplegia solution is infused into the aortic root. After the aorta is cross-clamped, no blood circulates through the coronary arteries, so the myocardium becomes ischemic. Cold cardioplegia solution at 4°C (39.2°F) is infused into the aortic root under pressure. As it circulates through the coronary arteries, the high potassium concentration causes immediate asystole and relaxation, and the cold produces myocardial hypothermia. Asystole and hypothermia protect against myocardial ischemia by decreasing the metabolic needs of myocardial tissue.[7] The inclusion of blood or oxygenated crystalloid in the cardioplegia solution lessens myocardial ischemia by supplying oxygen. Cardioplegia solution may be infused into the aortic root continuously or intermittently every 15 to 30 minutes and whenever cardiac electrical activity recurs.

Hypothermia is also created topically by pouring iced normal saline slush solution over the heart into the pericardial well. Several disadvantages to cold cardioplegia have been identified, including postoperative myocardial depression, ventricular dysrhythmias, decreased cerebral blood flow, irreversible platelet dysfunction, and shifts of the oxygen–hemoglobin dissociation so that blood delivers oxygen to the tissues less readily. A heart receiving cold crystalloid cardioplegia must have blood reintroduced into the coronary circulation (reperfusion). This reintroduction of oxygen may cause release of toxic substances that injure myocardial cells (reperfusion injury). To avoid these disadvantages, some cardiac surgeons use normothermic blood cardioplegia delivered at 37°C (98.6°F), which keeps the heart at a normal temperature. Patients who have undergone warm cardioplegia require less time on the ventilator and almost no rewarming technology in the ICU. This process varies, depending on the surgeon's preference.

After surgery is completed, the heat exchanger rewarms the blood to return the patient's core temperature to 37°C (98.6°F) if hypothermic techniques were used. After air is vented from the heart chambers and the aortic root, the aortic cross-clamp is removed so that blood again perfuses the coronary arteries, warming the myocardium. As perfusion and rewarming continue, a spontaneous cardiac rhythm may resume, ventricular fibrillation may develop (necessitating internal defibrillation), or pacing may be used to initiate a rhythm. After a reliable rhythm with a rate adequate to maintain the cardiac output and blood pressure is established, the patient is weaned from total cardiopulmonary bypass, and the cannulas are removed from the right atrium and aorta. Heparinization is reversed by the administration of protamine sulfate. If adequate cardiac output cannot be maintained during the weaning process, positive inotropic agents or intra-aortic balloon counterpulsation can be instituted.[1,7] (See Chapter 18 for more information about care of the patient on the intra-aortic balloon pump [IABP].)

## Completion of Surgery

If the need for postoperative cardiac pacing is anticipated, temporary pacing electrodes are placed on the epicardial surface of the heart and brought out through the chest wall on either side of the median sternotomy incision. Ventricular pacing electrodes are typically located to the left and atrial wires to the right of the sternum (Fig. 22-8) (see Chapter 18).

Chest tubes placed in the mediastinum and pericardial space for drainage are brought out through incision sites just below the median sternotomy. If the pleural space has been entered, pleural tubes are also placed. Once adequate hemostasis is obtained, the edges of the sternum are approximated with stainless steel wires, the incision is closed, and dressings are applied.

## Postoperative Phase

Patients are transported directly to the ICU, where they recover from anesthesia and usually remain for 24 hours after surgery. Patients arrive in the ICU with numerous lines and tubes (eg, endotracheal tube, hemodynamic monitoring lines). Immediate postoperative care involves cardiac monitoring and maintenance of oxygenation and hemodynamic stability, as described in Box 22-3.[1] Because cardiopulmonary bypass produces abnormal blood interface and altered blood flow patterns, it has profound physiologic effects (Table 22-2).

The postoperative course depends on the patient's preoperative condition. Factors that may increase mortality include age, male or female gender, previous sternotomy or heart surgery, preoperative occurrence of acute MI, and concomitant conditions such as diabetes mellitus, peripheral vascular disease, renal insufficiency, and chronic obstructive pulmonary disease (COPD).[1] Whether the surgery is elective or emergent may also influence outcome. Awareness of these conditions helps the critical care nurse anticipate problems. Accurate assessments, vigilant monitoring, and proper

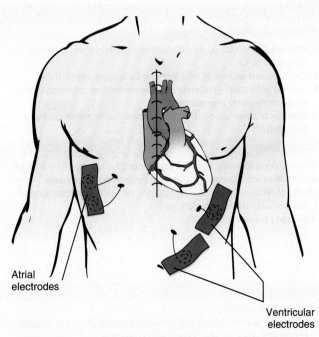

Atrial electrodes

Ventricular electrodes

FIGURE 22-8 Temporary epicardial pacing wires: position of atrial and ventricular wires on chest wall.

**BOX 22-3** Nursing Responsibilities in Caring for the Cardiac Surgery Patient in the Immediate Postoperative Period

**Priority Interventions Performed by the Critical Care Team on Arrival**

- Attach patient to bedside cardiac monitor and note rhythm.
- Attach pressure lines to bedside monitor (arterial and pulmonary artery); level and zero transducers and note pressure values and waveforms.
- Obtain cardiac output/index and note existing inotropic or vasoactive drips.
- After ventilator is connected to endotracheal tube, auscultate breath sounds bilaterally.
- Apply end-tidal carbon dioxide (ETCO$_2$) device to ventilator circuit and note waveform and value (best indicator of endotracheal tube placement).
- Apply pulse oximetry device to patient and note SpO$_2$ value and waveform.
- Check peripheral pulses and perfusion signs.
- Monitor chest tubes and character of drainage: amount, color, flow. Check for air leaks.
- Measure body temperature and initiate rewarming if temperature is less than 96.8°F (36°C).

**Once the Patient is Determined to be Hemodynamically Stable**

- Measure urine output and note characteristics.
- Obtain clinical data (within 30 minutes of arrival).
- Obtain chest radiograph.
- Obtain 12-lead ECG.
- Obtain routine blood work within 15 minutes of arrival; tests may include ABGs, potassium, glucose, PTT, and hemoglobin (varies with institution).
- Assess neurologic status.
- Test pacemaker function by assessing capture and sensing.

Data from South T: Coronary artery bypass surgery. Crit Care Nurs Clin North Am 23:573–585, 2011.

interventions are critical in stabilizing patients who have just undergone cardiac surgery.[2] Box 22-4 on page 404 presents a collaborative care guide for the patient after such surgery. Certain patient populations present special problems. Box 22-5 on page 406 lists factors to consider in managing older cardiac patients.

### Prevention of Hypothermia

Whether the cardiac procedure is performed on or off the cardiopulmonary bypass system, hypothermia is a common side effect. During rewarming on cardiopulmonary bypass, the patient's core temperature is returned to 98.6°F (37°C); however, as this warmed blood begins to circulate to the periphery, heat transfer to the surrounding tissues again causes the core temperature to decline. Patients frequently enter the ICU with a temperature in the 95° to 96.8°F (35° to 36°C) range. OPCABG surgery causes hypothermia because of heat loss secondary to prolonged exposure to cool operating room temperatures. Hypothermia causes peripheral vasoconstriction and a shift of the oxygen–hemoglobin dissociation curve to the left, which means that less oxygen is released from the hemoglobin to the tissues. Hypothermia can also impair coagulation because all enzyme systems in the body depend on a tight temperature range for optimal performance.[2,3,7]

The nurse assesses the patient's temperature on ICU admission using pulmonary artery or tympanic membrane temperature for the most accurate measurement. Increasing the room temperature and using radiant heat, blankets, or a warming blanket are effective techniques for increasing core temperature. Rewarming should occur slowly to prevent hemodynamic instability caused by rapid vasodilation.

It is important to prevent shivering, which occurs most often from 90 to 180 minutes after ICU admission. Shivering increases metabolic rate, oxygen consumption, carbon

**TABLE 22-2** Effects of Cardiopulmonary Bypass

| Effects | Clinical Implications |
|---|---|
| **Increased Capillary Permeability** | |
| Interface between blood and nonphysiologic surfaces or bypass circuit leads to<br>• Complement activation that increases capillary permeability<br>• Platelet activation—platelets secrete vasoactive substances that increase capillary permeability<br>• Release of other vasoactive substances that increase capillary permeability | Large amounts of fluid move from the intravascular to the interstitial space during and up to 6 h after cardiopulmonary bypass.<br>Patient becomes edematous. |
| **Hemodilution** | |
| Solution used to prime extracorporeal circuit dilutes patient's blood.<br>Secretion of vasopressin (antidiuretic hormone) is increased.<br>Levels of renin–angiotensin–aldosterone are increased because of nonpulsatile renal perfusion.<br>Total body water is increased. | Decreased blood viscosity improves capillary perfusion during nonpulsatile flow and hypothermia.<br>Hgb and Hct decrease.<br>Levels of coagulation factors are decreased because of dilution.<br>Intravascular colloid osmotic pressure is decreased, contributing to movement of fluid from intravascular to interstitial spaces.<br>Water is retained at collecting tubule of kidney.<br>Aldosterone causes retention of sodium and water at renal tubule.<br>Weight gain occurs. |
| **Altered Coagulation** | |
| Procoagulant effects:<br>• Interface between blood and nonendothelial surfaces of bypass circuit activates intrinsic coagulation cascade.<br>• Platelet damage activates intrinsic pathway. | Risk for microemboli is increased.<br>Platelet count decreases by 50%–70% of baseline.<br>Abnormal postoperative bleeding occurs.<br>Possibility of bleeding diathesis exists. |

| TABLE 22-2 Effects of Cardiopulmonary Bypass (*continued*) | |
|---|---|
| **Effects** | **Clinical Implications** |
| Anticoagulant effects:<br>• Interface between blood and nonendothelial surfaces of bypass circuit causes platelets to adhere to tubing and to clump; abnormal platelet function; activation of coagulation cascade, which depletes clotting factors; denaturation of plasma proteins, including coagulation factors.<br>• Coagulation factors are decreased as a result of hemodilution. | |
| **Damage to Blood Cells** | |
| Exposure of blood to nonendothelial surfaces causes mechanical trauma and shear stress.<br>• Platelet damage occurs.<br>• Red blood cell hemolysis occur<br>• Leukocytes are damaged. | Platelet count is decreased.<br>Free hemoglobin and hemoglobinuria are increased.<br>Hct is decreased<br>Immune response is diminished. |
| **Microembolization** | |
| Emboli form from tissue debris, air bubbles, platelet aggregation. | Microemboli to body organs (brain, lungs, kidney) are possible. |
| **Increased Systemic Vascular Resistance (SVR)** | |
| Catecholamine secretion is increased when cardiopulmonary bypass is initiated.<br>Renin secretion is due to nonpulsatile flow to kidney.<br>Hypothermia develops. | Hypertension is possible.<br>Increased SVR may decrease cardiac output. |

dioxide production, and myocardial workload. If left ventricular function is compromised, shivering should be managed with a neuromuscular blocker in combination with simultaneous sedation to avoid further cardiac compromise.

After rewarming, many patients experience an overshoot in body temperature. Narcotics and anesthetics administered during surgery may reset the hypothalamic regulatory center, altering peripheral blood flow and feedback.[2] A cold, constricted peripheral vascular bed may also be a factor in preventing heat dissipation. If the patient is bleeding after surgery, correction of temperature is imperative to aid in the return of normal coagulation enzyme function and clotting ability.[3]

### Monitoring for Systemic Inflammatory Response Syndrome

Any infectious or noninfectious insult to the body, including surgery, initiates the SIRS. An entire "body" inflammatory response may occur after CABG surgery, with symptoms that are similar to those of infectious processes. Symptoms and signs include fever, tachycardia, tachypnea, and an increased white blood cell count.

SIRS is a natural defense mechanism that is initiated when tissue or vessels are injured. A vascular injury, the inflammatory response, and the coagulation cascade are interrelated. An event that disrupts the integrity of the endothelium, such as trauma from cutting the vessel or hypoxia in a few endothelial cells, triggers the process. As a result of the endothelial damage, increased capillary permeability inevitably occurs.[2] Once the injury occurs, a local inflammatory reaction begins with the release of mediators called cytokines from "protector" cells (eg, lymphocytes, macrophages). These cytokines signal other cells (eg, neutrophils, monocytes) to move to the injured area, and these cells release other mediators. The endothelium then releases vasodilating mediators (eg, nitric oxide), which increase blood flow to the area, thereby increasing oxygen delivery. Counter-regulatory mediators cause vasoconstriction to balance vasodilatory actions. Platelets are attracted to the area to start coagulation. Nursing responsibilities focus on refining assessment skills to increase early detection of embolic events in any system, especially the nervous, cardiovascular, pulmonary, and renal systems.

Both on-pump and off-pump CABG initiate an SIRS response. Few interventions limit SIRS; the inflammatory process is so complex that it has been difficult to develop medications to counter all the numerous reactions. Steroids have been shown to decrease SIRS somewhat if given before surgery, but they should be used with caution, especially in patients with diabetes mellitus.[1] (See Chapter 54 for more detail on SIRS.)

### Controlling Pain

After cardiac surgery, the patient may experience pain resulting from the chest or leg incision, the chest tubes, rib spreading during surgery, and care activities. The ICU environment may accentuate the pain physiologically because of light and noise as well as psychologically because of separation and fear. Pain often stimulates the sympathetic nervous system, increasing heart rate and blood pressure, which can be detrimental to the patient's hemodynamic status. Discomfort can also result in diminished chest expansion, increased atelectasis, and retention of secretions.

Although pain perception varies from person to person, a median sternotomy incision is usually less painful than a thoracotomy incision, and most people report that the pain is most severe the first 3 to 4 days after surgery. Discomfort from the leg incision often worsens after the patient is ambulatory, especially if leg swelling occurs. Stretching of back and neck muscles as the ribs are spread and immobilization for several hours during surgery can cause back and neck discomfort. Patients who have internal mammary artery grafts may

**QSEN** BOX 22-4 *COLLABORATIVE CARE GUIDE for the Patient With DIC*

| Outcomes | Interventions |
|---|---|
| **Impaired Gas Exchange** | |
| Patient will have ABG values within normal limits and pulse oximeter value >92%. Pulmonary edema will be minimized on chest x-ray and demonstrated by improved breath sounds. | • Obtain ABG levels per protocol.<br>• Correlate pulse oximeter and end-tidal $CO_2$ with ABG results.<br>• Adjust ventilator settings after consulting with the respiratory therapist and physician.<br>• Wean from mechanical ventilation per protocol using the expertise of respiratory therapy.<br>• Extubate when patient is hemodynamically stable; able to protect airway.<br>• Provide supplemental oxygen after extubation. |
| Atelectasis will improve. | • Encourage use of incentive spirometer, cough, and deep breathe every 2–4 h after extubation.<br>• Encourage early, frequent ambulation for diaphragm expansion<br>• Minimize narcotic medications to prevent respiratory depression and sedation |
| Chest tubes will remain patent. | • Milk chest tubes if necessary to facilitate forward drainage movement. |
| **Decreased Cardiac Output**<br>**Ineffective Peripheral Tissue Perfusion** | |
| Patient will maintain adequate clinical perfusion.<br>Vital signs will be within normal limits, including MAP more than 70 mm Hg; cardiac index will be in a suitable range for the patient's left ventricular function. | • Monitor pulmonary artery pressure (PAP) and PAOP, CVP, cardiac output, SVR, and pulmonary vascular resistance (PVR) per protocol if pulmonary artery catheter is in place.<br>• Monitor ECG, ST segments, and arterial blood pressure continuously.<br>• Administer positive inotropic agents and reduce afterload with vasodilating agents guided by hemodynamic parameters and physician orders.<br>• Regulate volume administration as indicated by PAOP or CVP values.<br>• Evaluate effect of medications on BP, HR, and hemodynamic parameters.<br>• Monitor and treat dysrhythmias per protocol and physician orders.<br>• Anticipate need for temporary cardiac pacing; wires will be properly isolated for electrical safety.<br>• Prepare patient for IABP assist if necessary.<br>• Congestive heart failure from decreased cardiac output or perioperative MI will be minimized by collaborating with a physician.<br>• Assess for neck vein distention, pulmonary crackles, $S_3$ or $S_4$, peripheral edema, increased preload parameters, elevated "a" wave of CVP, or PAOP waveform. |
| Patient will be euthermic. | • Monitor 12-lead ECG if ECG changes are observed.<br>• Assess temperature every hour.<br>• Warm patient 1°C/h by using warming blankets, lights, and fluid warmer. |
| **Risk for Bleeding** | |
| Patient will have minimal bleeding and avoid cardiac tamponade. | • Chest tube drainage will be <200 mL/h.<br>• Monitor for signs of cardiac tamponade (hypotension, pulsus paradoxus, tachycardia, PA pressure equalization).<br>• Evaluate chest x-ray for widened mediastinum, consulting with a physician as needed.<br>• Monitor PT, PTT, CBC per protocol.<br>• Administer protamine, blood products, and other procoagulants per order or protocol.<br>• Monitor vasoactive drug need and report marked increase of drugs to physician immediately because this change may indicate possible tamponade. |
| **Risk for Imbalanced Fluid Volume**<br>**Risk for Electrolyte Imbalance** | |
| Patient will maintain or improve preoperative renal function. | • Renal function will be maintained as evidenced by urine output of approximately 0.5 mL/kg/h.<br>• Potassium will be replaced to maintain $K^+$ at 4.0 mEq/L.<br>• Monitor intake and output every 1 to 2 h.<br>• Monitor BUN, creatinine, electrolytes, magnesium, $PO_4$.<br>• Record daily weights.<br>• Administer fluid volume or diuretics as ordered. |

**BOX 22-4** *COLLABORATIVE CARE GUIDE for the Patient With DIC (continued)*

| Outcomes | Interventions |
|---|---|
| **Impaired Physical Mobility**<br>**Risk for Activity Intolerance**<br>**Risk for Impaired Tissue Integrity**<br>**Risk for Infection** | |
| Patient will maintain range of motion and muscle strength and will have intact skin integrity | • Turn patient side to side every 2 h while on bed rest and evaluate skin closely.<br>• Mobilize out of bed after extubation.<br>• Progress activity to chair for meals, bathroom privileges, increased distance walking, delegating to assistive personnel as indicated.<br>• Monitor vital signs, respiratory effort during activity. |
| Incisions will heal without evidence of infection. | • Check stability of sternotomy incision daily, especially with diabetic patients.<br>• Assess sternotomy and leg incision for redness, swelling, drainage.<br>• Apply compression hose and elevate legs to reduce edema.<br>• Caloric and nutrient intake meets metabolic requirements per calculation for long-term patients.<br>• Monitor prealbumin for trends on long-term patients. |
| **Impaired Comfort** | |
| Patient will have relief of surgical pain.<br>Patient will demonstrate no evidence of pain or anxiety such as increased heart rate, blood pressure, respiratory rate, or agitation during activity or procedures.<br>Timely administration of pain medication will be a priority. | • Assess quality, duration, location of pain. Use visual analog scale to assess pain quantity.<br>• Provide a calm environment. Provide for adequate periods of rest and sleep. |
| **Teaching/Discharge Planning** | |
| Patient and family will understand need for:<br>Tests, procedures, treatments.<br>Self-protective devices as indicated and per hospital policy.<br>In preparation for discharge to home, patient will understand activity levels, dietary restrictions, medication regimen, incision care. | • Consult nutritional support services.<br>• Make appropriate social work referrals early during hospitalization.<br>• Initiate family education regarding heart-healthy diet, physical activity limitations (eg, lifting over 10–15 pounds and driving restrictions), stress reduction strategies, management of pain, incision care. |

have increased pain because of increased stretching of the intercostal muscles and the incision into the parietal pleura, which is richly innervated.

Angina after CABG surgery may indicate graft failure; therefore, the nurse must be able to differentiate angina from incisional pain. Typical median sternotomy pain is localized, does not radiate, and can be sharp, dull, aching, or burning. It is often worse with deep breathing, coughing, or movement. Angina is usually precordial or substernal; not well localized; and frequently radiates to arms, neck, or jaw. It is often described as a pressure sensation and is not affected by respiration or movement.

Nursing management includes a thorough assessment of the patient's pain using a pain scale; administration of analgesics based on the reported pain intensity; provision of adequate pain relief as reported by the patient; and alleviation of factors that enhance pain perception, such as anxiety and fear. The common analgesic drugs used are morphine sulfate, fentanyl, and hydromorphone (Dilaudid), as needed. These drugs can be supplemented with nonsteroidal anti-inflammatory drugs (NSAIDs), such as ketorolac (Toradol), which decrease pain through a different mechanism. Caution should be used in administering NSAIDs to patients with compromised renal function and also when platelet counts are decreased (thrombocytopenia). Patient-controlled analgesia (PCA) pumps can be

used to allow the patient to control administration of pain medication. Interventions such as intercostal nerve blocks and spinal analgesia are less common. Regardless of the mechanism used, pain control is aggressively pursued to ensure comfort and rapid mobilization, which in turn can lessen complications. Alternative therapies, such as music therapy and guided imagery, may also be useful in controlling pain.

### Preventing Cardiovascular Complications

Many cardiovascular complications can be anticipated and prevented, which can lead to decreased length of stay and better patient outcomes. Astute nursing observations and appropriate interventions can contribute to better outcomes.

**VOLUME RESUSCITATION.** Adequate intravascular volume to provide preload is a primary concern. Increased capillary permeability resulting from SIRS causes intravascular volume to shift into the interstitial spaces. To maintain optimal cardiac performance and blood pressure, proper volume resuscitation is imperative. A variety of fluids may be used, including normal saline and hyperosmolar fluids (eg, 3% saline).[8,9] No fluid is definitively recommended. If the patient is bleeding, blood products should be the fluid of choice. If the patient's blood pressure is unresponsive to moderate infusion

**Physiologic Changes**

**Cardiovascular System**
- Increased stiffness of myocardial muscle
- Increased stiffness of peripheral vasculature and decreased ability to adjust to changes in blood volume
- Replacement of cells in conduction system with collagen and elastin
- Decreasing number of pacemaker cells in the sinoatrial (SA) and atrioventricular (AV) nodes
- Decreased cardiac responsiveness to β-adrenergic stimulation

**Pulmonary System**
- Breakdown of elastin and collagen that impairs elastic recoil of lung
- Thoracic cage less compliant
- Decreased expiratory muscle strength and mucociliary clearance

**Renal System**
- Progressive loss of cortical nephrons and decrease in cortico-medullary concentration gradient
- Impaired renal concentrating ability
- Decreased clearance of medications excreted by the kidneys (may be reduced by up to 40% by 80 years of age)

**Gastrointestinal System**
- Decreased and more variable gastrointestinal absorption of medications
- Decline in liver function, resulting in decreased hepatic breakdown of medications

**Musculoskeletal System**
- Skeletal osteoporosis

**Immune System**
- Immune response may be decreased, especially if concomitant malnutrition and decrease in serum proteins

**Neurologic System**
- Decline in neurotransmitters
- Increased risk for acute confusion

**Response to Medications**
- Decreased percentage of lean body tissue
- Increased percentage of body fat
- Decrease in body water

**Clinical Effect**
- Higher filling pressures (pulmonary artery diastolic [PAD] pressure and pulmonary artery occlusion pressure [PAOP])
- Decreased ability for vasoconstriction with position change, leading to orthostatic hypotension
- SA and AV node impairment
- Cardiac output maintained by increase in stroke volume
- Slowing of renal response to dehydration
- Decreased effectiveness of fluid conservation
- Toxic medication levels or abnormally prolonged duration of action
- Sensitive to drugs with narrow therapeutic range, such as digoxin
- More intense medication effect and longer duration of action for medications broken down in liver (eg, benzodiazepines)
- As a result of decreased body water, water-soluble medications concentrated in the bloodstream, resulting in higher serum drug levels
- Fat-soluble medications stored in fat; increase in fat tissue may result in slower therapeutic response and longer duration of action as drug is released slowly from fat

**Patient Teaching**
- Accommodate sensory deficits.
  - Ensure hearing aids are in and functional.
  - Speak loudly and face patient.
  - Use large print, easy-to-read materials.
- Teach one thing at a time and ensure that patient understands before moving on.
- Start with simple and progress to more complex information.
- Teach both patient and caregiver.

Adapted from Dixon V: Effects of vascular surgery on the elderly vascular patient. J Vasc Nurs 17:86–88, 1999.

rates, usually 500 mL is infused using a pressure bag and a large-bore catheter.[7] Hemodynamic parameters, including a low central venous pressure (CVP) (less than 8 to 10 mm Hg), low pulmonary artery diastolic pressure, and low pulmonary artery occlusion pressure (PAOP) (less than 14 to 18 mm Hg), in combination with a low cardiac index (less than 2.5 L/min/m[2]), help guide interventions.[7,9] Caution should be exercised in using these numerical values as absolute goals.

The preoperative condition of the heart must be considered. If the patient has had a recent MI or poor left ventricular performance, higher pressures may be required to maintain optimal cardiac work. The patient with a hypertrophied left ventricle, especially with valvular disease, is heavily dependent on volume resuscitation.[7]

The effectiveness of all interventions must be assessed against the patient's response. The combination of weak pulses and mottled extremities may indicate hypoperfusion. Resolution of these clinical findings, as well as improved pressure values, signals the return of adequate perfusion. Continuously monitoring the appearance of the extremities and the pulses is ongoing in the postoperative recovery.[2,7,9]

**MONITORING FOR DYSRHYTHMIAS.** Dysrhythmias are a major issue after CABG surgery. The hemodynamic response to a change in cardiac rhythm dictates the speed of the intervention in patients who have undergone CABG surgery, as in all critical care patients. In emergent situations, advanced cardiac life support (ACLS) algorithms are used. Knowledge of the patient's baseline rhythm is important. The types of dysrhythmias that may occur range from premature atrial contractions to ventricular fibrillation and asystole.[1,2,9,10]

Sinus tachycardia is common and may result from many factors. Some of the more common causes are sympathomimetic drugs, SIRS, hypovolemia, fever, and pain. Prolonged periods of tachycardia may be harmful because of decreased coronary artery filling time. Sinus bradycardia may occur, but it is not anticipated, because patients are in a sympathetically responsive state; in many cases, preoperative beta blockade may be the cause.

Causes of premature atrial contractions are usually electrolyte disturbances, ischemia, infarction, or hypoperfusion. Frequent premature atrial contractions may be a precursor to atrial fibrillation and occur very commonly, especially in patients with a previous history of pulmonary or valve disease in which the atria can be distended. The simple treatment for premature atrial contractions is repletion of potassium and magnesium. Maintenance of adequate serum potassium and magnesium may minimize premature atrial contractions.[2,7,10]

Atrial fibrillation may occur after CABG surgery, and prevention is a high priority. Cardiac decompensation or cerebrovascular accidents are the major risks associated with atrial fibrillation. Atrial fibrillation develops in up to 40% of patients who have undergone open heart procedures, which has led to prophylactic treatment with beta blockers before and after surgery in most patients.[1,3] For new-onset atrial fibrillation, the goal is conversion to sinus rhythm using antiarrhythmics, especially amiodarone (Cordarone).[10] Control of the ventricular response is a goal that can be achieved using diltiazem (Cardizem). Intravenous beta blockers including metoprolol are also used and administered in small boluses. Combination antiarrhythmics may be used but should be monitored carefully. If atrial fibrillation persists or reoccurs for more than 24 hours, warfarin (Coumadin) anticoagulation for 4 weeks may be needed.[1] For atrial fibrillation lasting longer than 48 hours, cardioversion is not a goal (unless the patient has received anticoagulants) because of the risk for atrial thrombus and possible embolization. If emergent cardioversion is required in the immediate postoperative period and anticoagulation is not an option, transesophageal echocardiography may be performed to check for thrombus formation in the left atrium.

Heart block dysrhythmias occur in patients with valve surgery secondary to the edema at the surgical site, near the conduction system. Resolution of this rhythm is usually attained 48 to 72 hours after surgery once the edema decreases. Myocardial ischemia and infarction also cause the heart block. Patients who have had cardiac surgery have an advantage due to the placement of epicardial pacing wires.[2,3,11] Use of these wires allows better control of ventricular response compared with the use of drugs such as atropine and isoproterenol (Isuprel).[10,11] Atrial pacing is preferred if the atrioventricular (AV) node is intact because it allows optimal hemodynamics with an atrial contraction. If the AV node is not functioning properly, AV sequential pacing may be required. Ventricular pacing is the last choice. If pacing is required for more than 72 hours, permanent pacemaker placement should be considered, especially in patients who have had valve surgery. (See pacers in Chapter 18.)

The occurrence of tachyarrhythmias may lead to emergent situations. If the patient is hemodynamically unstable in a fast rhythm, the first intervention is cardioversion, following ACLS guidelines. If ventricular dysrhythmias develop, electrical or pharmacologic interventions are necessary. If the patient develops polymorphic-ventricular tachycardia with a noninherited or acquired prolonged QT syndrome, IV magnesium may help this problem.[10] The current ACLS guidelines recommend amiodarone for patients who are unresponsive to CPR, defibrillation, and intravenous epinephrine.[10] Use of amiodarone prevents monomorphic ventricular tachycardia and other refractory ventricular arrhythmias, especially in patients with poor left ventricular function or coronary artery disease.[10] If ventricular tachycardia deteriorates into ventricular fibrillation or other rhythms with no pulse, cardiopulmonary resuscitation should be started

immediately; medical personnel should be prepared to open the chest at the bedside to determine and correct the cause of arrest.[7,11]

**IMPROVING CARDIAC CONTRACTILITY.** Contractility may be depressed because of the exposure of the heart muscle to manipulation, temperature change, and possible hypoperfusion. The first step taken to improve performance is to ensure optimal volume resuscitation; it will quickly become clear if volume does not increase the cardiac output and index. The addition and titration of sympathomimetic drugs is a common part of the care of patients with decreased contractility. Various drugs, including epinephrine, dobutamine, and milrinone, may be used. Dopamine is another drug that can increase contractility but may cause unwanted tachycardia. The choice of drugs varies with patient condition, institution formulary, and evidence-based decision making.

As the drug of choice is added, the cause of the ventricular dysfunction should be pursued. Myocardial ischemia and infarction typically cause decreased cardiac function, but other factors may be sources of the problem. Stunned myocardium, the transient depression of left ventricular function from a temporary reduction of myocardial blood flow, may cause transient dysfunction; it is usually associated with normally functioning myocardium.[12] Hibernating myocardium is chronically impaired yet viable myocardial tissue, which results in left ventricular dysfunction at rest because of persistently hypoperfused myocardium or repeated stunning.[12] This state can lead to more chronic dysfunction. The state of the right ventricle should also be considered. If right ventricular dysfunction develops after CABG surgery, use of nitric oxide is one of the more effective interventions.[6] Cardiac biomarkers can be used in the first 24 hours after CABG surgery. Troponin is a parameter that can be monitored to determine if the patient may have sustained myocardial damage.[1,7] In more complicated cases, sampling of mixed venous blood gases/mixed venous saturation ($SvO_2$) and the arterial–venous difference in oxygen may be useful; these values are indicators of oxygen transport and consumption and can help direct therapy. Although continuous $SvO_2$ monitoring may be used in patients with severe myocardial dysfunction, it is not a standard intervention; it is costly and has not been shown to make a difference in outcomes. Mechanical factors may lead to depressed cardiac function.

The IABP is a mechanical method used to improve coronary perfusion and reduce myocardial workload.[1] (See IABP in Chapter 18.) Whatever the cause, time and support of function are usually the major factors that improve cardiac performance. However, protracted periods of time with mechanical or pharmacologic support may be the signal to consider the placement of a ventricular assist device, usually as a bridge to heart transplantation.

**CONTROLLING BLOOD PRESSURE.** A reduction in SVR and blood pressure is another clinical maneuver that can increase cardiac performance and protect the integrity of bypass grafts. If the patient has adequate blood pressure (mean arterial pressure [MAP] exceeding 70 mm Hg or systolic blood pressure over 120 mm Hg), afterload reduction should be started even if the patient is on an inotropic agent for contractility. Various agents, including nitroprusside, nitroglycerin, hydralazine, labetalol, and angiotensin-converting enzyme (ACE) inhibitors, can be used. The necessary speed of response dictates the choice of drug. For example, IV drugs, especially nitroprusside, rapidly cause a reduction in afterload. ACE inhibitors can exacerbate renal dysfunction and should be used with caution in patients with impaired renal function.

## Preventing Pulmonary Complications

Postoperative pulmonary function depends on preoperative function. If the patient has a significant pulmonary history (eg, COPD, pulmonary hypertension), baseline pulmonary function tests and ABG values can be very helpful in setting goals in the postoperative period. These tests may help predict how the patient will respond to mechanical ventilation.

The causes of pulmonary dysfunction after cardiac surgery can be attributed to changes that occur with the inflammatory response. Various triggers, such as surgical trauma and regional myocardial ischemia, activate the complement system and release cytokines, leading to an egress of neutrophils and fluid across endothelium. These triggers can also cause end-organ dysfunction, including organs such as the lungs.[2,7,13] Such changes in the lungs can lead to alterations in microcirculation and gas exchange that ultimately result in ventilation–perfusion mismatching, shunting, and atelectasis.[13]

Mechanical ventilation is required to achieve adequate oxygenation and ventilation. Adequate oxygenation is achieved by adjusting the level of oxygen delivered by the ventilator; the usual starting point is 40% to 50% oxygen. Effective oxygenation is monitored using pulse oximetry with intermittent ABG sampling. Positive end-expiratory pressure (PEEP) is a standard intervention used to help keep the alveoli open and improve oxygenation. PEEP usually starts at 5 cm $H_2O$ but can be increased if hypoxemia is present. Care must be taken when increasing PEEP because it can decrease preload, thereby decreasing cardiac output and blood pressure. The initial mode for the ventilator is usually assist-control ventilation and is changed to continuous positive airway pressure (CPAP) when the patient is awake, stable, and ready to be weaned for extubation.

Adequate ventilation is maintained by selecting tidal volumes that are appropriate for body size as well as setting a sufficient rate for the ventilator tidal volumes. Monitoring of ventilation should include end-tidal carbon dioxide ($ETCO_2$) monitoring, which should be correlated with the partial pressure of carbon dioxide ($PaCO_2$) on an ABG analysis. $ETCO_2$ monitoring is also used to confirm proper endotracheal tube placement.

Weaning from mechanical ventilation is a quick process in patients who have undergone open heart surgery. Once the patient has displayed the ability to follow commands and the strength to protect the airway, a short CPAP trial is instituted. The patient can be extubated if (1) cardiac performance is good (cardiac index more than 2.2 L/min/m$^2$), (2) adequate oxygenation and ventilation are achieved without acidosis, and (3) chest tube bleeding is minimal. Aggressive use of incentive spirometry and physical mobility ensures proper pulmonary function. Auscultation of breath sounds should be performed at frequent intervals and as the patient's condition dictates. Diminished breath sounds, especially in

the left lower lobe, are common because left lower lobe atelectasis is an expected postoperative outcome after the lung is deflated during surgery. Observation of the work of breathing is also important, and signs such as tachypnea, use of accessory muscles, and prolonged expiratory time can indicate compromised pulmonary function. Bronchodilator therapy may be indicated and should be continued if the patient was using bronchodilators at home.

Prolonged mechanical ventilation may be a complication of cardiac surgery. Protracted poor cardiac function requires continued mechanical ventilation. Phrenic nerve damage due to cold preservation techniques for myocardial protection or physical transection is another cause of ventilatory failure due to diaphragm dysfunction.[3,13,14] Acute respiratory distress syndrome associated with SIRS, a hypoperfusion state, or both can also be a reason for prolonged ventilator days. A tracheostomy should be considered in patients with compromised pulmonary function because it can enhance the ventilator weaning process and promote patient comfort; however, infection risk of the sternal incision is a consideration with increased oral secretions that can contaminate the incision site.

## Preventing Neurologic Complications

Neurologic recovery of the cardiac surgery patient depends on several factors, such as preoperative neurologic state; age; renal function; presence of conditions such as aortic atherosclerosis, hypertension, and diabetes mellitus; and use of the IABP.[1] Because narcotics and benzodiazepines, with neuromuscular blockade, are now used more often than gases for anesthesia, the usual course of neurologic recovery is much faster.[7] There is little need for sedation when the patient is transported from the operating room unless hemodynamic instability is present; the patient is allowed to wake up and recover from the anesthesia as soon as possible. The elderly patient is not able to metabolize narcotics and paralytics as quickly as a younger patient and may require a longer recovery time. If the patient is difficult to arouse and has pinpoint pupils, reversal of narcotics with naloxone (Narcan) may be indicated. Naloxone diluted 0.4 mg in 10 mL normal saline solution and given 1 to 2 mL IV every 5 minutes is a delicate method of regaining level of consciousness that does not reverse pain control. If the patient does not have good muscle strength, reversal of neuromuscular blockade is indicated. Glycopyrrolate, 0.6 mg IV, and neostigmine, 3 mg IV (or more), are used. The patient in renal failure is not able to clear these drugs and probably needs reversal of both narcotic and neuromuscular blockade agents to expedite extubation.

Once the patient is awake, continual evaluation using standard neurologic examination to assess the level of consciousness and motor and sensory ability is essential. Postoperative neurologic deficits are divided into two categories: (1) major focal deficits (stroke), stupor, or coma and (2) deterioration in intellectual function.[3] The best predictor of stroke is proximal aortic atherosclerosis, which is the source of emboli that are released with the manipulation of the aorta, especially during cannulation or cross-clamping. Hypoxia, hypoperfusion, hemorrhage, and metabolic abnormalities may also cause strokes.[1,3] Cognitive changes are more difficult to detect because there may be deficits in memory, language, and psychomotor function; the family of the patient may be helpful in detecting any subtle changes. These changes are most noticeable immediately after surgery but may still be present 12 to 36 months after the procedure. Confirmation of a stroke can be performed with computed tomography or magnetic resonance imaging of the head, but these studies may need to be repeated; embolic events do not immediately appear on scans. If a patient has known carotid disease, maintaining higher blood pressure may help increase perfusion of the cerebral tissues. Thrombolytic therapy cannot be used for embolic stroke after surgery in the patient who has just had CABG surgery because of bleeding concerns.

## Monitoring Postoperative Bleeding

Postoperative bleeding is expected; the challenge is to know when and how to intervene. Chronic preoperative anticoagulation can confound bleeding problems in the patient who has had CABG surgery, especially in cases of emergent surgery when there has not been time to discontinue the drugs beforehand. Timely correction of bleeding problems can decrease both the occurrence of complications and the cost of patient care. Preoperative anticoagulation, such as therapy with thrombolytics and antiplatelet drugs, hampers coagulation, and the effects of these drugs are difficult to reverse; reversal may not even be an option, and postoperative bleeding may increase. It is recommended that if the patient is receiving clopidogrel, it should be stopped 5 to 7 days before surgery.[1]

Vigilant monitoring of chest tube drainage is imperative to anticipate impending bleeding events. Chest tube drainage is monitored hourly, and more frequently if the drainage is excessive. The usual chest tube output can range from 100 to 200 mL/h, with periods of increased drainage due to a change in position or temperature. If the chest tube output continues to be greater than 200 mL/h, intervention is necessary. Protamine, the first level of intervention, is given at 1 mg for every 100 units of heparin to reverse the effects of heparin, which is used in the surgical process.[2,3] PTT is commonly used to monitor the intrinsic pathway of the coagulation cascade, which heparin affects. Additional protamine may be necessary, especially if the patient is hypothermic, because a "rebound" phenomenon may occur. Aggressive rewarming is very important in a patient who has increased bleeding because the coagulation cascade, with its enzymatic reactions, cannot function properly at hypothermic temperatures. However, as the patient's temperature rises, heparin is reactivated, causing increased bleeding. Platelet infusion is used next to help decrease bleeding. It is important to remember that platelet infusion can cause a blood product reaction because each infusion may be from multiple donors. Causes of platelet dysfunction and postoperative bleeding include medications, such as aspirin; the bypass machine itself; the IABP, which mechanically destroys platelets; and heparin-induced thrombocytopenia, a phenomenon in which heparin exposure disables platelet function.

Follow-up coagulation studies act as a guide to the need for further infusions as well as monitoring blood loss, but they do not provide absolute parameters. If bleeding is increasing, a PT can be ordered to determine whether other factors need to be replaced. An elevated PT (more than 15 seconds) may indicate that bleeding is due to a lack of factors, such as fibrinogen, that can be replaced using fresh frozen plasma,

usually 4 to 6 units/infusion.[3] The overall goal is to determine whether bleeding is due to a coagulopathy or surgical bleeding. Chest tube bleeding that exceeds 500 mL/h is considered surgical bleeding and mandates surgical reexploration.

Other therapeutic interventions may also be used to decrease bleeding. Coagulation factors, such as cryoprecipitate (factors I and VIII) and factor VII, are indicated in severe bleeding.[2,3] Various drugs, such as aminocaproic acid (Amicar), a potent inhibitor of fibrinolysis, and desmopressin acetate (DDAVP), which influences factor VIII and enhances platelet adhesion, can be administered to promote coagulation.[15]

Intraoperative measures to prevent bleeding include minimizing hemodilution, minimizing autologous losses, and optimizing coagulation status with full rewarming.[2,3,15] Blood loss requires replacement, which should be considered carefully. Transfusion of red blood cells may not only increase exposure to infectious diseases, especially hepatitis and human immunodeficiency virus, but is also associated with increased immunosuppressive and microcirculatory complications.[1,15] The hemoglobin level indicated for transfusion is a controversial issue. A restrictive transfusion strategy (hemoglobin less than 7 g/dL) has demonstrated a lower mortality rate in patients who are less critically ill.[15] Autotransfusion of chest drainage also has been used, but there are no clear data that support improved outcomes with this intervention.

Cardiac tamponade is a serious complication of increased postoperative bleeding that occurs when excessive fluid or blood accumulates in the pericardial space, resulting in increasing pressure on the right atrium and ventricle that can lead to collapse of those structures. Tamponade may develop rapidly or slowly, depending on how fast blood accumulates in the pericardial sac. When a patient is treated for excessive bleeding, it is important to monitor the chest tube drainage closely and maintain patency.[3] The mechanism of cardiac tamponade is the collapse of the lower pressure chambers of the right heart as a result of the increasing of the CVP, pulmonary artery diastolic pressure, and the PAOP. This increase and equalization of the three values is classic evidence of cardiac tamponade. However, the clinical situation can be a late finding; decreasing cardiac performance and blood pressure, despite volume resuscitation and pressor support, are earlier indicators. An arterial line waveform with significant respiratory variation (best illustration of an increased pulsus paradoxus) is another warning sign that cardiac tamponade is pending, though this may be less prominent owing to positive pressure ventilation in intubated patients.[3,7] Definitive diagnosis is made with an echocardiogram.

Interventions to prevent tamponade include stripping and milking chest tubes when the blood begins to clot, although stripping the tubes can generate increased negative pressure. Because the chambers (atria and ventricles) are being compressed, cardiac pressures, especially CVP, may be elevated. Another useful intervention involves the infusion of volume even with increased pressure to keep the structures from collapsing.

## Preventing Renal Complications

The postoperative course of renal function is influenced by preoperative function. Preoperative risk factors are age, history of moderate-to-severe congestive heart failure, prior CABG surgery, and preexisting conditions including type 1 diabetes mellitus and renal disease (serum creatinine 1.4 to 2.0 mg/dL).[1,3] The usual postoperative course also depends on whether the surgery was performed on or off bypass. After on-bypass CABG surgery, brisk initial urine output is expected because of the priming of the bypass circuit with mannitol and the possible use of diuretics. The output diminishes as these effects decrease with time. After OPCABG surgery, there is a smaller urine volume because patients are not exposed to these interventions. As the inflammatory response diminishes within 24 to 48 hours, the leaky capillary membranes seal and extra interstitial fluid shifts into the intravascular space, increasing the need for pharmacologic diuresis with drugs, such as furosemide (Lasix).[7] Electrolyte repletion with potassium and magnesium after diuresis is also important to maintaining a regular cardiac rhythm.[3] A slight metabolic acidosis may be present in the patient with existing renal failure and may persist after surgery. If acidosis is present, the source (respiratory, metabolic, or combined) should be determined in order to intervene appropriately. The focus of interventions is to remove excess fluid while protecting metabolic and cardiac function.

**OLIGURIA.** Decreasing urine output (less than 0.5 mL/kg/h) is usually caused by decreased renal perfusion. Obvious causes, such as Foley catheter obstruction or malposition, may often be overlooked and should be considered initially, so that mechanical problems may be ruled out. Decreasing urine output may be a sign of aortic dissection following cardiac surgery.[3] Decreased cardiac function may also cause a decrease in urine output. Hypovolemia is a very common problem that can be addressed with fluid boluses, and monitoring pulmonary artery pressures and the cardiac output/cardiac index shortly after fluid infusions indicates whether the intervention was therapeutic.[2,7] Caution must be exercised when adding volume because excess fluid can cause decreased function in compromised myocardial muscle; in that situation, inotropic agents or vasoactive drugs may be required. Determining the patient's baseline blood pressure is important so that control of vasoactive drugs can be titrated according to a perfusion pressure (MAP or systolic blood pressure) that the patient's kidneys require.[7]

If none of these interventions are successful, diuresis may be necessary. Loop diuretics (eg, furosemide) are the usual first-line drugs.[7] If urine output does not increase, larger doses may be indicated, or other diuretics that act on other areas of the renal tubular system, such as thiazides like metolazone, may be added. Creatinine and BUN values are closely monitored.

**RENAL FAILURE.** If acute renal failure develops, dialysis is necessary. The method used depends on patient condition and practitioner preference. Continuous venovenous hemofiltration (CVVH) and hemodialysis are among the several methods that may be used.[7] CVVH is preferred in the patient who is severely hemodynamically compromised because it is more gradual and minimizes preload compromise, which could decrease cardiac performance. Patients who undergo dialysis require fluid restriction, nutrition modification for prolonged renal dysfunction, and other standard interventions, such as dietary modifications to decrease protein and potassium intake. Unfortunately, the mortality rate from acute renal failure in postoperative cardiac surgery patients is greater than 60%.[16] Chapter 31 provides a further discussion of renal failure, and Chapter 30 discusses dialysis.

## Preventing Endocrine Complications

Diabetes mellitus is one of the major risk factors for the development of cardiovascular disease. Diabetes mellitus affects almost all systems in the body and requires that the vigilant clinician continually monitor blood glucose and maintain strict glucose control. In the initial postoperative period, a blood glucose level less than 180 mg/dL is particularly important in managing wound healing and preventing infections or mediastinitis.[1] Intervention using an insulin drip initially may reduce the incidence of deep sternal wound infections by 50%.[1] Once good glucose control has been achieved, insulin is given subcutaneously, and glucose levels are followed closely. Such insulin therapy also decreases the incidence of diabetic ketoacidosis or hyperosmolar coma. It is important to remember that whereas hyperglycemia is detrimental, severe hypoglycemia can be fatal. The need for vigilant blood glucose monitoring cannot be overemphasized.

Adrenal insufficiency may occur, especially in patients who were receiving steroids at regular intervals before surgery. The administration of steroids can suppress adrenal function. To prevent suppression, postoperative stress doses of hydrocortisone (100 mg every 8 hours) should be given, and the patient's regular dose should be restarted. If the patient is taking vasoactive drugs and is not weaning off the drips, adrenal insufficiency is considered; this condition may be the result of hypoperfusion of the adrenal gland. Cortisol levels are low and confirm adrenal insufficiency.

Thyroid dysfunction, especially hypothyroidism, is common in elderly persons and women. Although perioperative effects do not result in dysfunction, preoperative function is an important consideration, and undiagnosed dysfunction may become apparent in the postoperative period because the thyroid hormones, especially triiodothyronine ($T_3$), can have cardiovascular effects.[1]

## Preventing Gastrointestinal Complications

Fortunately, the gastrointestinal aspects of the postoperative course are uneventful and similar to those of general surgery. After extubation, the patient takes nothing by mouth (NPO) for up to the first 8 hours, with a nasogastric tube in place to decompress the stomach. Then the patient is allowed to have small amounts of ice or water. This relatively simple aspect of nursing care is very important for the postoperative patient, who may experience significant thirst because of the anticholinergic drugs that were given before surgery. The use of ice pops and ginger ale can help with compliance and decrease the possibility of nausea, vomiting, and aspiration.

Complications such as cholecystitis, pancreatitis, and bowel infarction rarely occur. Their pathogenesis is not always clear but is attributed to splanchnic hypoperfusion and general gastrointestinal ischemia. Thorough assessment of the abdomen looking for pain, distention, or tympany may help discover subtle abnormalities. Lactate levels greater than 2.5 mmol/L may indicate splanchnic hypoperfusion. However, they may also be the result of nonpulsatile flow of the bypass machine, which may cause a release of angiotensin II, exacerbating splanchnic ischemia.[17] The need for further evaluation is dictated by the clinical presentation.

## Monitoring for Infection

In the early postoperative period, hypothalamic resetting is the cause of temperature derangement. Febrile reactions are usually attributed to SIRS and to overshoot from rewarming. If the fever (temperature more than 100.4°F [38°C]) persists for more than 48 to 72 hours, infection should be considered. The goal of infection prevention is achieved through the prudent use of prophylactic and empiric antibiotics, such as vancomycin or a cephalosporin (eg, cefuroxime cefazolin, ceftazidime), depending on the patient's previous known allergies or any history of resistant infections. Timing of antibiotic administration is pivotal; for optimal results, preoperative doses should be completely infused before the skin is cut. Antibiotic dosing depends on preoperative renal function. A short postoperative course should also be anticipated.[1]

Mediastinitis is the major infection in patients who have undergone CABG surgery and may be a devastating complication that increases the length of hospital stay and mortality. Risk factors associated with mediastinitis are obesity; prior cardiac surgery; preexisting type 1 diabetes mellitus; and perioperative factors, such as excessive electrocautery, transfusion of homologous blood, and use of both internal mammary arteries resulting in compromised blood flow to the chest wall.[1] Therapy is an extended antibiotic course and plastic surgery. The aggressive regulation of the blood glucose level using insulin drips initially instead of subcutaneous administration has been shown to decrease the occurrence of mediastinitis.[1] It is very important to instruct the patient not to use the arms excessively when moving and to use a "cough pillow" with coughing (a small pillow that is placed on the sternal incision and squeezed when coughing). Other interventions, such as having the patient sleep on his or her back, are also important. Following these instructions may help maintain the stability of the sternum.

## Patient Teaching and Discharge Planning

The usual length of hospitalization after cardiac surgery is 4 to 7 days. Discharge planning that begins at admission is imperative because of the short length of hospital stays. The patient should be discharged with the following medications, unless contraindicated: aspirin, a beta blocker, an ACE inhibitor (if the ejection fraction is less than 40%), and a statin.[1] If a medication is contraindicated, the rationale should be documented. Smoking cessation interventions, if applicable, should be included in discharge teaching.[1] Box 22-6 summarizes patient teaching about cardiac postoperative care.

## Carotid Endarterectomy

Stenosis or occlusion of the carotid arteries is usually due to atherosclerotic disease and may cause stroke, a leading cause of morbidity and mortality in the United States.[18] Carotid endarterectomy is the most common noncardiac vascular procedure performed to restore flow to the carotid arteries and is designed to decrease the risk for stroke and stroke-related death.[18]

The right carotid artery is a branch of the innominate artery that arises from the right side of the aortic arch. The left common carotid artery arises directly from the aortic arch.[18] At the level of the thyroid, the common carotids bifurcate into the external and internal carotids. Located near this bifurcation, in the carotid sinus, are the carotid chemoreceptors, which are sensitive to blood carbon dioxide and oxygen levels, and the baroreceptors, which help regulate blood pressure. The external carotid arteries supply blood to the structures in the head and neck, excluding the eyes and brain. The internal carotid arteries give rise to the ophthalmic arteries and the posterior communicating, anterior cerebral, and middle cerebral arteries, which help supply blood to the brain (Fig. 22-9).

Patients with carotid artery occlusive disease may have sudden dysphagia, unilateral motor weakness, expressive aphasia, dizziness, memory deficits, or monocular blindness.[18] They often exhibit signs of vascular disease in other parts of the body, such as the heart (CAD) or the legs (peripheral arterial disease). Risk factors for carotid artery occlusive disease are associated with stroke and should guide patient care. Hypertension is the most important risk factor for stroke,

---

**BOX 22-6** *TEACHING GUIDE* | *Recovering From Cardiac Surgery*

**General Instructions**

- Avoid lifting heavy objects (10 to 15 pounds or more) for first 3 months.
- Avoid strenuous arm movement, such as golf or tennis. When getting in and out of chair or bed, use legs. Arms should not bear weight and should be used only for balance.
- Do not drive for 6 weeks after surgery. (May ride in automobile.)
- Follow physician's instructions for activity progression.
- Resume sexual activity when you can climb two flights of stairs without stopping (with physician's recommendations).
- Use alternative positions for 3 to 4 months to decrease stress on sternum; avoid side-lying and prone positions.
- Inspect and cleanse surgical incisions daily with soap and water.
- Understand medications, including reason for taking, dosage, frequency, and side effects.
- Follow dietary restrictions.
- Understand how much pain to expect and how to manage it.

**Risk Factors**

- Follow instructions on individual risk factors, understand their impact on health after cardiac surgery, and learn how to modify them.
- Seek referrals as appropriate (eg, for a weight loss program or a smoking cessation program).

**Follow-Up With Physician**

- Know how and when to schedule follow-up appointments.
- Be alert for signs and symptoms of infection, such as fever, increased redness, tenderness, drainage, or swelling of incisions.
- Report palpitations, tachycardia, or an irregular pulse (if normally regular) to the physician immediately.
- Seek follow-up care if you experience dizziness or increased fatigue, sudden weight gain or peripheral edema, shortness of breath, or chest pain.

*Data from Hillis LD, Smith PK, Anderson JL: 2011 ACCF/AHA guideline for coronary artery bypass graft surgery. A report of the American College of Cardiology Foundation/American Heart Association Task Force on Practice Guidelines. Circulation 124:e652–e735, 2011.*

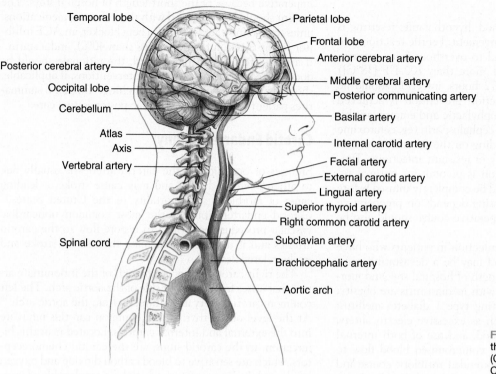

Temporal lobe
Parietal lobe
Frontal lobe
Anterior cerebral artery
Posterior cerebral artery
Middle cerebral artery
Occipital lobe
Posterior communicating artery
Cerebellum
Basilar artery
Atlas
Internal carotid artery
Axis
Facial artery
Vertebral artery
External carotid artery
Lingual artery
Superior thyroid artery
Right common carotid artery
Spinal cord
Subclavian artery
Brachiocephalic artery
Aortic arch

**FIGURE 22-9** Branches of the right external carotid artery. (Courtesy of Anatomical Chart Company.)

and blood pressure regulation is essential in the postoperative period.[1,18] Cigarette smoking, hyperlipidemia, alcohol consumption, and postmenopausal use of estrogen may also affect patient care.[18]

Patients with risk factors for carotid artery occlusive disease must be examined carefully. A carotid bruit can usually be auscultated over the artery because of turbulent flow through the narrowed artery.[18] Carotid Doppler ultrasonography is usually performed to estimate the presence and amount of stenosis, but angiography is the most reliable method to determine the exact amount of stenosis.[18] Magnetic resonance angiography, which is less invasive, may also be used.[18]

## Indications

Carotid artery occlusive disease is part of the systemic atherosclerotic process, which is reviewed in Chapter 21. Carotid endarterectomy (CEA) is indicated for recently symptomatic patients with 70% to 99% carotid artery stenosis.[18] This surgery should not be considered for symptomatic patients with less than 50% stenosis; these patients have better outcomes if treated medically.[18] Advanced age is not a limitation for proceeding with CEA in patients who are appropriate to undergo this procedure.[18]

## Surgical Procedure

A skin incision is made along the lower anterior border of the sternocleidomastoid muscle just below the angle of the jaw, and the common, internal, and external carotid arteries are isolated. The carotid arteries on the operative side must be clamped.[18] Clamping puts the ipsilateral cerebral

hemisphere and eye at risk for ischemia and infarct because the only perfusion to these areas occurs through the circle of Willis and collaterals, which may be inadequate. To prevent thromboembolus formation while the arteries are clamped, a heparin bolus may be given before clamping. Adequacy of circulation may be determined by continuous electroencephalographic monitoring in the operating room.[18] If circulation is determined to be inadequate, a temporary bypass or shunt may be placed from the common carotid artery to the distal portion of the internal carotid to provide continued intraoperative perfusion.[18] Patients treated with shunts often include those with contralateral carotid stenosis, neurologic deficits, history of cerebrovascular accidents, and stroke in evolution.

Endarterectomy or removal of the ulcerated or stenotic atheromatous plaque is then performed, and the artery is closed. If primary closure will cause a narrowing in the vessel, a patch may be used.[18]

## Postoperative Care

After extubation in the recovery room, patients are transferred to the ICU with ECG monitoring, an arterial line, CVP monitoring, and oxygen. Traditionally, patients stay in the ICU for 24 hours. However, patients can be monitored in an intermediate care unit with reduction of the hospital stay to 1 day.[19]

### Controlling Blood Pressure

Blood pressure is commonly labile up to 24 hours after surgery because of surgically induced abnormalities of the carotid baroreceptor sensitivity.[18] This is characterized as baroreflex failure syndrome and is usually associated with bilateral surgical procedures.[18] Preoperative hypertension is thought to be the most important determinant of postoperative hypertension, which means that the critical care nurse must be aware of the patient's preoperative blood pressure range. Increased blood pressure may also increase the risk for wound bleeding and possible hematoma formation.[18] The goal of blood pressure regulation is a blood pressure less than 140/80 mm Hg.[18,20] A systolic blood pressure greater than 170 mm Hg should be treated with nitroprusside or other IV agents, whereas one less than 120 mm Hg should be treated with IV fluid or a norepinephrine or phenylephrine drip if the patient is unresponsive to volume.[20]

## Wound Care

To minimize stress on the operative site, the patient's head and neck are kept in alignment. The dressing and the area behind the patient's neck and shoulders are assessed for the presence of blood. Persistent oozing from deep tissue, coughing, straining during extubation, and disruption of suture lines may all lead to bleeding into the operative site. The risk of bleeding can be further aggravated by anticoagulation with heparin, aspirin, or antiplatelet therapy.[18] The nurse assesses the neck size, comparing the operative side with the nonoperative side. Swelling could indicate hematoma formation. Any patient complaints of difficulty talking, swallowing, or breathing should be reported to the physician immediately. If a hematoma is suspected because of tracheal compression, surgical evacuation may be indicated. Wound hematomas occur in about 5.5% of patients.[18]

## Preventing Neurologic Complications

Brain injury, local nerve injury, or both may occur with carotid endarterectomy. Perioperative stroke occurs in approximately 3% of patients and may be due to embolization of atheromatous debris, air from the operative site, or low flow during carotid artery clamping.[18] Neurologic assessment includes monitoring level of consciousness, pupil reactivity, eye movement, orientation, appropriateness of response, and motor function (flexion, extension, and hand grips) for the first 24 hours. Abnormalities should be reported to the physician immediately.

Hyperperfusion syndrome occurs in patients with high-grade stenosis. Theoretically, the hemisphere distal to the stenotic area has suffered hypoperfusion that causes the small blood vessels to remain maximally dilated with a loss of autoregulation. Once the stenosis is repaired, autoregulation is still paralyzed, but a marked increase in blood flow occurs that cannot be controlled with vasoconstriction to protect the capillaries. Edema or hemorrhage to the area results.[18] Strict blood pressure control is imperative.

Several cranial nerves (CN) traverse the surgical area and can be exposed to trauma. The most commonly affected are CN VII (the facial nerve), CN X (the vagus nerve), CN XII (the hypoglossal nerve), and CN XI (the spinal accessory nerve).[18] Specific functional assessment for each nerve should be performed after surgery, including those listed in Table 22-3. If a deficit is present, the nurse should notify the physician, and explain to the patient how it occurred and that the deficit is usually temporary.

## Home Care Considerations

Patients are usually discharged on the first or second postoperative day. Aspirin (81 or 325 mg/d) should be prescribed postoperatively for at least 3 months to reduce the possibility of stroke, MI, or death.[18] Beta blockers, angiotensin inhibitors, and statins should also be taken to improve outcomes following carotid endarterectomy.

The critical care nurse plays an essential role in the care of the patient who has had a carotid endarterectomy. Although considered a vascular surgical procedure, postoperative complications usually manifest as neurologic symptoms, and the nurse must assess the patient for subtle neurologic changes. Patient education is also a key component of care. Patients and their families should understand that the patient has an underlying cardiovascular disease and that risk factor modification is necessary. Education should include the items listed in Box 22-7.

| **TABLE 22-3** | Postoperative Functional Assessment of Cranial Nerves Following Carotid Endarterectomy | | |
|---|---|---|---|
| **Nerve** | **Nerve Intervention** | **Functional Assessment** | **Functional Damage** |
| Facial nerve (VII) | Motor function of facial muscles | Ability to smile and frown | Asymmetrical contraction of the mouth |
| Vagus nerve (X) | Motor and sensory function of larynx and throat | Quality and tone of voice and ability to swallow | Difficult swallowing, hoarseness, speech problems, loss of gag reflex |
| Hypoglossal nerve (XII) | Muscles to tongue | Movement of tongue | Difficult swallowing, speech problems, deviation of tongue, sometimes airway damage |
| Spinal accessory nerve (XI) | Trapezius and sternocleidomastoid muscles | Ability to shrug shoulders and raise arm to horizontal position | Shoulder may sag, difficulty raising shoulder against resistance, difficulty raising arm to horizontal position |

---

**BOX 22-7** | **TEACHING GUIDE** | **Recovering From Carotid Endarterectomy**

**Risk Factor Reduction**
- Stop smoking.
- Eat a low-fat diet.
- Control hypertension if present.
- Control diabetes if present.

**Activity**
- There are usually no restrictions on activity. It is all right to move your neck in a normal manner.

**Incision Care**
- Bruising and discoloration are common.
- Wash the incision site with soap and water.

**General**
- Be familiar with signs and symptoms of incisional infection.
- Notify your physician of visual defects, changes in memory or sensation, or an inability to swallow or speak.
- Be knowledgeable about medication indications, including reason for taking, dosage, frequency, and side effects.
- Keep physician appointments.

*Data from Brott TG, Halperin JL, Abbara S: 2011 ASA/ACCF/AHA/AANN/AANS/ACR/ASNR/CNS/ SAIP/SCAI/SIR/SNIS/SVM/SVS guideline on the management of patients with extracranial ca- rotid and vertebral artery disease. Circulation 124:e54–e130, 2011.*

## Clinical Applicability Challenges

---

### CASE STUDY

Mr. B. is a 72-year-old man who underwent right-sided carotid endarterectomy; he returns to the ICU following 2 hours of surgery. He has a history of high blood pressure, cholesterol, and insulin-controlled diabetes for 5 years, and he smoked for 20 years but quit within the last year. His vital signs on arrival include a blood pressure of 162/85, heart rate of 99 beats/min, temperature of 96.6°F (35.9°C), and respiratory rate of 28 breaths/min.

1. What interventions will you provide to prevent complications in this patient?
2. What assessment findings would indicate that cranial nerve damage had occurred?
3. What assessment findings would you notify the surgical team providers about?

---

### WANT TO KNOW MORE?

A wide variety of resources to enhance your learning and understanding of this chapter are available on thePoint.

You will find:

- References
- Selected readings
- NCLEX-style review questions
- Internet resources
- And more!

**23**

# Anatomy and Physiology of the Respiratory System

MEGAN CECERE LYNN AND KAREN JOHNSON

**LEARNING OBJECTIVES**

*Based on the content in this chapter, the reader should be able to:*

1. Identify the major structures of the respiratory system that are located in the thorax.

2. Describe the movement of air through the airways from the nose to the alveoli.

3. Discuss the function of surfactant in maintaining alveolar inflation.

4. Differentiate the function of bronchial and pulmonary circulations.

5. Describe the mechanics of ventilation in terms of air movement into and out of the lungs, lung compliance, and airway resistance.

6. Explain four factors that affect the diffusion of gases across the alveolar–capillary membrane.

7. Identify physiologic and pathophysiologic conditions that produce a ventilation–perfusion mismatch.

8. Discuss conditions that affect the relationship described in the oxyhemoglobin dissociation curve and how these conditions affect oxygen exchange.

9. Describe the function of the chemoreceptors and lung receptors.

The structures of the respiratory system allow gases to move between the external environment and the internal environment. The cardinal function of the respiratory system is gas exchange, a process by which oxygen moves from the air into the blood and carbon dioxide moves out of the blood and is exhaled to the external environment. The respiratory system also has several other functions, including regulation of acid–base balance, metabolism of some compounds, and filtration of inhaled unwanted materials. Intact respiratory structures and proper functioning of the respiratory system are necessary for transport of gases in and out of the body. Knowledge of respiratory anatomy and physiology helps the nurse understand respiratory assessment techniques, principles of respiratory system management, and common disorders of the respiratory system.

## Anatomy of the Respiratory System

### The Thorax

The thorax contains the major structures of the respiratory system. These structures include the bony thoracic cage, the muscles of ventilation, the lungs, the pleural space, and the mediastinum (Fig. 23-1). The thoracic cage is a rigid, yet flexible, structure. Flexibility allows for inhalation/inflation and exhalation/deflation of the lungs. The thoracic cage consists of 12 vertebrae, each with a pair of ribs. Posteriorly, each rib is attached to a vertebra (Fig. 23-2). Anteriorly, the first seven ribs are attached to the sternum (Fig. 23-3). The 8th, 9th, and 10th ribs are attached by cartilage to the ribs above them. The 11th and 12th ribs are called "floating ribs," because they are not attached anteriorly to another structure.

### The Lungs, Mediastinum, and Pleural Space

Positioned within, and protected by, the thoracic cage, the lungs are located on either side of the chest. These air-filled, spongy structures are attached to the body only at the pulmonary ligament at the mediastinum. The right lung contains three lobes, and the left lung contains only two lobes. The base of each lung rests anteriorly at the level of the 6th rib at the mid-clavicular line and at the 8th rib at the mid-axillary line. The apices extend 2 to 4 cm above the inner aspects of the clavicles.

The space between the two lungs is the mediastinum. The mediastinum contains the heart, blood vessels, lymph nodes, thymus gland, nerve fibers, and esophagus.

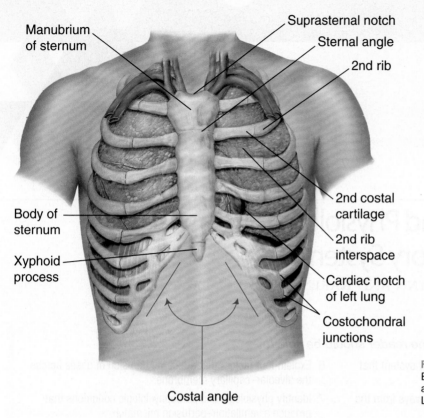

Manubrium of sternum

Suprasternal notch

Sternal angle

2nd rib

Body of sternum

Xyphoid process

2nd costal cartilage

2nd rib interspace

Cardiac notch of left lung

Costochondral junctions

Costal angle

**FIGURE 23-1**    Anatomy of the chest wall. (From Bickley LS: Bates' Guide to Physical Examination and History Taking, 11th ed. Philadelphia, PA: Lippincott Williams & Wilkins, 2013, p 293.)

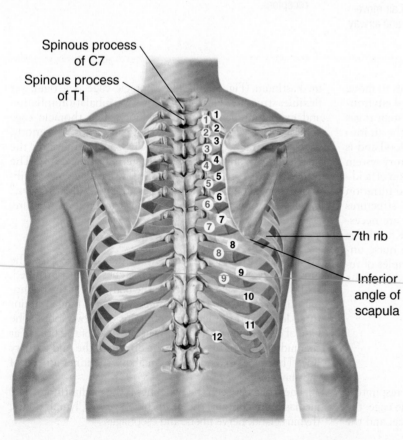

Spinous process of C7

Spinous process of T1

7th rib

Inferior angle of scapula

**FIGURE 23-2**    Posterior thoracic cage. (From Bickley LS: Bates' Guide to Physical Examination and History Taking, 11th ed. Philadelphia, PA: Lippincott Williams & Wilkins, 2013, p 295.)

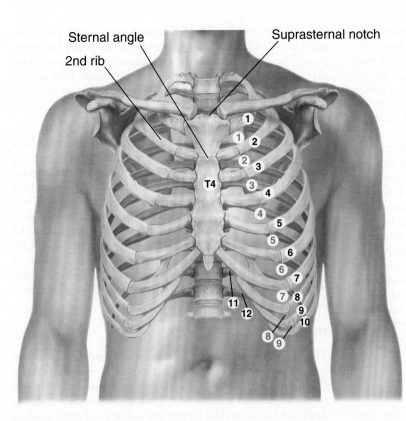

Sternal angle

2nd rib

Suprasternal notch

T4

FIGURE 23-3  Anterior thoracic cage. (From Bickley LS: Bates' Guide to Physical Examination and History Taking, 11th ed. Philadelphia, PA: Lippincott Williams & Wilkins, 2013, p 294.)

Pleural membranes surround the lungs and line the thoracic wall. The parietal pleura is the membrane lining the chest wall, and the visceral pleura overlays the lung parenchyma (Fig. 23-4). A thin layer of serous fluid in the small space between these two pleurae allows the parietal and visceral pleurae to slide over each other during inspiration and expiration. The pressure within the pleural space is called the intrapleural pressure and is normally less than the pressures within the lung. It is this negative pressure that keeps the lungs inflated. If the intrapleural space loses its negative pressure (by exposure to atmospheric pressure; eg, as a result

of chest trauma), the lung collapses, a condition known as a pneumothorax. The pleural space is also a potential space for the accumulation of fluid. An abnormal collection of fluid in the pleural space is a pleural effusion.

## The Respiratory Muscles

The muscles that elevate the thoracic cage are classified as *muscles of inspiration*.[1] The major muscle involved with inspiration is the diaphragm. The diaphragm is a thin, dome-shaped muscle that is innervated by the phrenic nerves. When it

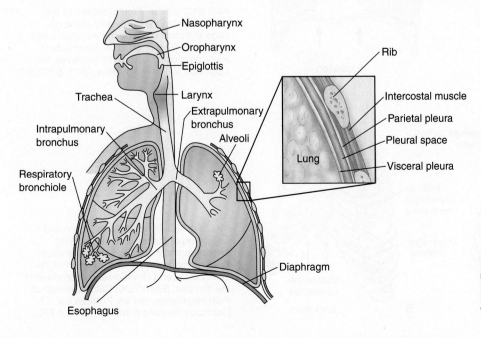

Nasopharynx

Oropharynx

Epiglottis

Trachea

Larynx

Extrapulmonary bronchus

Intrapulmonary bronchus

Alveoli

Respiratory bronchiole

Lung

Rib

Intercostal muscle

Parietal pleura

Pleural space

Visceral pleura

Diaphragm

Esophagus

FIGURE 23-4  Structures of the respiratory system. (From Porth CM: Essentials of Pathophysiology, 3rd ed. Philadelphia, PA: Lippincott Williams & Wilkins, 2011, p 514.)

contracts, the abdominal contents are forced downward, and the chest expands vertically (Fig. 23-5). In normal breathing, the level of the diaphragm moves about 1 cm, but on forced inspiration, a total excursion of up to 10 cm may occur.[2] The external intercostal muscles also assist with inspiration (Fig. 23-6). When the external muscles contract, the ribs are pulled forward and upward, and this increases the lateral and anterior–posterior diameters of the thoracic cage. The accessory muscles of inspiration include the scalene and sternocleidomastoid muscles. The scalene muscles elevate the first two ribs, and the sternocleidomastoid muscles raise the sternum.[2] During normal breathing, these muscles are not used, but during exercise, these muscles contract to aid in inspiration.

Muscles that depress the thoracic cage are classified as *muscles of expiration*.[1] Expiration is a largely passive process during normal breathing. During expiration, the diaphragm relaxes, and the elastic recoil of the lungs, chest wall, and abdominal structures compresses the lungs. The abdominal and intercostal muscles can increase expiratory effort (see Fig. 23-5). When the abdominal muscles contract, the intra-abdominal pressure increases and pushes the diaphragm upward. When the internal intercostal muscles contract, the ribs are pulled downward and inward, decreasing the thoracic volume.

## The Conducting Airways

The conducting airways include the nasopharynx, oropharynx, trachea, bronchi, bronchioles, and the terminal bronchioles (see Fig. 23-4). These airways warm, humidify, and filter air while channeling this air to the gas exchange region (Fig. 23-7). Because the conducting airways contain no alveoli and do not participate in gas exchange, they constitute the *anatomic dead space* which is approximately 150 mL.[3]

### Nasopharynx and Oropharynx

The nasopharynx is part of the upper airway structures and is the preferred route for entrance of air into the respiratory tract during normal breathing because it filters and warms inspired air.[4] The outer passages are lined with coarse hairs that filter large particles. The upper portion of the nasal cavity supplies warmth and moisture to the air inhaled. If nasal passages are plugged or when larger volumes of gases need to be exchanged, the oropharynx provides an alternate route. Obstruction of the oropharynx leads to immediate cessation of ventilation ("choking"). Foreign bodies and swelling of the pharyngeal airways from infection, injury, or allergic reaction can also cause airway obstruction.

### The Epiglottis

The epiglottis, also a part of the upper airway structures, is located posterior to the root of the tongue (see Fig. 23-4). During inhalation, the epiglottis moves upward to allow air to move through the trachea. During swallowing, it moves downward to cover the larynx and allow food and liquid to pass into the esophagus. Contraction of the intra-abdominal

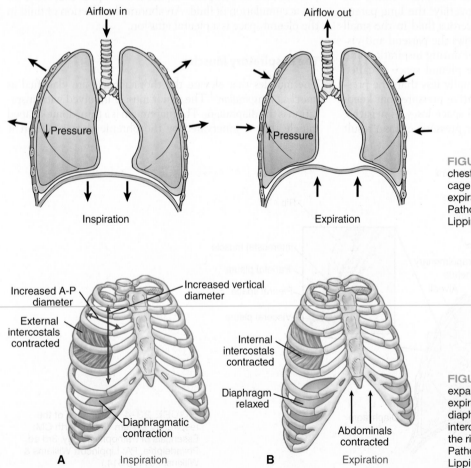

FIGURE 23-5    Frontal section of the chest showing the movement of the rib cage and diaphragm during inspiration and expiration. (From Porth CM: Essentials of Pathophysiology, 3rd ed. Philadelphia, PA: Lippincott Williams & Wilkins, 2011, p 522.)

FIGURE 23-6    **A, B:** Contraction and expansion of the thoracic cage during expiration and inspiration, demonstrating diaphragmatic contraction, function of the intercostals, and elevation and depression of the rib cage. (From Porth CM: Essentials of Pathophysiology, 3rd ed. Philadelphia, PA: Lippincott Williams & Wilkins, 2011, p 523.)

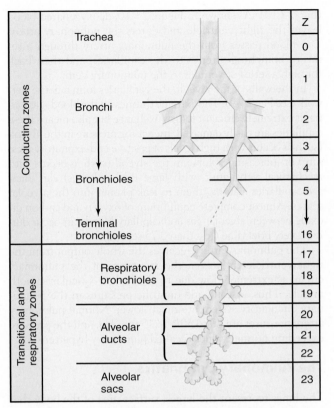

FIGURE 23-7    Idealization of the human airways. Note that the first 16 generations (Z) make up the conducting zone, and generations 17 to 23 make up the transitions and respiratory zones. Throughout childhood, the airways increase in diameter and length, and the number and size of the alveoli increase until adolescence, when respiratory development matures to that of an adult. (Adapted from West JB: Respiratory Physiology: The Essentials, 9th ed. Philadelphia, PA: Lippincott Williams & Wilkins, 2011, p 6.)

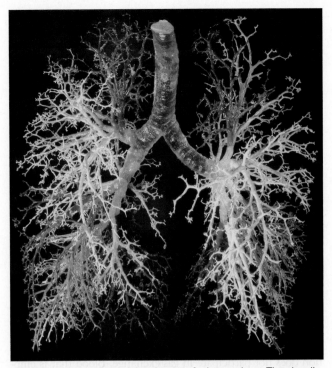

FIGURE 23-8    Cast of the airways of a human lung. The alveoli have been pruned away, allowing the conducting airways from the trachea to the terminal bronchioles to be seen. (From West JB: Respiratory Physiology: The Essentials, 9th ed. Philadelphia, PA: Lippincott Williams & Wilkins, 2011, p 5.)

muscles causes an increase in the intra-abdominal and intrathoracic pressures. These collective processes are called the *Valsalva maneuver*. The Valsalva maneuver can be dangerous because the abrupt increase in intrathoracic pressure can significantly reduce venous return and therefore cardiac output.

### The Tracheobronchial Tree

The tracheobronchial tree is part of the lower airway structures and consists of the trachea, bronchi, and bronchioles. The trachea connects the larynx and the major bronchi of the lungs (see Fig. 23-4). The trachea is primarily smooth muscle and is supported by horseshoe-shaped rings of cartilage that prevent the trachea from collapsing during coughing or bronchoconstriction of the smooth muscle.

The end of the trachea divides, forming the two large mainstem bronchi. The point at which the trachea divides is called the *carina*. When the carina is stimulated (eg, during tracheal suctioning), the cough reflex and bronchoconstriction are elicited. Because the right mainstem bronchus is wider and shorter than the left bronchus, it is the most common site of aspiration of foreign bodies. The right and left mainstem bronchi divide into lobar and segmental bronchi, which divide into bronchioles, which become terminal bronchioles (Fig. 23-8). The terminal bronchioles are the smallest airways without alveoli. The mainstem bronchi are supported by cartilage rings; however, as the bronchi extend

into the lungs, the cartilage rings become irregular and smaller until they disappear at about the level of the respiratory bronchioles. Here, smooth muscle wraps around the bronchioles. Contraction of these muscles (bronchospasm) causes narrowing of the bronchioles and impairs gas flow.[4]

## The Respiratory Airways

The terminal bronchioles branch into the respiratory airways. These airways include the respiratory bronchioles, the alveolar ducts, and the alveolar sacs (see Fig. 23-7). The respiratory zone makes up most of the lung, its volume being about 2.5 to 3 L.[5]

### The Respiratory Bronchioles

Each respiratory bronchiole forms a lobule which is the smallest functional unit of the lung and is where gas exchange takes place. A lobule consists of an arteriole, the pulmonary capillaries, and a venule (Fig. 23-9). Blood enters through a pulmonary artery and exits through a pulmonary vein. This is the only place in the body where highly oxygenated blood flows through a vein.

### The Alveoli

The alveolus is the end point of the respiratory tract, and it is here where gas exchange takes place (Fig. 23-9). The adult lung has a total alveolar surface area of 85 m$^{2}$.[5] The alveoli also contain macrophages that move from alveolus to alveolus, removing foreign substances and keeping the alveoli sterile.

*Type I alveolar cells* comprise approximately 90% of the total alveolar surface area and is where gas exchange takes place. *Type II alveolar cells* secrete pulmonary surfactant, a lipoprotein that decreases surface tension in the alveoli, prevents collapse of the smaller airways during expiration, and makes it easier to inflate the alveoli during inspiration. Injury to type II alveolar cells leads to alveolar collapse and impaired pulmonary gas exchange.

## The Lung Circulation

The lungs have a dual blood supply: the bronchial circulation and the pulmonary circulation. The bronchial circulation distributes blood to the airways, and the pulmonary circulation contributes to gas exchange.

### The Bronchial Circulation

The bronchial arteries that perfuse the left side of the thorax arise from the aorta, and the arteries that perfuse the right side of the thorax branch from the internal mammary, subclavian, and intercostal arteries. The capillaries of the bronchial circulation drain into the bronchial veins and eventually empty into the vena cava or the pulmonary vein. The bronchial circulation does not participate in gas exchange. Blood that is emptied into the pulmonary vein is unoxygenated blood and mixes with oxygenated blood flowing to the left side of the heart. This contributes to the "anatomic shunt" and is reason why arterial oxygen saturation is always less than 100%. The flow through the bronchial circulation is minimal, and the lung can function fairly well without it, such as after lung transplantation.[5]

### The Pulmonary Circulation

The pulmonary circulation arises from the pulmonary artery and provides for the gas exchange function of the lung

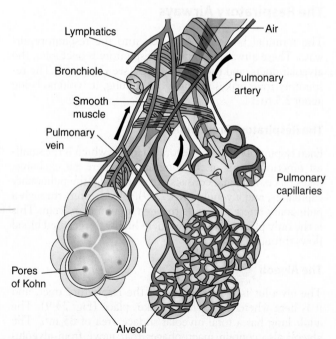

Lymphatics

Air

Bronchiole

Pulmonary artery

Smooth muscle

Pulmonary vein

Pulmonary capillaries

Pores of Kohn

Alveoli

**FIGURE 23-9** Lobule of the lung, showing the bronchial smooth muscle fibers, pulmonary blood vessels, and lymphatics. (From Porth CM: *Essentials of Pathophysiology*, 3rd ed. Philadelphia, PA: Lippincott Williams & Wilkins, 2011, p 518.)

(Fig. 23-10). As shown in Figure 23-10, deoxygenated blood leaves the right ventricle and enters the pulmonary artery. The blood passes from the pulmonary artery through a series of branching arteries to the capillaries, and then back through a series of venules to the pulmonary vein.

In the walls of the alveoli, the capillaries form a dense network (see Fig. 23-9). The extreme thinness of the blood–gas barrier is extremely efficient for gas exchange but also means these capillaries are easily damaged. Increasing pressure in the alveoli (such as occurs with high levels of positive end-expiratory pressure) or increasing volume in the alveoli (such as occurs with mechanical ventilation with large tidal volumes) can damage capillaries, causing them to leak plasma into the alveolar spaces. Almost complete equilibrium of oxygen and carbon dioxide between alveolar gas and capillary blood can occur during a very brief time (less than 0.75 second).[5]

The pulmonary artery receives the whole output from the right ventricle. However, the resistance of the pulmonary circuit is extremely low due to the lack of vascular smooth muscle. Thus, systolic and diastolic pressures in the pulmonary circulatory system are much lower. Normal pulmonary artery pressures are 20 to 30/8 to 15 mm Hg; and the pressure exceeding normal values is called pulmonary hypertension.

## The Pulmonary Lymphatics

The lungs represent the largest surface area of the body that is exposed to an increasingly hostile environment.[5] Fortunately, the lungs have multiple mechanisms to handle inhaled particles. The nose filters large particles. Particles that deposit in the conducting airways are removed by cilia that line the airways. The cilia brush the particles up toward the epiglottis, where they are then swallowed. By the process of phagocytosis, macrophages or leukocytes destroy foreign particles in the alveoli. Foreign materials that reach the alveoli are then removed by lymphatic tissue. The lymphatic vessels parallel the pulmonary vasculature (see Fig. 23-9). They surround the lobule and aid in the removal of particles and protein from the interstitial spaces. These vessels eventually drain into lymph nodes located at the hila of the lungs.

## Physiology of the Respiratory System

The goals of respiration are to provide oxygen to tissues and to remove carbon dioxide. The physiology of respiration involves the following three processes: (1) *ventilation*, or the movement of air between the atmosphere and the alveoli; (2) *diffusion* of oxygen and carbon dioxide between the pulmonary capillaries and the alveoli; and (3) *transport* of oxygen and carbon dioxide in the blood to and from the cells.[6]

### Ventilation

During ventilation, the movement of air into the lungs is known as *inhalation*, and the movement of air out of the lungs is known as *exhalation*. Air flows from a region of higher pressure to a region of lower pressure. To initiate a breath, a drop in pressure in the alveoli must precipitate airflow into the lungs.

### The Mechanics of Ventilation

Ventilation is a complex process with multiple variables, including the change in pressures and the integrity of the

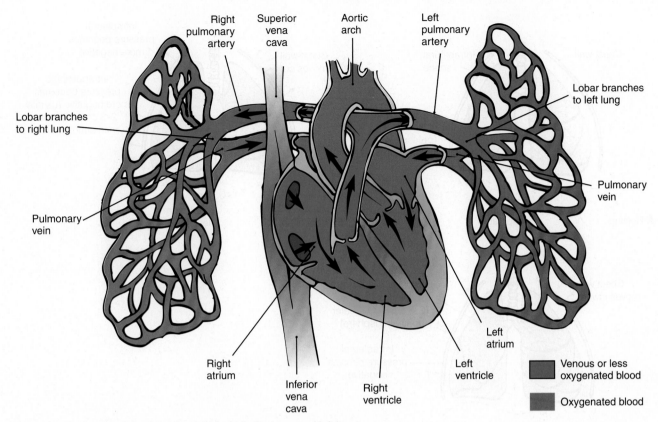

**FIGURE 23-10** Circulation from the right heart to the lungs and left heart.

muscles responsible for moving air in and out of the lungs, the compliance of the lungs, and the resistance afforded by the airways. Collectively, these variables are referred to as the *mechanics of ventilation*.

**MOVEMENT OF AIR INTO AND OUT OF THE LUNGS.** The movement of air in and out of the lungs requires muscles to expand and contract the chest cavity and a change in gas pressures to facilitate movement of air from one compartment to another. The lungs can be expanded and contracted by downward and upward movement of the diaphragm to lengthen and shorten the chest cavity and by elevation and depression of the ribs to increase and decrease the anterior–posterior diameter of the chest cavity.[1]

The movement of gases is always from an area of higher pressure to lower pressure. Several pressures are involved in the process of respiration (Fig. 23-11). The *airway pressure* is the pressure in the conducting airways. The *intrapleural pressure* is the pressure in the narrow space between the visceral and parietal pleurae. The *intra-alveolar pressure* is the pressure inside the alveoli. The pressure difference between the intra-alveolar pressure and the intrapleural pressure is called the *transpulmonary pressure*. The *intrathoracic pressure* is the pressure within the entire thoracic cavity.

The mechanics involved in ventilation are illustrated in Figure 23-12. Pressures in the resting state are shown in Figure 23-12A. Pleural pressure, a slightly negative pressure, creates a suction that holds the lungs open to their resting level. Without this negative pressure to hold the lungs against the chest wall, the elastic recoil properties of the lungs would cause them to collapse. When the glottis is open and no air is flowing, the pressure in the conducting airways

and alveoli equals atmospheric pressure. The pressures during inspiration are shown in Figure 23-12B. During inspiration, as the diaphragm and intercostal muscles contract, the volume of the chest cavity increases. Expansion of the chest wall pulls outward on the lungs, and the intrapleural pressure

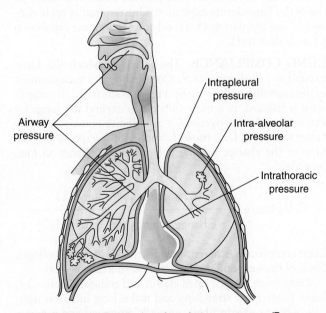

**FIGURE 23-11** Partitioning of respiratory pressures. (From Porth CM: Essentials of Pathophysiology, 3rd ed. Philadelphia, PA: Lippincott Williams & Wilkins, 2011, p 521.)

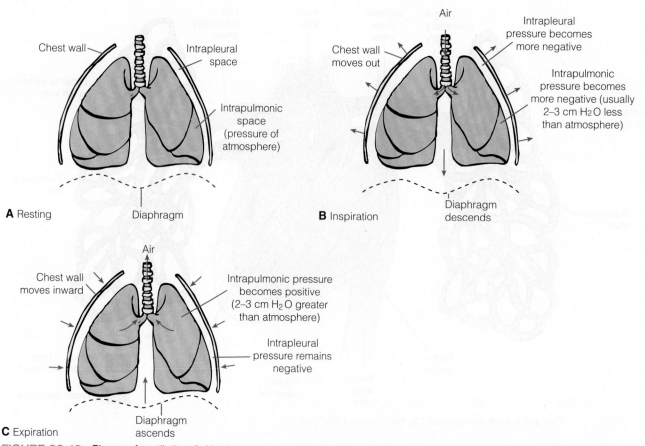

**FIGURE 23-12** Phases of ventilation. **A:** No air movement (resting). **B:** Air moves from the environment to the intrapulmonic space (inspiration). **C:** Air moves from the intrapulmonic space to the environment (expiration).

becomes more negative. As the alveolar pressure becomes more negative, air flows in from the atmosphere through the conducting airways to the alveoli. After inspiration, the muscles relax, and the chest cavity returns to its resting position. With this decrease in chest size and resultant compression of the lungs, the intra-alveolar pressure builds and forces air out of the lungs during expiration. One respiratory cycle consists of one inhalation (1 second at rest) and one exhalation (2 seconds at rest).

**LUNG COMPLIANCE.** The extent to which the lungs expand is called *compliance.* Compliance is a measurement of distensibility, or how easily a tissue is stretched. If compliance is reduced, it is more difficult to expand the lungs for inspiration. And conversely, if compliance is increased, it is easier to expand lung tissue. Compliance is expressed as the ratio of the change in lung volume to the change in lung pressure.

$$\text{Compliance} = \frac{\text{Change in lung volume (L)}}{\text{Change in lung pressure (cm } H_2O)}$$

Lung compliance is determined by the elastin and collagen fibers of the lung and the surface tension in the alveoli.

Lung tissue is made up of elastin and collagen fibers. Collagen fibers resist stretching and make lung inflation difficult, whereas elastin fibers are easily stretched and increase the ease of lung inflation. When elastin fibers are replaced

with scar tissue, such as that which occurs with pulmonary fibrosis or interstitial lung disease, the lungs become stiff and noncompliant.

The fluid lining the alveoli has a high surface tension. When the surface tension is high, the moist interior surfaces of an alveolus are difficult to separate from one another, and more energy is required to open and fill the alveolus with air during inspiration. When the surface tension is low, the alveoli walls separate more easily, requiring less effort for alveolar filling during inspiration. *Surfactant* decreases the surface tension of these fluids in the alveoli.

Surfactant has four important effects on lung inflation: it lowers the surface tension, increases lung compliance and ease of inflation, provides for stability and more even inflation of the alveoli, and assists in preventing pulmonary edema by keeping the alveoli dry.[4] Without surfactant, lung inflation is extremely difficult. Lack of surfactant or inefficient surfactant production may play a role in the development of *acute respiratory distress syndrome* (ARDS) in adults.

**AIRWAY RESISTANCE.** Airflow in the conducting airways is affected not only by pressure differences between the atmosphere and alveoli but also by the resistance that air encounters as it moves through the airways. According to Poiseuille's law, the resistance to flow is inversely proportional to the fourth power of the radius ($R = 1/r^4$). If the radius of the tube that gas is flowing through is cut in half, the resistance is increased 16-fold ($2 \times 2 \times 2 \times 2 = 16$). In the respiratory airways, small changes in airway diameter can have enormous effects on airflow resistance. Normally, airway resistance is so small that only small changes in pressure are needed to move large volumes of air into the lungs. But in conditions that decrease airway diameter, such as those caused by pulmonary secretions or bronchospasm, marked increases in airway resistance occur. To maintain the same rate of airflow as before the onset of increased airway resistance, people with these conditions must increase the driving pressure (or respiratory effort) to move air.

### Assessment of Ventilation

*Minute ventilation* is the volume of air inhaled and exhaled per minute. It is calculated by multiplying tidal volume ($V_T$) and respiratory rate. At rest, minute ventilation is approximately 7,500 mL/min.

Not all the air that enters the airways reaches the alveoli where gas exchange takes place. The part of $V_T$ that does not participate in alveolar gas exchange is called *dead space ventilation*. Dead space ventilation includes anatomical dead space volume and physiologic dead space volume. Anatomical dead space is the amount of air in the conducting airways and is normally about 2 mL/kg, or about 150 mL.[7] Anatomical dead space depends on body posture and disease states. In certain disease states, such as chronic obstructive pulmonary disease (COPD), anatomical dead space is larger than normal. Physiologic dead space occurs when ventilation is normal but perfusion to the alveoli is reduced or absent. This can occur with certain disease states, such as reduced cardiac output or pulmonary embolism. Dead space increases the partial pressure of arterial carbon dioxide ($PaCO_2$) because blood that is carrying carbon dioxide back from the tissues cannot reach the alveoli.

The *alveolar ventilation* is the volume of fresh gas entering the respiratory zone each minute. Alveolar ventilation is of key importance because it represents the amount of fresh inspired air available for gas exchange.[3] Alveolar ventilation is the minute ventilation minus dead space. It is inversely proportional to $PaCO_2$ levels. If one breathes excessively, alveolar ventilation is increased, and $PaCO_2$ decreases. If alveolar ventilation is decreased, $PaCO_2$ levels increase.

### Pulmonary Volumes and Capacities

The flow of air in and out of the lungs provides tangible measures of lung volumes. Although referred to as "pulmonary

**Anatomical and Physiologic Changes in the Respiratory System That Occur With Aging**

- The anterior–posterior diameter increases.
- Compliance is increased.
- Anatomical dead space is increased.
- The residual volume (RV) increases.
- Respiratory muscle strength decreases.
- The number of alveoli is reduced, resulting in decreased surface area for diffusion.
- Alveolar elasticity is decreased.
- Chest wall motility is decreased.
- The vital capacity (VC) decreases.
- Blood oxygen levels are decreased—subtract 1 mm Hg from a baseline arterial oxygen tension ($PaO_2$) of 80 mm Hg for every year over age 60.
- Anemia is common due to decreased hemoglobin and oxygen carrying capacity.

function" measures, in reality, these volumes represent "pulmonary anatomy" measures. In the evaluation of ventilation, structure or anatomy often determines function.

Ventilatory or pulmonary function tests measure the ability of the chest and lungs to move air into and out of the alveoli. Pulmonary function tests include volume measurements, capacity measurements, and dynamic measurements. These measurements are influenced by exercise and disease. Age, sex, body size, and posture are other variables that are taken into consideration when the test results are interpreted. (For a summary of age-related changes affecting the anatomy and physiology of the respiratory system, see Box 23-1.) Figure 23-13 illustrates pulmonary function tests showing normal lung volumes and capacity. Volume measurements show the amount of air contained in the lungs during various parts of the respiratory cycle. Measures of lung volume include $V_T$, inspiratory reserve volume (IRV), expiratory reserve volume (ERV), and residual volume (RV), as shown in Table 23-1. Capacity measurements quantify a part of the pulmonary cycle. They are measured as a combination of the previous volumes and include inspiratory capacity (IC), functional residual capacity (FRC), vital capacity (VC), and total lung capacity (TLC) (see Table 23-1).

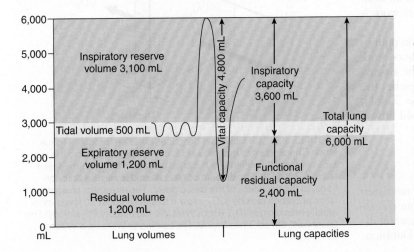

**FIGURE 23-13** Tracings of the respiratory volumes (**left**) and lung capacities (**right**) as they would appear if made using a spirometer. The tidal volume (*yellow*) represents the amount of air inhaled and exhaled during normal breathing; the inspiratory reserve volume (*pink*), the maximal amount of air in excess of the tidal volume that be forcefully inhaled; the maximal expiratory reserved (*blue*), the maximal amount of air that can be exhaled in excess of the tidal volume; and the residual volume (*green*), the air that continues to remain in the lung after maximal expiratory effort. The inspiratory capacity represents the sum of the inspiratory reserve volume and the tidal volume; the functional residual capacity, the sum of the maximal expiratory reserve and residual volumes; and the total lung capacity, the sum of all the volumes. (From Porth CM: Essentials of Pathophysiology, 3rd ed. Philadelphia, PA: Lippincott Williams & Wilkins, 2011, p 526.)

**TABLE 23-1**    **Lung Volumes and Lung Capacities**

| Term Used | Symbol | Description | Remarks | Normal Values (mL) |
|---|---|---|---|---|
| **Lung Volumes** | | | | |
| Tidal volume | $V_T$ | Volume of air inhaled and exhaled with each breath | Tidal volume may not vary, even with severe disease. | 500 |
| Inspiratory reserve volume | IRV | Maximum volume of air that can be inhaled after a normal inhalation | | 3,000 |
| Expiratory reserve volume | ERV | Maximum volume of air that can be exhaled forcibly after a normal exhalation | ERV is decreased with restrictive disorders, such as obesity, ascites, and pregnancy. | 1,100 |
| Residual volume | RV | Volume of air remaining in the lungs after a maximum exhalation | RV may be increased with obstructive diseases. | 1,200 |
| **Lung Capacities** | | | | |
| Vital capacity | VC | Maximum volume of air exhaled from the point of maximum inspiration | Decrease in VC may be found in neuromuscular disease, generalized fatigue, atelectasis, pulmonary edema, and COPD. | 4,600 |
| Inspiratory capacity | IC | Maximum volume of air inhaled after normal expiration | Decrease in IC may indicate restrictive disease. | 3,500 |
| Functional residual capacity | FRC | Volume of air remaining in lungs after a normal expiration | FRC may be increased with COPD and decreased in ARDS. | 2,300 |
| Total lung capacity | TLC | Volume of air in lungs after a maximum inspiration and equal to the sum of all four volumes ($V_T$, IRV, ERV, RV) | TLC may be decreased with restrictive disease (atelectasis, pneumonia) and increased in COPD. | 5,800 |

## The "Work" of Breathing

In normal quiet breathing, muscle contraction occurs during inspiration, and expiration is a passive process caused by elastic recoil of the lung. Thus, under normal resting conditions, muscle contraction (or work) is required only during inspiration. The work of inspiration can be divided into three categories: (1) work required to expand the lungs against lung and chest wall elastic forces, called *compliance work* or *elastic work*; (2) work required to overcome the viscosity of the lung and chest wall structures, called *tissue resistance work*; and (3) work required to overcome airway resistance during the movement of air into the lungs, called *airway resistance work*.[1] Normally during quiet respiration, only a small percentage of the total work is used to overcome tissue resistance, and a little more is used to overcome airway resistance; only 3% to 5% of the total energy expended by the body is required for ventilation. However, during heavy breathing when air must flow through the airways at a higher velocity, more work is used to overcome airway resistance.

All three types of work are frequently increased in pulmonary disease. Fibrosis of the lungs increases compliance work and tissue resistance work. Diseases that obstruct the airways increase airway resistance work. During heavy exercise, the amount of energy required can increase as much as 50-fold, especially if the person has any degree of increased airway resistance or decreased pulmonary compliance.[1]

## Diffusion

After the alveoli are ventilated with fresh air, the next step in the respiratory process is diffusion of oxygen from the alveoli to the pulmonary capillaries and diffusion of carbon dioxide from the pulmonary capillaries to the alveoli. Diffusion, or movement of molecules, occurs from an area of high to low concentration. Fick's law describes the diffusion of gases through the alveolar–capillary membrane (Fig. 23-14). Fick's law states that the rate of transfer of gas through a semipermeable membrane is proportional to the tissue surface area and the difference in gas pressures between the two sides, and inversely proportional to the tissue thickness. Recall that the surface area of the alveoli is very large (50 to 100 m$^2$) and that the thickness of the alveolar membrane is 0.3 µm, so the dimensions of the blood–gas barrier are ideal for diffusion of gases.[8] Different gases also cross the barrier at different rates

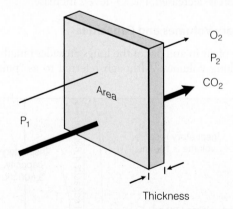

**FIGURE 23-14**    Fick's law describes diffusion through a tissue sheet. The amount of gas diffused is directly proportional to the surface area and the difference in partial pressures between the tissue sheets (P1 to P2). The amount of gas diffused is inversely proportional to the thickness of the tissue sheet. The molecular characteristics of carbon dioxide ($CO_2$) allow it to diffuse about 20 times more rapidly than oxygen ($O_2$). (From West JB: Respiratory Physiology: The Essentials, 9th ed. Philadelphia, PA: Lippincott Williams & Wilkins, 2011, p 26.)

| TABLE 23-2 | Factors Affecting Alveolar–Capillary Gas Exchange | |
|---|---|
| **Factors Affecting Gas Exchange** | **Examples** |
| Surface area available for diffusion | Removal of a lung or diseases, such as emphysema and chronic bronchitis, which destroy lung tissue or cause mismatching of ventilation and perfusion. |
| Thickness of the alveolar–capillary membrane | Conditions, such as pneumonia, interstitial lung disease, and pulmonary edema, which increase membrane thickness. |
| Partial pressure of alveolar gas | Ascent to high altitudes where the partial pressure of oxygen is reduced. In the opposite direction, increasing the partial pressure of a gas in the inspired air (eg, oxygen therapy) increases the gradient for diffusion. |
| Solubility and molecular weight of the gas | Carbon dioxide, which is more soluble in the cell membranes, diffuses across the alveolar–capillary membrane more rapidly than oxygen. |

From Porth CM: Pathophysiology: Concepts of Altered Health States, 7th ed. Philadelphia, PA: Lippincott Williams & Wilkins, 2005, p 650.

depending on their molecular characteristics. Carbon dioxide diffuses about 20 times more rapidly than oxygen. Thus, four factors affect alveolar–capillary gas exchange: (1) the surface area available for diffusion, (2) the thickness of the alveolar–capillary membrane, (3) the partial pressure of gas across the membrane, and (4) solubility and molecular characteristics of the gas (Table 23-2). Any condition or disease that affects one or more of these factors may impair diffusion of oxygen and carbon dioxide across the alveolar–capillary membrane.

## Perfusion

Once oxygen has diffused from the alveolus to the pulmonary capillary, it is carried away from the lung by the bloodstream. This gas exchange function of the lungs requires a constant flow of blood through the respiratory airways. The term *perfusion* is used to describe the flow of blood through the pulmonary capillary bed. The meshwork of the capillaries in the respiratory portion of the lungs is so dense that the flow in these vessels often is described as being similar to a "sheet" of blood.[4] When these blood vessels sense a low oxygen content in the alveoli, they vasoconstrict. The precise mechanism of this response, called *hypoxic vasoconstriction*, is not known.[9] Hypoxic vasoconstriction has the effect of directing blood flow away from hypoxic areas of the lung. By diverting blood flow from these areas, the deleterious effects on gas exchange are reduced.

## Relationship of Ventilation to Perfusion

### Distribution of Ventilation

Not all areas of the lung have the same ventilation. Body position affects distribution of ventilation. In a seated or standing position, lower regions of the lung ventilate better than upper zones. In a supine position, the apex and base of the lung ventilate about the same; however, ventilation in the lowermost (posterior) lung is greater than that of the uppermost (anterior) lung. In a lateral position, the dependent lung is best ventilated.[3]

### Distribution of Perfusion

As with ventilation, the distribution of pulmonary blood flow is affected by body position and gravity. For a person in the upright position, blood flow is better at the base of the lungs than the apex of the lungs. For a person in a supine position, the blood flow from apex to base is almost uniform, but blood flow in the posterior (dependent) regions of the lung exceeds that of the anterior regions. For a person in the prone position, the same holds true: blood flow in the dependent region (now the anterior chest) exceeds that of the posterior chest.

Considerable inequality of blood flow exists within the human lung (Fig. 23-15). The uneven distribution of blood flow can be explained by the hydrostatic pressure differences

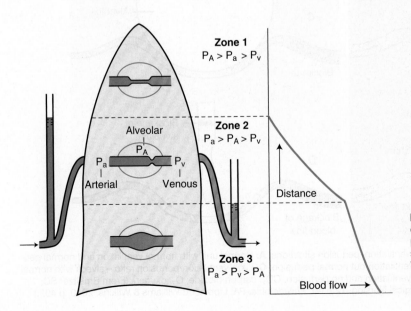

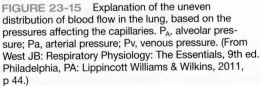

**FIGURE 23-15** Explanation of the uneven distribution of blood flow in the lung, based on the pressures affecting the capillaries. $P_A$, alveolar pressure; Pa, arterial pressure; Pv, venous pressure. (From West JB: Respiratory Physiology: The Essentials, 9th ed. Philadelphia, PA: Lippincott Williams & Wilkins, 2011, p 44.)

in the blood vessels. In zone 1, alveolar pressures exceed pulmonary arterial and pulmonary venous pressures. The capillaries are basically squashed flat by the pressure in the alveoli, and there is no blood flow. In zone 2, pulmonary arterial pressures are greater than alveolar pressures, so some blood flow occurs. Blood flow here is determined by the differences in arterial and alveolar pressures. In zone 3, there is minimal alveolar pressure influence on the pulmonary vasculature, and blood flow is determined in the usual way by the arteriovenous pressure difference.

### Matching of Ventilation to Perfusion

Effective pulmonary gas exchange depends on a balance or matching of ventilation to perfusion (Fig. 23-16A). Two factors may interfere with the matching of ventilation to perfusion: dead space and shunt. Dead space refers to areas in the respiratory system that do not participate in gas exchange. *Anatomical dead space* or the air in the conducting airways (about 150 mL) does not participate in gas exchange but increases with intubation. In zone 1 of the lung, the region is ventilated but not perfused, and this is referred to as *alveolar dead space*. Other areas of the lung may also contain alveolar dead space, such as that which occurs with collapsed alveoli from atelectasis or pneumonia. Shunt refers to blood that bypasses, or shunts by, alveoli without picking up oxygen. With an anatomical shunt, blood moves from the right side to the left side of the heart without passing through the lungs. Anatomical shunts occur with congenital heart diseases. With a physiologic shunt, blood is shunted past alveoli without picking up sufficient amounts of oxygen.

A ventilation–perfusion imbalance, known as a ventilation–perfusion mismatch, occurs when there is inadequate ventilation, inadequate perfusion, or both. Three types of ventilation–perfusion imbalances may occur:

- *Physiologic shunt* (low ventilation/perfusion ratio). When perfusion exceeds ventilation, the ratio is low, and a shunt is present. A shunt means that blood passes by alveoli without gas exchange occurring. A low ventilation–perfusion ratio is seen with pneumonia, atelectasis, tumor, or a mucous plug (see Fig. 23-16B).
- *Alveolar dead space* (high ventilation/perfusion ratio). When ventilation exceeds perfusion, the ratio is high and an alveolar dead space develops. The alveolus has inadequate perfusion available, and gas exchange cannot occur. A high ventilation/perfusion ratio is seen with a pulmonary embolus, pulmonary infarction, cardiogenic shock, and mechanical ventilation associated with high tidal volumes (see Fig. 23-16C).
- *Silent unit.* When both ventilation and perfusion are decreased, a silent unit occurs. A silent unit is seen with pneumothorax and severe ARDS (see Fig. 23-16D).

## Gas Transport

### Oxygen

Oxygen is carried in the blood in two forms: dissolved and attached to hemoglobin. The partial pressure of oxygen in arterial blood ($PaO_2$) represents the level of dissolved oxygen in plasma. Less than 3% of all oxygen is carried in this

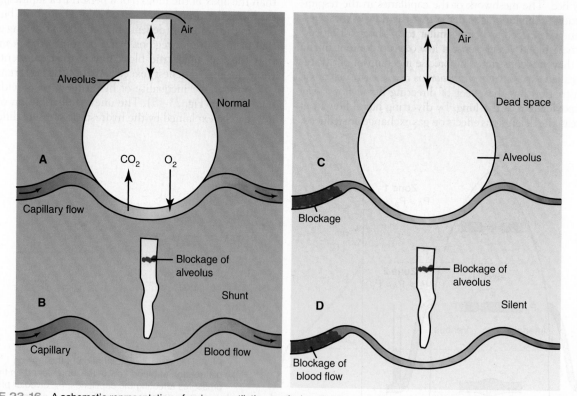

**FIGURE 23-16** A schematic representation of various ventilation–perfusion situations. **A:** Normal unit with normal ventilation and normal perfusion. **B:** Low-ventilation/perfusion ratio—alveoli with no ventilation but normal perfusion. **C:** High-ventilation/perfusion ratio—alveoli with normal ventilation but no perfusion. **D:** Silent unit—alveoli with no ventilation and no perfusion. $CO_2$, carbon dioxide; $O_2$, oxygen. (From Smeltzer SC, Bare BG: Brunner and Suddarth's Textbook of Medical Surgical Nursing, 12th ed. Philadelphia, PA: Lippincott Williams & Wilkins, 2010, p 492.)

form, whereas 97% of oxygen carried in the blood is bound to hemoglobin and is called *oxyhemoglobin*. Each gram of hemoglobin carries approximately 1.34 mL of oxygen when it is completely saturated. As oxygen diffuses across the alveolar–capillary membrane, it combines with hemoglobin in the red blood cell where it forms a reversible bond. Oxyhemoglobin is transported in arterial blood and made available to the tissues for use in cell metabolism. The saturation of oxygen in arterial blood ($SaO_2$) represents the percentage of hemoglobin molecules that are bound with oxygen.

The hemoglobin molecule is said to be fully saturated when oxygen is bound to all four of its oxygen-binding sites and only partially saturated when less than four molecules are bound to it. The term *affinity* is used to refer to the capacity of hemoglobin to combine with oxygen. When the affinity is high, hemoglobin binds readily with oxygen at the alveolar–capillary membrane. But, at the tissue level, hemoglobin does not readily release oxygen. When the affinity is low, hemoglobin does not bind readily with oxygen at the alveolar–capillary membrane. Instead, when affinity is low, hemoglobin releases oxygen more readily at the tissue level. The affinity of hemoglobin and oxygen is described by the oxyhemoglobin dissociation curve (Fig. 23-17).

The oxyhemoglobin dissociation curve is a graphic depiction of the relationship between oxyhemoglobin saturation (the percentage of hemoglobin combined with oxygen or the $SaO_2$) and the arterial oxygen tension ($PaO_2$) to which it is exposed. The initial part of the curve is very steep and then flattens at the top. The flat portion represents the binding of oxygen to hemoglobin in the lungs. The steep portion of the curve (between 40 and 60 mm Hg) represents the release of oxygen from the hemoglobin that occurs in the capillaries. At a $PaO_2$ of 40 mm Hg, hemoglobin molecules are still

about 70% to 75% saturated with oxygen. This provides a reserve supply of oxygen that can be given to the tissues in cases of emergency or strenuous exercise.

Hemoglobin's affinity for oxygen is influenced by pH, carbon dioxide concentration, temperature, and 2,3-diphosphoglycerate (2,3-DPG). 2,3-DPG is a metabolically important phosphate compound found in the blood in different combinations under different metabolic conditions.[10] Hemoglobin binds more readily with oxygen under conditions of increased pH, decreased carbon dioxide, decreased body temperature, and decreased 2,3-DPG. This is represented on the oxyhemoglobin dissociation curve as a shift to the left (see Fig. 23-17). With a shift to the left, there is higher oxygen saturation for any given $PaO_2$, increased affinity of hemoglobin for oxygen, and decreased release of oxygen to tissues. Hemoglobin more readily releases oxygen under conditions of decreased pH, increased carbon dioxide, increased body temperature, and increased 2,3-DPG. This relationship is represented on the curve by a shift to the right (see Fig. 23-17). With a shift to the right, there is lower oxygen saturation for any given $PaO_2$, decreased affinity of hemoglobin for oxygen, and increased release of oxygen to the tissues.

### Carbon Dioxide

Carbon dioxide is carried in the blood in three forms: as dissolved carbon dioxide (10%), attached to hemoglobin (30%), and as bicarbonate (60%).[4] Carbon dioxide is formed as a metabolic byproduct. It diffuses out of the cell and into the capillaries. Most of it diffuses into red blood cells, where it attaches to hemoglobin, and most of that is released from the red blood cell as bicarbonate. In the pulmonary capillaries, the concentration of carbon dioxide is greater in the capillaries than in the alveoli, so the carbon dioxide moves down this concentration gradient and diffuses into the alveoli and is exhaled. An increased rate of exhalation leads to greater elimination of carbon dioxide. The transport of carbon dioxide has a profound effect on the acid–base status of the blood and the body as a whole. The lung excretes more than 10,000 mEq of carbonic acid per day, compared with the kidney, which excretes less than 100 mEq of fixed acids per day.[11] Therefore, by altering alveolar ventilation (and subsequently, the elimination of carbon dioxide), the body is able to exert precise control over its acid–base balance.

### Regulation of Respiration

Breathing is controlled by both the nervous system and chemical regulation. Nervous system regulation is achieved by the respiratory centers, which are located in the medulla and pons (ie, the brainstem). Chemical regulation of breathing occurs through chemoreceptors, which respond to blood pH and the levels of oxygen and carbon dioxide in the blood. Chemoreceptors are located near the respiratory center in the medulla, in the carotid arteries, and in the aortic arch.

### Brainstem Centers and the Respiratory Cycle

Unlike the heart, the lungs have no spontaneous rhythm. Ventilation depends on rhythmic operation of brainstem centers and intact pathways to the respiratory muscles. There are two centers in the medulla: a center that stimulates inspiration by diaphragmatic contraction (by way of phrenic

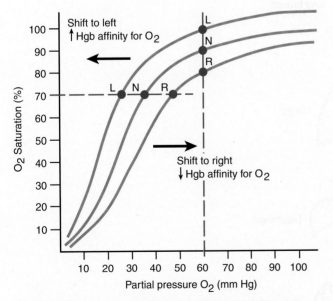

**FIGURE 23-17** Oxyhemoglobin dissociation curve. The shift to the left indicates a higher oxygen saturation at any given arterial oxygen tension ($PaO_2$), an increased affinity of hemoglobin for oxygen, and a decreased release of oxygen to the tissues. A shift to the right indicates a lower oxygen saturation at any given $PaO_2$, a decreased affinity of hemoglobin for oxygen, and an increased release of oxygen to the tissues. (From Smeltzer SC, Bare BG: Brunner and Suddarth's Textbook of Medical Surgical Nursing, 13th ed. Philadelphia, PA: Lippincott Williams & Wilkins, 2014, p 492.)

nerves) and another center that innervates both inspiratory and expiratory intercostal and accessory muscles (Fig. 23-18). The pons also contains two centers involved in controlling respiration: the pneumotaxic center and the apneustic center. The apneustic center produces sustained inspiration if stimulated. Voluntary control and involuntary control are further established by descending fibers from other brain centers. Neural control of ventilation is illustrated in Figure 23-18. In breathing at rest, the following sequence is thought to occur. The neurons innervating the inspiratory muscles fire bursts of impulses to these muscles, leading to inspiration. These neurons also stimulate the pneumotaxic center. This center, in turn, fires inhibitory impulses back to the inspiratory neurons, causing a halt in inspiration. Expiration follows passively. After expiration, the inspiratory neurons are again

stimulated to fire automatically. During exercise or other occasions when more vigorous ventilation occurs, the expiratory neurons of the medulla are postulated to participate in this sequence, causing active exhalation.

## Chemoreceptors

Chemoreceptors are like radar screens planted in the body to monitor blood levels of carbon dioxide and oxygen. Signals from these receptors are transmitted to the respiratory center, and ventilation is adjusted to maintain these gases in a normal range. There are two types of chemoreceptors: central chemoreceptors and peripheral chemoreceptors.

Central chemoreceptors sense changes in carbon dioxide content. They are located near the respiratory center in the

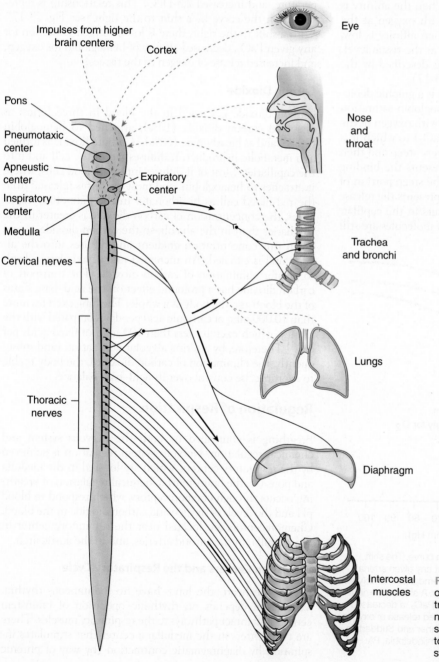

FIGURE 23-18 Schematic representation of activity in the respiratory center. Impulses traveling over afferent neurons activate central neurons, which activate efferent neurons that supply the muscles of respiration. Respiratory movements can be altered by a variety of stimuli.

medulla and are in close contact with cerebrospinal fluid (CSF). Carbon dioxide freely diffuses across the blood–brain barrier into the CSF. As the level of carbon dioxide in the CSF increases and the pH decreases, the nearby respiratory center is stimulated to increase respirations to "blow off" more carbon dioxide.

Peripheral chemoreceptors are located in the arch of the aorta and in the carotid arteries. These chemoreceptors are sensitive to changes in oxygen content in arterial blood. These receptors exert little control over respirations until the $PaO_2$ is below 60 mm Hg.[4] When this occurs, the respiratory center is stimulated to increase the rate and depth of respirations to inhale more oxygen.

### Lung Receptors

Lung and chest wall receptors provide information to the respiratory center on the status of airway resistance and lung expansion. There are three types of lung receptors: stretch, irritant, and juxtacapillary receptors. Stretch receptors, located in the smooth muscle layers of the conducting airways, respond to pressure changes in the airways. When the lungs are fully inflated, they inhibit further inspiration and trigger exhalation. These receptors are important because they establish respiratory patterns by adjusting respiratory rate and tidal volume in an attempt to respond to changes in airway resistance and lung compliance.

Irritant receptors, located in the airways, are stimulated by inhaled dust, smoke, chemicals, and cold air. Stimulation of these receptors triggers airway constriction and more rapid, shallow breathing. It is possible that these receptors play a key role in the bronchoconstriction that occurs with asthma.[4]

Juxtacapillary receptors are located in the alveolar wall close to the pulmonary capillaries. These receptors sense lung congestion. It may be stimulation of these receptors that produces the rapid, shallow breathing that is characteristic in patients with pneumonia and pulmonary edema.

## Clinical Applicability Challenges

### SHORT ANSWER QUESTIONS

1. Describe the process of inspiration and how it is defined as an "active" process.
2. Describe the three different types of ventilation/perfusion imbalances.
3. Discuss the central and peripheral chemoreceptors that are responsible for regulating respiration.

---

### WANT TO KNOW MORE?

A wide variety of resources to enhance your learning and understanding of this chapter are available on thePoint.

You will find:

- References
- Selected readings
- NCLEX-style review questions
- Internet resources
- And more!

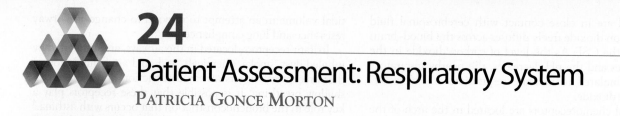

# 24

# Patient Assessment: Respiratory System

PATRICIA GONCE MORTON

## LEARNING OBJECTIVES

*Based on the content in this chapter, the reader should be able to:*

1. Describe the components of the history for respiratory assessment.
2. Explain the use of inspection, palpation, percussion, and auscultation for respiratory assessment.
3. Discuss the purpose of pulse oximetry and end-tidal carbon dioxide monitoring.
4. Explain the components of an arterial blood gas and the normal values for each component.
5. Compare and contrast the causes, signs, and symptoms of respiratory acidosis, respiratory alkalosis, metabolic acidosis, and metabolic alkalosis.
6. Analyze examples of an arterial blood gas result.
7. Describe the purpose of mixed venous oxygen saturation monitoring.
8. Discuss the purpose of respiratory diagnostic studies and associated nursing implications.

Nurses contribute significantly to the care of patients with respiratory problems by taking a comprehensive history and performing a thorough physical examination. This information allows the nurse to establish a baseline level of assessment of the patient's status and provides a framework for detecting rapid changes in the patient's condition. Assessments are valuable if made before, during, and after interventions that are likely to alter or improve respiratory status. High-quality assessments often uncover complications or changes that precede the information provided by other diagnostic tests.

## History

A thorough review of the patient's clinical history is an essential component of the overall physical assessment process. A properly conducted review of the patient's clinical history serves as a guide for the remainder of the physical examination. In many cases, obtaining a clinical history is the first step in developing a relationship with the patient. Patients often suppress information or underreport personal experiences that may be essential in identifying the underlying cause of illness. As a result, constant subjective evaluation of the patient's report should also serve to guide the clinical history. The interviewer must conduct the examination in such a way that the patient feels as comfortable as possible.

The clinical history of the respiratory system is divided into six components: (1) chief complaint, (2) history of present illness, (3) past health history, (4) family history, (5) personal and social history, and (6) review of systems (Box 24-1). The patient's history starts with the chief complaint and information about the present illness. Often, if the patient is very ill, a relative or friend provides information. Data about the present illness and any symptoms are thoroughly investigated using the mnemonic NOPQRST: normal (N), onset (O), precipitating and palliative factors (P), quality and quantity (Q), region and radiation (R), severity (S), and

time (T), as described in Box 17-1. Principal symptoms that are investigated in more detail commonly include dyspnea, chest pain, sputum production, and cough. An overview of the patient's past medical history and the family's respiratory history, as well as personal and social history, may uncover elements that are contributing to the patient's current health problem. Because smoking has a significant impact on the patient's respiratory health, the patient's use of tobacco is quantified by amount and how long the patient has smoked. Box 24-2 demonstrates the process for calculating this quantity, which is known as pack years.

## Dyspnea

Dyspnea is commonly seen in patients with pulmonary or cardiac compromise. Information about the onset of symptoms gives clues as to the source and duration of the problem. The nurse asks questions such as the following:

- Does the dyspnea occur when the patient is lying flat (therefore requiring the patient to sit up, as is seen more commonly in heart failure)?
- Does the dyspnea awaken the patient at night (paroxysmal nocturnal dyspnea)?
- Does the dyspnea occur only with exertion?

Paroxysmal nocturnal dyspnea and orthopnea often signify heart failure but may occur in a variety of pulmonary disorders. Description of the entire course of dyspnea, including exacerbating factors, length of episodes, and any relief measures attempted, is warranted.

## Chest Pain

Dyspnea that occurs with primary lung disease is associated with an anterior chest discomfort that must be distinguished from angina. First, the nurse determines whether the patient experiences more than one type of pain. For each type of

## BOX 24-1 Health History for Respiratory Assessment

**Chief Complaint**
- Patient's description of the problem

**History of the Present Illness**
- Complete analysis of the following signs and symptoms (using the NOPQRST format; see Chapter 17, Box 17-1).
- Dyspnea, dyspnea on exertion
- Shortness of breath
- Chest pain
- Cough
- Sputum production
- Hemoptysis
- Wheezing
- Orthopnea
- Clubbing
- Fatigue
- Cyanosis

**Past Health History**
- Relevant childhood illnesses and immunizations: whooping cough (pertussis), mumps, cystic fibrosis
- Past acute and chronic medical problems, including treatments and hospitalizations: streptococcal infection of the throat, upper respiratory infections, tonsillitis, bronchitis, sinus infection, emphysema, asthma, bronchiectasis, tuberculosis, cancer, pulmonary hypertension, heart failure, musculoskeletal and neurological diseases affecting the respiratory system
- Risk factors: age, obesity, smoking, environmental exposure such as asbestos, coal dust, chemicals, poison gas/vapors, dust, allergens
- Past surgeries: tonsillectomy, thoracic surgery, coronary artery bypass surgery, cardiac valve surgery, aortic aneurysm surgery, trauma surgery, tracheostomy
- Past diagnostic tests and interventions: tuberculin skin test, allergy tests, pulmonary function tests, chest radiograph, computed tomography scan, magnetic resonance imaging, bronchoscopy, cardiac stress test, ventilation–perfusion scanning, pulmonary angiography, thoracentesis, sputum culture

- Medications: use of oxygen, bronchodilators, antitussives, expectorants, mucolytics, anti-infectives, antihistamines, methylxanthine drugs, anti-inflammatory drugs
- Allergies and reactions
- Transfusions

**Family History**
- Health status or cause of death of parents and siblings: tuberculosis, cystic fibrosis, emphysema, asthma, malignancy

**Personal and Social History**
- Tobacco, alcohol, and substance use
- Family composition
- Occupation and work environment: asbestos, chemical, and coal dust exposure
- Living environment: exposure to allergens and toxic substances, type of heating and ventilation system
- Diet
- Sleep patterns: use of pillows
- Exercise
- Cultural beliefs
- Spiritual, religious beliefs
- Coping patterns and social support systems
- Leisure activities
- Sexual activity
- Recent travel

**Review of Systems**
- HEENT: strep throat, sinus infections, ear infection, deviated nasal septum, tonsillitis
- Cardiac: heart failure, dysrhythmias, coronary artery disease, valvular disease, hypertension
- Gastrointestinal: weight loss, nausea, vomiting
- Neuromuscular: Guillain–Barré syndrome, myasthenia gravis, amyotrophic lateral sclerosis, weakness
- Musculoskeletal: scoliosis, kyphosis

---

chest pain, the nurse asks the patient to describe the pain using the mnemonic NOPQRST. The detailed information obtained from using the mnemonic is key to determining the cause of the pain.

## Sputum Production

A pulmonary illness often results in the production (or a change in the production) of sputum. The nurse questions the patient about the amount (eg, tablespoonful, one-half cup) and color of the sputum produced in 24 hours. The color of the sputum provides important information about infection. An increase in either the color or the amount of sputum often means infection. Yellow, green, or brown sputum

## BOX 24-2 Steps for Calculating Pack Years

Pack years = (Number of packs smoked per day) × (Number of years smoking)
*Example*: The patient reports during the physical assessment that he has smoked two packs per day for 15 years.
  (2 packs/d) × (15 years) = 30 pack years

typically signifies bacterial infection; clear or white sputum may signify absence of bacterial infection. The color comes from white blood cells in the sputum. However, a yellow color may occur if there are many eosinophils in the sputum, thereby signifying allergy rather than infection. Rust-colored sputum (yellow sputum mixed with blood) may signify tuberculosis. Mucoid, viscid, or blood-streaked sputum is often a sign of a viral infection. Persistent slightly blood-streaked sputum is present in patients with carcinoma. Large amounts of clotted blood are present in the sputum of patients who have suffered a pulmonary infarction.

Occasionally, coughing does not yield sputum. Sometimes the patient with an infection is unable to cough up sputum. For example, a decrease in sputum production associated with worsening hypoxemia may signify bronchiolitis. A cough without sputum production usually means that the problem is not bacterial in origin.

It is important to know whether the sputum comes from the nose, the chest, or sinus postnasal drainage. Chronic sputum production may indicate chronic obstructive pulmonary disease (COPD).

Sometimes, the patient is afraid to mention that there has been blood in the sputum; it is essential to ask the patient, family members, and caregivers about the presence of blood. The amount of blood should be evaluated. Was it just streaks or specks, blood-colored mucus, or pure blood (bright red or dark)? Through careful questioning, the nurse determines whether the blood is associated with retching and vomiting or sputum production, as it often is in bronchitis and pneumonia, or whether it occurs alone, as is often true with a pulmonary embolus.

## Cough

A cough is a frequent respiratory symptom with varying significance. External agents, inflammation of the respiratory mucosa, or pressure on an airway caused by a tumor may stimulate a cough. Specifically, smoking, allergies, heartburn, asthma, and certain medications, including angiotensin-converting enzyme inhibitors and β-blockers, may cause a cough.

## Physical Examination

Physical assessment of the respiratory system is a reliable means of gathering essential data and is guided by the information obtained through the history. A thorough physical assessment includes inspection, palpation, percussion, and auscultation.

### Inspection

Inspection of the patient involves checking for the presence or absence of several factors (Box 24-3).

*Cyanosis* refers to a bluish discoloration of the skin or mucous membranes. Cyanosis is notoriously difficult to detect in a patient with anemia. The patient with polycythemia may have cyanosis in the extremities even if oxygen tension is normal. Peripheral cyanosis occurs in the extremities or on the tip of the nose or ears. Even with normal oxygen tensions, peripheral cyanosis may appear if there is diminished blood flow to these areas, particularly if they are cold or in a dependent position. Central cyanosis is apparent on the tongue or lips and usually means the patient has low oxygen tension. Unfortunately, the presence of cyanosis is a late and often ominous sign.

*Labored breathing* is an important marker of respiratory distress. As part of the inspection, the nurse determines whether the patient is using the accessory muscles of respiration (the scalene and sternocleidomastoid muscles). *Intercostal retractions* (ie, sucking in of the muscles and skin between the ribs during inspiration) usually mean that the patient is making a larger effort at inspiration than normal. The nurse also observes the patient for use of the abdominal muscles during the usually passive expiratory phase. Staccato speech, in which the patient's speech pattern is frequently interrupted as he or she gulps for air, may accompany labored breathing. Sometimes, the number of words a patient can say before having to gasp for another breath is a good measure of the degree of labored breathing.

The *anterior–posterior diameter of the chest* (ie, the size of the chest from front to back) is also checked (Fig. 24-1). Often, the cause of an increased anterior–posterior diameter is overexpansion of the lungs from obstructive pulmonary

---

**BOX 24-3** Components of the Inspection Process in the Physical Assessment of the Respiratory System

**General**
Mentation
Anxiety level
Speech
  • Staccato
  • Coherence
  • Aphasia
  • Articulation
  • Hoarseness
Skin turgor
Skin integrity
  • Scars
  • Rash
  • Wounds

Skin color
  • Pallor
  • Cyanosis
Weight
  • Obese
  • Malnourished
Body position
  • Leaning forward
  • Arms elevated

**Thorax**
Symmetry of thorax
Position of sternum
Anteroposterior diameter less than transverse by at least half
Rate, pattern, rhythm, and duration of breathing
Use of accessory muscles
Synchrony of chest and abdomen movement
Alignment of spine
Supernumerary nipples
Superficial venous patterns

**Head and Neck**
Nasal flaring
Pursed-lip breathing
Mouth breathing versus nose

Use of neck and shoulders
Tracheal position

**Extremities**
Clubbing
Edema
Peripheral cyanosis

---

disease. Patients with kyphosis (curvature of the spine) may also have an increase in anterior–posterior diameter.

*Chest deformities and scars* are important in helping to determine the reason for respiratory distress. A chest deformity, such as kyphoscoliosis or flail chest from trauma, may indicate why the patient has respiratory distress. A scar may signify recent or old injuries to the chest and provides clues to possible sources of distress. For example, evidence of recent trauma to the chest, such as a stabbing or compression injuries from an automobile collision, could be responsible for the present distress.

Observation of the *patient's posture* is necessary. Patients with obstructive pulmonary disease often sit and prop themselves up on outstretched arms or lean forward with their elbows on a table in an effort to elevate their clavicles. This posture gives the patient a slightly greater ability to expand the chest.

It is important to observe the *position of the trachea*. The nurse determines whether the trachea is in the midline as it should be or if it is deviated off to one side. Pleural effusion, hemothorax, pneumothorax, or a tension pneumothorax can deviate the trachea away from the affected side (toward the opposite side). However, atelectasis, fibrosis, and phrenic nerve paralysis often pull the trachea toward the affected side.

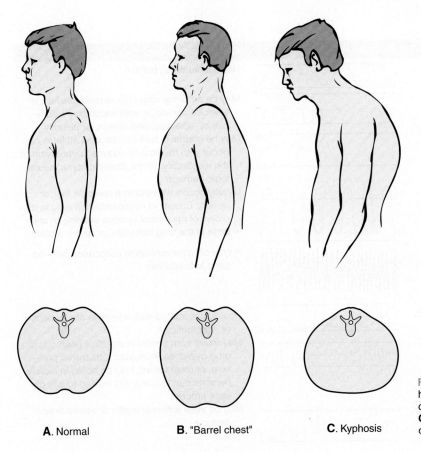

**A.** Normal          **B.** "Barrel chest"          **C.** Kyphosis

**FIGURE 24-1** Deformities and configurations of the human thorax. **A:** Normal chest. **B:** "Barrel chest," a chest deformity that typically results from emphysema. **C:** Kyphosis, a chest deformity that is most common in older adults.

The *respiratory rate* is an important parameter to follow. It should be counted over at least a 15-second period for stable patients and over a full minute for critically ill patients. The patient's rate must be compared with his or her usual rate. Breathing 24 to 26 times a minute may be normal in one patient but abnormal in another. The patient's family or friends may provide additional important information about the patient's usual rate of breathing.

The *respiratory effort* is often as meaningful as the respiratory rate. For instance, if a patient is breathing 40 times/min, the nurse might think a severe respiratory problem is the source of patient distress. However, the rate may be the result of Kussmaul respirations caused by diabetic acidosis. If a patient's respiration is shallow at a rate of 40 breaths/min (tachypnea), the indication may be severe respiratory distress from a primary pulmonary problem. Deep, rapid respirations, known as hyperventilation, may indicate compensation for acidosis. The pattern of respirations also should be noted because it may correlate with various disease processes. Table 24-1 provides a description of respiratory patterns and their clinical implications.

The *duration of inspiration versus the duration of expiration* helps determine the presence of obstructive lung disease. In patients with any of the obstructive lung diseases, expiration is more than one and a half times as long as inspiration.

Observation of *thoracic expansion* is an integral part of examining a patient. Normally, chest expansion of about 3 inches occurs from maximal expiration to maximal inspiration. Motion of the abdomen in breathing efforts (more likely to be normal in men than women) may be observed. Ankylosing spondylitis, a chronic condition resulting in painful, progressive inflammatory arthritis that typically affects the spine and sacroiliac joints, may be present. General chest expansion is limited in this condition. During the inspection, the nurse compares the expansion of the upper chest with that of the lower chest. The nurse also observes the movement of the diaphragm to determine whether the patient with obstructive pulmonary disease is concentrating on expanding the lower chest and using the diaphragm properly. Expansion of one side of the chest versus the other side is important to note: atelectasis, especially that caused by a plug of mucus, may cause unilaterally diminished chest expansion because the air cannot move equally through the pulmonary bed. Abnormal chest expansion may also occur with flail chest, in which the chest collapses instead of expanding during inspiration. Flail chest may result from broken or fractured ribs that cannot maintain the integrity of the chest wall during respiration. The nurse also notes whether the abdomen and chest rise and fall together as they should, or if the effort is not coordinated, and if there is symmetry of respiratory effort. Asynchronous respiratory effort decreases the quality of respiration at the cost of increased work of breathing and often precedes the need for ventilatory support.

A pulmonary embolus, pneumonia, pleural effusion, pneumothorax, or any problem associated with chest pain, such as fractured ribs, may lead to diminished chest expansion. An endotracheal or nasotracheal tube positioned beyond the trachea into one of the mainstem bronchi (usually the right) is a serious cause of diminished expansion of one side of the chest. If the tube slips into the right mainstem bronchus, the left lung is not expanded, and the patient may experience atelectasis on the left side and hypoxemia.

**TABLE 24-1** **Respiration Patterns**

| Type | Description | Pattern | Clinical Indication |
|---|---|---|---|
| Normal | 12–20 breaths/min and regular | | Normal breathing pattern |
| Tachypnea | More than 24 breaths/min and shallow | | May be a normal response to fever, anxiety, or exercise can occur with respiratory insufficiency, alkalosis, pneumonia, or pleurisy |
| Bradypnea | Less than 10 breaths/min and regular | | May be normal in well-conditioned athletes can occur with medication-induced depression of the respiratory center, diabetic coma, neurologic damage |
| Hyperventilation | Increased rate and increased depth | | Usually occurs with extreme exercise, fear, or anxiety. Causes of hyperventilation include disorders of the central nervous system, an overdose of the drug salicylate, or severe anxiety |
| Kussmaul | Rapid, deep, labored | | A type of hyperventilation associated with diabetic ketoacidosis |
| Hypoventilation | Decreased rate, decreased depth, irregular pattern | | Usually associated with overdose of narcotics or anesthetics |
| Cheyne–Stokes respiration | Regular pattern characterized by alternating periods of deep, rapid breathing followed by periods of apnea | | May result from severe congestive heart failure, drug overdose, increased intracranial pressure, or renal failure. May be noted in elderly persons during sleep, not related to any disease process |
| Biot respiration | Irregular pattern characterized by varying depth and rate of respirations followed by periods of apnea | | May be seen with meningitis or severe brain damage |
| Ataxic | Significant disorganization with irregular and varying depths of respiration | | A more extreme expression of Biot respirations indicating respiratory compromise |
| Air trapping | Increasing difficulty in getting breath out | | In COPD, air is trapped in the lungs during forced expiration |

Examination of the *patient's extremities* may provide additional information about the patient's respiratory status. Clubbing of the fingers, an enlargement of the distal portion of the fingers, is seen in many patients with respiratory and cardiovascular diseases (Fig. 24-2). Although the exact cause is not known, chronic hypoxia is a contributing factor. It is also important to assess the extremities for edema and peripheral cyanosis.

## Palpation

Chest palpation may indicate lung or chest abnormalities. To palpate the chest, the nurse places his or her hand flat against the patient's chest. When the patient speaks, sounds are generated by the larynx, and these sounds travel along the bronchial tree, resulting in a resonant motion of the chest wall. *Tactile fremitus* is the ability to feel the sound on

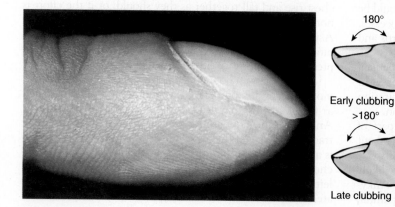

**FIGURE 24-2** In clubbing, the angle between the nail plate and the proximal nail fold increases to 180 degrees or more. Clubbing of the fingers is seen in patients with respiratory and cardiovascular disease. (Photo from Bickley LS: Bates' Guide to Physical Examination and History Taking, 10th ed. Philadelphia, PA: Lippincott Williams & Wilkins, 2009, p 193. Drawing from Weber J, Kelley J: Health Assessment in Nursing, 5th ed. Philadelphia, PA: Lippincott Williams & Wilkins, 2010, p 203.)

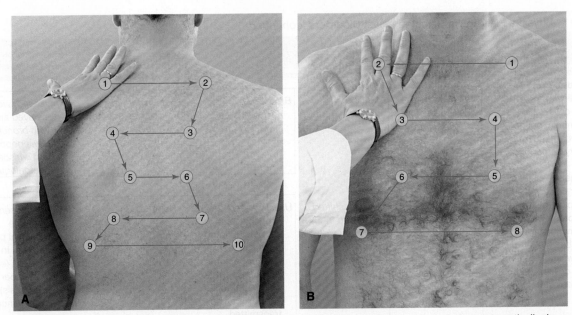

**FIGURE 24-3** Palpating the thorax is performed in a sequential fashion, starting near the neck and moving systematically downward. **A:** Posterior thorax. **B:** Anterior thorax. (Adapted from Weber J, Kelley J: Health Assessment in Nursing, 5th ed. Philadelphia, PA: Lippincott Williams & Wilkins, 2014, pp 382, 386.)

the chest wall. Tactile fremitus is more easily palpated over the large bronchi and is more difficult to palpate over the distant lung fields.

To assess tactile fremitus, the nurse asks the patient to say "ninety-nine" while moving his or her hands over the posterior surfaces of the chest wall (Fig. 24-3). Tactile fremitus should be symmetrical. Tactile fremitus may be diminished

or absent if there is an increase in air per unit volume of lung because air impedes the transmission of sound. For example, patients with emphysema have little or no tactile fremitus on physical examination. Tactile fremitus is slightly increased by the presence of solid substances, such as the consolidation of a lung from pneumonia. Other respiratory conditions causing an alteration in tactile fremitus are listed in Table 24-2.

**TABLE 24-2    Physical Findings in Selected Chest Disorders**

| Condition | Percussion Note | Trachea | Breath Sounds | Adventitious Sounds | Tactile Fremitus and Transmitted Voice Sounds |
|---|---|---|---|---|---|
| **Normal** The tracheobronchial tree and alveoli are clear; pleurae are thin and close together; mobility of the chest wall is unimpaired | **Resonant** | Midline | Vesicular, except perhaps bronchovesicular and bronchial sounds over the large bronchi and trachea, respectively | None, except perhaps a few transient inspiratory crackles at the bases of the lungs | Normal |
| **Chronic Bronchitis** The bronchi are chronically inflamed and a productive cough is present. Airway obstruction may develop | **Resonant** | Midline | Vesicular (normal) | None; or scattered coarse *crackles* in early inspiration and perhaps expiration; or *wheezes* or *rhonchi* | Normal |
| **Left-Sided Heart Failure** *(Early)* Increased pressure in the pulmonary veins causes congestion and interstitial edema (around the alveoli); bronchial mucosa may become edematous | **Resonant** | Midline | Vesicular | *Late inspiratory crackles* in the dependent portions of the lungs; possibly *wheezes* | Normal |

**TABLE 24-2** Physical Findings in Selected Chest Disorders (*continued*)

| Condition | Percussion Note | Trachea | Breath Sounds | Adventitious Sounds | Tactile Fremitus and Transmitted Voice Sounds |
|---|---|---|---|---|---|
| **Consolidation** Alveoli fill with fluid or blood cells, as in pneumonia, pulmonary edema, or pulmonary hemorrhage | **Dull** over the airless area | Midline | *Bronchial* over the involved area | *Late inspiratory crackles* over the involved area | *Increased* over the involved area, with *bronchophony, egophony,* and *whispered pectoriloquy* |
| **Atelectasis** *(Lobar Obstruction)* When a plug in a mainstem bronchus (as from mucus or a foreign object) obstructs air flow, affected lung tissue collapses into an airless state | **Dull** over the airless area | May be *shifted toward involved side* | *Usually absent* when bronchial plug persists. Exceptions include right upper lobe atelectasis, where adjacent tracheal sounds may be transmitted | None | *Usually absent* when the bronchial plug persists. In exceptions (eg, right upper lobe atelectasis) it may be increased |
| **Pleural Effusion** Fluid accumulates in the pleural space, separates air-filled lung from the chest wall, blocking the transmission of sound | **Dull** to flat over the fluid | *Shifted toward opposite side in a large effusion* | *Decreased to absent*, but bronchial breath sounds may be heard near top of large effusion | None, except a *possible pleural* rub | *Decreased to absent, but may be increased* toward the top of a large effusion |
| **Pneumothorax** When air leaks into the pleural space, usually unilaterally, the lung recoils from the chest wall. Pleural air blocks transmission of sound | **Hyperresonant** or tympanitic over the pleural air | *Shifted toward opposite side* if much air | *Decreased to absent* over the pleural air | None, except a *possible pleural* rub | *Decreased to absent* over the pleural air |
| **Chronic Obstructive Pulmonary Disease** Slowly progressive disorder in which the distal air spaces enlarge and lungs become hyperinflated. Chronic bronchitis is often associated | Diffusely **hyperresonant** | Midline | Decreased to absent | None, or the crackles, wheezes, and rhonchi of associated chronic bronchitis | Decreased |
| **Asthma** Widespread narrowing of the tracheobronchial tree diminishes air flow to a fluctuating degree. During attacks, air flow decreases further, and lungs hyperinflate | **Resonant** to diffusely **hyperresonant** | Midline | Often obscured by wheezes | Wheezes, possibly crackles | Decreased |

The black boxes in this table suggest a framework for clinical assessment. Start with the three boxes under Percussion. Note: resonant, dull, and hyperresonant. Then move from each of these to other boxes that emphasize some of the key differences among various conditions. The changes described vary with the extent and severity of the disorder. Abnormalities deep in the chest usually produce fewer signs than superficial ones, and may cause no signs at all. Use the table for the direction of typical changes, not for absolute distinctions.

From Bickley LS: Bates' Guide to Physical Examination and History Taking, 10th ed. Philadelphia, PA: Lippincott Williams & Wilkins, 2009, pp 320–321.

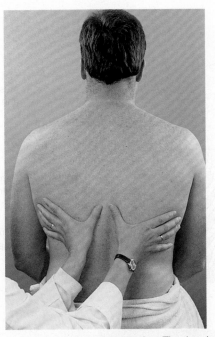

FIGURE 24-4 Palpating chest expansion. The thumbs are positioned at the level of the 10th rib. (From Weber J, Kelley J: Health Assessment in Nursing, 5th ed. Philadelphia, PA: Lippincott Williams & Wilkins, 2014, p 382.)

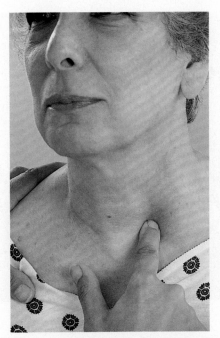

FIGURE 24-5 Palpating the trachea. The trachea should be midline, above the suprasternal notch. (Photograph B. Proud. From Weber J, Kelley J: Health Assessment in Nursing, 4th ed. Philadelphia, PA: Lippincott Williams & Wilkins, 2010, p 220.)

Palpation is also used to assess for subcutaneous emphysema, a condition in which air "leaks" out of the alveolus and moves through the subcutaneous tissue. By moving the fingers in a gentle rolling motion across the chest and neck, it is possible to feel the pockets of air underneath the skin. Feeling subcutaneous emphysema is often likened to the "crunch" of Rice Krispies under the skin. Subcutaneous emphysema may result from a pneumothorax, small pockets of alveoli that have burst with increased pulmonary pressure, or the use of positive end-expiratory pressure. In severe cases, the subcutaneous emphysema may spread into the lower thorax, arms, and face.

Evaluation of thoracic expansion during respiration also requires palpation. To perform this procedure, the nurse stands behind the patient, identifies the level of the 10th rib, and places his or her thumbs along the spine using the bony processes as a guide, letting the palms come in light contact with the posterolateral surface (Fig. 24-4). The nurse asks the patient to breathe normally and then deeply, both times watching as the thumbs diverge. Expansion of the chest wall should be symmetrical. Asymmetrical expansion may be indicative of a collapsed lung or unilateral disease. Retractions may be a sign of obstruction to inspiration and require immediate attention.

Palpation of the patient's trachea is an important element in the physical assessment of the respiratory system. To palpate the trachea to evaluate the midline position, the nurse positions his or her index finger in the suprasternal notch, feeling each side of the notch and palpating the tracheal rings (Fig. 24-5). The trachea should be in the midline position directly above the suprasternal notch.

## Percussion

Percussion of the chest results in slight motion of the chest wall and underlying structures, causing audible and tactile vibrations. To percuss a patient's chest, the nurse presses one finger from the nondominant hand flat against the chest and uses a fingertip from the dominant hand to strike the knuckle pressed against the chest (Fig. 24-6). Normally, the chest has a resonant or hollow percussion note. In diseases in which there is increased air in the chest or lungs, such as pneumothorax and emphysema, there can be hyperresonant percussion notes. However, these loud, low-pitched sounds are sometimes difficult to detect.

More important is a flat percussion note (eg, the sound that is heard when percussing over a part of the body that contains no air). A flat percussion note is a soft, high-pitched sound that is more easily distinguished by noting the change in sound when one moves from percussing an area with air to an area with no air. It is more likely to be heard if a large pleural effusion is present in the lung beneath the examining hand. A dull percussion note is medium in intensity and pitch. It is heard if atelectasis or consolidation resulting from pneumonia, pulmonary edema, or pulmonary hemorrhage is present. A tympanic drum-like sound is a high-pitched noise heard if asthma or a large pneumothorax is present. See Table 24-2 for a description of percussion sounds associated with various respiratory pathologies.

## Auscultation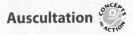

In chest auscultation, the diaphragm of the stethoscope is pressed firmly against the chest wall. The sequence for auscultating the posterior and anterior thorax is given in Figure 24-7. The nurse listens to the intensity or loudness of breath sounds. Normally, there is a fourfold increase in loudness of breath sounds when a patient takes a maximal deep breath as opposed to quiet breathing. Sounds are louder in the upper and central chest when listening to the larger

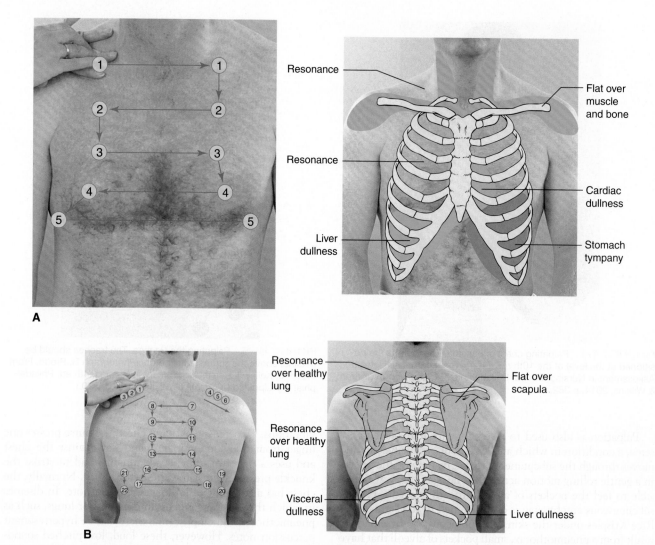

**A**

**B**

FIGURE 24-6 Percussing the thorax is performed in a sequential fashion, starting near the neck and moving systematically downward. **A:** Anterior thorax. **B:** Posterior thorax. (**A.** From Weber J, Kelley J: Health Assessment in Nursing, 5th ed. Philadelphia, PA: Lippincott Williams & Wilkins, 2014, pp 387, 388. **B.** From Weber J, Kelley J: Health Assessment in Nursing, 4th ed. Philadelphia, PA: Lippincott Williams & Wilkins, 2010, p 323.)

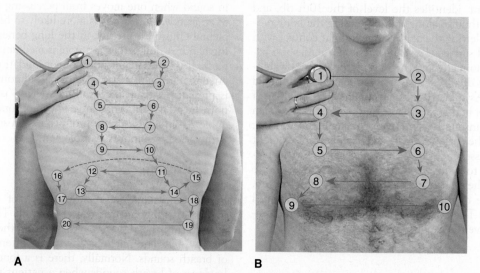

**A**

**B**

FIGURE 24-7 Auscultating the chest is performed in a sequential fashion, starting near the neck and moving systematically downward. **A:** Posterior thorax. **B:** Anterior thorax. (From Weber J, Kelley J: Health Assessment in Nursing, 5th ed. Philadelphia, PA: Lippincott Williams & Wilkins, 2014, pp 384, 388.)

bronchus and become quieter as the smaller airways are auscultated. The intensity of the breath sounds may be diminished because of decreased flow through the airways or the presence of substances between the lungs and the stethoscope. In pleural thickening, pleural effusion, pneumothorax, and obesity, an abnormal substance (fibrous tissue, fluid, air, or fat) lies between the stethoscope and the underlying lung; this substance insulates the breath sounds from the stethoscope, making the breath sounds seem less loud. In airway obstruction, such as COPD or atelectasis, the intensity of breath sounds is diminished. With shallow breathing, there is diminished air movement through the airways, and the breath sounds are not as loud. With restricted movement of the thorax or diaphragm, there are diminished breath sounds in the restricted areas.

In general, four types of sounds are heard in the normal chest (Table 24-3). *Vesicular breath sounds* are quiet, low-pitched sounds, and the inspiratory phase is longer than the expiratory phase. *Bronchovesicular breath sounds* are medium in pitch, and the inspiratory and expiratory phases are of equal length. *Bronchial breath sounds* are higher pitched and louder compared with vesicular sounds, and the expiratory phase is longer than the inspiratory phase. *Tracheal breath sounds* are loud, high-pitched sounds, and the inspiratory and expiratory phases are about equal in length.[1]

Bronchial breath sounds are heard over the manubrium not only in the normal state but when consolidation is present, as in pneumonia. Bronchial breath sounds are also heard above a pleural effusion in which the normal lung is compressed and sounds are transmitted through the tissue, which is not participating in airflow. Wherever there is bronchial breathing, there also may be two associated changes: E to A changes and whispered pectoriloquy.

An *E to A change* occurs when the patient says "E" and the nurse listening with a stethoscope actually hears an "A" sound rather than an "E" sound. This occurs if consolidation is present. *Egophony* is the term used to describe voice sounds that are distorted.

*Whispered pectoriloquy* is the presence of loud, clear sounds heard through the stethoscope when the patient whispers. Normally, the whispered voice is heard faintly and indistinctly through the stethoscope. The increased transmission of voice sounds indicates that air in the lungs has been replaced by fluid as a result of pneumonia, pulmonary edema, or hemorrhage.

*Adventitious sounds* are additional breath sounds heard with auscultation and include discontinuous sounds, continuous sounds, and rubs. Discontinuous sounds are brief, nonmusical, intermittent sounds and include fine and coarse *crackles*. (Crackles were formerly known as *rales*.) Fine crackles are soft, high-pitched, very brief popping sounds that occur most commonly during inspiration. Crackles result from fluid in the airways or alveoli, or from the opening of collapsed alveoli. Restrictive pulmonary disease results in crackles during late inspiration, whereas obstructive pulmonary disease results in crackles during early inspiration. Crackles become coarser as the air moves through larger fluid accumulations, as in bronchitis or pneumonia. Crackles that clear with coughing are not associated with significant pulmonary disease. When assessing crackles, the nurse also notes their loudness, pitch, duration, amount, location, and timing in the respiratory cycle.[2]

Continuous adventitious breath sounds are longer in duration than crackles and include wheezes and rhonchi. *Wheezes* are continuous musical sounds that are longer than crackles in duration and persist throughout the respiratory cycle. Wheezes (also known as sibilant wheezes) are continuous, high-pitched adventitious sounds that have a shrill quality. They are caused by the movement of air through a narrowed or partially obstructed airway, such as in asthma, COPD, or bronchitis.

*Rhonchi*, another type of continuous adventitious breath sound, are deep, low-pitched rumbling noises that are sometimes referred to as sonorous wheezes or gurgles. The presence of rhonchi indicates the presence of secretions in the large airways.[1] Conditions such as bronchitis cause sonorous wheezing. These sounds may clear somewhat with coughing.

A *friction rub* is a crackling, grating sound heard more often with inspiration than expiration. The sound of friction results from the visceral and parietal pleurae rubbing against each other. A friction rub can be heard with pleural effusion, pneumothorax, or pleurisy. It is important to distinguish a pleural friction rub from a pericardial friction rub. To determine the origin of the rub, the nurse asks the patient

---

**TABLE 24-3**    **Characteristics of Breath Sounds**

| | Duration of Sounds | Intensity of Expiratory Sound | Pitch of Expiratory Sound | Location Where Heard Normally |
|---|---|---|---|---|
| Vesicular | Inspiratory sounds last longer than expiratory ones | Soft | Relatively low | Over most of both lungs |
| Bronchovesicular | Inspiratory and expiratory sounds are about equal | Intermediate | Intermediate | Often in the first and second interspaces anteriorly and between the scapulae |
| Bronchial | Expiratory sounds last longer than inspiratory ones | Loud | Relatively high | Over manubrium, if heard at all |
| Tracheal | Inspiratory and expiratory sounds are about equal | Very loud | Relatively high | Over the trachea in the neck |

The thickness of the bars indicates intensity; the steeper their incline, the higher the pitch.
From Bickley LS: Bates' Guide to Physical Examination and History Taking, 10th ed. Philadelphia, PA: Lippincott Williams & Wilkins, 2009, p 303.

**Respiratory Assessment**

- Decreased ability to hold breath during examination
- Increased hyperresonance (caused by increased distensibility of the lungs)
- Decreased chest wall expansion
- Decreased use of respiratory muscles
- Increased use of accessory muscles secondary to calcification of rib articulations
- Less subcutaneous tissue
- Possible pronounced dorsal curvature
  - Kyphosis (abnormal convexity of the spine; see Fig. 24-1C)
  - Gibbus (severe kyphosis)
- Presence of basilar crackles in the absence of disease (should clear after a few coughs)

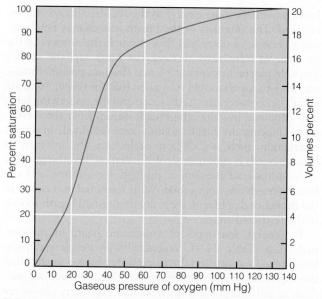

**FIGURE 24-8**   Oxyhemoglobin dissociation curve.

to hold his or her breath while the lungs are auscultated. If the sounds continue while the patient is holding his or her breath, it is most likely a pericardial friction rub; a pleural friction rub stops when breathing stops.

In elderly people, unique anatomical and physiological characteristics manifest in different assessment findings. Box 24-4 shows specific respiratory assessment findings in older patients.

## Respiratory Monitoring

### Pulse Oximetry

Approximately 3% of oxygen is dissolved in the plasma (Box 24-5). The partial pressure of oxygen dissolved in the arterial blood is measured by the $PaO_2$. The normal $PaO_2$ is 80 to 100 mm Hg at sea level. The remaining 97% of oxygen is attached to hemoglobin (Hgb) molecules in red blood cells. Each gram of Hgb can carry a maximum of 1.34 mL of oxygen. The percentage of saturation of Hgb is defined as the amount of oxygen that Hgb is carrying compared with the amount of oxygen that Hgb can carry, expressed as a percentage:

$$Percent\ O_2\ Saturation\ of\ Hgb =$$
$$\frac{Amount\ of\ O_2\ hemoglobin\ is\ carrying}{Amount\ of\ O_2\ hemoglobin\ can\ carry} \times 100$$

Because the amount of oxygen that Hgb can carry is a constant 1.34 mL/g,

$$1.34\ mL/g \times g\ Hgb \times \%\ saturation\ Hgb =$$
$$mL\ of\ O_2\ that\ Hgb\ is\ carrying$$

The arterial oxygen saturation of Hgb is known as the $SaO_2$. The normal $SaO_2$ ranges from 93% to 99%.

**BOX 24-5**   **How Oxygen Is Carried in the Blood**

| | |
|---|---|
| Oxygen dissolved in the plasma measured as $PaO_2$: | 0.3 mL/100 mL of blood |
| Oxygen combined with Hgb measured as $SaO_2$: | 19.4 mL/100 mL of blood |
| Total oxygen in blood: | 19.7 mL/100 mL of blood |

The relationship between $PaO_2$ and $SaO_2$ is depicted by the oxyhemoglobin dissociation curve (Fig. 24-8). The initial part of the curve is very steep and flattens at the top. The flattened part means that large changes in the $PaO_2$ result in only small changes in $SaO_2$. A critical point of the curve occurs when the $PaO_2$ drops below 60 mm Hg. At this point, the curve drops sharply, signifying that a small decrease in $PaO_2$ is associated with a large decrease in $SaO_2$.

When the curve shifts to the right, there is a reduced capacity for Hgb to combine with oxygen, resulting in more oxygen released to the tissues. When the curve shifts to the left, there is an increased capacity for Hgb to combine with oxygen, resulting in less oxygen released to the tissues. See Chapter 23 for a more detailed discussion of the oxyhemoglobin dissociation curve.

A pulse oximeter is a device used to measure a value known as $SpO_2$ (oxygen saturation as measured by pulse oximetry). The $SpO_2$ reflects the arterial oxygen saturation of Hgb. Through oximetry, light-emitting and light-receiving sensors quantify the amount of light absorbed by oxygenated/deoxygenated Hgb in arterial blood. The value displayed on the pulse oximeter is an average of numerous readings taken in a 3- to 10-second period. This reduces the effects of pressure waveform variation caused by patient activity. Usually, the sensors are in a clip placed on a finger or ear lobe and allow for evaluation of the quality of the pulsatile waveform. The oximeter sensor in some devices is placed on the forehead. For assessment of pulse oximetry in infants, flexible probes can measure saturation when placed on the palm, arm, penis, or foot.

Oximetry should not be used in place of arterial blood gas (ABG) monitoring. Instead, pulse oximetry may be used to assess trends in oxygen saturation when the correlation between arterial blood and pulse oximetry readings has been established. Values obtained by pulse oximetry are unreliable when vasoconstricting medications or intravenous dyes are used and when shock, cardiac arrest, or severe anemia is present. Pulse oximetry has limited usefulness in patients with known dyshemoglobins, such as carboxyhemoglobin, which is elevated in smokers, and methemoglobin, which is seen in patients undergoing nitrate and lidocaine therapy. These limitations should be considered when interpreting pulse oximetry readings in certain patients.

## End-Tidal Carbon Dioxide Monitoring

End-tidal carbon dioxide (ETCO$_2$) monitoring measures the level of carbon dioxide at the end of exhalation, when the percentage of carbon dioxide dissolved in the arterial blood (PaCO$_2$) approximates the percentage of alveolar carbon dioxide (PaCO$_2$). Therefore, samples of exhaled carbon dioxide measured at the end of exhalation (ETCO$_2$) can be used to approximate levels of PaCO$_2$. Levels of alveolar carbon dioxide and arterial carbon dioxide are similar; therefore, ETCO$_2$ can be used to estimate PaCO$_2$. Although PaCO$_2$ and ETCO$_2$ values are similar, ETCO$_2$ is usually lower than PaCO$_2$ by 2 to 5 mm Hg. The difference between PaCO$_2$ and ETCO$_2$ (PaCO$_2$–ETCO$_2$ gradient) may be attributed to several factors; pulmonary blood flow is the primary determinant.

ETCO$_2$ values are obtained by monitoring samples of expired gas from an endotracheal tube, an oral airway, or a nasopharyngeal airway. Because ETCO$_2$ provides continuous estimates of alveolar ventilation, its measurement is useful for monitoring the patient during weaning from a ventilator, in cardiopulmonary resuscitation, and in endotracheal intubation.

The accuracy of the ETCO$_2$ readings may be affected by high concentrations of oxygen and water vapor. The nurse using ETCO$_2$ technology must be aware of these conditions and their effect on the monitor being used. Impaired infrared absorption from the interaction of carbon dioxide and oxygen in high concentrations may cause falsely low ETCO$_2$ measurements, and the interference of water vapor with the absorption of infrared light may cause falsely elevated measurements. The nurse must combine ETCO$_2$ readings with a variety of other clinical data.

The exhaled carbon dioxide waveform is displayed on the monitor as a plot of ETCO$_2$ versus time called a capnogram, which provides the nurse with a continuous graphic reading of the patient's ETCO$_2$ level with each exhaled breath. Changes in the waveform indicate clinical abnormalities, mechanical abnormalities, or both and require immediate assessment by the nurse or other trained professional.

On a capnogram, the waveform is composed of four phases, each one representing a specific part of the respiratory cycle (Fig. 24-9):

1. The *first phase* is the baseline phase, which represents both the inspiratory phase and the very beginning of the expiratory phase, when carbon dioxide-free air in the anatomical dead space is exhaled. This value should be zero in a healthy adult.
2. The *second phase* is the expiratory upstroke, which represents the exhalation of carbon dioxide from the lungs. Any process that delays the delivery of carbon dioxide from the patient's lungs to the detector prolongs the expiratory upstroke. Conditions such as COPD and bronchospasm are known physiological causes of prolonged expiratory upstroke. Mechanical obstructions, such as kinked ventilator tubing, may also cause prolonged expiratory upstroke.

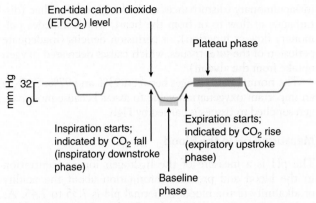

**FIGURE 24-9** Capnogram tracing, with four phases labeled. CO$_2$, carbon dioxide.

3. The *third phase* begins as carbon dioxide elimination rapidly continues; a plateau on the capnogram indicates the exhalation of alveolar gases. The ETCO$_2$ is the value generated at the very end of exhalation, indicating the amount of carbon dioxide exhaled from the least ventilated alveoli.
4. The *fourth phase* is known as the inspiratory downstroke. The downward deflection of the waveform is caused by the washout of carbon dioxide that occurs in the presence of the oxygen influx during inspiration.

## Arterial Blood Gases

In an ABG test, a sample of arterial blood is drawn and analyzed to help determine the quality and extent of pulmonary gas exchange and acid–base status. The ABG test measures PaO$_2$, SaO$_2$, PaCO$_2$, pH, and the bicarbonate (HCO$_3$) level. The procedure involves obtaining arterial blood from a direct arterial puncture or from an arterial line often placed in the radial artery. More recent technology allows the continuous monitoring of ABGs using a fiberoptic sensor placed in the artery. Normal ABG values are given in Box 24-6.

### Measuring Oxygen in the Blood

Oxygenation may be measured using an ABG by evaluating the PaO$_2$ and the SaO$_2$. As mentioned previously, only 3% of oxygen is dissolved in the arterial blood, and the remaining 97% is attached to Hgb in the red blood cells.

The normal PaO$_2$ is 80 to 100 mm Hg at sea level (barometric pressure of 760 mm Hg). For people living at higher altitudes, the normal PaO$_2$ is lower because of the lower barometric pressure. PaO$_2$ tends to decrease with age. For patients who are 60 to 80 years of age, a PaO$_2$ of 60 to 80 mm Hg is normal. An abnormally low PaO$_2$ is referred to as hypoxemia. Hypoxemia may result from many conditions, which are most commonly grouped according to their origin:

| BOX 24-6 | Normal Values for an Arterial Blood Gas |
| --- | --- |

**PaO$_2$:** 80 to 100 mm Hg
**SaO$_2$:** 93% to 99%
**pH:** 7.35 to 7.45
**PaCO$_2$:** 35 to 45 mm Hg
**HCO$_3$:** 22 to 26 mEq/L

intrapulmonary (disturbances in the lung), intracardiac (disturbance of flow to or from the heart, which impedes pulmonary flow or function), or perfusion deficits (inadequate perfusion of the lung tissues, which causes decreased oxygen uptake from the alveoli).

The normal $SaO_2$ ranges between 93% and 97%. $SaO_2$ is an important oxygenation value to assess because most oxygen supplied to tissues is carried by Hgb.

### Measuring pH in the Blood

The pH is a measure of the hydrogen ion concentration in the blood and provides information about the acidity or alkalinity of the blood. A normal pH is 7.35 to 7.45. As hydrogen ions accumulate, the pH drops, resulting in acidemia. Acidemia refers to a condition in which the blood is too acidic. Acidosis refers to the process that causes the acidemia.

A decrease in hydrogen ions results in an elevation of the pH and alkalemia. Alkalemia refers to a condition in which the blood is too alkaline. Alkalosis refers to the process that causes the alkalemia. Box 24-7 reviews the terms used in acid–base balance.

**ACIDS.** An acid is a substance that can donate a hydrogen ion ($H^+$) to a solution. There are two different types of acids: volatile acids and nonvolatile acids. Volatile acids are those that can move between the liquid and gaseous states. Once in the gaseous state, these acids can be removed by the lungs. The major acid in the blood serum is carbonic acid ($H_2CO_3$). This acid is broken down into carbon dioxide and water by an enzyme produced in the kidneys. Nonvolatile ("fixed") acids are those that cannot change into a gaseous form and therefore cannot be excreted by the lungs. They can only be excreted by the kidneys (a metabolic process). Examples of nonvolatile acids are lactic acid and ketoacids.

An acid–base disorder may be either respiratory or metabolic in origin. Table 24-4 lists the possible causes and signs and symptoms of acid–base disorders. An excess of either kind of acid results in acidemia. Also see Table 29-6 in Chapter 29. If carbon dioxide from volatile acids accumulates, then respiratory acidosis exists. If nonvolatile acids accumulate, then metabolic acidosis exists.

Alkalemia may be the result of losing too many acids from the serum. If too much carbon dioxide is lost, the result is respiratory alkalosis. If there are less than normal amounts of nonvolatile acids, the result is metabolic alkalosis.

**BASES.** A base is a substance that can accept a hydrogen ion ($H^+$), thereby removing it from the circulating serum.

---

**BOX 24-7** **Clinical Terminology**

**Acid:** A substance that can donate hydrogen ions ($H^+$)
*Example*: $H_2CO_3$ (an acid) $\rightarrow H^+ + HCO_3$
**Base:** A substance that can accept hydrogen ions, $H^+$; all bases are alkaline substances
*Example*: $HCO_3$ (base) $+ H^+ \rightarrow H_2CO_3$
**Acidemia:** Acid condition of the blood in which the pH is less than 7.35
**Alkalemia:** Alkaline condition of the blood in which the pH is greater than 7.45
**Acidosis:** The process causing acidemia
**Alkalosis:** The process causing alkalemia

---

The main base found in the serum is bicarbonate ($HCO_3$). The amount of bicarbonate that is available in the serum is regulated by the kidney (a metabolic process). If there is too little bicarbonate in the serum, the result is metabolic acidosis. If there is too much bicarbonate in the serum, the result is metabolic alkalosis.

Conditions leading to acidemia or alkalemia are influenced by a multitude of physiological processes (Table 24-4). Some of these processes include respiratory and renal function or dysfunction, tissue oxygenation, circulation, lactic acid production, substance ingestion, and electrolyte loss from the gastrointestinal tract. The identification of a pH abnormality should lead to the investigation of possible contributing factors.

### Measuring Carbon Dioxide in the Blood

The $PaCO_2$ refers to the pressure or tension exerted by dissolved carbon dioxide gas in arterial blood. Carbon dioxide is the natural byproduct of cellular metabolism. Carbon dioxide levels are regulated primarily by the ventilatory function of the lung. The normal $PaCO_2$ is 35 to 45 mm Hg. In interpretation of ABGs, $PaCO_2$ is thought of as an "acid." Elimination of carbon dioxide from the body is one of the main functions of the lungs, and an important relationship exists between the amount of ventilation and the amount of carbon dioxide in blood.

If a patient hypoventilates, carbon dioxide accumulates, and the $PaCO_2$ value increases above the upper limit of 45 mm Hg. The retention of carbon dioxide results in respiratory acidosis. Respiratory acidosis may occur even with normal lungs if the respiratory center is depressed and the respiratory rate or quality is insufficient to maintain normal carbon dioxide concentrations.

If a patient hyperventilates, carbon dioxide is eliminated from the body, and the $PaCO_2$ value decreases below the lower limit of 35 mm Hg. The loss of carbon dioxide results in respiratory alkalosis.

### Measuring Bicarbonate in the Blood

Bicarbonate ($HCO_3$), the main base found in the serum, helps the body regulate pH because of its ability to accept a hydrogen ion ($H^+$). The concentration of bicarbonate is regulated by the kidneys and is referred to as a metabolic process of regulation. The normal bicarbonate level is 22 to 26 mEq/L. Bicarbonate may be thought of as a "base" (alkaline). When the bicarbonate level increases above 26 mEq/L, a metabolic alkalosis exists. Metabolic alkalosis results from a gain of base (alkaline) substances or a loss of metabolic acids. When the bicarbonate level decreases below 22 mEq/L, a metabolic acidosis exists. Metabolic acidosis results from a loss of base (alkaline) substances or a gain of metabolic acids.

### Alterations in Acid–Base Balance

Disturbances in acid–base balance result from an abnormality of the metabolic or respiratory system. If the respiratory system is responsible, it is detected by the carbon dioxide in the serum. If the metabolic system is responsible, it is detected by the bicarbonate in the serum.

**RESPIRATORY ACIDOSIS.** Respiratory acidosis is defined as a $PaCO_2$ greater than 45 mm Hg and a pH of less than 7.35. Respiratory acidosis is characterized by inadequate

**TABLE 24-4     Possible Causes and Signs and Symptoms of Acid–Base Disorders**

| Condition | Possible Causes | Signs and Symptoms |
|---|---|---|
| **Respiratory Acidosis** | | |
| $PaCO_2$ greater than 45 mm Hg<br>   pH less than 7.35 | Central nervous system depression<br>Head trauma<br>Oversedation<br>Anesthesia<br>High cord injury<br>Pneumothorax<br>Hypoventilation<br>Bronchial obstruction and atelectasis<br>Severe pulmonary infections<br>Heart failure and pulmonary edema<br>Massive pulmonary embolus<br>Myasthenia gravis<br>Multiple sclerosis | Dyspnea<br>Restlessness<br>Headache<br>Tachycardia<br>Confusion<br>Lethargy<br>Dysrhythmias<br>Respiratory distress<br>Drowsiness<br>Decreased responsiveness |
| **Respiratory Alkalosis** | | |
| $PaCO_2$ less than 35 mm Hg<br>   pH greater than 7.45 | Anxiety and nervousness<br>Fear<br>Pain<br>Hyperventilation<br>Fever<br>Thyrotoxicosis<br>Palpitations<br>Salicylates<br>Gram-negative septicemia<br>Pregnancy | Light-headedness<br>Confusion<br>Decreased concentration<br>Paresthesias<br>Tetanic spasms in the arms and legs<br>Cardiac dysrhythmias<br>Central nervous system lesions<br>Sweating<br>Dry mouth<br>Blurred vision |
| **Metabolic Acidosis** | | |
| $HCO_3$ less than 22 mEq/L<br>   pH greater than 7.35 | *Increased acids*<br>Renal failure<br>Ketoacidosis<br>Anaerobic metabolism<br>Starvation<br>Salicylate intoxication<br>*Loss of base*<br>Diarrhea<br>Intestinal fistulas | Headache<br>Confusion<br>Restlessness<br>Lethargy<br>Weakness<br>Stupor/coma<br>Kussmaul respiration<br>Nausea and vomiting<br>Dysrhythmias<br>Warm, flushed skin |
| **Metabolic Alkalosis** | | |
| $HCO_3$ greater than 26 mEq/L<br>   pH greater than 7.45 | *Gain of base*<br>Excess use of bicarbonate<br>Lactate administration in dialysis<br>Excess ingestion of antacids<br>*Loss of acids*<br>Vomiting<br>Nasogastric suctioning<br>Hypokalemia<br>Hypochloremia<br>Administration of diuretics<br>Increased levels of aldosterone | Muscle twitching and cramps<br>Tetany<br>Dizziness<br>Lethargy<br>Weakness<br>Disorientation<br>Convulsions<br>Coma<br>Nausea and vomiting<br>Depressed respiration |

elimination of carbon dioxide by the lungs and may be the result of inefficient pulmonary function or excessive production of carbon dioxide.

**RESPIRATORY ALKALOSIS.** Respiratory alkalosis is defined as a $PaCO_2$ less than 35 mm Hg and a pH of greater than 7.45. Respiratory alkalosis is characterized by excessive elimination of carbon dioxide from the serum.

**METABOLIC ACIDOSIS.** Metabolic acidosis is a bicarbonate level of less than 22 mEq/L and a pH of less than 7.35. Metabolic acidosis is characterized by an excessive production of nonvolatile acids or an inadequate concentration of bicarbonate for the concentration of acid within the serum.

**METABOLIC ALKALOSIS.** Metabolic alkalosis is a bicarbonate level of greater than 26 mEq/L and a pH of greater than 7.45. Metabolic alkalosis is characterized by excessive loss of nonvolatile acids or excessive production of bicarbonate.

BOX 24-8 **Interpretation of Arterial Blood Gas Results**

Approach
1. Evaluate oxygenation by examining the $PaO_2$ and the $SaO_2$
2. Evaluate the pH. Is it acidotic, alkalotic, or normal?
3. Evaluate the $PaCO_2$. Is it high, low, or normal?
4. Evaluate the $HCO_3$. Is it high, low, or normal?
5. Determine whether compensation is occurring. Is it complete, partial, or uncompensated?

Examples:
Sample Blood Gas: Case 1
$PaO_2$: 80 mm Hg (normal)
$SaO_2$: 95% (normal)
pH $PaCO_2$: 7.30 (acidemia)
$PaO_2$: 55 mm Hg (increased—respiratory cause)
$HCO_3$: 25 mEq/L (normal)
Conclusion: Respiratory acidosis (uncompensated)

Sample Blood Gas: Case 2
$PaO_2$: 85 mm Hg (normal)
$SaO_2$: 90% (low saturation)
pH: 7.49 (alkalemia)
$PaCO_2$: 40 (normal)
$HCO_3$: 29 mEq/L (increased—metabolic cause)
Conclusion: Metabolic alkalosis with a low saturation (uncompensated)

## Interpreting Arterial Blood Gas Results

When interpreting ABG results, three factors must be considered: (1) oxygenation status, (2) acid–base status, and (3) degree of compensation. A suggested approach for interpreting ABG results is presented in Box 24-8, along with sample values for interpretation.

**EVALUATING OXYGENATION.** It is necessary to examine the patient's oxygenation status by evaluating the $PaO_2$ and the $SaO_2$. If the $PaO_2$ value is less than the patient's norm, hypoxemia exists. If the $SaO_2$ is less than 93%, inadequate amounts of oxygen are bound to Hgb.

**EVALUATING ACID–BASE STATUS.** The first step in evaluating acid–base status is the examination of the arterial pH. If the pH is less than 7.35, acidemia exists. If the pH is greater than 7.45, alkalemia exists.

The second step in evaluating acid–base status is examination of the $PaCO_2$. A $PaCO_2$ of less than 35 mm Hg indicates a respiratory alkalosis, whereas a $PaCO_2$ of greater than 45 mm Hg signifies a respiratory acidosis.

The third step in evaluating acid–base status is examination of the bicarbonate level. If the bicarbonate value is less than 22 mEq/L, metabolic acidosis is present. If the bicarbonate value is greater than 26 mEq/L, metabolic alkalosis exists.

Occasionally, patients present with both respiratory and metabolic disorders that together cause an acidemia or alkalemia. For example, alkalosis could result from an increase in bicarbonate and a decrease in carbon dioxide, or an acidosis could result from a decrease in bicarbonate and an increase in carbon dioxide. A patient with metabolic acidosis from acute renal failure could also have a very slow respiratory rate that causes the patient to retain carbon dioxide, creating a respiratory acidosis. Therefore, the ABG reflects a mixed respiratory and metabolic acidosis. Box 24-9 lists examples of ABGs in mixed respiratory and metabolic disorders.

BOX 24-9 **Arterial Blood Gases in Mixed Respiratory and Metabolic Disorders**

| Mixed Acidosis | Mixed Alkalosis |
|---|---|
| **pH:** 7.25 | **pH:** 7.55 |
| **$PaCO_2$:** 56 mm Hg | **$PaCO_2$:** 26 mm Hg |
| **$PaO_2$:** 80 mm Hg | **$PaO_2$:** 80 mm Hg |
| **$HCO_2$:** 15 mEq/L | **$HCO_3$:** 28 mEq/L |

**DETERMINING COMPENSATION.** If the patient presents with an alkalemia or acidemia, it is important to determine whether the body has tried to compensate for the abnormality. If the buffer systems in the body are unable to maintain normal pH, then the renal or respiratory systems attempt to compensate. If the problem is respiratory in origin, the kidneys work to correct it. If the problem is renal in origin, the lungs try to correct it. It may take as little as 5 to 15 minutes for the lungs to recognize a metabolic presentation and start to correct it. It may take up to 1 day for the kidneys to correct the respiratory-induced problem. One system will not overcompensate; that is, a compensatory mechanism will never make an acidotic patient alkalotic or an alkalotic patient acidotic.

The respiratory system responds to metabolic-based pH imbalances in the following manner:

- *Metabolic acidosis*: increase in respiratory rate and depth
- *Metabolic alkalosis*: decrease in respiratory rate and depth

The renal system responds to respiratory-based pH imbalances in the following manner:

- *Respiratory acidosis*: increase in hydrogen secretion and bicarbonate reabsorption
- *Respiratory alkalosis*: decrease in hydrogen secretion and bicarbonate reabsorption

ABGs are defined by their degree of compensation: uncompensated, partially compensated, or completely compensated. To determine the level of compensation, the pH, carbon dioxide, and bicarbonate are examined. First, it is determined whether the pH is acidotic or alkalotic. In some cases, the pH is not within the normal range, indicating an acidosis or alkalosis. If it is within the normal range, it is important to determine on which side of 7.40 (midpoint of the normal pH range) the pH lies. For example, a pH of 7.38 is tending toward acidosis, whereas a pH of 7.41 is tending toward alkalosis. Next, an evaluation is made to see whether carbon dioxide or bicarbonate has changed to account for the acidosis or alkalosis. Finally, it is determined whether the opposite system (metabolic or respiratory) has worked to try to shift back toward a normal pH. The primary abnormality (metabolic or respiratory) is correlated with the abnormal pH (acidotic or alkalotic). The secondary abnormality is an attempt to correct the primary disorder. By using the rules for defining compensation in Box 24-10, it is possible to determine the compensatory status of the patient's ABGs.

## Mixed Venous Oxygen Saturation

Mixed venous oxygen saturation ($SvO_2$) is a parameter that can be measured to evaluate the balance between oxygen supply and oxygen demand. Blood obtained from a vein in an extremity gives information mostly about that extremity;

**Compensatory Status of Arterial Blood Gases**

**Uncompensated:** pH is *abnormal* and *either* the $CO_2$ or $HCO_3$ is also abnormal. There is no indication that the opposite system has tried to correct for the other.

In the example below, the patient's pH is alkalotic as a result of the low (below the normal range of 35 to 45 mm Hg) $CO_2$ concentration. The renal system value ($HCO_3$) has not moved out its normal range (22 to 26 mEq/L) to compensate for the primary respiratory disorder.

**$PaO^2$:** 94 mm Hg (normal)
**pH:** 7.52 (alkalotic)
**$PaCO^2$:** 25 mm Hg (decreased)
**$HCO^3$:** 24 mEq/L (normal)

**Partially compensated:** pH is *abnormal*, and both the $CO_2$ and $HCO_3$ are also abnormal; this indicates that one system has attempted to correct for the other but has not been completely successful.

In the example below, the patient's pH remains alkalotic as a result of the low $CO_2$ concentration. The renal system value ($HCO_3$) has moved out its normal range (22 to 26 mEq/L) to compensate for the primary respiratory disorder but has not been able to bring the pH back within the normal range.

**$PaO^2$:** 94 mm Hg (normal)
**pH:** 7.48 (alkalotic)
**$PaCO^2$:** 25 mm Hg (decreased)
**$HCO^3$:** 20 mEq/L (decreased)

**Completely compensated:** pH is *normal* and both the $CO_2$ and $HCO_3$ are abnormal; the normal pH indicates that one system has been able to compensate for the other.

In the example below, the patient's pH is normal but is tending toward alkalosis (>7.40). The primary abnormality is respiratory because the $PaCO_2$ is low (decreased acid concentration). The bicarbonate value of 18 mEq/L reflects decreased concentration of base and is associated with acidosis, not alkalosis. In this case, the decreased bicarbonate has completely compensated for the respiratory alkalosis.

**$PaO^2$:** 94 mm Hg (normal)
**pH:** 7.44 (normal, tending toward alkalosis)
**$PaCO^2$:** 25 mm Hg (decreased, primary problem)
**$HcO^3$:** 18 mEq/L (decreased, compensatory response)

it can be quite misleading if the metabolism in the extremity differs from the metabolism of the body as a whole. This difference is accentuated if the extremity is cold or underperfused (eg, in shock), if the patient has performed local exercises with the extremity (eg, opening and closing the fist), or if there is local infection in the extremity.

Sometimes blood is sampled through a central venous pressure (CVP) catheter in the hope of obtaining mixed venous blood, but even in the superior vena cava or right atrium where a CVP catheter ends, there is usually incomplete mixing of venous return from various parts of the body. For complete mixing of the blood, it is necessary to obtain a blood sample from a pulmonary artery catheter. Use of the pulmonary artery catheter provides a sample of blood that has returned from the extremities and has been mixed in the right ventricle.

Oxygen measurements of mixed venous blood indicate whether the tissues are being oxygenated, but $SvO_2$ does not distinguish the independent contributions of the heart and the lungs. $SvO_2$ indicates the adequacy of the supply of oxygen relative to the demand for oxygen at the tissue levels. Normal $SvO_2$ is 60% to 80%; this means that supply of oxygen to the tissues is adequate to meet the tissue's demand. However, a normal value does not indicate whether compensatory mechanisms were needed to maintain the perfusion. For example, in some patients, an increase in cardiac output is needed to compensate for a low supply of oxygen.

A low $SvO_2$ may be caused by a decrease in oxygen supply to the tissues or an increase in oxygen use caused by a high demand. A decrease in oxygen supply results from low Hgb, hemorrhage, or low cardiac output. An increase in oxygen demand results from hyperthermia, pain, stress, shivering, or seizures. An $SvO_2$ of 40% to 60% may occur in heart failure, and values less than 40% may indicate profound shock. A decrease in $SvO_2$ often occurs before other hemodynamic changes and, therefore, is an excellent clinical tool in assessing and managing critically ill patients. The goals of interventions for a low $SvO_2$ include increasing the oxygen supply by blood transfusions or by increasing cardiac output. Treatment may also be aimed at eliminating the cause of the high demand.

A high $SvO_2$ value indicates that oxygen supply exceeds demand or a decrease in the demand. Elevated $SvO_2$ values are associated with increased delivery of oxygen (high fraction of inspired oxygen) or with decreased demand from hypothermia, hypothyroidism, or anesthesia. An elevated $SvO_2$ is also seen in the early stages of septic shock when the tissues are unable to use the oxygen. Table 24-5 summarizes possible causes of abnormalities in $SvO_2$.

A pulmonary artery catheter with an oximeter built into its tip that allows continuous monitoring of $SvO_2$ provides ongoing assessment of oxygen supply and demand imbalances. If a catheter with a built-in oximeter is not available, the nurse can draw blood from the pulmonary artery through a regular pulmonary artery catheter, send the sample to the laboratory for blood gas and $SvO_2$ analysis, and use the information in the same manner.

# Respiratory Diagnostic Studies

## Chest Radiography

Chest radiography is a valuable diagnostic tool that clinicians frequently use to assess anatomical and physiological features of the chest and to detect pathological processes. X-rays pass through the chest wall and make it possible to visualize various structures. Dense tissues, such as bones, absorb the x-ray beam and appear as opaque or white on the radiograph. Blood vessels and blood-filled organs, such as the heart, are moderately dense structures and appear as gray areas on the radiograph. During inspiration, normal lungs fill with air and appear black on the radiograph. When parts of the lungs fill with fluid, which is a more dense material, the lungs appear white.

The nurse uses the radiograph as an assessment parameter to validate clinical findings and suspected abnormalities. Using a systematic approach, the nurse examines the radiograph by comparing the film with previous films. The approach can be to examine the film starting in the periphery and then to move toward the center of the chest or to start centrally and move outward toward the soft tissue. Whatever the method, the objects of scrutiny are the soft tissue areas, the bony structures, the inner layers just under the bone, and

| TABLE 24-5 | Possible Causes of Abnormalities in Mixed Venous Oxygen Saturation (SvO$_2$) | |
|---|---|
| **Abnormality** | **Possible Cause** |
| Low SvO$_2$ (less than 60%) | **Decreased oxygen supply** |
| | • Low hematocrit from anemia or hemorrhage |
| | • Low arterial saturation and hypoxemia from lung disease, ventilation–perfusion mismatches |
| | • Low cardiac output from hypovolemia, heart failure, cardiogenic shock, myocardial infarction |
| | **Increased oxygen demand** |
| | • Increased metabolic demand, such as hyperthermia, seizures, shivering, pain, anxiety, stress, strenuous exercise |
| High SvO$_2$ (greater than 80%) | **Increased oxygen supply** |
| | • Supplemental oxygen |
| | **Decreased oxygen demand** |
| | • Anesthesia, hypothermia, early stages of sepsis |
| | **Technical problems** |
| | • False high reading because of wedged pulmonary artery catheter |
| | • Fibrin clot at end of catheter |

the internal structures. (See Figure 17-15 in Chapter 17.) The nurse examines the soft tissues on the radiograph by looking for homogeneity, beginning with lateral areas and moving medially. Air visualized in the lateral soft tissue may indicate a pneumothorax.

Bony structures inspected on the chest film include the ribs, clavicles, sternum, manubrium, spine, and vertebrae. Approximately eight to nine ribs should overlie lung tissue on the normal chest film. The nurse examines the ribs for fractures by following the curve of each rib, beginning anteriorly and moving around posteriorly. Like the ribs, the other bony structures are examined for correct position and intactness. The contour of the diaphragm is also visible on the radiograph. Normally, the diaphragm is rounded with sharp, pointed costophrenic angles. Pleural effusions may cause the angles to become blunted. The top of the diaphragm is apparent at about the sixth rib. A lowered diaphragm may indicate hyperinflation caused by emphysema.

The nurse assesses lung parenchyma by comparing right and left sides, moving top to bottom. Normal air-filled lungs should appear black or very dark compared with the bones and heart. It is important in the evaluation to look for symmetry. Abnormally high density on one side of the chest may indicate edema, a mass, pleural effusion, or pneumonia.

Interlobar fissures separate the lobes of the lungs. The minor fissure in the right lung is usually visible in the frontal film. Displacement of the normal fissures seen on the film may indicate atelectasis or lobar collapse.

The trachea should appear midline over the thoracic vertebrae. The trachea can shift toward areas of atelectasis and away from areas of pneumothorax or pleural effusion.

## Ventilation–Perfusion Scanning

Ventilation–perfusion scanning is a nuclear imaging test used to evaluate a suspected alteration in the ventilation–perfusion relationship. (See Chapter 23 for a discussion of ventilation–perfusion relationships.) A ventilation–perfusion scan is helpful in detecting the percentage of each lung that is functioning normally, diagnosing and locating pulmonary emboli, and assessing the pulmonary vascular supply.

The ventilation–perfusion scan consists of two parts: a ventilation scan and a perfusion scan. In the ventilation scan, the patient inhales radioactive gas, which follows the same pathway as air in normal breathing. In pathological conditions, the diminished areas of ventilation are visible on the scan. In the perfusion scan, a radioisotope is injected intravenously, enabling visualization of the blood supply to the lungs. When a pulmonary embolus is present, the blood supply beyond the embolus is restricted, revealing poor or no visualization of the affected area.

Ventilation–perfusion scans are often not useful in patients who depend on mechanical ventilation because the ventilation component of the scan is difficult to perform. Ventilation–perfusion mismatches may make interpretation of ventilation–perfusion scans difficult in patients with lung diseases, such as pneumonia. Because of these limitations, pulmonary angiography may be appropriate in the critically ill patient, especially if a pulmonary embolus is suspected.

## Pulmonary Angiography

Pulmonary angiography involves the rapid injection of a radiopaque substance for radiographic studies of the pulmonary vasculature. Suspected pulmonary embolus is the most common indication for pulmonary angiography. A radiopaque substance is injected into one or both arms, the femoral vein, or a catheter that has been placed in the pulmonary artery. A positive test result is indicated by the impaired flow of the radiopaque substance through a narrowed vessel or by the abrupt cessation of flow of the substance in a vessel.

## Bronchoscopy

Bronchoscopy involves the direct visualization of the larynx, trachea, and bronchi through a flexible fiberoptic bronchoscope. Bronchoscopy is used diagnostically to examine tissues, collect secretions, determine the extent and location of a pathologic process, and obtain a biopsy. In addition, bronchoscopy is used therapeutically as a means to remove foreign bodies or secretions from the tracheobronchial tree, treat postoperative atelectasis, and excise lesions.

In preparation for a bronchoscopy, a history and physical examination should be performed. A chest radiograph, clotting studies, and ABGs are also obtained. The patient often receives intravenous sedation or analgesia before the procedure. If the purpose of the bronchoscopy is therapeutic, medications that suppress a cough or diminish secretions are avoided (eg, intratracheal topical anesthetics, atropine, and codeine).

Careful monitoring of the patient is indicated after a bronchoscopy. The nurse assesses for any evidence of complications, which may include laryngospasm, fever, hemodynamic changes, cardiac dysrhythmias, pneumothorax, hemorrhage, or cardiopulmonary arrest.

## Thoracentesis

In thoracentesis, a needle is inserted into the pleural space to remove air, fluid, or both; obtain specimens for diagnostic evaluation; or instill medications. A chest radiograph, coagulation studies, and patient education are essential before a thoracentesis. Some patients may require medication to reduce anxiety. Unlike bronchoscopy, thoracentesis requires the cooperation of the patient; therefore, a local anesthetic, rather than moderate sedation, is used to minimize the pain and discomfort that accompanies the procedure. During the procedure, the patient is placed either in a chair or on the edge of the bed in an upright position with arms and shoulders raised so that the ribs lift and separate, allowing easier needle insertion. If a patient is unable to lift his or her arms, sitting on the bed with the arms placed above the head on a table is an alternative position.

During thoracentesis, the nurse's primary function is to provide comfort for the patient, perform ongoing assessment of the patient's respiratory system, dress the wound with sterile dressings on completion of the procedure, and send labeled specimens to the laboratory as ordered. Post-thoracentesis nursing care includes assessment for complications, including pneumothorax, pain, hypotension, and pulmonary edema.

## Sputum Culture

Sputum specimens are often part of the respiratory assessment. Because healthy patients do not produce sputum, obtaining a specimen requires the patient to cough to bring up sputum from the lungs. It is essential that the nurse distinguishes sputum from saliva before sending the specimen to the laboratory.

In most cases, sputum specimens are obtained for culture and sensitivity study. The specimen is examined for specific microorganisms and their corresponding drug sensitivities. In addition, sputum specimens are also required for studies of cytology and acid-fast bacilli. Culture of acid-fast bacilli requires serial collection (usually over 3 days) and is used to identify tuberculosis and mycobacteria.

## Pulmonary Function Tests

The flow of air in and out of the lungs provides tangible measures of lung volumes. Although these volumes are referred to as measures of "pulmonary function," in reality, they are measures of pulmonary anatomy. In the evaluation of ventilation, structure or anatomy often determines function. Ventilatory or pulmonary function tests measure the ability of the chest and lungs to move air into and out of the alveoli.

Pulmonary function tests include volume measurements, capacity measurements, and dynamic measurements. These measurements are influenced by exercise and disease. Age, sex, body size, and posture are other variables that are taken into consideration when the test results are interpreted. Figure 23-13 in Chapter 23 illustrates normal lung volumes and capacity.

### Volume Measurements

Volume measurements show the amount of air contained in the lungs during various parts of the respiratory cycle. Measures of lung volume include tidal volume ($V_T$), inspiratory reserve volume, expiratory reserve volume, and residual volume (see Chapter 23, Table 23-1).

### Capacity Measurements

Capacity measurements quantify part of the pulmonary cycle. They are a combination of the previous volumes and include inspiratory capacity, functional residual capacity (FRC), vital capacity, and total lung capacity (see Chapter 23, Table 23-1).

### Dynamic Measurements

The following measurements, called dynamic measurements, provide data about airway resistance and the energy expended in breathing (work of breathing).

- Respiratory rate or frequency is the number of breaths per minute. At rest, the respiratory rate is about 15 breaths/min.
- Minute volume, sometimes called minute ventilation, is the volume of air inhaled and exhaled per minute. It is calculated by multiplying tidal volume by respiratory rate. At rest, the minute volume is approximately 7,500 mL/min.
- Dead space is the part of the tidal volume that does not participate in alveolar gas exchange. The dead space (measured in milliliters) is the air contained in the airways (anatomical dead space) plus the volume of alveolar air that is not involved in gas exchange (physiological dead space; eg, air in an unperfused alveolus from pulmonary embolism or, more commonly, air in underperfused alveoli). Adult anatomical dead space is usually equal to the body weight in pounds (eg, 140 mL in a 140-pound person). In a healthy person, dead space is composed only of anatomical dead space. Physiological dead space occurs in certain disease states. Dead space is calculated by subtracting the partial pressure of arterial carbon dioxide ($PaCO_2$) from the partial pressure of alveolar carbon dioxide ($PaCO_2$). The normal value of dead space in healthy adults is typically less than 40% of the tidal volume. The dead space/tidal volume ratio is used to follow the effectiveness of mechanical ventilation.
- Alveolar ventilation, the complement of dead space, is expressed as the volume of tidal air that is involved in alveolar gas exchange. This volume is represented as volume per minute by the symbol $\dot{V}A$. $\dot{V}A$ is a measure of ventilatory effectiveness. It is more relevant to the blood gas values than either the dead space or tidal volume because these last two measures include physiological dead space.

$\dot{V}_A$ is calculated by subtracting the dead space ($V_D$) from the tidal volume ($V_T$) and multiplying the result by the respiratory rate (f):

$$\dot{V}_A = (V_T - V_D) \times f$$

About 2,300 mL of air (FRC) remains in the lung at the end of expiration. Each new breath introduces about 350 mL of air into the alveoli. The ratio of new alveoli air to total volume of air remaining in the lungs is

$$\frac{350 \text{ mL}}{2,300 \text{ mL}}$$

Therefore, new air is only about one seventh of the total volume contained in the lungs. The normal is 5,250 mL/min (350 mL/breath × 15 breaths/min = 5,250 mL/min). A normal breath ($V_T$) can replace 7,500 mL of air/min (500 mL/breath × 15 breaths/min = 7,500 mL/min), requiring 0.008 s/mL:

$$\frac{1 \text{ minute}}{7,500 \text{ mL}} \times \frac{60 \text{ seconds}}{1 \text{ minute}} = 0.008 \text{ s/mL}$$

Therefore, the FRC of the lungs can be completely replaced in 18.4 seconds (2,300 mL × 0.008 s/mL = 18.4 seconds) if air diffusion is uniform. This slow turnover rate prevents rapid fluctuations of gas concentrations in the alveoli with each breath.

## Clinical Applicability Challenges

### CASE STUDY

Mrs. T., age 86 years, has been admitted to the intensive care unit with a diagnosis of pneumonia. Her family tells you she has been short of breath and has had a sudden onset of confusion. On physical examination, her respiratory rate is 26 breaths/min, and she uses accessory muscles for breathing. Her mucous membranes are pale. You hear course crackles in the bases when you auscultate her lungs. Her ABGs are $PaO_2$, 65 mm Hg; $PaCO_2$, 33 mm Hg; $HCO_3$, 23 mEq/L; and pH 7.47.

1. Describe some of the differences in the respiratory assessment of the older adult.
2. Interpret the patient's ABGs.
3. Explain why crackles were heard when auscultating Mrs. T.'s lungs.

### WANT TO KNOW MORE?

A wide variety of resources to enhance your learning and understanding of this chapter are available on thePoint.

You will find:

- References
- Selected readings
- NCLEX-style review questions
- Internet resources
- And more!

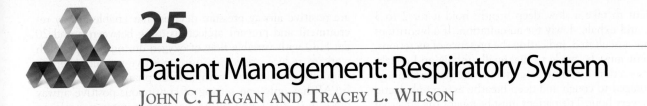

# 25

# Patient Management: Respiratory System

JOHN C. HAGAN AND TRACEY L. WILSON

**LEARNING OBJECTIVES**

*Based on the content in this chapter, the reader should be able to:*

1. Summarize the desired outcomes of the various bronchial hygiene therapies.
2. Describe the principles of chest physiotherapy.
3. Describe the nursing assessment and management of patients on oxygen therapy.
4. Compare and contrast indications for, and complications of, orotracheal intubation versus nasotracheal intubation.
5. Describe the principles governing chest tube drainage systems.
6. Discuss nursing management of the patient with a chest tube drainage system.
7. Discuss the pharmacologic agents used for the treatment of bronchospasm in asthma and chronic obstructive pulmonary disease.
8. Differentiate between the different types of positive-pressure ventilators.
9. Differentiate between pressure-cycled and volume-cycled ventilators in positive-pressure ventilation.
10. Compare and contrast the following ventilator modes: assist-control mode, synchronized intermittent mandatory mode, pressure-support ventilation, and pressure-controlled ventilation.
11. Summarize strategies to maximize oxygen delivery with the goal of achieving a nontoxic $FiO_2$ setting.
12. Summarize adverse effects of positive end-expiratory pressure, how they are identified, and the appropriate treatment.
13. Compare and contrast the advantages and disadvantages of tracheostomy versus endotracheal intubation.
14. Describe the nursing management of the ventilated patient, and explain how to prevent complications.
15. Discuss the differences between short-term and long-term ventilation liberation.

Respiration is necessary to sustain life, and the nurse plays an important role in helping the critically ill patient breathe. The nurse must be knowledgeable and skilled in assessing patient needs, providing quick and efficient care, evaluating results of intervention, and supporting and teaching the patient and family. Techniques, equipment, and procedures vary according to the patient's respiratory status.

## Bronchial Hygiene Therapy

Bronchial hygiene therapy (BHT), also known as pulmonary toilet, is helpful in preventing and treating pulmonary complications. The primary phases of lung function that BHT aims to improve are ventilation and diffusion (Fig. 25-1). These improvements are accomplished through the therapeutic goals of secretion mobilization and removal and improved gas exchange.

Specific BHT depends on existing pulmonary dysfunction. A healthy person's airway has a functioning mucociliary "escalator" with a cough reflex and normal mucus production. In contrast, the hospitalized patient may have pneumonia, atelectasis, or inability to perform deep breathing, cough, or clear mucus effectively because of weakness, sedation, or pain. The patient may also have a chronic condition such as chronic obstructive pulmonary disease (COPD), cystic fibrosis, pulmonary fibrosis, or quadriplegia.

The need for and the effectiveness of various methods of BHT are based on physical assessment, chest radiography, measurement of arterial blood gases (ABGs), and additional sources of information as indicated. Any one or a combination of the following measures is used: coughing and deep-breathing maneuvers, airway clearance adjunct devices, chest physiotherapy (CPT), and bronchodilator aerosol therapy. (Pharmacology is discussed later in the chapter.)

### Coughing and Deep Breathing

Effective coughing is necessary for the patient to clear secretions. The objectives of deep breathing and coughing are to promote lung expansion, mobilize secretions, and prevent the side effects of retained secretions (eg, atelectasis and pneumonia). These techniques are effective only if the patient is able to cooperate and has the strength to cough productively.

The patient is positioned seated and upright on the edge of the bed or chair with the feet supported. The nurse instructs

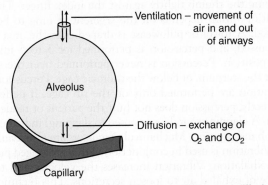

FIGURE 25-1   Primary lung functions: ventilation and diffusion.

Labels: Ventilation – movement of air in and out of airways; Alveolus; Diffusion – exchange of $O_2$ and $CO_2$; Capillary

the patient to take a slow, deep breath; hold it for 2 to 3 seconds; and exhale slowly for auscultation. If adventitious sounds are auscultated, indicating the presence of secretions, the patient must be made to maximally inhale and cough. Even if secretions are not auscultated, the patient should be encouraged to cough and deep breathe as a prophylactic measure every hour. The patient must be taught the effective use of the incentive spirometer (IS) to have immediate visual feedback on the breath depth, and coached to increase the volume. Ideally, the patient uses the IS hourly while awake, completing 10 breaths each session followed by coughing, and then the patient progressively increases breath volumes. The nurse coaches the patient to maximize the deep breaths, followed by coughing, and documents the IS volume results. IS, along with coughing and deep-breathing exercises, improves inhaled volumes and prevents atelectasis.

## Airway Clearance Adjunct Therapies

Various adjunct therapies may be useful for patients who require mucus removal—in particular, when coughing efforts are limited by a disease process, injury, or surgery. The Acapella and Flutter valves, two such methods of airway clearance, provide intermittent positive expiratory pressure (PEP) therapy, which improves mucus removal by causing airway vibration to loosen secretions, which can then be cleared with a cough.[1] The Acapella valve is just as effective as the Flutter valve and may be easier to use, especially in elderly patients. Both produce PEP and oscillatory vibrations in the airways to loosen mucus. The Acapella valve is available in two types: one for patients who can sustain a flow of 15 L/min or more, and one for patients whose sustained flow is equal to or less than 15 L/min. The nurse assists the patient to cough by using positive pressure on the abdominal costal margin during exhalation to increase the cough force (manually assisted cough). Various specialized BHTs are used for patients with cystic fibrosis and other chronic pulmonary diseases, including autogenic drainage (AD), which may be used with the huff cough.[1] AD is a series of controlled breaths and uses low-pressure cough with mini-coughs instead of one to two big coughs. The nurse teaches AD to patients who have reactive airway disease with likelihood of wheezing with normal cough.

The Vest® Airway Clearance System (Hill-Rom, Batesville, IN), another method of airway clearance, is a chest wall oscillation device that creates chest wall motion through a machine that rapidly alternates air into sections of a vest that is placed circumferentially around the chest. The method, called high-frequency chest wall oscillation, results in improved secretion removal. This is an alternative to traditional CPT. The Vest Airway Clearance System has been used in trials involving patients with bronchiectasis, cystic fibrosis, COPD, lung transplantation, and even spinal cord injury or quadriplegia, as well as in postoperative intensive care units (ICUs). The Vest Airway Clearance System has been shown to improve the removal of mucus and improve pulmonary function. It is well tolerated by surgical patients and can be self-administered at home.

Other therapies include the EzPAP® Positive Airway Pressure System (www.smithmedical.com), bilevel positive airway pressure (BiPAP), and IS, which may be given before any of the BHTs to improve mucus removal. EzPAP and BiPAP are positive airway pressure devices that enable airway recruitment and prevent atelectasis using between 5 and 20 cm $H_2O$ with variable flow of oxygen during therapy. Both work to reduce atelectasis using positive-pressure therapy, often in combination with aerosol pharmacology agents. EzPAP has only one setting of continuous positive airway pressure (CPAP), and BiPAP has both inspiratory peak airway pressure (IPAP) and expiratory airway pressure (EPAP). Both are used in patients when IS or other therapies are not sufficient to reduce or prevent atelectasis.

## Chest Physiotherapy

Postural drainage, positioning, and chest percussion and vibration are methods of CPT used to augment the patient's efforts and to improve pulmonary function. These may be used in sequence in different lung drainage positions and should be preceded by bronchodilator therapy and followed by deep breathing and coughing or other BHT. Changing the patient's position from supine to upright affects gas exchange, and positioning the patient in the lateral position may improve gas exchange, especially in unilateral lung disease. Positioning the patient with the "good" lung down improves oxygenation; this improvement occurs because shunting is decreased when the "good" lung is in the dependent position.

### Postural Drainage

Postural drainage positions facilitate gravitational drainage of pulmonary secretions into the main bronchi and trachea based on anatomy of the lung segments (Fig. 25-2). The focus of postural drainage should be on the lobes affected by atelectasis and on increasing mucus removal with suctioning or by cough effort. Postural drainage is not indicated in all positions for all critically ill patients. Contraindications are listed in Box 25-1. The nurse must closely monitor the patient who is in a head-down position for aspiration, respiratory distress, and dysrhythmias. Alternate techniques may include gentle percussion and using a mechanical percussor to stimulate mucus movement while avoiding surgical areas.

### Chest Percussion and Vibration

Chest percussion (tapotement) and vibration, performed by a trained health care professional, are used to dislodge secretions. Percussion involves striking the chest wall with the hands formed into a cupped shape by flexing the fingers and placing the thumb tightly against the index finger. The patient's position depends on the segment of lung to be percussed. A towel or pillowcase is draped over the area to be percussed, and percussion is performed for 3 to 5 minutes per position. Percussion is never performed over the spine, over the sternum, or below the thoracic cage. Percussion and vibration are performed only on the rib cage. If performed correctly, percussion does not hurt the patient or redden the skin. A clapping sound (as opposed to slapping) indicates correct hand position. Mechanical percussors are also available.

Vibration is used in conjunction with a prolonged pursed-lip exhalation. Vibration increases the velocity and turbulence of exhaled air to loosen secretions. This technique is accomplished by placing the hands side by side with fingers

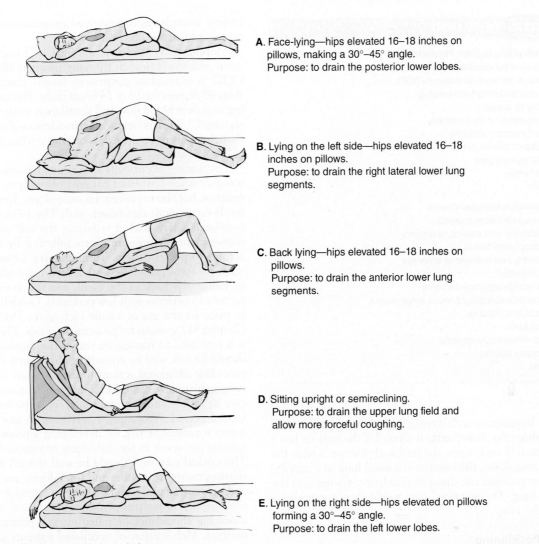

**A.** Face-lying—hips elevated 16–18 inches on pillows, making a 30°–45° angle.
Purpose: to drain the posterior lower lobes.

**B.** Lying on the left side—hips elevated 16–18 inches on pillows.
Purpose: to drain the right lateral lower lung segments.

**C.** Back lying—hips elevated 16–18 inches on pillows.
Purpose: to drain the anterior lower lung segments.

**D.** Sitting upright or semireclining.
Purpose: to drain the upper lung field and allow more forceful coughing.

**E.** Lying on the right side—hips elevated on pillows forming a 30°–45° angle.
Purpose: to drain the left lower lobes.

**FIGURE 25-2** Positions used in lung drainage.

extended and applying the flat of the palm over the affected chest area. The patient inhales deeply and then slowly exhales. While the patient exhales, the nurse vibrates the patient's chest by quickly contracting and relaxing the arm and shoulder muscles. Vibration is used instead of percussion if the chest wall is extremely painful.

Modern ICU beds have options to percuss, vibrate, or provide continuous lateral rotation therapy (CLRT), using either an added module or a system integrated into the bed. These bed features can be used to provide BHT to critically ill patients who may not tolerate manual therapy. The nurse assesses patients for tolerance to both position changes and the level of therapy; most bed systems allow variable settings of high to low frequency of percussion or vibration. Continuous lateral rotation is effective for certain patients, especially ventilated patients.[2]

## Contraindications and Adaptations

No single method of CPT has been shown to be superior, and there are many contraindications to using these techniques (see Box 25-1). Studies have questioned the efficacy of CPT, except in segmental atelectasis caused by mucus obstruction

and diseases that result in increased sputum production (at least 30 mL/d), such as cystic fibrosis and bronchiectasis.[3] Bronchoscopy is an alternative treatment to remove mucus plugs that result in atelectasis. CPT may produce bronchospasm in patients with asthma and spread infected material to uninfected lung tissue in patients with unilateral pneumonia.

The inclusion of CPT in the plan of care should be individualized and evaluated in terms of derived benefit versus potential risks. In addition, CPT should be discontinued when it fails to promote treatment goals. In patients who cannot tolerate CPT, turning the patient laterally every 2 hours aids in mobilizing secretions for removal with cough or suctioning. Progressive mobility from sitting up in a chair to weight bearing and to ambulation is used in all ventilated patients as part of pulmonary hygiene as well as to increase patient strength and endurance. Patients with an artificial airway or an ineffective cough may require suctioning after CPT.

To be effective, CPT must be accompanied by the postural drainage position specific to the affected area of the lung. Patients with unilateral disease are positioned with the healthy lung down for better ventilation and perfusion. Positioning the patient with the diseased lung down is likely

### Contraindications to Chest Physiotherapy

**Contraindications to Postural Drainage**

- Increased intracranial pressure (ICP)
- After meals/during tube feeding
- Inability to cough
- Hypoxia/respiratory instability
- Hemodynamic instability
- Decreased mental status
- Recent eye surgery
- Hiatal hernia
- Obesity

**Contraindications to Percussion/Vibration**

- Fractured ribs/osteoporosis
- Chest/abdominal trauma or surgery
- Bronchopleural fistula
- Pulmonary hemorrhage or embolus
- Coagulopathy
- Chest malignancy/mastectomy
- Pneumothorax/subcutaneous emphysema
- Cervical cord trauma
- Tuberculosis
- Pleural effusions/empyema
- Pulmonary edema
- Asthma

to cause hypoxemia with ventilation–perfusion mismatching and shunting. Positioning is altered if the patient has a lung abscess. In such cases, the preferred position is with the diseased lung down, because the abscessed lung in a gravity-dependent position can drain its purulent contents into the opposite lung. The abscessed lung would then contaminate the healthy lung.

### Patient Positioning

Studies have demonstrated improved oxygenation and an improvement in survival in 28- and 90-day mortality rates in patients with acute respiratory failure who were placed in the prone position.[4] Prone positioning is an advanced technique used with critically ill ventilated patients who have acute respiratory distress syndrome (ARDS). ARDS may be categorized as mild ($PaO_2/FiO_2$ greater than 200 mm Hg), moderate ($PaO_2/FiO_2$ 101 to 200 mm Hg) or severe ($PaO_2/FiO_2$ less than 100 mm Hg) acute lung injury (ALI).[5] The enhanced oxygenation is attributed to recruitment of collapsed lung areas related to body position change, allowing dependent lung regions to have improved perfusion and ventilation. Prone positioning involves multiple personnel and specialized beds or equipment, and it should be performed only by specially trained staff to prevent the many complications related to prone positioning.

Patients who are ventilated benefit from having the head of the bed (HOB) elevated 30 degrees at all times. The rationale is to promote lung expansion, prevent the aspiration that can occur in the recumbent position in intubated patients, and prevent ventilator-associated pneumonia (VAP). Keeping the HOB elevated 30 degrees, with the associated reduction in VAP, is included in the ventilator bundle to prevent VAP and is part of the Institute for Healthcare Improvement's 5 Million Lives Campaign. Mobilization of the

patient contributes to improved oxygenation, secretion removal, and airway patency.[6]

Mobilization of the patient using CLRT improves oxygenation and blood flow to the lung tissue in affected regions. CLRT is defined as continuous lateral positioning of less than 40 degrees for 18 of 24 hours daily. The lateral positioning improves blood flow and ventilation in the superior lung regions. CLRT may help reduce incidences of pneumonia, although it may not reduce days on the ventilator or the length of hospital stay.

Positioning of critically ill patients remains a nursing intervention for ventilated patients not only to improve oxygenation but also to prevent pressure ulcers. Turning by nurses has become more significant, with The Joint Commission–mandated safety goal of requiring the risk assessment and reassessment for pressure ulcers followed by implementing actions to prevent them. Turning every 2 hours allows the nurse to assess pressure points on the torso and extremities, including the back of the head, and this is even more important in patients with low perfusion. Guidelines should be in place for the use of a scale such as the Braden scale (see Chapter 51) to assess for pressure ulcer risk. The Braden scale is a tool used to reassess increased risk factors daily; its use should be followed by consulting the wound care team and providing additional actions to treat pressure ulcers. Repositioning manually, using CLRT or prone positioning, requires care to avoid causing tissue injury when positioning for extended periods. Prolonged positioning in any one position leaves a patient at risk for developing a pressure ulcer, and turning can result in the dislodging of various tubes or lines. The critical care staff should be well trained in prone positioning, monitoring tubes and lines during rotation therapy, and preventing prolonged pressure in lateral positions. Low-pressure airflow mattresses may help reduce skin ulcer occurrence but should not be relied on as a primary prevention method. Mobilization of ventilated patients using rotation therapy specialty beds is one method for nurses to improve patient outcomes of improved oxygenation; this technique also helps prevent VAP and skin ulcers. Ultimately, the critically ill patient should progress to weight-bearing positions, sitting up in a chair, and (with physical therapy) ambulation in order to improve overall physical reconditioning toward a return to independent functioning.

### Oxygen Therapy

The administration of oxygen therapy to a patient is designed to correct hypoxemia (low oxygen blood levels). When blood oxygen levels are decreased, it is referred to as hypoxemia. Hypoxia is a reduced oxygen supply, which can be generalized or region limited (eg, tissue hypoxia). If external or internal respiration is impaired, supplemental oxygen is vital to maintain the patient's cellular function. Oxygen therapy corrects hypoxemia, decreases the work of breathing, and decreases myocardial work. Any disease process that alters the gas exchange can cause hypoxemia.

Asthma, bronchitis, pneumonia, ARDS, COPD, and emphysema are disease processes that alter oxygen supply. Traumatic events that lead to pneumothorax or hemothorax, as well as surgical events such as pneumonectomy and lobectomy and events causing large pleural effusions, can significantly alter gas exchange. Oxygen delivery by nasal cannula may provide sufficient additional oxygen to reduce air hunger and shortness of breath. A patient with COPD may also need continuous oxygen because of permanent alterations in the lungs, which result in lowered oxygen delivery, especially with stress, illness, infection, and exercise. Patients with COPD and emphysema require close monitoring for carbon dioxide retention and narcosis or stupor associated with the delivery of too high a concentration of oxygen. These patients normally tolerate higher levels of carbon dioxide because their chemoreceptors no longer respond to the normally accepted partial pressure of carbon dioxide ($PCO_2$) levels and serum pH. These patients' primary drive to breathe comes from their oxygen levels rather than their carbon dioxide levels. The desired goals for all patients on oxygen therapy are stable arterial oxygen saturation ($SaO_2$) level, nonlabored respirations, and a decrease in anxiety and shortness of breath. These goals should be accomplished through delivery of the least amount of supplemental oxygen needed; therefore, the nurse continuously monitors the patient on oxygen for the desired result and complications (Box 25-2). Appropriate physician or advanced practice nurse orders are necessary to initiate this therapy.

## Patient Assessment

Assessment of the patient's oxygen need is based on the disease process and the severity of the hypoxemia. The nursing assessment considers the patient's level of consciousness, vital signs (including the rate and depth of breathing), nail bed color, airway patency or presence of an artificial airway, $SaO_2$, and ABGs. The use of accessory muscles or abdominal breathing may indicate severe distress, and the inability to speak (or the tendency to respond using only one-syllable words) is ominous. Accessory muscle use in any patient is usually a sign of respiratory fatigue. Laboratory data, including hemoglobin, hematocrit, electrolyte panel, ABGs, and chest radiographs, may be obtained to assist in correcting electrolyte and pH imbalances. A low phosphorus level, or hypophosphatemia, is associated with muscle weakness, including weakness of the diaphragm, that has an impact on ventilation. A low hemoglobin level affects oxygen transport and delivery to tissues. A full assessment, which may include collection of blood for blood gas analysis, takes time, whereas assessment of the person's vital signs, $SaO_2$, respiratory effort, and symptoms is possible to do quickly and repeatedly. To establish baseline activity tolerance and respiratory function, it may be necessary to involve the family if the patient

cannot communicate in complete sentences. The clinician should compare the usual symptoms exhibited by a patient who has asthma or COPD with the presenting symptoms to establish the severity of the patient's illness. The clinician should initiate oxygen therapy for distress and hypoxemia. After a thorough assessment, including laboratory data, it is necessary to adjust the oxygen delivery method to meet the therapeutic goal.

The patient's acuity and underlying disease process dictate the level of oxygen delivery required. The choice of oxygen delivery method is based on the assessment and presentation of the patient, the $SaO_2$ on room air, and the desired outcome. The desired oxygen level for a patient with COPD may be much lower than that for a patient with pneumonia who does not have COPD. The patient with pneumonia tolerates higher levels of oxygenation for longer periods than the patient with COPD, who is susceptible to carbon dioxide narcosis.

After giving oxygen, it is necessary to reassess the patient. Signs of improvement include reduced respiratory rate, a more comfortable breathing pattern, increased $SaO_2$, and the patient's own subjective statement of improved breathing with decreased anxiety or distress. Altered mental status may indicate hypoxemia but may also be due to pH, electrolyte, or carbon dioxide abnormalities. The nurse assesses the patient's respiratory status as often as needed until the desired results are achieved. ABG values guide therapy, especially in patients known to have carbon dioxide retention or continued lethargy or sedation, and in those unable to clear secretions. Ultimately, the ABG values indicate success or failure of efforts to correct the underlying hypoxemia.

## Oxygen Delivery Systems

Oxygen delivery systems are traditionally divided into high-flow and low-flow systems (Box 25-3). The choice of a delivery method depends on the patient's condition.

Low-flow oxygen devices work by supplying oxygen at flow rates less than the patient's inspiratory volume, usually 1 to 10 L/min. The rest of the volume is pulled from room air (entrained). Because of this oxygen and room air mixing (entrainment), the actual fraction of inspired oxygen ($FiO_2$) delivered to the patient is difficult to specify. Low-flow oxygen devices are suitable for patients with normal respiratory patterns, rates, and ventilation volumes. High-flow oxygen devices supply flow rates high enough to accommodate two to three times the patient's inspiratory volume, at 1 to 40 L/min. These devices are suitable for patients with high oxygen requirements because high-flow devices deliver 100% $O_2$ and maintain 100% humidification essential to prevent drying of the nasal mucosa.

Oxygen delivery devices all deliver different levels of oxygen. Device selection is based on the desired $FiO_2$. If increased distress, desaturation, or both are noted, more extreme interventions (such as intubation) may be necessary.

If lower concentrations of oxygen are needed, a nasal cannula may be used. The cannula can be used even with mouth breathers because oxygen fills the nasopharynx and, with inspiration, oxygen is entrained. The exact concentration of oxygen depends on the patient's inspired tidal volume ($V_T$). If the patient hypoventilates, the oxygen concentration

---

**QSEN BOX 25-2** *PATIENT SAFETY*

### Complications of Oxygen Therapy
- Respiratory depression/arrest
- Discomfort with skin breakdown from straps and masks
- Dry mucous membranes, epistaxis, or infection in the nares
- Oxygen toxicity (prolonged high levels seen in acute lung injury or acute respiratory distress syndrome [ARDS])
- Absorptive atelectasis
- Carbon dioxide narcosis (manifested by altered mental status, confusion, headache, somnolence)

---

**BOX 25-3** Oxygen Delivery Methods with Delivered Fraction of Inspired Oxygen (FiO₂)

Nasal Cannula—Low-Flow Device

| Flow (L/min) | FiO₂ |
|---|---|
| 1 | 21%–25% |
| 2 | 25%–28% |
| 3 | 28%–32% |
| 4 | 32%–36% |
| 5 | 36%–40% |
| 6 | 40%–44% |

High-Flow Nasal Cannula

| Flow (L/min) | FiO₂ |
|---|---|
| 1–40 | 21%–100% |

The high-flow nasal cannula (eg, AquinOx system or Vapotherm) is adjusted for the desired clinical effect depending on the arterial blood gas (ABG), SaO₂, and breaths per minute. These high-flow systems allow for humidification at 100%, with high levels of oxygen delivery maintaining nasal mucosa moisture not possible with a low-flow nasal cannula. The nurse should monitor the SaO₂ closely for at least 30 to 60 minutes when switching from another oxygen delivery device, evaluate ABG as needed, and assess patient tolerance. Be aware of clinical contraindications with increased oxygen delivery.

Face Mask—Low-Flow Device

| Flow (L/min) | FiO2 |
|---|---|
| 5–6 | 40% |
| 6–7 | 50% |
| 7–10 | 60% |

Face Tent—Low-Flow Device

Variable oxygen delivery of 21% to 50% depends on patient breathing (21% delivered with compressed air and up to 50% delivered with 10 L/min oxygen flow attached). Air is mixed with the oxygen flow in the mask, resulting in variable delivery with

humidification. This is often used for humidification as well as oxygen delivery in patients who do not like the claustrophobic feeling associated with more traditional masks.

Venturi Mask—Low-Flow Device

| Oxygen Flow (Minimal Rate) (L/min) | FiO₂ Setting* |
|---|---|
| 4 | 25% |
| 4 | 28% |
| 6 | 31% |
| 8 | 35% |
| 8 | 40% |
| 10 | 50% |
| 15 | 60% |

*FiO₂ setting is based on Venturi setting/adapter used and oxygen flow.

Nonrebreather Mask–Low-Flow Device

The nonrebreather mask is used in severe hypoxemia to deliver the highest oxygen concentration. The one-way valve on one side allows for the exhalation of carbon dioxide. The mask delivers 80% to 95% FiO₂ at a flow rate of 10 L/min depending on the patient's rate and depth of breathing, with some room air entrained through the open port on the mask. However, the mask should fit snugly to prevent additional entrainment of room air.

Tracheostomy Collar and T-Piece—Low-Flow Device

The T-piece is a T-shaped adapter used to provide oxygen to either an endotracheal or tracheostomy tube. The flow rate should be at least 10 L/min with humidification. Flow can also be provided by a ventilator. The tracheostomy collar may also be used and is generally the preferred method because it is more comfortable than the T-piece. The strap on the tracheostomy collar is adjusted to keep the collar on top of the tracheostomy. With both the T-piece and tracheostomy collar, the goal is to provide a high-enough flow rate to ensure that there is a minimal amount of entrained room air.

---

increases in the upper airway. In contrast, if the patient hyperventilates, the concentration of oxygen decreases because of large amounts of room air diluting the oxygen delivered. A simple calculation for nasal cannula delivery is to add another 4% for each liter of FiO₂ delivered to the room air value of 21% (see Box 25-3). Each of the other oxygen delivery devices delivers a variable FiO₂, based on breathing pattern and what device is used, as well as the oxygen flow in liters per minute.

If the oxygen concentration must be constant, Venturi systems (eg, the Venturi mask) are used. The Venturi mask delivers an exact percentage of oxygen regardless of the patient's tidal volume. Patients with COPD may require oxygen delivery by the Venturi system. These patients are "sensitive" to oxygen, and a small increase in the percentage of FiO₂ delivered may result in an elevated PaCO₂ and respiratory depression. The patient with COPD may have a respiratory drive based on his or her PaO₂; with this disease process, ventilation decreases with an increased FiO₂, resulting in hypercapnia. The carbon dioxide level can be detected through serial ABG monitoring, which may reveal large increases in PaCO₂ with small increases in oxygen flow.

When higher concentrations of oxygen are required, the nasal cannula is replaced by a mask system. A simple mask delivers the lowest concentrations of oxygen, and a nonrebreather mask delivers the highest concentration. The alternative to a nonrebreather for high FiO₂ delivery is high-flow oxygen via a humidified nasal cannula system. This system may be appropriate for patients who are just off the ventilator with low oxygen saturation for prevention of dry secretions with increased humidity (100%), those in pulmonary rehabilitation with decreased exercise tolerance, and those with COPD and asthma for whom high-flow nasal cannula systems improve breathing rate and dyspnea. Patients who have high oxygen requirements on mechanical ventilation should not be extubated until their clinical condition improves. A high flow nasal cannula allows high-liter oxygen flow through a nasal cannula with humidification at flows of 40 L/min. The high-flow nasal cannula may be more comfortable and allow improved tolerance by providing a constant temperature and high humidity, without the condensation and moisture buildup in the tubing that can occur and enter the nose in a low-flow nasal cannula. The other advantage of the high-flow nasal cannula is the ability to deliver a range of FiO₂—up to 100%—to meet patient oxygen demand. If a patient's $PaO_2$ and $SaO_2$ cannot be maintained using the nonrebreather mask or high-flow nasal cannula, respiratory failure, with the need for intubation and mechanical ventilation, is imminent.

## Complications of Oxygen Delivery

The delivery of oxygen can cause discomfort, skin breakdown, and other complications. Long-term oxygen by nasal cannula, even with humidification, can cause dry mucous membranes, epistaxis, and infection in the sinuses. Nasal cannula tubing, face masks (including the straps), and tracheostomy collars can cause skin breakdown along the face, bridge of the nose, back of the neck, and behind the ears. Oxygen delivery can fail if the tubing is disconnected from the wall, leading to hypoxemia with dysrhythmias or increased dyspnea. Contamination can occur with copious secretions coughed onto a tracheostomy collar or with mucus on any other device used. To prevent a fire-related injury, a "no smoking" rule must be enforced for all patients receiving oxygen therapy.

The nurse routinely inspects the skin and mucous membranes of the mouth and nares for signs of breakdown. For patients with a nasal cannula, the nurse inspects the ears, upper lip, and nares. Should skin injury occur, further breakdown can be prevented by providing skin barriers or cushions and possibly changing to another type of device. The mask may cause some patients anxiety, with feelings of suffocation, and, as with all devices, the nurse should ensure the patients' comfort. Finally, it is necessary to change disposable humidification systems according to manufacturer specifications to prevent system-related infections. Oxygen humidification sets for any device need routine changing at least every 72 hours. The key to preventing any complication, including hypoxemia, is accurate and timely assessment of oxygenation parameters and monitoring for complications of the therapies by the nurse.

Patients who are ventilated with high oxygen concentration for prolonged periods are at risk for oxygen toxicity. To prevent the pathologic cellular changes of oxygen toxicity, the patient's $FiO_2$ should be decreased as tolerated to the lowest possible setting as long as the $PaO_2$ remains greater than 60 mm Hg. The pathophysiologic changes that occur with oxygen toxicity occur at the alveolar level and may progress from capillary leaking to pulmonary edema and possibly to ALI if the high $FiO_2$ continues for several days. Once the oxygen concentration is decreased to safer levels, the pathophysiologic cellular changes may reverse, but if high $FiO_2$ levels continue, there may be permanent cellular changes and impairment of pulmonary function.

Carbon dioxide narcosis is a risk in patients with COPD who are "sensitive" to oxygen: an increased $FiO_2$ may result in an elevated $PaCO_2$, hypoventilation, and respiratory depression or respiratory arrest. Oxygen must therefore be administered with caution to patients with COPD, and often at low levels to prevent respiratory depression. Patients on high $FiO_2$ may develop absorptive atelectasis resulting from less nitrogen in the delivered gas mixture. Because nitrogen is not absorbed, it normally exerts a pressure within the alveoli, keeping the alveoli open. When nitrogen is "washed out," the oxygen replacing it is absorbed, resulting in alveolar collapse (atelectasis).

Respiratory arrest is a complication that can occur even in patients on oxygen therapy. Nurses prevent this complication by monitoring the patient's overall respiratory status, neurologic status, vital signs with $SaO_2$, and ABG values to evaluate for signs of impending respiratory failure. Respiratory arrest can also occur because of mucus plugging within the tracheobronchial airways or plugging of a tracheostomy or endotracheal tube (ETT). Respiratory failure from fatigue caused by the increased work of breathing can occur quickly in a patient with pulmonary compromise, such as a patient with COPD and new-onset pneumonia. Risk of aspiration of food or gastric contents can occur in hospitalized patients with dysphagia (eg, from a stroke, sedation, or secondary to prolonged intubation with vocal cord paralysis). The nurse must monitor the vulnerable patient more frequently when there is a clear comorbidity that may result in respiratory failure or arrest.

## Artificial Airways

Rigorous BHT and carefully monitored oxygen therapy may eliminate the need for an artificial airway or ventilatory support. However, if these measures fail to provide adequate oxygenation and removal of carbon dioxide, an artificial airway and ventilatory support become mandatory. Artificial airways have a fourfold purpose:

- Establishment of an airway
- Protection of the airway with the cuff inflated
- Provision of continuous ventilatory assistance with ETT and tracheostomy
- Facilitation of airway clearance

Knowledgeable, aggressive nursing care is required to maintain airway patency, maximize therapeutic effects, and minimize damage to the patient's natural airway.

The selection of the appropriate artificial airway is important. Because all artificial airways increase airway resistance, it is essential that the largest tube possible be used for intubation. The cuff on the endotracheal or tracheostomy tube must be very compliant (soft) so that trauma to the trachea, vocal cords, and subglottic area is minimized. The competency of the cuff must be established before intubation. Approximately 10 mL of air is injected into the cuff before use, and the clinician checks for leaks.

If a patient is sedated and lying supine or becomes unconscious, tongue and airway muscle tone is decreased, causing the tongue to occlude the airway. Although an oropharyngeal or nasopharyngeal airway will maintain the air passage, it will not eliminate the potential for aspiration. Figure 25-3 illustrates five frequently used artificial airways. The nasopharyngeal airway (nasal trumpet), a flexible tube that is inserted nasally past the base of the tongue to maintain airway patency, may be better tolerated than the oropharyngeal airway in patients with an intact gag reflex.

## Oropharyngeal Airway

An oropharyngeal airway is never placed in a conscious patient because it stimulates the gag reflex and can cause vomiting and aspiration.

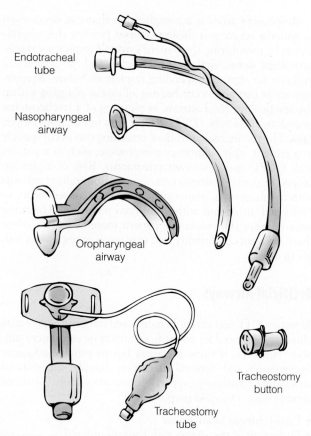

Endotracheal tube

Nasopharyngeal airway

Oropharyngeal airway

Tracheostomy tube

Tracheostomy button

**FIGURE 25-3** Five frequently used artificial airways.

Before placing an artificial airway, make sure any possible obstruction is cleared. Insert the oropharyngeal airway using the following three steps:

1. Gently open the patient's mouth using a crossed-finger technique or a modified jaw thrust.
2. Hold down the tongue with a depressor and guide the airway over the back of the tongue. (An optional method is to position the tip of the airway toward the roof of the mouth, with the curved end toward the roof, and gently advance the airway by rotating it 180 degrees.)
3. Monitor the patient frequently for airway patency by listening to breath sounds. Provide oropharyngeal suction as needed for emesis or oral secretions.

Oral suctioning is important to maintain oral hygiene when the patient is intubated because the patient's ability to swallow can be limited. Perform oral suctioning as needed for copious oral secretions and after suctioning the endotracheal or tracheostomy tubes to maintain oral hygiene and comfort.

To perform oral suctioning, use a Yankauer device (tonsil-tip suction apparatus). The larger openings on the Yankauer tip allow for suctioning of thick or copious secretions better than other suction catheters designed for suctioning through endotracheal or nasotracheal tubes, which are smaller in diameter. In addition, the smaller suction catheters are flexible, which may cause them to kink. The Yankauer device is angled to allow it to follow the contour of the oral cavity along the palate; this facilitates suctioning in the posterior oropharynx and the buccal pouches, where secretions may collect. After suctioning, rinse the tubing with tap water to

clear it of thick secretions and to ensure that the suction will continue to function in the future. To remove an oropharyngeal airway, suction the oropharynx and gently remove the airway.

## Nasopharyngeal Airway

Use the following steps to insert a nasopharyngeal airway:

1. Determine and select the correct tube length by measuring from the tip of the nose to the earlobe. Use a tube with the largest outer diameter that fits the patient's nostril.
2. Lubricate the tube with water, water-soluble jelly, or lidocaine jelly to alleviate discomfort.
3. Reassure the patient and familiarize him or her with the procedure.
4. Insert the airway into the nostril up to the end of the nasal trumpet.
5. Have the patient exhale with the mouth closed. (If the tube is in the correct position, air can be felt exiting from the tube opening.)
6. Open the patient's mouth, depress the tongue, and look for the tube's tip just behind the uvula.

In patients who require frequent nasotracheal suctioning, nasopharyngeal airways are frequently used to prevent patient discomfort and airway trauma from repeated suction catheter introduction through the nares.

Nasotracheal suctioning is best done using a red rubber suction catheter, which is more flexible and better tolerated than standard plastic catheters. Nasotracheal suctioning is done as a sterile procedure. The catheter is lubricated with water-soluble jelly and passed to the back of the nasopharynx initially. Supplemental oxygen is given before suctioning and in between each suction attempt. The oxygen can be given using a bag–valve–mask (BVM) apparatus or manual resuscitation bag (MRB) and gently bagging with each inspiration to provide a high $FiO_2$. Other high-flow devices, such as a Venturi mask, may also be used to provide more accurate concentrations of oxygen. The nurse or respiratory therapist then asks the patient to cough, which opens the epiglottis and allows the catheter to be advanced. A change in the sound of the cough and the return of sputum with suctioning indicates passage into the tracheal tree.

The technique of nasotracheal suctioning is difficult and should only be attempted by experienced practitioners. The nasopharyngeal airway may have to be gently rotated to withdraw it from the nares. It is important to be prepared for the potential of epistaxis with nasopharyngeal airway removal. Prior history of epistaxis or known coagulopathy should be carefully reviewed before placing a nasopharyngeal airway or performing nasotracheal suctioning that may lead to bleeding.

## Endotracheal Tubes

An ETT is inserted if the patient needs ventilation or protection of the airway from aspiration. Equipment listed in Box 25-4 is assembled before intubation. The ETT can be inserted nasally or orally.

To reduce the incidence of complications, personnel with specialized training must perform tracheal intubation. The

---

**BOX 25-4** **Equipment for Endotracheal Intubation**

- Laryngoscope with curved and straight blades and intact bulb
- Suction setup with Yankauer suction
- Correct size endotracheal tube (ETT) with stylet*
- 10-mL syringe for cuff inflation
- Adhesive tape, twill tape, or commercial ETT holder
- Magill forceps (may be used with nasal intubation)
- Pulse oximetry
- Oxygen source
- Manual resuscitation bag (MRB) with mask
- End-tidal $CO_2$ ($ETCO_2$) monitor or disposable detector
- Sedation and paralytic medication

*In adults, tube size is usually 8.0 initially unless the procedure is difficult, the patient is small, or a difficult intubation is anticipated, in which case smaller sizes are used. An ETT larger than 7.0 mm facilitates bronchoscopy.

---

**QSEN BOX 25-5** *PATIENT SAFETY*

**Complications of Intubation**

- Laryngospasm/bronchospasm
- Hypoxemia/hypercapnia during intubation
- Laryngeal edema resulting in stridor with extubation
- Trauma/bleeding to nasal, oral, esophageal, tracheal, or laryngeal sites
- Fractured teeth
- Nosocomial infection (pneumonia, sinusitis, abscess)
- Displacement of tube (right mainstem intubation, gastric intubation)
- Aspiration of oral or gastric contents
- Tracheal stenosis/tracheomalacia
- Laryngeal damage, paralysis, and necrosis
- Dysrhythmias, hypertension, hypotension

---

nurse explains the rationale for the procedure to the patient and family. The patient is positioned on his or her back with a small blanket under the shoulder blades to hyperextend the neck and open the airway. Air (10 mL) is injected into the endotracheal cuff before insertion to ensure an intact cuff, and then the cuff is deflated.

The nurse's role in intubation includes patient assessment; monitoring vital signs, pulse oximetry, and intubation and suction equipment; and collaborating with additional support staff as needed. Before the procedure, the nurse confirms that the suction is working properly. Using an MRB and mask, the nurse or respiratory therapist preoxygenates the patient. The health care provider may use a topical anesthetic, a sedative, or a short-acting neuromuscular blocking (NMB) agent to facilitate rapid and nontraumatic intubation. Newer short-acting intravenous (IV) anesthetics facilitate rapid intubation. Sedation with neuromuscular blockade must always be provided.

The nurse assists during intubation by providing suction as necessary and monitoring the patient's $SaO_2$ by pulse oximetry, as well as the patient's heart rate and blood pressure. If the $SaO_2$ falls below 90%, intubation attempts should be withheld and the patient oxygenated with the MRB. Hypoxemia during intubation may cause bradycardia, hypotension, dysrhythmias, cardiac arrest, and other complications.

After placement of the ETT, the cuff is inflated. It is necessary to auscultate the chest bilaterally for equal breath sounds, which may indicate a right mainstem intubation, and the abdomen for evidence of esophageal intubation. Waterproof tape is used to secure the ETT, and the centimeter mark is noted at the lips, teeth, or nostril for the nasotracheal tube. The level of the ETT must be noted to prevent changing of position, which could result in either right mainstem bronchus placement with left lung collapse or self-extubation. A portable chest radiograph is obtained immediately after the insertion to confirm proper tube placement, which is about 2 to 3 cm above the carina.

Complications of ETT placement are noted in Box 25-5. Initially during intubation, complications of hypoxemia, gastric intubation, mainstem intubation, and oral or tracheal tissue damage can occur. Vomiting during the procedure can lead to aspiration, which may result in lung injury. If the patient has prolonged hypoxemia and hypercapnia (as might occur with a difficult intubation), dysrhythmias such as bradycardia or tachycardia can occur, possibly leading to hemodynamic instability.

Once the patient is intubated, potential complications include disconnection, failure of the ventilator, tube obstruction, sinusitis, and tracheoesophageal fistula. Vocal cord paralysis or laryngeal or tracheal stenosis may present after extubation. Accidental extubation in a critically ill patient is a preventable complication. The most challenging cases involve confused patients who attempt to self-extubate. Orienting the patient to the need for the ETT and reassuring the patient that you will help make him or her more comfortable are the first interventions. Occasionally, physical or pharmacological restraints are necessary.

Many complications can be avoided by ensuring adequate fixation of the ETT, securing ventilator tubing properly, suctioning only as needed, and following other care maintenance protocols. These include providing oral care to remove secretions and maintaining the HOB elevated at 30 degrees to help prevent aspiration. Following aseptic policies decreases nosocomial infections, and maintaining proper cuff pressure helps prevent tracheal erosion. Ultimately, the long-term ventilated patient, intubated longer than 72 hours, may require a tracheostomy to continue ventilatory support and weaning.

### Suctioning

The presence of an artificial tube prevents glottic closure. As a result, the patient is unable to use the normal clearing mechanism (ie, effective coughing). Additionally, the foreign object increases production of secretions. Suctioning, therefore, becomes paramount to removing secretions and maintaining airway patency. Suctioning is not without risks and should be done only when needed. Possible complications of suctioning are listed in Box 25-6. Indications for

---

**QSEN BOX 25-6** *PATIENT SAFETY*

**Complications of Suctioning**

- Hypoxemia
- Dysrhythmias
- Vagal stimulation (bradycardia, hypotension)
- Bronchospasm
- Elevated ICP
- Atelectasis
- Tracheal mucosal trauma
- Bleeding
- Nosocomial infection

**BOX 25-7** **Procedure for Suctioning**

**Equipment**
Sterile suction catheter*
Sterile gloves
Sterile normal saline for irrigation, only when indicated
Sterile disposable container

**Technique**

1. Perform routine procedures before suctioning: administer medication, assemble equipment, explain the procedure to the patient, adjust bed to comfortable working position, prepare suction pressure, wash hands, prepare and open equipment and supplies, and don gloves.

2. Hyperoxygenate the patient with 100% oxygen using an MRB or the ventilator. If the ventilator method is used, preoxygenation must last at least 2 minutes. Return to the previous oxygen setting after suctioning is completed. In patients who do not tolerate suctioning with hyperoxygenation, a positive end-expiratory pressure (PEEP) attachment should be on the MRB at the appropriate setting, or in-line suctioning should be used to avoid loss of PEEP and desaturation.

3. Quickly but gently, insert the catheter as far as possible into the artificial airway without application of suction. For tracheostomy patients, limit the distance to just beyond the end of the tracheostomy device.

4. Withdraw the catheter 1 to 2 cm, and apply intermittent suction while rotating and removing the catheter. Limit suction pressure to 80 to 120 mm Hg. Aspiration should not exceed 10 to 15 seconds. (Prolonged aspiration can lead to severe hypoxemia, hemodynamic instability, and ultimately cardiac arrest.) Tracheostomy patients are usually suctioned for a briefer period of 3 to 5 seconds because of the very short device.

5. Do not instill sterile normal saline solution unless the patient has thick secretions and trial use has shown that it improves secretion removal. Routine instillation has been shown to decrease oxygenation and have other negative effects.[28-31]

6. Hyperoxygenate the patient before and after each subsequent pass of the catheter for at least 30 seconds, and before reconnection to the ventilator.

7. Monitor heart rate and rhythm and pulse oximetry during and after suctioning.

8. Discontinue the procedure if the patient does not tolerate it, as evidenced by dysrhythmias, bradycardia, or a drop in SaO2.

9. Remove equipment.

10. Perform oral hygiene. Cleanse suction tubing with a water rinse to remove secretions into the suction container.

11. Wash your hands.

12. Document procedure.

*Suction catheter sized for either ETT or tracheostomy; with tracheostomy, the red rubber or more flexible suction catheter brand is used to prevent tracheal bleeding.

suctioning include observing secretions in the airway, identifying secretions or mucus plugs by chest auscultation, coughing, increasing peak airway pressure, decreasing tidal volume during pressure ventilation, and deteriorating oxygenation as evidenced by decreased SaO2.

The procedure for suctioning is presented in Box 25-7. The nurse performs suctioning as a sterile procedure, using practices recommended by the Centers for Disease Control and Prevention (CDC). In-line suction catheters are available for use in patients on high levels of positive end-expiratory pressure (PEEP) who do not tolerate disconnection of the ventilator tubing for suctioning. Additionally, in-line suction catheters are used for patients with copious secretions who require frequent suctioning and for those with grossly bloody secretions. Patients who are identified as having the potential for long-term mechanical ventilation and patients who have been reintubated following a failed extubation are candidates for the use of the continuous aspiration of subglottic secretions (CASS) ETT. This device is used to prevent the subglottic accumulation of secretions above the ETT cuff that may lead to aspiration and is discussed in the section on VAP under Ventilatory Support, Complications of Mechanical Ventilation.

### Hyperoxygenation and Saline Instillation

The patient must be hyperoxygenated using the ventilator set to 100% if an in-line system is used. Patients not on ventilators also need to be hyperoxygenated before suctioning. The patient should be instructed to take deep breaths while connected to a 100% oxygen source. Patients incapable of taking a deep breath should be assisted using an MRB with mask; a squeeze on the MRB is timed with the patient's breath. The presence of epiglottitis or croup is an absolute contraindication to any kind of suctioning of patients without an artificial airway because this may worsen the patient's condition.

The routine instillation of normal saline solution has become increasingly questionable. In a test tube, saline and sputum act as oil and water: they do not form a mixture. Therefore, it is unlikely that saline instillation liquefies or increases the amount of sputum obtained during suction. ETT care and cuff pressure monitoring are discussed in more detail later in this chapter, under Ventilatory Support, Assessment and Management.

After the patient is intubated, the patient loses the ability to communicate easily. This inability to communicate can become a major stressor during the ventilated period.

## Chest Tubes

The chest tube is a drain. Its purposes are to remove air, fluid, or blood from the pleural space; restore negative pressure to the pleural space; reexpand a collapsed or partially collapsed lung (pneumothorax); and prevent reflux of drainage back into the chest. Chapter 23 provides a review of the anatomical and physiological principles of the lungs and chest that helps explain how chest tube systems work.

## Equipment for Chest Tube Insertion

Equipment needed for chest tube insertion is listed in Box 25-8.

Most chest tubes are multifenestrated transparent tubes with distance and radiopaque markers. The radiopaque markers enable the physician or other qualified health care professional to visualize the tube on chest radiograph and position it correctly in the pleural space. All openings in the tube must be placed within the rib cage to ensure that air leaks do not develop either in subcutaneous tissue or outside the chest wall. Chest tubes may be pleural or mediastinal, depending on distal tip location. Patients can have more than one tube in different locations, depending on the purpose of each tube.

Larger tubes (20 to 36 French) are used to drain blood or thick pleural drainage. Smaller tubes (16 to 20 French) are used to remove air.

- Chest tube tray or thoracotomy tray (with scalpel)
- Chest tube
- 1% lidocaine
- Syringe for lidocaine infiltration
- Topical antiseptic
- Sterile gloves
- Large curved hemostats
- Suture material (0-0 or 2-0 silk) on a cutting needle
- Bacteriostatic ointment or petrolatum gauze
- Sterile gauze with a slit
- Tape—both wide and narrow, or an occlusive dressing
- Chest tube drainage system and suction
- Sterile water for water seal systems
- Medication for pain and sedation

## Drainage Systems

To reestablish intrapleural negative pressure, a seal for the chest tube that prevents outside air from entering the system is necessary. The simplest way to accomplish this seal is to use an underwater system of drainage. A review of multichambered systems can provide a basis for understanding all the commonly used disposable drainage units. Knowledge of these systems enables the nurse to safely manage the most complex chest tube drainage setup.

Modern chest drainage systems are composed of disposable materials and may be configured in either two- or three-chamber system. The two-chamber system has a water seal and a collection chamber, whereas the three-chamber system

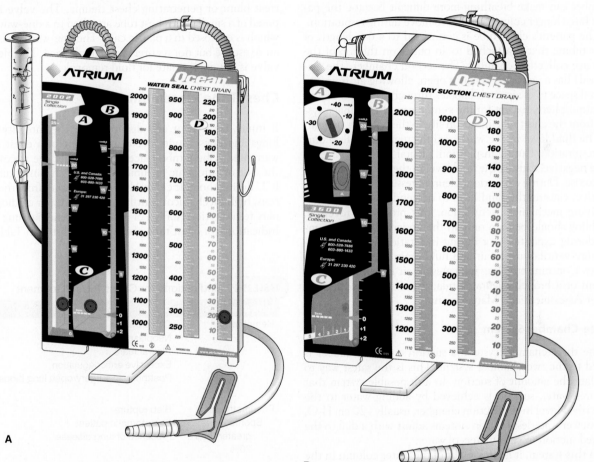

**FIGURE 25-4    Chest tube drainage systems.** The **Atrium Ocean** (*left*) is an example of a water seal chest drain system composed of a drainage chamber and water seal chamber. The suction control is determined by the height of the water column in that chamber (usually 20 cm). (**A**, suction control chamber; **B**, water seal chamber; **C**, air leak zone; **D**, collection chamber.) The **Atrium Oasis** (*right*) is an example of a dry suction water seal system that uses a mechanical regulator for vacuum control, a water seal chamber, and a drainage chamber. (**A**, dry suction regulator; **B**, water seal chamber; **C**, air leak monitor; **D**, collection chamber; **E**, suction monitor bellows.) (Courtesy of Atrium Medical Corporation, Hudson, New Hampshire.)

CDUs work with the same three chambers shown in the examples above. The collection chamber collects fluid with air passing through, the water seal prevents air going back into the patient, and a suction control chamber allows suction level settings depending on the medical condition. A collection chamber allows fluid volume up to 2,000 mL. This allows for assessment of type of drainage, amount of drainage, and rate changes, with some models having a sampling port. The water seal chamber is the one-way valve action that prevents air from returning to the chest while allowing air removal as in pneumothorax. The water seal chamber is filled to the –2 cm $H_2O$ level that maintains a slight negative pleural pressure and prevents air entering the pleural space when the CDU is off suction and on water seal. The suction control chamber is either the dry suction or a water-filled chamber. Water-filled suction is set by adjusting the water level. With continuous high suction, evaporation occurs, changing the volume of water that will change the suction level. Nursing care includes assessing the water level daily with suction off to refill the chamber to the desired level. Dry suction uses a mechanical system that allows the set suction level to be maintained regardless of the external suction level applied. The bellow window on dry suction systems allows a visual check that correct suction is applied; the colored indicator rises when sufficient suction is applied to maintain the set suction level from –10 to –40 cm $H_2O$. The wall suction regulator should be adjusted to –80 mm Hg, with a continuous gentle bubbling in the water seal chamber. All CDUs follow these same functions of collection, water seal, and suction regulation chambers, and the nurse adheres to manufacturer instructions concerning proper setup and monitoring of the system.

adds a suction control chamber. Figure 25-4 depicts disposable chest drainage systems.

## Two-Chamber System

In a two-chamber system, the first chamber is the collection receptacle and the second chamber is the water seal. In a disposable system that requires water, sterile water is added to the second chamber to the 2-cm level to achieve the seal. This level represents the negative pressure that is exerted on the pleural space as the water closes the chest drain to outside air, acting as a one-way valve. The water seal allows air to escape while preventing outside air from entering the pleural space. A fluid level higher than 2 cm $H_2O$ exerts a greater negative pressure on the pleural space and may prevent resolution of the air leak. In addition, a higher column of water in the water seal chamber can make breathing more difficult because the patient has a longer column of fluid to move during respiration.

The patient's chest tube is connected to a 6-ft length of latex tubing that is attached to an outlet on the top of the drainage collection chamber. The second chamber (the water seal) has a vent that remains open, allowing air from the pleural space to escape as it bubbles through the water seal to the atmosphere. Except for the vented cap, the drainage system from the chest tube insertion site to the bottle is airtight.

The fluid level in the water seal fluctuates ("tidals") during respiration. During inspiration, pleural pressures become more negative, causing the fluid level in the water seal chamber to rise. During expiration, pleural pressures become more positive, causing the fluid level to descend. If the patient is receiving mechanical ventilation, this process is reversed. Bubbling should be seen only in the underwater seal chamber during expiration (or during inspiration with positive-pressure ventilation) as air and fluid drain from the pleural cavity. Constant bubbling indicates an air leak in either the system or a bronchopleural fistula; this is discussed further under Assessment and Management.

## Three-Chamber System

In the three-chamber system, a suction control chamber is added to the two-chamber system. This is the safest way to regulate the amount of suction. In a disposable system that requires water, suction is achieved by adding water to the prescribed level in the suction chamber, usually –20 cm $H_2O$, and newer waterless suction systems adjust with a dial to the desired suction in centimeters of water.

In this system, it is the height of the water column in the third chamber, not the amount of wall suction, that determines the suction amount applied to the chest tube, most commonly –20 cm $H_2O$. Once the wall suction exceeds the force necessary to "lift" this column of fluid, any additional suction simply pulls air from a vented cap atop the chamber up through the water. The amount of wall suction applied to the third chamber should be sufficient to create a "gently rolling" bubble in the suction control chamber. Vigorous bubbling results in water loss through evaporation, changing suction pressure and increasing the noise level in the patient's room. It is important to assess for water loss and to add sterile water as necessary to maintain the prescribed level of suction. The bubbling should be assessed for gentle action, and the water level (–20 cm $H_2O$) should be assessed every 8 hours and when the patient's clinical status changes.

## Suction

Dry suction (waterless) systems use a spring mechanism to control the suction level and can provide higher levels of suction with easier setup than the two-chamber or three-chamber system. Dry suction systems can be easily adjusted for any setting between –10 and –40 cm $H_2O$ and are safer if the device is accidentally tipped over. If this happens, the drainage can be returned to the correct collection chamber without replacing the unit, resulting in cost savings. In addition, a dry suction system affords the patient a quieter environment. Dry suction systems that can deliver higher levels of suction may be necessary in patients with large bronchopleural fistulas, hemorrhage, or obesity.

Heimlich valves are reserved for treating pneumothoraces on an outpatient basis or by emergency medical providers to treat blunt or penetrating chest trauma. The valve is composed of a small-bore chest tube attached to a one-way valve, which is enclosed in a plastic case. The one-way valve allows air to escape but not reenter the pleural space. The Heimlich valve is not appropriate for fluid removal.

## Chest Tube Placement

If injury, surgery, or any disruption in the integrity of the lungs and chest cavity occur, placement of a chest tube is warranted. Chest tube placement may also be necessary in the case of iatrogenic pneumothorax, which can occur in the ICU during thoracic central line placement or from thoracentesis, high mechanical ventilation pressures, or cardiopulmonary resuscitation (CPR), or after transbronchial lung biopsy. Indications for chest tube placement are listed in Table 25-1.

**TABLE 25-1    Indications for Chest Tube Placement**

| Indication | Cause |
|---|---|
| Hemothorax | Chest trauma |
| | Neoplasms |
| | Pleural tears |
| | Excessive anticoagulation |
| | Postthoracic surgery/open lung biopsy |
| Pneumothorax Spontaneous: greater than 20% | Bleb rupture |
| | Symptomatic patient |
| | Presence of lung disease |
| Tension | Mechanical ventilation |
| | Penetrating puncture wound |
| | Prolonged clamping of chest tubes |
| | Lack of seal in chest tube drainage system |
| Bronchopleural fistula | Tissue damage |
| | Tumor (esophageal cancer) |
| | Aspiration of toxic chemicals |
| | Boerhaave syndrome (spontaneous rupture) |
| Pleural effusion | Neoplasms |
| | Cardiopulmonary disease, congestive heart failure |
| | Inflammatory conditions |
| | Recurrent infections/pneumonia |
| Chylothorax | Trauma or thoracic surgery |
| | Malignancy |
| | Congenital abnormalities |

Chest tube insertion can be accomplished in the operating room, in the emergency department, or at the bedside. Placement is based on the principle that, because of their different densities and weights, air rises and liquid sinks. The insertion site for air removal is near the second intercostal space along the midclavicular line. The insertion site for liquid drainage is near the fifth or sixth intercostal space on the midaxillary line. Fluid may occasionally become loculated (walled off), requiring ultrasound or computed tomography guidance for drainage tube placement. After cardiac surgery, placement may be in the mediastinum to drain blood from around the heart.

The nurse prepares the patient and family for the procedure, answering any questions they may have. The nurse also prepares the patient physically. Because parietal pleurae are innervated from the intercostal and phrenic nerves, this is a painful procedure, and administration of analgesics is indicated. The patient is placed in Fowler or semi-Fowler position. After the skin has been cleaned and anesthetized, the physician or other qualified health care professional makes a small skin incision. A hemostat is used to penetrate the pleural space (Fig. 25-5). The tract made by the hemostat is then dilated with a sterile, gloved finger. The proximal end of the tube is clamped with the hemostat and then inserted into the pleural space. If the placement is difficult, a metal trocar can be used to penetrate the chest wall, leaving the tube in place and removing the trocar.

After insertion, the external end of the tube is connected to a chest drainage unit (CDU). The ends of both the chest tube and the drainage system tubing must remain sterile as they are connected. To prevent the tube from dislodging, it is sutured to the skin around the insertion site. The ends of the suture are wrapped around the tube and tied off. Bacteriostatic ointment or petrolatum gauze can be applied to the incision site. Petrolatum gauze has been preferred because it is thought to prevent air leaks; however, it also has the potential to macerate the skin and predispose the site to infection. A 4″ × 4″ drain sponge is positioned over the tube and taped occlusively to the chest. All connections from the insertion site to the drainage collection system are securely taped to prevent air leaks as well as inadvertent disconnection. The proximal tube is taped to the chest to prevent traction on the tube and sutures if the patient moves.

A postinsertion chest radiograph is always ordered to confirm proper positioning. The lungs are auscultated, and the condition of the tissue around the insertion site is evaluated for the presence of subcutaneous air. This assessment provides a baseline for determining improvement or worsening of the patient's condition. Daily chest radiographs may be necessary to assess the clinical picture.

Pain management is an issue throughout the duration of chest tube use. Narcotics, nonsteroidal anti-inflammatory drugs, or a lidocaine transcutaneous patch may help reduce pain. The application of a lidocaine-infused patch proximal to the incision or at the chest tube incision site, which slowly releases medication over 12 to 24 hours, is an additional pain relief tool. Dressings are changed per institutional protocol, or as needed if soiled or loose. Chest tube output is assessed every 2 hours; the nurse looks for sudden cessation of drainage or an increase to more than 200 mL/h, or a sudden change in the character of the drainage.

## Assessment and Management

Nursing care is directed at maintaining patency and proper functioning of the chest tube drainage system. Vigilant and expert nursing care can prevent serious patient complications.

Drain the latex tubing frequently into the collection container. Coil the latex tubing loosely on the bed to prevent kinks and pooling of blood or drainage in a dependent loop hanging on the floor. Ensure that the patient does not inadvertently lie on the tubing. Never raise the chest tube drainage system above the chest, because the drainage will back up into the chest. At frequent intervals, check the chest tube drainage system for drainage, suction level, and water seal integrity. Secure the system to the foot of the patient's bed or tape it to the floor to avoid accidental overturning and possible reaccumulation of the pneumothorax. Inspect all tubing connections for leaks, and secure them with tape to prevent accidental disconnection.

To check for chest tube patency and respiratory cycle fluctuations, momentarily disconnect the suction (system placed only to water seal—not clamped). Use a step-by-step approach to evaluate and troubleshoot the system:

1. Assess cardiopulmonary status and vital signs every 2 hours and as needed.
2. Check and maintain tube patency every 2 hours and as needed.
3. Monitor type and amount of drainage.
4. Mark amount of drainage on collection chamber in hourly or shift increments and document in output record.
5. Prevent dependent loops from forming in tubing; ensure that the patient does not inadvertently lie on the tubing.
6. Refill water systems with sterile water to the water seal level and prescribed suction level (secondary to evaporation).
7. Assess for "tidaling" in the water seal chamber with respiration or mechanical ventilation breaths.

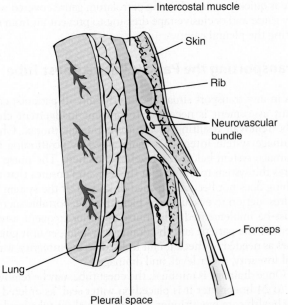

Intercostal muscle

Skin

Rib

Neurovascular bundle

Forceps

Lung

Pleural space

**FIGURE 25-5** Forceps penetrate the pleural space and are spread to create a track within the pleural space for the chest tube to be positioned. A gloved finger may also be used to create this track.

8. Assess for the location of air leaks (constant bubbling in the water seal chamber). Turn off the suction. Begin at the insertion site; occlude the chest tube or drainage tube (briefly) below each connection point until the drainage unit is reached.
9. Check that all tubing connections are securely sealed and taped. Another technique for sealing the connections is to use a banding gun that secures a plastic loop around the connections to prevent air leakage.
10. Assess the patient for pain and medicate as needed.
11. Assess the actual chest tube insertion site for signs of infection and subcutaneous emphysema with dressing changes.
12. Change the dressing twice daily or per unit guideline, when soiled, and when ordered.

### Drainage Monitoring

The nurse assesses and documents the color, consistency, and amount of drainage while remaining alert to significant changes. A sudden increase indicates hemorrhage or sudden patency of a previously obstructed tube. A sudden decrease indicates chest tube obstruction or failure of the chest tube or drainage system. The following nursing actions are recommended to reestablish chest tube patency:

- Attempt to alleviate the obstruction by repositioning the patient.
- If the clot is visible, straighten the tubing between the chest and drainage unit and raise the tube to enhance the effect of gravity.

Studies suggest that milking and stripping techniques may not be beneficial for maintaining chest tube patency.[8] These techniques may excessively increase intrapleural and intrapulmonary pressures, affecting ventricular function or causing trauma from aspiration of lung tissue into chest tube eyelets. However, under a health care practitioner's direction, this procedure may be necessary in cases of active bleeding to prevent blood clotting in the tubing that could lead to cardiac or pleural tamponade.

### Water Seal Monitoring

Monitoring the water seal of the chest tube drainage system is as important as observing the drainage. Visual checks are made to ensure water seal chambers are filled to the 2-cm water line. If suction is applied, the nurse ensures that the water line in a water-controlled suction chamber is at the ordered level (usually −20 cm $H_2O$), because water evaporates over time, decreasing the amount of suction being applied. It is important to add only sterile water to the system. If an Emerson pleural suction pump is used, the nurse checks the suction gauge for the desired suction level. It is essential that the air vent opening is never occluded. The suction tubing is disconnected briefly to accurately assess the water level in the chamber (water suction control) only after clamping the tubing. Then, the tubing is reattached and the clamp opened. The tubing should never be left clamped because this can result in pneumothorax or buildup of fluid in the chest, leading to respiratory distress.

Respiratory fluctuations are observed in the water seal chamber. The absence of fluctuations can indicate that the lung is reexpanded or that there is an obstruction in the system. Continuous vigorous bubbling in the water seal chamber, without suction, indicates continued pneumothorax, or it can indicate the tube has been displaced or disconnected, or that the drainage system is damaged. It is necessary to check the entire system for disconnections and to inspect the chest tube to see if it is displaced outside the chest. In the setting of mechanical ventilation at high volumes and pressures, bubbling in a chest tube system that persists may indicate a bronchopleural fistula when there is no pneumothorax or other known cause.

### Positioning

The ideal position for a patient with a chest tube is the semi-Fowler position. Turning the patient every 2 hours enhances air and fluid evacuation. The nurse teaches the patient how to support or "splint" the chest wall near the tube insertion site using a pillow, bath blanket, or arms placed firmly against the chest. The nurse also encourages coughing, deep breathing, and ambulation. Administration of pain medication before these exercises decreases pain and enhances lung expansion.

## Complications

The most serious complication resulting from chest tube placement is tension pneumothorax, which can develop if there is any obstruction in the chest tube drainage system. Clamping chest tubes as a routine practice predisposes patients to this complication. Clamping of chest tubes is recommended in only two situations:

- To locate the source of an air leak if bubbling occurs in the water seal chamber (*clamping is only momentary*)
- To replace the chest tube drainage unit (*clamping is only momentary*)

If the tube must be clamped, padded hemostats are used to avoid lacerating the vinyl chest tube.

Occasionally, the chest tube may become dislodged or be accidentally removed. In such a circumstance, the insertion site is quickly sealed off using petrolatum gauze covered with dry gauze and occlusive tape dressing to prevent air from entering the pleural cavity.

## Transporting the Patient With a Chest Tube

As in any transport situation for critically ill patients, constant assessment is necessary to prevent inadvertent chest tube removal, resulting in recurrent pneumothorax. Chest drainage system integrity is maintained by positioning the drainage system below the level of the chest. The nurse secures the system to the foot of the bed, and ensures that the tubing does not become crushed or kinked. If the system requires suction to evacuate the pleural space, portable suction must be implemented. The nurse performs frequent assessment of the patient and the drainage system per unit guidelines as needed to check for air leaks, dressing integrity, water seal integrity, water level, and drainage.

Once drainage is minimal, the chest tube may be removed 12 to 24 hours after it is placed on water seal, as ordered by the health care practitioner. Keeping the chest tube in place on water seal for a period of time allows for monitoring of

- One day after cessation of air leak
- Drainage of less than 50 to 100 mL of fluid/d
- One to three days after cardiac surgery
- Two to six days after thoracic surgery
- Obliteration of empyema cavity
- Serosanguineous drainage from around the chest tube insertion site
- Chest tube partially migrated out with holes visible (may require a new chest tube insertion)

persistent air leakage, which would indicate air in the pleural space and a need for continued chest tube suction. The presence of air in the pleural space can be confirmed by chest radiograph. Other indications for removal of the chest tube are listed in Box 25-9. When the tube is connected to water seal, disconnect the suction tube to facilitate atmospheric venting. Note that premature clamping or removal of the tube may cause reaccumulation of the pneumothorax.

## Chest Tube Removal

Before the chest tube is removed, the patient is placed in Fowler or semi-Fowler position (head of bed elevated 45 to 90 degrees). Premedication is recommended to alleviate pain and discomfort. The dressing over the insertion site is removed, and the area is cleaned. The suture is clipped. The tube is removed in one quick movement at end expiration with valsalva maneuver to prevent entraining air back into the pleural cavity through the chest tube eyelets. Immediately after tube removal, the lung fields are auscultated for any change in breath sounds, and an occlusive sterile dressing is applied over the site. A chest radiograph is usually obtained several hours later to look for the presence of residual air or fluid.

## Pharmacologic Agents

### Bronchodilator Therapy

Asthma is characterized by recurrent airway inflammation and increased hypersensitivity to a wide range of stimuli (noxious fumes and gases, air pollutants, animal dander, extreme cold, and exercise). The hypersensitivity leads to hyperreactivity of the airways with obstruction, with widely variable symptoms even in the same person. Asthma is an episodic disease with recurrent exacerbations and periods without symptoms. Management goals include symptom control to maintain normal activities, prevention of exacerbations, and minimization of pharmacologic side effects and toxicity. Pharmacologic therapy is designed around multiple classes of drugs and is aimed at reducing inflammation, treating acute symptoms, and maintaining a plan for the short-and long-term therapy. Bronchospasm may also be present in COPD and can be treated with the same pharmacologic agents.

Delivery of agents typically has been by propellant inhalers, with dosage dependent on the number of puffs per treatment using a metered-dose inhaler (MDI). The breath, depth, inspiratory flow rate, and use of a spacer (vs. administering just into the mouth) create variable medication

delivery. Cleaning and proper fitting together of the actuator to the valve stem, and onto a spacer (if used), are necessary. The preferred MDI method involves using a spacer—a tube attached to the inhaler to hold the medication until it is breathed in by the patient. For many patients, the spacer makes MDIs easier to use and deposits medications into the lungs more effectively. Dry powder inhalers (DPIs) allow some asthma medications to be taken in a dry powder form. The difference between DPIs and MDIs is that DPIs do not use a propellant, only the medication. Patient inhalation ensures delivery into the lungs. Patients must practice the proper use of these devices, maintain consistent inspiratory flow, and consistently use a spacer or aim the device directly into the mouth to achieve consistent medication dosage. These devices may be used by patients who range in age from 5 years to elderly, although they must be able to inhale forcefully enough to breathe in the medication. As with MDIs, patients need training to follow the directions and process for each form of DPI inhaler.

The Diskus inhaler is a version of the DPI. Usually, it contains a set number of metered doses of a long-acting $\beta_2$-agonist such as salmeterol (eg, Serevent) or a combination of fluticasone and salmeterol (eg, Advair). The Diskus inhaler is used to deliver medication for asthma control and not for an acute asthma attack; the medication is long acting, for daily use. A spacer is not used with the DISKUS inhaler. The patient must breathe in deeply and steadily, hold the breath for up to 10 seconds, and then slowly exhale. It is important to instruct the patient that the Diskus mouthpiece should never be washed in water, and that the inhaler should not be placed in water. In addition, the patient should be instructed not to breathe into the Diskus before inhaling.

### Bronchodilators

Bronchodilators act principally to dilate the airways by relaxing bronchial smooth muscles. The goals of bronchodilator therapy are to relax the airways, mobilize secretions, and reduce mucosal edema. Bronchodilator therapy can be delivered through an MDI, preferably with a spacer attachment, or via nebulization. Regardless of the mode of delivery, assessment before, during, and after the therapy is essential.

Assessment before and after treatment includes breath sounds, pulse, and respiratory rate. Pulse and respiratory rate commonly increase during bronchodilator therapy and can remain elevated for as long as 1 to 1.5 hours after treatment. (In people with asthma, the peak expiratory flow rate is measured with a peak flow meter before and after a treatment to determine whether the severity of airway obstruction has been reduced.) Objective evaluation is crucial, but subjective information is also valuable. Evaluation of patient response should be ascertained by asking about improvement in breathing, presence of wheezing, and side effects, such as tremor or palpitations.

Bronchodilators may be divided into three categories based on their mechanism and site of action. These are $\beta_2$-adrenergic agonists, anticholinergic agents, and methylxanthines.

**$\beta_2$-ADRENERGIC AGONISTS.** The bronchodilator effects of $\beta$-adrenergic agonists result from the stimulation of $\beta_2$-adrenergic receptors in the lung bronchial smooth muscle.

In addition, these agents may decrease the release of mediators from mast cells and basophils. $\beta_1$-Adrenergic receptors in the heart may also be stimulated, leading to undesired cardiac effects. Newer $\beta$-agonists are more specific for the $\beta_2$-receptor, although they retain some $\beta_1$ activity.

$\beta$-Agonists may be administered orally or inhaled. Aerosolized or inhaled therapy is preferred and has been shown to produce comparable bronchodilation and fewer systemic adverse effects.

$\beta$-Agonists are the bronchodilators of choice for treating acute exacerbation of asthma because of their rapid onset of action. They produce less bronchodilation in patients with COPD than in those with asthma. Albuterol (2.5 to 5 mg diluted in 3 mL normal saline solution) is the bronchodilator of choice in the acute setting and may be administered by continuous or intermittent frequent nebulization (every 15 to 20 minutes), then scheduled on an "as-needed" basis depending on patient response. Until recently, all available inhaled $\beta$-agonists, such as albuterol, had short durations of action (4 to 6 hours). Salmeterol is the first long-acting $\beta$-agonist, with duration of action of 12 hours. Salmeterol cannot be used for acute exacerbations of asthma because of its slow onset of action. The medication DuoNeb combines albuterol and ipratropium, allowing for a synergistic effect of both a bronchodilator and an anticholinergic agent, as discussed later. In addition, Advair Diskus combines a long-acting $\beta_2$-adrenergic agonist, Salmeterol, with fluticasone propionate, an inhaled corticosteroid, to provide twice-daily dosing for patients who do not achieve adequate control using other asthma medications.

**ANTICHOLINERGIC AGENTS.** Anticholinergic agents produce bronchodilation by reducing intrinsic vagal tone to the airways. They also block reflex bronchoconstriction caused by inhaled irritants.

Atropine is the prototype anticholinergic agent but is used infrequently because it is readily absorbed from the respiratory tract but produces unwanted systemic effects (eg, blurred vision, drying of respiratory secretions, tachycardia, and anxiety). Ipratropium, a quaternary amine that is not well absorbed from the respiratory tract, produces fewer systemic adverse effects and has taken the place of atropine. It is most effective in patients with COPD when used on a regular basis. It decreases submucosal gland secretion and relaxes bronchial smooth muscle. Ipratropium should not be used alone in acute exacerbations because of its slower onset of effect compared with $\beta$-agonists. It has been shown to be effective during status asthmaticus when administered through a nebulizer in combination with $\beta$-agonists, as in DuoNeb.

**METHYLXANTHINES.** Using methylxanthines for treating bronchospastic airway disease is controversial. The agents' mechanism of action is poorly understood. They inhibit phosphodiesterase, an enzyme that catalyzes the breakdown of cyclic adenosine monophosphate. They may also possess some degree of anti-inflammatory activity and may augment respiratory muscle contractility.

Theophylline, the prototype methylxanthine, may be used chronically in treating bronchospastic disease but is usually considered third- or fourth-line therapy. Some patients with severe disease that is not controlled with $\beta$-agonists, anticholinergics, or anti-inflammatory agents may benefit from theophylline. Aminophylline, the IV form of theophylline,

is rarely used in acute exacerbations because of the lack of evidence that it is beneficial in this situation.

Theophylline has a narrow therapeutic index. Depending on the clinical situation, serum drug concentration should be monitored to ensure efficacy and prevent toxicity. The accepted therapeutic range is 10 to 20 mcg/mL, although some references use 5 to 15 mcg/mL.[9] Theophylline interacts with a variety of other medications that may alter its serum concentration; these include erythromycin, ciprofloxacin, and cimetidine. Patients with liver disease or congestive heart failure eliminate theophylline more slowly and may be at an increased risk for toxicity. The level should be monitored 12 to 24 hours after the loading dose is administered and frequently as clinical condition and liver and renal function dictate.

### Anti-Inflammatory Agents

Anti-inflammatory agents interrupt the development of bronchial inflammation and have a prophylactic or preventive action. They may also reduce or terminate ongoing inflammation in the airway. Anti-inflammatory agents include corticosteroids, mast cell stabilizers, and leukotriene receptor antagonists.

**CORTICOSTEROIDS.** Corticosteroids are the most effective anti-inflammatory agents for treating reversible airflow obstruction. Corticosteroid therapy should be initiated simultaneously with bronchodilator therapy because the onset of action may be 6 to 12 hours. They may be administered parenterally, orally, or as aerosols. In acute exacerbations, high-dose parenteral steroids (eg, IV methylprednisolone) are used and then tapered as the patient tolerates. Short courses of oral therapy may be used to prevent the progression of acute attacks. Long-term oral therapy is associated with systemic adverse effects and should be avoided if possible. If chronic medication is necessary, inhaled corticosteroids, such as fluticasone (Flovent) or budesonide (Pulmicort), are preferred because of the decreased risk for systemic adverse effects.

**MAST CELL STABILIZERS.** The two available mast cell stabilizers are cromolyn and nedocromil. They are thought to stabilize mast cell membranes and prevent the release of mediators from mast cells. These agents are not indicated for acute exacerbations of asthma because they are used *prophylactically* to prevent acute airway narrowing after exposure to allergens (eg, exercise, cold air). A 4- to 6-week trial may be required to determine the efficacy in individual patients. The desired endpoint is to reduce the frequency and severity of asthma attacks and enhance the effects of concomitantly administered bronchodilator and steroid therapy. As a result, it may be possible to decrease the dose of bronchodilators or corticosteroids in patients who respond to mast cell stabilizers.

**LEUKOTRIENE RECEPTOR ANTAGONISTS.** Leukotriene receptor antagonists, such as montelukast, may be used in managing exercise-induced bronchospasm, asthma, allergic rhinitis, and urticaria. These agents block the activity of endogenous inflammatory mediators, particularly leukotrienes. These mediators cause increased vascular permeability, mucous secretion, airway edema, bronchoconstriction, and other inflammatory cell process activities. Leukotriene receptor antagonists are administered once daily and are usually well tolerated. They are not to be administered for acute conditions but as a part of an ongoing program of therapy.

### Cystic Fibrosis Agent (DNase)

DNase is used in cystic fibrosis patients to break down molecules in tenacious secretions to facilitate expectoration as well as decrease the amount of medium for bacterial growth. This also improves gas flow through airways. It is administered in an inhaled form either daily or twice daily.

## Antibiotics

Pneumonia is often treated empirically until the results of cultures and sensitivities are available, after which the antibiotic regimen is tailored to eradicate the specific pathogenic organism. Commonly, broad-spectrum antibiotics or combination therapy is used. The critically ill patient is at increased risk for developing pneumonia due to mechanical ventilation, decreased immune responses, use of corticosteroids, debilitated general health, and cross-infection by health care workers. Antibiotic therapy should be driven by institutional protocols to prevent antibiotic overuse and following guidelines for antimicrobial selection to limit resistance.

Empiric therapy for community-acquired pneumonia includes therapy directed toward the most common organisms associated with this type of pneumonia. These organisms include *Streptococcus pneumoniae* and *Haemophilus influenzae*. Methicillin-resistant *Staphylococcus aureus* should be suspected in patients admitted to the hospital from a nursing home. *Legionella* species should be suspected in patients with severe multilobar pneumonia. Patients infected with the human immunodeficiency virus require empiric treatment if there is suspected *Pneumocystis jiroveci* pneumonia (previously referred to as *Pneumocystis carinii* pneumonia).

Hospital-acquired pneumonia (HAP) or health care–associated pneumonia is often associated with Gram-negative bacilli, such as *Pseudomonas aeruginosa*, or it may be polymicrobial. HAP is the term for pneumonia that develops at least 48 hours after hospitalization; formerly, it was known as nosocomial pneumonia, and it includes VAP. Aspiration is a concern in mechanically ventilated patients or patients unable to protect their airways. Aspiration pneumonia is associated with anaerobic organisms (eg, *Actinomyces* species). Atypical organisms (*Mycoplasma pneumoniae*, *Chlamydia pneumoniae*, and *Legionella* species) should also be considered, as should viral infection. Patients should have a quantitative sputum culture to identify species on admission, and they may require bronchoscopy for specimen collection.

Consensus guidelines for pneumonia management are constantly under revision. The causes of pneumonia may stem from multiple factors that must be taken under consideration when treating the critically ill patient. Because of the prevalence of multidrug resistance and evolving antibiotic regimens, priority must be placed on obtaining a sputum culture and defining the susceptibility of the organism to several antibiotics. This will further ensure appropriate antibiotic use.

## Sedative Agents

Critically ill patients frequently require pharmacologic intervention for analgesia, sedation, control of anxiety, and

---

| BOX 25-10 | Etiologies of Agitation in Critically Ill Patients |
|---|---|

Pain
Mechanical ventilation
Dyspnea
Hypoxemia
Metabolic disarray
Withdrawal from alcohol or drugs
Anxiety
Sleep deprivation
Immobility
Sepsis
Age
Steroid administration
Alzheimer disease
Hearing or vision deficit (severe)

---

facilitation of mechanical ventilation. The selection of appropriate pharmacologic agents is based on the cause of the agitation (Box 25-10), underlying illness, possible adverse effects, history of previous drug use, and cost. Agents most commonly used in the ICU include opiates, benzodiazepines, haloperidol (Haldol), and propofol (Diprivan). Specifically, haloperidol is recommended for patients with delirium, and opiates are used synergistically to treat pain.

Several agents can be given as bolus doses, by continuous infusion, or by using a combination of the two approaches, although some drugs, such as haloperidol, are limited to bolus dosing. When administering these agents by continuous infusion, it is important to monitor the patient's response closely and adjust the dose to meet his or her individual needs. This is best accomplished by using an objective sedation rating scale for consistent assessment and documentation of the medication's efficacy. Such a protocol can help prevent the prolonged use of these agents and can lower the cumulative amount required for the control of pain or agitation. This can contribute to a decreased length of hospital stay and decreased length of mechanical ventilation.

When using a continuous infusion, if an increase in dosage is necessary, an additional small bolus dose should be given to facilitate rapid increase to the new desired blood level. To prevent withdrawal symptoms, dosages given to patients who have received large amounts of opiates or benzodiazepines for 2 or more weeks must be tapered gradually—for example, the dose may be decreased by 25% a day. Some protocols promote the conversion of benzodiazepine infusions to the enteral route before stopping the infusion. Enteral administration is performed to maintain an appropriate level of sedation and to wean patients who have required prolonged sedation, usually over 7 days. Protocols that include daily tapering or weaning of infusions along with daily sedation interruption are recommended. Another method of nurse-controlled monitoring, bispectral index monitoring, has been studied and found to be useful for controlling sedation in critically ill patients who are receiving sedation.[10]

## Neuromuscular Blocking Agents

If metabolic demands and work of breathing continue to compromise ventilatory or hemodynamic stability after maximization of sedation, NMB agents may be required. The goal of therapy with NMB agents is to maximize oxygenation and prevent complications such as barotrauma (alveolar rupture that can result in death), which can be caused by high ventilatory pressures.

The use of NMB agents is usually required if the pressure-controlled inverse ratio mode of ventilation is used. NMB drugs do *not* possess analgesic or sedative properties. When NMB agents are used, sedation and analgesia are required, along with patient and family education. *Do not leave a chemically paralyzed patient unattended.*

Recent reports of prolonged paralysis following use of NMB agents have prompted many institutions to initiate protocols for instituting, monitoring, and withdrawing these drugs. These range from the use of peripheral nerve stimulators to assess the level of neuromuscular blockade to the routine daily discontinuation of NMB agents to assess neurologic status and the need for continued administration.

Commonly used NMB agents are vecuronium (Norcuron), atracurium (Tracrium), and cisatracurium (Nimbex). Each has advantages and disadvantages related to concomitant drug effects, underlying illness, and cost. Both atracurium and cisatracurium have fewer side effects than other NMB agents. Both atracurium and cisatracurium are useful for patients with renal failure because metabolic breakdown of the drugs is in the plasma independent of renal or hepatic function. These two NMB agents are eliminated by ester hydrolysis and Hoffman elimination in the plasma, which is a spontaneous nonenzymatic degradation that is optimal with physiologic pH and temperature. Atracurium and cisatracurium may have prolonged duration in the setting of acute acidosis or hypothermia. Atracurium and cisatracurium are beneficial for patients with multisystem organ failure because other NMB drugs may have more prolonged effects with both renal and hepatic failure. Cisatracurium is less prone than atracurium to trigger histamine release.

## Ventilatory Support

When a patient is unable to maintain a patent airway, adequate gas exchange, or both, despite aggressive management with the interventions discussed previously, more invasive support with intubation and mechanical ventilation must be considered. This step carries risks and imposes significant physical and psychological burdens on the patient and family. Every effort should be made to avoid mechanical ventilation, but it is usually necessary at the point when respiratory distress becomes respiratory failure.

Respiratory failure is defined as the inability to maintain adequate respiration as measured by arterial blood pH, $PaCO_2$, and $PaO_2$. Respiratory failure may be categorized as hypoxemic or hypoxemic hypercapnia. Hypoxemic respiratory failure is when $PaO_2$ is less than 60 mm Hg. Hypoxemic hypercapnic respiratory failure is when $PaO_2$ is less than 60 mm Hg and $PaCO_2$ exceeds 55 mm Hg. If the ABG values deteriorate beyond these parameters, mechanical ventilatory support is often indicated. Patients are predisposed to developing acute respiratory failure if any of the systems involved in respiration are compromised or overwhelmed (Table 25-2). The degree of risk for developing respiratory failure depends on the patient's ability to move air, secretions, and oxygenated blood.

**TABLE 25-2**   **Possible Events Leading to Respiratory Failure**

| Body System | Event |
|---|---|
| Nervous system | |
|   Brainstem | Head trauma |
|   Spinal cord and nerves | Poliomyelitis |
| | Cervical (C1–C6) fractures |
| | Overdose |
| Muscular system | |
|   Primary—diaphragm | Myasthenia gravis |
|   Secondary—respiratory | Guillain–Barré |
| Skeletal system | |
|   Thorax | Flail chest |
| | Kyphoscoliosis |
| Respiratory system | |
|   Airways | Obstruction |
| | Laryngeal edema |
| | Bronchitis |
| | Asthma |
|   Alveoli | Emphysema |
| | Pneumonia |
| | Fibrosis |
|   Pulmonary circulation | Pulmonary embolus |
| Cardiovascular system | Congestive heart failure |
| | Fluid overload |
| | Cardiac surgery |
| | Myocardial infarction |
| Gastrointestinal system | Aspiration |
| Hematologic system | Disseminated intravascular coagulation |
| Genitourinary system | Renal failure |

The nurse plays a key role in recognizing the onset of acute respiratory failure. Identification of high-risk patients, serial monitoring and evaluation of respiratory status, and institution of appropriate measures may forestall or negate the need for ventilatory assistance. Before intubation and ventilation, the patient may have required increased $FiO_2$ to meet his or her oxygen demand.

When ventilatory assistance is required, the objective of mechanical ventilation is to support the patient through an episode of illness. Clinical goals of mechanical ventilation may include reversal of hypoxemia; reversal of acute respiratory acidosis; relief of respiratory distress; prevention or reversal of atelectasis; resting of ventilatory muscles; reduction in systemic oxygen consumption, myocardial oxygen consumption, or both; reduction in intracranial pressure (ICP); and stabilization of the chest wall. Mechanical ventilation is not curative and can actually cause complications (as discussed later in this chapter).

## Physiologic Principles

To understand the effects of modern mechanical ventilation, the reader is encouraged to review the physiology of normal respirations and lung compliance, as discussed in Chapter 23. The relationship between intrapulmonary pressures during inspiration and expiration is reversed during mechanical ventilation. The ventilator delivers air by pumping it into the patient; therefore, pressures during inspiration are positive. The positive pressure pumped into the lungs results in increased intrathoracic pressures and decreased venous return during inspiration. With the institution of PEEP, even greater pressures are generated during inspiration. During expiration, the pressure in the lungs decreases to the "baseline" PEEP level and continues to be positive throughout expiration. Most patients compensate for this hindrance to venous return by increasing peripheral venous tone. If conditions of decreased sympathetic response (eg, hypovolemia, sepsis, heart disease, drugs, or older age) are present, hypotension may develop. In addition, a large tidal volume (greater than 10 to 12 mL/kg) that generates pressures greater than or equal to 35 cm $H_2O$ not only reduces cardiac output but also increases the risk for pneumothorax.

Positive pressure can result in barotrauma. Barotrauma occurs when air leaks from the alveoli into the pleural space; this is called a pneumothorax. Another form of lung injury, called volutrauma, and is caused by delivery of large tidal volumes in patients with stiff, noncompliant lungs. With volutrauma, the alveoli develop fractures that allow fluid and protein to seep into the lungs. This phenomenon is a form of noncardiogenic pulmonary edema. Lung damage from either barotrauma or volutrauma can increase mortality, especially in susceptible patients (such as those with asthma or ARDS). To prevent lung injury, it is important to determine lung compliance so that the ventilator can be appropriately adjusted to minimize airway pressures.

*Ventilator-associated lung injury* (VALI) and *ventilator-induced lung injury* (VILI) are terms used to describe the damage to lungs from prolonged ventilation. Other causes of VALI and VILI are volutrauma resulting from the overexpansion of alveoli with high ventilation pressures, and atelectrauma, which is shear-induced injury from the repeated opening and closing of alveoli. In addition, prolonged high levels of $FiO_2$, high volumes and pressures leading to the loss of surfactant as well as inflammation of the lung tissue and alveoli, and the primary injury of pneumonia or aspiration result in lung injury while the patient's ventilator is on settings that lead to damage of the lung tissue. Vulnerable patients with ALI or ARDS may be more prone to VALI and VILI.

The medical community in the United States has developed a research system to study the diagnosis and treatment of ARDS, known as ARDSNet.[11] The ARDSNet protocols for protecting the lungs (from VALI and VILI) when the patient is on mechanical ventilation have recommended the following:

- Keep the plateau pressures lower than 30 cm $H_2O$.
- Reduce the $FiO_2$ to 50%.
- Maintain $V_T$ at 5 to 6 mL/kg ideal body weight or less.
- Maintain PEEP to avoid collapse of alveoli at the end of expiration.[11]

There has been an increased interest in comparing mortality and morbidity risk associated with the early use of extracorporeal $CO_2$ removal in ARDS to the conventional ARDS guidelines. Some studies have revealed no significant change in mortality and morbidity at 28 days, but this approach may have merit as a rescue strategy when other traditional therapies have failed.[11]

## Compliance

Compliance refers to the ability of the lung to distend. In terms of its compliance, the lung is frequently compared to a balloon. Initially, it is difficult to inflate (noncompliant) until it is stretched. After repeated inflations, this elastic resistance is lost (overly compliant), and the balloon becomes very easy to blow up. In conditions that reduce the lung's elasticity, such as inflammation, fibrotic changes, or edema, the lung requires more force to inflate. A patient who has normal lungs and who is on a ventilator should have compliance near 100 mL/cm $H_2O$ (normal). In contrast, a patient who has pulmonary disease that causes "stiff" lungs (eg, ARDS, sarcoidosis) and who is on a ventilator has a compliance as low as 20 to 30 mL/cm $H_2O$, indicating a severely compromised lung.

As the volume of gas is delivered to a patient on a mechanical ventilator, the ventilator's pressure gauge slowly rises from zero to peak inspiratory pressure (PIP). The rise in pressure is caused by airway resistance (to flow) as well as by lung and chest wall compliance (Box 25-11). A graph of pressure over time, depicting inspiration, would look like the example shown in Figure 25-6. Dynamic pressures and PIP can give an indication of both airway resistance and lung compliance.

## Static Pressure

One of the measurements used to obtain compliance is static pressure (SP) or plateau pressure. Plateau pressure is obtained by pressing the end-inspiratory hold button on a ventilator at the end of a maximal inspiration while on a volume mode of ventilation. This holds the volume of delivered air in the

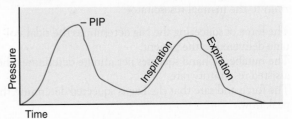

**BOX 25-11** **Factors Decreasing Compliance**

**Airway Factors**
Peak flow
Size of airways
Airway obstructions
External obstructions (kinked ventilator tubing or water in the tubing)

**Lung Factors**
Elasticity (stiffness) of the lung
Presence of auto-PEEP
Shunt (ARDS)

**Chest Wall Factors**
Chest wall deformities
Position of patient
External compression of chest wall or diaphragm (distended abdomen, obesity)

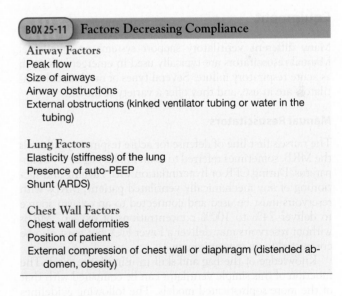

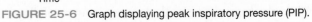

**FIGURE 25-6** Graph displaying peak inspiratory pressure (PIP).

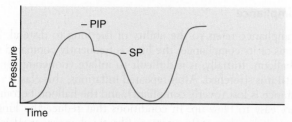
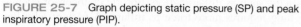

**FIGURE 25-7** Graph depicting static pressure (SP) and peak inspiratory pressure (PIP).

patient's chest by preventing exhalation. The PIP drops to a plateau pressure with this maneuver, which reflects the pressure necessary to hold the lungs open. A graph depicting SP and PIP can be seen in Figure 25-7. Static compliance is determined by dividing the tidal volume by the plateau pressure minus the total PEEP:

$$\text{Exhaled } V_T/[\text{plateau pressure} - \text{PEEP}] = \text{static compliance}$$

A higher compliance means that the lung is more easily distended, whereas a lower compliance means that the lung is stiffer and difficult to distend. In other words, a higher compliance is better. Low compliance may be due to stiff lungs as with ARDS, a restrictive chest wall (ie, kyphoscoliosis), or ventilation of only a small portion of lung, such as occurs with partial lung collapse from consolidation. Serial measurements of compliance performed by the respiratory care professional can alert the nurse to sudden decreases, which may be due to pneumothorax, mucus plugging, or pulmonary edema.

## Equipment

Many different ventilatory support systems are available. Manual resuscitators are typically used in emergencies, such as acute respiratory failure. Several types of mechanical ventilators are in use, and they offer a variety of modes.

### Manual Resuscitators

The nurse's first line of defense for acute respiratory failure is the MRB, sometimes referred to as an Ambu bag or BVM apparatus. During CPR or hyperinflation with bagging and suctioning of any mechanically ventilated patient, MRBs with reservoirs must be used and connected to an oxygen source to deliver 74% to 100% concentrations of oxygen. MRBs without reservoirs may deliver a lower FiO$_2$ but must also be connected to an oxygen source.

Knowledge of the bag and skill in using it are vital. The function of this simple ventilator can be compared with that of the more sophisticated models. The following guidelines pertain to the manual resuscitator:

- The force of squeezing the bag determines the tidal volume delivered to the patient.
- The number of hand squeezes per minute determines the assisted respiratory rate.
- The force and rate that the bag is squeezed determine the peak flow.

While the bag is being used, the nurse must carefully observe the patient's chest rise to determine whether the bag is ventilating properly and whether any gastric (abdominal) distention is developing. In addition, the amount of resistance encountered can roughly indicate lung compliance. If a patient becomes progressively more difficult to ventilate, an increase in secretions, pneumothorax, worsening bronchospasms, or other condition that might decrease the patient's compliance must be considered. Breaths delivered to a conscious patient must be timed to coincide with spontaneous inspiratory effort, or the discomfort of dyssynchronous breathing will create anxiety, and the patient will not tolerate the additional ventilation.

When delivering breaths with an MRB, the nurse allows time for complete exhalation between breaths to prevent air trapping (referred to as auto-PEEP), which can cause hypotension and barotrauma, especially in patients with obstructive airway disease.

## Mechanical Ventilators

The goal of mechanical ventilation is to maintain alveolar ventilation appropriate for the patient's metabolic needs and to correct hypoxemia and maximize oxygen transport. Ventilators are classified into two categories: negative-pressure ventilators and positive-pressure ventilators. Regardless of which type or model is used, the nurse must be familiar with the ventilator's function and limitations. The following discussion of ventilators is in order of evolution of ventilator technology and subsequent use in clinical practice.

### Positive-Pressure Ventilators

**VOLUME VENTILATORS.** The volume ventilator is commonly used in critical care settings. The basic principle of this ventilator is that a designated volume of air is delivered with each breath. The amount of pressure required to deliver the set volume depends on the patient's lung compliance and patient–ventilator resistance factors. Therefore, PIP must be monitored in volume modes because it varies from breath to breath. With this mode of ventilation, a respiratory rate, inspiratory time, and tidal volume are selected for the mechanical breaths.

**PRESSURE VENTILATOR.** The use of pressure ventilators is increasing in critical care units. A typical pressure mode delivers a selected gas pressure to the patient early in inspiration and sustains the pressure throughout the inspiratory phase. By meeting the patient's inspiratory flow demand throughout inspiration, patient effort is reduced and comfort increased. Although pressure is consistent with these modes, volume is not. Volume will vary based on changes in resistance or compliance. Therefore, exhaled tidal volume is the variable to monitor closely. With pressure modes, the pressure level to be delivered is selected, and with some mode options (described later), rate and inspiratory time are preset as well. Figure 25-8 shows a typical ventilator with computer-controlled system and multiple screens showing monitoring data and mode of ventilation.

**HIGH-FREQUENCY OSCILLATORY VENTILATOR.** The high-frequency ventilator accomplishes oxygenation by the diffusion of oxygen and carbon dioxide from high to low gradients of concentration. This diffusion movement is increased if the kinetic energy of the gas molecules is increased. High-frequency ventilators use small tidal volumes (1 to 3

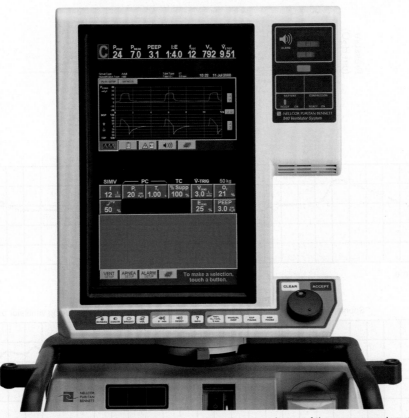

**FIGURE 25-8**  The Puritan-Bennett 840 (PB 840) Ventilator System. The close-up photos of the screens and controls are an example of the type of controls used with computer-controlled ventilators. The nurse should be familiar with the monitoring data, the alarm pause, and FiO$_2$ setting. He or she should know the alarm levels to respond immediately for high-urgency situations and be able to know the meaning of the alarm problem displayed in the upper screen for this ventilator. Familiarity with this and other ventilator manufacturers' alarm systems and controls is essential for every nurse who cares for ventilated patients.

mL/kg) at frequencies greater than 100 breaths/min measured in Hertz. The breathing pattern of a person on a high-frequency ventilator is somewhat analogous to the breathing pattern of a panting dog; panting entails moving small volumes of air at a very fast rate.

Theoretically, a high-frequency ventilator would be used to achieve lower peak ventilatory pressures, thereby reducing the risk of barotrauma and improving ventilation–perfusion matching because of its different flow delivery characteristics. Potential adverse effects associated with high-frequency ventilators include gas trapping and necrotizing tracheobronchitis when used in the absence of adequate humidification. The efficacy and safety of high-frequency oscillatory ventilation in critical care in patients with moderate to severe ARDS has been questioned; there is a lack of clear benefit, and it may increase in-hospital mortality.[12]

## Ventilator Modes

Several different modes of ventilatory control are available on ventilators; Figure 25-9 and Table 25-3 compare these modes. Volume modes include assist-control (A/C) mode and synchronized intermittent mandatory ventilation (SIMV) mode. Pressure modes include pressure-support ventilation (PSV) mode, pressure-controlled ventilation (PCV) mode, airway pressure release ventilation (APRV) mode, volume-guaranteed pressure options (VGPO) mode, CPAP/PEEP mode, and noninvasive BiPAP mode. There is no one best

mode for managing patients in respiratory failure, although each mode has its advantages and disadvantages.

### Volume Modes

**ASSIST-CONTROL MODE.** In assist control, or volume-control mode as it is often termed, a mandatory (or "control") rate is selected. If the patient wishes to breathe faster, he or she can trigger the ventilator and receive a full-volume breath. This mode of ventilation is often used to fully support a patient, such as when the patient is first intubated or when the patient is too weak to perform the work of spontaneous breathing (eg, when emerging from anesthesia).

**SYNCHRONIZED INTERMITTENT MANDATORY VENTILATION MODE.** In SIMV mode, the rate and tidal volume are preset. If the patient wants to breathe above this rate, he or she may. However, unlike the A/C mode, any breaths taken above the set rate are spontaneous breaths taken through the ventilator circuit. The tidal volume of these breaths can vary drastically from the tidal volume set on the ventilator because the tidal volume is determined solely by the patient's spontaneous effort. Adding pressure support (discussed in the next section) during spontaneous breaths can minimize the risk of increased work of breathing. In the past, SIMV was used as a popular weaning mode. To wean the patient, the mandatory breaths were gradually decreased, thereby allowing the patient to assume more and more of the work of breathing.

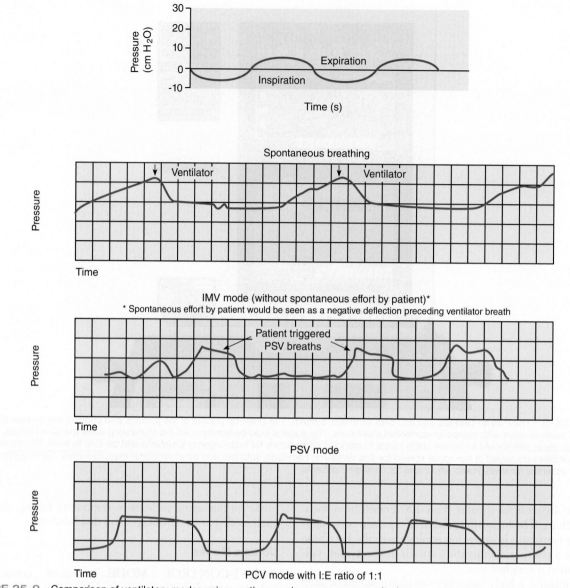

FIGURE 25-9 Comparison of ventilatory modes using continuous airway pressure monitoring.

## Pressure Modes

**PRESSURE-SUPPORT VENTILATION MODE.** PSV mode augments or assists spontaneous breathing efforts by delivering a high flow of gas to a selected pressure level early in inspiration and maintaining that level throughout the inspiratory phase. The patient's effort determines the rate, inspiratory flow, and tidal volume. When PSV mode is used as a stand-alone mode of ventilation, the pressure-support level is adjusted to achieve the approximate targeted tidal volume and respiratory rate. At high-pressure levels, PSV mode provides nearly total ventilatory support.

Specific uses of PSV are to promote patient comfort and synchrony with the ventilator, to decrease the work of breathing necessary to overcome the resistance of the ETT, and for weaning. As a weaning tool, PSV is thought to increase the endurance of the respiratory muscles by decreasing the physical work and oxygen demands during spontaneous breathing. Because the level of pressure support can be gradually decreased, endurance conditioning is enhanced.

In PSV mode, the inspired tidal volume and respiratory rate must be monitored closely in order to detect changes in lung compliance. Generally, if compliance decreases or resistance increases, tidal volume decreases and respiratory rate increases. PSV mode should be used with caution in patients with bronchospasm or other reactive airway conditions.

**PRESSURE-CONTROLLED VENTILATION MODE.** The PCV mode is used to control plateau pressures in conditions, such as ARDS, in which compliance is decreased and the risk for barotrauma is high. It is used when the patient has persistent oxygenation problems despite a high FiO$_2$ and high levels of PEEP. The inspiratory pressure level, respiratory rate, and inspiratory/expiratory (I:E) ratio must be selected. Tidal volume varies with compliance, and airway resistance must be closely monitored. Sedation and the use of NMB agents are frequently indicated because any patient–ventilator asynchrony usually results in profound drops in the SaO$_2$. This is especially true when inverse ratios

**TABLE 25-3** Comparison of Modes of Ventilation

| Ventilatory Mode | Indications | Advantages/Disadvantages | Special Monitoring |
|---|---|---|---|
| Assist-control (A/C) | Often used as initial mode of ventilation | *Advantages:* Ensures vent support during every breath. Each breath same tidal volume. *Disadvantages:* Hyperventilation, air trapping; may require sedation and paralysis | Work of breathing may be increased if sensitivity or flow rate is too low. |
| Synchronized intermittent mandatory ventilation (SIMV) | Often used as initial mode of ventilation and for weaning | *Advantages:* Allows spontaneous breaths (tidal volume determined by patient) between vent breaths; weaning is accomplished by gradually lowering the set rate and allowing the patient to assume more work. *Disadvantages:* Patient–ventilator asynchrony possible | |
| Pressure-support ventilation (PSV) | Intact respiratory drive in patient necessary. Used as a weaning mode, and in some cases of dyssynchrony | *Advantages:* Decreases work of breathing; increases patient comfort; can be combined with SIMV to allow a more comfortable mode. *Disadvantages:* Should not be used in patients with acute bronchospasm or with altered mental status with reduced spontaneous breathing | Adjust PSV level to maintain desired respiratory rate and tidal volume. Monitor for changes in compliance, which can cause tidal volume to change. Monitor respiratory rate and tidal volume at least hourly. |
| Pressure-controlled ventilation (PCV) | Used to limit plateau pressures that can cause barotraumas. Severe ARDS | *Disadvantages:* Patient–ventilator asynchrony possible, necessitating sedation/paralysis | Monitor tidal volume at least hourly. Monitor for barotrauma, hemodynamic instability. |
| Inverse ratio ventilation (IRV) | Usually used in conjunction with PCV | *Advantages:* Increases I:E ratio to allow for recruitment of alveoli and improve oxygenation. *Disadvantages:* Almost always requires paralysis | |
| Volume-guaranteed pressure options (VGPO) | Combines advantages of pressure ventilation with guaranteed tidal volume | *Advantages:* Ensures a delivered tidal volume. *Disadvantages:* Requires sophisticated knowledge of the mode and waveform analysis | Monitor for auto-PEEP, barotrauma, and hemodynamic instability. |
| Continuous positive airway pressure (CPAP) | Constant positive airway pressure for patients who breathe spontaneously | *Advantages:* Used in intubated or nonintubated patients. *Disadvantages:* On some systems, no alarm if respiratory rate falls | Monitor for increased work of breathing. |
| Noninvasive bilateral positive-pressure ventilation (BiPAP) | Nocturnal hypoventilation in patients with neuromuscular disease, chest wall deformity, obstructive sleep apnea, and COPD; to prevent intubation; to prevent reintubation initially after extubation | *Advantages:* Decreased cost when patients can be cared for at home; no need for artificial airway. *Disadvantages:* Patient discomfort or claustrophobia | Monitor for gastric distention, air leaks from mouth, aspiration risk. |

are used. The "unnatural" feeling of this mode often requires muscle relaxants to ensure patient–ventilator synchrony.

Most ventilators operate with a short inspiratory time and a long expiratory time (1:2 or 1:3 ratio). This promotes venous return and allows time for air to passively exit the lungs. Inverse ratio ventilation mode reverses this ratio so that inspiratory time is equal to, or longer than, expiratory time (1:1 to 4:1). Inverse I:E ratios are used in conjunction with pressure control to improve oxygenation in patients with ARDS by expanding stiff alveoli using longer distending times, thereby providing more opportunity for gas exchange and preventing alveolar collapse.

As expiratory time is decreased, the nurse must monitor for the development of hyperinflation or auto-PEEP. Regional alveolar overdistention and barotrauma may result from excessive total PEEP. When the PCV mode is used, the mean airway and intrathoracic pressures rise, potentially resulting in a decrease in cardiac output and oxygen delivery. Therefore, it is necessary to monitor the patient's hemodynamic status closely.

## Airway Pressure Release Ventilation Mode

APRV has been used in trauma and ARDS patients to reduce airway pressure and lower minute volume while allowing spontaneous breathing throughout the ventilator cycle, all with decreased sedation and NMB agent use. APRV mode allows lung protective strategies to be followed with limitation of plateau and peak pressures. The mode functions by having a time-triggered, pressure-limited, time-cycled mode of ventilation. It consists of a high-pressure setting and a low-pressure setting, with recruitment and oxygenation occurring during the high-pressure setting at a long set time interval (eg, 5 seconds) followed by a brief controlled release (eg, 0.6 second) to the low-pressure setting. What this means is that the patient spontaneously breathes both at a set high pressure with preset brief times and at low pressure, which is synchronized during exhalation. Because the patient is breathing spontaneously throughout both high-and low-pressure phases, sedation may be limited. Weaning from APRV is done by decreasing the high-pressure limit while increasing the time at high pressure. At the same time, the low-pressure limit may be dropped, allowing for reduced mean airway pressure. Usually, the low-pressure limit is reduced to 5 cm $H_2O$, and as the high pressure is lowered, this allows release to a PEEP level that prevents derecruitment. When the patient tolerates an $FiO_2$ of 50% or less, the patient can be switched to PSV and further weaning. This mode may improve oxygenation and prevent VALI and VILI in patients with ARDS or ALI.[13]

## Volume-Guaranteed Pressure Options Mode

VGPO mode ensures delivery of a prescribed tidal volume while using a decelerating flow pattern by means of a "pressure" breath. The options include both spontaneous and control rate parameters, and the volume guarantee is provided differently, depending on the ventilator. VGPO can be used in acutely ill patients as well as more stable, weaning patients. Some examples include the volume support and pressure-regulated volume-control options (Siemens Medical) as well as pressure augmentation (Bear Medical Systems).

In the acutely ill, unstable patient, this option may provide pressure ventilation while guaranteeing tidal volume and minute ventilation (MV) at a set rate. In the spontaneously breathing patient, the option is used as a "safety" when pressure ventilation is desired. The use of a volume guarantee in the spontaneously breathing patient may be especially important at night (when respiratory rates and volumes normally decrease) and in patients for whom secretions are a problem (because secretions increase resistance and result in decreased spontaneous volumes).

## Continuous Positive Airway Pressure/Positive End-Expiratory Pressure Mode

CPAP is the term used when PEEP is supplied during spontaneous breathing. PEEP is the term used to describe positive end-expiratory pressure with positive-pressure breaths. CPAP assists spontaneously breathing patients to improve their oxygenation by elevating the end-expiratory pressure in the lungs throughout the respiratory cycle. CPAP can be used for intubated and nonintubated patients. It may be used as a weaning mode and for nocturnal ventilation (nasal or mask CPAP) to splint open the upper airway, preventing upper airway obstruction in patients with obstructive sleep apnea.

PEEP is positive pressure exerted at the end of exhalation. It is common practice to use low levels of PEEP (2 to 5 cm $H_2O$) in the intubated patient. PEEP is increased in 2- to 5-cm $H_2O$ increments when $FiO_2$ levels are greater than 50% to attain an acceptable $SaO_2$ (greater than 90%) or $PaO_2$ (greater than 60 to 70 mm Hg). PEEP is most often necessary in patients with refractory hypoxemia (such as those with ARDS) in whom the $PaO_2$ deteriorates rapidly, despite greater concentrations of oxygen administration.

PEEP is used to keep alveoli stented open, and may recruit alveolar units that are totally or partially collapsed during any mode of ventilation. This end-expiratory pressure increases the functional residual capacity (FRC) by reinflating collapsed alveoli, maintains the alveoli in an open position, and improves lung compliance. This decreases shunt and improves oxygenation. In addition, there is some evidence that keeping the alveoli open enhances surfactant regeneration. High levels of PEEP should rarely be interrupted because it may take several hours to recruit alveoli again and restore the FRC; until this occurs, oxygenation may suffer. In the patient who does not have adequate circulating blood volume, institution of PEEP decreases venous return to the heart, decreases cardiac output, and decreases oxygen delivery to the tissues. If hypotension or decreased cardiac output results from PEEP application, restoring circulating intravascular volume with administration of IV fluids may correct the hypotension. Another serious complication of PEEP is barotrauma. It can occur in any mechanically ventilated patient but is most common when high levels of PEEP are used (10 to 20 cm $H_2O$ or more) in lungs with high ventilating pressures and low compliance and in patients with obstructive airway disease. The development of barotrauma is an emergency and usually requires placement of a chest tube in the event of pneumothorax.

## Noninvasive Bilevel Positive-Pressure Airway Pressure Ventilation Mode

BiPAP is a noninvasive form of mechanical ventilation provided by means of a nasal mask, nasal prongs, or a full face mask. It is used in the treatment of patients with chronic respiratory insufficiency to manage acute or chronic respiratory failure without intubation and conventional mechanical ventilation. It is also used as a bridge to weaning patients from mechanical ventilation and as an alternative to conventional mechanical ventilation in patients who are ventilated in their homes. The system allows the clinician to select two levels of positive-pressure support: an inspiratory pressure-support level (referred to as IPAP) and an expiratory pressure called EPAP (PEEP/CPAP level). Because BiPAP allows for the provision of assisted inspiration with ventilator rate set, application of this mode to those patients who hypoventilate as well as obstruct during sleep is possible.

BiPAP is beneficial in patients with worsening hypoventilation, obstructive apneic episodes, or both. It is also useful to prevent intubation in patients with respiratory failure and hypercarbia as well as to prevent reintubation following extubation in borderline cases. Use of a full face mask may increase the risk for aspiration and risk for rebreathing carbon dioxide; therefore, ventilation with a full face mask should be used cautiously. Thick or copious secretions and poor cough may be relative contraindications for BiPAP.

## Use of Mechanical Ventilators

### Setting Ventilator Controls

The nurse must know how to monitor the various ventilators, modes, and controls before giving mechanical ventilatory support to a patient. The following sections discuss these various controls and settings and their implications for nursing care. In some institutions, the respiratory therapists share or have complete responsibility for managing the ventilator, but the nurse still needs to be fully aware of the implications for the patient of the mode and level of mechanical support.

Ventilator settings must be frequently evaluated against patient response. Iatrogenically induced complications include overventilation (which causes respiratory alkalosis) and underventilation (which causes respiratory acidosis or hypoxemia). ABG studies determine the effectiveness of mechanical ventilation. Patients with chronic pulmonary disease, however, should be ventilated to stay relatively close to their normal ABG values. This usually means accepting relatively high carbon dioxide levels, lower-than-average oxygenation, or both.

**FRACTION OF INSPIRED OXYGEN.** Ventilators allow for adjustment of oxygen percentage ($FiO_2$) with in-circuit or external oxygen analyzers, thus allowing the nurse to ascertain the $FiO_2$ being delivered. Changes in $FiO_2$ are based on ABG values and the $SaO_2$. Usually, the $FiO_2$ is adjusted to maintain an $SaO_2$ of greater than 90% (roughly equivalent to a $PaO_2$ greater than 60 mm Hg). Oxygen toxicity is a concern when an $FiO_2$ of greater than 60% is required for more than 24 hours; therefore, most clinicians attempt to use strategies to allow for maintaining an $FiO_2$ of 60% or less.

**RESPIRATORY RATE.** The number of breaths per minute delivered to the patient can be directly set on most ventilator models. Ventilator monitoring should be performed frequently as to appropriate settings, patient response, and airway patency. In the pressure ventilator, the inspiratory time determines the duration of inspiration by regulating the gas flow rate. The higher the flow rate, the faster peak airway pressure is reached and the shorter the inspiration; conversely, the lower the flow rate, the longer the inspiration. A very high flow rate may produce turbulence, shallow inspirations, and uneven distribution of volume.

Respiratory rate times tidal volume equals minute ventilation (RR × VT = MV). In turn, minute volume determines alveolar ventilation. These two parameters are adjusted according to the $PaCO_2$. Increasing the minute volume decreases the $PaCO_2$; conversely, decreasing the minute volume increases the $PaCO_2$. In special cases, hypoventilation or hyperventilation is desired. For example, in a patient with a head injury, respiratory alkalosis may be required to promote cerebral vasoconstriction, with a resultant decrease in ICP. In this case, the tidal volume and respiratory rate are increased to achieve the desired alkalotic pH by manipulating the $PaCO_2$. In contrast, a patient with COPD whose baseline ABG values reflect an elevated $PaCO_2$ should not be hyperventilated; instead, the goal should be restoration

of the baseline $PaCO_2$. These patients usually have a large carbonic acid load, and lowering their carbon dioxide levels rapidly may result in seizures. Rate adjustments may also be necessary to enhance patient comfort or when rapid rates cause air trapping that results in auto-PEEP.

**TIDAL VOLUME.** In the volume ventilator, the number of milliliters of air to be delivered with each breath is set by the clinician. Traditionally, tidal volumes of 10 to 15 mL/kg of body weight were used. Research has identified a phenomenon of iatrogenic lung injury (VILI or VALI), in which forces produced in the lungs by the large tidal volumes may aggravate the damage inflicted on the lungs by the pathologic process that necessitated mechanical ventilation.[11] For this reason, lower tidal volume targets (5 to 8 mL/kg) are now recommended.

**PEAK FLOW.** Peak flow is the velocity of gas flow per unit of time and is expressed as liters per minute. On many volume ventilators, this is a separate setting. If auto-PEEP (owing to inadequate expiratory time) is present, peak flow is increased to shorten inspiratory time so that the patient may exhale completely. However, increasing peak flow increases turbulence, which is reflected in increasing airway pressures.

**INSPIRATORY PRESSURE LIMIT.** On volume-cycled ventilators, the inspiratory pressure limit (IPL) control limits the highest pressure allowed in the ventilator circuit. Once the high-pressure limit is reached, inspiration is terminated. Therefore, if the IPL is being constantly reached, the designated tidal volume is not being delivered to the patient. The cause of this can be coughing, accumulation of secretions, kinked ventilator tubing, pneumothorax, decreasing compliance, or a pressure limit alarm set too low. IPL is used with PSV to adjust the pressure during spontaneous breathing, providing reduced work of breathing. Weaning can be accomplished in the PSV mode, reducing IPL to low levels as the patient increases the work of breathing.

**POSITIVE END-EXPIRATORY PRESSURE.** The PEEP control adjusts the pressure that is maintained in the lungs at the end of expiration. PEEP and CPAP can be visualized on the respiratory pressure gauge or display. Instead of returning to zero (atmospheric pressure) at the end of expiration, the pressure value drops to the PEEP/CPAP level. PEEP reduction is considered if the patient has a $PaO_2$ of 80 to 100 mm Hg or an $FiO_2$ of 50% or less, is hemodynamically stable, and has stabilization or improvement of the underlying illness. To evaluate whether the effects of PEEP are beneficial, monitoring ABG values, $SaO_2$, compliance, and hemodynamic pressures (including cardiac output and blood pressure) is necessary. Baseline values are obtained before changes in PEEP are made. PEEP is usually increased in increments of 2 to 5 cm $H_2O$. The patient is monitored for adverse effects, such as hypotension and dysrhythmias. If these occur, the PEEP is reduced. If higher PEEP is tolerated, the patient is stabilized on the new PEEP settings for approximately 15 minutes. The monitored parameters are then repeated.

Hemodynamic measurements (cardiac output, pulmonary artery pressure [PAP], central venous pressure, and pulmonary artery occlusion pressure) are taken at end expiration with the patient on PEEP. Accuracy in selecting the point of end expiration on the waveform tracing is facilitated by using continuous airway monitoring (Fig. 25-10). PEEP does

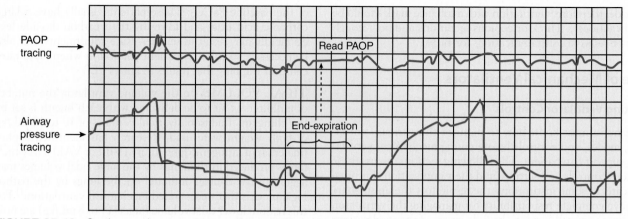

**FIGURE 25-10**    Continuous airway pressure monitoring assists in identifying point of end expiration.

not need to be discontinued before obtaining hemodynamic measurements. Hemodynamic measurements can be inaccurate (as an indicator of volume status) if a patient is on high PEEP or the position of the transducer is not leveled at the phlebostatic axis. The position of the catheter within the pulmonary circulation should also be verified on a chest radiograph.

Attempts are made to minimize removing the patient from the ventilator when using high levels of PEEP. Oxygenation can deteriorate and be slow to rebound because it takes a significant amount of time for the effects of PEEP to be reestablished. Therefore, if the patient is being oxygenated using an MRB, it must be equipped with a valve that allows levels of PEEP to be dialed in. An in-line suction apparatus may be helpful to prevent breaking the PEEP circuit to suction the patient.

**SENSITIVITY.** The sensitivity function controls the amount of patient effort needed to initiate an inspiration, as measured by negative inspiratory effort. Increasing the sensitivity (requiring less negative force) decreases the amount of work the patient must do to initiate a ventilator breath. Likewise, decreasing the sensitivity increases the amount of negative pressure that the patient needs to initiate inspiration and increases the work of breathing.

### Responding to Alarms

Mechanical ventilators are used to support life. Alarm systems are necessary to warn the nurse of developing problems. Alarm systems can be categorized according to volume and pressure, high and low. Low-pressure alarms warn of disconnection of the patient from the ventilator or circuit leaks. High-pressure alarms warn of rising pressures. Electrical failure alarms are necessary for all ventilators. A nurse or respiratory therapist must respond to every ventilator alarm. Alarms must never be ignored or disarmed. Some clinical troubleshooting guidelines are presented in Table 25-4.

Ventilator malfunction is a potentially serious problem. Nursing or respiratory therapists perform ventilator checks every 2 to 4 hours, and recurrent alarms may alert the clinician to the possibility of an equipment-related issue. When device malfunction is suspected, a second person manually ventilates the patient while the nurse or therapist looks for the cause. If a problem cannot be promptly corrected by ventilator adjustment, a different machine is procured so that

the ventilator in question can be taken out of service for analysis and repaired by technical staff.

### Ensuring Humidification and Thermoregulation

Mechanical ventilation bypasses the upper airway, thereby negating the body's protective mechanism for humidifying and warming inspired air. These two processes must be added to the ventilator circuit in the form of a humidifier with a temperature control. All air delivered by the ventilator passes through the water in the humidifier, where it is warmed and saturated, and this decreases insensible water loss. In most instances, the temperature of the air is about the same as body temperature. In some rare instances (severe hypothermia), the air temperatures can be increased. Caution is advised because prolonged inhalation of gas at high temperatures can cause tracheal thermal injury. An empty humidifier contributes to drying the airway, often with resultant mucus plugging and less ability to suction out secretions. A heat and moisture exchanger unit may be attached to the airway to act as an artificial nose in lieu of a humidifier.

As air passes through the ventilator to the patient, water condenses in the corrugated tubing. This moisture is considered contaminated and must be drained into a receptacle and not back into the sterile humidifier. If the water is allowed to build up, resistance is developed in the circuit, and PEEP is generated. In addition, if moisture accumulates near the ETT, the patient can aspirate the water. The nurse and respiratory therapist jointly are responsible for preventing this condensation buildup. The humidifier is an ideal medium for bacterial growth. Institutional policies should describe the frequency of ventilator circuit changes.

## Complications of Mechanical Ventilation

Complications that can occur with mechanical ventilation are listed in Box 25-12. Although all these adverse consequences occur over time in some ventilated patients, the incidence of these complications can be minimized by good preventive care practices.

### Aspiration

Aspiration can occur before, during, or after intubation. The potential for developing nosocomial pneumonia or ARDS

| TABLE 25-4 | Troubleshooting the Ventilator | |
|---|---|---|
| **Problem** | **Possible Causes** | **Action** |
| Volume or pressure alarm | ***Patient related*** | |
| | Patient disconnected from ventilator | Reconnect STAT. |
| | Loss of delivered $V_T$ | Auscultate neck for possible leak around ETT cuff. |
| | | Review chest radiograph for ETT placement—may be too high. |
| | | Check for loss of $V_T$ through chest tube. |
| | Decrease in patient-initiated breaths | Evaluate patient for cause: check respiratory rate, ABGs, last sedation. |
| | Increased compliance | May be due to clearing of secretions or relief of bronchospasms. |
| | ***Ventilator related*** | |
| | Leaks | Check all tubing for loss of connection, starting at patient and moving toward humidifier. |
| | | Check for change in ventilator settings. |
| | | (*Note:* If problem is not corrected STAT, use mandatory resuscitation bag until ventilator problem is corrected.) |
| High-pressure or peak-pressure alarm | ***Patient related*** | |
| | Decreased compliance | Suction patient. |
| | Increased dynamic pressures | Administer inhaled β-agonists. |
| | | If sudden, evaluate for pneumothorax. |
| | | Evaluate chest radiograph for ETT placement in right mainstem bronchus. |
| | | Sedate if patient is bucking the ventilator or biting the ETT. |
| | Increased SP | Evaluate ABG values for hypoxia, fluids for overload, chest radiograph for atelectasis. |
| | | Auscultate breath sounds. |
| | ***Ventilator related*** | |
| | Tubing kinked | Check tubing. |
| | Tubing filled with water | Empty water into a receptacle: Do not drain back into the humidifier. |
| | Patient–ventilator asynchrony | Recheck sensitivity and peak flow settings. |
| | | Provide sedation/paralysis if indicated. |
| Abnormal (ABGs) | ***Patient related*** | |
| Hypoxemia | Secretions | Suction. Increase $FiO_2$. |
| | Increase in disease pathology | Evaluate patient and chest radiograph. |
| | Positive fluid balance | Evaluate intake and output. |
| Hypocapnia | Hypoxia | Evaluate ABG values and patient. |
| | Increased lung compliance | Evaluate potential for weaning. |
| Hypercapnia | Sedation | Increase respiratory rate or $V_T$ settings. |
| | Fatigue | |
| | ***Ventilator related*** | |
| Hypoxemia | $FiO_2$ drift | Check ventilator with oxygen analyzer. |
| Hypocapnia | Settings not correct | Decrease respiratory rate, $V_T$, or minute ventilation (MV). |
| Hypercapnia | Settings not correct | Increase respiratory rate, $V_T$, or MV. |
| Heater alarm | Adding cold water to humidifier | Wait. |
| | Altered setting | Reset. |
| | Cold air blowing on humidifier | Redirect air flow. |

increases if aspiration occurs. The risk for aspiration after intubation can be minimized by maintaining appropriate cuff inflation, evacuating gastric contents and relieving distention with suction, suctioning the oropharynx (especially before cuff deflations), and elevating the head of the patient's bed 30 degrees or more at all times. Elevation of the HOB may be limited when the patient has femoral central venous catheters; however, the bed can be raised up to 15 to 20 degrees and then placed in slight reverse Trendelenburg to approximately 30 degrees of elevation.

## Barotrauma and Pneumothorax

Mechanical ventilation involves "pumping" air into the airway filling the chest, creating positive pressures during inspiration that may lead to barotrauma. If PEEP is added, the pressures are increased and continued throughout expiration. These positive pressures, especially with PEEP greater than 10 to 15 cm $H_2O$, can spontaneously rupture an alveolus or emphysematous bleb in the patient with COPD. Air then escapes into, and is trapped in, the pleural space, accumulating until it begins to collapse the lung. Eventually, the collapsing lung impinges on the mediastinal structures, compressing the trachea and eventually the heart; this is called tension pneumothorax. Signs and symptoms of tension pneumothorax are listed in Box 25-13. Signs of pneumothorax include extreme dyspnea, hypoxemia, and an abrupt increase in PIP. Breath sounds may be decreased or absent on the affected side; however, this sign may not be reliable in the patient on positive-pressure ventilation. Observation of the patient may reveal a tracheal deviation (to the opposite side) or the sudden development of subcutaneous emphysema. The PIP

## BOX 25-12 Complications of Mechanical Ventilation

**Airway**
- Aspiration
- Decreased clearance of secretions
- Ventilator-acquired pneumonia

**Endotracheal Tube**
- Tube kinked or plugged
- Rupture of piriform sinus
- Tracheal stenosis or tracheomalacia
- Mainstem intubation with contralateral lung atelectasis
- Cuff failure
- Sinusitis
- Otitis media
- Laryngeal edema

**Mechanical**
- Hypoventilation with atelectasis
- Hyperventilation with hypocapnia and respiratory alkalosis
- Barotrauma (pneumothorax or tension pneumothorax, pneumomediastinum, subcutaneous emphysema)
- Alarm "turned off"
- Failure of alarms or ventilator
- Inadequate nebulization or humidification
- Overheated inspired air resulting in hyperthermia

**Physiologic**
- Fluid overload with humidified air and sodium chloride retention
- Depressed cardiac function and hypotension
- Stress ulcers
- Paralytic ileus
- Gastric distention
- Starvation
- Dyssynchronous breathing pattern

## QSEN BOX 25-13 PATIENT SAFETY

### Signs and Symptoms of Tension Pneumothorax
- Tachycardia
- Tachypnea
- Agitation
- Diaphoresis
- Tracheal shift from midline
- Muffled heart tones
- Absent breath sounds over affected lung
- Hyperresonance to percussion over affected lung
- Elevation in peak airway pressures in ventilated patients
- Decrease in saturation of oxygen in arterial blood ($SaO_2$) or arterial oxygen tension ($PaO_2$)
- Hypotension
- Cardiac arrest

may become elevated and a ventilator alarm will be activated due to increased intrathoracic pressure. The most ominous signs of tension pneumothorax are hypotension and bradycardia that can deteriorate into a cardiac arrest without timely medical intervention. The physician or other qualified health care professional may decompress the chest by inserting a needle to evacuate the trapped air until a chest tube can be inserted.

## Ventilator-Associated Pneumonia

VAP is the second most common hospital-acquired infection.[14] The incidence of nosocomial pneumonia is increased tenfold in intubated patients, and the risk of developing VAP is especially great in critically ill patients who are mechanically ventilated. Factors that lead to nosocomial pneumonia are oropharyngeal colonization, gastric colonization, aspiration, and compromised lung defenses. Mechanical ventilation, reintubation, self-extubation, presence of a nasogastric tube, and supine position are a few of the associated risk factors for VAP. Maintenance of the natural gastric acid barrier in the stomach plays a major role in decreasing incidence and mortality from nosocomial pneumonia. The widespread use of antacids or histamine ($H_2$) blockers can predispose the patient to nosocomial infections because they decrease gastric acidity (increase alkalinity). These medications are used to guard against stress bleeding and may increase colonization of the upper gastrointestinal tract by bacteria that thrive in a more alkaline environment.

VAP is defined as hospital acquired nosocomial pneumonia in a patient who has been mechanically ventilated (by ETT or tracheostomy) for at least 48 hours at the time of diagnosis. A patient should be suspected of having a diagnosis of VAP if the chest radiograph shows new or progressive and persistent infiltrates. Other signs and symptoms can include a temperature higher than 100.4°F (38°C), leukocytosis, and at least two of the following: new-onset purulent sputum, new cough or dyspnea, bronchial breath sounds, and worsening gas exchange.[9]

There are numerous strategies for preventing VAP. The first step is to prevent colonization by pathogens of the oropharynx and gastrointestinal tract. Basic nursing care principles, such as meticulous handwashing and wearing gloves when suctioning patients orally or through the ETT, are essential. Gloves should also be worn when suctioning through closed-suction devices. In addition, critically ill patients have an increased risk for colonization by the microorganisms associated with poor oral hygiene. Oral care for a mechanically ventilated patient involves brushing the patient's teeth (at least every 8 hours), using antimicrobial solutions and alcohol-free mouthwash to cleanse the mouth, applying a water-based mouth moisturizer to maintain the integrity of the oral mucosa, and thoroughly suctioning oral and subglottic secretions. Chlorhexidine oral rinse is one agent that provides antimicrobial action and is used in many institutions. An oral care protocol should be in place for every adult critical care unit using the current evidence-based research and practice.

In patients receiving enteral feedings, the HOB should be elevated 30 to 45 degrees (unless contraindicated) to decrease the risk for aspiration.[15] Long-term nasally placed endotracheal and gastric tubes (ie, longer than 3 days) should be placed orally unless contraindicated or not tolerated by the patient. This intervention reduces the risk for the patient developing sinusitis, which is associated with the development of VAP. Sinusitis is relatively common in nasally intubated patients and can cause bacteremia and sepsis. Signs of sinusitis (fever, purulent nasal drainage) must be reported immediately. Lastly, the use of an ETT that provides a port for the CASS appears to prevent the development of VAP in the first week of intubation, and it may decrease the overall incidence of VAP but does not affect mortality or length of stay.[10] The use of the CASS ETT is typically reserved for those patients who can be identified as potentially requiring long-term ventilation.

The advent of the ventilator bundle of standard orders, which incorporates gastrointestinal and deep venous thrombosis prophylaxis, along with getting the patient out of bed, oral care, and keeping the HOB elevated 30 to 45 degrees, has reduced the incidence of VAP in many institutions. These procedures should be included as an integral part of the care of ventilated patients.[16]

### Decreased Cardiac Output

Decreased cardiac output, as reflected by hypotension, may be observed at the initiation of mechanical ventilation. Although this is often attributed to the drugs used for intubation (narcotics, sedatives, and NMB agents all reduce blood pressure), the most important contribution to this phenomenon is lack of sympathetic tone and decreased venous return due to the effects of positive pressure within the chest. In addition to hypotension, other signs and symptoms can include unexplained restlessness, decreased levels of consciousness, decreased urine output, weak peripheral pulses, slow capillary refill, pallor, fatigue, and chest pain. Increasing fluids to correct the relative hypovolemia usually treats hypotension. However, in this setting, vasopressors may be needed.

### Decreased Fluid Balance

The decreased venous return to the heart is sensed by the vagal stretch receptors located in the right atrium. This sensed hypovolemia stimulates the release of antidiuretic hormone from the posterior pituitary. The decreased cardiac output, leading to decreased urine output, compounds the problem by stimulating the renin–angiotensin–aldosterone response. A mechanically ventilated patient may be hemodynamically unstable and may require large amounts of fluid resuscitation. This patient can experience extensive edema, including limb, scleral, and facial edema.

### Complications Associated With Immobility

Many complications that contribute to the morbidity and mortality of mechanically ventilated patients are the result of immobility. These complications include muscle wasting and weakness, contractures, loss of skin integrity, pneumonia, and deep venous thrombosis that can result in pulmonary embolus, constipation, and ileus.

### Gastrointestinal Problems

Gastrointestinal complications associated with mechanical ventilation include distention (from air swallowing), hypomotility and ileus (from immobility and the use of narcotic analgesics), vomiting, and breakdown of the intestinal mucosa from the lack of normal nutritional intake. This breakdown allows translocation of bacteria from the gut into the bloodstream, leading to increased risk for bacteremia in patients who cannot be fed enterally. Maintenance of an adequate bowel elimination pattern is necessary to prevent abdominal distention with resulting impingement on diaphragmatic excursion.

---

| BOX 25-14 | Side Effects of Clinical Starvation |

- Atrophy of respiratory muscles
- Decreased protein
- Decreased albumin
- Decreased cell-mediated immunity
- Decreased surfactant production
- Decreased replication of respiratory epithelium
- Intracellular depletion of adenosine triphosphate
- Impaired cellular oxygenation
- Central respiratory depression

---

Many mechanically ventilated patients are already malnourished because of underlying chronic disease. Research verifies that the many side effects of clinical starvation can lead to pulmonary complications and death, as listed in Box 25-14. Early enteral nutrition is advocated for trauma and critically ill patients with either small-bore or Salem-sump tubes that end in the stomach or small intestine.[17] The advantage of small-bore feeding tubes is comfort, and with postpyloric placement, enteral feeding goal rates can be achieved sooner.

### Muscle Weakness

The muscles used in respiration, like other muscles, become deconditioned and may even atrophy with prolonged disuse. The ventilated patient's respiratory muscles may not be used (other than passive movement) while on the ventilator, especially if muscle relaxants, heavy sedation, or both have been part of the care plan. A retraining period to exercise and strengthen the respiratory muscles may be necessary before ventilatory support can be discontinued. Especially at risk for critical illness myopathies are patients who have been on corticosteroids in combination with NMB agents as well as those with multiorgan failure, sepsis, and ARDS.[18]

Muscle weakness also occurs as a result of muscle fatigue. Those patients requiring mechanical ventilation typically have one or more reasons for an increase in the work of breathing. These include an increase in carbon dioxide production, physiologic dead space (non–gas-exchanging air passages), or both; decreased lung compliance; and increased airway resistance, as with bronchospasm or thick secretions. When the work of breathing exceeds the capacity of weakened muscles, the patient begins to display abnormal respiratory mechanics with inefficient use of these muscles. This often occurs during a weaning trial after prolonged ventilation. The accepted intervention for fatigue in this setting is returning to muscle rest on the ventilator. However, this carries the risk for contributing further to muscle atrophy. The diaphragm muscle also requires sufficient electrolytes of calcium, magnesium, and phosphorus to optimize function during weaning. The nurse should review electrolyte values daily to ensure these diaphragm-essential electrolytes are kept normalized.

## Assessment and Management

The patient who needs ventilatory support also needs primary nursing care. One of the greatest contributions the nurse can make to decreasing costs, length of stay, and mortality in patients with respiratory problems is to implement interventions that will prevent or minimize complications. Because mechanical ventilation is supportive rather than curative, the focus of care for the mechanically ventilated patient is holistic. The nurse must interact effectively with each member of the health care team to achieve desired patient outcomes. Box 25-15 summarizes care of the patient on a ventilator. The mechanical ventilator, the artificial airway, and the care necessary to maintain mechanical ventilation require specialized nursing knowledge and skills, which are discussed in the following sections.

### Endotracheal Tube Care

To prevent tube movement, tube migration, or inadvertent extubation, ETTs must be anchored securely. Anchoring can be accomplished with adhesive tape or with commercially manufactured tube immobilization appliances. Usual practice is to retape the ETT every 1 to 2 days or when it is soiled or insecure. In orally intubated patients, the position of the ETT should be changed from side to side to facilitate oral care and to prevent areas of pressure necrosis on the lips, mouth, and tongue. The disadvantage of frequent retaping is that patients with fragile skin or prolonged intubation may incur skin breakdown. Twill tape can be substituted for adhesive tape in these situations and for patients with heavy beards. Retaping by two people is desirable to prevent accidental tube displacement. The final step in retaping is to check tube placement in comparison to placement before retaping. ETT placement is verified by radiography following initial intubation. The position in centimeters at the lips/teeth or nostril is recorded; this placement is verified every

---

**QSEN  BOX 25-15    COLLABORATIVE CARE GUIDE for the Patient on Mechanical Ventilation**

| Outcomes | Interventions |
|---|---|
| **Impaired Gas Exchange**<br>**Ineffective Breathing Pattern** | |
| A patent airway is maintained. Lungs are clear to auscultation.<br>Patient is without evidence of atelectasis.<br>Peak, mean, and plateau pressures are within normal limits.<br>ABG values are within normal limits. | • Auscultate breath sounds every 2 to 4 hours and as needed.<br>• Suction as needed for rhonchi, coughing, or oxygen desaturation.<br>• Hyperoxygenate and hyperventilate before and after each suction pass.<br>• Monitor airway pressures every 1 to 2 hours<br>• Monitor airway pressures after suctioning.<br>• Administer bronchodilators and mucolytics as ordered.<br>• Perform chest physiotherapy (CPT) if indicated by clinical examination or chest radiograph.<br>• Turn patient side to side every 2 hours<br>• Consider kinetic therapy or prone positioning as indicated by clinical scenario.<br>• Get patient out of bed to chair or standing position when stable.<br>• Monitor pulse oximetry and $ETCO_2$.<br>• Monitor ABG values as indicated by changes in noninvasive parameters, patient status, or weaning protocol. |
| **Decreased Cardiac Tissue Perfusion**<br>**Decreased Peripheral Tissue Perfusion**<br>**Risk for Shock** | |
| Blood pressure, heart rate, cardiac output, central venous pressure, and pulmonary artery pressure remain stable on mechanical ventilation. | • Assess hemodynamic effects of initiating positive-pressure ventilation (eg, potential for decreased venous return and cardiac output).<br>• Monitor electrocardiogram for dysrhythmias related to hypoxemia.<br>• Assess effects of ventilator setting changes (inspiratory pressures, $V_T$, PEEP, and fraction of inspired oxygen [$FiO_2$]) on hemodynamic and oxygenation parameters.<br>• Administer intravascular volume as ordered to maintain preload. |
| **Electrolyte Imbalance**<br>**Risk for Imbalanced Fluid Volume** | |
| Intake and output (I & O) measurements are balanced.<br>Electrolyte values are within normal limits. | • Monitor hydration status in relation to clinical examination, auscultation, amount, and viscosity of lung secretions.<br>• Assess patient weight, I & O totals, urine specific gravity, or serum osmolality to evaluate fluid balance.<br>• Administer electrolyte replacements (intravenous or enteral) per physician's order. |
| **Impaired Physical Mobility**<br>**Risk for Activity Intolerance** | |
| Patients will maintain/regain baseline functional status related to mobility and self-care.<br>Joint range of motion is maintained. | • Collaborate with physical/occupational therapy staff to encourage patient effort/participation to increase mobility.<br>• Progress activity to sitting up in chair, standing at bedside, ambulating with assistance as soon as possible.<br>• Assist patient with active or passive range-of-motion exercises of all extremities at least every shift.<br>• Keep extremities in physiologically neutral position using pillows or appropriate splint/support devices as indicated. |

**QSEN** BOX 25-15  *COLLABORATIVE CARE GUIDE for the Patient on Mechanical Ventilation (continued)*

| Outcomes | Interventions |
|---|---|

**Risk for Acute Confusion**
**Risk for Injury**

| | |
|---|---|
| ETT will remain in proper position.<br>Proper inflation of ETT cuff is maintained.<br>Ventilator alarm system remains activated. | • Securely stabilize ETT in position; use respiratory therapy expertise for best method.<br>• Note and record the "cm" line on ETT position at lip or teeth.<br>• Use patient self-protective devices or sedation per hospital protocol.<br>• Evaluate ETT position on chest radiograph daily (by viewing film or by report).<br>• Keep emergency airway equipment and MRB readily available, and check each shift.<br>• Inflate cuff using minimal leak technique or pressure less than 25 mm Hg by manometer.<br>• Monitor cuff inflation/leak every shift and as needed.<br>• Protect pilot balloon from damage.<br>• Perform ventilator setting and alarm checks every 4 hours (minimum) or per hospital protocol. |

**Impaired Tissue Integrity**

| | |
|---|---|
| Patient is without evidence of skin breakdown. | • Assess and document skin integrity at least every shift.<br>• Turn patient side to side every 2 hours; reassess bony prominences for evidence of pressure injury.<br>• When patient is out of bed to chair, provide pressure relief to sitting surfaces at least hourly.<br>• Remove self-protective devices from wrists, and monitor skin per hospital policy. |

**Imbalanced Nutrition**

| | |
|---|---|
| Nutritional intake meets calculated metabolic need (eg, basal energy expenditure equation).<br>Patient will establish regular bowel elimination pattern. | • Consult dietitian for metabolic needs assessment and recommendations.<br>• Provide early nutritional support by enteral or parenteral feeding.<br>• Monitor actual delivery of nutrition daily with I & O calculations.<br>• Weigh patient daily.<br>• Administer bowel regimen medications as ordered, along with adequate hydration. |

**Impaired Comfort**

| | |
|---|---|
| Patients will indicate/exhibit adequate relief of discomfort/pain while on mechanical ventilation. | • Document pain assessment, using numerical pain rating or similar scale when possible.<br>• Provide analgesia as appropriate, document efficacy after each dose.<br>• Prevent pulling and jarring of the ventilator tubing and endotracheal or tracheostomy tube.<br>• Provide meticulous oral care every 1 to 2 hours with oropharynx suctioning and mouth moisturizer as needed; teeth brushing scheduled at least three times daily, antimicrobial irrigation twice daily, oral assessment at least daily.<br>• Administer sedation as indicated. |

**Ineffective Coping**
**Impaired Individual Resilience**

| | |
|---|---|
| Patient participates in self-care and decision making related to own activities of daily living (ADLs) (eg, turning, bathing).<br>Patient communicates with health care providers and visitors. | • Encourage patient to move in bed and attempt to meet own basic comfort/hygiene needs independently.<br>• Establish a daily schedule for bathing, time out of bed, treatments, and so forth, with patient input.<br>• Provide a means for patient to write notes and use visual tools to facilitate communication.<br>• Encourage visitor conversations with patient in normal tone of voice and subject matter.<br>• Teach visitors to assist with range of motion and other simple care delivery tasks to facilitate normal patterns of interaction. |

**Teaching/Discharge Planning**

| | |
|---|---|
| Patient cooperates with and indicates understanding of need for mechanical ventilation.<br>Potential discharge needs are assessed. | • Provide explanations to patient/significant others regarding:<br>Rationale for use of mechanical ventilation<br>Procedures such as suctioning, airway care, CPT<br>Plan for and progress toward weaning and extubation<br>• Initiate early social worker involvement to screen for needs, resources, and support systems. Potential discharge needs are assessed. |

shift to detect inadvertent position changes. Tube placement is checked, following retaping, by comparing the centimeter markings at the lips/teeth or nostril with the last radiologic documentation of position. Placement of an oral bite block can prevent biting on the tube, which can cause airway narrowing or tube displacement. The use of a swivel connector (connecting the tube to the ventilator circuit), along with anchoring a large loop of tubing to the bed, facilitates patient movement without ETT movement. Oral inspection and hygiene are of paramount importance when a bite block is used.

Persistent coughing may suggest that the ETT has migrated to touch the carina, requiring the tube to be withdrawn to an appropriate level. The pilot cuff balloon is protected from inadvertent disruption; cuff rupture or ETT occlusion with a mucus plug usually requires reintubation. If a patient is prematurely extubated for any reason, the airway must be kept patent. Oxygenation and ventilation may be provided with an MRB and mask until reintubation can be accomplished.

## Tracheostomy Care

In patients requiring long-term mechanical ventilation, the airway is converted to a tracheostomy at some point to prevent the complications of endotracheal intubation, such as tracheal stenosis and vocal cord paralysis. The preferred method of airway management is the tracheostomy tube for long-term ventilation. Past practice involved tracheostomy after 11 and up to 21 days on the ventilator. Current practice promotes earlier tracheostomy at 72 hours after intubation. Earlier tracheostomy (eg, after 3 to 7 days on the ventilator) is performed to facilitate earlier weaning, particularly if the patient has multiple comorbidities and demonstrates difficulty weaning or has trauma or neurologic diagnoses associated with prolonged need for an artificial airway. Tracheostomy is also performed for patient comfort and safety when mobilizing the patient and may lead to decreased ventilator weaning time. In addition to long-term ventilation, indications for tracheostomy include upper airway obstruction, airway edema from anaphylaxis, failed intubation, multiple intubations (high risk for complications), complications of ETT intubation, absence of protective reflexes, home care, conditions in which ETT intubation is not possible (eg, facial trauma, cervical fractures), and the desire for improved patient comfort.

The advantages of tracheostomy over endotracheal intubation include faster weaning (at least in part because of decreased dead space), enhanced patient comfort, enhanced communication, and the possibility of oral feeding. The tracheostomy is inserted into the trachea, thereby avoiding the mouth, upper airway, and glottis, and this decreases problems of airway resistance and occlusion.

Tracheostomy is not without disadvantages. These include hemorrhage, infection, pneumothorax, and the need for an operative procedure that is itself a risk. Box 25-16 presents complications of tracheostomy. The most serious complication is erosion into the innominate artery, which can result in exsanguination. If bleeding occurs, the cuff can be hyperinflated in an attempt to control bleeding until emergency surgery can be performed. The practice of bedside percutaneous tracheostomy using a progressive dilation technique has been touted to decrease the morbidity and cost incurred with

---

**QSEN BOX 25-16** *PATIENT SAFETY*

### Complications of Tracheostomy
- Acute hemorrhage at the site
- Air embolism
- Aspiration
- Tracheal stenosis
- Erosion into the innominate artery with exsanguination
- Failure of the tracheostomy cuff
- Laryngeal nerve damage
- Obstruction of tracheostomy tube
- Pneumothorax
- Subcutaneous and mediastinal emphysema
- Swallowing dysfunction
- Tracheoesophageal fistula
- Infection
- Accidental decannulation with loss of airway
- False placement of cannula (not in trachea)
- Weak voice/hoarseness

---

an operative procedure because it is often earlier than surgical tracheostomy. Although there is no major difference in mortality risk, it has been found that early tracheostomy resulted in decreased ventilator days. Less infection and bleeding have also been given as advantages over the standard procedure performed in the operating room. The ability to predict extubation as short or extended (more than 10 days) is limited.[19]

The nurse can prevent complications by assessing for them with each patient interaction and during tracheostomy care. Proper fixation of the tracheostomy tube reduces the movement of the tube in the airway and limits friction injury to the tracheal wall or larynx. Maintaining the cuff pressure at the minimum required to prevent air leak on the ventilator reduces the risk for tissue breakdown due to excessive pressure on the trachea wall. The tracheostomy tube must be firmly secured. The ventilator tubing should have enough length to allow movement without pulling on the tracheostomy and to allow for procedures. A tracheostomy swivel connector, with or without flex tubing, reduces the tension on the tracheostomy while the patient is on the ventilator. A confused or very mobile patient can easily self-decannulate; patient restraints may be needed to prevent accidental decannulation. Orienting the patient to the need for an artificial airway and providing pain control and sedation are measures that are taken before resorting to restraint application. If restraints are needed, it is necessary to obtain a physician's order, with regular review of continued need. The nurse must monitor the patient closely for potential injury and must perform circulatory checks with removal of restraints frequently.

Tracheostomy care includes frequent changing of tracheal ties and dressing, although initial ties are not changed until at least 24 to 48 hours after placement to allow for hemostasis of the site. The sutures from either a percutaneous or surgical tracheostomy are left in place for 48 to 72 hours or even up to a week (per hospital protocol) to prevent decannulation. As with retaping of the ETT, changing of tracheostomy ties should be a two-person procedure. The ties should be tied so that one to two fingers can be inserted between the ties and the skin, allowing minimal movement of the tracheostomy tube but maintaining comfort. It is mandatory to maintain a midline position for the tracheostomy to prevent pressure on surrounding tissue. The stoma is cleansed with half-strength hydrogen peroxide, followed by rinse with sterile saline solution, and observed for wound healing, bleeding, and signs of infection The routine practice of inner cannula cleaning or changes may not be necessary with a disposable inner cannula that can be changed daily. The routine care for tracheostomy is cleaning the tracheostomy site at least every 8 to 12 hours and as needed, changing the inner cannula daily (or according to facility policy), and changing soiled tracheostomy ties as needed, progressing to daily and as-needed care. This longer care interval usually occurs after 7 to 10 days or when secretion and tracheostomy drainage are minimal. The routine care of tracheostomies is always performed as a sterile procedure while in the hospital.

If decannulation occurs within the first 7 days of tracheostomy insertion, the patient may be reintubated with an ETT if emergent tracheostomy tube replacement cannot be done safely. An obturator and a new, appropriately sized tracheostomy tube are kept at the bedside. If inadvertent decannulation occurs after a tract has developed, the tube is carefully replaced using the obturator.

### Tube Cuff Pressure Monitoring

Tube cuff pressures are monitored every shift to prevent overdistention and excess pressure on the tracheal wall mucosa, which can cause complications such as tracheal stenosis. If a patient is on the ventilator, the best pressure is the lowest possible pressure without having a loss of inspiratory volume. Physiologically, pressures of about 20 to 30 mm Hg obliterate capillary circulation to the tracheal mucosa. If a cuff leak is suspected, auscultation at the neck for the sound of air escaping above the cuff can determine whether the seal is adequate.

One method used to inflate a cuff is called the minimal occluding volume. Air is injected slowly into the pilot balloon during ventilator inspiration while auscultation is performed over the trachea. When the harsh "squeak" of air escaping is no longer audible, the minimal occluding volume has been reached, and the tube cuff is occluding the airway without excessive pressure on the trachea. Extra air should not be added. In the ICU, the best practice is actual measurement of cuff pressure using a manometer. This device is attached to the ETT pilot balloon to obtain a reading, which should ideally be 20 to 25 mm Hg. If a leak is still present above this level of inflation, slight repositioning of the ETT within the patient's airway may correct the problem. Changing to a larger or longer ETT may be necessary with increasing pressures to seal the airway. The cuff pressure is assessed with the manometer every 6 to 8 hours and, when a leak is noted, to help prevent aspiration of subglottic secretions. Whenever a cuff leak is found, the medical team and respiratory care practitioner should be notified. Recurrent cuff leaks may indicate the need for an extra-long tube or a larger size to provide for ventilation.

### Discharge Planning and Patient Teaching

Discharge planning is necessary for patients who will be discharged to home with tracheostomies. Rationales for tracheostomy care include promotion of ostomy healing, prevention of infection, maintenance of a patent airway, and increased patient comfort.

Teaching the patient and family care giver tracheostomy care allows for independence and self-care. This is an essential component of discharge teaching. Communication about the procedure and reassurance during the training process reduce anxiety and improve cooperation.

### Nutritional Support

Respiratory muscles, like all other body muscles, need energy to work. If energy needs are not met, muscle fatigue occurs, leading to discoordination of respiratory muscles and a decrease in tidal volume. Hypomagnesemia and hypophosphatemia have been implicated in muscle fatigue caused by depleted levels of adenosine triphosphate. Electrolyte imbalances must be corrected and monitored daily for optimal muscle functioning during ventilator weaning. In prolonged starvation, the body cannibalizes the intercostal and diaphragmatic muscles for energy.

Metabolic needs in critically ill patients are much higher than in normal subjects. Basic caloric requirements are usually increased by 25% for hospital activity and stress associated with treatment. Adequate nutrition is a prerequisite for weaning from mechanical ventilation; nutritional support should be instituted early. If the gastrointestinal tract is intact, enteral nutrition is preferred and can be provided through a small-bore feeding tube.

Initial tube feeding is started slowly, with close monitoring of blood glucose and electrolyte levels. The nurse observes the patient for signs of intolerance, such as diarrhea and hyperosmolar dehydration. If the patient tolerates feedings, the rate is gradually increased until the goal rate is achieved. If tube feedings cannot be tolerated, parenteral hyperalimentation should be considered (see Chapter 40).

Patients who require long-term mechanical ventilation typically need additional protein and calories per day. When available, metabolic cart testing (also called indirect calorimetry) or a 24-hour urine nitrogen test can assess individual nutritional requirements. The monitoring of the prealbumin level may give an indication of recent nutritional state. Nutritionists are invaluable in determining the caloric needs of critically ill patients.

### Eye Care

Eye care of the ventilator patient is important. Many patients in the ICU are comatose, sedated, or chemically paralyzed and therefore have lost the blink reflex or ability to close their eyelids completely. This can lead to corneal dryness and ulceration. Increase PEEP on the ventilator can lead to increase water retention and sclera edema. Patients requiring proning will also develop sclera edema.[14]

Eye care hygiene and care should be scheduled and not on an as-needed basis to ensure 24-hour application. For eye hygiene, clean the lid with sterile water soaked gauze. Swab in one direction from inside to outside. If eye dryness is present or the patient at risk following eye hygiene, apply 1 cm of approved lubricant to the "V" pocket between eyeball and lower lid every 4 hours. Cover the eye with transparent polyethylene covers for best protection. Elevate the HOB at least 30 degrees to prevent or minimize scleral edema. It is recommended to cover eyes during suctioning of patient to prevent cross contamination.[14] The use of a lubricating ointment in addition to covering the affected eye(s) protects from dryness and corneal damage.

### Oral Care

Frequent oral care must be performed on all mechanically ventilated patients. Oral care not only increases comfort but also preserves the integrity of the oropharyngeal mucosa. An intact mucosa helps prevent infection and colonization of organisms that leads to VAP. The oropharynx is colonized with potential pathogens such as *Staphylococcus aureus*, *Streptococcus pneumoniae*, *Prevotella* species, *Bacteroides fragilis*, and many more.[16]

As noted in the VAP discussion, evidence-based studies note the use of oral care protocols for ventilated adult patients in preventing VAP. Nursing skill manuals do present guidelines for oral care in patients with and without teeth as well as in those who are incapacitated. However, these general oral care guidelines are not suitable for patients with an ETT and do not prevent VAP. The current literature includes oral care guidelines using every 2-, 4-, and 8-hour interventions with specific interventions of tooth brushing, oral and subglottic suctioning, moisturizer, and oral rinses.[10] The CDC recommends that every ICU implement a complete oral care program with use of an antimicrobial oral rinse to prevent oral colonization.[10] The Cochrane Oral Health Group recently reviewed 17 oral hygiene care RCTs which provided moderate-quality evidence for using either chlorhexidine mouthwash or gel. The results of these studies demonstrated a 40% reduction in the odds of VAP. No evidence existed to show a decrease in ICU mortality rate, the number of ventilator days, or duration in ICU days. The combination of using chlorhexidine and toothbrushing did not demonstrate a difference from using chlorhexidine alone.[15]

What is still needed is a definitive research study regarding the optimal frequency, products, type of oral rinse, and materials to provide oral care for adult ventilated patients. Including the oral care guideline as part of VAP prevention may help reduce VAP by educating nurses and implementing practice changes, along with continuing quality improvement by monitoring the effectiveness of oral care and VAP protocols. Every ICU should either review its oral care guideline or create one with the current evidence-based research and available protocols. ICUs should follow the recent findings of the Cochrane Collaboration on oral care in the critically ill to prevent ventilator associated pneumonia.[15] Suggested guidelines may include the following:

- Systematic assessment of the oral mucosa performed daily and with each cleaning
- Handwashing before and after every nursing intervention
- Routine brushing of teeth to remove dental plaque every 8 hours
- Cleansing of the mouth every 2 hours and as needed
- Use of an alcohol-free or antimicrobial (chlorhexidine) oral rinse every 8 or 12 hours to reduce oropharyngeal colonization
- Suctioning the mouth and subglottic pharynx to minimize aspiration risk and provide a cover for the suction set with replacement every 8 or 24 hours
- Applying a water-based mouth moisturizer to prevent mucosal drying and maintain integrity of the oral mucosa

Commercial kits are available that provide the suction catheters, covered tonsil-tip suction, toothbrushes with suction, and toothpaste for brushing in individually wrapped sets to prevent contamination.

### Psychological Care

The ventilated patient is subjected to extreme physical and emotional stress in the ICU environment. Psychological distress can be caused by sleep deprivation, sensory overstimulation, sensory deprivation for familiar cues, pain, fear, inability to communicate, and commonly used pharmacologic agents. Common ICU treatments can often be perceived as dehumanizing.

Feelings of helplessness and lack of control can be overwhelming. The patient may exhibit signs of agitation, delirium, and anxiety; these reactions may be exacerbated in patients with a history of psychiatric problems or drug or alcohol abuse. If the patient is incapable of dealing with stress through coping mechanisms, he or she may exhibit depression, apathy, and lack of emotional involvement.[20] Nursing interventions aimed at decreasing the psychological effects are numerous. These include promoting sleep–wake cycles, minimizing sedation to achieve Richmond Agitation Sedation Scale (RASS) to light or negative one, optimizing nutrition, preventing glucose fluctuations, and providing frequent updates to the patient.[21] Other interventions include music therapy, pet therapy, massage or Reiki therapy, encouraging family and friends to visit, being out of bed with ambient sunlight, and restarting home antidepressants or antipsychotics if indicated.

Assisted ventilation can precipitate a psychological dependence in those with primary respiratory disorders. If, for the first time in years, a patient is receiving enough oxygen to meet metabolic needs and does not have to struggle for air, he or she may be reluctant to give up the ventilator. Weaning can become even more stressful for this patient.

### Facilitating Communication

A number of interventions can facilitate communication with the patient who has an endotracheal or tracheostomy tube. Before assessing the patient's ability to communicate, provide the patient with his or her eyeglasses or hearing aid (if applicable). Complete explanations from staff members regarding any procedures may help decrease the patient's stress. The care giver can use verbal and nonverbal communication skills. Nonverbal communication may include sign language, gestures, or lip reading. If the patient is unable to use these forms of nonverbal communication, helpful devices include pencil and paper, clipboard or dry erase boards, picture or alphabet boards, electronic communication boards, and even a computer.

Once the patient is off the ventilator and tolerating the tracheostomy collar, the tracheostomy patient can communicate by using a cap or speaking valves that occlude the tracheostomy tube. These allow for the passage of air around the tracheostomy to the vocal chords as long as the cuff is deflated. The tracheostomy may be capped for 24 to 48 hours before decannulation, and the patient breathes and speaks around the tracheostomy. The cap is the final test to ensure airway protection by the patient.

Two other options to the cap are the Passy-Muir valve and the Shiley speaking valve. The Passy-Muir and Shiley speaking valves are one-way valves that allow air to enter during inspiration and then close to allow the air to flow over the vocal chords with exhalation. These valves each have a side port for oxygen tubing to be attached, providing oxygen support in addition to the humidified air from a tracheostomy collar. The tracheostomy collar should be used nearly continuously to prevent the accumulation of secretions and the drying of the airway mucosa. Neither speaking valve should be used during sleep to prevent aspiration with a deflated cuff. Patients with copious secretions are at risk for obstruction of these valves. They must be monitored very closely. In addition, patients at high risk for aspiration, especially those with laryngeal or pharyngeal dysfunction, should be carefully assessed before one of these devices is used. The nurse should store these valves in a container clearly identified with the patient's name for safekeeping because each type of valve is relatively costly. The patient should be taught to remove the valve with excessive sputum during cough and call for assistance to clean the valve before reuse. The tracheostomy patient with a speaking valve is at increased risk for aspiration because the cuff must be deflated for the patient to communicate.

### Caring for the Family

Having a loved one in an ICU setting can create stress and anxiety for family members.[21] Family members must deal with a strange environment, a critically ill loved one, and the financial strain imposed by the illness. Nursing support is given by familiarizing the family with the physical surroundings, supplying information about visitation policies, and providing frequent progress reports on the patient's condition. The nurse establishes open communication with the patient and family, proactively arranges for visits, and provides the family with information. Promoting spiritual and cultural support, scheduled family communication conferences, patient care education, and open communication assists the family with coping and reduces stress.[21]

## Mechanical Ventilation Liberation

As soon as mechanical ventilation starts, plans begin for weaning the patient from mechanical support. The process to achieve this goal includes correcting the cause of respiratory failure, preventing complications, and restoring or maintaining physiologic and psychological functional status. Patients requiring prolonged mechanical ventilation will need a different, often individualized, approach to ventilator weaning. The terms *weaning* and *liberation from the ventilator* are often used interchangeably but have two different meanings: weaning implies a slower process whereas liberation implies a faster process. Earlier evidence supported a more gradual approach to extubation (ie, weaning), but newer evidence supports a faster approach (ie, liberation).[22]

Each patient is evaluated daily for readiness to wean by performing a spontaneous breathing trial. Box 25-17 presents guidelines for ventilator liberation. It is important to perform this assessment and address weaning impediments before initiating weaning trials. Many weaning indices have been advocated for use in predicting weaning readiness. Some look exclusively at respiratory factors, such as muscle strength and endurance (eg, negative inspiratory pressure [NIP], PEP

---

### BOX 25-17 Guidelines for Ventilator Liberation

In patients requiring mechanical ventilation for more than 24 hours, reversing all possible ventilatory and nonventilatory issues should be an integral part of the ventilator discontinuance process. A formal assessment of discontinuation potential should be made if the patient meets the following criteria:

- Evidence of reversal or improvement of the underlying cause of respiratory failure
- Adequate oxygenation (eg, $PaO_2/FiO_2$ greater than 150 to 200 mm Hg) on low PEEP (5 to 8 cm $H_2O$ or less) and pH 7.25 or higher
- Hemodynamic stability: no active myocardial ischemia, no clinically significant hypotension
- Capability to initiate an inspiratory effort
- Spontaneous breathing trial needs to be coordinated with sedation awakening trial
- Spontaneous breathing trial settings include pressure support and PEEP of 5 or less
- The criteria for SBT tolerance include respiratory pattern, adequacy of gas exchange, hemodynamic stability, and subjective comfort.
- SBT tolerance lasting 30 to 120 minutes should prompt consideration for permanent ventilator discontinuation. After passing the SBT, artificial airway removal should be based on assessment of airway patency and ability of patient to protect the airway.
- If failing an SBT, cause for failure should be determined. After reversing cause for failure, if patient meets SBT criteria, SBTs should be performed every 24 hours.
- Patients failing an SBT should receive a stable, non-fatiguing, comfortable form of ventilator support.
- Anesthesia/sedation strategies and ventilator management aimed at early extubation should be used in postsurgical patients.
- Protocols aimed at optimizing sedation also should be developed and implemented.
- Discontinuation protocols designed for nonphysician healthcare providers should be developed and implemented by ICUs.
- Tracheostomy should be considered after an initial period of stabilization on the ventilator, when it becomes apparent the patient will require prolonged ventilator assistance.

---

weaning index, or rapid shallow breathing index as the ratio of frequency to tidal volume). Others are integrated indices that look at a broad range of physiologic factors that influence weaning readiness. Many of these factors individually lack predictability, and often several factors are assessed for weaning readiness.

The performance of the diaphragm, as well as accessory muscles of respiration, depends on both the endurance and strength of the muscles. The effectiveness of diaphragmatic contraction is a function of both the resting length of muscle fibers and the speed with which they contract. Both of these factors are affected by physiologic changes that change the resting position of the diaphragm. For example, patients with COPD will demonstrate a shorter rest length (weakening force of contraction). In patients with diaphragmatic distention, such as abdominal ascites or morbid obesity, the diaphragm must push down abdominal contents as it contracts. Reactive airway disease, such as asthma, increases the resistance to airflow, with increased workload for muscles of respiration. Any of these abnormalities can lead to significant fatigue of these muscles and respiratory distress.

Respiratory muscle fatigue impedes weaning. It may take as long as 24 hours of complete rest (the mechanical ventilator assumes all of the work of breathing for the patient) for recovery of fatigued respiratory muscles. Therefore, it is common practice to increase ventilatory support at night to ensure rest. This can be accomplished with any of the "resting" modes, as long as the patient's respiratory rate is less than 20 breaths/min. The intent is to promote and simulate the normal decrease in rate and work of breathing that occurs during each person's sleep–rest cycle.

Weaning trials are discontinued if signs of fatigue or respiratory distress develop. The weaning tolerance criteria and observations are summarized in Boxes 25-18 and 25-19. During physical therapy and activities, it is necessary to monitor the patient for fatigue with use of accessory muscles, increased respiratory rate, and decreased oxygen saturation that indicates respiratory muscle fatigue. The use of sedatives and narcotics during weaning should be limited to only the level of medication clearly needed to control pain or anxiety.[20]

Regardless of the mode or approach, certain factors have been found to positively influence weaning success. These include the use of collaborative, multidisciplinary teams to formulate comprehensive plans of care based on assessment of individual patients; the use of standardized weaning protocols that are assigned to each patient based on individual assessment; and the use of critical pathways. The interplay of these strategies, all designed to promote consistency of and rationale for practice, truly leads to outcomes showing that the whole (process) is greater than the sum of its parts.

## Extubation Criteria

Whichever mode or combination of modes is used for weaning, extubation cannot occur until several criteria are met based on short-term or long-term ventilation (see Boxes 25-18 and 25-19). Before extubation, the patient must be able to maintain his or her own airway, as evidenced by an appropriate level of consciousness and the presence of cough and gag reflexes. In all patients, but especially in those with a history of difficult intubation or reactive airway disease, the cuff-leak test should be performed before extubation. This entails deflation of the tube cuff (after suctioning of the oropharynx) and a brief period of occluding the ETT in order to demonstrate an air leak with patient inspiration. Absence of a leak can indicate edema and may predict laryngeal stridor after extubation. A direct visualization of the trachea with a bronchoscope may be performed before extubation to determine whether the edema has resolved.

Extubation should never occur unless a qualified person is available to reintubate emergently if the patient does not tolerate extubation.

After explaining the procedure and preparing the patient, the nurse or respiratory therapist suctions the patient's tube and posterior oropharynx. Equipment includes an MRB and mask at bedside. The ETT securing device or tape is loosened and the

---

**BOX 25-18** **Guidelines for Weaning from Short-Term Ventilation**

Patients are often intubated electively for surgical or other procedures or more urgently owing to respiratory distress related to underlying pulmonary disease or traumatic injury. The other common reason for intubation is the need for airway protection because of airway swelling (eg, as a result of acute inhalation injury) or significant change in mental status (eg, as with cerebrovascular accident or head injury). Once the procedure is completed or the patient is stabilized, the goal should be extubation as soon as the patient is able to protect the airway. The weaning process in this setting may proceed rapidly, based on individual patient response to reducing ventilator support.

Readiness Criteria
- Hemodynamically stable, adequately resuscitated, and not requiring vasoactive support
- $SaO_2$ greater than 90% on $FiO_2$ 40% or less, PEEP 5 cm $H_2O$ or less
- Chest radiograph reviewed for correctable factors; treated as indicated
- Metabolic indicators (serum pH, major electrolytes) within normal range
- Hematocrit more than 25%
- Core temperature more than 36°C and less than 39°C
- Adequate management of pain/anxiety/agitation
- No residual neuromuscular blockade
- ABG values normalized or at patient's baseline

Weaning Intervention
- Reduce ventilator rate, then convert to pressure-support ventilation (PSV) only.
- Wean PSV as tolerated to 10 cm $H_2O$ or less.

- If patient meets tolerance criteria for at least 2 hours on this level of support *and* meets extubation criteria (see later), may extubate.
- If patient fails tolerance criteria, increase PSV or add ventilator rate as needed to achieve "rest" settings (consistent respiratory rate less than 20 breaths/min) and review weaning criteria for correctable factors.
- Repeat wean attempt on PSV 10 cm after rest period (minimum, 2 hours). If patient fails second wean trial, return to rest settings and use "long-term" ventilation weaning approach.

Tolerance Criteria
If the patient displays any of the following, the weaning trial should be stopped and the patient returned to "rest" settings.
- Sustained respiratory rate greater than 35 breaths/min
- $SaO_2$ less than 90%
- Tidal volume 5 mL/kg or less
- Sustained minute ventilation greater than 200 mL/kg/min
- Evidence of respiratory or hemodynamic distress:
  Labored respiratory pattern
  Increased anxiety, diaphoresis, or both
  Sustained heart rate greater than 20% higher or lower than baseline
  Systolic blood pressure exceeding 180 mm Hg or less than 90 mm Hg

Extubation Criteria
- Mental status: alert and able to respond to commands
- Good cough and gag reflex and able to protect airway and clear secretions
- Able to move air around ETT with cuff deflated and end of tube occluded

## BOX 25-19 Guideline for Liberation from Long-Term Ventilation

Patients on mechanical ventilation for longer than 72 hours or those having failed short-term weaning often display significant deconditioning as a result of acute or chronic complex illness, or both. These patients usually require a period of "exercising" respiratory muscles to regain the strength and endurance needed for successful return to spontaneous breathing. Goals for this process are:

- To have the patient tolerate two to three daily weaning trials of reduction in ventilatory support without exercising to the point of exhaustion
- To rest the patient between weaning trials and overnight on ventilator settings that provide diaphragmatic rest, with minimal or no work of breathing for the patient

### Readiness Criteria
- Same as for short-term ventilation (see Box 25-18), with emphasis on hemodynamic stability, adequate analgesia/sedation (record scores on flow sheet), and normalizing volume status

### Liberation Intervention
- Transfer to PSV mode, adjust support level to maintain patient's respiratory rate at less than 35 breaths/min.
- Observe for 30 minutes for signs of early failure (same tolerance criteria as with short-term ventilation; see Box 25-18).
- If tolerated, continue trial for 2 hours, then return patient to "rest" settings by adding ventilator breaths or increasing PSV to achieve a total respiratory rate of less than 20 breaths/min.
- After at least 2 hours of rest, repeat trial for 2 to 4 hours at same PSV level as previous trial. If the patient exceeds the tolerance criteria (listed in Box 25-18), stop the trial and return to "rest" settings. In this case, the next trial should be performed at a higher support level than the "failed" trial.
- Record the results of each weaning episode, including specific parameters and the time frame if "failure" observed, on the bedside flow sheet.

- The goal is to increase the length of the trials and reduce the PSV level needed on an incremental basis. With each successive trial, the PSV level may be decreased by 2 to 4 cm $H_2O$, the time interval may be increased by 1 to 2 hours, or both, while keeping the patient within tolerance parameters. The pace of weaning is patient specific, and tolerance may vary from day to day. Review readiness criteria for correctable factors daily *and* each time the patient "fails" a weaning trial.
- Ensure nocturnal ventilation at "rest" settings (with a respiratory rate of less than 20 breaths/min) for at least 6 hours each night until the patient's weaning trials demonstrate readiness to discontinue ventilator support.

### Discontinuing Mechanical Ventilation
The patient should be weaned until ventilator settings are $FiO_2$ 40% or more, PSV 10 cm $H_2O$ or less, and PEEP 5 cm $H_2O$ or less. Once these settings are well tolerated, the patient should be placed on continuous positive airway pressure 5 cm $H_2O$ or (if tracheostomy in place) on tracheostomy collar. If the patient meets tolerance criteria over the first 5 minutes, the trial should be continued for 1 to 2 hours. If clinical observation and ABG values indicate that the patient is maintaining adequate ventilation and oxygenation on this "minimal" support, the following options should be considered:

- If the patient meets extubation criteria (see Box 25-18), this step should be attempted.
- If the patient is on tracheostomy collar, the trials should be continued two to three times per day with daily increases in time on tracheostomy collar by 1 to 2 hours per trial until total time off the ventilator reaches 18 h/d. At this point, the patient may be ready to remain on tracheostomy collar for longer than 24 hours unless the tolerance criteria are exceeded.
- Ventilator weaning is considered successful once the patient achieves spontaneous ventilation (extubated or on tracheostomy collar) for at least 24 hours.

---

cuff is deflated. The ETT is removed quickly while having the patient cough. The patient's mouth is suctioned, and humidified oxygen is applied immediately. The patient is evaluated for immediate signs of distress: stridor, dyspnea, and decrease in $SaO_2$. Treatment of stridor includes inhaled racemic epinephrine and sometimes administration of IV steroids; if these interventions fail, immediate reintubation may be necessary.[22]

### Long-Term Ventilation Weaning for Prolonged Mechanical Ventilated Patients

The process of long-term weaning often takes weeks. It incorporates gradual and progressive conditioning for respiratory and body muscles using a multidisciplinary team approach. Whole body conditioning, with emphasis on upper body strength and respiratory muscle function, has been successful in improving ventilator liberation results; aggressive physiotherapy is necessary. The entire process is typically complicated, involving multiple delays and setbacks. During long-term weaning, the patient may fail a weaning trial and should then be rested on the ventilator up to 24 hours before another trial is attempted. The rest period allows for recovery of the respiratory muscles. Patients who fail a weaning trial often exhibit rapid, shallow breathing patterns consistent with their respiratory muscle weakness. Regular reevaluation of the weaning plan by the multidisciplinary team, coupled

with continuous communication with the patient and family, is necessary (see Box 25-19).

### Methods of Ventilator Weaning

Various methods for weaning from the ventilator have been studied, and controversies exist about which methods are best. Some of the most common weaning methods include T-piece, CPAP trials, and gradual PSV reduction to minimal settings. Comprehensive assessment of the patient's needs and progress toward weaning, monitoring of the weaning parameters, and following established goals promote successful weaning. Multidisciplinary and comprehensive approaches to weaning based on health care professionals monitoring and implementing a weaning plan with continuity promote positive outcomes.

**T-PIECE TRIAL.** The T-piece is connected to the patient at the desired $FiO_2$ (usually slightly higher than the previous ventilator setting). The patient's response and tolerance to the trial are continuously observed. The duration of T-piece trials is not standardized, and some clinicians extubate if an initial trial of 30 minutes ends with acceptable ABG values and patient response. Increasing frequency and duration of T-piece trials builds the patient's endurance, with periods of rest on the ventilator between extended trials. When the latter method is used, the patient is generally deemed ready to be extubated after 24 successive hours on a T-piece.

## SYNCHRONIZED INTERMITTENT MANDATORY VENTILATION MODE.

The SIMV mode was initially heralded as the optimal weaning mode, allowing some spontaneous breathing (to prevent respiratory muscle atrophy) while providing a backup rate. Weaning with the SIMV method entails a gradual reduction in the number of delivered breaths until a low rate is reached (usually 4 breaths/min). The patient is then extubated if all other weaning criteria are met. However, low levels of SIMV (fewer than 4 breaths/min) may result in a high level of work and fatigue. SIMV plus PSV, called synchronized pressure-support ventilation (SPSV), may be used to decrease the work of breathing associated with spontaneous breaths. Use of the SPSV mode can easily progress to PSV alone when the patient initiates all breaths by dialing down the ventilator breaths. As a result, PSV "stand-alone" mode is often preferred for weaning trials.

## CONTINUOUS POSITIVE AIRWAY PRESSURE METHOD.

CPAP entails breathing through the ventilator circuit with a small amount of (or zero) positive pressure. The use of CPAP rather than a T-piece for weaning remains controversial. Often, the decision to use one over the other is determined by observing the patient's response or is simply based on the clinician's preference.

## PRESSURE-SUPPORT VENTILATION MODE.

Low levels of PSV decrease the work of breathing associated with ETTs and ventilator circuits. Weaning using the PSV mode entails a progressive decrease in IPL to 5 to 10 cm $H_2O$ based on the patient maintaining an adequate tidal volume (6 to 12 mL/kg) and a respiratory rate of fewer than 25 breaths/min. PSV is associated with less work of breathing than with volume modes, so longer weaning trials may be tolerated. The 5-cm $H_2O$ IPL is thought to overcome the work of breathing through the ETT and ventilator tubing. Typically, the IPL is reduced by 2 cm $H_2O$ daily, or twice daily following the patient's response to the ventilator change. Tolerance of PSV weaning is assessed as with any weaning mode: by evaluating the patient's response to changes in respiratory rate, $SaO_2$, and heart rate, along with observing for fatigue (see Boxes 25-18 and 25-19). There is support for use of CPAP, T-piece, or even PSV during a spontaneous breathing trial before extubation because each is an effective method for the weaning readiness trial.[22]

## Adjuncts to Weaning

Several adjuncts to long-term weaning are used to improve weaning tolerance and patient comfort. The mode on newer ventilators that allows for the regulation of pressure support for the size and type of tube (endotracheal or tracheostomy) adjusts for the type of tube resistance to allow less work of breathing. Called automatic tube compensation (ATC) on some ventilators, this is another tool to consider during weaning. The fenestrated tracheostomy tube provides for communication during weaning periods, improving patient interaction. The fenestrated tracheostomy tube has an opening in the outer cannula but not the inner cannula. With the inner cannula in place and the cuff inflated, mechanical ventilation is easy. During the weaning process, the inner cannula is removed, the cuff deflated, the outer cannula capped, and supplemental oxygen supplied by nasal cannula. This system permits air to pass the vocal cords, allowing verbal communication by the patient. The cuff should never be inflated while the inner cannula is capped because the patient will be unable to breathe. The speaking valves provide communication during weaning periods for patients with nonfenestrated tracheostomy tubes, which are generally used more frequently. These valves provide less resistance than the fenestrated tracheostomy tube, and each type of speaking valve allows for supplemental oxygen through a side port. Humidified air with a tracheostomy collar is required to keep the airway moist and prevent secretions from drying, especially at night when speaking valves should be removed for sleep. Use of a large ETT (greater than 7.0 mm) decreases resistance to breathing and decreases the work of breathing. A larger ETT also supports bronchoscopy and the removal of secretions when needed. Tracheostomy in many instances is more comfortable for patients and allows for improved oral care, better communication, and tracheostomy collar trials for weaning.

Considerations for weaning the older patient can be found in Box 25-20.

---

**BOX 25-20** **CONSIDERATIONS for the Older Patient**

**Overcoming Barriers to Ventilator Liberation**

An elderly patient on mechanical ventilation poses a unique challenge to care givers. Successful weaning requires effective nursing interventions to address the patient's basic care needs.

- **Sleep Deprivation:** Learn the patient's normal sleep habits, establish a restful environment, and minimize interruptions for at least 6 hours each night and 2 hours of midday rest. Consult the pharmacist or doctor for sleep medication as needed at bedtime.
- **Imbalanced Nutrition: Less Than Body Requirements; and Risk for Fluid Volume Imbalance:** Consult the registered dietitian and begin delivery of recommended nutrition as soon as possible. Assess patient tolerance and increase to goal rate per order. Evaluate fluid balance each shift (input and output, weight, clinical examination) and discuss changes in intake and the possible need for diuretics with the physician.
- **Acute Pain; Anxiety; and Acute Confusion:** Administer analgesia per order, assessing need and effect of intervention by pain scale or physiologic parameters. Carefully evaluate possible etiology of anxiety or agitation; when pharmacologic intervention is indicated, titrate to achieve desired response using standardized sedation scale to limit sedation. Interventions are essential in the elderly patient (eg, orientation to place, date, and time; spiritual; massage). Adjust care for hearing impairment or for other sensory limitations that may contribute to confusion or anxiety.
- **Risk for Constipation; and Diarrhea:** Learn the patient's "usual" elimination pattern if possible; start with similar intervention and add more aggressive bowel regimen as needed to establish regular bowel movements. Evaluate factors (eg, medications or narcotics) that may alter bowel function, and ensure adequate hydration by enteral route if possible.
- **Risk for Activity Intolerance; and Impaired Bed Mobility or Impaired Physical Mobility:** Consult the physical or occupational therapist to evaluate functional capacity and initiate appropriate therapy. Begin getting patient out of bed as soon as possible, and encourage active range-of-motion exercises and participation in activities of daily living.

## Out-of-Hospital Mechanical Ventilation

Certain patients requiring invasive mechanical ventilation may be candidates for home care, chronic ventilator dependent facilities, or ventilator weaning rehabilitation. These patients may require full or partial invasive mechanical ventilation because of neuromuscular weakness, neurogenic hypoventilation, or cardiopulmonary diseases that result in ineffective gas exchange. The following conditions may warrant ventilator management post–acute stay:

- Neurologic disorders (eg, amyotrophic lateral sclerosis, Guillain–Barré syndrome, multiple sclerosis, muscular dystrophy, myasthenia gravis, poliomyelitis, polymyositis, spinal cord injury)
- Restrictive disorders (eg, interstitial pulmonary fibrosis, kyphoscoliosis, obesity, sarcoidosis)
- Obstructive disorders (eg, bronchiectasis, bronchiolitis obliterans, bronchopulmonary dysplasia, chronic bronchitis and emphysema, cystic fibrosis, obesity, sleep apnea syndromes)

## Clinical Applicability Challenges

---

### CASE STUDY

Mr. J. M. is a 32-year-old male who presents to the hospital with a 1-day history of dyspnea, fever, and chills. While being evaluated in the emergency department, he went into acute decompensated heart failure with hypoxia and increased work for breathing. He required emergent intubation and mechanical ventilation. His workup revealed positive influenza B and methicillin-resistant *Staphylococcus* aureus (MRSA) community-acquired pneumonia. His condition continued to worsen, resulting in adult respiratory distress syndrome (ARDS).

1. What are common complications associated with mechanical ventilation?
2. What factors will reduce complication risk of ventilator-associated pneumonia (VAP) in the patient receiving mechanical ventilation?
3. Identify common physiologic issues associated with mechanical ventilation and appropriate nursing interventions.

---

### WANT TO KNOW MORE?

A wide variety of resources to enhance your learning and understanding of this chapter are available on thePoint.

You will find:

- References
- Selected readings
- NCLEX-style review questions
- Internet resources
- And more!

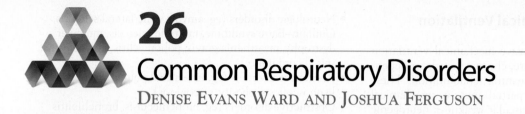

# 26

# Common Respiratory Disorders

### DENISE EVANS WARD AND JOSHUA FERGUSON

## LEARNING OBJECTIVES

**Based on the content in this chapter, the reader should be able to:**

1. Compare the etiology, pathophysiology, assessment, management, and prevention of community-acquired, hospital-acquired, and health care–associated pneumonia.
2. Discuss the pathophysiology, assessment, and management of pleural effusion.
3. Describe the pathophysiology, assessment, and management associated with pneumothorax.
4. Discuss the pathophysiology, assessment, management, and prevention of pulmonary embolism.
5. Explain the pathophysiology, assessment, management, and prevention of chronic obstructive pulmonary disease.
6. Describe the pathology, assessment, and management of a patient at various points on the asthma continuum, from mild attack to severe asthma.
7. Explain the key characteristics of hypoxemic acute respiratory failure and hypercapnic acute respiratory failure in terms of pathophysiology, assessment, and management.

Symptoms associated with common respiratory disorders can mimic or exacerbate other disease processes. Understanding the pathophysiology of the different respiratory disorders, in conjunction with an adequate physical assessment and patient history, will enhance the ability of the nurse to quickly assess and initiate the appropriate therapy. Prompt treatment often prevents complications for the patient and possibly saves the patient's life.

## Pneumonia

Pneumonia remains a common infection found in both the community and hospital, even though there have been advances in identifying people at risk and implementing preventive measures. Critical care nurses encounter pneumonia when it complicates the course of a serious illness or leads to acute respiratory distress.

Pneumonia is an infection involving the lower respiratory tract, caused by any class of organism (ie, bacteria, viruses, fungi, amoebae, or parasites) associated with human infections. Pneumonia is the leading cause of death worldwide in the United States; pneumonia combined with influenza is the ninth leasing cause of death.[1] In most cases, the diagnosis of community-acquired pneumonia (CAP) is straightforward; however, in the older population, other common disease such as cardiovascular disease can present with similar symptoms. Also, the older populations can present with atypical symptoms.[2] In the outpatient setting, CAP is typically a mild form of pneumonia; patients requiring hospitalization usually have a severe form of CAP.

Hospital admission behaviors for pneumonia can be inconsistent and often do not actually reflect disease severity, as there are no cardinal hallmarks of pneumonia.[2] A number of risk stratification tools have been developed to assist in objectively identifying actual pneumonia severity. Both the Infectious Disease Society of America (IDSA) and the American Thoracic Society (ATS) recommend either using the Pneumonia Severity Index (PSI) or the CURB-65 Score

(Box 26-1) as an adjunct tool to guide the initial treatment for adults with CAP. The PSI was developed as part of the Pneumonia Patient Outcomes Research Team (PORT) cohort study for the purpose of identifying patients with CAP at low risk for mortality. The PSI stratifies patients into five risk categories: the higher the score, the higher the risk of death, admission to the intensive care unit (ICU), or readmission, and the longer the length of stay.[3] Patients in risk classes I, II, and III are at low risk for death and can most likely be treated safely in the outpatient setting. Patients in risk classes IV and V should be hospitalized, with those in class V being admitted to the ICU.[3] While the PSI is a tool that has been validated, one of the significant drawbacks of this tool is that it requires a score to be based upon 20 different variables. Because of the complexity of calculating a score, the CURB-65 score is often preferred. The CURB-65 uses five easily measurable variables (see Box 26-1). Patients with a score of 0 or 1 can most likely be treated in the outpatient setting. Patients with a score of 2 should be hospitalized, those with a

---

**BOX 26-1** | **CURB-65 Tool for Determining the Initial Treatment of Adults with CAP**

**CURB-65 (one point is given for each positive finding)**
- **C**onfusion, disorientation to person, place, or time
- **U**rea greater than 7 mm/L
- **R**espiratory rate greater than 30 breaths/min
- **B**lood pressure SBP less than 90 mm Hg or DBP less than 60 mm Hg
- Age 65 years or older

**Score**
- 0–1 = outpatient management
- 2–3 = hospital admission (consider ICU admission with score of 3)
- 4–5 = ICU admission

From Jones BE, Jones J, Bewick T, et al: CURB-65 pneumonia severity assessment adapted for electronic decision support. Chest 140(1):156–163, 2011.

score of 3 should be assessed for possible ICU admission, and those with a score of 4 or 5 should be admitted to the ICU.[2]

Nosocomial pneumonia (NP), which includes hospital-acquired pneumonia (HAP), health care–associated pneumonia (HCAP), and ventilator-associated pneumonia (VAP), is the second most common form of nosocomial infections.[4] NP is defined as a pneumonia occurring 48 hours following admission and not incubating at the time of admission.[5,6] Box 26-2 lists current definitions of HAP, HCAP, and VA. The need for an HCAP category is currently being reevaluated. Researchers argue that there is often an overgeneralization of risk factors and an assumption that all patients who have criteria for HCAP will have an increased risk for multiple drug resistant (MDR) pathogens. Treating patients who have HCAP criteria leads to an underutilization of broad-spectrum antibiotics and patient risk. HAP and VAP, occurring at a rate of 5 to 20 cases per 1,000 hospital admissions, are significant causes of morbidity and mortality despite advances in antimicrobial therapy and advanced supportive measures.[2,7] In addition to increased morbidity and mortality, VAP is associated with poor clinical and economic outcomes.[8]

The American Thoracic Society HAP guidelines state that the criteria defining severe CAP can also be used to define severe HAP.[5] Severe HAP may occur in the ICU, with patients receiving mechanical ventilation being at the greatest risk, or it may precipitate admission to the ICU.[5] HAP and VAP independently contribute to mortality in critically ill patients; the attributable mortality rate is 33% to 50%.[8]

## Etiology

The specific etiology of a pneumonia varies greatly depending on host factors, geographical location, and underlying existing disease processes.[9] Of the four million cases of pneumonia every year in the United States, *Streptococcus pneumoniae* (pneumococcus) is the predominant pathogen[9] and the most common cause in patients requiring hospitalization for pneumonia. Other organisms frequently considered to be causative agents include *Haemophilus influenzae*, *Staphylococcus aureus*, and other gram-negative bacilli.[3,9] Drug-resistant *S. pneumoniae* is frequently seen in individuals older than 65 years of age.[3] Pathogens that should be considered in severe CAP requiring admission to the ICU

include *S. pneumoniae, Chlamydia pneumoniae, S. aureus, Mycobacterium tuberculosis, Legionella* species, respiratory viruses, and endemic fungi.[3]

Etiologic factors may be used to classify pneumonia as typical or atypical. Typical pneumonia is usually caused by a pathogen such as *S. pneumoniae, Streptococcus pyrogenes*, and *Staphylococcus aureus*. Atypical pneumonia is caused by pathogens such as *Mycoplasma pneumoniae, C. pneumoniae*, influenza virus, adenovirus, and *Legionella* species.[9] However, clinical symptoms usually do not help to distinguish between typical or atypical pneumonia.[9] In addition to the patient presentation, patient history (ie, exposure, recent travel, underlying health condition) often aids clinicians in identifying potential causative agents.[9] When evaluating for NP, timing of onset is an important factor in determining potential pathogens and associated outcomes in patients with HAP or VAP.[5] HAP or VAP occurring within 4 days of admission is more likely to be caused by bacteria sensitive to antibiotics; conversely, HAP or VAP occurring beyond this time period is likely to a MDR pathogen(s).[5] HAP may be polymicrobial; common causative pathogens include aerobic gram-negative bacilli, such as *Escherichia coli, Klebsiella pneumoniae*, and *Pseudomonas aeruginosa*; and gram-positive cocci such as *S. aureus*.[5] Polymicrobial pathogens are particularly common (greater than 50%) in patients receiving mechanical ventilation (VAP). Highly resistant gram-negative organisms (eg, *P. aeruginosa, Acinetobacter* species) and methicillin-resistant *S. aureus* are frequently seen in late-onset HAP but may occur in early-onset HAP in patients with risk factors for these pathogens.[4-6] The spectrum of potential pathogens can be defined by assessment of a variety of factors, including pneumonia severity, comorbidities, prior therapy (including antibiotics), and length of hospitalization.[5]

## Pathophysiology

Pneumonia is an inflammatory response to inhaled or aspirated foreign material or the uncontrolled multiplication of microorganisms invading the lower respiratory tract. This response results in the accumulation of neutrophils and other proinflammatory cytokines in the peripheral bronchi and alveolar spaces.[4] The body's defense system, which includes anatomical, mechanical, humoral, and cellular defenses, is designed to repel and remove organisms entering the respiratory tract. Many systemic diseases increase the patient's risk for pneumonia by altering the respiratory innate defense mechanism. Pneumonia develops when normal pulmonary defense mechanisms are impaired or overwhelmed, allowing microorganisms to multiply rapidly. The severity of pneumonia depends on the amount of material aspirated, the virulence of the organism, the amount of bacteria in the aspirate, and the host defenses.[4]

### Risk Factors

The means by which pathogens enter the lower respiratory tract include aspiration, inhalation, hematogenous spread from a distant site, and translocation. Risk factors that predispose an individual to one of these mechanisms may be categorized as conditions that enhance colonization of the oropharynx, conditions favoring aspiration, conditions requiring prolonged intubation, and host factors.[5]

**COLONIZATION OF THE OROPHARYNX.** Colonization of the oropharynx (colonization is the presence of microorganisms other than the normal flora in the absence of clinical evidence of infection) has been identified as an independent factor in the development of HAP. Gram-positive bacteria and anaerobic bacteria normally live in the oropharynx, and they occupy bacterial binding sites in the oropharyngeal mucosa. When normal oropharyngeal flora is destroyed, these binding sites are susceptible to colonization by pathogenic bacteria. Risk factors associated with oropharyngeal colonization include previous antibiotic therapy, increased age, dental plaque, smoking, and chronic diseases, such as chronic obstructive pulmonary disease (COPD), gastroesophageal reflux disease, alcoholism, diabetes mellitus, and malnutrition.[4]

The exact role the stomach plays in the development of pneumonia is controversial. In healthy individuals, the stomach is normally sterile because of the bactericidal activity of hydrochloric acid. However, when gastric pH increases above normal (pH greater than 4), as occurs with the use of proton pump inhibitors (PPI), histamine-2 antagonists, and antacids for stress ulcer prophylaxis, microorganisms are able to multiply.[5] Gastric colonization increases retrograde colonization of the oropharynx and increases the risk for pneumonia. Individuals at risk for gastric colonization include the elderly; those with achlorhydria, ileus, or upper gastrointestinal disease; and those receiving PPI, antacids, histamine-2 antagonists, or enteral feedings.[5] The gram-negative or pathogenic gram-positive organisms that have colonized the oropharynx are readily available for aspiration into the tracheobronchial tree.

**ASPIRATION.** Aspiration occurs frequently in healthy individuals while they are sleeping. The risk for clinically significant aspiration is increased in individuals unable to protect their airways—for example, patients with alcohol abuse, depressed level of consciousness, or dysphagia. (Dysphagia often occurs in patients who were recently intubated or had surgery on or around the vocal cords, and in the frail elderly.) Aspiration of bacteria found in dental plaques is receiving increased attention as a significant source of pneumonia.

**PROLONGED INTUBATION.** Prolonged intubation is associated with an increased risk of of pneumonia due to a patient's inability to clear secretions and microaspiration of secretions around the cuff of the endotracheal tube or tracheostomy. Ocasionally, the condensate that collects in the ventilator tubing can become contaminated with secretions and serve as a reservoir for bacterial growth.[10] Inhalation is an effective entry mechanism for *Legionella* species, M. tuberculosis, certain viruses, and fungi. Organisms are carried through small inhaled droplets from the tracheobronchial tree into the lower respiratory tract.[10]

**HOST FACTORS.** Hematogenous spread serves as a mechanism for the development of pneumonia; the pulmonary circulation provides a potential portal of entry for microbes. The pulmonary capillaries form a dense network in the walls of the alveoli that is ideal for gas exchange. Hematogenous microbes from distant sites of infection can migrate through this network and cause pneumonia. (Pneumonia can also cause bacteremia. Secondary bacteremia after pneumonia has been reported in 6% to 20% of pneumonia cases.)

Translocation of bacterial toxins from the bowel lumen to the mesenteric lymph, nodes, and eventually to the lungs, may possibly cause bacterial pneumonia. However, translocation has not yet been confirmed as a pathophysiologic mechanism.[5]

## Assessment

### History

A patient's history is extremely important in determining the correct treatment for pneumonia. Hemoptysis implies tissue necrosis, and is more common with pyogenic streptococcal pneumonia, anaerobic lung abscesses, *S. aureus*, necrotizing gram-negative organisms, and invasive *Aspergillus* species.[4] Extrapulmonary symptoms may indicate specific pathogens; for example, diarrhea and abdominal discomfort are present with *Legionella* species, and otitis media and pharyngitis are present with M. *pneumoniae*.[9,10] The clinical presentation in the older adult may vary somewhat from what is "typical" in a younger person (Box 26-3).[7]

A detailed social history provides further helpful information. It is important to determine whether the patient has had contact with animals, especially birds, bats, rats, and rabbits; this information can assist with the diagnosis of histoplasmosis, psittacosis, tularemia, and plague. In addition, a complete history, including dental hygiene history and place of residence, may assist in the differential diagnosis.[5]

Presenting features and findings of pneumonia are similar to those of a number of noninfectious conditions, necessitating a differential diagnosis. These conditions include heart failure, atelectasis, pulmonary thromboembolism, drug reactions, pulmonary hemorrhage, and acute respiratory distress syndrome (ARDS), malignancy, alveolar hemorrhage, and hypersensitivity pneumonitis.

### Physical Findings

The physical exam should include a focus on the respiratory, cardiovascular, neurologic, and renal systems. The nurse should assess for signs of hypoxemia (duskiness or cyanosis) and dyspnea. Patients presenting with new-onset respiratory symptoms (eg, cough, sputum production, dyspnea, pleuritic chest pain, presence of hemoptysis) usually have an accompanying fever and chills. Inspection of the chest includes assessing respiratory pattern and respiratory rate, observing the patient's posture and work of breathing, and inspecting for the presence of intercostal retractions. Percussion of the

---

**BOX 26-3** | *CONSIDERATIONS for the Older Patient: Pneumonia*

- **Presentation.** The usual symptoms (fever, chills, increased white blood count) may be absent. Confusion and tachypnea are common presenting symptoms in older patients with pneumonia. Other symptoms in the older patient include weakness, lethargy, failure to thrive, anorexia, abdominal pain, episodes of falling, incontinence, headache, delirium, and nonspecific deterioration.
- **Prevention.** People 65 years of age and older should recieve both the pneumococcal and influenza vaccines based upon CDC recommendations.

chest frequently reveals dullness with lobar pneumonia. Decreased breath sounds are heard on auscultation; egophony and tactile fremitus may also be present. Crackles or bronchial breath sounds are heard over the area of consolidation.

Extrapulmonary symptoms of pneumonia may include myalgia, new-onset seizures, periodontal disease, gastrointestinal symptoms, nonexudative pharyngitis, and splenomegaly. Confusion may be a subtle symptom in elderly patients.[9]

### Diagnostic Studies

Diagnostic tests are ordered for two reasons: to determine whether the pneumonia is the cause of the patient's symptoms and to determine the pathogen when pneumonia is present.[5] Table 26-1 summarizes the current ATS recommendations. The diagnostic evaluation must be performed rapidly to prevent delays in initiation of antibiotic therapy.

All patients should have a chest radiograph (posteroanterior and lateral views) to identify both the presence and location of infiltrates. The chest radiograph helps with differentiating pneumonia from other conditions and in identifying severe pneumonia, which is indicated by the presence of multilobular, rapidly spreading, or cavitary infiltrates.[9]

Microbiologic studies should be considered based upon the patient's pneumonia severity and underlying medical conditions. The value of examining lower respiratory secretions with Gram stain and culturing sputum is controversial; it is complicated by the quality of the specimen, transport, the rapidity and effectiveness of processing, and the timing in obtaining the specimen with administration of antibiotics. A negative sputum culture result does not necessarily rule out the presence of a bacterial pathogen. The ATS does not recommend routine use of Gram stain and sputum culture and advises that results must be interpreted cautiously;[3,5] on the other hand, the Infectious Diseases Society of America (IDSA) recommends routine Gram stain and culture of deep-cough specimens.[3] Lower respiratory secretions can be easily obtained in intubated patients using endotracheal aspiration. Nonquantitative endotracheal aspiration cultures may assist in excluding certain pathogens and may be helpful in modifying initial empirical treatment.[3] Routine use of quantitative invasive diagnostic techniques (mini bronchoalveolar lavage [mini-BAL], bronchoscopy with protected specimen brush [PSB] or bronchoalveolar lavage [BAL]) in severe pneumonia is not recommended by the ATS, the Centers for Disease Control and Prevention (CDC), or IDSA.[3,5] Current guidelines suggest that BAL or PSB be used only in selected circumstances, such as in nonresponse to antimicrobial therapy, immunosuppression, suspected tuberculosis in the absence of a productive cough, pneumonia with suspected neoplasm or foreign body, and conditions that require lung biopsy.[3,4] The IDSA recommends HIV testing for people age 15 to 54 years who have risk factors.[3] Urinary antigen testing for *Streptococcus pneumoniae* and *Legionella pneumophila*

**TABLE 26-1** Diagnostic Studies in Patients With Severe Community-Acquired Pneumonia or Severe Hospital-Acquired Pneumonia

| Study | Rationale |
|---|---|
| Chest radiograph (anterior–posterior and lateral) | For evaluation of patient who are likely to have pneumonia, to aid in differentiating diagnosis<br>To assess for pleural effusion |
| Pretreatment blood samples for culture (two sets of blood cultures from separate sites): Not necessary for community-acquired pneumonia (CAP), except for those with intensive care unit (ICU) admission, failure of outpatient antibiotic therapy, cavitary infiltrates, leukopenia, active alcohol abuse, severe liver disease, asplenia, positive pneumococcal urinary antigen test (UAT) result, and pleural effusion | To evaluate possible cause of severe CAP because of higher yield, great possibility of the presence of pathogen not covered by the usual empirical antibiotic therapy, and to narrow antibiotic treatment to treat the pathogen |
| Complete blood count | To document the presence of multiple-organ dysfunction |
| Serum electrolytes | To evaluate for leukopenia that is associated with high incidence of bacteremia |
| Renal and liver function | To help define severity of illness |
| Arterial blood gases (ABGs) | To define severity of illness<br>To determine need for supplemental oxygen and mechanical ventilation |
| Thoracentesis (if pleural effusion is 10 mm identified on lateral decubitus film) Pleural fluid studies, including:<br>White blood count with differential<br>Gram stain and acid-fast stain<br>Culture for bacteria, fungi, and mycobacteria | To rule out empyema |
| Pretreatment Gram stain and culture of expectorated sputum | Gram stain results will help broaden initial empirical coverage for less common pathogens and validate sputum culture results. |
| Obtain UA Trinary Antigen Testing for *Legionella pneumophila* and *Streptococcus pneumonia* | To rule out *Legionella* and *Streptococcus* |
| Respiratory Viral Testing | To rule out viral pathogens including influenza A (including subtypes), influenza B, RSV, parainfluenza, adenovirus, metapneumovirus, enterovirus/rhinovirus, *Bordetella pertussis*, *Mycoplasma* |

From data in Mandell LA, et al: Infectious Disease Society of America/American Thoracic Society consensus guidelines on the management of community-acquired pneumonia in adults. Clin Infect Dis 44(Suppl 2):S27–S72, 2007.

infections is routinely recommended based on the pneumonia severity. The advantage of this test is the rapidity with which results are obtained and their strong predictive value.[3] Viral polymerase chain reaction (PCR) testing for typical viral pneumonia pathogens are routinely recommended based on the rapidity in obtaining results and in providing additional information to support antibiotic de-escalation and tailoring of correct therapy.

## Management

### Antibiotic Therapy

Antibiotic therapy is the cornerstone of treatment for CAP, HAP, and VAP. Patients should initially be treated empirically, based on the disease severity, suspected causative pathogen, and corresponding antibiotic sensitivity.[5] Table 26-2 presents ATS guidelines for treatment of severe CAP, and Table 26-3 presents guidelines for treatment of HAP and VAP. According to the 2012 Surviving Sepsis Campaign, initial therapy should be instituted within 3 hours of initial hospital presentation.[11,12] Data suggest a reduced 30 day mortality in hospitalized patients with CAP who received their first dose of antibiotic therapy within 4 to 8 hours of arrival.[13]

Initial therapy should not be changed within the first 48 to 72 hours unless progressive deterioration is evident or initial microbiologic (blood or respiratory) cultures indicate a need to modify therapy.[3,5] De-escalation of antibiotic therapy occurs typically within 48 to 72 hours as the patient begins to improve clinically and as microbiology results are reported.

Factors to consider when determining the duration of therapy include concurrent illness, bacteremia, severity of pneumonia at the onset of antibiotic therapy, infecting pathogens, risk for MDR, and rapidity of clinical response.[5,7,9] Recommended duration of therapy is 7 to 10 days for *S. aureus* and *H. influenzae*; 10 to 14 days for *M. pneumoniae* and *C. pneumoniae*; and 8 to 14 days for *P. aeruginosa*, *Acinetobacter*

species, multilobar involvement, malnutrition, and a necrotizing gram-negative bacillus.[4]

### Supportive Therapy

Oxygen therapy may be required to maintain adequate gas exchange. Mechanical ventilation to correct hypoxemia is frequently required in both severe CAP and HAP. Humidified oxygen should be administered by mask or endotracheal tube to promote adequate ventilation. Aggressive pulmonary toilet is indicated to mobilize secretions, open closed alveoli, and promote oxygenation. Adequate nutritional support is critical. In addition, a nutritional consult should be initiated with implementation of appropriate enteral or parenteral therapy.

## Prevention

A complete understanding of the pathogenesis of HAP enables the critical care nurse to develop interventions to prevent the onset of pneumonia. The CDC, IDSA, and ATS consider education the cornerstone of an effective infection control program and the prevention of HAP.[3,5] Targets of opportunity in the prevention of HAP include strict infection control, hand washing using an alcohol-based disinfectant, surveillance for pathogens, and early removal of invasive lines.[5] The American Association of Critical-Care Nurses (AACN) has published guidelines for preventing VAP as part of their AACN Practice Alerts (see Chapter 25). According to the evidence-based directive from AACN, in all patients receiving mechanical ventilation as well as those at high risk for aspiration, the head of the bed should be elevated at 30 to 45 degrees unless medically contraindicated; endotracheal tubes should have dorsal lumens above the cuff to allow drainage and continuous tracheal secretions; and patient ventilator circuits should be changed based on need because of contamination rather than by routine.[14] In addition

| TABLE 26-2 | Recommended Therapy for Community-Acquired Pneumonia, Inpatients* |
|---|---|
| **Type of Patient** | **Therapy†,‡** |
| Non-ICU inpatient | A respiratory fluoroquinolone<br>A β-lactam *plus* macrolide |
| ICU patient | Intravenous β-lactam (cefotaxime, ceftriaxone, or ampicillin/sulbactam) *plus* either azithromycin or a respiratory fluoroquinolone (for penicillin-allergic patient, a respiratory fluoroquinolone and clindamycin are recommended) |
| At risk for *Pseudomonas aeruginosa* | Selected intravenous antipneumococcal, antipseudomonal β-lactam (cefepime, imipenem, meropenem, piperacillin/tazobactam) *plus* intravenous antipseudomonal fluoroquinolone (ciprofloxacin or levofloxacin)<br>or<br>Intravenous antipneumococcal, antipseudomonal β-lactam (cefepime, imipenem, meropenem, piperacillin/tazobactam) *plus* intravenous macrolide (azithromycin) and aminoglycoside<br>or<br>Intravenous antipneumococcal antipseudomonal β-lactam (cefepime, imipenem, meropenem, piperacillin/tazobactam) *plus* aminoglycoside and intravenous antipneumococcal fluoroquinolone (for penicillin-allergic patients, substitute aztreonam for above β-lactam |
| At risk for CA-methicillin-resistant *Staphylococcus aureus* (MRSA) | Add vancomycin or linezolid to current antibiotic regime if positive or at risk for MRSA. |

*Excludes patients at risk for HIV.
†Combination therapy required.
‡In no particular order.
Reprinted with permission from the Infectious Disease Society of America/American Thoracic Society consensus guidelines on the management of community-acquired pneumonia in adults. Clin Infect Dis 44(Suppl 2):s27–s72, 2007.

TABLE 26-3 Antibiotic Therapy for Patients With Hospital-Acquired or Ventilator-Associated Pneumonia

| Initial Empiric Antibiotic Therapy for Hospital-Acquired Pneumonia or Ventilator-Associated Pneumonia in Patients With No Known Risk Factors for Multidrug-Resistant Pathogens, Early Onset, and Any Disease Severity | |
|---|---|
| **Potential Pathogen** | **Recommended Antibiotic** |
| Streptococcus pneumoniae* <br> Haemophilus influenzae <br> Methicillin-sensitive Staphylococcus aureus <br> Antibiotic-sensitive enteric gram-negative bacilli <br> Escherichia coli <br> Klebsiella pneumoniae <br> Enterobacter species <br> Proteus species <br> Serratia marcescens | Ceftriaxone <br> or <br> Levofloxacin, moxifloxacin, or ciprofloxacin <br> or <br> Ampicillin/sulbactam <br> or <br> Ertapenem |

| Initial Empiric Therapy for Hospital-Acquired Pneumonia, Ventilator-Associated Pneumonia, and Health Care–Associated Pneumonia in Patients With Late-Onset Disease or Risk Factors for Multidrug-Resistant Pathogens and All Disease Severity | |
|---|---|
| **Potential Pathogens** | **Combination Antibiotic Therapy**[†] |
| Pathogens listed in above table and MDR pathogens | Antipseudomonal cephalosporin (cefepime, ceftazidime) <br> or |
| Pseudomonas aeruginosa <br> Klebsiella pneumoniae (ESBL+)‡ <br> Acinetobacter species§ | Antipseudomonal carbapenem (imipenem or meropenem) <br> or <br> β-Lactam/β-lactamase inhibitor (piperacillin/tazobactam) plus <br> Antipseudomonal fluoroquinolone+(ciprofloxacin or levofloxacin) <br> or <br> Aminoglycoside(amikacin, gentamicin, or tobramycin) plus‡ |
| MRSA <br> Legionella pneumophila+‡ | Linezolid or vancomycin |

*The frequency of penicillin-resistant S. pneumoniae and multidrug-resistant S. pneumoniae is increasing; levofloxacin and moxifloxacin are preferred to cipro-floxacin, and the role of other new quinolones, such as gatifloxacin, has not been established.
†Initial antibiotic therapy should be adjusted or streamlined on the basis of microbiologic data and clinical response to therapy.
‡If MRSA risk factors are present or there is a high incidence locally.
§If an ESBL+ strain, such as K. pneumoniae, or an Acinetobacter species is suspected, a carbapenem is a reliable choice. If L. pneumophila is suspected, the combination antibiotic regimen should include a macrolide (eg, azithromycin) or a fluoroquinolone (eg, ciprofloxacin or levofloxacin) should be used rather than an aminoglycoside.
Reprinted with permission from the Infectious Diseases Society of America/American Thoracic Society consensus guidelines for the management of adults with hospital-acquired, ventilator-associated, and health care–associated pneumonia. Am J Respir Crit Care Med 171:388–416, 2005.

to these guidelines, the AACN has also published guidelines for aggressive oral care in patients with mechanical ventilation. These guidelines include frequent oral care and use of oral moisturizing agents.[14] The CDC has published comprehensive guidelines on the prevention of HAP.[5] Internet access to the CDC guidelines is available at http://www.cdc.gov.

# Pleural Effusion

## Pathophysiology

The pleural space is the space that exists between the visceral pleura, which lines the lungs, and the parietal pleura, which lines the interior chest wall. It is normal to have a small amount of fluid in the pleura space; this fluid allows for sliding between the lung and chest wall during normal inspiration and expiration.[15] The vessels in the parietal pleura are responsible for most of the production of pleural fluid under normal conditions.

The lymphatics of the parietal pleura assist with resorption of the fluid.[12] Under normal conditions, the fluid produced by the vessels in the pleura is a small amount and the lymphatics are able to maintain a constant rate of reabsorption to prevent excessive fluid in the space. However, some pathologic conditions can cause an excess of fluid to accumulate in the

pleural space, causing a pleural effusion. A pleural effusion is the presences of fluid within that space that exceeds the normal amount. This can be caused by excessive fluid production, alteration in the pleural membranes, or the inability of the lymphatics to drain the excessive fluid.[15]

Pleural effusions are caused by one of the following mechanisms:[16]

- Increased pressure in pulmonary capillaries (eg, heart failure, massive PE)
- Increased capillary permeability (eg, pneumonia, malignancy, infection, pancreatitis)
- Decreased plasma osmotic pressure (eg, hypoalbuminemia, hypoproteinemia, cirrhosis)
- Increased intrapleural negative pressure (eg, atelectasis, trapped lung)
- Impaired lymphatic drainage of the pleural space (eg, pleural malignancy or infection)

## Transudates

Transudative pleural effusions, unilateral or bilateral, are ultrafiltrates of plasma, indicating that the pleural membranes are not diseased.[17] Systemic factors cause the fluid accumulation in transudative pleural effusion. Almost half the pleural effusions diagnosed in ICU patients will be transudative.[14] In heart failure, an increase in pulmonary venous pressure contributes to the formation of pleural effusions. Treatment focuses on reducing afterload and improving cardiac output with diuretics, inotropes, or both.[17] Another cause of transudative pleural effusions is atelectasis, which may cause pleural fluid to accumulate because of a decrease in pleural pressure. The fluid continues to accumulate until the pleural–parietal pleural interstitial pressure gradient returns to normal.[18] Other causes of transudative pleural effusions include cirrhosis, nephrotic syndrome, malignancy blocking the lymphatic outflow, and peritoneal dialysis.

### Exudates

Exudative pleural effusions result from local factors, such as parapneumonic effusions caused by bacteria, virus, tuberculosis, pulmonary embolism, infection, drugs, trauma and malignancy.[19] Exudative pleural effusions satisfy any one of the following criteria, known as Light's criteria:[16,20]

- Pleural fluid-to-serum protein ratio greater than 0.5
- Pleural fluid-to-serum LDH ratio greater than 0.6
- Pleural fluid LDH that is two thirds of the upper normal limit for serum LDH

Four million Americans are affected by bacterial pneumonia, 20% of whom require hospitalization. Forty percent of these hospitalized patients develop effusions.[19] Malignancies are the second most common cause of exudative pleural effusions. If a massive effusion opacifies, an entire hemithorax, metastatic disease, or chylothorax should be suspected. Other causes of exudative pleural effusion are tuberculosis, trauma, pancreatitis, mesotheliomas, and esophageal perforation.[17]

A hemothorax, which is often associated with either blunt or penetrating chest trauma, is an example of an exudative pleural effusion that is bloody (see Chapter 55).[12,15] Other causes are invasive procedures (placement of central venous catheter, thoracentesis) and anticoagulation therapy. Empyema refers to gross pus in the pleural cavity and requires drainage with a chest tube or surgery. Chylothorax refers to the presence of chyle or a fatty substance in the pleural space and is usually caused by disruption or obstruction of the thoracic duct outlet.[15] Malignancies, surgery, trauma, intra-abdominal process, and connective tissues disease can also cause an exudative pleural effusion.[15]

## Assessment

### History and Physical Findings

Subjective findings include shortness of breath and pleuritic chest pain, depending on the amount of fluid accumulation. Objective findings include tachypnea and hypoxemia if ventilation is impaired, dullness to percussion, and decreased breath sounds over the involved area.

### Diagnostic Studies

Diagnosis can be made by chest radiograph, ultrasound, or a CT scan. When a pleural effusion is suspected on the basis of physical examination and is confirmed radiologically, obtaining a sample of pleural fluid is necessary to determine whether the pleural effusion is transudative or exudative and infectious. Aspiration of pleural fluid from the pleural space is called thoracentesis. The laboratory tests performed on the pleural fluid obtained by thoracentesis are listed in Table 26-4.

## Management

Treatment of the underlying cause of the pleural effusion is necessary. Drainage of the pleural effusion by thoracentesis, chest tube placement, or surgery may be indicated depending on the severity of patient symptoms and size of effusion.

## Pneumothorax

A pneumothorax occurs when air enters the pleural space between the visceral and parietal pleurae, producing partial or complete lung collapse.

**TABLE 26-4** Assessment of Pleural Fluid

| Test | Comment |
|---|---|
| Red blood cell count <100,000/mm$^3$ | Trauma, malignancy, pulmonary embolism |
| Hematocrit >50% of peripheral blood | Hemothorax |
| White blood cell count (WBC) >50,000–100,000/mm$^3$ | Grossly visible pus, otherwise total WBC less useful than WBC differential |
| >50% neutrophils | Acute inflammation or infection |
| >50% lymphocytes | Tuberculosis, malignancy |
| >10% Eosinophils | Most common: hemothorax, pneumothorax; also benign |
| >5% Mesothelial cells | Asbestos effusions, drug reaction, paragonimiasis; tuberculosis less likely |
| Glucose <60 mg/dL | Infection, malignancy, tuberculosis, rheumatoid, hemothorax, Paragonimiasis, Churg–Strauss syndrome |
| Amylase >200 units/dL | Pleuritis, esophageal perforation, pancreatic disease, malignancy, ruptured ectopic pregnancy Isoenzyme profile: salivary–esophageal disease, malignancy (especially lung) |
| pH <7.0 | Complicated Parapneumonic effusion |
| pH <7.2 | Systemic acidosis, esophageal rupture, rheumatoid pleuritis, tuberculous pleuritis, malignant pleural disease, hemothorax, paragonimiasis, or Churg–Strauss syndrome. |
| Triglyceride >110 mg/dL | Chylothorax |
| Microbiologic studies | Etiology of infection |
| Cytology | Diagnostic of malignancy (adenocarcinoma, benign or malignant mesothelial cells) |

Adapted from Light RW: Physiology of pleural fluid production. In: Shield TW, LoCicero J, Reed CE, et al (eds): General Thoracic Surgery, 7th ed. Philadelphia, PA: Lippincott Williams & Wilkins, 2009, pp 763–770.

## Pathophysiology

Air or gas enters the pleural space as a result of a rupture in either the visceral or partial pleura and chest wall. When this occurs, air in the lung parenchyma enters the pleural cavity during inspiration, but is unable to escape during expiration. The accumulation of the air in the pleural cavity will eventually cause an interruption in the normal physiology between the lung and the chest wall, preventing the normal expansion of the lung (Fig. 26-1).[21] When the pleural pressure rises, elasticity of the lung causes it to collapse, and the mediastinum shifts to the contralateral side, which can cause compression of the great vessels and eventually compression of the contralateral lung if not treated.[22] The main consequence of lung collapse is a decrease in both vital capacity and arterial $PO_2$. In addition, patients with low arterial $PO_2$ also have an increase in the alveolar–arterial partial pressure of oxygen ($PAO_2$–$PaO_2$) gradient, a decreased ventilation–perfusion ratio, and an intrapulmonary shunt resulting in hypoxemia.[22]

There are two types of pneumothorax: spontaneous and traumatic. Spontaneous pneumothorax is any pneumothorax that develops without any trauma. In the past, spontaneous pneumothorax was divided into two classifications: primary and secondary pneumothorax. The pneumothorax was designated as primary when the patient did not have evidence of an underlying lung disease, and as secondary when there was evidence of an underlying lung disease such as COPD, asthma, Marfan syndrome, lung cancer, necrotizing tuberculosis, or cystic fibrosis. Recent publications suggest that spontaneous pneumothorax should not be classified as primary or secondary, but instead should be viewed on a continuum based on the presentations of patient's symptoms.[23]

The most common causes of a traumatic pneumothorax in critically ill patients are invasive procedures and barotrauma.[20,22] (See Chapter 55 for a discussion of blunt and penetrating trauma as causes of pneumothorax.) Barotrauma can be a complication of positive pressure mechanical ventilation. Pulmonary interstitial gas or emphysema is the initial radiographic indication of barotrauma. The mechanically ventilated patient is at risk for development of a tension pneumothorax. A tension pneumothorax occurs when the pressure of air in the pleural space exceeds atmospheric pressure. As pressures in the thorax increase, the mediastinum shifts to the contralateral side, placing torsion on the inferior vena cava and decreasing venous return to the right side of the heart (see Fig. 26-1).[22]

## Assessment

### History and Physical Findings

The patient complains of sudden onset of acute pleuritic chest pain localized to the affected lung. The pleuritic chest pain is usually accompanied by shortness of breath, increased work of breathing, and dyspnea. Chest wall movement may be uneven because the affected side does not expand as much as the healthy side. Breath sounds are distant or absent. Chest percussion produces a hyperresonant sound. Tachycardia occurs frequently in all types of pneumothorax. Tension pneumothorax is a life-threatening condition manifested by respiratory distress (Box 26-4).

### Diagnostic Studies

A chest radiograph is done to confirm the diagnosis of simple pneumothorax.

A chest CT scan is sometimes used to help with diagnosis, depending on the area and size of the pneumothorax. The diagnosis of tension pneumothorax should be made by physical exam alone. Physical symptoms of a tension pneumothorax would include absent or decrease breath sounds, tracheal deviation away from the affected lung, severe hypoxemia, and hypotension. Obtaining a chest film in such cases would only

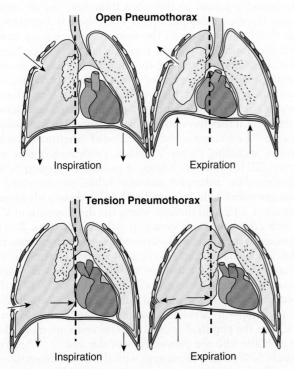

**Open Pneumothorax**

Inspiration            Expiration

**Tension Pneumothorax**

Inspiration            Expiration

**FIGURE 26-1**   Open or communicating pneumothorax (**top**) and tension pneumothorax (**bottom**). In an open pneumothorax, air enters the chest during inspiration and exits during expiration. There may be slight inflation of the affected lung due to a decrease in pressure as air moves out of the chest. In tension pneumothorax, air can enter but not leave the chest. As the pressure in the chest increases, the heart and great vessels are compressed, and the mediastinal structures are shifted toward the opposite side of the chest. The trachea is pushed from its normal midline position toward the opposite side of the chest, and the unaffected lung is compressed. (From Porth C: Essentials of Pathophysiology, 3rd ed. Philadelphia, PA: Lippincott Williams & Wilkins, 2011, p 571.)

---

**QSEN  BOX 26-4   *PATIENT SAFETY***

**Signs and Symptoms of Tension Pneumothorax**
- Hypoxemia (early sign)
- Apprehension
- Respiratory distress (severe tachypnea)
- Increasing peak and mean airway pressures, decreasing compliance, and auto–positive end-expiratory pressure (auto-PEEP) in patients receiving mechanical ventilation
- Cardiovascular collapse (heart rate >140 beats/min with any of the following: peripheral cyanosis, hypotension, pulseless electrical activity)

delay urgent treatment, which is the immediate placement of a chest tube on the affected side.

## Management

Supplemental oxygen should be administered to all patients with pneumothorax because oxygen accelerates the rate of air resorption from the pleural space.[21] If the pneumothorax is 15% to 20%, no medical intervention is required.[24] If the pneumothorax is greater than 20%, a chest tube is placed in the apical and anterior aspect of the pleural space to assist air removal. Connecting the chest tube to underwater seal drainage alone is usually adequate to resolve the pneumothorax. If the pneumothorax persists after 12 to 24 hours of underwater seal drainage, 15 to 20 cm $H_2O$ suction should be applied to facilitate closure.[24]

When treating tension pneumothorax, if a chest tube is not immediately available, a large-bore (16-or 18-gauge) needle should be placed into the anterior second intercostal space. After needle insertion, a chest tube is placed and connected to underwater seal drainage. When the tension pneumothorax is relieved, the effect is rapid and is evidenced by an improvement in oxygenation, a decrease in heart rate, and an increase in blood pressure.

## Pulmonary Embolism

Venous thromboembolism (VTE) includes both pulmonary embolism (PE) and deep vein thrombosis. If this condition is not quickly recognized and treated immediately, it can have deadly consequences, including sudden death when a thrombus breaks loose and enters into the pulmonary circulation. Current estimates suggest that 1 to 2 per 1000 people will be affected by VTE disease. Approximately 10% to 30% of the people with VTE will die within 1 month of diagnosis.[25] It has been determined that illnesses and surgeries requiring hospitalization are a major risk factor for the development of VTE. Hospitals must now have aggressive prevention guidelines because the Institute of Medicine has declared the development of a VTE while hospitalized is a medical error.[26]

## Etiology

There are number of environmental and genetic factors that contribute to the risk of developing VTE. Acquired risk factors include age, recent surgery, cancer, and thrombophilia. Risk factors that increase the incidence of VTE are listed in Box 26-5. Most incidents of PE occur when a thrombus (clot) breaks loose and migrates to the pulmonary arteries, obstructing part of the pulmonary vascular tree (Fig. 26-2). Nonthrombotic causes of PE include fat (from long bone fracture), air (during neurosurgery, or from central venous catheters), and amniotic fluid (occurs during active labor), but these are much less common than thromboembolism.[27]

Thrombus formation usually occurs in a large deep vein. Lower extremities are a common area for the formation of deep vein thrombosis (DVT) Other sites for thrombus formation include the right side of the heart (as in untreated atrial fibrillation) and the veins in the pelvic region.[27]

---

| BOX 26-5 | Risk Factors for Thromboembolism |
| --- | --- |

**Risk Factors**
Cancer
Major surgery or trauma
Prolonged immobilization, including long distance flights or recent hospital stay
Pregnancy and puerperium
Contraceptives and hormone replacement therapy
Inherited blood clotting disorders
Previous venous thromboembolism
Atrial fibrillation
Heart Failure
Obesity
Smoking

Data from Bauersachs, RM: Clinical presentation of deep vein thrombosis and pulmonary embolism. Best Pract Res Clin Haematol 25(3):243–251, 2012.

## Pathophysiology

A cascade of events begins the process of thromboembolus development. Virchow's triad of factors, which include venous stasis, hypercoagulability, and vascular endothelium damage, has long been believed to contribute to venous thromboembolism. The development of venous stasis occurs when there is slowing of blood flow return to the heart. Immobility, heart failure, and varicose veins are conditions that predispose a person to thrombus formation due to venous stasis. Hypercoagulability occurs when there is disruption in the fine balance between the activation of clotting factors and the fibrinolytic system that prevents thrombus formation. Common reasons for this disruption include trauma, surgery, malignancy, pregnancy, oral contraceptive use, and hormone replacement therapy.[27] Patients with cancer have a greater risk if they are receiving chemotherapy or radiation therapy, or if they have undergone surgery or have metastatic disease.[26] Less common factors included inherited thrombophilias, including Factor V Leiden, prothrombin gene mutation 20210, and deficiencies of protein C, protein S, and antithrombin. Inherited thrombophilias are suspected in younger individuals diagnosed with VTE, those with a family history of VTE, and those in whom the development of VTE is not correlated with common risk factors (Box 26-5).[28] Damage to the vessel wall causes adhesion and aggregation of platelets and contributes to the activation of clotting factors. Common reasons for damage vessels include local trauma, infection, surgical incisions, and atherosclerosis.[28] DVTs that form in the calf are considered stable clots because only 20% of patients will develop a pulmonary embolus. However, DVTs in the popliteal and ileofemoral veins are more likely to embolize into the pulmonary vascular system.[28] Approximately 50% to 70% of patients with the initial diagnosis of a PE will subsequently be diagnosed with a DVT in the lower extremity.[27] Occlusion in the pulmonary vascular artery by an embolus can produce both pulmonary and hemodynamic changes.

Respiratory dead space within the pulmonary system occurs when the alveoli are ventilated but not perfused by the blood that normally flows through the pulmonary arteries and capillaries. This produces areas of mismatched ventilation and perfusion. As a result, well-ventilated alveoli are underperfused, and gas exchange is compromised. Pulmonary

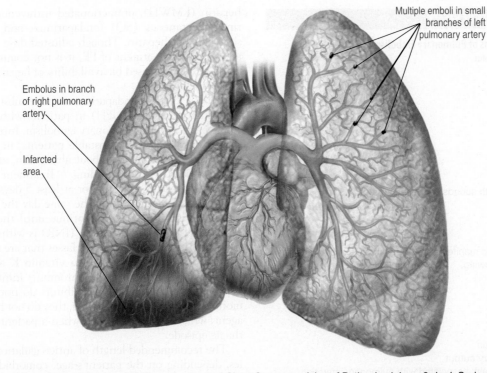

Multiple emboli in small branches of left pulmonary artery

Embolus in branch of right pulmonary artery

Infarcted area

**FIGURE 26-2**   Sites of pulmonary emboli. (From Anatomical Chart Company: Atlas of Pathophysiology, 3rd ed. Springhouse, PA: Lippincott Williams & Wilkins, 2010, p 107.)

vascular constriction resulting from decreased carbon dioxide, which is normally present in pulmonary arterial blood. Blood flow is shunted from the under-perfused alveoli to alveoli that are being perfused. This causes a state where perfusion is now greater than normal ventilation. When this occurs, a percentage of the blood will not be perfused and will return to the left side of the heart without having experienced gas exchange, leading to hypoxemia. Direct physiologic pulmonary changes to adapt to the decreased gas exchange include increased minute ventilation, decreased vital capacity, increased airway resistance, and decreased diffusing capacity.[29]

The severity of hemodynamic change in pulmonary embolism depends on the size of the embolus and degree of pulmonary vascular obstruction as well as on the preexisting status of the cardiopulmonary system. In patients with no previous cardiopulmonary disease, there is a relationship between the degree of pulmonary artery obstruction and the pulmonary artery pressure. Increased right ventricular afterload results from obstruction of the pulmonary vascular bed by embolism. In patients with no preexisting cardiopulmonary disease, obstruction of less than 20% of the pulmonary vascular bed produces compensatory events that minimize adverse hemodynamic consequences.[29] Cardiac output is maintained by increases in both right ventricular stroke volume and heart rate, and recruitment and distention of pulmonary vessels occur, producing normal or near-normal pulmonary artery pressure and pulmonary vascular resistance.[29] When the degree of pulmonary vascular obstruction exceeds 30% to 40%, increases in pulmonary artery pressure occur, followed by modest increases in right atrial pressure.[29] As the degree of pulmonary artery obstruction exceeds 50% to 60%, compensatory mechanisms are overcome, producing

a decrease in cardiac output and dramatic increases in right atrial pressure.[29] Patients with preexisting cardiopulmonary disease have degrees of pulmonary hypertension that are disproportionate to the degree of embolic obstruction.[29] Severe pulmonary hypertension may develop from a relatively small reduction of pulmonary blood flow.

## Assessment

Pulmonary embolism is often call "the great masquerader" because of its nonspecific signs and symptoms.[30] It is common for other diagnosis, such as pneumonia or heart failure, be ruled out before considering a pulmonary embolus.[31] However, pulmonary embolism should be suspected in a patient with new onset of dyspnea, tachycardia, or sustained hypotension without other explanations. Other symptoms include chest pain, coughing with or without hemoptysis, clinical signs of deep vein thrombosis, and syncope.[30] It is also common that a DVT or embolus produces no significant symptoms and may be an incidental finding when the patient undergoes imaging for other reasons.[2] Signs and symptoms of pulmonary embolism are listed in Box 26-6.

Clinical evaluation may indicate a need for further studies but is not reliable for confirmation or exclusion of the diagnosis of pulmonary embolism.[29] Computed pulmonary angiography (CTPA) is recommended for confirming the diagnosis in patients with suspected pulmonary embolus. However, CTPA uses contrast dye, which may be contradicted for patients with acute kidney disease or in patients with an allergy to contrast dye. Ventilation–perfusion (VQ) scans will be used in such patients to help with the diagnosis, even though VQ scans are not as sensitive as the CTPA for confirming a diagnosis.[31] Transthoracic echocardiogram is often

### Signs and Symptoms of Pulmonary Embolism

**Small to Moderate Embolus**
- Dyspnea
- Tachypnea
- Tachycardia
- Chest pain
- Mild fever
- Hypoxemia
- Apprehension
- Cough
- Diaphoresis
- Decreased breath sounds over affected area
- Rales
- Wheezing

**Massive Embolus**

A more pronounced manifestation of the above signs and symptoms, plus the following:
- Cyanosis
- Restlessness
- Anxiety
- Confusion
- Hypotension
- Cool, clammy skin
- Decreased urinary output
- Pleuritic chest pain: associated with pulmonary infarction
- Hemoptysis: associated with pulmonary infarction

**Signs of Pulmonary Embolism in Intensive Care Patients**
- Worsening hypoxemia or hypocapnia in a patient on spontaneous ventilation
- Worsening hypoxemia and hypercapnia in a sedate patient on controlled mechanical ventilation
- Worsening dyspnea, hypoxemia, and a reduction in $PaCO_2$ in a patient with chronic lung disease and known carbon dioxide retention
- Unexplained fever
- Sudden elevation in pulmonary artery pressure or central venous pressure in a hemodynamically monitored patient

used to determine if there is associated cardiac dysfunction related to a PE.

Deep vein thrombosis (DVT) is often associated with acute pulmonary embolism. It is important to assess for a DVT when patients presents with symptoms of an acute PE or unilateral leg swelling and tenderness. Common studies used to assist with the diagnosis of DVT include the D-dimer blood test and ultrasonography. However, a positive D-dimer does not necessarily indicate a DVT/PE. The clinician should always follow-up with an ultrasound of the lower extremities when suspecting a DVT in a patient that has positive D-dimer.

## Management

Heparin and thrombolytic agents are used to treat pulmonary embolism. Guidelines developed by the American College of Chest Physicians (ACCP) for the treatment of venous thromboembolism are shown in Table 26-5.[32]

Patients with DVT or pulmonary embolism should immediately start treatment with parenteral anticoagulant therapy. Options include subcutaneous low molecular weight

heparin (LMWH), unfractionated intravenous (IV) heparin, subcutaneous (SQ) fondaparinux, and adjusted-dose subcutaneous heparin. Though adjusted-dose SQ heparin is an option for treatment of PE, it is not commonly used because of the decreased bioavailability of heparin when given subcutaneously.

LMWH or SQ fondaparinux can be substituted for unfractionated heparin (UFH) in patients with DVT and in stable patients with pulmonary embolism. Intravenous UFH should only be used in unstable patients, in obese patient when there are concerns about absorption, and in patients with increased risk of bleeding.[32] Treatment with heparin or LMWH should continue for at least 5 days. Oral anticoagulation, should be started the same day the initial IV/SQ treatment is initiated and continue until the patient's international normalization ratio (INR) is within therapeutic treatment range. Current drug classes that are recommended for oral anticoagulation include vitamin K antagonist (ie, warfarin) and factor X a/IIa (thrombin) inhibitors. Unlike Warfarin, the factor Xa/IIa inhibitors do not require close monitoring of the INR. However, they do not have a reversal agent, which could be needed when a patient has a hemorrhagic episode.[33]

The recommended length of anticoagulation therapy varies, depending on the patient's age, comorbidities, and the likelihood of recurrence of pulmonary embolism or DVT. In most patients, anticoagulation therapy with warfarin should be continued for 3 to 6 months.[33] The first episode of an unprovoked DVT should be treated for at least 3 months. After 3 months, the patient should be evaluated for potential risks versus benefits before extending therapy.[32] Patients with new-onset DVT and a risk factor (eg, cancer, inhibitor deficiency state) or recurrent venous thrombosis should be treated indefinitely.[32] Patients with massive pulmonary embolism or severe iliofemoral thrombosis may require a longer period of heparin therapy.[32] Anticoagulation using LMWH for several months is effective in patients who have contraindications to warfarin (eg, pregnant women) but who can safely take heparin.[32]

Thrombolytic therapy is only recommended for patients with acute massive pulmonary embolism who are hemodynamically unstable and not prone to bleeding.[33] All thrombolytic agents act systemically and have the potential to lyse a fresh platelet–fibrin clot anywhere and cause bleeding at that site.[32] Intracranial disease, recent intracranial or spinal surgery, trauma, history of hemorrhagic stroke, and hemorrhagic diseases are contraindications to thrombolytic therapy. Urokinase, streptokinase, and recombinant tissue plasminogen activator are the thrombolytic agents approved for treating pulmonary embolism and venous thromboembolism. Heparin therapy is not administered concurrently with thrombolytics; however, thrombolytic therapy is followed by administration of heparin, then oral anticoagulation.

An inferior vena cava filter is recommended to prevent pulmonary embolism in patients with contraindications to heparin therapy (risk for major bleeding or drug sensitivity).[32] Placement of an inferior vena cava filter is also recommended in patients with recurring thromboembolism despite adequate anticoagulation, chronic recurrent embolism and pulmonary hypertension, and concurrent surgical pulmonary embolectomy or pulmonary endarterectomy procedure.[32]

**TABLE 26-5**    American College of Chest Physicians Recommendations for Treatment of Venous Thromboembolism

| Anticoagulation Guidelines for | Recommended Therapy |
| --- | --- |
| **Unfractionated Heparin (UFH)** | |
| Suspected VTE | • Obtain baseline aPTT, PT, CBC.<br>• Check for contraindications to heparin therapy.<br>• Give heparin 5,000 units IV.<br>• Order imaging study. |
| Confirmed VTE | • Re-bolus with heparin 80 units/kg IV or 5,000 units, and start maintenance infusion at 18 units/kg/h or 1,300 units/h.<br>• Check aPTT at 6 h; maintain a range corresponding to a therapeutic heparin level.<br>• Start warfarin therapy on day 1 at 5 mg; adjust subsequent daily dose according to INR. (do not give a bolus dose)<br>• Stop heparin after 3–5 d of combined therapy, when INR is 2.0 (2.0–3.0) for 24 h.<br>• Anticoagulate with warfarin for at least 3 mo (target INR 2.5; 2.0–3.0). |
| **Low-Molecular-Weight Heparin (LMWH)** | |
| Suspected VTE | • Obtain baseline aPTT, PT, CBC.<br>• Check for contraindication to heparin therapy.<br>• Give UFH, 5,000 units IV.<br>• Order imaging study. |
| Confirmed VTE | • Give LMWH (enoxaparin), 1 mg/kg subcutaneously every 12 h or 1.5 mg/kg daily<br>• Start warfarin therapy on day 1 at 5 mg; adjust subsequent daily dose according to the INR.<br>• Consider checking platelet count between days 3 and 5.<br>• Stop LMWH after at least 4–5 d of combined therapy, when INR is 2.0 on 2 consecutive days.<br>• Anticoagulate with warfarin for at least 3 mo (goal INR 2.5; 2.0–3.0), then it is recommended to continue with low intensity therapy (INR range 1.5–1.9) with less frequent monitoring over stopping treatment. |

VTE, venous thromboembolism; aPTT, activated partial thromboplastin time; PT, prothrombin time; INR, international normalized ratio; CBC, complete blood count.
From American College of Chest Physicians: Ninth ACCP consensus conference on Antithrombotic and Thrombolytic Therapy. Chest 41(2)(suppl)e419s–e494s2012;1412supple: e419S–e12.

## Prevention

Prevention of venous thromboembolism is essential to decreasing the morbidity and mortality associated with pulmonary embolism. Prophylactic measures are based on the patient's specific risk factors.[32] See Table 26-6 for preventive measures recommended by the ACCP.

## Chronic Obstructive Pulmonary Disease

In the past, the two terms associated with chronic obstructive pulmonary disease (COPD) were *chronic bronchitis* (disease of the small airways) and *emphysema* (parenchymal destruction), which were often discussed as two different disease processes. However, COPD is a combination of both the disease of the small airways and destruction of the lung parenchymal along with other several structural abnormalities (Fig. 26-3).[34] The current COPD guideline suggest not using these specific terms when describing COPD, because they do not completely describe the pathologic processes associated with COPD. Currently, COPD is defined as an airflow limitation that is not fully reversible. The airflow limitation is usually progressive and associated with an abnormal chronic inflammatory response of the lungs to noxious particles or gases (primarily cigarette smoke) or an inherited deficiency of $\alpha_1$-antitrypsin (see Spotlight on Genetics 26-1).[34] Refer to the Global Initiative for Chronic Obstructive Lung Disease (GOLD) Global Strategy for the Diagnosis, Management, and Prevention of Chronic Obstructive Pulmonary Disease for current updates (www.goldcopd.org).

## Pathophysiology

COPD is a major cause of chronic morbidity and mortality, ranking as the third leading cause of death in the United States. This number is expected to increase because of the aging population.[35]

In COPD, pathologic changes occur in the central airways, peripheral airways, lung parenchyma, and pulmonary vasculature.[34] As the disease progresses, pathophysiologic changes usually occur in the following order: mucous hypersecretion, ciliary dysfunction, airflow limitation, pulmonary hyperinflation, gas exchange abnormalities, pulmonary hypertension, and cor pulmonale.[34] The peripheral airways become the major site of obstruction in patients with COPD. The structural changes in the airway wall are the most important cause of the increase in peripheral airway resistance. Inflammatory changes such as airway edema and hypersecretion of mucus, also contribute to narrowing of the peripheral airways.[34] Hypersecretion of mucus is caused by the stimulation of the enlarged mucus-secreting glands and the increased number of goblet cells by inflammatory mediators such as leukotrienes, interleukins, and tumor necrosis factor.[34] Ciliated epithelial cells undergo squamous metaplasia, leading to impaired mucociliary clearance, which is usually the first physiologic abnormality to occur in COPD.[34] This abnormality may be evident for many years before any other abnormalities develop.[34]

Airway obstruction is caused by inflammation of the major and small airways (Fig. 26-4). Subsequently, edema and hyperplasia of submucosal glands and excess mucus excretion

**TABLE 26-6** American College of Chest Physicians Recommendations for Prevention of Venous Thromboembolism

| Patient Population | Recommended Therapy | |
|---|---|---|
| Low-risk general surgery | Early and frequent ambulation | B1 |
| Moderate-risk general surgery | LMWH, LDUH, or mechanical prophylaxis, preferably with IPC | 2B, 2C |
| Higher-risk general surgery | LMWH, LDUH three times a day, or mechanical prophylaxis | |
| High-risk general surgery with multiple risk factors | LDUH three times a day, LMWH, combined with graduated compression stockings, and/or intermittent pneumatic compression | 1B, 2C |
| Total hip replacement or total knee replacement surgery | Use one of the following for a minimum of 10–14 days: LMWH, fondaparinux, apixaban, dabigatran, rivaroxaban, LDUH, adjusted dose VKA, ASA, or intermittent pneumatic compression device (IPCD) LMWH: started more than 12 h before surgery or more than 12 h after surgery; duel prophylaxis with an antithrombotic agent and IPCD recommended during hospitalization | 1B, 1C, 2C |
| Major trauma, traumatic brain injury, acute spinal injury, traumatic spine injury | Intermittent pneumatic Compression Device when not contraindicated. LMWH and LDUH when risk of bleeding diminishes. | 2C |
| Myocardial infarction | UFH or LMWH or bivalirudin or fondaparinux | A |
| | Intermittent pneumatic compression or elastic stockings when heparin is contraindicated | C |
| Ischemic stroke with restricted mobility | UFH or LMWH or intermittent compression devices over no prophylaxis | 2B |
| Medical patients with risk factors for VTE (including heart failure and chest infections) | LDUH TID, LMWH BID, or fondaparinux | 1B |
| Patients with long-term indwelling central vein catheters | Suggest against routine prophylaxis with LMWH or LDUH and suggest against the prophylactic use of VKAs (Coumadin) | 2B, 2C |
| Patients receiving a spinal puncture or epidural catheter placement | Use appropriate patient selection and caution when using anticoagulant thromboprophylaxis | |

*1A1: Methods strong, results consistent—randomized clinical trials (RCTs), no heterogeneity, effect clear that benefits do (or do not) outweigh risks. 2A: Methods strong, results consistent—RCTs, no heterogeneity, effect equivocal—uncertain whether benefits outweigh risks. 1B: Methods strong, results inconsistent—RCTs, heterogeneity present, effect clear that benefits do (or do not) outweigh risks. 2B2: Methods strong, results inconsistent—RCTs, heterogeneity present, effect equivocal—uncertain whether benefits outweigh risks. 1C: Methods weak—observational studies, effect clear that benefits do (or do not) outweigh risks. 2C: Methods weak—observational studies, effect equivocal—uncertain whether benefits outweigh risks.
LDUH, low-dose unfractionated heparin; LMWH, low-molecular-weight heparin.
From American College of Chest Physicians: Ninth ACCP Conference on Antithrombotic and Thrombolytic Therapy. Prevention of venous thromboembolism. Chest 133(412 Suppl):7S–47S, 2012. Retrieved from http://http://chestjournal.chestpubs.org/content/141/2_suppl.

into the bronchial tree occur, resulting in a chronic productive cough.[34] Cigarette smoking is the major causal factor in the development of airway obstruction caused by inflammation.[34] Other causes of chronic airway irritation include air pollutants and occupational exposure to nitrogen, sulfur oxides, or endotoxin.[34] Nonspecific pathologic changes in the lung, including infiltration of airway mucosa and submucosa with neutrophils and mononuclear cells, smooth muscle hypertrophy, and enlargement of the submucosal secretory glands, may also contribute to the development of COPD.[34]

Once the airway lumina are occluded by secretions and narrowed by a thickened wall, patients develop airflow

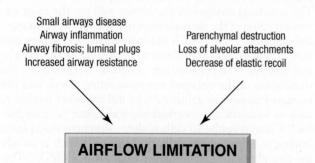

**FIGURE 26-3** Mechanisms underlying airflow limitation in COPD. (From Global Strategy for Diagnosis, Management and Prevention of COPD 2015. © Global Initiative for Chronic Obstructive Lung Disease (GOLD), all rights reserved. Available from http://www.goldcopd.org.)

---

🧬 **SPOTLIGHT ON GENETICS**

**α1-ANTITRYPSIN DEFICIENCY**

- α₁-antitrypsin deficiency affects about 1 in 1,500 to 3,500 individuals with European ancestry. It is uncommon in people of Asian descent but is commonly observed in COPD patients.
- Mutations in the *SERPINA1* gene cause α₁-antitrypsin deficiency. This gene provides instructions for making a protein called α₁-antitrypsin, which protects the body from a powerful enzyme called neutrophil elastase.
- Leads to a deficiency of α₁-antitrypsin or an abnormal form of the protein that cannot control neutrophil elastase. Without enough functional α₁-antitrypsin, neutrophil elastase destroys alveoli and causes lung disease.
- There are numerous genetic tests available for the detection of α₁-antitrypsin deficiency.

Data from Genetic Home Reference. Retrieved August 10, 2015, from http://ghr.nlm.nih.gov; and Franciosi AN, McCarthy C, McE Ivaney NG: The efficacy and safety of inhaled human α-1 antitrypsin in people with α-1 antitrypsin deficiency-related emphysema. Expert Rev Respir Med 9(2):143–151, 2015.

obstruction. Acute bacterial or viral infection in patients with existing COPD can increase airway and parenchymal damage, impair mucociliary clearance, obstruct bronchioles, and contribute to chronic epithelial damage and bacterial colonization that further exacerbate symptoms and airway obstruction.[34] Common bacteria isolated from the secretions of

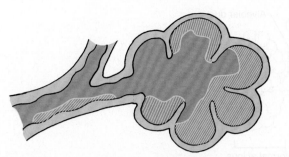

**FIGURE 26-4** Small airway changes in COPD: inflammation and thickening produce narrowing of airways. *Lined areas* indicate secretions.

patients with COPD include *H. influenzae, Haemophilus parainfluenzae, S. pneumoniae,* and *Moraxella catarrhalis.*[34] Even in nonsmoking patients, acute viral infection may lead to the chronic airway inflammation and chronic sputum production characteristic of COPD.[34] In these patients, the symptoms may have a reversible component if the source of chronic infection or irritation is treated. These patients normally do not have hyperinflation or abnormal diffusion test results.

Parenchyma destruction includes the loss of lung elasticity and abnormal, permanent enlargement of the airspaces distal to the terminal bronchioles with destruction of the alveolar walls and capillary beds without obvious fibrosis (Fig. 26-5).[34] There are three areas of destruction: centrilobular, panacinar, and paraseptal (Fig. 26-6). Centrilobular emphysema is common in smokers and often localizes in the upper lung zones. Paracinar emphysema is frequently found in patients with $\alpha_1$-protease inhibitor deficiency and is often

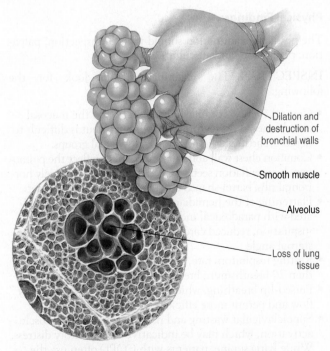

Dilation and destruction of bronchial walls

Smooth muscle

Alveolus

Loss of lung tissue

**FIGURE 26-5** Parenchymal changes in COPD. Airspaces are enlarged in the emphysematous lung. (From Anatomical Chart Company: Atlas of Pathophysiology, 3rd ed. Springhouse, PA: Lippincott Williams & Wilkins, 2010, p 91.)

localized in the lower lobes. Paraseptal emphysema is also common in smokers and is localized peripherally, with possible formation of large bullae.[36]

The enlargement of the airspaces in COPD results in hyperinflation of the lungs and increased total lung capacity.[36] This is believed to result from the breakdown of elastin by enzymes, called proteases, which digest proteins. These proteases, especially elastase, are released from neutrophils, alveolar macrophages, and other inflammatory cells.[36] Two recognized conditions that cause these changes are smoking and inherited $\alpha_1$-antitrypsin deficiency. Smoking contributes to increased inflammatory cells in the alveoli, enhanced release of elastase from neutrophils, increased elastase activity in macrophages, and activation of mast cells that release mast cell elastases.[36] $\alpha_1$-Antitrypsin usually protects the lung from the destructive inflammatory cells; however, the elastic tissue–destructive process continues unabated in patients with an inherited $\alpha_1$-antitrypsin deficiency.[36]

Almost all people who develop COPD before 40 years of age have an $\alpha_1$-antitrypsin deficiency. Evidence has shown that cigarette smoking decreases levels of $\alpha_1$-antitrypsin and increases the number of macrophages in the alveolar walls. This vicious cycle promotes increased numbers of neutrophils. A hereditary deficiency in $\alpha_1$-antitrypsin is responsible for about 1% of all cases of COPD.[36] Smoking and repeated respiratory tract infections further decrease $\alpha_1$-antitrypsin levels, adding to the risk for COPD in people with low $\alpha_1$-antitrypsin levels.[36]

A common phenomenon in COPD is spontaneous pneumothorax related to rupture of thinned parenchyma.[36] Patients may experience acute severe dyspnea and respiratory failure depending on the amount of pulmonary reserve (see the discussion of barotrauma in the section on Pneumothorax). In advanced COPD, peripheral airway obstruction, parenchymal destruction, and pulmonary vascular irregularities reduce the lung's capacity for gas exchange, resulting in hypoxemia (low blood oxygen) and hypercapnia (high blood carbon dioxide).[34] A VQ ratio mismatch is the driving force behind hypoxemia in patients with COPD, regardless of the stage of the disease. Chronic hypercapnia usually indicates inspiratory muscle dysfunction and alveolar hypoventilation.[34] As hypoxemia and hypercapnia progress late in COPD, pulmonary hypertension often develops, which causes hypertrophy of the right ventricle, better known as cor pulmonale.[34] Right-sided heart failure leads to further venous stasis and thrombosis that may potentially result in pulmonary embolism and further compromise the pulmonary circulation. Last, COPD is associated with systemic inflammation and skeletal muscle dysfunction that may result in limitation of exercise capacity and decline of health status.[34]

## Assessment

A physical examination is rarely diagnostic in COPD, although it remains an important aspect of patient care. When evaluating a patient, key indicators to consider include the following: dyspnea that is progressive and persistent, chronic cough that may be intermittent and nonproductive, or cough with sputum production, history of smoking, or occupational exposures to dusts and chemical for a significant period of time.[34]

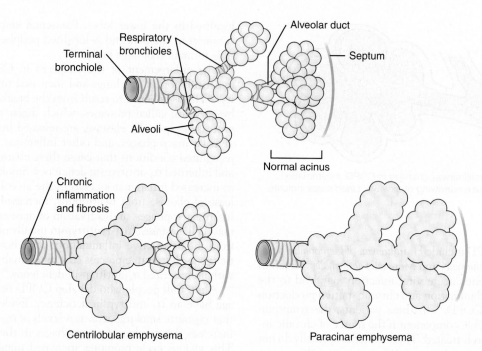

**FIGURE 26-6** Types of emphysema. The acinus, the gas-exchanging structure of the lung distal to the terminal bronchiole, consists of the terminal bronchiole, respiratory bronchioles, alveolar ducts, alveolar sacs, and alveoli. In centrilobular (proximal acinar) emphysema, the respiratory bronchioles are mainly involved. In paraseptal (distal acinar) emphysema, the alveolar ducts are mainly affected. In panacinar (panlobular) emphysema, the acinus is uniformly damaged.

## History

A detailed medical history of a new patient with known or suspected COPD should include the following:

- Exposure to risk factors, such as smoking, and occupational or environmental exposures to pollutants
- Past medical history, including asthma, allergy, sinusitis or nasal polyps, respiratory infections in childhood, and other respiratory diseases
- Family history of COPD or other chronic respiratory disease
- Pattern of symptom development. COPD typically develops in adults, and most patients are aware of the occurrence of increased breathlessness, increased frequency of winter "colds," and some social restriction for a number of years before seeking medical attention.
- History of exacerbations or previous hospitalizations for respiratory disorder. Patients may be conscious of periodic worsening of symptoms even if these episodes have not been identified as acute exacerbations of COPD. Indications for hospital assessment or admission for acute exacerbation of COPD include a marked increase in intensity of symptoms; severe underlying COPD or other serious comorbidities; onset of new physical signs; frequent exacerbations, or failure of exacerbations to respond to medical management; older age; and insufficient home support.[34]
- Comorbidities such as cardiovascular disease, skeletal muscle dysfunction, metabolic syndrome, osteoporosis, depression, and lung cancer may also contribute to restriction of activity or treatments.
- Appropriateness of current medical treatments, such as β blockers, commonly prescribed for heart disease. β blockers are usually contraindicated in COPD.

- Impact of disease on patient's life, including limitation of activity, missed work and economic consequences, effect on family routines, or feelings of depression or anxiety
- Social and family support
- Possibilities for reducing risk factors, especially smoking cessation[34]

### Physical Findings

The physical examination should include inspection, palpation, percussion, and auscultation.

**INSPECTION.** The examiner should look for the following:

- Central cyanosis or bluish discoloration of the mucosal membranes. This feature may be present but is difficult to detect in artificial light and in many racial groups.
- Common chest wall abnormalities, which reflect the pulmonary hyperinflation seen in COPD, including relatively horizontal ribs, barrel-shaped chest, and protruding abdomen
- Flattening of the hemidiaphragms, which may be associated with paradoxical indrawing of the lower rib cage on inspiration, reduced cardiac dullness, and widening xiphisternal angle
- Resting respiratory rate, which is often increased to more than 20 breaths/min; breathing may be shallow.
- Pursed-lip breathing, which may serve to slow expiratory flow and permit more efficient lung emptying
- Supraclavicular wasting and nasal flaring; resting muscle activation, which may be indicative of respiratory distress. While lying supine, patients with COPD often use the scalene and sternocleidomastoid muscles.
- Ankle or lower leg edema, which may be an indication of right-sided heart failure

**PALPATION AND PERCUSSION.** Palpation and percussion are often unhelpful in COPD. The examiner should be alert for the following:

- Heart apex beat, which may be difficult to detect because of pulmonary hyperinflation
- Pulmonary hyperinflation, which also leads to downward displacement of the liver and an increase in the ability to palpate this organ without it actually being enlarged

**AUSCULTATION.** Upon auscultation, the examiner may find the following:

- Reduced breath sounds
- Wheezing. Occurrence during quiet breathing is a useful indicator of airflow limitation; however, wheezing heard only after forced expiration is of no diagnostic significance.
- Inspiratory crackles, which occur in some patients with COPD but are of little assistance diagnostically
- Heart sounds heard over the xiphoid area
- Evidence of right heart failure secondary to COPD; includes an increased second heart sound, jugular venous distention, and right ventricular heave

Indications for ICU admission for patients with acute exacerbation of COPD include severe dyspnea with inadequate response to therapy; changes in mental status; persistent or worsening hypoxemia; severe or worsening respiratory acidosis in spite of supplemental oxygen; hemodynamic instability; and the need for invasive mechanical ventilation.[34]

## Diagnostic Studies

Laboratory and diagnostic tests in COPD are summarized in Table 26-7

**SPIROMETRY.** Patients with a history of a dyspnea and chronic cough with or without sputum production and who are considered high risk (ie history of smoking) should be evaluated for COPD. Spirometry measures the maximal volume of air forcibly exhaled from the point of maximal inspiration (forced vital capacity, or FVC) and the volume of air exhaled during the first second of this exercise (forced expiratory volume in 1 second, or $FEV_1$). The ratio of these two measurements ($FEV_1$/FVC ratio) is then calculated. This is usually done before and after a patient has been given a bronchodilator. Spirometry measurements are evaluated by comparison of the results with appropriate reference values based on age, height, sex, and race.[34] $FEV_1$/FVC ratio less than 70% confirms the presence of airflow limitation that is not fully reversible; this is considered the gold standard for diagnosing COPD (Table 26-8).[34] After the diagnosis of COPD has been confirmed, repeated measurements of the $FEV_1$ are used to help document the progression and severity of the disease.[34]

As the disease process progresses, $FEV_1$ and FVC decrease; this is related to the increased thickness of the airway wall, loss of alveolar attachments, and loss of lung elastic recoil.[34] In severe COPD, air is trapped in the lungs during forced expiration, leading to an abnormally high functional residual capacity (FRC). Increasing FRC leads to pulmonary hyperinflation.[34]

---

**TABLE 26-7  Laboratory and Diagnostic Tests for Patients With Chronic Obstructive Pulmonary Disease**

| Test | Rationale |
|---|---|
| Spirometry | Measures FVC and $FEV_1$; gold standard for diagnosing disease and monitoring progression |
| Diffusing capacity | Measures the degree of lung function, and provides information on the functional impact of emphysema related changes in COPD |
| Bronchodilator reversibility | Performed once during diagnosis stage and useful for the following reasons:<br>• To rule out an asthma diagnosis (If $FEV_1$ returns to predicted normal range after administration of bronchodilator, airflow limitation is likely due to asthma.)<br>• To establish a patient's best attainable lung function at that point in time |
| Chest radiography | • To exclude alternative diagnoses<br>• Evaluation of bullous disease<br>Radiologic changes seen include:<br>• Flattened diaphragm on lateral chest film<br>• Increased volume of retrosternal air space (signs of hyperinflation)<br>• Hyperlucency of the lungs<br>• Rapid tapering of vascular markings |
| Computed tomography | Not routinely recommended except when doubt about the diagnosis of COPD or pending lung reduction surgery |
| ABGs | • Performed if $FEV_1$ is <35% predicted or if signs of respiratory failure or right-sided heart failure are present<br>• Performed if peripheral saturation is <92%. |
| α1-antitrypsin deficiency screening | Indicated for patients in whom COPD develops at 45 years of age or who have a strong family predisposition (α1-antitrypsin serum level below 15%–20% of normal value is highly suggestive of homozygous α1-antitrypsin deficiency) |
| Exercise testing | • Used to assess health status impairment and predictor of prognosis<br>• Assess effectiveness of pulmonary rehabilitation |

$FEV_1$, forced expiratory volume in 1 s; FVC, forced vital capacity.
Data from Global Initiative for Chronic Lung Disease (GOLD): Global Strategy for the Diagnosis, Management, and Prevention of Chronic Obstructive Pulmonary Disease. Updated 2015. Retrieved from http://www.goldcopd.org/uploads/users/files/GOLD_Report_2015_Sept2.pdf.

| TABLE 26-8 | Classification of Severity of Airflow Limitation in COPD (Based on Post-Bronchodilator FEV$_1$) | |
|---|---|---|
| **In Patients With FEV$_1$/FVC <0.70** | | |
| GOLD 1 | Mild | FEV$_1$ ≥80% predicted |
| GOLD 2 | Moderate | 50% ≤ FEV$_1$ <80% predicted |
| GOLD 3 | Severe | 30% ≤ FEV$_1$ <50% predicted |
| GOLD 4 | Very Severe | FEV$_1$ <30% predicted |

From Global Initiative for Chronic Obstructive Pulmonary Disease (GOLD): Global Strategy for the Diagnosis, Management, and Prevention of Chronic Obstructive Pulmonary Disease: Updated 2015, p 14. Retrieved from http://www.goldcopd.org/uploads/users/files/GOLD_Report_2015_Sept2.pdf.

In addition to spirometry testing, another measurement of significant value from a pulmonary function test is the DLCO, or the diffusion capacity of the lung for carbon monoxide. This value is indicative of the amount of gas exchange that is occurring in the lung. When one takes the data from the FEV$_1$ and the DLCO, one can determine the true respiratory status of a patient. Figure 26-7 demonstrates a normal spirogram and a spirogram characteristic of a patient with COPD with mild to moderate airflow limitation. Patients with COPD have decreased FEV$_1$ and FVC, and the degree of spirometric abnormality generally reflects the severity of the disease.[34,37]

**ARTERIAL BLOOD GASES.** ABG measurements should be performed in all patients in moderate and severe stages of the disease (FEV$_1$ less than 40% predicted) or when clinical signs of respiratory failure or right-sided heart failure are present (ie, central cyanosis, ankle swelling, increase in jugular venous pressure).[34] Respiratory failure is indicated by a partial pressure of arterial oxygen (PaO$_2$) of 60 mm Hg with or without a partial pressure of arterial carbon dioxide (PaCO$_2$) of 45 mm Hg while breathing air at sea level.[34] Several precautions must be taken to ensure accurate results. First, it should be noted whether the patient is currently receiving oxygen and the amount of oxygen delivered to the patient during the blood gas sample time. Second, if the fraction of inspired oxygen (FiO$_2$) has been changed, a period of 20 to 30 minutes should elapse before gas tensions are rechecked.[34]

**CHEST RADIOGRAPH.** The chest x-ray is not routinely used to help confirm the diagnosis of COPD, but it helps to exclude other causes of the presenting symptoms. Radiologic changes associated with COPD include the following:

- Flattened diaphragm on lateral chest film
- Increased volume of retrosternal air space
- Hyperlucency of the lungs
- Rapid tapering of vascular markings

## Management

Several different treatment modalities, ranging from exercise training, nutrition counseling, and education to drug therapy, oxygen use, and surgery, may be effective in COPD treatment. Box 26-7 provides a collaborative care guide for the patient with COPD.

### Nonpharmacologic Therapy

The main goals of pulmonary rehabilitation are to decrease symptoms, improve quality of life, and increase physical and emotional participation in day-to-day activities.[34] The 2015 GOLD guidelines for the diagnosis, management, and prevention of COPD recommend a comprehensive pulmonary rehabilitation program.

**PULMONARY REHABILITATION.** In recent years, the value of pulmonary rehabilitation in managing COPD is being realized. Studies have shown that muscle fatigue rather than dyspnea is likely the primary cause of deconditioning in patients with COPD.[34] Pulmonary rehabilitation does not improve lung function but rather helps patients optimize their functional status as well as their quality of life within the limitations of their pulmonary disease process. Pulmonary rehabilitation has been shown to increase exercise tolerance, reduce dyspnea, decrease anxiety and depression, improve quality of life, improve cognitive function, provide the patient with a feeling of empowerment, and decrease hospitalizations and days in the hospital.[34,36] Pulmonary rehabilitation programs consist of three to four supervised sessions per week lasting for 6 to 12 weeks. If a patient is unable to participate in a pulmonary rehab program, the physician will recommend a structured exercise program such as walking 20 minutes daily.

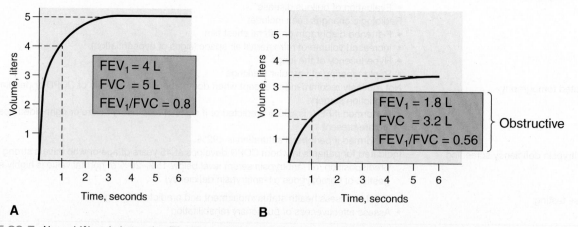

**FIGURE 26-7** Normal (**A**) and obstructive (**B**) patterns of a forced expiration. (FVC, forced vital capacity; FEV, forced expiratory volume. (From Global Strategy for Diagnosis, Management and Prevention of COPD 2015. © Global Initiative for Chronic Obstructive Lung Disease (GOLD), all rights reserved. Available from http://www.goldcopd.org.)

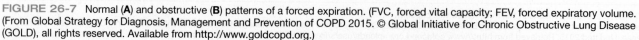

**QSEN BOX 26-7** *COLLABORATIVE CARE GUIDE for the Patient With Chronic Obstructive Pulmonary Disease*

| Outcomes | Interventions |
| --- | --- |
| **Impaired Gas Exchange** **Ineffective Breathing Pattern** | |
| Patient has arterial blood gases (ABGs) within normal limits and pulse oximeter value >90% | • Assess respiratory rate, effort, and breath sounds every 2 to 4 hours. • Obtain ABGs per order or signs of respiratory distress. • Monitor arterial saturation by pulse oximeter. • Provide supplemental oxygen by nasal cannula or face mask using lowest possible $FiO_2$ and flow rate. • Provide humidification with oxygen. • Provide intubation and mechanical ventilation as necessary (refer to Collaborative Care Guide for the Patient on Mechanical Ventilation, Chapter 25 on pages 478 to 479). |
| Patient maintains normal rate and depth of respiration. Patient has clear chest x-ray. Patient has clear breath sounds | • Monitor respiratory rate, pattern, and effort (eg, use of accessory muscles). • Assess respirations during sleep; note sleep apnea or Cheyne-Stokes patterns. • Obtain chest x-ray daily • Monitor breath sounds for crackles, wheezes, or rhonchi every 2 to 4 hours. • Administer diuretics per order. • Administer bronchodilators and mucolytics as indicated. |
| There is no evidence of atelectasis or pneumonia. | • Encourage nonintubated patients to use incentive spirometer, cough, and deep breathe every 2 to 4 hours and PRN. • Assess quantity, color, and consistency of secretions. • Turn side to side every 2 hours. • Mobilize out of bed to chair. |
| **Decreased Cardiac Perfusion** **Decreased Peripheral Perfusion** **Decreased Cardiac Output** | |
| Blood pressure, heart rate, and hemodynamic parameters are within normal limits. | • Monitor vital signs every 1 to 2 hours. • Monitor pulmonary artery pressures and right atrial pressure every 1 hour and cardiac output, systemic venous resistance, and peripheral venous resistance every 6 to 12 hours if pulmonary artery catheter is in place. • Assess for signs of right ventricular dysfunction (eg, increased central venous pressure, neck vein distention, peripheral edema). |
| Patient is free of dysrhythmias. | • Maintain patent intravenous access. • Monitor for atrial dysrhythmias due to right atrial dilation and ventricular dysrhythmias due to hypoxemia and hypoxia. |
| Serum lactate will be within normal limits. | • Monitor lactate daily until it is within normal limits. • Administer red blood cells, positive inotropic agents, colloid infusion as ordered to increase oxygen delivery. |
| **Electrolyte Imbalance** **Risk for Imbalanced Fluid Volume** | |
| Renal function is maintained as evidenced by urine output more than 30 mL/h, normal laboratory values. | • Monitor intake and output every 1 to 2 hours. • Monitor blood urea nitrogen, creatinine, electrolytes, Mg, $PO_4$. • Replace potassium, magnesium, and phosphorus per order or protocol. • Weigh daily. |
| Patient is euvolemic. | • Administer fluid volume and diuretics based on vital signs, physical assessment, secretion viscosity as ordered. |
| **Impaired Physical Mobility** **Risk for Activity Intolerance** **Risk for Infection** | |
| There is no evidence of loss of muscle tone or strength. | • Promote standing at bedside, sitting up in chair, ambulating with assistance as soon as possible. • Establish activity program. • Monitor response to activity. |
| Patient maintains joint flexibility. | • Consult with physical therapist. • Use passive and active range of motion every 4 hours while awake. |
| There is no evidence of evidence of infection. | • Monitor systemic inflammatory response syndrome criteria: increased WBC count, increased temperature, tachypnea, tachycardia. |
| WBC counts are within normal limits. | • Use strict aseptic technique during procedures and monitor others. • Maintain invasive catheter tube sterility. • Per hospital protocol, change invasive catheters, culture blood, line tips, or fluids. |

*(continued)*

| Outcomes | Interventions |
|---|---|
| There is no evidence of deep vein thrombosis (DVT). | • Initiate DVT prophylaxis within 24 hours of admission.<br>• Monitor for leg pain, redness, or swelling. |
| **Impaired Tissue Integrity** | |
| There is no evidence of skin breakdown. | • Turn side to side every 2 hours.<br>• Remove self-protective devices from wrists, and monitor skin per hospital policy.<br>• Assess risk for skin breakdown using objective tool (eg, Braden scale). Consider pressure relief/reduction mattress. |
| **Imbalanced Nutrition** | |
| Caloric and nutrient intake meets metabolic requirements per calculation (eg, Basal Energy Expenditure). | • Provide parenteral, enteral, or oral nutrition within 48 hours.<br>• Consult dietitian or nutritional support service.<br>• Avoid high-carbohydrate load if patient retains $CO_2$.<br>• Monitor albumin, prealbumin, vitamin D level, transferrin, cholesterol, triglycerides, glucose. |
| **Impaired Comfort** | |
| Patient is comfortable and evaluates pain as 4 on the pain scale. | • Assess pain/comfort every 4 hours.<br>• Administer analgesics and sedatives cautiously, closely monitoring respiratory rate, depth, and pattern.<br>• Differentiate between agitation caused by discomfort or caused by hypoxia before medication administration.<br>• Elevate head of bed to improve breathing comfort. |
| **Ineffective Coping**<br>**Impaired Individual Resilience** | |
| Patient demonstrates decreased anxiety. | • Assess vital signs during treatments, discussions, and so forth.<br>• Cautiously administer sedatives.<br>• Consult social services, clergy as appropriate.<br>• Provide for adequate rest and sleep.<br>• Provide support during periods of dyspnea. |
| **Teaching/Discharge Planning** | |
| Patient/significant others understand procedures and tests needed for treatment.<br>Significant others understand the severity of the illness, ask appropriate questions, anticipate potential complications.<br>In preparation for discharge to home, patient understands activity levels, dietary restrictions, medication regimen, metered inhaler. | • Prepare patient/significant others for procedures such as chest physical therapy, bronchoscopy, pulmonary artery catheter insertion, or laboratory studies.<br>• Explain the causes and effects of COPD and the potential for complications, such as pneumonia or cardiac dysfunction.<br>• Encourage significant others to ask questions related to the ventilator, pathophysiology, monitoring, treatments, and so forth.<br>• Make appropriate referrals and consults early during hospitalization.<br>• Initiate family education regarding proper use of metered inhaler, signs and symptoms of respiratory failure, and appropriate actions. |

**NUTRITIONAL COUNSELING.** Malnutrition is a common problem in patients with COPD and is present in more than 50% of patients with COPD admitted to the hospital. The incidence of malnutrition varies with the degree of gas exchange abnormality. Malnutrition results in wasting of respiratory muscles and further respiratory muscle weakness.[34] A complete nutritional assessment should be conducted to identify strategies to maximize the patient's nutritional status. Improving the nutritional state of weight-losing patients with COPD can lead to increased respiratory muscle strength.[34]

**SMOKING CESSATION.** Smoking cessation is the single most effective method of reducing the risk of developing COPD. The value of smoking cessation cannot be underestimated in slowing the progression of COPD. Every smoker should have such a counseling session at every visit to a health care provider.[34] The effectiveness of smoking cessation depends upon the patient being mentally ready to stop smoking. Numerous effective pharmacotherapies exist today

for smoking cessation, including nicotine replacement products in various forms (inhalation, oral, sublingual, or transdermal). Some of the most effective pharmacotherapies for smoking cessation are varenicline, bupropion, and nortriptyline. However, studies have shown that the effectiveness of these medications is enhance when they are used in conjunction with other supportive intervention programs, such as counseling or group therapy.[34]

### Pharmacologic Therapy

The goal of pharmacotherapy for COPD is to prevent and decrease symptoms and to reduce the frequency and severity of exacerbations, as well as to improve exercise tolerance and improve health status. According to the 2015 GOLD guidelines, pharmacologic treatment for stable patients with COPD consists of bronchodilators, β-2 agonists, anticholinergics, inhaled corticosteroids, and occasional use of methylxanthines and phosphodiesterase-4 inhibitors.[34] These medications can be administered alone or in combination depending on the response to therapy as well as the severity of the disease. A combination of agents may produce greater effects than single-agent therapy, and the inhaled route is the preferred route of delivery.[34] Other pharmacologic treatments that have been used in the past, such as systemic glucocorticoid, mucoactive agents, and chronic antibiotic therapy, are no longer being used to treat stable COPD patients.[34,38]

**BRONCHODILATORS.** Bronchodilators, primarily β-2 agonists, improve dyspnea by stimulation of the β-2 adrenergic receptors, and by causing the relaxation of the airway smooth muscle. β-2 agonists and anticholinergics, along with inhaled glucocorticoids,[34] are the mainstay of pharmacologic management of stable COPD. These medications are sometimes used as single agents or in combination. Bronchodilators offer long-term improvement in symptoms, exercise capacity, and quality of life. However, these medications, as well as any other pharmacologic agents, have not been shown to reverse the progression of COPD. Patients are usually on a combination of a long-acting bronchodilator such as tiotropium bromide (Spiriva), which is a long-acting anticholinergic, and a short-acting bronchodilator such as albuterol (Ventolin), which is a β-2 agonist, for a rescue inhaler.[34] Long-acting anticholinergics are preferred over long-acting β-2 agonists because they have been shown to decrease hyperinflation, decrease COPD exacerbation, and improve dyspnea.[34] They increase the $FEV_1$ by widening the smooth muscle tone of the airways rather than by altering the elastic recoil properties of the lung.[34] Long-acting bronchodilators are the most convenient. The choice of the particular form of bronchodilator therapy depends on availability and the patient's response in terms of symptom relief and side effects. Combination therapy, rather than an increased dose of a single agent, may lead to improved efficacy and a decreased risk of side effects.[34]

**CORTICOSTEROIDS.** COPD is a disease that is characterized by systemic and airway inflammation.[34] The aim of inhaled glucocorticoids is to reduce the inflammation. Studies have shown that inhaled glucocorticoids decrease COPD exacerbations but have little to no impact on overall mortality or improvement of lung function.[34] Inhaled glucocorticoids should always be used in conjunction with long-acting bronchodilators and never as a single agent.[1,34] Regular treatment with inhaled glucocorticosteroids for COPD is appropriate only for patients who have $FEV_1$ less than 60% predicted value.[34]

Oral corticosteroids are usually given for a short time and are reserved for patients with a COPD exacerbation. Steroid myopathy, which is associated with muscle weakness and decreased function, is a side effect associated with long-term use. Muscle function decline contributes to respiratory status decline in patients with severe COPD.[34]

**OTHER PHARMACOLOGIC AGENTS.** Several other drugs may be useful for COPD but are not universally recommended. One such medication is theophylline. Studies have shown that theophylline decreases dyspnea and improves gas exchange.[34] However, several problems exist with using theophylline.[34] Theophylline is a medication that requires monitoring of blood levels. It is metabolized by the liver, so anything that interferes with an individual's liver function may cause changes in the theophylline blood level, which

leads to toxicity. Theophylline also interacts with a number of other medications. For these reasons, theophylline is not used in the standard management of COPD, except in cases when inhaled long-acting bronchodilators are not available or affordable.[34] Phosphodiesterase-4 inhibitors reduce inflammation and promote smooth muscle relaxation with subsequent bronchodilation.[38] However, the use of these medications is limited because the adverse side effects, and they should always be used with a long-acting bronchodilator.[34] Antibiotics should not be used in COPD except for treating infectious exacerbations and other bacterial infections.[34] Current research indicates that mucolytic agents, such as N-acetylcysteine, have minimal overall benefits, and their widespread use is not recommended.[34]

### Oxygen Therapy

Oxygen therapy is one of the principal nonpharmacologic treatments for patients with severe COPD. Oxygen therapy improves the quality of life and cognitive performance, as well as long-term survival of patients in a hypoxic state.[34] Oxygen therapy can be administered as long-term continuous therapy, during exercise, nocturnally, and in the relief of acute dyspnea. The goal of long-term oxygen therapy is to produce an oxygen saturation as measured by pulse oximetry ($SpO_2$) of at least 88% at rest and sleep.[34] Supplemental oxygen therapy is recommended for individuals who are hypoxic as a result of COPD progression or in individuals recovering from an exacerbation with a $PaO_2$ at or below 55 mm Hg or an $SaO_2$ at or less than 88%, with or without hypercapnia.[34] Supplemental oxygen therapy is also indicated in individuals when $PaO_2$ is below 60 mm Hg or when $SaO_2$ is below 88% and there is evidence of cor pulmonale or polycythemia (hematocrit greater than 55%) despite optimal medical management.[34]

Noninvasive mechanical ventilation (NIMV) can be used in a stable patient with severe COPD. The combination of supplement oxygen and NIMV, especially in patient with daytime hypercapnia, can improve survival but necessarily quality of life.[34]

### Surgical Therapy

Surgical intervention may include lung volume reduction surgery (LVRS), bullectomy, and lung transplantation. The potential benefit of these procedures for a select group of patients with COPD is improvement in lung volumes, exercise tolerance, dyspnea, pulmonary function tests, quality of life, and survival.[34]

**LUNG VOLUME REDUCTION SURGERY.** LVRS is a surgical procedure in which parts of the nonfunctioning or scarred lung, usually the upper lobes, are resected, thereby reducing the lung volume. LVRS can be performed via a median sternotomy or video-assisted thoracoscopic surgery. A rationale as to why LVRS works is that removal of the nonfunctioning or scarred part of the upper lung lobes improves the mechanical functioning of the diaphragm and intercostal muscles. This is achieved by decreasing the FRC and returning the diaphragm to its more normal curvature and lengthening configuration.[34,38] Therefore, this surgery improves the mechanics of breathing and potentially decreases the work of breathing, but it is mainly successful in patients with upper lobe involvement.

OTHER SURGICAL PROCEDURES. Patients with severe COPD (stage III) may also consider bullectomy and lung transplantation.[34] Bullectomy is a surgical procedure for bullous emphysema, which is effective in alleviating dyspnea and improving overall lung function.[34] Appropriately selected patients with advanced COPD are potential candidates for lung transplantation. Lung transplantation has been shown to improve quality of life, exercise capacity, and functional capacity. Aside from potential postoperative complications, there are concerns about acute rejection, bronchiolitis obliterans, and opportunistic infections such as rare bacterial and fungal infections. The option of lung transplantation is limited by the available donors.[34]

## COPD Exacerbations

COPD exacerbation is an acute episode of increased symptoms beyond the patient's normal daily limitations (Box 26-8). These exacerbations are often precipitated by a viral upper and possible lower respiratory tract infection.[34] Changes include increased dyspnea and cough, with or without sputum production. Physical presentation may include increased use of accessory respiratory muscles, central cyanosis, mental confusion, paradoxical chest wall movement, and hemodynamic instability. Patients may require hospitalization, but most can be treated as outpatients.[34]

Treatment may require immediate stabilization, including airway management, but most patients will require only an immediate change in medications to treat the presenting symptoms and supplemental oxygen for the hypoxemia. Antibiotics should only be given in an acute exacerbation when there is compelling evidence the patient has a bacterial infection. This includes using antibiotics for patients with moderate or severe COPD exacerbation who also present

---

| BOX 26-8 | **Manifestations and Severe Exacerbations of COPD** |

**Constitutional Signs**
Temperature frequently subnormal
White blood cell count varies—may be slightly ↑, normal, or ↓

**Central Nervous System Disturbances**
Headache
Confusion
Hallucinations
Depression
Drowsiness
Somnolence
Coma
Papilledema

**Cardiovascular Signs**
Diaphoresis
Tachycardia
Blood pressure varies: normal, ↑, or ↓
Vasoconstriction initially followed by vasodilation

**Neuromuscular Signs**
Fine tremors
Asterixis
Flaccidity
Convulsions

---

with increased cough and sputum purulence, or who require mechanical ventilation.[34]

## Palliative Care, End of Life, and Hospice Care

Palliative care, end of life, and hospice need to be considered for advanced COPD patients who experience frequent hospitalizations for acute exacerbations.[34] Palliative care focuses on symptom management, supportive care, and enhancing the quality of life rather than stopping the progression of the disease. Hospice is incorporated when patients have less than 6 months to live.[34]

## Acute Asthma

Asthma is a chronic respiratory disease with varying symptoms, including wheezing, shortness of breath, chest tightness, and cough, that contribute to expiratory airflow limitations.[39] The symptoms associated with asthma can be triggered by several variables, such as exercise, exposure to an allergen, change in weather, or a viral respiratory infection.[39] Symptoms of asthma often resolve with medications, and sometimes resolve spontaneously without medical intervention.[39] However, in some cases, asthma can be life-threatening and require immediate medical attention beyond just giving the standard oral or inhaled medications.

The prevalence of asthma is increasing in many countries and it is considered a global health problem.[39] Currently, asthma affects 7.7% of the total population in the United States. With 7.4% affecting adults and 8.6% affecting children.[40] The incidence of asthma is increasing in the younger population, lower social economic populations, minorities, and especially in children living in the inner cities.[37] Recent research classifies asthma as a heterogeneous disease with different underlying disease processes contributing to the symptoms of asthma. Asthma phenotypes are classified by clinical or pathophysiologic characteristics. The following list includes the most recognized asthma phenotypes:

- *Allergic asthma*: This is the most common type of asthma; it may be associated with eczema, allergic rhinitis, or food or drug allergy.
- *Nonallergic asthma*: This type of asthma is not associated with an allergen.
- *Late-onset asthma*: This type is more common in women; it usually presents in adulthood and is often the nonallergic type.
- *Asthma with fixed airflow limitation*: Patients with long-standing asthma can develop a fixed airflow limitation.
- *Asthma with obesity*: Obese asthma patients have prominent respiratory symptoms that are not associated with eosinophilic airway inflammation.[39]

## Pathophysiology

Inflammation may be present throughout the bronchial tree, from large airways to the alveoli. This inflammation is characterized by mast cell activation, inflammatory cell infiltration, edema, denudation and disruption of the bronchial epithelium, collagen deposition beneath the basement

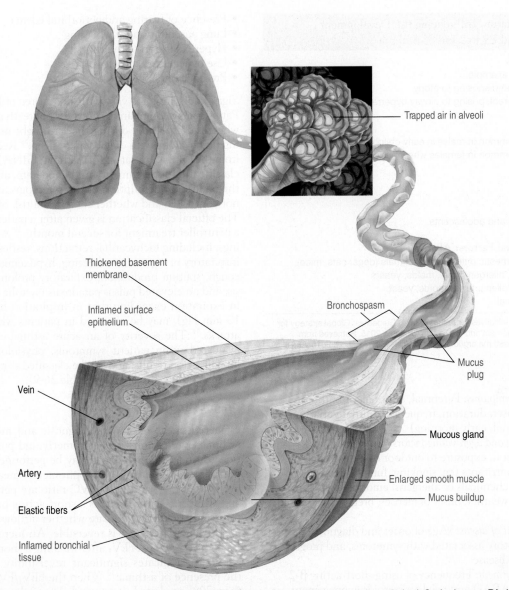

Trapped air in alveoli

Thickened basement
membrane

Inflamed surface
epithelium

Bronchospasm

Mucus
plug

Vein

Artery

Elastic fibers

Inflamed bronchial
tissue

Mucous gland

Enlarged smooth muscle

Mucus buildup

**FIGURE 26-8** Asthmatic bronchus. (From Anatomical Chart Company: Atlas of Pathophysiology, 3rd ed. Springhouse, PA: Lippincott Williams & Wilkins, 2010, p 85.)

membrane, goblet cell hyperplasia (which contributes to mucous hypersecretion), and smooth muscle thickening (Fig. 26-8). This inflammatory process contributes to airway hyperresponsiveness, airflow limitation, pathologic damage, and associated respiratory symptoms (ie, wheezing, shortness of breath, and chest tightness.[10]

Factors contributing to the airflow limitation in asthma include acute bronchoconstriction, airway mucosal edema, chronic formation of mucous plugs, and airway remodeling.[10]

The T lymphocytes (helper T [Th] cells) are believed to play a crucial role in the inflammation process.[37] Th1 cells serve a protective role against airway inflammation, and Th2 cells promote development of chronic airway inflammation. Recent studies suggest the possibility that early childhood viral and bacterial infections may contribute to Th2 cell stimulation and result in asthma pathogenesis.[39]

The etiology and pathogenesis of asthma are not fully understood. Inhaled irritants, such as cigarette smoke, inorganic dusts, and environmental pollutants, are common precipitants. These irritants stimulate the irritant receptors in the walls of the larynx and large bronchi, which initiate a reflex arc that travels to the central nervous system and back through the vagus nerve. This in turn induces bronchoconstriction.[10] The most common precipitant of an acute asthmatic exacerbation is an upper respiratory tract viral infection. This can induce increased airway inflammation, reduce lung function, and increase bronchial hyperresponsiveness that can last for days to a few weeks.[37] Factors influencing the development and expression of asthma are listed in Box 26-9.

## Assessment

### History and Physical Findings

The medical history should address the following areas: [41]

- *Symptoms*: Cough, wheezing, shortness of breath, chest tightness, sputum production.

## BOX 26-9 | Factors Influencing the Development and Expression of Asthma

**Host Factors**

Genetic—for example:
- Genes predisposing to atopy
- Genes predisposing to airway hyperresponsiveness

Obesity

Sex
- More common in males in early childhood
- More common in females when diagnosed in adulthood.

Depression

Anxiety

Age-related
- Elderly
- Children and adolescents

**Environmental Factors: Allergens**

- Indoor: Domestic mites, furred animals (dogs, cats, mice), cockroach, allergen, fungi, molds, yeasts
- Outdoor: Pollens, fungi, molds, yeast
- Occupational

Data from Global Initiatives for Asthma (GINA) Guidelines: Global strategy for asthma management and prevention. Updated 2015. Retrieved from http://www.ginasthma.org/local/uploads/files/GINA_Report_2015_Aug11 .pdf.

- *Pattern of symptoms:* Perennial, seasonal, or both; intermittent; onset, duration, frequency; diurnal variations (eg, nocturnal, early morning)
- *Precipitating and aggravating factors:* Upper respiratory viral infection, exposure to outdoor or indoor allergens, exposure to irritants (eg, smoking, fumes), exercise, occupational chemicals or allergens, emotions, stress, drugs, changes in weather, onset of menses, pregnancy, thyroid disease
- *Development of disease:* Age of onset and diagnosis, past medical history associated with symptoms, and progression of the disease
- *Current treatment:* Frequency of using short-acting β-2 agonists (SABAs) and need for steroids; management plans for exacerbations
- *Effect of symptoms* on activities of daily living
- *Impact of asthma on the patient and family:* Number of episodes requiring medical evaluations, number of missed days for work or school, disruptions in family routines, activities, or dynamics, and economic impact
- *Perceptions of the disease by the patient and family:* Beliefs regarding use of prescribed management including medications.

The physical examination should focus on the following areas:[39]

- Vital signs
- Height, weight, and a comparison of normal values for age
- Inspection of skin for evidence of atopic dermatitis or eczema
- Mouth breathing
- Dark discoloration beneath the lower eyelids ("allergic shiners")
- Edematous or pale nasal mucosa
- Clear nasal discharge
- Hypertrophy of tonsils and adenoids

- Presence of tearing and periorbital edema
- Lung auscultation for wheezing
- Hyperexpansion of the thorax
- Use of accessory muscles
- Presence of tachypnea

Signs and symptoms vary with the degree of bronchospasm. Patients may complain of shortness of breath associated with wheezing, especially during the late night and early morning hours, along with disruption of sleep.[39] Recent guidelines from the Global Initiative for Asthma (GINA) simplified the classification for asthma to mild, moderate, and severe, with the additional description of the symptoms as controlled or not controlled and whether there was a risk of exacerbation. The official classification is given after a patient has been on a controller treatment for several months.[39] Additional findings, including tachycardia, retractions, restlessness, anxiety, inspiratory or expiratory wheezing, hypoxemia, hypercapnia, cough, sputum production, expiratory prolongation, cyanosis, and an elevated pulsus paradoxus (systolic blood pressure in expiration exceeding that in inspiration by greater than 10 mm Hg), may be observed in patients who have severe attacks.[41] The severity of an acute asthma exacerbation is evaluated using patient symptoms, physiologic signs, and lung function results. and can be classified as mild, moderate, severe, and life-threatening (Table 26-9).

### Diagnostic Studies

Objective measures in the diagnosis and measurement of asthma severity consist of spirometry and pulmonary function testing. Allergy testing may be performed to ascertain precipitating allergens.[39,42] Spirometry measurements of the FVC, $FEV_1$, and $FEV_1$/FVC ratio are performed before and after the patient inhales a short-acting bronchodilator; these measurements indicate whether airflow obstruction is present and whether it is reversible. An increase of at least 12% and 200 mL in $FEV_1$ after inhaling a short-acting bronchodilator indicates significant reversibility and confirms the presence of asthma.[39] When the $FEV_1$/FVC ratio is less than 70% predicted, it can indicate an increase in airway obstruction, because the $FEV_1$ is significantly reduced when compared to the FVC measurement. For example, a person with asthma can have an $FEV_1$ of 2.5 L with a FVC of 4 L; the ratio will be 2.5/4.0, which equals 63%. The FVC is near normal, but the person has a low $FEV_1$. Airway resistance is increased, so $FEV_1$ is reduced out of proportion to FVC reduction.

Portable peak flow meters are used to monitor ongoing lung function. Patients are instructed how to measure peak expiratory flow, an indicator of the degree of airflow obstruction in the large airways, by using the peak flow meter on a regular basis.[39]

### Management

The level of treatment is based on the patient's level of asthma severity, which changes with time, age, and compliance with treatment.[39] Frequent reassessments of the level of severity are necessary to provide adequate therapy. The overall goals of therapy are to prevent chronic and troublesome symptoms, prevent exacerbations of symptoms, maintain normal activity levels, maintain normal pulmonary function,

| TABLE 26-9 | Classification of Severity of Asthma Exacerbations | | |
|---|---|---|---|
| | **Mild or Moderate** | **Severe** | **Impending Respiratory Failure** |
| Breathlessness | Walking Prefers sitting or lying. | At rest Hunched forward | At rest |
| Talks in: | Phrases | Words | |
| Alertness | Not agitated | agitated | Confused or drowsy |
| Respiratory rate | Increased | Often more than 30 breaths/min | |
| Use of accessory respiratory muscles | Usually not | Usually | Paradoxical thoracoabdominal movement |
| Breath sounds | Moderate wheezing, often end expiratory | Usually loud wheezes | Absence of wheezes |
| Heart rate (beats/min) | 100–120 bpm | >120 | Bradycardia |
| Pulsus Paradoxus (mm Hg) | Absent or <10 | Often present, >25 | Often absent |
| PEF (% predicted or personal best) | >50% | <50% predicted or personal best or response to therapy lasts <2 h | |
| $SaO_2$ (%, room air) | 90%–95% | <90 | |
| $PaO_2$ (mm Hg, room air) | Normal | <60 | |
| $PaCO_2$ (mm Hg) | <45 | >45 | |

Data from Global Initiative for Asthma (GINA): Global Strategy for Asthma Management and Prevention. Updated 2015. Retrieved from http://www.ginasthma .org/local/uploads/files/GINA_Report_2015_Aug11.pdf.

optimize pharmacotherapy and minimize side effects, and satisfy the patient's and the family's expectations and goals for asthma care.[39] A stepwise pharmacologic approach is recommended in treating patients with asthma. The main goal is to gain control quickly and to "step down" to the lowest medication level required to maintain asthma control.[39] A flow chart outlining the stepwise approach to the management of asthma exacerbations in the acute care setting is shown in Figure 26-9.

Asthma education and self-management training are critical to helping the asthmatic patient control airway inflammation. The 2015 Global Initiatives for Asthma guidelines describe the critical components of asthmatic patient education.[39] An important aspect of asthmatic patient education programs is training in the necessary management skills. These skills include inhaler technique, adherence to medication, knowing the early warning signs of an asthma attack, making decisions on the basis of self-monitoring of symptoms and peak flow results, and maintaining control of environmental asthma triggers (ie, dust mites, fur-bearing animals).[39] Recent studies have confirmed that appropriate therapy, coupled with structured asthma education, significantly improves short-term compliance with therapy and decreases asthma morbidity.[39] Long-term asthma management requires regular follow-up care with a clinician experienced in long-term asthma to maintain optimal asthma control and avoid preventable complications.[39]

## Acute Severe Asthma

Patients with severe persistent symptoms of asthma after receiving repeated courses of β-2 agonist therapy or subcutaneous epinephrine are classified as having acute severe asthma (formerly known as status asthmaticus). This is considered a medical emergency because it can become a life-threatening condition.[39] Patients present with a dramatic picture of acute agitation, markedly labored breathing,

tachycardia, $O_2$ saturations less than 90%, and diaphoresis. Deterioration of pulmonary function results in alveolar hypoventilation with subsequent hypoxemia, hypercapnia, and acidemia. A rising $PaCO_2$ in a patient with an acute asthmatic attack is often the first objective indication of severe asthma.[39] The treatment of acute severe asthma involves the institution of multiple therapeutic modalities. Patients should be placed on supplemental oxygen immediately. Treatment with a short-acting β-2 agonist and ipratropium bromide should be continued, and a high dose of oral or IV corticosteroids should be given. IV magnesium can also be given. Treatments with the short-acting β-2 agonist may need to be repeated several times. If the patient does not respond to the standard therapy, a trial of helium and oxygen therapy may be considered.[39] If pulmonary function does not improve and respiratory failure ensues, the patient may require intubation and assisted ventilation (see Chapter 25). A spontaneous pneumothorax may occur during severe acute asthmatic attacks, as well as during positive-pressure mechanical ventilation (see section on Pneumothorax, Management).

## Acute Respiratory Failure

Acute respiratory failure is defined as the rapid onset of inadequate gas exchange, demonstrated by hypoxemia in which $PaO_2$ is 50 mm Hg or less, or hypercapnia in which $PaCO_2$ is 50 mm Hg or greater with a pH of 7.25 or less.[12] Acute respiratory failure may occur in individuals with normal respiratory systems and in those with chronic pulmonary diseases. Causes of respiratory failure may include injury to the chest wall, lungs, and airways, or as a result of pulmonary disease (Box 26-10). Respiratory failure can occur as a complication to surgery, especially surgeries involving the chest, thorax, or upper abdomen. The most common pulmonary complications from surgery include atelectasis, pulmonary edema, pneumonia, and pulmonary emboli, all of which can precipitate acute respiratory failure.[12]

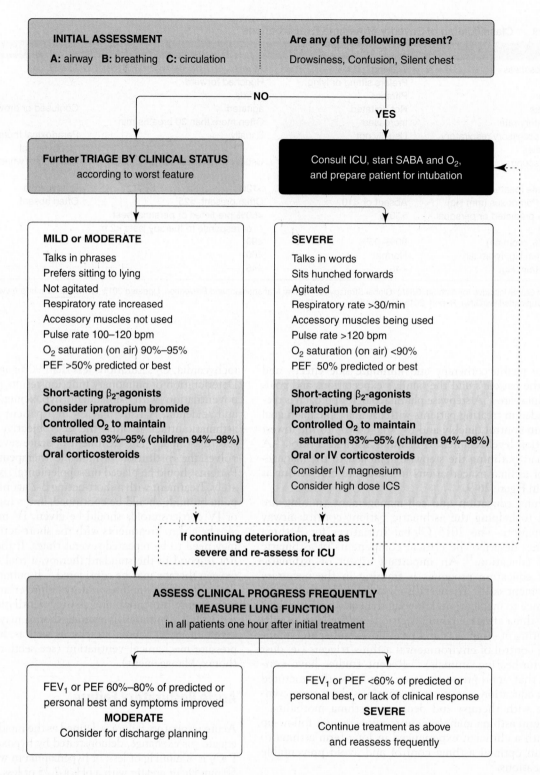

INITIAL ASSESSMENT

**A:** airway   **B:** breathing   **C:** circulation

Are any of the following present?

Drowsiness, Confusion, Silent chest

NO

YES

**Further TRIAGE BY CLINICAL STATUS**
according to worst feature

Consult ICU, start SABA and $O_2$, and prepare patient for intubation

**MILD or MODERATE**

Talks in phrases
Prefers sitting to lying
Not agitated
Respiratory rate increased
Accessory muscles not used
Pulse rate 100–120 bpm
$O_2$ saturation (on air) 90%–95%
PEF >50% predicted or best

**Short-acting $\beta_2$-agonists**
**Consider ipratropium bromide**
**Controlled $O_2$ to maintain**
  **saturation 93%–95% (children 94%–98%)**
**Oral corticosteroids**

**SEVERE**

Talks in words
Sits hunched forwards
Agitated
Respiratory rate >30/min
Accessory muscles being used
Pulse rate >120 bpm
$O_2$ saturation (on air) <90%
PEF  50% predicted or best

**Short-acting $\beta_2$-agonists**
**Ipratropium bromide**
**Controlled $O_2$ to maintain**
  **saturation 93%–95% (children 94%–98%)**
**Oral or IV corticosteroids**
Consider IV magnesium
Consider high dose ICS

**If continuing deterioration, treat as
severe and re-assess for ICU**

**ASSESS CLINICAL PROGRESS FREQUENTLY
MEASURE LUNG FUNCTION**
in all patients one hour after initial treatment

$FEV_1$ or PEF 60%–80% of predicted or
personal best and symptoms improved
**MODERATE**
Consider for discharge planning

$FEV_1$ or PEF <60% of predicted or
personal best, or lack of clinical response
**SEVERE**
Continue treatment as above
and reassess frequently

ICS: inhaled corticosteroids; ICU: intensive care unit; IV: intravenous; $O_2$: oxygen; PEF: peak expiratory flow; $FEV_1$: forced expiratory volume in 1 second

**FIGURE 26-9**   Management of asthma exacerbation in acute care settings. PEF, peak expiratory flow. (From Global Initiative for Asthma [GINA]: Global Strategy for Asthma Management and Prevention. Updated 2015. Retrieved from http://www.ginasthma.org/local/uploads /files/GINA_Report_2015_Aug11.pdf. )

**BOX 26-10** Causes of Acute Respiratory Failure

**Intrinsic Lung/Airway Diseases**

Large Airway Obstruction
- Congenital deformities
- Acute laryngitis, epiglottitis
- Foreign bodies
- Intrinsic tumors
- Extrinsic pressure
- Traumatic injury
- Enlarged tonsils and adenoids
- Obstructive sleep apnea

Bronchial Diseases
- Chronic bronchitis
- Asthma
- Acute bronchiolitis

Parenchymal Diseases
- Pulmonary emphysema
- Pulmonary fibrosis and other chronic diffuse infiltrative diseases
- Severe pneumonia
- Acute lung injury from various causes (acute respiratory distress syndrome)

**Cardiovascular Disease**
- Cardiac pulmonary edema
- Massive or recurrent pulmonary embolism
- Pulmonary vasculitis

**Extrapulmonary Disorders**

Diseases of the Pleura and the Chest Wall
- Pneumothorax
- Pleural effusion

- Fibrothorax
- Thoracic wall deformity
- Traumatic injury to the chest wall: flail chest
- Obesity

Disorders of the Respiratory Muscles and the Neuromuscular Junction
- Myasthenia gravis and myasthenia-like disorders
- Muscular dystrophies
- Polymyositis
- Botulism
- Muscle-paralyzing drugs
- Severe hypokalemia and hypophosphatemia

Disorders of the Peripheral Nerves and Spinal Cord
- Poliomyelitis
- Guillain–Barré syndrome
- Spinal cord trauma (quadriplegia)
- Amyotrophic lateral sclerosis
- Tetanus
- Multiple sclerosis

Disorders of the Central Nervous System
- Sedative and narcotic drug overdose
- Head trauma
- Cerebral hypoxia
- Cerebrovascular accident
- Central nervous system infection
- Epileptic seizure: status epilepticus
- Metabolic and endocrine disorders
- Bulbar poliomyelitis
- Primary alveolar hypoventilation
- Sleep apnea syndrome

## Pathophysiology

Acute respiratory failure is defined as a $PaO_2$ of 55 mm Hg or less, a $PaCO_2$ greater than 50 mm Hg, and an arterial pH less than 7.35.[42,43] This definition is valid only in cases in which baseline ABG values are assumed to be normal.[42] In patients with established chronic hypoxemia or hypercapnia, acute respiratory failure is indicated by the acute deterioration of blood gases relative to their previous levels rather than their absolute values.[42] In patients with chronic lung disease, ABG values associated with classical acute respiratory failure may not be present because these patients have adapted to blood gas levels outside this range, consistent with their disease process.[42]

Acute respiratory failure may be caused by a variety of pulmonary and nonpulmonary diseases. Respiratory failure may result from malfunction of the respiratory center, abnormal respiratory neuromuscular system, chest wall diseases, airway obstruction, or parenchymal lung disorders.[44] Many factors may precipitate or exacerbate acute respiratory failure such as, medications, cardiovascular disorders, trauma, chest muscle fatigue, recreational drug use, and infection.

A vicious positive feedback mechanism characterizes the deleterious effects of continued hypoxemia and hypercapnia. Hypoxemia affects every organ and tissue, and hypercapnia impairs cellular functions.[42] Hypoxemia in respiratory failure may be caused by any number of the

conditions, separately or in various combinations.[42–44] Hypercapnia results from alveolar hypoventilation and ventilation–perfusion mismatching when there is no compensation by increased ventilation of well-perfused regions.[44] In acute hypercapnia, arterial blood pH is decreased, indicating acute respiratory acidosis. Patients with advanced COPD and chronic hypercapnia may exhibit an acute rise of $PaCO_2$ to a high level, a decrease of blood pH, and a significant increase in serum bicarbonate during the onset of acute respiratory failure.[44]

## Classification

Acute respiratory failure is classified as acute hypoxemic respiratory failure, acute hypercapnic respiratory failure, or combined hypoxemic and hypercapnic respiratory failure.[44] Acute hypoxemic respiratory failure is a direct defect in oxygenation. Acute hypercapnic respiratory failure is a direct defect in ventilation.

### Acute Hypoxemic Respiratory Failure

Hypoxemia is qualified by a reduction in the oxygenation of arterial blood. It is caused by alterations in respiration and is evidenced by a low $PaO_2$.[12] Hypoxemia can lead to tissue hypoxia, but hypoxia can also be caused by a low cardiac output or cyanide poisoning that is not associated with pulmonary function. Manifestations of hypoxemia may include cyanosis, confusion, tachycardia, edema, and decreased renal output.

Hypoxemia results from problems with one or more of the major mechanisms of oxygenation:[12]

1. Oxygen delivery to the alveoli
   a. Oxygen content of the $FiO_2$
   b. Ventilation of the alveoli
2. Diffusion of oxygen from the alveoli into the blood
   a. Balance between alveolar ventilation and perfusion
   b. Diffusion of oxygen across the alveolocapillary membrane
3. Perfusion of capillary membranes

Hypoxemia can result in widespread tissue dysfunction and organ infarction.[12] The major causes of this type of failure are listed in Table 26-10.

### Acute Hypercapnic Respiratory Failure

Acute hypercapnic respiratory failure is caused by hypoventilation of the alveoli and is manifest by an increase in $CO_2$ in the arterial blood. There are many causes of hypercapnia, including depression of the respiratory center by drugs, diseases of the medulla, infections or trauma of the central nervous system, abnormalities of the spinal conducting pathways (as in spinal cord injury or poliomyelitis), diseases of the respiratory muscles or the neuromuscular junction, thoracic cage abnormalities (such as chest injury or congenital deformity), large airway obstruction, increased work of breathing, and physiologic dead space.[12]

Manifestations of hypercapnia can result in several conditions, such as electrolyte imbalance, that occur in response to a low pH and may cause dysrhythmias. High levels of $CO_2$ can create somnolence or even coma because of changes in intracranial pressure resulting in increased cerebral vasodilation.[12,45]

## Assessment

### History

A complete medical and social history should be obtained from the patient or a family member to determine the patient's baseline respiratory status on admission. This information can be used in determining interventions to ensure proper medical care.

### Physical Findings

Presentation of acute respiratory failure may vary, depending on the underlying disease, precipitating factors, and degree of hypoxemia, hypercapnia, or acidosis.[42,44,45] Typically, intubation and ventilation are necessary in patients with depressed mental status or coma, severe respiratory distress, extremely low or agonal respiratory rate, obvious respiratory muscle fatigue, peripheral cyanosis, or impending cardiopulmonary arrest.[44]

The classical symptom of hypoxemia is dyspnea, although this may be completely absent in ventilatory failure resulting from depression of the respiratory center.[45] Other presenting symptoms of hypoxemia include cyanosis, restlessness, confusion, anxiety, delirium, tachypnea, tachycardia, hypertension, cardiac dysrhythmias, and tremor.[45] The cardinal

symptoms of hypercapnia are dyspnea and headache.[45] Other clinical manifestations of hypercapnia include peripheral and conjunctival hyperemia, hypertension, tachycardia, tachypnea, impaired consciousness, papilledema, and asterixis.[45] Other physical findings on examination may include use of accessory muscles of respiration, intercostal or supraclavicular retraction, and paradoxical abdominal movement if diaphragmatic weakness or fatigue is present.[45]

### Diagnostic Studies

Because the signs and symptoms of acute respiratory failure are nonspecific and insensitive, the physician must request an ABG analysis to determine the exact level of $PaO_2$, $PaCO_2$, and blood pH in cases of suspected acute respiratory failure. Only determination of the blood gases and pH can confirm the diagnosis.[45] Other diagnostic tests necessary to determine the etiology of acute hypoxemic respiratory failure include chest radiography, sputum examination, angiography, ventilation–perfusion scanning, CT, toxicology screen, complete blood count, serum electrolytes, cytology, urinalysis, bronchoscopy, electrocardiography, echocardiography, and thoracentesis.[45] See Table 26-10 for more details about the use of these diagnostic tests in acute respiratory failure.

## Management

Acute respiratory failure warrants immediate intervention to correct or compensate for the gas exchange abnormality and identify the cause.[45] Although the recommended therapeutic intervention may vary according to the specific disease's pathologic process, general management principles are applicable to every patient with acute respiratory failure. See Table 26-11 for specific therapies for managing common causes of acute respiratory failure.[45]

If alveolar ventilation is inadequate to maintain $PaO_2$ or $PaCO_2$ levels related to respiratory or neurologic failure, endotracheal intubation and mechanical ventilation may be lifesaving.[42,45] The initial assessment and the decision to initiate mechanical ventilation should be performed rapidly to minimize the life-threatening complications associated with extended hypoxemia (eg, cardiac dysrhythmias, anoxic encephalopathy).[42,45] See Chapter 25 for further information on airway management and care of the patient on a ventilator.

Patients with acute hypoxemic respiratory failure should receive immediate treatment with rapidly increased $FiO_2$ and continuous pulse oximetry monitoring until an $SaO_2$ of 90% or higher is obtained.[45] Once hypoxemia is reversed, oxygen is titrated to the minimum level necessary for correction of hypoxemia and prevention of significant carbon dioxide retention.[45]

Patients with acute hypercapnic respiratory failure should be immediately assessed for either an impaired central respiratory drive associated with sedative or narcotic therapy or for underlying bronchospasm secondary to an asthma exacerbation or COPD.[45] Reversal agents (opiate antagonists; eg, naloxone) are used in the case of impaired central respiratory drive, and inhaled bronchodilators and systemic corticosteroids are used in the case of underlying bronchospasm.[45]

**TABLE 26-10**  **Evaluation and Management of Causes of Acute Respiratory Failure**

| Etiology | Key Clinical Findings | Key Diagnostic Tests | Specific Therapy |
|---|---|---|---|
| **Respiratory Failure Caused by Central Nervous System Dysfunction*** | | | |
| **CNS-depressant drugs** | History of drug overdose, head trauma, or anoxic encephalopathy<br>Pupillary changes, needle marks | Response to naloxone<br>Toxicology screen<br>Electrocardiogram | Antidotes for the drugs taken<br>Neurologic evaluation |
| **Hypothyroidism** | Myxedema | Thyroid function test | Cautious thyroid replacement |
| **Starvation** | Cachexia<br>Diarrhea | ↓Albumin<br>↓Cholesterol | Nutrition |
| **Metabolic alkalosis** | Lethargy<br>Confusion | ABGs<br>Serum electrolytes | Treat underlying causes |
| **Structural brain stem damage** | Localizing neurologic findings<br>Headache | CT, MRI, cerebrospinal fluid cytology | Radiation, chemotherapy |
| **Neoplasm** | Headache, fever | CT, MRI, cardiac echo | Antimicrobial therapy |
| **Infection** | | | |
| **Primary alveolar hypoventilation (Ondine's curse)** | Daytime hypersomnolence, headache, rarely dyspneic, polycythemia, cor pulmonale | Blunted or absent ventilatory response to ↑$CO_2$, ↓$O_2$ in inspired gas<br>Normal pulmonary function test | Nighttime ventilatory support<br>Electrophrenic pacing<br>Medroxyprogesterone acetate<br>Supplemental oxygen |
| **Central sleep apnea** | Same as primary alveolar hypoventilation | Polysomnography: apnea without respiratory effort<br>Normal $CO_2$,$O_2$ response curves while awake | Nighttime ventilatory support<br>Electrophrenic pacing<br>Supplemental oxygen |
| **Respiratory Failure Caused by Peripheral Nervous System Dysfunction*** | | | |
| **Spinal cord disease** | Above C5, diaphragm, intercostal, and abdominal activity abolished | Spinal x-ray film, CT, MRI | Supportive, vital capacity tends to improve more than 3 mo in traumatic lesions C5 and below |
| **Traumatic** | Below C5, diaphragm preserved, intercostal and abdominal activity abolished | | Phrenic nerve pacing for high cervical cord lesions with intact phrenic nerve |
| **Strychnine** | Intense muscle spasms<br>Apnea<br>Metabolic acidosis | Toxicology screen<br>Clinical picture | Supportive<br>Gastric lavage, charcoal |
| **Hyperthyroidism** | Thyrotoxicosis heat intolerance, tachycardia, hyperreflexia | TSH, TFT | Propylthiouracil, methimazole |
| **Hypothyroidism** | Myxedema, cold intolerance<br>Hyporeflexia, bradycardia | TSH, TFTs | Replace thyroid hormone |
| **Respiratory Failure Caused by Respiratory Muscle Dysfunction*** | | | |
| **Muscle dystrophies** | Proximal muscle weakness and atrophy | Muscle biopsy<br>Elevated CPK<br>Genetic analysis | Supportive<br>Duchenne: prednisone |
| **Periodic paralyses** | Hypokalemic, hyperkalemic, or normokalemic<br>Genetic<br>Muscle weakness associated with exercise, emotional upset, cold, alcohol | Serum potassium<br>Family history | Avoid precipitating factors<br>Carbonic anhydrase inhibitor |
| **Respiratory Failure Caused by Chest Wall, Pleural, and Upper Airway Diseases*** | | | |
| **Kyphoscoliosis** | Spinal curvature ≥120 degrees<br>Progressive dyspnea on exertion over several years | Spinal x-ray films<br>Restriction on PFTs | Nighttime ventilatory support |
| **Flail chest** | Multiple rib fractures, paradoxical respiration ± pleuritic chest pain | Chest film | Mechanical positive-pressure ventilation |
| **Ankylosing spondylitis** | Limited chest expansion<br>Apical pulmonary fibrosis<br>Limited lumbar mobility<br>Chronic lower back pain | PFTs (↓functional residual capacity, ↓total lung capacity)<br>HLA-B27<br>Spine and sacroiliac x-ray films | Anti-inflammatory agents<br>Flexibility exercises |
| **Angioedema/anaphylaxis** | Stridor in setting of Hymenoptera sting, contrast media, or drug administration | Other evidence of angioedema/anaphylaxis; complement levels | Epinephrine parenterally<br>Cricothyroidotomy |

*(continued)*

**TABLE 26-10** Evaluation and Management of Causes of Acute Respiratory Failure (*continued*)

| Etiology | Key Clinical Findings | Key Diagnostic Tests | Specific Therapy |
|---|---|---|---|
| **Foreign body aspiration** | Unable to speak<br>Stridor or apnea | X-ray film helpful when foreign body below vocal cords | Heimlich maneuver<br>Bronchoscopy<br>Cricothyroidotomy |
| *Respiratory Failure by Intrapulmonary Causes* | | | |
| **Cardiogenic pulmonary edema**[†] | Rales, diaphoresis | Chest x-ray: pulmonary edema<br>Echocardiogram | Fluid management for adequate peripheral perfusion(diuresis/fluid)<br>Reduce LVEDP |
| **Adult respiratory distress syndrome**[†] | Rales<br>$PaO_2$ <55 mm Hg with $FiO_2$ more than 60%<br>$PaO_2/FiO_2$ 200 mm Hg or less (regardless of PEEP)<br>Fever | CXR: bilateral infiltrates<br>CBC<br>Pulmonary artery catheter: PAOP 18 mm Hg or less when measured OR no clinical evidence of left atrial hypertension | Treat underlying cause<br>Pulmonary vasodilators<br>Corticosteroids<br>Lung protective mechanical ventilation |
| **Acute lung injury** (caused by sepsis, blood transfusion, pneumonia, aspiration, and/or multiple traumas)[†] | Dyspnea<br>$PaO_2/FiO_2$ ≤300 mm Hg (regardless of PEEP) | CXR: Bilateral airspace disease,<br>CT: Pulmonary edema from increased permeability<br>ABG<br>Pulmonary artery catheter: PAOP 18 mm Hg or less when measured OR no clinical evidence of left atrial hypertension | Increase $FiO_2$<br>PEEP<br>Bronchodilation<br>Inhaled nitric oxide<br>Antibiotics |
| **COPD**[‡] | Dyspnea on exertion<br>Prolonged forced expiratory time<br>Wheezing<br>Decrease in breath sounds<br>Hyperinflation<br>New onset of paradoxical respiratory motion or respiratory alternans | PFTs<br>ABG<br>CXR<br>CT scan | Oxygen therapy<br>Bronchodilators<br>Antibiotics<br>Corticosteroids<br>Nutritional supports<br>Smoking cessation |

CNS, central nervous system; CBC, complete blood cell count; CT, computed tomography; CPK, creatinine phosphokinase; CXR, chest x-ray; HLA-B27, human leukocyte antigen-B27; LVEDP, left ventricular end-diastolic pressure; MRI, magnetic resonance imaging; PAOP, pulmonary artery occlusion pressure; PFTs, pulmonary function tests; TFT, thyroid function text; TSH, thyroid stimulating hormone.
*Data from Hollingsworth HM, Pratter MR, Irwin RS: Respiratory failure Part V: Extrapulmonary causes of respiratory failure. In: Irwin RS, Rippe JM (eds): Irwin and Rippe's Intensive Care Medicine, 6th ed. Philadelphia, PA: Lippincott Williams & Wilkins, 2008, pp 541–555.
†Data from Allen GB, Parsons PE: Respiratory failure Part II: Acute respiratory failure due to acute respiratory distress syndrome and pulmonary edema. In: Irwin RS, Rippe JM, (eds): Irwin and Rippe's Intensive Care Medicine, 6th ed. Philadelphia, PA: Lippincott Williams & Wilkins, 2008, pp 497–515.
‡Data from Balter MS, Grossman RF: Respiratory failure Part IV: Chronic obstructive pulmonary disease. In: Irwin RS, Rippe JM (eds): Irwin and Rippe's Intensive Care Medicine, 6th ed. Philadelphia, PA: Lippincott Williams & Wilkins, 2008, pp 531–540.

**TABLE 26-11** Acute Respiratory Failure Management

| Management Outcomes | Therapeutic Intervention |
|---|---|
| Establishment and maintenance of an adequate airway | • *Oropharyngeal airway*: Used to secure and maintain an open airway in patients with a decrease or loss of consciousness. The person cannot have an intact gag reflux if these devise are going to be used.<br>• *Nasopharyngeal airway*: Used in patients at risk for obstruction or in patients with trismus. It also helps with secretion control by facilitating suctioning. Tracheal intubation may be necessary to prevent aspiration, maintain airway patency, and provide effective suctioning.<br>• Strictly adhere to adequate tracheobronchial toilet (ie, deep breathing, coughing, tracheobronchial suctioning). |
| Oxygenation | • Increase ($FiO_2$) concentration by administration of supplemental oxygen to increase oxygen at a cellular level and improve tissue perfusion.<br>• Use of mechanical ventilator indications includes apnea, acute hypercapnia, severe hypoxemia, and progressive patient fatigue despite current interventions. |
| Ventilation | • Use of noninvasive positive pressure ventilation (NPPV) in cooperative patients with COPD exacerbation, altered level of consciousness or Do Not Resuscitation (DNR) orders needing support for a short period of time. |

**TABLE 26-11** **Acute Respiratory Failure Management** (*continued*)

| Management Outcomes | Therapeutic Intervention |
|---|---|
| Correction of acid–base disturbance | • Correct pH disturbances: Increased ventilation from mechanical or NPPV will promote alveolar ventilation and:<br>  • Help with compensation for metabolic acidosis associated with fever, sepsis, or cardiac failure.<br>  • Reverse acute hypercapnia or respiratory acidosis in conditions which are associated with decreased ventilation include drug overdoses, decrease or loss of consciousness, severe asthma, and COPD exacerbation. |
| Restoration of fluid and electrolyte balance | • Monitor for excessive intravenous fluid administration or decrease oral intake.<br>• Monitor daily fluid intake and output closely.<br>• Prevent and treat promptly hypokalemia and hypophosphatemia.<br>• It can promote hypoventilation due to respiratory muscle weakness. |
| Optimization of cardiac function | • Maintain adequate cardiac output.<br>• Bedside Echocardiogram for measurement of cardiac function and fluid status. |
| Identification and treatment of underlying correctable conditions and precipitating causes | • Prevent or treat respiratory tract infections (viral, bacterial, or fungal).<br>• Prevent potential airway obstruction by maintenance of proper tracheobronchial hygiene; recognize increased tracheobronchial secretions, changes in their characteristics, or difficulty in their elimination due to various factors.<br>• Identify and treat heart failure appropriately.<br>• Recognize and treat bronchospasm with bronchodilators and corticosteroids.<br>• Assess for organic or metabolic disorder affecting the central nervous system or neuromuscular function.<br>• Assess tolerance to sedative, hypnotic, and narcotic drugs in patients with chronic ventilatory insufficiency. In case of a narcotic drug overdose, a proper antidote may be administered.<br>• Remove air or fluid in the pleural cavity.<br>• Prevent and treat abdominal distention by insertion of a nasogastric tube.<br>• For trauma and surgical patients, assess limitation of the thoracic wall movement, ineffective cough, immobility, and lack of deep breathing.<br>• Control fever and other causes of increased metabolism.<br>• Assess diaphragmatic fatigue; if present, mechanical ventilatory support is indicated to rest these muscles and restore their contractility.<br>• Promptly identify and adequately treat hypophosphatemia, hypokalemia, and hypocalcemia. |
| Prevention and early detection of potential complications | • Most of these complications occur in mechanically ventilated patients (see Chapter 25).<br>• Keep HOB > 30 degrees-to avoid aspiration<br>• DVT prophylaxis<br>• Stress ulcer prophylaxis<br>• Skin care to prevent pressure ulcers<br>• Psychological and emotional support for patient and family members<br>• Sedation vacation to reduce overuse of sedatives to prevent delirium and decrease ventilator days.<br>• Promote early mobility when hemodynamically stable |
| Nutritional support | • Enteral alimentation is preferred over parenteral feeding because bowel wall integrity is maintained.<br>• Avoid over feeding, especially with high-lipid formulas over high carbohydrates because it can increase $CO_2$ production and worsen or induce hypercapnia. |
| Periodic assessment of the course, progress, and response to therapy | • ABG measurements as indicated by patient condition<br>• Monitor arterial oxygen saturation by pulse oximetry. |
| Determination of a need for mechanical ventilatory support | • Continuously assess the patient's respiratory status and need for ventilator support (see Chapter 25). |

Data from Farzan S: Respiratory failure. In: Farzan S (ed): A Concises Handbook of Respiratory Diseases, 4th ed. Stamford, CT: Appleton & Lange, 1997, pp 371–386; and Papadakis MA, McPhee SJ: Current Medical Diagnosis and Treatment, 54th ed. Columbus, OH: McGraw-Hill Education, 2015, pp 315–317.

# Clinical Applicability Challenges

## CASE STUDY

S.H. is a 67-year-old woman admitted to the ICU with an acute onset of dyspnea and fever following an endoscopy procedure. S.H. has a history of ovarian cancer, which was treated with debulking surgery, chemotherapy, and radiation 5 years ago. Despite the aggressive treatment, S.H.'s disease continue to progress. Two months ago, she presented to the ED with a complaint of urinary retention. S.H. was evaluated and found to have metastatic cancer with ureteral obstruction. The obstruction was managed with a left nephrostomy tube and right ureteral stent. However, while in the hospital, S.H. also developed a left DVT, which required inpatient anticoagulation therapy.

Eventually S.H. was discharged to home and instructed to follow up with her primary care physician for management of her oral anticoagulation therapy. Within a few weeks, S.H. returned to the hospital with the complaint of increased abdominal pain and severe constipation. She was diagnosed with colon obstruction secondary to metastatic disease. S.H. was transferred to endoscopy for placement of a colonic stent. In addition to the colon obstruction they found extensive liver metastasis and multiple pulmonary nodules consistent with metastasis.

During the endoscopy procedure, S.H. had an episode of vomiting with possible aspiration; however, she did not show immediate signs of distress following the episode. The procedure was completed without further complications, and S.H. was transferred to the floor for further management. A few hours later, S.H. became more short of breath and developed a fever. Eventually she was transferred to the ICU because of her increased dyspnea and mild hypoxia. At that time, S.H. was requiring 6 L/min of oxygen to keep her oxygen saturations greater than 90%. Her blood pressure was 130/70 mm Hg, heart rate 115, and respiratory rate 38. She also had a temperature of 39.9°C (103.8°F). Portable chest radiograph showed low lung volumes with atelectasis and nodules in the upper left lung.

1. What additional diagnostic tests would be helpful?
2. Depending on the diagnosis, what medical options are available for S.H?
3. What part of Virchow's triad might contribute to S.H.'s current symptoms?Want to Know More?

## WANT TO KNOW MORE?

A wide variety of resources to enhance your learning and understanding of this chapter are available on thePoint.

You will find:

- References
- Selected readings
- NCLEX-style review questions
- Internet resources
- And more!

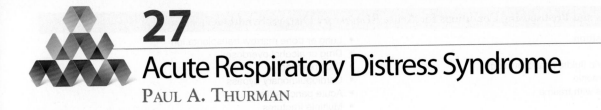

# 27

# Acute Respiratory Distress Syndrome

PAUL A. THURMAN

**LEARNING OBJECTIVES**

*Based on the content in this chapter, the reader should be able to:*

1. Relate the causes, assessment findings, and outcomes of acute respiratory distress syndrome (ARDS) to the care of the critically ill.
2. Assess patients with ARDS based on international definitions.
3. Relate the assessment and diagnostic findings of ARDS to the pathophysiologic processes.
4. Describe mechanical ventilation strategies used to prevent ventilator-induced lung injury.
5. Explain the management of patients with ARDS and rationales for the interventions.
6. Discuss potential complications of ARDS and the related interventions.
7. Review the use of critical care "bundles" as they relate to the care of patients with ARDS.

Acute respiratory distress syndrome (ARDS) represents a complex clinical syndrome rather than a single disease process, and carries a high risk of mortality. The severity of the clinical course, the uncertainty of the outcome, and the reliance on the full spectrum of critical care resources require the collaborative practice of the entire health care team. Since the 1960s, researchers and clinicians have investigated the nature of the pathologic process and explored treatment options with the goal of improving outcome. Through this application of research to practice, we know that some previous strategies have been ineffective, and innovations in mechanical ventilation, sedation, nutrition, pharmacologic intervention, and extracorporeal support remain important research initiatives. A key role for the critical care nurse is early detection and prevention of lung injury, making it essential to be knowledgeable about risk factors, assessment tools and protocols, and prevention strategies in relation to the pathophysiology of lung injury.

ARDS was first described in 1967 and was termed *adult* (rather than *acute*) respiratory distress syndrome because of a misconception that the syndrome occurred only in adults. Recognition of the prevalence of this syndrome in younger patients led to the current terminology. ARDS is at the extreme end of a continuum of hypoxic lung injury that results in respiratory failure. In 1994, the American–European Consensus Conference (AECC) members issued definitions of acute lung injury (ALI) and ARDS that have been widely used; however, in 2012 the definitions were revised to improve the identification of patients with ALI and ARDS.[1] The Berlin Definition addresses some of the limitations of the AECC definition, including clarification of the exclusion of hydrostatic edema and adding minimum ventilator settings, and provides slight improvement in predictive validity. ALI was removed from the definition in favor of having three severity categories of ARDS: mild, moderate, and severe.[1]

## Etiology, Diagnostic Criteria, and Incidence

ARDS may be precipitated by direct or indirect pulmonary injury, possibly in previously healthy people who are exposed to an insult (Box 27-1). ARDS is acute in onset, and symptoms typically develop over 4 to 48 hours after the inciting insult, making a cause-and-effect association somewhat difficult. Recently, several related respiratory disorders have been found presenting with clinical signs of ALI. These disorders may ultimately lead to development of ARDS and include influenza, severe acute respiratory syndrome (SARS), and transfusion-related acute lung injury (TRALI).

TRALI is the leading cause of transfusion-related mortality in the United States.[2] It is theorized that an interaction occurs between the recipient's blood and the donor's, among the bioactive compounds produced during blood storage, or a combination of both.[3] Clinical presentation is the sudden onset of respiratory distress within 1 to 2 hours after a transfusion of red blood cells or thawed plasma.[2,3] Peak airway pressures are elevated, airway secretions may be frothy, and the chest radiograph shows patchy infiltrates. Management of the patient is supportive and involves the same principles of mechanical ventilation used in ARDS and avoidance of aggressive diuresis. The blood bank should be notified of a TRALI case, and the patient should not receive further blood products from that donor.

Diagnostic criteria for ARDS have been difficult to define because ARDS closely resembles other conditions. Diagnostic testing is used to "rule out" these conditions, yet the final diagnosis of ARDS is largely based on clinical presentation. No one test, including radiographic evidence, a plasma brain natriuretic peptide less than 500 pg/mL, or a pulmonary artery occlusion pressure (PAOP, formerly known as pulmonary artery wedge pressure) less than 18 cm $H_2O$, is truly indicative of ARDS. An early feature of ARDS is diffuse alveolar damage. Biomarkers of inflammation may provide earlier

---

**BOX 27-1** **Causes and Predisposing Conditions for Acute Respiratory Distress Syndrome**

Genetic Predisposition

Direct Injury

- Aspiration (gastric fluids, near-drowning)
- Infectious pneumonia
- Lung contusions with trauma
- Toxic inhalation
- Upper airway obstruction (relieved)
- SARS coronavirus
- Neurogenic pulmonary edema
- Acute eosinophilic pneumonia*
- Bronchiolitis obliterans with organizing pneumonia*
- Miliary tuberculosis*

Indirect Pulmonary Injury

- Sepsis
- Burns
- Trauma
- Blood transfusion (TRALI)

- Lung or bone marrow transplantation
- Drug or alcohol overdose
- Drug reaction
- Cardiopulmonary bypass
- Acute pancreatitis
- Multiple fractures
- Venous air embolism
- Amniotic fluid embolism
- Pancreatitis

Systemic Inflammatory Response Syndrome Criteria

SIRS is manifested by two or more of the following:

- Temperature greater than 100.4°F (38°C) or less than 96.8°F (36°C)
- Heart rate greater than 90 beats/min
- Respiratory rate greater than 20 breaths/min or an arterial carbon dioxide tension ($PaCO_2$) less than 32 mm Hg
- White blood cell count greater than 12,000 cells/mm³ or less than 4,000 cells/mm³ OR more than 10% immature (band) forms.

*Specific treatment required.

---

recognition of ARDS before deterioration is seen in the clinical presentation. Currently work is underway to identify these biomarkers in plasma,[4] bronchoalveolar lavage,[5] and the patient's exhaled breath.[6]

ARDS occurs between 33.8 and 75 patients per 100,000 of the population in the United States with a 40% to 50% mortality rate.[7] The patients most at risk for development of ARDS are older than 65 years, with a severe acute illness on presentation, such as sepsis or a preexisting chronic disorder. Although sepsis is the most common cause of ARDS, any person with one of the potential precipitating causes of ARDS is susceptible, and nurses need to be vigilant for early warning signs (see Box 27-1). Most patients with ARDS require a period of mechanical ventilation support for days to weeks.

## Pathophysiology

ARDS was first described in case reports of patients presenting with acute tachypnea, decreased lung compliance, diffuse pulmonary infiltrates on chest radiograph, and hypoxemia.[8] Researchers have used histologic examination of lungs showing lung fibrosis and that pathologic processes are not limited to the lung endothelium but also a result of alterations of lung epithelium and vascular tissue as well as the development of hyaline membranes. Pathologic changes in lung vascular tissue, increased lung edema, and impaired gas exchange are hallmarks of ARDS and directly related to a

cascade of events resulting from release of cellular and biochemical mediators.

## Pathologic Changes in ARDS

Mediators released as a result of either direct or indirect injury can precipitate ARDS. There is a relationship between clinical presentation (hypoxemia resistant to supplemental oxygen, tachypnea, and dyspnea), mediator release (interleukins [ILs], tumor necrosis factor-α [TNF-α], and platelet-activating factor [PAF]), and pathologic changes (microvascular permeability, pulmonary hypertension, and pulmonary endothelial damage). Some primary mediators responsible for lung damage in ARDS and their major actions as they relate to ARDS are listed in Table 27-1.[9-12]

Adequate pulmonary gas exchange depends on open, air-filled alveoli, intact alveolar-capillary membranes, and normal blood flow through the pulmonary vasculature. Diffuse alveolar-capillary membrane damage occurs and increases membrane permeability allowing fluids to move from the vascular space into the interstitial and alveolar space (Fig. 27-1). Air spaces fill with bloody proteinaceous fluid and debris from degenerating cells, causing interstitial and alveolar edema, impairing oxygenation. Inflammatory mediators cause vasoconstriction of the pulmonary vascular bed inducing pulmonary hypertension and reduced blood flow to portions of the lung. Because of the reduced blood flow and decreased hemoglobin (Hgb) in capillaries, there

---

**TABLE 27-1** **Examples of Pathologic Responses to Biologic Mediators**

| Response | Biologic Mediators |
| --- | --- |
| Persistent inflammatory response | Cytokines: IL-1, IL-6, interferon-γ (INF-γ), TNF-α, complement, thromboxane |
| Endothelial membrane disruption | Complement, thromboxane, kinins, TNF-α, toxic oxygen metabolites, leukotrienes, prostaglandins ($PGE_1$ and $PGE_2$) |
| Selective vasoconstriction | Thromboxane, TNF-α, PAF, toxic oxygen metabolites |
| Systemic vasodilation | Complement, prostaglandins, TNF-α, IL-1, IL-6 |
| Myocardial depression | Complement, leukotrienes, TNF-α, myocardial depressant factor |
| Bronchoconstriction | Complement, thromboxane, leukotrienes, PAF |

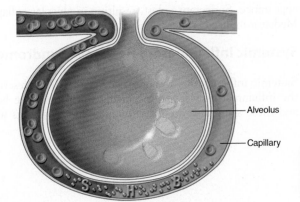

**Phase 1.** Injury reduces normal blood flow to the lungs. Platelets aggregate and release histamine (H), serotonin (S), and bradykinin (B).

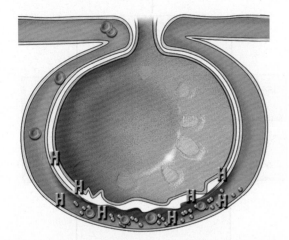

**Phase 2.** Those substances, especially histamine, inflame and damage the alveolar–capillary membrane, increasing capillary permeability. Fluids then shift into the interstitial space.

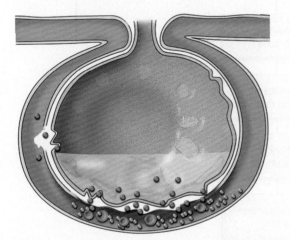

**Phase 3.** As capillary permeability increases, proteins and fluids leak out, increasing interstitial osmotic pressure and causing pulmonary edema.

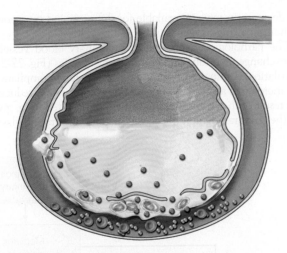

**Phase 4.** Decreased blood flow and fluids in the alveoli damage surfactant and impair the cell's ability to produce more. As a result, alveoli collapse, impeding gas exchange and decreasing lung compliance.

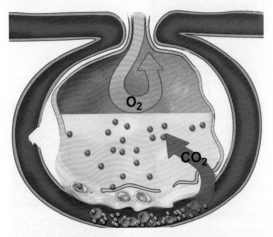

**Phase 5.** Sufficient oxygen cannot cross the alveolar–capillary membrane, but carbon dioxide ($CO_2$) can and is lost with every exhalation. Oxygen ($O_2$) and $CO_2$ levels decrease in the blood.

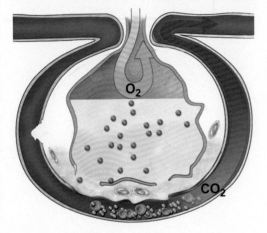

**Phase 6.** Pulmonary edema worsens, inflammation leads to fibrosis, and gas exchange is further impeded.

**FIGURE 27-1**    Pathogenesis of ARDS. Changes in lung epithelium and vascular endothelium result in fluid and protein movement, changes in lung compliance, and disruption of the alveoli with accompanying hypoxia. (From Anatomical Chart Company: Atlas of Pathophysiology, 3rd ed. Ambler, PA: Lippincott Williams & Wilkins, 2010, pp 81, 83.)

is a decrease in oxygen available for diffusion and transport, further impairing oxygenation.

The pathologic changes affect pulmonary blood vessels, gas exchange, and lung and bronchial mechanics (Fig. 27-2). Ventilation is impaired from a decrease in lung compliance and increase in airway resistance. Lung compliance is reduced as a result of the stiffness of fluid-filled, nonaerated lung, giving the chest radiograph the classic "patchy" or "ground glass"

appearance. Surfactant is lost, resulting in alveolar collapse. Mediator-induced bronchoconstriction restricts air flow.

## Systemic Inflammatory Response Syndrome

Systemic inflammatory response syndrome (SIRS) describes the inflammatory response occurring throughout the body and these symptoms are often manifested in patients with

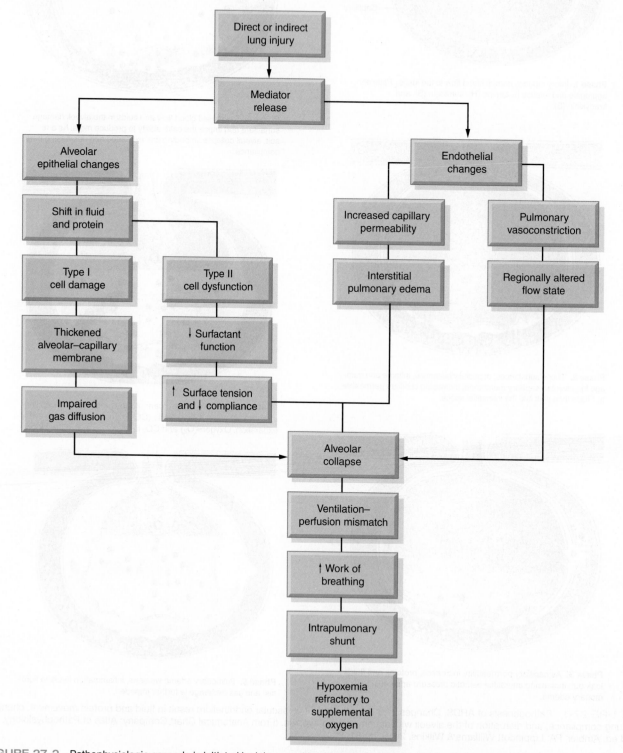

**FIGURE 27-2** Pathophysiologic cascade is initiated by injury resulting in mediator release. The multiple effects result in changes to the alveoli, vascular tissue, and bronchi. The ultimate effect is ventilation–perfusion mismatching and refractory hypoxemia.

ARDS (see Box 27-1). The respiratory system may be the earliest and most common organ system to be involved in the systemic response. Thus, an understanding of the pathophysiology of SIRS and knowledge of the interventions used for SIRS are important in relation to ARDS. Often, patients with SIRS develop multisystem organ dysfunction (MODS). As endothelial damage progresses and tissue hypoxia ensues, the inflammatory response is perpetuated, and the cascade intensifies (upregulates) with the release of more mediators. ARDS and MODS are therefore part of a vicious cycle in the continuum of SIRS. Determination of the triggers for SIRS and ARDS that are present in some individuals but not others and investigations of how to stop the cascade pathways are the subjects of ongoing research. For a more detailed discussion of SIRS and MODS, see Chapter 54.

## Stages of ARDS

The pathologic changes associated with ARDS start with increasing pulmonary edema and progress to inflammation, fibrosis, and impaired healing in the later stages (Table 27-2). Recognizing the dynamic nature of ARDS enables the nurse to understand the changes in physical assessment, mechanical ventilation strategies, treatment, and management that occur throughout the patient's critical care stay.

In stage 1, diagnosis is difficult because the signs of impending ARDS are subtle. Clinically, the patient exhibits increased dyspnea and tachypnea, but there are few radiographic changes. At this point, neutrophils are sequestering; however, there is no evidence of cellular damage. Within 24 hours (a critical time for early treatment), the symptoms of respiratory distress increase in severity, with cyanosis, coarse bilateral crackles on auscultation, and radiographic changes consistent with patchy infiltrates. A dry cough or chest pain may be present. It is at this point (stage 2) that the mediator-induced disruption of the vascular bed results in increased interstitial and alveolar edema. The endothelial and epithelial beds are increasingly permeable to proteins. This is referred to as the "exudative" stage. The hypoxemia is resistant to supplemental oxygen administration, and mechanical ventilation is required for worsening ratio of arterial oxygen to fraction of inspired oxygen ($PaO_2$:$FiO_2$ ratio).

Stage 3, the "proliferative" stage, develops from the 2nd to the 10th day after injury. Evidence of SIRS is now present, with hemodynamic instability, generalized edema, possible onset of nosocomial infections, increased hypoxemia, and lung involvement. Air bronchograms may be evident on chest radiography as well as decreased lung volumes and diffuse interstitial markings.

Stage 4, the "fibrotic" stage, develops after 10 days and is typified by few additional radiographic changes. There is increasing multiorgan involvement, SIRS, and increases in the arterial carbon dioxide tension ($PaCO_2$) as progressive lung fibrosis and emphysematous changes result in increased dead space. Fibrotic lung changes result in ventilation management difficulties, with increased airway pressure and development of pneumothoraces.

## Assessment

### History

Obtaining an accurate and thorough history may provide information that allows for removal of the precipitating cause and interrupting the ensuing mediator response. The history may be difficult to obtain because of the critical presentation of the patient and problems associating a remote event with the ALI. Because the outcome is uncertain and often involves a long critical care admission, the health care team plays a large role in providing support to both the patient and the family. Developing a relationship early (eg, by taking the time to obtain a thorough history) may assist with care throughout the course of admission.

All health care team members contribute information to the history. Information about past relevant incidents (medications, blood transfusions, radiographic contrast agents), the use of medical and complementary therapies, and social factors may be helpful for the person's care. Items of importance include assessment of risk factors for the development of ARDS (see Box 27-1), a social history to assess risk behaviors (eg, human immunodeficiency virus status, smoking, substance abuse), medications (including over-the-counter medications), environmental exposures (chemicals or biologic), and complementary therapies (all exogenous

| TABLE 27-2 | Clinical Presentation and Pathologic Changes During Acute Respiratory Distress Syndrome |  |
|---|---|---|
| **Radiographic Change** | **Clinical Presentation** | **Pathologic Change** |
| *Stage 1* (first 12 h):<br>Normal chest x-ray | Dyspnea, tachypnea | Neutrophil sequestration, no evidence of cellular damage |
| *Stage 2*—Exudative (24 h):<br>Patchy alveolar infiltrate, primarily in dependent lung areas; normal heart size | Dyspnea, tachypnea, cyanosis, tachycardia, coarse crackles, hypoxemia | Neutrophil infiltration, vascular congestion, fibrin strands, increased interstitial and alveolar edema |
| *Stage 3*—Proliferative (2–10 d):<br>Diffuse alveolar infiltrates, possibly air bronchograms, decreased lung volume, normal heart size | Hyperdynamic hemodynamic parameters, SIRS presentation | Type II cell proliferation, microemboli formation, increased interstitial and alveolar inflammatory exudate, early deposition of collagen |
| *Stage 4*—Fibrotic (more than 10 d):<br>Persistent infiltrates, new pneumonic infiltrates, recurrent pneumothorax | Multiple organ involvement, difficulty maintaining adequate oxygenation, sepsis, pneumonia | Type II cell hyperplasia, thickening of interstitial wall with fibrosis, macrophages, fibroblasts, remodeling of arterioles, cyst formation |

Adapted from van Soeren MH, Diehl-Jones WL, Maykut RJ, et al: Pathophysiology and implications for treatment of acute respiratory distress syndrome. AACN Clin Issues 11(2):179–197, 2000.

substances, including inhalations). This information is obtained in addition to the history of the present illness and presenting signs and symptoms.

## Physical Examination

Acute respiratory failure initially may present within a few hours to several days, depending on the initial insult, and does not always progress to ARDS. Monitoring patients who meet the SIRS criteria (see Box 27-1) may aid identification of those who are at risk for development of ARDS. There are few reliable early indicators of impending ARDS and subtle changes may go unnoticed. Vital signs throughout the progression of ARDS vary, but the general trend is hypotension, tachycardia, and hyperthermia or hypothermia. Respiration, initially rapid and labored, varies once mechanical ventilation is instituted.

Early signs and symptoms of respiratory failure include tachypnea, dyspnea, and tachycardia. Breath sounds often are clear in this phase (Table 27-3). Patients with acute respiratory failure may exhibit neurologic changes, such as restlessness and agitation associated with impaired oxygenation and decreased perfusion to the brain. Use of accessory respiratory muscles is evident. The cardiovascular response is tachycardia to improve cardiac output as compensation for poor tissue oxygenation. These attempts to reduce hypoxia represent an adaptive sympathetic nervous system response. These attempts to reduce hypoxia are likely to be ineffective because mediators are already circulating and triggering a cascade of systemic responses.

As ARDS progresses, lung auscultation may reveal crackles secondary to an increase in secretions and narrowed airways; however, the bubbling crackles of cardiogenic pulmonary edema may be minimal. Assessment must be considered in the context of the presenting or initiating disease. For example, pneumonia, one risk factor for ARDS, may confound the ability to diagnose early-stage lung sound changes. The patient may be increasingly restless and confused secondary to hypoxia. Decreases in arterial oxygen saturation ($SaO_2$) are early signs of impending decompensation.

The ability to compensate decreases with increasing pathologic changes. Dependent lung fields have decreased breath sounds as fluid accumulates and alveoli collapse. Agitation may give way to unresponsiveness, an ominous sign in which interventions to support ventilation and oxygenation are required quickly. Other later stages of progression result from tissue hypoxia and include dysrhythmias, chest pain, decreased renal function, and decreased bowel sounds. These are indications of multisystem involvement as highly perfused organ systems respond to decreased oxygen delivery with diminished function.

In the later stages of ARDS, mechanical ventilation support is required. Consolidation of the lungs with fluid reduces breath sounds. Lung compliance decreases, and increasing difficulties maintaining ventilation in the face of increasing resistance ensue. Changes in ventilation (such as decreased $PaO_2$ or increased peak inspiratory pressure) cannot be minimized because development of spontaneous pneumothoraces is a frequent complication of ARDS in the later stages. Transmitted sounds, poor air entry throughout all lung fields, and diffuse crackles coupled with ventilation make breath sounds difficult to assess. Cardiac output decreases despite

**TABLE 27-3  Integrated Assessment of the Patient With Acute Respiratory Distress Syndrome**

| Stage | Physical Examination | Diagnostic Test Results |
|---|---|---|
| Stage 1 (first 12 h) | • Restlessness, dyspnea, tachypnea<br>• Moderate to extensive use of accessory respiratory muscles | • *ABG:* Respiratory alkalosis<br>• *CXR:* No radiographic changes<br>• *Chemistry:* Blood results may vary depending on precipitating cause (eg, elevated white blood cell count, changes in Hgb)<br>• *Hemodynamics:* Elevated PAP, normal or low PAOP |
| Stage 2 (24 h) | • Severe dyspnea, tachypnea, cyanosis, tachycardia<br>• Coarse bilateral crackles<br>• Decreased air entry to dependent lung fields<br>• Increased agitation and restlessness | • *ABG:* Decreased Sao₂ despite supplemental oxygen administration<br>• *CXR:* Patchy bilateral infiltrates<br>• *Chemistry:* Increasing acidosis (metabolic) depending on severity of onset<br>• *Hemodynamics:* Increasingly elevated PAP, normal or low PAOP |
| Stage 3 (2–10 d) | • Decreased air entry bilaterally<br>• Impaired responsiveness (may be related to sedation necessary to maintain mechanical ventilation)<br>• Decreased gut motility<br>• Generalized edema<br>• Poor skin integrity and breakdown | • *ABG:* Worsening hypoxemia<br>• *CXR:* Air bronchograms, decreased lung volumes<br>• *Chemistry:* Signs of other organ involvement: decreased platelets and Hgb, increased white blood cell count, abnormal clotting factors<br>• *Hemodynamics:* Unchanged or becoming increasingly worse |
| Stage 4 (more than 10 d) | • Symptoms of MODS, including decreased urine output, poor gastric motility, symptoms of impaired coagulation<br>**OR**<br>• Single-system involvement of the respiratory system with gradual improvement over time | • *ABG:* Worsening hypoxemia and hypercapnia<br>• *CXR:* Air bronchograms, pneumothoraces<br>• *Chemistry:* Persistent signs of other organ involvement: decreased platelets and Hgb, increased white blood cell count, abnormal clotting factors<br>• *Hemodynamics:* Unchanged or becoming increasingly worse |

CXR, chest radiograph; PAP, pulmonary artery pressure.

persistent tachycardia, due to inflammatory mediators, resulting in hypotension.

## Diagnostic Studies

Throughout the stages of ARDS, the reliance on diagnostic tests is important (see Table 27-3). In the early stages, the need to establish cause may require specific tests, such as blood cultures, bronchoalveolar lavage cultures, and computed tomography (CT). As hypoxemia worsens, instability may preclude transport for diagnostic studies. In later stages, further vigilance is required to intervene for early management of any nosocomial infections. Ongoing monitoring of routine blood gas values, chemistry, and hematology is performed to ensure stability in metabolic parameters and optimization of existing function. Other laboratory studies are generally nonspecific and may include leukocytosis and lactic acidosis.

### Blood Gas Analysis

Deterioration of arterial blood gas (ABG) values, despite interventions, is a hallmark of ARDS. Initially, hypoxemia (an arterial oxygen tension, or $PaO_2$, of less than 60 mm Hg) may improve with supplemental oxygen; however, hypoxemia becomes refractory with a persistently low $SaO_2$. Early in acute respiratory failure, dyspnea and tachypnea are associated with a decreased $PaCO_2$ inducing a respiratory alkalosis (pH greater than 7.45). As gas exchange and ventilation become increasingly impaired, carbon dioxide levels increase. Hypercarbia and elevated lactate from tissue hypoxia and anaerobic metabolism induced by hypoxemia result in a mixed respiratory and metabolic acidosis. Measurement of arterial lactate is commonly ordered as an indication of tissue hypoxia and anaerobic metabolism. Any elevated blood lactate concentration is common in early ARDS and resolves as oxygenation improves. Monitoring lactate levels can aid in ensuring adequate perfusion to tissues despite hypoxemia through manipulation of oxygen delivery, cardiac output, and Hgb. Base excess and deficit follow a similar trend, depending on the degree of tissue and organ hypoxia.

### Radiographic Studies

In the early phase of ARDS, the chest radiographic changes are usually negligible. Within a few days, the chest radiographic findings show patchy bilateral alveolar infiltrates, usually in the dependent lung fields. This may be mistaken for cardiogenic pulmonary edema. Over time, these patchy infiltrates progress to diffuse infiltrates, consolidation, and air bronchograms. CT of the chest also shows areas of infiltrates and consolidation of lung tissue. Daily chest radiographs are important in the continuing evaluation of the progression and resolution of ARDS and for ongoing assessment of potential complications, especially pneumothoraces.

### Intrapulmonary Shunt Measurement

An intrapulmonary shunt is a type of ventilation–perfusion mismatch defined as the percentage of cardiac output that is not oxygenated owing to pulmonary blood flowing past collapsed or fluid-filled and nonventilated alveoli (a physiologic shunt), absence of blood flow to ventilated alveoli (alveolar dead space), or a combination of both of these conditions (silent unit [alveoli with no ventilation and no perfusion]; see Chapter 23, Fig. 23-16). An intrapulmonary shunt of 3% to 5% is present in all people; however, advanced respiratory failure and ARDS are associated with a shunt of 15% or more due to changes in blood flow, endothelial disruption, and alveolar collapse. As the intrapulmonary shunt increases to 15% and greater, more aggressive interventions, including mechanical ventilation, are required because this level of shunt is associated with profound hypoxemia.

Measurement of intrapulmonary shunt requires the use of a pulmonary artery catheter, which may be used in more severe cases. The intrapulmonary shunt fraction (Qs/Qt) is calculated using the arterial oxygen content ($CaO_2$), the mixed venous oxygen content ($CvO_2$), and the capillary oxygen content ($CcO_2$). Oxygen content is determined by Hgb, oxygen saturation ($SO_2$), and partial pressure of oxygen, measured by calculating the oxygen content in the pulmonary capillary bed, in the systemic arterial system, and in the mixed venous blood from the pulmonary artery.

The intrapulmonary shunt fraction may also be estimated using the ratio of arterial oxygen to inspired oxygen (ie, $PaO_2$:$FiO_2$ ratio). In general, a $PaO_2$:$FiO_2$ ratio greater than 300 is normal. Values less than 200 are associated with an intrapulmonary shunt of 15% to 20%, and a value of 100 or less is associated with an intrapulmonary shunt of more than 20%.

### Lung Compliance, Airway Resistance, and Pressures

Lung compliance, or distensibility, decreases as the alveoli fill with fluid or collapse. More effort and greater pressure are required to move air into the lungs as they become increasingly "stiff." In addition, the resistance to airflow into and out of the lungs increases with the accumulation of secretions and mediator-induced bronchoconstriction. Because the patient with ARDS requires mechanical ventilation, lung compliance and airway resistance can be evaluated by assessing ventilator pressures and tidal volume changes. Increases in these pressures as tidal volumes are maintained to achieve a normal $PaCO_2$ indicate reduced compliance and increased resistance to airflow. As airway pressures rise, the lung epithelium is traumatized, resulting in further lung tissue damage. Volutrauma (lung epithelial damage) from persistently elevated airway pressures thus has additional deleterious effects on ventilation and oxygenation.

## Management

Therapeutic modalities to actually treat ARDS have remained elusive. Although there are multiple potential causes of ARDS, management principles are similar. Treatment is supportive, that is, contributing factors are minimized, corrected, or reversed, and while the lungs heal, care is taken so that treatment does no further damage.

In addition, extensive work has gone into creating "bundles," which are elements of care considered core to the management and treatment of specific critical illnesses in intensive care units (ICUs). Box 27-2 lists essential critical care bundles that apply to managing ARDS. These treatments span prevention at early stages of disease onset, such as early goal-directed fluid resuscitation and longer-term prevention

Ventilator-associated pneumonia "bundle" basics
- Elevated head of the bed 30 to 45 degrees
- Daily weaning assessment (spontaneous breathing trials)
- Daily sedation withholding
- Weaning protocol
- DVT prophylaxis
- Peptic ulcer prophylaxis

Sepsis "bundle" basics
- Appropriate antibiotic therapy
- Early goal-directed fluid resuscitation
- Steroid administration
- Activated protein C
- DVT prophylaxis
- Peptic ulcer prophylaxis

Other protocols that may be added
- Tight glucose control
- Postpyloric feeding
- Subglottic suctioning
- Electrolyte replacement

of complications, such as sedation protocols. Regardless, one of the most important roles for critical care nurses is ensuring attention to all these elements to prevent mortality, complications, and to promote recovery.

## Oxygenation and Ventilation

### Oxygen Delivery

Patients with ALI and ARDS develop refractory hypoxemia. Strategies have attempted to optimize normal oxygen delivery parameters, including Hgb, cardiac output, and $SO_2$. Oxygen delivery ($DaO_2$), as determined by Hgb, arterial oxygenation, and cardiac output, is the amount of oxygen delivered to the tissues every minute. Adequate $DaO_2$ (greater than 800 mL $O_2$/min) is essential to meet tissue requirements for oxygen, thereby preventing anaerobic metabolism and hypoxia, which can trigger and perpetuate SIRS. Critically ill patients with ARDS have high demands for oxygen to maintain organ function.

Sufficient amounts of Hgb are necessary to carry oxygen to the cells. There is little research to support the intuitive concept that normal or increased Hgb is required to promote oxygen delivery in patients with SIRS or ARDS. Studies on transfusion requirements indicate that values of approximately 8.0 g/dL are sufficient for critically ill patients, except for those with cardiac disease.

Cardiac output may be altered in ARDS because of SIRS, the effect of hypoxemia on the myocardium, and the decrease in venous return induced by mechanical ventilation. Evaluation of the cardiac output is important so that oxygen delivery can be assessed and appropriate interventions initiated. Therapies to optimize cardiac output are directed toward enhancing preload and contractility and normalizing afterload. The use of a thermodilution pulmonary artery catheter to assess oxygen delivery and consumption for patients with ARDS is rare, but may be used to ensure that appropriate interventions are instituted. There are other less-invasive methods to measure cardiac output utilizing the patient's transduced arterial blood pressure, as well as utilizing

the patient's central venous catheter to measure the venous oxygen content. These methods provide data that can be trended over time without the need for placement of additional catheters.

Fluid management has been used for many years in an effort to balance the type of fluid needed to manage the hallmark edema and decompensation associated with ARDS. At the onset of the disease, early goal-directed fluid resuscitation is recommended. Diuretics and reduced fluid administration have been studied to reduce lung edema. Conservative fluid management with diuresis, plus albumin for hypoproteinemic patients, is associated with modest improvements in oxygenation.[13]

Positive inotropic agents, such as dobutamine or milrinone, are used to enhance contractility and increase cardiac output; however, care must be taken with these agents as they may cause systemic vasodilation worsening hypotension. Vasoconstrictors, such as norepinephrine, may be added to the therapies to counteract the vasodilation induced by SIRS. Vasoconstricting agents must be administered cautiously because many vascular beds, especially in the lungs, are constricted, also as a result of SIRS mediators and hypoxia. Patients receiving inotropic or vasoactive medications require continuous arterial blood pressure monitoring and may require evaluation of cardiac output and other hemodynamic measures.

### Mechanical Ventilation

Methods to deliver appropriate levels of oxygen and allow for removal of carbon dioxide include types of mechanical ventilation and positioning. Lung-protective ventilation strategies limit ventilator-induced lung injury (VILI); these include low tidal volumes (less than 6 mL/kg predicted body weight), the use of adequate positive end-expiratory pressure (PEEP) to reduce the risk of using a high $FiO_2$ and precipitating oxygen toxicity, and limiting plateau pressures to 30 cm $H_2O$.[14,15]

Multiple modes of mechanical ventilation are available to support the patient with respiratory failure. (See Chapter 25 for a complete discussion of mechanical ventilation.) In general, the principle of "do no harm" includes use of the lowest $FiO_2$ to achieve adequate oxygenation and use of small tidal volumes to minimize airway pressures, thus preventing or reducing lung damage (volutrauma). Permissive hypercapnia may be necessary to prevent an increased respiratory rate in the face of lower tidal volumes. PEEP prevents collapse and recruits alveoli, allowing diffusion of gases across the alveolar-capillary membrane. Recommended values for PEEP are 10 to 15 cm $H_2O$, but values in excess of 20 cm $H_2O$ are acceptable to reduce inspired oxygen requirements or maintain adequate oxygenation.[14-18]

Permissive hypercapnia is a strategy that allows the $PaCO_2$ to rise slowly above normal through reduction of tidal volume, therefore limiting the plateau and peak airway pressures. A $PaCO_2$ between 55 and 60 mm Hg and a pH of 7.25 to 7.35 are tolerated when achieved gradually. It is necessary to monitor the increase in $PaCO_2$ to prevent too rapid a rise, and overall values should be no greater than 80 to 100 mm Hg because of the potential effects on cardiopulmonary function. These techniques are not used for patients with cardiac or neurologic involvement.

Several modes of mechanical ventilation are directed toward minimizing airway pressures and iatrogenic lung injury, associated with conventional volume-controlled mechanical ventilation. Pressure-controlled ventilation limits the peak inspiratory pressure to a set level (as opposed to volume-controlled ventilation, which delivers a set tidal volume despite the pressure required to move the set volume into the lungs). Pressure-controlled ventilation also uses a decelerating inspiratory airflow pattern to minimize the peak pressure while delivering the necessary tidal volume. Patients on pressure-controlled ventilation mode may require sedation to prevent dyssynchrony with the ventilator.

### Novel Ventilation Strategies

Inverse-ratio ventilation is another strategy thought to improve alveolar recruitment. Reversal of the normal inspiratory–expiratory ratio (I:E ratio) to 2:1 or 3:1 prolongs inspiration time, preventing complete exhalation. An inverse I:E ratio is achieved through manipulation of the mechanical ventilator. This increased end-expiratory volume creates auto-PEEP (intrinsic PEEP) that is added to the applied extrinsic PEEP. The theoretical advantages include reduced alveolar pressures and overall PEEP levels. This therapy requires sedation and paralytics to improve tolerance.

Airway pressure release ventilation (APRV) similarly inverses the I:E ratio but with the advantage of allowing the patient to initiate breaths. These patients do not require the same level of sedation or paralysis to achieve pressure-limited ventilation and may have improved recruitment of alveoli.

High-frequency oscillatory ventilation (HFOV) uses very low tidal volumes (1 to 4 mL/kg) delivered at rates of 3 to 15 Hz or cycles/s rather than breaths/min, resulting in lower airway pressures and reduced volutrauma. Deleterious effects of HFOV include increased trapping of air in the alveoli (auto-PEEP) and increased mean airway pressures to high levels in some patients. HFOV requires sedation and paralysis as any change in airway pressure will cause oscillation to cease. While there is evidence demonstrating the safety of this approach and improvements in oxygenation, there is no evidence from randomized trials demonstrating mortality benefits over volume assist control, the primary mode used in major ARDS trials, and one study was associated with increased in-hospital mortality.[15,19-21]

Partial ventilatory modes with preserved spontaneous breathing activity during mechanical ventilation have gained use in patients with ARDS. These modes may include assist control (A/C), synchronized intermittent mandatory ventilation, pressure support ventilation, proportional assist ventilation, APRV, biphasic positive airway pressure, or neurally adjusted ventilatory assist. Traditionally these modes were reserved for use in weaning patients from mechanical ventilation, but are now used in all phases of mechanical ventilation. These modes adjust the degree of mechanical support provided to patient need, preserving diaphragmatic contraction and allowing spontaneous breathing efforts. It is unclear whether partial ventilatory support modalities improve survival, but have been shown to alleviate patient–ventilator asynchrony more efficiently than others and decrease the use of sedatives and neuromuscular blockade.[22] Additional studies are needed to support the use of these modes in ARDS.

### Extracorporeal Therapies

Extracorporeal lung support (ECLS) technology involves the use of large vascular cannulas to remove blood from the patient. A pumping device and circuit circulate the blood, and one or two "artificial lungs" remove carbon dioxide and oxygenate the blood. Extracorporeal membrane oxygenation (ECMO) and extracorporeal carbon dioxide removal may potentially be effective in managing ARDS. These highly invasive, high-risk technologies allow the lungs to "rest," because near-apneic ventilation or ventilation with small tidal volumes and slow respiratory rates greatly reduce airway pressures while gas exchange takes place in the artificial membrane lungs.

ECLS gained considerable attention following the 2009 H1N1 influenza pandemic. In these patients, ECMO was used as rescue oxygenation therapy. Several randomized clinical trials and observational studies suggested that ECMO associated with protective mechanical ventilation could improve outcome, but its efficacy remains uncertain. Technological advances have improved the size, safety, and simplicity of ECLS, and may lead to an important advance in the management and outcome of patients with ARDS. Rigorous evidence on the optimum timing, disease characteristics, and indications for ECLS in patients with severe ARDS, and its ability to improve short-term and long-term outcomes, are needed. ECLS should be considered for patients with life-threatening hypoxemia or hypercapnia refractory to conventional mechanical ventilation.[21,23-28] ECLS may generate ethical concerns within the care team. Goal-directed care with a clear plan should be developed at the outset with the care team, patient (when able), and their family.

### Positioning

Frequent position change is well established as a means to prevent and reverse atelectasis and to facilitate removal of secretions from the airways. Although not a treatment for ARDS, elevating the head of the bed greater than 30 degrees is considered necessary care for preventing ventilator-associated pneumonia (VAP).

Prone positioning, either in the patient's bed, using a Stryker frame or Roto-Prone™ therapy system, improves pulmonary gas exchange, facilitates pulmonary drainage in the dorsal lung regions, and aids resolution of consolidated dependent alveoli (in the supine position), particularly in the dorsal lung regions. The evidence for the effectiveness of prone positioning, now a common intervention with ARDS, is variable. Data indicate that carefully performed prone positioning offers an absolute survival advantage of 10% to 17%, making this intervention highly recommended in this specific population.[29-31] Associated risks include loss of airway control through accidental extubation, loss of vascular access, facial edema and development of pressure areas, and difficulties with cardiopulmonary resuscitation. Recommendations on the steps involved in prone positioning appear in Box 27-3.

### Pharmacologic Therapy

Antibiotic therapy is appropriate in the presence of a known microorganism but should not be used prophylactically. The

**BOX 27-3** Summary of Key Steps to Consider for Prone Positioning

1. Evaluate with the interdisciplinary team the patient's condition and determine whether a trial of prone positioning is warranted.
2. Organize the team to ensure familiarity with the procedure and patient care while prone.
   - Use your hospital's evidence-based procedure.
   - Equipment on site.
   - Assign and clarify team roles during prone positioning.
3. Prepare the patient for the procedure.
   - Provide explanation to patient and family.
   - Consider insertion of feeding tube, nasogastric tube, or both as necessary.
4. Assess and document the patient's pre-prone positioning status.
   - Hemodynamic and ventilatory parameters, skin or wound condition, and so forth
5. Protect and maintain the patient's airway.
   - Secure endotracheal tube.
   - Apply in-line suction if not already in place.
6. Use safety precautions to ensure body position will be maintained during the prone positioning procedure.
7. Administer adequate sedation and analgesic medication.
8. Complete the procedure as per protocol. Note: Risks for inadvertent extubation or line displacement are high during the procedure.
9. Assess, evaluate, and monitor the patient's condition.
10. Implement preventive care for pressure areas, eyes, and skin.

signs of SIRS are similar to those of infection (ie, tachycardia, fever, increased white blood cell count), thus creating the temptation to treat with antimicrobial therapy. It is essential to identify a source of infection (isolation of specific bacteria through blood, wound, pulmonary, and other cultures) before initiating antibiotics. Prophylactic antibiotic therapy has not been shown to improve outcome. Emphasis is on prevention of infection, especially nosocomial infection related to the use of invasive vascular catheters and ventilators (eg, VAP).

Bronchodilators and mucolytics are useful in ARDS to assist in maintaining airway patency and reducing the inflammatory reaction and accumulation of secretions in the airways. The response to therapy is evaluated by monitoring airway resistance and pressures and lung compliance.

Administration of intravenous corticosteroids at low doses has been shown to improve survival and reduce morbidity in patients with ARDS; however, the results from recent randomized controlled trials failed to show improved outcomes. Early use of high-dose corticosteroids may increase mortality and cause adverse effects in patients with ARDS and is therefore not recommended. The effectiveness of corticosteroid treatment may largely depend on the underlying diseases and the timing during the course of ARDS.[32]

Nitric oxide is an inhaled gas that causes selective pulmonary vasodilation and therefore reduces the deleterious effects of pulmonary hypertension. To date, nitric oxide has not been shown to improve mortality or oxygenation beyond the first 24 hours of therapy. Nitric oxide should be reserved for those patients with life-threatening refractory hypoxemia after mechanical ventilation has been maximized. Inhaled prostacyclin has also produced pulmonary vasodilation similar to nitric oxide and may be considered.[32]

## Sedation

Effective use of sedation to promote comfort and reduce respiratory effort, thus decreasing oxygen demand, is an important consideration for nurses dealing with patients with ARDS. Neuromuscular blocking agents (NMBAs) and general anesthetics, such as propofol, although not sedatives, are frequently used in these patients to facilitate patient–ventilator synchrony, decreasing the work of breathing and facilitating ventilation, especially when high airway pressures or prone position is applied. Patients with severe ARDS that had early administration of the NMBAs improved the survival rate in a randomized controlled trial.[32,33] NMBAs require concurrent use of sedation to prevent patients who are chemically paralyzed from being alert but unable to move. Frequent assessment of adequacy of both neuromuscular blockade and sedation is an important nursing intervention. NMBAs have been associated with critical illness polyneuropathy and polymyopathy, especially when concurrently administered with corticosteroids.

Pain, anxiety, and delirium are all possible reasons for needing pharmacologic treatment, and it is important to distinguish between them because each requires a different pharmacologic intervention. It is vital to understand why each is being given, what the goals of therapy are, and what the long-term implications of overuse can be. These considerations are balanced with the need to decrease oxygen demand and provide comfort for patients requiring intensive ventilation management and undergoing potentially uncomfortable procedures.

## Nutritional Support

Early initiation of nutritional support is essential for patients with ARDS because nutrition plays an active therapeutic role in recovery from critical illness. There are two major theoretical reasons to use early enteral feeding as a therapeutic intervention in SIRS and ARDS. Mediators (TNF-$\alpha$ and IL-1 in particular) stimulate release of proteolytic enzymes that stimulate protein catabolism from skeletal muscle. Persistent protein loss is compounded by interstitial loss through capillary leak and downregulation of messenger RNA production of intravascular proteins, such as albumin. Earlier in this chapter, reference was made to changes in circulatory patterns resulting from hypoxic sympathetic nervous system reactions. In this way, there is decreased perfusion to the gut. After resuscitation, increases in release of neutrophils further damage the injured, reperfused colon through increased vascular endothelial permeability, thus releasing normal gut bacteria into the systemic circulation and leading to increases in the incidence of peritonitis, pneumonia, and sepsis. The mechanism through which enteral feeding improves outcome remains unproved, but the reduction in mortality in the critically ill who receive enteral feedings indicates that this practice is of general benefit.

A diet with a balanced caloric, protein, carbohydrate, and fat intake is calculated based on metabolic needs, with particular attention paid to specific amino acids, lipid, and carbohydrate intake. Patients with SIRS or ARDS usually require 35 to 45 kcal/kg/d. High-carbohydrate solutions are avoided to prevent excess carbon dioxide production. Recent innovations in amino acid supplementation are being reviewed because of the role of amino acids in the immune response. The role of antioxidants and omega-3 fatty acids is still being investigated as to their use in improving outcomes in ARDS patients.[14,32]

The problem facing the practitioner is the ability to deliver enteral nutrition in the face of decreased gut motility. Insertion of small bowel feeding tubes may be considered.

The role of total parenteral nutrition is controversial, and some clinicians rarely use it, either alone or in combination with enteral nutrition. The risk for aspiration associated with enteral feeding needs to be appreciated, and careful monitoring of absorption and gut function is essential.

A collaborative care guide for the patient with ARDS is given in Box 27-4.

---

**QSEN BOX 27-4** | *COLLABORATIVE CARE GUIDE for the Patient With Acute Respiratory Distress Syndrome*

| Outcomes | Interventions |
|---|---|
| **Impaired Gas Exchange** | |
| Patent airway will be maintained. A $PaO_2$:$FiO_2$ ratio of 200 to 300 or more will be maintained, if possible | • Auscultate breath sounds every 2 to 4 hours and as required<br>• Intubate to maintain oxygenation and ventilation and to decrease work of breathing<br>• Suction endotracheal airway when appropriate (see Chapter 25, Box 25-16, Collaborative Care Guide for the Patient on Mechanical Ventilation)<br>• Hyperoxygenate before and after each suction pass |
| Lung-protective ventilation strategies will be used. Maintain a low tidal volume (<6 mL/kg), a plateau pressure ≤30 cm $H_2O$, and PEEP levels titrated to pressure–volume curve | • Monitor airway pressures every 1 to 2 hours<br>• Monitor airway pressures after suctioning<br>• Administer bronchodilators and mucolytics<br>• Obtain a PEEP study to determine optimal oxygen delivery<br>• Consider a change in ventilator mode to prevent volutrauma |
| The risk for atelectasis, VAP, and volutrauma will be reduced and oxygenation will be improved | • Turn patient side-to-side every 2 hours<br>• Perform chest physiotherapy every 4 hours, if tolerated<br>• Elevate head of bed 30 degrees<br>• Monitor chest x-ray daily |
| Oxygenation will be maximized (a $PaO_2$ of 55 to 80 mm Hg or an $SaO_2$ of 88% to 95%) | • Monitor pulse oximetry and end-tidal carbon dioxide<br>• Monitor ABG values as indicated by changes in noninvasive parameters<br>• Monitor intrapulmonary shunt (Qs/Qt and $PaO_2$:$FiO_2$ ratio)<br>• Increase PEEP and $FiO_2$ to decrease intrapulmonary shunting, using lowest possible $FiO_2$<br>• Consider permissive hypercapnia to maximize oxygenation<br>• Monitor for signs of volutrauma, especially pneumothorax<br>• Consider risk for prolonged hyperoxia and decrease $FiO_2$ to <65% as soon as able |
| **Decreased Cardiac and Peripheral Tissue Perfusion** | |
| Blood pressure, cardiac output, central venous pressure, and pulmonary artery pressures remain stable related to mechanical ventilation | • Assess hemodynamic effects of initiation of mechanical ventilation (eg, decreased venous return and cardiac output)<br>• Monitor electrocardiogram for dysrhythmias related to hypoxemia<br>• Assess hemodynamic effects of changes in inspiratory pressure settings, tidal volume, PEEP, and ventilatory modes<br>• Assess effects of ventilator setting changes on cardiac output and oxygen delivery<br>• Administer intravascular volume to maintain preload |
| Blood pressure, heart rate, and hemodynamic parameters are optimized to therapeutic goals | • Monitor vital signs every 1 to 2 hours<br>• Monitor pulmonary artery pressures and right atrial pressure every hour and cardiac output, systemic vascular resistance, peripheral vascular resistance, $DaO_2$, and oxygen consumption ($VO_2$) every 6 to 12 hours, if pulmonary artery catheter is in place<br>• Administer intravascular volume agents as indicated by real or relative hypovolemia, and evaluate response |
| Serum lactate level will be within normal limits | • Monitor lactate level as required until it is within normal limits<br>• Administer red blood cells, positive inotropic agents, and colloid infusion as ordered to increase oxygen delivery |
| **Risk for Ineffective Renal Perfusion**<br>**Risk for Imbalanced Fluid Volume**<br>**Risk for Electrolyte Imbalance** | |
| Patient is euvolemic. Urine output is >0.5 mL/kg/h | • Monitor hydration status to reduce viscosity of lung secretions<br>• Monitor intake and output<br>• Avoid use of nephrotoxic substances and overuse of diuretics<br>• Administer fluids and diuretics to maintain intravascular volume and renal function |

*(continued)*

**QSEN BOX 27-4** *COLLABORATIVE CARE GUIDE for the Patient With Acute Respiratory Distress Syndrome (continued)*

| Outcomes | Interventions |
| --- | --- |
| There is no evidence of electrolyte imbalance or renal dysfunction | • Replace electrolytes as ordered<br>• Monitor urine output, blood urea nitrogen, creatinine, creatinine clearance, serum osmolarity, and urine electrolytes as required |

**Impaired Physical Mobility**
**Risk for Infection**

| | |
| --- | --- |
| There is no evidence of complications related to bed rest and immobility | • Initiate DVT prophylaxis<br>• Reposition patient frequently<br>• Mobilize patient to chair when hemodynamic stability and hemostasis are achieved<br>• Consult physiotherapist<br>• Conduct range-of-motion and strengthening exercises when able |
| Physiologic changes are detected and treated without delay | • Monitor mechanical ventilator alarms and settings and patient parameters (eg, tidal volume) every 1 to 2 hours<br>• Ensure appropriate settings and narrow limits for hemodynamic, heart rate, and pulse oximetry alarms |
| There is no evidence of infection; white blood cell count is within normal limits | • Monitor for SIRS criteria (increased white blood cell count, increased temperature, tachypnea, tachycardia)<br>• Use strict aseptic technique during procedures, and monitor others<br>• Maintain sterility of invasive catheters and tubes<br>• Change chest tube and other dressings and invasive catheters<br>• Culture blood and other fluids and line tips when they are changed |

**Impaired Tissue Integrity**

| | |
| --- | --- |
| Skin will remain intact | • Assess skin every 4 hours and each time patient is repositioned<br>• Turn patient every 2 hours<br>• Consider pressure relief/reduction mattress, kinetic therapy bed, or prone positioning<br>• Use Braden Scale to assess risk for skin breakdown |

**Imbalanced Nutrition**

| | |
| --- | --- |
| Caloric and nutrient intake will meet metabolic requirements per calculation (eg, basal energy expenditure) | • Provide enteral nutrition within 24 hours<br>• Consult dietitian or nutritional support service<br>• Consider small bowel feeding tube if gastrointestinal motility is an issue for enteral feeding<br>• Monitor lipid intake<br>• Monitor albumin, prealbumin, transferrin, cholesterol, triglyceride, and glucose levels |

**Impaired Comfort**

| | |
| --- | --- |
| Patient will be as comfortable as possible as evidenced by stable vital signs or cooperation with treatments or procedures | • Objectively assess comfort/pain using a pain scale<br>• Provide analgesia and sedation as indicated by assessment<br>• Monitor patient cardiopulmonary and pain response to medication<br>• If patient is receiving neuromuscular blockade for ventilatory control:<br>• Use peripheral nerve stimulator to assess pharmacologic paralysis<br>• Provide continuous or routine (every 1 to 2 hours) intravenous sedation and analgesia |

**Ineffective Coping**

| | |
| --- | --- |
| Patient demonstrates decreased anxiety | • Assess vital signs during treatments, discussions, and the like<br>• Cautiously administer sedatives<br>• Consult social services, clergy, as appropriate<br>• Provide for adequate rest and sleep |

**Teaching/Discharge Planning**

| | |
| --- | --- |
| Patient/significant others understand procedures and tests needed for treatment | • Prepare patient/significant others for procedures, such as bronchoscopy, pulmonary artery catheter insertion, or laboratory studies<br>• Explain the causes and effects of ARDS and the potential for complications, such as sepsis, volutrauma, or renal failure |
| Significant others understand the severity of the illness, ask appropriate questions, and anticipate potential complications | • Encourage significant others to ask questions related to the ventilator, the pathophysiology of ARDS, monitoring, and treatments |

## Prevention of Complications

Complications of ARDS are primarily related to SIRS, VILI, and immobility imposed by critical illness. The most serious of these is the development of MODS due to hypoxemia, hypoxia, and the persistent inflammatory response. An entire spectrum of potential complications exists for the critically ill patient. Critical care forums have compiled evidence-based protocols into bundles for two major critical care situations: VAP and sepsis (see Box 27-2). The introduction of care bundles into critical care supports application of evidence to reduce major complications. The implementation of care bundles has been shown effective in reducing length of stay and reducing ventilator days, but consistent application requires teamwork and monitoring.

Mechanical ventilation with high levels of PEEP, high tidal volumes, and volume-controlled modes predisposes the patient with ARDS to volutrauma, as previously described. Volutrauma may present as a pneumothorax, pneumomediastinum, or subcutaneous or interstitial emphysema. Prompt chest tube insertion is required for a pneumothorax. Prevention of volutrauma by maintaining the lowest possible airway pressures, PEEP, and tidal volumes may be achieved through the use of pressure-limiting modes of mechanical ventilation.

Prevention or reduction in the incidence of VAP can be accomplished by using in-line suction catheters. The use of endotracheal tubes that allow for the removal of pooled subglottic secretions has been shown to reduce VAP. Sinusitis is also associated with VAP. The critical care nurse needs to monitor for nasal secretions and ensure that devices such as nasotracheal or feeding tubes are removed from the nose when these occur. Oral care is an essential component in the prevention of VAP, as it decreases the amount of organisms in the mouth, which may migrate to the lungs (see Chapter 25, Evidence-Based Practice Highlight 25-2). Elevating the head of the bed 30 degrees and feeding the critically ill patient with a postpyloric feeding tube have been shown to reduce microaspiration and VAP.

Immobility caused by bed rest, sedation, or pharmacologic paralysis has multisystem effects. Not infrequently, nosocomial pneumonia develops from accumulated secretions in the airways and atelectasis secondary to immobilization, with bacterial access through and around the endotracheal tube. As discussed, frequent repositioning accompanied by chest physiotherapy will help to reduce stasis of secretions and facilitate removal.

Deep venous thrombosis (DVT) and subsequent pulmonary embolus may be life-threatening complications of immobility. Initiation of DVT prophylaxis within 48 hours of admission minimizes the risk for development of DVT. Low-dose heparin, graded elastic stockings, external pneumatic compression devices, frequent mobilization, and ambulation have been useful in reducing DVT formation.

The physiologic aging process compounds the severity of the metabolic insults and complications of ARDS (Box 27-5).

Patient with ARDS may require transport to areas outside the critical care unit for diagnostic or operative procedures. Careful planning is necessary to ensure that the patient receives the same level of care during the procedure. This is a coordinated multidisciplinary process that includes the nurse,

---

**BOX 27-5**   *CONSIDERATIONS for the Older Patient*

**Acute Respiratory Distress Syndrome**

- People who are 65 years of age or older are at increased risk for multisystem organ involvement with less chance of recovering from ARDS; therefore, the mortality rate rises in this population.
- Because of increased immunosuppression with aging, the elderly are at greater risk for infection; therefore, nosocomial infections, such as urinary tract infections and VAP, are more common.
- Hemodynamic instability adds metabolic insults to already-decreased renal function, thus predisposing this group to renal failure.
- Decreased stroke volume; possible coronary artery disease (CAD), atherosclerosis, or both; and increased systolic blood pressure and peripheral vascular resistance alter hemodynamic recovery.
- Decreased maximal oxygen uptake associated with decreased lung volumes puts elderly patients at greater risk for ventilator-associated lung injury.
- Decreased muscle mass associated with aging makes recovery from prolonged immobility more difficult. Therefore, an elderly person with ARDS may require prolonged rehabilitation.
- Generalized peripheral edema, multiple invasive tests, and prolonged bed rest, combined with the decreased skin integrity associated with old age, increase the elderly patient's potential for development of pressure ulcers and skin tears.
- Elderly patients with ARDS are at risk for not receiving the same quality and quantity of treatment and care as younger patients, due to the effects of ageism. The patient's age is one factor to consider in outcome and prognosis, but not the only one.
- The incidence of comorbid conditions, especially non-insulin-dependent diabetes mellitus and CAD, increases with age. Research findings indicate that comorbid conditions increase the risk for death in patients with ARDS.
- Based on previously expressed wishes, the patient and family may request no initiation of, or early removal from, life support. A person's life experience or vision of risk related to prolonged illness with high possibility of mortality may influence this decision, and these wishes should be respected.

---

respiratory therapist, provider, perfusionist, and receiving department. Loss of an endotracheal tube or ECLS cannula could be fatal. The nurse should map out the shortest direct route to the destination and ensure that all necessary personnel and equipment will fit within the elevator if the route involves changing floors. Make sure that all diagnostic tests needed are ordered prior to the transport to minimize the number of transports.

## Outcomes and Conclusion

Patients who survive their critical illness may have significant disability, both physical and psychologic. Some survivors develop pulmonary fibrosis with chronic lung disease. Recent evidence demonstrates that mechanical ventilation, particularly where significant overstretch occurs, may drive the pathogenesis of fibrosis in patients with ARDS.[34] Survivors may have significant muscle wasting and weakness, which could have profound impact on their rehabilitation and long-term outcome. A study of ARDS survivors showed that at 3-month follow-up almost 40% of patients screened positive for general anxiety symptoms—over twice that of the general population. These symptoms were associated with impaired physical functioning and lower health-related quality of life. Critical care nurses can affect not only the survival of these patients, but their long-term functioning should they survive, by preventing the complications associated with ARDS.

## Clinical Applicability Challenges

### CASE STUDY

A.D., a 36-year-old man, is admitted to the hospital for pneumonia after having influenza. He progresses to sepsis with shock. He is transferred to the ICU.

After arrival in the ICU, the patient develops cardiorespiratory failure, and is intubated and placed on vasoactive support of vasopressin, 0.04 units/min, and norepinephrine, 10 mcg/min. He is having multiple episodes of oxygen desaturation requiring an $FiO_2$ of 1.00. He is placed on A/C ventilation of 20 breaths/min and a tidal volume of 6 mL/kg with PEEP of 10 cm $H_2O$. His breath sounds are clear with no crackles or wheezes. His temperature is 101.1°F (38.4°C).

As the day progresses, A.D. becomes difficult to ventilate and is sedated with a fentanyl infusion and propofol (Diprivan) infusion. He also requires neuromuscular blockade with cisatracurium (Nimbex) for patient–ventilator dyssynchrony. His cardiac index is 4.0, heart rate is 120 beats/min, central venous pressure is 8 mm Hg, PAOP is 10 mm Hg, and systemic vascular resistance index is 900 dynes/s/m²/cm⁵. ABG values show $PaO_2$ of 68 mm Hg, $PaCO_2$ of 39 mm Hg, pH of 7.36, $HCO_3$ of 18 mEq/L, and $O_2$ saturation of 95.5%.

The following day, A.D. continues to decline on 100% $FiO_2$. He has developed a mild to moderate bilateral wheeze in his chest. Chest radiography shows small bilateral effusions but is otherwise clear. $PaO_2$ remains low at 50 mm Hg. Blood, sputum, and urine specimens are sent to the laboratory for culture. Empiric broad-spectrum antibiotics are started. With no improvement in the ABGs and the rising pulmonary arterial pressures (47/16 mm Hg), nitric oxide is started at 10 ppm. CT of the thorax is performed and shows bilateral airspace opacity. A.D. is placed in the prone position with moderate improvement in oxygenation. Before proning,

A.D. has a postpyloric feeding tube placed to begin enteral feeding.

Three days after admission, $FiO_2$ remains at 100%, nitric oxide continues at 10 ppm, and prone position with no improvement in oxygenation. Temperature remains elevated at 102°F (39.1°C) with a white blood cell count of 12,000/mm³. All cultures remain negative. Chest radiography shows fluffy white opacities bilaterally and an opacified right upper lung lobe. A bronchoscopy is performed to examine the right upper lobe, and copious secretions are removed. Several short attempts at lung recruitment to expand the lungs are performed, and because there is still no improvement, A.D. is placed on ECLS.

Over the next few days, A.D. makes small steps forward with his oxygenation, yet continues to require full ECLS support. A transbronchial biopsy is performed and demonstrates DAD and organizing pneumonia. After 10 days, he has made improvement and ECLS is being weaned.

After almost 4 months in hospital, P.F. is discharged home. On a follow-up examination, he had recovered to about 60% of his prehospital status. His pulmonary function test shows mild impairment. CT of his thorax shows scarring and fibrosis in nondependent lung zones and some bronchiectasis in dependent lung zones. This is interpreted as ventilator-acquired (induced) lung injury with stretch injury in the nondependent areas and airway trauma in the dependent airways.

1. What symptoms were presented early in A.D. that indicated the onset of ARDS?
2. Early enteral feeding was used to support A.D. For what other care should the nurse advocate to reduce complications?
3. What is the evidence that NMBAs have a positive benefit in treating a patient with ARDS?

### WANT TO KNOW MORE?

A wide variety of resources to enhance your learning and understanding of this chapter are available on thePoint.

You will find:

- References
- Selected readings
- NCLEX-style review questions
- Internet resources
- And more!

# PART 7

# Renal System

# **28**

# Anatomy and Physiology of the Renal System

Kara Adams Snyder

*Based on the content in this chapter, the reader should be able to:*

1. Describe the impact of afferent and efferent blood supply on renal function.
2. Discuss the structures comprising the nephron: glomerulus, proximal tubule, loop of Henle, and distal and collecting tubules.
3. Differentiate the functions of the nephron, including glomerular filtration, active and passive transport, and tubular secretion.
4. Compare normal fluid pressures in the nephron and how they affect glomerular filtration rate.
5. Explain the relationship of antidiuretic hormone, rennin, and aldosterone to fluid regulation by the kidneys.
6. Explain the mechanisms used by the kidneys to help achieve clearance of substances and maintain homeostasis.
7. Describe the physiologic roles of the predominant electrolytes.

With each contraction of the heart, the kidneys receive 21% of the cardiac output. This means that approximately 1.2 L of blood passes through the kidneys each minute, and the body's entire blood volume is filtered through the kidneys 340 times/d.[1] Given this large volume of blood, the kidneys have a dominant role in filtration and a minor role in metabolism. Therefore, the kidneys have a large requirement for pressure and a relatively smaller requirement for oxygen. The regulation and maintenance of the concentration of solutes in the extracellular fluid (ECF) of the body are the primary functions of the kidney. The kidneys remove metabolic waste products and excess concentrations of constituents and conserve substances present in normal or low quantities.

## Macroscopic Anatomy of the Renal System

The kidneys are bean-shaped organs that lie in a retroperitoneal position in the abdomen (Fig. 28-1). The kidneys are partially protected by the last pair of ribs, with the right kidney slightly lower than the left because of the location of the liver. The adrenal glands, which are discussed in more detail in Chapter 42, cap the kidneys.

The adult kidneys are approximately 12 cm long, 6 cm wide, and 2.5 cm thick. The kidney weighs about 150 g, the size of a clenched fist. The size and weight of the kidneys are clinically valuable indicators in ultrasound-guided differential diagnosis of renal failure (see Chapter 29).

There are two distinct layers of the kidney: the renal cortex and the renal medulla (Fig. 28-2). The renal cortex is the outer portion of the kidney and has two regions: the cortical region and the juxtamedullary "next to the medulla" region (Fig. 28-2). The cortex contains the glomeruli, the proximal tubules, the cortical loops of Henle, the distal tubules, and the cortical collecting ducts. The inner layer, the medulla, in addition to the cortical structures, contains the renal pyramids. The renal cortex receives 90% of the total renal blood flow and only 5% to 10% reaches the outer medulla. The pyramids contain the medullary loops of Henle and the medullary portions of the collecting ducts, which join to form a minor calyx. Minor calyces come together to form a major calyx. The renal calyces further join to become the conduit for directing urine into the ureter.

Urine exits the kidney at an oblique angle through a fibromuscular structure, the ureter. Peristalsis helps maintain the flow of urine through the ureter. The ureter enters the bladder in the trigone region. The trigone region of the bladder is so called for the three structures that form the shape of a triangle: the two ureters and the urethra. The peristaltic actions in the ureter and the angle of entry at the bladder help prevent the reflux of urine. Urine exits the bladder through the urethral orifice via the urethra. The male urethra is about 20 cm long; the female urethra is about 3 to 5 cm long.[1] On the medial aspect of each kidney, there is an indentation known as the hilum. It is through this indentation that the renal arteries and nerves enter and the renal veins, lymphatics, and ureters exit (see Fig. 28-2). The kidneys receive their blood supply from the renal artery, a branch of the descending aorta. The renal artery divides into several smaller branches and eventually

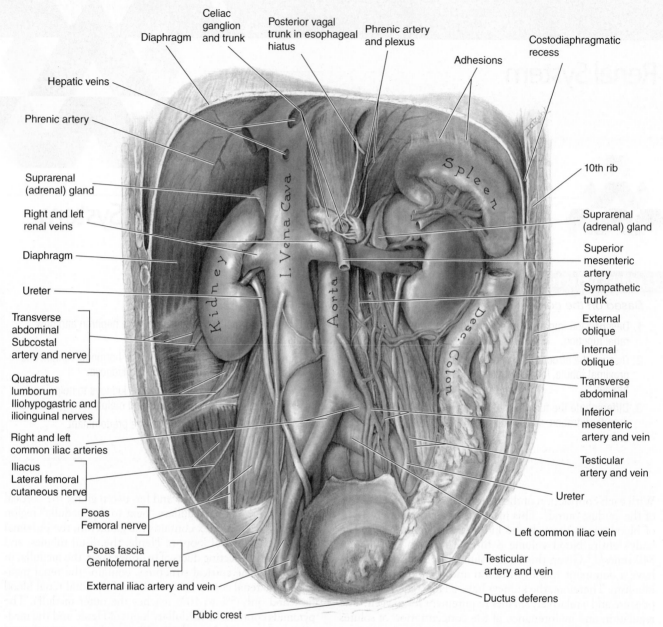

Celiac
ganglion
and trunk

Posterior vagal
trunk in esophageal
hiatus

Phrenic artery
and plexus

Adhesions

Costodiaphragmatic
recess

Diaphragm

Hepatic veins

Phrenic artery

Suprarenal
(adrenal) gland

Right and left
renal veins

Diaphragm

Ureter

Transverse
abdominal
Subcostal
artery and nerve

Quadratus
lumborum
Iliohypogastric and
ilioinguinal nerves

Right and left
common iliac arteries

Iliacus
Lateral femoral
cutaneous nerve

Psoas
Femoral nerve

Psoas fascia
Genitofemoral nerve

External iliac artery and vein

Pubic crest

10th rib

Suprarenal
(adrenal) gland

Superior
mesenteric
artery

Sympathetic
trunk

External
oblique

Internal
oblique

Transverse
abdominal

Inferior
mesenteric
artery and vein

Testicular
artery and vein

Ureter

Left common iliac vein

Testicular
artery and vein

Ductus deferens

Kidney — I. Vena Cava — Aorta — Desc. Colon — Spleen

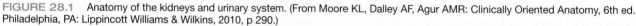

**FIGURE 28.1** Anatomy of the kidneys and urinary system. (From Moore KL, Dalley AF, Agur AMR: *Clinically Oriented Anatomy*, 6th ed. Philadelphia, PA: Lippincott Williams & Wilkins, 2010, p 290.)

into numerous afferent arterioles (Fig. 28-3). Each afferent arteriole forms a tuft of capillaries, known as the glomerulus, where blood is filtered. The efferent (leaving the glomerulus) arteriole branches to form a second capillary bed, known as the peritubular capillaries (see Fig. 28-3). The peritubular capillaries surround the loop of Henle to reabsorb more water and solutes as needed for homeostasis. Reconnecting, this vast network of vessels eventually returns to the central circulation through the renal veins. The renal blood flow per weight unit is higher than any other major organ in the body.

The glomerular filtration rate (GFR) is relatively stable over a wide range of arterial blood pressures. The concept of "autoregulation" offers the kidneys such stability: the afferent arterioles adjust their diameter in response to the pressure of blood coming to them. If the blood pressure decreases, the smooth muscles of the afferent arterioles relax, vasodilation

occurs, and perfusion increases, thereby maintaining the GFR at its normal rate. Conversely, with an increase in blood pressure, these vessels constrict. In healthy persons, autoregulation maintains homeostasis quite nicely when mean blood pressure falls approximately within a range of 80 to 180 mm Hg. Outside of this range, autoregulation is limited and GFR is proportional to renal perfusion. For example, if the systemic blood pressure falls greatly, such as in shock, the GFR falls to near zero, thereby producing near anuria.

## Microscopic Anatomy of the Renal System and Normal Renal Physiology

Urine, the end product of kidney function, is formed from the blood by the smallest unit of the kidney, the nephron

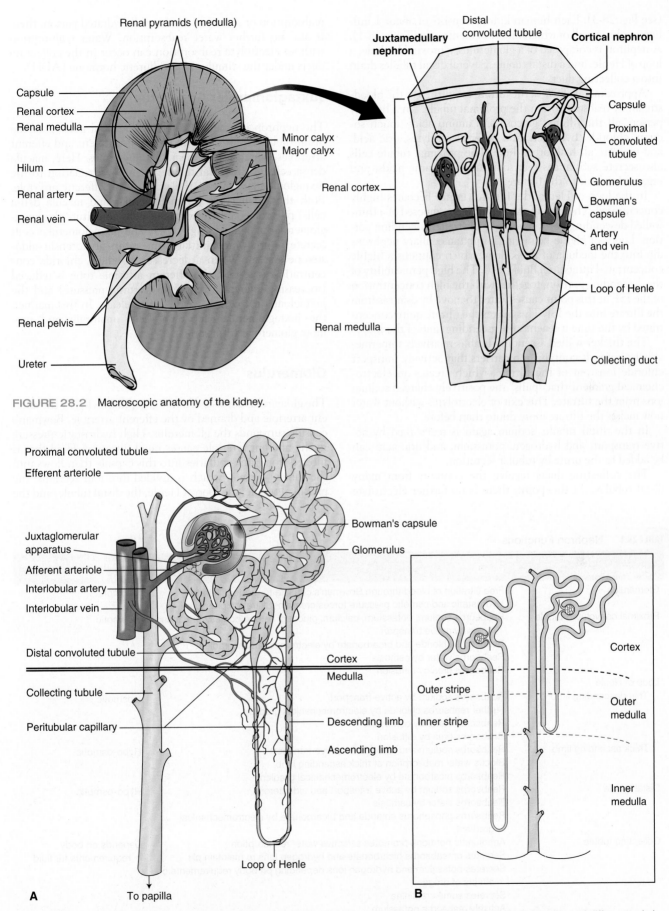

**FIGURE 28.2** Macroscopic anatomy of the kidney.

**FIGURE 28.3** **A:** Nephron, showing the glomerular and tubular structures along with the blood supply. **B:** Comparison of differences in location of tubular structures of the cortical and juxtamedullary nephrons. (From Porth CM: Pathophysiology: Concepts of Altered Health States, 9th ed. Philadelphia, PA: Lippincott Williams & Wilkins, 2013, p 743.)

(see Fig. 28-3). Each human kidney consists of about 1 million nephrons, all of which function identically (Table 28-1). A nephron is composed of a glomerulus, a proximal tubule, a loop of Henle, and a distal tubule. Several distal tubules drain into a collecting duct.

Approximately 80% of the filtrate is returned to the bloodstream by reabsorption in the proximal tubule.[1] In a healthy person, all the filtered glucose and amino acids, much sodium, chloride, hydrogen, and other electrolytes, uric acid, and urea are all reabsorbed here. The proximal tubule cells also secrete substances (eg, some drugs, organic acids, and organic bases) into the filtrate.

In the loop of Henle, the filtrate (urine) becomes highly concentrated. This part of the nephron is composed of a thin-walled descending portion and a thick-walled ascending portion. Loops of Henle belonging to juxtamedullary nephrons dip into the medulla of the kidney, which contains a highly concentrated interstitial fluid (ISF). The high permeability of the descending portion, together with the high concentration of the ISF, at this point causes water to move by osmosis from the filtrate into the ISF. This makes the filtrate quite concentrated by the time it reaches the ascending limb of the loop.

The thicker-walled ascending limb is relatively impermeable to water. It contains ion carriers that actively transport chloride ions out of the filtrate, which creates an electrochemical gradient that "pulls" the positively charged sodium ions from the filtrate. This exit of electrolytes without water now makes the filtrate more dilute than before.

In the distal tubule, sodium again is reabsorbed by active transport, and hydrogen, potassium, and uric acid can be added to the urine by tubular secretion.

The collecting ducts receive the contents from many distal tubules. At this point, there is no further electrolyte reabsorption or secretion. In the well-hydrated person, there is also no further water reabsorption. Water reabsorption without electrolyte reabsorption can occur in the collecting ducts under the stimulus of antidiuretic hormone (ADH).

## Juxtaglomerular Apparatus

The nephron is arranged so that the initial portion of the distal tubule lies at the juncture of the afferent and efferent arterioles, which is very near the glomerulus. Here, macula densa cells of the distal tubule lie in approximation to the juxtaglomerular cells of the wall of the afferent arteriole. Both these cell types (juxtaglomerular and macula densa cells) plus some connective tissue cells constitute the juxtaglomerular apparatus (Fig. 28-4). The juxtaglomerular cells secrete renin, which initiates the renin–angiotensin–aldosterone system. When a decrease in sodium chloride concentration is sensed, the afferent arteriole tone is reduced (increasing afferent arteriole hydrostatic pressure) and the juxtaglomerular cells increase renin release. In this manner, the juxtaglomerular apparatus helps maintain and promote glomerular filtration.

## Glomerulus

The glomerulus consists of a tuft of capillaries fed by the afferent arteriole and drained by the efferent arteriole. Bowman's capsule surrounds the glomerulus. High hydrostatic pressure in the afferent arteriole causes rapid filtration. Fluid that is filtered from the capillaries into this capsule then flows into the tubular system, which is divided into four sections: the proximal tubule, the loop of Henle, the distal tubule, and the

**TABLE 28.1** **Nephron Functions**

| Nephron Structure | Function | Concentration of Filtrate Along the Nephron |
|---|---|---|
| Glomerulus | Free filtration of blood through Bowman's capsule to produce filtrate | Isosmotic |
| | Hydrostatic and osmotic pressure forces create net filtration pressure | |
| Proximal convoluted tubule | Reabsorbs sodium, potassium, calcium, glucose, ketone bodies, and amino acids by active transport | Isosmotic |
| | Reabsorbs chloride and bicarbonate by electromechanical gradient | |
| | Reabsorbs water by osmosis | |
| | Reabsorbs urea by diffusion | |
| Loop of Henle | | |
| Thin descending limb | Reabsorbs sodium by active transport | Isosmotic |
| | Further reabsorbs chloride by electromechanical gradient | |
| | Reabsorbs water by osmosis | |
| | Reabsorbs urea by diffusion | |
| Thick ascending limb | Reabsorbs sodium and chloride by active transport | Hypo-osmotic |
| | Blocks water reabsorption at thick ascending limb | |
| | Reabsorbs bicarbonate by electromechanical gradient | |
| Distal tubule | Reabsorbs sodium by active transport and aldosterone | Hypo-osmotic |
| | Reabsorbs water by osmosis | |
| | Reabsorbs phosphorus chloride and bicarbonate by electromechanical gradient | |
| Collecting tubule | Antidiuretic hormone promotes selective water reabsorption | Depends on body requirements for fluid |
| | Secretes or reabsorbs bicarbonate and hydrogen ions to maintain pH | |
| | Secretes potassium and hydrogen ions depending on body requirements or effects of drugs | |
| | Secretes some creatinine | |
| | Actively reabsorbs potassium | |

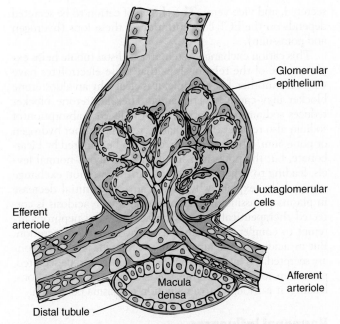

**FIGURE 28.4** The juxtaglomerular apparatus. The macula densa cells lie in close proximity to the afferent and efferent arterioles, which help to regulate nephron functions.

collecting duct (see Fig. 28-3). Lower hydrostatic pressure in the efferent circulation allows reabsorption. Most of the water and electrolytes are reabsorbed into the blood in the peritubular capillaries that surround the tubular structures. The end products of metabolism remaining in the tubules pass into the urine.

Glomerular filtration is determined by net filtration pressure. Hydrostatic pressure and osmotic pressure forces are major factors. Hydrostatic pressure is driving or "pushing" pressure. Osmotic pressure is the pressure exerted by water (or any solvent) on a semipermeable membrane as it attempts to cross the membrane into an area containing more molecules that cannot cross the semipermeable membrane. The pores in the glomerular capillary make it a semipermeable membrane that permits smaller molecules and water to cross but prevents larger molecules (eg, plasma proteins) from crossing. Protein concentrations are the greatest factors in determining an osmotic pressure, and therefore, osmotic pressure is often referred to as colloid osmotic pressure. Four forces are considered when determining net filtration of fluid (Fig. 28-5).

The rate at which the filtrate is formed is the GFR. Major clinical factors that influence the GFR are the blood hydrostatic pressure and the filtrate osmotic pressure. Hypoproteinemia, as in starvation, lowers filtrate osmotic pressure and increases the GFR. The GFR decreases with severe hypotension because of a drop in blood hydrostatic pressure, when autoregulatory control may be lost. Other factors that decrease the hydrostatic pressure, (and therefore the GFR) are afferent arteriole constriction and renal artery stenosis.

From the 20% to 25% of the cardiac output that goes to the kidneys in a resting adult, about 125 mL of filtrate is produced each minute. This totals 180 L/d and is about 4.5 times the total amount of fluid in the body. Obviously, not all this filtrate can be excreted as urine. As this filtrate passes from Bowman's capsule through the remainder of the nephrons, 178.5 L is reabsorbed into the bloodstream and about 1.5 L/d is excreted as urine. Similarly, at plasma glucose levels of less than 200 mg/dL, none of the filtered glucose is found in the urine when it enters the collecting tubules. The volume and content of the urine are the result of tubular reabsorption and tubular secretion.

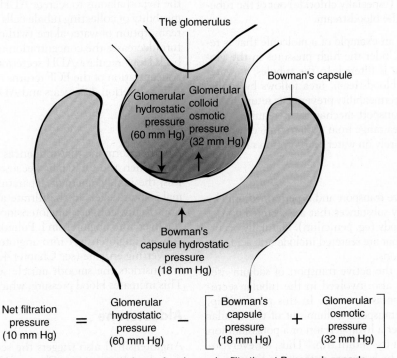

**FIGURE 28.5** Interaction of hydrostatic and osmotic forces for glomerular filtration at Bowman's capsule.

## Tubules

### Tubular Reabsorption

Reabsorption is accomplished by active transport, osmosis, and diffusion. It occurs in all parts of the nephron as substances moving from the lumen into the peritubular capillaries.

**ACTIVE TRANSPORT.** Active transport involves the binding of a molecule of a substance to a carrier, which then, acting as a pump, moves the molecule from one side of the membrane to the other against the concentration gradient of that substance. Many processes for active transport use the sodium–potassium pump. Therefore, the small oxygen requirements of the kidneys are closely linked to the active transport processes that occur in the nephron.

In the nephrons, reabsorption by active transport removes molecules from the filtrate (urine) back to the bloodstream.

Because active transport involves carrier molecules and energy exchanges, there is an upper limit to the number of molecules of a substance that can be transported at one time. This maximal limit for reabsorption rates is called $T_{max}$. Glucose is an example of a molecule that appears in the same concentrations that it appears in the blood. As serum glucose rises, filtrate glucose also rises. The renal tubules reabsorb the filtered glucose at faster and faster rates, until all of this molecule's active transport mechanisms are being used. At this $T_{max}$ more glucose is appearing in the filtrate than can be reabsorbed, and glucose is excreted in the urine. This "spilling" of glucose into the urine indicates serum levels higher than $T_{max}$.

**OSMOSIS.** The active transport of sodium is responsible for the osmotic reabsorption of water from the filtrate in the proximal (and later, in the distal) tubule. Water is osmotically "pulled out" of the tubular fluid. Both water and sodium then diffuse into peritubular capillaries and are returned to the bloodstream. This movement of positively charged sodium ions also creates an electrochemical gradient that draws negatively charged ions (especially chloride) out of the tubular fluid and back into the bloodstream.

**DIFFUSION.** Urea is an example of a molecule that is reabsorbed by diffusion. Under the high pressures in the glomerular capillaries, urea is filtered. In the tubules, as water is reabsorbed into the bloodstream, urea follows by simple diffusion. No selective permeability prevents its return to the bloodstream, and no transport mechanism is required. The reabsorption rates of urea range from 40% to 60% of what is filtered and depend entirely on water reabsorption rates.

### Tubular Secretion

Secretion involves active transport and is performed only by distal tubule cells. Many substances that are secreted do not occur naturally in the body (eg, penicillin). Naturally occurring bodily substances that are secreted include uric acid, potassium, and hydrogen ions.

In the distal tubule, the active transport of sodium uses a carrier system that is also involved in the tubular secretion of hydrogen and potassium ions. In this relationship, every time the carrier transports sodium out of the tubular fluid, it also carries either a hydrogen ion or a potassium ion into the tubular fluid on its "return trip." Thus, for every sodium ion reabsorbed, a hydrogen or potassium ion must be secreted, and vice versa. The choice of cation to be secreted depends on the ECF concentration of these ions (hydrogen and potassium).

This cation exchange system in the distal tubule helps explain some of the relationships that these electrolytes have with one another. For example, it is clear why an aldosterone blocker may cause hyperkalemia. The aldosterone blocker reduces sodium reabsorption. Such reduced reabsorption of sodium also reduces the tubular secretion of either hydrogen or potassium. The hydrogen excess can be buffered by bicarbonate, but the potassium simply rises to above-normal levels, leading to hyperkalemia. Similarly, the cation exchange system helps explain why there can be an initial decrease in plasma potassium in alkalosis or as severe acidosis is corrected therapeutically. In severe acidosis, the nephrons attempt to compensate by increasing hydrogen ion secretion. But as acidosis is therapeutically corrected, potassium ions are secreted. As hydrogen ions no longer need to be secreted, potassium ions become the sole exchange for sodium ions, leading, it is thought, to a reduction in plasma potassium.

## Hormonal Influences

Through the reabsorption of sodium and the passive "following" of water and chloride, it is possible to make urine of the same osmolality as blood. However, under conditions of dehydration, urine is very concentrated, whereas if a great deal of water is consumed, urine is more dilute than blood. This final regulation of urine is under the influence of three hormones: ADH, rennin, and aldosterone.

### Antidiuretic Hormone

Osmoreceptors in the hypothalamus are sensitive to serum osmolality. During dehydration, when serum osmolality rises, osmoreceptors in the hypothalamus respond by stimulating the hypothalamus to secrete ADH, which increases the permeability of collecting tubule cells to water. This permits the reabsorption of water alone (without electrolytes), which in turn decreases the concentration of the ECF. Negative feedback loops regulate ADH secretion. This means that as the concentration of the ECF returns to normal, the stimulus for ADH secretion disappears and ADH secretion stops.

### Renin

Another hormone that influences urine concentration is renin. When the GFR falls because of dehydration or blood loss, the juxtaglomerular apparatus secretes renin.[1] Subnormal sodium levels in the filtrate also stimulate renin secretion. Renin converts angiotensinogen, which is secreted by the liver, into angiotensin I. Pulmonary capillary cells in turn convert angiotensin I into angiotensin II with angiotensin-converting enzyme (see Chapter 42, Fig. 42-9). Angiotensin II constricts the smooth muscle surrounding the arterioles. This increases blood pressure, which increases the GFR.

### Aldosterone

Angiotensin II also triggers the secretion of aldosterone by the adrenal cortex (see Chapter 42, Fig. 42-9). Aldosterone is the third substance that influences urine osmolality. By increasing sodium reabsorption in distal tubule cells, aldosterone causes an increase in renal water reabsorption. This increases blood pressure and decreases serum osmolality. Simultaneously, potassium is excreted in the urine in exchange for the sodium reabsorption. Therefore, aldosterone also is secreted in response to subnormal serum sodium and elevated potassium levels.

## Functions of the Renal System

### Renal Clearance

From the previous discussion, an important concept in renal function emerges: clearance. As the filtrate moves along the nephron, it contains a large proportion of metabolic end products. These products are removed from the blood and exit the body in the urine. For each 125 mL of glomerular filtrate formed per minute, about one half, or 60 mL, returns to the blood without urea, and about one half is excreted with urea. In normally functioning kidneys 60 mL of plasma is cleared of urea each minute as well as creatinine, uric, acid, potassium, sulfate, phosphate, and so forth. It is possible to calculate renal clearance by simultaneously sampling urine and plasma. By dividing the quantity of substance found in each milliliter of plasma into the quantity found in the urine, the milliliters cleared per minute can be calculated and used to test kidney function.

Other methods of assessing renal function involve chemicals that are known to be filtered only, or both filtered and secreted. The polysaccharide, inulin, for example, is filtered only and neither absorbed nor secreted. Therefore, the clearance of inulin provides a measure of glomerular filtration.

The sodium concentration in the urine can also serve as an index of tubular health in certain situations. For example, in acute renal failure, an increased clearance of sodium can indicate acute tubular necrosis. Accordingly, supernormal blood levels of filtered substances (creatinine and other nitrogenous wastes) indicate a decrease in glomerular filtration and therefore in nephron health.

### Regulation

In addition to excreting nitrogenous wastes as urea and other by-products of metabolism, the kidneys help regulate the electrolyte concentration and the pH of the ECF (ie, the blood and ISF of the body).

#### Electrolyte Concentration

Electrolytes are substances that, when in water, disassociate and become charged. When charged, the solution is capable of carrying an electrical current. Positively charged electrolytes are cations; negatively charged electrolytes are anions.

Despite the complex physiology associated with electrolytes they have four main functions in homeostasis:

1. Cell metabolism and contribution to body structures
2. Facilitation of water movement between body compartments
3. Help in the maintenance of acid–base balance
4. Maintenance and production of membrane potentials in nerve and muscle cells.

The functions of individual electrolytes are given in Table 28-2. For normal functions to occur, the concentration of electrolytes must be carefully maintained. Energy, usually in the form of adenosine triphosphate, is often required to maintain

| TABLE 28.2 | Electrolyte Functions | |
|---|---|---|
| **Electrolyte** | **Normal Range** | **Functions** |
| Sodium (Na$^+$) | 135–145 mEq/L | Exerts an extracellular osmolality thereby regulating movement of body fluids |
| | | Facilitates nerve impulses through active transport and the sodium–potassium pump |
| Potassium (K$^+$) | 3.5–5 mEq/L | Maintains nervous impulse conduction in the heart |
| | | Promotes skeletal muscle function |
| | | Plays small role in osmotic regulation |
| | | Assists with acid–base regulation |
| Chloride (Cl$^-$) | 100–110 mEq/L | Maintains electroneutrality by passively following the positively charged ions |
| | | Helps regulate osmotic pressure differences between intracellular and extracellular fluid compartments |
| | | Regulates body water balance with sodium |
| | | Combines with H$^+$ in gastric mucosal cells to make hydrochloric acid |
| Calcium (Ca$^{2+}$) | 8.5–10.0 mg/dL (total) | Major structural component of bones and teeth |
| | 4.4–5.4 mg/dL (ionized) | Plays role in blood coagulation |
| | | Promotes muscle contraction and nervous impulse transmission |
| | | Decreases neuromuscular irritability |
| Phosphorus (PO$_4^-$) | 2.5–4.5 mg/dL | A structural component of bones and teeth |
| | | Helps maintain acid–base balance |
| | | Energy production (adenosine triphosphate) |
| | | Delivery of oxygen to tissues as a component of 2,3-diphosphoglycerate |
| Magnesium (Mg$^{2+}$) | 1.8–2.5 mEq/L | Ensures the cross-membrane transport of sodium and potassium in the sodium–potassium pump |
| | | Promotes neuromuscular excitability |
| | | Plays role in heart contraction |
| | | Facilitates transmission of central nervous system impulses |
| | | Part of many enzymatic reactions for carbohydrate and protein metabolism |

this balance. As described earlier in this chapter, the kidneys play a crucial role in electrolyte balance. In addition to being lost in the urine, electrolytes are lost from the gastrointestinal tract in the stool and emesis and through the skin in sweat.

**SODIUM.** The kidneys, with influences of aldosterone and ADH, carefully regulate the balance of sodium. Regulation occurs primarily through reabsorption (or excretion) in the proximal tubule under the influence of aldosterone.

**POTASSIUM.** Although some potassium may be lost in sweat and feces the kidneys excrete approximately 80% to 90% of the potassium lost by the body. In cases of hyperkalemia, aldosterone release facilitates increased potassium excretion. Potassium also assists with acid–base regulation through the cellular exchange with hydrogen ions.

**CHLORIDE.** Chloride is the most abundant extracellular anion. Negatively charged chloride passively follows the positively charged sodium to maintain electroneutrality. A large amount of chloride is also found in the gastric mucosal cells in the form of hydrochloric acid.

**CALCIUM.** Calcium has both structural and functional roles in homeostasis. Unlike the other electrolytes, calcium is absorbed from the small intestine under the influence of vitamin D, with the remaining ingested calcium lost in the feces. Excretion also occurs in the proximal convoluted tubule of the kidneys.

A low calcium concentration stimulates the release of parathyroid hormone (PTH) from the parathyroid glands. PTH facilitates the shift of calcium in its solid form (calcium phosphate, found in the bones) to its ionized form. PTH also increases the calcium absorbed from the intestine by signaling the kidneys to activate vitamin D. Reabsorption of calcium at the renal tubules is also increased under the influence of PTH. Calcitonin, secreted by the thyroid gland, is another hormone that plays a comparatively small role in calcium regulation. Calcitonin acts in opposition to PTH in an effort to reduce plasma calcium levels.

**PHOSPHORUS.** PTH regulates phosphorus, with effects directly opposite to those of calcium. PTH causes an increase in calcium plasma concentration and promotes excretion of phosphorus. PTH also causes release of phosphorus in the bones and shifts it to the ECF. Presumably, this would cause an increase in phosphorus; however, PTH also decreases the transport of phosphate ions by the kidney tubules, so more phosphate ions are lost in the urine.

**MAGNESIUM.** Magnesium ensures the cross-membrane transport of sodium and potassium in the sodium–potassium pump. It also plays a role in enzymatic reactions for carbohydrate and protein metabolism. Often, reactions requiring calcium require magnesium as well.

**pH.** If respiratory buffers for pH regulation are insufficient, the kidneys begin to take part, although much more slowly than the lungs. Although respiratory control of carbon dioxide, and therefore hydrogen ion level, can take only seconds to achieve, 48 to 72 hours may pass before the renal system can change the serum acid–base balance significantly.

Alkalosis occurs as a result of too few hydrogen ions or too many bicarbonate ions. To compensate, the body must conserve hydrogen ions. In renal compensation for alkalosis, tubular reabsorption of hydrogen ions is increased and secretion is decreased. This increases the hydrogen ion concentration of the ECF and thereby decreases the alkalosis.

Acidosis occurs as a result of too many hydrogen ions or too few bicarbonate ions. To compensate, the body must secrete hydrogen ions. Renal compensation for acidosis involves increasing the hydrogen ion secretion of the tubule cells, especially in the distal tubule cells. In this case, bicarbonate and sodium ions are continually being filtered from the glomerulus. Also, hydrogen ion secretion by distal tubule cells causes an increase in sodium reabsorption. Such sodium reabsorption can increase bicarbonate reabsorption electrochemically. Therefore, as hydrogen ions are being eliminated from the ECF, sodium and bicarbonate ions are being added to it. Both serve to decrease the acidosis (Fig. 28-6).

Urine can be acidified (by hydrogen ion secretion) only to a pH level of 4.0 to 4.5. If the tubular secretion of hydrogen ions was the only mechanism operating, only a few hydrogen ions could be secreted before the critical shut-off level of 4.0 was reached. This would occur because hydrogen would combine with urinary chloride to make hydrochloric acid. Not many of these strong hydrochloric acid molecules are needed to make the urine pH 4.0. The formation of hydrochloric acid would then stop tubular hydrogen ion secretion before sufficient compensation for acidosis could be obtained. This does not occur because tubule cells deaminate certain amino acids and secrete the nitrogenous component as ammonia. This ammonia combines with hydrogen in the urine to form

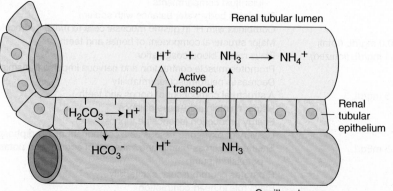

**FIGURE 28.6** Renal compensation for acidosis. Hydrogen ($H^+$) is moved from blood into the filtrate by active transport and exits in the urine as ammonium ($NH_4^+$). $HCO_3^-$, bicarbonate; $NH_3$, ammonia.

ammonium. Because tubule membranes are not permeable to ammonium, much of it is secreted in this form. Some ammonia combines with chloride to form ammonium chloride.

## Fluid Balance

The body contains about 60% water in most individuals. This percentage may vary between 50% and 70%, depending on a person's fat content. Adipose tissue has very low water, and therefore people with more fat have a lower percentage of body weight as water.

Water is distributed between the two main compartments in the body: intracellular fluid (ICF) and ECF. The ICF is the amount of volume within the cell and makes up about two thirds of the total-body water, or about 40% of the body weight. The ECF represents the remaining one third of the body water, or about 20% of the body weight. The solution primarily contains sodium chloride and bicarbonate. Figure 28-7 illustrates the different body water compartments.

There are three subcompartments to the ECF: the ISF, the plasma, and the transcellular fluid. ISF surrounds the cells but does not circulate. This subcompartment makes up about three fourths of the ECF. The second subcompartment of the ECF is the plasma, which circulates as the extracellular component of blood. Plasma makes up about one fourth of the ECF.

The third subcompartment of ECF is called transcellular fluid. This fluid is neither in the plasma nor in the interstitium; instead, it is the fluid that makes up the digestive juices, cerebrospinal fluid, synovial fluid, pericardial fluid, and mucus. Although the transcellular fluid is only about 1 to 2 L in total (<1 pound), it plays a very important role in homeostasis. Transcellular fluid helps cushion the heart with each beat, makes joint movement smooth, carries critical oxygen and glucose to the brain, and removes bacteria and antigens from the respiratory tract.

There is a constant movement of water between body compartments. For example, in diseases in which there is a lack of plasma oncotic pressure (eg, liver disease), there

may be excessive movement of fluid from the plasma to the interstitium. The lymph for recirculation reabsorbs this additional ISF; however, the volume that the lymph system is capable of holding becomes overwhelmed. This then causes edema formation. During times of dehydration, hormonal influences are recruited to pull additional ICF, ISF, and transcellular water into the plasma to maintain effective circulating volume.

Several factors may influence body water. Body water moves between compartments and is regulated by hormones, such as ADH, aldosterone, and atrial natriuretic peptide. Approximately 2.5 L of water is lost each day through normal bodily functions, such as urination, defecation, respiration, and sweating. This volume of water lost must be replaced. As people age, there is a decrease in total-body water as the ratio of muscle to fat changes. As fat increases, total-body water decreases. In part, this physiologic change accounts for the older adult's propensity for dehydration.

## Other Renal Functions

Renal interstitial (not nephron) cells manufacture and secrete two hormones, calcitriol (vitamin D) and erythropoietin, the actions of which are unrelated to urine formation. Calcitriol is a hormone that increases plasma calcium concentration by increasing intestinal absorption of calcium, promoting bone resorption, and stimulating the renal tubular reabsorption of calcium. Erythropoietin is a glycoprotein hormone that stimulates the bone marrow to produce red blood cells. Any process that decreases the oxygen content in the blood, such as bleeding or hypoxemia, is sensed by the kidney, and it initiates the release of erythropoietin. This increases the arterial oxygen content required to maintain cell integrity.

The kidneys also activate vitamin D. Ingested with food, vitamin D is absorbed in an inert form. The kidneys activate vitamin D so that it may assist in the absorption of calcium, which occurs in the intestines. Calcium has many functions as discussed earlier in this chapter. If renal failure occurs,

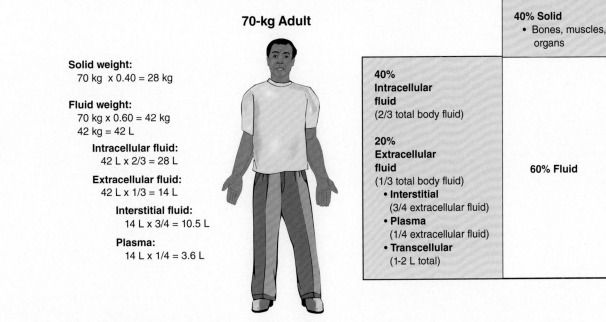

**FIGURE 28.7**  Body water compartments.

there is a marked reduction in vitamin D and subsequently bioavailable calcium, thereby putting the patient at risk for bone diseases (such as osteoporosis) and bleeding.

## Clinical Applicability Challenges

### SHORT ANSWER QUESTIONS

1. Mr. Jones has been admitted to the Intensive Care Unit after a motor vehicle accident. In addition to his injuries, he shows evidence of dehydration and hypotension. When a patient is dehydrated, the urine is very concentrated. The final regulation of urine is under the influence of three hormones. What are these hormones and what are their functions?

2. You are caring for Ms. Lopez in the Intensive Care Unit. Her laboratory values indicate she has a low potassium level. What is the normal level and what is the role of potassium in the body?

3. Mrs. Lopez weighs 65 kg. What is the weight of her intracellular and extracellular fluid?

### WANT TO KNOW MORE

A wide variety of resources to enhance your learning and understanding of this chapter are available on thePoint.

You will find:

- References
- Selected readings
- NCLEX-style review questions
- Internet resources
- And more!

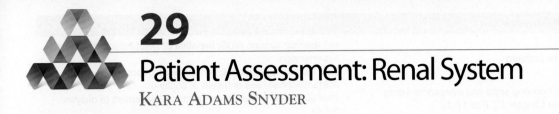

# 29

# Patient Assessment: Renal System

KARA ADAMS SNYDER

## LEARNING OBJECTIVES

*Based on the content in this chapter, the reader should be able to:*

1. Formulate a plan for collecting history and physical examination data for patients with renal disorders and fluid and electrolyte imbalance.

2. Describe diagnostic and laboratory blood tests used to evaluate renal and electrolyte status.

3. Discuss methods to evaluate fluid balance.

Assessment of the renal system involves determining how well the kidneys perform their many functions. It also includes gathering information about other systems. A careful assessment of the history and physical findings, with interpretation of laboratory and diagnostic test results, provides early clues to the diagnosis of disorders of water and volume imbalance and other complications of renal dysfunction in the critically ill patient.

## History

The patient history provides important information that helps determine the cause, severity, treatment, and management of renal dysfunction. It involves gathering information about the present illness, past health history, family history, personal history, and social history. A good history can help uncover the medical conditions that can predispose patients to acute or chronic kidney injury and fluid and electrolyte disturbances. In addition, relevant information about the status of other body systems is gathered through a review of systems. Box 29-1 presents a guide for renal assessment.

## Physical Examination

The physical examination provides objective data that are used to substantiate and clarify the history. The nurse begins the physical examination by observing the patient's overall appearance, including facial expression, height and weight, position in bed, grooming, personal hygiene, and signs of distress. The nurse observes the patient's level of responsiveness, cognition, and interaction with people, including positive, negative, or unusual responses.

Because patients with renal problems usually have significant problems with fluid and electrolyte balance, the nurse evaluates the patient's volume status throughout the examination. The nurse begins by taking the vital signs. Particular attention is paid to the blood pressure, noting pulse pressure and presence of a positive pulse paradoxus. An elevated temperature may indicate an infection.

Throughout the physical examination, the nurse inspects the skin on the extremities and trunk for color and evidence of excoriation, bruising, or bleeding; palpates for moistness, dryness, temperature (using the back of the fingers), and edema; and checks mobility and turgor by lifting a fold of skin and noting the ease (mobility) and speed with which it returns into place (turgor). To assess hydration further, the nurse inspects the tongue and mucous membranes in the mouth and looks for a saliva pool under the tongue. Additional volume status assessment is done when examining the neck, as the nurse observes for jugular vein distention and determines the need to measure jugular venous pressure.

The anterior and posterior chest is inspected for respiratory rate, rhythm, depth, and effort. Deformities of the thorax, shape of chest, or bulging of interspaces during expiration are noted. The precordial area is observed and palpated for heaves, pulsations, and thrills. The nurse listens for heart rate and rhythm, extra heart sounds, murmurs, clicks, and pericardial friction rub. Fluid overload often results in the presence of a third or fourth heart sound.

The nurse auscultates anterior and posterior lung fields, noting the quality of vesicular breath sounds and the presence of adventitious breath sounds (crackles, wheezes, rubs), which may indicate volume overload.

After auscultating the posterior chest, the nurse assesses kidney tenderness. First the nurse places one hand over the posterior costovertebral angle (CVA). Then, using the fist of the second hand, the nurse gently percusses the CVA (Fig. 29-1) and notes whether the patient has discomfort, which is known as CVA tenderness.

The nurse inspects the abdomen and then listens for bowel sounds. In addition to auscultating bowel sounds, the nurse auscultates the renal arteries for bruits by placing the stethoscope above and to the left and right of the umbilicus (Fig. 29-2). A bruit is an abnormal sound that resembles a blowing or swishing noise, similar to the sound of a cardiac *murmur*. The presence of a renal bruit may indicate renal artery stenosis, which means there may be diminished blood flow to the kidney. This diminished blood flow may result in acute or chronic renal dysfunction.

Next, the nurse percusses and palpates the abdomen and then palpates the liver border to determine enlargement. If ascites is suspected, the nurse measures abdominal girth and may check for a fluid wave or shifting dullness. During

**BOX 29-1** *Health History for Renal Assessment*

**Chief Complaint**
- Patient's description of the problem

**History of the Present Illness**
- Complete analysis of the following signs and symptoms (using the NOPQRST format, see Chapter 17, Box 17-1):
  - Frequency
  - Urgency
  - Hesitancy
  - Burning
  - Dysuria
  - Hematuria
  - Incontinence
  - Lower back pain
  - Pain with urination
  - Change in color, odor, or amount of urine
  - Thirst
  - Change in weight
  - Edema

**Past Health History**
- Relevant antenatal history and immunizations: prematurity; antenatal use of angiotensin-converting enzyme inhibitors, angiotensin-receptor blockers, or nonsteroidal anti-inflammatory drugs (NSAIDs; eg, ibuprofen); ensuring antenatal vaccination against rubella; screening for cytomegalovirus or toxoplasmosis
- Past acute and chronic medical problems, including treatments and hospitalizations: renal failure; renal calculi; renal cancer; glomerulonephritis; Wegener granulomatosis; polycystic kidney disease; dialysis, including type, frequency, and duration; urinary tract infections; systemic lupus erythematosus; sickle

cell anemia; cancer; AIDS; hepatitis C; heart failure; diabetes; hypertension
- Risk factors: age; trauma; heavy use of ibuprofen, naproxen, or acetaminophen; use of heroin or cocaine
- Past surgeries: kidney transplantation, placement of dialysis fistula
- Past diagnostic tests and interventions: urinalysis, cystoscopy, IV pyelography, ultrasound of kidneys, renal biopsy, magnetic resonance imaging, diagnostic tests that have used contrast dyes
- Medications: diuretics, aminoglycosides, antibiotics, NSAIDs
- Allergies and reactions: radiographic contrast media
- Transfusions

**Family History**
- Health status or cause of death of parents and siblings: hereditary nephritis, polycystic kidney disease, diabetes, high blood pressure

**Personal and Social History**
- Tobacco, alcohol, and substance use
- Family composition
- Occupation and work environment: exposure to nephrotoxic substances such as organic acids, pesticides, lead, and mercury
- Living environment: exposure to nephrotoxic substances such as organic acids, pesticides, lead, mercury
- Diet: salt consumption, fluid intake

**Review of Systems**
- Skin: dryness, itching
- HEENT: periorbital edema
- Neurologic: numbness, tingling, burning, tremors, memory loss
- Musculoskeletal: rhabdomyolysis, muscle weakness

the abdominal examination, the right and left kidneys are palpated by placing one hand under the patient's flank and placing the other examining hand in the quadrant just below the costal margin at the midclavicular line (Fig. 29-3). The kidneys are normally not palpable, although an enlarged kidney may be palpable; the enlargement may be due to a cyst, tumor, or hydronephrosis. If indicated by history, the nurse may palpate and percuss the bladder. The bladder cannot be palpated unless it is distended above the symphysis pubis. When palpated, the dome of the distended bladder feels smooth and round. For palpation and percussion of the bladder, the nurse begins at the symphysis pubis and moves upward and outward to estimate the bladder size. A full bladder is dull to percussion.

If the patient is at risk for excess vascular volume, the nurse looks for hypertension; pulmonary edema; crackles; engorged, elevated neck veins; liver congestion and enlargement; heart failure; and shortness of breath. Signs and symptoms related to excess extravascular volume include pitting edema of feet, ankles, hands, and fingers; periorbital edema; sacral edema; and ascites. Table 29-1 presents a scale used to document levels of pitting edema.

While examining the extremities, the nurse can check the quality of the peripheral pulses; observe for tremors; test for paresthesia, numbness, and weakness; and palpate fingernails and toenails, checking for color, shape, and capillary refill time.

If the patient has an arteriovenous graft or fistula for dialysis, the nurse assesses it for patency and for adequate circulation to the extremity distal to the access. Palpating for a thrill and auscultating for a bruit help to assess patency of the graft. If assessment reveals a change, the physician or practitioner must be notified urgently because the graft may be saved through radiologic or surgical intervention. If the patient has temporary dialysis access, the exit site is inspected for signs of inflammation or infection. Often the lumens of the temporary access have high doses of heparin to maintain patency, so flushing or use of the device is clarified with the physician or practitioner before any manipulation or use of the catheter.

Patients with renal impairment may be at risk for hypocalcemia, hypomagnesemia, or both. Physical assessment of these electrolyte changes can be achieved by checking for Chvostek and Trousseau signs. Chvostek sign occurs when there is facial irritability after tapping the facial nerve in front of the auditory meatus with the finger. Trousseau sign occurs when there is spasm of the hands and feet (carpopedal spasm) in response to arm compression (eg, as with a blood pressure cuff).

During the history and examination, the critical care nurse continuously observes the patient's level of consciousness and mental status. If more data are needed, the nurse may use tools such as the Glasgow Coma Scale and Folstein Mini-Mental Examination.

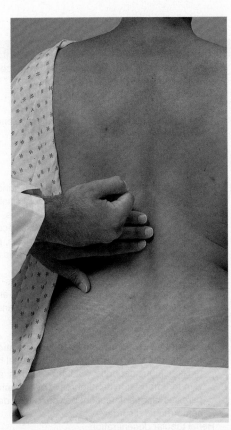

FIGURE 29-1 Assessing CVA tenderness. (From Bickley LS: Bates' Guide to Physical Examination, 11th ed. Philadelphia, PA: Lippincott Williams & Wilkins, 2013, p 464.)

## Assessment of Renal Function

### Laboratory Studies

#### Urine Studies

**URINALYSIS.** The nurse inspects the urine for color, clarity, and odor. Normally, the urine is clear and yellow to straw-colored and smells of ammonia. Changes in the characteristics of the urine can indicate kidney damage, infection, excretion of drugs, or the kidney's compensation for systemic homeostatic imbalance. Cloudy urine may indicate infection, whereas very clear and colorless urine may be a sign of diuresis, either induced pharmacologically or by diabetes insipidus.[1] Blood in the urine may appear bright red or dark brown. If hematuria is present, additional evaluation and follow-up with specialists may be considered to investigate the presence of a malignancy.[2] Urinalysis is used to identify more specifically the components of the urine. Table 29-2 summarizes the components of the urinalysis.

**URINE VOLUME.** The difference between the amount of blood filtered by the kidney, or the glomerular filtration rate (GFR) (see Chapter 28), and the amount of water reabsorbed determines the urine volume. A patient with normal renal function filters 180 L daily and must reabsorb approximately 179 L. This is the equivalent of roughly greater than 99% of filtered volume. Patients with renal disease and impairment may actually excrete an appropriate amount of urine.

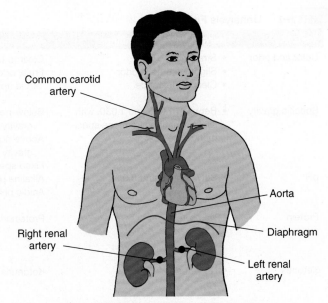

FIGURE 29-2 Sites for auscultation of renal bruits.

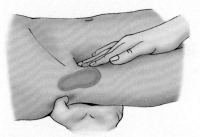

FIGURE 29-3 Palpating the right and left kidney. (Adapted from Weber J, Kelley J: Health Assessment in Nursing, 5th ed. Philadelphia, PA: Lippincott Williams & Wilkins, 2014, p 620.)

**TABLE 29-1 Assessing Pitting Edema**

| Value | Description | Indentation (in mm) | Time to Return to Baseline |
|---|---|---|---|
| 1+ | Trace | 2 or less | Returns to normal rapidly |
| 2+ | Mild | 4 | Under 30 s |
| 3+ | Moderate | 6 | 1 or 2 min |
| 4+ | Severe | 8 | 2 min or longer |

For example, a patient with severe renal disease may have a GFR of 10 L but still filter 1 L or 90% reabsorption. Thus, urine volume is of little diagnostic importance in this setting. However, urine volume is important in the setting of acute anuria. In acute anuria, a patient may be making normal volume and experience an abrupt change in pattern. Causes of acute anuria include the following:

• Complete bilateral obstruction (ie, abdominal compartment syndrome)
• Glomerulonephritis
• Bilateral vascular occlusion.

However, trends in urine production can provide important clues to the body's recruitment of important compensatory

**TABLE 29-2   Urinalysis Findings**

| Test | Normal Values or Findings | Abnormal Findings | Possible Causes of Abnormal Findings |
|---|---|---|---|
| Color and odor | • Straw color<br>• Slightly aromatic odor<br>• Clear appearance | Clear to black<br>Fruity odor<br>Turbid appearance | Dietary changes; use of certain drugs, metabolic inflammatory, or infectious disease<br>Diabetes mellitus, starvation, dehydration<br>Renal infection |
| Specific gravity | • Between 1.005 and 1.030, with slight variations from one specimen to the next | Below-normal specific gravity<br>Above-normal specific gravity<br>Fixed specific gravity | Diabetes insipidus, glomerulonephritis, pyelonephritis, acute kidney injury, alkalosis<br>Dehydration, nephrosis<br>Severe renal damage |
| pH | • Between 4.5 and 8.0 | Alkaline pH (above 8.0)<br>Acidic pH (below 4.5) | Fanconi syndrome (chronic renal disease) urinary tract infection, metabolic or respiratory alkalosis<br>Renal tuberculosis, phenylketonuria, acidosis |
| Protein | • No protein | Proteinuria | Renal disease (such as glomerulosclerosis, acute or chronic glomerulonephritis, nephrolithiasis, polycystic kidney disease, and acute or chronic renal failure) |
| Ketones | • No ketones | Ketonuria | Diabetes mellitus, starvation, conditions causing acutely increased metabolic demands and decreased food intake (such as vomiting and diarrhea) |
| Glucose | • No glucose | Glycosuria | Diabetes mellitus |
| RBCs | • 0–3 RBCs/high-power field | Numerous RBCs | Urinary tract infection, obstruction, inflammation trauma, or tumor; glomerulonephritis; renal hypertension; lupus nephritis; renal tuberculosis; renal vein thrombosis; hydronephrosis; pyelonephritis; parasitic bladder infection; polyarteritis nodosa; hemorrhagic disorder |
| Epithelial cells | • Few epithelial cells | Excessive epithelial cells | Renal tubular degeneration |
| WBCs | • 0–4 WBCs/high-power field | Numerous WBCs<br><br>Numerous WBCs and WBC casts | Urinary tract inflammation, especially cystitis or pyelonephritis<br>Renal infection (such as acute pyelonephritis and glomerulonephritis, nephrotic syndrome, pyogenic infection, and lupus nephritis) |
| Casts | • No casts (except occasional hyaline casts) | Excessive casts<br>Excessive hyaline casts<br>Epithelial casts<br>Fatty, waxy casts<br>RBC casts | Renal disease<br>Renal parenchymal disease, inflammation, glomerular capillary membrane trauma<br>Renal tubular damage, nephrosis, eclampsia, chronic lead intoxication<br>Nephrotic syndrome, chronic renal disease, diabetes mellitus<br>Renal parenchymal disease (especially glomerulonephritis), renal infarction, subacute bacterial endocarditis, sickle cell anemia, blood dyscrasias, malignant hypertension, collagen disease |
| Crystals | • Some crystals | Numerous calcium oxalate crystals<br>Cystine crystals (cystinuria) | Hypercalcemia<br>Inborn metabolic error |
| Yeast cells | • No yeast crystals | Yeast cells in sediment | External genitalia contamination, vaginitis, urethritis, prostatovesiculitis |
| Parasites | • No parasites | Parasites in sediment | External genitalia contamination |
| Creatinine clearance | • Male (age 20): 90 mg/min/173 m² of body surface<br>• Female (age 20): 84 mL/min/1.73 m² of body surface<br>• Older patients: normally decreased concentrations by 6 mL/min/decade | Above-normal creatinine clearance<br>Below-normal creatinine clearance | Little diagnostic significance<br>Reduced renal blood flow (associated with shock or renal artery obstruction), acute tubular necrosis, acute or chronic glomerulonephritis, advanced bilateral renal lesions (as in polycystic kidney disease, renal tuberculosis, and cancer), nephrosclerosis, heart failure, severe dehydration |

From *Critical Care Nursing Made Incredibly Easy*, 3rd ed. Philadelphia, PA: Lippincott Williams & Wilkins, 2012, pp 523–524.

responses, as in hypovolemia. The body initiates the renin–angiotensin–aldosterone system to maintain the crucial water balance (see Chapter 28).

**URINE pH.** Urinary pH is normally acidic, with a range between 5.0 and 6.5, depending primarily on dietary intake. The kidneys play a tremendous role in acid–base balance (see Chapter 28). Clinically, urinary pH is important in two settings. First, an alkaline urinary pH (above 7.5) suggests the presence of a urinary tract infection. Second, a low, or acidic, pH indicates that the kidney may be compensating for a serum acidosis. Physiologically, in this state, the kidneys reabsorb more bicarbonate and excrete more hydrogen ions to buffer the serum acidosis. The urine becomes increasingly acidic (lower pH) when the body is attempting to conserve sodium, as in states of dehydration.

**URINE PROTEIN.** Most proteins are large molecules and under normal conditions should not penetrate Bowman capsule. Urinary protein levels, therefore, are typically zero to trace. Proteinuria usually indicates damage to the capillary structures, as in the case of glomerular diseases (glomerulonephritis) and intrarenal acute kidney injury. For diagnostic purposes, a 24-hour sample of urine is used to assess for proteinuria. Single dipstick measurements are not as sensitive and may lead to false-positive values.

**URINE GLUCOSE AND KETONES.** Glucose, like most proteins, is not present in the urine under normal conditions. Unlike proteins, however, glucose is freely filtered but is reabsorbed in the proximal tubule. Glucose becomes detectable if the serum glucose is elevated (greater than 200 mg/dL) as the filtered load exceeds the kidney's reabsorptive abilities. Findings of glucosuria should be confirmed with serum or capillary blood glucose measurement.

Ketone bodies are by-products of fat metabolism and are formed in states of insulin deficiency. Three ketone bodies are formed: β-hydroxybutyric acid (the primary ketone formed), acetoacetic acid, and acetone. The latter two ketone bodies are detected in the urine. Acetone may be measured in the serum. A urine sample that is positive for ketones may indicate diabetic ketoacidosis.

**URINARY SEDIMENT.** Sediment is a particulate matter that, when examined, can reveal certain physiologic conditions in the renal system. Sediment in general refers to casts, red cells, white cells, epithelial cells, and crystals. Casts are the breakdown products of cellular material formed in the collecting tubules. Urinary stasis, as in prerenal disease, may promote cast formation. Casts can be made up of different types of cells, and thus, the shape, composition, and size of the casts can help in identifying the presence and etiology of a disease.

**Red Blood Cells.** Red blood cells (RBCs) may be microscopic (microscopic hematuria) or grossly visible (macroscopic hematuria). RBCs enter the urine anywhere along the urinary tract. Any injury or damage to the structures making up the urinary tract can cause hematuria. Kidney stones, trauma, and prostatic disease are examples of extrarenal causes of hematuria (ie, not related to the kidneys).

Microscopic bleeding can be present in glomerular diseases, such as glomerulonephritis. When assessing the results of the urinalysis, take note of the presence of RBC casts and the RBC morphology. Glomerular bleeding is often associated with some type of fragmentation of the RBC, whereas extrarenal bleeding often leaves the cell intact. The presence of RBC casts is virtually diagnostic of glomerulonephritis.

Myoglobin in the urine makes the urine appear red; however, when the urine is inspected under the microscope, there is no evidence of RBCs. Myoglobin is a component of skeletal muscle breakdown, or rhabdomyolysis. Crush injuries or protracted down times are the greatest predictors of this disease. When muscle begins to break down, it releases the myoglobin, which is similar in chemical structure to hemoglobin. Because of its large molecular size, myoglobin blocks the renal tubules, placing patients at very high risk for intrarenal acute kidney injury.

**White Blood Cells.** White blood cells (WBCs) in the urine (pyuria) usually indicate infection anywhere along the urinary tract. Leukocyte esterase is an enzyme produced by WBCs along the urinary tract that can be detected in the urine. This enzyme is present along the urinary tract as a component of the local immune response. High levels of this enzyme can indicate infection. The presence of nitrites may also aid in the diagnosis of a bacterial infection along the urinary tract.

**SPECIFIC GRAVITY AND OSMOLALITY.** The specific gravity of the urine tests the kidneys' ability to concentrate and dilute the urine. The specific gravity measures the buoyancy of a solution compared with water and depends on the number of particles in the solution and their size and weight.

The normal kidney has the capacity to dilute the urine to a specific gravity of 1.001 and to concentrate the urine to at least 1.022. For reference, the specific gravity of water is 1.000. Normally, a person's water balance determines whether the urine is concentrated or dilute; dilute urine is an indicator of water excess, and concentrated urine indicates water deficit. In many renal diseases, the ability of the kidneys to form concentrated urine is lost, and the specific gravity can become "fixed" at approximately 1.010. Often, this finding is seen in acute tubular necrosis, acute nephritis, and chronic renal disease. A falsely high specific gravity can be seen when high-molecular-weight substances, such as protein, glucose, mannitol, and radiographic contrast material, are present in the urine. Therefore, a greater degree of accuracy can be obtained by checking the urine osmolality in these cases.

Osmolality measures the osmoles of solute particles present per kilogram of solvent. The main determinants of osmolality are the sodium, urea, and glucose. In states of volume depletion or excess, several neuroendocrine responses interact to maintain homeostasis, thereby affecting the urinary osmolality. Because of this dynamic interaction, particularly in critical illness, single measurements of the osmolality are of little diagnostic importance. The urinary osmolality is often followed for the evaluation of patients with hyponatremia.

Normal urine osmolality ranges from 300 to 900 mOsm/kg/24 h. Because of this wide range, more information about renal function is obtained when simultaneous serum and urine samples are collected and interpreted. In renal disease, one of the first functions to be lost is the ability to concentrate urine. This can result in the urine osmolality becoming fixed within 150 mOsm of the simultaneously determined serum osmolality.

**URINARY SODIUM CONCENTRATION.** The urinary sodium excretion is used as an indicator of renal function in differentiating the oliguria associated with acute kidney injury from other prerenal causes. States of poor kidney perfusion are usually associated with a decrease in urinary sodium concentration (usually less than 10 mEq/L). This is a compensatory reaction generated by the activation of the renin–angiotensin–aldosterone system. Activation of this neuroendocrine response allows for increased reabsorption of sodium (reduced excretion) with a subsequent increase in water reabsorption. The root cause of kidney hypoperfusion can be anything that causes a reduction in effective circulating volume; volume depletion and heart failure are two examples. Acute kidney injury may develop if hypoperfusion persists. In acute kidney injury, urine sodium concentration is usually greater than 30 to 40 mEq/L despite oliguria because of damage to the tubular transport mechanisms. However, when the urine pH is alkaline, urine sodium concentration does not reflect sodium balance accurately, and the chloride concentration becomes a better indicator of volume status.

**FRACTIONAL EXCRETION OF SODIUM TEST.** The fractional excretion of sodium ($FE_{Na}$) test gives a more precise estimation of the amount of filtered sodium that remains in the urine and is more accurate in predicting tubular injury than the urinary sodium concentration.[3] One benefit of the $FE_{Na}$ compared with the urinary sodium is that it removes the confounding effect of water. It can be calculated by using the following formula:

$$FE_{Na} = \frac{U_{Na} \times P_{Cr}}{P_{Na} \times U_{Cr}}$$

where $U$ and $P$ are the urinary and plasma concentrations of sodium and creatinine, respectively. (Although volume measurements are necessary to derive the absolute urinary excretion of both sodium and creatinine, these cancel out in deriving the formula.)

The $FE_{Na}$ test requires the determination of both serum and urinary sodium and creatinine concentrations on simultaneously obtained samples. Values less than 1% indicate transient acute kidney injury, typically caused by underperfusion. Values greater than 1% (and frequently greater than 3%) are indicative persistent acute kidney injury. Some situations render a falsely low (less than 1%) $FE_{Na}$, including glomerulonephritis, myoglobinuric renal failure, contrast nephropathy, renal transplant rejection, acute interstitial nephritis, and acute urinary tract obstruction. $FE_{Na}$ is also a poor indicator of renal function in patients who have received diuretic therapy.[3]

### Blood Studies

**CREATININE AND CREATININE CLEARANCE.** Creatinine is a by-product of normal muscle metabolism and is excreted in the urine primarily as the result of glomerular filtration, with a small percentage secreted into the urine by the kidney tubules. Therefore, creatinine is currently the most useful indicator of GFR. The amount of creatinine excreted in the urine is directly related to muscle mass and normally remains constant unless significant muscle wasting (a catabolic state) occurs. Normal serum values for creatinine are 0.6 to 1.2 mg/dL.

The creatinine clearance can be defined as the amount of blood that is cleared of creatinine in 1 minute and is an excellent clinical indicator of renal function. As renal function diminishes, creatinine clearance decreases. To obtain an accurate creatinine clearance, the nurse collects all urine made in a 24-hour period and obtains a blood specimen at some point during the urine collection. Thus, it is essential for the nurse to communicate to other team members that a 24-hour collection is in progress. For consistency, the blood sample is usually collected at the midpoint of the urine collection. It is important to note the exact beginning and ending times of the urine collection.

The actual creatinine clearance is calculated by the following formula:

$$CrCl = \frac{U_{Cr} \times V}{P_{Cr}}$$

where $U$ is the urine creatinine concentration, $V$ the urine volume, and $P$ the plasma creatinine concentration.

The product $U$ multiplied by $V$ tells how much creatinine appears in the urine during the period of collection. This can be converted readily to milligrams per minute, which is the standard reference point. Dividing this value by the plasma creatinine concentration (which must be converted from milligrams per 100 mL to milligrams per milliliter) tells the minimal number of milliliters of plasma that must have been filtered by the glomeruli to produce the measured amount of creatinine in the urine. The final result is usually expressed in milliliters per minute. The normal range varies between 80 and 120 mL/min, depending on the person's size, age, and sex. The results can be adjusted to a standard body size of 1.73 m² (body surface area [BSA]), which can be derived from standard tables if the patient's height and weight are known; it averages between 120 and 125 mL/min/1.73 m² BSA. After age 40 years, normal creatinine clearance values generally decrease 6.5 mL/min per decade because of a decline in GFR.

There are also formulas that estimate creatinine clearance based on a single serum creatinine level. An estimate may be made when there is difficulty collecting a 24-hour urine sample or when spot-checking the creatinine clearance will assist prompt treatment (as in the case of drug nephrotoxicity). The estimate may be accurate only in patients with chronic renal failure with stable renal function who are not edematous or extremely overweight. The following is the Cockcroft–Gault formula for estimating creatinine clearance:

$$\text{Creatinine Clearance} = \frac{(140 - \text{age}) \times \text{weight (kg)}}{72 \times xP_{Cr}\ \text{(mg/dL)}}$$

where $P_{Cr}$ is plasma creatinine; for women, the final result is multiplied by 0.85. Many labs are now routinely reporting the GFR using estimate formulas for creatinine clearance.

When the kidneys are damaged by a disease process, the creatinine clearance decreases, and the serum creatinine concentration rises. The urine creatinine excretion decreases initially until the blood level rises to a point at which the amount of creatinine appearing in the urine is equal to the amount being produced by the body. Because men tend to have a higher proportion of muscle than women, the creatinine and creatinine clearance can be higher in men than women. A healthy person with a serum creatinine concentration of 1 mg/dL and a creatinine excretion of 1 mg/min has a creatinine clearance of 100 mL/min. When the person experiences a 50% loss of renal function, the serum creatinine rises to 2 mg/dL, and the person will continue to excrete 1 mg/min of creatinine in the urine when balance is restored. When the person has rapidly changing renal function and oliguria (eg, acute kidney injury), the creatinine clearance is less reliable. Until renal function stabilizes, serum creatinine levels provide a better indication of the rate and direction of change. In patients with rhabdomyolysis, the serum creatinine is elevated out of proportion to the reduction of GFR as the result of chemical conversion of muscle creatine to creatinine. In this situation, the serum creatinine is less reliable as an indicator of renal function.

**BLOOD UREA NITROGEN.** The blood urea nitrogen (BUN) level has been used for many years as an indicator of kidney function, but unlike the serum creatinine, the BUN level can be influenced by many factors. At low urine flow rates, more sodium and water, and consequently more urea, are reabsorbed. Therefore, when the patient is volume depleted, the BUN tends to increase out of proportion to any change in renal function. A normal value for the BUN is considered to be 8 to 20 mg/dL.

Increased urea production can result from increased protein intake (tube feedings and some forms of hyperalimentation), increased tissue breakdown (as with crush injuries), febrile illnesses, steroid or tetracycline administration, and reabsorption of blood from the intestine in a patient with intestinal hemorrhage. The BUN may also be elevated in the dehydrated patient, because the lack of fluid volume causes a concentrated value. The patient in shock and the patient with heart failure may have an elevated BUN secondary to decreased renal perfusion. The opposite is true for patients with decreased protein intake or liver disease (both of which reduce urea production) and for patients with large urine volumes secondary to excessive fluid intake. However, the BUN can be of significant value when used as a comparison with the serum creatinine concentration. Normally, there is a urea/creatinine ratio of 10:1. Discrepancies in this ratio might suggest a potentially correctable situation, as Box 29-2 shows.

**OSMOLALITY.** The osmolality of a solution is an expression of the total osmoles per kilogram (Osm/kg) of solvent and is independent of the size, molecular weight, and electrical charge of the molecules. All substances in solution contribute to the osmolality. The total concentration of particles in a solution equals the osmolality and is normally reported in

units of osmoles per kilogram of solvent. In the clinical setting (because of much smaller concentrations), the osmolality is reported in milliosmoles (thousandth of an osmole, abbreviated mOsm) per kilogram of solvent (plasma or serum).

The normal serum osmolality consists primarily of sodium and its accompanying anions, with urea and glucose contributing about 5 mOsm each. Therefore, when the serum sodium, urea, and glucose concentrations are known, the osmolality of plasma can be calculated by the following formula:

$$Osmolality = 2(Na) + \frac{Glucose}{18} + \frac{BUN}{2.8}$$

The normal adult average osmolality is 280 to 290 mOsm/kg and remains quite constant. Because water can move freely between the blood, interstitial fluid, and tissues, any change in the osmolality of one body compartment produces a shift in body fluids. Therefore, the osmolality of the plasma is the same as that of other body compartments except in rapidly changing conditions, when a slight lag may occur.

A decrease in the serum osmolality can occur only when the serum sodium is decreased. An increase in the serum osmolality can occur whenever the serum sodium, urea, or glucose is elevated or when abnormal compounds are present in the blood, such as drugs, poisons, or metabolic waste products, such as lactic acid. Symptoms usually do not occur until the osmolality exceeds 350 mOsm/kg. Coma can occur when the osmolality is 400 mOsm/kg or greater.

The calculated osmolality is normally within 10 mOsm of the measured osmolality. Comparing the calculated and measured osmolality can be useful in determining potential substances present. An elevated osmolar gap provides evidence for the presence of a significant amount of abnormal solutes. Ethanol, methanol, and ethylene glycol are three examples of solutes that, when present in appreciable amounts, cause an elevated osmolar gap. If ingestion of one of these substances is suspected, calculate the osmolar gap.

**NONSPECIFIC STUDIES.** Changes in hematocrit, hemoglobin, platelets, and uric acid levels may be indications of a disorder.

**Hematocrit and Hemoglobin.** The normal hemoglobin for men is 13.5 to 17.5 g/dL and is 12 to 16 g/dL for women. The normal hematocrit should be 40% to 52% for adult men and 37% to 48% for adult women. False elevations of hematocrit can be seen with dehydration or after dialysis. Low hematocrits may be a dilutional value due to hypervolemia. The kidney is the primary site for the production of erythropoietin. It stimulates the bone marrow to release mature RBCs. Many patients with chronic kidney disease produce insufficient amounts of erythropoietin, which can result in chronic anemia.

**Platelets.** Patients with uremia are particularly susceptible to platelet dysfunction. Gastrointestinal (GI) bleeding may be a presenting symptom. The bleeding time, indicative of platelet function, may be prolonged. One mechanism of platelet dysfunction is that uremic platelets tend to synthesize less thromboxane-A2, the chemical that gives platelets their sticky function.

**Uric Acid.** Uric acid is a nitrogenous end product of protein and purine metabolism. Humans produce only small

---

**BOX 29-2** | **Factors Affecting the Serum Urea: Creatinine Ratio**

Decreased Urea/Creatinine Ratio (<10:1)
- Liver disease
- Protein restriction
- Excessive fluid intake

Increased Urea/Creatinine Ratio (>10:1)
- Volume depletion
- Decreased "effective" blood volume
- Catabolic states
- Excessive protein intake

quantities of uric acid under normal conditions, and the normal uric acid serum level is between 2 and 8.5 mg/dL. Uric acid is excreted primarily by the kidneys, with some in the stool. The value may be elevated because of excessive production from cell breakdown or inadequate excretion by the kidney.

## Diagnostic Studies

### Radiologic Studies

Radiologic studies of the kidneys that may be useful in evaluating renal abnormalities include roentgenography, ultrasonography, and radionuclide studies. Table 29-3 summarizes these studies and their purposes.

### Renal Biopsy

Renal biopsy is the most invasive diagnostic test and has been shown to have excellent sensitivity and specificity for malignancy.[4] It is used to define the histologic counterpart of the clinical picture, provide etiologic clues for diagnosis, assess prognosis, and guide therapy. Table 29-4 lists the indications for renal biopsy. Contraindications to biopsy include serious bleeding disorders, excessive obesity, and severe hypertension.

**TABLE 29-3**    **Radiologic Study of Kidneys**

| Diagnostic Test | Definition | Purpose |
|---|---|---|
| Radiograph of kidney/ ureter/bladder | Also known as abdominal x-ray. Standard x-rays capture image | Detects abnormal calcifications and renal size |
| Tomography | Standard x-rays capture series of cross-sectional scans made along single axis of bodily structure or tissue. Computer software is used to construct three-dimensional image of that structure. Delayed contrast administration can show collecting system anatomy | Determines renal outlines and abnormalities |
| Intravenous pyelography (IVP) | X-ray of renal structures using contrast material. Images are captured on real-time basis. Contrast material is injected intravenously and then collected in renal system; this turns areas bright white, allowing assessment of anatomy and function of kidneys and lower urinary tract | Detects anatomical abnormalities of kidneys and ureters |
| Retrograde pyelography | Similar to IVP, with use of x-ray and contrast material. Contrast material is injected through urinary catheter. This test is typically performed at the same time as cystoscopy | Assesses renal size, evaluates ureteral obstruction, and localizes and diagnoses tumors as well as obstructions |
| Antegrade pyelography | Similar to IVP and retrograde pyelography, this x-ray test uses contrast material to visualize structures of urinary tract. Contrast dye, however, is injected into ureter. Thus, structures of upper urinary tract are well visualized | Distinguishes cysts from hydronephrosis |
| Renal arteriography and venography | Vessel (artery or vein) is accessed and contrast dye is injected to visualize structures "downstream" | Evaluates possible renal arterial stenosis, renal mass lesions, renal vein thrombosis, and venous extension of renal cell carcinoma |
| Digital subtraction angiography | X-ray with a computer technique that compares x-ray image of kidney vessels before and after contrast dye is injected. Tissues and blood vessels on first image are digitally subtracted from second image, leaving clear picture of artery, which can then be studied independently from rest of the body | Visualizes major arterial vessels |
| Ultrasonography | Imaging technique that is excellent means of visualizing tissues and organs to assess their size, structure, and possible pathology. Images are created by emission and receiving of sound waves | Delineates renal outlines. Measures longitudinal and transverse dimensions of the kidneys. Evaluates mass lesions. Examines perinephric area. Detects and grades hydronephrosis |
| Radionuclide scintillation imaging (renal scan) | Nuclear medicine test that uses small amounts of radioactive materials (radioisotopes) to measure kidney function | Used to evaluate kidney function and determine blood flow through the kidney |
| Static imaging | Gives information about the size, shape, and position of the kidneys; and whether there are scars on the kidney from a previous infection | Evaluates location, size, and contour of functional renal tissue; may reveal areas of inhomogeneity or filling defects |
| Dynamic imaging | Gives information about the blood flow to the kidneys and how well each kidney is functioning for the production of urine | Monitors passage of radiopharmaceutical agent through vascular, renal parenchymal, and urinary tract compartments; also indicates whether there are any obstructions in urine output |
| Magnetic resonance imaging | Uses nonionizing radiofrequency signals (as opposed to computed tomography, which uses ionizing radiation) to acquire its images and is best suited for noncalcified tissue | Determines anatomical abnormalities |

**TABLE 29-4** Indications for Renal Biopsy

| Clinical Condition | Biopsy Indicated | Expected Gain |
|---|---|---|
| Orthostatic proteinuria | No | — |
| Isolated hematuria and/or proteinuria | No* | — |
| Hematuria and/or proteinuria with ↓ GFR | Yes | D, P, T |
| Nephrotic syndrome | Yes | D, P, T |
| Systemic disease with renal abnormalities | Yes† | D, P, T |
| Classic ARF | No | — |
| ARF with | Yes | D, T |
| 1. Azotemia for >3 wk | Yes | D, P |
| 2. Moderate proteinuria | Yes | D, T |
| 3. Anuria | Yes | D, T |
| 4. Eosinophilia or eosinophiluria | | D, T |
| Posttransplant ↓ in GFR | Yes | D, P, T |

*Biopsy may be indicated for insurance, administrative reasons, and so forth.
†Biopsy may or may not be indicated, depending on clinical picture.
D, diagnosis; P, prognosis; T, therapy; ARF, acute renal failure.

Renal biopsies are usually performed percutaneously with a biopsy needle, and occasionally under ultrasound guidance. Preparation for a renal biopsy includes obtaining informed consent, prebiopsy clotting studies, preoperative blood typing, and sedation (usually diazepam, 5 to 10 mg). While complications of renal biopsy are less than 2%, it is still necessary to establish intravenous (IV) access to anticipate treatment of any complications.[4] After the biopsy, the patient's vital signs are checked frequently for the first 24 hours as the patient is monitored during the emergency from sedation and for signs of bleeding. The patient's urine is examined for blood. The major complication is bleeding, which can occur either retroperitoneally or into the urinary tract. Other complications that can occur are biopsy of other abdominal viscera such as bowel, pancreas, liver, spleen, or vessels, and tears in the diaphragm or pleura.

### Renal Angiography

Assessment of the renal vasculature may be accomplished by ultrasonography. When precise measurements are required, evaluation of renal blood flow through angiography may be used. This procedure may be performed in conjunction with cardiac catheterization. Access is obtained by percutaneous technique: an introducer, or sheath, is inserted into the femoral artery, and a small catheter is passed to the bifurcation of the renal arteries. Contrast medium is injected to provide radiologic visualization of blood flow. Preparation for a renal angiogram is similar to that for renal biopsy; it includes obtaining informed consent, preprocedure clotting studies, preoperative blood typing, and sedation, as well as establishing IV access to prevent or treat complications. After the angiogram, the patient's vital signs are checked frequently for the first 24 hours as the patient is monitored for emergence from sedation and for bleeding. Pressure is applied locally when the arterial access is removed. Because the artery has been accessed, life-threatening bleeding can ensue. Therefore, the access site is assessed for bleeding with the same frequency as the vital signs are assessed. Diligence in application of pressure to the site and conducting site assessment is imperative. Watch for development of bradycardia, because pressure applied to the groin area may stimulate the vagus nerve.

## Assessment of Electrolytes and Acid–Base Balance

The role of the kidney is central in maintaining fluid volume and ionic composition of body fluids. When the kidneys properly regulate the excretion of water and ions, homeostasis is achieved. When the kidneys fail to adapt adequately, imbalances occur. Table 29-5 summarizes electrolyte values and signs and symptoms of imbalance. The critical care nurse needs to monitor closely all of the electrolytes because minor shifts can be lethal.

### Sodium Balance

Serum sodium concentration is normally 135 to 145 mEq/L. It is regulated by the kidneys and depends on the sodium concentration in the extracellular fluid (ECF). When the concentration of sodium rises, antidiuretic hormone (ADH) is secreted from the posterior pituitary gland, and the kidneys retain water in response. When the concentration falls, aldosterone promotes sodium retention by the kidneys (see Chapter 42, Fig. 42-9). When the kidneys malfunction, this balance is not maintained. Low serum sodium usually indicates water intake in excess of sodium and is characterized by an increase in body weight. High serum sodium usually indicates water loss in excess of sodium and is reflected in weight loss. Sodium is essential for maintaining the osmolality of ECFs, neuromuscular function, acid–base balance, and various other cellular chemical reactions.

Hyponatremia is important because it can produce a wide range of neurologic symptoms, including death. The severity of symptoms depends on the degree of hyponatremia and the rate at which it has developed. Usually, symptoms do not occur until the serum sodium level is below 120 mEq/L.[2] For patients with hyponatremia, the severity of symptoms encountered depends on how rapidly the sodium concentration was lowered, as well as the value. Hyponatremia requires further evaluation. Figure 29-4 illustrates the etiologies and evaluation for hyponatremia.

Symptoms of hypernatremia are generally the same as those of hyperosmolality and result from central nervous system dehydration. Mental confusion, stupor, seizures, coma, and death may occur, in addition to other signs of dehydration, such as fatigue, muscle weakness and cramps, and anorexia. The serum osmolality is usually above 350 mOsm/L before significant symptoms are noted. This corresponds to a serum sodium level of 165 to 170 mEq/L.

### Potassium Balance

Potassium is essential for regulating nerve impulse conduction and muscle contraction and is involved in numerous other body functions, including intracellular osmolality and acid–base balance. The normal serum potassium concentration is 3.5 to 5 mEq/L. Potassium balance is maintained by dietary intake and renal excretion. Ninety-eight percent of potassium is located in the skeletal muscle; therefore, the balance of this electrolyte is also strongly tied to the exchanges between the intracellular and extracellular compartments in the body.

Hypokalemia can result from inadequate potassium intake, excessive potassium loss through the kidneys, GI loss, and extracellular-to-intracellular potassium shifts. Also,

## TABLE 29-5  Disorders of Electrolyte Balance

| Electrolyte Imbalance | Signs and Symptoms | Diagnostic Test Results |
|---|---|---|
| Hyponatremia | • Muscle twitching and weakness<br>• Lethargy, confusion, seizures, and coma<br>• Hypotension and tachycardia<br>• Nausea, vomiting, and abdominal cramps<br>• Oliguria or anuria | • Serum sodium <135 mEq/L<br>• Decreased urine specific gravity<br>• Decreased serum osmolality<br>• Urine sodium >100 mEq/24 h<br>• Increased RBC count |
| Hypernatremia | • Agitation, restlessness, fever, and decreased level of consciousness<br>• Muscle irritability and convulsions<br>• Hypertension, tachycardia, pitting edema, and excessive weight gain<br>• Thirst, increased viscosity of saliva, and rough tongue<br>• Dyspnea, respiratory arrest, and death | • Serum sodium >145 mEq/L<br>• Urine sodium <40 mEq/24 h<br>• High serum osmolality |
| Hypokalemia | • Dizziness, hypotension, dysrhythmias, electrocardiogram (ECG) changes, and cardiac and respiratory arrest<br>• Nausea, vomiting, anorexia, diarrhea, decreased peristalsis, abdominal distention, and paralytic ileus<br>• Muscle weakness, fatigue, and leg cramps | • Serum potassium <3.5 mEq/L<br>• Coexisting low serum calcium and magnesium levels not responsive to treatment for hypokalemia usually suggest hypomagnesemia<br>• Metabolic alkalosis<br>• ECG changes, including flattened T waves, elevated U waves, depressed ST segment |
| Hyperkalemia | • Tachycardia changing to bradycardia, ECG changes, and cardiac arrest<br>• Nausea, diarrhea, and abdominal cramps<br>• Muscle weakness and flaccid paralysis | • Serum potassium >5 mEq/L<br>• Metabolic acidosis<br>• ECG changes, including tented and elevated T waves, widened QRS complex, prolonged PR interval, flattened or absent P waves, depressed ST segment |
| Hypochloremia | • Muscle hyperexcitability and tetany<br>• Shallow, depressed breathing<br>• Usually associated with hyponatremia and its characteristic symptoms, such as muscle weakness and twitching | • Serum chloride <96 mEq/L<br>• Serum pH >7.45, serum $CO_2$ <32 mEq/L (supportive values) |
| Hyperchloremia | • Deep, rapid breathing<br>• Weakness<br>• Lethargy, possibly leading to coma | • Serum chloride >108 mEq/L<br>• Serum pH <7.35, serum $CO_2$ <22 mEq/L (supportive values) |
| Hypocalcemia | • Anxiety, irritability, twitching around the mouth, laryngospasm, seizures, positive Chvostek and Trousseau signs<br>• Hypotension and dysrhythmias due to decreased calcium influx | • Serum calcium <8.5 mg/dL<br>• Low platelet count<br>• ECG changes: lengthened QT interval, prolonged ST segment, and dysrhythmias |
| Hypercalcemia | • Drowsiness, lethargy, headaches, irritability, confusion, depression, apathy, tingling and numbness of fingers, muscle cramps, and convulsions<br>• Weakness and muscle flaccidity<br>• Bone pain and pathologic fractures<br>• Heart block<br>• Anorexia, nausea, vomiting, constipation, dehydration, and abdominal cramps<br>• Flank pain | • Serum calcium >10.5 mg/dL<br>• ECG changes: signs of heart block and shortened QT interval<br>• Decreased parathyroid hormone level<br>• Calcium stones in urine |
| Hypomagnesemia | • Nearly always coexists with hypokalemia and hypocalcemia<br>• Hyperirritability, tetany, leg and foot cramps, positive Chvostek and Trousseau signs, confusion, delusions, and seizures<br>• Dysrhythmias, vasodilation, and hypotension | • Serum magnesium <1.8 mEq/L<br>• Coexisting low serum potassium and calcium levels |
| Hypermagnesemia | • CNS depression, lethargy, and drowsiness<br>• Diminished reflexes, muscle weakness to flaccid paralysis<br>• Respiratory depression<br>• Heart block, bradycardia, widened QRS, and prolonged QT interval<br>• Hypotension | • Serum magnesium >2.5 mEq/L<br>• Coexisting elevated potassium and calcium levels |
| Hypophosphatemia | • Muscle weakness, tremor, and paresthesia<br>• Tissue hypoxia<br>• Bone pain, decreased reflexes, and seizures<br>• Weak pulse<br>• Hyperventilation<br>• Dysphagia and anorexia | • Serum phosphate <2.5 mg/dL<br>• Urine phosphate >1.3 g/24 h |
| Hyperphosphatemia | • Usually asymptomatic unless leading to hypocalcemia, then evidenced by tetany and seizures<br>• Hyperreflexia, flaccid paralysis, and muscular weakness | • Serum phosphate >4.5 mg/dL<br>• Serum calcium <8.5 mg/dL<br>• Urine phosphate <0.9 g/24 h |

From Anatomical Chart Company: Atlas of Pathophysiology, 3rd ed. Ambler, PA: Lippincott Williams & Wilkins, 2010, pp 32–33.

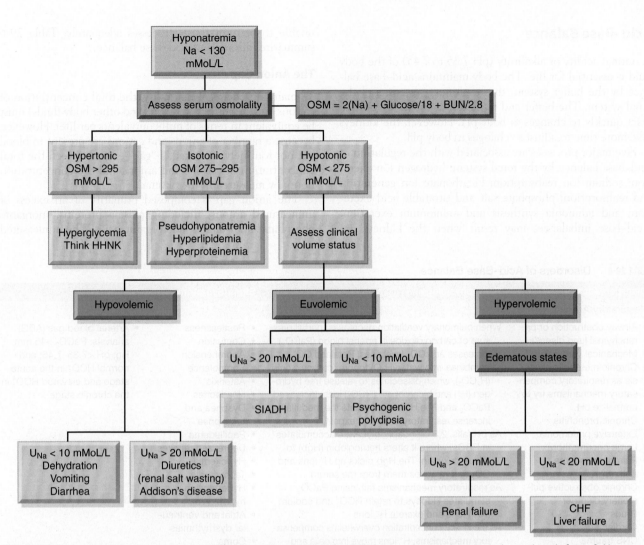

**FIGURE 29-4** Assessing hyponatremia. (CHF, congestive heart failure; HHNK, hyperglycemic hyperosmolar nonketotic [coma]; Na, sodium; OSM, osmolality; SIADH, syndrome of inappropriate antidiuretic hormone secretion; U$_{Na}$, urine sodium.)

diuretic therapy can contribute to potassium excretion, further compounding the problem.

Hyperkalemia may be caused by a decrease in the renal excretion of potassium or transcellular shifts of potassium. This is seen most often in acidosis, cell injury or destruction, and hyperglycemia.

## Calcium and Phosphate Balance

Calcium and phosphate are regulated reciprocally in the body by vitamin D, parathyroid hormone, and calcitonin. The calcium and phosphate salts are normally deposited in bone. When calcium levels are high, phosphate levels are low. Because in renal failure, the kidneys are unable to eliminate phosphate, patients with renal failure often have high phosphate and low calcium levels.

Calcium's primary function is maintenance of bone and tooth strength. It also plays an important role in myocardial and skeletal contractility. Calcium also maintains cellular permeability and assists in blood coagulation. The normal serum concentration of calcium is 8.5 to 10.5 mg/dL. The total serum calcium is composed of two major fractions: the diffusible or ultrafiltrable (or ionized) calcium and the nondiffusible or

protein-bound (primarily to albumin) calcium. Many critically ill patients have low albumin, which will result in low serum calcium. This result does not necessarily mean that the patient's calcium is low. It is necessary to either assess the ionized calcium (if available) or to correct the serum calcium for the albumin level, using the following formula:

$$\text{Corrected calcium} = [0.8 \times (\text{normal albumin} - \text{patient's albumin})] + \text{serum}$$

Phosphate is essential for the formation of adenosine triphosphate. Phosphate also assists in maintaining cell membrane structure, oxygen delivery, and cellular immunity. The normal phosphate level is 3 to 4.5 mg/dL.

## Magnesium Balance

The magnesium ion is the second major intracellular ion. The normal serum concentration is 1.4 to 2.1 mEq/L. Magnesium balance is necessary for the functional integrity of the neuromuscular system. The parathyroid glands regulate both magnesium and calcium. Sodium is necessary for magnesium reabsorption. Magnesium can accumulate in the serum, bone, and muscle in renal failure, causing numerous problems.

## Acid–Base Balance

A normal acidity or alkalinity (pH 7.35 to 7.45) of the body fluid is essential for life. The body maintains acid–base balance by the buffer system, the respiratory system, and the renal system. The buffer and respiratory systems are able to react quickly to changes in body pH. However, the kidneys take more time to adjust to changes in body pH.

Five major processes are associated with the regulation of acid–base balance by the renal system: hydrogen ion excretion; sodium ion reabsorption; bicarbonate ion generation and reabsorption; phosphate salt and titratable acid excretion; and ammonia synthesis and ammonium excretion. Acid–base imbalances may result when the kidneys are

unable to perform those processes adequately. Table 29-6 summarizes disorders of acid–base balance.

### The Anion Gap

To maintain chemical neutrality, the total concentration of cations and anions in the blood (and other body fluids) must be equivalent in terms of milliequivalents per liter. However, because a number of anions and cations are present in blood but not routinely measured, a "gap" exists between the total concentration of cations and anions and the concentration normally measured in the plasma.

The anion gap is composed primarily of an excess of unmeasured anions, including plasma proteins, inorganic phosphates and sulfates, and organic acids. The unmeasured

**TABLE 29-6   Disorders of Acid–Base Balance**

| Disorder/Causes | Pathophysiology | Signs/Symptoms | Diagnosis |
|---|---|---|---|
| **Respiratory Acidosis** | | | |
| • Airway obstruction or parenchymal lung disease<br>• Mechanical ventilation<br>• Chronic metabolic alkalosis as respiratory compensatory mechanisms try to normalize pH<br>• Chronic bronchitis<br>• Extensive pneumonia<br>• Large pneumothorax<br>• Pulmonary edema<br>• Asthma<br>• Chronic obstructive pulmonary disorder<br>• Drugs<br>• Cardiac arrest<br>• CNS trauma<br>• Neuromuscular diseases<br>• Sleep apnea | When pulmonary ventilation decreases, partial pressure of carbon dioxide in arterial blood ($PaCO_2$) increases and $CO_2$ level rises. Retained $CO_2$ combines with water ($H_2O$) to form carbonic acid ($H_2CO_3$), which dissociates to release free hydrogen ($H^+$) and bicarbonate ($HCO_3^-$) ions. Increased $PaCO_2$ and free $H^+$ ions stimulate the medulla to increase respiratory drive and expel $CO_2$<br>As pH falls, 2,3-diphosphoglycerate accumulates in RBCs, where it alters hemoglobin (Hgb) to release oxygen. The Hgb picks up $H^+$ ions and $CO_2$ and removes them from the serum<br>As respiratory mechanisms fail, rising $PaCO_2$ stimulates kidneys to retain $HCO_3^-$ and sodium ($Na^+$) ions and excrete $H^+$ ions<br>As the $H^+$ ion concentration overwhelms compensatory mechanisms, $H^+$ ions move into cells and potassium ($K^+$) ions move out. Without enough oxygen, anaerobic metabolism produces lactic acid | • Restlessness<br>• Confusion<br>• Apprehension<br>• Somnolence<br>• Asterixis<br>• Headaches<br>• Dyspnea and tachypnea<br>• Papilledema<br>• Depressed reflexes<br>• Hypoxemia<br>• Tachycardia<br>• Hypertension/hypotension<br>• Atrial and ventricular dysrhythmias<br>• Coma | • Arterial blood gas (ABG) analysis: $PaCO_2$ >45 mm Hg; pH <7.35–7.45; and normal $HCO_3^-$ in the acute stage and elevated $HCO_3^-$ in the chronic stage |
| **Respiratory Alkalosis** | | | |
| • Acute hypoxemia, pneumonia, interstitial lung disease, pulmonary vascular disease, or acute asthma<br>• Anxiety<br>• Hypermetabolic states such as fever and sepsis<br>• Excessive mechanical ventilation<br>• Salicylate toxicity<br>• Metabolic acidosis<br>• Hepatic failure<br>• Pregnancy | As pulmonary ventilation increases, excessive $CO_2$ is exhaled. Resulting hypocapnia leads to reduction of $H_2CO_3$, excretion of $H^+$ and $HCO_3^-$ ions, and rising serum pH<br>Against rising pH, the hydrogen–potassium buffer system pulls $H^+$ ions out of cells and into blood in exchange for $K^+$ ions. $H^+$ ions entering blood combine with $HCO_3^-$ ions to form $H_2CO_3$, and pH falls<br>Hypocapnia causes an increase in heart rate, cerebral vasoconstriction, and decreased cerebral blood flow. After 6 h, kidneys secrete more $HCO_3^-$ and less $H^+$<br>Continued low $PaCO_2$ and vasoconstriction increases cerebral and peripheral hypoxia. Severe alkalosis inhibits calcium ($Ca^{++}$) ionization; increasing nerve/muscle excitability | • Deep, rapid breathing<br>• Light-headedness or dizziness<br>• Agitation<br>• Circumoral and peripheral paresthesias<br>• Carpopedal spasms, twitching, and muscle weakness | ABG analysis showing $PaCO_2$ <35 mm Hg; elevated pH in proportion to decrease in $PaCO_2$ in the acute stage but decreasing toward normal in the chronic stage; normal $HCO_3^-$ in the acute stage but less than normal in the chronic stage |
| **Metabolic Acidosis** | | | |
| • Excessive acid accumulation<br>• Deficient $HCO_3^-$ stores<br>• Decreased acid excretion by the kidneys<br>• Diabetic ketoacidosis<br>• Chronic alcoholism<br>• Malnutrition or a low-carbohydrate, high-fat diet | As $H^+$ ions begin accumulating in the body, chemical buffers (plasma $HCO_3^-$ and proteins) in cells and ECF bind them. Excess $H^+$ ions decrease blood pH and stimulate chemoreceptors in the medulla to increase respiration. Consequent fall of partial pressure of $PaCO_2$ frees $H^+$ ions to bind with $HCO_3^-$ ions. Respiratory compensation occurs but is not sufficient to correct acidosis | • Headache and lethargy progressing to drowsiness, CNS depression, Kussmaul respirations, hypotension, stupor, and coma and death | • Arterial pH <7.35; $PaCO_2$ normal or <35 mm Hg as respiratory compensatory mechanisms take hold; $HCO_3^-$ may be <22 mEq/L |

**TABLE 29-6** Disorders of Acid–Base Balance (*continued*)

| Disorder/Causes | Pathophysiology | Signs/Symptoms | Diagnosis |
|---|---|---|---|
| • Anaerobic carbohydrate metabolism<br>• Underexcretion of metabolized acids or inability to conserve base<br>• Diarrhea, intestinal malabsorption, or loss of sodium bicarbonate from the intestines<br>• Salicylate intoxication, exogenous poisoning, or, less frequently, Addison disease<br>• Inhibited secretion of acid | Healthy kidneys compensate, excreting excess $H^+$ ions, buffered by phosphate or ammonia. For each $H^+$ ion excreted, renal tubules reabsorb and return to blood one $Na^+$ ion and one $HCO_3^-$ ion<br>Excess $H^+$ ions in ECF passively diffuse into cells. To maintain balance of charge across cell membrane, cells release $K^+$ ions. Excess $H^+$ ions change the normal balance of $K^+$, $Na^+$, and $Ca^{++}$ ions, impairing neural excitability | • Associated GI distress leading to anorexia, nausea, vomiting, diarrhea, and possibly dehydration<br>• Warm, flushed skin<br>• Fruity-smelling breath | • Urine pH <4.5 in the absence of renal disease<br>• Elevated plasma lactic acid in lactic acidosis<br>• Anion gap >14 mEq/L in high–anion gap metabolic acidosis, lactic acidosis, ketoacidosis, aspirin overdose, alcohol poisoning, renal failure, or other disorders characterized by accumulation of organic acids, sulfates, or phosphates<br>• Anion gap 12 mEq/L or less in normal anion gap metabolic acidosis from $HCO_3^-$ loss, GI or renal loss, increased acid load, rapid IV saline administration, or other disorders characterized by $HCO_3^-$ loss |
| **Metabolic Alkalosis** | | | |
| • Chronic vomiting<br>• Nasogastric tube drainage or lavage without adequate electrolyte replacement<br>• Fistulas<br>• Use of steroids and certain diuretics (furosemide [Lasix], thiazides, and ethacrynic acid [Edecrin])<br>• Massive blood transfusions<br>• Cushing disease, primary hyperaldosteronism, and Bartter syndrome<br>• Excessive intake of bicarbonate of soda, other antacids, or absorbable alkali<br>• Excessive amounts of IV fluids, high serum concentrations of bicarbonate or lactate<br>• Respiratory insufficiency<br>• Low serum chloride<br>• Low serum potassium | Chemical buffers in ECF and intracellular fluid bind $HCO_3^-$ in the body. Excess unbound $HCO_3^-$ raises blood pH, depressing chemoreceptors in the medulla, inhibiting respiration, and raising $PaCO_2$. $CO_2$ combines with $H_2O$ to form $H_2CO_3$. Low oxygen limits respiratory compensation<br>When blood $HCO_3^-$ rises to 28 mEq/L, the amount filtered by renal glomeruli exceeds reabsorptive capacity of the renal tubules. Excess $HCO_3^-$ is excreted in urine, and $H^+$ ions are retained. To maintain electrochemical balance, $Na^+$ ions and water are excreted with $HCO_3^-$ ions<br>When $H^+$ ion levels in ECF are low, $H^+$ ions diffuse passively out of cells and extracellular $K^+$ ions move into cells. As intracellular $H^+$ ion levels fall, calcium ionization decreases, and nerve cells become permeable to $Na^+$ ions. $Na^+$ ions moving into cells trigger neural impulses in peripheral nervous system and in CNS | • Irritability, picking at bedclothes (carphology), twitching, and confusion<br>• Nausea, vomiting, and diarrhea<br>• Cardiovascular abnormalities due to hypokalemia<br>• Respiratory disturbances (such as cyanosis and apnea) and slow, shallow respirations<br>• Possible carpopedal spasm in the hand, due to diminished peripheral blood flow during repeated blood pressure checks | • Arterial blood pH >7.45; $HCO_3^-$ >26 mEq/L<br>• Low potassium (<3.5 mEq/L), calcium (<8.9 mg/dL), and chloride (<98 mEq/L) |

From Anatomical Chart Company: Atlas of Pathophysiology, 3rd ed. Ambler, PA: Lippincott Williams & Wilkins, 2010, pp 34–35.

cations that exist in smaller concentrations are primarily calcium and magnesium.

The anion gap is usually calculated by subtracting the anions (chloride and bicarbonate) from the cations (sodium and potassium) using the following formula:

$$\text{Anion gap} = ([Na^+] + [K]) - ([Cl^-] + [HCO_3])$$

The normal mean is approximately 12 mEq/L (range, 8 to 16 mEq/L). However, departures from this "normal" anion gap may have important diagnostic significance in acid–base disorders, especially metabolic acidoses.

The most common abnormality of the anion gap is an increase that is associated with increased concentrations of lactate, ketone bodies, or inorganic phosphate and sulfate that are found in lactic acidosis, ketoacidosis, and uremia, respectively.

Other forms of acidosis associated with ingestion of toxins, such as ethylene glycol, methanol, paraldehyde, and salicylates, also may produce significant increases in the anion gap.

Decreases in the anion gap are less common but equally important. They can occur because of increases in unmeasured cations or because of decreases in unmeasured anions. Table 29-7 lists the causes of altered anion gap.

## Assessment of Fluid Balance

The nurse's role in the assessment of problems of fluid balance includes accurate measurement of intake and output, weight, and vital signs. Although vital signs can provide supporting data, they may not be abnormal until significant

**TABLE 29-7** Causes of an Altered Anion Gap

| Increased Anion Gap | Decreased Anion Gap |
|---|---|
| **Increased Unmeasured Anions** | **Increased Unmeasured Cations** |
| Endogenous metabolic acidosis | Normal cations |
|   Lactic acidosis |   Hypercalcemia |
|   Ketoacidosis |   Hyperkalemia |
|   Uremic acidosis |   Hypermagnesemia |
| Exogenous anion ingestion | Abnormal cations |
|   Ethylene glycol |   Increased globulins |
|   Methanol |   (eg, myeloma) |
|   Paraldehyde |   Lithium |
|   Salicylates | |
|   Penicillin | |
|   Carbenicillin | |
| Increased plasma proteins | |
|   Hyperalbuminemia | |
| **Decreased Unmeasured Cations** | **Decreased Unmeasured Anions** |
| Hypokalemia | Hypoalbuminemia |
| Hypocalcemia | |
| Hypomagnesemia | |

volume or water deficits occur. Assessment of fluid imbalance needs to be based on keen observation and recognition of pertinent symptoms.

## Weight

Weight is one of the single most important tests for critically ill patients. The admission weight is compared with that obtained in the history. Of note is whether the weight has changed significantly over the past 1 to 2 weeks. Weights should be carefully measured at the same time, with the same scale, and with the same linens and clothing daily. Variations in the procedure should be noted and made known to the physician. One liter of fluid equals 1 kg of body weight, equivalent to 2.2 pounds. A kilogram scale provides for greater accuracy because drug, fluid, and diet measurements can be calculated easily using the metric system. An increase in weight does not specify where the weight is gained. For example, a patient may be intravascularly volume depleted yet show an increase in weight because of third spacing of fluid (ie, movement of water to the interstitial space).

Rapid daily gains and losses of weight are usually associated with changes in fluid volume and not nutritional factors. Critically ill patients often experience unmeasured insensible losses, such as ventilation and wound losses. Fever can increase the amount of fluid lost through the skin and lungs by as much as 75 mL/1°F above baseline. Serial weights are often more reliable, and weight changes usually detect imbalances before any symptoms are apparent. In addition to the fluid balance perspective, body weights are also used to calculate drug dosages and, for the patient receiving dialysis, determine the amount of fluid to be removed during therapy.

## Intake and Output

An accurate intake and output record provides valuable data for evaluating and treating fluid and electrolyte imbalances.

It is important that the nurse teach the patient or visitors to assist in this assessment. Intake and output are measured and recorded as they occur and totaled at the end of every shift. In the presence of excessive losses or deterioration of cardiac, hepatic, renal, or respiratory function, more detailed recording of every source of fluid intake and output is necessary, and calculations may be required every 1 to 4 hours.

In the critically ill patient, intake and output are monitored every 1 to 2 hours. The intake and output values are summed to provide an overall balance at the end of a 24-hour period. A net balance is calculated by subtracting the output from the intake:

$$\text{Fluid balance} = \text{total fluid intake} - \text{total fluid output}$$

Depending on the patient's condition, daily therapeutic goals, and response to interventions, the net balance may be neutral, positive, or negative. The 24-hour balance is compared with the daily weight to assess overall balance. If the net daily balance is positive, but the daily weight reflects a loss over the past 24 hours, insensible losses may be the cause of the discrepancy.

Intake should include all liquids, such as water, juices, or soup, and any foods that are high in water content (eg, oranges, grapefruit, gelatin, and ice cream). It is useful to keep a list of equivalents for fruits, ice cubes and chips, and other sources of fluid. Output should include urinary and intestinal losses and estimates of respiratory and cutaneous losses when the patient's temperature or the ambient temperature is high. Also recorded are other sources of fluid loss that are present, such as ileostomy or other enteric drainage, wound drainage, or thoracic drainage.

In severe electrolyte and fluid imbalances, the time and type of fluid intake and the time and amount of each voiding must be recorded. In the event that renal function decreases, this information may aid immeasurably in the diagnosis and possible prevention of prerenal azotemia or acute kidney injury. Box 29-3 gives risk factors for excessive fluid loss.

## Hypovolemia and Hypervolemia

The critical care nurse must be continually on the alert to detect early changes in the patient's volume status. Seldom is the diagnosis made on the basis of one parameter. The first clue may be the patient's general appearance; after observing this, the nurse seeks and notes more specific parameters.

Symptoms vary with the degree of imbalance; some are seen early in imbalance states, and others are not evident until severe imbalances are present. Table 29-8 lists the signs and symptoms of hypovolemia and hypervolemia.

In volume depletion, the patient may complain of orthostatic light-headedness when assuming the sitting or standing position (this also can occur from inactivity and autonomic dysfunction). Development of tachycardia on assuming the upright position and a decrease in blood pressure (orthostatic hypotension), as opposed to the normal rise, are frequent early findings. Later, the pulse may become rapid, weak, and thready. There may be early dryness of the skin, with loss of elasticity, sunken eyes, loss of axillary sweating, and a dry, coated tongue. When severe volume depletion occurs, thirst, decreased urine volume, and weight loss may be noted; however, weight loss and orthostatic blood pressure and pulse changes may be the only findings.

**BOX 29-3**  *Patient Safety*

**Risk Factors for Excessive Fluid Loss**

- **Fever:** A patient with a body temperature of 40°C (104°F) and a respiratory rate of 40 breaths/min can lose as much as 2,500 mL of fluid in a 24-hour period from the respiratory tract and from the skin.
- **Environment:** Hot, dry climates can increase evaporative sweat losses to 1,500 mL/h to maintain body evaporative heat loss. This can increase to between 2 and 2.5 L/h for short times in acclimatized people exercising in hot climates.
- **Hyperventilation:** Hyperventilation can increase respiratory water losses as a result of either disease or use of nonhumidified respirators or oxygen delivery systems.
- **GI tract:** Vomiting, nasogastric suction, diarrhea, and enterocutaneous drainage or fistulas can increase GI losses.
- **Third spacing:** Formation of pleural or peritoneal effusions and edema from liver, renal, or hepatic disease or from the diffuse capillary leak syndrome can result in a loss of effective intravascular volume. Drainage of peritoneal or pleural fluid, when formation of these third spaces is still occurring, can result in further effective intravascular losses because of continued fluid shifts from the vascular compartment to the third space.
- **Burns:** Fluid loss into burned tissues can result in a significant decrease in effective intravascular volume. Because both evaporative and transudative losses through the burned skin can result in very large losses of fluid daily, the burned patient requires special attention to maintain fluid and electrolyte balance. Formulas for determining burn area and fluid resuscitation are discussed in Chapter 53.
- **Renal losses:** Inappropriate solute and fluid loss from the kidneys can occur because of renal salt wasting. This is seen in the diuretic phase of acute tubular necrosis, in some rare patients with true renal salt wasting, and as a result of excessive diuretic administration. It may also occur as a result of solute diuresis from high-protein or high-saline enteral and parenteral alimentation and from administration of osmotic agents, such as mannitol and radiocontrast agents. Finally, fluid can be lost during the generation phase of metabolic alkalosis, in which compensatory urinary bicarbonate excretion obligates renal sodium excretion. This frequently results in volume depletion.

Laboratory studies, such as a high urine osmolality and low urinary sodium, may facilitate the diagnosis. Other guidelines, such as elevated hematocrit, decreased central venous pressure, and decreased pulmonary wedge pressure, may corroborate the diagnosis.

In fluid overload, the patient, if alert, may complain of puffiness or stiffness in the hands and feet. Later, periorbital edema or puffiness, followed by pitting edema of the dependent parts (feet and ankles if upright; sacral area and posterior thighs if supine), will occur, followed by dyspnea or ascites, depending on etiology (ie, cardiac decompensation and systemic fluid overload versus hepatic disease). Urine volume and urine sodium may be normal, increased, or decreased, depending on the etiology. In most diseases with fluid retention, except for the syndrome of inappropriate ADH secretion, urine sodium is reduced. The hematocrit is decreased, reflecting hemodilution.

The pulse may be rapid, and auscultation of the heart may reveal a third heart sound ($S_3$), fourth heart sound ($S_4$), or murmur secondary to volume overload. Respirations may be increased because of pulmonary congestion, and auscultation of the chest may reveal rales. A chest film may reveal pulmonary vascular congestion, increased alveolar lung markings, cardiac dilation, frank pulmonary congestion, and pleural effusions.

All data should be evaluated in the light of other evidence. Trends are usually more significant than isolated values. For example, when a decrease in urine output is noted, a systematic assessment should be done to determine why this is happening and what nursing interventions are most appropriate. Depending on the stability of the patient, the health care team may use advanced physiologic monitoring (eg, pulmonary artery catheter) to guide assessment and management. Box 29-4 lists factors affecting water balance.

## Hemodynamic Monitoring

Hemodynamic monitoring offers the clinician an improved assessment of the patient's overall status. For a detailed discussion, refer to Chapter 17. Although physical assessment may provide insight into the volume status, changes in physical assessment are reflected later than changes in hemodynamic assessment parameters, such as central venous pressure. Through improved monitoring, interventions are guided by information on a real-time basis. Table 29-9 provides an overview of the causes of altered parameters for the assessment of preload.

Based on the data from the history, physical examination, and laboratory and diagnostic tests, nursing diagnoses are developed for the patient with renal problems.

**TABLE 29-8**  **Signs and Symptoms of Hypovolemia and Hypervolemia**

| Parameters | Hypovolemia | Hypervolemia |
|---|---|---|
| Skin and subcutaneous tissues | Dry, less elastic | Warm, moist, pitting edema over bony prominences; wrinkled skin from pressure of clothing |
| Face | Sunken eyes (late symptom) | Periorbital edema |
| Tongue | Dry, coated (early symptom); fissured (late symptom) | Moist |
| Saliva | Thick, scanty | Excessive, frothy |
| Thirst | Present | May not be significant |
| Temperature | May be elevated | May not be significant |
| Pulse | Rapid, weak, thready | Rapid |
| Respirations | Rapid, shallow | Rapid dyspnea, moist rales, cough |
| Blood pressure | Low, orthostatic hypotension; small pulse pressure | Normal to high |
| Weight | Loss | Gain |

---

**BOX 29-4** **Factors Affecting Water Balance**

**Water Excess**

**Intake: Thirst**
Decreased thirst threshold
Increased osmolality
Potassium depletion
Hypercalcemia
Fever
Dry mucous membranes
Poor oral hygiene
Unmisted $O_2$ administration
Hypotension
Psychiatric disorders

**Intake: Parenteral Fluids**
Excessive $D_5W$

**Output: Renal Excretion**
Inappropriate ADH release
Appropriate ADH release
Congestive failure
Decompensated cirrhosis
Volume depletion
• Adrenal insufficiency
• Renal salt wasting
• Hemorrhage
• Diuretics
Burns
Hypothyroidism
Renal disease
ARF
Chronic renal failure
Nephrotic syndrome
Acute glomerulonephritis
Nonsteroidal anti-inflammatory agents

**Water Deficiency**

**Intake: Thirst**
Increased thirst threshold
Decreased osmolality
Lack of access
Psychiatric disorders

**Intake: Parenteral Fluids**
Deficient replacement
Osmotic loads
Parenteral nutrition
Hyperglycemia
Mannitol
Radiographic contrast agents

**Output: Sweating**
High ambient temperature
High altitude
Fever

**Output: Renal Excretion**
Excess excretion
Central
Nephrogenic
• Potassium depletion
• Hypercalcemia
• Lithium administration
• Demeclocycline (Declomycin)
Methoxyflurane (Penthrane)

$D_5W$, dextrose 5% in water; ARF, acute renal failure.

---

**TABLE 29-9** **Etiologies of Altered Preload**

| Hemodynamic Parameter | Increased | Decreased |
|---|---|---|
| Preload | Renal failure | Hemorrhage |
| | Volume or blood administration | Diuresis |
| | Vasopressors | Diaphoresis |
| | Cardiogenic shock | Vomiting |
| | Bradycardia | Diarrhea |
| | Cardiac tamponade | Poor intake |
| | Constrictive pericarditis | Third spacing |
| | | Vasodilators |
| | | Septic shock |
| | | Neurogenic shock |
| | | Anaphylactic shock |
| | | Tachycardia |
| | | Loss of atrial kick |
| Right-sided preload | Right ventricular failure | |
| | Tricuspid/pulmonic valve disease | |
| | Ventricular septal defect | |
| | Right ventricular papillary muscle dysfunction | |
| Left-sided preload | Left ventricular failure | |
| | Mitral/aortic valve disease | |
| | Left ventricular papillary muscle dysfunction | |

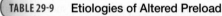

## Clinical Applicability Challenges

**CASE STUDY**

Mr. S. is a 41-year-old man with a history of pulmonary hypertension, hypertension, obstructive sleep apnea, and morbid obesity. Five days ago, Mr. S. presented to the emergency department complaining of difficulty breathing, chest pain, and scrotal swelling. His vital signs upon arrival to the emergency department were as follows: temperature, 97.9°F (36.6°C); pulse rate, 101 beats/min; blood pressure, 148/94 mm Hg; respiratory rate, 23 breaths/min; oxygen saturation by pulse oximetry ($SpO_2$), 92% to 97% (on 4 L/min of inspired oxygen per nasal cannula). Laboratory tests on admission to the medical/surgical unit included the following: $Na^+$, 134 mEq/L; $K^+$, 5.3 mEq/L; $Cl^-$, 94 mEq/L; $CO_2$, 31 mmol/L; BUN, 14 mg/dL; creatinine, 1.1 mg/dL; phosphorus, 6.6 mg/dL; glucose, 114 mg/dL.

On Day 6, Mr. S. is noted to have gained 2.2 kg since his last daily weight. He has bilateral 2+ pitting edema in his ankles, bibasilar crackles are auscultated during his lung assessment.

1. What questions would you ask Mr. S. to determine his baseline renal function?
2. Based on your knowledge of abnormal electrolyte values, what symptoms would you expect Mr. S. to exhibit?
3. What are Mr. S.'s risk factors for developing renal insufficiency?
4. Why do the physical assessments on Day 6 indicate Mr. S. is going into renal failure?
5. What other physical assessment findings and lab values would you expect if Mr. S. developed acute renal failure?

**WANT TO KNOW MORE?**

A wide variety of resources to enhance your learning and understanding of this chapter are available on thePoint.

You will find:

- References
- Selected readings
- NCLEX-style review questions
- Internet resources
- And more!

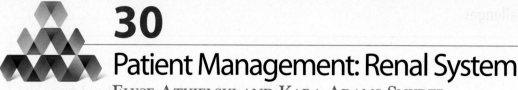

# 30

# Patient Management: Renal System

ELYSE ATKIELSKI AND KARA ADAMS SNYDER

## LEARNING OBJECTIVES

*Based on the content in this chapter, the reader should be able to:*

1. Explain the physiologic principles involved in renal replacement therapies: hemodialysis, continuous renal replacement therapies, and peritoneal dialysis.
2. Describe the differences in equipment and procedures used in renal replacement therapy.
3. Explain the types of vascular access used in hemodialysis and continuous renal replacement therapies.
4. Compare and contrast the indications, assessment and management, and complications for each renal replacement therapy.
5. Discuss the psychosocial and teaching needs surrounding renal replacement therapy for patients and their families.
6. Describe the nursing assessments and interventions for patients receiving fluid therapy.
7. Analyze the specific fluid therapies chosen based on physiologic alterations.
8. Explain the nursing management for patients with selected electrolyte disorders.

Renal function may be replaced by a process called dialysis, which is a life-maintaining therapy used in acute kidney injury and chronic kidney disease (also known as chronic renal failure). Critical care nurses may encounter patients suffering from the effects of acute kidney injury or patients already on some form of chronic dialysis who subsequently become critically ill. Critical care nurses must be familiar with various dialysis therapies to help care for patients with complex illnesses. This chapter discusses the three most common forms of renal replacement therapy: hemodialysis, continuous renal replacement therapies (CRRTs), and peritoneal dialysis. Common management strategies for fluid and electrolyte imbalances experienced by critically ill patients are also explored.

## Physiology of Dialysis

All forms of dialysis make use of the principles of osmosis and diffusion to remove waste products and excess fluid from the blood. A semipermeable membrane is in the dialysis circuit between the blood and the dialysate. Dissolved substances, such as urea and creatinine, diffuse across the membrane from an area of greater concentration (blood) to an area of lesser concentration (dialysate). Water molecules move across the membrane by osmosis to the solution that contains fewer water molecules. Dialysate is formulated with varying concentrations of dextrose or sodium to produce an osmotic gradient, thereby pulling excess water from the circulatory system. This process of fluid moving across a semipermeable membrane in relation to forces created by osmotic and hydrostatic pressures is called *ultrafiltration*.

These basic principles are the foundation of any dialysis therapy. The manner in which dialysis is accomplished varies depending on the therapy.

## Extracorporeal Therapies

Hemodialysis and the CRRTs use an extracorporeal (outside the body) circuit. Therefore, they may require access to the patient's circulation and anticoagulation of the circuit.

### Access to Circulation

The three most common methods used to access a patient's circulation are vascular catheter, arteriovenous fistula, and synthetic vascular graft. Patients who suddenly need hemodialysis or CRRT have a venous catheter, whereas patients already receiving chronic hemodialysis typically have either an arteriovenous fistula or a synthetic vascular graft. Box 30-1 lists nursing interventions for the patient with dialysis vascular access.

#### Venous Catheters

Dual-lumen catheters inserted into large central veins are used for acutely ill patients who need hemodialysis, continuous venovenous hemofiltration (CVVH), or continuous venovenous hemofiltration with dialysis (CVVH/D). These catheters are also used for hemodialysis when there is no other means of access to the circulation. Veins commonly used are the femoral, internal jugular, and subclavian. The site chosen depends on the patient's anatomy and vein accessibility and the physician's experience and preference.

Dual-lumen venous catheters are also used temporarily for patients on acute dialysis who are critically ill or patients on chronic dialysis who are waiting for a more permanent access (eg, an arteriovenous fistula or graft) to mature. Tunneled dual-lumen central venous catheters are often used as a permanent means of access for patients in whom all other means of entry into the circulatory system have been

## BOX 30-1 | Nursing Interventions

### For the Patient with Dialysis Vascular Access

**Dual-Lumen Venous Catheter**

- If in upper torso, such as subclavian or internal jugular position, verify central line catheter placement radiographically before use.
- Do not inject IV fluids or medication into the catheter. Both lumens of the catheter may be filled with concentrated heparin.
- Do not unclamp the catheter unless preparing for dialysis therapy. This can cause blood to fill the lumen and clot.
- Maintain sterile technique in handling vascular access.
- Observe catheter exit site for signs of inflammation or catheter kinking.

**Arteriovenous Fistula or Graft**

- Do not take blood pressure or draw blood from the access limb.
- Listen for bruit and palpate for thrill regularly (such as every shift) and before and after accessing for dialysis treatment.
- Make sure there is no tight clothing or restraints on the access limb.
- Check access patency more frequently when patients are hypotensive. Hypotension can predispose the blood to clotting.
- In the event of postdialysis bleeding from the needle site, apply just enough pressure to stop the flow of blood and hold the pressure until bleeding stops. Do not occlude the vessel.

exhausted. The tunneled catheter has an implantable cuff around which tissue grows and acts as a barrier against infection. If possible, the catheter should be placed in the right or left internal jugular vein, because catheters placed in the subclavian vein increase the risk of vessel stenosis. Such stenosis can cause increased venous pressure and edema that may thwart future efforts to create an arteriovenous fistula or place a graft.

Whenever venous catheters are used, care must be taken to avoid accidental slippage and dislodgment during hemodialysis. For safety, catheters are usually secured with sutures as well as a sterile dressing to avoid movement. The length of time catheters are left in place depends on catheter function and institutional policy. In general, central venous catheters may be used for up to 3 to 4 weeks. Placement of tunneled dialysis catheters is a suggested strategy for reducing central line–associated bloodstream infection in the guidelines from the Centers for Disease Control if hemodialysis is expected to last longer than 3 weeks.[1] Tunneled or long-term dialysis catheters should not be used for any purpose other than hemodialysis without first checking with dialysis clinicians. Cleansing and dressing of the insertion site are the same as with other central lines using strict aseptic technique.

Pressure is applied to the puncture site when dialysis catheters are removed (ie, when dialysis treatment is no longer needed or another form of permanent access has been established). Dialysis catheters tend to be larger in diameter than other standard central lines and therefore have an increased tendency to bleed when removed. The site is checked for several hours thereafter so that any recurrent bleeding can be detected. Removal of the more permanent tunneled catheter requires use of local anesthetic at the exit site and careful dissection around the cuff to free it from the attached subcutaneous tissue. To remove any dialysis catheter, a nurse must have specialized training and competency assessment.

Catheter patency must be maintained. Thrombolytics may be used to dissolve clots in venous catheters. Thrombolytics are enzymes derived from streptococcal bacteria that are capable of activating the fibrinolytic system and dissolving intravascular thrombi. These agents can help preserve vascular access and reduce the need for surgery or catheter reinsertion; however, their use is associated with inherent risks and side effects, including bleeding and an allergic response. The key element in catheter patency is proper and routine flushing to prevent the formation of thrombosis. Catheters left in place between dialysis treatments are filled with a concentrated heparin-saline solution or 0.9% normal saline solution (dependent on end cap used and institutional policy) after dialysis to prevent clotting.

In the early days of dialysis, vascular access was created at every treatment by cannulating an artery to remove blood from the body and a vein to return dialyzed blood to the patient. The lines carrying blood to the dialyzer were called arterial lines, and the lines returning blood to the body were called venous lines. The two lumens of the venous catheter used in dialysis are still designated "arterial" and "venous." The arterial lumen is longer than the venous lumen, so it can pull the venous blood flowing by and allow it to be pumped out of the body to the dialyzer. Blood is returned upstream from the arterial lumen, thereby avoiding dialyzing blood already returned. The lumens are distinguished by the presence of colored ends: red on the arterial lumen and blue on the venous lumen.

### Arteriovenous Fistulas

The arteriovenous fistula technique was developed in 1966 in an effort to provide long-term access for hemodialysis. To create the arteriovenous fistula, a surgeon anastomoses an artery and a vein, creating a fistula or artificial opening between them (Fig. 30-1A). Arterial blood flowing into the venous system results in a marked dilation of the vein, which

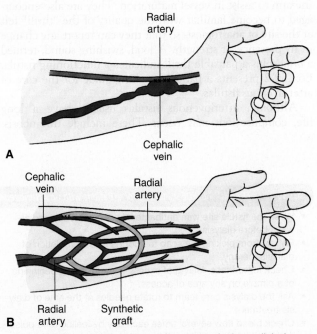

**FIGURE 30-1** Methods of vascular access for hemodialysis. **A:** Arteriovenous fistula. **B:** Synthetic graft.

can then be punctured easily with a 15-, 16-, or 17-gauge dialysis needle. Two venipunctures are made at the time of dialysis: one for blood outflow and one for blood return. Fistulas have several advantages over vascular catheters, not the least of which is the avoidance of inserting a foreign object into the body. Infectious complications are reduced for patients with fistulas, though special precautions are taken to maintain functioning of the arteriovenous fistula long term.

Maintaining blood flow through the fistula is the priority of care. Specific site care is unnecessary; in fact, after the arteriovenous fistula incision has healed, the site is cleansed by normal bathing or showering. To avoid scar formation, excessive bleeding, or hematoma of the arteriovenous fistula, care is taken to avoid traumatic venipuncture, excessive manipulation of the needles, and repeated use of the same site for venipuncture. Adequate pressure must be put on the puncture sites after the needles are removed. Blood pressure measurements and venipunctures should not be performed on the arm with the fistula. To ensure communication regarding the fistula precautions, it is advisable to place a sign regarding these precautions above the patient's hospital bed.

Vein preservation strategies are considered for patients receiving (or potentially receiving) dialysis in order to offer patients all options for vascular access. Peripherally inserted central catheters (PICCs) and central lines placed in the subclavian vein have been shown to have a high association with central vein stenosis and thrombosis. It is recommended that PICCs and subclavian vein catheterization not be used in patients with kidney disease who may require future fistula placement. Patients should be educated about the importance of vascular preservation to ensure successful fistula construction.[2]

Most arteriovenous fistulas are developed and ready to use 1 to 3 months after surgery, and should be placed at least 6 months prior to the anticipated start of hemodialysis. After initial healing has occurred, patients are taught to exercise the arm to assist in vessel maturation. They are also encouraged to become familiar with the quality of the "thrill" felt at the site of anastomosis so that they can report any change in its presence or strength. A loud, swishing sound, termed a *bruit*, plus a palpable thrill indicates a functioning fistula. Box 30-2 presents a patient teaching guide for the care of arteriovenous fistulas.

Although arteriovenous fistulas usually have a long life, complications may occur. These include thrombosis, aneurysm or pseudoaneurysm, or distal hypoperfusion ischemic syndrome, also known as "steal syndrome." Steal syndrome occurs when shunting of blood from the artery to the vein produces ischemia of the hand, causing pain or coldness in the hand. Surgical intervention can remedy these problems and restore adequate fistula flow.

### Synthetic Grafts

The synthetic graft is made from polytetrafluoroethylene (PTFE), a material manufactured from an expanded, highly porous form of Teflon. The graft is anastomosed between an artery and a vein and is used in the same manner as an arteriovenous fistula (see Fig. 30-1B).

For many patients whose own vessels are not adequate for fistula formation, PTFE grafts are extremely valuable. PTFE segments are also used to patch areas of arteriovenous grafts or fistulas that have stenosed or developed areas of aneurysm. It is best to avoid venipuncture in new PTFE grafts for 2 to 4 weeks while the patient's tissue grows into the graft. When tissue growth progresses satisfactorily, the graft has an endothelium and wall composition similar to the patient's own vessels.

The procedures for preventing complications in grafts are the same as those used for arteriovenous fistulas. However, certain complications are seen more frequently with grafts than with fistulas, including thrombosis, infection, aneurysm formation, and stenosis at the site of anastomosis.

## Anticoagulation

Blood in the extracorporeal system, such as the dialyzer and blood lines, clots rapidly unless some method of anticoagulation is used. Heparin is most commonly used because it is simple to administer, it increases clotting time rapidly, it is monitored easily, and its effect may be reversed with protamine. Citrate solutions may also be used for anticoagulation during dialysis; these agents chelate calcium, thereby inactivating the clotting cascade. Evidence suggests that the use of citrate in CRRTs is associated with fewer life-threatening bleeding complications than heparin.[3]

Specific anticoagulation procedures vary, but the primary goal of all methods is to prevent clotting in the dialyzer with the least amount of anticoagulation. Two methods of heparinization commonly used are intermittent and continuous infusion. Regardless of the type of anticoagulation used, close

---

**BOX 30-2**    *TEACHING GUIDE*    *Caring for a Patient with an Arteriovenous Fistula*

- Wash the fistula site with antibacterial soap each day and always before dialysis.
- Refrain from picking the scab that forms after completion of dialysis therapy.
- Check for redness, feeling of excess warmth, or the beginning of a pimple on any area of access.
- Ask the dialysis care team to rotate needles at the time of dialysis treatment.
- Check blood flow several times each day by feeling for a pulse or thrill. If this is not felt, or if there is a change, call your health care provider or dialysis center.

- Refrain from wearing tight clothes or jewelry on the access arm. Also avoid carrying anything heavy or doing anything that will put pressure on the access site.
- Avoid sleeping with your head on the arm where the access site is located.
- Remind care givers and staff not to use a blood pressure cuff on, or draw blood from, the arm where the access site is located.
- Apply only gentle pressure to the access site after the needle is removed. Too much pressure stops flow of blood to the access site.

monitoring of appropriate laboratory values is necessary to ensure patient safety.

## Systemic Anticoagulation

Typically, the circuit is initially primed with a dose of heparin, followed by smaller intermittent doses of anticoagulant or heparin administered at a constant rate by an infusion pump. This results in systemic anticoagulation, in which the clotting times of the patient and the dialyzer are essentially the same. Definitive guidelines are difficult to provide because methods and dialyzer requirements vary. The normal clotting time of 6 to 10 minutes may be increased to 30 to 60 minutes. The effect of heparin is generally monitored by the activated partial thromboplastin time (aPTT).

The patient's need for heparinization and an appropriate beginning heparin dose should be assessed routinely before dialysis, especially in the critically ill patient who may be actively bleeding or at risk for bleeding. In addition, there is also a need to assess for the development of heparin-induced thrombocytopenia with the administration of all heparin products (refer to Chapter 49 for a discussion of hematologic abnormalities). The patient's platelet count, serum calcium level, and results of coagulation studies are valuable in assessing current function of the clotting process. Often, little or no heparin may be used when the patient has serious alterations in one or more factors needed for effective clotting.

## Regional Anticoagulation

Regional anticoagulation is another option to maintain blood flow during extracorporeal therapies. Regional anticoagulation is where the patient's clotting time is kept normal while the clotting time of the dialyzer is increased. Regional anticoagulation is accomplished by infusing an anticoagulant at a constant rate into the dialyzer and simultaneously neutralizing its effects with its antidote before the blood returns to the patient. Typical combinations include heparin/protamine sulfate or trisodium citrate/calcium.

Regional anticoagulation has no associated standard ratios of anticoagulants to antidotes. Frequent monitoring of the clotting times with adjustment of the antidote rate is the best way to achieve effective regional anticoagulation. One patient safety concern is bleeding secondary to over-anticoagulation. Causes of over-anticoagulation include infusion pump malfunction, errors in setting delivery rates, and infrequent monitoring of clotting times. Because of these hazards, anticoagulation delivery must be monitored carefully and frequently, with meticulous checking of pump rates.

Another way to prevent dialyzer clotting and reduce the risk of bleeding from anticoagulation is to administer the anticoagulant with intermittent boluses and use frequent normal saline flushes. Occasionally, saline flushes are used alone, which dilutes the patient's blood (and clotting factors) before it enters the dialyzer.

When regional citrate anticoagulation is used, citrate is infused into the system before the dialyzer binds calcium, obstructing the normal clotting pathway. The patient's sodium levels may rise because the citrate is administered in the form of sodium citrate.[4] Citrate has a higher pH, and therefore patients may also develop metabolic alkalosis.

## Intermittent Hemodialysis

In hemodialysis, water and excess waste products are removed from the blood as it is pumped by the dialysis machine (Fig. 30-2) through an extracorporeal circuit (Fig. 30-3) into a device called a dialyzer or artificial kidney. The blood is in one compartment and the dialysate is in another compartment. The blood flows through a semipermeable membrane, a thin, porous sheet made of cellulose or a synthetic material. The pore size of the membrane permits diffusion of low-molecular-weight substances such as urea, creatinine, and uric acid. In addition, water molecules are small and move freely through the membrane, but most plasma proteins, bacteria, and blood cells are too large to pass through the pores of the membrane. The difference in the concentration of the substances in the two compartments is called the concentration gradient.

The blood, which contains waste products such as urea and creatinine, flows into the blood compartment of the dialyzer, where it comes into contact with the dialysate, which contains no urea or creatinine. A maximal gradient is established so that these substances move from the blood to the dialysate. These waste products fall to more normal levels in the blood as the blood passes through the dialyzer repeatedly at a rate ranging from 200 to 400 mL/min over 2 to 4 hours. Excess water is removed by a pressure differential created between the blood and fluid compartments. This pressure

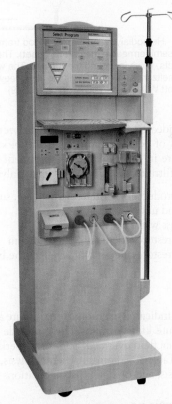

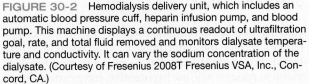

**FIGURE 30-2** Hemodialysis delivery unit, which includes an automatic blood pressure cuff, heparin infusion pump, and blood pump. This machine displays a continuous readout of ultrafiltration goal, rate, and total fluid removed and monitors dialysate temperature and conductivity. It can vary the sodium concentration of the dialysate. (Courtesy of Fresenius 2008T Fresenius VSA, Inc., Concord, CA.)

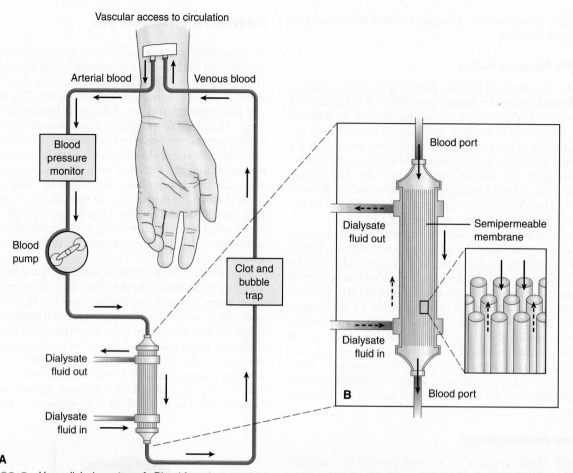

Vascular access to circulation

Arterial blood

Venous blood

Blood pressure monitor

Blood pump

Clot and bubble trap

Dialysate fluid out

Dialysate fluid in

**A**

Blood port

Dialysate fluid out

Semipermeable membrane

Dialysate fluid in

Blood port

**B**

**FIGURE 30-3** Hemodialysis system. **A:** Blood from an artery is pumped into a dialyzer (**B**), where it flows through the cellophane tubes, which act as the semipermeable membrane (**inset**). The dialysate, which has the same chemical composition as the blood except for urea and waste products, flows in around the tubules. The waste products in the blood diffuse through the semipermeable membrane into the dialysate. (From Smeltzer SC, Bare BG, Hinkle JL, Cheever KH: Brunner & Suddarth's Textbook of Medical-Surgical Nursing, 13th ed. Philadelphia, PA: Lippincott Williams & Wilkins, 2014, p 1549)

differential is aided by the action of the dialyzer pump, and usually consists of positive pressure in the blood path and negative pressure in the dialysate compartment. This is the process of ultrafiltration. In summary, hemodialysis

- removes by-products of protein metabolism, such as urea, creatinine, and uric acid
- removes excess water
- maintains or restores the body's buffer system
- maintains or restores electrolyte levels in the body.

## Indications

Hemodialysis is indicated in chronic renal failure and for complications of acute kidney injury. These include but are not limited to uremia, fluid overload, acidosis, hyperkalemia, and drug overdose. Table 30-1 compares hemodialysis, CRRT, and peritoneal dialysis, and Box 30-3 lists indications for dialysis.

## Contraindications

Hemodialysis may be contraindicated in patients with coagulopathies, because the extracorporeal circuit needs to be heparinized. Intermittent hemodialysis may also be difficult to perform in patients who are hypotensive, have extremely low

cardiac output, or are sensitive to abrupt changes in volume status. For critically ill patients in these situations, CRRT may be the optimal choice. In addition, intermittent hemodialysis may not keep up with the metabolic needs of a highly catabolic patient. In this case, CRRT would likely be chosen as the dialysis method. Patients treated chronically for renal failure may be given the choice to undergo hemodialysis or peritoneal dialysis.

## Assessment and Management

The degree and complexity of problems arising during hemodialysis vary among patients and depend on many factors. Important variables are the patient's diagnosis, stage of illness, age, other medical problems, fluid and electrolyte balance, prior experience with hemodialysis, and emotional state. Because an increasing number of older adults are receiving dialysis, it is also important to consider the normal renal and urinary system changes resulting from the aging process (Table 30-2).

### Preprocedure

A predialysis assessment is the first step in managing the patient receiving hemodialysis. It consists of a review of the

**TABLE 30-1  Comparison of Hemodialysis, Continuous Renal Replacement Therapy, and Peritoneal Dialysis**

| | Hemodialysis | CRRT | Peritoneal Dialysis |
|---|---|---|---|
| Access | Arteriovenous fistula or graft; dual-lumen venous catheter | Dual-lumen venous catheter | Temporary or permanent peritoneal catheter |
| Anticoagulation requirements | Systemic heparinization or frequent saline flushes | Systemic anticoagulation with heparin or trisodium citrate may be indicated depending on patient's coagulation studies before starting therapy | May only need heparin intraperitoneally. Not absorbed systemically |
| Length of treatment | 3–4 h, three or more times per week, depending on patient acuity and need | Continuous throughout day; may last as many days as needed | Continuous (cycled) or intermittent exchanges; time between exchanges = 1–6 h |
| Advantages | Quick, efficient removal of metabolic wastes and excess fluid<br>Useful for drug overdoses and poisonings | Best choice for patient who is hemodynamically unstable because less blood is outside body than with hemodialysis and blood flow rates are slower; amount of fluid removed can still be achieved but over a much longer period of time<br>Good for hypercatabolic patients who receive large amounts of IV fluids | Continuous removal of wastes and fluid<br>Better hemodynamic stability<br>Fewer dietary restrictions |
| Disadvantages | May require frequent vascular access procedures<br>Places strain on a compromised cardiovascular system<br>Potential blood loss from bleeding or clotted lines<br>Requires specially skilled staff to perform therapy<br>Risk of bloodstream infection | Requires vascular access procedures; potential blood loss from clotting or equipment leaks; uses an extra piece of equipment<br>Requires specially skilled staff to perform therapy<br>Costly<br>Risk of bloodstream infection | Contraindicated after abdominal surgery or in presence of many scars<br>Waste products may be removed too slowly in a catabolic patient<br>Danger of peritonitis<br>Abdominal discomfort |

patient's history and clinical findings, response to previous dialysis treatment, laboratory results (such as electrolytes), consultation with other caregivers, and the nurse's direct assessment of the patient.

The nurse evaluates fluid balance before dialysis so that corrective measures may be initiated at the beginning of the procedure. Blood pressure, pulse, weight, intake and output, tissue turgor, and other factors assist the nurse in estimating fluid overload or depletion. Monitoring tools, such as pulmonary artery catheters and central venous pressures, also help determine cardiovascular fluid load.

The term *dry weight* or *ideal weight* is used to express the weight at which fluid volume is in a normal range for a patient who is free of the symptoms of fluid imbalance. It provides a guideline for fluid removal or replacement. The figure is not absolute: it requires frequent review and revision, especially in patients receiving dialysis in whom frequent weight changes occur.

After reviewing the data and while consulting with the physician and the bedside nurse (as applicable), the dialysis nurse establishes objectives regarding fluid removal and

restoration of electrolyte balance for the dialysis treatment. The objectives vary from one dialysis to the next in the patient whose condition may change rapidly. For example, fluid removal may take precedence over correction of an electrolyte imbalance, or vice versa.

### Procedure

The nurse begins the procedure by checking the equipment (Box 30-4). After predialysis preparation, a safety check of equipment, and checking physician orders, the nurse is ready to begin hemodialysis. Access to the circulatory system is gained by a dual-lumen catheter, an arteriovenous fistula, or a graft. The dual-lumen catheter is opened under aseptic conditions according to institutional policy. Two large-gauge (15-, 16-, or 17-gauge) needles are needed to cannulate a graft or fistula.

Figure 30-3 illustrates the hemodialysis circuit. After vascular access is established through strict aseptic technique, blood begins to flow, assisted by the blood pump. The part of the disposable circuit before the dialyzer is designated the arterial line, both to distinguish the blood in it as blood that has not yet reached the dialyzer and in reference to needle placement. The arterial needle is placed closest to the arteriovenous anastomosis in a graft or fistula to maximize blood flow. A clamped bag of saline solution is always attached to the circuit just before the blood pump. In episodes of hypotension, blood flow from the patient can be clamped while the bag of saline solution is opened and allowed to infuse rapidly to correct blood pressure. Blood transfusions and plasma expanders also can be attached to the circuit at this point and allowed to drip in, assisted by the blood pump. Heparin infusions may be located either before or after the blood pump, depending on the equipment in use.

---

**BOX 30-3  Indications for Dialysis**

- Anuria secondary to acute/chronic kidney failure
- Symptomatic pulmonary edema unresponsive to diuretic therapy
- Severe electrolyte disturbances (ie, hyperkalemia and hyperphosphatemia refractory to medical therapy)
- Metabolic acidosis
- Uremic complications involving other organs (ie, pericarditis, encephalopathy)
- Drug/toxin overdoses that are dialyzable (ie, salicylates)
- Evolving use of hemodialysis in the literature: treatment of sepsis

**TABLE 30-2** Renal and Urinary System Changes Resulting From the Aging Process

| Pathophysiologic Changes | Physiologic Effects | Nursing Implications |
|---|---|---|
| Decrease in number and function of nephrons | Decreased ability to concentrate urine and conserve water. At risk for dehydration; dry mouth | Provide routine oral care and offer fluids liberally (as ordered) |
| Decreased GFR | Decreased secretion of sodium, water, urea, ammonia, and drugs. Increased risk for confusion, dry skin, and thirst. Less clearance of renally eliminated drugs leading to toxicity | Fall precautions as needed. Thorough skin assessments with position changes every 2 h. Review medications/prescriptions with multidisciplinary team to ensure appropriate medications and doses for age |
| Decline in kidney efficiency | Predisposes to hypernatremia, fluid overload, drug reactions | Routine assessment for heart failure symptoms (crackles, edema, S3 heart tones). Daily weights and intake and output as ordered |
| Reduction in bladder tonicity and capacity | Increased residual urine, nocturnal urination. Risk for incontinence and associated skin breakdown. Increased risk of falls associated with incontinence | Monitor for incontinence and skin breakdown. Provide skin protection as appropriate. Offer toileting program. Call bell in reach at all times. Teach Kegel exercises |
| Decreased regulatory functions such as sensation of thirst, secretion of aldosterone, calcium absorption, response to vasopressin | Increased risk for dehydration. Less ability to conserve sodium and excrete potassium. Altered bone formation. Risk for injury. Increased needs for supplements. Risk for hypotensive episodes | Provide adequate fluid intake and encourage as appropriate. Monitor for fluid and electrolyte imbalances. Assess gait and balance, place on fall precautions if indicated |

The dialyzer is the next important component of the circuit. Blood flows into the blood compartment of the dialyzer, where exchange of fluid and waste products takes place. Blood leaving the dialyzer passes through an air detector that shuts down the blood pump if any air is detected in the circuit. At this point in the pathway, any medications that can be given during dialysis are infused through a medication port. However, unless otherwise ordered, most medications are withheld until after dialysis.

Blood that has passed through the dialyzer returns to the patient through the venous (post-dialyzer) line. After the prescribed treatment time, dialysis is terminated by clamping off blood from the patient, opening the line for saline solution, and rinsing the circuit to return the patient's blood.

A dialysis nurse is in constant attendance during acute hemodialysis. Blood pressure and pulse are recorded at least every half hour when the patient's condition is stable. All machine pressures and flow rates are checked and recorded on a regular basis. The nurse assesses the patient's responses to fluid and solute removal and the condition and function of the patient's vascular access. Gloves are always worn by the nurse performing hemodialysis because of the risk for exposure to blood. The dialysis nurse and critical care nurse work together to care for the patient because they must coordinate their specific patient care responsibilities.

### Postprocedure

The results of a dialysis treatment can be determined by assessing the amount of fluid removed (as assessed by postdialysis

weight) and the degree to which electrolyte and acid–base imbalances have been corrected. Blood drawn immediately after dialysis may show falsely low levels of electrolytes, urea nitrogen, and creatinine; the process of equilibration is thought to continue for some time after dialysis because these substances move from inside the cell to the plasma. To ensure accuracy of laboratory data after dialysis, a minimum of 2 to 3 hours should elapse before samples for laboratory tests are taken from the patient.

## Complications

### Dialysis Dysequilibrium

Uremia must be corrected slowly to prevent dysequilibrium syndrome, which is a set of signs and symptoms ranging from headache, nausea, restlessness, and mild mental impairment to vomiting, confusion, agitation, and seizures. This complication is seen most commonly when patients begin dialysis treatment for the first time. It is thought to occur as the plasma concentration of solutes, such as urea nitrogen, is lowered. Blood urea and nitrogen play a role in calculating the serum osmolarity. Because of the blood–brain barrier, solutes are removed much more slowly from brain cells; therefore, plasma becomes hypotonic in relation to the brain cells. This results in a shift of water from plasma to the brain cells and causes cerebral edema and symptoms of dysequilibrium syndrome. This syndrome can be avoided by dialyzing patients for short periods, such as 1 to 2 hours on 3 or 4 consecutive days.

### Hypovolemia

Fluid overload is treated during dialysis by removing excess water. Because this removal depends on shifting fluid from other body compartments to the vascular space, clinicians must take care to avoid removing fluid so rapidly during dialysis that it leads to volume depletion. Excessive fluid removal may lead to hypotension, and little is gained if intravenous (IV) fluids are given to correct the problem. Therefore, it is better to reduce the volume overload over two or three

**BOX 30-4** Nursing Interventions

For Checking Hemodialysis and CVVH/D With Dialysis Equipment
- Prime lines and dialyzer or filter to expel all air before starting treatment
- Test all alarms before connecting the patient to the circuit.
- Respond to all alarms immediately.
- Replace wet pressure transducers if they interfere with transmission of pressure reading.
- Inspect and tighten all connections before initiating treatment.

dialyses, unless pulmonary congestion is life threatening. Dialysis nurses regularly use monitors to aid in the assessment of patient's plasma refill during dialysis treatment.

### Hypotension

Generally, normal saline solution in bolus amounts of 100 to 200 mL is used to correct hypotension. Dialysis machines now aid in preventing hypotension because the amount of ultrafiltration is controlled at the push of a button. It is also possible to vary the sodium concentration of dialysate. A higher sodium level in the dialysate means that less sodium is removed from the blood. A higher serum sodium assists the body as it shifts fluid from the interstitial to the intravascular compartment. Blood volume expanders, such as albumin, are sometimes used in patients with a low serum protein.

The use of antihypertensive drugs in patients who undergo dialysis may precipitate hypotension during dialysis. To avoid this, standard practice in many dialysis units is to omit antihypertensive drugs 4 to 6 hours before dialysis. Restriction of fluids and sodium before and during the dialysis phases is a more desirable method for controlling hypertension. Sedatives and tranquilizers also may cause hypotension and should be avoided, if possible.

### Hypertension

Fluid overload, dysequilibrium syndrome, renin response to ultrafiltration, and anxiety are the most frequent causes of hypertension during dialysis. Hypertension during dialysis is usually caused by sodium and water excess. This can be confirmed by comparing the patient's present weight to his or her ideal or dry weight. If fluid overload is the cause of hypertension, ultrafiltration usually brings about a reduction in the blood pressure.

Some patients who may be normotensive before dialysis become hypertensive during dialysis. The blood pressure rise may occur either gradually or abruptly. The cause is not well understood, but it may be the result of renin production in response to ultrafiltration and an increase in renal ischemia. Patients must be carefully monitored because the vasoconstriction caused by the renin response is limited. Once a decrease in blood volume surpasses the ability to maintain blood pressure through vasoconstriction, hypotension can occur precipitously.

### Muscle Cramps

Muscle cramps may occur during dialysis as a result of excess fluid removal, which results in diminished intravascular volume and reduced muscle perfusion. During dialysis, cramps may be treated by lowering the rate of ultrafiltration and administering hypertonic solutions, normal saline solution boluses, mannitol, or glucose in an attempt to increase perfusion to the muscles.

### Dysrhythmias and Angina

Dysrhythmias and angina may occur in patients with underlying cardiac disease in response to fluid and electrolyte removal. Decreasing the rate of fluid removal may help. Medication may be needed to control the patient's cardiac rhythm.

## Continuous Renal Replacement Therapies

In CRRT, blood circulates outside the body through a highly porous filter similar to that used with hemodialysis. The process is similar to hemodialysis in that water, electrolytes, and small- to medium-sized molecules are removed by ultrafiltration. CRRT occurs continuously for an extended period and is accompanied by a simultaneous reinfusion of a physiologic solution. A pump, slightly different from that used in hemodialysis, is used and often incorporates a weighing system so that fluids can be intricately balanced hour to hour (Fig. 30-4).

The most common types of CRRTs include CVVH, CVVH/D, and slow continuous hemofiltration (Table 30-3). This discussion focuses primarily on CVVH and CVVH/D because these therapies are replacing previous arteriovenous procedures. Access to the circulation for CVVH and CVVH/D is generally a large-bore dual-lumen central venous catheter designed for hemodialysis. The extracorporeal circuit is similar to the hemodialysis circuit (Fig. 30-5). A pump is added to assist blood flow. The rate of blood flow is typically much slower than in hemodialysis (mimicking the patient's natural blood flow). The ultrafiltration rate is titrated to reach an hourly goal and is based on the patient's cardiac and pulmonary status, as well as hourly intake and output.

When CVVH is used, a replacement fluid is ordered and is connected either before or after the filter, depending on patient characteristics and institutional practice. When dialysis is added to the CVVH process, it is called CVVH/D. Adding the dialysate increases the ability to remove wastes; therefore, it is used when uremia must be aggressively managed, such as with the highly catabolic patient. CVVH and

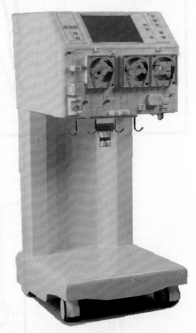

**FIGURE 30-4** PRISMAFLEX. This device for administering CRRT offers an integrated fluid warmer for the heating of infusion and dialysate fluids, a weighing system to reduce the possibility of error in assessing fluid balance, and a battery backup that allows treatments to continue when the patient is moved. (Courtesy of Gambro Renal Products, Inc.)

**TABLE 30-3** **Continuous Renal Replacement Therapies**

| Type of Therapy | Mechanism of Action | Indications |
| --- | --- | --- |
| CVVH/D | Blood is driven from the access port through the low-permeability dialysis filter; there is a countercurrent flow of dialysis solution into the dialysate compartment and to the ultrafiltrate bag<br>There is hydrostatic pressure pushing molecules (electrolytes and toxins) and fluid and osmotic pressure pulling additional molecules (electrolytes and toxins) across the filter. Both actions create the effluent that drains into the ultrafiltrate collection bag<br>Solute clearance is mainly achieved by diffusion; replacement solution is not needed<br>Efficiency of clearance is limited to small molecules | Fluid and solute clearance |
| CVVH | Blood is driven from the access port through the high-permeability dialysis filter; replacement fluid is added to the system, typically just prior to the filter. This results in a "push-only" phenomena: there is hydrostatic pressure pushing molecules (electrolytes and toxins) and fluid across the filter. The addition of replacement fluid will increase this hydrostatic pressure to help facilitate clearance. The effluent created then drains into the ultrafiltrate collection bag<br>Fluid removed may or may not be replaced depending on the needs of the patient<br>Ultrafiltration is in excess of patient weight loss; replacement solution is needed | Fluid and solute clearance |
| CVVH/D | Both replacement fluid and dialysate are used<br>Blood is driven through highly permeable dialyzer, and countercurrent flow of dialysis solution is delivered on the dialysate compartment. Replacement fluid is added typically just prior to connection to the filter<br>Solute clearance is obtained both by diffusion and convection; replacement solution is needed to obtain fluid balance (sometimes referred to as "push–pull" dialysis) | For combined convection and diffusion clearance |

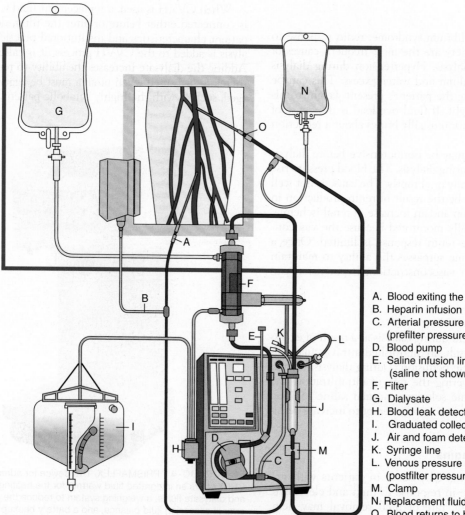

A. Blood exiting the body
B. Heparin infusion
C. Arterial pressure monitor (prefilter pressure)
D. Blood pump
E. Saline infusion line (saline not shown here)
F. Filter
G. Dialysate
H. Blood leak detector
I. Graduated collection device
J. Air and foam detector
K. Syringe line
L. Venous pressure monitor (postfilter pressure)
M. Clamp
N. Replacement fluid
O. Blood returns to body

**FIGURE 30-5** CVVH with dialysis. (Courtesy of Baxter Health Care Corporation, Renal Division, McGaw Park, IL.)

CVVH/D can be performed and managed by the critical care nurse. Typically, didactic training, competency assessment, and validation occur before the nurse cares for patients receiving CRRT.

## Indications

CRRT is indicated in patients with a high risk of hemodynamic instability who do not tolerate the rapid fluid shifts that occur with intermittent hemodialysis; in those who require large amounts of hourly IV fluids or parenteral nutrition; and in those who need more than the usual 3- to 4-hour hemodialysis treatment to correct the metabolic imbalances of acute renal failure. Examples of diagnoses where CRRT is applied include sepsis, systemic inflammatory response syndrome (SIRS), multiorgan failure, adult respiratory distress syndrome, heart failure, liver failure, toxic ingestions or exposures, and rhabdomyolysis. CVVH is used when patients primarily need excess fluid removed, whereas CVVH/D is used when patients also need waste products removed because of uremia. For a comparison of CRRT with hemodialysis and peritoneal dialysis, see Table 30-1.

## Contraindications

CRRT is contraindicated when patients become hemodynamically stable or no longer require continuous therapy; intermittent hemodialysis should be used for these patients. It may be difficult to achieve access to circulation in some patients with coagulopathies, which may prolong initiation of therapy.

## Equipment

A typical CVVH/D setup is shown in Figure 30-5. Blood exits the body through the arterial limb of the vascular access. The first infusion line shown is for anticoagulation. Located just before the blood pump is a line that measures pressure in the prefilter portion of the circuit, known as the arterial pressure. The blood pump, which propels blood into the filter, is next. An infusion port just after the blood pump is usually connected to normal saline solution for flushing the circuit or for attaching the replacement fluid. A bag of dialysate is shown flowing through the filter and surrounding the hollow fibers in which the blood travels. As the dialysate exits the filter, it passes through a sensor that detects microscopic amounts of blood, thereby warning of filter rupture. The dialysate and excess fluid removed from the patient are collected in a graduated/weighed collection device for easy measurement. Meanwhile, the blood exits the filter and passes into a drip chamber, where air and foam are trapped instead of entering the patient's circulation. The drip chamber also contains a line that measures pressure in the post-filter section of the circuit, known as venous pressure. A clamp is located after the drip chamber and automatically engages if air tries to pass through it to the patient. The arterial and venous pressure transducers are protected by a disposable filter. As blood returns to the body, replacement fluid is infused. In some systems, the line for replacement fluid is placed before the blood pump so that it can be infused before the blood reaches the filter. The total amount of blood in the circuit is about 150 to 200 mL.

## Assessment and Management

### Preprocedure

Baseline hemodynamics, vital signs, laboratory values (ie, electrolytes and coagulation results), and weight are obtained before initiation of therapy. The potential exists for uncontrolled losses of a large amount of fluid; therefore, an hourly fluid balance goal is set for the patient after careful evaluation of fluid volume balance. Fluid is either removed or replaced each hour in varying amounts to achieve the fluid balance goal (Box 30-5).

### Procedure

Before therapy is initiated, the equipment is checked as well as the physician's orders, to ensure patient safety (see Box 30-4). The lines and filter are primed to expel air from the circuit. Arterial and venous lines are connected to the corresponding port of the access catheter, and the blood pump is turned on. Blood starts to flow through the tubing. Ultrafiltration begins to produce plasma water (ultrafiltrate) that starts to flow into the collection device. Blood flow rates through the circuit average 30 to 60 mL/min and up to 200 mL/min for optimal clearance. Substances are adequately cleared when ultrafiltration produces 500 to 600 mL/h of ultrafiltrate.

Anticoagulation, if indicated, is administered as therapy begins. Low-dose heparin is the standard anticoagulant used, and aPTT values should be monitored frequently. It may also be used along with saline flushes to prevent circuit clotting, which is the most common mechanism for interruption of CRRT. Saline flushes without low-dose heparin may be used when the patient has a low platelet count. A typical protocol is to flush 50 to 100 mL through the circuit every hour. Another method of anticoagulation is to infuse citrate before the filter; this anticoagulates only the extracorporeal part of the circuit. It chelates calcium, which is then replaced through an infusion through the venous return line or peripherally to

---

**BOX 30-5** **Example Showing Hourly Fluid Goal With Intake and Output in Fluid Replacement in CVVH/D**

1. The patient needs to have 100 mL of fluid removed per hour.
2. The patient receives 450 mL/h of IV fluid (eg, a blood transfusion and IV medications).
3. The patient has 100 mL of chest tube drainage and 50 mL of nasogastric drainage in 1 hour.
4. Dialysate is added at the rate of 1,000 mL/h to increase clearance.
5. The total amount of fluid in the collecting bag at the end of 1 hour is 1,500 mL. (Remember, 1,000 mL is 1 L dialysate, so 500 mL has been filtered from the patient's plasma.)

To calculate the amount of replacement fluid, add the input fluid of 450 mL of IV fluid and 1,000 mL of dialysate. Output is the 500 mL that has been filtered from the patient's plasma, 50 mL of nasogastric drainage, and the 100 mL of chest tube drainage. Total output is 1,650 mL and the total input is 1,450 mL. The difference is 200 mL. The hourly fluid removal goal of 100 mL is subtracted, indicating 100 mL has been removed in excess of the goal and needs to be replaced this hour.

**For Monitoring Fluid and Electrolyte Balance During CVVH/D**

- Monitor and record patient weight daily—preferably with the same scale and at the same time.
- Draw blood for electrolyte, blood urea nitrogen, and creatinine analysis before initiating treatment and then at least twice daily.
- Assess vital signs, central pressure readings (if available), intake, and output before initiating treatment and at least every hour during treatment.
- Collaborate with nephrologist to determine hourly fluid balance.
- Record all intake and output when calculating replacement fluid for the next hour.
- Administer replacement fluid tailored to the patient's electrolytes or obtain custom-mixed dialysate from the pharmacy.
- If hypotension occurs, administer boluses of saline solution as ordered (100 to 200 mL), reduce ultrafiltration and, if necessary, obtain an order for 5% albumin.
- Observe patient for signs of electrolyte imbalances (ie, electrocardiographic changes and muscle weakness, as with hypokalemia).

maintain normal ionized calcium levels.[4] Therefore, the patient needs to be closely monitored to prevent hypercalcemia or hypocalcemia.

Hourly maintenance of the CVVH/D system includes measuring blood and dialysate flows, calculating net ultrafiltration and replacement fluid, titrating anticoagulants, assessing the integrity of the vascular access, and monitoring hemodynamic parameters and blood circuit pressures. In consultation with the interdisciplinary team, the nephrologist sets a goal for hourly fluid balance, and the critical care nurse is responsible to see that it is met. Box 30-6 lists nursing interventions in monitoring fluid and electrolyte balance. By comparing total intake and output, the hourly net fluid balance is calculated. The amount of replacement fluid is determined by the difference between desired and net fluid balance. Fluid balance and replacement should be carefully documented in the patient's intake and output record.

In CVVH, replacement fluid may be infused before or after the filter. Both techniques have advantages and disadvantages. Fluid given before the filter decreases blood viscosity and increases blood flow through the filter. This enhances ultrafiltrate (plasma fluid) production and solute removal and decreases the frequency of clotting. The disadvantage is the increased need for fluid replacement. If replacement fluid is given after the filter, there is less total fluid loss and less need for replacement fluid. However, there is an increased incidence of filter clotting and decreased filter life. The method chosen depends on the system used and institutional preference.

Electrolytes, urea nitrogen, creatinine, and glucose levels are measured before the procedure is started and then at least every 6 to 12 hours. Electrolyte imbalances can be corrected by altering the composition of the replacement fluid or by custom-mixing the dialysate. Anticoagulation is monitored by checking activated clotting times or prothrombin time and PTT. Although frequency is determined by each

institution, it is not unusual to check clotting times every 1 or 2 hours to prevent clotting of the filter and blood lines.

No one policy delineates the optimal time to change the circuit. Many institutions put a 24- to 48-hour limit on circuit life, although there are reports of filters lasting an average of 4 days. System performance is monitored by checking the amount of urea nitrogen in the filtrate compared with the amount of urea nitrogen before the filter. A decreasing ratio indicates inadequate performance. A decreasing rate of ultrafiltration and increases in the venous pressure indicate clotting in the filter.

Treatment may be interrupted to transport the patient for a diagnostic test or to fix a mechanical problem with the circuit or vascular access. Treatment may be terminated if the patient shows signs of recovering renal function. When it is determined that continuous therapy can be terminated, the blood is returned to the patient. First, the ultrafiltrate outlet is clamped, and the dialysate is turned off. Then, anticoagulation is turned off, and the blood is returned to the patient through a saline flush. Once the lines are clear, they are disconnected from the vascular access. Then, the vascular access is flushed and locked per unit policy. Documentation includes fluid balance, condition of the access, and the patient's response to treatment. The tubing and filter are disposable. When working with the circuit and ultrafiltrate, the nurse uses standard precautions.

## Technical Complications

### Access Problems

Blood flows used in CVVH/D are much lower than for intermittent hemodialysis, making it more likely that a catheter will provide adequate flow. However, poorly functioning access can jeopardize the entire CVVH/D procedure. Depending on the location of the access catheter (especially femoral or internal jugular), the position of the patient can affect blood flow. An obstruction, such as a clot or kink in the arterial lumen of the catheter, results in less blood being delivered to the circuit and manifests as lowered arterial and venous pressures. Clots or kinks in the venous lumen of the catheter raise venous pressures as blood tries to return against an obstruction. The treatment may be temporarily halted while the nurse manually flushes each lumen to determine patency. If blood flow still cannot be established, the physician is notified for further intervention, such as administration of a thrombolytic to restore patency to the dialysis catheter or to replace the catheter.

### Clotting

An early sign of filter clotting is a reduced rate of ultrafiltration that cannot be corrected by increasing blood flow. As clotting progresses, venous pressure rises, arterial pressure drops, and the blood lines appear dark. Clotting times are low. A bolus of saline solution may help determine the location and extent of clotting. It may be possible to return some of the patient's blood before changing the circuit, but if clotting is extensive, this should not be attempted. Box 30-7 lists some nursing interventions for maintaining blood flow through a CVVH/D circuit.

- Check clotting times at initiation and at the prescribed intervals throughout treatment.
- Flush system as often as needed with saline solution to assess appearance of filter and circuit.
- Monitor ultrafiltration rates, venous and arterial pressure, and color of blood in circuit.
- If system is clotting, return as much blood as possible to the patient before changing the system.

## Air in the Circuit

If the connections are loose, or a prefilter infusion line runs dry, air disrupts the system by collecting in the drip chamber and setting off the air detector alarm, triggering the clamp on the venous (return) line to close. The nurse assesses the circuit's integrity to detect the source of air. Before resetting the line clamp, the nurse makes sure all bubbles have been tapped out of the drip chamber, all connections are tight, and there is no danger of air getting into the patient's bloodstream.

## Blood Leaks

Blood appears in the ultrafiltrate if there is any rupture inside the filter. The blood leak alarm sounds, and the blood pump stops. Testing the ultrafiltrate by sending a specimen to the lab can verify a microscopic leak. Blood can be safely returned to the patient as long as there is no gross blood in the ultrafiltrate; then the circuit should be changed. A gross leak is readily identifiable; blood should not be returned to the patient, and the patient's hematocrit should be checked to determine the need for transfusion.

## Physiologic Complications

### Hypotension

If blood pressure and intravascular filling pressures fall below optimal, the nurse can increase the infusion rate of replacement fluid, decrease the amount of fluid removal, give a normal saline bolus, or titrate existing vasoactive IV drips per physician order. An infusion of 5% albumin may also help stabilize blood pressure. If this situation persists, the physician is consulted to adjust the net ultrafiltration goal.

### Hypothermia

Some patients experience chills and lowered body temperature while their blood is circulating outside the body. If this happens, it may be advisable to use a blood warmer to warm blood in the venous line as it returns to the patient. A warming blanket may also be used if a blood warmer is not available. Advancements in the technologies used to perform CRRT have improved the precision of fluid balance and reduced the hypothermia that can develop with any extracorporeal therapy. Close monitoring of the patient's temperature along with interventions to achieve normothermia is essential, because hypothermia can mask important signs of infection as well as cause clotting deficiencies, dysrhythmias, and calorie loss through shivering.[5]

## Psychological Aspects

The psychological impact of short-term renal replacement therapy is different from that of lifelong therapy. Although the patient depends on a machine in both situations, in short-term therapy there is usually hope that the patient may recover renal function. Therefore, concerns usually focus on the discomfort associated with insertion of the temporary vascular access and the dialysis treatment. Once these concerns are addressed, the patient and family then must cope with the uncertainty of how long renal failure will last and how long dialysis will be necessary.

Patients who develop chronic renal failure must deal with the fact that renal replacement therapy will be necessary for the rest of their lives. At first, patients usually deny a great deal of what is happening to them. This may continue for some time and prevent some patients from accepting necessary aspects of their treatment regimen. Other patients who feel considerably better after starting dialysis may enter a "honeymoon phase" and appear quite euphoric for a while. Patients should progress through the normal grieving stages and develop healthy coping mechanisms to deal with their long-term treatment.

Patient consent is necessary prior to initiation of any dialysis treatment. Patients who do not wish to undergo the procedure after they have been fully educated about risks and benefits should not receive dialysis. Patient and family discussion is imperative before initiation of therapy. Patients may not wish to receive CRRT because of the need to have 24-hour access to the patient's blood. It is essential that patient wishes be considered.

### Anxiety

Anxiety and apprehension, especially during the first dialysis, may contribute to change in blood pressure, restlessness, and gastrointestinal (GI) upset. The presence of a competent and caring nurse during dialysis may increase the patient's sense of security enough to avoid the need for an antianxiety drug that might precipitate changes in vital signs. A basic explanation of the procedure and its place in the total plan of care for the patient may also allay some of the anxiety experienced by the patient and family. They must understand that dialysis is being used to support normal body function rather than to "cure" the kidney disease process.

### Depression

Depression is the most common psychosocial complication in patients with end-stage renal disease (ESRD).[6] Patients with depression and ESRD have a lower quality of life, decreased adherence to the dialysis therapies, greater comorbidities, and decreased survival as compared with patients who have ESRD alone.[7] It has been suggested that more than two thirds of dialysis patients may experience depressive-type symptoms.[6] Medications for depression have had variable results, and psychosocial interventions, such as chair-side discussions, are yielding promising results.[7] The nurse caring for a patient with ESRD is well positioned to screen for depression symptoms and provide pre- and post-therapy counseling.[8] The most promising treatments for the ESRD patient group are cognitive-behavioral therapy, exercise, treatment of anxiety, and music therapy.[9] All members

### BOX 30-8  Examples of Medications Commonly Hemodialyzed

Acetaminophen, acyclovir, allopurinol, amoxicillin, ampicillin, aspirin, atenolol

Captopril, cefazolin, cefepime, cefoxitin, ceftazidime, cimetidine, ciprofloxacin

Enalapril, esmolol

Ferrous sulfate, fluconazole

Ganciclovir, gentamicin

Imipenem

Lisinopril, lithium

Mannitol, meropenem, metformin, methotrexate, methylprednisolone, metoprolol, metronidazole, morphine

Nitroprusside

Penicillin, phenobarbital, piperacillin, procainamide

Salsalate, sotalol, streptomycin, sulfamethoxazole

Theophylline, tobramycin

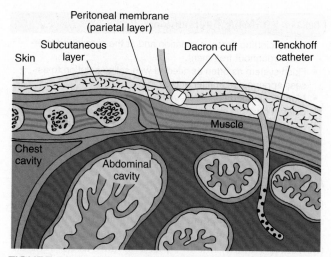

**FIGURE 30.6**    A Tenckhoff (peritoneal) catheter is used to access the peritoneal cavity. A Dacron cuff wrapped around the catheter helps to reduce complications related to infection.

of the interprofessional team must ensure that resources are provided when depressive symptoms are recognized. At hemodialysis visits, the nurse monitors the patient's response to pharmacologic and nonpharmacologic treatments.

## Hemodialysis Applied to Other Therapies

The technical equipment and knowledge needed to perform hemodialysis are often applied to other therapies that involve an extracorporeal blood process, such as hemoperfusion and therapeutic apheresis. Hemoperfusion is used primarily for treating drug overdose. Blood is pumped from the body and perfused through a column of charcoal or other absorbent materials that bind the drug. This leads to a rapid reduction in serum levels and avoids potential tissue damage caused by an abnormally high drug level. This therapy is particularly useful for drugs that are fat-bound or whose molecular structure is too large to be removed by hemodialysis. With this in mind, critical care nurses may need to take the hemodialysis schedules of their patients into consideration when timing administration of medications. For a list of medications that are removed during dialysis, see Box 30-8.

Therapeutic plasma exchange, or apheresis, is another therapy that may be performed using standard hemodialysis equipment in conjunction with a plasma separator cell and replacement fluids. Apheresis is used to treat diseases caused or complicated by circulating immune complexes or their abnormal proteins. During the procedure, the patient's whole blood is separated into its major components, and the offending components are removed.

## Peritoneal Dialysis

Peritoneal dialysis and hemodialysis accomplish the same objective and operate on the same principle of diffusion. However, in peritoneal dialysis, the peritoneum is the semipermeable membrane, and osmosis, rather than the pressure differentials used in hemodialysis, is used to remove fluid. To access the peritoneal cavity, a Tenckhoff (peritoneal) catheter is inserted (Fig. 30-6). Intermittent peritoneal dialysis (IPD) is an effective alternative method of treating acute

renal failure when hemodialysis is not available or when access to the bloodstream is not possible. It is sometimes used as an initial treatment for renal failure while the patient is being evaluated for a hemodialysis program. For a comparison of peritoneal dialysis with hemodialysis and CRRT, see Table 30-1.

Peritoneal dialysis has the following advantages over hemodialysis:

- The required technical equipment and supplies are less complicated and more readily available.
- There is less training required by personnel.
- The adverse effects associated with the more efficient hemodialysis are minimized. This may be important for patients with severe cardiac disease, who cannot tolerate rapid hemodynamic changes.
- Patients can learn to manage their own peritoneal dialysis at home.

Peritoneal dialysis also has a few disadvantages, which are as follows:

- It requires more time to remove metabolic wastes adequately and to restore electrolyte and fluid balance.
- Repeated treatments may lead to peritonitis.
- Long periods of immobility may result in complications, such as pulmonary congestion and venous stasis.

Because fluid is introduced into the peritoneal cavity, peritoneal dialysis is contraindicated in patients who have existing peritonitis, in those who have undergone recent or extensive abdominal surgery, and in those who have abdominal adhesions. In the event of a cardiac arrest, the patient's abdomen is drained immediately to maximize the efficiency of chest compressions.

## Equipment

### Solutions

As in hemodialysis, peritoneal dialysis solutions contain "ideal" concentrations of electrolytes but lack urea, creatinine, and other substances that are to be removed. Unlike dialysate used in hemodialysis, solutions must be sterile. Dextrose concentrations of the solutions vary; a 1.5%, 2.5%, or 4.25% dextrose solution can be used. Use of 2.5% or 4.25% solutions is usually reserved for more fluid removal and occasionally for better solute clearance. Cornstarch-based solutions (eg, Extraneal) are commonly used for patients with diabetes since these solutions do not contain dextrose. The starch in the solution acts as the osmotic agent instead of dextrose. If peritoneal dialysate does not contain potassium, a small amount of potassium chloride may have to be added to the dialysate to prevent hypokalemia. The patient's serum potassium must be monitored closely to regulate the amount of potassium to be added.

### Automated Peritoneal Dialysis Systems

Automated peritoneal dialysis systems have built-in monitors and a system of automatic timing devices that cycle the infusion and removal of peritoneal fluid. For this reason they are called cyclers, and they may be used in the intensive care setting. They are convenient because they eliminate the need to change solution bags constantly and can be set to cycle throughout the night, minimizing disruption patient's daily activities. Most cyclers also have a log that retains cycle-by-cycle information on ultrafiltration. Setting up the cycler requires attaching the appropriate strength of large-volume (5 L) solution bags to the cycler tubing, using aseptic technique. The cycler is programmed to deliver a set amount of dialysate per exchange for a certain length of time. When the time is up, the patient is automatically drained and then refilled. Cyclers are usually used when patients have a permanent peritoneal access device.

## Assessment and Management

### Preprocedure

Before peritoneal dialysis begins, the nurse must perform the following interventions:

1. If a new catheter is required, prepare the patient for catheter insertion and the dialysis procedure by giving a thorough explanation of the procedure. Depending on hospital policy, a signed consent form may be necessary.
2. Ask the patient to empty his or her bladder just before the procedure.
3. Give a preoperative medication, as ordered, to enhance relaxation during the procedure.
4. Warm the dialyzing fluid to body temperature or slightly warmer, using a device manufactured solely for this purpose. Avoid warming peritoneal dialysate in microwave ovens because of uneven heating of the fluid and inconsistency from one microwave to another.
5. Take and record baseline vital signs, such as temperature, blood pressure, pulse, respirations, and weight. An in-bed scale is ideal for frequent monitoring of the patient's weight.
6. Take the patient's history, identifying abdominal surgery or trauma.
7. Examine the abdomen before catheter insertion.
8. Follow specific orders, obtained before the procedure, regarding fluid removal, replacement, and drug administration.

### Procedure

The following items are needed for the catheter placement procedure:

- Peritoneal dialysis administration set
- Peritoneal dialysis catheter set, which includes the catheter, a connecting tube for connecting the catheter to the administration set, and a metal stylet
- Trocar set of the physician's choice
- Ancillary drugs: local anesthetic solution (2% lidocaine), aqueous heparin (1,000 units/mL), potassium chloride, broad-spectrum antibiotics.

The physician makes a small midline incision just below the umbilicus under sterile conditions. A trocar is inserted through the incision into the peritoneal cavity. The obturator is removed, and the catheter is inserted and secured. The placement of the peritoneal dialysis catheter is ideally performed in a special procedures department or in the operating room.

The dialysis solution flows into the abdominal cavity by gravity as rapidly as possible (5 to 10 minutes; Fig. 30-7). If it flows in too slowly, the catheter may need to be repositioned. When the solution is infused, the tubing is clamped, and the solution remains in the abdominal cavity for 30 to 45 minutes. Next, the solution bottles or bags are placed below the abdominal cavity, and the fluid drains out of the peritoneal cavity by gravity. If the system is patent and the catheter well placed, the fluid drains in a steady, forceful stream. Drainage should take no more than 20 minutes.

This cycle is repeated continuously for the prescribed time, which varies from 12 to 36 hours, depending on the purpose of the treatment, the patient's condition, and the proper functioning of the system. Dialysis effluent is considered a contaminated fluid, and personal protection equipment is worn while handling it.

### Postprocedure

After the procedure, the nurse must perform the following interventions:

1. Maintain accurate records of intake and output and weights obtained from the same scale for the assessment of volume depletion or overload.
2. Monitor blood pressure and pulse rate. Orthostatic blood pressure changes and increased pulse rate are valuable clues that help the nurse evaluate the patient's volume status.
3. Detect signs and symptoms of peritonitis early. Low-grade fever, abdominal pain, and cloudy peritoneal fluid all are possible signs of infection.
4. Maintain sterility of the peritoneal system. Masks and sterile gloves must be worn while the abdominal dressing is being changed and when the catheter is being accessed or discontinued from the exchange. Solution bags or bottles are changed in as controlled a physical environment as possible to avoid contamination (eg, avoiding areas of high traffic and high air flow).
5. Detect and correct technical difficulties early before they result in physiologic problems. Slow outflow of the peritoneal fluid may indicate early problems with the patency of the peritoneal catheter.

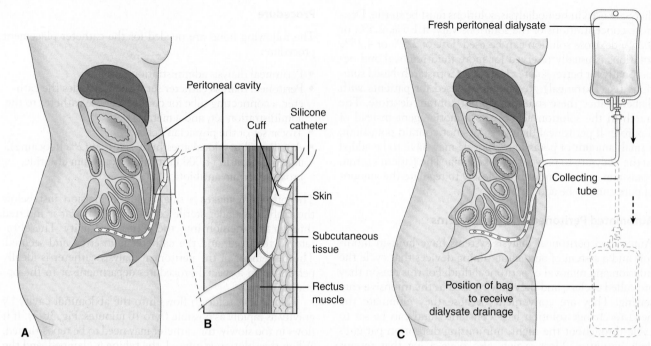

**FIGURE 30-7** Continuous ambulatory peritoneal dialysis. **A:** The peritoneal catheter is implanted through the abdominal wall. **B:** Dacron cuffs and a subcutaneous tunnel provide protection against bacterial infection. **C:** Dialysate flows by gravity into the peritoneal catheter and then into the peritoneal cavity. After a prescribed period of time, the fluid is drained by gravity and discarded. New solution is then infused into the peritoneal cavity until the next drainage period. Dialysis thus continues on a 24-hour-a-day basis during which the patient is free to move around and engage in his or her usual activities. (From Smeltzer SC, Bare BG, Hinkle JL, et al: Brunner & Suddarth's Textbook of Medical–Surgical Nursing, 13th ed. Philadelphia, PA: Lippincott Williams & Wilkins, 2014, p 1556)

6. Prevent complications of bed rest and provide an environment that helps the patient in accepting bed rest for prolonged periods.

7. Prevent constipation. Difficult or infrequent defecation decreases the clearance of waste products and causes the patient more discomfort and distention.

## Technical Complications

### Incomplete Recovery of Fluid

The fluid that is removed should equal or exceed the amount infused. Commercially prepared dialysate contains about 1,000 to 2,000 mL of fluid. If, after several exchanges, the volume drained is less (by 500 mL or more) than the amount infused, an evaluation must be made. Signs of fluid retention include abdominal distention or complaints of fullness. The most accurate indication of the amount of unrecovered fluid is weight.

If the fluid drains slowly, the catheter tip may be buried in the omentum or clogged with fibrin. Turning the patient from side to side, elevating the head of the bed, and gently massaging the abdomen may facilitate drainage. If fibrin or blood exists in the outflow drainage, heparin needs to be added to the dialysate. The specific dose, which is ordered by the physician, is 500 to 1,000 units/L.

### Leakage Around the Catheter

Superficial leakage after surgery may be controlled with extra sutures and a decrease in the amount of dialysate instilled into the peritoneum. Increases in intra-abdominal pressure

may also cause dialysate leaks. Therefore, continued vomiting, coughing, and jarring movements should be avoided during the initial postoperative period. The abdominal dressing must be checked frequently to detect leakage. Dialysate leaks can be distinguished from other clear fluids by checking with a dextrose test strip. Dialysate tests positive because of its dextrose content. A leaking catheter must be corrected because it acts as a pathway for bacteria to enter the peritoneum.

### Blood-Tinged Peritoneal Fluid

Blood-tinged peritoneal fluid is expected in the initial outflow but should clear after a few exchanges. Gross bleeding at any time is an indication of a more serious problem and must be investigated immediately.

## Physiologic Complications

### Peritonitis

Peritonitis is a serious but manageable complication of peritoneal dialysis. Signs of peritonitis include low-grade fever, abdominal pain when fluid is being inserted, and cloudy peritoneal drainage fluid. Early detection and treatment reduce the patient's discomfort and prevent more serious complications.

Treatment begins as soon as a sample of peritoneal fluid is obtained for culture and sensitivity. The patient is started on a broad-spectrum antibiotic, which is usually added to the dialysate solution, although it also can be given intravenously. Depending on the severity of the infection, the patient's condition should improve dramatically after 8 hours of antibiotic therapy.

### Catheter Infection

During the daily dressing change, the nurse examines the exit site closely for signs of infection, such as tenderness, redness, and drainage around the catheter. In the absence of peritonitis, a catheter infection is usually treated with an oral, broad-spectrum antibiotic. Box 30-9 lists nursing interventions for preventing infections during peritoneal dialysis.

### Hypotension

Hypotension may occur if excessive fluid is removed. Vital signs are monitored frequently, especially if a hypertonic solution is used. Lying and sitting blood pressure readings are especially useful for evaluating fluid status. Progressive drops in blood pressure and weight are signs of fluid deficit.

### Hypertension and Fluid Overload

If all the dialysate solution is not removed in each cycle, hypertension and fluid overload may occur. If there is hypertension and a weight increase, the nurse assesses catheter patency and notes the exact amount of fluid in the dialysate bag. Some manufacturers add 50 mL to a 1,000-mL bag; over a period of hours, this can make a considerable difference.

The nurse also observes the patient for signs of respiratory distress and pulmonary congestion. In the absence of other symptoms of fluid overload, hypertension may be the result of anxiety and apprehension. Nonpharmacologic measures to reduce anxiety are preferable to administering sedatives and tranquilizers.

### High Blood Urea Nitrogen and Creatinine Levels

Blood urea nitrogen and creatinine levels are closely monitored because they help evaluate the effectiveness of the dialysis. When levels remain high, it indicates inadequate clearance of these waste products.

### Hypokalemia

The serum potassium is monitored closely because hypokalemia is a common complication of peritoneal dialysis since dialysate does not typically contain potassium. When the serum potassium level is low, potassium chloride is added to the dialysate.

### Hyperglycemia

Supplemental insulin can be added to the dialysate to control hyperglycemia. Blood glucose levels should be monitored closely in patients with diabetes mellitus and hepatic disease.

### Pain

Patients may experience mild abdominal discomfort at any time during the procedure. It is probably related to the constant distention or chemical irritation of the peritoneum. If a mild analgesic does not provide relief, injecting 5 mL of 2% lidocaine directly into the catheter may help. The patient may be more comfortable if nourishment is given in small amounts, when the fluid is draining out rather than when the abdominal cavity is distended.

Severe pain may indicate more serious problems of infection or paralytic ileus. Infection is not likely in the first 24 hours. Aseptic technique and prophylactic antibiotics minimize the risk for infection. Periodic cultures of the outflowing fluid help in the early detection of pathogenic organisms.

### Immobility

Immobility may lead to hypostatic pneumonia, especially in the debilitated or older patient. Deep breathing, turning, and coughing should be encouraged during the procedure. Leg exercises and the use of elastic stockings may prevent the development of venous thrombi and emboli.

### Discomfort

Peritoneal dialysis results in slower clearance of waste products than hemodialysis; therefore, it is rarely associated with the dysequilibrium seen with hemodialysis. However, boredom is a frequent problem because the treatment is longer. Nursing measures are directed toward making the patient as comfortable as possible. Diversions such as reading, watching television, and visitors should be encouraged. Educating the patient about peritoneal dialysis and involving the patient in the care may reduce some of the anxiety and discomfort.

## Peritoneal Dialysis as a Chronic Treatment

IPD has been used for chronic therapy for some time, but it requires the patient to remain stationary for up to 10 to 14 hours, three times per week. Because of this inconvenience to the patient and increased staff time needed if this therapy is performed in-center, IPD is seldom used and is not available in many dialysis centers.

Peritoneal dialysis has gained popularity as a chronic form of dialysis therapy, especially since continuous ambulatory peritoneal dialysis (CAPD) has become available. CAPD is easily taught to patients and does not limit ambulation between dialysate fluid exchanges. It uses the dialysis fluid that is continuously present in the peritoneal cavity 24 hours a day, 7 days a week. Dialysis fluid is drained by the patient and replaced with fresh solution three to five times per day. The number of solution exchanges needed per day depends on the patient's individual needs. Although the patient is required to perform dialysis techniques every day, CAPD is attractive to many patients with ESRD because they can accomplish it easily and independently. CAPD may also be preferred in patients who benefit from a slow, continuous removal of sodium and water, such as in those with refractory congestive heart failure.

Continuous cyclic peritoneal dialysis (CCPD) is another variation of chronic peritoneal dialysis therapy. CCPD uses an automated system previously described in this chapter. Patients who choose this form of therapy perform IPD at night during sleep using a cycling machine and in the morning instill dialysis fluid, which remains in the abdomen during the entire day. This is most convenient for patients who require the help of working family members to perform their exchanges.

As with acute peritoneal dialysis, peritonitis is the greatest potential problem associated with chronic forms of dialysis. Peritoneal catheters are permanent and inserted in the operating room. Such catheters have one or two Dacron cuffs that the surgeon sutures to the abdominal wall, subcutaneous tissue, or both to anchor the catheter and provide a permanent seal against invading bacteria. Patients are taught how to recognize any potential problem associated with the catheter or treatment and to seek help from the CAPD team when needed.

Patients who perform IPD, CAPD, or CCPD at home usually visit the dialysis unit every 4 to 8 weeks. At this time, a nursing assessment is performed, techniques are reviewed, and required blood studies are obtained. All health team members, including the physician, nurse, dietitian, and social worker, work together with the patient and family to ensure successful adaptation to the chosen mode of treatment.

## Pharmacologic Management of Renal Dysfunction

When the kidneys fail, treatment such as dialysis may be used to achieve fluid and electrolyte balance. Pharmacologic treatment may be initiated to enhance an already functional kidney, attempt to recover renal function, or optimize fluid balance.

### Diuretics

Diuretics are drugs that promote fluid removal through increased urine production. There are three major classes of diuretics: loop, thiazide, and potassium sparing. In addition, acetazolamide (a carbonic anhydrase inhibitor) and mannitol (an osmotic diuretic) may be used to promote fluid removal. It may be necessary to use combination therapy to achieve the desired therapeutic end point. Drugs from different classes are chosen to maximize urine production in combination therapy.

Diuretics may be administered orally or intravenously. The effect is more immediate with IV therapy. The patient is monitored for breath sounds, hemodynamic value changes, weight, and peripheral edema to determine his or her response to therapy. Careful laboratory assessment of the blood urea nitrogen and creatinine level is required to monitor for development or worsening of acute renal failure. Ideally, the

patient's pulmonary status and fluid balance improve while the glomerular filtration rate remains normal.

Diuretics have both desirable and undesirable effects. Overdiuresis is the most common side effect. The nurse must monitor for fluid volume depletion, especially when diuretic regimens are altered or initiated. Signs of volume depletion are discussed in Chapter 29. Other side effects include hyponatremia, hypokalemia, hyperkalemia, hypocalcemia, hypercalcemia, hypomagnesemia, and acid–base disturbances. A reduction in volume from vomiting, third-spacing of fluid, diuretic therapy, or other conditions may have the same consequences.

Hypokalemia is another common side effect of diuretics, particularly the loop and thiazide diuretics. In general, hypokalemia is a benign condition that can be managed effectively with potassium supplementation. If left untreated, patients may experience harmful, sometimes life-threatening, cardiac dysrhythmias.

### Vasoactive Drugs

Sometimes, the cause of decreased effective circulatory volume is reduced cardiac contractility. In such a case, an inotropic agent (eg, dobutamine or milrinone) may be added to the plan of care to improve the forward flow of the heart, thereby improving the effective circulatory volume and stopping the cascade of counterproductive compensatory mechanisms. A failing heart, such as in congestive heart failure, can cause reduced blood flow to the kidney and potentiate acute renal failure. The same compensatory mechanisms used in volume depletion operate in an attempt to restore renal function. Namely, the renin–angiotensin–aldosterone system is activated to increase sodium and water retention and achieve renal and peripheral vasoconstriction.

Dopamine is a vasoactive drug at higher doses but can stimulate dopaminergic receptors in the kidneys when infused at lower doses (1 to 3 mcg/kg/min). Stimulation of dopamine receptors increases renal blood flow and promotes natriuresis. Although this practice may still be used to prevent or treat acute renal failure in some settings, several studies have found that there is no improvement in clinical outcome and a lack of sufficient clinical evidence to support its routine use.[5,10]

### Disorders of Fluid Volume

Critically ill patients often have imbalances in fluid homeostasis related to their primary underlying disease. Fluid imbalance occurs when there is an excess or deficit of fluid and may be either absolute or relative. Medications such as diuretics put patients at increased risk for fluid imbalance. Infection increases metabolic demand and insensible loss, and fluid volume deficits may develop. Regardless of patient diagnosis, assessment of fluid balance (see Chapter 29) and careful management are mainstays of patient care in the critical care setting.

### Fluid Volume Deficit

When fluid loss exceeds intake, a fluid volume deficit exists. A fluid volume deficit is a physiologic situation in which fluids are lost in an isotonic fashion (both fluid and electrolytes are lost together). Dehydration is the loss of water alone, resulting in a hyperosmolar state. Although the critically ill patient typically can have both a fluid volume deficit and dehydration states simultaneously, this discussion is limited strictly to disorders of fluid volume deficit.

Several patient populations are particularly vulnerable to the development of fluid volume deficits. Young children at prespeech developmental levels cannot communicate thirst; therefore, during times when fluid requirements increase, they do not increase their fluid intake of their own accord. Debilitated patients—for example, patients affected by stroke—may have difficulty communicating their needs or have swallowing disturbances and cannot manage their own intake of fluid. Elderly patients are at particular risk for a fluid volume deficit because of the multisystem changes associated with aging. For a review of the changes associated with aging and nursing implications for fluid volume assessment and management, see Table 30-2.

## Causes

**GASTROINTESTINAL LOSS.** Physiologically, the body produces approximately 5 L of GI fluid. In the GI tract, fluids help act as a carrier of important enzymes and buffers to aid in digestion. In the distal small intestine and large intestine, fluid is reabsorbed, leaving only approximately 150 mL lost through the stool daily.

Excess loss from any site from which fluids are ordinarily lost may cause a fluid imbalance. Conditions such as vomiting and diarrhea may cause an increase beyond the typical 150 mL and result in a fluid volume deficit. In addition, surgically placed drainage tubes and nasogastric tubes used for suction may cause such a deficit.

**INFECTION.** Infection causes fluid deficits in several ways as follows:

- Infection can increase metabolic demand, increasing insensible water loss. When patients are not critically ill, they often mitigate this imbalance by increasing fluid intake. When they have widespread infections or a self-care deficit, which may occur in elderly people, fluid intake may not be sufficient to restore fluid balance.
- Mediators are released as part of the immune response. These mediators cause a loosening of the capillary tight junctions, resulting in the third-spacing of fluids.
- Carbon dioxide production increases due to increased metabolism. To maintain pH balance, tachypnea may develop. Although only a very small amount of fluid is lost daily through the respiratory tract, water loss may become clinically significant when the respiratory rate is greater than 35 breaths/min.

**RENAL LOSS.** The kidneys filter approximately 180 L/d. However, urine output is only 1% to 2% of total blood volume filtered. Reabsorption of fluid is influenced by a complex regulatory system that includes the actions of aldosterone, angiotensin, and antidiuretic hormone (ADH). A defect in any one of the regulatory functions can cause a disruption in renal fluid balance.

Several endocrine disorders may disrupt the renal regulatory system. Adrenal insufficiency, the absence of glucocorticoids and aldosterone, can reduce the absorption of sodium, thereby promoting water loss. Diabetes insipidus is

a profound reduction in ADH, which reduces the amount of fluid reabsorbed at the distal convoluted tubule. Water loss predominates in diabetes insipidus, and therefore, volume imbalance is related to dehydration (see Chapter 44).

Serum osmolarity is predicted by sodium, glucose, and blood urea nitrogen. Normally, glucose does not influence the overall osmolarity. However, in profound hyperglycemia, the influence of glucose increases greatly. Serum osmolarity increases and is sensed by the osmoreceptors, thereby pulling fluids into the vascular space and initiating an osmotic diuresis. Two conditions that pathologically increase glucose are diabetic ketoacidosis (DKA) and hyperglycemic hyperosmolar nonketotic coma. Both of these disorders are discussed in more detail in Chapter 44.

Diuretic therapy is intended to treat fluid volume excess. However, overadministration of diuretics may result in a fluid volume deficit. It is important to recognize the immediate onset that diuretics can have when administered intravenously, initiated for the first time, or adjusted in dosage.

**THIRD-SPACING OF FLUID.** Third-spacing of fluid is the movement of fluid from the vascular space to the interstitial space. To create a movement of fluid between body compartments, there is an alteration in capillary permeability because of inflammation, ischemia, or injury. Causes of third-spacing of fluids are numerous and include infection; SIRS, such as in pancreatitis; hypoalbuminemia, such as in liver failure; burns; intestinal obstruction; and surgery. The amount of fluid lost depends on the degree of the pathophysiologic alteration. Regardless of cause, the fluid lost is not functioning to maintain vascular volume, and therefore, a fluid volume deficit exists. When fluid leaks out of the vascular space, daily weights can increase, paradoxically, despite intravascular volume depletion.

## Management: Fluid Volume Replacement

To correct a fluid volume deficit, it is necessary to treat the underlying cause and replace the lost fluid. The main purposes of fluid administration include replacement of lost fluid, maintenance of fluid balance, and replacement of lost electrolytes. Several types of fluids, which have different physiologic effects, are available. Administration of fluids may occur using the GI tract or an IV or intraosseous route. When chronic replacement is required, such as in patients with long-term tube feeding, the GI approach is used. Enteral access is required when patients cannot take fluids by mouth. When rapid restoration of fluid balance is required, the IV route is preferred. Occasionally, both routes are used.

**MAINTENANCE FLUIDS.** Under normal conditions, the average healthy adult requires about 2.5 L/d. This volume replaces fluids lost through the feces, the respiratory tract, sweating, and the urine. Patients who are unable to consume their usual intake of fluid are often prescribed IV maintenance fluids of 2 to 3 L/d. When determining the rate of administration of maintenance fluid, factors such as medical history (renal failure), age (young or old), confounding water excesses (heart failure), and ongoing assessment parameters (edema formation) must be considered.

**REPLACEMENT FLUIDS.** Critically ill patients are often unable to consume the additional fluid required to replace the lost fluid. In this case, IV administration beyond baseline maintenance fluids is required for homeostasis. This is achieved either by administering a bolus of fluid or by increasing the total daily fluid intake. When fluid loss occurs acutely, the loss must be replaced immediately to maintain tissue perfusion. The type of fluid given depends on the type of fluid lost. When whole blood is lost, such as in trauma or surgery, blood may be administered. When intravascular volume is depleted, such as in diarrhea, isotonic solutions may be administered. The rate of administration depends on the patient's medical history and amount of volume lost.

**Crystalloids.** Crystalloid solutions are prepared with a specified balance of water and electrolytes. Box 30-10 provides a description of commonly used crystalloid solutions, and although here they are described separately, they are most commonly used in combination. Fluids are classified as hypotonic (osmolarity less than 250 mEq/L), isotonic (osmolarity approximately 310 mEq/L), or hypertonic (osmolarity greater than 376 mEq/L).

Dextrose solutions are given to provide free water and some calories to prevent protein catabolism. The 5% solution contains 50 g of dextrose for every liter of fluid and provides approximately 170 cal/L. When pure dextrose solutions, such

---

**BOX 30-10** | **Common Crystalloid Solutions**

**5% dextrose in water (D$_5$W):** no electrolytes, 50 g dextrose
- Supplies about 170 cal/L and free water to aid in renal excretion of solutes
- Should not be used in excessive volumes in patients with increased ADH activity or to replace fluids in hypovolemic patients

**0.9% NaCl (isotonic saline):** Na$^+$ 154 mEq/L, Cl$^-$ 154 mEq/L
- Isotonic fluid commonly used to expand the extracellular fluid in presence of hypovolemia
- Because of relatively high chloride content, it can be used to treat mild metabolic alkalosis

**0.45% NaCl (1/2 strength saline):** Na$^+$ 77 mEq/L, Cl$^-$ 77 mEq/L
- A hypotonic solution that provides sodium, chloride, and free water (sodium and chloride provided in fluid allow kidneys to select and retain needed amounts)
- Free water desirable as aid to kidneys in elimination of solutes

**0.33% NaCl (1/3 strength saline):** Na$^+$ 56 mEq/L, Cl$^-$ 56 mEq/L
- A hypotonic solution that provides sodium, chloride, and free water
- Often used to treat hypernatremia (because this solution contains a small amount of sodium, it dilutes the plasma sodium while not allowing the level to drop too rapidly)

**3% Saline Solution**
- Grossly hypertonic solution used only to treat severe hyponatremia
- This solution used only in settings where the patient can be closely monitored

**Lactated Ringer solution:** Na$^+$ 130 mEq/L, K$^+$ 4 mEq/L, Ca$^{2+}$ 3 mEq/L, Cl$^-$ 109 mEq/L, lactate (metabolized to bicarbonate) 28 mEq/L
- Approximately isotonic solution that contains multiple electrolytes in about same concentrations as found in plasma (note that this solution is lacking magnesium and phosphate)
- Used in treating hypovolemia, burns, and fluid lost as bile or diarrhea
- Useful in treating mild metabolic acidosis

---

as 5% dextrose in water (D$_5$W), are administered, the dextrose is metabolized, resulting in the administration of free water. When given intravenously, free water decreases the plasma osmolarity, thereby promoting the movement of water evenly into all body compartments. Free water does not stay in the vascular space; therefore, pure dextrose solutions should not be used when intravascular replacement of fluids is required.

Saline solutions are commonly used and are available in different strengths, such as 0.9% and 0.45%. Normal saline, or 0.9% saline, is an isotonic solution. Approximately one fourth of the fluid administered remains in the vascular space, and the remaining fluid moves into the extracellular space 1 hour after administration. During critical illness, the amount that exits into the extracellular space can increase as a result of increased capillary permeability.

Half-strength (0.45%) saline solution, in comparison, is a hypotonic solution. Additional free water is administered with this solution, making it an ideal maintenance fluid. Occasionally, half-strength saline solution is administered to replace fluids lost when there is concurrent hypernatremia.

Saline solutions, such as 3% saline, are hypertonic and may be given to treat symptomatic hyponatremia. The hypertonicity pulls fluid from the extravascular space to the vascular space. Hypertonic solutions should be administered only when patients may be closely monitored because fluid volume excess can develop rapidly. Some studies have shown that hypertonic saline solutions, such as 3% or 7.5% saline, may be beneficial during resuscitation.[11,12]

**Colloids.** Colloids are high-molecular-weight substances and therefore do not cross the capillary membrane under normal conditions. Table 30-4 describes commonly prepared colloid solutions.

Albumin is the most abundant circulating protein in the body and accounts for 80% of the colloidal oncotic pressure. For therapeutic uses, albumin is prepared from donor plasma. With albumin, there is no risk of bloodborne diseases, such as hepatitis or human immunodeficiency virus infection. Albumin is available in two concentrations, 5% and 25%, and both preparations contain some sodium. The 5% solution is similar in osmolarity to plasma. In contrast, the 25% solution is hypertonic, thereby pulling extravascular water into the vascular space. Both preparations of albumin can cause the intravascular volume to expand beyond the volume of albumin infused because of the increased oncotic pressure generated. Care must be taken when administering albumin to patients at high risk for volume overload. The use of albumin as a resuscitation fluid across a variety of conditions has been the source of profound debate in the literature and recommendations on selection of albumin versus crystalloids remain mixed.[13,14]

The starches dextran and hetastarch, which differ from each other only slightly, have an oncotic pressure similar to albumin. Both substances are used to expand plasma volume by exerting an oncotic pressure and thereby pulling water from the extravascular space to the vascular space. Hetastarch is metabolized by both the kidneys and liver. The diuresis that may occur with hetastarch is an osmotic diuresis and does not reflect an increase in effective renal circulatory volume. Both dextran and hetastarch may cause

**TABLE 30-4** Common Colloid Solutions

| Solution | Contents | Indications | Comments |
|---|---|---|---|
| Albumin | Available in two concentrations: 5%: oncotically similar to plasma 25%: hypertonic<br>Both 5% and 25% solutions contain about 130–160 mEq/L of sodium | Used as volume expander in treatment of shock<br>May be useful in treating burns and third-spacing shifts | Cost is 25–30 times more than for crystalloid solutions<br>Increased interstitial oncotic pressure in disease states in which there is increased capillary leaking (eg, burns, sepsis) may occur; this may result in increased vascular space loss of fluid<br>Use caution with rapid administration; watch for volume overload |
| Hetastarch | Synthetic colloid made from starch (6%) and added to sodium chloride solution | May be used to expand plasma volume when volume is lost from hemorrhage, trauma, burns, and sepsis | Plasma volume expansion effects decrease over 24–36 h<br>Starch is eliminated by kidneys and liver; therefore, use caution in patients with liver and kidney impairment<br>Mild, transient coagulopathies may occur<br>Transient rise in serum amylase may occur |
| Dextran | Glucose polysaccharide substance, available as low-molecular-weight dextran (dextran 40) or high-molecular-weight dextran (dextran 70)<br>No electrolyte content | May be used to expand plasma volume when volume is lost from hemorrhage, trauma, burns, and sepsis | Has been associated with greater risk for allergic reaction than albumin or hetastarch<br>Interference with blood cross-matching may occur<br>May cause coagulopathy; has more profound effect on coagulation than hetastarch |

coagulopathies; however, dextran has a more profound effect on coagulation.

## Fluid Volume Excess

Fluid volume excess occurs when there is retention of sodium, resulting in the reabsorption of water. Electrolytes typically remain unchanged when there is an increase in total-body water and electrolytes increase in parallel. Many critically ill patients may have mixed disturbances with manifestations of the confounding compensatory mechanisms. Causes of fluid volume excess include overadministration of fluids, edematous disorders (eg, congestive heart failure, kidney, or liver failure), excessive sodium intake, and medications (eg, steroids, desmopressin acetate [DDAVP]).

When the kidneys are functioning normally and regulating fluid balance, the body typically rids itself of excess fluid, and fluid overload is not manifested clinically. When the kidneys sense a decrease in effective circulatory volume, the compensatory mechanisms prevent the excretion of excess water, such as in congestive heart failure.

Management of fluid volume excess is directed toward correcting the underlying disorder. If this is not feasible, efforts are geared to preventing pulmonary compromise by attempting to rid the body of the excess sodium and water. In cases of volume overload, there is an increase in pulmonary hydrostatic pressure, which promotes movement of water into the alveoli, thereby impeding gas exchange. Sodium restriction reduces the amount of water reabsorption but does contribute to acute correction of volume overload. Diuretics are the mainstay of treatment for acute resolution of fluid volume excess.

## Management of Electrolyte Imbalances

Electrolyte disorders commonly occur in critically ill patients, typically in combination with other conditions. Management of the underlying problem ensures long-term restoration of balance. However, acute management of electrolyte disorders is often required to maintain cellular integrity.

## Sodium

Sodium is the major extracellular cation. It is a major predictor of serum osmolarity and controls movement of water. Disorders of sodium are typically associated with water disorders (Table 30-5).

Hyponatremia may be associated with volume excess, such as in edematous disorders (eg, heart, kidney, or liver failure), or with volume deficit, such as when volume loss is exceeded by sodium loss (eg, in GI fluid, diuretic overuse, or adrenal insufficiency). Low sodium with euvolemia is manifested as the syndrome of inappropriate antidiuretic hormone secretion (SIADH; see Chapter 44). Pseudohyponatremia may occur in association with hyperlipidemia and hypoproteinemia; the total-body sodium remains unchanged, but the actual sodium measurement is altered.

Management of hyponatremia is aimed at correcting the underlying cause (see Table 30-5). When the hyponatremia is associated with hypervolemia, diuretics may be beneficial. When the disorder is associated with euvolemia, such as in SIADH, water restriction may be useful. In conditions in which there is both sodium loss and water loss, administration of hypertonic saline solution, typically started in symptomatic patients, at slow rates may help improve this clinically significant hyponatremia.

Hypernatremia may occur as an isolated condition when there is a loss of free water, which raises the sodium level. Increased insensible loss of fluid, such as that occurs in sweating, hyperventilation, or fever, is the most common cause of this type of hypernatremia. The fluid volume deficit associated with the hypernatremia depends almost entirely on the degree of insensible loss. Endocrine disorders, such as hyperaldosteronism or Cushing disease, can result in hypernatremia and are associated with total-body water excess. Administration of hypertonic fluids, such as sodium bicarbonate, 3% saline solution, or albumin, may also cause hypernatremia.

**TABLE 30-5** Management of Electrolyte Disorders

| Electrolyte | Selected Medical Conditions Associated With Disturbance | Collaborative Interventions |
|---|---|---|
| **Sodium** | | |
| *Hyponatremia* | Congestive heart failure<br>Liver failure<br>Kidney failure<br>Hyperlipidemia<br>Hypoproteinemia<br>SIADH<br>GI loss<br>Adrenal insufficiency<br>Thiazide diuretics<br>Drugs: nonsteroidal anti-inflammatory drugs, tricyclic antidepressants, selective serotonin reuptake inhibitors, chlorpropamide, omeprazole<br>Tumors associated with ectopic excessive ADH production: oat cell carcinoma, leukemia, lymphoma<br>Pulmonary disorders: pneumonia, acute asthma<br>Acquired immunodeficiency syndrome | Review medication profile and patient history<br>Monitor for sites of fluid losses or gains<br>Monitor fluid balances and for signs and symptoms of electrolyte disturbance<br>Attempt to manage underlying cause<br>Correction of electrolyte may require sodium replacement (3% saline solution) or water restriction, depending on etiology of disorder |
| *Hypernatremia* | Profound dehydration, usually in patients not able to ask for water (eg, debilitated elderly or children), in those with impaired thirst regulation (eg, elderly), or in those with heat stroke<br>Hypertonic tube feedings without water supplementation<br>Increased insensible water loss (eg, excessive sweating, second- and third-degree burns, hyperventilation)<br>Excessive administration of sodium-containing fluids (3% saline, sodium bicarbonate)<br>Diabetes insipidus | Assess in patients at particular risk for hypernatremia, including debilitated or elderly patients, acutely or critically ill children, and patients receiving tube feedings<br>Monitor laboratory values closely in patients with insensible fluid losses and in those receiving parenteral administration of sodium-containing fluids<br>For comprehensive review of management of diabetes insipidus, see Chapter 44<br>Administer therapeutic medications, including vasopressin, DDAVP<br>Administer hypotonic fluids (1/2 saline to free water, $D_5W$) |
| **Potassium** | | |
| *Hypokalemia* | GI loss: diarrhea, laxatives, gastric suction<br>Renal loss: potassium-losing diuretics, hyperaldosteronism, osmotic diuresis, steroids, some antibiotics<br>Intracellular shifts: alkalosis, excessive secretion or administration of insulin, hyperalimentation<br>Poor intake: anorexia nervosa, alcoholism, debilitation | Monitor laboratory values closely in patients at particular risk for hypokalemia<br>Pay particular attention to potassium level in patients receiving digoxin<br>Administer potassium either orally or IV (see Box 30-11)<br>Monitor magnesium levels in patients who are refractory to potassium replacement |
| *Hyperkalemia* | Pseudohyperkalemia: prolonged tight application of tourniquet; fist clenching and unclenching immediately before or during blood draws; hemolysis of blood sample<br>Decreased potassium excretion: oliguric renal failure, potassium-sparing diuretics, hypoaldosteronism<br>High potassium intake: improper use of oral potassium supplements; rapid IV potassium administration<br>Extracellular shifts: acidosis, crush injuries, tumor cell lysis after chemotherapy | Ensure that minimal negative pressure is used to obtain all laboratory samples, particularly when drawn through small-gauge needles<br>Restrict potassium-sparing diuretics<br>Promote excretion: sodium polystyrene sulfonate orally or rectally, dialysis, potassium-losing diuretics (eg, furosemide)<br>Emergency management measures: calcium IV, sodium bicarbonate, IV insulin with glucose, β2-adrenergic agonists |
| **Calcium** | | |
| *Hypocalcemia* | Surgical hypoparathyroidism<br>Primary hypoparathyroidism<br>Malabsorption (alcoholism)<br>Acute pancreatitis<br>Excessive administration of citrated blood<br>Alkalotic states<br>Drugs (loop diuretics, mithramycin, calcitonin)<br>Hyperphosphatemia<br>Sepsis<br>Hypomagnesemia<br>Medullary carcinoma of thyroid<br>Hypoalbuminemia | Monitor for signs and symptoms associated with low calcium, especially for seizures, and stridor<br>Administer calcium IV for acute replacement (see Box 30-11)<br>Ensure adequate dietary intake for patients at particular risk |

**TABLE 30-5   Management of Electrolyte Disorders (*continued*)**

| Electrolyte | Selected Medical Conditions Associated With Disturbance | Collaborative Interventions |
|---|---|---|
| Hypercalcemia | Hyperparathyroidism<br>Malignant neoplastic disease<br>Drugs (thiazide diuretics, lithium, theophylline)<br>Prolonged immobilization<br>Dehydration | Administer bisphosphonates, such as etidronate or mithramycin, especially when disorder is related to malignancy<br>Administer diuretics, such as loop diuretics, to promote renal excretion<br>Provide fluid replacement with 0.9% saline solution |
| **Magnesium** | | |
| Hypomagnesemia | Inadequate intake: starvation, total parenteral nutrition without adequate Mg2+ supplementation, chronic alcoholism<br>Increased GI loss: diarrhea, laxatives, fistulas, naso-gastric tube suction, vomiting<br>Increased renal loss: drugs (loop and thiazide diuretics, mannitol, amphotericin B), diuresis (uncontrolled diabetes mellitus, hypoaldosteronism)<br>Changes in magnesium distribution: pancreatitis, burns, insulin, blood products | Monitor for hypokalemia in patients with low magnesium because kidneys are not able to conserve potassium when magnesium level is low<br>Administer magnesium IV for acute replacement (see Box 30-11)<br>Administer PO preparations for long-term replacement |
| Hypermagnesemia | Renal failure<br>Excessive intake of magnesium-containing compounds (eg, antacids, mineral supplements, laxatives | Avoid administration of magnesium-containing compounds to patients in renal failure<br>In extreme cases, dialysis may be indicated |
| **Phosphorus** | | |
| Hypophosphatemia | Refeeding syndrome<br>Alcoholism<br>Phosphate-binding antacids<br>Respiratory alkalosis<br>Administration of exogenous insulin IV<br>Burns | Ensure nutritional intake<br>Monitor phosphorus for the first few days after initiation of enteral or parenteral nutrition<br>Administer by oral supplementation (Neutra-Phos capsules) or IV (see Box 30-11) |
| Hyperphosphatemia | Renal failure<br>Chemotherapy<br>Excessive administration of phosphate compounds | Prevention is mainstay of therapy; avoid administration of phosphorus to patients in renal failure<br>Administer calcium acetate<br>Administer IV fluids to promote renal excretion<br>In severe cases, administration of high levels of glucose with insulin may help shift phosphorus intracellularly |

Management of hypernatremia is primarily aimed at restoring fluid balance (see Table 30-5). Correcting the underlying cause of the increased sodium is also important.

## Potassium

Potassium is the major intracellular ion. Potassium plays a key role in neuromuscular functioning, and high or low levels may result in alterations in the cardiac rhythm. Because of the narrow range of extracellular potassium balance, renal function is essential to regulation of potassium. In critically ill patients, disorders of potassium are common and have numerous causes (see Table 30-5).

Hypokalemia is most commonly caused by an absolute deficiency in potassium. Losses of potassium occur through the kidneys, GI tract, sweat, and intracellular shifting. Although relative deficiencies may occur, such as in metabolic alkalosis, they are rare compared with the absolute deficits. Management of hypokalemia involves replacing depleted potassium to restore potassium balance. It may be necessary to check the magnesium level in patients who do not respond to potassium replacement. Box 30-11 presents nursing considerations in potassium replacement.

Hyperkalemia is caused by reduced renal excretion, excessive administration of potassium replacements, transcellular shifts, and measurement error. Patients with chronic renal failure or acute kidney injury are at particular risk. Dialysis is typically used to manage hyperkalemia in patients with ESRD. Noncompliance with dialysis can certainly cause hyperkalemia and is a frequent reason for hospital admission. Potassium replacement therapy, although performed frequently in critical care settings, must be performed carefully; particular attention should be paid to cardiac signs and laboratory reassessments. Acidosis of any cause can potentiate hyperkalemia; therefore, patients who are acidotic must be carefully monitored for potassium shifts. In this situation, the primary goal of management is resolution of the acidosis. Clinically significant hyperkalemia must be resolved using the measures described in Table 30-5. Temporizing measures for hyperkalemia center on stabilization of cell membrane (calcium) and shifting potassium from the extracellular to the intracellular spaces (bicarbonate, insulin). These measures resolve the potassium imbalance temporarily and give clinicians time to address the underlying problem. If it is anticipated that correction of this problem will take some time, the interprofessional team may consider administering

## BOX 30-11   Nursing Interventions

### For Intravenous Electrolyte Replacement

#### Potassium

*Dilution*

- Do not administer undiluted potassium directly IV.
- Keep all vials of undiluted potassium away from patient care area.
- Dilution of potassium depends on the amount of fluid the patient can tolerate. Highly concentrated potassium solutions can cause irritation, pain, and sclerosing of vein.
- Typical concentrations of potassium are 10 to 40 mEq/100 mL. Premixed bags are available.

*Peripheral IV Administration*

- In collaboration with prescribing provider, consider the addition of small volume of lidocaine to minimize pain.
- Administer in central vein if available.
- For mild to moderate hypokalemia, rates of 10 to 20 mEq/h are recommended.
- Rates exceeding 40 mEq/h are not recommended.
- Use infusion pump to administer replacement.

*Monitoring*

- Monitor urinary output, blood urea nitrogen, and creatinine in patients receiving potassium replacement. Patients with impaired renal function or oliguric renal failure may experience transient hyperkalemia. Consider smaller replacement dosages and periodic reevaluation.
- When rate of administration exceeds 10 mEq/h, monitoring of cardiac rhythm is recommended.
- Assess magnesium level because correction of potassium may be refractory to potassium replacement with concurrent hypomagnesemia.

#### Calcium

*Dilution*

- Calcium can be delivered as calcium gluconate (4.5 mEq of elemental $Ca^{2+}$) or calcium chloride (13.5 mEq of elemental $Ca^{2+}$).

- Calcium can be irritating to veins. If peripheral administration is required, calcium gluconate is recommended because damage can occur to surrounding soft tissues.

*Administration*

- Administer by slow IV push through central vein or administer by mixing with compatible IV fluids.
- Administer slowly (over 1 to 2 hours) for patients receiving digoxin.

#### Magnesium

*Administration*

- Administer with caution to patients with renal failure because magnesium is primarily excreted by the kidneys.
- During emergencies, such as torsades de pointes, magnesium may be injected directly.
- In mild to moderate hypomagnesemia, a rate of infusion of 1 to 2 g over 1 hour is advisable.

*Monitoring*

- Monitor for hypotension or flushing during administration.
- Monitor deep tendon reflexes periodically during administration.

#### Phosphorus

- Phosphorus IV replacement is available as sodium or potassium phosphate. Note that phosphorus is dosed in millimoles, whereas sodium and potassium are dosed in milliequivalents.
- Administer sodium phosphate for patients with renal failure.
- Do not administer with calcium.
- Administer over several hours, typically 15 to 30 mmol phosphorus over 4 to 6 hours.

---

sodium polystyrene, dialysis, and diuretics. Drawing laboratory samples can cause hemolysis of cells, which causes liberation of the abundant intracellular potassium. Evaluating trends and assessing the overall clinical picture prevent unnecessary treatment and therefore prevent hypokalemia.

## Calcium

Almost all of the calcium in the body is contained in the bone, and the remaining 1% is either bound to albumin (50% plasma calcium) or in an ionized form. The primary function of calcium is promotion of the neuromuscular impulse. Several clotting factors also depend on calcium.

Hypocalcemia has numerous causes (see Table 30-5). Most hypocalcemia is a relative deficiency; causes include intracellular shifting, decreased circulating protein, and binding with fatty acids (pancreatitis). The relative hypocalcemia that occurs with a massive transfusion of blood is common in the critical care setting. The blood is mixed with citrate to prevent coagulation; when the blood is infused, the citrate binds to calcium, causing a relative calcium deficiency. Citrate used for anticoagulation in CRRT also results in hypocalcemia. Other causes of hypocalcemia include increased renal excretion (loop diuretics) or decreased absorption (malabsorption syndromes).

Calcium is transported in its ionized form, provides some of the structural components in bone, and is also bound to albumin. A low albumin level can therefore be one cause of a low calcium level. The calcium level should be corrected for the low albumin before considering calcium replacement. Replacement of calcium is required to prevent complications of bleeding and decreased impulse transmission. For a review of nursing considerations in calcium replacement, see Box 30-11.

Hypercalcemia, which is less common in the critical care setting, is most often caused by malignancy. Treatment is supportive and involves administration of diuretics and IV fluids, sometimes simultaneously.

## Magnesium

About two thirds of the magnesium in the body is in the skeletal system, and the remaining one third is in the intracellular space. About 1% circulates in the extracellular space. Magnesium is a catalyst for hundreds of enzymatic reactions and plays a role in neurotransmission and cardiac contraction. Magnesium is primarily excreted by the kidneys.

Hypomagnesemia is caused by loss of magnesium through the GI tract or (less commonly) the kidneys. Alcoholism is a significant cause. The etiologic mechanism is not completely understood, but it is thought that decreased dietary intake due to malnutrition, decreased absorption, and increased GI losses (due to periodic emesis) all play a role. Several drugs may also cause hypomagnesemia, including loop diuretics, aminoglycosides, amphotericin B, *cis*-platinum, cyclosporine, and citrate. For a review of the causes of hypomagnesemia, see Table 30-5.

Magnesium is available in a variety of preparations, including 50%, 20%, or 10% solutions. It is important to pay particular attention to how the replacement preparation is ordered; the replacement solution should be "dosed" in grams instead of milliliters. For a review of nursing considerations in magnesium replacement, see Box 30-11.

## Phosphorus

Phosphorus is the major intracellular anion. The source of adenosine triphosphate (ATP), phosphorus is implicated in many life-sustaining processes, such as muscle contraction, neuromuscular impulse conduction, and the regulation of several intracellular and extracellular electrolyte balances.

Hypophosphatemia may be caused by several metabolic disorders, including refeeding syndrome and alcoholism, intracellular shifting due to respiratory alkalosis, binding by medications, such as phosphate-binding magnesium-containing antacids, and excessive excretion of phosphate, such as in DKA (see Table 30-5). Refeeding syndrome occurs when the patient is fed, either enterally or parenterally, after some time of starvation. During starvation, protein catabolism occurs, depleting all of the intracellular phosphorus. When a large glucose load is administered, as occurs with refeeding, it is thought that the insulin response shifts the phosphorus intracellularly.

Management of hypophosphatemia may be problematic, particularly for patients on a mechanical ventilator. Contraction of all muscles, including the diaphragm, depends on ATP. Replacement of phosphorus is indicated in critically ill patients to achieve adequate pulmonary function. Once the critical illness abates, the hypophosphatemia typically resolves as well. However, replacement with either sodium or potassium phosphate is indicated in the meantime. For a review of nursing considerations in phosphorus replacement, see Box 30-11.

Hyperphosphatemia is commonly associated with renal failure due to reduced elimination of phosphorus. Because of the inverse relationship with calcium, the high phosphorus may also be associated with hypocalcemia. Administration of phosphate binders and calcium supplementation are indicated.

## Clinical Applicability Challenges

### CASE STUDY

Mrs. G. is a 74-year-old woman with a history of diabetes and hypertension. Two years ago she was diagnosed with an abdominal aortic aneurysm (AAA). Four days ago she was admitted to the cardiovascular intensive care unit postoperatively for repair of her AAA. Immediate postoperative data are as follows: temperature, 97.3° F (36.3°C); pulse rate, 120 beats/min; blood pressure, 87/50 mm Hg; respiratory rate, 18 breaths/min; and oxygen saturation by pulse oximetry (SpO$_2$), 98% (on 50% fraction of inspired oxygen [FiO$_2$]). Laboratory test on admission included Na$^+$, 130 mEq/L; K$^+$, 3.5 mEq/L; Cl$^-$, 100 mEq/L; CO$_2$, 18 mmol/L; blood urea nitrogen, 28 mg/dL; creatinine, 1.4 mg/dL; and glucose, 162 mg/dL. This morning, the data included temperature, 101.5° F (38.5°C); pulse rate, 80 beats/minute; blood pressure, 127/85 mm Hg; respiratory rate, 16 breaths/min; oxygen saturation by pulse oximetry (SpO$_2$), 96% (on 2 L/min by nasal cannula); Na$^+$, 132 mEq/L; K$^+$, 4.5 mEq/L; Cl$^-$, 105 mEq/L; CO$_2$, 17 mmol/L;

blood urea nitrogen, 45 mg/dL; creatinine, 2.1 mg/dL; and glucose, 122 mg/dL.

1. Explain the pathophysiologic basis of the changes in Mrs. G.'s blood urea nitrogen and creatinine values before and after surgery.
2. What are Mrs. G.'s risk factors for developing acute kidney injury?
3. What are some of the nursing care priorities for Mrs. G.? What treatments could you anticipate for her?
4. It is postoperative day 3 and Mrs. G. has developed acute kidney injury, with lab values now as follows: Na$^+$, 138 mEq/L; K$^+$, 5.2 mEq/L; Cl$^-$, 1,109 mEq/L; CO$_2$, 15 mmol/L; blood urea nitrogen, 67 mg/dL; creatinine, 3.9 mg/dL; and glucose, 154 mg/dL. What is the pathophysiologic basis for the change in Mrs. G's CO$_2$? Her potassium?
5. An arterial blood gas has been requested. What do you suspect the results will demonstrate?

### WANT TO KNOW MORE?

A wide variety of resources to enhance your learning and understanding of this chapter are available on thePoint.

You will find:
- References
- Selected readings
- NCLEX-style review questions
- Internet resources
- And more!

# 31

# Acute Kidney Injury and Chronic Kidney Disease

## DORENE M. HOLCOMBE AND NANCY KERN FEELEY

### LEARNING OBJECTIVES

*Based on the content in this chapter, the reader should be able to:*

1. Explain the causes of acute kidney injury (AKI).
2. Identify interventions used to reduce the risk of contrast-induced nephropathy.
3. Differentiate between the three types of AKI based on history and physical examination, laboratory values, and diagnostic tests.
4. Discuss the major causes and the clinical stages of chronic kidney disease (CKD).
5. Explain factors that can contribute to the progression of CKD.
6. Discuss the clinical manifestations and management of renal failure.

## Acute Kidney Injury

Acute kidney injury (AKI) occurs in up to 2% to 20% of non–intensive care unit (ICU) hospitalized patients and in as many as 67% of patients treated in ICUs.[1-4] Regardless of the underlying etiology, AKI is associated with increased in-hospital morbidity, mortality, and costs as well as increased long-term mortality and morbidity.[1-6] Patients with AKI who are treated with renal replacement therapy (RRT) have a mortality rate between 40% and 70% despite advances in technology and RRT.[3,4,6] Evidence suggests that even in patients who survive AKI and approach normal kidney function by hospital discharge are at increased risk for later development of chronic kidney disease (CKD) and should have longitudinal monitoring of their kidney function.[5,7]

AKI is a common clinical syndrome in which there is a sudden onset of reduced renal function that can result in derangements in fluid and electrolyte balance, acid–base homeostasis, calcium and phosphate metabolism, blood pressure (BP) regulation, and erythropoiesis. The hallmark of AKI is a decreased glomerular filtration rate (GFR), reflected by an accumulation of blood urea nitrogen (BUN) and serum creatinine—a condition termed azotemia. Serum creatinine is the better marker because increases in serum creatinine are relatively unaffected by metabolic factors.

AKI was previously known as acute renal failure (ARF). More than 35 different definitions of ARF were contained in the medical literature. The lack of a standard definition resulted in variations in the reported incidence of ARF and conflicting reports regarding morbidity and mortality. This situation had an adverse effect on research studies.[1] Consequently, in 2004, a group of expert intensivists and nephrologists formed the Acute Dialysis Quality Initiative (ADQI) to develop a consensus definition for ARF/AKI. The consensus definition formulated by the ADQI is known as the Risk, Injury, Failure, Loss of kidney function, and End-stage kidney disease (RIFLE) classification. As defined by the RIFLE

classification[1] (Table 31-1), there are three increasing grades of severity of AKI—risk, injury, and failure—based on a relative increase in serum creatinine or a period of decreased urine output. Also, two outcome criteria—loss and end-stage kidney disease—are defined by duration of loss of kidney function, 4 weeks and 3 months, respectively.[1]

In 2007, the RIFLE criteria were modified by the Acute Kidney Injury Network (AKIN), which included the ADQI group as well as other representatives from nephrology and intensive care societies. The AKIN-proposed diagnostic criteria for AKI are an abrupt (within 48 hours) increase in the serum creatinine of 0.3 mg/dL or more from baseline, a percentage increase in the serum creatinine concentration of 50% or more, or a urine output of less than 0.5 mL/kg/h for more than 6 hours.[1] Most recently, the Kidney Disease/Improving Global Outcomes (KDIGO) *Clinical Practice Guideline for Acute Kidney Injury* further revised the definition of AKI. KDIGO is a nonprofit international foundation established in 2003 with the mission to develop global practice guidelines to improve kidney disease care and outcomes. The main change in the KDIGO definition is the extension of the timeframe for a 50% or more increase in serum creatinine to 7 days (see Table 31-1).[8] In the future, it is likely that functional markers of renal failure (urine output and serum creatinine) will be replaced or augmented by biologic injury markers, analogous to how troponin is now used to help diagnose an acute myocardial infarction (MI). It is hoped that such markers of kidney cellular injury will not only define AKI but will also offer the potential to diagnose the disorder before functional decline.

Urine output patterns in AKI can manifest as oliguria (less than 500 mL/d), nonoliguria (greater than 500 mL/d), or anuria (less than 50 mL/d). Categorization of AKI as oliguric or nonoliguric is diagnostically significant because the oliguric form is associated with higher morbidity and mortality rates. This may be mediated in part by the more pronounced fluid retention in oliguric versus nonoliguric patients.[9-11] Anuria is rare and is most often seen in two conditions: shock and

**TABLE 31-1** Acute Kidney Injury Staging Criteria

| Stage | Creatinine Criteria | Urine Output Criteria |
|---|---|---|
| **RIFLE Criteria** | | |
| Risk | Creatinine increase of 1.5–2 times baseline value | <0.5 mL/kg/h × 6 h |
| Injury | Creatinine increase of 2–3 times baseline value | <0.5 mL/kg/h × 12 h |
| Failure | Creatinine increase of 3 or more times baseline value or a creatinine value >4 mg/dL with an acute increase of 0.5 mg/dL or more | <0.3 mL/kg/h × 24 h or anuria × 12 h |
| Loss | Persistent ARF for >4 wk | |
| End-stage kidney disease | Persistent ARF for >3 mo | |
| **AKIN Criteria*** | | |
| 1 | Creatinine increase of 1/5–2 times baseline value or increases in creatinine of 0.3 or more mg/dL | <0.5 mL/kg/h × 6 h |
| 2 | Creatinine increase of 2–3 times baseline value | <0.5 mL/kg/h × 12 h |
| 3 | Creatinine increase of 3 or more times baseline value or a creatinine value >4 mg/dL with an acute increase of 0.5 mg/dL or more | |
| **KDIGO Criteria** | | |
| 1 | Creatinine increase of 1.5–1.9 times baseline** or ≥0.3 mg/dL*** | <0.5 mL/kg/h × 6 h |
| 2 | Creatinine increase of 2–2.9 times baseline | <0.5 mL/kg/h × 12 h |
| 3 | Creatinine increase of 3 or more times baseline or a creatine value of ≥4 mg/dL or initiation of RRT | <0.3 mL/kg/h × 24 h or anuria × 12 h |

*Reduction in renal function must occur within 48 h.
**Serum creatinine increase is known or presumed to have occurred within the prior 7 days.
***Serum creatinine increase within any 48-h period.

complete bilateral urinary tract obstruction. Any sudden and complete cessation of urinary flow in a patient with a Foley catheter should alert the nurse to inspect, flush, or change the urinary catheter.

## Causes of Acute Kidney Injury

Many pathophysiologic pathways may lead to the syndrome of AKI. To aid in establishing a diagnostic and management plan, AKI is organized into three general categories according to precipitating factors and the symptoms manifested (Box 31-1).

### Prerenal Acute Kidney Injury

Prerenal AKI is characterized by any physiologic event that results in renal hypoperfusion. Most commonly, precipitating events include hypovolemia and cardiovascular failure; however, any other event that leads to an acute decrease in "effective renal perfusion" can fall into this category (see Box 31-1). For example, in sepsis, a systemic inflammatory response triggers a cascade of events that results in a vasodilated hypotensive state despite no net loss in body fluids.

### Intrarenal Acute Kidney Injury

The intrarenal category of AKI is characterized by actual damage to the renal parenchyma, and has many possible associated causes. One way to categorize these causes is by anatomical compartment: glomerular, vascular, interstitial, and tubular. The glomerular etiologies, which result in acute glomerulonephritis, include immune complex–mediated causes (eg, as seen with poststreptococcal glomerulonephritis) and diseases that cause vasculitis, such as Wegener granulomatosis and antiglomerular basement membrane disease.

Interstitial causes include acute allergic interstitial nephritis, usually caused by pharmacologic agents, and infectious causes such as pyelonephritis. Vascular etiologies include malignant hypertension as well as microangiopathic processes, such as atheroembolic disease or hemolytic–uremic syndrome (HUS) and thrombotic thrombocytopenic purpura (TTP). Finally, the tubules of the kidney can be primarily affected because of obstruction or acute tubular necrosis (ATN). Obstructive causes include multiple myeloma and acute urate nephropathy.

A common cause of intrarenal hospital-acquired AKI is ATN. ATN results from either a prolonged prerenal condition (ischemic ATN) or the effects of toxins on the tubules (toxic ATN). Examples of potential toxins to the tubules include pharmacologic agents, such as aminoglycosides, amphotericin B, and chemotherapeutic agents; heavy metals; organic solvents; heme pigments (eg, myoglobin and hemoglobin); and radiocontrast media (Box 31-2).

### Postrenal Acute Kidney Injury

Any obstruction in the flow of urine from the collecting ducts in the kidney to the external urethral orifice can result in postrenal AKI. Postrenal obstruction can result from ureteral blockage (as with bilateral renal stones), urethral blockage (as from stricture and benign prostatic hypertrophy), or an extrinsic source, such as a retroperitoneal tumor or fibrosis. Another source of postrenal AKI is a dysfunctional bladder (eg, as might be caused by ganglionic blocking agents that interrupt autonomic supply to the urinary system). Elderly men and the young are populations particularly susceptible to postrenal AKI. Children are at risk secondary to congenital anomalies, and elderly men are at risk because of the high prevalence of benign or malignant prostatic hypertrophy.

---

**BOX 31-1** **Precipitating Causes of Acute Kidney Injury**

**Prerenal**

Decreased intravascular volume
- Dehydration
- Hemorrhage
- Hypovolemic shock
- Hypovolemia (gastrointestinal losses, diuretics, diabetes insipidus)
- Third-spacing (burns, peritonitis)

Cardiovascular failure
- Heart failure
- Myocardial infarction
- Cardiogenic shock
- Valvular heart disease
- Renal artery stenosis or thrombosis

Drugs
- ACE inhibitors
- NSAIDs—inhibit prostaglandin-mediated afferent arteriolar vasodilation
- Calcineurin inhibitors (eg, tacrolimus, cyclosporine)—cause pre-glomerular vasoconstriction

Decreased "effective renal perfusion"
- Sepsis
- Cirrhosis
- Neurogenic shock

**Intrarenal**

Acute glomerulonephritis
- Immune complex–mediated (postinfectious, lupus nephritis, cryoglobulinemia, immunoglobulin A nephropathy)
- With vasculitis (Wegener's granulomatosis, antiglomerular basement membrane disease, polyarteritis nodosa)

Vascular disease
- Malignant hypertension
- Microangiopathic HUS
- TTP

- Scleroderma
- Eclampsia
- Atheroembolic disease
- Acute cortical necrosis

Acute interstitial disease
- Allergic interstitial nephritis
- Acute pyelonephritis

Tubular obstruction
- Multiple myeloma
- Acute urate nephropathy
- Ethylene glycol or methanol toxicity

Acute tubular necrosis
- Ischemia
- Nephrotoxins (contrast dye, drugs, heme pigments)
- Kidney transplant rejection

**Postrenal**

Ureteral obstruction
- Intrinsic (stones, transitional cell carcinoma of the ureter, blood clots, stricture)
- Extrinsic (ovarian cancer; lymphoma; metastatic cancer of the prostate, cervix, or colon; retroperitoneal fibrosis)

Bladder problems
- Tumors
- Blood clots
- Neurogenic bladder (spinal cord injury, diabetes mellitus, ischemia, drugs)
- Stones

Urethral obstruction
- Prostate cancer or benign prostatic hypertrophy
- Stones
- Stricture
- Blood clots
- Obstructed indwelling catheter

---

**BOX 31-2** **Common Causes of Acute Tubular Necrosis**

**Ischemic Causes**
Hemorrhagic hypotension
Severe volume depletion
Surgical aortic cross-clamping
Cardiac surgery
Defective cardiac output
Septic shock
Pancreatitis
Immunosuppression (cyclosporine, tacrolimus)
NSAIDs

**Nephrotoxic Causes**
Drugs, including antimicrobials (aminoglycosides, amphotericin), cyclosporine, anesthetics, chemotherapeutic agents
Heavy metals (mercury, lead, cisplatinum, uranium, cadmium, bismuth, arsenic)
Radiologic contrast agents
Heme/pigments (myoglobin, hemoglobin)
Organic solvents (carbon tetrachloride)
Fungicides and pesticides
Plant and animal substances (mushrooms, snake venom)

## Pathophysiology of Acute Kidney Injury

### Prerenal Acute Kidney Injury

The pathophysiology of prerenal AKI is centered on the kidneys' response to inadequate perfusion. A decrease in renal perfusion results in the release of the enzyme renin from juxtaglomerular cells in the walls of the afferent arterioles. This activates the renin–angiotensin–aldosterone cascade, the end result being the production of angiotensin II and the release of aldosterone from the adrenal cortex. Angiotensin II causes profound systemic vasoconstriction, and aldosterone induces sodium and water retention. These effects help the body preserve circulatory volume to maintain adequate blood flow to essential organs such as the heart and brain. In the kidneys, angiotensin II also helps maintain the GFR by increasing efferent arteriolar resistance and by stimulating intrarenal vasodilator prostaglandins (which dilate the afferent arteriole), increasing hydrostatic pressure in the glomeruli.[12] In this way, the kidneys can preserve the GFR over a wide range of mean arterial pressures. However, when renal perfusion is severely compromised, the capacity for autoregulation is overwhelmed, and the GFR decreases.

Even with moderate hypovolemia or congestive heart failure, certain drugs, such as angiotensin-converting enzyme (ACE) inhibitors, angiotensin receptor blockers (ARBs), and nonsteroidal anti-inflammatory drugs (NSAIDs), can overwhelm the kidney's ability to autoregulate. These drugs disrupt some of the autoregulatory mechanisms, such as prostaglandin-mediated afferent arterial vasodilation, in the case of NSAIDs, and increased efferent arteriolar resistance, in the case of ACE inhibitors and ARBs. Predisposing factors for NSAID- and ACE inhibitor–induced prerenal failure are hypovolemia, baseline renal insufficiency, liver disease, heart failure, and diseases of the renal arteries. Concomitant use of diuretics, ACEI, or ARBS with NSAIDS may also increase the risk of NSAID-induced AKI, even in the absence of other risk factors.[12]

In prerenal AKI, once autoregulatory capacity is overwhelmed and the GFR decreases, changes in urinary composition and volume occur in a predictable pattern. When the GFR decreases, the amount of tubular fluid is reduced, and the fluid travels through the tubule more slowly. This results in increased sodium and water reabsorption. Because of the reduced renal circulation, the solutes reabsorbed from the tubular fluid are removed more slowly than normal from the interstitium of the renal medulla. This results in increased medullary tonicity, further augmenting water reabsorption from the distal tubular fluid. As a result of these events, the urinary volume is reduced to less than 400 mL/d (less than 17 mL/h), the urine specific gravity is increased, and the urine sodium concentration is low (usually less than 5 mEq/L; Fig. 31-1). Because of these characteristic changes associated with renal underperfusion, measurement of urinary volume, urinary sodium, and specific gravity is a simple method for determining the effect of management on renal perfusion.

An increase in systemic BP does not necessarily imply improvement in renal perfusion. This may be especially evident when drugs such as norepinephrine are used to correct the hypotension associated with states of volume depletion. These drugs may be associated with further reduction in renal blood flow as a consequence of constriction of the renal arteries. This is manifested by a further fall in urinary volume and rise in specific gravity. In turn, if the hypoperfusion state is more appropriately and specifically treated by replacement of volume, improvement of cardiac output, correction of dysrhythmias, or a combination of these approaches, the improved renal perfusion is manifested as an increased urinary volume and urine sodium concentration and as a decreased specific gravity of the urine. This ability to reverse prerenal AKI is the key to its diagnosis.

## Intrarenal Acute Kidney Injury

Just as there are many causes of intrarenal AKI, there are also many pathophysiologic mechanisms that lead to it (Fig. 31-2). Because ATN is the most common hospital-acquired form of intrarenal AKI, this discussion focuses on the pathophysiology of ATN, which is complex, but intense and ongoing research has increased understanding of the factors contributing to this condition. Ischemia and nephrotoxicity are two major underlying causes of ATN (Fig. 31-3).

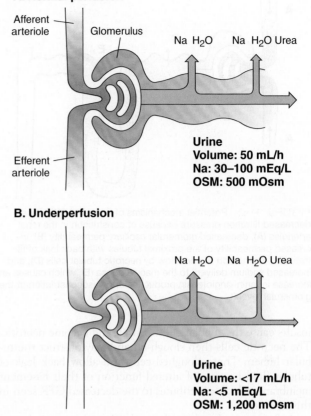

**A. Normal perfusion**

Afferent arteriole — Glomerulus

Na H₂O    Na H₂O Urea

Efferent arteriole

**Urine
Volume: 50 mL/h
Na: 30–100 mEq/L
OSM: 500 mOsm**

**B. Underperfusion**

Na H₂O    Na H₂O Urea

**Urine
Volume: <17 mL/h
Na: <5 mEq/L
OSM: 1,200 mOsm**

**FIGURE 31-1** Normal perfusion of the kidney compared with underperfusion as seen in prerenal AKI. Underperfusion of the kidney results in decreased renal blood flow and glomerular filtration, an increase in the fraction of filtrate reabsorbed in the proximal tubule, and low urine flow with low sodium (Na) content and increased concentration. H₂O, water; OSM, osmolarity.

## Ischemic Acute Tubular Necrosis

Ischemic ATN results from prolonged hypoperfusion. Thus, prerenal AKI and ischemic ATN are actually a continuum, a fact that underscores the importance of prompt recognition and treatment of the prerenal state. When renal hypoperfusion persists for a sufficient time (the exact duration of which is unpredictable and varies with clinical circumstances), renal tubular epithelial cells become hypoxic and sustain damage to the point that restoration of renal perfusion no longer causes an improvement in glomerular filtration.

Ischemia results in an inflammatory response and decreased adenosine triphosphate production in renal cell mitochondria. Inflammatory mediators produced by activated leukocytes and tubular epithelial cells promote inflammation in a positive feedback loop, causing further kidney injury. Decreased adenosine triphosphate production robs the cells of a needed energy supply. Part of this energy is used to keep the proper concentration of electrolytes in the cell through electrolyte exchange channels. Some of the cellular electrolyte disturbances from ischemia are decreased intracellular potassium, magnesium, and phosphate and increased intracellular sodium, chloride, and calcium. Increased intracellular calcium specifically has been shown to predispose the cells to injury and dysfunction.[13]

During reperfusion, cellular insults also occur from the formation of oxygen free radicals. Eventually, these cellular

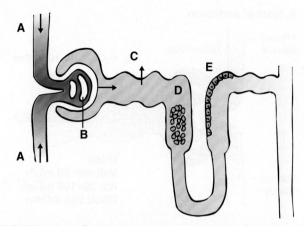

**FIGURE 31-2** Potential mechanisms of intrarenal AKI include decreased filtration pressure because of constriction in the renal arterioles (**A**), decreased glomerular capillary permeability (**B**), increased permeability of the proximal tubules with back leak of filtrate (**C**), obstruction of urine flow by necrotic tubular cells (**D**), and increased sodium delivery to the macula densa (**E**), which causes an increase in renin–angiotensin production and vasoconstriction at the glomerular level.

insults cause the tubular cells to swell and become necrotic. The necrotic cells then slough off and may obstruct the tubular lumen. These sloughed cells also allow back leak of tubular fluid because of altered function of their basement membrane, which contributes to the decreased GFR seen in this disorder.

A final contributor to the pathophysiology of ischemic ATN is profound renal vasoconstriction and reduced renal blood flow. These hemodynamic disturbances further compromise renal oxygen delivery and add to the ischemic damage. Vasoconstrictors involved include norepinephrine from sympathetic nervous system activation, angiotensin II, thromboxane $A_2$, adenosine, leukotrienes C4 and D4, prostaglandin $H_2$, and endothelin. Release of endothelin, a powerful vasoconstrictor, by damaged vascular endothelial cells of the kidney results in profound reductions in GFR. Oxygen free radicals augment renal vasoconstrictor responses, and cellular swelling can further compromise renal blood flow.[13]

### Toxic Acute Tubular Necrosis

The pathophysiology of toxic ATN begins with a concentration of a nephrotoxin in the renal tubular cells, which causes necrosis. These necrotic cells then slough off into the tubular lumen, possibly causing obstruction and impairing glomerular filtration in a manner similar to that of ischemic ATN. However, there are significant differences between toxic ATN and ischemic ATN. In toxic ATN, the basement membrane of the renal cells usually remains intact, and the injured necrotic areas are more localized. In addition, nonoliguria occurs more often with toxic ATN, and the healing process is often more rapid.

Although the potential nephrotoxins in toxic ATN are many (see Box 31-2), aminoglycoside antibiotics and radiocontrast dye deserve special mention because of the frequency with which they are seen as causes of toxic ATN in hospitalized patients. Nephrotoxicity occurs in 10% to 25% of patients treated with aminoglycosides.[8,14,15] The onset of AKI secondary to aminoglycosides is usually delayed, often

beginning 5 to 10 days after the onset of therapy. The toxicity of these agents is dose dependent, and because these agents are primarily eliminated by the kidneys, dosage must be adjusted in patients with preexisting renal impairment. To ensure that the correct therapeutic range is being achieved, blood is drawn frequently for peak and trough level analysis. Several studies have suggested that a single daily dose of an aminoglycoside may result in less nephrotoxicity than giving the same total amount of medication in three daily doses.[8,15,16] Accordingly, the KDIGO Practice Guideline for AKI recommends both once-daily dosing and close monitoring of drug levels.[8] Other risk factors for aminoglycoside toxicity are volume depletion, advanced age, diabetes, concurrent use of other nephrotoxic agents, and hepatic dysfunction.[14,15] If feasible, using alternative antibiotics with decreased associated nephrotoxicity is the best prevention of aminoglycoside-induced nephrotoxicity.

Contrast-induced nephropathy (CIN), the sudden decline of renal function following intravascular injection of contrast media, accounts for a significant number of hospital-acquired cases of AKI. In critically ill patients, the frequency of CIN is 2% to 23%.[17,18] It usually begins within 24 to 48 hours of intravenous (IV) radiocontrast administration and peaks within 3 to 7 days. Typically, CIN is nonoliguric, transient, and reversible; however, in high-risk patients, dialysis may be required on an intermittent or permanent basis. Patients at greatest risk for CIN are those with diabetes and those with underlying renal impairment. In these patients, the incidence of CIN may be as high as 50%.[18] Other patients at risk are elderly patients; those with intravascular volume depletion, heart failure, therapy, or concomitant use of nephrotoxic drugs; and those who receive a large contrast load.[17]

The only proven way to reduce the risk for CIN is by aggressive volume expansion with isotonic crystalloids (normal saline solution) before and after contrast agent administration.[5,19] Because CIN is believed to involve the production of oxygen free radicals, it is postulated that alkalinization of the urine with sodium bicarbonate may confer greater protection than IV fluids alone. However, multiple trials comparing the use of sodium bicarbonate with normal saline for prophylaxis have yielded inconsistent results, and meta-analyses have been inconclusive.[5,8,19] Accordingly, the KIDGO AKI Guideline recommends volume expansion with either isotonic sodium chloride or sodium bicarbonate solutions in patients with increased risk of CIN-AKI. Recently, there has been increased clinical trial activity revolving around the concept of forced diuresis (combining diuretics to augment urine output while given crystalloids to maintain euvolemia) for CIN prevention.[5,20,21] Although some studies have shown promise, further research is needed.

Other interventions to reduce the incidence of CIN include using the minimal necessary dose of contrast media, using low or iso-osmolar nonionic contrast media instead of ionic hyperosmolar agents, stopping the intake of nephrotoxic drugs 24 hours before contrast media injection, and avoiding short intervals between contrast procedures. N-Acetylcysteine (NAC), an antioxidant and a potent vasodilator, is part of the protocol in many hospitals to prevent CIN based on clinical trials demonstrating its renoprotective effects in patients receiving IV contrast media. However, NAC has been the subject of many trials and meta-analyses, and overall there has been insufficient evidence to support

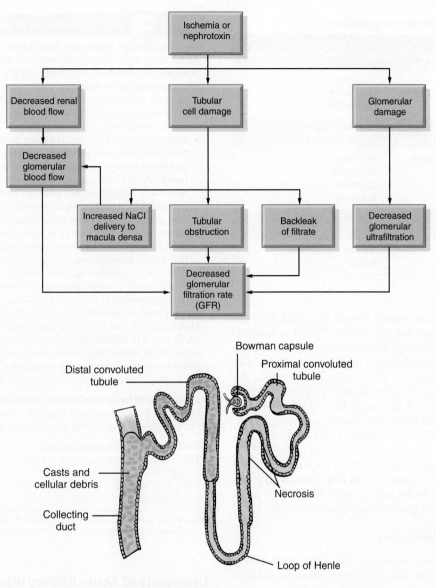

FIGURE 31-3 Ischemic ATN results from prolonged hypoperfusion. A sequence of pathophysiologic processes results in the sloughing off of necrotic cells that block the tubular lumen. Toxic ATN occurs when a nephrotoxin becomes concentrated in the renal tubular cells and causes necrosis. The necrotic cells slough off and obstruct the tubular lumen, similar to ischemic ATN. In toxic ATN, the basement membrane of the renal cells usually remains intact, and the necrotic areas are more localized.

the use of NAC to prevent CIN.[5,18,22,23] However, despite lack of evidence of benefit, it remains a popular approach to CIN-AKI prevention, presumably owing to its low cost and negligible potential for harm. Studies have shown that other pharmacologic interventions, such as calcium-channel blockers, dopamine, mannitol, and atrial natriuretic peptide, do not consistently reduce the incidence of CIN and may even be harmful.

Of course, avoiding any use of iodinated contrast media in high-risk patients is the best prevention; alternative studies, such as ultrasonography, computerized tomography (CT) scanning without contrast, and contrast-enhanced magnetic resonance imaging (MRI), should be considered. The MRI contrast agents in use are mostly chelates of gadolinium and are less nephrotoxic than iodinated

radiocontrast, particularly when used in small doses. This has led to the use of gadolinium-based contrast agents (GB-CAs) as alternatives to iodinated contrast agents for digital subtraction angiography or interventional procedures, especially in patients with iodinated contrast allergies. However, one important caveat regarding the use of GBCA in patients with AKI or severe CKD (GFR <30 mL/min) is the rare but serious risk for developing nephrogenic systemic fibrosis (NSF). NSF, a fibrosing disorder seen only in patients with kidney disease, is characterized by thickening and hardening of the skin overlying the extremities and trunk. Occasionally, fibrosis of deeper structures (such as joints, muscles, the testes, dura, kidneys, and the heart) occurs as well. Because the condition can be devastating to a patient (resulting in significant loss of mobility and

**TABLE 31-2** **ACR Classifications of GBCAs**

| GBCA | Trade Name |
|---|---|
| **Group I: Agents with greatest number of NSF cases** | |
| Gadodiamide | Omniscan |
| Gadopentetate dimeglumine | Magnevist |
| Gadoversetamide | OptiMARK |
| **Group II: Agents associated with few, if any, unconfounded cases of NSF** | |
| Gadobenate dimeglumine | MultiHance |
| Gadoteridol | ProHance |
| Gadoteric acid | Dotarem |
| Gadobutrol | Gadovist |
| **Group III: Agents that have only recently appeared on the market in the United States** | |
| Gadofosveset | Ablavar |
| Gadoxetic acid | Eovist |

even death), gadolinium agents should be avoided in patients with a GFR less than 30 mL/min.[24-26] If it is determined that a study using a GBCA must be performed, the American College of Radiology (ACR) recommends that the lowest possible dose of GBCA needed to conduct the study be used, and that there be allotted a sufficient period of time for elimination of the agent from the body before readministration. In addition, for patients receiving hemodialysis, prompt hemodialysis following GBCA administration is recommended to enhance elimination of the GBCA.

Finally, the ACR has classified GBCA into three different groups based on their association with NSF cases, with group I agents associated with the highest rates (Table 31-2). All group I GBCAs are contraindicated in high-risk patients.[24,27,28]

## Postrenal Acute Kidney Injury

Obstruction can occur at any point in the urinary tract. When urine cannot get around the obstruction, resulting congestion causes retrograde pressure through the collecting system and nephrons. This slows the rate of tubular fluid flow and lowers the GFR. As a result, the reabsorption of sodium, water, and urea is increased, leading to a lowered urine sodium concentration and increased urine osmolality and BUN. Serum creatinine levels also increase. With prolonged pressure from urinary obstruction, the entire collecting system dilates, compressing and damaging nephrons. This results in dysfunction of the concentrating and diluting mechanism, and the urine osmolality and urine sodium concentration become similar to that of plasma. This circumstance can be avoided by prompt removal of the obstruction.

Because a single well-functioning kidney is adequate to maintain homeostasis, the development of AKI from obstruction requires blockage of both kidneys (ie, urethral or bladder neck obstruction or bilateral ureteral obstruction) or unilateral ureteral obstruction in patients with a single kidney. After relief of the obstruction, there is often a profound diuresis of greater than 4 L/d. Postobstructive diuresis in postrenal AKI ICU patients may be predictive of complete renal recovery.[29] However, if electrolytes and water are not replenished as needed, this diuresis can lead to hemodynamic compromise, dysrhythmias, and ATN.

**BOX 31-3** *CONSIDERATIONS for the Older Patient*

**Physiologic Changes Affecting the Renal System**

As the body ages, physiologic systemic and kidney-specific changes occur that are important to take into consideration when addressing the kidney.

- Vascular changes: At 30 years of age, arteriosclerosis starts to develop, including in the renal arteries; this can result in significant damage.
- Musculoskeletal changes: In elderly people, there is a decreased muscle mass and body weight. These changes must be kept in mind when assessing renal function because of the possibility of a consequent decreased baseline serum creatinine value. A minimum rise in serum creatinine value in elderly patients, which may be within normal limits for a young adult, may actually signify major renal impairment.
- Kidney-specific changes: With aging, there is a decrease in the total number of functioning glomeruli, a decrease in renal blood flow, and a decrease in GFR of about 0.75 mL/min/1.73 m² per year after 30 years of age.[24]

In view of these systemic and kidney-specific changes, an accurate assessment of GFR using a 24-hour urine study or an isotopic study is essential. The Cockroft–Gault formula or the Modification of Diet in Renal Disease (MDRD) formulas below, which take into account gender and age, can also be used. It is important to realize that these formulas are not extensively validated in patients older than 70 years. After true GFR is realized, therapy (eg, drug dosages) can be guided more safely.

**Cockcroft–Gault Formula for Creatinine Clearance (mL/min)**

Men = (140 − age) × weight in kg/72 × serum creatinine
Women = 0.85 × creatinine clearance for men

**MDRD Formula for GFR (adults; mL/min)**

175 × Serum creatinine concentration$^{-1.154}$
× Age$^{-0.203}$
× 0.742 (if female)
× 1.210 (if black)

Websites are available to aid in the calculation of the GFR through these formulas. These include http://www.kidney.org and http://www.nephron.com.

## Diagnosis of Acute Kidney Injury

Diagnosis of AKI begins with a determination of whether the AKI is prerenal, intrarenal, or postrenal. The assessment tools used to make this determination include the history and physical examination, laboratory tests, and diagnostic studies. Special considerations for assessing renal function in older patients are given in Box 31-3.[30]

### History and Physical Examination

Essential to any assessment is the health history and physical examination. By taking a detailed history, clues to the categorization and exact cause of the AKI can be obtained. Important indications in the history that suggest prerenal AKI include any event or condition that may have contributed to decreased renal perfusion (eg, acute MI, cardiovascular surgery, cardiac arrest, high fever, any shock state, and the use of certain drugs, such as NSAIDs). Also, a history of atherosclerotic disease may be a clue to renal artery stenosis, another precipitant of prerenal AKI. Clues to an intrarenal cause provided by the history include any prolonged prerenal event or condition as well as exposure to nephrotoxins, especially aminoglycoside antibiotics and radiocontrast media. It is

**TABLE 31-3** Acute Kidney Injury: Comparison of Laboratory Findings in Prerenal Failure, Postrenal Failure, and Acute Tubular Necrosis

| Value | Prerenal | Postrenal | Acute Tubular Necrosis |
|---|---|---|---|
| Urine volume | Oliguria | May alternate between anuria and polyuria | Anuria, oliguria, or nonoliguria |
| Urine osmolality | Increased (>500 mOsm/kg H$_2$O) | Varies, increased, or equal to serum | 250–300 mOsm/kg H$_2$O |
| Urine specific gravity | Increased (>1.020) | Varies | Approximately 1.010 |
| Urine sodium | <20 mEq/L | Varies | >40 mEq/L |
| Urine sediment | Normal, few casts | Normal, may be crystals | Granular casts, tubular epithelial cells |
| FE$_{Na}$ | <1% | >1% | >1% (often >3%) |
| BUN:Cr | >20:1 | 10:1 to 15:1 | 10:1 to 15:1 |

FE$_{Na}$, fractional excretion of sodium; BUN:Cr, blood urea nitrogen/creatinine ratio.

also important to collect information about systemic diseases such as lupus or vasculitis, recent streptococcal infections, and causes of heme pigment toxicity, such as rhabdomyolysis (eg, a history of trauma or a patient found unconscious for an unknown amount of time). In addition, a history of cardiac catheterization, anticoagulation, and thrombolytic therapy increases the possibility of atheroembolic intrarenal diseases. Findings that may point to postrenal AKI include any history of abdominal tumors or calculi, and especially a history of benign prostatic hypertrophy in elderly men. A family history of urolithiasis or benign prostatic hypertrophy may be contributory.

The physical examination, particularly regarding fluid status, is critical to the diagnosis of AKI. In prerenal AKI, a state of decreased renal perfusion related to dehydration or hypovolemia is heralded by poor skin turgor, dry mucous membranes, weight loss, and reduced jugular venous distention. In contrast, when decreased perfusion is related to vasodilation, third spacing, cardiovascular disease (eg, heart failure), liver disease, or a combination of these factors, findings of increased extracellular fluid may be manifested by edema, ascites, and weight gain. For critical care patients, hemodynamic monitoring values help determine intravascular fluid status as well as cardiac functioning. Surveillance values include central venous pressure (CVP), pulmonary artery occlusion pressure (PAOP), and cardiac output (or cardiac index). By correlating physical examination findings with the history, hemodynamic values, and laboratory tests, potential prerenal etiologies can be narrowed down.

Although no specific physical examination finding prompts consideration of intrarenal AKI, many examination findings are helpful clues to potential causes of intrarenal AKI. For example, signs of a streptococcal throat infection, lupus (eg, a butterfly mask rash), or embolic phenomena (eg, discolored toes and livedo reticularis, a semipermanent bluish mottling of the skin in the extremities) may all suggest an intrarenal cause. Again, correlation with the history and laboratory studies helps narrow the list of potential causes. Findings on physical examination that may suggest a postrenal cause include a distended bladder, an abdominal mass, an enlarged or nodular prostate gland, and, most obviously, a kinked or obstructed Foley catheter.

## Laboratory Studies

Laboratory assessment, critical to the diagnosis and categorization of AKI, includes both serum and urinary values.

For a basic comparison of laboratory values in prerenal AKI, postrenal AKI, and ATN, see Table 31-3. In addition to helping differentiate between prerenal, intrarenal, and postrenal AKI, blood and urine tests are also helpful for diagnosing the underlying etiology of the AKI (Box 31-4).

**URINARY VALUES.** Obtaining a urine specimen for diagnostic evaluations is invaluable in establishing the diagnosis and determining the type of AKI. The urine specimen should be obtained before a diagnostic challenge dose of

**BOX 31-4** Diagnostic Clues in Acute Kidney Injury

Urine
- Urate crystals: Tumor lysis, especially lymphoma (urate nephropathy)
- Oxalate crystals: Ethylene glycol nephrotoxicity, methoxyflurane nephrotoxicity
- Eosinophils: Allergic interstitial nephritis, especially methicillin
- Positive peroxidase test without red blood cells: Hemoglobinuria or myoglobinuria
- Pigmented casts: Hemoglobinuria or myoglobinuria
- Massive proteinuria: Acute interstitial nephritis, thiazide diuretics, hemorrhagic fevers (eg, Korean, Scandinavian)
- Abnormal urine protein electrophoresis: Multiple myeloma
- Anuria: Renal cortical necrosis, bilateral obstruction, renal vascular catastrophe

Plasma
- Marked hyperkalemia: Rhabdomyolysis, tissue necrosis, hemolysis
- Marked hypocalcemia: Rhabdomyolysis
- Hypercalcemia: Hypercalcemic nephropathy
- Hyperuricemia: Tumor lysis, rhabdomyolysis, toxin ingestion
- Marked acidosis: Ethylene glycol, methyl alcohol
- Elevated creatine kinase or myoglobin levels: Rhabdomyolysis
- Low complement levels: Systemic lupus erythematosus (SLE), postinfectious glomerulonephritis, subacute bacterial endocarditis
- Abnormal serum protein electrophoresis: Multiple myeloma
- Positive antibody/glomerular basement membrane ratio: Goodpasture's syndrome
- Positive antineutrophilic cytoplasmic antibody: Small vessel vasculitis (Wegener's granulomatosis or polyarteritis nodosa)
- Positive antinuclear antibody or antibody to double-stranded DNA: SLE
- Positive antibodies to streptolysin O: Poststreptococcal glomerulonephritis
- Elevated lactate dehydrogenase level, elevated serum bilirubin level, or decreased haptoglobin level: HUS or TTP

diuretics is administered because these agents may alter the urine's chemical composition. The urine sodium concentration, osmolality, and specific gravity are especially helpful in distinguishing between prerenal AKI and ATN because these values reflect the concentrating ability of the kidney. In prerenal failure, the hypoperfused kidney actively reabsorbs sodium and water in an attempt to increase circulatory volume. Consequently, the urine sodium level and the fractional excretion of sodium ($FE_{Na}$) are low (less than 20 mEq/L and less than 1%, respectively), whereas the urine osmolality and concentration of nonreabsorbable solutes are high. In contrast, in ATN in which parenchymal damage affects the kidney, the tubular cells can no longer effectively reabsorb sodium or concentrate the urine. As a result, the urine sodium concentration is often greater than 40 mEq/L, the $FE_{Na}$ is greater than 1%, and the urine osmolality is close to that of plasma (isosthenuria). Unfortunately, there is a limit to the usefulness of these indices because of overlap in these values for prerenal AKI and ATN (ie, urine sodium concentration values in the 20 to 40 mEq/L range). Values at the extremes are thus the most useful.

The sediment in a urinalysis is also very helpful in diagnosing and distinguishing the types of AKI. In prerenal AKI, the urinary sediment is normal with only a few hyaline casts, whereas in ATN, coarse, muddy-brown granular casts and tubular epithelial cells are typically found. In postrenal AKI, the sediment is often normal but can be helpful in diagnosing kidney stones.

**BLOOD UREA NITROGEN AND CREATININE LEVELS.** Serum tests for BUN and creatinine are essential not only for diagnosing AKI but also for helping to distinguish between prerenal AKI and ATN or postrenal AKI. In prerenal AKI, the BUN-to-creatinine ratio is increased from the normal ratio of 10:1 to more than 20:1. This finding is caused by a state of dehydration and by the fact that, as the tubules become more permeable to sodium and water in prerenal AKI, urea is also passively reabsorbed. In ATN and postrenal AKI, when the concentrating ability of the kidneys is impaired, both the BUN and creatinine increase proportionally, maintaining the normal 10:1 ratio.

### Diagnostic Studies

Renal ultrasonography, an important diagnostic test in the evaluation of AKI, is especially useful in ruling out an obstruction, and has the advantage of being noninvasive. With a high-grade obstruction, dilation of the urinary collecting system is detectable on ultrasonography within 1 to 2 days of the onset of the obstruction. Ultrasonography may also reveal proximal renal calculi as a cause of postrenal obstruction. In addition, it can be used to estimate renal size, which is helpful in distinguishing between AKI and advanced CKD. Often in advanced CKD, the kidneys are small (less than 9 cm) and echogenic.

Other studies that may be useful in diagnosing AKI are CT and MRI to evaluate for masses, vascular disorders, and filling defects in the collecting system, and renal angiography to evaluate for renal artery stenosis. It is notable that the iodinated contrast media used in some studies are allergenic and nephrotoxic, and that GBCAs can cause NSF in patients with severe kidney disease (GFR < 30 mL/min). For any

diagnostic test, the benefits of the study must be weighed against potential risks. If available, alternative technology, such as the use of carbon dioxide gas in digital subtraction angiography, should be considered for patients allergic to iodinated agents or with advanced kidney failure.[31,32] Finally, renal biopsy may be helpful in patients thought to have intrarenal AKI that is not ATN, especially if significant proteinuria or unexplained hematuria is revealed on urinalysis. In addition to having diagnostic value, the results of a biopsy may help determine prognosis and therapy.

## Chronic Kidney Disease

CKD is a slow, progressive, irreversible deterioration in renal function that results in the kidney's inability to eliminate waste products and maintain fluid and electrolyte balance. Ultimately, it leads to end-stage renal disease (ESRD) and the need for RRT or renal transplantation to sustain life.

Currently, there are more than 615,000 dialysis and renal transplant recipients in the United States, which is a 26% increase in prevalence since the year 2000. In 2011 alone, more than 115,000 patients were newly diagnosed with ESRD. Among ESRD patients, incidence rates are higher in men than in women and are higher with increasing age. The incidence rates in the African American population are 3.4 times greater than in the white population. Hispanics and Native Americans also have higher incidence rates than whites, but the difference in rates is not as dramatic.[33] These differences in incidence rates are important when considering patient risk factors and target populations for health education.

Factors postulated to contribute to the increasing prevalence of ESRD include changes in the demographics of the population, differences in disease burden among racial groups, under-recognition and undertreatment of earlier stages of CKD, under-recognition of the risk factors for CKD, and increased survival of patients with ESRD.[33] Increasing evidence shows that early detection and treatment of CKD may prevent, or at least delay, progression to ESRD.[34,35] Consequently, it is important that opportunities to prevent and treat CKD are not lost secondary to underdiagnosis or undertreatment.

### Definition and Classification

In an effort to address the growing public health problem of CKD, the National Kidney Foundation Kidney Disease Outcome Quality Initiative (NKF KDOQI) published clinical practice guidelines for CKD in 2002. The goals of the working group that developed these guidelines were to define CKD and classify its stages, to evaluate laboratory measurements for clinical assessment of kidney disease, to associate the level of kidney function with the complications of CKD, and to stratify risk for the loss of kidney function and the development of cardiovascular disease.[36]

The KDOQI defines CKD as either kidney damage with or without decreased GFR for 3 or more months *or* a GFR of less than 60 mL/min/1.73 $m^2$ for greater than 3 months (Box 31-5). Markers of damage include abnormal findings in the blood or urine tests or imaging studies. Examples are proteinuria, abnormalities in the urine sediment, increased serum creatinine, and multiple renal cysts detected on ultrasound in a patient with a family history of polycystic kidney

> **BOX 31-5** | **Definition of Chronic Kidney Disease**
>
> 1. Kidney damage for greater than or equal to 3 months as defined by structural or functional abnormalities of the kidney, with or without decreased GFR, manifested by *either:*
>    a. Pathologic abnormalities; *or*
>    b. Markers of kidney damage, including abnormalities in the composition of the blood and urine, or abnormalities in imaging tests
> 2. GFR less than 60 mL/min/1.73 m$^2$, with or without kidney damage
>
> From National Kidney Foundation: K/DOQI clinical practice guidelines for chronic kidney disease: Evaluation, classification, and stratification. Am J Kidney Dis 39(2 Suppl 1):S1–S266, 2002.

disease (see Spotlight on Genetics 31-1). A GFR (considered to be the best overall measure of kidney function) of less than 60 mL/min/1.73 m$^2$ was chosen for two reasons: (1) it represents a loss of half or more of the adult level of normal kidney function, and (2) below this level, the prevalence of complications from CKD increases.

Because predictable complications and management issues are based on the level of kidney dysfunction, regardless of the specific underlying etiology of CKD, the KDOQI working group also developed a classification system for CKD based on the measured GFR. This classification system had five stages based on GFR (Table 31-4). In 2013, *KDIGO 2012 Clinical Practice Guideline for the Evaluation and Management of CKD* was released, updating CKD staging. KDIGO recommended a classification based on cause of CKD, GFR category, and albumin category (referred to as CGA). Etiology of CKD was added because it provides important prognostic information and influences treatment decisions. The KDIGO Guideline recommends cause of CKD be based on the presence or absence of systemic disease, such as diabetes or lupus, and the anatomic location of the pathologic abnormality within the kidney. For GFR, KDIGO maintained the prior KDOQI stages, except that stage 3 was divided into 3a and 3b. This subdivision of stage 3 was in response to the great disparity in complications seen in patients in this stage. Lastly, KDIGO added the level of albuminuria in the staging. Albuminuria is assessed using the albumin-to-creatinine ratio (ACR) in an untimed spot urine. The threshold for an abnormally elevated ACR is 30 mg/g or greater. This addition was made in response to mounting evidence that there is an increase in mortality and progression of CKD to ESRD with higher levels of albuminuria, independent of GFR.[34] Consequently, patients now have a "G-stage" based on GFR and an albuminuria or "A-stage," both identifying a patient's risk for CKD progression and complications (Fig. 31-4). This classification system provides a common language for practitioners and patients to improve communication, enhance education, and promote research. Most importantly, it also provides a framework for evaluation and development of a treatment plan for patients with various stages of CKD.

## G-Stages

- G1 is characterized by the lack of a clear filtration deficit and is defined as normal or increased kidney function (GFR ≥ 90 mL/min/1.73 m$^2$) in association with evidence of kidney damage.

> **SPOTLIGHT ON GENETICS 31-1**
>
> ### POLYCYSTIC KIDNEY DISEASE
>
> - Polycystic kidney disease is one of the most common disorders caused by mutations in a single gene. It affects about 500,000 people in the United States. The autosomal-dominant form of the disease is much more common than the autosomal-recessive form. Autosomal-dominant polycystic kidney disease affects 1 in 500 to 1,000 people, while the autosomal-recessive type occurs in an estimated 1 in 20,000 to 40,000 people. Clusters of fluid-filled sacs, called cysts, develop in the kidneys and interfere with their ability to filter waste products from the blood.
> - Mutations in the *PKD1*, *PKD2*, and *PKHD1* genes cause polycystic kidney disease.
> - Mutations in either the *PKD1* or *PKD2* gene can cause autosomal-dominant polycystic kidney disease. These genes provide instructions for making proteins whose functions are not fully understood. Researchers believe that they are involved in transmitting chemical signals from outside the cell to the cell's nucleus. The two proteins work together to promote normal kidney development, organization, and function. Mutations in the *PKD1* or *PKD2* gene lead to the formation of thousands of cysts, which disrupt the normal functions of the kidneys and other organs.
> - Genetic tests for autosomal-dominant and autosomal-recessive type of polycystic kidney disease are available.
>
> Genetic Home Reference. Retrieved August 10, 2015, from http://ghr.nlm.nih.gov.
> Mochizuki T, Tsuchiya K, Nitta K: Autosomal dominant polycystic kidney disease: Recent advances in pathogenesis and potential therapies. Clin Exp Nephrol 17:317–326, 2013.

- G2 is defined as a mild reduction in kidney function (GFR 60 to 89 mL/min/1.73 m$^2$) that occurs in association with kidney damage.
- G3a is defined as mildly to moderately decreased kidney function (GFR 45 to 59 mL/min/1.73 m$^2$).
- G3b is defined as moderately to severely decreased kidney function (GFR 30 to 44 mL/min/1.73 m$^2$).
- G4 is defined as severely decreased kidney function (GFR 15 to 29 mL/min/1.73 m$^2$).
- G5 is defined as a GFR of less than 15 mL/min/1.73 m$^2$ or the need for dialysis therapy. The term ESRD, widely used in regulatory and administrative circles, correlates to G5 CKD and represents those patients receiving or eligible for RRT by dialysis or transplantation.

## Albuminuria—A Stages

- A1 is defined as an ACR < 30 mg/g.
- A2 is defined as an ACR 30 to 299 mg/g.
- A3 is defined as an ACR ≥ 300 mg/g.

## Causes

The causes of CKD are numerous (Box 31-6). By far, the two most common causes are diabetes mellitus and hypertension, which account for more than 44% and 28% of incident cases of ESRD, respectively.[33] Other causes include glomerulonephritis (both primary and secondary to systemic diseases),

**TABLE 31-4** 2002 National Kidney Foundation Kidney Disease Outcome Quality Initiative Stages of Chronic Kidney Disease

| Stage | Description | GFR (mL/min/1.73 m²) |
|---|---|---|
| 1 | Kidney damage with normal or increased GFR | 90 or more |
| 2 | Kidney damage with mild or decreased GFR | 60–89 |
| 3 | Moderately decreased GFR | 30–59 |
| 4 | Severely decreased GFR | 15–29 |
| 5 | Kidney failure | <15 or dialysis |

interstitial nephritis, congenital malformations, genetic disorders, neoplasms, hepatorenal syndrome, obstructive uropathy, and microangiopathic etiologies, such as scleroderma and atheroembolic disease.

## Pathophysiology

Although many diseases can cause CKD, there appear to be common pathophysiologic pathways for disease progression. The outstanding common morphologic features seen in CKD include fibrosis, loss of native renal cells, and infiltration by monocytes and macrophages. The mediators of the process are many and include abnormal glomerular hemodynamics, hypoxia, proteinuria, and vasoactive substances such as angiotensin II.[34,35]

In discussing glomerular hemodynamics, it is important to understand intact nephron theory. Because each of the more than 1 million nephrons in each kidney is an independent functioning unit, as renal disease progresses nephrons can lose function at different times. When an individual nephron becomes diseased, nephrons in close proximity increase their individual filtration rates by increasing the rate of blood flow and hydrostatic pressure in their glomerular capillaries. This hyperfiltration response in the nondiseased nephrons enables the kidneys to maintain excretory and homeostatic functions, even when up to 70% of the nephrons are damaged. Eventually, however, the intact nephrons reach a point of maximal filtration, and any additional loss of glomerular mass is accompanied by an incremental loss in GFR and subsequent accumulation of filterable toxins.

Although hyperfiltration is an adaptive measure to nephron loss, over time it can actually accelerate the loss of nephrons, because the hyperfiltration causes endothelial injury, stimulation of profibrotic cytokines, infiltration by monocytes and macrophages, and detachment of glomerular epithelial cells. In addition, hypertrophy of the nondiseased nephrons caused by hyperfiltration leads to increased wall stress and even more injury.[37] This is why many interventions to slow down the progression of renal failure involve measures that reduce glomerular hydrostatic pressure. One such example is the use of ACE inhibitors and ARBs, which prevent angiotensin II–mediated efferent arteriolar vasoconstriction and subsequent nephron hyperfiltration.

Other possible mediators of CKD progression are hypoxia and angiotensin II. In CKD, the loss of peritubular capillaries by various causes results in reduced capillary perfusion of the tubules. The resultant hypoxia favors the release of proinflammatory and profibrotic cytokines, leading to fibrosis and cell injury. Angiotensin II stimulates growth factors and cytokines that contribute to fibrosis aside from its hemodynamic effects on the glomerulus.[38,39]

Proteinuria, the result of glomerular hypertension and abnormal glomerular permeability, also contributes to CKD progression. Abnormally filtered protein is reabsorbed by proximal tubular cells through endocytosis and accumulates in the cells, causing the production of cytokines. These proinflammatory factors ultimately cause fibrosis and scarring of the tubulointerstitium.[40] Proteinuria is a very strong predictor of CKD progression, consistent with its role in the

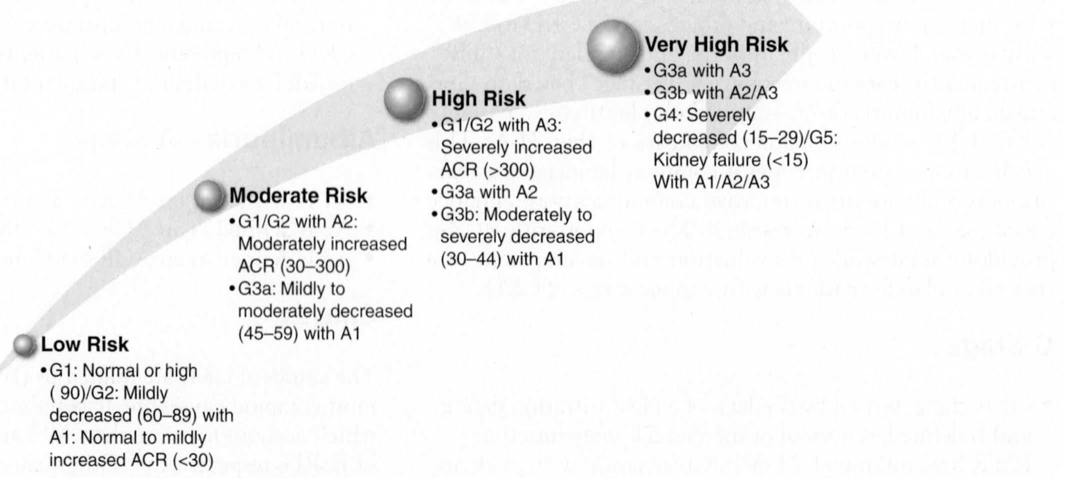

**Very High Risk**
- G3a with A3
- G3b with A2/A3
- G4: Severely decreased (15–29)/G5: Kidney failure (<15) With A1/A2/A3

**High Risk**
- G1/G2 with A3: Severely increased ACR (>300)
- G3a with A2
- G3b: Moderately to severely decreased (30–44) with A1

**Moderate Risk**
- G1/G2 with A2: Moderately increased ACR (30–300)
- G3a: Mildly to moderately decreased (45–59) with A1

**Low Risk**
- G1: Normal or high ( 90)/G2: Mildly decreased (60–89) with A1: Normal to mildly increased ACR (<30)

**FIGURE 31-4** Risk of CKD progression according to KDIGO staging.

Diabetes mellitus
Hypertension
Glomerulonephritis
- Primary (immunoglobulin A nephropathy, postinfectious glomerulonephritis)
- Secondary (HIV nephropathy, lupus, cryoglobulinemia, Wegener's granulomatosis, Goodpasture's syndrome, polyarteritis nodosa, amyloidosis)

Interstitial nephritis (allergic interstitial nephritis, pyelonephritis)
Microangiopathic vascular disease (atheroembolic disease, scleroderma)
Congenital disease
Genetic disease (polycystic kidney disease, medullary cystic kidney disease)
Obstructive uropathy
Neoplasms or tumors
Transplant rejection
Hepatorenal syndrome

pathophysiology of CKD and as evidenced by its inclusion in the new KDIGO CKD staging.

## Diabetic Nephropathy

Because of the extremely high prevalence of diabetes and hypertension as causes of CKD, an understanding of the renal pathophysiology specific to these entities, and knowledge of interventions designed to slow down or even prevent progression to stage G5 CKD, is imperative. Diabetic nephropathy is a major complication of diabetes, with an incidence of approximately 20% to 40%.[41]

In diabetes, the microvasculature in the organ systems of the body, including the kidneys, is damaged. In the kidneys, primarily the afferent and efferent arterioles and the glomerular capillaries are affected. Glomerular changes include thickening of the basement membrane, mesangial expansion from overproduction and underdegradation of extracellular matrix proteins, and diffuse glomerulosclerosis. Late in diabetic nephropathy, tubular atrophy and interstitial fibrosis also occur. The exact physiologic mechanism for these structural alterations is unclear, but hyperglycemia is a major contributor. In the classic Diabetes Control and Complications Trial (DCCT)—a prospective, randomized, multicenter trial performed to assess the effectiveness of tight blood glucose control on the complications of type 1 diabetes—researchers found that strict blood glucose control delayed, and possibly even prevented, the progression of diabetic nephropathy.[42] The follow-up study to the DCCT, called the Epidemiology of Diabetes Interventions and Complications (EDIC) study, revealed that the benefits of tight control persist for a number of years.[43] Most recently, it has also been shown that intensive diabetes therapy in type 1 diabetics improve renal outcomes even after the development of persistent microalbuminuria (urine albumin excretion rate of 30 to 300 mg/24 h).[44] In addition, the classic United Kingdom Prospective Diabetes Study (UKPDS) reached conclusions about people with type II diabetes that were similar to those of the DCCT.[45]

At the onset of diabetic nephropathy, patients may have an increased GFR (as high as 140 mL/min) because of hyperfiltration, slightly enlarged kidneys, and microalbuminuria

(30 to 300 mg/d of albumin in the urine). Over the course of approximately 10 to 15 years, hypertension and protein leakage increase. Eventually, protein leakage is massive, with consequent hypoalbuminemia and edema as well as mild azotemia. At this point kidney damage is extensive, often requiring dialysis therapy within a few years.

### Hypertensive Nephrosclerosis

Systemic hypertension may result in a condition known as nephrosclerosis. Hypertensive nephrosclerosis involves the development of sclerotic lesions in the renal arterioles and glomerular capillaries that cause them to become thickened, narrowed, and eventually necrotic. Hypertensive nephrosclerosis can be benign or malignant. In benign nephrosclerosis, associated with chronic mild or moderate hypertension, renal impairment occurs over many years. Malignant nephrosclerosis, associated with malignant hypertension, can lead to permanent renal failure rapidly if BP is not immediately reduced. Often, symptoms such as blurred vision and a severe headache accompany this crisis situation.

Because hypertensive nephrosclerosis is directly caused by hypertension, its incidence is greater in populations with a higher incidence of primary hypertension (eg, elderly people, African Americans). Among African Americans younger than 75 years, the incidence rate for hypertension-induced ESRD is between 6 and 11 times that of Caucasians.[33] The signs of hypertensive nephrosclerosis vary depending on the severity of the renal damage and the acuteness of the hypertension. Some signs that may be present include proteinuria, azotemia, and hematuria with red blood cell casts. Unfortunately, like those with hypertension, patients often remain asymptomatic until extensive damage has occurred. To prevent or delay the progression of hypertensive nephropathy, BP control is essential, and often multiple antihypertensive medications are required. This is an area in which patient education can have a great impact in decreasing the incidence of ESRD. Educating patients about the complications of uncontrolled hypertension is particularly important and may foster the patient's active involvement in controlling his or her BP.

## Preventing the Progression of Chronic Kidney Disease

An important characteristic of CKD is continuous progression. Slowing the rate of progression after CKD is diagnosed is a focus of extensive and ongoing research. Regardless of the primary cause of CKD, specific identifiable secondary insults to the kidney can rapidly accelerate the loss of nephrons. Such secondary insults include an alteration in renal perfusion, as observed in congestive heart failure or intravascular volume depletion; the administration of nephrotoxic agents; urinary obstruction; and urinary infections. Consequently, monitoring for and avoiding these insults and aggressively treating them if they occur are paramount.

It is also important to educate patients and their families about the dangers of these insults. Patients and families should be instructed, for instance, about the signs and symptoms of urinary infections and the need for prompt treatment, as well as common nephrotoxic drugs to avoid. Common over-the-counter and prescription analgesics, such as NSAIDs, can cause rapid deterioration in renal function and should be avoided in patients with CKD.

Strict control of blood glucose levels is critical to preventing and retarding the progression of renal failure in people with diabetes. The targets for key parameters of glucose control set by the American Diabetes Association for people with diabetes are a glycosylated hemoglobin of less than 7.0%, a preprandial plasma glucose of 70 to 130 mg/dL, and a peak postprandial plasma glucose of less than 180 mg/dL.[41]

BP control is also essential for preventing the progression of renal failure from almost any primary etiology, not just hypertension or diabetes. According to the *KDIGO Clinical Practice Guideline for the Management of Blood Pressure in Chronic Kidney Disease* and the Eighth Joint National Committee (JNC 8) *2014 Evidence-Based Guideline for the Management of High Blood Pressure in Adults*, the target of therapy is a BP of less than 140/90 mm Hg.[35,46] KDIGO, however, recommends a lower target of less than 130/80 mm Hg in CKD patients with an ACR ≥ 30 mg.[35] Control of hypertension entails lifestyle changes, such as exercise, salt restriction, smoking cessation, and avoidance of excessive alcohol, as well as pharmacologic therapy if necessary. ACE inhibitors and ARBs have been shown to offer a selective advantage in slowing the progression of diabetic and other proteinuric syndromes. Both drugs have been proved to lower BP, reduce proteinuria, and slow the progression of kidney disease, presumably because of their ability to decrease intraglomerular pressure by blocking the effect of angiotensin II on the afferent and efferent arterioles. Combination therapy with an ARB and an ACE inhibitor has not been shown to decrease proteinuria or delay progression of CKD.[34,35,46,47]

A protein-restricted diet as a means to slow the progression of renal failure is controversial. The KDIGO Clinical Practice Guideline recommends lowering protein to 0.8 g/kg/d in adults with diabetes or in adults with a GFR < 30. KDIGO also suggested that a high-protein diet (1.3 g/kg/d) be avoided in any CKD patient at risk for progression.[35] A more severe protein restriction of 0.6 to 0.8 g/kg/d is recommendation by some renal nutritionists, providing that signs of malnutrition are absent.[48] However, it is important to proceed cautiously with protein restriction, especially in critically ill patients who are in a catabolic state. Malnutrition itself is a major determinant of morbidity and mortality in patients with renal failure.[48,49] Ways to avoid malnutrition include providing protein with high biologic value, ensuring that adequate caloric requirements are met, and closely monitoring nutritional assessment parameters (ie, body weight, serum albumin and prealbumin levels, and total protein levels). Because of the complexity of nutritional requirements in critically ill patients, collaboration with a dietitian is essential.

Finally, increased sodium intake and obesity are modifiable risk factors that can potentially alter CKD progression. Increased sodium intake is associated with worsening albuminuria and GFR reduction. Current recommendations are to restrict sodium intake to less than 2 g/d unless contraindicated.[35] Contradictions include patients with salt-wasting kidney diseases and patients prone to hypotension and volume contraction. Obesity, as with the non-CKD population, can contribute to hypertension, increased insulin resistance, and result in the production of inflammatory cytokines. Patients should be counseled to achieve and maintain a healthy weight (body mass index of 20 to 25).[34,50]

# Management of Renal Failure

Although some distinct differences exist in how AKI and CKD are managed, many of the clinical manifestations and complications encountered are the same. Thus, the general management of renal failure is addressed here, noting any differences between AKI and CKD as necessary. In either type of renal failure, management begins with treating the primary insult. An overview of the management of patients with AKI is provided in the accompanying Collaborative Care Guide (Box 31-7).

## Managing Fluid Balance Alterations

Clinical management of fluid balance is of primary importance in patients with renal failure, and is the area in which differences in the management of AKI and CKD are perhaps most dramatic.

### Fluid Balance Changes in Acute Kidney Injury

In prerenal AKI and the early stages of ischemic ATN, the cause of the renal failure is inadequate renal perfusion, often from intravascular volume deficits. After using laboratory, physical assessment, and hemodynamic clues to make a rapid diagnosis of intravascular volume depletion, therapy involves prompt administration of replacement fluids, such as blood and crystalloids. The replacement solutions used should reflect the type of losses (eg, for a patient with a hemorrhagic condition, blood would be the replacement fluid of choice). Often in AKI, even if signs and symptoms of intravascular volume deficits are not present, large boluses of IV fluids are given. Reversal of AKI after such a bolus is therapeutic as well as diagnostic of prerenal AKI.

Fluid administration in AKI is also indicated for the prevention or alleviation of tubular obstruction seen in obstructive causes of AKI, including ATN and many postrenal etiologies. However, in any oliguric state, caution must be taken to prevent fluid overload. In a sustained oliguric state, such as the oliguric stage of ATN, fluid is restricted to the previous day's urine output amount plus 500 to 800 mL to account for insensible losses.

Diuretics are often used in AKI to increase urinary flow and thereby help alleviate conditions of fluid overload or to prevent tubular obstruction. Furosemide, a loop diuretic, and mannitol, an osmotic diuretic, are often used with hydration to prevent tubular obstruction in certain obstructive causes of AKI, such as acute urate nephropathy, and in heme pigment nephropathy, such as rhabdomyolysis. In states of fluid overload, such as pulmonary edema and heart failure, diuretics are also useful. Often in these situations, furosemide is administered every 6 hours, with the initial dose ranging between 20 and 100 mg depending on whether the patient has taken furosemide regularly. If within an hour the response is inadequate, the dose may then be doubled. This process may be repeated until adequate urine output is achieved. Sometimes even a continuous furosemide drip is required. In addition, a thiazide diuretic, such as chlorothiazide, may be administered with furosemide because of the synergistic action of these diuretics in promoting urinary excretion.

With the use of diuretics, caution must be taken to avoid complications of dehydration, electrolyte imbalances, and

**QSEN BOX 31-7** *COLLABORATIVE CARE GUIDE for the Patient With Acute Kidney Injury*

| Outcomes | Interventions |

**Coordination of Care**

| | |
|---|---|
| All appropriate team members and disciplines will be involved in the plan of care | • Develop the plan of care with the patient, family, primary physician, nephrologist, pulmonologist, cardiologist, registered nurse, advanced practice nurse, social worker, respiratory therapist, physical therapist, occupational therapist, dietitian, chaplain, and dialysis staff |

**Ineffective breathing pattern**
**Impaired gas exchange**

| | |
|---|---|
| Patient will have adequate gas exchange as evidenced by: <br> • ABGs within normal limits <br> • Functional oxygen saturation (SpO$_2$) >92% <br> • Clear breath sounds <br> • Normal respiratory rate and depth <br> • Normal chest x-ray | • Monitor ABGs and continuous pulse oximetry <br> • Monitor acid–base status <br> • Monitor for signs and symptoms of pulmonary distress from fluid overload <br> • Provide routine pulmonary toilet, including the following: <br>    • Airway suctioning <br>    • Chest percussion <br>    • Incentive spirometer <br>    • Frequent turning <br> • Mobilize out of bed to chair <br> • Support patient with oxygen therapy, mechanical ventilation, or both as indicated. Involve respiratory therapist |

**Decreased cardiac and peripheral tissue perfusion**

| | |
|---|---|
| Patient's BP, heart rate, and hemodynamic parameters will be within normal limits. <br> Patient will have adequate tissue perfusion as evidenced by: <br> • Adequate hemoglobin levels <br> • Euvolemic status <br> • Optimal urine output depending on phase of AKI <br> • Appropriate level of consciousness | • Monitor vital signs every 1 to 2 hours <br> • Monitor PAOP, right atrial pressure, cardiac output, systemic vascular resistance, and peripheral vascular resistance every 4 hours or as ordered if pulmonary artery catheter is in place <br> • Assess vital signs continuously or every 15 minutes during dialysis <br> • Monitor hemoglobin and hematocrit levels daily <br> • Assess evidence of tissue perfusion (pain, pulses, color, temperature, and signs of decreased organ perfusion such as an altered level of consciousness, ileus, and decreasing urine output) <br> • Administer intravascular crystalloids or blood products as indicated |

**Excess fluid volume related to decreased kidney function**
**Ineffective renal perfusion**

| | |
|---|---|
| Patient will be euvolemic <br> Patient will achieve normal electrolyte balance <br> Patient will achieve optimal renal function | • Monitor fluid status, including input and output (fluid restriction), daily weight, urine output trends, vital signs, CVP, and PAOP <br> • Monitor for signs and symptoms of hypervolemia (hypertension, pulmonary edema, peripheral edema, jugular venous distention, and increased CVP) <br> • Monitor serum electrolytes daily <br> • Monitor renal parameters, including urine output, BUN, serum creatinine, acid–base status, urine electrolytes, urine osmolality, and urine specific gravity <br> • Administer fluids and diuretics to maintain intravascular volume and renal function, per order <br> • Replace electrolytes as ordered <br> • Treat patient with, and monitor response to, dialysis therapies if indicated <br> • Monitor and maintain dialysis access for chosen intermittent or continuous dialysis method: <br> *Continuous Veno–Veno Dialysis* <br> • Monitor and regulate ultrafiltration rate hourly based on patient's response and fluid status <br> • Provide fluid replacements as ordered <br> • Assess and troubleshoot hemofilter and blood tubing hourly <br> • Protect vascular access from dislodgment <br> • Change filter and tubing per protocol <br> • Monitor vascular access for infection <br> *Peritoneal Dialysis* <br> • Slowly infuse warmed dialysate <br> • Drain after appropriate dwell time <br> • Assess drainage for volume and appearance <br> • Send cultures daily or as ordered <br> • Assess access site for infection <br> *Intermittent Hemodialysis* <br> • Assess shunt for thrill and buzzing sound (bruit) every 12 hours <br> • Avoid constrictions (ie, BPs), phlebotomy, and IV fluid administration in arm with shunt <br> • Assess for infection <br> • Monitor perfusion of related extremity |

*(continued)*

**BOX 31-7** *COLLABORATIVE CARE GUIDE for the Patient With Acute Kidney Injury (continued)*

| Outcomes | Interventions |
|---|---|
| **Impaired physical mobility** | |
| Patient will remain free of complications related to bed rest and immobility | • Initiate deep venous thrombosis prophylaxis<br>• Reposition frequently<br>• Mobilize to chair when possible<br>• Consult physical therapist<br>• Conduct range-of-motion and strengthening exercises |
| **Risk for injury**<br>**Risk for falls** | |
| Patient will be protected from possible harm | • Assess need for wrist restraints if patient is intubated, has a decreased level of consciousness, is unable to follow commands, or is acutely agitated, or for affected extremity during hemodialysis. Explain need for restraints to patient and family members. If restrained, assess response to restraints and check every 1 to 2 hours for skin integrity and impairment in tissue perfusion. Follow hospital protocol for use of restraints<br>• Use siderails on bed and safety belts on chairs as appropriate<br>• Follow seizure precautions |
| **Impaired skin integrity** | |
| Patient will have intact skin | • Assess skin integrity and all bony prominences every 4 hours<br>• Turn every 2 hours<br>• Consider a pressure relief/reduction mattress. Use Braden Scale to assess risk for skin breakdown<br>• Use superfatted or lanolin-based soap for bathing and apply emollients for pruritus<br>• Treat pressure ulcers according to hospital protocol. Involve enterostomal nurse in care |
| **Imbalanced nutrition**<br>**Electrolyte imbalance** | |
| Patient will be adequately nourished as evidenced by:<br>• Stable weight not <10% below, or >20% above, ideal body weight<br>• An albumin level of 3.5 to 4.0 g/dL<br>• A total lymphocyte count of 1,000 to 3,000 × $10^6$/L<br>• A total protein level of 6 to 8 g/dL | • Consult dietitian to direct and coordinate nutritional support<br>• Observe sodium, potassium, protein, and fluid restriction as indicated<br>• Provide small, frequent feedings<br>• Provide parenteral or enteral feeding as ordered<br>• Monitor albumin, prealbumin, total protein, hematocrit, hemoglobin, and white blood cell counts, and monitor daily weights to assess effectiveness of nutritional therapy |
| **Impaired comfort** | |
| Patient will be as comfortable and as pain free as possible as evidenced by:<br>• No complaints of discomfort<br>• No objective indicators of discomfort | • Monitor for signs and symptoms of respiratory distress related to fluid overload and support oxygenation as needed. Keep head of bed elevated and teach breathing techniques to minimize oxygen distress, such as pursed-lip breathing<br>• Plan fluid restrictions over 24 hours, allowing for periodic sips of water and ice chips to minimize thirst<br>• Provide frequent mouth and skin care<br>• Assess quantity and quality of discomfort<br>• Provide a quiet environment and frequent reassurance<br>• Observe for complications that may cause discomfort, such as infection of vascular access device, peritonitis or inadequate draining during peritoneal dialysis, and gastrointestinal disturbances (nausea, vomiting, diarrhea, constipation)<br>• Administer analgesics, antiemetics, antidiarrheals, laxatives (non–magnesium and non–phosphate containing), stool softeners, antihistamines, sedatives, or anxiolytics as needed and monitor response |
| **Ineffective coping** | |
| Patient will demonstrate a decrease in anxiety as evidenced by:<br>• Vital signs within normal limits<br>• Level of consciousness within normal limits<br>• Subjective reports of decreased anxiety levels<br>• Objective assessment of decreased anxiety level | • Assess vital signs<br>• Explore patient and family concerns<br>• If the patient is intubated, develop interventions for effective communication<br>• Arrange for flexible visitation to meet needs of the patient and family<br>• Provide for adequate rest and sleep<br>• Provide frequent information and updates on condition and treatment, and explain equipment. Answer all questions<br>• Consult social services and clergy as appropriate<br>• Administer sedatives and antidepressants as appropriate and monitor response |

| Outcomes | Interventions |
|---|---|
| **Teaching/Discharge Planning** | |
| Patient and family members will understand procedures and tests needed for treatment during the acute phase and maintenance of a patient with chronic disease <br><br> Patient and family members understand the severity of the illness, ask appropriate questions, and anticipate potential complications <br><br> In preparation for discharge to home, the patient and family members will demonstrate an understanding of RRT, fluid and dietary restrictions, and the medication regimen | • Prepare the patient and his or her family members for procedures, such as insertion of dialysis access, dialysis therapy, or laboratory studies <br> • Explain the causes and effects of renal failure and the potential for complications, such as hypertension and fluid overload <br> • Encourage family members to ask questions related to the pathophysiology of renal failure, dialysis, and dietary or fluid restrictions <br> • Make appropriate referrals and consults early during hospitalization <br> • Initiate family education regarding home care of the patient on dialysis, what to expect, maintenance of renal function, and when to seek medical attention |

side effects. Tinnitus and hearing impairment (reversible and irreversible) have been reported after IV furosemide administration. Ototoxicity is associated with rapid injection, excessively high doses, or concomitant therapy with other ototoxic drugs. The manufacturer recommends controlled IV infusion (not to exceed 4 mg/min) for high-dose parenteral furosemide therapy.

The use of diuretics to convert oliguria to nonoliguria, unlike the aforementioned uses of diuretics, has not been substantiated in medical research and may even be harmful. Additionally, research has not shown that the use of loop diuretics in AKI reduces mortality, shortens the duration of renal failure, or helps avoid or reduce the requirements for RRT.[51–53] Hence, based on the literature, it is reasonable to use diuretics for a short time for volume control but not for therapy for established oliguric AKI.

Dopamine is another agent that has been traditionally used in AKI because of its ability to theoretically cause renal vasodilation at "renal doses" (1 to 3 mcg/kg/min), thereby increasing renal perfusion. However, the efficacy of this agent to affect the course of AKI has not been substantiated despite many clinical trials, and some studies have even shown deleterious effects.[52,54] Thus, based on current evidence, there is no current role for dopamine in preventing AKI.

If fluid complications arise and cannot be controlled by fluid restrictions and pharmacologic agents, dialysis (discussed in detail in Chapter 30) or isolated ultrafiltration may be necessary. This is often the case in oliguric patients who are receiving large amounts of IV fluids hourly in the form of medications and nutritional supplements. People in whom AKI develops secondary to hypoperfusion or tubular injury may have a delayed recovery time, necessitating maintenance dialysis until the tissue repairs itself and normal function returns. For these patients, discharge planning should take into consideration the need for outpatient dialysis therapy (which may last for several weeks to months), the need to modify the person's diet and consumption of fluids, and the psychosocial implications of these measures for the patient and family members.

### Fluid Balance Changes in Chronic Kidney Disease

In CKD, fluid and salt restriction is a mainstay of therapy to prevent fluid overload. Sodium is restricted to less than 2,000 mg/d, and fluid intake is limited to 500 mL plus the patient's previous day's 24-hour urine output. Diuretics are also used to manage volume overload. Patients are usually able to respond to diuretics until their GRF falls below 10 to 15, at which point extensive renal damage prevents an adequate response. By the time CKD progresses to stage G5, oliguria is typically manifested, and signs and symptoms of fluid overload, such as edema, hypertension, pulmonary edema, heart failure, and jugular vein distention, occur unless dialysis therapy is instituted. In these patients, an ongoing assessment of fluid status, including obtaining accurate intake and output measurements with daily weights and monitoring for fluid complications, is imperative.

### Managing Acid–Base Alterations

AKI and CKD typically result in metabolic acidosis because of the nephrons' inability to secrete and excrete hydrogen ions and reabsorb bicarbonate ions as renal failure progresses. In critically ill patients, this acid–base disturbance may be intensified because of concurrent conditions, such as lactic acidosis or diabetic ketoacidosis, and because such patients are in a high-catabolic state, which increases the release of intracellular acids into the circulation. Clinical manifestations of metabolic acidosis include headaches, nausea and vomiting, deep and rapid respirations (Kussmaul respirations), altered mental status, hyperkalemia, and tachycardia. In severe metabolic acidosis, bradycardia and hypotension may manifest because of myocardial depression and vasodilation. There is also a dramatic depression of the patient's level of consciousness, often resulting in stupor or coma.

In CKD, metabolic acidosis begins to manifest as the patient reaches G stage 3A and the GFR falls below 60 mL/min/1.73 m². Although the metabolic acidosis associated with CKD is usually mild ($CO_2$, 16 to 22 mEq/L), it is associated with many adverse consequences, including fatigue, protein catabolism, and bone demineralization. The bones become demineralized because bone phosphate and carbonate are used as buffers against excess hydrogen ions.

Laboratory assessments of acid–base status using arterial blood gas (ABG) values and venous carbon dioxide content guide therapy. Patients with a plasma bicarbonate level less than 22 mEq/L warrant treatment. Therapy involves the administration of alkaline medications (eg, Bicitra, sodium bicarbonate tablets), dialysis, or both. When using citrate-containing medications, such as Bicitra, it is important that these medications not be given with aluminum-containing phosphate binders. Using these agents together would put the patient at risk for aluminum toxicity because citrate significantly increases aluminum absorption from the gastrointestinal tract.

The use of IV sodium bicarbonate is reserved for severe acidosis (evidenced by a blood pH < 7.2 or a plasma bicarbonate level less than 12 to 14 mEq/L) because of potential complications of extracellular volume excess, metabolic alkalosis, and hypokalemia. Intractable acidosis is an indication for dialysis, which removes excess hydrogen ions and adds a buffer to the body. In hemodialysis the buffer is bicarbonate, and in peritoneal dialysis it is lactate, which is metabolized to bicarbonate. When correcting metabolic acidosis, caution is advised. Rapid correction may result in a suppressed respiratory drive and hypoventilation. Rapid correction can also lead to acute hypocalcemia and tetany, because the amount of ionized calcium decreases in an alkalotic state owing to increased binding of calcium with albumin and inorganic substances such as phosphate. Throughout any kind of acid–base therapy, it is necessary to monitor serum bicarbonate, pH, and calcium and potassium levels closely.

## Managing Cardiovascular Alterations

Alterations in the cardiovascular system can cause or accelerate AKI and CKD. In addition, cardiovascular complications can arise as a result of renal failure itself. Common cardiovascular complications in AKI and CKD include hypertension and hyperkalemia. Pericarditis, another cardiovascular complication of renal disease, is primarily seen with CKD.

### Hypertension

Hypertension as a complication of renal failure results from excess retention of water and sodium, overactivation of the sympathetic nervous system, and stimulation of the renin–angiotensin–aldosterone system. Because controlling BP is essential to prevent end-organ damage and reduce the risk for life-threatening cardiovascular events, adequate treatment is essential. Management may include fluid and sodium restrictions, diuretic administration, antihypertensive therapy, and dialysis to remove excess fluid. Extensive patient teaching regarding nonpharmacologic and pharmacologic treatment and the potential complications of uncontrolled hypertension is an integral part of management.

### Hyperkalemia

Hyperkalemia is a life-threatening condition seen in patients with AKI and CKD. As the GFR decreases, the ability of the kidneys to excrete excess potassium diminishes. In critically ill patients, this renal impairment is frequently compounded by states of increased catabolism, acidosis, cellular injury, administration of potassium-based medications, and blood transfusions, all of which can raise serum potassium levels. If not recognized and treated, hyperkalemia leads to fatal dysrhythmias.

Assessment of hyperkalemia involves close monitoring of serum potassium levels as well as monitoring the effects of potassium on the electrical conduction system of the heart. Characteristically, electrocardiogram (ECG) changes occur as potassium levels rise (Fig. 31-5). The first ECG changes that occur, usually when serum potassium is in the range of 6 to 7 mEq/L, are the appearance of tall, tented T waves and a prolonged PR interval. Next, there is a loss of the P wave and a slight widening of the QRS complex. At this point, the serum potassium is usually in the range of 8 to 9 mEq/L. From here, the QRS complex continues to widen until a sine wave (wavy line) pattern develops. This ominous sign is closely followed by ventricular fibrillation or standstill.

When evaluating hyperkalemia, note that patients with long-standing elevations in serum potassium are more refractory to its effects on the heart than patients in whom hyperkalemia develops suddenly. Thus, potassium and ECG changes must be evaluated together to determine the acuteness of the situation. Other effects of hyperkalemia that are monitored include paresthesias, hyporeflexia, and muscle weakness (which typically begins in the lower extremities and ascends to the trunk and upper extremities).

Mild hyperkalemia (a serum potassium level less than 6 mEq/L without ECG changes) may be treated with dietary potassium restriction, diuretics, and potassium-binding resins (eg, sodium polystyrene sulfate [SPS]). SPS is given orally,

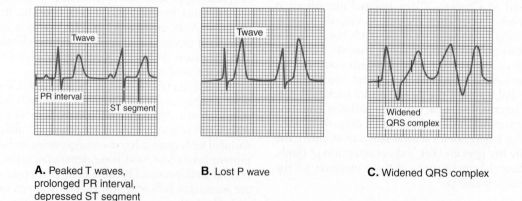

**A.** Peaked T waves, prolonged PR interval, depressed ST segment

**B.** Lost P wave

**C.** Widened QRS complex

FIGURE 31-5  Typical ECG findings indicative of various degrees of hyperkalemia. **A:** When the serum potassium (K+) level is about 6 to 7 mEq/L, the T waves become peaked, the PR interval is prolonged, and the ST segment is depressed. **B:** At about 8 to 9 mEq/L, the P wave is lost. **C:** At about 10 to 11 mEq/L, the QRS complex widens.

with or without sorbitol, or as an enema without sorbitol. The oral dose is 15 to 30 g every 4 to 6 hours as needed. The rectal dose is 50 g in 150 mL of tap water; it should be retained in the colon for at least 30 to 60 minutes. This drug must be used with extreme caution in critically ill patients with decreased colonic motility, such as postsurgical patients and patients taking large amounts of opiates, because of its association with colonic necrosis in this population. The risk of colonic necrosis may be increased when SPS is mixed with sorbitol.[55] Use should be discontinued in patients who develop constipation, and repeated doses should not be administered if a patient has not passed stool. It is recommended that a cleansing enema with 250 to 1,000 mL tap water at body temperature be given after rectal administration. Sodium polystyrene should never be used in a patient with a gastrointestinal obstruction or ileus, and bowel sounds should always be assessed before its administration.

Treatment of life-threatening hyperkalemia entails taking steps to antagonize the effects of potassium on the heart, promote intracellular shifting of potassium, and remove potassium from the body. Antagonizing the effects of potassium on the heart is achieved with IV calcium gluconate or chloride, and is the first priority for patients with substantial ECG changes. Intracellular shifting of potassium is done next to bridge the gap until potassium removal from the body can be executed. Means to shift potassium into the cell include IV insulin and dextrose administration and IV bicarbonate administration. $\beta_2$-Adrenergic therapy can also effect transcellular potassium shifting, but is less commonly used because of the requirement for 10 to 20 times the dose used for reactive airway disease. Removal of potassium from the body entails, as previously mentioned, diuretic administration and the use of potassium exchange resins. If these measures do not control hyperkalemia, dialysis must be initiated. Obviously, in a patient who has stage G5 CKD, and who is likely already receiving dialysis therapy, dialysis is initiated immediately along with other emergent therapy in life-threatening hyperkalemia.

## Pericarditis

Pericarditis resulting from uremia (uremic pericarditis) is a complication that can be seen primarily in stage G5 CKD. This type of pericarditis is characterized by an inflammation of the pericardial membrane, which causes the pericardial capillaries to become permeable to fluid, red blood cells, fibrinogen, and albumin. In most cases, the inflammation is aseptic, although it may also result from bacterial or viral infections. The consequent serous or serosanguineous fluid in the pericardial cavity (pericardial effusion) can increase the intrapericardial pressure and compromise ventricular contractility, stroke volume, and cardiac output. Pericardial tamponade, which results when the accumulation of pericardial fluid is so large that adequate cardiac output cannot be maintained, is a life-threatening emergency. The exact etiology of uremic pericarditis is unknown, but it is associated with prolonged inadequate dialysis therapy, uremic toxins, infectious agents, treatment with the antihypertensive agent minoxidil, and heparin administration.

Chest pain, fever, and a pericardial friction rub are the classic triad of findings associated with pericarditis. The chest pain is characteristically sharp and steady, and is relieved by sitting forward and intensified by breathing deeply. The pericardial friction rub (a harsh, leathery sound heard over the precordium) may precede the pain, may persist after the pain has subsided, and may disappear when the volume of effusion increases. The typical ECG changes in pericarditis are new-onset atrial dysrhythmias and widespread ST elevations with an upward concavity (versus the upward convexity typical in an acute MI). However, the widespread ST wave elevations are not consistently present in uremic pericarditis because its etiology is metabolic in nature, and injury is uncommon. In a large pericardial effusion, signs and symptoms are more dramatic and include dyspnea, tachycardia, mental confusion, weakness, increased jugular vein distention, peripheral edema, and a paradoxical pulse greater than 10 mm Hg during inspiration. Tamponade results in distended neck veins, tachypnea, a narrowed pulse pressure, an increased PAOP, muffled heart sounds, diminished peripheral pulses, and a decreased level of consciousness.

Therapy for uremic pericarditis includes aggressive dialysis therapy, usually daily, until symptoms disappear. Also, because anticoagulation during dialysis may precipitate or enhance bleeding into the pericardial space, low-dose, regional, or no heparin may be prescribed. Systemic steroids and NSAIDs, such as indomethacin, may also be used but have had variable results. Cardiac tamponade is an emergency that requires urgent pericardiocentesis to relieve the pressure on the heart. For the patient in whom recurrent pericarditis develops or in whom the pericardium becomes constrictive, surgical creation of a pericardial window or pericardiectomy may be necessary.

## Cardiovascular Disease in Chronic Kidney Disease

CKD is associated with high cardiovascular morbidity and mortality. In fact, patients with CKD are much more likely to suffer from cardiac disease resulting in cardiovascular death than to eventually require RRT.[35,50] The predominant cardiac disorders in CKD are left ventricular hypertrophy, coronary artery disease, dysrhythmias, cardiomyopathy, congestive heart failure, and valvular dysfunction.

Because most of these cardiovascular disorders develop over a period of at least a few years, they usually present early in CKD and continue to progress as renal function declines. This association between CKD and cardiovascular disease may occur for the following reasons: (1) cardiovascular disease causes renal dysfunction (ie, heart failure); (2) CKD causes an increased risk for cardiovascular disease; or (3) other factors (eg, hypertension, diabetes mellitus, anemia, or hyperlipidemia) cause or accelerate both renal dysfunction and cardiovascular disease. In any case, monitoring for cardiovascular disease, reducing modifiable risk factors, and treating specific cardiovascular conditions when present are essential to decrease mortality in patients with CKD.

Diagnostic tests useful in assessing for cardiovascular disease in these high-risk patients include routine ECGs, echocardiography, and cardiac stress testing. Pharmacologic rather than exercise stress testing is the stress test of choice because patients with CKD are often unable to attain the level of exercise needed to make exercise stress tests useful. More invasive tests for symptomatic patients include a thallium scan and coronary angiography. Regarding blood testing, in patients with a GFR < 60, cardiac biomarkers (troponins and

B-type natriuretic peptides) must be interpreted with caution as their diagnostic value becomes less reliable.[35]

Modifiable risk factors that can contribute to cardiovascular disease, and that should be addressed as part of managing patients with CKD, include hypertension, obesity, hyperlipidemia, hypervolemia, anemia, smoking, hyperglycemia, calcium and phosphate imbalances, vitamin D deficiency, and metabolic acidosis. Statin therapy is recommended for lipid lowering in CKD, to decrease all-cause and cardiovascular mortality for patients not yet on dialysis; benefits are less clear for patients already on dialysis.[34] As with the general population, disease-specific treatment (eg, antiplatelet therapy and β-blocker administration for coronary artery disease) must be instituted as appropriate.

## Managing Pulmonary Alterations

A frequent complication in patients with oliguric AKI or stage G5 CKD is the development of pulmonary edema. This complication results from fluid overload, heart failure, or both. Clinical manifestations include dyspnea; crackles on auscultation; the production of pink, frothy sputum; tachypnea; tachycardia; decreased arterial oxygen saturation ($SaO_2$); and evidence of fluid overload on chest radiograph. Management involves fluid and sodium restriction, treating underlying cardiac disease, and possibly diuretic medications if the patient's kidneys can respond to them. Frequently, pulmonary edema becomes life threatening, necessitating intubation, emergent dialysis, or both to improve arterial oxygenation and restore fluid balance.

Other pulmonary complications in renal failure include pleural effusions, pleuritic inflammation and pain, uremic pneumonitis, and pulmonary infections. Pleuritic inflammation and uremic pneumonitis occur more frequently with stage G5 CKD and are due to the effect of uremic toxins on the lungs and inadequate dialysis. Pulmonary infections, on the other hand, are common in both AKI and CKD, especially in critically ill patients. Factors associated with renal failure that contribute to pulmonary infections include decreased pulmonary macrophage activity, a generalized immunocompromised state, tenacious sputum, and a depressed cough reflex. Collaborative management includes culturing sputum, administering broad-spectrum antibiotics until organism-specific sensitivities are available, and teaching and encouraging pulmonary hygiene measures (ie, coughing and deep breathing).

## Managing Gastrointestinal Alterations

A potentially life-threatening gastrointestinal complication in both AKI and CKD is gastrointestinal bleeding. Proposed etiologies for gastrointestinal bleeding as it relates to renal failure include platelet and blood-clotting abnormalities; anticoagulation with dialysis, access patency, or both; ingestion of irritating drugs (eg, NSAIDs, aspirin); arteriovenous malformations (with CKD), and increased ammonia production in the gastrointestinal tract from urea breakdown. Ammonia is known to be irritating to mucosal surfaces. CKD patients with high urea levels are prone to develop gastritis, ulcerative esophagitis, and duodenitis as evidenced by biopsy.[56] Physiologic stress, especially in critically ill patients, is another proposed contributor. Assessment parameters include

examining all vomit and stool for gross and occult blood; monitoring iron, hemoglobin, hematocrit, and red blood cell indices; and paying close attention to signs of intravascular volume depletion. If gastrointestinal bleeding is suspected, radiographic and endoscopic examinations are often required to diagnose and treat specific lesions. Management depends on the specific lesion, but often includes volume restoration with crystalloids and blood products as well as administration of histamine-2 receptor ($H_2$) blockers, proton-pump inhibitors (PPIs), or both.

Other gastrointestinal complications associated with renal failure occur primarily in CKD and include anorexia, nausea, vomiting, diarrhea, constipation, gastroesophageal reflux disease (GERD), and oral cavity alterations, such as stomatitis, a metallic taste in the mouth, and uremic fetor (the smell of urine and ammonia on the breath). Oral alterations and symptoms of anorexia, nausea, and vomiting are partially attributable to high levels of uremic toxins, which affect the intestinal mucosa and stimulate vomiting centers in the brain. The reason GERD is common is unclear, but it may be due to delayed gastric emptying, increased gastrin production, and use of medications that affect lower esophageal sphincter tone (ie, calcium-channel blockers).[57] Collaborative management involves initiating (or providing) adequate dialysis, providing prophylactic antacids and $H_2$ blockers or PPIs, and administering antiemetics. Good oral hygiene is also essential.

The complication of constipation is seen frequently in patients with renal failure owing to decreased bulk and fluid in the diet and the administration of oral iron supplements and calcium-based phosphate binders. Diarrhea may also occur as a result of intestinal irritation from uremia. Collaborative management includes increasing dietary bulk; administering bulk-forming laxatives, stool softeners, or both; administering antidiarrheal agents; or a combination of these therapies. For patients with stage G5 CKD, magnesium-containing medications, including cathartics such as magnesium citrate, should be avoided because of the risk of hypermagnesemia in these patients. In addition, Fleet enemas, which contain large amounts of phosphate that could be absorbed systemically, should not be used.

## Managing Neuromuscular Alterations

Neuromuscular alterations include sleep disturbances, cognitive process disturbances, lethargy, muscle irritability, and peripheral neuropathies, including restless leg syndrome and burning feet syndrome. Restless leg syndrome is characterized by a discomfort in the legs, especially at night, which is sometimes relieved by continuous movement of the extremities. Burning feet syndrome consists of paresthesias and numbness in the soles of the feet and lower parts of the legs. These neuromuscular complications are associated primarily with stage G4 and G5 CKD and are thought to be the result of electrolyte imbalances, metabolic acidosis, and the effect of uremic toxins on motor and sensory nerves. Cognitive process disturbances, such as difficulty concentrating and impaired short-term memory, are linked to elevations of BUN in the cerebral vasculature, which can result in cerebral edema. Extensive cerebral edema can result in seizures, projectile vomiting, and even coma or death.

Frequent assessments for cognitive disturbances, seizure activity, and other neuromuscular alterations are important. In addition to thorough neuromuscular examinations, nerve conduction studies and diagnostic tests, including electroencephalograms and head CT scans, may be used. Collaborative management involves implementing emergency treatment, as in the case of sustained seizure activity; maintaining electrolyte balance; correcting metabolic acidosis; using regular dialysis; and providing extensive patient teaching. Specific points that need to be included during patient teaching are the importance of preventing injury to the extremities by heat or trauma when paresthesias are present, and that alterations in neuromuscular function often improve with regular dialysis or transplantation. However, if components of the patient's neuropathies are due to other comorbid conditions, such as diabetes, the problem may respond only minimally to dialysis or renal transplantation.

It is important to be aware of possible cognitive alterations during patient teaching. Because the patient may have difficulties concentrating and impairments in short-term memory, teaching should be provided in short, frequent sessions with reinforcement of material, and should include the family as much as possible. This is especially true for critically ill patients who are, by definition, in a crisis situation.

## Managing Hematologic Alterations

Hematologic system alterations are major complications in AKI and CKD. These alterations include an increased bleeding tendency, an impaired immune system, and anemia.

### Increased Bleeding Tendency

The increased bleeding tendency in renal failure is attributable to impaired platelet aggregation and adhesion and an altered platelet–vessel wall interaction. These alterations are thought to be due to uremia, but their exact pathophysiologic mechanisms are unknown. Assessment involves the monitoring of platelet counts, coagulation studies, and assessing for bleeding, especially gastrointestinal bleeding. Collaborative management includes administering blood products as needed, protecting the patient from injury, and avoiding medications that alter platelet function, such as NSAIDs and aspirin. Often heparin (for dialysis) and aspirin (for MI prevention) are indicated in patients with renal failure; in such cases, the effects of these medications on platelets must be closely monitored. One potential and serious complication of heparin is heparin-induced thrombocytopenia; the development of this complication mandates discontinuation of the drug.

### Impairments in the Immune System

Patients with renal failure are in an immunocompromised state, which sets the stage for infections (a major cause of mortality in AKI and CKD). The impairments in the immune system are thought to be due to malnutrition and the effects of uremia on white blood cells. These effects include depressed T cell–mediated and antibody-mediated immunity, impaired phagocytosis, and decreased chemotaxis and adherence of white blood cells.[58]

Assessing the patient for infection and monitoring laboratory indicators of infection must be done continuously. The baseline body temperature in uremic patients is decreased, and thus any increase in temperature above baseline is significant as a gauge of infection. Collaborative management includes frequent hand washing, removing invasive catheters as soon as possible (or avoiding their use altogether), and culturing blood and other body fluids that may be infected to identify specific organisms and determine appropriate antimicrobial therapy.

### Anemia

Anemia associated with renal failure is attributable to three main mechanisms: erythropoietin deficiency, decreased red blood cell survival time, and blood loss from an increased bleeding tendency. Of these three mechanisms, erythropoietin deficiency has the most dramatic effect.

More than 90% of the hormone erythropoietin is produced in the kidneys. It is a glycoprotein that stimulates red blood cell production in response to hypoxia, and it is essential to maintaining normal red blood cell counts. As kidney disease progresses and nephrons are damaged, this hormone is inadequately synthesized, and a hypoproliferative anemia occurs, resulting in normocytic normochromic red blood cells. Before the production of erythropoietin by human recombinant techniques, this hormone deficiency caused most patients with CKD to be in a severely anemic state, requiring frequent blood transfusions.

Decreased red blood cell survival time in renal failure occurs in the form of a mild hemolysis. The exact mechanism for this hemolysis is unclear, but it may be related to dialysis therapy or the effect of uremia on red blood cells. The average survival of red blood cells in uremia is only 70 days, which contrasts with the normal 120-day life span of a red blood cell in the general population.

In addition to the three aforementioned mechanisms of anemia, other factors can contribute to anemia in patients with renal failure, particularly those who are critically ill. Examples are malnutrition, frequent laboratory blood sampling, dialyzer malfunction and sequestration of blood in the dialyzer, and infectious states. Treating anemia in patients with renal failure is extremely important for many different reasons, including increasing the oxygen-carrying capacity of the blood, increasing intravascular volume, and preventing the negative consequences of anemia on the cardiovascular system. Anemia exacerbates myocardial, cerebral, and peripheral ischemia and increases the risk for development (or acceleration) of left ventricular hypertrophy. Correcting anemia has also been shown to have a positive impact on quality-of-life issues in patients with renal failure, including increases in appetite, energy, and work capacity.[59] A thorough evaluation of anemia involves diagnostic studies and a history and physical examination. Diagnostic metabolic parameters that should be obtained and monitored include hemoglobin, hematocrit, red blood cell indices, and reticulocyte counts. In addition, the stool or vomit should be tested for occult blood. Iron studies also need to be obtained, because iron deficiency itself can cause anemia, and because adequate iron stores are needed for erythropoietin to be effective. Specific iron indices that should be obtained include total serum iron, total iron-binding capacity, and serum ferritin levels. Finally, nutritional parameters and levels of folic acid, pyridoxine, and vitamin $B_{12}$, all of which affect red blood cell production, need to be monitored.

A thorough history and physical examination involve questioning patients about potential sites of bleeding (eg, by asking about stool color), assessing for signs and symptoms of anemia (eg, angina, tachycardia, skin and mucous membrane pallor, appetite suppression, weight loss, decreased energy levels, fatigue), assessing for sources of blood loss, assessing for inflammation or infection, and assessing for other diseases that can cause anemia (eg, lupus, sickle cell anemia).

Collaborative management of anemia includes minimizing blood loss, administering oral or IV iron supplements, providing vitamin supplementation, aggressively treating infections, ensuring adequate nutrition, and administering erythropoietin-stimulating agents (ESAs), such as human erythropoietin or darbepoetin, blood products, or both. The KDIGO Guideline suggests iron administration in CKD patients when transferrin saturation is ≤30% and serum ferritin level is ≤500 ng/mL.[60] Goals for ESA therapy are less concrete owing to potential cardiovascular risks when targeting normal hemoglobin levels. These cardiovascular risks prompted the Federal Drug Administration (FDA) to issue a warning in all package inserts of ESAs. Hemoglobin goals should be individualized, based on patient symptoms and comorbidities, using the lowest ESA dose to reduce the need for red blood cell transfusions. The KDIGO Guideline advises not to use ESAs to intentionally increase Hgb concentration greater than 11.5 mg/dL, or recommend against their use in patients with active cancer or a recent history of malignancy.[35]

Certain points regarding ESA therapy and the management of anemia deserve special mention. One is that the full effect of these medications takes weeks to achieve, and hence in patients with profound anemia, blood administration is indicated. In addition, ESA administration may result in an elevation of BP; in some cases, modification of antihypertensive therapy may be needed. When there is an inadequate response to ESAs despite increased dosages, reasons for erythropoietin resistance need to be explored. These include occult infections, inflammatory states, human immunodeficiency virus infection, hyperparathyroidism, aluminum toxicity, malnutrition, iron deficiency, and bone marrow malignancy.

Important clinical features regarding iron preparations should also be considered. Oral iron is poorly absorbed if taken with phosphate binders, antacids, $H_2$ blockers, or PPIs, all of which are commonly prescribed to patients with renal failure. On the other hand, IV iron has much better bioavailability but carries the risk of an allergic, sometimes life-threatening, reaction. This risk has significantly decreased with newer, more biocompatible IV preparations.

Extensive patient teaching about anemia is crucial. At minimum, teaching should include information about medication therapy; timing of iron supplements; potential causes, signs, and symptoms of worsening anemia; and energy conservation techniques. Instruction about measures to decrease bleeding, such as use of a soft toothbrush and avoidance of NSAIDs, is also helpful.

## Managing Alterations in Drug Elimination

Because many pharmacologic agents, their metabolites, or both are excreted by the kidneys, extreme caution must be used when administering medication to patients with renal failure. Depending on the patient's GFR, adjustments may need to be made in drug dosage, the interval between drug dosages, or both. Important to consider, especially in AKI, is that the GRF is often unstable, and thus the GFR must be monitored frequently to determine dosages accurately. As in patients without renal failure, monitoring serum levels of certain medications to be sure they are within the therapeutic range is essential. For patients receiving dialysis, the health care team must be cognizant of which drugs are removed during dialysis therapy to ensure appropriate timing of drug administration.

## Managing Skeletal Alterations

In renal failure, disturbances in calcium and phosphate balance set the stage for secondary hyperparathyroidism and high-turnover renal osteodystrophy (renal bone disease). As the GFR declines, glomerular filtration of phosphate also decreases, and serum phosphate levels begin to rise. This results in decreased serum ionized calcium levels because of binding of the calcium with the phosphate. Calcium levels also decrease because of the failing kidneys' inability to convert vitamin D to its active form (1,25-dihydroxycholecalciferol, or vitamin $D_3$), which is needed for adequate intestinal absorption of calcium. In response to decreased ionized calcium levels, elevations in serum phosphorus levels, and reduced vitamin $D_3$ synthesis, the parathyroid glands secrete parathyroid hormone (PTH). Over time, the continuous PTH stimulation leads to hyperplasia and proliferation of the parathyroid cells, resulting in secondary hyperparathyroidism. PTH causes the reabsorption of calcium and phosphate salts from bones, thus increasing the serum calcium level at the expense of bone density and mass. PTH also causes calcium reabsorption and phosphate excretion in the kidneys; however, as renal failure progresses, this effect of PTH is not realized. Eventually, as calcium and phosphate continue to be reabsorbed from bones, both levels rise in the serum concomitantly. This results in an elevation in the normal calcium–phosphate product (serum calcium multiplied by serum phosphate) of less than 40 mg/dL. When the product exceeds 55 mg/dL, calcium phosphate crystals can form and precipitate in various parts of the body (a condition known as metastatic calcifications), including the brain, eyes, gums, valves of the heart, myocardium, lungs, joints, blood vessels, and skin. Other insults to bones that can occur in renal disease include bone demineralization in response to metabolic acidosis and low-turnover renal osteodystrophy from aluminum deposits in the bone or overuse of vitamin $D_3$ therapy. The events related to high-turnover renal osteodystrophy in renal failure are summarized in Figure 31-6.

Complications from renal bone disease include bone pain, fractures, pseudogout from deposits of calcium oxalate in synovial fluid, periarthritis from calcifications of the joints, proximal muscle weakness, spontaneous tendon rupture, and pruritus. Metastatic calcifications can result in calcified blood vessels and valves, skin lesions, red-eye syndrome from crystal deposition in the conjunctiva, and, most seriously, ischemic ulcers. Laboratory data, including levels of calcium, phosphate, aluminum, alkaline phosphatase, and intact PTH, help make the diagnosis. Radiographic findings also may be helpful, particularly in high-turnover bone disease; images may reveal subperiosteal bone thinning, most easily

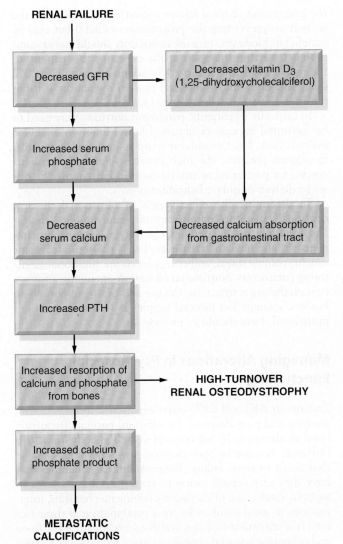

FIGURE 31-6   Effects of renal failure on the skeletal system.

seen in the hands and clavicles. A bone biopsy, considered the gold standard for obtaining a definitive diagnosis of renal bone disease, is not routinely performed because of patient discomfort and controversy surrounding the indications for this invasive test.

Management involves phosphate regulation, maintenance of normal calcium levels, treatment of vitamin D deficiency, suppression of PTH, prevention of aluminum toxicity, and control of metabolic acidosis. Measures to control phosphate levels include dietary restrictions and phosphate-binding medications. Commonly used phosphate binders are calcium acetate (Phos-lo), calcium carbonate (Tums), sevelamer hydrochloride (Renagel), and lanthanum carbonate (Fosrenol). Sevelamer and lanthanum carbonate are calcium-free phosphate binders and are preferred over calcium-based binders in patients with high calcium levels because they lessen the risk for hypercalcemia and further elevations in the calcium–phosphate product. Aluminum hydroxide binders, once a mainstay of therapy, are now infrequently used because of the effects of aluminum toxicity on the bones as well as the nervous system. Aluminum toxicity causes erythropoietin resistance as well.

According to the KDIGO Clinical Practice Guideline, calcium levels should be maintained in the normal range.[61] This is accomplished with diet and calcium supplements. If calcium levels exceed 10.2 mg/dL, therapies that may be contributing to hypercalcemia (eg, administering calcium or vitamin D supplements) should be adjusted to reduce the risk for extraskeletal calcifications.

Vitamin D supplements are administered to suppress PTH secretion. Besides causing a decrease in PTH indirectly through the elevation of serum calcium, active vitamin D also directly inhibits PTH secretion by binding to vitamin D receptors on the parathyroid gland. Active vitamin D may be given orally (calcitriol) or intravenously (Calcijex). In either case, caution must be exercised with the administration of these agents to avoid hypercalcemia and hyperphosphatemia as well as to avoid oversuppression of the parathyroid gland. Two synthetic analogs of active vitamin D that can also be used are paricalcitol (Zemplar) and doxercalciferol (Hectorol). These drugs have the advantage of causing less dramatic increases in serum calcium and phosphate levels while still causing PTH suppression.

The most recent therapeutic agents developed to help suppress PTH and the development of secondary hyperparathyroidism are calcimimetics, which work by increasing the sensitivity of the calcium-sensing receptor in the parathyroid gland to extracellular calcium. In the United States, the Food and Drug Administration approved the calcimimetic cinacalcet hydrochloride (Sensipar) for patients with ESRD. It has been shown to be both safe and effective, with the most common side effects being nausea and vomiting and hypocalcemia. Rarely, a parathyroidectomy may be necessary for patients who are refractory to available treatments for secondary hyperparathyroidism, including vitamin D therapy and calcimimetics.

Patient teaching concerning bone disease and its management is complex and needs to be continually reinforced. Particular areas that should be included are the purpose and timing of medications (eg, phosphate binders must be given with meals to be effective), dietary modifications, and the complications of untreated bone disease.

## Managing Integumentary Alterations

Alterations in the integumentary system in renal failure include xerosis (dryness), pruritus, pallor, ecchymosis and purpura, and pigmentation changes. Pigment changes include hyperpigmentation, especially at sun-exposed sites, or a yellow discoloration to the skin. CKD is also associated with hair loss and nail changes, such as the absence of the lunula, splinter hemorrhages, Beau lines (white lines across the fingernails), and onychomycosis. Possible contributing factors to these alterations are iron deficiency anemia, decreased activity of sweat and sebaceous glands, retained skin pigments, platelet dysfunction and capillary fragility, deposition of calcium phosphate crystals into the skin, hyperparathyroidism, hyperphosphatemia, increased vitamin A levels in the epidermis, and impaired cellular immunity.[62] Uremic frost, a white powdery substance composed of urates on the skin, is due to crystallization of urea; it is usually seen only in severely uremic patients for whom needed dialytic therapy is being withheld. These skin alterations, particularly pruritus and xerosis, may lead to localized infection from excoriation and secondary skin changes, such as lichen simplex and keratic papules. In addition, substantial patient discomfort and psychological disturbances from skin disfigurement may occur.

Collaborative management for skin alterations includes phosphate regulation, nutritional supplementation, correction of anemia, antihistamine medications, and meticulous skin care and turning to prevent skin breakdown. Dialysis therapy helps as well by removing metabolic waste products. However, because of potential allergies to the dialysis system components, dialysis therapy can also aggravate some conditions, such as pruritus. Patient education should include information on factors contributing to skin alterations, the importance of keeping the skin clean and well moisturized, and ways to avoid excoriation (such as keeping the fingernails trimmed).

## Managing Alterations in Dietary Intake

The goals of nutritional therapy in renal failure are to minimize uremic symptoms; reduce the incidence of fluid, electrolyte, and acid–base imbalances; minimize symptoms of anemia; decrease the patient's vulnerability to infections; and limit catabolism. Dietary restrictions related to managing comorbid conditions and reducing cardiovascular risk also need to be considered. Because of the complexity of achieving a nutritional therapy plan that meets these goals, a collaborative health care team approach, including the ongoing participation of a dietitian, is essential. This is particularly the case in critical care, where patients are usually in a catabolic state and are at risk for substantial malnutrition.

Renal diet prescriptions include restrictions in fluid, sodium, potassium, and phosphate intake, and may include supplementations of iron, vitamins, and calcium. Calorically, critically ill patients with renal disease need a high-calorie diet with a total of 20 to 30 kcal/kg/d, most of which should come from a combination of carbohydrates and lipids. In addition, adequate protein intake must be administered to prevent catabolism, and at least 50% of protein intake should be of high biologic value to ensure that the minimal intake requirements of essential amino acids are met. Protein restriction to decrease symptoms of uremia and slow the progression of renal failure is controversial (refer to the section on preventing the progression of CKD) but may be beneficial. However, protein restriction should never compromise meeting anabolic goals, exposing the patient to the risk of malnutrition. In AKI patients, the KDIGO 2012 Guideline does not recommend protein restriction as it has not been shown to delay the need for RRT.

In critically ill patients, parenteral nutrition may need to be instituted because of impaired bowel function or severe malnutrition, but the enteral route is preferred if feasible. In oliguric patients, the high hourly volume requirements needed for parenteral or enteral nutrition often must be offset by dialysis or isolated ultrafiltration.

To determine the effectiveness of nutritional therapy, continual laboratory monitoring of serum protein, cholesterol, albumin and prealbumin, electrolytes, hemoglobin, hematocrit, and urea and creatinine levels is essential. Patient weight, volume status, and energy levels are additional monitoring parameters. Nutritional education, including information on dietary restrictions, the use and timing of phosphate binders, vitamin and mineral supplements, and measures of nutritional status should be provided.

## Managing Alterations in Psychosocial Functioning

Patients in AKI and CKD often experience feelings of fear, anxiety, and powerlessness. In addition, patients frequently have an alteration in self-concept as well as body image disturbances because of both physical and functional changes that occur in renal failure. Patients and their families may have difficulty coping owing to stress, limited resources or support, inadequate or ineffective coping mechanisms, interruptions in usual family roles, or a combination of these factors. It is important that the health care team attend to these and other psychosocial complications of renal failure to treat the patient and family holistically. Specific interventions include thorough patient and family teaching, active involvement of the patient and family members in managing the condition, ensuring adequate rest and sleep for the patient, exploring the patient's and family's feelings and concerns, providing support, and obtaining the active involvement of social services and clergy as appropriate.

## Clinical Applicability Challenges

### CASE STUDY

Mr. X., a 63-year-old white man, was admitted for ST elevation MI. He was in his normal state of health until 6 hours before admission, when he developed substernal chest pain (SSCP) with radiation to his left arm. Pain was accompanied by mild diaphoresis. After self-administering antacids without relief, he asked his wife to take him to the emergency department (ED).

In the ED, he was found to be anxious and diaphoretic, and he complained of dyspnea and 9/10 SSCP. Initial vital signs were as follows: temperature 37.5°C, BP 90/60, pulse 105, respiratory rate 24, peripheral capillary oxygen saturation 92% on 4 L nasal cannula. The physical exam was significant for an elevated jugular venous pressure and pulmonary crackles halfway up bilaterally. Mr. X. did not have any peripheral edema. His past medical history included hypertension for 22 years with variable control, hyperlipidemia, CKD (baseline serum creatinine of 1.8 mg/dL), and type II diabetes mellitus for 15 years.

Initial labs in the ED were notable for a serum creatinine of 1.9 mg/dL, an elevated troponin, and 2+ protein on urinalysis. EKG revealed 3 mm ST elevation in leads II and AVF. Chest x-ray revealed moderate pulmonary artery prominence. Home medications include aspirin 81 mg QD, Lisinopril 20 mg QD, Lantus 15 units QHS, Lasix 20 mg, and atorvastatin 20 mg QHS. Aside from supplemental oxygen, Mr. X received aspirin 325 mg and nitroglycerin SL 0.4 mg in the ED. Post SL nitroglycerin, his chest pain remained unchanged and his BP decreased to 85/50; HR 110.

The patient was evaluated by the cardiology department and emergently taken to the catheterization laboratory; coronary angiography revealed a 95% stenotic lesion in the mid-right coronary artery. The remaining arteries showed no flow limiting. The patient underwent percutaneous transluminal angioplasty and placement of a bare metal stent. He received 175 mL of IV contrast dye. Following the procedure, the patient started on Plavix, SSI, beta-blocker therapy, and continued on daily aspirin.

On postprocedure day 1, the patient was feeling well and chest pain free. BP was 140/85, HR 70, SPO$_2$ 95% on RA. Urine output was 1,100 mL and serum creatinine was 1.8 mg/dL. On postprocedure day 2, urine output had decreased to 600 mL. Serum creatinine was 1.9 mg/dL. By postprocedure day 3, the patient was oliguric with a total urine output of 200 mL and required 4 L nasal cannula supplemental oxygen to maintain SPO$_2$ over 92%. Serum creatinine was 2.7 mg/dL. Chest x-ray revealed pulmonary edema, and retained contrast could be seen in the visible portion of the kidneys.

1. What information supports the diagnosis of AKI in Mr. X. versus progression of his CKD?
2. What makes Mr. X. at risk for contrast-induced nephropathy?
3. In caring for Mr. X., what fluid and electrolyte and acid–base alterations may be anticipated?

**WANT TO KNOW MORE?**

A wide variety of resources to enhance your learning and understanding of this chapter are available on thePoint.

You will find:

- References
- Selected readings
- NCLEX-style review questions
- Internet resources
- And more!

# 32

# Anatomy and Physiology of the Nervous System

DONNA MOWER-WADE AND REBECCA E. MACINTYRE

## LEARNING OBJECTIVES

*Based on the content in this chapter, the reader should be able to:*

1. Describe the cellular units of the nervous system.
2. Explain the characteristics of neurons and nerve regeneration.
3. Describe the components of the central nervous system.
4. List areas of the brain and their corresponding function.
5. Define briefly the sensory system and the motor system.
6. Explain the baroreceptor reflex and three spinal cord reflexes.
7. Explain the anatomy and physiology of pain.
8. Explain the concept of homeostasis.
9. Describe the acute stress response.
10. Describe age-related changes that can occur to the nervous system.

The brain is a central organ that coordinates activity of most, if not all, body systems through its influence on the endocrine and immune systems as well as its more generally appreciated influence on skeletal muscle and autonomic function. Its influence is modulated by sensory perceptions that convey a picture of the external and internal environments and also by internal circuits having to do with emotional state and levels of arousal. Therefore, the brain can be thought of as the integrative organ that drives our responses to environmental influence. Moreover, separation of the brain and spinal cord from the periphery is more anatomical than conceptual, and modern nurses must always keep in mind that the brain has a profound influence on almost everything that happens in the periphery, and vice versa.

Traditionally, the nervous system is discussed with reference to both anatomical and functional divisions. Anatomical components are the central nervous system (CNS), comprising the brain and spinal cord, and the peripheral nervous system (PNS), comprising the cranial and spinal nerves. The nervous system is functionally separated into the sensory, integrative, and motor (somatic and autonomic) divisions. Content in this chapter is ordered according to both divisions. However, cell anatomy and physiology are discussed first.

## Cells of the Nervous System

The cellular units are the neuron—the basic functional unit—and its attendant cells, the neuroglia.

### Neuroglia

Neuroglia constitute the supportive tissue associated with the neurons. In the CNS, there are four types of neuroglia: microglia, astrocytes, ependymal cells, and oligodendroglia. The microglia are phagocytic cells of the nervous system similar to macrophages in the periphery. The astrocytes are supportive cells of the nervous system and make up the blood–brain barrier. The ependymal cells line the ventricles and aid in the production and circulation of the cerebrospinal fluid (CSF). The oligodendroglia are mostly found in the white matter and produce the myelin that covers nerve fibers in the CNS. In the PNS, the counterpart of the myelin-producing oligodendroglial cell is the Schwann cell.

Under most circumstances, neurons lose their ability to undergo mitosis early in the life of the individual. However, neuroglia retain mitotic abilities throughout a person's life span. Because of this, malignant or benign proliferative lesions originating in the CNS involve neuroglia rather than neurons. However, as the neuroglial tumor enlarges, it adversely affects adjacent neurons—early by exerting pressure and later by promoting an inflammatory reaction along with the pressure.

## Neurons

The basic functional unit of the nervous system is the neuron (or nerve cell), and all information and activity, whether sensory, motor, or both, is accomplished by neurons. The neuron consists of a nerve cell body or soma that contains nuclear and cytoplasmic material and processes, either axons or dendrites, which arise from the soma (Fig. 32-1). Axons normally carry nerve impulses away from the cell body, whereas dendrites conduct impulses toward the cell body. Axons and dendrites may be merely microscopic knobs or areas on the cell body surface, or they may be cylindrical processes that can extend to more than 1 m (3.25 ft) long. A specialized structure at the end of the axon is called the axon terminal. This is a bulbous ending (sometimes called a bouton) that forms a synapse with another neuron. The axon

terminal contains vesicles of neurotransmitter that is released into the synapse, diffuses across to the postsynaptic neuron, and binds to specific receptors on the membrane of the postsynaptic cell. Binding of a particular neurotransmitter to its specific receptor on the postsynaptic neuron either depolarizes or hyperpolarizes the postsynaptic neuron in the area of the synapse. Axons and dendrites are referred to collectively as nerve fibers. A bundle of nerve fibers together with their coverings is called a tract in the CNS and a nerve in the periphery.

Some nerve fibers are covered with a white lipid–protein sheath termed the myelin sheath. This covering is what differentiates white matter from gray matter in the CNS. The myelin sheath is formed in the CNS by the oligodendrocytes. Other fibers remain unmyelinated. All nerve fibers in the PNS are covered by a neurilemma. This is a sheath formed by the Schwann cells, which wrap themselves around the fiber. Some Schwann cells around particular fibers secrete myelin; others do not (see Fig. 32-1). The neurilemma of a myelinated fiber comes in contact with the axon at periodic intervals. These periodic constrictions of the neurilemmal sheath are termed the nodes of Ranvier. The nodes of

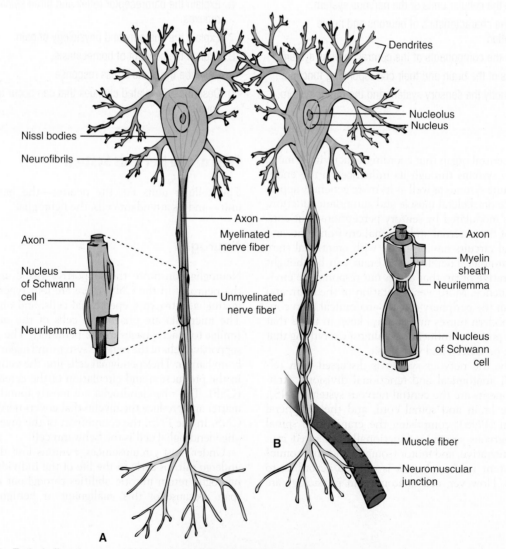

**FIGURE 32-1**   Typical efferent neurons. **A:** Unmyelinated fiber. **B:** Myelinated fiber.

Ranvier produce faster nerve impulse conduction by allowing the impulse to jump from one node to the next (saltatory conduction).

Neurons are very diverse, with many specialized anatomical features that are important to their function. Some neurons are extremely large or may give rise to extremely long nerve fibers. Transmission velocities in long, myelinated fibers may be as high as 100 m/s, whereas unmyelinated neurons with very short, unmyelinated processes demonstrate velocities of 1 m/s. Some neurons connect to many different neurons, perhaps thousands of other neurons, in a "network," whereas others have relatively few connections to other cells of the nervous system.

It is estimated that the human CNS has one hundred billion neurons. Three fourths of these neurons are located in the cerebral cortex, where conscious thought and feeling reside, along with integrative processing and smoothing of planned motor movements. This processing includes not only the determination of appropriate and effective responses but also the storage of memory and the development of associative motor and thought patterns.

## Characteristics of Neurons

### Resting Membrane Potential

The neuronal cell membrane contains sodium–potassium pumps that keep the inside of the neuron more negatively charged than the outside interstitial fluid. The cytoplasm of all cells contains anions (negatively charged ions) that are too large to leave the cell. Many ions, including sodium, potassium, and chloride, are small enough to diffuse through tiny pores in the cell membrane. Concentrations of these ions would be equal on the inside of the cell compared with the outside if not for the sodium–potassium pump. The sodium–potassium pump in the cell membrane pumps sodium ions out of the cell almost as fast as they enter. For every two sodium ions that are pumped out, one potassium ion is pumped into the cell. Because of this, there is a net positive charge leaving the cell, and the large anions cannot be counterbalanced. Thus, under resting conditions when no impulse is being conducted, the inside of the neuron is negative with respect to the outside. This internal relative negativity is the resting membrane potential of the neuron and typically measures about –70 mV.

In addition, as a result of activity of the sodium–potassium pump, sodium ion concentration inside the cell is much lower than outside, and potassium ion concentration is much higher inside the cell than outside. These concentration gradients are important for depolarization produced by synaptic transmission and for conduction of the action potential down the axon (Fig. 32-2).

### Synaptic Transmission

Submicroscopic spaces between the axon (or axons) of one neuron and the dendrite (or dendrites) or soma of another are called synapses. Axons or dendrites may branch, enabling the axon of one neuron to synapse with dendrites or somas of several neurons. A synapse consists of a presynaptic axon terminal, a postsynaptic neuron, and the synaptic cleft

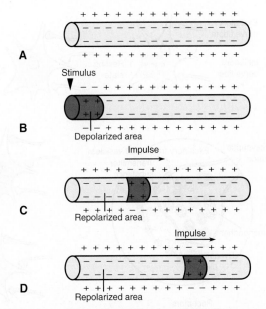

**FIGURE 32-2** Propagation of impulses. **A:** Resting membrane. **B:** Action potential, first stage: stimulation of fiber results in depolarization. **C:** Action potential, second stage: repolarization occurs as the resting potential is restored. **D:** Propagation of impulses continues in direction of *arrow*.

(Fig. 32-3A). When an action potential is conducted down the presynaptic axon and depolarizes the axon terminal, vesicles of neurotransmitter fuse with the plasma membrane, releasing neurotransmitter into the synaptic cleft. The molecules of neurotransmitter diffuse across the cleft and bind to specific receptors on the postsynaptic cell membrane. The binding of neurotransmitter to its receptor causes a change in the membrane potential of the postsynaptic cell, either a depolarization or a hyperpolarization.

In very short time (millionths of a second), the neurotransmitter detaches from the receptor site and may reattach or be inactivated. Inactivation can occur either by the neurotransmitter returning back into the axon terminal by specific reuptake pumps and repackaging it in vesicles to be reused or it can be destroyed by an enzyme in the synaptic cleft. Rapid, repetitive, discrete stimulation of neurons is necessary for activity of a neural pathway to continue. Neural pathways can be stimulated over prolonged periods by repeated depolarizations of presynaptic neurons, or activity of a specific pathway can be turned on or off almost instantaneously.

Synaptic transmission is a one-way street—from the axon across the synaptic cleft to the dendrite or soma of the next neuron. It cannot proceed in the opposite direction. Moreover, decreased destruction or decreased reuptake of a transmitter can increase the effect of this transmitter on the postsynaptic membrane. Similarly, increased destruction or increased reuptake of a transmitter reduces its postsynaptic effects. Several classes of pharmacologic agents take advantage of these facts. For instance, acetylcholinesterase inhibitors such as pyridostigmine bromide increases the amount of acetylcholine remaining in the synapse of the neuromuscular junction. This is used to counteract the effects of paralytic drugs given during anesthesia, or for the treatment of myasthenia gravis. Serotonin or norepinephrine reuptake pump inhibitors increase the amount of serotonin or

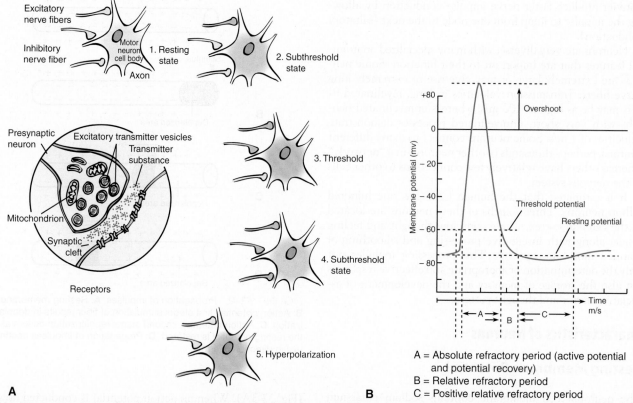

**FIGURE 32-3**    Conduction at synapses. **A**: A neuron may be excited or inhibited by transmitter substances liberated by presynaptic nerve fiber endings. Two excitatory fibers and one inhibitory fiber are shown. (1) During the resting state, no impulses are received. (2) During the subthreshold state, impulses from only one excitatory fiber cannot cause the postsynaptic neuron to mount an action potential. (3) The threshold is reached by the addition of impulses from a second excitatory fiber. This enables the postsynaptic neuron to mount an action potential. (4) The subthreshold state is restored by impulses from an inhibitory fiber. (5) When the inhibitory fiber alone is carrying impulses, the postsynaptic neuron is in a state of hyperpolarization and is unable to fire. **B**: The time course of a neural action potential.

norepinephrine in the synapse and have therapeutic effects in depressed patients.

It was thought that each neuron synthesizes and stores only one major neurotransmitter in its axon terminal but research now suggests that some neurons can store and release more than one neurotransmitter. Major neurotransmitters include serotonin, acetylcholine, gamma-aminobutyric acid (GABA), glycine, glutamate, and the catecholamines, dopamine, norepinephrine, and epinephrine. Examples of neuropeptide neurotransmitters are the endogenous opioids (endorphins and enkephalins) and substance P, all of which appear to be involved in pain sensation. The endorphins and enkephalins, often described as the body's own morphine, contribute to a decrease in pain sensation. Substance P excites sensory neurons that respond to painful stimuli, so it is thought to be involved in transmission of pain information from the periphery to the CNS.

Each major neurotransmitter has multiple receptors.[1] For instance, epinephrine can bind to $\alpha_1$, $\alpha_2$, $\beta_1$, $\beta_2$, and $\beta_3$ receptors, and acetylcholine can bind to neuronal nicotinic, skeletal muscle nicotinic, or muscarinic receptors, which are further subdivided into $m_1$, $m_2$, and $m_3$. The postsynaptic membrane of each synapse contains only one receptor type for the particular neurotransmitter synthesized by the presynaptic neuron. The receptor subtype dictates the effects of a neurotransmitter in a particular synapse on the postsynaptic cell (hyperpolarization or depolarization). All GABA receptor types are hyperpolarizing, and GABA is the most important inhibitory neurotransmitter in the nervous system. Likewise, glutamate and glycine are always depolarizing (excitatory) neurotransmitters.

## Neuronal Thresholds and the Action Potential

A depolarizing impulse that reaches a neuron's dendrites or soma through action of a neurotransmitter binding to its receptors causes the membrane to depolarize locally through action of the receptor. The depolarization causes voltage-sensitive sodium channels to open, and sodium ions are transmitted down their concentration gradient from outside the neuron to inside, causing further depolarization. If enough sodium channels open, the resulting depolarization is large enough to open sodium channels in adjacent areas, depolarizing a larger area of the membrane. Conversely, release of an inhibitory neurotransmitter, such as GABA, at a synapse may cause hyperpolarization of the postsynaptic neuron through receptor action.

For a given nerve cell, typically there are many other neurons that synapse with its soma or dendrites. Some of these synapsing neurons release an excitatory neurotransmitter that interacts with the nerve cell's receptors to depolarize the postsynaptic neuron. Other synapsing neurons release inhibitory neurotransmitters that interact with their receptors to hyperpolarize the postsynaptic neuron. If the depolarizing influences outweigh the hyperpolarizing influences, the membrane potential of the nerve cell body may reach a value called threshold. At that point, an action potential is generated at the point where the axon leaves the soma. The action potential is propagated down the axon by the process of sodium channel openings in the area of the advancing action potential, followed by complete depolarization of that area. After this process, sodium channels close, and the membrane repolarizes through activity of the sodium–potassium pump and through openings of voltage-sensitive potassium channels. As potassium accumulates within the cell, either by entry through the voltage-sensitive potassium channels or the sodium–potassium pump, the membrane potential is reestablished.

The action potential normally propagates down the entire length of the axon to the axon terminal. At that point, depolarization of the axon terminal causes neurotransmitter to be released, which diffuses across the synapse and binds to specific receptors, causing a depolarizing or hyperpolarizing change in the postsynaptic neuron.

Figure 32-3B depicts the time course of a neuronal action potential as monitored by electrodes inserted into an axon. Compared with cardiac action potentials, neuronal action potentials are quite short, with durations of approximately 5 to 15 ms. Like the cardiac action potential, there are absolute and relative refractory periods during which the neuron cannot easily be reexcited. These refractory periods are very short because repeated impulse conduction is necessary to maintain tonic activity of particular neural pathways. For instance, the motor pathways that supply muscles of posture must be tonically active to maintain a steady contraction in these muscles that keep us erect. Other pathways that have tonic activity include the autonomic motor pathways (sympathetic and parasympathetic), as discussed later in this chapter.

The electrical activity of the action potential can be monitored in certain clinical situations. For example, the electroencephalogram depicts multiple action potentials from surface neurons of the brain and nerve conduction studies can be performed on peripheral nerves to diagnose areas of compression or entrapment.

## Remodeling of Connections in the Nervous System

Neurons in adults, and all but the youngest children, do not divide to form more neurons, and in fact neurons die throughout our life span. Our CNS is in a constant state of remodeling (often referred to as *plasticity*), with formation of new connections between neurons (synapses) and regression of previous connections. This is an area of continuing research, but evidence suggests that sensory information that is communicated to the brain as a result of our experiences is responsible for the remodeling. These alterations in brain circuitry may explain phenomena, such as emotional maturation and motor learning. They may also explain the development of mental illness at certain times in a person's life or the intense cravings that appear with substance abuse disorders.

## Nerve Regeneration

If a nerve fiber is severed, the portion distal to the cut dies, and the part still attached to the cell body regenerates. In peripheral nerves, the neurilemma itself provides a channel that can be followed by a regenerating fiber so that it may become reattached to its original anatomical connection (Fig. 32-4). Regeneration also occurs in the absence of a neurilemma, as in the case of CNS neurons. Because there is no channel to ensure correct anatomical reconnection, regenerations do not produce recovered function due to the regrowing stump winding aimlessly among other structures or curling into a useless tangle.

Note that nerve processes, axons, or dendrites that are cut may regenerate, but if the soma is damaged or the nerve cell is killed by lack of oxygen or a neurotoxin, there will be no regeneration. Moreover, under ordinary circumstances,

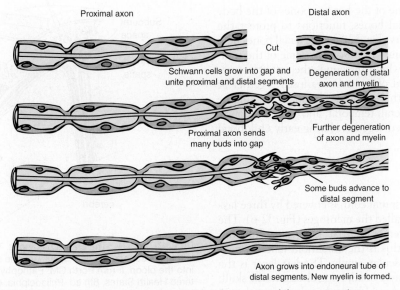

Proximal axon

Distal axon

Cut

Schwann cells grow into gap and unite proximal and distal segments

Degeneration of distal axon and myelin

Proximal axon sends many buds into gap

Further degeneration of axon and myelin

Some buds advance to distal segment

Axon grows into endoneural tube of distal segments. New myelin is formed.

**FIGURE 32-4** Diagram of changes that occur in a nerve fiber that has been cut and then regenerates.

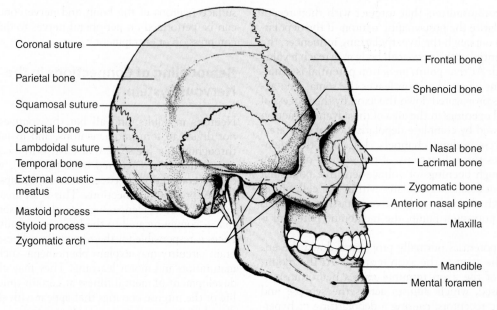

**FIGURE 32-5** Lateral view of the skull. (From Hickey JV: The Clinical Practice of Neurological and Neurosurgical Nursing, 6th ed. Philadelphia, PA: Lippincott Williams & Wilkins, 2009, p 47.)

a neuron that dies cannot be replaced because neurons do not normally undergo mitosis in people older than age 2.

## Central Nervous System

The CNS comprises the brain and spinal cord. It receives sensory input through sensory neurons whose dendrites run within spinal and cranial nerves, and it sends out motor impulses through axons of motor neurons that run in these same nerves. The CNS also contains large numbers of neurons that are entirely contained within it. These neurons are termed internuncial neurons, or interneurons, and exist inside the brain or the spinal cord or connect one with the other.

## Skull

The skull (cranium) is one of the hardest bones of the body and, along with the facial bones, functions to protect the brain from traumatic injury (Fig. 32-5). The facial bones help protect the brain from injury by absorbing some of the traumatic forces. The skull, which surrounds the soft structures of the brain, is composed of eight bones fused together at suture lines. The bones that compose the main part of the skull are the frontal, parietal, temporal, and occipital bones, and these bones are joined together during early childhood (see Fig. 32-5).

## Meninges

The CNS, including the spinal cord, is covered by three layers of tissue collectively called the meninges (Fig. 32-6). The pia mater is a delicate membrane that adheres to the brain and spinal cord. Above this is the arachnoid mater, which contains a substantial vascular supply. The last layer is the dura mater, the thickest layer of all, lying closest to the skull. Between the pia and arachnoid layers lies the subarachnoid space. CSF circulates through the subarachnoid space. In addition, the subarachnoid space contains the cerebral vasculature. When a cerebral vascular abnormality rupture occurs, it bleeds into the subarachnoid space, causing a subarachnoid hemorrhage. The space between the arachnoid and dura mater is named the subdural space. The space between the dura mater and skull bone is known as the epidural space. The epidural space that surrounds the spinal cord is used for epidural pain management.

The CNS is richly supplied with blood vessels that bring oxygen and nutrients to the cells. However, many substances cannot easily be exchanged between the blood and the brain

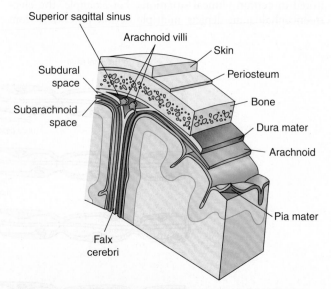

**FIGURE 32-6** The cranial meninges. The arachnoid villi, shown within the superior sagittal sinus, are one site of passage of CSF into the blood. (From Porth CM: Pathophysiology: Concepts of Altered Health States, 8th ed. Philadelphia, PA: Wolters Kluwer Health | Lippincott Williams & Wilkins, 2009, p 1211.)

because the endothelial cells of the vessels and the astrocytes of the CNS form extremely tight junctions collectively referred to as the blood–brain barrier. In particular, polar molecules and large molecules, such as proteins, do not cross the blood–brain barrier, but lipid-soluble molecules cross with ease. Many drugs penetrate the brain poorly because they do not have sufficient lipid solubility to cross the blood–brain barrier.

The space between the arachnoid layer and the pia mater, termed the subarachnoid space, contains CSF, which is another means of supplying nutrients, but not oxygen, to the CNS. CSF also serves a protective function by cushioning the brain and spinal cord.

## Cerebrospinal Fluid

CSF, a clear, colorless fluid, flows in the ventricles of the brain and the subarachnoid space of the brain and spinal cord. Functioning as a fluid shock absorber, CSF keeps the delicate CNS tissues from being mechanically injured by surrounding bony structures. CSF is actually a plasma filtrate that is exuded by the capillaries in the roofs of each of the four ventricles of the brain. As such, it is similar to plasma without the large plasma proteins, which stay behind in the bloodstream. Red blood cells, which contain the hemoglobin that is responsible for most oxygen transport in blood, are not present in CSF. Therefore, the CSF is a poor source of oxygen, although it contains glucose, amino acids, and other nutrients that might be needed by the cells of the CNS.

Most of the CSF is produced in the lateral ventricles, which are located in each cerebral hemisphere. The choroid plexus, which is located within the ventricles, produces approximately 500 mL of CSF each day, or 25 mL/h. The CSF moves from there through ducts into the third ventricle of the diencephalon (Fig. 32-7). From there, it travels through

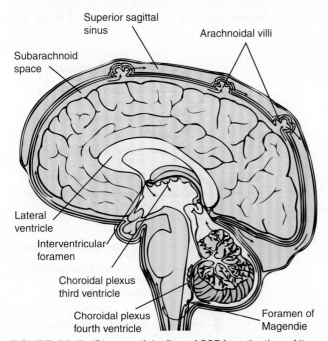

**FIGURE 32-7** Diagram of the flow of CSF from the time of its formation from blood in the choroid plexuses until its return to the blood in the superior sagittal sinus. (Adapted from Hickey JV: The Clinical Practice of Neurological and Neurosurgical Nursing, 6th ed. Philadelphia, PA: Lippincott Williams & Wilkins, 2009, p 52.)

the aqueduct of Sylvius of the midbrain and enters the fourth ventricle in the medulla oblongata. Most of it then passes through holes (foramina) in the roof of this ventricle and enters the subarachnoid space. A small amount passes down into the spinal canal. In the subarachnoid space, the CSF is reabsorbed into the bloodstream at certain structures called the arachnoid villi.

The formation and reabsorption of CSF is governed by the same hydrostatic and colloid osmotic forces that regulate the movements of fluid and small molecules between the plasma and interstitial fluid compartments. Briefly reviewed, the action of these forces is as follows. Two opposing push–pull forces influence the movement of water and small molecules through the semipermeable capillary membranes. One force is composed of plasma oncotic pressure and CSF hydrostatic pressure. It favors movement of water and small molecules from the CSF compartment into the plasma. The movement of water and small molecules in the opposite direction is influenced by the force of plasma hydrostatic pressure and CSF oncotic pressure. These two opposing forces are exerted simultaneously and continually. In the lateral ventricles, the flow of CSF out of the ventricles reduces CSF hydrostatic pressure. This tips the influence in favor of the movement of water and small molecules from plasma to the ventricles. The low plasma hydrostatic pressure of blood in the venous sinuses next to the arachnoid villi tips the scales in favor of the movement of water and solute from the CSF compartment back into the bloodstream. These forces are modulated by death of cells lining the CSF compartment, which releases proteins into the CSF. This elevates CSF oncotic pressure and retards reabsorption (while also hastening CSF formation if the damage is in ventricle walls). Increased CSF proteins from this or other causes can provoke or exacerbate a condition of excess CSF called hydrocephalus. If at any time the arachnoid villi become blocked or the flow of CSF is otherwise disrupted, hydrocephalus occurs.

Because the CSF is formed in the ventricles and must travel through the subarachnoid space to be reabsorbed, any impediment to its flow impairs its absorption. The aqueduct of Sylvius or the foramina in the roof of the fourth ventricle may become clogged by adhesions from an infection (meningitis), clots from a subarachnoid hemorrhage, a tumor, or a congenital abnormality. This produces an obstructive hydrocephalus with increased pressure in the CSF. Communicating hydrocephalus, caused by infection or subarachnoid hemorrhage, occurs when CSF cannot be reabsorbed by the arachnoid villi.

## Cerebral Vasculature

Because the brain requires a continuous supply of oxygen and glucose to survive, it receives about 20% of the cardiac output at a rate of approximately 750 mL/min. Two major sets of vessels supply the brain with blood: the two internal carotid arteries and the two vertebral arteries. The left common carotid artery arises from the aortic arch, and the right common carotid artery is formed from the bifurcation of the short brachiocephalic trunk, which arises from the aorta. Each carotid artery bifurcates to form the internal and external carotid arteries. The internal carotid arteries supply most of the cerebrum and upper portion of the diencephalon, and the external carotid artery supplies the face and scalp.

The vertebral arteries arise from the subclavian arteries. After entering the foramen magnum, the vertebral arteries join to form the basilar artery, which sends branches to the cerebellum, brainstem, and posterior diencephalon. The basilar artery joins the circle of Willis by bifurcating to form the two posterior cerebral arteries.

The circle of Willis, located in the subarachnoid space, is the area in which the branches of the basilar and internal carotid arteries unite (Fig. 32-8). This area is composed of the two anterior cerebral arteries, the anterior communicating artery, the two posterior cerebral arteries, and the two posterior communicating arteries. These arteries send branches to supply the various lobes of the cerebral cortex. This circular network permits blood to circulate from one hemisphere to the other and from the anterior to the posterior areas of the brain. The anterior circulation consists of the middle and anterior cerebral arteries and one anterior communicating cerebral artery. The posterior circulation consists of posterior and posterior communicating cerebral arteries and one basilar artery. This system allows for collateral circulation if one vessel is occluded.

It is not unusual for a vessel in the circle of Willis to be atrophic or even absent. This accounts for different clinical presentations among patients with the same lesion. For example, a person with an occluded carotid artery and a fully patent circle of Willis may be totally asymptomatic, but a patient in whom the circle of Willis is incomplete may demonstrate a massive cerebral infarction.

## Brain

The basic anatomy of the brain is illustrated in Figure 32-9. The parts of the brain, in descending order, are the cerebral hemispheres (the cerebrum), diencephalon, midbrain, pons varolii (usually called the pons), medulla oblongata (usually called the medulla), and cerebellum.[2] The general appearance of the brain can be viewed as a stem extending upward from the spinal cord with an inferior small flowering overgrowth (cerebellum) covering the lower part of the stem and a large superior flowering overgrowth (cerebrum) covering most of the upper portion of the stem. The medulla, pons, and midbrain compose the brainstem.

## Cerebrum

Each of the two cerebral hemispheres (left and right) has a layer of cortex covering the surface. This cortical layer consists of several different types of neurons with accompanying neuroglia arranged in six distinctive layers according to cell type and function. Some of these neurons project myelinated axons deeper into the cortex with ultimate destinations lower in the CNS or in the opposite cortex. Areas of myelinated axons appear as white matter. Gray matter is made up of nerve cell bodies that are vascular in nature and have a gray appearance. Deep within each hemisphere is a lateral ventricle containing CSF, along with several collections of nerve cell bodies, termed the basal ganglia. The left and right hemispheres are connected and communicate with each other by a transverse band of white matter termed the corpus callosum, formed by myelinated axons traveling between each side of the cortex. For the most part, each hemisphere serves the contralateral side of the body (fibers cross over in the CNS). However, one notable exception is Broca's speech area. This area of the cortex subserves all motor speech functions and is located in a posterolateral area of the left frontal lobe for all right-handed and most left-handed people. Damage to this area in an adult produces motor dysphasia, which includes dysarthria (difficulty with spoken words) and dysgraphia (difficulty with written words).

Each hemisphere has four lobes that are named for the skull bones that cover them: frontal, parietal, temporal, and occipital. Primary functions of each lobe are as follows. The

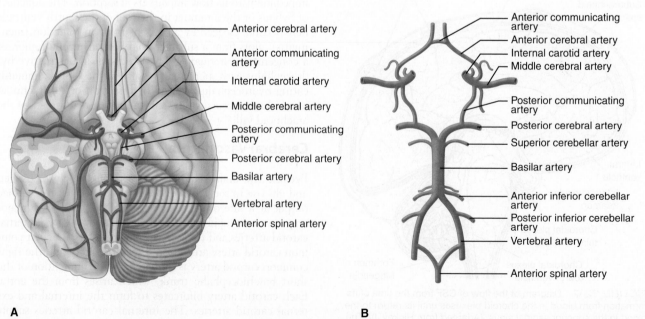

**A**

Anterior cerebral artery

Anterior communicating artery

Internal carotid artery

Middle cerebral artery

Posterior communicating artery

Posterior cerebral artery

Basilar artery

Vertebral artery

Anterior spinal artery

**B**

Anterior communicating artery

Anterior cerebral artery

Internal carotid artery

Middle cerebral artery

Posterior communicating artery

Posterior cerebral artery

Superior cerebellar artery

Basilar artery

Anterior inferior cerebellar artery

Posterior inferior cerebellar artery

Vertebral artery

Anterior spinal artery

**FIGURE 32-8** Circle of Willis (arterial blood supply to the brain). **A:** The circle of Willis seen from below the brain. **B:** Schematic of the circle of Willis.

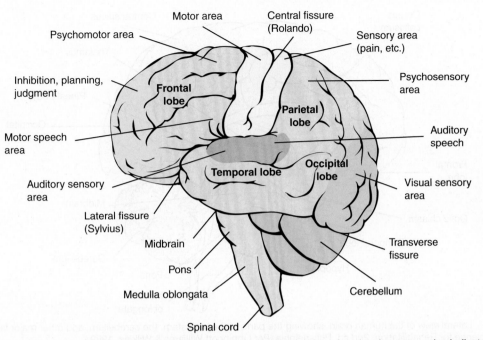

Psychomotor area

Motor area

Central fissure (Rolando)

Sensory area (pain, etc.)

Inhibition, planning, judgment

**Frontal lobe**

Psychosensory area

**Parietal lobe**

Motor speech area

Auditory speech

**Temporal lobe**

**Occipital lobe**

Auditory sensory area

Visual sensory area

Lateral fissure (Sylvius)

Midbrain

Pons

Transverse fissure

Medulla oblongata

Cerebellum

Spinal cord

FIGURE 32-9  The human brain, showing the lobes and fissures of the cerebrum. Major functional areas are also indicated. The cortex is composed of the frontal lobe, the parietal lobe, the temporal lobe, and the occipital lobe.

frontal lobes perform high-level cognition, memory, and voluntary motor movement. The parietal lobes deal mostly with sensation. The temporal lobes are primarily responsible for a variety of sensory functions such as learning, memory, emotion, and visual stimuli. The occipital lobes primarily function to interpret.

Many areas of the cerebrum operate together to produce coordinated human function. The process of communication provides a good example of this coordination. Verbal communication depends on the ability to interpret speech and translate thought into speech. Ideas are usually communicated between people by either the spoken or the written word. With the spoken word, the input of sensory information occurs through the primary auditory cortex. In auditory association areas, the sounds are interpreted as words and the words as sentences. These sentences are then interpreted by a common integrative area of the cortex as thoughts.

The common integrative area also develops thoughts to be communicated. Letters seen by the eyes are associated with words and sentences in the visual association areas and then integrated into thought in the common integrative area. Operating in conjunction with facial regions of the somesthetic sensory area, the common integrative area initiates a series of impulses, each representing a syllable or word, and transmits them to the secondary motor area controlling the larynx and mouth. The speech center, in addition to controlling motor activity of the larynx and mouth, sends impulses to the respiratory center of the secondary motor cortex to provide appropriate breath patterns for the speech process.

## Cortex

As mentioned, the cortex is the most superficial layer of the cerebrum. It is responsible for all higher mental

functions, such as judgment, language, memory, creativity, and abstract thinking. It also functions in the perception, localization, and interpretation of all sensations and governs all voluntary motor activities (see Fig. 32-9). Various areas of the cortex have been identified as having different motor and sensory functions, but some of these areas are being implicated in other functions as well. For example, the occipital area, which usually takes sensory impulses from the eyes and integrates them into visual images, is now known to function in some learning processes of blind people.

## Basal Ganglia

The basal ganglia function in cooperation with other lower brain parts in providing circuitry for basic and subconscious bodily movements. They provide the necessary background muscle tone for discrete voluntary movements, smoothness and coordination in functions of muscle antagonists, and the basic automatic subconscious rhythmic movements involved in walking and balance. Lesions of the basal ganglia produce various clinical abnormalities, such as chorea, hemiballismus, and Parkinson's disease.

## Diencephalon

The diencephalon, a major division of the cerebrum, lies below the cerebral hemispheres. The diencephalon is a paired structure on each side of the third ventricle, directly above the brainstem. The most important areas of the diencephalon are the thalamus and the hypothalamus, described in the following sections. The subthalamus is the ventral portion of the thalamus, and the epithalamus is an area that contains the pineal gland, thought to play an important role in diurnal rhythms (Fig. 32-10).

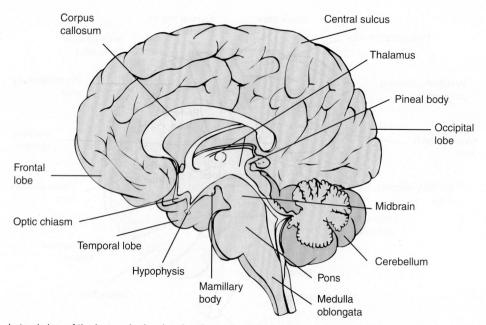

**FIGURE 32-10**  Lateral view of the human brain, showing the parts of the brainstem, the cerebellum, and other major landmarks. (From Cohen H: Neuroscience for Rehabilitation, 2nd ed. Philadelphia, PA: Lippincott Williams & Wilkins, 1999.)

## Thalamus

The thalamus (see Fig. 32-10) functions as a sensory and motor relay center. Its neurons receive sensory impulses from synapsing neurons that originate at lower levels in the spinal cord or brainstem and relay sensory input, including sight, sound, and touch, to the sensory cortex. The thalamus also functions in the gross awareness of certain sensations, most notably pain. Discrete localization and the finer perceptual details of sensations are cortical functions, but awareness occurs at the thalamic and even midbrain areas. Finally, the thalamus is involved in the reticular activating system (RAS), the neural system that promotes wakefulness and consciousness and possibly some aspects of attention.

## Hypothalamus

The hypothalamus is the seat of neuroendocrine interaction. It has a part in controlling visceral, autonomic, endocrine, and emotional function. It is connected to the reticular formation of the brainstem as well as the diencephalon, the cortex, and the pituitary gland. This area of the brain also contains some of the centers for coordinated parasympathetic and sympathetic stimulation, as well as those for temperature regulation, appetite regulation, regulation of water balance by antidiuretic hormone (ADH), and regulation of certain rhythmic psychobiologic activities (eg, sleep).

## Brainstem

A major subdivision of the brain, the brainstem consists of the midbrain, pons, and medulla and contains respiratory and autonomic control centers, as well as many tracts of myelinated motor axons that are passing through on their way down to the spinal cord or sensory axons passing through on their way up to the thalamus. In addition, areas of the brainstem are important in coordinating activity of the cerebellum with the rest of the brain. Also, 10 of the 12 cranial nerves originate from this area (Fig. 32-11).

## Midbrain

The midbrain lies between the diencephalon and the pons. It contains the aqueduct of Sylvius, many ascending and descending nerve fiber tracts (white matter), and centers for auditory and visually stimulated nerve impulses. The Edinger–Westphal nucleus in the midbrain contains the autonomic reflex centers for pupillary accommodations to light. It receives sensory fibers from the retina through cranial nerve II and sends motor impulses by way of sympathetic and parasympathetic fibers (cranial nerve III) to the smooth muscles of the iris. Impaired pupillary accommodation means that at least one of these inputs or outputs is damaged or that the midbrain is suffering insult (often from tentorial herniation or stroke). Cranial nerve IV also originates in the midbrain.

## Pons

The pons lies between the midbrain and the medulla and has cell bodies of fibers contained in cranial nerves V, VI, VII, and VIII. It contains respiratory centers and fiber tracts connecting higher and lower centers, including the cerebellum.

## Medulla Oblongata

The medulla lies between the pons and the spinal cord. It contains centers that regulate vital functions, such as breathing, heart rate, and vasomotor tone, as well as centers for swallowing, vomiting, gagging, coughing, and sneezing reflex behaviors. It also contains the fourth ventricle. Cranial nerves IX, X, XI, and XII originate in the medulla. Impairment of any of the vital functions or reflexes involving these cranial nerves suggests medullary damage.

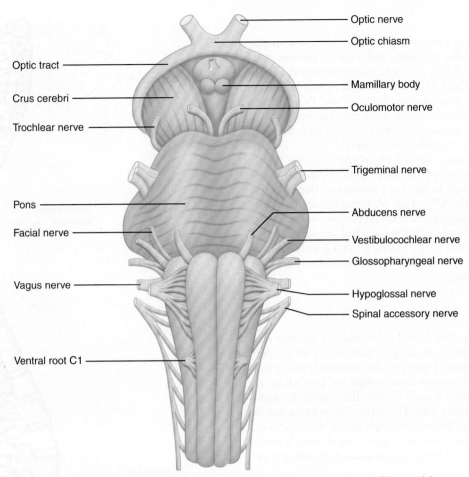

**FIGURE 32-11**    Anterior surface of the brainstem, showing the emergence and entrance of most of the cranial nerves.

## Functionally Integrated Brainstem Systems

Four networks of neurons in the brainstem should be mentioned. They are the integrated systems responsible for posture and equilibrium, consciousness, emotional reactions, and sleep.[3]

### Bulboreticular Formation

The bulboreticular formation is a network of neurons in the brainstem that helps maintain balance and erect posture. This area receives sensory information from a variety of sources, including the peripheral sensory receptors that are relayed from the spinal cord, the cerebellum, the inner ear vestibular apparatus, the motor cortex, and the basal ganglia. Therefore, the bulboreticular formation is an integrative network for sensory information and motor information that has to do with body posture and balance. Output from the bulboreticular formation travels down descending fibers to internuncial neurons in the spinal cord, which synapse with motor neurons. This output alters the tonus of muscles maintaining balance and erect posture and positions of major body parts (trunk, appendages) necessary for the performance of discrete actions (eg, writing at a table, walking).

### Reticular Activating System

The RAS is an ascending nerve fiber system originating in the midbrain and thalamus. The RAS is stimulated by sensory impulses from various sources. These include input from the optic and acoustic cranial nerves, somesthetic impulses from the dorsal column and spinothalamic pathways, and fibers from the cortex. Therefore, the RAS is an integrative system that receives sensory information concerning light, sound, and touch that may indicate a need for alertness. Excitatory output of the RAS extends to a variety of higher centers, including the cortex. In this way, the RAS can stimulate these centers to maintain alertness. The stimulation of the cortex by the RAS seems to be the major physiologic basis for consciousness, alertness, and attention to various environmental stimuli. Decreased activity of the RAS produces decreased alertness or levels of consciousness, including stupor and coma. Inactivation of the RAS can result from anything that interrupts the entry of a critical amount of sensory input or from any damage that prevents the RAS fibers from sending impulses to the cortex.

### Limbic System

The hypothalamus, the cingulate gyrus of the cortex, the amygdala and hippocampus in the temporal lobes, and the septum and interconnecting nerve fiber tracts among these areas compose a functional unit of the brain called the limbic system. This system provides a neural substrate for emotions (eg, terror, intense pleasure, eroticism). This region of the brain is involved in emotional experience and in the control of emotion-related behavior. Also, it is here that neural pathways provide a connection between higher brain functioning and endocrine or autonomic activities.

### Sleep Centers

The release of stored serotonin from axon terminals in the diencephalon, medulla, thalamus, and a small forebrain area, collectively called DMTF, results in inactivation of the RAS and activation of the DMTF. DMTF activity results in the four stages of sleep. During sleep stages III and IV, parasympathetic activity (with decreased heart rate, respiratory rate, and so forth) predominates, and this is when sleepwalking, sleep talking, and nocturnal enuresis occur.

Rhythmic discharges (about four to eight times per night, from 10 to 20 minutes per episode) from the pontine nuclei during sleep result in rapid eye movement sleep, during which approximately 80% of all dreaming occurs and sympathetic nervous system activity predominates. Based on circadian rhythmicity and decreasing cerebral serotonin levels, the RAS is reactivated in the morning, after 6 to 8 hours of sleep. See Chapter 2, Box 2-2 for a review of the stages and characteristics of sleep.

## Cerebellum

The cerebellum (see Fig. 32-10) is located just superior and posterior to the medulla. It receives "samples" of all ascending somesthetic sensory input and all descending motor impulses. Use of these connections enables the cerebellum to match intended motor stimuli (before they reach the muscles) with actual sensory data. This ensures an optimal match for voluntary motor "intention" with actual motor action, with time to alter the motor message in case of error. It sends its own messages to the basal ganglia and cortex and to parts of the brainstem.

The cerebellum functions to produce smooth, steady, harmonious, and coordinated skeletal muscle actions; maintain equilibrium; and control posture without any jerky or uncompensated movements or swaying. The cerebellum is also involved in motor learning and is responsible for reflexive activities that occur when motor learning is complete, such as correcting one's balance when riding a bike. Cerebellar disease can produce typical symptoms, the most prominent of which are disturbances of gait, equilibrium ataxia (overstability or understability of the walk), inability to perform rapid repetitive movements, and characteristic intention tremors.

## Spinal Cord

The spinal cord lies within the neural canal of the vertebral column for protection from traumatic injury. The bony structures of the spine, along with those of the skull, are one mechanism for protection of the delicate structures of the CNS (see Figs. 32-5 and 32-12). The vertebral column of the spine is composed of 33 vertebrae: 7 cervical, 12 thoracic, 5 lumbar, 5 sacral (fused into one), and 4 coccygeal (fused into one). Each vertebra is composed of two essential parts, an anterior body and a posterior arch, which form a protective ring (vertebral foramen) around the spinal cord. The arch has two pedicles and two laminae to support seven processes (four articular, two transverse, and one spinous), on which muscles and ligaments can attach (Fig. 32-13). The first cervical vertebra, the atlas, supports the weight of the head by articulating with the occiput of the skull. The second cervical vertebra, the axis, has a perpendicular projection called

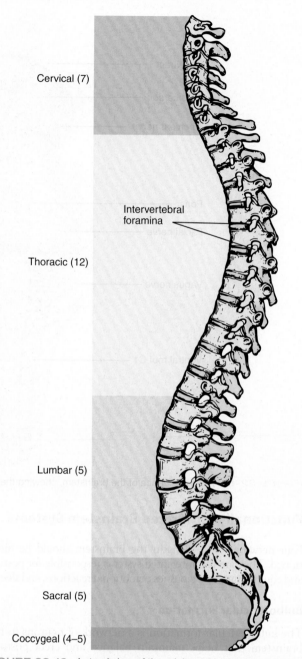

**FIGURE 32-12** Lateral view of the adult vertebral column. (From Hickey JV: The Clinical Practice of Neurological and Neurosurgical Nursing, 6th ed. Philadelphia, PA: Lippincott Williams & Wilkins, 2009, p 48.)

Cervical (7)

Intervertebral foramina

Thoracic (12)

Lumbar (5)

Sacral (5)

Coccygeal (4–5)

the odontoid process that the atlas sits on; this allows for lateral rotation of the head (Fig. 32-14).

In addition to the bony structures of the spinal column, ligaments and the intervertebral disks also protect the spinal cord by providing support and stability to the vertebral column. The anterior longitudinal ligament and the posterior longitudinal ligament hold the disks and vertebral bodies in position. The intervertebral disks are fibrocartilaginous, disk-shaped structures located between the vertebral bodies from the second cervical vertebra to the sacrum. These disks, which act as shock absorbers between the vertebrae, have a central core known as the nucleus pulposus surrounded by a fibrous capsule known as the anulus fibrosus (Fig. 32-15).

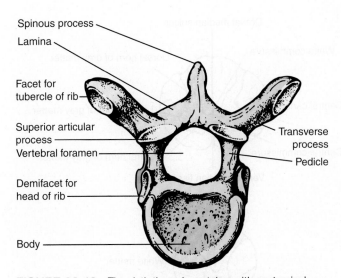

FIGURE 32-13 The sixth thoracic vertebra with anatomical markings. The vertebral foramen is the site of the spinal cord, and the spinous and transverse processes serve as places for attachments for muscles. The articular processes form synovial joints between the vertebrae. The vertebral body is opposed to superior and inferior intervertebral disks. (From Hickey JV: The Clinical Practice of Neurological and Neurosurgical Nursing, 6th ed. Philadelphia, PA: Lippincott Williams & Wilkins, 2009, p 416.)

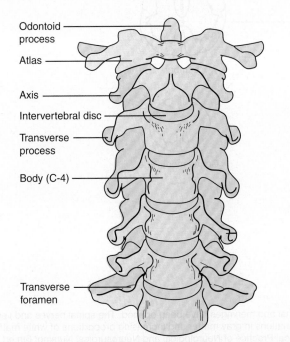

FIGURE 32-14 The cervical spine. Note odontoid process of C2 and the atlas, C1, positioned on top of C2. (Adapted from Hickey JV: The Clinical Practice of Neurological and Neurosurgical Nursing, 6th ed. Philadelphia, PA: Lippincott Williams & Wilkins, 2009, p 50.)

The spinal cord extends down and fills the neural canal to the level of about the second lumbar vertebra in an adult. Over the entire length of the vertebral column, a pair of spinal nerves exits between adjacent vertebrae at its respective level (eg, C5, T11, L1, S1). However, because the cord is shorter than the spinal column, the level of the cord that gives rise to a particular pair of spinal nerves is above the vertebra of that level. For instance, the two spinal nerves

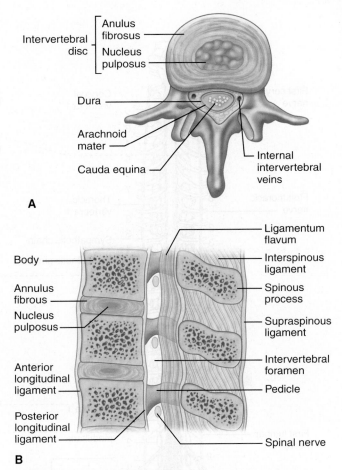

FIGURE 32-15 **A:** Third lumbar vertebra seen from above, showing the intervertebral disk. **B:** Sagittal section through three lumbar vertebrae, showing the ligaments and the intervertebral disks. (Adapted from Hickey JV: The Clinical Practice of Neurological and Neurosurgical Nursing, 6th ed. Philadelphia, PA: Lippincott Williams & Wilkins, 2009, p 49.)

that leave the spinal column between the L4 and L5 vertebrae have to travel down the neural canal from the cord level L4, which is actually up at about vertebral level T12. Below the point at which the cord terminates, the neural canal is filled with descending spinal nerves collectively known as the cauda equina (horse's tail), which exit the neural canal at the vertebra that corresponds to the cord level from which they arose (Fig. 32-16). Because neurons occupy less space in the canal at lower lumbar levels, it is here that spinal taps may be performed safely. This anatomical fact also explains why injuries to lumbar and lower thoracic vertebrae can produce impairment at disproportionately lower body levels.

Within the cord lie ascending sensory fibers and descending motor fibers, many of which are myelinated and appear as white matter. Interneurons, and the nerve cell bodies and dendrites of the second-order somatic (voluntary) and first-order autonomic motor neurons, are not myelinated and appear as gray matter. The central area of the cord contains nerve cell bodies and internuncial neurons (ie, nerve cells contained entirely within the cord) and also appears as gray matter. The gray matter has left and right dorsal and ventral projections (Fig. 32-17). Nerve cell bodies of motor neurons supplying skeletal muscles lie in the ventral horns. Nerve cell

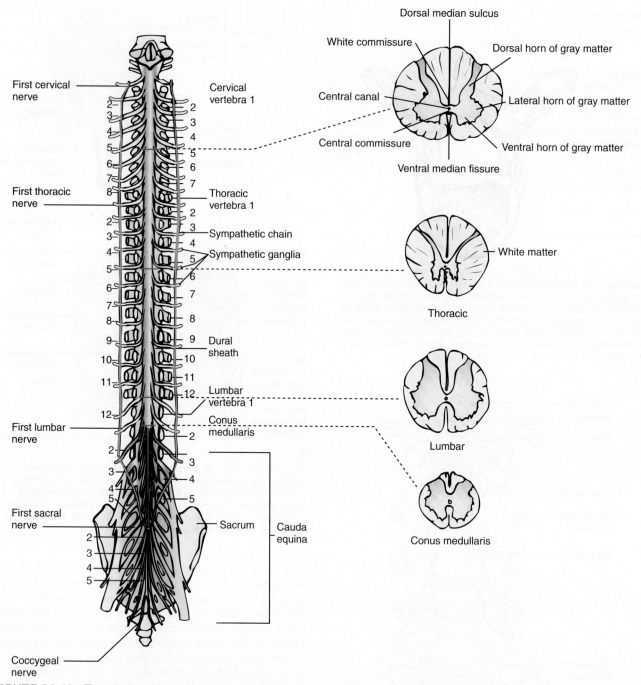

First cervical nerve

Cervical vertebra 1

First thoracic nerve

Thoracic vertebra 1

Sympathetic chain

Sympathetic ganglia

Dural sheath

Lumbar vertebra 1

First lumbar nerve

Conus medullaris

First sacral nerve

Sacrum

Cauda equina

Coccygeal nerve

Dorsal median sulcus

White commissure

Central canal

Central commissure

Ventral median fissure

Dorsal horn of gray matter

Lateral horn of gray matter

Ventral horn of gray matter

White matter

Thoracic

Lumbar

Conus medullaris

**FIGURE 32-16** The spinal cord within the vertebral canal. The spinal canal and meninges have been opened. The spinal nerves and vertebrae are numbered on the left. Cross (transverse) sections with regional variations in gray matter and increasing proportions of white matter as the cord ascends appear on the right. (Adapted from Hickey JV: The Clinical Practice of Neurological and Neurosurgical Nursing, 6th ed. Philadelphia, PA: Lippincott Williams & Wilkins, 2009, p 69.)

bodies of the sympathetic preganglionic neurons lie in left and right lateral projections or horns of gray matter referred to as the intermediolateral cell column in the thoracic and upper lumbar cord.

It is important to realize that the spinal cord is really an extension of the brain and contains many integrative and processive functions. For instance, the substantia gelatinosa contains nerve terminals of descending neurons, and also interneurons, which function to moderate ascending pain impulses (see later section on Pain, pp. 25–27).

## Peripheral Nervous System

The PNS consists of 12 pairs of cranial nerves and 31 pairs of spinal nerves and includes all neural structures lying outside the pia mater of the spinal cord and brainstem. The parts of the PNS inside the neural canal and attached to the ventral and dorsal surfaces of the cord are called the spinal nerve roots. Those attached to the ventrolateral surface of the brainstem are the cranial nerve roots.

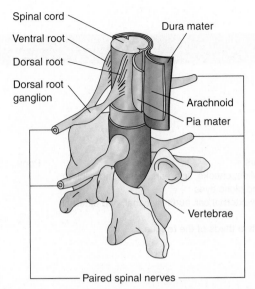

Spinal cord

Ventral root

Dorsal root

Dorsal root
ganglion

Dura mater

Arachnoid

Pia mater

Vertebrae

Paired spinal nerves

**FIGURE 32-17** Spinal cord and meninges. (From Porth CM: Pathophysiology: Concepts of Altered Health States, 8th ed. Philadelphia, PA: Wolters Kluwer Health: Lippincott Williams & Wilkins, 2009, p 1211.)

Functionally, the PNS is separated into sensory and motor divisions. The sensory division includes sensory neurons that innervate the skin, muscles, joints, and viscera and provide sensory information about the environment outside and inside the body to the CNS. The motor division includes motor neurons that innervate skeletal muscles and the autonomic nervous system (ANS) that innervates smooth and cardiac muscle and glands. The ANS is responsible for regulating the ongoing functions of many organ systems, such as blood pressure, heart rate, and gastrointestinal activity.

## Cranial Nerves

The 12 pairs of cranial nerves supply motor and sensory fibers mostly to the structures of the head, neck, and upper back, although cranial nerve X, the vagus nerve, supplies the viscera to about the level of the waist (Table 32-1). Most cranial nerves originate in the brainstem (see Fig. 32-11), except cranial nerves I and II, which originate in the diencephalon. Cranial nerves are classified as either sensory, motor, or mixed (carrying both sensory and motor signals). They bring input from the special senses (vision, hearing, smell)

**TABLE 32-1  The Cranial Nerves**

| Cranial Nerve | Tract(s) | Function | Location of Origin |
|---|---|---|---|
| I. Olfactory | Sensory | Sense of smell | Diencephalon |
| II. Optic | Sensory | Vision | Diencephalon |
| III. Oculomotor | Parasympathetic | Pupillary constriction | Midbrain |
|  | Motor | Elevation of upper eyelid and four of six extraocular movements |  |
| IV. Trochlear | Motor | Downward, inward movement of the eye (superior oblique) | Midbrain |
| V. Trigeminal | Motor | Muscles of mastication and opening jaw | Pons |
|  | Sensory | Tactile sensation to the cornea, nasal and oral mucosa, and facial skin |  |
| VI. Abducens | Motor | Lateral deviation of eye (lateral rectus) | Pons |

(continued)

**TABLE 32-1** **The Cranial Nerves** (*continued*)

| Cranial Nerve | Tract(s) | Function | Location of Origin |
|---|---|---|---|
| 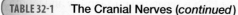 VII. Facial | Parasympathetic | Secretory for salivation and tears | Pons |
| | Motor | Movement of the forehead, eyelids, cheeks, lips, ears, nose, and neck to produce facial expression and close eyes | |
| | Sensory | Tactile sensation to parts of the external ear, auditory canal, and external tympanic membrane | |
| | | Taste sensation to the anterior two thirds of the tongue | |
| VIII. Vestibulocochlear (also known as acoustic or cochlear) | Sensory | *Vestibular branch:* Equilibrium *Cochlear branch:* Hearing | Pons |
| IX. Glossopharyngeal | Parasympathetic | Salivation | Medulla |
| | Motor | Voluntary muscles for swallowing and phonation | |
| | Sensory | Sensation to pharynx, soft palate, and posterior one third of tongue | |
| | | Stimulation elicits gag reflex | |
| X. Vagus | Parasympathetic | Autonomic activity of viscera of thorax and abdomen | Medulla |
| | Motor | Involuntary activity of visceral muscles of the heart, lungs, and digestive tract | |
| | | Innervation of striated muscles of the soft palate, pharynx, and larynx for voluntary swallowing | |
| | Sensory | Sensation to the auditory canal, pharynx, larynx, and viscera of the thorax and abdomen | |
| XI. Spinal accessory | Motor | Sternocleidomastoid and trapezius muscle movements | Medulla |
| XII. Hypoglossal | Motor | Tongue movements | Medulla |

Artwork from Evans MJ: Neurologic Neurosurgical Nursing, 2nd ed. Springhouse, PA: Springhouse, 1995, pp 7–8.

and somatic sensory input from the face and head into the brain. They also send motor commands out to the muscles and glands of the head and neck to control facial expression, eye movements, movements of the structures in the mouth and throat, movements of the head and neck, and autonomic functions of the eyes, salivary glands, and viscera in the chest and upper abdomen. Most cranial nerves contain fibers of more than one functional type; thus, most cranial nerves are associated with more than one nucleus in the brainstem (see Table 32-1).

## Spinal Nerves

Spinal nerves are attached to the spinal cord in pairs; there are 8 cervical, 12 thoracic, 5 lumbar, 5 sacral, and 1 coccygeal pair of spinal nerves (see Fig. 32-16). In the cervical spine, the spinal nerves exit above the vertebrae. At C7, an extra spinal nerve exists below C7, giving rise to the C8 spinal nerve. All of the rest of the spinal nerves (ie, the thoracic, lumbar, sacral, and coccygeal spinal nerves) exit below the vertebrae. Spinal nerves contain both sensory and motor fibers. Each spinal nerve attaches to the cord by a dorsal and a ventral root. The dorsal root houses the nerve cell bodies of sensory neurons. Motor axons, whose nerve cell bodies lie in the gray matter of the ventral horn of the cord, traverse the ventral root. Thus, damage to the dorsal root may impair sensory function without impairing motor function, and vice versa. However, a spinal nerve injury distal to the roots could damage both sensory and motor functioning. A dermatome is the area of skin innervated by sensory fibers from a particular spinal nerve emanating from a particular segment of the spinal cord (see Chapter 37, Fig. 37-3).

## Sensory Division

The sensory division of the nervous system is composed of sensory receptors, sensory neurons whose axons form sensory pathways, and perceptive areas of the brain.

### Sensations and Sensory Receptors

Sensations are often divided into the special senses (eg, vision, hearing, and smell) and those termed somesthetic sensations (eg, pain, touch, and stretch). In this section, only somesthetic sensations are discussed. Such sensations provide information about, for example, body position and conditions of the external and internal environment. These are called proprioceptive, exteroceptive, and visceral sensations, respectively.

Proprioceptive sensations describe the physical position state of the body, such as muscle tension, joint flexion or extension, tendon tension, and deep pressure in dependent parts, such as the feet while one is standing or the buttocks while one is sitting. Exteroceptive sensations monitor conditions on the body surface, such as temperature and pain.

Visceral sensations are similar to exteroceptive sensations, except that they originate from within the body and monitor pain, pressure, and fullness from internal organs.

The sensory receptors for somesthetic sensations are basically dendrites, which can have the form of free nerve endings or specialized receptors. Free nerve endings are nothing more than small, filamentous branches of dendrites. They detect crude sensations of touch, pain, heat, and cold. The precision is crude because different neurons have overlapping distributions of their dendrites. These nerve endings are the most widely distributed and most numerous of sensory receptors and perform the general discriminatory functions. The more specialized sensory receptors discriminate between very slight differences in degrees of touch, pain, heat, and cold. Indeed, the special exteroceptive end organs for detecting light touch, warmth, and cold differ structurally from one another and are specific in their function. The physiologic

basis for this specific function has not been determined but is presumed to be based on some specific physical effect on the receptor itself.

Sensation from the internal organs may come from specialized sensory receptors, such as baroreceptors and chemoreceptors that reside in arterial walls, or stretch receptors in sphincters. In contrast, visceral pain is the result of stimulation of unmyelinated, raw sensory nerve endings, usually by stretch, as might happen during swelling or distention, or by pressure on the organ as might happen from compression by a tumor. For both specialized and unspecialized visceral receptors, the sensory fibers run within the autonomic nerves (sympathetic or parasympathetic) back to CNS centers that are closely associated with autonomic motor responses. For this reason, these sensory fibers are sometimes referred to as autonomic afferent fibers. This is a somewhat misleading name because the ANS is purely a motor system (see later), and the name refers only to the anatomical location of sensory fibers within the nerves that also carry autonomic motor fibers.

Stimulation of a sensory receptor initiates an electrical charge (generator potential) that depolarizes the sensory dendrite, causing a series of nerve impulses to travel along the sensory dendrite to the cell body. As mentioned, the sensory neuron cell body is contained in the dorsal root ganglion just outside the spinal cord. The sensory neuron sends axons into the spinal cord (or brain in the case of cranial nerves), where it synapses with projection neurons in either brain or spinal cord that carry impulses to the appropriate centers in the brain, including the thalamus, where the sensation finally may be perceived consciously. The projection neuron may synapse in the thalamus with another neuron, which relays the sensory impulse to the sensory cortex.

When the sensation first stimulates the sensory receptor in the periphery, there is a burst of impulses; if the stimulus persists, the frequency of impulses transmitted begins to decrease. All sensory receptors show this phenomenon of adaptation to varying degrees and at different rates. Adaptations to light touch and pressure occur in a few seconds, whereas pain and proprioceptive sensations adapt very little, if at all, and at a very slow rate. This adaptation results in our being unaware of the touch of our clothing to our skin or the pressure on our buttocks while we are seated. Determination of the intensity of the sensation is made on a relative rather than an absolute basis.

Although there are structurally different receptors for detecting each type of sensation, the area of the brain to which the information is transmitted determines the modality, or type of sensation, a person feels. The thalamus and sensory cortex operate together to attribute various sensory qualities and intensities to nerve impulse information they receive.

### Sensory Pathways

As mentioned, sensory neurons that enter the cord synapse with projection neurons that carry the sensory information up the spinal cord. There are a number of pathways by which sensory information is transmitted up the cord by axons of the projection neurons. Depending on the type of somesthetic receptor involved, fibers of sensory neurons may, on entering the cord, do one of three things.

First, they may send axons up the cord to the medulla on the same side of the body as the sensory receptor. This tract of myelinated axons (white matter) is called the dorsal column. In the medulla, the sensory neurons synapse with projection neurons that cross over to the opposite side of the brain and travel to the thalamus. This tract is called the medial lemniscus (Fig. 32-18). It is used for conducting impulses originating from stimulation of joint, muscle, and tendon

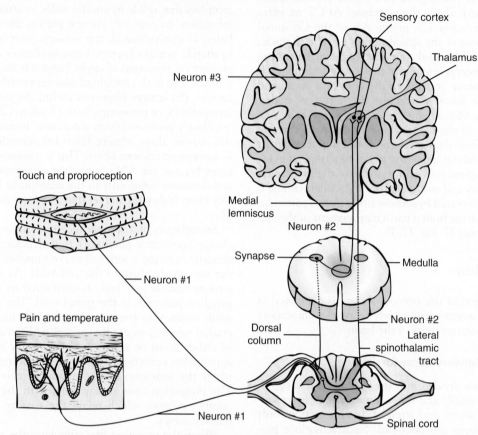

**FIGURE 32-18** Pathways of ascending tracts. Sensory neurons enter the cord at the dorsal horn. Axons of sensory neurons for touch and proprioception ascend in the dorsal columns to the medulla, where they synapse with second-order projection neurons that cross (decussate) to the opposite side before ascending to the thalamus in the tract called the medial lemniscus. First-order neurons for pain and temperature enter the dorsal gray matter of the cord, where they synapse with second-order projection neurons that cross to the opposite side and ascend in the lateral spinothalamic tract to the thalamus. Third-order neurons connect both pathways from thalamus to the sensory cortex.

| Motor system | | Peripheral nervous system | | | Effector organ (receptors) |
|---|---|---|---|---|---|
| Somatic nervous system | Spinal cord or brain | Acetylcholine | | | Skeletal muscle (nicotinic receptors) |
| Autonomic nervous system — Parasympathetic | Sacral cord or brain | Acetylcholine | Ganglion (nicotinic receptors) | Acetyl-choline | Smooth muscle, cardiac nodes, and glands (muscarinic receptors) |
| Autonomic nervous system — Sympathetic | Thoracic and high lumbar cord | Acetyl-choline | Ganglion (nicotinic receptors) | Norepinephrine | Smooth muscle, cardiac nodes and muscle, and glands ($\alpha$ or $\beta_1$ receptors) |
| | Thoracic and high lumbar cord | Acetylcholine | Adrenal medulla (nicotinic receptors) | Norepinephrine / Epinephrine | Smooth muscle, cardiac nodes and muscle, and glands ($\alpha$ or $\beta_1$, or $\beta_2$ receptors) |

**FIGURE 32-19** A comparison between the divisions of the motor systems. The somatic nervous system (*pink*) sends cholinergic motor axons from the spinal cord or brain to the skeletal muscles. Acetylcholine released from these axon terminals binds to nicotinic receptors on skeletal muscles to cause contraction. The ANS is composed of parasympathetic (*blue*) and sympathetic (*green*) divisions. For both divisions, preganglionic cholinergic neurons originate in the brain or spinal cord and send their axons to ganglia in the periphery, where they synapse with postganglionic neurons having ganglionic nicotinic receptors. Postganglionic neurons of the parasympathetic division are cholinergic and synapse with muscarinic receptors on end organs. Postganglionic neurons of the sympathetic division are noradrenergic and synapse with $\alpha$ or $\beta_1$ receptors on end organs. The adrenal medulla is innervated by preganglionic sympathetic neurons. Acetylcholine released by these neurons binds to ganglionic nicotinic receptors on cells of the adrenal medulla, causing them to release norepinephrine and epinephrine into the bloodstream.

proprioceptors; vibration-sensitive receptors; and receptors in the skin involved in precise localization of touch.

Second, the sensory neurons may synapse immediately on entering the cord with projection neurons that immediately cross over to the opposite side of the cord. Fibers from these projection neurons then travel up the white matter of the cord to the thalamus. This is called the spinothalamic pathway (see Fig. 32-18). It conducts impulses concerned with pain, temperature, poorly localized touch, and sex organ sensations. Both the dorsal column–medial lemniscus pathway and the spinothalamic pathway involve crossing of the sensory information from each side of the body to the opposite side of the CNS. Therefore, sensations on each side of the body are perceived by the thalamus and sensory cortex on the opposite side. In the thalamus, neurons of both the dorsal column pathway and the spinothalamic pathway synapse with other neurons that transmit impulses to the appropriate area of the sensory cortex. Because of their final destination in the cortex, impulses from either pathway give rise to consciously perceived sensations.

Third, certain sensory neurons may synapse with a projection neuron belonging to the spinocerebellar pathway. Spinocerebellar neurons do not cross over. They carry impulses only as far as the cerebellum (and possibly lower brainstem). This pathway carries impulses originating from stimulation of joint, muscle, and tendon proprioceptors. Because this pathway ends at the cerebellum, it transmits sensory information that is not perceived consciously. Instead, these data are used in reflex postural adjustments.

## Motor Division and the Neuromuscular Junction

The motor division comprises the areas of the brain, descending fiber tracts, and motor neurons involved in producing or altering movement or adjusting tonus of skeletal, cardiac, and smooth muscles and in regulating the secretions of the various exocrine and certain endocrine gland cells. Muscle and glandular tissues are referred to as the effector organs of this system.

The motor division can be divided on the basis of motor neurons and effector organs into somatic and autonomic subdivisions (Fig. 32-19). The former involves skeletal muscles and the motor neurons innervating them. The latter is composed of smooth muscle, cardiac muscle, and gland cells plus the sympathetic and parasympathetic fibers innervating them.

### Somatic Motor Division

Figure 32-20 depicts the major descending fiber tracts from motor areas of the cortex. The most prominent of these tracts is the corticospinal tract, often called the pyramidal tract because it originates from pyramid-shaped nerve cell bodies in the cortex. The corticospinal tract is heavily myelinated and appears as white matter in the brain and spinal cord. The fibers cross to the opposite side in an area of the medulla referred to as the decussation (crossing over) of the pyramids. Several other motor tracts originate in the cortex or in the cerebellum. These tracts may cross over in the brain or in cord centers. Motor fibers from the brain ultimately stimulate

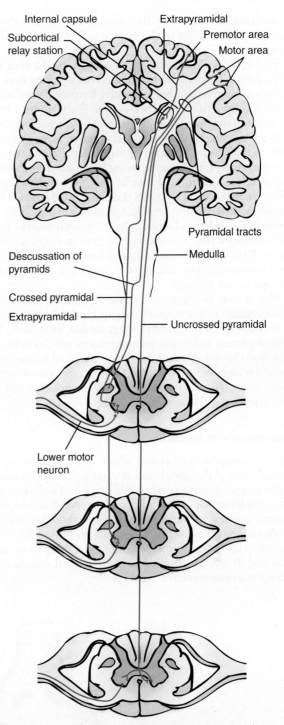

**FIGURE 32-20** Diagram of motor pathways between the cerebral cortex, one of the subcortical relay centers, and lower motor neurons in the spinal cord. Decussation (crossing) of fibers dictates that each side of the brain controls skeletal muscles on the opposite side of the body.

somatic motor neurons, the nerve cell bodies of which lie in the anterior (ventral) horn of the gray matter in the cord. The axons of these motor neurons travel within spinal nerves and terminate at the neuromuscular junction, the synapse between the somatic motor neuron axon and the muscle cell. When a motor neuron depolarizes, acetylcholine is released into the synapse at the neuromuscular junction. It binds to nicotinic receptors on the skeletal muscle membrane, causing depolarization of the muscle cell, which stimulates contraction.

Figure 32-20 also shows several extrapyramidal (not part of the pyramidal [corticospinal] tracts) tracts arising from the brainstem centers (eg, bulboreticular formation, midbrain). Some of these cross over; others do not. Fibers in these tracts descend the cord and ultimately stimulate either somatic motor neurons, which stimulate skeletal muscle contraction, or other motor neurons (gamma efferent) that alter the tensions of stretch receptor organelles (muscle spindles) in the skeletal muscles. Alteration of spindle tension provokes a spinal reflex arc that efficiently alters skeletal muscle tonus. These extrapyramidal pathways conduct impulses that produce the automatic coordinated alterations in skeletal muscle tonus and movement that are necessary for gross motor movements (eg, walking) and for appropriate posture for conduction of finer movements (eg, sitting at a desk with arm flexed in preparation for writing).

Not shown in Figure 32-20 are descending fiber tracts that stimulate motor neurons responsible for the movement of skeletal muscles of the head (eg, tongue, face, jaw). The general pattern and myoneural transmitter are the same, except that the somatic motor neuron nerve cell bodies lie in particular areas of the brain and exit through cranial nerves. These fibers must also cross over from the opposite side before synapsing with the motor neurons.

## Neuromuscular Junction

As mentioned, motor neurons whose cell bodies are in the ventral horn of the spinal cord at each level send axons out of the ventral root into each spinal nerve and innervate specific skeletal muscles. Similarly, cranial nerves that innervate skeletal muscles of the head, neck, and shoulders contain axons of motor neurons that originate in the nuclei of the brainstem and pons. The axon terminals of these motor neurons end in specialized synapses with skeletal muscle cells, termed the neuromuscular junction.

Motor neurons may innervate several muscle fibers. The combination of axon terminals and the corresponding muscle fibers innervated by one motor neuron is referred to as a motor unit. The axon terminals reach into invaginations on the skeletal muscle fiber, called motor end plates, and form the highly structured synapses that compose the neuromuscular junctions (Fig. 32-21). The cell membrane of the skeletal muscle contains abundant nicotinic skeletal muscle receptors concentrated in the area of the motor end plate. These receptors bind acetylcholine, which is released from the motor neuron in response to an arriving action potential. These nicotinic receptors are slightly different from those located at ganglionic synapses of the ANS, making it possible to design drugs that bind only to skeletal muscle nicotinic receptors, not ganglionic ones. These drugs, such as cisatracurium and vecuronium, are used for neuromuscular blockade during anesthesia or in the intensive care unit.

Also located within the neuromuscular junction, similar to other cholinergic synapses, are many molecules of acetylcholinesterase, an enzyme that degrades acetylcholine into acetate and choline with great rapidity. This enzyme is responsible for terminating the activity of acetylcholine in the synapse. Following the degradation of acetylcholine, choline is quickly taken back up into the motor nerve terminal and used to resynthesize acetylcholine. Acetate can be used for fuel by body cells by conversion to acetyl coenzyme A. Acetylcholinesterase inhibitors are drugs that can be used to prolong the activity of acetylcholine. This may be helpful, as in the reversal of neuromuscular blockade or the treatment of myasthenia gravis.

Myasthenia gravis is a disease of the neuromuscular junction in which antibodies develop to nicotinic skeletal muscle receptors (see Chapter 35). Immune attack of these receptors decreases the number available for activation by acetylcholine, rendering the muscle contraction weaker than normal. Lambert–Eaton syndrome, a similar condition prevalent in cancer patients, is due to decreased release of acetylcholine into the neuromuscular junction.

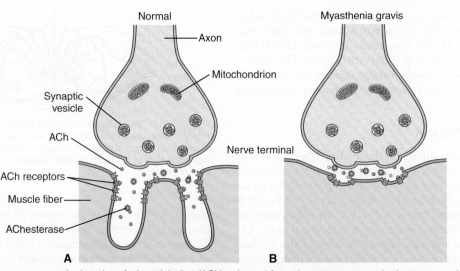

**FIGURE 32-21** The neuromuscular junction. **A:** Acetylcholine (ACh), released from the motor neurons in the myoneural junction, crosses the synaptic space to reach receptors that are concentrated in folds of the endplate of the muscle fiber. Once released, ACh is rapidly broken down by the enzyme acetylcholinesterase (AChesterase). **B:** Decrease in Ach receptors in myasthenia gravis. (From Porth CM: Essentials of Pathophysiology, 3rd ed. Philadelphia, PA: Lippincott Williams & Wilkins, 2011, p 901.)

## Autonomic Motor Division

The autonomic division contains both sympathetic and parasympathetic motor fibers. They are responsible for contraction and relaxation of smooth muscle, rate and strength of contraction of cardiac muscle, secretion by exocrine glands, and secretion by the adrenal medulla. They also influence the secretion by the islets of Langerhans in the pancreas.

The sympathetic and parasympathetic sections differ on the basis of the anatomical distribution of nerve fibers, the secretion of two different neurotransmitters by the postganglionic fibers of the two divisions, and the antagonistic effects of the two divisions on some of the organs they innervate. Figure 32-22 shows the anatomy of the sympathetic and parasympathetic nervous systems. The CNS center

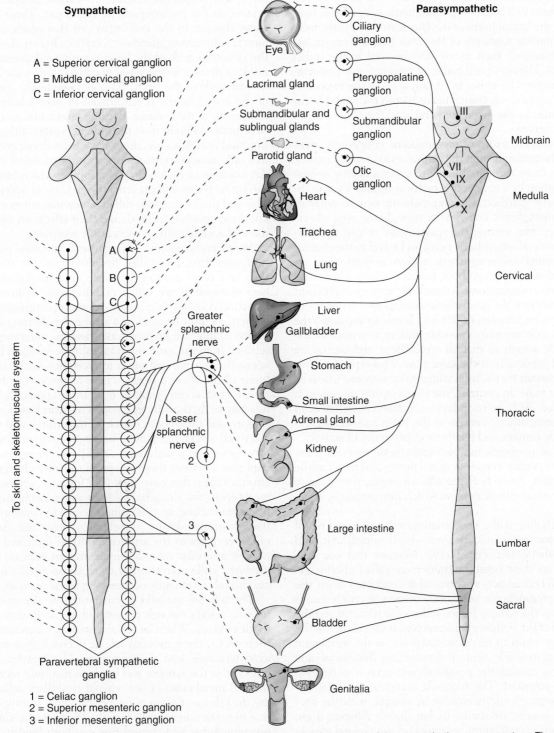

**FIGURE 32-22**  The ANS and the organs it affects. The *left side* illustrates the actions of the sympathetic nervous system. The *right side* illustrates the parasympathetic nervous system. (From Porth CM: Pathophysiology: Concepts of Altered Health States, 8th ed. Philadelphia, PA: Lippincott Williams & Wilkins, 2009.)

immediately responsible for sympathetic outflow resides in the thoracic cord. In contrast, 80% of parasympathetic activity originates in the brain and travels through cranial nerve X (the vagus nerve), and approximately 20% originates in the sacral cord and travels through pelvic nerves.

Both the sympathetic and parasympathetic motor pathways are composed of a chain of two neurons carrying nerve impulses from the CNS to the effector organ. The first neuron in the chain is the preganglionic neuron; the second is the postganglionic neuron. (A ganglion is a group of cell bodies.) Nerve cell bodies of preganglionic sympathetic neurons lie in the lateral horns of the gray matter of the thoracic and high lumbar segments of the cord (the intermediolateral cell columns); their axons exit the cord in the spinal nerve roots. The nerve cell bodies of preganglionic parasympathetic neurons lie either in certain areas of the brain and send their axons down cranial nerve X or in the lateral horns of gray matter in the sacral cord and send their axons down the pelvic nerves.

As mentioned, axons of preganglionic sympathetic neurons exit the cord and enter the ventral roots of spinal nerves. They then leave the spinal nerve to enter a nearby sympathetic ganglion by a connecting pathway termed a ramus. In a sympathetic ganglion, the preganglionic neuron synapses with a postganglionic one. The postganglionic sympathetic neuron then may reenter the spinal nerve or exit the ganglion by a special sympathetic nerve and travel to the effector organ. Preganglionic sympathetic neurons may also send axons up or down the sympathetic ganglion chain, where they synapse with postganglionic sympathetic neurons at different levels. In this way, the sympathetic nervous system maintains communication between its different levels up and down the cord. This anatomy makes possible unitary activation of the sympathetic system so that all sympathetic end organs are stimulated maximally at the same time. This type of activation is important for the total sympathetic response involved in flight or fight. In contrast, the parasympathetic system is more diffuse, with more indirect communication between vagal parasympathetic centers in the brain and sacral parasympathetic centers, and relative independence of activity.

Axons of preganglionic parasympathetic neurons leave the CNS by certain cranial or spinal nerves and travel to the effector organ. At or near the effector organ, they synapse with the postganglionic neuron, which innervates the effector organ.

Acetylcholine is the neurotransmitter synthesized by all preganglionic autonomic neurons—both sympathetic and parasympathetic (see Fig. 32-19). Neurons that use acetylcholine as their neurotransmitter are called cholinergic neurons. When an action potential is conducted down the axon of a preganglionic autonomic neuron, acetylcholine is released into the synapse between the axon terminal and the membrane of the postganglionic neuron. It diffuses across the synapse and binds to nicotinic receptors on the membrane of the postganglionic neuron, depolarizing that membrane and possibly causing the postganglionic neuron to develop an action potential. The nicotinic acetylcholine receptors on the postganglionic neuron at its synapse with the preganglionic neuron are similar to, but slightly different from, the nicotinic acetylcholine receptors on the skeletal muscle membrane at the neuromuscular junction. This is why drugs such as cisatracurium and vecuronium are able to block the

skeletal muscle nicotinic receptors without affecting ganglionic nicotinic receptors at normal doses.

Acetylcholine is also the neurotransmitter synthesized by the axons of postganglionic parasympathetic neurons (see Fig. 32-19). An action potential conducted down the axon of a postganglionic parasympathetic neuron as the result of a strong depolarizing influence received from the preganglionic neuron causes acetylcholine to be released from the axon terminal into the synapse. The acetylcholine diffuses across the synapse and binds to muscarinic acetylcholine receptors on the parasympathetic end organ. These receptors cause changes in the end-organ cell that result in smooth muscle contraction, glandular secretion, hyperpolarization of the sinoatrial node of the heart (causing a decrease in heart rate), or slowing in the speed of conduction in the atrioventricular node of the heart. As noted previously, the activity of the acetylcholine is terminated by acetylcholinesterase, an enzyme in the synapse. Because muscarinic receptors are structurally different from nicotinic receptors, although both can bind acetylcholine, drugs have been developed that affect only muscarinic receptors and not nicotinic receptors. An example of such a drug is atropine, which blocks muscarinic receptors and prevents the binding of acetylcholine. This and similar drugs are called muscarinic antagonists (also known as anticholinergics), and their effects are opposite to those of acetylcholine at muscarinic receptors.

Most postganglionic sympathetic neurons synthesize norepinephrine, also called noradrenaline. For this reason, they and other neurons that use norepinephrine as their neurotransmitter are called noradrenergic neurons. When an action potential is conducted down a postganglionic sympathetic neuron because of a strong depolarizing influence received from the preganglionic neuron, norepinephrine is released from the axon terminal into the synapse. It diffuses across the synapse and binds to receptors on the cell membrane of the effector organ. These receptors may be $\alpha$ or $\beta$ receptors; $\alpha$ receptors may be $\alpha_1$ or $\alpha_2$ receptors, and $\beta$ receptors may be $\beta_1$, $\beta_2$, or $\beta_3$ receptors. The heart has mostly $\beta_1$ receptors, and the smooth muscle of the arteries and veins has mostly $\alpha_1$ and $\alpha_2$ receptors. The sympathetic nervous system innervates organs with $\alpha_1$, $\alpha_2$, and $\beta_1$ receptors, and norepinephrine activates these receptors to cause changes in the effector organs that have them. For instance, activation of $\beta_1$ receptors in the sinoatrial node by norepinephrine released from sympathetic axon terminals results in depolarization of the sinoatrial node and an increase in heart rate. Activation of $\alpha_1$ receptors in the arteries results in increased contraction by arteriolar smooth muscle and an increase in blood pressure, while activation of $\alpha_2$ receptors results in arterial smooth relaxation and a decrease in blood pressure.

The adrenal medulla is innervated by the sympathetic nervous system through preganglionic (cholinergic) sympathetic neurons. When an action potential is conducted down their axons, these neurons release acetylcholine from their axon terminals into their synapses. The acetylcholine diffuses across the synapse and binds to nicotinic receptors on the cell membranes of the adrenal medullary cells, triggering the release of some norepinephrine but mostly epinephrine from the adrenal cells into the bloodstream. Circulating norepinephrine and epinephrine can both bind to $\alpha$ and $\beta$ receptors on sympathetic effector organs, similar to synaptic norepinephrine that is released from sympathetic nerve terminals. However, there is one important difference between norepinephrine and epinephrine. As mentioned, $\beta_2$ receptors are not innervated by the sympathetic nervous system, and norepinephrine does not bind or activate $\beta_2$ receptors to any degree. However, epinephrine is a powerful stimulator of $\beta_2$ receptors, which it reaches through the bloodstream after being secreted by the adrenal medulla. Thus, dilation of bronchiolar smooth muscle and dilation of blood vessels in skeletal muscles are important effects of $\beta_2$ receptors that are mediated by circulating epinephrine rather than by norepinephrine released from sympathetic nerve terminals or the adrenal medulla.

Although the sympathetic nerves originate in the thoracic and high lumbar cord, and parasympathetic nerves originate with nuclei that send axons down various cranial nerves or sacral spinal nerves, inputs into the patterns of autonomic function are regulated or triggered by centers in the hypothalamus, medulla, and bulboreticular formations. These centers in the CNS send impulses along descending fibers to the appropriate preganglionic autonomic neuron. In the cord, such fibers travel by special descending tracts in the white matter until they reach the appropriate level of the cord. Thus, any interruption of these descending fibers (eg, transection of cervical tracts) impedes or prevents stimulation of preganglionic autonomic neurons in the thoracic, lumbar, and sacral regions of the cord.

Inputs into the centers in the brainstem and hypothalamus that regulate sympathetic or parasympathetic outflow come from diffuse areas throughout the brain, including visual or auditory centers and areas of the brain associated with conscious thought or planning. Therefore, when we see an alarming sight, such as a car bearing down on us, or hear a frightening noise, sympathetic centers are stimulated and sympathetic outflow increases. Conversely, if we smell food, parasympathetic outflow might increase to prepare the digestive glands for secretion.

In many organ systems, the sympathetic and parasympathetic systems are antagonistic. For instance, the sympathetic system increases the rate of firing of the sinoatrial node and increases the speed of conduction in the atrioventricular node of the heart, whereas the parasympathetic system does the opposite. The parasympathetic system activates the gastrointestinal tract, whereas the sympathetic system inhibits it. Although this is a recurring theme, it is not an absolute rule. Thus, sympathetic stimulation constricts blood vessels (through $\alpha_1$ receptors), but blood vessels are not innervated by the parasympathetic system, so an opposite effect is not produced by the parasympathetic system. The sympathetic system stimulates cardiac ventricular contractility (through $\beta_1$ receptors), but the ventricles are not innervated by the parasympathetic system, so contractility is not affected by it. The two systems actually work together in the male genitalia, where the parasympathetic system mediates erection while the sympathetic system mediates ejaculation.

Both the sympathetic and parasympathetic systems are tonically active most of the time. One or the other may be more active at a given time, but it is rare that either of them is completely silent. Therefore, a person's heart rate at any given time is a summation of the positive effects of the sympathetic system and the negative effects of the parasympathetic system. At rest, parasympathetic influence is strongest, and the heart rate is slow. With exertion or strong emotion, sympathetic activation increases, and the heart rate speeds up.

## Reflexes

A reflex is a motor response to a sensory input. Reflexes have three components. There is a sensory component, which may consist of only one sensory input or multiple inputs. There is an integrative CNS component that processes the sensory component and "decides" whether it is strong enough to warrant a motor response. Finally, the motor component executes the response. The motor component can consist of one motor nerve and one muscle, or several motor nerves and several muscles. The three components together constitute a "reflex arc." Reflexes are mediated by lower areas of the brain or by the spinal cord, so that they happen without conscious thought. We become aware of the sensory input and the motor response when they are communicated to our cortex, but by then, the reflex is over. However, if we know that a reflexive action is likely, such as when we see someone about to strike our knee with a reflex hammer, we can often suppress a reflex by willing ourselves not to perform the motor action. This capability illustrates that the cortex has input into the integrative CNS component of the reflex. If higher centers are damaged, the reflex still occurs. For example, people with spinal cord transections still have reflexes in areas supplied by spinal nerves below the transection. Of course, they are unaware that these reflexes are taking place because they cannot receive sensory input to their cortex from below the level of the transection.

## Brain Reflexes

Brain reflexes include those involving the cardioregulatory and vasomotor centers of the medulla, plus the pupillary adjustment center, which involves the midbrain. Additional reflexes mediated by brain centers include the gag reflex, blink reflex, vomiting, and swallowing.

Because of its importance to critical care, the baroreceptor reflex will be used as an illustration of a brain reflex. The sensory components of the baroreceptor reflex are stretch receptors in various arteries, the most important of which are in the carotid sinuses and the aortic arch. These stretch receptors are actually specialized dendrites of sensory nerves that sense the stretch in the arterial wall produced by the pulse. If the blood pressure is high, the stretch receptors are highly stimulated, whereas if the blood pressure is low, the stretch receptors are not stimulated very much. The stretch receptors send nerve impulses down their dendrites to sensory ganglia near the brain in their respective nerves (cranial nerve IX—the glossopharyngeal nerve—in the case of the carotid sinuses, and cranial nerve X—the vagus nerve—in the case of the aortic arch) that are proportional to the degree of stretch. This information is communicated by sensory axons to autonomic centers in the medulla that process the information and compare it with a "set point" that represents the degree of stimulation they should receive if blood pressure were normal. If the medullary centers receive too little stimulation from the baroreceptors, they send impulses to sympathetic centers to increase sympathetic outflow. This stimulates sympathetic nerves supplying the heart to increase their release of norepinephrine, which binds to $\beta_1$ receptors in the sinoatrial node to increase heart rate and $\beta_1$ receptors in the ventricles to increase contractility. Sympathetic nerves supplying the veins release norepinephrine, which binds to $\alpha$ receptors, causing constriction of the veins, which increases venous return to the heart. Sympathetic nerves supplying the arteries release norepinephrine, which binds to $\alpha$ receptors, causing constriction of the arteries, which raises the blood pressure. The combination of increased venous return to the heart, increased heart rate, and increased contractility raises the cardiac output, which also increases the blood pressure. Finally, sympathetic nerves supplying the juxtaglomerular apparatus in the kidney release norepinephrine, which binds to $\beta_1$ receptors there, stimulating renin release. Through a series of events, renin stimulates the formation of angiotensin II, which is a potent arterial constrictor, increasing blood pressure directly; it also acts on the kidney (through aldosterone) to cause sodium and water retention. Increased retention of sodium and water further increases venous return to the heart, causing additional increased cardiac output and blood pressure. Therefore, activation of the sympathetic nervous system in response to decreased stimulation of the baroreceptors produces many consequences at the effector organs, all of which separately and together cause a rise in blood pressure. If the stretch on the baroreceptors is too high (according to the normal set point), the sympathetic nervous system is inhibited, sympathetic outflow decreases, and consequences at the effector organs are diminished.

## Spinal Cord Reflexes

In one type of cord reflex, the sensory component of the reflex is the sensory neurons that send their axons to the cord through one of the spinal nerves, the CNS integrative component is the spinal cord, and the motor component is the motor neurons that supply skeletal muscles. Deep tendon reflexes belong in this classification, as does the withdrawal reflex (Fig. 32-23A). These reflexes are present at each level of the spinal cord, bilaterally.

The sensory component of the withdrawal reflex is pain that originates in nociceptors, specialized dendrites of sensory neurons. Impulses are conducted through dendrites of the sensory neurons to the dorsal root ganglia next to the spinal cord and from there along sensory axons into the cord. These impulses stimulate cord interneurons, which, if the sensory input is strong enough, stimulate motor neurons whose axons innervate skeletal muscles, causing contraction. When contracted, the skeletal muscles produce withdrawal of the body part from the painful stimulus. The withdrawal reflex depends on the appropriate anatomical connections between sensory neurons, interneurons, and motor neurons in the cord. If these become nonfunctional (eg, spinal shock or physical trauma), this and other spinal reflexes do not occur.

The withdrawal reflex of one foot is associated with another reflex, the crossed extensor reflex (see Fig. 32-23B). This reflex involves stimulation of various extensor muscles

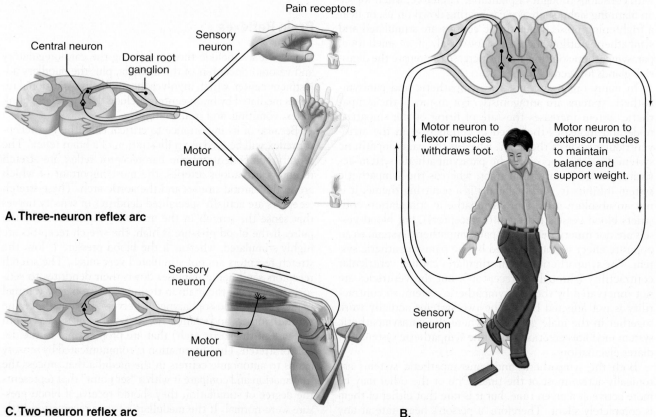

**FIGURE 32-23** Reflex arcs showing pathways of impulses in response to a stimulus. **A:** The withdrawal reflex involves a three-neuron reflex arc: sensory, central, and motor neurons. **B:** The flexor and crossed extensor reflexes. **C:** Example of a stretch reflex, involving only a two-neuron reflex arc: sensory and motor neurons.

in the opposite leg so that a person's weight is fully supported by the other leg while one lower extremity is withdrawn from a painful stimulus. Such a reflex is complex and involves many levels of the cord. Any imbalance, however slight, during the operation of this reflex in a normal person triggers the occurrence of additional reflexes involving the bulboreticular formation, cerebellum, and various muscles of arms and trunk to maintain balance and posture.

Another cord reflex is the stretch reflex or deep tendon reflex, most commonly illustrated by the clinical test of the knee jerk response (see Fig. 32-23C). In the deep tendon reflex, the sensory component is a specialized sense organ, the muscle spindle, which sends its signals along a spinal nerve to the dorsal horn of the spinal cord. The CNS component is a single synapse of the sensory axon terminal with the motor nerve cell body. The motor component is the motor axon supplying the skeletal muscle. In the knee jerk test, a reflex hammer blow stretches the quadriceps tendon, which stretches the muscle spindle, which sends impulses through the dendrite and axon of its nerve cell to release neurotransmitter from the axon terminal. This causes the motor neuron cell body in the spinal cord to depolarize. If the depolarization is strong enough, an action potential is conducted down the axon of the motor neuron to depolarize the muscle through release of acetylcholine into the synapse at the neuromuscular junction, as discussed previously. This causes contraction of the quadriceps, which causes the lower leg to kick forward. Other deep tendon reflexes of clinical importance are the ankle jerk and the biceps and triceps reflexes. All work similar to the knee jerk.

An important feature of all cord reflexes involving skeletal muscles is reciprocal inhibition, which occurs in the antagonist muscle of the one stimulated. For example, when a flexor reflex stimulates the biceps, it also inhibits its antagonist, the triceps, and provides for more efficient performance of motor activities in the upper arm.

Spinal cord activities also include autonomic reflex circuits, which aid in the control of visceral functions of the body. Sensory input arises from visceral sensory receptors and is transmitted to the spinal cord, where reflex patterns appropriate to the sensory input are determined. The signals are then transmitted to autonomic motor neurons in the gray matter of the spinal cord, which send impulses to the sympathetic nerves innervating visceral motor end organs.

A most important autonomic reflex is the peritoneal reflex. Tissue damage in any portion of the peritoneum results in the activation of this reflex, which slows or stops all motor activity in the nearby viscera, such as the intestine. Other autonomic cord reflexes are capable of modifying local blood flow in response to cold, pain, and heat. This vascular control by autonomic reflexes in the spinal cord can operate as a backup mechanism for the usual brainstem control patterns in patients with transectional injuries at the brainstem. Alternatively, because the autonomic reflexes arising lower in the cord of a patient with a cervical transectional injury are not modulated by brainstem centers as they are in patients without a transection, sensory input to autonomic centers in the cord can cause extreme motor responses, similar to the development of clonus with unmodulated deep tendon reflexes. However, these motor reflexes are sympathetic, and their out-of-control state in spinal injury patients is called autonomic hyperreflexia.

Also included in the autonomic reflexes of the spinal cord are those causing the emptying of the urinary bladder and the rectum. These reflexes are mediated by the sacral parasympathetic system. When the bladder or bowel becomes distended, sensory signals from stretch receptors in the bladder or bowel wall are transmitted by sensory neurons to the internuncial neurons of the upper sacral and lower lumbar segments of the cord. These neurons in turn stimulate parasympathetic motor neurons innervating the smooth muscle in the wall of the bladder or bowel, and their respective internal smooth muscle sphincters are also reflexively inhibited by the internuncials. The result is a reflex contraction of bladder or bowel and an opening of the respective smooth muscle sphincter, thereby permitting micturition or defecation.

In addition to their smooth muscle sphincters, both the bladder and bowel have skeletal muscle sphincters that are controlled by motor neurons. Descending motor fibers from the cortex synapse with the motor neurons, and, in toilet-trained people, keep the skeletal muscle sphincters in a state of contraction, inhibiting the reflex emptying of bladder or bowel at times or places deemed inappropriate. When an appropriate time and place is reached, the person can consciously relax the skeletal muscle sphincter and either void or defecate reflexively. Toilet training of infants must await the functional maturation of these descending motor fibers. Cord transection or other damage above the level of the cord housing the neurons for the bladder or bowel evacuation reflexes interrupts some or all of these descending fibers. This produces a condition in which the patient cannot consciously control (prevent) the emptying of the bladder or bowel, or both. As long as the sacral cord and associated spinal nerves are functioning, voiding or defecation proceeds reflexively in such a patient. Damage to or interrupted function of the level of the cord housing the anatomical neuronal connections for these reflexes (as in, eg, spina bifida, spinal shock, or severe injuries to the lower sacral or lumbar cord) or damage to the spinal nerves supplying the bladder or rectum prevents reflex evacuation of bladder or bowel, or both. Such a patient may exhibit retention with overflow and does not possess any effective mechanism for emptying the bladder or bowel.

## Pain

The sensation of pain warrants special consideration because it plays such an important protective role. Whenever there is tissue damage, pain receptors, called nociceptors, are stimulated and send impulses back to the spinal cord. These impulses are transmitted up to the brain, where they are perceived, as previously explained. Stimulation of the nociceptors is caused by the release of substances from damaged tissue and from activation of the inflammatory response. Damaged cells release potassium and hydrogen ion, both of which can stimulate nociceptors. However, the inflammatory response that is evoked in response to tissue damage is responsible for much of the stimulation of nociceptors. For instance, histamine can stimulate nociceptors and prostaglandins, and leukotrienes can sensitize nociceptors to other stimuli. All of these substances are released by inflammatory cells (macrophages, neutrophils, and other white blood cells) that are attracted to the area of tissue injury. In addition, activated platelets that participate in clot formation in response to tearing of blood vessels release serotonin, which also stimulates nociceptors. Finally, the nociceptor itself may release substance P when it is stimulated, which sensitizes it to other activating substances. Thus, pain may be due to actual tissue injury or the inflammatory response evoked by the injury.

## Pain Pathways and Their Modulation

The sensation of pain is transmitted to the spinal cord and up to the brain in the same manner as previously described for sensations in general. To review, the nociceptor is actually a specialized dendrite of a sensory neuron, whose cell body is in the dorsal root ganglion of the spinal nerve. When the nociceptor is stimulated enough to mount an action potential, the impulse travels to the dorsal root ganglion, and then down the sensory nerve's axon into the dorsal horn, where it synapses with one or more projection neurons. The projection neurons carry the pain message to the thalamus, where pain is first perceived. The projection neurons synapse in the thalamus with neurons that carry the message to the sensory cortex, where the pain is perceived as a localized sensation.

However, there is an important difference in how pain messages are transmitted to the thalamus and cortex compared with other sensations. This difference is in the way the pain impulse can be modulated by spinal influences before it ascends the cord. In brief, gating mechanisms exist in an area in the gray matter called the substantia gelatinosa at all levels of the dorsal cord. These mechanisms are capable of regulating the number of pain impulses that can enter the ascending tracts and travel to the brain.

To regulate ascending pain impulses, an area of the brainstem called the periaqueductal gray sends axons to the nucleus raphe magnus in the medulla. These axons synapse with neurons that send axons from the nucleus raphe magnus back down to all levels of the cord in the substantia gelatinosa. These neurons regulate the ability of pain-stimulated sensory neurons to stimulate projection neurons of the spinothalamic tract. Thus, the descending fibers of the substantia gelatinosa control the entry of pain impulses into the spinal pain conduction system at the level of the cord where the particular sensory neuron enters (Fig. 32-24). Sensory stimuli cannot be conducted and, at least to the thalamus, cannot be perceived.

How do the descending fibers modulate stimulation of the projection neurons by the sensory neurons? When researchers answered this question, we also obtained the answer to another perplexing question: How do the opioid drugs relieve pain? The neurons that descend from the nucleus raphe magnus in the medulla, as well as the modulating internuncial neurons, use previously undiscovered small protein neurotransmitters collectively referred to as the endogenous opioid peptides:[3]

- Leucine-enkephalin
- Methionine-enkephalin
- β-Endorphin
- Dynorphin
- α-Neoendorphin.

When the endogenous opioid peptides are released into a synapse and bind to their receptors on the postsynaptic cell, they produce hyperpolarization of the postsynaptic cell. As explained previously, this makes the postsynaptic cell less likely to be able to conduct an action potential along its axon.

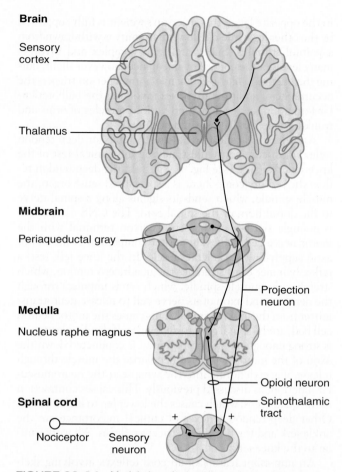

**FIGURE 32-24** Modulation of ascending pain impulses by descending opioid neurons with origins in the nucleus raphe magnus and input from the periaqueductal gray. The sensory neuron's influence on the projection neuron is stimulatory (depolarizing), designated by the plus sign, but the influence of the opioid neuron is inhibitory (hyperpolarizing), designated by the minus sign. Therefore, if the strength of impulses descending in the opioid neuron is high, the projection neuron will experience fewer action potentials and send fewer pain impulses up to the thalamus.

Therefore, the descending fibers that synapse with the projection neurons can produce hyperpolarization in the projection neurons, lessening or perhaps even eliminating the pain messages that would otherwise be conducted upward by the projection neurons. Therefore, the endogenous opioid neurotransmitters, by binding to their receptors on the projection neurons, lessen the perception of pain in the thalamus and cortex. Under extreme circumstances, these descending pathways may be so inhibitory to projection neurons that they eliminate all ascending pain messages, producing complete analgesia to pain. This phenomenon is sometimes seen in victims of automobile crashes or in wounded soldiers, who continue to function, oblivious to their wounds.

What stimulates areas of the periaqueductal gray and nucleus raphe magnus to send these descending inhibitory messages to the substantia gelatinosa, resulting in the release of opioid neurotransmitters and diminution of ascending pain signals? Unfortunately, very little is known about this, but it is possible that acupuncture and electrical stimulation devices for pain control are stimulating these pathways, causing inhibition of the projection neurons by the descending neurons' release of opioid neurotransmitters.

The opioid drugs work in the same way as the endogenous opioid neurotransmitters. They bind to opioid receptors on the projection or internuncial neuron, producing hyperpolarization and a decrease in the amount of pain stimulus reaching the thalamus and the cortex. There are neurons that use the endogenous opioids as neurotransmitters in the brain as well, and opioid drugs also bind to the receptors that these neurons supply. These effects may increase the analgesic effects of the drug, or they may be responsible for other effects, such as the somnolence or dizziness that opioid drugs produce. In addition, there are opioid receptors in the intestinal tract that are stimulated by endogenous opioids and by opioid drugs. These receptors inhibit peristalsis in the intestinal tract, and this effect is responsible for the constipation and nausea often seen with opioid drugs.

Pain is a complex sensation. There is great variation in pain thresholds among different people and within the same person at different times. These variations can partly be explained by the modulation of pain pathways by endogenous opioid neurotransmitters. In addition, the amount of tissue injury and presence of chemical mediators can increase the pain experience qualitatively, quantitatively, temporally, and spatially. However, pain perception is also influenced by expectations and by cultural influences. It is helpful to remember that pain is a perception and that we have to take a person's word in describing that perception to us. It is impossible to judge a patient's pain by his or her appearance or actions, or physical or laboratory signs. The complexity of the pain pathways can make the clinical management of pain difficult, but every patient's description of his or her pain should be taken seriously. Opioid addiction is practically unknown in patients without a history of drug abuse who receive opioids for pain relief. Pain medication should be administered to most patients based on their own self-report of their pain.

## Referred Pain

Referred pain is pain perceived as arising from a site that is different from its true point of origin. The "true point of origin" for this type of pain is usually some visceral organ or deep somatic structure, and the "point of reference" is some area of the body surface. Well-known examples include the referring of pain from severe cardiac ischemia to the left arm or the referring of diaphragmatic pain to the neck and shoulder.

The most generally accepted theory for referred pain is that the two sensory neurons, one from the region of the true point of origin and one from the point of reference, enter the same segment of the spinal cord and synapse with the same projection neuron. There is no way for the cortex to know whether a given projection neuron was originally stimulated by pain from the true point of origin or from the referred area. In localizing the source of the pain stimulus, the cortex relies on prior experience regarding the person's geographical knowledge of his or her own body. Because surface areas are more familiar to a person than the locations of the visceral or deep somatic structures, the referred locale is used preferentially over the more unfamiliar but true point of origin (Fig. 32-25).

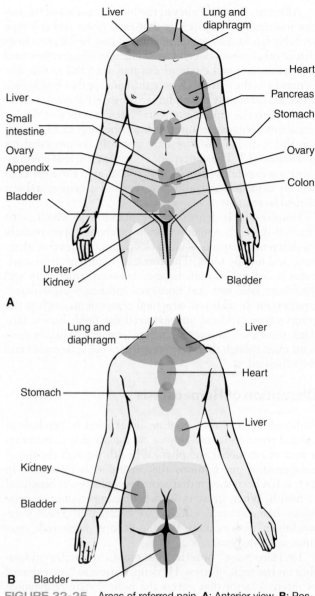

**FIGURE 32-25**  Areas of referred pain. **A:** Anterior view. **B:** Posterior view.

## The Neurohormonal Stress Response

### Homeostasis

In the middle of the 19th century, the French physiologist Claude Bernard (1813–1878) coined the term milieu intérieur to mean the internal environment to which body cells are exposed. He stated that to maintain proper cell functioning, the milieu intérieur must be constant and proper.[4,5]

The living body, though it has need of the surrounding environment, is nevertheless relatively independent of it. This independence that the organism has of its external environment derives from the fact that in the living beings, the tissues are in fact withdrawn from direct external influences. The tissues are also protected by a veritable internal environment that is constituted, in particular, by the fluids circulating in the body.

Although Bernard believed the blood constituted the milieu intérieur, we now realize that each tissue and cell type probably has its own environment that may be different from that of other tissues or cell types. The idea of a constant and appropriate internal environment remains valid to this day. Bernard was the first to advance the concept that bodily processes are constantly responding to the external environment to maintain the milieu intérieur: "The constancy of the internal environment requires such a perfection in the organism that external variations are instantly compensated for and balanced."[4] The concept of a constant internal environment was expanded upon by Walter Canon in the early 20th century to include all bodily processes and structures and was termed *homeostasis*.

Homeostasis is defined as the situation in which attributes of the body remain constant or change appropriately for different situations, such as blood pressure, level of alertness, and muscle tone,. The constant nature of these attributes is due to the right balance between stimulatory and inhibitory neuronal and hormonal influences—a dynamic equilibrium. In addition, structural components, such as the composition of blood and extracellular fluid, bones, tendons, muscles, and internal organs, remain essentially constant even though their components are being degraded and resynthesized.

## Disruption of Homeostasis

Although each of us is continually exposed to psychological and physiologic stressors, we are usually able to maintain a state of emotional and physical health through the use of compensatory mechanisms that maintain homeostasis. In fact, it has been shown that some level of stress is beneficial to health. When stressors overwhelm compensatory mechanisms, homeostasis is lost and we become ill. These overwhelming stressors occur because of large magnitude over time, or sudden onset.

Dr. Hans Selye[6,7] was the most prolific researcher and author on the topic of stress. He defined stress as "any external or internal factor that affects the normal state of dynamic equilibrium in an individual." These factors, or stressors, can be either physical or psychological. Regardless of whether the person consciously perceives a threat, the body responds with certain intrinsic reactions. One person may have compensatory mechanisms with a large capacity to handle stressors, whereas another person may not. Therefore, exposure to a given stressor does not elicit the same response in all people. This difference may be based on internal conditioning factors, such as age, sex, and genetics, or on external factors, such as culture, previous life events, exposure to similar stressors, diet and nutrition, and medications.

### General Adaptation Syndrome

Selye and his collaborators noted commonalities in responses to different stressors in different individuals. They termed these commonalities the general adaptation syndrome. Although this term has fallen from favor, and the changes they noted are probably not as general as they thought, the concept of a generalized response to stress remains. They defined three basic stages of the stress syndrome—the alarm reaction, stage of resistance, and stage of exhaustion.

- *Alarm reaction.* During this initial stage, the threat is perceived, either consciously or subconsciously, and body processes are modified to counteract it. The sympathetic nervous system is stimulated by the stressor, and there is a subsequent response through the release of norepinephrine and epinephrine. Additionally, adrenocorticotropic hormone (ACTH) and ADH are released by the anterior and posterior pituitary. Stimulation of the sympathetic nervous system raises heart rate and blood pressure and stimulates the renin–angiotensin–aldosterone system, which results in sodium and water retention, increasing the blood pressure. ACTH stimulates the release of cortisol by the adrenal cortex, which produces numerous adaptations to stress, outlined below. ADH raises blood pressure mainly by causing the kidney to retain water.
- *Stage of resistance.* During the second stage, the stress is being compensated for by increased activity of the stress responses evoked during the alarm phase. Cortisol secretion, the sympathetic nervous system, and other mechanisms triggered in the alarm reaction may continue to be activated at a lower, more constant level. This phase may continue for a long time, even years, if the increased levels of stress response mechanisms are maintained. However, the increased levels of stress response mechanisms come at a price—the use of additional resources of energy and nutrients. It is during this stage that symptoms of disease may become chronic if the compensatory responses are not adequate to control them.
- *Stage of exhaustion.* The ability to mount a stress response has limits. The stress response can be activated only for a finite time or to a finite degree. If the stressor is not removed or adaptation does not occur, the person is no longer able to resist the stressor and homeostasis is no longer achievable. A shock state may occur (see Chapter 54), and without appropriate intervention, organ failure and death may rapidly ensue.

## The Stress Response

### Acute Stress

Consider a prehistoric man walking on the African grasslands. Suddenly, a lion springs from behind some vegetation. The man's eyes capture an image of the lion, which is communicated to the visual areas in his occipital cortex, which is sent to and processed by his prefrontal and frontal cortex and perceived as a threat. This threat is communicated to many centers in the brain, including those supplying the ANS. Immediately, sympathetic outflow is increased by activation of brainstem sympathetic centers and through unitary activation of the sympathetic nervous system increasing the rate of firing of the sympathetic nerves, releasing norepinephrine into sympathetic synapses. At the same time, parasympathetic outflow is inhibited, decreasing activity of the gastrointestinal system and the need for blood to those organs. The heart rate and cardiac contractility ($\beta_1$ receptors) are greatly increased, both of which increase cardiac output, and arteriolar constriction ($\alpha$ receptors) thus raising the blood pressure. The adrenal medulla is stimulated by sympathetic outflow (neuronal nicotinic receptors) to secrete some norepinephrine, but mostly epinephrine, into the bloodstream. The epinephrine stimulates $\alpha$ and $\beta_1$ receptors causing the same effects as norepinephrine and $\beta_2$ receptors on bronchiolar smooth muscle, causing relaxation and dilation of the bronchioles. It also stimulates $\beta_2$ receptors on arterioles in skeletal muscle beds, causing profound dilation, increasing the capacity of these beds for blood flow. Blood flow to the brain is also increased because arterioles supplying the brain have few $\alpha$ receptors, so they remain fully dilated. Stimulation of $\beta_1$ receptors in the juxtaglomerular apparatus of the kidney by norepinephrine (from sympathetic nervous system nerve terminals and the adrenal medulla) and epinephrine (from the adrenal medulla) causes the release of renin, which activates the renin–angiotensin–aldosterone system. Renin acts on circulating angiotensinogen to angiotensin I, which is further converted to angiotensin II by angiotensin-converting enzymes. Angiotensin II causes additional arteriolar constriction, increasing blood pressure still further. It also causes the release of aldosterone, which causes the kidney to retain sodium and water. Sodium and water retention increases the preload to the heart further increasing cardiac output.

In addition, communication of the threatening sight to the hypothalamus activates neurohormonal mechanisms controlled by the pituitary. The hypothalamus increases its synthesis and release of ADH from the posterior pituitary. ADH causes the kidney to retain water, further increasing the preload and thereby the cardiac output. The hypothalamus also increases its secretion and release of corticotropin-releasing hormone, which causes the anterior pituitary to secrete additional ACTH, which in turn causes the adrenal cortex to release increased quantities of cortisol. Cortisol has far-reaching effects on many organs that increase their ability to respond to stress. Growth hormone (GH) synthesis and release by the anterior pituitary is also increased. Like cortisol, GH has many far-reaching effects on many organs, but its overall effect is to increase the activity of tissue repair mechanisms and utilization of nutrients.

Finally, the immune system is activated by the stress response. This activation is achieved by multiple influences. First, GH increases the ability of many cells of the immune system, such as neutrophils and T and B lymphocytes, to carry out their functions, including phagocytosis, antigen presentation, and antibody production. In addition, the physiologically high levels of cortisol affect the immune system's ability to respond to foreign antigens. (Levels produced by pharmacologic doses of corticosteroids are much higher than those produced by stress and are immunosuppressive.) The effects of physiologically elevated levels of cortisol in response to stress on immune function are complex and may involve effects on the ability of immune cells to exit the circulation and go to sites of tissue injury, or their ability to respond to antigen presentation. Catecholamines affect the immune system's ability to respond to tissue injury or foreign antigens. The net response of the immune system to acute influences of the stress is generally considered to be the ability to mount an inflammatory response and respond to a foreign antigen. Figure 32-26 summarizes the effects on various body systems.

Returning to our prehistoric man threatened by a lion, the changes produced in his body by the threatening sight of a lion all have the effect of increasing the ability to help him run faster or fight harder to escape the lion and increase his ability to respond to tissue injury that might result from this encounter. These changes constitute the alarm reaction characterized by Selye. The lion threat represents an acute stressor that would end very quickly, because the man either escaped or was killed. If the man was successful in escaping the lion,

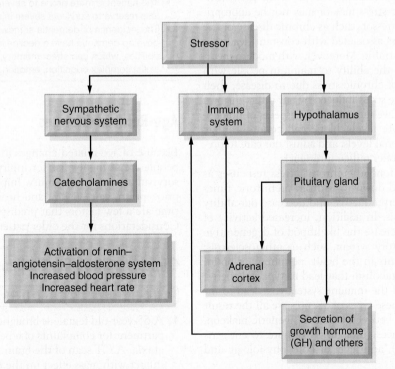

**FIGURE 32-26** The stress response induces increased activity in the sympathetic nervous system, including the adrenal medulla, which activates the renin–angiotensin–aldosterone system and increases the blood pressure and heart rate, among other things. The stress response also activates the pituitary gland, which secretes increased GH; the adrenal cortex, which secretes increased cortisol; and the immune system.

the stress response would extinguish itself very rapidly, and his physiologic state would gradually return to normal.

The question that arises for modern humans is, "How are the changes of the alarm reaction beneficial for stresses encountered in modern times?" If one is running to get away from a dangerous situation or to catch a bus, is injured in an automobile crash, or contracts an acute illness, the acute stress response is very likely still beneficial. However, if one undergoes an acute emotional stress, such as an intense argument or the death of a loved one, the alarm reaction is invoked, the same as it would be for a more physiologically oriented stress. In such circumstances, we do not need increased ability to fight or run away, decreased activity of our gastrointestinal system, or increased ability for tissue repair. Therefore, in these circumstances, the acute stress response is at best superfluous and at worst consumes resources and unnecessarily creates wear and tear on body systems.

## Chronic Stress

Selye's "stage of resistance" describes our ability to handle chronic stress. Chronic stressors that affected prehistoric humans included starvation or extreme heat or cold. Responses to these stressors included some of the same mechanisms as outlined earlier for acute stress but at diminished levels that are more sustainable over a long period. However, responses to these stressors also included additional mechanisms that conserve body stores of nutrients and energy. These responses include cortisol, but also insulin, glucagon, and GH. The chronic stress response in prehistoric times probably did not include response to diseases. Because disease processes could not be treated, affected people quickly died during the acute stress response. The mechanisms that evolved prehistorically to handle chronic stress may or may not be appropriate to handle modern stressors such as chronic disease or the chronic emotional stress associated with constant deadlines or commuting in heavy traffic. Moreover, with modern medical care, we now have the ability to maintain people with extremely high levels of chronic stress due to disease, their emotional state, and the stress induced by our interventions. In intensive care units, we measure many aspects of homeostasis, such as electrolyte levels, blood cell counts, cardiac functioning, and hormonal levels, and adjust our care to preserve homeostasis (a proper milieu intérieur).

In many such situations, the chronic stress responses as they have been handed down to us from prehistoric times may actually be counterproductive and decrease our ability to maintain homeostasis. In addition, increased activity of stress responses may increase the likelihood of degenerative diseases of the circulatory system, such as atherosclerosis, leading to vascular events in the heart, periphery, or brain; disorders of glucose metabolism that lead to type 2 diabetes; or, perhaps, disorders of the immune system that lead to inflammatory diseases. These types of diseases are all the result of a complex interplay between a person's genetic makeup, his or her life experiences (including exposure to antigens and infectious diseases), and level of both physiologic and psychological stress.

---

**BOX 32-1** *Considerations for the Older Patient*

**Anatomical and Physiologic Changes in the Nervous System That Occur With Aging**

- Cerebral atrophy results in a decrease in total brain weight and volume, especially in the frontal and temporal lobes; enlargement of the ventricles; and a loss of gray matter.
- Cerebral atrophy causes the dura mater and bridging veins to become tightly adherent to the skull; thus, they are easily torn with significant movement of the cranial contents, leading to subdural hematoma formation.
- Cerebral atrophy creates more space for intracranial blood to be concealed, so the older patient may manifest only subtle symptoms, which may lead to a delay in diagnosis.
- Axonal loss or decreases in myelination result in a loss of white matter.
- There is atrophy of the hippocampus, which correlates with a decline in learning and memory and cognitive impairments.
- A decreased number of neuronal cells and degeneration of dendrites and dendritic spines in cortical pyramidal cells lead to declining synaptic transmission and slowed impulse conduction.
- There is decreased production, release, and metabolism of neurotransmitters.
- Altered circulation in the inner ear and fewer functional cochlear cells lead to reduced hearing.
- A decreased number of olfactory cells in nasal mucosa lead to a reduced sense of smell.
- There is an increase in wakefulness and arousal from sleep and a decrease in slow-wave sleep, leading to changes in sleep patterns.
- The odontoid process in the cervical spine is most commonly fractured because of osteoporosis and degenerative joint disease.
- Central cord syndrome occurs more frequently because of spinal stenosis.
- The patient is more prone to severe brain injury and may have less reserve to survive a severe injury.
- The incidence of dementia somewhat increases. Those who develop dementia have a decline in cognitive and emotional abilities, which can affect memory, language, visuospatial skills, complex cognition, emotion, and personality.

---

## Age-Related Changes

Because of age-related changes in the nervous system, older people are at higher risk for injury and have less chance for survival after a severe injury. Impairment of sensation, proprioception, gait, vision, and hearing and delayed response time are a few factors that predispose older people to injury. Considerations for the older patient are given in Box 32-1.

## Clinical Applicability Challenges

### SHORT ANSWER QUESTIONS

1. A 65-year-old female is brought to the emergency department for complaints of a persistent headache and ataxia. A CT scan of the brain reveals a left cerebellar infarct with mass effect on the brain stem and fourth

ventricle. Describe the symptoms this patient is at risk for developing.

2. A 54-year-old man with a history of myasthenia gravis is admitted to the hospital with a myasthenia exacerbation. The patient is ordered plasmapheresis. Discuss the purpose of plasmapheresis and how it works. Explain the importance of monitoring fatigability and vital capacity. Define myasthenic crisis.

3. A 22-year-old male is admitted after sustaining a severe traumatic brain injury. An ICP monitor is placed and the initial reading is 28 mm Hg. What nursing measures can be instituted initially to treat the elevated ICP? What would be the next steps pharmacologically and operatively to decrease the ICP? Describe early and late signs of increased ICP.

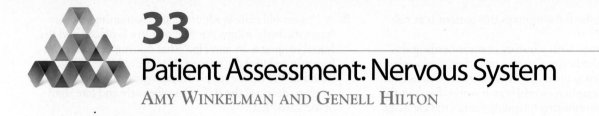

# 33

# Patient Assessment: Nervous System

## AMY WINKELMAN AND GENELL HILTON

### LEARNING OBJECTIVES

*Based on the content in this chapter, the reader should be able to:*

1. Perform a comprehensive neurologic assessment.
2. Describe abnormal assessment findings consistent with neurologic compromise.
3. Analyze assessment findings and identify potential nursing diagnoses.
4. Evaluate the effect of neurologic dysfunction on the patient.
5. Discuss preprocedure and postprocedure nursing interventions appropriate to selected neurodiagnostic tests.

Assessment and care of a patient with a neurologic problem constitutes one of the biggest challenges for critical care nurses. Basic nursing education and critical care courses may not address the assessment of the nervous system to the depth or complexity observed with other body systems. In addition, a comprehensive neurologic assessment involves the use of techniques not commonly performed in the assessment of other body systems. Therefore, it is not uncommon for even the experienced nurse to feel uncertain when gathering data about the nervous system.

There are four major objectives in the nursing assessment of a patient with a real or potential neurologic problem. The first objective is to gather data about the functioning of the nervous system in an unbiased and orderly manner, avoiding inconsistencies in data collection or inadequate data collection. It is essential that examination results be recorded clearly so that changes in findings can be easily identified. A standard neurologic documentation tool, with clearly delineated grading scales and definition of terms, should be used by all the nursing staff.

The second objective of neurologic assessment is to follow the data over time, discovering correlations and trends. For such correlations to be of value, it is necessary to interrelate the results of history, physical assessment, and diagnostic tests. Use of a patterned format helps establish medical and nursing diagnoses and guides the nurse in choosing and evaluating therapy.

The third objective of neurologic assessment is to analyze the data to develop a list of potential or actual diagnoses. Minor changes in neurologic status may be the first indication that the patient's physical condition is worsening. The nurse providing care to the patient is responsible to recognize these changes, correlate these findings to the pathophysiologic process, and intervene appropriately.

The fourth objective of the neurologic nursing assessment is to determine the effect of dysfunction on the patient's daily living and ability to perform self-care. Up to this point, the goals of physicians and nurses in the care of a patient with a neurologic problem have been similar. Each discipline uses many of the same questions and techniques to determine normal and abnormal nervous system functioning. The focus of nursing is to help patients cope with real or potential changes in daily living and self-care.

These objectives of neuroassessment are the same for all patients. In older patients, it is necessary to take the normal changes of aging into account when assessing for neurologic problems. Older adults are at increased risk for certain medical conditions that predispose them to neurologic problems. These same medical conditions or their prescribed treatment may also alter neurologic assessment findings. Special considerations for older adults are given in Box 33-1.

## History

Neurologic assessment begins with the first patient encounter. Conversation with the patient and family is a vital source of the data needed to evaluate overall functioning. The nurse ascertains the reason for the patient's visit, obtains information about symptoms, and evaluates the patient's past medical history, family history, and personal and social history (Box 33-2). A comprehensive review of systems is also performed as part of the initial assessment.

---

**BOX 33-1**    *CONSIDERATIONS for the Older Patient*

**Neuroassessment**

When assessing an older adult, it is necessary to ascertain the person's previous level of functioning to adequately assess the person's status. The following should be taken into consideration when the nurse assesses an older adult's neurologic function:

- Motor function may be affected by decreased strength, alterations in gait, changes in posture, and increased tremors.
- Vision may be decreased, pupils may be less reactive, color discrimination may be decreased, gaze may be impaired, and night vision may be diminished.
- Hearing may be diminished and changes in Rinne test findings may be noted. The nurse should bear in mind that an undetected hearing impairment can lead to the erroneous assumption that a person has more neurologic deficits than he or she actually has.
- Changes in sensory function may include decreased reflexes, decreased vibratory and position sense, and decreased two-point discrimination.
- Older adults are at increased risk for depression, nutritional abnormalities, stroke, transient ischemic attacks, and dementia.
- Older adults may have impaired sleep patterns.

BOX 33-2 *HEALTH HISTORY for Neurologic Assessment*

**Chief Complaint**
- Patient's description of the problem

**History of Present Illness**
- Complete analysis of the following signs and symptoms (using the NOPQRST format; see Chapter 17, Box 17-1)
- Dizziness, syncope, or seizures
- Headaches
- Vision or auditory changes, including sensitivity to light and tinnitus
- Difficulty swallowing or hoarseness
- Slurred speech or word finding difficulty
- Confusion, memory loss, or difficulty concentrating
- Gait disturbances
- Motor symptoms, including weakness, paresthesia, paralysis, decreased range of motion, and tremors

**Past Health History**
- Relevant childhood illnesses and immunizations: Febrile seizures, birth injuries, physical abuse or trauma, meningitis
- Past acute and chronic medical problems, including treatments and hospitalizations: Tumors, traumatic head injuries, hypertension, thrombophlebitis or deep venous thrombosis, coagulopathies, sinusitis, meningitis, encephalitis, seizures, diabetes, cancer, psychiatric disorders
- Risk factors: Diabetes, smoking, hypercholesterolemia, hypertension, drug use, alcohol use, cardiovascular disease
- Past surgeries: Peripheral vascular surgeries; carotid endarterectomy; aneurysm clipping; evacuation of hematoma; head, eyes, ears, nose, or throat (HEENT) procedures
- Past diagnostic tests and interventions: Electroencephalography, brain scan, carotid Doppler, head and neck computed tomography, magnetic resonance imaging, thrombolytic therapy, cardiac catheterization

- Medications: Anticonvulsants, anticoagulants, psychotropic agents, oral contraceptives, β-blockers, calcium channel blockers, antihyperlipidemics, hormone replacement therapy
- Allergies and reactions: Contrast medium, medications
- Transfusions including type and date

**Family History**
- Health status or cause of death of parents and siblings: Coronary artery disease, peripheral vascular disease, cancer, hypertension, diabetes, stroke, hyperlipidemia, coagulopathies, seizures, psychiatric disturbances

**Personal and Social History**
- Tobacco, alcohol, and substance use
- Family composition
- Occupation and work environment: Exposure to chemicals and toxins
- Living environment: Physical, verbal, and emotional abuse
- Diet
- Sleep patterns
- Exercise and leisure activities
- Cultural, spiritual, and religious beliefs
- Sources of stress, coping patterns, and social support systems
- Travel: Especially overseas

**Review of Systems**
- HEENT: Visual changes, tinnitus, headache
- Cardiovascular: hypertension, syncope, palpitations, intermittent claudication
- Respiratory: Shortness of breath, infections, cough, dyspnea
- Gastrointestinal: Weight loss, change in bowel habits, nausea/vomiting/diarrhea
- Genitourinary: Change in bladder habits, painful urination, sexual dysfunction
- Musculoskeletal: Sensitivity to temperature changes, varicosities, loss of hair on extremities, change in sensation

# Physical Examination

A comprehensive neurologic evaluation of the critically ill patient includes assessment of mental status, motor function, pupillary response, cranial nerve function, reflexes, and sensation. Findings are correlated with the vital signs.

## Mental Status

The mental status examination includes tests to evaluate level of consciousness and arousal, orientation to the environment, and thought content.

The quality of a patient's level of consciousness is the most basic and critical parameter requiring assessment. Level of consciousness indicates the functioning of the cerebral hemispheres as well as that of the reticular activating system, which is responsible for arousal. The degree of a patient's awareness of, response to, and interaction with the environment is the most sensitive indicator of nervous system dysfunction. Responsiveness may be categorized according to the patient's arousal to external stimuli, and gradations of response include terms such as lethargic, stuporous, and semicomatose (Box 33-3).

Orientation to the environment involves not only the patient's ability to respond but also the content of his or her response. Orientation is assessed by asking the patient

BOX 33-3 Clinical Terminology for Grading Responsiveness

**Alert (full consciousness):** Normal
**Awake:** May sleep more than usual or be somewhat confused on first awakening, but fully oriented when aroused
**Lethargic:** Drowsy but follows simple commands when stimulated
**Obtunded:** Arousable with stimulation; responds verbally with a word or two; follows simple commands; otherwise drowsy
**Stuporous:** Very hard to arouse; inconsistently may follow simple commands or speak single words or short phrases; limited spontaneous movement
**Semicomatose:** Movements are purposeful when stimulated; does not follow commands or speak coherently
**Comatose:** May respond with reflexive posturing when stimulated or may have no response to any stimulus

questions such as, "What is your name? Where are you right now? What is the month/year/date/time? Why are you in the hospital?" An increase in the number of wrong answers indicates increasing confusion and possible deterioration in neurologic status. Likewise, an increase in the number of correct answers may indicate neurologic improvement.

In instances in which brain injury is suspected, the Glasgow Coma Scale (GCS) has proved a reliable tool for assessing arousal and level of consciousness (Box 33-4). The

## BOX 33-4    The Glasgow Coma Scale

| Best Eye-Opening Response | Score |
|---|---|
| Spontaneously | 4 |
| To speech | 3 |
| To pain | 2 |
| No response | 1 |

| Best Verbal Response | Score |
|---|---|
| Oriented | 5 |
| Confused conversation | 4 |
| Inappropriate words | 3 |
| Garbled sounds | 2 |
| No response | 1 |

| Best Motor Response | Score |
|---|---|
| Obeys commands | 6 |
| Localizes stimulus | 5 |
| Withdrawal from stimulus | 4 |
| Abnormal flexion (decorticate) | 3 |
| Abnormal extension (decerebrate) | 2 |
| No response | 1 |

A total score of 3 to 8 suggests severe impairment, 9 to 12 suggests moderate impairment, and 13 to 15 suggests mild impairment.

GCS allows the examiner to record objectively the patient's response to the environment in three major areas: eye opening, verbalization, and movement. In each category, the best response is scored. The GCS uses two responses, best eye-opening response and best verbal response, to assess arousal and level of consciousness. Best eye-opening response is scored from 1 to 4, with 1 as no response and 4 as spontaneous eye opening. Best verbal response addresses orientation and ranges from 1 to 5, with 1 again indicating no response and 5 indicating a fully oriented patient. The intubated patient is usually noted to have a verbal score of 1T, which should be added into the total score. In this way, recognition is given to the patient's inability to speak secondary to the presence of the endotracheal tube. Best motor response ranges from 1 to 6, with 1 indicating no motor response and 6 representing a patient with movement of all extremities to command. The maximal total score for a fully awake and alert person is 15. A minimum score of 3 is consistent with complete lack of

responsiveness. An overall score of 8 or below is associated with coma, and the likely inability to protect one's airway. If maintained over time, a low GCS score may be a predictor of poor functional recovery.

The GCS was designed as a guide for rapid evaluation of the acutely ill or severely injured patient whose status may change quickly. It is not useful as a guide for evaluation of patients in long-standing comas or during prolonged recovery from severe brain injury. More complex information about nervous system functioning can be obtained by gathering data about the patient's ability to integrate attention, memory, and thought processes (Table 33-1). Such a mental status examination also may uncover clues about additional problems affecting the patient's lifestyle. The Mini-Mental State Examination (MMSE) is a widely used cognitive assessment tool that is easy and quick to administer, and has good interrater reliability. It is frequently used to monitor disease progression in patients with dementia or other progressive disease states. The MMSE is composed of questions related to orientation, recall/memory, attention, calculation, language, and spatial insight. Points are assigned for correct answers, with a maximum of 30 points. A score of less than 20 may indicate neurologic disease. Examples of specific deficits are presented in Table 33-2.

When gathering such a wealth of data, assessment of the patient's ability to communicate becomes paramount. Use of language requires comprehension of verbal and nonverbal symbols and the ability to use those symbols to communicate with others. Evaluation of the patient's understanding normally is accomplished through the spoken word. However, speech dysfunctions (Table 33-3) can make such evaluations exceedingly difficult. In patients whose primary language is not English, use of an interpreter to ensure accurate assessment of orientation may be indicated.

## Motor Function

Evaluation of motor function includes assessment of motor response to stimuli, as well as motor strength and coordination. Assessment of motor response involves evaluating the type of stimuli necessary to elicit a motor response. This gives the health care team information about the level of awareness

## TABLE 33-1    Mental Status Examination

| Functions | Test | Implications |
|---|---|---|
| Orientation | Time: State year, month, date, season, day of week<br>Place: Indicate state, county, city of residency; state hospital name, floor or room number | May be altered by a multitude of neurologic conditions |
| Attention | Digit span; serial 7's; recitation of months of the year in reverse order | May be impaired in delirium, frontal lobe damage, and dementia |
| Memory | Short-term: Recall of three items after 5 min<br>Long-term: Recall of such items as mother's maiden name, events of previous day | May be impaired in conditions such as dementia, cerebrovascular accident, and delirium |
| Language | Naming: Point to three objects and have patient name them<br>Comprehension: Give simple and complex commands<br>Repetition: Repeat phrases such as "no ifs, ands, or buts"<br>Reading: Have patient read and explain a short passage<br>Writing: Have patient write a brief sentence | Requires integration of visual, semantic, and phonologic aspects of knowledge<br>Dysfunction may be associated with lesions of Broca area; may be dependent on educational level |
| Spatial/perceptual | Copy drawings such as cross or square; draw a clock face<br>Point out right and left side of self<br>Demonstrate such actions as putting on a coat or blowing out a match | May be associated with parietal lobe lesions |

**TABLE 33-2  Selected Deficits in Higher Intellectual Function**

| Type | Characteristics |
|---|---|
| Anomia | Inability to name objects or recognize written or spoken names of objects |
| Phonemic paraphasia | Substitutes parts of words (eg, pan opener instead of can opener) |
| Semantic paraphasia | Substitutes whole words (eg, apple for orange) |
| Dyslexia | Inability to recognize and comprehend written words |
| Alexia | Reading letter by letter instead of whole words |
| Neglect dyslexia | Omissions or substitutions of letters confined to initial part of the word |
| Surface dyslexia | Difficulty reading words with irregular spelling |
| Dysgraphia | Difficulty with writing |
| Central dysgraphia | Affects both written and oral spelling |
| Neglect dysgraphia | Misspelling the initial part of the word |
| Agnosia | Failure to recognize objects despite intact sensory input; may be visual, auditory, or sensory |
| Prosopagnosia | Inability to recognize familiar faces |
| Achromatopsia | Inability to discriminate colors |
| Acalculia | Inability to read, write, and comprehend numbers |

necessary to obtain a motor response as well as the patient's ability to follow commands. Evaluation of motor strength and coordination assesses motor neuron pathways within the brain, from the primary motor cortex to the spinal cord, as well as multiple other areas involved in coordination, such as the cerebellum and basal ganglia.

**Motor Response to Stimuli**

The nurse first attempts to elicit a motor response by asking the patient to move an extremity against gravity. If no response is forthcoming, the patient may be unable to comprehend or to respond to verbal commands. In this instance, noxious stimuli should be used to elicit a motor response.

When noxious stimuli are needed to evoke a response, the nurse pays careful attention to where the painful stimulus is applied. Noxious stimuli can involve either central or peripheral stimulation. Central stimulation involves pinching of the trapezius muscle, or pressure on the supraorbital ridge, while peripheral stimulation response may be elicited by compression of the nail bed. However, be aware that a misplaced examiner's hand may cause serious skin or tissue injury. Areas to avoid include the skin of the nipples and genital area. Also, the commonly used sternal rub can cause severe bruising, and does not elicit a clear response. When stimulating the supraorbital ridge, the nurse should take care not to compress the eye itself.

Localization to painful stimuli is characterized by an organized attempt to remove the central stimulus (ie, the examiner's hand), and entails movement of an upper extremity to a location above the clavicle (Fig. 33-1A). This is in contrast to withdrawal, in which the patient simply pulls away from the noxious stimulus, rather than attempting to remove it (Fig. 33-1B). Localization is a response that indicates a higher level of cerebral function than withdrawal. Appropriate responses, such as localization or withdrawal, infer that the sensory and corticospinal pathways are functioning. There may be monoplegia or hemiplegia, indicating that the corticospinal pathways are interrupted on one side.

Inappropriate responses include decorticate rigidity and decerebrate rigidity. Flexion of the arms, wrists, and fingers; adduction of the upper extremities; and extension, internal rotation, and plantar flexion of the lower extremities characterize decorticate rigidity (Fig. 33-1C). Such rigidity results from lesions of the internal capsule, basal ganglia, thalamus, or cerebral hemisphere, interrupting corticospinal pathways. Decerebrate rigidity consists of extension, adduction, and hyperpronation of the upper extremities and extension of the lower extremities, with plantar flexion of the feet (Fig. 33-1D). The person may also have clenched teeth. Injury to the midbrain and pons results in decerebration. At times, the inappropriate responses of decortication and decerebration may switch back and forth. If there is no response to noxious stimuli or only very weak flexor responses (ie, flaccidity), the patient likely has extensive brainstem dysfunction (Fig. 33-1E). Additional abnormal motor responses in a comatose patient include tonic contraction, which is consistent muscular

**TABLE 33-3  Patterns of Speech Deficits**

| Type | Deficit Locations | Speech Patterns |
|---|---|---|
| Fluent dysphasia | Left parietal–temporal lobes (Wernicke area) | • Fluent speech that lacks coherent content<br>• Impaired understanding of spoken word despite normal hearing<br>• May have normal-sounding speech rhythm but no intelligible words<br>• May use invented, meaningless words (neologism), word substitution (paraphasia), or repetition of words (perseveration, echolalia) |
| Nonfluent dysphasia | Left frontal area (Broca area) | • Slow speech with poor articulation<br>• Inability to initiate sounds<br>• Comprehension usually intact<br>• Usually associated with impaired writing skills |
| Global dysphasia | Diffuse involvement of frontal, parietal, and occipital areas | • Nonfluent speech<br>• Inability to understand spoken or written words |
| Dysarthria | Corticobulbar tracts; cerebellum | • Loss of articulation, phonation<br>• Loss of control of muscles of lips, tongue, palate<br>• Slurred, jerky, or irregular speech but with appropriate content |

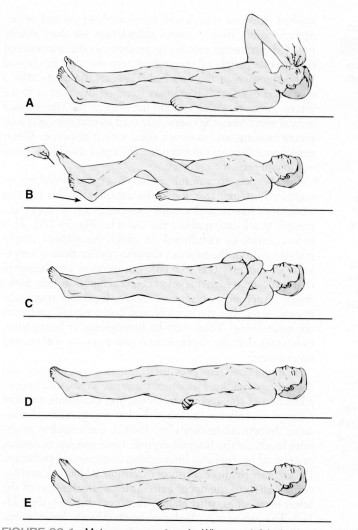

(A) Localizing pain: An appropriate response is to reach up above shoulder level toward the stimulus. Remember, a focal motor deficit such as hemiplegia may prevent a bilateral response.

(B) Withdrawal: An appropriate response is to pull the extremity or body away from the stimulus. As brainstem involvement increases, your patient may respond by assuming one of the following postures. Each one shows more advanced deterioration.

(C) Decorticate posturing: One or both arms in full flexion on the chest. Legs may be stiffly extended.

(D) Decerebrate posturing: One or both arms stiffly extended. Possible extension of the legs.

(E) Flaccid: No motor response in any extremity.

**FIGURE 33-1** Motor responses to pain. When a painful stimulus is applied to an unconscious patient's supraorbital notch, the patient responds in one of these ways.

contraction, and clonus, which is alternating muscle spasticity and relaxation.

## Motor Strength and Coordination

The second component of the motor assessment addresses strength and coordination. Muscle weakness is a cardinal sign of dysfunction in many neurologic disorders. The nurse tests extremity strength by offering resistance to various muscle groups, using his or her own muscles or gravity. As a quick test to detect weakness of the upper extremities, the nurse asks the patient to hold the arms straight out with palms upward and eyes closed, and observes for any downward drift or pronation of the forearms (referred to as pronator drift). A similar test for the lower extremities involves having the patient lie in bed and raise the legs, one at a time, straight off the bed against the examiner's resistance. Weakness noted in any of these tests can indicate damage to the motor neuron pathways of the pyramidal system, which transmits commands for voluntary movement. Motor function for each extremity is reported as a fraction, with 5 as the denominator, as shown in Box 33-5.

Muscle groups are assessed individually, initially without resistance and then against resistance, to obtain a thorough evaluation. Upper extremity muscle strength is evaluated by asking the patient to shrug the shoulders (trapezius and levator scapulae muscles), raise the arms (deltoid muscle), flex the elbow (biceps muscle), extend the arm (triceps muscle), and extend the wrist (extensor carpi radialis longus muscle). Lower extremity muscle strength is evaluated by asking the patient to raise the leg (iliopsoas muscle), extend the knee (quadriceps muscle), dorsiflex and plantarflex the foot (anterior tibialis and gastrocnemius muscles, respectively), and flex the knee (hamstring muscle group consisting of the biceps femoris, semitendinosus, and semimembranosus muscles).

Assessment of movement and strength in a patient who cannot follow commands or is unresponsive can be difficult because participating in muscle strength testing against gravity requires the patient's understanding and cooperation. If the patient is unable to mount a motor response to painful stimuli, the nurse may not have the opportunity to test for muscle strength in a reliable manner. Therefore, for comatose patients, it is important to note what, if any, stimuli

| BOX 33-5 | A Motor Function Scale |
|---|---|
| **Score** | **Interpretation** |
| 0/5 | No muscle contraction |
| 1/5 | Flicker or trace of contraction |
| 2/5 | Moves but cannot overcome gravity |
| 3/5 | Moves against gravity but cannot overcome resistance of examiner's muscles |
| 4/5 | Moves with some weakness against resistance of examiner's muscles |
| 5/5 | Normal power and strength |

initiate a response, and to describe or grade the type of response obtained.

The nurse may also assess each extremity for size, muscle tone, and smoothness of passive movement. Abnormal responses may indicate problems in the basal ganglia (also called the extrapyramidal system). These pathways normally suppress involuntary movements through controlled inhibition. Assessment findings may include the "clasp-knife" phenomenon, in which initially strong resistance to passive movement suddenly decreases. Alternatively, "lead-pipe" rigidity may be present, which is steady, continuous resistance to passive movement and is characteristic of diffuse hemispheric damage. "Cogwheel" rigidity, which is a series of small, regular, jerky movements felt on passive movement, is characteristic of Parkinson disease. The nurse also should be alert to involuntary movements, from mild fasciculation (muscle twitching) to violent, flailing movement of an extremity. Descriptive terms for involuntary movements are given in Box 33-6.

Hemiparesis (weakness) and hemiplegia (paralysis) are unilateral symptoms resulting from a lesion contralateral to the corticospinal tract. Paraplegia results from a spinal cord lesion below the first thoracic vertebrae or from peripheral nerve dysfunctions. Quadriplegia (also known as tetraplegia) is associated with cervical spinal cord lesions, brainstem dysfunction, and large bilateral lesions in the cerebrum.

| BOX 33-6 | Types of Voluntary Movements |
|---|---|

**Tremor:** Purposeless movement
- Resting: Lesion in basal ganglia
- Intention: Lesion in cerebellum
- Asterixis: Metabolic derangement
- Physiologic: Due to fatigue or stress

**Fasciculation:** Twitching of resting muscles due to peripheral nerve or spinal cord lesion or to metabolic influences such as cold or anesthetic agents

**Clonus:** Repetitive movement; elicited with stretch reflex and implies lesion of the corticospinal tracts

**Myoclonus:** Nonrhythmic movement; single jerk-like movements; symmetrical; unknown etiology

**Hemiballismus:** Flailing movement of extremity; violent movement; not present during sleep; lesion in subthalamic nuclei of basal ganglia

**Chorea:** Irregular movements; involves limbs and facial muscles; asymmetrical movements at rest; involuntary movements may increase when purposeful movement is attempted

**Athetosis:** Slow, writhing movements

The cerebellum is responsible for smooth synchronization, balance, and ordering of movements. It does not initiate any movements, so a patient with cerebellar dysfunction is not paralyzed. Instead, ataxia, dysmetria, and lack of synchronization of movement are common manifestations. Some of the more common tests for cerebellar synchronization of movement with balance include the following:

- **Romberg test:** This test is performed by having the patient stand with his or her feet together, first with the eyes open, then with the eyes closed. The nurse looks for sway or direction of falling and is prepared to catch the patient if necessary.
- **Finger-to-nose test:** This test is performed by having the patient touch one finger to the examiner's finger, then touch his or her own nose. Overshooting or past-pointing the mark is called dysmetria. Both sides are tested individually.
- **Rapidly alternating movement (RAM) test:** The patient's ability to perform RAMs is checked on each side by having the patient oppose each finger and thumb in rapid succession or by performing rapid pronation and supination of the hand on the leg. Inability to perform RAMs is termed adiadochokinesia; performing RAMs poorly or clumsily is termed dysdiadochokinesia.
- **Heel-to-shin test:** This test is performed by having the patient extend the heel of one foot down the anterior aspect of the shin, moving from the knee to the ankle. Inability to complete this movement, or a lack of smooth motor movement, is an indicator of cerebellar dysfunction.

## Pupillary Changes

Assessment of pupillary response is an important component of the neurologic examination. Pupils are examined for size (specified in millimeters; Fig. 33-2) and shape. The patient focuses on a distant point in the room. To isolate the eye being examined, the examiner places the edge of one hand along the patient's nose. A bright light is directed into one eye, and the briskness of pupillary constriction (direct response) is noted. The other pupil also should constrict (consensual response). The procedure is then repeated with the other eye. Anisocoria (unequal pupils) is normal in a small percentage of the population but can also indicate neural dysfunction. If it is a normal variant, the difference in pupil size should be less than 1 mm.

Pupil reactivity is also assessed with respect to accommodation. To test accommodation, an object is held 8 to

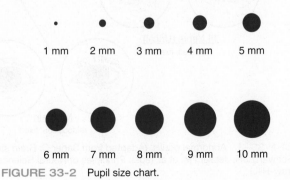

FIGURE 33-2  Pupil size chart.

12 inches in front of the patient's face. The patient focuses on the object as the examiner moves it toward the patient's nose. The pupils should constrict as the object gets closer, and the eyes should turn inward to maintain a clear image.

The normal response to testing is documented as PER-RLA, or **p**upils **e**qual, **r**ound, **r**eactive to **l**ight and **a**ccommodation. Some important pupillary abnormalities are shown in Figure 33-3. Causes of small, reactive pupils include metabolic abnormalities and bilateral dysfunction in the diencephalon. Large, fixed pupils (5 to 6 mm) that may show slight rhythmic constriction and dilation when stimulated may indicate midbrain damage. Midposition, fixed pupils (4 to 5 mm) also may indicate midbrain dysfunction, involving interruption of the sympathetic and parasympathetic pathways. Pinpoint, nonreactive pupils are seen after damage to the pons area of the brainstem (thus the phrase "pontine pupils are pinpoint"), with selected eye medications, and with opiate administration. A unilaterally dilated, nonreactive ("blown") pupil is seen with third cranial (oculomotor) nerve damage when the uncal portion of the temporal lobe herniates through the tentorium. When structures are compressed around the opening in the tentorium or fold of dura that separates the cerebrum from the cerebellum and brainstem, loss of functioning of the parasympathetic nerves to the pupil on that side results in ipsilaterally (same side) dilated pupils. A quick guide to causes of pupil size changes is given in Box 33-7.

The assessment of pupillary response for comatose patients is the same as for conscious patients. Pupil reactivity to light, by direct and consensual response, is easily obtained. It may be impossible to ascertain reactivity to accommodation because the patient may be unable to cooperate.

## Cranial Nerve Function

Cranial nerve assessment varies depending on whether the patient is conscious or unconscious. Assessment of the cranial nerves in the unconscious patient is important because it provides data regarding brainstem function; however many components may need to be eliminated or adapted. For specific physiologic information about the cranial nerves, see Chapter 32.

### Cranial Nerve I (Olfactory Nerve)

The first cranial nerve contains sensory fibers for the sense of smell. Testing of this nerve is usually deferred unless the patient complains of an inability to smell. The nurse tests the nerve, with the patient's eyes closed, by placing aromatic substances near the nose for identification. Items that have

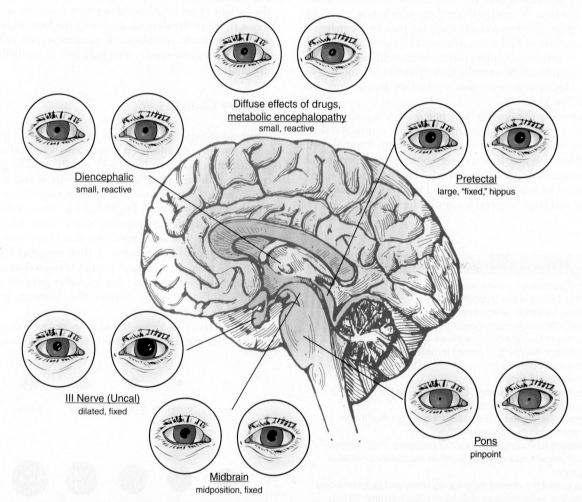

Diffuse effects of drugs, metabolic encephalopathy
small, reactive

Diencephalic
small, reactive

Pretectal
large, "fixed," hippus

III Nerve (Uncal)
dilated, fixed

Midbrain
midposition, fixed

Pons
pinpoint

**FIGURE 33-3**   Abnormal pupils. (Adapted from Saper C: Brain stem modulation of sensation, movement, and consciousness. In: Kandel ER, Schwartz JH, Jessel TM, et al. (eds): Principles of Neural Science, 5th ed. New York, NY: McGraw-Hill, 2012, p 1054, with permission from McGraw-Hill.)

**Quick Guide to Causes of Pupil Size Change**

**Pinpoint Pupils**
- Drugs: Opiates
- Drops: Medications for glaucoma
- "Nearly dead": Damage in the pons area of the brainstem

**Dilated Pupils**
- Fear: Panic attack, extreme anxiety
- "Fits": Seizures
- "Fast living": Cocaine, crack, phencyclidine

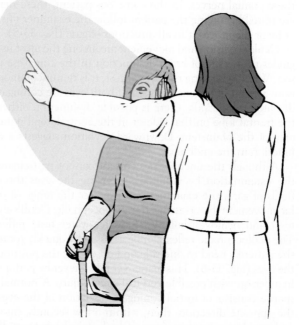

**FIGURE 33-4**   Confrontational method of testing visual fields.

a distinct smell (eg, soap, coffee, cinnamon) should be used. Ammonia should not be used because the patient will respond to irritation of the nasal mucosa rather than to the odor. Each nostril is checked separately by closing off one nostril at a time. Loss of smell may be caused by a fracture of the cribriform plate or a fracture in the ethmoid area. The patient may also have anosmia (loss of sense of smell) from a shearing injury to the olfactory bulb after a basilar skull fracture or from cerebrospinal fluid (CSF) leak.

### Cranial Nerve II (Optic Nerve)

Assessment of the optic nerve involves evaluation of visual acuity and visual fields. Gross visual acuity is checked by having the patient read ordinary newsprint, noting the patient's preinjury need for corrective lenses. Visual fields are tested by having the patient look straight ahead with one eye covered. The examiner moves a finger from the periphery of each quadrant of vision toward the patient's center of vision. The patient should indicate when the examiner's finger is seen. This is done for both eyes, and the results are compared with the examiner's visual fields, which are assumed to be normal (Fig. 33-4). Damage to the retina produces a blind spot. An optic nerve lesion produces partial or complete blindness on the same side. Damage to the optic chiasm results in bitemporal hemianopsia, blindness in both lateral visual fields. Pressure on the optic tract can cause homonymous hemianopsia, half-blindness on the opposite side of the lesion in both eyes. A lesion in the parietal or temporal lobe may produce contralateral blindness in the upper or lower quadrant of vision, respectively, in both eyes (quadrant deficit). Damage in the occipital lobe can cause homonymous

hemianopsia with central vision sparing. Table 33-4 depicts visual field defects.

### Cranial Nerves III (Oculomotor Nerve), IV (Trochlear Nerve), and VI (Abducens Nerve)

Cranial nerves III, IV, and VI are assessed together because they all innervate extraocular muscles involved in eye movement. The parasympathetic fibers of the oculomotor nerve are responsible for lens accommodation and pupil size through control of the ciliary muscles. This is the nerve tested when a nurse elicits a pupillary response. The motor fibers of the oculomotor nerve innervate the muscles that elevate the eyelid and those that move the eyes up, down, and medially. These include the superior rectus, inferior oblique, inferior rectus, and medial rectus muscles. The trochlear nerve innervates the superior oblique muscle to move the eyes down and in. The lateral rectus muscle moves the eyes laterally and is innervated by the abducens nerve. Diplopia, nystagmus, conjugate deviation, and ptosis may indicate dysfunction of

**TABLE 33-4**   **Visual Field Defects Associated With Defects of the Visual System**

| Visual Field Defect | Left | Right | Description |
|---|---|---|---|
| Anopsia | ○ | ● | Blindness in one eye; due to complete lesion of the right optic nerve |
| Bitemporal hemianopsia (central vision) | ◖ | ◗ | Blindness in both lateral visual fields; due to lesions around the optic chiasm such as pituitary tumors or aneurysms of the anterior communicating artery. Affected fibers originate in the nasal half of each retina |
| Homonymous hemianopsia | ◖ | ◖ | Half-blindness involving both eyes with loss of visual field on the same side of each eye; due to lesion of temporal or occipital lobe with damage to the optic tract or optic radiations (blindness occurs on the side opposite the lesion; here, the lesion occurred in the right side of the brain, resulting in loss of vision in the left visual field of both eyes) |
| Quadrant deficit | ◔ | ◔ | Blindness in the upper or lower quadrant of vision in both eyes, resulting from a lesion in the parietal or temporal lobe |

these cranial nerves. In the conscious patient, these nerves are tested by having the patient follow the examiner's finger as he or she moves it in all directions of gaze (Fig. 33-5).

Ocular position and movement are among the most useful guides to the site of brain dysfunction in the comatose person. When observing the eyes at rest, it is not uncommon to note a slight divergence of gaze. If both eyes are conjugately deviated to one side, there is possible dysfunction either in the frontal lobe on that side or in the contralateral pontine area of the brainstem. Downward deviation suggests a dysfunction in the midbrain.

Although the unconscious patient cannot participate in the examination by voluntarily moving the eyes through fields of gaze, the examiner still can test the range of ocular movement by assessing the oculocephalic ("doll's eyes" test) and oculovestibular (caloric ice-water test) reflexes. The oculocephalic reflex can be assessed by quickly rotating the patient's head to one side and observing the position of the eyes (Fig. 33-6). This maneuver must never be performed in a person with possible cervical spine injury. A normal response consists of initial conjugate deviation of the eyes in the opposite direction, then, within a few seconds, smooth and simultaneous movement of both eyes back to midline position. This response indicates an intact brainstem. An abnormal reflex response occurs when one eye does not follow the normal response pattern. Absence of any ocular movement when the head is rotated briskly to either side or up and down indicates an absent reflex and portends severe brainstem dysfunction.

The examiner tests the oculovestibular reflex by elevating the patient's head 30 degrees and irrigating each ear separately with 30 to 50 mL of ice water (Fig. 33-7). This test should never be performed in a patient who does not have an intact eardrum or who has blood or fluid collected behind the eardrum. Also, the external ear canal should be unobstructed by cerumen or debris. In an unconscious patient with an intact brainstem, the eyes exhibit horizontal nystagmus with

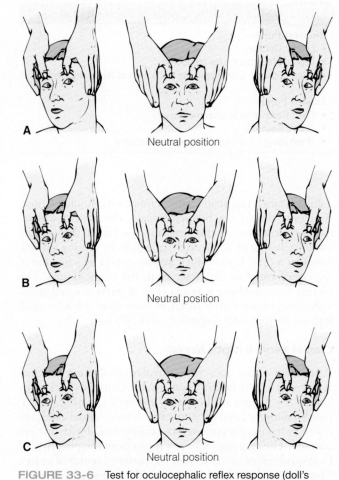

**A** Neutral position

**B** Neutral position

**C** Neutral position

**FIGURE 33-6** Test for oculocephalic reflex response (doll's eyes phenomenon). **A:** Normal response—when the head is rotated, the eyes turn together to the side opposite to the head movement. **B:** Abnormal response—when the head is rotated, the eyes do not turn in a conjugate manner. **C:** Absent response—as head position is changed, eyes do not move in the sockets.

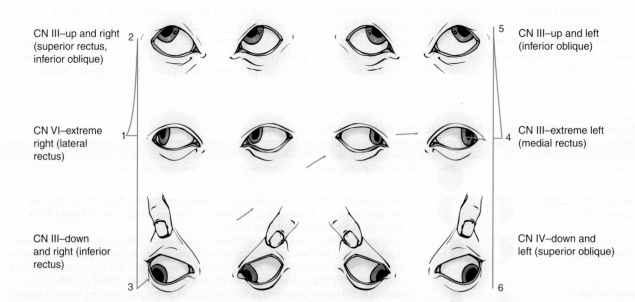

CN III—up and right (superior rectus, inferior oblique)

CN III—up and left (inferior oblique)

CN VI—extreme right (lateral rectus)

CN III—extreme left (medial rectus)

CN III—down and right (inferior rectus)

CN IV—down and left (superior oblique)

**FIGURE 33-5** Muscles used in conjugate eye movements in the six cardinal directions of gaze. Lead the patient's gaze in the sequence numbered 1 through 6. CN III, oculomotor nerve; CN IV, trochlear nerve; CN VI, abducens nerve.

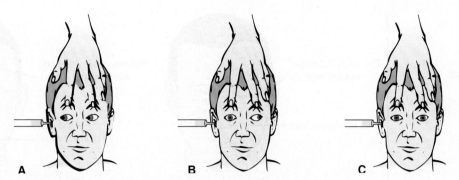

**FIGURE 33-7** Test for oculovestibular reflex response (caloric ice-water test). **A:** Normal response—ice-water infusion in the ear produces conjugate eye movements. **B:** Abnormal response—infusion produces disconjugate or asymmetrical eye movements. **C:** Absent response—infusion produces no eye movements.

slow, conjugate movement toward the irrigated ear followed by rapid movement away from the stimulus. When the reflex is absent, both eyes remain fixed in midline position, indicating midbrain and pons dysfunction.

### Cranial Nerve V (Trigeminal Nerve)

Cranial nerve V has three divisions: ophthalmic, maxillary, and mandibular. The sensory portion of this nerve controls sensation to the cornea and face. The motor portion controls the muscles of mastication. This nerve is partially tested by checking the corneal reflex; if it is intact, the patient blinks when the cornea is stroked with a wisp of cotton or when a drop of normal saline is placed in the eye. Care must be taken not to stroke the eyelash because this can cause the eye to blink regardless of a corneal reflex. Facial sensation can be tested by comparing light touch and pinprick on symmetrical sides of the face. The ability to chew or clench the jaw also is observed.

### Cranial Nerve VII (Facial Nerve)

The sensory portion of cranial nerve VII is concerned with taste on the anterior two-thirds of the tongue. The motor portion controls muscles of facial expression (Fig. 33-8). Testing is performed by asking the patient to raise the eyebrows, smile, or grimace. With a central (supranuclear) lesion, there is muscle paralysis of the lower half of the face on the side opposite the lesion; the muscles around the eyes and forehead are unaffected. With a peripheral (nuclear or infranuclear) lesion, there is complete paralysis of facial muscles on the same side as the lesion.

The most common type of peripheral facial paralysis is Bell palsy, which consists of ipsilateral facial paralysis. There is drooping of the upper lid with the lower lid slightly everted. Facial lines on the same side are obliterated, with the mouth drawn toward the normal side.

### Cranial Nerve VIII (Acoustic Nerve)

Cranial nerve VIII is divided into the cochlear and vestibular branches, which control hearing and equilibrium, respectively. The cochlear nerve is tested by air and bone conduction. There are two distinct auditory tests: the Weber test and the Rinne test. For the Rinne test, a vibrating tuning fork is placed on the mastoid process and the patient is asked to listen to the sound and to indicate when it disappears.

The tuning fork is then placed in front of the ear; a normal result occurs when the patient can still hear sound transmitted through air. The Weber test involves placement of the tuning fork on the patient's forehead. A normal response would be equal hearing of the sound in both ears. The patient may complain of tinnitus or decreased hearing if this nerve is damaged. The vestibular nerve may not be evaluated routinely. However, the nurse should be alert to complaints of dizziness or vertigo from the patient.

### Cranial Nerves IX (Glossopharyngeal Nerve) and X (Vagus Nerve)

Cranial nerves IX and X usually are tested together. The glossopharyngeal nerve supplies sensory fibers to the posterior third of the tongue and the uvula and soft palate. The vagus nerve innervates the larynx, pharynx, and soft palate and conveys autonomic responses to the heart, stomach, lungs, and small intestine. These nerves can be tested by eliciting a gag reflex, observing the uvula for symmetrical movement when the patient says "ah," or observing midline elevation of the uvula when both sides are stroked. Inability to cough forcefully, difficulty with swallowing, and hoarseness may be signs of dysfunction. Autonomic vagal functions usually are not tested because they are checked during the general physical examination.

### Cranial Nerve XI (Spinal Accessory Nerve)

Cranial nerve XI controls the trapezius and sternocleidomastoid muscles. The examiner tests this nerve by having the patient shrug the shoulders or turn the head from side to side against resistance.

### Cranial Nerve XII (Hypoglossal Nerve)

Cranial nerve XII controls tongue movement. This nerve can be checked by having the patient protrude his or her tongue. The examiner checks for deviation from midline, tremor, and atrophy. If deviation is noted secondary to nerve damage, it will be to the side of the cerebral lesion.

### Quick Screening Test

Testing cranial nerve function completely is time consuming and exacting. A partial, quicker screening assessment may be performed, focusing on nerves in which dysfunction may

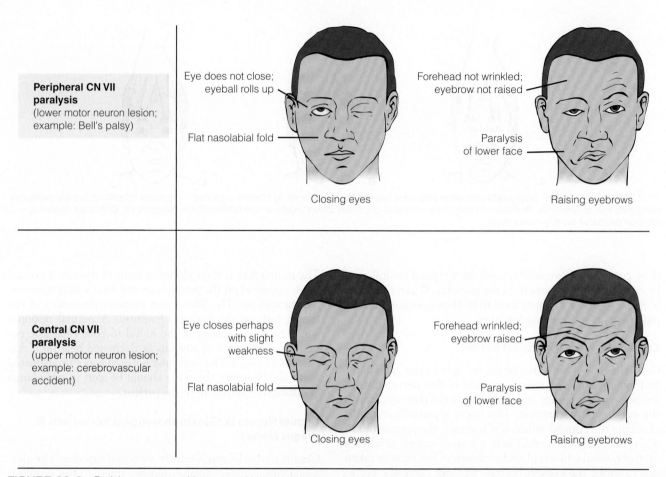

**Peripheral CN VII paralysis**
(lower motor neuron lesion; example: Bell's palsy)

Eye does not close; eyeball rolls up

Flat nasolabial fold

Closing eyes

Forehead not wrinkled; eyebrow not raised

Paralysis of lower face

Raising eyebrows

**Central CN VII paralysis**
(upper motor neuron lesion; example: cerebrovascular accident)

Eye closes perhaps with slight weakness

Flat nasolabial fold

Closing eyes

Forehead wrinkled; eyebrow raised

Paralysis of lower face

Raising eyebrows

**FIGURE 33-8** Facial movements with upper and lower motor neuron facial paralysis. CN VII, facial nerve. In the comatose patient, motor function of the facial muscles and jaw can be ascertained by observing spontaneous muscle activity such as yawning, grimacing, or chewing. Symmetry of movement may be assessed, and facial droops may be observed.

**TABLE 33-5** A Quick Screening Test for Cranial Nerve Function

| | Nerve | Reflex | Procedure |
|---|---|---|---|
| II | Optic | Pupil constriction (protection of the retina) | Shine a light into each eye and note if the pupil on that side constricts (direct response). Next, shine a light into each eye and note if the opposite pupil constricts (consensual response). |
| III | Oculomotor | | |
| V | Trigeminal | Corneal reflex (protection of the cornea) | Approaching the eye from the side and avoiding the eyelashes, touch the cornea with a wisp of cotton. Alternatively, a drop of sterile water or normal saline may be used. A blink response should be present. |
| VII | Facial | | |
| IX | Glossopharyngeal | Airway protection | Touch the back of the throat with a tongue depressor. A gag or cough response should be present. |
| X | Vagus | | |

indicate serious problems or interfere with activities of daily living. The cranial nerves of primary importance in a screening examination are the optic, oculomotor, trigeminal, facial, glossopharyngeal, and vagus nerves (Table 33-5).

## Reflexes

A reflex occurs when a sensory stimulus evokes a motor response. Cerebral control and consciousness are not required for a reflex to occur. Superficial and deep reflexes are tested on symmetrical sides of the body and compared by noting the strength of contraction elicited on each side.

Cutaneous, or superficial, reflexes occur when certain areas of skin are lightly stroked or tapped, causing contraction of the muscle groups beneath. Such reflexes are graded simply as normal, abnormal (pathologic), or absent. An example is the plantar reflex. A sensory stimulus is applied by briskly stroking the outer edge of the sole and across the ball of the foot with a dull object, such as a tongue blade or key. The normal motor response is downward or plantar flexion of the toes. An abnormal response (Babinski sign) is upward or dorsiflexion of the big toe, with or without fanning of the other toes. A positive Babinski sign can indicate a lesion in the pyramidal tract. It should be noted, however, that a positive Babinski sign is normal in children under the age of 2.

Muscle stretch reflexes, also called deep tendon reflexes, are elicited by a brisk tap with a reflex hammer on the appropriate tendon insertion site. The target for this sensory stimulus is a stretched tendon of a muscle group. Deep tendon reflexes are tested on the biceps, brachioradial, triceps, patellar, and Achilles tendons. The desired motor response is contraction of the stimulated muscle group. Deep tendon reflexes are commonly graded on a scale of 0 to 4:

4+: A very brisk response; evidence of disease, electrolyte imbalance, or both; associated with clonic contractions
3+: A brisk response; possibly indicative of disease
2+: A normal response
1+: A response in the low-normal range
0: No response; possibly evidence of disease or electrolyte imbalance.

Hyperreflexia is associated with upper motor neuron disease, whereas areflexia (absence of reflexes) is associated with lower motor neuron dysfunction, such as spinal cord lesions. Reflexes can be tested on the comatose patient. It is anticipated that, depending on the severity and location of the neuronal damage, either hyperreflexia or areflexia will be present.

## Sensation

The last component of the neurologic examination, other than vital signs, involves a sensory assessment. Normal sensory findings require that the spinal cord, sensory pathways, and peripheral nervous system are intact. The primary forms of sensation are tested first. These include perception of touch (cotton wisp), pain (pinprick), temperature (hot, cold), proprioception (limb position), and vibration. With the patient's eyes closed, multiple and symmetrical areas of the body are tested, including the trunk and extremities.

The nurse assesses the perception of touch by asking the patient to close the eyes and identify when and where he or she feels a cotton wisp or cotton swab on the skin. Pain is assessed with the use of a pin or the sharp edge of a cotton swab, moving in a head-to-toe direction on both sides of the body. If temperature is tested, the nurse uses glass tubes of hot and cold water and proceeds in the manner described previously. Two-point discrimination may also be tested;

this refers to the patient's ability to distinguish between two closely located points. Discrimination of sharp versus dull is also a commonly used test.

Proprioception is tested by asking the patient, again with the eyes closed, to identify the direction of movement (eg, moving a finger upward and then asking the patient if the finger is up or down). The same test is performed on the other hand, as well as both lower extremities. The nurse assesses vibration using a tuning fork placed over a bony prominence. The patient is asked to identify when vibration is felt.

The patient's ability to perceive the sensation is noted, with distal areas compared with proximal areas and right and left sides compared at corresponding points. The nurse also determines whether sensory change involves one entire side of the body. Abnormal results may indicate damage somewhere along the pathways of the receptors in the skin, muscles, joints and tendons, spinothalamic tracts, or sensory area of the cortex (Table 33-6).

Cortical forms of sensation also should be tested. When primary sensation is intact, but interpretation of the sensory input is altered, then damage to the parietal lobe may be anticipated. Problems with discriminative sensation include those involving stereognosis, graphesthesia, and point localization. The ability to recognize and identify objects by touch is called stereognosis, and is a function of the parietal lobe. The inability to recognize objects by touch, sight, or sound is termed agnosia. This may be tested by placing an object in a patient's hand and asking him or her, with the eyes closed, to identify the object solely based on touch. Identification of an object by the sense of sight is a function of the parieto-occipital junction. The temporal lobe is responsible for identification of objects by sound. Each of these senses should be tested separately. For example, a patient may not be able to identify a whistle by its sound but may recognize it immediately if he or she holds it or looks at it.

Graphesthesia is the ability to recognize numbers or letters traced lightly on the skin. Bilateral sides are compared. Point localization refers to the ability to locate the precise spot on the body touched by the examiner. One version of

### TABLE 33-6 Testing Superficial and Deep Sensations

| Sensation | Stimuli | Dysfunction |
| --- | --- | --- |
| **Spinothalamic Tracts Carry Impulses for** | | |
| Pain | Alternate sharp and dull ends of a pin, asking patient to discriminate between the two (superficial pain). Squeeze nail beds; apply pressure on the orbital rim; rub sternum (deep pain). | • Ipsilateral sensory loss implies a peripheral nerve lesion.<br>• Contralateral sensory loss is seen with lesions of the spinothalamic tract or in the thalamus. |
| Light touch | Use a wisp of cotton on skin and ask patient to identify when it touches. | • Bilateral sensory loss may indicate a spinal cord lesion.<br>• Paresthesia is an abnormal sensation, such as itching or tingling. |
| Temperature | Use test tubes filled with hot and cold water or use small metal plates of varying temperatures. (Test only if pain and light touch sensations are abnormal.) | • Causalgia is a burning sensation that can be caused by peripheral nerve irritation. |
| **Posterior Columns Carry Impulses for** | | |
| Vibration | Apply a vibrating tuning fork on bony prominences, and note patient's ability to sense and locate vibrations bilaterally. | Ipsilateral sensory loss may be due to spinal cord injury or to peripheral neuropathy. |
| Proprioception | Move the patient's finger or toe up and down and ask patient to identify final resting position. | Contralateral loss may occur from lesions of the thalamus or of the parietal lobes. |

dysfunction in this area is called extinction phenomenon, the inability to recognize bilateral sensations when the examiner simultaneously touches two symmetrical areas on opposite sides of the body.

In a comatose patient, it is impossible to perform a complete test for sensation because patient cooperativeness is required. However, use of painful stimuli to elicit a response gives a gross indication that some degree of sensory function remains intact. More detailed data would be unavailable, however.

## Vital Signs

Vital sign assessment is crucial to the neurologic examination. Changes in temperature, heart rate, and blood pressure are considered late findings in neurologic deterioration. Changes in respiratory rate, on the other hand, can indicate progression of neurologic impairment and are frequently seen early in neurologic deterioration.

### Respirations

Variations in respiratory pattern are commonly associated with neurologic injury. Shallow, rapid respirations can indicate a problem with maintenance of a patent airway or the need for suctioning. Snoring respirations or stridor can also indicate a partially obstructed airway. The inability to maintain an effective airway may be associated with a high cervical spinal cord lesion or progressive diaphragmatic paralysis (seen with neurodegenerative diseases), or it may be seen with a decreasing level of consciousness.

Changes in respiratory pattern can also be a direct indication of increasing intracranial pressure (ICP) (see Chapter 36, Fig. 36-6). Cheyne–Stokes respirations (crescendo–decrescendo respirations alternating with periods of apnea) are frequently noted in neurologic disease.

Hypoventilation after cerebral trauma can lead to respiratory acidosis. As the blood carbon dioxide increases and blood oxygen decreases, cerebral hypoxia and edema can result in secondary brain injury, thereby extending the degree of damage. Hyperventilation after cerebral trauma produces respiratory alkalosis with decreased blood carbon dioxide levels. This causes vasoconstriction of cerebral vessels, contributing to decreased cerebral blood flow.

### Temperature

Normal regulation of temperature occurs in the hypothalamus; therefore, diffuse cerebral damage that includes the hypothalamus can result in loss of temperature control, leading to hyperthermia. Fevers caused by damage to the hypothalamus may be very high, and differentiate themselves from other causes of fever by their resistance to antipyretic therapy. Hypothermia occurs with metabolic causes, pituitary damage, and spinal cord injuries; it is not the result of hypothalamic injury.

### Pulse

Variations in heart rate and rhythm may be associated with neurologic injury. An increase in ICP may lead to episodes of tachycardia and can predispose the patient to alterations in electrocardiogram pattern, such as ventricular or atrial

dysrhythmias. As the ICP increases, bradycardia results, and the combination of the two is indicative of impending herniation.

### Blood Pressure

Blood pressure is controlled at the level of the medulla. Therefore, specific damage to this area or encroaching edema secondary to injury in other areas results in alterations in blood pressure. Hypotension is not normally associated with neurologic injury. On the other hand, hypotension must be avoided in the postinjury stage because it can lead to decreased cerebral perfusion, hypoxia, and extension of the initial injury.

Hypertension is much more commonly seen. In the intact brain, the mechanism of cerebral autoregulation maintains constant blood flow to the brain, despite wide variations in systemic pressure. However, after injury, autoregulatory mechanisms fail, and cerebral blood flow varies dramatically with variations in systemic pressure. As blood pressure increases, cerebral blood flow increases, resulting in an increase in ICP. Likewise, as blood pressure decreases, cerebral blood flow decreases, resulting in ischemia.

## Signs of Trauma or Infection

Signs of trauma or infection may be evident on examination:

- **Battle sign** (bruising over the mastoid areas) suggests a basilar skull fracture.
- **Raccoon eyes** (periorbital edema and bruising) suggests a frontobasilar fracture.
- **CSF rhinorrhea** (drainage of CSF from the nose) suggests fracture of the cribriform plate with herniation of a fragment of the dura and arachnoid through the fracture.
- **CSF otorrhea** (drainage of CSF from the ear) usually is associated with fracture of the petrous portion of the temporal bone.
- **Signs of meningeal irritation** include nuchal rigidity (ie, pain and resistance to neck flexion), fever, headache, and photophobia. A positive Kernig sign (ie, pain in the neck when the thigh is flexed on the abdomen and the leg is extended at the knee) also may be present. Brudzinski sign (involuntary flexion of the hips when the neck is flexed toward the chest) is another indication of meningeal inflammation. Kernig sign and Brudzinski sign are shown in Figure 33-9.

## Signs of Increased Intracranial Pressure

The prevention of increased ICP, or intracranial hypertension, is of key importance to the nurse's role when caring for a patient with a neurologic injury. It is first essential for the nurse to establish a baseline neurologic assessment of the patient to which further deterioration or improvement can be compared. In general terms, increased ICP is manifested by deterioration in all aspects of neurologic functioning.

Level of consciousness decreases as ICP rises. Initially, the patient may present with evidence of restlessness, confusion, and combativeness. This then decompensates into lower levels of consciousness, ranging from lethargy to obtundation to coma. Pupillary reactions begin to diminish, with

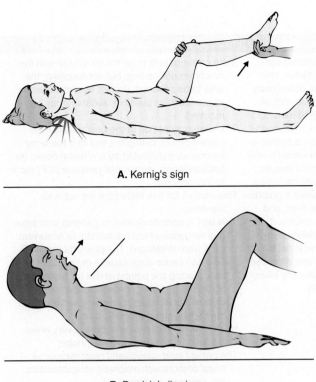

**A.** Kernig's sign

**B.** Brudzinksi's sign

FIGURE 33-9 Two signs of meningeal irritation.

sluggishly reactive pupils and eventually fixed, dilated pupils. Frequently, because of the potential for injury to be ipsilateral, one pupil dilates before the other one does, resulting in unequal pupils.

Motor function also declines with increased ICP, and the patient begins to show abnormal motor activity. For example, the patient who initially may have shown a localized response to painful stimuli (ie, moved an upper extremity above the clavicle in order to remove the stimuli) now shows either abnormal flexion or extension. Changes in vital signs are considered a late finding. Variations in respiratory patterns occur, eventually resulting in complete apnea. Cushing triad is considered a sign of impending herniation (see Chapter 36); this triad consists of an increased systolic pressure (resulting in an increased pulse pressure), bradycardia, and decreased irregular respirations.

## Evaluation of Dysfunction in the Patient's Living Patterns

Neurologic nursing assessment would be incomplete if the process consisted solely of gathering data and identifying abnormal functions. The scope of nursing care includes an evaluation of the impact of dysfunction on the patient's living patterns and ability to care for self. For example, diplopia (double vision) is an abnormal finding and may be an indicator of problems with the ocular muscles or with the nervous system; however, the nurse will also recognize that diplopia will make it difficult for the patient to perform daily activities, and will incorporate this knowledge into the plan of care.

## Neurodiagnostic Studies

Neurodiagnostic tests benefit the patient in an acute setting by shortening the time required to arrive at a diagnosis and institute therapy. The choice of which investigative test to perform should be based on the examiner's ability to integrate the findings with neurologic assessment and locate the cause of the abnormality. The nurse's role in neurodiagnostic testing involves patient and family preparation and monitoring the critically ill patient for potential complications during and after the procedure. Although there has been a definite increase in the number of tests that can be performed at the bedside, many still require that the patient be transported to the imaging department or even out of the institution, further expanding the role of the critical care nurse. Table 33-7 provides a summary of neurodiagnostic tests and outlines nursing implications.

## Neuroradiologic Techniques

Conventional radiographs of the skull and spine are used to identify fractures, dislocations, and other bony anomalies, especially in the setting of acute trauma. The use of plain films has decreased in recent years as computed tomography (CT) and magnetic resonance imaging (MRI) have proved to be better diagnostic tools.

Spinal films may still be used as an initial screening in suspected vertebral or spinal cord trauma; however, designated trauma centers rely increasingly on cervical spine CT scans. If plain films are to be taken, visualization of the cervical spine through C7 is indicated to rule out a cervical spine injury. Further visualization of C1 to C2 may require an odontoid or Waters view; this film is taken through the open mouth of the patient and necessitates patient cooperation. The nurse's role involves monitoring the patient and attendant equipment during the procedure and being alert for complications related to patient position and the length of the procedure. In the spinal cord injured–patient, care should be taken to ensure stabilization of the neck by a hard cervical collar and logrolling during testing.

## Computed Tomography

CT scans have been in use in the United States since 1973. CT scanning uses intersecting x-ray beams through the brain and skull to measure the density of tissues through which the x-ray beams pass. The denser the material (ie, skull), the whiter it appears on the film (Fig. 33-10). The less dense the material (ie, air), the darker it appears on the film. With mathematical reconstruction, multiple views or slices of the brain can be seen, which allows for a very precise, detailed picture of the brain and its contents. For example, cerebral edema appears less dense and therefore is of a lighter color than normal tissue.

The value of this technique is illustrated best in the trauma setting, where the ability to rapidly and accurately image the intracranial contents and position of the vertebrae and spinal cord has dramatically changed the treatment of patients with neurologic problems. CT scans are recommended in the initial workup of seizures, headache, and loss of consciousness and for the diagnosis of suspected hemorrhage, tumors, and

**TABLE 33-7** Neurodiagnostic Tests

| Diagnostic Test | Description | Information Obtained | Nursing Considerations and Interventions |
| --- | --- | --- | --- |
| Computed tomography, or CT scan (invasive and noninvasive) | A scanner takes a series of radiographic images all around the same axial plane. A computer then creates a composite picture of various tissue densities visualized. The images may be enhanced with the use of IV contrast dye. | CT scans give detailed outlines of bone, tissue, and fluid structures of the body. They can indicate shift of structures due to tumors, hematomas, or hydrocephalus. A CT scan is limited in that it gives information only about structure of tissues, not about functional status. | Instruct the patient to lie flat on a table with the machine surrounding, but not touching, the area to be scanned. Patient also must remain as immobile as possible; sedation may be required.<br>The scan may not be of the best quality if the patient moves during the test or if the x-ray beams were deflected by any metal object (ie, traction tongs, intracranial pressure [ICP] monitoring devices). |
| Magnetic resonance imaging (MRI) | A selected area of the patient's body is placed inside a powerful magnetic field. The hydrogen atoms inside the patient are temporarily "excited" and caused to oscillate by a sequence of radiofrequency pulsations. The sensitive scanner measures these minute oscillations, and a computer-enhanced image is created. | An MRI scan creates a graphic image of bone, fluid, and soft tissue structures. It gives a more defined image of anatomical details and may help one diagnose small tumors or early infarction syndromes. | Risk factors for this technique are not well identified.<br>This test is contraindicated in patients with previous surgeries where hemostatic or aneurysm clips were implanted. The powerful magnetic field can cause such clips to move out of position, placing the patient at risk for bleeding or hemorrhage. Other contraindications include cardiac pacemakers, prosthetic valves, bullet fragments, and orthopedic pins.<br>Inform patient that the procedure is very noisy.<br>Use caution if patient is claustrophobic.<br>The patient (and care givers) must remove all metal objects with magnetic characteristics (eg, scissors, stethoscope). |
| Positron emission tomography (PET)<br>Single-photon emission computed tomography (SPECT) | The patient either inhales or receives by injection radioactively tagged substances, such as oxygen or glucose. A gamma scanner measures the radioactive uptake of these substances, and a computer produces a composite image, indicating where the radioactive material is located, corresponding to areas of cellular metabolism. | These diagnostic tests are the only ones to measure physiologic and biochemical processes in the nervous system. Specific areas can be identified as to functioning and nonfunctioning. Cerebral metabolism and cerebral blood flow can be measured regionally. PET and SPECT scans help diagnose abnormalities (tumors, vascular disease) and behavioral disturbances, such as dementia and schizophrenia, that may have a physiologic basis. | The patient receives only minimal radiation exposure because the half-life of the radionuclides used is from a few minutes to 2 h.<br>Testing may take a few hours.<br>Procedure is very expensive.<br>Inform the patient that remaining very still and immobile will produce best test results. |
| Cerebral angiography (invasive) | This is a radiographic contrast study in which radiopaque contrast medium is injected by a catheter into the patient's cerebral arterial circulation. The contrast medium is directed into each common carotid artery and each vertebral artery, and serial radiographs are then taken. | The contrast medium illuminates the structure of the cerebral circulation. The vessel pathways are examined for patency, narrowing, and occlusion, as well as structural abnormalities (aneurysms), vessel displacement (tumors, edema), and alterations in blood flow (tumors, arteriovenous malformations). | In preparation for this test, inform the patient as to the location of the catheter insertion (femoral artery is a common site) and that a local anesthetic will be used. Also warn that a warm, flushed feeling will occur when the contrast medium is injected.<br>After this procedure, assess the puncture site for swelling, redness, and bleeding. Also check the skin color, temperature, and peripheral pulses of the extremity distal to the site for signs of arterial insufficiency due to vasospasm or clotting.<br>A large amount of contrast medium may be needed during this test, with resulting increased osmotic diuresis and risk for dehydration and renal tubular occlusion. Other complications include temporary or permanent neurologic deficit, anaphylaxis, bleeding or hematoma at insertion site, and impaired circulation to the extremity used for injection. |

**TABLE 33-7** Neurodiagnostic Tests (*continued*)

| Diagnostic Test | Description | Information Obtained | Nursing Considerations and Interventions |
|---|---|---|---|
| Digital subtraction angiography (invasive) | In this test, a plain radiograph is taken of the patient's cranium. Then, radiopaque contrast medium is injected into a large vein, and serial radiographs are taken. A computer converts the images into digital form and "subtracts" the plain radiograph from the ones with the contrast medium. The result is an enhanced radiographic image of contrast medium in the arterial vessels. | Extracranial circulation (arterial, capillary, and venous) can be examined. Vessel size, patency, narrowing, and degree of stenosis or displacement can be determined. | There is less risk to the patient for bleeding or vascular insufficiency because the injection of contrast medium is intravenous rather than intra-arterial. The patient must remain absolutely motionless during the examination (even swallowing will interfere with the results). |
| Radioisotope brain scan (noninvasive) | In this test, radioactive isotope is usually injected intravenously. The scanning device produces films of areas of concentration of the isotope within the patient's head. | Because damaged brain tissue absorbs more isotope, the presence of an intracranial lesion can be diagnosed as well as cerebral infarction or contusion. Lack of uptake of the isotope may indicate brain death. | Minimal patient preparation is required. The isotope may not be readily available within the institution. Movement will make the test difficult to interpret. This test is less commonly used than CT scan or MRI. |
| Myelography (invasive) | A myelogram is a radiographic study in which a contrast medium (either air or dye) is injected into the lumbar subarachnoid space. Fluoroscopy, conventional radiographs, or CT scans are used to visualize selected areas. | The spinal subarachnoid space is examined for partial or complete obstructions due to bone displacements, spinal cord compression, or herniated intervertebral disks. | Instruct the patient as for a lumbar puncture. In addition, advise that a special table will tilt up or down during the procedure. Postprocedure care is determined by the type of contrast medium used: *Oil-based contrast dye:* • Flat in bed for 24 h. • Force fluids. • Observe for headache, fever, back spasms, nausea, and vomiting. *Water-based contrast dye:* • Head of bed elevated for 8 h. • Keep patient quiet for first few hours. • Do not administer phenothiazines. • Observe for headache, fever, back spasms, nausea, vomiting, and seizures. |
| Electroencephalogram, or EEG (noninvasive) | An EEG is a recording of electrical impulses generated by the brain cortex that are sensed by electrodes on the surface of the scalp. | Analysis of the resulting tracings helps detect and localize abnormal electrical activity occurring in the cerebral cortex. It aids in seizure focus detection, localization of a source of irritation such as a tumor or abscess, and diagnosis of metabolic disturbances and sleep disorders. | Reassure the patient that he or she will not feel an electrical shock or pain during this test. You also may need to clarify for the patient that the machine cannot "read minds" or indicate the presence of mental illness. The patient's scalp and hair should be free of oil, dirt, creams, and sprays because they can cause electrical interference and thus an inaccurate recording. Inform the EEG technician of electrical devices around the patient that may cause interference during the procedure (eg, cardiac monitor, ventilator). |
| Cortical evoked potentials (noninvasive) • Somatosensory evoked potentials • Brainstem auditory evoked response • Visual evoked potentials | In this test, a specialized device senses central or cortical cerebral electrical activity by skin electrodes in response to peripheral stimulation of specific sensory receptors. The sensory receptors stimulated can be those for vision, hearing, or tactile sensation. The signals are graphically displayed by a computer and characteristic peaks, and the intervals between them, are measured. | Cortical evoked potentials provide a detailed assessment of neuron transmission along particular pathways. It has value in determining the integrity of visual, auditory, and tactile pathways in patients with multiple sclerosis and spinal cord injury. This test also may be used in the assessment of a sensory pathway before, during, and after surgery. | This test may be used in conscious as well as unconscious patients and can be performed at the bedside. The patient must be as motionless as possible during some phases of this test to minimize musculoskeletal interference. Depending on the sensory pathway being tested, the patient may be instructed to watch a series of geometric designs or listen to a series of clicking noises. |

(*continued*)

**TABLE 33-7** Neurodiagnostic Tests (*continued*)

| Diagnostic Test | Description | Information Obtained | Nursing Considerations and Interventions |
|---|---|---|---|
| Transcranial Doppler sonography | This is a test in which high-frequency ultrasonic waves are directed from a probe toward specific cerebral vessels. The ultrasonic energy is aimed through cranial "windows," areas in the skull where the bony table is thin (temporal zygoma) or where there are small gaps in the bone (orbit or foramen magnum). The reflected sound waves are analyzed for shifts in frequency, indicating flow velocity. | The speed or velocity at which blood travels through cerebral vessels is an indicator of the size of the vascular channel and the resistance to blood flow. An approximation of cerebral blood flow may be determined. Cerebral autoregulation can be monitored by observing the response of intracranial vessels to changes in arterial carbon dioxide and to the partial occlusion of the proximal vessels, as may occur in vasospasm. | The test is noninvasive and may be performed at the bedside by the physician or ultrasound technician in 30–60 min. There are no known adverse effects, and the procedure may be repeated as often as necessary. The testing is accomplished with the patient initially supine, and later on his or her side, with the head flexed forward. |
| Lumbar puncture (invasive) | A hollow needle is positioned in the subarachnoid space at L3–L4 or L4–L5 level, and cerebrospinal fluid (CSF) is sampled. The pressure of the CSF also is measured. Normal pressure varies with age from 45 mm $H_2O$ in full-term newborns to 120 mm $H_2O$ in adults. | The CSF is examined for blood and for alterations in appearance, cell count, protein, and glucose. The opening pressure is roughly equivalent to the ICP for most patients, if the patient is recumbent and no block is present. | This test is contraindicated in patients with suspected increased ICP because a sudden reduction in pressure from below may cause brain structures to herniate, leading to death. In preparation for this test, position the patient on side with knees and head flexed. Explain to the patient that some pressure may be felt as the needle is inserted and not to move suddenly or cough. After this procedure, keep the patient flat for 8–10 h to prevent headache. Encourage liberal fluid intake. |

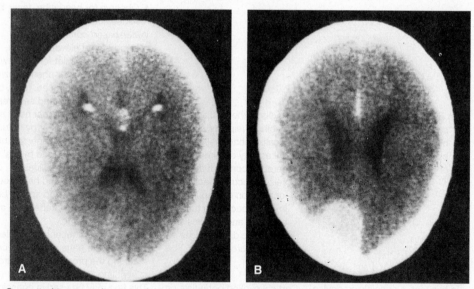

**FIGURE 33-10**  Computed tomography scan of the brain. **A:** Normal scan. **B:** Scan showing a large mass in the left frontal lobe. (Reprinted from Hickey J: The Clinical Practice of Neurological and Neuroscience Nursing, 6th ed. Philadelphia, PA: Lippincott Williams & Wilkins, 2009, p 92, with permission.)

other lesions. CT scanning can reliably detect conditions such as skull fractures, tissue swelling, hematomas, tumors, and abscesses. However, it has been noted that some vascular lesions are not as reliably documented using CT scan as they are with MRI. Therefore, MRI is indicated if these lesions are suspected.

Use of a contrast medium can enhance a CT scan. Using radiographic contrast material allows better visualization of

vascular areas and enhances lesions previously seen on noncontrast films. Care should be taken in the patient with renal failure or renal insufficiency because contrast medium clearance by the kidneys may be impaired.

Nursing management focuses on patient education to obviate any potential complications, such as poor patient tolerance. The patient should be aware that he or she must lie very still during the procedure, and that he or she may experience feelings of claustrophobia. In addition, the nurse ascertains whether the patient has any preexisting allergies, particularly if contrast medium is to be used. The nurse may need to remain with the patient during the procedure to continue to monitor neurologic status and vital signs.

## Magnetic Resonance Imaging

MRI has become widely available in medium and large medical centers. This modality uses nonionizing forms of radiation to produce computerized cross-sectional images in much the same fashion as a CT scan. However, since the radiation reacts differently to different soft tissue densities, it provides more finely detailed images that look remarkably like anatomical slices of the body. MRI is superior to a CT scan in the early diagnosis of cerebral infarction and the detection of demyelinating disorders. It is also helpful in diagnosing small lesions, such as tumors and hemorrhages, that might not appear on a CT scan, or in evaluation of ligamentous injury of the spinal cord.

Although superior in many ways to CT scanning, MRI has its limitations. Its powerful magnetic fields interfere with the functioning of devices such as cardiac pacemakers. Patients with surgical clips and prosthetic implants made of ferrous metal cannot be scanned. It is also difficult to study patients on life-support equipment because most ventilators and monitors are constructed in part of ferrous metal. If emergency therapy is needed, the patient must be removed from the scanning chamber and the imaging suite before resuscitation can begin.

## Positron Emission Tomography and Single-Photon Emission Computed Tomography

Positron emission tomography (PET) is a process in which molecules labeled with radioactive isotopes are located in the brain and recorded by radiation-sensitive detectors outside the head. PET has the capacity to measure cerebral blood flow and cerebral metabolism as the isotope-labeled glucose or oxygen is used in the body. It is superior to previous technologies that could image structure only, not function. It currently assists in diagnosing Alzheimer disease, which shows a characteristic pattern of glucose consumption, as well as in Parkinson disease, Huntington disease, and Tourette syndrome. However, the complexity of the testing, the comparatively high cost per scan, and the need to have a cyclotron nearby to produce the short-lived radioactive isotopes make this modality impractical and unwieldy in the clinical setting.

Single-photon emission computed tomography (SPECT) combines the imaging ability of conventional nuclear medicine scanners with the technology of transaxial CT scanning to overcome some of the limitations of PET. Using more stable radioisotopes, SPECT scanning can detect diminished perfusion in an area of stroke before there is conventional CT evidence of infarction. SPECT can also detect alterations in regional blood flow in patients with Alzheimer disease.

## Angiography and Digital Subtraction Angiography

Cerebral angiography (Fig. 33-11) remains the study of choice for evaluating cerebrovascular problems. It is the only test that can reveal large and small aneurysms and arteriovenous malformations and their relationship to adjacent structures and vessels. It involves the passage of a radiographic catheter through a large artery (usually femoral) to each of the arterial vessels bringing blood to the brain and spinal cord. Radiopaque contrast (a dye-like medium) is then injected into each vessel. A rapid sequence of images is taken after the contrast agent has passed through small arterial branches and capillaries and into the venous circulation. In this way, the vessel lumen and size and the presence of any occlusions can be visualized. Cerebral angiography has been used before surgery to help decide the appropriateness of medical versus surgical management. It has also been combined with balloon angioplasty in instances of vascular occlusion or coiling in the treatment of aneurysms.

Digital subtraction angiography makes use of radiographic contrast to illuminate the cerebral circulation, but in considerably smaller quantities than required for conventional angiography. The contrast medium may be injected into the arterial or the venous systems. Films are taken before and after the injection and converted into digital information in the accompanying computer. The images are "subtracted" from each other, removing all images in common. The resultant image displays only the enhanced circulatory system, free of other anatomical distortion.

The major complications associated with angiography include stroke, vasospasm, and renal failure secondary to the contrast load. Contraindications to angiography include identified allergies to the contrast medium, anticoagulant therapy, and kidney and liver disease.

## Cerebral Blood Flow Studies

In the diagnostic setting, cerebral blood flow is evaluated most commonly by a radioisotope brain scan. A radioactive

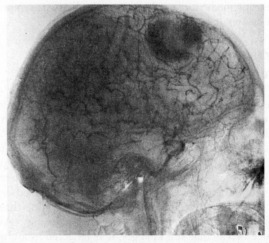

**FIGURE 33-11** Cerebral angiogram showing an abnormal, large, space-occupying lesion at 1 o'clock. (Reprinted from Hickey J: The Clinical Practice of Neurological and Neuroscience Nursing, 6th ed. Philadelphia, PA: Lippincott Williams & Wilkins, 2009, p 103, with permission.)

isotope is injected intravenously; in unusual circumstances, the isotope can be administered orally or intra-arterially. The brain is then scanned to determine which areas show an accumulation of the radioactive substance. If there is blood flow to the brain, damaged areas absorb more of the isotope than areas without damage. A newer technique, perfusion CT, involves scanning before, during, and after infusion of the contrast agent to obtain "real time" data with respect to blood flow. Cerebral blood flow studies are indicated in the detection of either increased or decreased blood flow during surgical procedures or to assess for vasospasm. They may also be used after carotid endarterectomy. The test may be used to determine brain death, which is evidenced if there is no flow to the cerebral hemispheres. In certain disorders, such as carbon monoxide poisoning, there may be increased blood flow to the brain, yet anoxic brain death may still occur. The measurement of cerebral flow assists in decision making regarding treatment and in the identification of complications.

## Myelography

Myelography is a contrast study of the spinal cord and surrounding structures. It involves the introduction of water-soluble material into the CSF through a lumbar or cisternal puncture, performed under fluoroscopy, after about 10 mL of CSF has been removed. Myelography is indicated in evaluating herniated intervertebral disks, spinal cord tumors, and congenital problems, and in assessing spinal cord trauma. It allows for better visualization of nerve roots and surrounding structures because it uses a contrast agent that is lighter than CSF. However, the agent disperses rapidly into the subarachnoid space, which means that the patient's position cannot be adjusted. The contrast agent does not require removal; therefore, the patient should be kept well hydrated to facilitate the agent's excretion. A heavier, oil-based contrast agent is sometimes used, and it must be removed at the end of the procedure.

The contrast agents are potentially toxic to cerebral tissue and may cause grand mal seizures. Thus, the patient must remain with the head up at least 30 to 45 degrees, and phenothiazine medications, which increase the toxic symptoms, must be avoided.

## Ultrasonography and Noninvasive Cerebrovascular Studies

Transcranial Doppler ultrasonographic studies are a noninvasive means of monitoring intracranial hemodynamics at the bedside. The examination is performed through cranial "windows," areas in the skull where the bone is relatively thin, such as the temporal area, or where there are small spaces between bones, such as the orbit. The ultrasonic probe transmits sound waves at certain frequencies to a specified depth. The resultant reflected signal from blood traveling through cerebral vessels is interpreted for speed or velocity. As resistance or vascular size changes, it is reflected as a change in blood flow velocities. The data may be used to monitor therapy, aid in determining prognosis, and provide early recognition of cerebral vasospasm in patients after subarachnoid hemorrhage or severe head injury. Serial Doppler studies in

patients with an aneurysm provide data on postoperative vasospasm and alleviate the need for repeat angiograms.

Carotid and vertebral artery duplex scans provide anatomical imaging of blood vessels combined with hemodynamic information. Doppler studies at the cranial window provide information about direction of flow, pulsatile rhythmicity, and resistance to flow of the cerebral vasculature. Carotid duplex scans are routinely used as a screening tool in patients at risk for atherosclerotic disease. The nurse should be aware of whether the patient has any history of dysrhythmias or cardiac disease, because these may alter the hemodynamic profile and findings of the test.

## Electrophysiologic Studies

### Electroencephalography

Using electroencephalography (EEG), a record is made of the brain's electrical activity. Small plate electrodes are placed in specific locations on the patient's scalp, and 16 to 21 channels transcribe the electrical potentials generated by the brain. Waveforms are classified in terms of voltage and amplitude. EEG is most valuable in the diagnosis and treatment of patients with seizures. In addition, it may help localize structural abnormalities, such as tumors and abscesses, and aid in the differentiation of structural and metabolic abnormalities. It also may provide confirmatory criteria in the diagnosis of brain death. In recent years, a modified form of EEG has been used at the bedside in critical care to monitor the effects of pharmacologic agents that reduce cerebral blood flow and hence reduce electrical activity. This continuous EEG monitoring is rapidly becoming a standard of care in many facilities. It is intended to detect subclinical or nonconvulsive seizure activity in patients who are taking medications that suppress electrical activity.

A computerized technique that dramatically compresses standard EEG data and converts them into a more easily interpreted and colorized form is compressed spectral array. This technique is also seen at the bedside in neurologic intensive care units to monitor patients with severe head injuries.

### Evoked Potentials

An evoked potential is an electrical manifestation of the brain's response to an external stimulus: auditory, visual, somatic, or a combination of these. The measurement of such a response provides an assessment of the function of neuropathways from the periphery through the spinal cord and brainstem and finally to cortical structures. This technique has been most helpful in diagnosing multiple sclerosis and Guillain–Barré syndrome, and in determining the prognosis for reversibility of coma in the brainstem-injured patient. It also may be used during surgery to monitor potential injury during manipulations of spinal nerves and structures.

The three most frequently used techniques in head trauma evaluation are somatosensory evoked potentials (SSEPs), which use electrical shock as a stimulus; brainstem auditory evoked response (BAERs), which uses click or sound stimulus; and visual evoked potentials (VERs), which use light stimulus. SSEPs assess neurologic function in specific neural pathways postinjury and detect further central nervous system insults from secondary processes, such as hypoxia and hypertension.

**TABLE 33-8** Normal and Abnormal Values for Cerebrospinal Fluid

| Characteristic | Normal | Abnormal |
|---|---|---|
| Color | Clear, colorless | Cloudy, often due to presence of WBC or bacteria<br>Xanthochromic due to presence of RBCs |
| White blood cell (WBC) | 0–5/mm³, all mononuclear | Elevated count accompanies many conditions (tumor, meningitis, subarachnoid hemorrhage, infarct, and abscess) |
| Red blood cell (RBC) | None | Presence may be due to traumatic tap or subarachnoid hemorrhage |
| Chloride | 120–130 mEq/L | Low concentration associated with meningeal infection and tuberculosis meningitis<br>Elevated level not neurologically significant |
| Glucose | 50–75 mg/100 mL<br>Normal CSF glucose is 2/3 blood glucose level | Decreased level associated with presence of bacteria in CSF<br>Elevated level not neurologically significant |
| Pressure | 70–180 mm H₂O | Low pressure associated with inaccurate placement of needle, dehydration, or block along subarachnoid space or at foramen magnum<br>Elevated pressure associated with benign intracranial hypertension; cerebral edema; central nervous system tumor, abscess, or cyst; hydrocephalus; muscle tension or abdominal compression; or subdural hematoma |
| Protein | 14–45 mg/100 mL | Decreased level not neurologically significant<br>Increased level associated with demyelinating or degenerative disease, Guillain–Barré syndrome, hemorrhage, infection, and spinal block tumor |

From Bader M, Littlejohns L (eds): Core Curriculum for Neuroscience Nursing, 5th ed. Chicago, IL: American Association of Neuroscience Nurses, 2010.

## Lumbar Puncture for Cerebrospinal Fluid Examination

A lumbar puncture for CSF analysis may be performed to help diagnose autoimmune disorders or infections. Occasionally, it is performed to verify subarachnoid hemorrhage, although a CT scan is the procedure of choice and is safer for such a patient. The fluid is sent for content analysis and for culture, sensitivity, and other serologic tests (Table 33-8). Pressure readings may also be obtained for diagnostic use.

If a lumbar puncture is performed in a patient with elevated ICP, herniation can be a life-threatening complication. Complications that can result from a CSF leak include a postprocedure headache, nuchal rigidity, fever, and difficulty voiding. Treatment involves the injection of blood into the dura, called a blood patch, to stop the leak.

## Clinical Applicability Challenges

---

### CASE STUDY

Mrs. Q is a 63-year-old woman who collapsed at home after complaining of a severe headache. Her husband reported that she suddenly stopped talking to him and lost consciousness. Per Emergency Medical System report her Glasgow Coma Scale on arrival was 10 (E3V3M4), pupils PERRL, BP 190/78, P 87, RR 20. Your initial assessment reveals that she now requires physical stimulation to open her eyes, she localizes with her left arm but only withdraws with her right, and her verbalizations are becoming garbled. Her respiratory rate has decreased to 10, and she remains hypertensive at 194/82.

1. What interventions do you anticipate if Mrs. Q's neurologic status continues to decline?
2. What past medical history items are most important for diagnosing Mrs. Q's condition and determining the safety of the diagnostic testing she may require?
3. After Mrs. Q is stabilized in the ED, you are transferring her to the ICU. Why is it important to provide a detailed neurologic exam as opposed to simply stating a GCS score?

---

### WANT TO KNOW MORE?

A wide variety of resources to enhance your learning and understanding of this chapter are available on thePoint.

You will find:

- References
- Selected readings
- NCLEX-style review questions
- Internet resources
- And more!

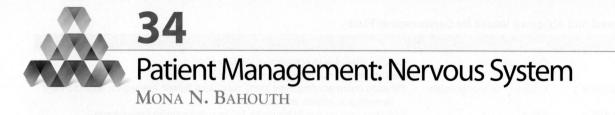

# 34

# Patient Management: Nervous System

MONA N. BAHOUTH

## LEARNING OBJECTIVES

*Based on the content in this chapter, the reader should be able to:*

1. Define intracranial pressure (ICP) and intracranial hypertension.
2. Discuss several physiologic principles affecting ICP, including the Monro–Kellie doctrine, compliance, autoregulation, and cerebral perfusion.
3. Discuss indications for ICP monitoring.
4. Describe currently available methods of monitoring ICP.
5. Explain three possible complications associated with ICP monitoring and discuss troubleshooting strategies.
6. Identify various strategies used to manage increased ICP.
7. Discuss three general principles when selecting a sedating agent for use in the patient with neurologic injury.

Caring for a critically ill patient with neurologic injury requires an understanding of three general principles: (1) the evolving neurologic examination; (2) concepts of intracranial pressure (ICP); and (3) available treatments (pharmacologic and nonpharmacologic strategies) in this population of patients.

ICP is defined as the pressure in the cranial vault relative to atmospheric pressure. Understanding general principles regarding the concepts of ICP provides the critical care nurse with a framework that he or she can then apply to multiple neurologic conditions. In addition, a working knowledge of the pharmacologic agents used in neurologic emergencies, such as osmotic treatments, steroids, antihypertensive agents, diuretics, analgesics, sedatives, barbiturates, and anticonvulsants, better prepares the nurse to handle these situations.

## Physiologic Principles

### Intracranial Dynamics

Concepts of ICP and its management are based on the principle that the skull is a rigid box, a nonexpansile, noncontractile space. Its contents are divided into three intracranial sections: blood maintained in the blood vessels, cerebrospinal fluid (CSF), and brain parenchyma. The brain's ability to self-regulate is based on the Monro–Kellie doctrine of fixed intracranial volume. This doctrine states that the volume of the intracranium is equal to the volume of the intravascular cerebral blood (3% to 10%) plus the volume of the CSF (8% to 12%) plus the volume of brain tissue, which itself consists of more than 80% water. As long as the total intracranial volume remains the same, ICP remains constant. To maintain equilibrium, there cannot be any increase in volume of one of these components without a compensatory decrease in the other two. Any alterations in the volume of any of these three components within the cranial vault, without a response from the other two components, may lead to a change in ICP. A normal ICP measurement ranges between 0 and 15 mm Hg. An ICP measurement greater than 15 mm Hg is considered intracranial hypertension or increased ICP. Numerous conditions can lead to changes within the intracranial vault and thus intracranial pressure (Table 34-1).

### Cerebral Blood Flow

Autoregulation is defined as the ability of an organ to maintain consistent blood flow despite marked changes in arterial circulatory and perfusion pressures. The normal brain has the ability to autoregulate cerebral blood flow (CBF) via ongoing arterial and venous modifications responsive to metabolic, neurogenic, and myogenic influences. Normally, autoregulation ensures a constant blood flow through the cerebral vessels over a range of perfusion pressures by changing the diameter of vessels in response to changes in arterial pressures. This mechanism is the brain's protective device against the constantly fluctuating changes of blood pressure. When autoregulation is impaired, the CBF fluctuates in direct correlation with the systemic blood pressure. In patients with impaired autoregulation, any activity that causes an increase in blood pressure, such as coughing, suctioning, or restlessness, can cause an increase in CBF that could also increase ICP.

The first of three components that may undergo changes as the body attempts to maintain a consistent intracranial volume is the CBF. Normal CBF is provided by a cerebral perfusion pressure (CPP) in the range of 60 to 100 mm Hg. The brain receives approximately 750 mL/min of arterial blood (15% to 20% of total cardiac output when at rest). For autoregulation to be functional, hemodynamic must be within acceptable range: CPP greater than 60 mm Hg, mean arterial pressure (MAP) less than 160 mm Hg, systolic pressure between 60 and 140 mm Hg, and ICP less than 30 mm Hg.[1] Factors that alter the ability of the cerebral vessels to constrict or dilate, such as hypoxia, hypercapnia, and brain trauma, also interfere with autoregulation. Carbon dioxide is a potent vasodilator of cerebral vessels, causing increased CBF and increased volume, leading to increased ICP.

**TABLE 34-1** Potential Causes of Increased Intracranial Pressure

| Contributing Physiology | Intracranial Component Involved | Potential Cause | Potential Treatment |
|---|---|---|---|
| Overproduction of CSF | CSF space | Choroid plexus papilloma | Surgical removal, diuretics |
| Inadequate CSF reabsorption (communicating hydrocephalus) | CSF space | Subarachnoid hemorrhage, infection | Drainage of CSF from lumbar intrathecal site, shunt placement |
| Blockage of CSF circulation (obstructive hydrocephalus) | CSF space | Posterior fossa tumor, brain injury, birth defects (spina bifida) | Ventricular drainage, surgical removal of obstruction |
| Edema (vasogenic, cytotoxic) | Brain tissue | Tumor, infection, infarction, hypoxia, arteriovenous malformation | Drainage of CSF, removal of lesion, adequate oxygenation |
| Expansile mass | Brain tissue | Tumor, abscess, intracerebral hemorrhage | Surgical removal, steroids |
| Vasospasm | Intracranial circulation | Subarachnoid hemorrhage | Hypervolemia, hypertensive therapy, calcium channel antagonists |
| Vasodilation | Intracranial circulation | Elevated $PaCO_2$, systemic vasodilators ($\alpha$-adrenergic agents) | Hyperventilation, removal of offending agent |

## Cerebrospinal Fluid Circulation

Cerebrospinal fluid (CSF) also contributes to fluctuations in intracranial hemodynamics. CSF is a clear fluid produced predominantly in the choroid plexus in the lateral, third, and fourth ventricles. It fills the ventricles and subarachnoid space and protects the brain and spinal cord from injury. Circulation of CSF occurs in a closed system; it is predominantly reabsorbed by the arachnoid villi located in the subarachnoid space and dispersed into the venous system through the superior sagittal sinus (see Chapter 32, Fig. 32-6). Along the entire CSF cycle, potential disturbances in production, circulation, and absorption can contribute to changes in ICP. For instance, overproduction of CSF in the choroid plexus overwhelms the circulatory system. Obstruction of CSF circulation through the ventricles leads to dilation of the ventricular system (obstructive hydrocephalus). Marked slowing of absorption in the arachnoid villi caused by blood or infectious debris interferes with the reabsorption of CSF, thereby leading to systemic overload (communicating hydrocephalus).

## Parenchyma

The third and most difficult intracranial component to manipulate without surgical intervention is the brain parenchyma. However, the brain tissue does respond to increased ICP and changes within the other two intracranial components. The brain can accommodate for increased ICP by making changes in volume via partial collapse of the cisterns, ventricles, and vascular systems, in turn decreasing production and increasing reabsorption of CSF. Compensatory mechanisms to maintain normal ICP include the following:

- Shunting of CSF into the spinal subarachnoid space
- Increased CSF absorption
- Decreased CSF production
- Shunting of venous blood out of the skull

During the compensatory period, ICP remains fairly constant. However, when these compensatory mechanisms have been exhausted, pressure increases rapidly until shifting of brain tissue toward open spaces in the skull (brain herniation) occurs, and the blood supply to the medulla is cut off. The ability of the intracranial content to compensate depends on the location of the lesion, the rate of expansion, and cranial compliance.

## Volume–Pressure Curve

The intracranial volume–pressure curve, also called a pressure–volume index (PVI), demonstrates the relationship between changes in intracranial volume and changes in ICP. An awareness of the patient's position on this curve is useful in monitoring and selecting appropriate interventions. The rate at which ICP increases in response to a change in intracranial volume depends on the compliance of the brain. *Compliance* is defined as the ability to change volume related to a change in pressure. When compliance in the intracranial compartment is low, a small volume change causes a large increase in ICP. In Figure 34-1, the curve illustrates compliance, as the compensatory mechanisms maintain ICP in the normal range during increases in intracranial volume. Little change occurs in ICP during the initial increase in volume because the volume added to the cranium is compensated for by volume displacement. As the compensatory mechanisms become exhausted, the volume added becomes greater than the volume displaced, and there is a larger increase in ICP with any incremental volume increase. Free communication of CSF between the lateral ventricles and infratentorium is lost as a result.

A major reason for controlling and decreasing ICP is the maintenance of cerebral oxygenation by adequate CBF, which is estimated clinically by the measurement of CPP. Many factors contribute to increased ICP along the volume–pressure curve. Drastic increases in ICP may result from hypercarbia, hypoxia, rapid eye movement sleep, pyrexia, or the administration of certain anesthetics. Additionally, ICP is affected by environmental stimulation and increased metabolic rates.[2]

## Cerebral Perfusion Pressure

Cerebral perfusion pressure (CPP) is the blood pressure gradient across the brain. CPP is calculated by subtracting the mean ICP from the MAP: CPP = MAP – ICP. When the CPP is greater than 100 mm Hg, there is a potential for hyperperfusion and increased ICP. When the CPP is less than

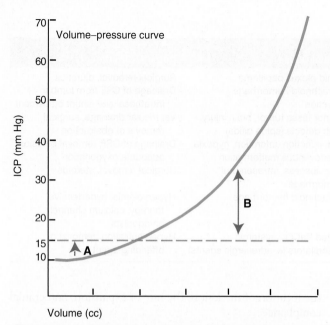

**FIGURE 34-1** Volume–pressure curve. Volume–pressure response (VPR), also referred to as the pressure–volume index (PVI), provides a method of estimating the compensatory capacity of the intracranial cavity. Note that the intracranial pressure (ICP) remains within the normal limit of 0 to 15 mm Hg as long as compliance is normal and fluid can be displaced by the additional volume (**A**). Once the compensatory system is exhausted, a small additional volume causes a greater increase in pressure (**B**). Acute changes can cause serious and sometimes fatal neurologic deterioration.

60 mm Hg, blood supply to the brain is inadequate, and neuronal hypoxia and cell death may occur. If MAPs and ICPs are equal, CPP is zero, indicating no CBF. CBF may also cease totally at pressures somewhat greater than zero. Patients with hypotension, such as postcardiac resuscitation or trauma patients, with normal ICPs (0 to 15 mm Hg), may have impaired CPP.

Autoregulation is an active, energy-requiring process to constrict or dilate vessels in order to maintain a steady state of intravascular blood flow based in changing ICPs. The autoregulation system for maintenance of constant blood flow does not function at pressures less than 40 mm Hg. Because an acutely injured brain requires a higher CPP than a normal brain, a minimum CPP of 70 mm Hg is required for maintenance of adequate cerebral perfusion and potentially improved outcomes in patients with brain injuries.[2] When CPP decreases, the cardiovascular system responds by increasing systemic pressure. If CPP is below the lower level of autoregulation oligemia ensues.

When brain damage is severe, as with widespread brain edema or when blood flow has been arrested in the brain, CBF may be reduced at relatively normal levels of CPP. The cause is impedance to the flow of blood across the cerebrovascular bed. If autoregulation is impaired, CBF may not increase despite increases in CPP. Increased ICP leads to ischemia, anoxic injury, decreased compliance, and possible herniation.[3]

## Increased Intracranial Pressure

Signs of increased intracranial pressure can include restlessness, nausea, headache, somnolence, and pupillary changes.

Pupillary changes that can be seen range from slight ovoid shape to complete loss of pupillary tone and reactivity. Knowledge of the patient's baseline status, including the presence of a surgical pupil, is essential to avoid unnecessary testing or treatment.

## Cushing Triad

The Cushing response is a protective reflex to respond to increased ICPs. Cushing triad is the classical syndrome of increased ICP and includes increased pulse pressure, decreased pulse, and change in respiratory pattern with pupillary changes. This syndrome usually occurs only in association with posterior fossa lesions and seldom with the more commonly observed supratentorial mass lesions, such as expanding tumors or subdural hematomas. When these classical signs do accompany a supratentorial lesion, they are associated with a sudden pressure increase and usually herald a state of decompensation. Brain damage usually is irreversible if prolonged, and death is imminent without rapid intervention.

## Cerebral Edema

Cerebral edema leading to increased ICP is a process common to multiple neurologic illnesses including hepatic failure, brain trauma, central nervous system (CNS) infections, brain tumors, stroke, etc. Its presence leads to secondary complications related to the expansion of brain tissue within the closed space of the cranium, including impaired circulation leading to secondary hypoxia. Independently, cerebral edema can cause marked increases in ICP and must be treated aggressively. In general, once edema begins, its progression is rapid and difficult to control.

Treatment of cerebral edema may include using corticosteroids as well as osmotic diuretics directed at reducing ICP. These agents work by increasing plasma osmolarity, which draws fluid out of the brain tissue and into the circulating blood. The goal of therapy is to maintain plasma osmolarity up to 320 mOsm/L. See Chapter 36 for further information about cerebral edema.

### Vasogenic Edema

The most common type of cerebral edema is vasogenic edema, which is characterized by a disruption in the blood–brain barrier and the inability of the cell walls to control movement of water in and out of the cells. Capillary permeability is affected, and fluid and protein are allowed to leak from the plasma into the extracellular space, resulting in increased extracellular fluid volume predominantly in the white matter. Common processes leading to vasogenic edema include brain tumors and cerebral abscess.

### Cytotoxic Edema

Cytotoxic edema is characterized by swelling of the individual neurons and endothelial cells, which increases fluid in the intracellular space and reduces available extracellular space, affecting the gray matter. Eventually, the cell membrane cannot maintain an effective barrier, and both water and sodium enter the cell, causing swelling and loss of function. Cytotoxic edema occurs after injuries such as anoxia or hypoxic injury. Ischemic stroke leads to a combination of both types of edema. Cytotoxic edema occurs early in the stroke process due to energy failure and anoxic membrane depolarization of the ischemic core. Later, vasogenic edema predominates due to disruption of the blood–brain barrier and increased permeability.[4]

## Herniation

Herniation is defined as the displacement of tissue through structures within the skull and is the result of increased ICP. Transtentorial or uncal shifting of brain tissue through rigid openings in the skull or dura leads to displacement of midline brain structures and compression of structures in the CNS, causing traditional clinical herniation syndromes. See Chapter 36 for more information about herniation syndromes.

## Intracranial Pressure Monitoring

Monitoring ICP provides information that facilitates earlier interventions to prevent secondary cerebral ischemia and brainstem distortion. For ICP monitoring to be safe and effective, the indications for monitoring, methods of monitoring, and ethical considerations for patient care and nursing practice must be taken into account for each patient. Factors that affect patient selection include the potential benefit from invasive ICP monitoring and therapy, the patient's diagnosis and prognosis, and the availability of the appropriate level of critical care. ICP monitoring helps improve patient outcome by providing information about the likelihood of cerebral herniation and facilitating calculation of CPP. It is also helpful in guiding the use of potentially harmful treatments, such as hyperventilation, mannitol, and barbiturates.

## Indications

ICP monitoring is primarily used for guiding therapy. General guidelines exist to provide direction in therapy for patients at risk for and with increased ICP. Potential diagnostic indications for ICP measurement include brain injury, stroke, brain tumors, cardiac arrest, and surgery. The decision to use ICP monitoring should be based on clinical and radiographic evaluation as well as computed tomography (CT) diagnosis.

Currently, ICP monitoring is not indicated for patients with mild to moderate brain injury, defined as a Glasgow Coma Scale (GCS) score of 9 to 15. However, ICP monitoring may be appropriate for comatose patients or patients with severe brain injury with or without abnormalities on a CT scan of the head. Severe brain injury is defined as a GCS score of 3 to 8 with abnormal CT scan findings such as hematoma, contusion, edema, or compressed basal cisterns. ICP monitoring is also appropriate for patients who have brain injury with a normal CT scan and who have two or more of the following criteria: age greater than 40 years, any motor posturing, or systolic blood pressure less than 90 mm Hg.[5]

The upper limit of normal ICP is defined typically as 15 mm Hg. Although no prospective, randomized trial has been completed, a summary of the literature suggests that ICP monitors are beneficial in

- limiting indiscriminate use of therapies with potentially harmful consequences
- reducing ICP through CSF drainage, thereby improving CPP
- assisting in determining a prognosis
- possibly improving outcomes.[4]

Nontraumatic neurologic disorders that may benefit from ICP monitoring are subarachnoid hemorrhage, intracerebral hemorrhage, large territory ischemic infarction, infection, hydrocephalus, and, rarely, brain tumors with associated edema or with significant lesion volume. Coagulopathy, systemic infection, CNS infection, and infection at the site of device insertion are relative contraindications to the placement of ICP monitors.

## Devices

Various devices, such as intraventricular catheters, fiberoptic devices, and epidural monitors, are used to monitor ICP. Use of external ventricular drainage systems are commonplace in the neuroscience intensive care unit (ICU); these systems have seen numerous changes since its first use in 1744.[6] A chosen ICP device should have pressure range capability of 0 to 100 mm Hg, accuracy within the ICP range of 0 to 20 $\pm$ 2 mm Hg, and a maximal error of 10% in the range of 20 to 100 mm Hg of ICP.[5] The type of monitor used depends on several clinical factors, the type of neurologic process, and the patient's symptoms on presentation (Fig. 34-2). A variety of advantages and disadvantages exist with each of the devices; therefore, an awareness of potential complications is essential in the bedside management of the patient undergoing such monitoring (Table 34-2).

Intraventricular catheters provide accurate, low-cost, and reliable ICP monitoring, and they are widely used. The catheter is a tubular instrument that is placed inside fluid-filled cavities in the ventricles. CSF is synthesized in these cavities and flows out to circulate over the surface of the brain. IVCs allow for simultaneous monitoring and treatment of

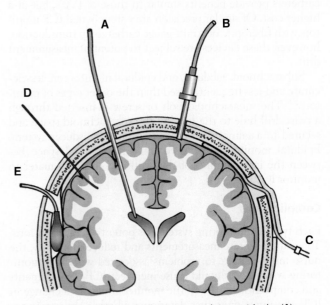

FIGURE 34-2 ICP monitoring systems: intraventricular (**A**); subarachnoid (**B**); subdural (**C**); parenchymal (**D**); and epidural (**E**).

**TABLE 34-2** Advantages and Disadvantages of Intracranial Pressure Monitoring Devices

| Monitoring Site | Advantages | Disadvantages |
|---|---|---|
| Intraventricular (ventriculostomy) | • Very accurate<br>• True central direct measure of ICP<br>• Can withdraw CSF to decrease ICP or measure compliance<br>• Ease of CSF sampling | • Need transducer repositioned with every change in head position<br>• High risk for serious infection<br>• Difficult insertion in patients with small or displaced ventricles<br>• Risk for intracerebral bleeding or edema along the cannula track |
| Intraventricular (fiberoptic catheter) | • Versatile; may be placed in ventricle or subarachnoid space<br>• No adjustment of transducer with head movement | • Separate monitoring system required<br>• Fragile catheter<br>• Unable to recalibrate once device is placed |
| Intraparenchymal | • Ease of insertion<br>• True brain pressures | • Infections rare, but serious |
| Lumbar/subarachnoid | • Simple-to-do single readings<br>• No penetration of the brain parenchyma<br>• Decreased risk for infection<br>• Can sample CSF<br>• Direct pressure management | • Contraindicated with evidence of increased ICP<br>• Requires intact skull<br>• Transducer repositioned with head movement |
| Subdural<br>Epidural | • Ease of insertion<br>• Low risk for infections<br>• No transducer adjustment with head movement | • Risk for serious infection<br>• Imperfect correlation with intradural pressure (sensing through dura)<br>• Operating room for placement<br>• Unable to recalibrate once device is placed<br>• Unable to drain CSP |

ICP by intermittently draining CSF (Fig. 34-3). IVCs can be inserted under sterile conditions at the bedside in the ICU or in the operating room during surgery. Unlike parenchymal monitors, the IVC can be recalibrated *in situ*. Additionally, the IVC can have an added use in clearance of intraventricular blood products in patients with primary or secondary intraventricular hemorrhage.[7]

Fiberoptic monitors use fiberoptic technologies to measure ICP. The tip of the fiberoptic probe has a transducer, which is inserted into brain parenchyma, the ventricles it surrounds, or the subdural space. Fiberoptic monitors are easily inserted, and their use is increasing. Fiberoptic ventricular catheters provide benefits similar to those of IVCs, but at a higher cost. Of similar precision are parenchymal ICP monitors with fiberoptic or strain-gauge catheter-tip transduction; however, these devices are subject to potential measurement drift.

Subarachnoid, subdural, and epidural monitors are less accurate and less frequently used than the other types of monitors.[5,8] The subarachnoid bolt or screw is inserted through a twist drill hole to the level of the subarachnoid space and secured to a saline-filled pressure tubing transducer system. Epidural monitors are placed into the epidural space between the inner surface of the skull and the dura mater to monitor ICP.

## Complications

Each type of monitoring system has potential complications. To ensure accurate measurements and reduce morbidity, the nurse must be alert to problems associated with ICP monitoring systems that could cause incorrect ICP measurements and complications. When the monitor indicates a change in ICP, the nurse must first determine whether the reading is accurate. If the reading is accurate, an attempt is then made

to determine the reason for the pressure change. Table 34-3 provides a guide to troubleshooting ICP lines.

As with any invasive procedure, complications may occur. In critically ill patients with neurologic problems, the risk/benefit ratio for any therapy must be considered before the implementation of that therapy. For instance, IVCs carry the potential risks for catheter misplacement, obstruction, infection, and hemorrhage. Use of antibiotic-impregnated IVCs is on the rise as a promising technology for reducing device-related infection rates though controversies persist.

Because drainage holes responsible for the collection of excessive CSF are very small, it is easy for the catheter to become obstructed; the nurse must monitor for this complication, which is evidenced by either poor drainage of the system or change in the patient's neurologic status. Malfunction or obstruction occurs at a rate of 6% to 10% in patients with an IVC and is significantly higher in patients with parenchymal or ventricular fiberoptic catheter-tip devices, at a rate of 9% to 40%.[9] Higher rates of obstruction have been correlated with malignant elevations of ICP greater than 50 mm Hg. A reduction in catheter infections has been reported with recent changes in insertion techniques, antibiotic prophylaxis, and improved CSF sampling methods.[9] Hemorrhage associated with IVC placement is poorly described in the literature, prompting the reporting of a 1.1% to 2.8% risk for hematoma formation. The hemorrhage rate is highly dependent on the choice of device.

### Intracranial Pressure Waveforms

Waveforms of ICP provide an index of ICP dynamics, such as changes in intracerebral compliance. The appearance of ICP waveforms varies according to the measurement technique being used, the patient's pathologic status and activities, interventions, and environmental changes. Hemodynamic and

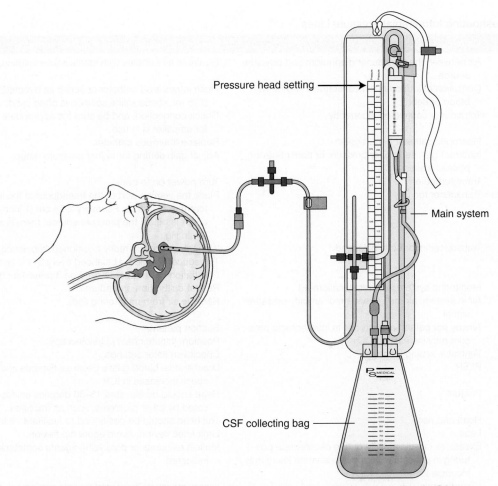

Pressure head setting

Main system

CSF collecting bag

FIGURE 34-3    Intraventricular catheter system. (Courtesy of Medtronic Neurologic Technologies, Goleta, CA.)

respiratory oscillations can be observed in ICP traces. Computerized systems are being developed to analyze waveforms and integrate ICP, CPP, and other relevant parameters.

Sometimes, the waveforms closely resemble arterial pressure waveforms; at other times, they resemble central venous pressure waveforms. To varying degrees, oscillations corresponding to intracranial arterial pulsations with retrograde venous pulsations are seen with each heartbeat (Fig. 34-4). In patients with ICP less than 20 mm Hg, a slower waveform, synchronous with respiration and caused by changes in intrathoracic pressure, can be seen (see Fig. 34-4, middle). Alterations in arterial driving force, disturbance of venous outflow, and cerebral vasodilation correlate with changes in waveform appearances. At times, a small "A" wave is superimposed on diastole, reflecting right arterial pressure.

Some patients exhibit waveform variation, most commonly A, B, and C waves. A waves, also known as plateau waves, are spontaneous, rapid increases of pressure ranging from 50 to 200 mm Hg, occurring at variable intervals (see Fig. 34-4, bottom). They tend to occur in patients with moderate elevations of ICP, last 5 to 20 minutes, and fall spontaneously. Plateau waves usually are accompanied by a temporary increase in neurologic deficit.

Although the mechanism of A waves has not been established firmly, it is thought that they indicate decreased intracranial compliance; therefore, these waveforms should be identified and treated quickly. They may result from an increase in blood volume with a simultaneous decrease in blood flow. The sudden reversal of high pressure may be caused by increased CSF absorption. Falls in CPP with intact autoregulation and low intracranial compliance have been correlated with the initiation of plateau waves. Plateau waves may also be set off by a vasodilating stimulus or by nonspecific stimuli, such as hypoventilation or hyperventilation, pain, and aroused mental activities.

B waves are small, sharp, rhythmic waves with ICPs up to 50 mm Hg, occurring at a frequency of 0.5 to 2 per minute. They correspond to changes in respiration, providing clues to periodic respiration related to poor cerebral compliance or pulmonary dysfunction. B waves often are seen with Cheyne-Stokes respirations (see Chapter 36). They may precede A waves and increase as compliance decreases. At times, they occur in patients with normal ICP and no papilledema. They may be secondary to oscillations of cerebral blood volume.

C waves are small, rhythmic waves with ICPs up to 20 mm Hg, occurring at a rate of approximately 6 per minute. They are related to blood pressure. Like A waves, they indicate severe intracranial compression, with limited remaining volume residual in the intracranial space.

## Measurements

Normal measurements of ICP range between 0 and 10 mm Hg, with an upper limit of 15 mm Hg. During coughing or

**TABLE 34-3** Troubleshooting Intracranial Pressure Lines

| Problem | Cause | Nursing Considerations and Interventions |
|---|---|---|
| No ICP waveform | Air between the transducer diaphragm and pressure source | Eliminate air bubbles with sterile saline solution. |
| | Occlusion of intracranial measurement device with blood or debris | Flush intracranial catheter or screw as directed by physician: 0.25 mL sterile saline solution is often used. |
| | Transducer connected incorrectly | Check connection, and be sure the appropriate connector for amplifier is in use. |
| | Fiberoptic catheter bent, broken | Replace fiberoptic catheter. |
| | Incorrect gain setting for pressure or patient having plateau waves | Adjust gain setting for higher pressure range. |
| | Trace turned off | Turn power on to trace. |
| False high-pressure reading | Transducer too low | Place the venting port of the transducer at the level of the foramen of Monro. For every 2.54 cm (1 inch) the transducer is below the pressure source, there is an error of 2 mm Hg. |
| | Transducer incorrectly balanced | With transducer correctly positioned, rebalance. Transducer should be balanced every 2–4 h and before the initiation of treatment based on a pressure change. |
| | Monitoring system incorrectly calibrated | Repeat calibration procedures. |
| | Air in system: air may attenuate or amplify pressure signal | Remove air from monitoring line. |
| High-pressure reading | Airway not patent: an increase in intrathoracic pressure may increase $PaCO_2$ | Suction patient. Position. Initiate chest physiotherapy. |
| | Ventilator setting incorrect | Check ventilator settings. |
| | PEEP | Draw arterial blood gases because hypoxia and hypercarbia cause increases in ICP. |
| | Posture | Head should be elevated 15–30 degrees unless contraindicated by other problems, such as fractures. |
| | Head and neck | The head should be positioned to facilitate venous drainage. |
| | Legs | Limit knee flexion. Avoid acute hip flexion. |
| | Excessive muscle activity during decerebrate posturing in patients with upper brainstem injury may increase ICP | Muscle relaxants or paralyzing agents sometimes are indicated. |
| | Hyperthermia | Initiate measures to control muscle movement, infection, and pyrexia. |
| | Excessive muscle activity | |
| | Increased susceptibility to infection | |
| | Fluid and electrolyte imbalance secondary to fluid restrictions and diuretics | Draw blood for serum electrolytes, serum osmolality. Note pulmonary artery pressure. Evaluate input and output with specific gravity. |
| | Blood pressure: vasopressor responses occur in some patients with elevating ICP. | Use measures to maintain adequate continuous positive pressure. |
| | Low blood pressure associated with hypovolemia, shock, and barbiturate coma may increase cerebral ischemia. | |
| False low-pressure reading | Air bubbles between transducer and CSF | Eliminate air bubbles with sterile saline. |
| | Transducer level too high | Place the venting port of the transducer at the level of the foramen of Monro. For every 2.54 cm (1 inch) the transducer is above the level of the pressure source, there will be an error of approximately 2 mm Hg. |
| Low-pressure reading | Zero or calibration incorrect | Re-zero and calibrate monitoring system. |
| | Collapse of ventricles around catheter | If ventriculostomy is being used, there may be inadequate positive pressure. Check to make sure a positive pressure of 15–20 mm Hg exists. Drain CSF slowly. |
| | Otorrhea or rhinorrhea | These conditions cause a false low-pressure reading secondary to decompression. Document the correlation between drainage and pressure changes. |
| | Leakage of fluid from connections | Eliminate all fluid leakage. |
| | Dislodgment of catheter from ventricle into brain | Contact physician regarding appropriate diagnostic studies and intervention. Use soft catheter designed for intraventricular measurement. |
| | Occlusion of the end of a subarachnoid screw by the necrotic brain | In most cases, remove screw. |

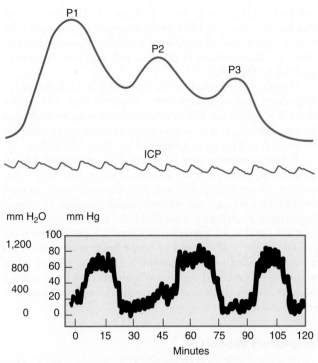

**FIGURE 34-4**  Intracranial pressure (ICP) waveforms. **Top:** A normal ICP pulse waveform may demonstrate three or more descending peaks. P1, the pressure wave, originates from choroid plexus pulsations. P2, the tidal wave, is more variable in shape and amplitude and ends on the dicrotic notch. P3, the dicrotic wave, follows the dicrotic notch and tapers down to the diastolic position unless retrograde venous pulsations cause a few more peaks. The P2 portion of the waveform most directly reflects the state of intracerebral compliance. As mean ICP rises, P2 progressively elevates, causing the pulse wave to appear more rounded. When a state of decreased compliance exists, the P2 component is equal to or higher than P1. **Middle:** An ICP waveform demonstrating hemodynamic and respiratory oscillations. Note the vascular pressure-type notches in the waveforms and the baseline variations that reflect respirations. **Bottom:** "A," or plateau, waves, associated with decreased intracranial compliance, may be secondary to an increase in blood volume with a simultaneous decrease in blood flow.

straining, a normal ICP may increase to 100 mm Hg. A patient's tolerance of a change in ICP varies with the acuteness of its onset. A patient with a slower buildup of ICP (eg, as the result of an expanding brain tumor) is typically more tolerant of elevations in ICP than a patient whose ICP increases rapidly (eg, as the result of an acute subdural hematoma). Uncontrolled ICP between 20 and 25 mm Hg is considered extremely dangerous for the patient with brain injury. Sustained ICP greater than 60 mm Hg usually is fatal. ICP may rise to the level of the MAP. The greater the variations in the mean ICP, the more nearly exhausted are the compensatory mechanisms for intracranial volume increases.

CPP is the main indicator of the circulatory system's ability to infuse the brain. However, CPP has limitations; it measures only a single parameter that influences oxygen delivery and the neurons' ability to sustain injury. Neuronal demand for oxygen is governed by the cell's metabolic needs, which increase during neuronal activity or injury. Therefore, to understand the metabolic status of the neuron, both CBF and oxygen content in the blood must be measured. The equation CBF $\times$ OEF $\times$ SaO$_2$ is commonly used to

calculate the cerebral metabolic rate for oxygen (CMRO$_2$). The oxygen extraction fraction (OEF), which is measured using both the arterial and venous oxygen content, describes how much oxygen is extracted. SaO$_2$ represents the oxygen saturation in the arterial blood. Necessary information can be obtained using multimodality monitoring, including blood flow studies, such as jugular venous bulb oximetry, as well as positron emission tomography and single-photon emission CT.

### Multimodal Monitoring

Multimodal neuromonitoring allows for tracking of the metabolic balance of the injured brain when combined with ICP information. CBF can be estimated based on flow velocities using transcranial Doppler; local metabolic biomarkers can be trended using invasive microdialysis; and the utilization of oxygen can be measured using jugular venous bulb oximetry. These technologies may prove useful to improve patient survival through the acute brain injury period.[8,10]

### Jugular Venous Bulb Oximetry

Jugular venous bulb oximetry is an invasive technique that involves placing a sampling catheter in the internal jugular vein, with the tip of the jugular venous bulb at the base of the brain. Blood samples from this location measure the mixed venous oxygen saturation (SjO$_2$) of blood leaving the brain; this is normally 50% to 75%. The SjO$_2$ decreases when there is an imbalance between oxygen consumption and delivery. If the SjO$_2$ decreases to less than 50% (without a decrease in SaO$_2$), this implies either a decrease in CBF or an increase in oxygen utilization (higher CMRO$_2$). If CPP is maintained, a decrease in CBF is due to an increase in cerebrovascular resistance (CVR). Vascular spasm and an increase in CVR are very common after brain injury and are significantly worsened by hyperventilation; therefore, this technique is discouraged. An increase in SjO$_2$ greater than 85% implies either a hyperemia with an increase in CBF, shunting of blood away from neurons, or a decrease in CMRO$_2$ (impending cell death or brain death). It should be emphasized that SjO$_2$ is a measure of global cerebral oxygenation and is not sensitive to small areas of focal ischemia. However, SjO$_2$ may be of assistance in guiding some therapies for the patient with brain injury, including barbiturate-induced cerebral metabolic suppression and the rare use of induced hyperventilation.

### Transcranial Doppler Ultrasound

Transcranial Doppler ultrasound is a noninvasive method of assessing the state of the intracranial circulation. The velocity of flow can be measured in the middle, anterior, and posterior cerebral arteries, the ophthalmic artery, and internal carotid artery. Flow cannot be measured from velocity because the cross-sectional area of the arteries cannot be measured directly. However, the Doppler shift measured is inversely proportional to the diameter of the vessel, so that if all other factors remain constant, vascular narrowing leads to an increase in flow velocity. Doppler waveform analysis can provide further information about the state of blood flow, but the value and utility of these and other multimodality techniques are as yet unknown.

## Management of Increased Intracranial Pressure

In the stage between the onset of increased ICP and herniation, many treatments are available to reduce ICP and maintain adequate cerebral perfusion. No single management routine is appropriate for all patients. In addition to clinical pathways and protocols, algorithms for the incremental application and weaning of ICP management have been developed. First-tier therapy includes ventricular CSF drainage, administration of osmotic therapy, respiratory support, and sedation and analgesia. Second-tier therapy includes hypothermia, barbiturate coma, optimized hyperventilation, hypertensive CPP therapy, and decompressive craniectomy.

Treatment goals for the patient with increased ICP are as follows: reduce ICP, optimize CPP, maintain adequate tissue oxygenation, and avoid brain herniation. Most management techniques are oriented toward control of cerebral blood volume and CSF circulation, the two major mechanisms responsible for the regulation of ICP. Measures to reduce ICP are usually initiated when the patient's ICP increases to approximately 15 mm Hg.

## Clinical Management

### Hyperosmolar Therapy

Intracranial hypertension can be managed through the administration of hypertonic saline or mannitol, a hypertonic crystalloid solution.

**HYPERTONIC SALINE.** Hypertonic saline is a mainstay for the treatment of patients with intracranial edema. Induced hypernatremia has been demonstrated to both increase CPPs and decrease intracerebral pressure in the setting of multiple pathologies (stroke, subarachnoid hemorrhage, mass lesions). Timing of the initiation of such therapies continues to be debated, and clear recommendations have yet to be provided. Therefore, treatment with hypertonic saline varies both in the concentration of the hypertonic solution and in the method of delivery. Induced hypernatremia can be achieved with solutions ranging from 2% to 23.4%. Additionally, agents can be administered via bolus dosing or continuous infusion.

Peripheral intravenous access can be used if administering 2% hypertonic saline. However, giving a more hyperosmolar agent (greater than 3%) requires central venous access to avoid infusion phlebitis or regional necrosis. A 250-mL bolus of 3% hypertonic saline can be expected to raise serum sodium by nearly 5 mEq/L.[11] Central pontine myelinolysis remains a theoretical concern though has yet to be proven in the literature as a reality.

**MANNITOL.** Mannitol, a hypertonic crystalloid solution that decreases cerebral edema, is also used as first-tier therapy for reducing ICP after brain injury. It is typically administered as a bolus intravenous (IV) infusion over 10 to 30 minutes in doses ranging from 0.25 to 2 g/kg body weight. Studies have demonstrated the effect of mannitol on ICP, CPP, CBF, and brain metabolism, and have also shown a beneficial effect on long-term neurologic outcome. The immediate plasma-expanding effect of mannitol, which reduces blood viscosity, increases CBF and cerebral oxygen metabolism, permitting

cerebral arterioles to decrease in diameter. This lowers cerebral blood volume and ICP while maintaining constant CBF. Use of hypertonic saline follows a similar pharmacodynamic effect in the treatment of elevated ICP and may provide an alternative therapy.[12–15]

Mannitol is excreted in the urine. If it is administered in large doses and serum osmolarity is greater than 320 mOsm, there is a significant risk of acute tubular necrosis and renal failure. Therefore, it is customary to measure serum osmolarity every 6 to 8 hours to a target of less than 320 mOsm.

A Foley catheter must be inserted when mannitol is administered. When mannitol is used during the early resuscitation phase in hypovolemic patients with brain injuries, crystalloid solutions are infused simultaneously to correct hypovolemia. Adjunct crystalloid fluid administration facilitates rapid renal excretion of mannitol, preventing renal failure. In the early phases of acute brain injury, mannitol is recommended as monotherapy. Caution is advised when mannitol is combined with furosemide because there is a risk of over-diuresis, depletion of intravascular volume, and electrolyte imbalance.

### Respiratory Support

There are several considerations when managing the respiratory status of a critically ill patient with neurologic injury. Mean airway pressure is the leading factor affecting ICP in the patient who is receiving ventilation therapy. Positive airway pressure is transmitted to the intracranial cavity through the mediastinum by preventing jugular venous outflow. Therefore, any condition decreasing pulmonary compliance or use of positive end-expiratory pressure (PEEP) increases the mean airway pressure and decreases the MAP and CPP.

Normocapnia is essential for maintaining stable ICP because carbon dioxide directly affects the degree of vasodilation in the cerebral blood vessels. Hyperventilation is a temporary strategy for the treatment of malignant ICP. Hyperventilation decreases the arterial carbon dioxide tension ($PaCO_2$) and results in cerebral vasoconstriction. As a result, the CBF is reduced because of the strong vasoconstrictive effect of hypocarbia on the cerebral arteries. The $PaCO_2$ should be lowered gradually to avoid a rebound effect of vasodilation from overcorrection. When hyperventilation is discontinued, ventilation rates should be gradually returned to normal. In the absence of a malignant increase in ICP, hyperventilation therapy ($PaCO_2$ less than 25 mm Hg) should be avoided after a traumatic brain injury. Also, the use of prophylactic hyperventilation therapy ($PaCO_2$ less than 35 mm Hg) during the first 24 hours after a traumatic brain injury should be avoided because it can compromise cerebral perfusion during a time of critically reduced CBF.[5,16] Severe, prolonged hyperventilation has been conclusively shown to worsen the outcome of patients with a severe brain injury and should be reserved for those cases in which all other therapies have failed. Severe hyperventilation is defined as a $PaCO_2$ of less than 25 mm Hg by jugular venous oxygen saturation monitor. Extreme hyperventilation is believed to cause secondary ischemia by constricting cerebral vasculature.[5]

Increasing intrathoracic pressure directly increases ICP; therefore, suctioning should be approached thoughtfully. Limiting the duration of passes of the suction catheter to no more than 5 to 10 seconds avoids hypoxia. Limiting the number of passes to one or two avoids overstimulation of the cough reflex and decreases the incidence of increased intrathoracic pressure and ICP.

## Pharmacologic Therapy

### Analgesics, Sedatives, and Paralytics

In patients with a severe brain injury (GCS score less than 8), pain medications and sedatives are used to

- reduce agitation, discomfort, and pain
- facilitate mechanical ventilation by suppressing coughing
- limit responses to stimuli, such as suctioning, which may increase ICP.

Before starting patients on analgesics or sedatives, every effort should be made to implement nonpharmacologic management techniques for pain, agitation, anxiety, and confusion. When medication is required, the agent should be selected based on both desired mechanism of action as well as half-life of the medication, because restoration of the neurologic function is critical for the care of these patients. The treatment of pain lowers energy expenditures and thereby facilitates healing. Furthermore, analgesics and sedatives may potentiate each other, allowing patients to achieve comfort and sedation.[17]

**ANALGESICS.** Opioid narcotics primarily affect the CNS. Fentanyl and morphine are two of the most frequently used opiate narcotics for brain-injured patients. These agents:

- limit pain caused by injuries and nursing interventions
- facilitate mechanical ventilation
- potentiate the effect of sedatives.[17]

Potentially life-threatening adverse effects of narcotics include respiratory depression, depression of the cough reflex, mood changes, nausea, and vomiting. Vital signs and pulse oximetry values must be monitored diligently when a patient receives IV pain medication. When preparing for such complications, the critical care nurse should ensure that resuscitation and intubation equipment are readily available in case respiratory depression occurs. Naloxone, which reverses CNS depression that can occur with the administration of fentanyl and morphine, may be required. With proper dosing and diligent nursing observation, narcotic analgesics can be used effectively in the critically ill patient.

The basic principles of narcotic administration are adequate pain relief and safe administration. It is especially important to begin with the lowest possible dose when treating a patient with neurologic illness, especially the older patient, because the injured brain's response to medication is unpredictable. When a patient with a brain injury also has severe pain caused by multiple traumatic injuries, a continuous infusion of fentanyl or morphine is indicated and can be titrated every 15 to 30 minutes until pain control is achieved. For a patient with moderate pain, a 24-hour regimen of opiate narcotic administration has proved to provide increased pain relief versus an "as-needed" schedule of opiate dosing.

For the patient who can communicate, a verbal pain scale is used to assess pain. Standardized rating scales, such as a 1 to 10 pain scale, should be used to quantify and evaluate

pain status and response to therapy. In addition to location, quality, and duration of pain, the nurse must document the effectiveness of analgesics after initial administration and with dose changes. It is exceedingly important to observe for sedating effects that hinder monitoring of the neurologic examination. All hospitals have a pain management protocol that identifies analgesics that should be used, dosing titration guidelines, and documentation requirements.

For the patient who is unable to communicate, physiologic parameters are used to determine the effectiveness of pain management. The nurse assesses heart rate, respiratory rate, use of accessory muscles for breathing, and blood pressure. Adequate pain management leads to less patient movement (eg, thrashing) that increases metabolic activity. The following clues can be used to determine whether adequate pain relief has been obtained for the patient who cannot communicate:

- ease of breathing
- mechanically ventilated patient whose breathing is synchronous with the ventilator
- possible decrease in heart rate
- less agitation, as indicated by restful sleep state
- cooperation with nursing interventions without excessive physical activity.

The nurse must be aware that narcotics decrease gastric motility and may cause constipation. Patients with neurologic illness in the critical care setting are often immobilized or confined to bed, and thus are especially prone to constipation. All patients on narcotic therapy should be on a bowel regimen to avoid this complication, and the quality and frequency of bowel movements should be monitored closely. Straining increases ICP and could possibly be avoided with strict bowel regimens. Patients may also be susceptible to nausea and vomiting with the administration of narcotics. Protection of the airway is especially important in the patient with a neurologic diagnosis. Mechanically ventilated patients require the insertion of a nasogastric or orogastric tube to decompress the stomach and prevent vomiting.

**SEDATIVES.** The most commonly used sedatives in the ICU are benzodiazepines, which cause little change in CBF, ICP, and cerebral metabolic rate, and potentiate the effects of analgesic agents. Midazolam, diazepam, and lorazepam are used frequently for sedation before ICU procedures and as needed to treat anxiety. Lorazepam is frequently used for alcohol withdrawal and anticonvulsant therapy. Midazolam, in combination with fentanyl, is most often used for sedation before procedures to produce amnesia of immediate events. Side effects of sedatives include respiratory depression, hypotension, and somnolence. It is mandatory that resuscitation equipment be available at all times when IV benzodiazepines are used. Benzodiazepines should be administered at the lowest possible dose that produces effective sedation, without causing somnolence. As with analgesic agents, frequent vital signs must be obtained with the administration of sedatives. Recommended minimal documentation of vital signs should be after administration of the sedative and every hour for 4 hours.

Various scales may be used to document the patient's response to sedation. The target sedation level for a patient with a critical neurologic illness is one that allows easy arousal of the patient with light touch or voice. For the patient who cannot communicate (as discussed earlier with analgesic use), the assessment of physiologic parameters can be used to determine the patient's response to sedation in order to achieve maximal comfort. Pharmacologic management of sedation is only one strategy to treat anxiety. Nursing measures to provide comfort must be offered in addition to medications.

**ANESTHETICS.** Propofol is a fat-soluble anesthetic that is administered as a continuous infusion to decrease agitation in the critically ill patient. Studies have shown that propofol may decrease CBF, ICP, CPP, and cerebral metabolic function.[18] Propofol is easily titrated based on patient response. It also has a short half-life and can be discontinued for neurologic assessments. Propofol can decrease the level of consciousness in 2 minutes. A common side effect is hypotension; therefore, frequent blood pressure monitoring must be performed, especially if the patient has increased ICP. Since this anesthetic agent causes loss of respiratory drive, diligent airway protection must be provided for the patient receiving propofol. To prevent respiratory depression, the patient must be intubated and mechanically ventilated when propofol is administered. For these reasons, the patient who receives a continuous infusion of propofol must be cared for in the ICU, with constant surveillance by the critical care nurse. In most states, an anesthesia provider may administer an IV bolus dose of propofol.

Propofol infusion syndrome is a rare but significant adverse drug event associated with prolonged propofol use (more than 48 hours) at high doses (more than 4 mg/kg/h). This syndrome is characterized by hypotension, severe metabolic acidosis, rhabdomyolysis, hyperkalemia, renal failure, hepatomegaly, and cardiovascular collapse. Therefore, duration of propofol therapy should be monitored and limited when possible.

Other considerations with propofol are related to the handling of the drug. Propofol is manufactured by using a fat emulsion, making it a powerful medium for bacterial growth. Propofol must be handled meticulously to prevent the risk for bacterial or fungal infection associated with its use. The fat calories provided by propofol should be included when calculating nutritional supplementation for the patient receiving this infusion. It may be necessary to monitor the triglyceride level for patients receiving propofol longer term.

Dexmedetomidine (Precedex) is an α-adrenergic receptor agonist that provides sedation, antianxiolysis, and analgesia without respiratory depression.[18,19] This IV medication may be a good alternative in the critical care setting, since patients can be weaned from the ventilator and extubated while receiving this medication. The most common side effect is hypotension.[18] This medication is especially useful for the patient with neurologic injury, because respiratory changes (especially manipulation of carbon dioxide levels) can have significant effect on intracranial pressure, and less effect on the mental status is desirable. Cost is a consideration when using this medication.

**NEUROMUSCULAR BLOCKADE.** Neuromuscular blockading (NMB) agents are used to induce muscle paralysis in cases of refractory ICP. An NMB agent blocks the transmission of acetylcholine at the motor end plate, producing skeletal muscle paralysis. Reversal of NMB agents is provided by acetylcholinesterase inhibitors such as neostigmine, edrophonium, and pyridostigmine. The use of an NMB agent

requires mechanical ventilation with full support. Resuscitation equipment must be present at all times when a patient is treated with an NMB agent. For a conscious patient, the inability to move and communicate is frightening; therefore, concurrent administration of analgesia and sedation is mandatory.[20] Analgesia and sedation provide the added benefit of producing amnesia.

Complications common with most NMB agents are tachycardia, hypotension, and dysrhythmias. Cardiac medications such as antidysrhythmics, diuretics, and calcium channel and β-blockers can potentiate the action of NMB drugs. Certain antibiotics, such as aminoglycosides and clindamycin, can potentiate the action of paralytic agents. Alterations in body temperature or acid–base balance and electrolyte disturbances also alter the action of NMB agents.[20]

A troubling complication of paralytic therapy is prolonged polymyopathy.[21] A condition known as acute quadriplegic myopathy syndrome, or postparalytic quadriparesis, is one of the most devastating complications of prolonged use of an NMB agent.[20,21] This condition is manifested by prolonged weakness of the upper and lower extremities. The extraocular motor muscles are usually spared in this condition. A patient may also experience painful muscle fasciculations. To avoid these complications, the smallest dosage of an NMB agent should be used to obtain adequate respiratory support.

Peripheral nerve stimulation monitoring is mandatory with NMB therapy;[20] its use every 4 hours, with a dosage change as necessary, may help prevent complications associated with NMB therapy. A peripheral nerve stimulator is a small handheld device used in the ICU to monitor the depth of NMB in the patient receiving prolonged paralytic therapy. This device delivers a small jolt of energy to the ulnar surface of the wrist, causing the thumb to twitch. The train-of-four method is used to measure the efficacy and depth of NMB. The peripheral nerve stimulator delivers four 2-Hz stimuli of 0.2 millisecond at intervals of 0.5 second to the ulnar nerve at the wrist. Normally, the thumb twitches four times when the peripheral nerve stimulator is activated. The nurse observes thumb movements after peripheral nerve stimulation. If the thumb twitches two or three times, NMB dosing is usually sufficient. If four thumb twitches occur, paralysis is ineffective. If no twitches occur, paralysis is excessive, and the dose of the NMB agent must be reduced.

Excellent nursing care also can help prevent some of the complications caused by NMB agents. A patient repositioning schedule must be rigidly maintained to prevent the development of pressure ulcers. Aspiration precautions and excellent pulmonary toilet must be maintained at all times to avoid pneumonia. Also, deep venous thrombosis prophylaxis must be implemented before induction of paralysis.

**BARBITURATE COMA.** For the patient with severe and refractory elevated ICP, an induced barbiturate coma may be attempted to decrease systemic metabolic activity in an attempt to preserve brain function. In cases of malignant ICP elevations, "putting the brain to sleep" to reduce the metabolic demand and decrease ICP may be of benefit. Criteria for inducing a barbiturate coma includes a GCS score of less than 7, ICP greater than 25 mm Hg at rest for 10 minutes, and failed maximal interventions, including drainage of CSF, mannitol, analgesia, and sedation. Barbiturate coma is typically used for less than 72 hours because longer use leads to accumulation of medication in the adipose tissue, making weaning difficult.

In addition to reducing cerebral metabolic activity and cerebral oxygen demand, barbiturates have an additional benefit of suppressing seizure activity. These combined effects, along with metabolic demand, electroencephalographic (EEG) activity, and systemic hemodynamics, may decrease CBF by 50%. Barbiturate therapy appears to have a direct restrictive effect on cerebral vasculature by diverting small amounts of blood from well-perfused areas to ischemic areas, thereby improving cerebral pressure.

Before the administration of barbiturates, the following must be provided for the patient: a secure airway with mechanical ventilation; ICP, blood pressure, cardiac, and pulmonary artery monitoring; and continuous EEG monitoring. An EEG is obtained before administration of a barbiturate so that spontaneous electrocortical activity is documented. The EEG pattern of burst suppression is the most common method to establish barbiturate dosing: the barbiturate dose is adjusted until EEG burst suppression is achieved. The initial dose may be supplemented by an IV bolus to achieve burst suppression. Barbiturate serum levels alone are poor measures of therapeutic efficacy and systemic toxicity.

Barbiturates should be discontinued with any of the following clinical findings:

- ICP less than 15 mm Hg for 24 to 72 hours
- systolic blood pressure less than 90 mm Hg despite the use of vasopressors
- progressive neurologic impairment, as evidenced by deterioration of brainstem auditory evoked responses
- cardiac arrest.

At the time of discontinuation, the barbiturate dosage is gradually reduced over 24 to 72 hours. Arousal is gradual and prolonged, even after blood levels have been zero for several days. The patient must be weaned slowly and carefully from mechanical ventilation because residual muscle weakness may occur. Patients may experience facial weakness for several days after the barbiturate has been discontinued. Occasionally, the patient may experience dysarthria, related to weakness of the muscles of speech. During the first 24 hours of barbiturate withdrawal, slow, abnormal muscle movements may be observed.

### Blood Pressure Management

The regulation of blood pressure is an important aspect of managing the patient with increased ICP. Blood pressure is directly related to cerebral blood volume, perfusion pressure, ischemia, and compliance. For patients with brain injuries, the preservation of CPP and maintenance of systemic oxygenation are two important goals. Also, patients with the most severe brain injuries are at risk for secondary injury caused by hypotension and hypoxia. Patients with brain injury may have increased metabolic oxygen consumption, mild hypertension, and increased cardiac indices. Invasive blood pressure monitoring is routinely used to provide continuous and accurate blood pressure measurement during the acute management phase of patients with brain injuries. MAP is the parameter used for evaluating CPP and the efficacy of antihypertensive or vasopressor therapies. See Chapter 17 for further description of hemodynamic monitoring.

Drug therapies to manage blood pressure may cause a precipitous increase or decrease in cardiac output. When the cardiac output is low, patients with neurologic injuries are in jeopardy of further ischemic injury since the protective mechanisms of autoregulation are disturbed. The cardiac index is usually maintained at 3 L/min/m$^2$ because patients with head injuries frequently have increased metabolic needs. The pulmonary artery capillary wedge pressure is usually maintained at 12 to 15 mm Hg in patients with head injuries. In addition, noninvasive continuous pulse oximetry and arterial blood gas measurement are used to determine arterial oxygen content.

Different classes of antihypertensive medications can be used to treat systemic hypertension in the critically ill patient.[22] For patients with acute ischemic stroke, acute hypertension is defined as a systolic blood pressure greater than 185 mm Hg and a diastolic blood pressure greater than 110 mm Hg. These patients are especially dependent on systemic blood pressure to maintain perfusion through a partially occluded intracranial vessel. IV hydralazine or labetalol are frequently used for elevated blood pressure and should be titrated slowly to avoid sudden episodes of hypotension. If the patient remains hypertensive after hydralazine or labetalol administration, nicardipine or nitroprusside may be used. Both nicardipine and nitroprusside are potent vasodilators and can lower the blood pressure quickly. They are administered as continuous infusions, are easily titrated, and have relatively short half-lives. These medications must be used in the ICU or emergency department where continuous blood pressure monitoring can be provided. Hypotension may occur if the infusion is increased too quickly.

For patients with hemorrhagic brain injury, a more rigorous blood pressure range is maintained. An MAP greater than 110 mm Hg is avoided in these patients.[23] Angiotensin-converting enzyme (ACE) inhibitors and β-blockers are often used to treat hypertension in the head-injured patient with systemic hypertension. β-Blockers are most often used because of their safe side effect profile, although they may cause bradycardia. Calcium channel blockers are usually avoided in head-injured patients because of their potential to exacerbate cerebral edema.

### Seizure Prophylaxis

Patients with neurologic injury are often prone to seizure activity, which markedly elevates the cerebral metabolic rate and CBF, and may lead to hypoxia. In patients with traumatic brain injury, use of antiepileptic agents for 7 days has been shown to decrease the incidence of early seizure activity, but it does not prevent development of later seizures. However, the practice of using antiepileptic agents varies, because there are no compelling data suggesting improved outcome with their use. Anticonvulsant therapy may be used to prevent early posttraumatic seizure, especially in patients with a reduced seizure threshold (eg, brain tumor, cortical lesions, temporal lobe pathologies). Phenytoin, levetiracetam, and carbamazepine are considered treatment agents for preventing early (less than 7 days) posttraumatic seizure activity. Levetiracetam may be more convenient to administer but can cause agitation in some patients.

The treatment of choice for acute-onset seizures (such as tonic–clonic seizures) in the critically ill patient remains diazepam. The patient should be positioned on his or her side and an oxygen mask applied. There should be no attempt to restrain a seizing patient, because this may lead to joint dislocation or fracture. When seizure activity has subsided, the nurse should obtain a serum glucose analysis to determine whether hypoglycemia is a contributing cause. An EEG may also be ordered to determine whether the patient is continuing to experience subclinical seizures and to determine seizure focus.

## Other Management Methods

### Hypothermia

Hypothermia continues to be explored as a means of reducing the brain's metabolic demands during peak times of cerebral edema and brain injury. It is recommended for patients with fulminant hepatic failure leading to cerebral edema.[24] One difficulty is cooling the patient adequately to achieve optimal neuroprotection without shivering, which can raise intracranial pressure.[25] To date, the optimal degree of coolness has not been established, although it continues to be investigated in multicenter clinical trials. However, control of fever is essential and is being more aggressively addressed using different types of cooling devices (both surface cooling and intravascular cooling devices).[25–27]

### Decompressive Craniectomy

Another strategy used for managing refractory intracranial hypertension is decompressive craniotomy. This surgery is based on the theory that ICP can be reduced through surgical release of the rigid skull. Although surgical decompression remains an option for patients with uncontrollable ICPs, studies have shown varying results on mortality based on the etiology of the raised intracranial pressure. Early decompressive hemicraniectomy for younger patients with malignant edema after ischemic stroke demonstrate a mortality benefit in numerous trials.[27–35]

There continues to be debate in the traumatic brain injury literature.[36] However, the procedure remains widely used for patients with malignant cerebral edema after traumatic brain injury. Long-term morbidity and mortality as well as the best timing for this procedure continues to be evaluated and debated.[36–41] Surgical intervention has been shown to be life-saving, but impact on functional outcome is yet to be confirmed.

Suboccipital craniotomy for clinically deteriorating patients with cerebellar pathologies is a mainstay in therapy, because the posterior fossa does not allow for any increased volume without brainstem herniation. There are no prospective data specific to this intervention, although observational case series and practice recommendations for patients with cerebellar infarction with swelling support surgical treatment for this population of patients who are at risk for rapid herniation.[42,43]

## Patient Care Considerations

Nursing care activity can compound primary and secondary intracranial insults, contributing to rapid deterioration in the unstable patient who has lost intracranial compliance, autoregulation, and vasomotor tone.[23] Patient positioning, agitation, pain, hemodynamic and respiratory status, and seizures can all contribute to a patient's elevated ICP. The following sections describe a few patient management strategies for reducing ICP; see also Table 34-4.

---

**TABLE 34-4** Nursing Considerations for Patients at Risk for Increased Intracranial Pressure

| Problem | Nursing Action | Rationale |
|---|---|---|
| Adequate ventilation | • Assess respiratory patterns and rate<br>• Suctioning: Preoxygenate with 100% $O_2$, one or two catheter passes, no more than 10 s per catheter insertion<br>• Monitor continuous pulse oximetry and blood gases | • Indicates neurologic changes, pain status, and patency of airway<br>• Prevents increased $CO_2$ (vasodilator that increases ICP); decreases coughing stimulation and increased intrathoracic pressure<br>• Alerts nurse to airway problems; good indicator of hemodynamics of respiration |
| Neurologic assessment | • Evaluate patient baseline neurologic status at beginning of shift (preferably with previous shift RN)—mental status; pupil shape, size, and response; motor function<br>• Assess vital signs—note trends (review ordered parameters for notification of physician)<br>• Review nursing actions and emergency algorithm for neurologic deterioration (available medications, mannitol, hyperventilation, etc.) | • Subtle changes from baseline indicate deterioration and the need for early intervention<br>• MAP directly correlates with ICP in patient with loss of autoregulation<br>• Ensures optimal benefit to patient and decreases secondary injury from prolonged ICP |
| Positioning | • Place head of bed flat or at 30 degrees elevation per orders<br>• Maintain head in neutral position<br>• Avoid hip flexion<br>• Assess agitation in restrained patients<br>• Turn patient every 2 h, instructing patient to exhale with turn<br>• Carry out passive range-of-motion exercises<br>• Avoid clustering of patient activities (eg, turning, bathing, suctioning) | • Promotes cerebral perfusion or facilitates venous drainage; orders based on physiologic process<br>• Promotes jugular outflow<br>• Decreases intrathoracic pressure<br>• Increases ICP<br>• Prevents skin breakdown and avoids Valsalva maneuver during repositioning<br>• Prevents contractures while avoiding Valsalva-inducing isometric contractions |

**TABLE34-4   Nursing Considerations for Patients at Risk for Increased Intracranial Pressure (*continued*)**

| Problem | Nursing Action | Rationale |
|---|---|---|
| Transport of patient with invasive ICP monitor | • Use therapeutic interventions for emotional upset—speak with soft voice, use caution with unpleasant conversations, decrease noxious stimuli (noise), use therapeutic touch<br>• Confirm time of test or possibility of completing as portable study<br>• Prepare respiratory therapy and other assistants during transport<br>• Gather transport supplies (sedation if ordered, transport monitor, antihypertensives)<br>• Assist with transfer of patient to diagnostic table with RN at head of bed monitoring device<br>• Monitor and record hemodynamics and ICP dynamics during study | • Produces prolonged ICP spikes<br>• Causes elevations in ICP; comatose patients still respond to unpleasant environmental stimuli<br>• Avoids excessive delays in uncontrolled and potentially overstimulating environment<br>• Adequate oxygenation remains a priority; multiple lines necessitate additional manpower<br>• Prepare for intervention with any adverse patient response during travel specific to contributors of increased ICP<br>• Ensures patient protection and provides for monitor equipment recalibration for accuracy of monitoring<br>• Monitors patient response to procedure |
| Temperature control | • Frequent temperature checks (oral or rectal preferred if no contraindications)<br>• Confirm orders for early treatment of fever and aggressively treat | • Cerebral metabolic rate increases with elevated body temperature<br>• Increased CBF increases ICP<br>• Provide gradual cooling with cooling blanket, closely monitored<br>• Shivering increases ICP |
| Glycemic control | • Monitor serum glucose and fingersticks as ordered (every 4–6 h); adhere closely to sliding scale protocols in nondiabetic patients<br>• Maintain euvolemia with normal saline | • Alterations in glucose can produce neurologic changes (ie, changes in metabolic rate)<br>• Hypotonic glucose IV solutions should be avoided |
| Bowel and bladder regimens | • Administer daily stool softeners as ordered<br>• Avoid enemas<br>• Assess patency of Foley catheters<br>• Document strict intake and output | • Reduces risk for straining and increased intra-abdominal pressure, which increases ICP<br>• Prevents Valsalva maneuver<br>• Important to monitor amount of diuresis, especially in patients treated with osmotic diuretics<br>• Important to maintain euvolemia |
| Seizure precautions | • Seizure precautions per hospital protocol (padding, etc.)<br>• Monitor serum anticonvulsant drug levels | • Prevents injury in high-risk patients<br>• Maintains therapeutic levels |

## Positioning

Primary positioning strategies for the patient with impending or active increased ICP include placement of the head and neck in a neutral position. Extreme neck flexion, extension, or rotation restricts venous drainage from the head through the internal jugular venous system and the vertebral venous plexus, increasing the total intracranial content. Decerebrate or decorticate posturing may also increase ICP. In addition, head-of-bed elevation has been shown to promote venous drainage and decrease ICP. The head is elevated 15 to 30 degrees, unless contraindicated by spine or limb fractures.

Tracheostomy ties and cervical collars are frequently checked for proper fit. Flexion of the hips greater than 90 degrees is avoided because it contributes to intra-abdominal and thoracic pressures and also impairs venous outflow.

## Environmental Stimuli

Environmental stimuli contribute to pain, stress, and anxiety, which can increase cerebral metabolic rates and blood flow, confounding the management of increased ICP. To reduce environmental overload in the critically ill patient, pain control and sedation are essential, but the resulting need for serial neurologic assessments must be considered as well. Anxiety and discomfort in the ICU cannot be underestimated in the patient who is neurologically impaired. Periods of uninterrupted sleep and rest should be provided between activities. Only essential interventions should be performed during times of poor intracranial compliance, and activities should be spaced to avoid a cumulative effect. It is also helpful to avoid unnecessary painful procedures, such as frequent blood draws.

# Clinical Applicability Challenges

---

### CASE STUDY

Mr. R., a 44-year-old man with history of hypertension and tobacco use, was admitted to the hospital after being found down. The patient was in his usual state of health, although he reported a headache for 1 week. On the day of presentation, he had been preparing for work in the AM as usual, but was found on the floor by his wife 30 minutes later. Emergencey Medical Services (EMS) was activated; in the field, blood pressure was noted to be 242/132 and heart rate 88 and regular.

Mr. R.'s past medical/surgical history is as follows:

- Hypertension and hyperlipidemia
- *Allergies*: None
- *Social history*: Works in sales, married with supportive wife, two children; social ingestion of alcohol; smoking history 1 pack per day for 29 years
- *Medications*: Lisinopril (Zestril), 20 mg/d; atorvastatin (Lipitor), 10 mg/d

CT scan performed in the emergency department reveals a 30-cc intracerebral hemorrhage in the basal ganglia with noted intraventricular extension. After treatment of elevated blood pressure, Mr. R. is admitted to the neuroscience ICU for additional management, hemodynamic monitoring, and treatment of potential complications.

Later that evening, Mr. R. becomes increasingly restless, and his left pupil demonstrates an ovoid shape. Mr. R.'s nurse is concerned that increasing intracranial pressure may be the cause of these subtle changes. The nurse elevates the head of the bed and notified the on-call provider of the change in Mr. R.'s condition. A CT scan is obtained urgently and demonstrates increased cerebral edema with a 6-mm midline shift.

Upon return to the unit, Mr. R. is more somnolent. He is intubated for airway protection and hyperventilated for the first minute postintubation. He is treated with a bolus of mannitol. An intraventricular drainage device is placed under sterile conditions at the bedside, with initial ICP recorded at 32 mm Hg. Mr. R.'s nurse activates strict interventions to avoid increased ICP, including maintaining a quiet environment, limiting nursing activities, and avoiding flexion and extension of the neck. Mr. R.'s blood pressure normalizes and he does not require antihypertensive or sedating medications. He demonstrates good response to the single bolus of mannitol and is monitored closely.

On day 2 of his hospital stay, Mr. R.'s nurse observes a 30-second tonic–clonic seizure, which is treated with diazepam and a phenytoin load, with daily phenytoin ordered. CT scan reveals no change in the intracerebral hemorrhage or amount of edema. He is started on an antiepileptic medication to avoid additional seizures, which would contribute to increased intracranial pressure. On day 5, Mr. R. is extubated. He is alert and interactive, and begins physical, occupational, and speech therapy.

Mr. R. is at risk for complications of immobility related to his stroke, and therefore receives prophylactic deep venous thrombosis. He remains on lisinopril for hypertension and is educated about the importance of medication adherence. Diagnostic studies to determine the etiology of the bleeding do not reveal any vascular malformation or aneurysm. It is suspected that poorly controlled hypertension is the etiology of the hemorrhage.

Until discharge, Mr. R.'s vital signs and clinical status remain stable. Mr. R. is transferred to a stroke rehabilitation facility for aggressive treatment of persistent hemiparesis and dysarthria.

1. How does intracerebral hemorrhage lead to increased intracranial pressure?
2. Describe the rationale for rapid blood pressure reduction in patients with intracerebral hemorrhage.
3. What benefit is there for the placement of an intraventricular catheter in this scenario?

---

### WANT TO KNOW MORE

A wide variety of resources to enhance your learning and understanding of this chapter are available on thePoint.

You will find:

- References
- Selected readings
- NCLEX-style review questions
- Internet resources
- And more!

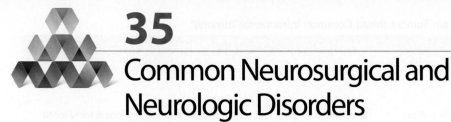

# 35

# Common Neurosurgical and Neurologic Disorders

STEPHANIE GIRE AND ERIN WICE

## LEARNING OBJECTIVES

**Based on the content in this chapter, the reader should be able to:**

1. Discuss the surgical management of the patient with a brain tumor.
2. Explain the care for the patient with a cerebral aneurysm or arteriovenous malformation.
3. Compare and contrast the classifications of stroke.
4. Discuss the nursing management of a patient who has experienced a stroke.
5. Differentiate between partial and generalized seizures.
6. Describe the clinical manifestations and management of the patient with Guillain–Barré syndrome.
7. Describe the clinical manifestations and management of the patient with myasthenia gravis.

During the course of illness, many patients with neurologic diseases require critical care management. Routine neurosurgical procedures may involve a short intensive care unit (ICU) admission for monitoring in the immediate postoperative period. Complications of tumor or related treatments may necessitate readmission. ICU admission may follow use of thrombolytic therapy for stroke and may be required to treat the patient with stroke complicated by increased intracranial pressure (ICP). Patients with myasthenia gravis or Guillain–Barré syndrome may require ICU level of care for cardiorespiratory consequences of their disease. The critical care nurse is better prepared to manage the acute and chronic needs of this patient population when armed with understanding of the course of the disease, as well as available medical and surgical tools. This chapter provides an overview of the etiology, clinical manifestations, diagnostic tests, and current management of the neurosurgical and neurologic disorders most often encountered in the ICU environment.

## Neurologic Surgery

Surgery is indicated for several neurologic disorders. Neurologic surgery is a common and integral part of the management of patients with intracranial tumors, arteriovenous malformations (AVMs), and aneurysms. Craniotomy is the most common procedure performed for these problems. The following section reviews the etiology and pathophysiology of these conditions and describes surgical approaches used for the management of these patients.

## Brain Tumors

A brain tumor is broadly described as any neoplasm arising within the intracranial space. Tumors may originate in the brain (primary) or seed in the brain from other organs (metastatic).[1,2] Through pathologic examination, the tumor can be classified by cell type. Tumors are further graded based on

the degree of malignancy. Classification and grade are used to predict patient outcome.[1,2] Table 35-1 outlines common brain tumor descriptions, symptoms, prognosis, and treatments and includes the World Health Organization (WHO) grading system.[5] Other predictors of outcome include patient age and general health, early detection, treatment choice, and tumor location.[2,3]

Although many brain tumors are low grade or "benign," their location may impede surgical removal and cause brain edema as well as shifting of the surrounding structures. This causes increased ICP. Untreated ICP can lead to brain herniation and can be fatal. Early diagnosis, symptom management, and histologic diagnosis are important prognostic factors.[1–3]

### Etiology

The cause of most brain tumors is still unknown. As research advances in the area of genetics, there is increased interest in identifying chromosomal abnormalities in many types of cancer, including brain tumors. Cytogenetic studies of glioblastoma, the most common primary brain tumor, have shown multiple chromosomal changes, with both gain and loss of certain chromosomes.[3,4] It is hypothesized that this information will, at the very least, aid in the development of individualized therapies for patients with primary brain tumors. Some hereditary diseases, such as neurofibromatosis and polyposis, are associated with the development of certain types of brain tumors.

An environmental factor currently being studied for an association with intracranial tumors is ionizing radiation. Some examples of ionizing radiation are x-rays, ultraviolet light, infrared light, microwaves, and radio waves. Environmental factors that have been recently studied but show no definitive association with intracranial tumors include foods (particularly those that are broken down in the stomach or bladder to form N-nitroso compounds) and cell phone use.[2–4] High-dose ionizing radiation has been shown to increase the occurrence of some brain tumors (nerve sheath tumors,

**TABLE 35-1    Classification and Grading of Brain Tumors (Most Common Intracranial Tumors)***

| Classification/Grade | Description | Symptoms | Treatment/Prognosis |
|---|---|---|---|
| **Neuroepithelial (approximately 30% of primary tumors)** | | | |
| *Gliomas* | | | |
| **Astrocytic** | | | |
| WHO grade I—pilocytic—astrocytoma | Pediatric; 85% cerebellar; slow growing; well circumscribed; cystic; benign | Increased ICP; focal neurologic signs | Curable with surgery (craniotomy for tumor removal) |
| WHO grade II—astrocytoma | Infiltrative; slow growing | Seizures; acute or subtle onset of symptoms | Radiation therapy (RT) for residual tumor; may withhold RT after gross total resection; young age is good prognostic factor |
| WHO grade III—anaplastic—astrocytoma | Hypercellular; anaplasia | May have acute onset of symptoms | RT with or without chemotherapy; high recurrence rate; age and overall health affect prognosis |
| WHO grade IV—glioblastoma—multiforme | Poorly differentiated, with high mitotic rate; highly malignant; most common glioma in adults | Rapid onset of symptoms; increased ICP or focal signs | Infiltrative nature: complete removal of all cells not possible; RT with chemotherapy; experimental protocols; recurrence in virtually all cases; median survival: 12–18 mo |
| **Oligodendroglioma** | Well differentiated; calcified; infiltrative; slow growing; some tumors are malignant (anaplastic) | Seizures; headaches; subtle onset of symptoms | RT with residual tumor; may withhold after gross total resection; RT with or without chemotherapy for anaplastic oligodendroglioma |
| **Mixed glioma—(oligoastrocytoma)** | May behave more or less aggressively, depending on features | Dependent on location and degree of malignancy | Variable outcome |
| **Ependymoma** | Pediatric and young adult patients; originates from lining of the ventricles; frequently in posterior fossa; usually benign | May present with hydrocephalus; symptoms related to location | RT for residual or recurrent disease; craniospinal RT for evidence of spinal disease only; good prognosis |
| *Embryonal (primitive neuroectodermal tumor) medulloblastoma, most common* | Primarily pediatric; malignant; occurs mainly in posterior fossa; CSF metastasis in 33% of patients | Symptoms by location; hydrocephalus common | Craniospinal RT; poor prognosis, particularly with CSF dissemination |
| **Peripheral Nerve Tumors** | | | |
| **Vestibular schwannoma (acoustic neuroma)** | Cerebellopontine angle; benign; encapsulated; seen in association with neurofibromatosis, type 2 | Decreased hearing; tinnitus; balance problems; may have other cranial nerve deficits | Curable with surgery; excellent prognosis; cranial nerve deficits may be permanent or temporary; affect quality of life |
| **Meningeal Tumors (approximately 27% of primary brain tumors)** | | | |
| **Meningioma** | Composed of arachnoid cells; attached to dura; usually benign; well circumscribed; may be vascular; common locations: falx convexity; olfactory groove; sphenoid ridge; parasellar region; optic nerve | Headaches may occur from dural stretching; seizures and focal neurologic signs | Degree of resection (and recurrence) associated with location; excellent prognosis with gross total resection; atypical and malignant—meningiomas have more aggressive features and less favorable outcomes |
| **Lymphomas and Hematopoietic Tumors** | | | |
| **Malignant CNS lymphoma** | Arise in CNS without systemic lymphoma; commonly suprasellar; diffuse brain infiltration; may be periventricular and may involve leptomeninges; solitary or multiple | Neurologic or neuropsychiatric symptoms | Diagnosis commonly via stereotactic biopsy or CSF cytology; steroids may decrease or temporarily obliterate lesion on CT or MRI; RT with or without chemotherapy; high-dose methotrexate used as single medication; some studies defer RT; increasing incidence in immunocompetent persons; decreasing in patients with AIDS |

**TABLE 35-1** Classification and Grading of Brain Tumors (Most Common Intracranial Tumors)* (*continued*)

| Classification/Grade | Description | Symptoms | Treatment/Prognosis |
|---|---|---|---|
| **Germ Cell Tumors** | | | |
| | Developmental tumors—from gonads and extragonadal sites; germinoma (solid, enhancing on MRI) and teratoma (cystic, with fat and calcification) most common | Symptoms are location dependent; germinomas are often suprasellar—diabetes insipidus | Treatment and prognosis dependent upon many factors including histology, location, and ability to resect |
| **Sellar Tumors** | | | |
| **Pituitary adenoma** | 6.3% of sellar tumors; benign; originate from adenohypophysis; classification by hormonal content; microadenoma 1 cm or less; macroadenoma 1 cm or more | Hypersecretion:<br>• *Prolactin*: amenorrhea, galactorrhea<br>• *Growth hormone*: acromegaly<br>• *Adrenocorticotropic hormone*: Cushing syndrome<br>• Thyroid-stimulating hormone: hyperthyroidism (rare)<br>Hyposecretion caused by compression of the pituitary gland<br>Visual field deficits (bitemporal hemianopia); headache; pituitary apoplexy: acute hemorrhage or infarct of gland—emergency treatment indicated | *Surgical*: transsphenoidal for approximately 95% of surgical cases *Medical*: appropriate in some cases of prolactin-secreting and growth hormone–secreting tumors; RT for recurrence or for hypersecretory tumors, when medical management has failed |
| **Craniopharyngioma** WHO grade I | Benign, calcified, cystic tumors | Endocrine abnormalities; visual impairment; cognitive and/or personality changes; may have increased ICP | Gross total resection affects prognosis; RT for residual tumor |
| **Metastatic Tumors (approximately 150,000 new cases yearly; occur in 20%–40% of cancer patients)** | | | |
| | Originate from primary systemic tumors; discrete, round, ring-enhancing; 50% are solitary; lung and breast are most common primary sites | Symptoms are location dependent | Prognosis dependent on number of tumors, tumor location, systemic disease, and patient age; improved prognosis with gross total resection and RT |

*For all tumors, biopsy or craniotomy for tumor removal is necessary to establish a definitive diagnosis.
Data From: U.S. Department of Health and Human Services, National Institutes of Health, National Cancer Institute: Adult brain central nervous system tumors treatment: Health professionals version. Updated January 15, 2016. Retrieved January 18, 2016, from http://www.cancer.gov/types/brain/hp/adult-brain-treatment-pdq; Goldblum JR, Folpe AL, Weiss SW: Enzinger & Weiss's Soft Tissue Tumors, 6th ed. Philadelphia, PA: Saunders, 2014; National Cancer Institute: Primary CNS Lymphoma Treatment—For Health Professionals (PDQ). Bethesda, MD: National Cancer Institute. Updated April 2, 2015. Retrieved December 12, 2015, from http://www.cancer.gov/types/lymphoma/hp/primary-cns-lymphoma-treatment-pdq; and National Cancer Institute: Pituitary Tumors Treatment—For Health Professionals (PDQ). Bethesda, MD: National Cancer Institute. Updated May 14, 2015. Retrieved December 21, 2015, from http://www.cancer.gov/types/pituitary/hp/pituitary-treatment-pdq.

meningiomas, and gliomas).[2,4] The same effect has not been shown definitively for low-dose radiation exposure, which is a topic of discussion and controversy.

## Epidemiology

There are approximately 238,000 newly diagnosed primary brain tumors worldwide each year.[5] There is a significantly higher incidence of metastatic brain tumors diagnosed in the United States each year.

Epidemiologic studies have confirmed certain patterns of brain tumor incidence. There has been a significant increase in the incidence of brain tumors in developed countries over the past several decades. Some of this increase can be attributed to improved diagnostic techniques, access to medical care, and an increasing elderly population. However, it is suspected that some of these increases are also attributable to environmental and lifestyle factors, as previously discussed.

Other patterns of incidence have been documented by age, ethnicity, and sex.[2,4] For example, the incidence of pilocytic astrocytoma and medulloblastoma decreases with age, while glioblastoma incidence increases with age.

Glioblastomas are diagnosed more often in the white population and in men. African Americans and women have higher rates of meningiomas.[2]

## Pathophysiology

The brain has its own distinct protective mechanism in the form of the blood–brain barrier. This highly selective barrier limits the transport of molecules, including drugs, into the cerebrum.[1] Tumors are able to disrupt this blood–brain barrier, as evidenced by computed tomography (CT) and magnetic resonance imaging (MRI) scans, which show contrast uptake at the site of many tumors.[1,3,4] Disruption of the blood–brain barrier may relate to increasing permeability of the tumor blood supply at the capillary level with higher levels of malignancy.

Vasogenic edema, caused by increased capillary permeability and commonly seen in association with brain tumors and other brain lesions, is the direct result of blood–brain barrier disruption.[1-3] As outlined in the Monro–Kellie doctrine, the contents of the cranial vault—brain, CSF, and blood—have a fixed volume. Any addition to this volume must be balanced by reduction in one of the other components. When this compensatory mechanism can no longer function, edema develops and ICP increases.[1] In Figure 35-1, an MRI scan shows brain edema and mass effect (shifting of brain structures) caused by a glioblastoma. Some slow-growing tumors (eg, meningiomas) can become quite large as a result of this compensatory mechanism and the brain's plasticity. This plasticity allows the brain to accommodate to slow tumor growth over a long period of time.

## Clinical Manifestations

The patient with a brain neoplasm may present with one or more signs of tumor growth. The signs may be general or focal. The most common general signs of brain tumors are headaches, seizures, or mental status changes. These are related to increasing ICP.[1-3]

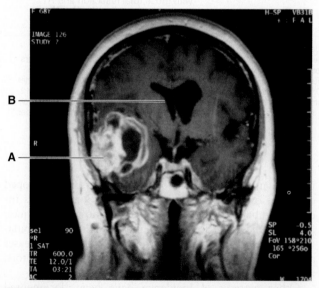

**FIGURE 35-1** Coronal MRI view of ring-enhancing glioblastoma **(A)** with evidence of mass effect **(B)**. (Courtesy of Henry Brem, MD, Johns Hopkins University, Baltimore, MD.)

The triad of symptoms associated with increased ICP includes headache, nausea with or without vomiting, and papilledema (swelling of the optic disks). Symptoms are typically treated with corticosteroids, which are discussed later in this chapter.[2-4] Clinical evidence of herniation (shifting of brain tissue by masses, increased ICP, or both) often requires critical care management using fluid restriction, hyperventilation, osmotic drugs, and diuretics. Some situations necessitate the use of CSF drainage through an intraventricular catheter (see Chapter 34).

The frequency of seizures depends on tumor location as well as tumor histology. Many patients experience seizures over the course of their disease.[1,2,4] Seizure activity is more common in patients with low-grade tumors. Tumors in the cerebral hemispheres are much more likely to cause seizure activity than posterior fossa tumors. Seizures may be focal or generalized, as discussed later in this chapter.

Mental status changes occur as the result of mass effect on the brain caused by increased ICP or hydrocephalus. Patients may become drowsy and mentally slower as ICP increases. Cognitive changes occur in the form of problems concentrating, memory difficulties, personality changes, confusion, or disorientation. Although mental status changes are associated with frontal lobe tumors, they are also the result of increased ICP.[1]

Focal neurologic deficits may be the temporary result of tumor compression, or may be permanent, as a result of tumor destruction. These deficits are directly related to tumor location. Figure 35-2 outlines site-specific signs and symptoms of brain tumors.

## Diagnosis

History taking is a key element in the process of diagnosing a brain neoplasm. The duration, frequency, and severity of symptoms are ascertained. It is important to assess whether there is a particular time of day or series of activities that initiate symptoms. Are symptoms intermittent or continuous? Do they resolve with pharmacologic management? The physical examination aids in further localizing the lesion. Patients may minimize or are often unaware of subtle neurologic deficits. Family involvement in this discussion is useful.

Imaging studies, such as CT scans and MRI, are typically ordered to localize the lesion and assess the amount of edema and mass effect on surrounding structures. CT scans are often performed to establish a differential diagnosis when a patient is seen in the emergency department.[1,2,5] Because MRI shows tumors in three dimensions (axial, coronal, and sagittal), it is the preferred diagnostic tool. An electroencephalogram (EEG) is used to confirm the presence of seizure discharges, which may be useful in determining whether anticonvulsants are needed. Magnetic resonance angiography (MRA) images the vascular anatomy and vessels that feed certain tumors. It can be a noninvasive alternative to the angiogram, which is an invasive study that may be needed to identify and perform embolization of feeding vessels to the tumor with the use of glue preparations. In some cases, angiography and embolization are performed within 24 to 48 hours of surgery for large tumors such as meningiomas.

Functional MRI (fMRI) is a type of imaging used for tumors in the dominant hemisphere or motor strip. It is believed

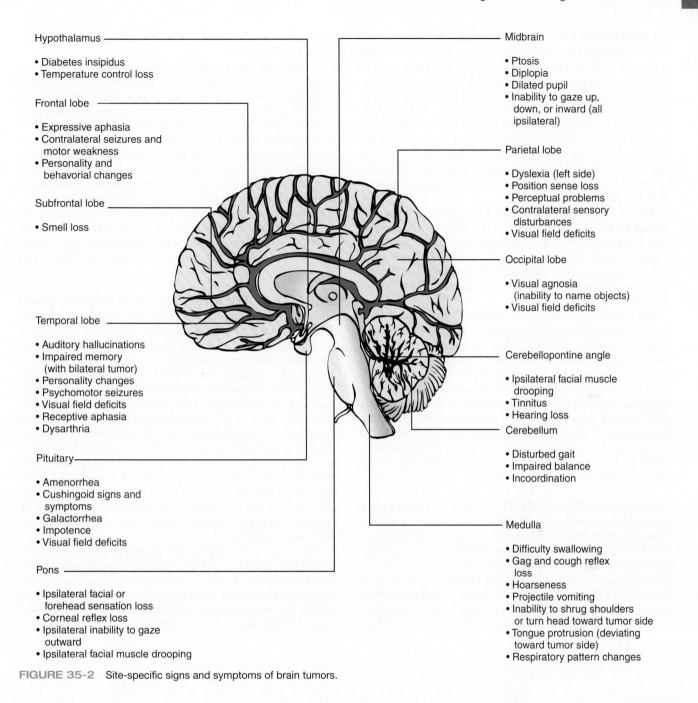

Hypothalamus

- Diabetes insipidus
- Temperature control loss

Frontal lobe

- Expressive aphasia
- Contralateral seizures and motor weakness
- Personality and behaviorial changes

Subfrontal lobe

- Smell loss

Temporal lobe

- Auditory hallucinations
- Impaired memory (with bilateral tumor)
- Personality changes
- Psychomotor seizures
- Visual field deficits
- Receptive aphasia
- Dysarthria

Pituitary

- Amenorrhea
- Cushingoid signs and symptoms
- Galactorrhea
- Impotence
- Visual field deficits

Pons

- Ipsilateral facial or forehead sensation loss
- Corneal reflex loss
- Ipsilateral inability to gaze outward
- Ipsilateral facial muscle drooping

Midbrain

- Ptosis
- Diplopia
- Dilated pupil
- Inability to gaze up, down, or inward (all ipsilateral)

Parietal lobe

- Dyslexia (left side)
- Position sense loss
- Perceptual problems
- Contralateral sensory disturbances
- Visual field deficits

Occipital lobe

- Visual agnosia (inability to name objects)
- Visual field deficits

Cerebellopontine angle

- Ipsilateral facial muscle drooping
- Tinnitus
- Hearing loss

Cerebellum

- Disturbed gait
- Impaired balance
- Incoordination

Medulla

- Difficulty swallowing
- Gag and cough reflex loss
- Hoarseness
- Projectile vomiting
- Inability to shrug shoulders or turn head toward tumor side
- Tongue protrusion (deviating toward tumor side)
- Respiratory pattern changes

**FIGURE 35-2**   Site-specific signs and symptoms of brain tumors.

that increased cerebral blood flow (CBF) is recognized as an increased signal on the fMRI. The patient performs a particular task, and the fMRI indicates which part of the brain is activated. This noninvasive procedure is currently used in some centers as part of the preoperative assessment of language, motor, and sensory function in relation to tumor location. Positron emission tomography (PET) uses radionuclides to measure CBF and brain metabolism. It is used to differentiate low-grade from high-grade (and more metabolically active) tumors. PET is also used to differentiate radiation necrosis from high-grade tumors in previously treated patients. Magnetic resonance spectroscopy (MRS) is a noninvasive radiographic technique that measures metabolite levels in brain tumors. Biologic compounds, such as choline, can be quantitated in brain tumors. Because MRS is obtained at the same time as MRI, the anatomic and metabolic characteristics of the tumor are obtained with little additional inconvenience to the patient.

## Clinical Management

Once the differential diagnosis of brain tumor is obtained through history, physical examination, and imaging studies, decisions are made regarding appropriate treatment modalities. A medical and surgical plan of care is developed with the patient and family members.

**PHARMACOLOGIC MANAGEMENT.** Tumors and tumor treatments are known to cause increased ICP, which is treated with corticosteroids.[2-4] Corticosteroids such as dexamethasone reduce brain edema by reducing the permeability of tumor capillaries and possibly by shifting some of the fluid into the ventricular system. A dose of 16 mg daily is standard in the perioperative period. It is usually given in two to four divided doses, spaced over the course of the day. Resolution of symptoms can be quite rapid. Steroids also increase the safety of the surgical procedure. They are, however, associated with significant side effects, as outlined in Table 35-2.[1,2]

Type 2 histamine receptor ($H_2$) blockers are often prescribed for the patient taking steroids. They are used to prevent gastrointestinal (GI) symptoms that can be associated with prolonged steroid use. Steroids used alone have a low risk for causing peptic ulcers and GI bleeding, but the risk increases in patients taking nonsteroidal anti-inflammatory drugs (NSAIDs).[1,2]

Anticonvulsant therapy is initiated when the patient presents with a seizure. Many surgeons also use prophylactic antiepileptic drugs (AEDs) during the perioperative period. Because studies have shown little difference in the occurrence of postoperative seizures in patients receiving AEDs compared with control groups without such drugs, some physicians are limiting the use of postoperative and prophylactic AED therapy. However, 70% of members of the American Association of Neurological Surgeons who responded to a survey stated that they continue to prescribe prophylactic AEDs for their patients with brain tumors. Seizures are extensively discussed later in this chapter.

**SURGICAL MANAGEMENT.** Clinical and radiographic evaluations are useful in obtaining a differential diagnosis. However, pathologic examination of tumor tissue produces the definitive diagnosis. There are two distinct surgical approaches to diagnosing and treating brain tumors. Stereotactic biopsy is used to obtain small samples of tumor tissue under CT or MRI guidance. Craniotomy is performed when tumor removal is feasible and provides both a pathologic diagnosis and surgical resection of the lesion.[1,2,5] These approaches are discussed in the "Surgical Approaches" section of this chapter.

During the past several decades, improvements in anesthesia, microsurgical equipment, intraoperative monitoring techniques, and pharmacologic management have significantly improved intraoperative mortality rates. Postoperative morbidity has also significantly decreased. The perioperative management of the patient with a brain tumor involves a multidisciplinary team approach, as outlined in Table 35-3.

Despite substantial improvements in the management of the patient with a brain tumor, surgical complications may be severe and require critical care monitoring and management. The most common complications include brain edema, infection, hyponatremia or other electrolyte imbalances, hemorrhage, venous thromboembolism (including deep venous thrombosis [DVT] and pulmonary embolism [PE]), and seizures (Box 35-1).[2,3]

**RADIATION THERAPY.** Many brain tumors are treated with adjuvant therapies, either because they cannot be surgically resected or because of their aggressive nature. For most brain tumors, radiation therapy (RT) is the first-line treatment after biopsy or craniotomy. The energy produced by radiation damages tumor DNA at the time of cell division.[2,5] Three-dimensional conformal radiation is generally used to treat those tumor cells that are not surgically resectable. This form of RT treats the shape and the volume of tumor while normal brain tissue is protected. A standard dose of up to 6,000 centigray (cGy; also referred to as radiation absorbed dose, or rad) is administered to primary brain tumors 5 days a week over a period of 6 weeks. Multiple metastatic tumors receive a dose of approximately 3,000 cGy divided over 10 treatments. Some metastases may be treated with higher radiation doses with or without a boost of focused radiation.[2-4]

There are other approaches to applying RT. Intensity-modulated radiation therapy (IMRT) modifies the radiation beam so that a more focused dose can be given, without exposing surrounding brain tissue. Stereotactic radiosurgery (SRS) (eg, gamma knife and linear accelerator) is applied under MRI guidance. A three-dimensional image is obtained,

| TABLE 35-2 | Complications of Corticosteroid Therapy |
|---|---|
| **System** | **Complications** |
| Neurologic | *Common:* Behavior changes, insomnia, myopathy, hallucinations, hiccups, tremor, cerebral atrophy |
| | *Uncommon:* Psychosis, dementia, seizures, dependence, paraparesis (epidural lipomatosis) |
| General | Weight gain, cushingoid features (moon facies, buffalo hump, centripetal obesity), opportunistic infections (eg, candidiasis, Pneumocystis carinii pneumonitis), night sweats, hypersensitivity reactions, peripheral edema |
| | *Note:* Steroid taper may cause recurrence of preexisting conditions (eg, arthritis, allergic reaction) |
| Cardiovascular | Hypertension, atherosclerosis, increased cardiovascular and cerebrovascular disease |
| Dermatologic | Thin skin, ecchymoses, purpura, acne, striae, inhibited wound healing, hirsutism |
| Endocrinologic | Hyperglycemia, hypokalemia, hyperlipidemia, fluid retention |
| Gastrointestinal | Increased appetite, abdominal bloating, GI bleeding, peptic ulcers, pancreatitis, liver hypertrophy |
| Genitourinary | Polyuria, menstrual irregularities, infertility |
| Hematologic | Neutrophilia, lymphopenia |
| Ophthalmologic | Visual blurring, cataracts, glaucoma, uveitis |
| Rheumatologic | Osteoporosis, avascular necrosis |

Data from Hickey JV: The Clinical Practice of Neurological and Neurosurgical Nursing. Philadelphia, PA: Wolters Kluwer/Lippincott Williams & Wilkins, 2014; and Stummer W: Mechanisms of tumor-related brain edema. Neurosurg Focus, 2007. Retrieved August 7, 2015, from http://www.medscape.com/viewarticle/559000_6.

**TABLE 35-3**  Multidisciplinary Management Guide for the Patient With a Brain Tumor

| Stage | Management Team | Interventions | Nursing Considerations |
|---|---|---|---|
| **Preoperative** | | | |
| **History and physical** | Neurosurgeon, nurse practitioner, RN | • Baseline history and physical examination<br>• Neurologic evaluation: mental status, cranial nerves, motor and sensory function, coordination, reflexes | • Preoperative teaching to begin<br>• Involve family as much as possible |
| **Medications** | Physician, pharmacist, nurse practitioner, RN | • Steroids; histamine type 2 receptor (H2) blockers, as needed; anticonvulsants for supratentorial lesions<br>• Prescribe new medications; medication review; discuss interactions or contraindications | • Anticoagulants, NSAIDs to be discontinued (with consent of prescribing physician) |
| **Diagnostic testing** | Neuroradiologist | • Baseline MRI or CT scan<br>• ECG, chest x-ray<br>• Other diagnostic studies as indicated | • Most preoperative testing performed within 1 wk of surgery |
| **Preoperative teaching** | By specialty: RN, neurosurgeon, neuroanesthesiologist | • Informed consent<br>• Obtain all test results before admission day | • A written teaching pamphlet is recommended for patient and family use |
| **Hospital admission** | Admitting office, OR staff | • Obtain/confirm demographics | • Most patients are admitted on the day of surgery |
| **Intraoperative** | | | |
| **Stereotactic biopsy** | OR team, surgeon, anesthesiologist, radiologist, pathologist | • Stereotactic frame placed; samples taken through catheter inserted under MRI/CT guidance<br>• Histologic evaluation | • May be performed in radiology suite or<br>• Teaching regarding stereotactic frame<br>• May also be done as a frameless procedure |
| **Craniotomy** | OR team, surgeon, anesthesiologist, pathologist | • Tumor tissue obtained for biopsy; tumor resected<br>• Histologic evaluation | • Teaching regarding general anesthesia |
| **Postoperative** | | | |
| **Critical care unit** | Critical care staff, neurosurgeon | • Hemodynamic monitoring; frequent neurologic evaluations | • If possible, it is useful for patient and family to see the unit before surgery |
| **Nursing unit** | Floor nurses, surgeon, consulting physicians, rehabilitation medicine, pharmacist, clergy, nutritionist | • Postoperative care to include vital signs, neurologic exam, wound care, cough, and deep breathing; increase activity as tolerated; advance diet as tolerated<br>• Rehabilitation medicine consult<br>• Evaluate for deficits and complications and provide consultations, as indicated | • More family participation in care when possible<br>• Patients are usually out of bed within 24 h of surgery<br>• Recently, short hospital stays cause increased family involvement and responsibility; begin teaching while patient is on the nursing unit |
| **Discharge planning** | Social worker, nursing staff, consulting physicians, radiation oncologist, medical oncologist (when indicated) | • Inpatient/outpatient rehabilitation as needed (occupational therapy, physical therapy, speech, cognitive)<br>• Outpatient therapies as needed (eg, radiation, chemotherapy)<br>• Hospice care (inpatient or home hospice) may be indicated, particularly in cases of recurrent malignant gliomas, refractory to conventional treatments | • Ideally, planning begins as soon as the patient arrives on the nursing unit<br>• Family takes on greater role because patient is often discharged from the hospital 2–3 d postoperatively, particularly in cases of highly malignant tumors where home hospice is indicated |

Adapted from Bohan E, Macenka DG: Surgical management of patient with brain tumors. Semin Oncol Nurs 20(4):240–252, 2004.

and radiation is given in one large dose to residual tumor, sparing normal brain tissue.[6,7] Brachytherapy uses radioactive isotopes in seeds or liquid-filled balloons inserted into residual tumor.[5] Radiosensitizers are agents given in addition to RT. It is postulated that some substances increase oxygen delivery to hypoxic tumors. The oxygen enhances the effects of radiation. Hyperthermia is also being applied with the

same goal of increasing oxygen to tumors to maximize the effects of radiation.[5]

**CHEMOTHERAPY.** Malignant brain tumors require multiple treatment modalities. Chemotherapy is given in conjunction with radiation or at the time of tumor recurrence. Drugs may be administered orally or intravenously but can

| BOX 35-1 | Critical Care Management of the Patient With Brain Tumor Complications |

**Increased ICP**
- Corticosteroids and antacids or histamine type 2 receptor ($H_2$) blockers
- IV fluids: Avoid hypotonic solutions
- Elevate head of bed and maintain adequate body alignment
- Avoid hypotension and control hypertension; arterial line useful; if ICP monitor is available, titrate fluid therapy and vasoactive/inotropic drugs as ordered and clinically appropriate to maintain MAP between 70 and 80 mm Hg to maintain CPP. Elevated ICP may require higher MAP to maintain CPP 60 to 70 mm Hg.
- Keep well oxygenated; may need to intubate
- Judicious use of osmotic therapy: mannitol to expand plasma volume and draw fluid out of the brain
- Sedation to reduce activity and decrease hypertension
- Intraventricular catheter may be necessary to monitor ICP and drain CSF
- Cautious use of hyperventilation for short periods only to reduce arterial carbon dioxide pressure ($PCO_2$) (6 to 24 hours)
- May require surgical intervention for hematoma

**Wound Infection, Intracranial Abscess, or Bone Flap Infection**
- Blood work, including complete blood count and blood cultures
- CT scan, MRI, and in some cases MRS to identify abscess
- Surgical removal of abscess or bone flap, when feasible
- Appropriate wound cultures, when possible
- Antibiotic therapy
- Infectious disease consultation for appropriate drug, dose, and duration

**Hyponatremia or Hypernatremia**
- Possible diabetes insipidus, salt-wasting syndrome, or syndrome of inappropriate antidiuretic hormone secretion
- For hyponatremia: fluid restriction, hypertonic saline
- For hypernatremia: fluids, free water

**Intracranial Hemorrhage**
- Immediate CT scan to evaluate for early signs of a bleed
- Monitor BP
- Check laboratory values: prothrombin time, partial thromboplastin time, platelets, INR
- Management of increased ICP, as described above
- May need to intubate and ventilate
- Surgery may be necessary to remove blood clot

**Thromboembolism: DVT and Pulmonary Embolus (PE)**
- Diagnosed through TCD study or ventilation-perfusion scan
- Heparinization *only after* CT scan has ruled out intracranial blood
- Alternatively, vena cava filter (IVC) may be used
- Large PEs require ICU care for further medical treatment

**Seizures**
- Potential for status epilepticus
- Protect patient from injury
- Titrate antiepileptics to therapeutic levels

cause systemic toxicities and have difficulty crossing the blood–brain barrier in sufficient amounts to provide benefit. An approach using RT in conjunction with temozolomide chemotherapy has shown survival benefit in the most malignant primary brain tumor, glioblastoma.[2–5]

Chemotherapy can also be placed in the tumor resection cavity at the time of craniotomy. A biodegradable polymer wafer that delivers a continuous infusion of carmustine (BCNU) chemotherapy over a period of 2 to 3 weeks is being used for primary malignant and metastatic brain tumors. The wafer is surgically implanted at the time of initial diagnosis or when the tumor recurs.[3,5]

### Nursing Management

**ASSESSMENT.** Some tumors are cured with surgery, whereas others have a protracted course involving adjuvant therapies and treatment for recurrent disease. As part of the multidisciplinary team, the nurse plays a central role in patient care and family support throughout the course of the patient's illness. The nurse participates in the diagnosis, treatment, and follow-up care of the patient with a brain tumor.[1,2,5] Ongoing assessment of medical decision-making capacity is an essential part of care because of the potential for mental status changes in the patient with a brain tumor; such changes, however subtle, may compromise decision-making capacity.[5]

**PLAN.** Careful history taking and symptom evaluation contribute to the accurate diagnosis of a brain tumor. Once medications are prescribed, patient education includes discussion of dose, side effects, and contraindications. The results of tests leading to a differential diagnosis are reviewed with the patient and family. When a decision has been made to proceed with surgery, extensive teaching is required in the perioperative period. Table 35-3 outlines the nurse's role in the plan of care for this patient population. Box 35-1 provides information about the management of the patient with brain tumor complications.

Surgery and follow-up therapies are disruptive to patient and family activities. It is important to encourage a return to normalcy as soon as possible. Continuing with activities of daily living that encourage a positive and motivated attitude contributes to recovery.

**HOSPICE.** Multiple surgical procedures and adjuvant therapies are often successful in containing malignant brain tumors for a period of time. Inevitably, these tumors recur and become resistant to all treatment modalities. In addition, patient quality of life may be so compromised that further therapy is not feasible. Palliative care services are now available in many hospitals. Home and inpatient hospice are available in most communities and provide dedicated and supportive end-of-life care.

## Aneurysms

An aneurysm is a weakening in the arterial wall that causes either a ballooning effect or overall distention of the affected vessel. Aneurysms may be congenital or degenerative arterial lesions. Concern arises if the outpouching of the vessel wall ruptures or becomes large enough to exert pressure on surrounding brain structures.[6–8] Approximately 10% to 15% (and in some references up to 30%) of patients die from the initial bleeding of the aneurysm before reaching medical care.[8] An additional 50% die within 1 month from the initial hemorrhage.[6,8] Rebleeding is the leading cause of death in patients with a history of ruptured aneurysm. Of those who survive the initial bleeding, 25% die within 24 hours, and 40% to 49% die within 3 months.[7] Rebleeding most often occurs around the seventh day after the original bleed. Some recent data suggest that the overall mortality rate from aneurysmal subarachnoid hemorrhage (SAH) is as high as 65%.[7] Predictors of good recovery by 1 month after the bleed include a high score on the admission Glasgow Coma Scale (GCS) and an absence of blood on the first CT scan.[6–8]

### Etiology

The etiology of aneurysms is unclear but is probably a combination of congenital and degenerative factors. Carmichael described the combination hypothesis of aneurysm formation. Of the three layers of an artery—tunica intima (innermost), tunica media (middle), and tunica adventitia (outer layer)—he found that congenital focal defects of the tunica media are common. However, degenerative changes are also necessary for the formation of aneurysms. Histologic investigation of the normal vessel wall into the aneurysmal sac shows that the tunica media usually ends at the neck of the aneurysm and the internal elastic lamina becomes fragmented as it enters the sac. Consistent with this hypothesis, aneurysms are rare in childhood but are common into late adulthood.[6–8]

Although the exact cause of intracranial aneurysms is not understood, there is evidence to support that acquired and genetic factors contribute to their development. Genetic factors include heredity and genetically transmitted diseases. Acquired factors include traumatic brain injury, sepsis, cigarette smoking, and hypertension.[6–8] Multiple concurrent clinical conditions, including Marfan syndrome, coarctation of the aorta, polycystic kidney disease, and systemic lupus erythematosus, are associated with cerebral aneurysms, supporting a genetic component to aneurysm development.[6–8]

### Epidemiology

Intracranial aneurysms are common lesions, with autopsy reports indicating a prevalence of 1% to 6% in the adult population.[6] In the United States, approximately 30,000 new cases of SAH each year are attributed to aneurysmal rupture.[7]

Aneurysm may also be associated with other pathologic processes, such as polycystic kidney disease.[6–8] Screening with MRI is warranted for patients who have two immediate relatives with a history of intracranial aneurysm, and for all patients with autosomal dominant polycystic kidney disease. The incidence of aneurysms increases with age, with peak incidence occurring between 55 and 60 years.[6–8] Aneurysms occur more often in women than in men. as noted earlier, they can be linked to cigarette smoking. Clinicians observed that there may be a seasonal variability, with increases occurring in spring and fall.

The Cooperative Study of Intracranial Aneurysms and Subarachnoid Hemorrhage reported that in 32% of cases, the hemorrhage occurred during physical activity. The study also reported that a similar proportion occurred during sleep. In summary, the incidence of SAH in relation to activity can be roughly divided into thirds: sleeping, active, and at rest.

### Pathophysiology

Arterial vessels are composed of three layers: endothelial lining, smooth muscle, and connective tissue. A defect in the smooth muscle layer, or tunica media, allows the endothelial lining to bulge through, creating an aneurysm. Most aneurysms arise from larger arteries around the anterior section of the circle of Willis (Fig. 35-3). The most common sites of occurrence in the anterior circulation are the anterior communicating artery, the posterior communicating artery (PCA), the middle cerebral artery (MCA) bifurcation, and the internal carotid artery bifurcation.[6–8] In the posterior circulation, the most common locations are the basilar artery apex and the posterior inferior cerebellar artery.[6–8]

As the intimal layers of the vessel weaken, high-velocity blood begins to flow, creating a whirlpool effect that stretches the wall of the vessel; this creates an abnormal pocket or sac of blood. As the wall of the vessel expands, it begins to weaken and may eventually rupture. Compression by the sac on surrounding brain structures may result in focal neurologic deficits. Rupture of the aneurysm may result in subarachnoid, intracerebral, or intraventricular hemorrhage.[6–8]

Aneurysms may be classified according to shape. *Saccular aneurysms* are also known as "berry" aneurysms because of their well-defined stem and the berry-like outpouching of the medial layer of the arterial wall. Berry aneurysms are usually located on major cerebral arteries at the apex of branch points, which is where maximal hemodynamic stress occurs in the vessel (see Fig. 35-3). *Fusiform aneurysms* occur more commonly in the vertebrobasilar system. Fusiform aneurysms are dilated circumferentially and usually occur secondary to atherosclerosis. A third type of aneurysm, known as a *mycotic aneurysm*, is due to infection.[6–8]

Aneurysms may also be categorized according to size. A small aneurysm is smaller than 10 mm, a large aneurysm is 10 to 20 mm, and a giant aneurysm is larger than 25 mm. Giant aneurysms are a cause for great concern because they may compress surrounding brain tissue or compromise the existing circulation to the area. Controversy exists about size and relationship to rupture. The average size of a ruptured

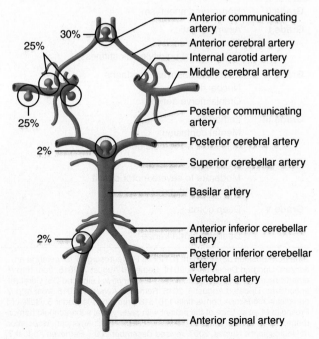

**FIGURE 35-3** Circle of Willis with common aneurysm sites.

aneurysm is 7 mm, but smaller lesions routinely hemorrhage.[6–8] Hemorrhage from an aneurysm usually occurs in the subarachnoid space, because aneurysm-forming vessels usually lie in the space between the arachnoid layer of the meninges and the brain. The force of the rupturing vessel can be so great that it can push blood through the pia mater and into the brain substance, causing an intracerebral hemorrhage. It can also push through the arachnoid into the subdural space, causing a subdural hemorrhage.[6,7]

### Clinical Manifestations

Many aneurysms are silent and never cause a problem but may be discovered on postmortem examination. An aneurysm that does cause problems typically does so in patients between ages 35 and 60 years.

Use of a grading scale can enhance the ability to determine clinical outcome. Aneurysmal SAHs are graded according to their severity on the Hunt and Hess scale. In this grading system, grade 0 is the unruptured aneurysm, and grade V is a hemorrhage with severe neurologic sequelae (Table 35-4). The World Federation of Neurological Surgeons grading scale is also used for SAHs. The Fisher scale is another grading scale that is used to estimate the density of subarachnoid blood on CT scan at the time of a patient's admission to the hospital (Table 35-5).[6–8] A score of 3 or 4 on the Fisher scale has been found to increase the likelihood of poor clinical outcomes. A score of 1 to 2 has not been shown to increase mortality rates.

Approximately half of patients have some warning signs before an aneurysm ruptures. These signs may include headache, lethargy, neck pain, a "noise in the head," and optic, oculomotor, or trigeminal cranial nerve dysfunction.[6–8]

After an aneurysm has bled or ruptured, the patient usually complains of a horrific headache. The classic description

**TABLE 35-4** Hunt and Hess Grading Scale for Aneurysms

| Grade 0 | Unruptured aneurysm |
|---|---|
| Grade I | Asymptomatic<br>Minimal headache<br>Slight nuchal rigidity (neck stiffness) |
| Grade II | Moderate to severe headache<br>Nuchal rigidity<br>Cranial nerve deficits |
| Grade III | Lethargy<br>Mental confusion<br>Mild focal neurologic deficit |
| Grade IV | Stupor<br>Moderate to severe motor deficit<br>Possible posturing |
| Grade V | Deep coma<br>Posturing<br>Declining appearance |

Data from Brisman JL, Abraham K, Norvin P: Neurosurgery for cerebral aneurysm. Updated December 4, 2014. Retrieved August 7, 2015, from http://emedicine.medscape.com/article/252142-overview; Leibskind DS: Cerebral aneurysms. Updated August 6, 2015. Retrieved August 7, 2015, from http://emedicine.medscape.com/article/1161518-print; and Alexander S, Gallek M, Prescuitti M, et al: Care of the patient with aneurysmal subarachnoid hemorrhage. AANN Clinical Practice Guideline. Glenview, IL: American Association of Neuroscience Nurses, 2007, revised December 2009. Retrieved August 7, 2015, from http://www.aann.org/pdf/cpg/aannaneurysmalsah.pdf.

**TABLE 35-5** Fisher Grading Scale

| Fisher Group | Blood on CT |
|---|---|
| 1 | No blood detected |
| 2 | Diffuse thin layer of subarachnoid blood |
| 3 | Localized thrombus or thick layer of subarachnoid blood |
| 4 | Intracerebral or intraventricular hemorrhage with diffuse or no SAH |

Data from Brisman JL, Abraham K, Norvin P: Neurosurgery for cerebral aneurysm. Updated December 4, 2014. Retrieved August 7, 2015, from http://emedicine.medscape.com/article/252142-overview; Leibskind DS: Cerebral aneurysms. Updated August 6, 2015. Retrieved August 7, 2015, from http://emedicine.medscape.com/article/1161518-print; and Alexander S, Gallek M, Prescuitti M, et al: Care of the patient with aneurysmal subarachnoid hemorrhage. AANN Clinical Practice Guideline. Glenview, IL: American Association of Neuroscience Nurses, 2007. Revised December 2009. Retrieved August 7, 2015, from http://www.aann.org/pdf/cpg/aannaneurysmalsah.pdf

is "the worst headache of my life," often abbreviated as WHOL in the medical record. Other symptoms that may accompany SAH or aneurysms that present with mass effect are nausea, vomiting, focal neurologic deficits, and coma. Aneurysms presenting with mass effect typically show symptoms associated with increased ICP. With an SAH, there are also signs of meningeal irritation, such as a stiff and painful neck, photophobia, blurred vision, irritability, fever, positive Kernig sign, and positive Brudzinski sign. Exactly which deficits are present depends on the location of the aneurysm, the subsequent hemorrhage, and the severity of the bleeding.[6–8]

Bleeding stops because ICP in the subarachnoid space reaches mean arterial pressure (MAP) quickly, resulting in a tamponade effect that stops the bleeding long enough for the rupture to seal. If this does not occur, the patient dies.[6–8]

When there is blood in the subarachnoid space, it irritates the brainstem, causing abnormal activity in the autonomic nervous system, often with cardiac dysrhythmias and hypertension. Hypertension can also result from elevated ICP. Another complication of blood in the subarachnoid space is hydrocephalus. Blood in the subarachnoid space impedes reabsorption of CSF by the arachnoid villi. Hydrocephalus results in enlargement of the lateral and third ventricles.[6–8]

### Diagnosis

The diagnosis of a cerebral aneurysm usually is made on the basis of history, physical examination, CT scan, lumbar puncture, and cerebral angiogram. When the nurse takes the patient's history, he or she identifies risk factors such as genetic predisposition, hypertension, and cigarette smoking. Patients with an SAH may present with a headache, neck discomfort, or both without any neurologic signs. The headache may range in severity from mild to severe. A CT scan reveals hemorrhage in most cases when it is obtained within 24 hours of the hemorrhage; it has the most sensitivity when obtained within 24 hours of onset.[6–8] There is a steady decline over ensuing days, with approximately 50% of CTs being positive 5 days after an SAH occurs.

If the results of a CT scan are negative and there are signs and symptoms indicating that a patient has experienced an SAH, a lumbar puncture is typically performed to confirm the diagnosis. After positive lumbar puncture results, a cerebral angiogram is obtained to determine the source of the SAH. Different types of angiography may be used for this purpose, including CT angiography, MRA, or digital subtraction angiography (DSA). Although all of these studies can determine vascular anatomy, DSA is the gold standard if surgery is planned. Transcranial Doppler (TCD) ultrasonography can also be used to diagnose and treat vasospasm, a common complication of an SAH.[6–8]

### Clinical Management

Before repair, the management of a patient with a ruptured or leaking aneurysm focuses on minimal stimulation of the patient. Some institutions initiate "aneurysm precautions" as precautionary measures to prevent rebleeding. These measures include providing a quiet environment, establishing a bowel regimen to prevent straining (Valsalva maneuver), and limiting visitors.[8]

**PHARMACOLOGIC MANAGEMENT.** Antihypertensive medications may be used to manage blood pressure (BP) before procedures or surgery. Plasma volume should not be allowed to fall. Patients frequently have abnormalities of electrolytes—notably hyponatremia, which is usually associated with cerebral salt wasting rather than syndrome of inappropriate antidiuretic hormone; it is managed with sodium replacement and euvolemia.[6–9]

Stool softeners are used in managing patients with an aneurysm to prevent straining. Mild analgesics can be used to relieve headaches. An antipyretic, usually acetaminophen, and hypothermia blankets can be used to manage fever typically caused by blood in the subarachnoid space. Acetaminophen can be used without masking neurologic signs.

## SURGICAL MANAGEMENT

**Clipping.** Surgical clipping may be considered if the aneurysm is in an accessible area. The goal of surgery is complete obliteration of the aneurysm. Aneurysms of the vertebrobasilar system often present the problem of surgical inaccessibility. The accepted surgical treatment is the placement of a clip across the neck of the aneurysm (Fig. 35-4). These clips, which are made of titanium, come in a variety of shapes and sizes. For larger or wider aneurysms, more than one clip can be used to ensure complete occlusion of the neck of the aneurysm. Once clipped, the aneurysm may be punctured to allow it to collapse and relieve mass effect if present.[6–8]

Some aneurysms may be wrapped in a gauze-like material or coated with an acrylic substance that gives the aneurysm support. Although wrapping or coating should not be the goal of surgery, there may be conditions, as with a fusiform aneurysm, in which there is no other option.

Controversy continues about when surgical intervention should occur. The current thinking is that surgery should occur sooner rather than later. Thus, surgery may generally be performed 24 to 48 hours after the rupture and initial bleed occur.[6–9]

After aneurysm clipping, the patient is managed in a critical care environment. Maintenance of an adequate airway is vital. If the patient is intubated and suctioning is needed, it is important that the suction catheter be passed and removed quickly; this is necessary in order to prevent oxygen desaturation as well as surges in ICP that may occur as a result of stimulation of the cough reflex, which increases intrathoracic pressure.

Signs of vasospasm, such as hemiparesis, visual disturbance, seizures, or a decreasing level of consciousness (LOC),

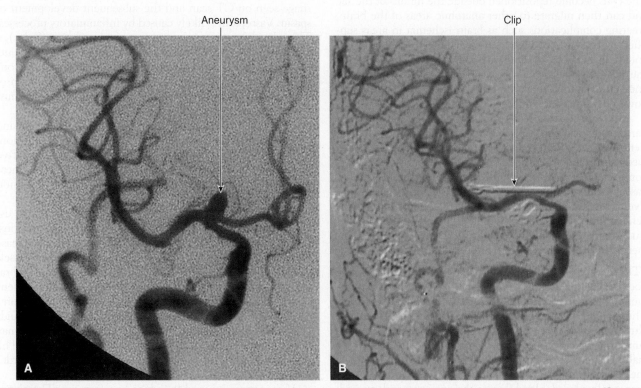

**FIGURE 35-4** Preoperative (**A**) and postoperative (**B**) angiography: clipping of right internal carotid artery termination aneurysm. (Courtesy of Rafael Tamargo, MD, and Richard Clatterbuck, MD, Johns Hopkins University, Baltimore, MD.)

should be noted and reported so that medical interventions can be rapidly implemented. Control of ICP is a collaborative effort. Nurses should keep the head of the patient's bed elevated and ensure that there is no neck flexion or severe rotation. Nursing care activities should be spaced to avoid causing a sharp rise in ICP.[6-8]

**Coiling.** One of the most valuable recent developments in aneurysm management has been the technique of endovascular thrombosis of aneurysms with Guglielmi detachable coils (GDCs). These thrombogenic platinum alloy microcoils are soft, allowing the coil to conform to the shape of the aneurysm. Coils are available in various shapes, dimensions, lengths, and diameters to provide maximal occlusion.[6,7,9]

The procedure used to introduce the coil into the aneurysm is similar to that for a cerebral angiogram, using the femoral artery and fluoroscopic equipment. In this procedure, a microcatheter is passed through the aorta, around the aortic arch, and then into the vessel specific to the aneurysm. Once the catheter is in position, the coil system is advanced through the catheter into the aneurysm sac. The coil is then in position, and if placement is satisfactory, a low-voltage current is applied. The current causes the coil to detach. If the coil is successfully placed, it occludes the aneurysm and separates it from the cerebral circulation. The number of coils placed is individualized to the patient. Through this coiling procedure, the risk for hemorrhage or re-hemorrhage is reduced.[6,7,9]

Complications of this treatment are embolic stroke, coil migration, failure to obliterate the aneurysm, and aneurysm rupture. Stroke may occur because the parent artery feeding the aneurysm becomes occluded or because of the introduction of air or particles into the catheter system. Coil migration occurs because of reintroduction of blood into the sac. The coils become repositioned outside the fundus of the sac and can then migrate to other anatomic areas of the brain, creating complications such as brain ischemia in areas supplied by the affected blood vessel. Failure to obliterate the aneurysm is also a possibility. If the coils fail to obliterate the aneurysm, the sac may grow larger, cause more symptoms, and may even rupture. Further intervention with another endovascular procedure or surgery is then warranted.[6,7]

Although clipping is the preferred treatment or gold standard for most aneurysms, GDC coiling is an option for patients who are considered to be surgically high-risk because of medical instability, or those who would otherwise be treated conservatively. With the rapidly evolving technology, endovascular embolization of cerebral aneurysms is a safe alternative to surgical clipping in treating ruptured and unruptured cerebral aneurysms.[6,7,9] Long-term outcomes require further study. Some experts consider coiling to be the preferred treatment, although this is still a matter of controversy.

**"The Pipeline": A New Treatment Option.** In 2014, the Food and Drug Administration (FDA) approved a new treatment option for aneurysms, referred to as the "pipeline." The pipeline is a tube made of platinum and nickel–cobalt chromium alloy that is used to stop blood flow to larger aneurysms located in the internal carotid artery (ICA). A specially trained surgeon places the pipeline into the ICA via the femoral artery under fluoroscopy. Once the pipeline is successfully placed, blood flow to the aneurysm is decreased; this allows a clot to form and reduces the chances of the aneurysm rupturing or enlarging. In the study conducted as part of the approval process, 70% of patients with large or giant aneurysms showed complete blockage without stenosis at 1 year postprocedure.[10]

**MEDICAL MANAGEMENT OF COMPLICATIONS.** As previously noted, vasospasm can occur after, as well as before, surgery in the patient with an aneurysm. Angiographic vasospasm is seen early. Vasospasm may be recognized clinically through frequent neurologic assessment. The patient's signs and symptoms can fluctuate but may include changes in LOC, headache, language impairment, hemiparesis, and seizures.[6-9]

Vasospasm usually occurs 3 to 12 days after an SAH; the peak incidence is between postbleed days 7 and 10. Although the aneurysm may have been clipped successfully, vasospasm can cause the development of a large area of ischemia or infarcted brain, with severe deficits. Vasospasm is of clinical significance because it decreases CBF, depriving brain tissue of oxygen and promoting accumulation of metabolic waste products, such as lactic acid. The reduced size of the vessel lumen restricts blood flow to the brain tissue, causing brain ischemia and possible permanent neurologic consequences.[6-9]

TCD imaging is a valuable noninvasive technique used to diagnose vasospasm. This technique, which can be performed at the bedside, measures the velocity of blood flow through segments of the arterial vessels. Monitoring trends in flow velocity allows prompt identification of early indications of vasospasm and patients at risk for developing vasospasm. The results of the neurologic examination can be correlated with TCD findings for prompt diagnosis and treatment of vasospasm.

The exact etiology of vasospasm is not clear. Apparently, there is a positive correlation between the size of the hemorrhage seen on CT scan and the subsequent development of spasm. Vasospasm is likely caused by inflammatory processes. There has been some success in using nimodipine (Sular), a calcium antagonist, after an SAH to improve patient outcomes. It is recommended that nimodipine be used from onset through day 21. Nimodipine reduces the contraction of smooth and cardiac muscles without affecting skeletal muscles. The dose is 60 mg every 4 hours.

"Triple H" therapy is the standard for preventing and treating vasospasm. It consists of hypervolemic expansion, hemodilution, and induced hypertension in postoperative patients. Nimodipine is used with this therapy. These measures reduce smooth muscle spasm and maximize perfusion when spasm does occur.[6-9]

Hypervolemia is accomplished by volume expansion, using both intravenous (IV) colloid and crystalloid solutions. They are given to increase intravascular volume and decrease blood viscosity. Through hypervolemia, the cerebral vessels dilate and the MAP increases, thereby improving cerebral perfusion pressure (CPP). During this therapy, the patient should be monitored for pulmonary edema and heart failure.

Hemodilution through the administration of IV fluids decreases blood viscosity, increases regional CBF, and may decrease infarction size and increase oxygen transport. The goal of hemodilution is to decrease blood viscosity in order to improve cerebral blood flow.[9]

Vasopressors are used to induce hypertension. The objective is to maintain systolic BP at greater than 20 mm Hg over normal. Vasopressors raise the patient's BP and brain perfusion to the point where neurologic deficit improves.[6-9]

When conventional medical therapy is not effective, acute arterial vasospasm secondary to an SAH can be managed by balloon angioplasty in centers where this technology is available. Recent advances in microballoon technology now allow access to the cerebral vasculature with soft, flexible angioplasty balloons, which mechanically dilate and improve CBF through the major arterial segments affected by vasospasm. Balloon angioplasty allows direct widening of the stenotic segment.[6,7,9] Intra-arterial administration of verapamil or nicardipine to selectively treat cerebral vasospasm is an additional technique that can be used. Increasing vasopressor dosing may be required to maintain systemic arterial pressure but has been noted to be well-tolerated.[9]

Another complication after aneurysmal rupture is hydrocephalus. Hydrocephalus indicates an imbalance between the production and absorption of CSF; it may occur in patients who have experienced an SAH. When there is blood in the subarachnoid space, the red blood cell clots and possible brain edema can occlude the very small channels leading from one ventricle to another. If this occurs, an obstructive hydrocephalus develops and obstructs the normal flow of CSF, often between the third and fourth ventricles, or at the exits from the fourth ventricle. There is also the potential for a reabsorption problem, whereby red blood cells and their breakdown products occlude the arachnoid villi, impeding reabsorption and resulting in a communicating hydrocephalus. The patient may require a shunt. With a ventriculoperitoneal shunt, the proximal tip of the catheter is placed in a lateral ventricle, and the distal tip is placed in the peritoneum. The shunt drains CSF into the peritoneal cavity to treat the hydrocephalus and prevent dangerous ICP elevations.[6-8]

Seizures may occur from blood in the subarachnoid space acting as an irritant to neurons. Typically, patients receive an anticonvulsant to minimize seizure risk.[6-8]

Rebleeding is another complication in patients with an SAH if the aneurysm is not repaired. There is a 2% to 4% risk of aneurysmal rebleeding within the first 24 hours of initial hemorrhage. The risk for rebleeding increases dramatically during the first year after the initial hemorrhage.[9]

### Nursing Management

**ASSESSMENT.** One of the nurse's primary responsibilities is to obtain a baseline neurologic assessment and perform subsequent assessments to monitor for changes. After surgery, the nurse must be alert to the development of new deficits or a worsening of preoperative deficits. The severity and duration of any postoperative disability depend largely on the location and extent of the vascular lesion and resultant ischemia. The patient must also be carefully monitored for the development of cerebral edema.[8]

**PLAN.** Before surgery, the nurse implements aneurysm precautions by providing a quiet environment with limited stimulation. The nurse does a bowel assessment and implements individualized interventions.

A patent airway is required. Management of the patient's fluid and electrolytes includes careful monitoring for hyponatremia, which can cause an increase in cerebral edema. Accurate intake and output measurements are imperative.[8]

The nurse also monitors vital signs to rapidly identify any changes in BP and initiate corrective action to maintain BP within the target range. Hypotension must be treated immediately to prevent a drop in cerebral perfusion. Cardiac dysrhythmias may be present, especially if there was bleeding into the subarachnoid space. Dysrhythmias require prompt management because they may precipitate a drop in cardiac output and a consequent drop in cerebral perfusion.[6-8]

Continuous fluids are a part of the management of vasospasm. A patent IV site is maintained for hydration; maintaining two IV accesses may be appropriate as a matter of clinical judgment. The IV site is monitored frequently, and fluids are not interrupted for any reason. In the event of an infiltrate, the nurse restarts the line immediately.[8] Measures also need to be taken to manage increased ICP elevation if it develops; this would be noted initially as a decline in LOC. In the event the ICP elevation is severe enough to markedly reduce the LOC, endotracheal intubation and controlled ventilation should be initiated. Hyperventilation may be done as an initial emergent measure to lower dangerous ICP elevations pending initiation of additional therapies, such as osmotic diuretics and ventricular drainage, which are valuable tools in managing ICP elevations.

Emotional support is a crucial part of the overall nursing care of the patient with a ruptured aneurysm. Because of an aneurysm's abrupt onset, the hospital admission cannot be planned. Often the rupture suddenly interrupts the patient's daily life and may leave the patient with neurologic impairment. The patient's support system needs to be reorganized to tend to daily activities and responsibilities in his or her absence. Families require assistance when confronting the financial, physical, and emotional burden of caring for a patient after an SAH. A social worker can be instrumental in helping to organize the support of friends and family.[8]

**PATIENT EDUCATION AND DISCHARGE PLANNING.** Smoking and hypertension are both preventable risk factors associated with intracranial aneurysm and SAH. Patients can be instructed that cessation of smoking and control of hypertension can reduce the incidence of aneurysm formation and rupture.

Patients who have undergone clipping of cerebral aneurysms should be carefully screened before MRI. Although titanium clips used after 1996 are "MRI friendly," it is necessary to determine the composition of the clip before the patient undergoes MRI.

If a patient has experienced a seizure and is being maintained on anticonvulsant therapy, instructions should be given about medication monitoring and the need for compliance. In addition, the patient should be instructed about seizure safety.

Patients who have experienced SAH face a lengthy recovery. Rehabilitation for specific deficits should begin early.[8] Family participation in the rehabilitation plan is encouraged. Members of the health care team, including physical, occupational, and speech therapists, can help in restoring the patient's independence, and such services can be coordinated either for inpatient or outpatient settings, depending on the extent of impairment and financial circumstances.

### Arteriovenous Malformations

Arteriovenous malformations (AVMs) are lesions consisting of dilated arteries and veins without a capillary system, in which arterial blood flows directly into the venous system. AVMs are usually described as a "tangle" of blood vessels with a well-defined nidus that does not involve brain parenchyma.[11–13] AVMs are usually congenital, and they typically enlarge with age.[11] Although they are found throughout the central nervous system (CNS), approximately 90% of AVMs are located in the cerebrum, most commonly in the frontal and temporal lobes and supplied by the MCA.

## Epidemiology

AVMs are relatively uncommon brain lesions. Population-based studies have estimated a prevalence of less than 1% of the general population.[11] There is no statistically significant predisposition by sex. AVMs are diagnosed most often in young adults, with the majority being diagnosed in patients younger than age 40.[14] In cases in which the patient has both an AVM and an aneurysm (7%), the symptomatic lesion is treated initially. In some instances, both can be surgically treated at the same time. The aneurysms are more likely to be the cause of the hemorrhage.

## Pathophysiology

AVMs are most likely to arise between 4 and 8 weeks of embryo development, when cells begin to differentiate and when capillary components of the brain develop. (See the accompanying box, Spotlight on Genetics: Cerebral Arteriovenous Malformation.)

AVMs occur in locations where the primitive vasculature fails to develop an adequate capillary system. In an AVM, blood is shunted directly from the arterial to the venous circulation without benefit of a capillary bed; thus, there is less resistance, and as a result AVMs receive significant blood

flow. Arteries and veins enlarge to carry this increased flow, and their walls are characteristically quite thin. Arteries providing blood to the malformation and draining veins also become enlarged with increased flow volume in the lesion.[1,11,13]

## Clinical Manifestations

Hemorrhage, the most common presenting sign of AVMs, occurs in more than 50% of affected patients.[11] The hemorrhage may be intracerebral, subdural, or subarachnoid. A small lesion may be associated with an increased risk for hemorrhage because of higher flow and pressure from the feeding vessels. Increased risk of hemorrhage is also seen in AVMs located in the basal ganglia and posterior fossa; in lesions with deep venous drainage; and in lesions having only a few draining veins or a single draining vein, which causes high pressures within the arterial vessels feeding the AVM.[11]

There is an approximate 10% to 15% mortality rate after a hemorrhage.[11] The risk for rebleeding is higher in the first year after the initial hemorrhage and declines over subsequent years.[11] Cerebral AVMs cause about 2% of SAHs.[13] An SAH caused by an AVM is less lethal than one caused by an aneurysm rupture but is associated with significant neurologic morbidity.

Seizures, another common presenting sign of an AVM, occur in 20% to 25% of affected patients.[11] The risk of a seizure increases with the size of the lesion: seizures are more likely to occur in patients who have large and more superficial AVMs.[12] Patients who present with a seizure are treated with AEDs, but AEDs are not routinely used prophylactically for AVMs.

Other presenting signs of AVM include headache, increased ICP, neurologic deficits referable to the location of the lesion (5% to 7%), bruit, and visual symptoms.[11,13] Cognitive decline is seen, particularly in older patients with large AVMs; this may be related to "cerebral steal," in which arterial blood is diverted away from normal brain tissue to the AVM, causing ischemic changes.[12]

AVMs are graded based on features, location, and venous drainage. The Spetzler–Martin grading system, used to estimating the risk of neurosurgery for a patient with an AVM, assigns 1 point to lesions smaller than 3 cm, 2 points for 3- to 6-cm lesions, and 3 points for lesions larger than 6 cm. If the AVM is located in an eloquent area of the brain (sensory, motor, speech, visual, brainstem), it is given 1 additional point; no points are given for noneloquent areas. If deep venous drainage associated with the malformation, it is allotted 1 additional point, with no points for superficial venous drainage. A low score is associated with better surgical outcomes and a higher score with increased morbidity from surgery.[12,14]

## Diagnosis

CT and MRI are used to evaluate the presence of an AVM. The lesion is differentiated from tumors and other brain lesions by the presence of a hemosiderin ring around the lesion. Three-dimensional imaging is useful in establishing the malformation in relation to the surrounding anatomy. MRA is a noninvasive method of evaluating feeding and draining vessels in relation to the nidus of the AVM. Although MRA does provide useful information, it cannot consistently replace the more invasive angiography that is also used to evaluate feeding arteries and draining veins. Rarely, the AVM is

---

### SPOTLIGHT ON GENETICS 35-1

#### CEREBRAL ARTERIOVENOUS MALFORMATION

- Single nucleotide polymorphism (SNP) in the promoter region of the *IL6* gene has been associated with brain arteriovenous malformation (BAVM) and intracerebral hemorrhage. The *IL6* gene provides instructions for making a protein termed interleukin 6 (IL6). IL6 expression may modulate downstream inflammatory and angiogenic targets that contribute to intracranial hemorrhage in BAVM.
- The *IL6* mutation that is associated with BAVM involves a DNA segment known as promoter region of the *IL6* gene, specifically at (−174G/C). In brain tissue from patients with BAVM, researchers found that the highest IL6 protein and mRNA levels were associated with the *IL6 −174GG* genotype compared to the GC and CC genotypes. IL6 protein levels were increased in BAVM tissue from patients with hemorrhagic presentation compared to those without hemorrhage.
- Genetic testing for single nucleotide polymorphism (SNP) is available.

Data from Online Mendelian Inheritance in Man (OMIM). Retrieved August 10, 2015, from http://omim.org; Chen Y, Pawlikowska L, Yao JS, et al: Interleukin-6 involvement in brain arteriovenous malformations. Ann Neurol 59:72–80, 2006; and Weinsheimer SM, Xu H, Achrol AS, et al: Gene expression profiling of blood in brain arteriovenous malformation patients. Transl Stroke Res 2(4):575–587, 2011.

not angiographically evident; this may be true of lesions that have bled, have small feeding and draining vessels, or have low flow. TCD, single-photon emission computed tomography (SPECT), and PET are also used to image blood flow changes. To identify the AVM in relation to eloquent areas of the brain, fMRI is useful.[11,13]

## Clinical Management

AVMs are managed based on the patient's age and medical condition, flow associated with the malformation, history of hemorrhage, other symptoms, and the location of the lesion.

**INTERVENTIONAL MANAGEMENT.** Endovascular embolization of feeding arteries is used for small, low-grade malformations. The cure rate is low (10% to 15%), and one or more procedures may be needed to occlude the abnormal vessels. Embolization is used as an adjunct to surgery and radiosurgery. In this procedure, particles, liquids (such as acrylic glue), balloons, or coils are inserted into the AVM nidus before surgery or radiosurgery.[11-13] Endovascular treatment of intracranial micro-AVMs can be accomplished immediately, with good patient selection, and may be an alternative to open operative resection of the lesion.[12]

**RADIOSURGICAL MANAGEMENT.** SRS by gamma knife, linear accelerator, or heavy ion radiation provides good outcomes for relatively small lesions. When radiosurgery is used for lesions less than 3 cm in diameter, studies indicate an approximate 96% cure rate; however, complete obliteration of the malformation takes 2 to 3 years, and there is a risk for hemorrhage during this time.[14,15] Very large cerebral AVMs may be successfully treated by staged radiosurgical procedures. Given the time required to achieve obliteration of the lesion, long-term follow-up remains necessary.[15]

**SURGICAL MANAGEMENT.** Surgery is the preferred treatment for most AVMs. Surgery can reduce the risk for both hemorrhage and seizure. Brain mapping, fMRI, and intraoperative evoked potentials may be used in surgical planning for lesions in eloquent areas of the brain. Outcomes are positive, particularly in the case of Spetzler–Martin grade I and II lesions. Moreover, neurologic complications are low; surgery also provides an immediate cure. Intraoperative angiography is recommended.[12-14]

**MULTIMODAL MANAGEMENT.** Treatment approaches vary between surgery and radiosurgery for Spetzler–Martin grade III lesions. For large AVMs or lesions in eloquent areas of the brain, multimodality therapy with embolization, radiosurgery, or microsurgery is preferred. The most appropriate treatment approach for Spetzler–Martin grade IV and V lesions is a matter of controversy; some practitioners recommend the multimodality approach, whereas others opt for no treatment.

In addition to intracranial hemorrhage as a presenting event of AVM, hydrocephalus may occur, possibly as a consequence of the AVM acting as a space-occupying lesion interfering with CSF flow. Cerebral hydrodynamics may also be affected by mechanical obstruction by a draining vein associated with the lesion. If this causes acute hydrocephalus and ICP elevation, ventricular drainage may be necessary; if chronic, ventriculoperitoneal shunt may be necessary for long-term management. Definitive management of hydrocephalus should be prioritized during management of the AVM.[12,13]

## Nursing Management

**ASSESSMENT.** The nursing management of the patient with an AVM is similar to that described for a patient with a cerebral aneurysm. Baseline and follow-up neurologic assessments are necessary to monitor for subtle changes or evidence of hemorrhage.

**PLAN.** Careful evaluation of focal neurologic signs or evidence of cerebral edema minimizes significant postoperative morbidity.

**PATIENT EDUCATION AND DISCHARGE PLANNING.** Patients who have experienced a hemorrhage or seizures secondary to an AVM are managed in much the same way as patients with aneurysms. Patient and family education includes signs of increased ICP, seizure control and safety, anticonvulsant therapy, postoperative complications, and side effects of radiation, when appropriate.

## Surgical Approaches

Neurologic surgery may be performed in a number of situations as follows:

1. To obtain tissue for pathologic diagnosis
2. To remove an abnormal mass or space-occupying lesion (eg, tumor, cyst, hemorrhage) and, consequently, to reduce mass effect
3. To repair an abnormality (eg, aneurysm)
4. To place a device (eg, shunt, reservoir)

A number of factors are considered when making the appropriate surgical decision. Diagnostic studies are first performed to establish a differential diagnosis. Patient age, neurologic status, and concurrent medical conditions are factors in the decision to proceed with surgery and the decision regarding the appropriate approach. The most commonly used surgical procedures are briefly described in the following sections.

### Stereotactic Biopsy

A stereotactic biopsy is used to obtain tissue for definitive pathologic diagnosis. It is often used when a tumor is suspected but the lesion is too small or deep for surgical removal. It is used for tumors in eloquent areas of the brain, lesions crossing the corpus callosum, and multiple lesions that are not resectable.[2,16-18] A stereotactic biopsy is also used to confirm the diagnosis of previously treated tumors for example, when a malignant glioma has been treated with multiple therapies, tissue is obtained and analyzed to differentiate active tumor from treatment effect (ie, necrosis). In addition, some patients may have multiple medical problems and be too ill to proceed with a craniotomy. Others may opt to have the less invasive biopsy.[2]

The goal of stereotactic surgery is to locate a target using a trajectory. Stereotactic biopsies with a frame require placement of a rigid head frame to establish the appropriate coordinates. Next, a contrast-enhanced CT scan or MRI is obtained by using the localizing frame. An axial image of the tumor is displayed, with a number of coordinates to indicate entry points. The biopsy can be performed under general or local anesthesia in the Operating Room (O.R.).[1,2,16] After the skin is shaved and prepared, a small hole (twist drill or burr hole) is made, a needle is passed to the lesion, and one or more biopsies are obtained and immediately evaluated by a pathologist. Once sufficient tissue or cyst fluid is obtained for diagnostic purposes, the procedure is complete.

A stereotactic biopsy may also be performed without a frame. Frameless stereotaxy is a navigational system used to generate a three-dimensional tumor image. A CT or MRI scan is taken before the procedure, and markers (fiducials) are placed on the scalp. The markers are evident on the scan and are used to determine the actual target. A computer image is then generated from the imaging data.[2,16]

### Craniotomy

A craniotomy is performed to remove a space-occupying abnormality such as a tumor, cyst, or vascular malformation. This procedure may also be needed on an emergency basis to evacuate a hematoma or reverse a herniation syndrome. When appropriate, a craniotomy is used to clip an aneurysm.[1,6–8]

In this procedure, the surgeon makes a skin incision, elevates the bone flap, opens the dura, and obtains tissue from the lesion for biopsy or performs resection. The neurosurgical patient has quite distinct intraoperative pharmacologic needs. The neuroanesthesiologist administers drugs that provide the needed anesthetic effect while minimizing risks for increasing ICP or lowering seizure threshold. Rapid reversibility is also particularly important in patients receiving a craniotomy because their postoperative neurologic status needs to be assessed quickly.[1,18]

In addition to the equipment used during surgery to maximize safety and efficiency, specific tools for intraoperative monitoring may enhance the outcome for these patients. During the past 15 to 20 years, significant advances have taken place. Ultrasonography has been a standard of neurosurgical monitoring for some years because it can distinguish abnormal lesions from normal brain tissue and edema. Residual abnormal tissue may be identified before closing the surgical site. Frameless stereotaxy, as described previously, is also used during craniotomy. It is thought that this procedure enhances surgical safety and effectiveness by reducing craniotomy size, minimizing brain manipulation, and maximizing tumor resection.[16,17] Cortical mapping is used for masses in eloquent areas of the brain. Somatosensory evoked potentials are recorded during surgery under general anesthesia to assess the relationship between the motor strip and the lesion to be resected. Direct cortical stimulation provides for localization of the sensorimotor cortex and is also used to minimize neurologic deficits and maximize tumor removal. In some cases, greater seizure control is accomplished with these procedures. Direct cortical stimulation requires local anesthesia and the patient to be conscious during much of the procedure.[2,17,18]

Postoperative management of the patient who has undergone a craniotomy or stereotactic biopsy for a brain tumor focuses on assessment of and intervention for a number of potential complications. In the immediate postoperative period, patients may be slow to respond because of the effects of general anesthesia. Temporary changes in mental status or new focal neurologic signs should resolve rather quickly in this situation.[2] If there is a significant change from the baseline examination, radiographic documentation of hemorrhage or cerebral edema is performed. A CT scan or MRI is obtained to rule out postoperative complications. Edema is expected and can often be treated with corticosteroids. If significantly increased ICP occurs, the patient is medically managed in an ICU under close observation. Occasionally, surgical intervention is required for acute postoperative hemorrhage.

Other postoperative monitoring includes ongoing evaluation of vital signs and neurologic status; early ambulation to avoid pulmonary and cardiovascular complications; physical and occupational therapy evaluations; speech and cognitive assessment when indicated; DVT and PE prophylaxis; and wound evaluation and care.

### Transsphenoidal and Transnasal Surgeries

Transsphenoidal and transnasal surgeries are being used in many centers to remove pituitary tumors and cysts. The transnasal and transsphenoidal approaches replace transcranial surgery, when appropriate. An estimated 75% to 95% of cases are treated in this way. The patient is positioned on the operating table under general anesthesia. The sphenoid sinus is opened, the sella is opened, and the tumor is removed using the surgical microscope. If there is evidence of a CSF leak at the time of surgery, the sellar cavity is packed with fat tissue, typically taken from the patient's abdomen. The mucosal incision is closed with reabsorbable sutures. Nasal packing is often placed postoperatively and removed in 3 to 4 days.[1,2]

This procedure is usually well tolerated. Postoperative care is aimed at increasing mobility, monitoring respiration, evaluating fluid and electrolyte balance, and observing for evidence of CSF leak. The patient should be advised to avoid coughing, sneezing and nose blowing in order to avoid an increase in ICP and dislodgement of nasal packing.[2]

### Neuroendoscopy as a Surgical Tool

Endoscopic microsurgical techniques are being used with increasing frequency. This surgical tool improves visualization of normal anatomy and of abnormal lesions. It is most often used for smaller, avascular lesions of soft consistency. Colloid and choroid plexus cysts, ependymomas, some skull base tumors, and certain gliomas are amenable to this approach. The technique involves the use of an angled, flexible endoscope, thus enhancing the approach to tumor removal and aneurysm clipping.[19] Additionally, it allows for improved visualization during transsphenoidal surgery, providing closer evaluation of the pituitary tumor.[19]

## Neurologic Disorders

### Stroke

Cerebrovascular disease includes any pathologic process that involves the blood vessels of the brain. It is the most frequent neurologic disorder that affects adults. Most cerebrovascular disease is caused by thrombosis, embolism, or hemorrhage. The mechanism of each of these etiologies is different, but the ultimate result is damage to a focal area of the brain.[20–22]

A stroke may be defined as a neurologic deficit that has a sudden onset, results in permanent damage to the brain, and is caused by cerebrovascular disease. A stroke occurs when there is a disruption of blood flow to a region of the brain.

Blood flow is disrupted because of an obstruction of a vessel, a thrombus or embolus, or the rupture of a vessel. The apparent clinical features depend on the location of the event and region of the brain perfused by the vessel.[20-22]

A stroke is now referred to as a "brain attack" to encourage health care professionals and the public to think about stroke with the same urgency as a "heart attack." A "brain attack" must be viewed as a medical emergency. To reverse cerebral ischemia, patients must be evaluated promptly. Ischemic brain injury occurs when arterial occlusion lasts longer than 2 to 3 hours. Delay in seeking medical care may eliminate the potential for tissue-saving therapy with thrombolytic drugs. Stroke is the fourth leading cause of death in the United States.[22] Even when stroke is not fatal, it can result in serious long-term disability.[20-22]

Advances have been made in the treatment of stroke. Early recognition and prompt entry into the emergency medical system (EMS) are essential to reduce death and disability from stroke. Media campaigns have been launched to increase public awareness about the signs and symptoms of stroke so that care may be sought promptly.

An innovation in the way stroke care is delivered involves the establishment of the Joint Commission's certified stroke centers. The Joint Commission implemented a Disease-Specific Care Certification program in 2002, and stroke was one of the disease-specific categories in which program certification could be achieved. In this voluntary program, organizations have disease management programs reviewed by the Joint Commission. Criteria for the program include compliance with consensus-based national standards, effective use of established clinical practice guidelines to manage and optimize care, and an organized approach to monitor performance improvement activities. Achievement of Primary Stroke Center certification denotes clinical excellence in the management of stroke provided by a multidisciplinary team from several departments. This designation is attractive to many institutions that aspire to be recognized for their care of stroke patients.[22,23]

### Etiology

Approximately 75% of strokes in the United States are due to vascular obstruction (thrombi or emboli), resulting in ischemia and infarction. About 25% of strokes in the United States are hemorrhagic, resulting from hypertensive vascular disease (which causes an intracerebral hemorrhage), a ruptured aneurysm, or an AVM.[20,24,25] Figure 35-5 outlines stroke classification.

### Epidemiology

Approximately 795,000 people have a new or recurrent stroke each year, with a mortality rate of 35%.[24] Even though the average age of stroke is 70 years, 40% of all strokes occur in people younger than 60 years. Women have overtaken men in stroke incidence, with about 60,000 more women than men experiencing strokes annually. With longer life expectancies for women, more women actually die of stroke, accounting for 61% of stroke deaths. It is estimated that there are 3 million stroke survivors and that stroke is a leading cause of disability and a leading diagnosis for long-term

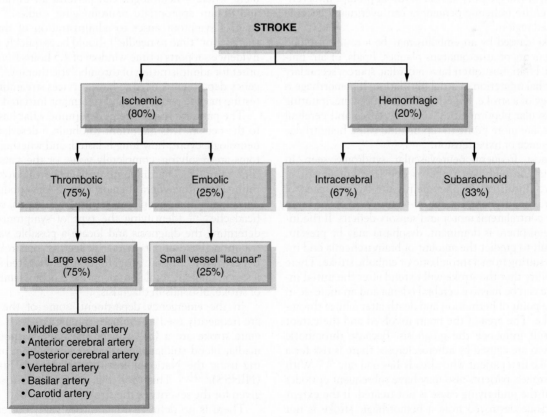

Note: Generated/simplified data

FIGURE 35-5   Classification of stroke. (Courtesy of Eric Aldrich, MD, PhD, The Johns Hopkins University, Baltimore, MD.)

care.[24] Risk factors for stroke include smoking, hypertension, obesity, cardiac disease, hypercholesterolemia, diabetes, cancer, use of birth control pills, and patent foramen ovale with atrial septal aneurysm. Prevention efforts focus on lifestyle changes that can modify risk factors. In addition, the appropriate use of anticoagulants (warfarin, apixaban, dabigatran, and rivaroxaban) in patients at risk for cardiac sources of emboli (eg, atrial fibrillation) and use of aspirin in patients at risk for thrombotic stroke constitute primary prevention.[21,22,26]

### Pathophysiology

When blood flow to any part of the brain is impeded as a result of a thrombus or embolus, oxygen and substrate deprivation of the cerebral tissue begins. Deprivation for 1 minute can lead to reversible symptoms, such as loss of consciousness. Oxygen deprivation for longer periods can produce microscopic necrosis of the neurons. The necrotic area is then said to be infarcted.[1,26]

The initial oxygen deprivation may be caused by general ischemia (from cardiac arrest or hypotension) or hypoxia (from an anemic process or high altitude). If the neurons are ischemic only and have not yet necrosed, they may be saved. This ischemic tissue may be either salvaged with appropriate treatment or killed by secondary events.[1,26]

Cerebral ischemia is a complex process that depends on the severity and duration of the decline in CBF. The ischemic cascade begins within seconds to minutes after perfusion failure, creating a zone of irreversible infarction and a surrounding area of potentially salvageable "ischemic penumbra." The goal of acute stroke management is to salvage the ischemic penumbra, or the territory at risk. Without prompt intervention, the entire ischemic penumbra can eventually become an infarcted region.[1,26]

A stroke caused by an embolus may be a result of blood clots, fragments of atheromatous plaques, lipids, or air. Emboli to the brain most often have a cardiac source, secondary to myocardial infarction or atrial fibrillation. If hemorrhage is the etiology of a stroke, hypertension often is a precipitating factor. Vascular abnormalities, such as AVMs and cerebral aneurysms, are more prone to rupture and cause hemorrhage in the presence of hypertension.[25]

The most frequent neurovascular syndrome seen in thrombotic and embolic strokes is due to involvement of the MCA. This artery supplies mainly the lateral aspects of the cerebral hemisphere. Infarction to that area of the brain can cause contralateral motor and sensory deficits. If the infarcted hemisphere is dominant, dysphasia may be present. It is difficult to predict the amount of brain ischemia and infarction resulting from a thrombotic or embolic stroke. There is a possibility that the stroke will extend after the initial insult. There can be massive cerebral edema and an increase in ICP to the point of herniation and death after a huge thrombotic stroke. The area of the brain involved and the extent of the insult influence the prognosis. Because thrombotic strokes often are caused by atherosclerosis, there is risk for a future stroke in a patient who already has had one.[24,26] With embolic strokes, patients also may have subsequent episodes of stroke if the underlying cause is not treated. If the extent of brain tissue destroyed from a hemorrhagic stroke is not excessive and is in a nonvital area, the patient may recover with minimal deficits. If the hemorrhage is large or in a vital

area of the brain, the patient may not recover; however, if the intracerebral hemorrhage is less massive, survival is possible. For the purposes of this discussion, the focus is on the diagnosis and management of ischemic stroke.

### Clinical Manifestations

A stroke is usually characterized by the sudden onset of focal neurologic impairment. The patient may experience signs such as weakness, numbness, visual changes, dysarthria, dysphagia, or aphasia. The manifestations of a stroke depend on the anatomical location of the lesion; an infarct in a certain portion of the brain results in loss of function of the body part that it controlled or skill for which it was responsible.[1,25,26] Table 35-6 presents the correlation of blood supply to symptomatology in a brain attack.

If symptoms resolve in less than 24 hours, the event is classified as a transient ischemic attack (TIA), which is defined as a "neurologic deficit lasting less than 24 hours that is attributed to focal cerebral or retinal ischemia." Most TIAs last for only minutes to less than an hour, which further clouds recognition and prompt treatment. A TIA precedes approximately 15% of all strokes.[24] An aggressive workup following TIA is encouraged.

### Diagnosis

Rapid diagnosis of a stroke is essential so that appropriate patients can receive thrombolytic therapy, the goal of which is to save damaged brain tissue and minimize permanent deficits. The patient should be taken to an emergency department where a neurologist can perform an initial screening and obtain appropriate neuroimaging studies.[20,22,27,28] The time of symptom onset to administration of thrombolytic therapy (or "time to needle") should be as quickly as possible. Evidence supports a time window of 4.5 hours from symptom onset for administration of thrombolytic therapy.[22,26,27] Emergency departments need to have services streamlined so that testing may be performed and treatment initiated promptly.

The patient's history helps determine what has happened to the person. It is important to obtain a description of the neurologic event; how long it lasted; and whether the symptoms are resolving, completely gone, or the same as at the time of onset. The differential diagnosis of stroke includes ruling out intracerebral hemorrhage, SAH, subdural or epidural hematoma, neoplasm, seizure, meningitis, or migraine headache.[25,26] Identifying the type of symptoms can help determine the diagnosis and locate a possible vascular distribution. Determination of risk factors for stroke, such as hypertension, chronic atrial fibrillation, elevated serum cholesterol, smoking, oral contraceptive use, or a familial history of stroke, also aids in diagnosis.

In the emergency department, some of the tests that are frequently used to evaluate the patient with acute ischemic stroke are a CT scan of the brain without contrast media, blood studies, neurologic examination, and screening using the National Institutes of Health Stroke Scale (NIHSS).[22,25-28] This tool (Fig. 35-6) allows a score to be given for the severity of the stroke.

There is no definitive laboratory study currently available that determines whether a patient has experienced a stroke. Rather, the results are viewed in conjunction with

**TABLE 35-6** Stroke: Correlation of Blood Supply to the Brain with Symptomatology

| Artery | Brain Structure | Signs/Symptoms of Occlusion |
|--------|-----------------|----------------------------|
| **Anterior Blood Supply** | | |
| **Anterior cerebral artery** | Medial, frontal, and parietal lobe, caudate head, globus pallidus, anterior limb of internal capsule | • Amnesia<br>• Flat affect, slowness, distractibility<br>• Impaired judgment<br>• Disinhibition and speech perseveration<br>• Contralateral sensory and motor deficits greater in leg than arm<br>• Incontinence<br>• Primitive reflexes (grasping, sucking)<br>• Gait apraxia<br>• Slow or delayed response |
| **Middle cerebral artery** | Lateral frontal and parietal lobes, lateral and anterior temporal lobe, globus pallidus and putamen, internal capsule | • Contralateral hemiparesis and sensory deficits<br>• Weakness in arm and face worse than leg<br>• Contralateral hypesthesia<br>• Ipsilateral hemianopsia<br>• Gaze preference toward the side of the lesion<br>• Agnosia<br>• Receptive or expressive aphasia—lesion in dominant hemisphere<br>• Neglect and inattention—lesion in nondominant hemisphere |
| **Posterior Blood Supply** | | |
| **Posterior cerebral artery** | Occipital lobes, medial and posterior temporal and parietal lobes, brainstem, posterior thalamus, and midbrain | • Contralateral homonymous hemianopsia<br>• Cortical blindness<br>• Visual agnosia<br>• Altered mental status<br>• Impaired memory<br>• Vertigo<br>• Nausea and vomiting<br>• Nystagmus<br>• Diplopia<br>• Visual field deficits<br>• Dysphagia<br>• Dysarthria<br>• Facial hypesthesia<br>• Syncope<br>• Ataxia |

Data from Hickey JV: The Clinical Practice of Neurological and Neurosurgical Nursing. Philadelphia, PA: Wolters Kluwer/Lippincott Williams & Wilkins, 2014; and Jauch EC: Ischemic stroke. Updated July 30, 2015. Retrieved August 7, 2015, from http://emedicine.medscape.com/article/1916852-print.

the history, neurologic examination, and neuroimaging studies. Laboratory tests, including complete blood cell count, electrolytes, glucose, and coagulation parameters, are obtained.

An urgent CT scan should be performed to rule out intracerebral hemorrhage. Ideally, the CT scan is obtained within 60 minutes of arrival in the emergency department so that treatment decisions can be made. A CT scan can be useful in differentiating between cerebrovascular and nonvascular lesions. For example, a subdural hemorrhage, brain abscess, tumor, SAH, or intracerebral hemorrhage is visible on the CT scan.[1,20,29] However, an area of infarction may not show on the CT scan for 24 to 48 hours.

Newer neuroimaging techniques also provide valuable information. MRI, including T1- and T2-weighted, fluid-attenuated inversion recovery (FLAIR), and diffusion-weighted techniques, has become widely available and is better at detecting infarction than a CT scan.[21,22,27] The earliest changes normally appear within the first 24 hours.

Other studies that may be performed, based on availability of the technology, are MRI diffusion-weighted imaging (DWI) and perfusion-weighted imaging (PWI). These techniques help identify the infarct core and penumbra, which is important because the presence of viable tissue directs interventions such as reperfusion. The ischemic penumbra surrounds the infarcted tissue. It is the marginally perfused area of the brain that has been damaged by the insult but is potentially salvageable. DWI detects acute infarction as early as a few hours after the onset of symptoms. It can reveal changes associated with infarcted tissue hours before a CT scan or conventional MRI can detect any abnormality. It also differentiates acute from chronic ischemic changes. PWI shows the regional abnormalities of CBF. The difference between the diffusion defect and the perfusion defect represents the ischemic penumbra, or the "territory at risk."[22] DWI–PWI identifies patients who are ideal candidates for thrombolytic therapy.

Cerebral angiography has been the gold standard for evaluating cerebral vasculature. There is an estimated 1.5% to 2% associated risk for morbidity or mortality with this procedure. However, it can demonstrate an arterial occlusion or embolus. Because of the time that it takes to perform cerebral angiography, the window of opportunity to treat a patient with IV thrombolytics may be missed. However, angiography is necessary for intra-arterial thrombolysis in which tissue plasminogen activator (t-PA) or another thrombolytic

# NIH STROKE SCALE

Patient Identification ___ ___-___ ___ ___-___ ___ ___

Pt. Date of Birth ___ ___/___ ___/___ ___

Hospital _____ (___ ___-___ ___)

Date of Exam ___ ___/___ ___/___ ___

Interval: [ ] Baseline    [ ] 2 hours post treatment    [ ] 24 hour post onset of symptoms ±20 minutes    [ ] 7-10 days

[ ] 3 months    [ ] Other _____

Time: ___ ___:___ ___  [ ] am [ ] pm

Person Administering Scale _____

Administer stroke scale items in the order listed. Record performance in each category after each subscale exam. Do not go back and change scores. Follow directions provided for each exam technique. Scores should reflect what the patient does, not what the clinician thinks the patient can do. The clinician should record answers while administering the exam and work quickly. Except where indicated, the patient should not be coached (i.e., repeated requests to patient to make a special effort).

| Instructions | Scale Definition | Score |
|---|---|---|
| **1a. Level of Consciousness:** The investigator must choose a response if a full evaluation is prevented by such obstacles as an endotracheal tube, language barrier, orotracheal trauma/bandages. A 3 is scored only if the patient makes no movement (other than reflexive posturing) in response to noxious stimulation. | 0 = **Alert;** keenly responsive. <br> 1 = **Not alert;** but arousable by minor stimulation to obey, answer, or respond. <br> 2 = **Not alert;** requires repeated stimulation to attend, or is obtunded and requires strong or painful stimulation to make movements (not stereotyped). <br> 3 = Responds only with reflex motor or autonomic effects or totally unresponsive, flaccid, and areflexic. | |
| **1b. LOC Questions:** The patient is asked the month and his/her age. The answer must be correct - there is no partial credit for being close. Aphasic and stuporous patients who do not comprehend the questions will score 2. Patients unable to speak because of endotracheal intubation, orotracheal trauma, severe dysarthria from any cause, language barrier, or any other problem not secondary to aphasia are given a 1. It is important that only the initial answer be graded and that the examiner not "help" the patient with verbal or non-verbal cues. | 0 = **Answers** both questions correctly. <br> 1 = **Answers** one question correctly. <br> 2 = **Answers** neither question correctly. | |
| **1c. LOC Commands:** The patient is asked to open and close the eyes and then to grip and release the non-paretic hand. Substitute another one step command if the hands cannot be used. Credit is given if an unequivocal attempt is made but not completed due to weakness. If the patient does not respond to command, the task should be demonstrated to him or her (pantomime), and the result scored (i.e., follows none, one or two commands). Patients with trauma, amputation, or other physical impediments should be given suitable one-step commands. Only the first attempt is scored. | 0 = **Performs** both tasks correctly. <br> 1 = **Performs** one task correctly. <br> 2 = **Performs** neither task correctly. | |
| **2. Best Gaze:** Only horizontal eye movements will be tested. Voluntary or reflexive (oculocephalic) eye movements will be scored, but caloric testing is not done. If the patient has a conjugate deviation of the eyes that can be overcome by voluntary or reflexive activity, the score will be 1. If a patient has an isolated peripheral nerve paresis (CN III, IV or VI), score a 1. Gaze is testable in all aphasic patients. Patients with ocular trauma, bandages, pre-existing blindness, or other disorder of visual acuity or fields should be tested with reflexive movements, and a choice made by the investigator. Establishing eye contact and then moving about the patient from side to side will occasionally clarify the presence of a partial gaze palsy. | 0 = **Normal.** <br> 1 = **Partial gaze palsy;** gaze is abnormal in one or both eyes, but forced deviation or total gaze paresis is not present. <br> 2 = **Forced deviation,** or total gaze paresis not overcome by the oculocephalic maneuver. | |
| **3. Visual:** Visual fields (upper and lower quadrants) are tested by confrontation, using finger counting or visual threat, as appropriate. Patients may be encouraged, but if they look at the side of the moving fingers appropriately, this can be scored as normal. If there is unilateral blindness or enucleation, visual fields in the remaining eye are scored. Score 1 only if a clear-cut asymmetry, including quadrantanopia, is found. If patient is blind from any cause, score 3. Double simultaneous stimulation is performed at this point. If there is extinction, patient receives a 1, and the results are used to respond to item 11. | 0 = **No visual loss.** <br> 1 = **Partial hemianopia.** <br> 2 = **Complete hemianopia.** <br> 3 = **Bilateral hemianopia** (blind including cortical blindness). | |
| **4. Facial Palsy:** Ask – or use pantomime to encourage – the patient to show teeth or raise eyebrows and close eyes. Score symmetry of grimace in response to noxious stimuli in the poorly responsive or non-comprehending patient. If facial trauma/bandages, orotracheal tube, tape or other physical barriers obscure the face, these should be removed to the extent possible. | 0 = **Normal** symmetrical movements. <br> 1 = **Minor paralysis** (flattened nasolabial fold, asymmetry on smiling). <br> 2 = **Partial paralysis** (total or near-total paralysis of lower face). <br> 3 = **Complete paralysis** of one or both sides (absence of facial movement in the upper and lower face). | |
| **5. Motor Arm:** The limb is placed in the appropriate position: extend the arms (palms down) 90 degrees (if sitting) or 45 degrees (if supine). Drift is scored if the arm falls before 10 seconds. The aphasic patient is encouraged using urgency in the voice and pantomime, but not noxious stimulation. Each limb is tested in turn, beginning with the non-paretic arm. Only in the case of amputation or joint fusion at the shoulder, the examiner should record the score as untestable (UN), and clearly write the explanation for this choice. | 0 = **No drift;** limb holds 90 (or 45) degrees for full 10 seconds. <br> 1 = **Drift;** limb holds 90 (or 45) degrees, but drifts down before full 10 seconds; does not hit bed or other support. <br> 2 = **Some effort against gravity;** limb cannot get to or maintain (if cued) 90 (or 45) degrees, drifts down to bed, but has some effort against gravity. <br> 3 = **No effort against gravity;** limb falls. <br> 4 = **No movement.** <br> UN = **Amputation** or joint fusion, explain: _____ <br> **5a. Left Arm** <br> **5b. Right Arm** | |
| **6. Motor Leg:** The limb is placed in the appropriate position: hold the leg at 30 degrees (always tested supine). Drift is scored if the leg falls before 5 seconds. The aphasic patient is encouraged using urgency in the voice and pantomime, but not noxious stimulation. Each limb is tested in turn, beginning with the non-paretic leg. Only in the case of amputation or joint fusion at the hip, the examiner should record the score as untestable (UN), and clearly write the explanation for this choice. | 0 = **No drift;** leg holds 30-degree position for full 5 seconds. <br> 1 = **Drift;** leg falls by the end of the 5-second period but does not hit bed. <br> 2 = **Some effort against gravity;** leg falls to bed by 5 seconds, but has some effort against gravity. <br> 3 = **No effort against gravity;** leg falls to bed immediately. <br> 4 = **No movement.** <br> UN = **Amputation** or joint fusion, explain: _____ <br> **6a. Left Leg** <br> **6b. Right Leg** | |

**FIGURE 35-6**   National Institutes of Health Stroke Scale. (From National Institute of Neurological Disorders and Stroke [NINDS], National Institutes of Health [NIH], Bethesda, MD. Retrieved from http://www.ninds.nih.gov/doctors/nih_stroke_scale.pdf.)

# NIH STROKE SCALE

Interval: [ ] Baseline    [ ] 2 hours post treatment    [ ] 24 hour post onset of symptoms ±20 minutes    [ ] 7-10 days
[ ] 3 months    [ ] Other _____

Patient Identification ___ ___-___ ___-___ ___ ___
Pt. Date of Birth ___ ___/___ ___/___ ___
Hospital _____ (___ ___-___ ___)
Date of Exam ___ ___/___ ___/___ ___

| Instructions | Scale Definition | Score |
|---|---|---|
| **7. Limb Ataxia:** This item is aimed at finding evidence of a unilateral cerebellar lesion. Test with eyes open. In case of visual defect, ensure testing is done in intact visual field. The finger-nose-finger and heel-shin tests are performed on both sides, and ataxia is scored only if present out of proportion to weakness. Ataxia is absent in the patient who cannot understand or is paralyzed. Only in the case of amputation or joint fusion, the examiner should record the score as untestable (UN), and clearly write the explanation for this choice. In case of blindness, test by having the patient touch nose from extended arm position. | 0 = **Absent.** <br> 1 = **Present in one limb.** <br> 2 = **Present in two limbs.** <br> UN = **Amputation** or joint fusion, explain: _____ | |
| **8. Sensory:** Sensation or grimace to pinprick when tested, or withdrawal from noxious stimulus in the obtunded or aphasic patient. Only sensory loss attributed to stroke is scored as abnormal and the examiner should test as many body areas (arms [not hands], legs, trunk, face) as needed to accurately check for hemisensory loss. A score of 2, "severe or total sensory loss," should only be given when a severe or total loss of sensation can be clearly demonstrated. Stuporous and aphasic patients will, therefore, probably score 1 or 0. The patient with brainstem stroke who has bilateral loss of sensation is scored 2. If the patient does not respond and is quadriplegic, score 2. Patients in a coma (item 1a=3) are automatically given a 2 on this item. | 0 = **Normal**; no sensory loss. <br> 1 = **Mild-to-moderate sensory loss**; patient feels pinprick is less sharp or is dull on the affected side; or there is a loss of superficial pain with pinprick, but patient is aware of being touched. <br> 2 = **Severe to total sensory loss**; patient is not aware of being touched in the face, arm, and leg. | |
| **9. Best Language:** A great deal of information about comprehension will be obtained during the preceding sections of the examination. For this scale item, the patient is asked to describe what is happening in the attached picture, to name the items on the attached naming sheet and to read from the attached list of sentences. Comprehension is judged from responses here, as well as to all of the commands in the preceding general neurological exam. If visual loss interferes with the tests, ask the patient to identify objects placed in the hand, repeat, and produce speech. The intubated patient should be asked to write. The patient in a coma (item 1a=3) will automatically score 3 on this item. The examiner must choose a score for the patient with stupor or limited cooperation, but a score of 3 should be used only if the patient is mute and follows no one-step commands. | 0 = **No aphasia**; normal. <br> 1 = **Mild-to-moderate aphasia**; some obvious loss of fluency or facility of comprehension, without significant limitation on ideas expressed or form of expression. Reduction of speech and/or comprehension, however, makes conversation about provided materials difficult or impossible. For example, in conversation about provided materials, examiner can identify picture or naming card content from patient's response. <br> 2 = **Severe aphasia**; all communication is through fragmentary expression; great need for inference, questioning, and guessing by the listener. Range of information that can be exchanged is limited; listener carries burden of communication. Examiner cannot identify materials provided from patient response. <br> 3 = **Mute, global aphasia**; no usable speech or auditory comprehension. | |
| **10. Dysarthria:** If patient is thought to be normal, an adequate sample of speech must be obtained by asking patient to read or repeat words from the attached list. If the patient has severe aphasia, the clarity of articulation of spontaneous speech can be rated. Only if the patient is intubated or has other physical barriers to producing speech, the examiner should record the score as untestable (UN), and clearly write an explanation for this choice. Do not tell the patient why he or she is being tested. | 0 = **Normal.** <br> 1 = **Mild-to-moderate dysarthria**; patient slurs at least some words and, at worst, can be understood with some difficulty. <br> 2 = **Severe dysarthria**; patient's speech is so slurred as to be unintelligible in the absence of or out of proportion to any dysphasia, or is mute/anarthric. <br> UN = **Intubated** or other physical barrier, explain:_____ | |
| **11. Extinction and Inattention (formerly Neglect):** Sufficient information to identify neglect may be obtained during the prior testing. If the patient has a severe visual loss preventing visual double simultaneous stimulation, and the cutaneous stimuli are normal, the score is normal. If the patient has aphasia but does appear to attend to both sides, the score is normal. The presence of visual spatial neglect or anosognosia may also be taken as evidence of abnormality. Since the abnormality is scored only if present, the item is never untestable. | 0 = **No abnormality.** <br> 1 = **Visual, tactile, auditory, spatial, or personal inattention** or extinction to bilateral simultaneous stimulation in one of the sensory modalities. <br> 2 = **Profound hemi-inattention or extinction to more than one modality;** does not recognize own hand or orients to only one side of space. | |

**FIGURE 35-6**  *(continued)*

is administered at the site of the clot by catheter into the artery.[22] The time window may be as long as 6 hours from symptom onset for intra-arterial thrombolysis, 8 hours from symptom onset for mechanical thrombolysis, and 24 hours for intravascular intervention for basilar artery stroke. The vasculature can be evaluated noninvasively by the use of TCD, ultrasonography, MRA, or CT angiography.

An electrocardiogram (ECG) should be obtained to assess for evidence of dysrhythmia or cardiac ischemia. The ECG helps determine whether a dysrhythmia is present, which may have caused the stroke. Atrial fibrillation is a dysrhythmia in which clots form in the heart and may travel to the brain (hence a cardioembolic etiology). Other changes that might be found on an ECG are an inverted T wave, ST elevation or depression, and QT prolongation.

In summary, prompt performance of a CT scan and subsequent interpretation are crucial to acute stroke management. Head CT provides vital information to allow the physician to make the decision to use thrombolytic therapy. An alternate approach is urgent MRI with PWI and DWI.

## Clinical Management

The management of an ischemic stroke has four primary goals: restoration of CBF (reperfusion), prevention of recurrent thrombosis, neuroprotection, and supportive care. The timing of each element of clinical management should be implemented in a decisive manner.

Optimally, patients are initially evaluated at a center that has a stroke program, perhaps even a Joint Commission Primary Stroke Center. Decisions in the emergency department determine the patient's treatment plan. Emergency departments may have standardized orders, clinical pathways, or protocols that have been developed by a multidisciplinary team to guide care.[23,28]

The focus of initial treatment is to save as much of the ischemic area as possible. Three ingredients necessary to this area are oxygen, glucose, and adequate blood flow. The oxygen level can be monitored through arterial blood gas analyses or pulse oximetry, and oxygen can be given to the patient if indicated. Hypo/hyperglycemia can be evaluated with serial checks of blood glucose levels. Reperfusion may be accomplished by the use of IV t-PA.[22,26,27]

CPP is a reflection of the systemic BP and ICP. Regional perfusion is influenced by autoregulation in the brain, and MAP is influenced by cardiac output and heart rate (CPP = MAP – ICP). The parameters most easily controlled externally are the BP and cardiac rate and rhythm.[1] Dysrhythmias can reduce cardiac output and BP but usually can be corrected. There is a loss of autoregulation in the ischemic penumbra, so that reducing BP can further reduce blood flow in the penumbra and can lead to infarction.[26]

If the patient is a candidate for IV thrombolytic therapy, treatment with t-PA begins in the emergency department, and he or she is then moved to the ICU or other specialized monitored setting such as a neuroscience step-down or dedicated stroke unit for further monitoring. If the patient is not a candidate for thrombolytic therapy, the complexity of the patient's problems determines his or her placement in the ICU, medical unit, or stroke specialty unit.

Currently, two emergency treatments are available for stroke management: IV t-PA and embolus removal by use of mechanical device. IV t-PA is an approved US FDA treatment.

**THROMBOLYTIC DRUGS.** Thrombolytic medications are exogenous drugs that dissolve clots. IV t-PA dissolves the clot and permits reperfusion of the brain tissue. IV thrombolytic therapy should be initiated as quickly as possible from symptom onset. The maximal time window is 4.5 hours or less from the onset of neurologic symptoms.[22,26,27] The clock begins for the patient from the time he or she was last seen well. For example, a patient retires to bed at 11:00 PM and awakens at 5:00 AM to go to the bathroom. As he attempts to rise from the bed, he feels weak and has difficulty standing up. As he calls out for his wife's help, his speech is garbled. The last time he was awake and functioning normally was at 11:00 PM. Even if his symptoms started only a few minutes ago, the time he was last seen well was 6 hours ago. Therefore, he is already outside of the treatment window for IV t-PA.

Candidate selection for IV t-PA must be done carefully. The neurologic examination, NIHSS score, and results of neuroimaging studies assist the physician with the decision to offer thrombolytic therapy. Box 35-2 outlines eligibility criteria for this treatment. The standards for the administration of IV t-PA to treat stroke are a result of the National Institute of Neurologic Disorders and Stroke t-PA Stroke Study. A dose of IV t-PA, 0.9 mg/kg (maximal dose, 90 mg), is administered as 10% of the total dose as a bolus over 1 to 2 minutes, with the remainder infused over 60 minutes. The t-PA activates plasminogen, a naturally occurring enzyme present in the intravascular endothelium that protects against excessive clotting. Activating plasminogen initiates the process of dissolving the clot through fibrinolysis. No other antithrombotic therapy should be given for the next 24 hours. A major risk of this therapy is intracerebral hemorrhage.[1,22,26] However, it is encouraging that this agent may prove effective in reversing a neurologic deficit and improving quality of life after a stroke.

The direct administration of a thrombolytic into an artery is an alternative to IV t-PA. Such administration is effective in acute ischemic stroke and can be given up to 6 hours after the onset of symptoms. A limiting factor is that the

**BOX 35-2** **Eligibility Criteria for Thrombolytic Therapy**

**Inclusion Criteria**
1. Symptom onset of less than 4.5 hours
2. Clinical diagnosis of ischemic stroke with measurable deficit on the NIHSS
3. Older than 18 years
4. CT criteria: No evidence of multilobar infarction (high hypodensity over one-third hemisphere) or intracerebral hemorrhage

**Exclusion Criteria**
1. Stroke or serious head trauma within past 3 months
2. Systolic BP more than 185 mm Hg or diastolic BP more than 110 mm Hg that is refractory to IV medications.
3. Conditions that could precipitate or suggest parenchymal bleeding (subarachnoid and intracerebral hemorrhage; recent-onset myocardial infarction; seizures at onset; GI or urinary tract hemorrhage within previous 21 days; and arterial puncture of a noncompressible site or lumbar puncture within previous 7 days)
4. Glucose less than 50 mg/dL; INR greater than 1.7; platelet count less than 100,000/mm³
5. Recent treatment with IV or subcutaneous heparin within past 48 hours and elevated partial thromboplastin time
6. Relative Exclusion Criteria: Women of childbearing age who have a positive pregnancy test result; major surgery or serious trauma within past 14 days; seizure at onset with postictal neurologic impairments; acute myocardial infarction within past 3 months; rapidly improving stroke symptoms or only minor symptoms.

Data from Liebeskind DS: Hemorrhagic stroke. Medscape. Updated January 8, 2015. Retrieved January 16, 2015, from http://emedicine.medscape.com/article/1916662-print; and Jauch EC: Ischemic stroke. Medscape. Updated July 30, 2015. Retrieved August 7, 2015, from http://emedicine.medscape.com/article/1916852-print.

patient must be admitted to a specialty center in which localized intra-arterial infusion of thrombolytic drugs is possible. Through this approach, an occluded cerebral artery can be reopened. For intra-arterial therapy, a femoral arterial sheath is usually inserted, through which a microcatheter can be threaded, under fluoroscopy. The catheter tip is positioned into the clot and advanced as the clot dissolves. The femoral sheath usually remains in place for 24 hours in case of recurrent vessel occlusion. The advantage of this approach is that the medication can be delivered directly to its target.[22,26]

**MECHANICAL DEVICES.** There are four mechanical devices approved by the FDA for clot removal.[26] These devices can be used for up to 8 hours after stroke onset to remove blood clots from vessels. If a patient arrives at the hospital too late to receive IV t-PA or is ineligible for intravenous fibrinolytics, these devices present another treatment option.[26]

Mechanical devices work like a corkscrew to retrieve the clot. During cerebral angiography, an interventional radiologist passes the microcatheter into the femoral artery. It is advanced into the carotid until it reaches the clot. A wire is then pushed through the catheter, causing it to return to a corkscrew shape. It then snares the embolus.[30,31]

Potential hazards from use of a mechanical retriever include bleeding and vascular dissection or perforation. The patient needs to be closely monitored for the first 24 hours to detect adverse effects. The nurse, who plays a key role in postprocedure monitoring, performs neurologic assessments and carefully monitors the patient for signs of intracranial hemorrhage, new stroke, or myocardial infarction.[1]

**ANTICOAGULATION.** Aside from thrombolytic therapy and mechanical clot retrieval, secondary treatment options for stroke include anticoagulation with antithrombotic and antiplatelet drugs. If a patient experiences atrial fibrillation, anticoagulation medication may be warranted. Education includes the purpose of the medication and instruction about bleeding precautions. If the patient is prescribed warfarin (Coumadin) information about moderate consumption of leafy green vegetables containing vitamin K and the importance of having blood drawn regularly to monitor prothrombin time and the INR is indicated.[22]

Antiplatelet drugs include dipyridamole-ER, ticlopidine, clopidogrel, and aspirin. These drugs deter platelets from adhering to the wall of an injured blood vessel or other platelets and are given to prevent a future thrombotic or embolic event. Although several antiplatelet drugs exist, the most commonly prescribed is Aspirin. Aspirin limits platelet adhesion and aggregation. The suggested dose of aspirin is 81 to 325 mg/d. The administration of all antiplatelet drugs plays a role in stroke prevention by decreasing the risk for future strokes.[1,22,26]

**CONTROL OF HYPERTENSION AND INCREASED INTRACRANIAL PRESSURE.** The control of hypertension, increased ICP, and CPP takes the efforts of the nurse and the physician. The nurse must assess for these problems, recognize them and their significance, and advocate for the patient, ensuring that medical interventions are initiated.

Patients with moderate hypertension usually are not treated acutely. If their BP decreases after the brain becomes accustomed to the hypertension needed for adequate perfusion, the brain's perfusion pressure falls along with the BP. If the diastolic BP is above approximately 105 mm Hg, it needs to be lowered gradually. This can be accomplished effectively with labetalol as well as calcium channel blockers.[1,22,27]

If ICP is elevated in a patient who has had a stroke, it usually occurs after the first day. Although this is a natural response of the brain to some cerebrovascular lesions, it is destructive to the brain. The usual methods of controlling increased ICP can be instituted: hyperventilation (in a patient receiving controlled ventilation in the short term only to control critical ICP elevations pending institution of additional therapies); fluid restriction; head elevation; avoidance of neck flexion or severe head rotation that would impede venous outflow from the head; and the use of osmotic diuretics (mannitol) to decrease cerebral edema.

**SURGICAL MANAGEMENT.** In patients with carotid stenosis, carotid endarterectomy may be performed to prevent a stroke. Carotid endarterectomy is a surgical procedure in which atherosclerotic plaque that has accumulated inside the carotid artery is surgically removed. Once the plaque is removed, blood flow is restored. Although the use of carotid endarterectomy has increased over the years for emergent stroke treatment a systematic review of 47 studies concluded that the procedure is high risk for patient with unstable neurologic status.[22] During aggressive clinical management for stroke, brain edema and ICP elevation may become refractory to measures such as controlled/short-term hyperventilation

and osmotic diuresis. A subset of patients may benefit from hemicraniectomy, allowing additional space for edematous brain to expand and relieving ICP elevations pending resolution of brain edema. Additionally, extracranial–intracranial bypass surgery, with careful patient selection in limited case series, has been effective in arresting stroke progression and has resulted in rapid improvement in neurologic assessment findings.[22]

**NONSURGICAL MANAGEMENT.** Although the gold standard for managing carotid artery stenosis has been carotid endarterectomy, another management option, carotid stenting, is available. This newer, minimally invasive procedure is attractive for patients in whom traditional surgery is contraindicated, such as those with severe cardiac or pulmonary disease. Carotid artery stenting opens vessels that have been narrowed by plaque accumulation. An interventional radiologist passes a catheter along the femoral artery to the narrowed artery. Once the catheter crosses the area of stenosis, a small filter may be deployed to catch any pieces of plaque that may be dislodged during the procedure. Angioplasty, in which plaque is pressed against the artery wall, may be performed, and a stent is placed in the artery. Research has shown that both carotid artery stenting and carotid endarterectomy are performed in order to prevent stroke rather than in acute stroke treatment.[22]

Following carotid stenting, there is a risk for stroke and hyperperfusion syndrome. Postprocedure, the nurse monitors the patient's neurologic status and assesses the groin site for bleeding and hematoma formation.

Additional options under study and potentially on the treatment horizon for stroke patients include therapeutic hypothermia. Hyperthermia after a stroke has a direct correlation with additional neuronal death and further neurologic deficits. Aggressive control of fever (aggressive normothermia) in the stroke patient may be accomplished using acetaminophen as well as convective and conductive cooling devices. Therapeutic hypothermia has been studied after cardiac arrest and is under study poststroke for neuroprotection. Pharmacologic neuroprotective agents are being studied with no clear benefit obtained at this stage.[22]

**INTRACEREBRAL HEMORRHAGIC STROKE.** Intracerebral hemorrhagic (ICH) stroke is a potentially devastating consequence of cerebrovascular disease. It may occur, as noted earlier, consequent to cerebral aneurysm or AVM rupture. It may also occur consequent to prolonged hemodynamic stress within arterial vessels in the brain parenchyma. With vessel rupture, blood, under arterial pressure, flows from a high-pressure arterial system into the low-pressure system of the intracranial space and brain parenchyma. Expanding hematoma formation acts as a space-occupying lesion, displacing internal structures and promoting brain edema as an additional mechanism of injury. Additionally, if hemorrhage extends to the ventricles or causes obstruction of CSF pathways, obstructive or communicating hydrocephalus may result. Figure 35-7, a CT scan of the brain, shows a severe ICH stroke with resulting hematoma formation and progressive displacement of intracranial structures.

Intracerebral hemorrhage accounts for 8% to 13% of all strokes. The 30-day mortality rate for hemorrhagic stroke is 44%. Those with brainstem intracerebral hemorrhage show a 75% mortality rate within the first 24 hours.[32] In addition

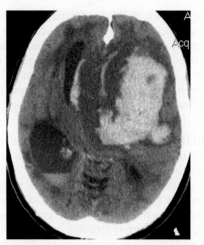

**FIGURE 35-7** Large hypertensive hemorrhagic stroke. CT of head illustrating expanding hematoma with mass effect, brain edema, displacement of brain structures with midline shift and hemorrhage extending into the ventricular system. (Courtesy of Richard Arbour, MSN, RN, FAAN, Albert Einstein Healthcare Network, Philadelphia, PA.)

to aneurysmal and AVM hemorrhage, ICH may be caused by coagulopathies, vasculitis, and abuse of cocaine or other sympathomimetic drugs.[32] Clinical assessment findings are determined by location of hemorrhage and affected vessel watershed within the brain as well as degree and rate of ICP elevation.[32] Diagnostics include clinical neurologic examination and CT of the brain. Based on clinical state and LOC, airway control and ICU admission may be necessary for aggressive, mechanism-based care.[32]

Aggressive, mechanism-based care for managing ICH may include airway control and mechanical ventilation to prevent hypercarbia. Controlled ventilation may also be utilized for short-term hyperventilation (PaCO$_2$ 25 to 30 mm Hg) to modulate CBF in the short term only while other therapies for ICP control are being maximized. Osmotic diuresis with agents, such as mannitol or hypertonic saline solution, may be utilized to draw water from edematous brain tissue. Ventricular drainage may be utilized to remove CSF and decrease ICP as well as provide an ICP monitoring device. Metabolic suppression using drugs such as sedatives/analgesics, propofol or barbiturates decreases brain metabolism, blood flow and ICP in a dose-related manner.[32] Surgical intervention, as clinically appropriate, for clot removal as well as aggressive BP control may be utilized.[8,32]

### Nursing Management

**ASSESSMENT.** A thorough neurologic assessment is essential to identify deficits the patient is experiencing. As previously discussed, the NIHSS is a valuable tool that can be used in the emergency department to rate severity of the stroke and determine whether the patient is a candidate for t-PA (see Box 35-2). The brevity and reliability of the tool make it ideal for use in the emergency department. The NIHSS is also helpful for making subsequent assessments and should be performed in conjunction with the neurologic examination.

As a member of a large multidisciplinary team, the nurse must be prepared to assume a critical role to assist with the administration of thrombolytic therapy, optimize acute patient care, and move the patient to rehabilitation quickly to maximize the patient's opportunity for an improved outcome. The nurse is in the unique position to identify problems and collaborate with the physician to initiate appropriate referrals to rehabilitation medicine specialists, social workers, speech-language pathologists, and dietitians. Because of the nature of the patient's problems, the multidisciplinary approach provides comprehensive care by addressing all needs.

In addition, the nurse must carefully monitor the patient for infection, changes in temperature, and changes in glucose level, all of which have potentially deleterious effects in people who have had a stroke. Hyperglycemia in acute stroke patients increases cerebral infarction size and worsens neurologic outcomes with and without preexisting diabetes mellitus. In a critical care unit, the upper limit of glycemic control should be 110 mg/dL. Strict glycemic control in the intensive care setting may be achieved with a continuous insulin infusion or sliding-scale regimen.

**PLAN.** The nurse plays a significant role in preventing complications associated with immobility, hemiparesis, or any neurologic deficit produced by a stroke. Preventive measures are particularly important in the areas of urinary tract infections, aspiration, pressure ulcers, contractures, and thrombophlebitis. Patients in critical care units are at risk for DVT and its resultant complications. Mechanical prophylactic measures for DVT prevention include range-of-motion exercises, antiembolism stockings, and pneumatic compression devices. Additionally, pharmacologic measures such as unfractionated heparin, low-molecular-weight heparin, or warfarin may be ordered to prevent blood coagulability. Effective interventions for treating acute stroke help lower the mortality rate and reduce the morbidity of patients who have had a stroke. The Collaborative Care Guide (Box 35-3) delineates the specific outcomes and interventions for the patient who has had a stroke.

**EMOTIONAL AND BEHAVIORAL MODIFICATION.** Patients who have experienced a stroke may display emotional problems, and their behavior may be different from baseline. Emotions may be labile without explanation or control. Tolerance to stress may also be reduced. A minor stressor in the prestroke state may be perceived as a major problem after the stroke. Families may not understand the behavior. Patients may show frustration or agitation with the nursing staff or their family members.

It is the nurse's role to help the family understand these behavioral changes. The nurse can help modify the patient's behavior by controlling stimuli in the environment, providing rest periods throughout the day to prevent fatigue, giving positive feedback, and providing repetition when the patient is trying to relearn a skill.

**COMMUNICATION.** Patients can demonstrate much frustration with their deficits. Probably no deficit produces more frustration for the patient and those trying to communicate with him or her than the one involving the production and understanding of language. Dysphasia can involve motor abilities, sensory function, or both. If the area of brain injury is in or near the left Broca area, the memory of motor patterns of speech is affected. This results in an expressive or nonfluent dysphasia, in which the patient understands language but is unable to use it appropriately.

**QSEN BOX 35-3** *COLLABORATIVE CARE GUIDE for the Patient Who Has Experienced a Stroke*

| Outcomes | Interventions |
|---|---|
| **Impaired Gas Exchange** **Ineffective Breathing Pattern** | |
| Adequate airway is maintained. Oxygen saturation (SpO₂) is maintained within normal limits. Atelectasis is prevented. | • Monitor breath sounds every shift. • Check oxygen saturation every shift. • Instruct to cough and deep-breathe and use incentive spirometry every 2 hours while awake. • Assist with removal of airway secretions as needed. |
| **Risk for Decreased Cardiac Tissue Perfusion** **Risk for Decreased Cardiac Output** | |
| Patient is free of dysrhythmias. | • Monitor vital signs closely. • Manage BP carefully; avoid sharp drops in BP that could result in hypotension and cause an ischemic event secondary to hypotension. • During cardiac monitoring, identify dysrhythmias. • Treat dysrhythmias to maintain adequate perfusion pressure and reduce chance of neurologic impairment. |
| **Risk for Inadequate Cerebral Tissue Perfusion** **Risk for Impaired Verbal Communication** | |
| Adequate perfusion pressure is maintained. | • Obtain vital signs and perform a neurologic assessment to establish a baseline and to monitor for the development of additional deficits. • Use the NIHSS for detection of early changes suggesting cerebral edema or extension of stroke. • Position head of bed at 30 degrees to promote venous drainage. |
| Effective communication is established. | • Assess ability to speak and to follow simple commands. • Arrange for consultation with speech-language pathologist to differentiate language disturbances. • Use communication aids such as picture cards, pantomime, erase board, or computer to enhance communication. • Provide a calm, unrushed environment. Listen attentively to the patient. Speak in a normal tone. |
| **Risk for Imbalanced Fluid Volume** **Risk for Electrolyte Imbalance** | |
| Electrolytes are within normal limits. | • Monitor laboratory results, especially glucose. • Monitor intake and output. |
| **Risk for Impaired Physical Mobility** **Risk for Falls** **Risk for Injury** | |
| Safety is maintained. Complications of immobility are avoided. | • Initiate DVT precautions to include TED hose, sequential compressive devices, and subcutaneous heparin, as ordered. • Perform fall risk assessment. • Consult with physical therapy. • Provide active or passive range-of-motion exercises to all extremities every shift. • Establish splinting routine for affected limbs. • Instruct in use of mobility aids and fall prevention strategies. • For visual field cuts, teach scanning techniques. |
| **Risk for Impaired Skin Integrity** | |
| Skin is intact. | • Perform skin assessment using the Braden scale. • Provide pressure relief mattress as indicated by Braden scale. • Turn and reposition patient every 2 hours. • Consult with wound nurse specialist for skin issues and concerns. |
| **Imbalanced Nutrition** | |
| Patient has adequate caloric intake and does not experience decrease in weight from baseline. Patient is free from aspiration. | • Obtain admission weight. • Perform cranial nerve assessment (including ability to swallow) to identify deficits. • Obtain consultation from speech-language pathologist to determine whether patient is safe to eat orally. • Provide proper diet and assist with feeding as needed. • Monitor calorie intake; implement calorie count, if necessary. • Obtain dietary consultation to obtain recommendation for nutritional supplements. |
| **Ineffective Coping** | |
| Support network is established. | • Use picture boards or aids to facilitate communication. • Assess for family support systems. • Screen for poststroke depression. |
| **Teaching/Discharge Planning** | |
| Risk factors are modified. Secondary preventive measures have been taken. | • Provide education about BP management. • Provide dietary instructions. |

**TABLE 35-7**  Comparison of Expressive and Receptive Dysphasia

| Expressive Dysphasia | Receptive Dysphasia |
| --- | --- |
| Hemiparesis is present because motor cortex is near Broca's area. | Hemiparesis is mild or absent because lesion is not near motor cortex. |
| | Hemianopsia or quadrantanopsia may be present. |
| Speech is slow, nonfluent; articulation is poor; speaking requires much effort. Total speech is reduced in quantity. Patient may use telegraphic speech, omitting small words. | Speech is fluent; articulation and rhythm are normal. Content of speech is impaired; wrong words are used. |
| Patient understands written and verbal speech. | Patient does not understand written and verbal speech. |
| Patient writes dysphasically. | Content of writing is abnormal. Penmanship may be good. |
| Patient may be able to repeat single words with effort. Phrase repetition is poor. | Repetition is poor. |
| Object naming is often poor, but it may be better than attempts to use spontaneous speech. | Object naming is poor. |
| Patient is aware of deficit, often experiencing frustration and depression. | Patient is often unaware of deficit. |
| Curses or other ejaculatory speech may be well articulated and automatic. Patient may be able to hum normally. | Patient may use wrong words and sounds. |

Receptive or fluent dysphasia usually is a result of injury to the left Wernicke area, which is the control center for recognition of spoken language. The patient therefore is unable to understand the meaning of the spoken word (and usually the written word). Having both expressive and receptive dysphasia is referred to as global dysphasia. Table 35-7 summarizes differences between expressive and receptive problems.

It is important for the nursing staff to inform families that having dysphasia does not mean that a person is intellectually impaired. Communication at some level should be attempted, whether it is by writing, using picture boards, or gesturing.

**PATIENT EDUCATION AND DISCHARGE PLANNING.** Education provides information to patients about modifying risk factors and teaches people to recognize the signs and symptoms of a stroke. Information can be presented regarding medication and other lifestyle modifications to manage BP. Patients can be referred to smoking cessation programs. Teaching about glucose control, weight management, and exercise programs is also valuable. Compliance with medication regimens should be stressed as well.

A stroke is often a life-altering experience for the patient and family. Depending on the outcome, family members may require education about how to provide care for the patient at home. Instruction about mobility, nutrition, safety, sleep, and eliminative care must occur, along with referrals for home care, if appropriate. With support, the patient will be able to achieve maximal quality of life and reintegrate into the community.

## Seizures

A seizure is an episode of abnormal and excessive discharge of cerebral neurons. It can result in altered sensory, motor, or behavioral activities and can be associated with changes in the LOC. Specific symptoms depend on the location of the discharge in the brain. Some seizures are so mild that only the patient is aware of them. Others are quite severe. The actual period of the seizure (the ictal period) may be followed by a postictal phase of lethargy and disorientation, which varies with the severity of the seizure.

Epilepsy is a condition in which seizures are spontaneous and recurrent. Status epilepticus is defined as a condition of either continued seizure activity or repetitive seizures without interictal recovery, over a period exceeding 30 minutes. Status epilepticus can be associated with tonic–clonic, complex–partial, or absence seizures. It is a neurologic emergency and requires immediate treatment.[33–35]

Psychogenic nonepileptic seizures, which emulate epileptic seizures, are events that involve either motor activity or physical collapse.[35] Pseudoseizures can often be clinically differentiated from epilepsy because they may involve asymmetrical motor activity, side-to-side head movements, and purposeful activity. They also may be gradual in onset. The motor activity can last for many minutes, unlike epilepsy. There is usually a brief or no "postictal" phase. Patients, who are likely to have either emotional or psychological disorders, may require antidepressants, counseling, and psychiatric intervention. In about 20% of cases, patients also suffer from true epilepsy. Childhood abuse is not uncommon in these patients, although the episodes are usually signs of abnormal coping and can have many causes.

### Etiology

Many generalized seizures may have a genetic basis and are termed "idiopathic" or primary seizures. They have no specific underlying cause. Symptomatic or secondary seizures have a known cause.[35]

Idiopathic seizures account for about 50% of all epileptic seizures. They occur most often in children younger than 10 years. Congenital and genetic causes of epilepsy are seen in approximately 10% of the population. Although inherited epilepsy is more often idiopathic, it is also associated with other conditions.[35]

Symptomatic seizures have numerous causes, including vascular disease, alcohol, cerebral tumors, trauma, infection or fever, metabolic disturbances, anoxia, and degenerative diseases. Developmental abnormalities, such as cortical dysgenesis (abnormal development of the cerebral cortex), are common causes of childhood-onset epilepsy.[1,34]

A number of other variables affect seizure frequency and intensity. Fatigue and sleep deprivation may lower the seizure threshold.[1] Emotional and physical stresses correlate with seizure onset but are difficult to quantify. Many women who keep records of seizure activity discover that they are cyclic, occurring more frequently or increasing in severity during menstruation, pregnancy, or menopause. Alcohol and drug abuse as well as electrolyte disturbances cause seizures and may provoke epileptic seizures.[34,35] Many medications have the effect of lowering seizure threshold, although most patients with controlled epilepsy on medications are not affected. Patients keeping a diary of seizure activity, warning signs, and any precipitating factors, such as sleep deprivation or emotional upset, may potentially lead to effective preventive treatment.[1]

Common causes of new-onset status epilepticus are cerebrovascular disease, brain tumors, intracranial infections, fevers, head trauma, and metabolic disorders. Status epilepticus is also associated with drug withdrawal, metabolic disturbances, or concurrent illness in patients with known epilepsy.[35]

## Epidemiology

Approximately 200,000 new cases of seizure occur each year. Between 40% and 50% of those will recur and be classified as epilepsy. Infants and young children are most likely to experience seizures, followed by elderly people.[1,33] Populations in developing countries are at greater risk for seizures or epilepsy, probably because of compromised hygiene, poor nutrition, increased risk for infection, and the high percentage of children. Single seizures are much less common than epileptic seizures (epilepsy or seizure disorder) (20 per 100,000 versus 50 per 100,000, respectively). Five percent of patients who develop epilepsy present with status epilepticus. Of epileptic seizures, partial seizures account for approximately 57%, and generalized seizures account for 40%. Medical treatment completely controls seizures in approximately 70% of patients.

## Pathophysiology

Nerve cells (neurons) in the brain possess an electrical charge that reflects a balance between intracellular and extracellular charged ions. The electrical activity of the neuronal membrane is determined by the flow of ions between these spaces. Ions, such as sodium ($Na^+$), potassium ($K^+$), calcium ($Ca^{2+}$), and chloride ($Cl^-$), are regulated by receptor channels and flow across the membrane when receptors are activated by voltage changes and neurotransmitter modulation. If the permeability of the cells is altered, their excitability can change, making the neuron more likely to discharge. Hyperexcitability can result in increased random neuronal firing. When this is combined with a certain pattern of neuronal firing (synchronization), epileptogenic properties in the neuron exist.[33,34]

Although it is not known exactly how the mechanisms of abnormal neuronal excitation and synchronization lead to epileptiform activity, continued exploration of cell membrane activity, environmental variables, and pharmacologic responses has led to increased understanding and management of epilepsy.

## Clinical Manifestations

Clinical features of epilepsy are based on the location of the epileptiform discharge and the type of event.[33,34] Box 35-4 describes specific seizures and resulting clinical characteristics.

---

**BOX 35-4** | **Classification of Seizure Types**

1. **Generalized:** involves both hemispheres; loss of consciousness; no local onset in the cerebrum
   a. *Tonic-clonic* (grand-mal)—loss of consciousness; stiffening; forced expiration (cry); rhythmic jerking
   b. *Clonic*—symmetrical, bilateral semirhythmic jerking
   c. *Tonic*—sudden increased tone and forced expiration
   d. *Myoclonic*—sudden, brief body jerks
   e. *Atonic* ("drop attacks")—sudden loss of tone; falls
   f. *Absence* (petit mal)—brief staring, usually without motor involvement
2. **Partial:** involves one hemisphere
   a. *Simple partial seizure*—no change in LOC, Jacksonian
      i. Motor—frontal lobe
      ii. Somatosensory—parietal lobe
      iii. Visual—occipital lobe
      iv. May involve: autonomic (eg, respiratory changes, tachycardia, flushing); psychic (eg, déjà vu); cognitive (without change in LOC)
   b. *Complex partial seizures*—altered LOC; with or without automatisms: lip smacking, swallowing, aimless walking, verbalizations
      i. Simple partial followed by change in LOC
      ii. Starts with change in consciousness
      iii. Typically of temporal lobe origin
   c. Partial with secondary generalization
      i. Simple partial generalization
      ii. Complex partial generalization
      iii. Simple partial complex partial generalization
      iv. Continuous EEG monitoring may be necessary to differentiate from generalized seizures
3. **Unclassified**

---

## Diagnosis

The patient who presents with a seizure is initially evaluated to ascertain the cause of the seizure and establish a diagnosis of epilepsy.[1,36] History taking begins with a description of the event by the patient or witnesses. This description should include the following:

1. What the patient was doing at the time of the seizure
2. Duration of the episode
3. Unusual symptoms or behaviors before the seizure
4. Specific features, including movements, sensations, sounds, tastes, smells, and incontinence
5. LOC during and after the event
6. Duration and description of symptoms after the seizure
7. Reporting of any similar previous episodes and age of onset

Inquiry should be made about the following:

1. Sleep patterns
2. Alcohol or drug abuse
3. History of illnesses or injuries
4. Family seizure history
5. Other possible variables: menstrual cycle, stress, fevers, metabolic disorders
6. If other seizures have occurred, similarities in symptoms, duration, frequency, and time of day

After the first seizure occurrence, a CT scan or MRI is obtained to assess for a structural lesion. An EEG is obtained to screen for interictal seizure discharges (electrical abnormalities present in between seizures) and to measure cerebral excitability. These techniques can help determine whether the seizures have focal origins or are more generalized. During the EEG, scalp electrodes are placed to measure neuronal membrane activity in the underlying cerebral cortex. Rhythms may be obtained when the patient is both awake and asleep. The EEG localizes the region from which the patient's seizure arises at one time point.[36,37]

If additional information regarding seizure patterns and characteristics is needed, an inpatient hospital stay may be recommended in an epilepsy monitoring unit, as discussed in the following section. Also, continuous EEG monitoring is now being used in the ICU, where it has helped identify subtle seizures in critically ill patients. Because it is not uncommon for these patients (eg, brain injured or comatose patients) to suffer nonconvulsive seizures, use of EEG is becoming more widespread in the ICU.[35,36]

### Epilepsy Monitoring Unit

Patients who require more detailed seizure characterization or localization are admitted for video EEG monitoring to an appropriate unit, where scalp electrodes are placed. Video EEG monitoring is continuous and involves audiovisual observations. Monitoring occurs while the patient is awake and asleep. Medication dosages may be slowly reduced or withdrawn during these observations. Because video EEG monitoring captures ictal, postictal, and interictal data, seizures are documented and localized, and the patient's clinical symptoms are observed. Video EEG can often localize seizures for possible epilepsy surgery. It is also very helpful for identifying pseudoseizures and other disorders that are mistaken for epileptic disorders. Neuropsychological and psychiatric evaluations may be part of the assessment, particularly if surgery is being anticipated.[1]

In situations in which localization is not obtained or is questionable, a more invasive approach using surgical electrodes to localize seizure activity may be necessary. Three different types of electrodes can be implanted for intracranial recording.

Depth electrodes are typically placed bilaterally, targeting the hippocampus and other common seizure sites in the amygdala and frontal lobes. Multiple electrodes are placed under local or general anesthesia through twist drill or burr holes for simultaneous recording. The electrode cables exit the skull, and patients have continuous video monitoring over several days in the epilepsy monitoring unit. Hemorrhage, headache, and infection are possible complications. This procedure is most often used to show which regions are involved at seizure onset.[37]

Subdural and epidural electrodes are typically placed unilaterally, under general anesthesia. Strips are placed through burr holes. Grids require a craniotomy and allow for a larger region to be monitored (Fig. 35-8). They are secured to the dura, and the electrode leads exit through an incision for continuous monitoring. Infection, hemorrhage, and mass effect from cerebral edema are possible risks. The bone flap can be replaced at the end of the procedure or after the strips or grids are removed. Intracranial monitoring may be initiated before seizure surgery.[37]

### Clinical Management

**PHARMACOLOGIC MANAGEMENT.** In most cases, the patient with epilepsy can be treated medically. Certain AEDs are known to be more appropriate for specific classes

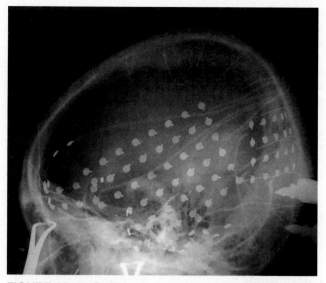

**FIGURE 35-8** Radiograph of a grid for seizure monitoring. (Courtesy of Frederick Lenz, MD and Ira Garonzik, MD, The Johns Hopkins University, Baltimore, MD.)

of seizures. Some AEDs are preferred as monotherapy, and others are more appropriate as adjunctive therapy with other drugs.[33]

Status epilepticus is an emergency situation and requires rapid pharmacologic management. Parenteral drugs are given to provide fast absorption. Drugs are given intravenously or intramuscularly. In emergent circumstances benzodiazepines such as diazepam (Valium) may be administered rectally in an emergency in the absence of intravenous access.[33] Many fast-acting drugs are lipid soluble and have a tendency to redistribute from the plasma to the fat and muscle, thereby leading to an initial drop in blood and brain concentrations. This may lead to seizure recurrences. Repeat boluses or a continuous infusion must be administered judiciously because the drugs saturate fat, and muscle and plasma levels will increase. This may result in prolonged decreased mental status, obtundation, and even death. Although seizure related mortality is low the risk of injury is greater than in the general population with the most common injuries being to the face and neck.[34] Emergency management of status epilepticus is summarized in Box 35-5.

**SURGICAL MANAGEMENT.** There are situations in which AEDs are unable to control epilepsy. Attempts at monotherapy and adjunctive therapy have been exhausted and multiple drug regimens have failed; seizure activity has compromised a patient's quality of life. In these cases, seizures are intractable, and surgery is considered to obtain seizure control. It may also be considered in situations in which the side effects of therapy are so debilitating that the patient is unable to function at an acceptable capacity.[34]

In many cases, the patient is monitored before surgery in an epilepsy monitoring unit using a video EEG. Surgery for grid or strip placement to localize seizure focus and identify functional areas is often performed. After surgery, the nurse performs regular, intermittent neurologic examinations and has the patient attempt to perform certain tasks. Language deficits and motor weakness are observed. The goals of this procedure are to localize epileptiform discharges in relation

**BOX 35-5** **Emergency Treatment of Status Epilepticus**

**Goals:** maintain airway, breathing, circulation; stop seizures; stabilize patient; identify and treat cause

**Treatment:** airway; $O_2$; intubation, if necessary; EEG monitoring; monitor ECG and BP; catheter for incontinence; CT scan; lumbar puncture if CNS infection is suspected; CPR if needed

**Blood work:** electrolytes; magnesium; calcium; anticonvulsant levels; blood gases; complete blood count; renal and liver function studies; coagulation studies; toxicology studies may be needed

**Medications:**
- Benzodiazepines (lorazepam, 1 to 2 mg/min as a starting dose over 8 minutes or diazepam to total of 20 mg). These are short-acting drugs, and simultaneous loading with phenytoin at 50 mg/min or fosphenytoin at equivalent of 150 mg phenytoin/min is necessary; may total 20 mg/kg
- For persistent seizures, add 5 to 10 mg/kg phenytoin *or* phenobarbital at 50 to 100 mg/min to total of 20 mg/kg
- If ineffective, barbiturate anesthesia: pentobarbital and intubation. Benzodiazepines (eg, midazolam) may be attempted prior to barbiturate anesthesia. Continuous EEG monitoring in ICU environment.

**TABLE 35-8** **Clinical Applications of Seizure Surgery**

| Procedure | Indications |
|---|---|
| **Temporal lobectomy:** removal of 6 cm of temporal lobe in the nondominant hemisphere and 4–5 cm in the dominant hemisphere | Intractable anterior—temporal lobe—seizures >5 y duration<br>Significant quality-of-life compromise |
| **Lesionectomy:** surgical removal of structural anomalies | Pediatric patients |
| **Vagal nerve stimulator:** implanted programmable signal generator in the chest with stimulating electrodes to the left vagus nerve | Refractory to medication<br>Often partial seizures |
| **Deep brain stimulator:** Electrodes placed in deep brain structures (thalamus, hippocampus, internal capsule) and programmed to activate when seizure activity is recorded | Uncontrolled epilepsy |

Data from Ko DY: Epilepsy and seizures. Medscape. Updated November 19, 2015. Retrieved January 15, 2016, from http://emedicine.medscape.com/article/1184846-print.

to speech, memory, and sensory or motor function. It is also useful in identifying the relationship between seizure discharges and a focal lesion, such as a tumor, when present. This enhances the safety and accuracy of tumor surgery.[34,37]

The decision to proceed with surgery depends on a thorough discussion among the multidisciplinary team members. The neurologist, neurosurgeon, patient, and family review the medical treatment used to date and establish that therapy has been maximized. They evaluate the likelihood of seizure control with surgery. Preoperative neuropsychological testing is obtained, and other appropriate testing is established and discussed. Some or all of the diagnostic studies previously outlined may be indicated.

The goal of seizure surgery is to remove or disrupt the seizure focus. Patients are often maintained on AEDs for 2 years postoperatively because seizure recurrence is most likely during this period. Table 35-8 summarizes the most commonly performed surgical procedures and indications for these procedures.

### Nursing Management

**ASSESSMENT.** Careful history taking is a central component of the accurate diagnosis and management of epilepsy. Family history, age at onset, frequency, and a description of symptoms and their duration all aid in the development of a plan of care tailored to the patient's particular situation. AEDs are prescribed based on all these data. Changes in severity or frequency of symptoms require modification of the treatment regimen. Drug therapy may last indefinitely; therefore, treatment should address both efficacy and tolerability. Side effects can compromise quality of life, necessitating the use of different, and possibly less effective, medications or multiple AEDs.[1,34]

**PLAN.** Inpatient nursing care includes monitoring the patient during the seizure (the patient is never left alone) and providing support and protection without attempting to restrain the individual. Turning the patient to his or her side during a generalized seizure, if possible, helps maintain a patent airway.

**PATIENT EDUCATION AND DISCHARGE PLANNING.** Patient education should provide instructions for independent functioning. The following patient education points are critical parts of discharge planning:

1. Make the home environment safe, particularly in the case of tonic–clonic epilepsy.
2. Assess for injury after each seizure.
3. Keep a log to record a description of the seizure and postictal period, duration, time of day, severity, and any new characteristics.
4. Be aware of state laws on driving restrictions related to epilepsy.
5. Wear a medical identification bracelet.
6. Monitor serum AED levels when appropriate.
7. Be aware of circumstances when emergency treatment is required.
8. Consult seizure experts for intractable epilepsy.

## Guillain–Barré Syndrome

Guillain–Barré syndrome, also known as acute inflammatory demyelinating polyneuropathy, is a rapidly evolving illness that commonly presents as symmetrical weakness, sensory loss, and areflexia. This condition is an inflammatory peripheral neuropathy in which lymphocytes and macrophages strip myelin from axons. The diffuse inflammatory reaction may be seen in the peripheral nervous system, cranial nerves, and spinal nerve roots. It is referred to as a syndrome, as opposed to a disease, because of the combination of signs and symptoms seen in the patient.[38]

### Etiology

Guillain–Barré syndrome is an immune-mediated neuropathy that is associated with a broad range of symptoms, severity, and length of progression. This disorder follows an antecedent infection in some patients.[38–41] Approximately half of the people in whom Guillain–Barré syndrome develops have a mild febrile illness 2 to 3 weeks before the onset of symptoms. The febrile infection is usually respiratory or GI. *Campylobacter jejuni* and cytomegalovirus are causes of the most frequent antecedent infections, which usually occur 1 to 4 weeks before the onset of symptoms of Guillain–Barré syndrome.[38,39,41] Some studies show a potential association between vaccinations and increased risk of Guillain–Barré syndrome.[41] Although previously administered vaccinations, including H1N1 and rabies vaccines, have been linked to the development of Guillain–Barré syndrome,[41] a strong causal relationship has not been demonstrated. Currently, no recent vaccine has been conclusively demonstrated to induce the disease.

The attack on the immune system is extensive and occurs proximally at the nerve roots and distally at the motor axon terminal. Both cellular and humoral immune mechanisms appear to be implicated. Lymphocytes and macrophages are the effector cells that result in damage to myelin and adjacent axons. Motor, sensory, and autonomic nerves are involved. Weakness and sensory disturbances result from blockage of nerve fiber action potentials (secondary to demyelination or axon damage).[38,40,41]

In affected patients, the immune system most likely is first primed as it responds to a virus or bacteria. Then, the immune system inappropriately attacks host tissue that shares an epitope (surface portion of an antigen capable of triggering an immune response). This process is referred to as molecular mimicry.[41]

### Epidemiology

Guillain–Barré syndrome occurs with equal frequency in both sexes and all races. It can develop at any age. The annual incidence is approximately 1 to 2 cases per 100,000 population in the United States.[38,40,41]

### Pathophysiology

In Guillain–Barré syndrome, the myelin sheath surrounding the axon is lost. The myelin sheath is susceptible to injury by many agents and conditions, including physical trauma, hypoxemia, toxic chemicals, vascular insufficiency, and immunologic reactions. Demyelination is a common response of neural tissue to any of these adverse conditions.[38,40,41]

Myelinated axons conduct nerve impulses more rapidly than unmyelinated axons. Along the course of a myelinated fiber are interruptions in the sheath (nodes of Ranvier), where there is direct contact between the cell membrane of the axon and the extracellular fluid. The membrane is highly permeable at these nodes, resulting in especially good conduction. The movement of ions into and out of the axon can occur rapidly only at the nodes of Ranvier; therefore, a nerve impulse along a myelinated fiber may jump from node to node (known as saltatory conduction) quite rapidly. Loss of the myelin sheath makes saltatory conduction impossible, and nerve impulse transmission is aborted.[40–42]

A current theory regarding the disease process of Guillain–Barré syndrome speculates that a primary lymphocytic T-cell mechanism is the cause of the inflammation. Cells migrate through the vessel walls to the peripheral nerve. The result is edema and perivascular inflammation. Macrophages then break down the myelin.[40,41] A potential secondary process is that demyelination is initiated by an antibody attack on the myelin early in the course of the disease. Demyelination causes axon atrophy, which results in slowed or blocked nerve conduction.[41]

### Clinical Manifestations

Guillain–Barré syndrome may develop rapidly over the course of hours or days, or it may take up to 3 to 4 weeks to develop. Most patients demonstrate the greatest weakness in the first weeks of the disorder and are weakest by the third week of the illness.[38,39,41]

In the beginning, a flaccid, ascending paralysis develops quickly. The patient is most commonly affected in a symmetrical pattern. The patient may first notice weakness in the lower extremities that may quickly extend to include weakness and abnormal sensations in the arms. Deep tendon reflexes are usually lost, even in the earliest stages. The trunk and cranial nerves may become involved. Respiratory muscles can become affected, resulting in respiratory compromise.[38,39,41] Autonomic disturbances such as urinary retention and orthostatic hypotension may also occur. Some patients experience tenderness and pain on deep pressure or movement of some muscles.[38,41]

Sensory symptoms of paresthesias, including numbness and tingling, may occur. Pain is a complaint in many patients. It is aching in nature and often compared with the feeling of muscles that have been overexerted. If there is cranial nerve involvement, cranial nerve VII, the facial nerve, is most often affected. Guillain–Barré syndrome does not affect LOC, pupillary function, or cognitive functioning.[38,41]

Symptoms may progress for several weeks. The level of paralysis may stop at any point. Progression usually occurs in three stages: acute, plateau, and recovery. The acute stage starts at the onset of symptoms and rapidly progresses until no additional deterioration occurs. The plateau stage, during which patients are symptomatic, lasts for a few days up to a few weeks. The recovery phase can take up to 2 years. It is thought that the recovery phase coincides with remyelination and axonal regeneration. Although demyelination occurs rapidly, the rate of remyelination is approximately 1 to 2 mm/d. Motor function returns in a descending fashion.[38,41]

### Diagnosis

The diagnosis of Guillain–Barré syndrome depends greatly on the patient's history and clinical progression of symptoms. As noted, onset is usually sudden, and the history often reveals an upper respiratory or GI disorder occurring 1 to 4 weeks before onset of the neurologic manifestations. The history of the onset of symptoms can be revealing because symptoms of Guillain–Barré syndrome usually begin with weakness or paresthesias of the lower extremities and ascend in a symmetrical pattern.[38,40,41]

A lumbar puncture may be performed and reveals increased protein. However, negative results from this test should be interpreted cautiously because only 50% of patients in the first week of illness have increased protein. By 3 weeks, this percentage increases to greater than 90%. Also, nerve conduction studies record impulse transmission along the nerve fiber. In the patient with Guillain–Barré syndrome, the velocity of conduction is reduced.[38,40,41]

Pulmonary function tests are performed when Guillain–Barré syndrome is suspected to establish a baseline for comparison as the disease progresses. Declining pulmonary function capacity may indicate the need for mechanical ventilation and management in an ICU.[38,41] Severe respiratory failure consequent to Guillain–Barré syndrome requiring mechanical ventilation is a predictor of mortality in the hospitalized patient.

## Clinical Management

Because of the risks associated with respiratory failure, bulbar symptoms, and autonomic dysfunction, all patients with Guillain–Barré syndrome, except those with mild disease, should be admitted to a hospital that has specialized ICUs. Progression to mechanical ventilation is expected in patients with rapid disease progression, bulbar involvement, bilateral facial weakness, or dysautonomia. ICU admission is recommended for patients with vital capacity below 20 mL/kg, vital capacity checks that are required more than every 4 hours, aspiration, autonomic instability, or rapid progression or weakness.[38,41]

Certain strategies can lessen the severity of the illness and hasten recovery. A useful clinical sign of respiratory compromise is the strength of the neck flexor muscles. When the head cannot be lifted against gravity, the phrenic nerves are also affected, causing diaphragm paralysis and reduction of the forced vital capacity (FVC) the amount of air a patient can forcefully exhale after maximal inhalation. Under these circumstances, the airway cannot be successfully managed without intubation.

Preventive measures need to be established so that DVT and subsequent PE do not develop. DVT prophylaxis includes subcutaneous heparin, 5,000 units twice daily, along with antiembolism stockings and sequential compression devices. Also, autonomic nervous system fluctuations need to be evaluated by checking BP and monitoring for cardiac dysrhythmias.[38,41]

Plasmapheresis was the first therapy proved to benefit patients with Guillain–Barré syndrome. It is the only therapy that has been proved superior to supportive treatment alone. This procedure mechanically removes humoral factors. Currently, it is recommended that patients with Guillain–Barré syndrome receive plasmapheresis. A dual-lumen central vascular access device and trained team specialists are needed to perform the plasmapheresis treatments. The physician may order plasmapheresis when the patient's condition is worsening in an attempt to reduce the severity of the disease.[38,39,41] Of note, two prominent risks associated with plasmapheresis are catheter-related infections and hemorrhage during catheter placement.

Intravenous immunoglobulin (IVIG) is also useful in managing Guillain–Barré syndrome. A blood product that has been derived from large pools of plasma donors, IVIG has the potential to bind many common pathogens and modulate a wide range of effectors in autoimmune disease, such as Guillain–Barré syndrome. The major component is immunoglobulin G, with a trace amount of immunoglobulin A. Immunoglobulins can be infused easily, even in the home setting, without expensive equipment. The optimal dosages and frequency of administration are individualized. Immunoglobulin, which binds to receptors on T cells or receptors on nerves, induces only a temporary improvement because of the turnover of T cells or the loss of antibodies from the receptors. Daily treatments with IVIG may be helpful in acute Guillain–Barré syndrome when the patient is rapidly deteriorating.[38,40,41]

The dose of IVIG is set at 2 g/kg, and usually the total dose is divided into five daily infusions of 400 mg/kg each. Neurologists who use IVIG for Guillain–Barré syndrome are familiar with the side effects, which include low-grade fever, chills, myalgia, diaphoresis, fluid overload, hypertension, nausea, vomiting, rash, headaches, aseptic meningitis, and neutropenia.[38,41] The most serious adverse effect is acute tubular necrosis, which occurs with any concomitant disease that compromises renal glomerular filtration.

Currently, there are no efficacy data that favor IVIG rather than plasmapheresis in managing Guillain–Barré syndrome. IVIG and plasma exchange have a similar ability to speed a patient's recovery. The individual patient's circumstances, such as availability of resources to perform plasmapheresis and underlying medical conditions, dictate the specific treatment for each patient. IVIG is an attractive treatment because it can be easily administered in the critical care setting.[38,41]

## Nursing Management

**ASSESSMENT.** For the patient with Guillain–Barré syndrome, careful assessment and the resultant plan help minimize the complications of immobility and move the patient toward rehabilitation without deficits. Although patients are critically ill, their chances of returning to a productive life are good if they survive the acute stages and avoid the complications of immobility. Most deaths are due to preventable respiratory complications or autonomic dysfunction.

Once Guillain–Barré syndrome is suspected, the patient is hospitalized so that frequent assessments can be performed to monitor the patient for deterioration. Because of the progressive nature of the disease, assessment should focus on the neurologic examination (ie, cranial nerve involvement, motor weakness, and sensory changes). Cranial nerve deficits identify if the patient is at risk for aspiration. The patient's motor and sensory function should be monitored frequently.[1]

Cardiovascular assessment is done to monitor BP and heart rate. The autonomic nervous system is frequently involved in Guillain–Barré syndrome. Dysautonomia manifests itself as sinus tachycardia but may result in other cardiac dysrhythmias or labile BPs that require close monitoring because they may be life-threatening. The patient's respiratory status should be monitored, and FVC should be assessed at least once every shift. GI and urinary function should come under surveillance as well. The patient is at risk for constipation and urinary tract infections resulting from urinary retention. Other complications of immobility are the potential for pressure ulcers and DVT.[38,39,41]

**PLAN.** When caring for a patient with Guillain–Barré syndrome, the major goals are to prevent infections and complications of immobility, provide functional maintenance of the body systems, treat life-threatening crises promptly, and provide psychological support for the patient and family. In terms of the patient's neurologic status, weakness results in impaired mobility.

Also, steps are taken to maintain proper body alignment. Measures such as splint placement are implemented to prevent wrist hyperflexion and footdrop.[1,38] Physical therapy is initiated early in the course of hospitalization and continued throughout the recovery period.

Cranial nerve involvement places the patient at risk for aspiration, and adequate nutrition must be maintained. If the patient is unable to take oral feedings, enteral tube feedings are initiated. A nutritional consultation with a registered dietitian should occur to provide adequate calories for remyelination as well as rehabilitation activities. Enteral nutritional support that supplies at least 1,500 to 2,000 kcal/d should be instituted if the patient is unable to receive food by mouth.[38,41]

Additionally, because of intubation or impaired verbal communication, alternate methods to facilitate communication are important. Alternate ways to communicate are established using communication boards as well as nonverbal means such as gestures and eye blinking. Inability to communicate can be frustrating for the patient and cause undue anxiety.

Respiratory failure is the most severe complication of Guillain–Barré syndrome. Weakened respiratory muscles put the patient at great risk for hypoventilation and repeated pulmonary infections. Fifty percent of patients with Guillain–Barré syndrome have some respiratory compromise, resulting in reduced tidal volume and vital capacity or perhaps complete respiratory arrest. A tracheostomy may be indicated if the patient requires long-term mechanical ventilation.[38]

If there is autonomic nervous system involvement, drastic changes in BP (hypotension or hypertension), heart rate, or both can occur. Labile hypertension and dysrhythmias occur frequently, prompting admission and management in the ICU. Cardiac monitoring allows quick identification and treatment of dysrhythmias. Because Valsalva maneuver, coughing, and suctioning may trigger an autonomic nervous system disturbance, the patient needs to be monitored closely.[38,41]

Comfort measures, such as frequent position changes, may be helpful. When remyelination occurs, it is often uncomfortable, and the patient may complain of numbness and pain. This can be an encouraging sign to the patient because the disease process is reversing.

Although the patient is incapacitated physically, he or she is fully aware of the surroundings. The patient may experience a sense of fear, loss of control, as well as helplessness and hopelessness. Frequent explanations of the interventions and of progress are useful.[1] The patient should be allowed to participate in care as much as functionally possible. It is essential that the nurse in the critical care setting provide empathy, compassion, sensitivity, and active listening to the patient with Guillain–Barré syndrome so that his or her emotional concerns can be addressed.

**PATIENT EDUCATION AND DISCHARGE PLANNING.** Education of the patient and family about all issues of care is important The nurse can provide information about the disease process, course, and recovery.[1] Patients need to know that the disease may progress to the point at which mechanical ventilation is required. In addition, they should understand that they may be discharged to a rehabilitation facility where recovery can continue. Many months of rehabilitation may be required for them to regain strength and previous level of functioning. Patients may continue to show improvement for up to 2 years. The nurse can tell patients and their families about the Guillain–Barré Syndrome International Foundation, which provides information and resources. Before discharge to home, the patient can be referred to resources for support so that he or she can interact with other people who have had Guillain–Barré syndrome.[1]

## Myasthenia Gravis

Myasthenia gravis is an autoimmune disorder of the neuromuscular junction transmission that presents with fatigue and muscle weakness in the ocular, bulbar, diaphragm, or limb muscles. Myasthenia is derived from the Greek words for "muscle" and "weakness," whereas gravis means "grave" in Latin. Because of the high mortality related to diaphragmatic muscle weakness, the disorder was called "grave muscle weakness."[1] However, myasthenia gravis is not a grave disease today because of advancements with immunomodulatory treatments and the ability to manage respiratory failure.

### Etiology

Myasthenia gravis is an autoimmune disorder characterized by weakness and fatigability of skeletal muscles. The disease involves a reduction in the number of acetylcholine receptors (AChRs) at the neuromuscular junction caused by antibodies against the AChR.[42-44] The factors that trigger the autoimmune process are not known, but the thymus gland plays an important role. The thymus gland lies behind the sternum and may extend down to the diaphragm and up to the neck. This gland plays a role in the responsiveness of T cells to foreign antigens. Most patients display abnormalities related to the thymus.[43]

### Epidemiology

Myasthenia gravis is seen more often in women than in men at a ratio of 3:2. It is primarily a disease of young women and older men. Symptoms most commonly appear in the third decade of life, although any age group may be affected.[42] During the past 50 years, prevalence has increased because of improved recognition of the disorder, medical management, and survival. Myasthenia gravis is not hereditary in the Mendelian sense; however, there may be a history of autoimmune disorders in the family, including thyroid disorders or lupus. It should be remembered that approximately 10% of women with myasthenia gravis may transmit a transient type of neonatal myasthenia to the infant that resolves within days after birth.

### Pathophysiology

Myasthenia gravis is a result of circulating antibodies directed toward the AChRs in the skeletal muscle.[42-44] The AChR is a protein composed of five subunits situated in a specialized surface of the muscle membrane termed the end plate. When acetylcholine is released from the nerve after depolarization, it binds to the AChR and causes the ion channel to open. This passage of ions moving through the channel leads to depolarization of the end plate, action potential generation, and subsequent muscle fiber contraction. With this process, the depolarization of the end plate is three to four times greater than what is required for action potential generation. Therefore, fluctuations in end plate depolarization do not affect action potential generation or the overall strength of muscle contraction.[42]

The AChR antibodies in myasthenia gravis lead to the loss of AChRs by increased internalization of the receptor and complement-based lysis of the muscle membrane. Compromise of ion flow through AChR occurs, leading to a decrease in end plate depolarization, which may be insufficient to generate an action potential. This results in a failure of the muscle to contract. Often, at rest, the compromise of neuromuscular transmission is mild, and action potentials are still generated. However, with exercise or with repetitive nerve stimulation, the end plate potential is further reduced, the action potential is not generated, and muscle weakness occurs. In summary, antibodies attack the AChRs of the neuromuscular junction, thereby blocking the transmission of nerve impulses to muscle.[42–44]

## Clinical Manifestations

Myasthenia gravis can be characterized as ocular myasthenia or generalized myasthenia, depending on whether the symptoms are limited to the eye muscles or are spread elsewhere. In ocular myasthenia, patients may present with problems such as droopy eyelids or double vision. More than 90% of patients have ocular symptoms. In only 16% of the patients, the symptoms remain confined to the eye muscles. In the rest, the symptoms spread to other muscles (bulbar, limb, diaphragm) within a year of the onset of eye symptoms.[42,43]

In generalized myasthenia gravis, patients may demonstrate ocular manifestations as well as bulbar symptoms, presenting as difficulty with chewing, swallowing, talking, and handling secretions, and neck weakness. The voice may have a nasal quality. Prolonged talking brings on slurred speech. Weakness of jaw closure (masseter muscle) may lead to the jaw hanging open. Muscle weakness in the limbs is also apparent and can vary among patients. Patients often demonstrate more proximal than distal weakness. They often report increased weakness with sustained activity and improvement with rest. Patients may also demonstrate respiratory compromise due to weakness of the respiratory muscles. The most serious potential complication of myasthenia gravis is respiratory failure (myasthenic crisis) secondary to intercostal and diaphragmatic muscle weakness.[42,43] Respiratory failure may result in death. With earlier diagnosis and intervention for patients with myasthenia gravis, in-hospital mortality is low. Respiratory failure consequent to myasthenia gravis and advanced age are predictors of increased mortality.[42]

## Diagnosis

Similar to other neurologic disorders, the patient's history along with other diagnostic tests aids in an accurate diagnosis. Patients may present with complaints of double vision or drooping eyelids. Also, myasthenia gravis causes weakness of the shoulder girdle muscles. Therefore, the patient may complain of the inability to perform a variety of self-care activities, such as drying the hair with a blow dryer.

The neurologic examination is also valuable in making the diagnosis. The cranial nerve examination may reveal ptosis and diplopia as well as other cranial nerve involvement. Motor weakness may be exhibited.[42,43] In addition, laboratory studies indicate that AChR antibodies are present in approximately 90% of patients.[43]

Repetitive nerve conduction study during electromyography (EMG) is helpful in the diagnosis of myasthenia gravis. In EMG, a needle electrode is inserted into a skeletal muscle, and a recording of the electrical activity at rest, during voluntary activity, and with electrical stimulation is displayed on an oscilloscope. The patient should be informed that the needle causes some discomfort. In myasthenia gravis, the loss of functional AChRs results in a decrease in action potential size with repeated stimulation. Repetitive muscle stimulation produces a rapid decline in muscle action potential because of the deficient numbers of AChRs. Single-fiber EMG is a very sensitive test to assess the functioning of neuromuscular junction transmission.[42,43]

The Tensilon, or edrophonium, test is a classical diagnostic tool for confirming a diagnosis of myasthenia gravis. A positive test result lends strong support for the diagnosis of myasthenia gravis. In this test, 10 mg of IV Tensilon, a short-acting anticholinesterase agent, is given over approximately 1 minute. When injected, it transiently inhibits the breakdown of acetylcholine at the neuromuscular junction. A response is anticipated within 2 to 3 minutes. The test is most useful if there is improvement of ptosis or strength of the extraocular muscles. Limb strength or improved bulbar function may be difficult to interpret. When Tensilon is administered, atropine should be readily available in the event that the patient develops bradycardia. Because there have been reports of ventricular tachycardia and death as well, Tensilon should be administered in a monitored setting.[42,43]

A CT scan or MRI of the chest may also be performed to rule out thymoma or thymic hyperplasia. As noted earlier, patients with myasthenia gravis may have thymic tumors and should be screened. Thyroid function tests and vitamin $B_{12}$ levels should also be checked, along with antinuclear antibodies, parietal cell antibodies, and antimicrosomal antibodies.[42]

## Clinical Management

The clinical management of myasthenia gravis includes the following strategies: use of medications to enhance neuromuscular transmission; long-term immunosuppression with corticosteroids, mycophenolate mofetil (CellCept), azathioprine (Imuran), or cyclosporine; cyclophosphamide (Cytoxan); short-term immunomodulation with plasmapheresis or IVIG; or thymectomy.[42,43,45]

**PHARMACOLOGIC MANAGEMENT.** Pharmacologic management includes the use of anticholinesterases, steroids, or other immunosuppressive drugs. Pyridostigmine (Mestinon) is available in three formulations: liquid, a 60-mg tablet, or a 180-mg time-span formula. This drug inhibits the enzymatic elimination of acetylcholine, thus prolonging its action at the postsynaptic membrane and enhancing neuromuscular transmission. As a result of this action, more acetylcholine is available at the neuromuscular junction, and the patient has improved muscle strength. Medication onset of action is 30 minutes after administration, peaks in 1 hour, and lasts for 3 to 6 hours.[1,42]

Pyridostigmine should always be administered promptly as prescribed. It should be given every 3 to 4 hours when the patient is awake. If there is difficulty with chewing and swallowing, timing the medication 30 minutes before meals is helpful. The 180-mg time-span tablet is administered at bedtime and should never be crushed. Because the medication is given at night, the patient will have the benefit of sleep. Muscarinic side effects include diarrhea, abdominal cramping, increased salivation, blurred vision, bradycardia, and increased perspiration. Nicotinic side effects include muscle twitching, weakness, and fatigue.[1]

If the patient cannot take oral pyridostigmine because of fasting, or NPO status, or intubation, a comparable approach is to use IV neostigmine. IV neostigmine bromide 1 mg is equivalent to pyridostigmine 60 mg. Neostigmine can be infused as a continuous infusion, and care should be taken to ensure the patency of the IV access. Cardiac monitoring is essential.[43]

Steroids and other immunosuppressive medications may be used with pyridostigmine in managing myasthenia gravis.[42,43]

The patient should not receive some medications. For example, D-penicillamine is contraindicated in patients with myasthenia gravis. Other drugs, including some antibiotics, can cause an increase in myasthenic weakness (Box 35-6).[42,43] Both patients and health care professionals need to be cognizant of these medications. Although physicians and nurses working in the neuroscience arena are often familiar with these drugs, patients may face potential difficulties in settings, such as the emergency department or surgery, where health care professionals do not encounter patients with myasthenia gravis on a regular basis and may not be familiar with these medications.[42,43]

**PLASMAPHERESIS.** Plasmapheresis may be indicated for patients in crisis or who are otherwise refractory to treatment. Plasmapheresis is initiated to remove circulating anti-AChR antibodies from the plasma, which results in clinical improvement. This procedure is performed through a dual-lumen central vascular access device, which is similar to a dialysis catheter. Plasmapheresis is generally performed as an emergent procedure but can also be utilized on an outpatient basis.[43,45] The patient's circulating blood volume is removed through one of the lumens, filtered, and then returned through the second lumen. The patient's plasma is removed and albumin is returned, along with the solid components of the patient's blood. The procedure takes several

---

**OSEN** **BOX 35-6** *PATIENT SAFETY*

**Medications to Avoid in Myasthenia Gravis**
**Antibiotics:** Aminoglycosides, "mycins," tetracycline, polymyxin B and E, colistin
**Antiepileptic Drugs:** Phenytoin, mephenytoin, trimethadione
**Cardiovascular Medications:** Quinidine, procainamide, β-blockers
**Psychotropic Drugs:** Lithium carbonate, phenothiazines
**Muscle Relaxants:** Curare, succinylcholine
**Others:** Magnesium preparations, quinine, d-penicillamine, chloroquine

---

hours, and the patient is monitored for hypotension. Electrolytes and clotting factors are evaluated after each treatment.

The catheters must be managed appropriately because they are a potential source of infection. They can pose a special challenge because the patient with myasthenia gravis may be receiving steroids or other immunosuppressive therapy. The nurse must also be aware that plasmapheresis removes medications, including pyridostigmine, which the patient has taken. The nurse must obtain an order from the physician to withhold the medication.

**INTRAVENOUS IMMUNOGLOBULIN.** Another treatment in place of plasma exchange is IVIG. It is used either for acute disease management or as a long-term treatment for patients with myasthenia gravis who do not respond to other types of treatments. It is often used before thymectomy to stabilize the patient. The patient's dose is individualized. Patients may exhibit clinical improvement in 2 to 4 days, and it may last for varying intervals. The mechanism of action of IVIG is unknown. The patient needs to be monitored for fever and chills, leukopenia, headache, fluid overload, and renal failure.[1,43]

**THYMECTOMY.** Thymectomy is a standard treatment for patients younger than 56 years with generalized myasthenia gravis. This surgical procedure promotes sustained remission and improvement, although no controlled studies have been performed. However, the fall in antibody titers after surgery supports the use of thymectomy. Patients must be aware that this procedure is performed for its long-term benefit so that they do not expect a dramatic improvement immediately after surgery. Clinical improvement may not be realized for 6 to 12 months after thymectomy. In some cases, benefit may not be seen for several years.[42,43] Patients may demonstrate enough improvement so that their medications may be reduced, thereby reducing adverse effects.

Post-thymectomy care involves a short stay in the ICU. Epidural analgesia is used to manage pain after the procedure. The patient is usually extubated immediately after the surgery. Intermittent positive-pressure breathing may be used to minimize postoperative respiratory complications. After the critical care stay, patients are transferred to an inpatient setting, where they are monitored for complications. Multiple effective surgical approaches for performing a thymectomy exist including trans-sternal, video-assisted, and robotic-assisted.[46]

**MANAGEMENT OF MYASTHENIC VERSUS CHOLINERGIC CRISIS.** Factors such as stress, respiratory infection, too rapid a steroid taper, or medication affecting the neuromuscular junction may predispose the patient to a crisis. A myasthenic crisis needs to be differentiated from a cholinergic crisis because the management of each is different.[43]

A myasthenic crisis is characterized by respiratory failure along with sudden exacerbation of weakness in other muscle groups. It is usually caused by lack of medication or lack of responsiveness at the neuromuscular junction to cholinergic treatment, as well as a worsening of the disease process. The patient is unresponsive to an increase in anticholinesterase medications and can experience severe weakness, dysphagia, and respiratory compromise. Frequent FVC checks should be performed, and when FVC falls below 15 mL/kg, the patient should be intubated. Any patient with myasthenia gravis with uncertain respiratory status should be admitted to an ICU to permit close monitoring of FVC, negative inspiratory force, and anxiety, as well as to facilitate a physical examination.[42,43]

The hallmarks of cholinergic crisis are muscarinic or nicotinic side effects, namely, increased perspiration, abdominal cramping, and diarrhea. Cholinergic crisis results from too much medication that causes neuromuscular blockage (which prevents muscle depolarization because of excess acetylcholine). The patient may also experience respiratory failure. Indeed, respiratory failure may be seen in both types of crises.[1,43,45]

Patients should be managed intensively. Admission to the ICU includes DVT prophylaxis and ulcer prevention. Providers need to be aware that patients in myasthenic crisis are not intubated due to lung or systemic problems, but rather to difficulties with muscle strength.[42,43,45] Given the hazards of intubation and controlled ventilation, including airway injury as well as lung injury and ventilator-associated pneumonia, measures to avoid intubation should be considered as clinically appropriate. One option is noninvasive positive pressure ventilation (NIPPV). Vigilant assessment and early recognition of impending respiratory failure may identify appropriate candidates for NIPPV. Using NIPPV in patients with myasthenic crisis before hypercapnia develops may prevent intubation and prolonged mechanical ventilation as well as decrease hospital length of stay and reduce risk of pulmonary complications.[1,47]

In the past, the Tensilon test was used to determine whether the patient was in a myasthenic or cholinergic crisis. If there was an improvement in muscle strength when Tensilon was administered, it indicated a myasthenic crisis.[1,42] If there was no improvement or further deterioration of muscle strength, the patient was most likely experiencing a cholinergic crisis. This test is no longer required because the withdrawal of cholinesterase drugs is necessary for improvement in both crises. Respiratory and nutritional support is provided in both situations.

### Nursing Management

**ASSESSMENT.** The nurse must focus the neurologic assessment on cranial nerve involvement, motor strength, and the extent of respiratory involvement. The patient should be monitored for ptosis and double vision. The patient's motor strength should be evaluated by the use of arm abduction times up to 5 minutes. One valuable tool for monitoring respiratory function is a handheld spirometer to measure FVC. The nurse must be vigilant in monitoring the patient's respiratory status because the patient's diaphragm and intercostal muscles may become weak. If the patient's FVC falls below 1 liter, it usually indicates respiratory failure, and intubation and mechanical ventilation are necessary. An easy bedside test involves counting out numbers in one breath. Most patients should be able to count out up to 50 in one breath. In summary, useful clinical assessment involves arm abduction times, FVC, range of eye movements, and time to the development of ptosis on upward gaze. Muscle strength testing is also valuable.

**PLAN.** The patient with myasthenia gravis may need assistance with activities of daily living. Adaptive equipment can help him or her perform self-care activities. Short rest periods are planned throughout the day, to help reduce patient fatigue and conserve energy.

Nutrition also needs to be addressed. Meals should be planned when pyridostigmine is at its peak. Aspiration precautions should be established. Thin liquids should be given only if the patient can tolerate them well. If the patient chokes when swallowing water, oral intake should cease. If the patient has a wet, gurgling voice or respiratory sounds or develops stridor, intubation may be necessary for airway protection, and nutrition may need to be offered through the enteral route. Caloric intake must be sustained to prevent a negative energy balance that interferes with weaning from the ventilator.

Skin care also needs to be incorporated into the care routine, and measures should be taken to avoid pressure ulcers. Pressure relief devices can be used in bed or on chairs.

An effective method of communication should also be developed, particularly if it becomes difficult to understand the patient because of the nasal quality of the voice. A communication board may be helpful as an alternate communication device.

**PATIENT EDUCATION AND DISCHARGE PLANNING.** Support and education about myasthenia gravis are crucial for the successful management of the disease. The patient needs to learn about the purpose of medications, medication schedules, and side effects. Doses of medication should be kept at home and work so that they are readily available. During travel, the patient should always carry his or her medication (eg, in a purse or camera case) so that it does not become lost with luggage.

It is also helpful for the patient to obtain a medical identification bracelet and card so that rapid identification can occur in the event of a medical emergency. If the patient is unable to communicate, successful management may hinge on health care professionals recognizing that the person has myasthenia gravis.

The patient and family are taught to recognize signs and symptoms of a crisis. In addition, the importance of avoiding potential triggers for a crisis, such as respiratory infection or undue stress, is emphasized. During the winter months, when colds and flu are prevalent, the patient should be instructed to stay away from places where large groups of people gather, such as movies or concerts.

The patient should also be educated about community support groups. The Myasthenia Gravis Foundation can provide valuable resources. Long-term outcomes in myasthenia gravis have improved markedly because of the availability of immune-modulating therapies, and patients need to be educated on how to live with their disease.

# Clinical Applicability Challenges

## CASE STUDY

H.B. is a 38-year-old man who was admitted to the neuro critical care unit through the ED. H.B. was at work in his job as an electrician when he noticed decreased strength in his left hand to the point where he was unable to complete his task. He drove himself to the nearest emergency department.

On admission to the ED, H.B.'s neuro exam revealed the following: A & O × 4 (oriented to self, situation, place, and date), PERRLA, facial sensation and shoulder shrug equal and intact, full strength and sensation in the right upper and lower extremities, and decreased strength on the left. H.B. was unable to extend the fingers on his left hand, demonstrated a pronator drift, and had difficulty with depth perception. In addition, he had weakness in plantar and dorsiflexion of his left ankle.

A CT scan of the head showed a 4.3 × 2.6 cm mass along the parietal bone consistent with a meningioma. There was also associated underlying mass effect with subcortical edema within the adjacent brain with a right-to-left midline shift of 5 mm. There was no evidence of hydrocephalus.

H.B. is scheduled for resection of his right parietal tumor for tomorrow. A corticosteroid and a type 2 histamine receptor blocker are administered, and H.B. is placed on a sliding scale for blood glucose control.

1. For patients with cerebral edema, a corticosteroid is often administered to reduce edema. Why are type 2 histamine receptor blockers prescribed in conjunction with a corticosteroid?
2. Why would H.B. be placed on an insulin sliding scale for blood glucose control?
3. H.B.'s tumor lies in the right parietal lobe. If the tumor had been located within the cerebellum, what symptoms might H.B. have experienced?
4. Because of H.B.'s increased intracranial pressure (ICP), what type of fluid would the nurse anticipate infusing?

## WANT TO KNOW MORE?

A wide variety of resources to enhance your learning and understanding of this chapter are available on thePoint.

You will find:

- References
- Selected readings
- NCLEX-style review questions
- Internet resources
- And more!

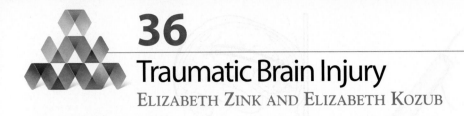

# 36

# Traumatic Brain Injury

### ELIZABETH ZINK AND ELIZABETH KOZUB

## LEARNING OBJECTIVES

*Based on the content in this chapter, the reader should be able to:*

1. Explain the significance of the mechanism of injury when assessing the patient with traumatic brain injury.

2. Compare and contrast various types of head injuries and typical patient presentation.

3. Differentiate between primary and secondary brain injury.

4. Explain the importance of and technique for serial neurologic assessment in the patient with traumatic brain injury.

5. Discuss the rationale for medical and nursing management in the care of the patient with a traumatic brain injury.

6. Describe the roles of multidisciplinary health care team members in caring for the patient with traumatic brain injury.

Traumatic brain injury (TBI) is a leading cause of disability and death in the United States and has devastating effects on patients and their families.[1] There are approximately 1.7 million TBIs each year, with 80% of those being evaluated and discharged from emergency departments (EDs); 275,000 are admitted to hospitals and 52,000 die. It is suspected that a large number of people who sustain TBI do not seek health care. However, over the past decade, with increased awareness about head injury, ED visits increased by 70%, while hospitalizations increased by 11% and death rates decreased by 7%.[2]

Falls are the leading cause of TBI, constituting 35% of all cases, followed by unknown causes (21%), unintentional blunt trauma (16.5%), and motor vehicle-related injuries (17%).[1] The incidence of TBI is greater in males than females, and TBI occurs most frequently in children younger than age 5 years and in adolescents between ages 15 and 19 years.[1] TBI in adults older than age 65 years most often results from falls (61%). Critical care nurses play an important role in reducing the incidence of head injury through patient and family teaching as well as participation in primary prevention efforts (eg, helmet safety, violence prevention, fall prevention, and drug and alcohol awareness). Box 36-1 lists nursing interventions for preventing falls in older adults.

TBI can have a profound and lasting effect on the patient and family. Neurologic deficits may affect the patient's ability to resume his or her chosen career or to return to work at all. Emotional and behavioral changes may affect interpersonal relationships and family roles. A thorough understanding of the pathophysiology of TBI enables the critical care nurse to individualize nursing care and positively affect patient and family outcomes. Critical care nurses play a key role in planning and implementing the multidisciplinary care of these complex patients and their families.

## Mechanisms of Traumatic Brain Injury

Typical mechanisms of injury include acceleration, acceleration–deceleration, coup–contrecoup, rotational injury, and penetrating injury (Fig. 36-1).

- **Acceleration injuries** occur when a moving object strikes the stationary head (eg, a bat striking the head or a missile fired into the head).

- **Acceleration–deceleration injuries** occur when the head in motion strikes a stationary object. For example, a motor vehicle crash in which the head strikes the windshield produces an acceleration–deceleration injury. Acceleration–deceleration injuries can also occur with falls or physical assaults.

- **Coup–contrecoup injuries** occur when the brain "bounces" back and forth within the skull, striking both poles of the brain (ie, front and back or right side and left side). Coup refers to the area of brain tissue initially making forceful contact with the inside of the skull, and contrecoup refers to the second impact of brain tissue with the inside of the skull, usually on the opposite side. When assessing a patient struck in the back of the head, the clinician evaluates for injury to posterior structures (ie, the occipital lobes and cerebellum) as well as anterior brain structures (ie, the frontal lobes).

- **Rotational forces** cause the brain to twist within the meninges and the skull, resulting in stretching and tearing

---

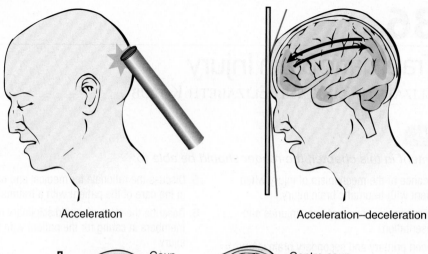

Acceleration

Acceleration–deceleration

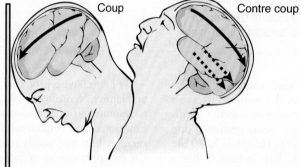

Coup

Contre coup

Coup-contre coup

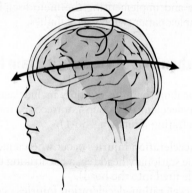

Rotation

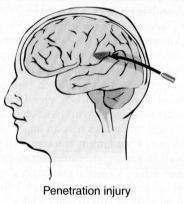

Penetration injury

FIGURE 36-1   Typical mechanisms of head injury.

of blood vessels and shearing of neurons. Physical assaults and motor vehicle crashes are examples of situations in which rotation and torsion may be a mechanism of injury.

- **Penetration injuries** may be caused by a bullet, shrapnel, or another sharp object traveling at a velocity substantial enough to disrupt the integrity of the skull. Depending on the speed and trajectory of the object, underlying brain structures may or may not be injured.

Cervical spine injury must be automatically assumed and systematically excluded with all types of TBI before immobilization devices are removed. TBI is categorized by severity based on radiographic injury and the Glasgow Coma Scale (GCS) (Table 36-1).

**TABLE 36-1   Defining the Severity of Head Injury**

| Severity | Description |
|---|---|
| Mild | GCS score 13–15 |
| | Loss of consciousness or amnesia for 5–60 min |
| | No abnormality on CT scan and length of hospital stay >48 h |
| Moderate | GCS score 9–12 |
| | Loss of consciousness or amnesia for 1–24 h |
| | May have abnormality on CT scan |
| Severe | GCS score 3–8 |
| | Loss of consciousness or amnesia for >24 h |
| | May have a cerebral contusion, laceration, or intracranial hematoma |

GCS, Glasgow Coma Scale.

# Primary and Secondary Brain Injury

The term *primary brain injury* describes an injury occurring at the time of trauma. Injury to the brain beginning immediately after the traumatic event is referred to as *secondary brain injury*. The initial injury causes immediate disruption of the skull, brain structures (ie, meninges, blood vessels, brain tissues, neurons), and functions (blood flow, oxygenation, cellular metabolism). Secondary injury describes the physiologic response to brain injury, including cerebral edema, cerebral ischemia, and biochemical changes. Care of the patient with TBI is aimed at preventing and mitigating secondary brain injury to maximize chances for positive functional outcomes.

## Primary Brain Injury

### Scalp Laceration

A scalp laceration frequently causes significant bleeding owing to the vascularity of the scalp, and may be associated with other underlying injuries to the skull and brain. The scalp should be carefully palpated, assessing for deformation. Skull fractures may be present even if deformities are not palpable; therefore, care must be exercised in applying pressure to scalp wounds. Scalp lacerations can be sutured at the bedside or may require surgical repair, depending on the size and extent of injury. Avulsion of areas of the scalp may require surgical reimplantation to address injured vascular structures.

### Skull Fracture

The skull protects the brain by distributing forces outward, lessening direct impact to the brain. Skull fractures are categorized by location; the fractured bones may be located in the anterior, middle, or posterior fossae (bony compartments or regions of the skull), or at the base of the skull. Skull fractures may be compound (ie, occurring with an open wound), displaced (closed wound in which the edges of the fracture no longer meet), or linear. Depressed skull fractures are fractures in which bone fragments are driven into the underlying meninges of brain tissue; this often presents as a depression or dip when palpating the scalp. Patients with depressed skull fractures may require surgical management to remove bone fragments, repair the skull or dura, evacuate a hematoma, or repair other adjacent structures, such as blood vessels.[3] Blood vessels travel along bony grooves on the inside surface of the skull; as a result, they are vulnerable to injury during a direct blow to the skull. Injury to the dura may cause a breach in a typically watertight sterile compartment, placing a patient at risk for meningitis; therefore, careful monitoring for signs and symptoms of infection, such as fever, neck pain and stiffness, and headache, is important.

Basilar skull fractures occur at the base or floor of the skull, typically in the areas of the anterior and middle fossae. Basilar skull fractures may be linear or displaced. Assessment of extraocular movements is important in detecting impingement of cranial nerves that pass through foramina in the skull (outlets within the skull that allow for blood vessels and nerves to travel through the skull). Nasogastric and nasotracheal intubation are avoided to reduce the risk of passing the tube through fractured areas of the skull into the brain.

Drainage of cerebrospinal fluid (CSF) from the ear or nose indicates injury to the dura. Drainage from the ear (otorrhea) typically signifies a fracture in the middle fossa. Ecchymosis (bruising) behind the ear (Battle sign) is a delayed sign of a basilar skull fracture in the middle fossa. Rhinorrhea (CSF drainage from the nose) occurs with a fracture in the anterior fossa; "raccoon eyes," a ring-like pattern of bruising around the eyes, is a late sign of this type of fracture.

Drainage from the ear or nose may be mixed with blood, making identification of CSF difficult. A layering of fluids, with blood on the inside and CSF in a yellowish ring on the outside (the "halo sign"), may appear when the area is wiped with gauze; however, a more definitive test of the fluid for a substance called β-2 transferrin is more effective in distinguishing between CSF and other body fluids. Patients may also report a sweet or salty taste if CSF is draining into the pharynx.

CSF leaks typically heal on their own with rest; however, when a CSF leak persists, diversion of CSF into an external drainage device may be necessary to reduce pressure on the dural tear and allow time for healing. In some cases, surgical repair of the damaged region of dura must be performed. A loose gauze dressing can be applied to the ear or nose to quantify the amount and character of drainage while allowing unobstructed drainage of the fluid. The skin around the site of drainage is kept clean, and the patient is instructed not to blow his or her nose.

### Concussion

A concussion is defined as any alteration in mental status resulting from trauma. The patient may or may not lose consciousness. Loss of consciousness may last up to 30 minutes. Often patients are unable to recall events leading up to the traumatic event, and occasionally short-term memory is affected. Concussions are not associated with structural abnormalities on radiographic imaging; however, a growing body of research suggests that neuronal injury does occur with concussions and is associated with a metabolic crisis at the cellular level.[4] This cellular metabolic crisis may cause the symptoms attributed to postconcussive syndrome.[4]

Recovery after a concussion is usually quick and complete; however, some patients exhibit symptoms that last longer, particularly with repetitive concussive injuries.[4] Symptoms may include headaches, decreased attention span and concentration, sleep disturbances, anxiety, short-term memory impairment, dizziness, irritability, emotional lability, fatigue, visual disturbances, noise and light sensitivity, and difficulties with executive functions.[5] These symptoms may last for months to years and can be alarming to the patient and family. If postconcussion symptoms last longer than 3 months, the patient is described as having a postconcussive syndrome. Discharge teaching must include a review of the signs and symptoms of postconcussive syndrome as well as criteria for obtaining medical follow-up. In a recent systematic review, Nygren–deBoussard et al.[6] found that early education and counseling interventions may confer benefit in reducing postconcussive symptoms, and that prolonged bedrest does not contribute to improved recovery. Furthermore, emphasis on preventive strategies to avoid reinjury is necessary to prevent future chronic and catastrophic brain injury.[4]

### Contusion

Contusions in the brain are the result of laceration of the microvasculature. They are focal and superficial, occasionally spreading to deeper layers of the brain. Cerebral contusions can range from mild to severe depending on the location, size, and extent of brain tissue injury. Cerebral contusions are most often located in the frontal and temporal lobes. Contusions are often associated with other brain injuries, including subdural hematoma, subarachnoid hemorrhage, and cranial fractures.[7]

The diagnosis of cerebral contusion is made using computed tomography (CT). Small lesions may result in focal neurologic deficits, whereas multiple or large contusions may result in a depressed level of consciousness and coma. Complications of a cerebral contusion include expansion of the hematoma and cerebral edema.[7] Cerebral edema peaks 24 to 72 hours after injury, causing increased intracranial pressure (ICP). The patient's clinical condition may progressively deteriorate over the first 72 hours; therefore, the patient requires intensive anticipatory monitoring (serial neurologic assessments) to identify signs and symptoms of increased ICP quickly and prevent further brain injury.

### Epidural Hematoma

An epidural hematoma is a collection of blood between the dura and inside surface of the skull, often caused by laceration of the middle meningeal artery (Fig. 36-2). Although this type of hemorrhage is often associated with injury to an artery, injury to a vein or venous sinus located above the dura may also produce an epidural hematoma. Prompt recognition and expeditious surgical intervention to evacuate the hematoma result in improved outcomes. Patients may present in a coma or fully conscious.

### Subdural Hematoma

A subdural hematoma is an accumulation of blood below the dura and above the arachnoid layer covering the brain

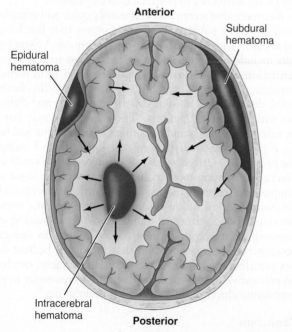

**FIGURE 36-2** Cerebral hematomas. (From Smeltzer: Brunner & Suddarth's Textbook of Medical-Surgical Nursing, 13th ed. Philadelphia, PA: Lippincott Williams & Wilkins, 2014, p 1999.)

(see Fig. 36-2). Tearing of the surface veins or disruption of venous sinuses can cause a subdural hematoma. The risk of subdural hematoma is higher in the elderly and in people with alcoholism.[8] Cortical atrophy in these two populations causes tension on bridging veins leading from the surface of the brain to the inner surface of the dura. An increased incidence of falls also compounds the risk for subdural hematoma in these populations. Up to half of elderly patients do not recall a specific traumatic injury that may have caused a subdural hematoma.[8] In patients who do not report a fall or trauma, the initial injury has been found to be an average of 49 days prior to symptom development. Patients who are on anticoagulant medications are at increased risk for subdural hematoma.[8]

Subdural hematomas can be separated into three categories based on the time from injury to the onset of symptoms: acute, subacute, and chronic. The size and location of the hematoma, the degree of neurologic dysfunction, imaging results, presence of mass effect, and increased ICP are considered in making the decision to surgically evacuate the hematoma.[9]

Patients with *acute subdural hematomas* manifest symptoms within 24 to 48 hours after injury depending on the rate and amount of blood accumulation. Symptoms include headache, focal neurologic deficit, unilateral pupillary abnormalities, and a decreasing level of consciousness.

Patients with *subacute subdural hematomas* have a delayed onset of symptoms, 2 days to 2 weeks after injury. The delay in symptom onset may be explained by a slower accumulation of blood from disruption of smaller blood vessels. In some cases, cerebral atrophy may allow for a greater amount of fluid to collect before symptoms of increased ICP manifest.

Patients with *chronic subdural hematomas* may initially experience a small bleed that does not cause symptoms. Over time, the small collection of blood breaks down to a proteinaceous fluid and becomes encapsulated by a fibrous membrane. Slow capillary leaking of fluid causes expansion of the mass and produces symptoms of increased ICP. Chronic subdural hematomas are often seen in elderly patients with a history of falling or in patients with alcoholism. The slow accumulation of fluid accounts for delayed presentation of signs and symptoms of increased ICP.[9] Common symptoms include headache, lethargy, confusion, and seizures. A drain may be placed intraoperatively to prevent reaccumulation of fluid. Some practitioners elect to position the head of the patient's bed flat to decrease tension on bridging veins in an attempt to prevent rebleeding.

### Intracerebral Hematoma

An intracerebral hematoma is a collection of blood within brain tissue caused by disruption of blood vessels (see Fig. 36-2). Traumatic causes of intracerebral hematoma include depressed skull fractures and penetrating injuries. Surgical management of intraparenchymal hematomas is indicated in patients with deteriorating neurologic status referable to the injured region of brain tissue, and in patients with increased ICP that is uncontrolled with maximal medical therapies (eg, osmotic therapy, hyperventilation, and sedation). Medical therapy aims to manage cerebral edema and promote adequate cerebral perfusion.

## Traumatic Subarachnoid Hemorrhage

Traumatic subarachnoid hemorrhage occurs with tearing or shearing of microvessels in the arachnoid layer where CSF flows around the brain. A traumatic subarachnoid hemorrhage often accompanies other severe brain injuries and has been suggested to be associated with poor neurologic outcome and increased mortality.[10] Additional complications, such as hydrocephalus and cerebral vasospasm, add to the complexity of the injury. The onset of vasospasm after TBI may occur within 1 to 2 days after the initial injury and peaks at 5 to 7 days.[10] There are several theories for the mechanism of vasospasm in traumatic subarachnoid hemorrhage, but the precise mechanism is not known.

## Diffuse Axonal Injury

Diffuse axonal injury (DAI) is characterized by direct microscopic tearing or shearing of axons, leading to edema during the first 12 to 24 hours. DAI prolongs or disables signal conduction from the white matter to gray matter in the brain, and is thought to occur with rotational and acceleration–deceleration forces, or unrestricted head movements that create the shearing of the axons.[11] After the initial injury, secondary injury causing axonal swelling may affect axons that were not initially damaged, resulting in further degeneration of axons.[11]

DAI can be classified as mild, moderate, or severe based on length of coma and degree of neurologic dysfunction. Mild DAI is associated with a coma lasting no longer than 24 hours. Moderate DAI is characterized by a coma lasting longer than 24 hours with transient flexor or extensor posturing. Severe DAI is characterized by prolonged coma, fever, diaphoresis, and severe extensor posturing.

DAI is not easily identified through radiographic imaging in the first 24 hours; however, small punctate hemorrhages may be visualized deep in the white matter, a finding that increases suspicion that DAI has occurred. Magnetic resonance imaging (MRI) may be helpful in identifying neuronal damage after 24 hours. Unfortunately, not all patients with DAI will have radiographic changes; therefore diagnosis is often made by excluding other clinical conditions.[12]

## Cerebrovascular Injury

Carotid or vertebral artery dissection must be considered in situations in which a patient presents with neurologic deficits unexplained by other brain injuries, particularly those patients who have suffered blunt trauma.[13] Arterial dissection is caused by shearing of the innermost or middle vessel layers, the intima and media. Damage to the intima can result in clot formation or an intimal flap, either of which can occlude the vessel, resulting in an ischemic stroke.

The key to preventing stroke in these patients is early identification of the injury, exclusion of concomitant hemorrhage, and initiation of anticoagulation therapy in some cases. To detect this type of injury, cerebral angiography or cerebral computerized tomographic angiography (CTA) may be performed in patients who have sustained injury to the neck or unexplained focal neurologic deficits.[13] Damage to the intima or media allows blood to leak between the blood vessel layers, resulting in a ballooning of the outermost vessel layers and creating an aneurysm. This type of aneurysm is referred to as a traumatic intracerebral aneurysm or pseudoaneurysm.

## Secondary Brain Injury

Secondary brain injuries occur after the initiating traumatic event and cause additional damage to brain tissue. Examples of conditions causing or exacerbating secondary brain injury are uncontrolled ICP, cerebral ischemia, hypotension, hypoxemia, and local or systemic infection. Secondary brain injury occurs as a function of the inflammatory response, reduced cerebral blood flow, and dysfunctional cerebral autoregulation causing damage to neurons. These secondary processes can result in cerebral infarction (stroke), coma, and increased cerebral edema. Prevention of hypotension, hypercarbia, hypoxemia, hyperthermia, and seizures is extremely important in attempting to prevent further injury.[14]

Understanding intracranial dynamics and cerebral blood flow is essential to preventing and treating secondary brain injury. (See Chapter 34 for a complete discussion of intracranial dynamics and the Monro-Kellie doctrine.)

Compensation for increased volume in the cranium occurs when CSF is channeled through the foramen magnum into the spinal canal, CSF production is decreased, and venous blood is channeled out of the cranium into the jugular veins. The compliance curve (Fig. 36-3) illustrates the body's ability to compensate for the addition of water, CSF, or blood into the cranial vault and the point at which intracranial compliance is maximized. Decreased intracranial compliance results in a small addition of volume, causing disproportionate increases in ICP. Examples of conditions causing decreased intracranial compliance are cerebral edema (an increase in brain water), expansion of a hematoma (an increase in blood), and hydrocephalus (an increase in CSF). An understanding of pressure–volume relationships allows the nurse to anticipate deterioration of the patient's clinical

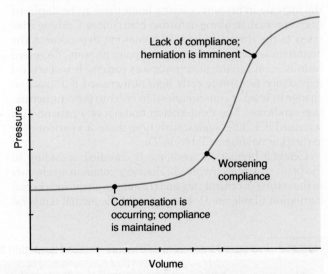

**FIGURE 36-3** The compliance curve. The body is able to compensate for the addition of water, blood, or CSF to the cranial vault until a critical point is reached where compensation has been maximized. At this point, the addition of a small amount of volume will cause a disproportionate increase in ICP. Biochemical mechanisms also play a significant role in causing secondary brain injury. The inflammatory response has been implicated as a potential cause or exacerbating factor in secondary brain injury.

condition, tailor nursing interventions, and anticipate potential medical or surgical treatments.

Cerebral autoregulation is a protective mechanism that enables the brain to receive constant blood flow over a range of systemic blood pressures (see Chapter 34 for a complete discussion). Several studies have suggested that regional cerebral blood flow may decrease to 70% of normal on the same side (ipsilateral) of the injury.[14]

### Cerebral Edema

Cerebral edema commonly occurs in patients with TBI 24 to 48 hours after the primary insult, and was originally thought to peak at 3 days; however, emerging research shows that cerebral edema resulting in increased ICP may remain present for 3 to 7 days after injury.[15] Patients require increased observation during this period because of the increased risk of neurologic deterioration. If cerebral edema is not quickly and aggressively treated, herniation syndrome may occur. The treatment of cerebral edema is discussed in Chapter 34.

### Ischemia

Cerebral ischemia, a type of secondary brain injury and a major cause of morbidity and mortality, may be a result of direct vascular injury or cerebral edema that causes compression or occlusion of blood vessels within the brain. Ischemia in the brain may occur at the time of injury or during the period subsequent to the injury. Cerebral ischemia occurs whenever blood flow is inadequate to meet metabolic demands of the brain. If the cause of cerebral ischemia is not controlled, cerebral infarction (stroke) may result. (See Chapter 35 for further information on cerebral ischemia and stroke.)

### Herniation Syndrome

Herniation syndrome occurs when pressure builds within the cranium that exceeds the brain's ability to compensate for the increase in pressure, causing brain tissue to be displaced or compressed, resulting in further brain injury. Cushing triad refers to the three late signs of herniation that occur as the brainstem is compressed: increased pulse pressure, decreased heart rate, and an irregular respiratory pattern. It is of critical importance to identify early signs of increased ICP (such as change in level of consciousness) in order to prevent herniation syndrome. The examination findings of a patient with increased ICP differ significantly from those of a patient with herniation syndrome (Table 36-2).

Cerebral herniation syndrome is classified according to the brain structures involved. The most common syndromes in the setting of critical care and trauma are uncal and central herniation (Table 36-3). Herniation of the medial temporal lobe (uncus) through the tentorium and into the brainstem is called uncal herniation, and results in ipsilateral (same side) pupillary dilation and contralateral hemiparesis. Central or tonsillar herniation describes the downward displacement of the cerebellar tonsils through the foramen magnum, causing compression of the brainstem. Clinical signs of central herniation syndrome include loss of consciousness, bilateral pupillary dilation, respiratory pattern changes or respiratory arrest, and flaccid paralysis (Fig. 36-4).

Patients at risk for herniation syndrome must be closely monitored by performing serial neurologic examinations, taking into account subtle changes. Once thought to be immediately fatal, herniation syndrome may be reversible in certain circumstances if it is identified early and aggressive therapies are applied in a systematic manner, much like advanced cardiac life support is applied in the setting of cardiac arrest.[16]

### Coma

Coma is an alteration in consciousness caused by damage to both hemispheres of the brain or the brainstem. Coma results from disruption of the reticular activating system (RAS), which is a physiologic region encompassing nuclei from the medulla to the cerebral cortex. The RAS is responsible for wakefulness, heightened arousal, and alertness. Consciousness spans a continuum from full consciousness to coma (see Chapter 33, Box 33-3). The states of coma can be subdivided into light coma, coma, and deep coma.

### Persistent Vegetative State

Several terms describe a persistent vegetative state, such as irreversible coma or coma vigil. A persistent vegetative state is characterized by a period of sleeplike coma followed by a return to the awake state with an inability to respond to the environment. In a persistent vegetative state, higher cortical functions of the cerebral hemispheres have been damaged permanently, but the lower functions of the brainstem remain intact. The patient's eyes open spontaneously and may appear as if they are opening in response to verbal stimuli. Sleep–wake cycles exist, and the patient maintains normal cardiovascular and respiratory control. Also seen are involuntary lip smacking, chewing, and roving eye movements. Persistent vegetative state should not be diagnosed until 12 months after onset of TBI and coma; the chance of regaining consciousness is extremely low at that point.[17]

For the patient in a persistent vegetative state, the critical care nurse organizes resources for family and patient support such as pastoral care and social services. Support groups and assistance programs are often available for families of patients

---

**TABLE 36-2** Increased Intracranial Pressure versus Herniation Syndrome

| | Increased Intracranial Pressure | Herniation Syndrome |
|---|---|---|
| Level of arousal | Increased stimulus required | Unarousable |
| Motor function | Subtle motor weakness or pronator drift | Dense motor weakness, posturing or absent response |
| Pupillary response | Sluggish pupillary response | Unilateral dilated and fixed pupil ("blown pupil") |
| Vital signs | May be stable or labile | Cushing triad (increased systolic blood pressure, decreased heart rate, irregular respiration) |

Used with permission from an unpublished lecture, Lower J. 2002. Facing Neuro Assessment Fearlessly. Nursing; 32(2):58–64.

**TABLE 36-3** Herniation Syndromes

| Name | Tissue Displaced | Common Causes | Clinical Signs |
|---|---|---|---|
| Central (transtentorial) herniation | Supratentorial | Compression and impaired blood flow to the brainstem | Early altered alertness |
| | | Chronic increases in ICP | Respiratory sighs, yawns, pauses |
| | | Tumor in frontal, parietal, occipital lobes | Roving eyes, small pupils |
| | | | Late sign: decorticate or decerebrate posturing |
| Uncal herniation | Supratentorial | Rapidly expanding lesions—hematoma | Early unilateral dilating pupil |
| | | | Once brainstem signs begin, deterioration is rapid |
| Upward cerebellar herniation | Infratentorial | Posterior fossa mass | Coma |
| | | | Cerebellar infarct if superior cerebellar arteries occluded |
| | | | Hydrocephalus with involvement of sylvian aqueduct |
| Tonsillar herniation | Infratentorial | Elevated ICP | Cranial nerve abnormalities |
| | | Expanding mass | Respiratory changes (apneustic/cluster breathing) |
| | | | Change in level of consciousness (rapid) |

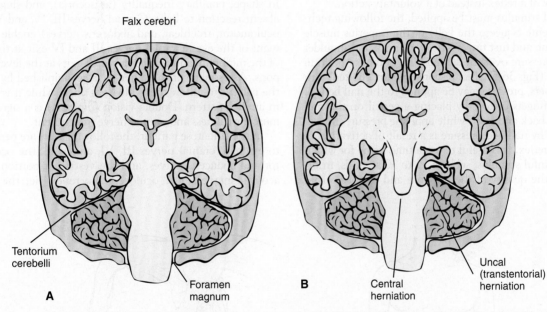

**FIGURE 36-4** **A:** Normal brain. **B:** Herniated brain. Herniation associated with brainstem compression is called *central herniation*, whereas herniation associated with the supratentorial structures is called *uncal (transtentorial) herniation*.

with TBI. Supporting the family in the process of gathering information and making decisions is an essential role of the multidisciplinary critical care team.

## Assessment

### Physical Examination

Two essential tenets of neurologic assessment are as follows:

1. Level of consciousness is the most sensitive indicator of increased ICP.
2. Maximal stimulus must be applied to achieve the maximal patient response.

Performing serial neurologic examinations that include evaluation of level of consciousness and motor and cranial nerve function is necessary to identify increased ICP and prevent

herniation syndrome. The GCS (see Chapter 33, Box 33-4) is useful for assessing trends of neurologic function over time; however, focal motor deficits are not taken into consideration. The advantages of the GCS are ease of use and proven consistency across evaluators.

### Assessment of Cognitive Function

Cognitive function is usually assessed by asking three orientation questions regarding person, place, and time. However, it is necessary to elicit an "embroidered" or specific history from the patient to facilitate the detection of subtle changes over time. Patients may learn to answer the same questions correctly because of repetition, but may continue to appear confused when questioned further. Instead of asking the patient to state his or her location, the nurse may ask the patient to recall what type of place he or she is in, or ask the name of the hospital, the city, and the state.

## Assessment of Level of Arousal

Assessment of arousal determines a patient's capacity for wakefulness. A maximum stimulus must be applied in a systematic and escalating fashion to effectively elicit the patient's best, or maximal, response. A patient should be stimulated first by calling his or her name (in the same manner as you would try to wake a person who is sleeping), then by shouting the name (as you would to wake a "sound sleeper"), next by shaking, and finally by applying central pain. This staged approach affords the patient the opportunity to demonstrate increasing wakefulness or his or her best response. If the patient awakens readily, the ability to follow simple commands is assessed by asking the patient to move his or her extremities or "show two fingers." When asking a patient to grip or squeeze the evaluator's hand, it is important to make sure that the person can squeeze and release the grip. Patients with injury to the frontal lobe may have damaged the area of grasp inhibition, which develops in infancy. In this instance, the patient grasps because of a reflex instead of a voluntary action.

If a painful stimulus must be applied, the following techniques are useful: Squeeze the belly of the trapezius muscle with the thumb and first finger where the neck and shoulder meet, apply pressure over the supraorbital notch, or perform a sternal rub (Fig. 36-5). If a response is not elicited with these maneuvers, pressure may be applied to the nail beds of the patient's fingers or toes by placing a pencil on the nail and rolling it back and forth while applying pressure. Movement elicited by nail bed pressure is a result of activation of a spinal cord reflex. It is useful to use a time frame for which to apply a painful stimulus, such as 15 to 30 seconds, in order to trend the quality of the response and to ensure that

the injured brain is given adequate time to respond. Patients with brain injury may exhibit delayed responses to stimuli.

## Assessment of the Eyes

Assessment of the eyes includes evaluation of the pupils and extraocular movements, which assists in localizing cranial nerve dysfunction. Testing of cranial nerve II (the optic nerve) involves detection of gross visual field defects and visual acuity. Visual fields can be adequately assessed by the patient's ability to detect movement of the evaluator's finger in each field of vision (see Chapter 33 for technique). Visual acuity can be grossly assessed by asking the patient to read printed words on a page or by using a Snellen eye chart. If there is concern about optic nerve impairment, a full evaluation by an ophthalmologist is recommended.

Evaluation of cranial nerve III (the oculomotor nerve) involves inspection of the pupil, including size, shape, equality, and reaction to light. Increased ICP can cause irregularities in shape, pupillary inequality (anisocoria), and sluggish or absent reaction to light. Cranial nerves III, IV, and VI (the oculomotor, trochlear, and abducens nerves) enable movement of the eyes. Cranial nerves III and IV exit at the level of the midbrain, and cranial nerve VI exits at the level of the pons. Assessment of these nerves is accomplished by asking the patient to follow the evaluator's finger while it is moved in an "H" pattern. Double vision (diplopia) is a sign of eye muscle weakness and cranial nerve impairment.

In the comatose patient, the following tests are performed to evaluate cranial nerves III, VI, and VIII (the oculomotor and abducens nerves, and the vestibular portion of the acoustic nerve). The oculocephalic reflex (ie, the "doll's

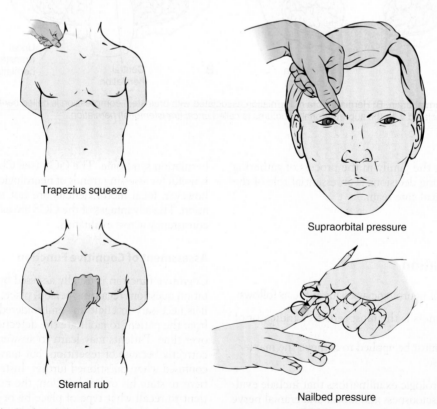

Trapezius squeeze

Supraorbital pressure

Sternal rub

Nailbed pressure

FIGURE 36-5 Methods of applying a painful stimulus.

eyes" phenomenon; see Chapter 33, Fig. 33-6) is tested by moving the head from side to side in a horizontal plane (after confirming the absence of cervical spinal fracture). If the oculocephalic response is present, the eyes move together in the opposite direction of the head as it is turned from side to side. Absence of eye movement on head turning reflects brainstem dysfunction. The oculovestibular reflex (see Chapter 33, Fig. 33-7) is tested by instilling cold water into each ear and observing the eyes for movement. A normal oculovestibular response is characterized by movement of the eyes toward the stimulus with nystagmus. The absence of movement signals loss of function of the vestibular portion of the eighth cranial nerve as well as the brainstem.

### Assessment of Brainstem Responses

The brainstem can be further assessed in the unconscious patient by testing corneal, cough, and gag reflexes. The corneal reflex reflects function of cranial nerves V and VII (the trigeminal and facial nerves), which exit the brain at the level of the pons. This reflex is tested by stimulating the lower lid of each eye by applying a drop of saline or passing a wisp of cotton over the inside of the lower lid. A blinking motion of the lower eyelid indicates the presence of the reflex. Sensation of the irritating stimulus represents gross function of one branch of the trigeminal nerve, and movement of the lower eyelid represents motor function of the facial nerve. Care must be taken in testing the corneal reflex to avoid corneal abrasions.

Cranial nerves IX and X (the glossopharyngeal and vagus nerves) exit at the level of the medulla and are responsible for the cough and gag reflexes and protection of the airway from aspiration. The cough and gag reflexes should be evaluated in the awake and unconscious patient.

### Assessment of Motor Function

Motor function is evaluated by using the staged approach described earlier. The awake and cooperative patient can be further assessed by having the patient move the extremities against gravity and with passive resistance; the movement is graded on a scale of 1 to 5 (see Chapter 33).

The unresponsive patient may exhibit localization, withdrawal, flexor posturing, or extensor posturing in response to noxious stimuli. Localization of a painful stimulus is observed as a purposeful response in which the patient is able to locate the source of pain and move toward it with one or both extremities crossing the midline of the body. A patient may try to remove the evaluator's hand when he or she performs a trapezius squeeze, or the patient may attempt to grab medical equipment (eg, catheters or endotracheal tubes). A withdrawal response is characterized by movement away from a painful stimulus. Flexor (decorticate) posturing is indicative of diffuse cortical injury and is characterized by the bending or flexing of the upper extremities and extension of the lower extremities and feet. Extensor (decerebrate) posturing indicates injury to the brainstem and is observed as extension and internal rotation of the upper extremities and extension of the lower extremities and feet (see Chapter 33, Fig. 33-1). It is possible that a patient may exhibit one type of movement in one extremity and another type of movement in another extremity. Presence of the Babinski reflex may also be observed in the patient with severe TBI.

### Assessment of Respiratory Function

Assessment of respiratory patterns is important in detecting worsening neurologic injury and the need for airway management and mechanical ventilation. Numerous locations in both cerebral hemispheres regulate voluntary control over the muscles used in breathing. The cerebellum synchronizes and coordinates the muscles involved in respiration. The cerebrum controls the rate and rhythm of respiration. The pons and midbrain regulate the automaticity of respiration.

Abnormal respiratory patterns may be correlated with injured regions of the brain, as shown in Figure 36-6. Cheyne-Stokes breathing is periodic breathing in which the depth of each breath increases to a peak and then decreases to apnea; the hyperpneic phase usually lasts longer than the apneic phase. This breathing pattern may be seen in patients with bilateral lesions located deep in the cerebral hemispheres. Compression in the area of the midbrain and pons can cause central neurogenic hyperventilation. Hyperventilation is sustained, regular, rapid, and deep. Apneustic breathing is characterized by a long pause at full inspiration or full expiration. The etiology of this pattern is loss of all cerebral and cerebellar control of breathing, with respiratory function at the brainstem level only. Cluster breathing may be seen in a patient when the lesion is high in the medulla or low in the pons. This pattern of respiration is seen as gasping breaths with irregular pauses.

The critical centers of inspiration and expiration are located in the medulla oblongata. Rapidly expanding intracranial lesions, such as cerebellar hemorrhage, can compress the medulla, resulting in ataxic breathing. This irregular breathing consists of both deep and shallow breaths with irregular pauses; it signals the need for endotracheal intubation.

### Assessment of Other Body Systems

In addition to thorough assessment of the central nervous system, comprehensive assessment of all other body systems is crucial in the early identification of complications in patients with TBI. Organ dysfunction, particularly respiratory failure, is common in patients with severe TBI.

## Diagnostic Testing

CT is performed as an initial diagnostic test to identify structural injuries in the brain and intracranial bleeding. A CT scan can be obtained quickly. One disadvantage of the CT scan is that it does not provide adequate views of the cerebelli and brainstem. An initial CT scan is performed without contrast. CT scans performed with intravenous contrast are used to investigate suspected masses (ie, tumors or abscesses). MRI is useful to assess structures in the posterior fossa and spinal cord. Magnetic resonance angiography may be used to evaluate cerebral vascular injuries such as carotid or vertebral dissection.[18]

Cerebral angiography is the gold standard diagnostic test to investigate injuries to cerebral blood vessels. A cerebral angiogram may also be obtained to confirm the absence of cerebral blood flow in brain death.

Transcranial Doppler (TCD) ultrasonography indirectly evaluates cerebral blood flow and autoregulatory mechanisms by measuring the speed with which blood travels through blood vessels. TCD may also be used to document cessation of blood flow to the brain.

| Type | Respiratory Pattern | Neuroanatomical Lesion |
|------|--------------------|------------------------|

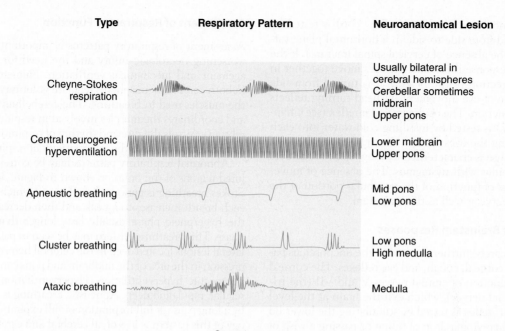

| | | |
|------|--------------------|------------------------|
| Cheyne-Stokes respiration | | Usually bilateral in cerebral hemispheres Cerebellar sometimes midbrain Upper pons |
| Central neurogenic hyperventilation | | Lower midbrain Upper pons |
| Apneustic breathing | | Mid pons Low pons |
| Cluster breathing | | Low pons High medulla |
| Ataxic breathing | | Medulla |

├─One minute─┤

**FIGURE 36-6**   Injury to the brainstem can result in various abnormal respiratory patterns.

Other diagnostic tests are used to assess electrical impulse transmission in the brain. These tests are often obtained to provide information for patient prognosis. Neurophysiologic tests include the electroencephalogram (EEG), brainstem auditory evoked responses (BAERs), and somatosensory evoked potentials (SSEPs). The EEG measures electrical activity in all regions of the cortex and is useful in identifying seizures and correlating the abnormal neurologic examination with abnormal cortical function. The EEG is necessary in ruling out subclinical or nonconvulsive seizures in the comatose patient. It may also be used as a confirmatory test in brain death to demonstrate cessation of electrical conduction to the cerebral cortex. A common finding in a patient with TBI is slowing of electrical activity in the area of injury. BAER and SSEP are useful prognostic tests in a patient with TBI. Abnormal results of either of these tests may help confirm a diagnosis of severe brainstem or cortical dysfunction.

## Management

Guidelines for the management of severe TBI have been developed by the Brain Trauma Foundation and the American Association of Neurological Surgeons to disseminate evidence-based recommendations.[19] The goal of these guidelines is to create a consistent standard for the care and treatment of patients with severe TBI. Specific guidelines for managing severe TBI in infants, children, and adolescents are available, outlining the unique needs of the pediatric population.[20] The focus of the discussion in this chapter is the management of severe TBI in adults.

### Initial Management

Initial assessment and treatment of the patient with TBI begins immediately after the insult, often with prehospital care providers. Prehospital treatment of the patient with a head injury focuses on rapid neurologic assessment, definitive airway management, and treatment of hypotension.[21] Guidelines for prehospital management emphasize early correction of hypoxia and hypercarbia, which have been shown to affect morbidity and mortality in patients with TBI (Fig. 36-7).

Airway management is a crucial initial step to prevent hypoxia and hypercarbia, which exacerbate secondary brain injury. Initial mechanical ventilation strategies aim to maintain normal ventilation or a partial pressure of carbon dioxide ($PaCO_2$) within normal limits (35 to 45 mm Hg). Signs of cerebral herniation may necessitate hyperventilation therapy ($PaCO_2$, 30 to 35 mm Hg). The goal of hyperventilation in TBI is to decrease $PaCO_2$, causing constriction of cerebral blood vessels and decreased cerebral blood volume. Decreased blood volume in the brain results in decreased ICP. Global cerebral vasoconstriction places healthy regions of brain tissue at risk for developing ischemia and should not be used prophylactically.[22] Continuous monitoring of end tidal carbon dioxide ($EtCO_2$) or frequent assessment of $PaCO_2$ (obtained in an arterial blood gas) is essential to prevent excessive vasoconstriction and cerebral ischemia. Monitoring cerebral oxygenation (ie, $SjO_2$ or $PbtO_2$) is an option for identifying cerebral ischemia. Research suggests that the brain experiences decreased blood flow in the first 24 hours after injury; therefore, hyperventilation should be avoided during this period.[19]

Diagnostic testing is performed subsequent to the initial resuscitation to evaluate the need for immediate surgical intervention. Typical tests include radiographs of the cervical spine and a CT scan of the brain, which is useful in diagnosing intracranial bleeding that may require surgical intervention. Additional imaging and blood tests may be obtained to rule out systemic injuries and assist in treating complications.

INITIAL MANAGEMENT OF SEVERE BRAIN INJURY

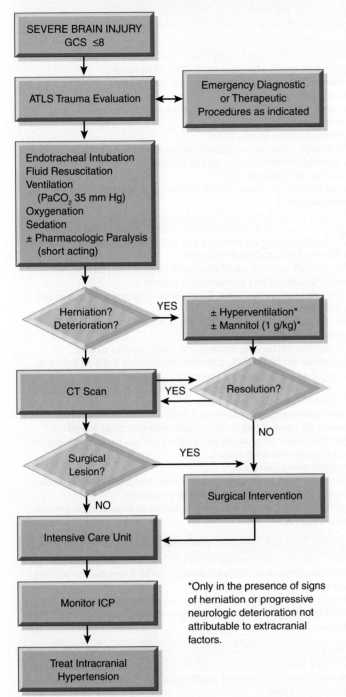

FIGURE 36-7 Flowchart for resuscitation of the patient with a severe head injury before ICP monitoring. (© 2000 Brain Trauma Foundation, Inc. Used with permission.)

The mechanism of injury helps determine appropriate diagnostic testing.

Continuing management seeks to control ICP, promote cerebral perfusion, and correct the primary pathologic process. General management of the patient with TBI requires a holistic, multisystem, multidisciplinary approach, taking into consideration the unique physiologic and psychosocial characteristics of the patient (Box 36-2).

## Monitoring and Controlling Intracranial Pressure

ICP monitoring, which is discussed in depth in Chapter 34, allows the health care team to make rapid treatment decisions based on pressure displays and ICP waveform analysis. The ICP monitor is typically inserted by a neurosurgeon at the bedside or in the operating room. ICP monitoring is recommended for patients with severe head injury (GCS score lower than 8) and CT scan abnormalities on admission.[19] ICP monitoring may also be considered when the CT scan is normal but the patient meets two or more of the following criteria: older than 40 years, posturing, or a systolic blood pressure less than 90 mm Hg.[19] Determining precise thresholds for treatment of increased ICP must be individualized for each patient by the healthcare team using neurologic assessment information and, in some circumstances, other monitoring parameters (discussed below) as evidence of a patient's positive or negative response to a particular value of ICP or cerebral perfusion pressure (CPP).[23,24] The impact of ICP monitoring on patient outcome is under investigation, in particular identification of patients with TBI who would benefit from ICP guided treatment. Elevation in ICP can occur within 24 hours after the initial injury, remaining elevated up to 7 days.[25]

Nursing interventions to manage increased ICP include maintaining body alignment as well as avoiding sharp turning of the head to one side and sharp hip flexion. Turning the head to one side causes compression of the jugular vein, preventing drainage of venous blood from the head, resulting in increased ICP. Sharp hip flexion increases intra-abdominal pressure, decreasing venous outflow and causing an increase in ICP.

## Maintaining Cerebral Perfusion

Management of cerebral perfusion involves control of ICP and maintenance of mean arterial pressure (MAP). CPP is calculated by subtracting ICP from MAP: CPP = MAP − ICP. Maintenance of CPP within the range of 50 to 70 mm Hg prevents cerebral ischemia at the lower end and mitigates the risk for acute respiratory distress syndrome (ARDS), which has been shown to occur more frequently when CPP is pushed over the upper limit of 70 mm Hg.[19]

## Multimodal Monitoring: Brain Oxygenation and Cerebral Microdialysis

Monitoring brain tissue oxygenation using a catheter placed through a drilled opening in the skull into the brain tissue (parenchyma) allows healthcare providers to evaluate oxygen supply and utilization of oxygen in bran tissue.[26] Interpretation of brain tissue oxygenation values typically requires concomitant ICP monitoring. The PbtO$_2$ catheter also allows direct measurement of brain temperature. A normal PbtO$_2$ level ranges between 25 and 35 mm Hg, while brain hypoxia occurs at 15 mm Hg, severe brain hypoxia at 10 mm Hg, and neuronal cell death at lower than 5 mm Hg.[26] Challenges with PbtO$_2$ monitoring include cost, interpretation of the readings, and management strategies. Controversy exists regarding catheter placement in uninjured

**QSEN BOX 36-2** *COLLABORATIVE CARE GUIDE for the Patient With a Head Injury*

| Outcomes | Interventions |
| --- | --- |
| **Impaired Gas Exchange** **Ineffective Breathing Pattern** | |
| Patient will maintain a patent airway. Lungs will be clear to auscultation. Arterial pH, $PaO_2$, and $SaO_2$ will be maintained within normal limits. $ETCO_2$ or $PCO_2$ will be maintained within prescribed range. There will be no evidence of atelectasis or pneumonia on chest x-ray. | • Auscultate breath sounds every 2–4 h and as needed. • Hyperoxygenate before and after each suction pass. • Avoid suction passes >10 s. • Monitor ICP and CPP during suctioning and chest physiotherapy. • Provide meticulous oral hygiene. • Monitor for signs of aspiration. • Encourage nonintubated patients to use incentive spirometer, cough, and deep breathe every 4 h and as needed. • Turn side-to-side every 2 h. • Move patient out of bed to chair one to two times daily when ICP has been controlled. |
| **Decreased Cardiac and Peripheral Tissue Perfusion** | |
| Patient will exhibit normal sinus rhythm without ectopy or ischemic changes. Patient will not experience thromboembolic complications. | • Monitor for myocardial ischemia and dysrhythmias due to sympathetic activation and catecholamine surges. • Prevent DVT with the use of pneumatic compression devices, antiembolism stockings, and subcutaneous heparin. • Implement early mobilization. Facilitate moving to a chair one to two times daily. • Monitor blood pressure continuously by arterial line or frequently by noninvasive cuff. • Monitor oxygen delivery (hemoglobin, $SaO_2$, cardiac output). • Administer red blood cells, inotropes, intravenous fluids as indicated. |
| **Risk for Impaired Cerebral Perfusion** | |
| CPP will be >60 mm Hg. ICP will be <20 mm Hg. Patient will not experience seizure activity. | • Monitor ICP and CPP every hour. • Perform neurologic checks every 1 to 2. • Elevate the head of bed to 30 degrees unless contraindicated. • Maintain proper body alignment, keeping the head in a neutral position, and avoiding sharp hip flexion. • Maintain normothermia. • Maintain a quiet environment, cluster care, and provide rest periods. • Provide sedation as necessary and as prescribed. • Administer prophylactic antiepileptic agents as prescribed to prevent seizure activity. |
| **Electrolyte Imbalance** **Risk for Imbalanced Fluid Volume** | |
| Serum electrolytes will be within normal limits. Serum osmolality will remain within prescribed range. | • Strict documentation of input/output; consider insensible losses from intubation, fever, and the like. • Monitor serum electrolytes, glucose, and osmolality as ordered. • Consider need for electrolyte replacement therapy and administer per physician order or protocol. |
| **Risk for Injury** **Risk for Falls** | |
| There will be minimal and transient changes in ICP/CPP during treatments or patient care activities. ICP/CPP will return to baseline within 5 min. Patient will not experience complications related to prolonged immobilization (eg, DVT, pneumonia, ankylosis). Patient will not harm self by dislodging medical equipment or falling. | • Provide range of motion and functional splinting for paralyzed limbs or patients in a coma. • Position patient off of pressure points at least every 2 h. • Consider use of specialty mattresses based on skin and risk factor assessments. • Keep bed rails in the upright position. • Provide restraints if necessary to prevent dislodgment of medical devices as policies permit. |

y tissue providing information on global oxygenation rain versus injured but potentially salvageable tissue, y allow more focused therapy.[26] It is important to treatment strategies targeting $PbtO_2$ alone have rated an influence functional outcomes. Global nation can be measured using jugular venous oxygen saturation ($SjO_2$), which is determined by inserting an intravenous catheter into the internal jugular vein and directing it upward toward the brain. The $SjO_2$ is indicative of oxygen extraction in the brain; in the healthy brain, $SjO_2$ is 55% to 70%.[13] If $SjO_2$ is less than 55%, cells are not extracting oxygen from the hemoglobin molecule efficiently (see

Chapter 17 for discussion of oxygen consumption). If $SjO_2$ is greater than 70%, the rate of oxygen extraction is increased. An increase in cerebral oxygen extraction often occurs as a result of cerebral ischemia.

Cerebral microdialysis is another adjunctive strategy for treating patients with severe TBI. During cerebral microdialysis, a specific catheter with a semi-permeable membrane is inserted into the brain.[27] A cerebrospinal fluid–like solution flows through the catheter, allowing for diffusion of solutes between the catheter and the surrounding brain tissue. The solution can be sampled periodically to assess for biochemical substrates such as lactate and pyruvate, which may indicate brain tissue ischemia and cell death. Cerebral microdialysis may be used as an adjunctive monitoring method to evaluate the effects of interventions used to modulate ICP and CPP.[27] Limits to cerebral microdialysis include the time delay in reporting data, catheter placement, and the lack of data suggesting positive functional outcomes in patients. At this point, cerebral microdialysis still remains under investigation as a treatment strategy in TBI patients.[28]

## Preventing and Treating Seizures

Seizures during the early stages of TBI can have severe negative effects on ICP and cerebral metabolic demands. Evidence-based guidelines support the use of antiseizure medication in the first 7 days after TBI to prevent early posttraumatic seizures.[19,29] Seizures after the first initial period are called late posttraumatic seizures and are not prevented by prophylactic administration of antiseizure medications.[19] Seizures that occur during the initial first 7 days are correlated with more severe TBI.[29] It is estimated that in patients with severe TBI (GCS less than 8), 20% to 25% will experience at least one seizure.[29] The Brain Trauma Foundation (BTF) guidelines recommend the use of phenytoin during the acute period.

Phenytoin is usually given as a bolus dose intravenously, followed by a maintenance dosing schedule. The patient is monitored closely for hypotension, bradycardia, rashes, and IV infiltration during and after administration. Hypotension can be mitigated by administering the drug slowly (no greater than 50 mg/min). Truncal rashes with varying severity, including Stevens-Johnson syndrome, can occur with administration of phenytoin. The drug should be discontinued at the appearance of rash. The pro-drug of phenytoin, fosphenytoin, is administered IV or IM and is metabolized in the body to phenytoin. Fosphenytoin can be administered rapidly without the infusion site reactions associated with phenytoin. Other more recent studies suggest that levetiracetam (Keppra) may be as effective in preventing seizures in TBI patients as phenytoin.[29,30,31]

## Maintaining a Normal Body Temperature

Hyperthermia (body temperature higher than 37.5°C [99.5°F]) in a patient with severe TBI increases cerebrometabolic demands and may compound secondary brain injury, and should be avoided. Frequent monitoring of body temperature is necessary to maintain normothermia (35°C to 37.5°C [95°F to 99.5°F]). Infection must be ruled out as the cause of fever, and cooling methods are used as needed to maintain a

normal body temperature. Inducing hypothermia (32°C to 35°C [89.6°F to 95°F]) in patients with TBI has shown mixed to no benefit in improving functional outcome.[19,32,33]

## Identifying and Managing "Sympathetic Storming"

Patients with severe TBI may experience a condition known as paroxysmal sympathetic hyperactivity (also known as "sympathetic storming"). This condition is characterized by diaphoresis; agitation, restlessness, or flexion or extension posturing; hyperventilation; tachycardia; and fever. Sympathetic storming occurs as a result of an imbalance of the sympathetic and parasympathetic nervous systems. The precise cause of this imbalance is poorly understood. An average of 10% of TBI patients will develop paroxysmal sympathetic hyperactivity.[34]

Triggers of a storming episode may include any stressful event, such as endotracheal suctioning, turning, development of fever, or alarm sounds in the patient's room. The diagnosis of sympathetic storming is typically based on the appearance of the common signs and symptoms and exclusion of other conditions, such as infection.[35] Symptoms of sympathetic storming can last from 2 to 127 days, with an average of 15 days.[35]

Treatment focuses on finding a medication regimen that suppresses the sympathetic nervous system while avoiding adverse effects such as hypotension and bradycardia.[36] Medication regimens may include one or more of the following drug classes: α-adrenergic blockers, β blockers, opiates, sedatives, gamma-aminobutyric acid agonists, and dopamine agonists. Nursing management of the patient with sympathetic storming includes monitoring and assessing the patient to determine the effectiveness of the medication regimen, reducing environmental stimuli to reduce triggers of storming episodes, and preventing complications such as skin breakdown or injury from restlessness or agitation. Patients experiencing sympathetic storming may appear uncomfortable and evoke concern in family members; therefore, family education is important.

## Monitoring Fluid and Electrolyte Status

Administration of osmotic diuretics, insensible fluid loss, and pituitary gland dysfunction may be responsible for fluid and electrolyte disturbances in patients with TBI. Strict monitoring of intake and output, as well as hemodynamic monitoring, guides the healthcare team in prescribing adequate fluid replacement. Routine monitoring of serum osmolality is helpful in preventing excessive systemic dehydration when administering osmotic diuretics such as mannitol or hypertonic saline. Surveillance of serum electrolytes allows for early identification and treatment of electrolyte abnormalities.

Disorders of sodium imbalance are common in the patient with TBI (Table 36-4). Hyponatremia most commonly occurs as a result of the syndrome of inappropriate antidiuretic hormone secretion (SIADH), in which antidiuretic hormone (ADH) is released in excessive amounts, resulting retention of water and hemodilution.[37] Hemodilution leads to a lower concentration of sodium in the blood. SIADH often is a transient phenomenon that can be treated with fluid restriction.

**TABLE 36-4** Disorders of Sodium Imbalance: Comparison of Diabetes Insipidus, SIADH, and Cerebral Salt-Wasting Syndrome

|  | Diabetes Insipidus | SIADH | Cerebral Salt-Wasting Syndrome |
|---|---|---|---|
| Urinary output | Increased | Decreased | Increased |
| Specific gravity | Decreased | Increased | Decreased |
| Volume status | Decreased | Mildly increased | Decreased |
| Serum sodium | Increased | Decreased | Decreased |
| Treatment | Administration of exogenous vasopressin, fluid replacement | Fluid restriction, judicious sodium replacement | Fluid and sodium replacement |

SIADH, syndrome of inappropriate antidiuretic hormone secretion.

Cerebral salt-wasting syndrome may also cause hyponatremia. The precise physiologic mechanism of cerebral salt-wasting syndrome is poorly understood but involves a primary loss of sodium and free water through the kidneys. Treatment of this disorder requires fluid and sodium replacement in amounts that equal losses and may include the administration of hypertonic saline.[37]

Diabetes insipidus (DI) is a cause of hypernatremia and hypovolemia that occurs commonly in patients with injury or ischemia in or around the pituitary gland. Herniation syndrome often causes direct compression of the pituitary gland or compression to the supplying blood vessels. Damage to the pituitary gland prevents or decreases the secretion of ADH. DI is diagnosed by increasing serum sodium level, low urine specific gravity, and increased urine output.[38] Treatment of DI includes aggressive fluid replacement that matches hourly fluid losses and the administration of exogenous ADH (vasopressin). Vasopressin may be given intravenously, subcutaneously, or intranasally, depending on the severity of the disorder.

## Managing Cardiovascular Complications

Myocardial stunning and a transient decrease in cardiac function may occur in severe TBI. Inversion of T waves and ST-segment elevation or depression may be noted. Serum cardiac enzyme levels, electrocardiography, and echocardiography may be used to evaluate myocardial function. In one study, 22% of patients with TBI had an abnormal echocardiogram; this was associated with increased in-hospital mortality.[39] Hemodynamic monitoring devices, such as arterial and central lines and pulmonary artery catheters, may be used to guide medical therapies during the critical phases of TBI.

Disorders of coagulation, causing the release of large amounts of thromboplastin in response to brain injury, are a significant concern in patients with TBI. Furthermore, TBI patients often have imbalances of coagulation and lysis, either leading to hypercoagulation with microthrombosis or hypocoagulation with bleeding.[40] Disseminated intravascular coagulation may result. Treatment options for coagulopathy after TBI should be targeted to address the primary cause and to reduce hemorrhage, and may include administering fresh frozen plasma, platelets, or recombinant factor VIIa.[40]

Prophylaxis of deep venous thrombosis (DVT) is an essential component in the care of patients with head injuries, who are often immobile for extended periods and thus at high risk for venous thromboembolic events. Prophylactic anticoagulation in patients with TBI remains a challenge, and evidenced-based clinical practice guidelines are lacking.[41] Recent studies suggest that initiation of subcutaneous injections of low-dose unfractionated heparin for thromboprophylaxis does not increased the risk of intracranial hemorrhage in patients with TBI when neuroimaging is deemed stable.[41,42]

## Managing Pulmonary Complications

Pulmonary complications in the patient with TBI include pneumonia, ARDS, neurogenic pulmonary edema, and pulmonary embolus. Pulmonary toilet, vigilant oral hygiene, and monitoring of endotracheal tube cuff pressure are necessary to prevent nosocomial pneumonia and mitigate pulmonary complications in patients with head injuries who require prolonged mechanical ventilation. (See Chapter 25 for a discussion of the causes and prevention of ventilator-associated pneumonia.) See Chapter 27 for a complete discussion of ARDS management.

Early mobility is critical in facilitating pulmonary toilet, preventing atelectasis, and preventing pulmonary emboli due to DVT. Early consideration of extubation to reduce the number of days on mechanical ventilation, as well as early planning for tracheostomy in patients unable to protect their airway, may prevent additional pulmonary complications.[19]

Neurogenic pulmonary edema may result from injury to the brainstem, increased ICP, or an increase in sympathetic tone that causes a catecholamine surge at the time of trauma. Neurogenic pulmonary edema often presents as "flash pulmonary edema," characterized by a sudden onset and demonstration of large amounts of fluid suctioned from the lungs. This type of pulmonary edema is thought to be caused by massive vasoconstriction due to an acute increase in ICP causing activation of the sympathetic nervous system. Consequently, there is marked increase in systemic afterload resulting in left ventricular failure. Pulmonary edema resulting from left ventricular failure is exacerbated by an increase in pulmonary capillary permeability, causing further edema.[43] Treatment includes judicious use of low-dose diuretics. The condition is typically self-limiting in patients without cardiac disease.

Multidisciplinary care of the patient with TBI with respect to pulmonary complications requires the involvement of the nursing and the physician teams; the respiratory therapist; the occupational therapist; the physical therapist (for early mobilization); and the speech–language pathologist (to address issues with aspiration).

## Managing Nutrition and Maintaining Glycemic Control

Head injury is thought to cause hypermetabolic and hypercatabolic states as well as a decrease in immune competence.[44] Morbidity and mortality may significantly increase if nutritional requirements are not met. Indirect calorimetry is useful in determining resting energy expenditure (REE).[45] Current recommendations suggest replacement of 140% of REE in patients who are not paralyzed, and 100% of REE in patients who are paralyzed.[19] Recognition of the importance of nutrition and multidisciplinary collaboration with a nutrition support team are essential to optimize patient outcome. Research suggests a detrimental effect of hyperglycemia and hypoglycemia on morbidity and mortality of patients with TBI; however, specific treatment thresholds have not been established. Hyperglycemia with a blood glucose exceeding 200 mg/dL and hypoglycemia should be avoided in patients with TBI.[19,46]

## Managing Musculoskeletal and Integumentary Complications

Comprehensive assessment of the musculoskeletal and integumentary systems is necessary to prevent skin breakdown and other complications, such as contractures. A recent study suggested a relationships between development of a pressure ulcer and mortality within 21 days of TBI, as well as poor neurologic outcome.[47] Collaboration with other disciplines, such as occupational and physical therapy, is essential in developing a plan of care to prevent or mitigate the effects of immobility on the skin and musculoskeletal systems. Splinting of the hands and feet in an unresponsive patient is necessary to preserve musculoskeletal function and ensure the best conditions for future rehabilitation.

## Caring for the Family

Caring for families in crisis, as well as coordinating available services (such as social work and pastoral care), is an important function of the critical care nurse. Bond and colleagues surveyed the needs of family members of patients with severe TBI and found the following four needs[48]:

- The need for specific truthful information
- The need for information to be consistent
- The need to be actively involved in care
- The need to make sense of the entire experience

Critical care nurses have an opportunity to meet all of these specific needs and to change unit culture to meet these needs. Encouraging family members to touch the patient and allowing family members to assist in providing sensory stimulation (Box 36-3) may be helpful and comforting to some family members. Finding opportunities to involve family members in the patient's plan of care may also be therapeutic for the patient and the family. The Ranchos Los Amigos Scale can be used by the critical care nurse to describe the stages of coma as they relate to rehabilitative methods and interventions (Table 36-5). Attention is given to including both spiritual and cultural needs in the plan of care.

---

**BOX 36-3**  **Nursing Interventions**

**For Sensory Stimulation**

Sound
- Explain to the patient what you are going to do.
- Play the patient's favorite television or radio program for 10 to 15 minutes. Alternatively, play a recording of a familiar voice of a friend or family member.
- During the program, do not converse with others in the room or perform other activities of patient care. The goal is to minimize distractions so the patient may learn to attend to the stimulus selectively.
- Another approach is to clap your hands or ring a bell. Do this for 5 to 10 seconds at a time, moving the sound to different locations around the bed.

Sight
- Place a brightly colored object in the patient's view. Present only one object at a time.
- Alternatively, use an object that is familiar, such as a family photo or favorite poster.

Touch
- Stroke the patient's arm or leg with fabrics of various textures. Alternatively, the back of a spoon can simulate smooth texture and a towel rough texture.
- Rubbing lotion over the patient's skin will also stimulate this sense. For some, firm pressure may be better tolerated than very light touch.

Smell
- Hold a container of a pleasing fragrance under the patient's nose. Use a familiar scent, such as perfume, aftershave, cinnamon, or coffee.
- Present this stimulation for very short periods (1 to 3 minutes maximum).
- If a cuffed tracheostomy or endotracheal tube is in place, the patient will not be able to appreciate this stimulation fully.

---

A patient with TBI may be discharged to home, a rehabilitation program, or a nursing facility depending on the severity of his or her neurologic deficits. Families must be informed and educated about the expected course of events and potential scenarios for continued care after the acute hospitalization, especially when the patient has severe TBI. Family resources, as well as other support systems and services available to the patient, should be assessed early in all patients with TBI to facilitate a smooth transition into the next stage of care. Social workers and case managers play an integral role in obtaining information and communicating with the patient, the family, and the multidisciplinary team.

## Brain Death

A patient's condition may be so severe that brain death is the final outcome. In the past, the declaration of brain death was controversial with regard to the standardization of tests needed to make the decision and ethical considerations. The Uniform Determination of Death Act was developed in 1981 by the President's Commission for the Study of Ethical Problems in Medicine and Biomedical Behavior Research and adopted by all 50 states. This act states: "An individual, who has sustained either (1) irreversible cessation of circulatory and respiratory functions, or (2) irreversible cessation of

**TABLE 36-5** Ranchos Los Amigos Scale

| Level | Guidelines for Interacting With Patient |
|---|---|
| 1. **No response** to any stimuli occurs. | • Assume that the patient can understand all that is said. Converse with, not about, the patient.<br>• Do not overwhelm the patient with talking. Leave some moments of silence between verbal stimuli. |
| 2. **Generalized response:** Stimulus response is incoherent, limited, and nonpurposeful with random movements or incomprehensible sounds. | |
| 3. **Localized response:** Stimulus response is specific but inconsistent; patient may withdraw or push away, may make sounds, may follow some simple commands, or may respond to certain family members. | • Manage the environment to provide only one source of stimulation at a time. If talking is taking place, the radio or television should be turned off.<br>• Provide short, random periods of sensory input that are meaningful to the patient. A favorite television program or recording or 30 min of music from the patient's favorite radio station will provide more meaningful stimulation than constant radio accompaniment, which becomes as meaningless as the continual bleep of the cardiac monitor. |
| 4. **Confused–agitated:** Stimulus response is primarily to internal confusion with increased state of activity; behavior may be bizarre or aggressive; patient may attempt to remove tubes or restraints or crawl out of bed; verbalization is incoherent or inappropriate; patient shows minimal awareness of environment and absent short-term memory. | • Be calm and soothing when handling the patient. Approach with gentle touch to decrease the occurrence of defensive emotional and motor reflexes.<br>• Watch for early signs that the patient is becoming agitated (eg, increased movement, vocal loudness, resistance to activity).<br>• When the patient becomes upset, do not try to reason with him or her or "talk him or her out of it." Talking will be an additional external stimulus that the patient cannot handle.<br>• If the patient remains upset, either remove him or her from the situation or remove the situation from him or her. |
| 5. **Confused, inappropriate–nonagitated:** Patient is alert and responds consistently to simple commands; however, patient has a short attention span and is easily distracted; memory is impaired and patient exhibits confusion of past and present events; patient can perform previously learned tasks with maximal structure but is unable to learn new information; may wander off with vague intention of "going home." | • Present the patient with only one task at a time. Allow time to complete it before giving further instructions.<br>• Make sure that you have the patient's attention by placing yourself in view and touching the patient before talking.<br>• If the patient becomes confused or resistant, stop talking. Wait until he or she appears relaxed before continuing with instruction or activity.<br>• Use gestures, demonstrations, and only the most necessary words when giving instructions. |
| 6. **Confused–appropriate:** Patient shows goal-directed behavior but still needs external direction; can understand simple directions and reasoning; follows simple directions consistently and requires less supervision for previously learned tasks; has improved past memory depth and detail and basic awareness of self and surroundings. | • Maintain the same sequence in routine activities and tasks. Describe these routines to the patient and relate them to time of day. |
| 7. **Automatic–appropriate:** Patient is able to complete daily routines in structured environment; has increased awareness of self and surroundings but lacks insight, judgment, and problem-solving ability. | • Supervision is still necessary for continued learning and safety.<br>• Reinforce the patient's memory of routines and schedules with clocks, calendars, and a written log of activities. |
| 8. **Purposeful–appropriate:** Patient is alert, oriented, and able to recall and integrate past and recent events; responds appropriately to environment; still has decreased ability in abstract reasoning, stress tolerance, and judgment in emergencies or unusual situations. | • The patient should be able to function without supervision.<br>• Consideration should be given to job retraining or a return to school. |

all functions of the entire brain, including the brainstem, is dead. A determination of death must be made in accordance with accepted medical standards."[48]

The brain death examination seeks to confirm the following three cardinal findings: coma or unresponsiveness, absence of brainstem reflexes, and apnea.[49,50] Tests specific for brain death include, but are not limited to, motor testing; evaluation of pupillary responses; evaluation of the oculocephalic reflex ("doll's eyes" phenomenon); evaluation of the oculovestibular reflex (caloric ice-water test); evaluation of the corneal, cough, and gag reflexes; and apnea testing. Electrolyte abnormalities, hypothermia or hyperthermia, severe hypotension, or the presence of medications in amounts that could cause coma must be resolved before brain death testing can be performed. Apnea testing is performed by removing

the patient from the ventilator, inspecting the chest for spontaneous respiratory effort while providing supplemental oxygen, and monitoring for an increase in $PaCO_2$. Baseline acid–base balance is established with an arterial blood gas (ABG) measurement prior to removal from the ventilator, and then serial ABG measures are obtained. A $PaCO_2$ greater than 60 mm Hg or an increase in the $PaCO_2$ of 20 mm Hg or more above the patient's baseline $PaCO_2$ is regarded as a positive test, supporting the diagnosis of brain death.[51] The patient is simultaneously observed for spontaneous respiration and hemodynamic instability, which may cause the test to be aborted. An increased $PaCO_2$ is the single strongest stimulus for the initiation of breathing; therefore, the absence of respiratory effort in the presence of severe hypercarbia constitutes strong evidence of brain death. Confirmatory tests for brain death, such as cerebral angiography (to test for the absence of cerebral blood flow), TCD ultrasonography, EEG, BAER, and SSEP, can be used if any doubt exists after a full clinical examination has been completed.

The American Academy of Neurology recommends repeating the clinical evaluation for brain death after 6 hours.[49] Time of death is recorded at the time that brain death is declared. Different institutions specify requirements based on state laws and statutes for physicians declaring brain death. Brain death determination in pediatric patients differs from that in adults because of the increased viability of the immature brain.[51]

The concept of brain death is often confusing for families, because death is typically associated with cardiopulmonary death. Therefore, the language used in discussions is very important. Some family members may interpret the term "brain dead" to mean that the rest of the body can continue to live, so care must be taken to assess the understanding and coping behaviors of family members. Family presence during examinations used to determine brain death has been associated with an increased understanding of the concept without an increase in psychological distress.[52]

The discussion of brain death is typically separated in time from conversations regarding organ donation. It is essential to work closely with an organ procurement organization to provide the most complete and accurate information regarding organ donation.

## Clinical Applicability Challenges

### CASE STUDY

Mr. H. is a 30-year-old man who was involved in a motor–pedestrian collision: he was struck by a vehicle traveling at 35 miles per hour. EMS took the patient to the ED. Upon arrival, the patient was comatose with a GCS of 7 (eye opening to pain [E2], incomprehensible sounds [V], motor flexion to painful stimuli [3]). The patient had a visible skull fracture with extruding brain matter. Owing to the patient's altered mental status and evidence of head injury on exam, he was intubated using rapid sequence intubation and placed on mechanical ventilation.

A head, thoracic, abdominal, and pelvic CT was done and revealed left frontal contusion, left temporal intracerebral hemorrhage, right subdural hematoma, depressed skull fracture, multiple facial and orbital fractures, multiple rib fractures, pulmonary contusions, hemothorax and pneumothorax, and pelvic fracture. Mr. H had an ICP monitor, chest tube, central venous catheter, and arterial line placed.

Over the next 4 days, Mr. H.'s ICPs ranged from 9 to 35 mm Hg, requiring multiple boluses of mannitol 50 g to treat the elevated ICP. His neurologic exam revealed localization to pain, eye opening to pain, and brisk pupillary response. The patient was on a fentanyl infusion at 25 mcg/h for analgesia. Once Mr. H.'s ICP stabilized on ICU day 5, he went to the operating room for a cranioplasty to repair the depressed skull fracture. After the skull fracture was repaired, Mr. H. was moved out of bed to a cardiac chair daily to facilitate pulmonary drainage.

On ICU day 7, Mr. H. continued to have acute respiratory failure, and a percutaneous tracheostomy was placed at the bedside to facilitate prolonged mechanical ventilation.

During the first week of hospitalization, Mr. H. required multiple bronchoscopies because of mucus plugging and went to the operative room for repair of the rib fractures, repair of facial fractures, and skin debridement. On ICU day 10, Mr. H started to open eyes to voice and began following simple commands. Physical therapy was started, and he ambulated on ICU day 13. Ventilator weaning occurred with spontaneous breathing trials and tracheostomy collar trials over 6 days. Once he was successfully tolerating tracheostomy collar, Mr. H. had a speaking valve placed to facilitate speaking. On hospital day 16, Mr. H was transferred to the progressive care unit, passed a swallow evaluation, and started eating.

Mr. H. was discharged to home on hospital day 24, alert and oriented × 4, GCS 15, with an intact neuro assessment. He had outpatient physical therapy and was back to work 2 months later.

1. Based on the radiologic findings and your knowledge of the pathophysiology of head injury, explain why Mr. H. has a decreased level of consciousness.
2. Name at least three multisystem complications from having a severe TBI that Mr. H. may experience.
3. Using the description of the patient's neurologic status at the beginning and end of the case study, place the patient into the appropriate level on the Ranchos Los Amigos Scale (see Table 36-5).
4. Name two interventions that could be used when interacting with patients in these categories.

### WANT TO KNOW MORE?

A wide variety of resources to enhance your learning and understanding of this chapter are available on thePoint.

You will find:

- References
- Selected readings
- NCLEX-style review questions
- Internet resources
- And more!

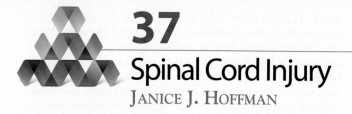

# 37

# Spinal Cord Injury

JANICE J. HOFFMAN

**LEARNING OBJECTIVES**

*Based on the content in this chapter, the reader should be able to:*

1. Discuss the various classification systems for spinal cord injuries.
2. Differentiate central cord syndrome, Brown–Séquard syndrome, anterior cord syndrome, and posterior cord syndrome.
3. Differentiate spinal shock, neurogenic shock, and orthostatic hypotension.
4. Perform an assessment of a patient with an SCI.
5. Develop a collaborative plan of care for a patient with an acute SCI.
6. Describe immediate nursing actions when the patient develops autonomic dysreflexia.
7. Explain other typical complications that occur after an SCI.

Spinal cord trauma is often a devastating injury resulting in permanent paralysis and disability. The estimated annual incidence of spinal cord injury (SCI) in the United States is 54 cases per million, or approximately 17,000 new cases, and these numbers do not include those individuals who die at the accident scene.[1] According to the National Spinal Cord Injury Database (2016), there are about 282,000 (range of 243,000–347,000) people living with SCI in the United States.

SCI most often affects young adults, with nearly half of all injuries occurring in those between the ages of 16 and 30 years, but as the age of the general population has increased by approximately 9 years since the mid-1970s, so has the average age of the population with SCI.[1] Since 2010, the average age at time of injury has increased from 29 to 42 years of age.[1] Males are overwhelmingly most often affected, representing 80% of those with injuries in the national database. An analysis of race and ethnicity reveals that since 2010, 63.5% were non-Hispanic white, 22% were non-Hispanic black, 11% were of Hispanic origin, 2% were Asian, 0.5% were Native American, and 1% were other.

Motor vehicle crashes are the most common etiology of SCI (38%), followed by falls (30.5%), acts of violence (13.5%), which are primarily gunshot wounds, and sports (9%).[1] Although the life expectancy of persons with SCI has significantly increased since the 1980s, it is still below that of those without SCI. Renal failure was a leading cause of death in patients with SCI for many years; however, with advancements in urologic management there has been a shift, with pneumonia and septicemia being the leading causes of death. The mortality rates are highest during the first year after injury, and greater in those with higher-level spinal cord injuries.[1]

In 2016, the National Spinal Cord Injury Statistical Center (NSCISC) reported that the average length of stay in acute care settings for patients after SCI was 11 days. Patients were then usually transferred to a rehabilitation unit or facility, where the average length of stay was 35 days. The cost of care differed significantly based upon the level of injury. Estimated first-year costs for patients with high tetraplegia (quadriplegia, C1–C4) was $1,065,980; for those with low

tetraplegia (C5–C8), $770,264; and for those with paraplegia, $519,520. For succeeding years, the estimated annual cost was $185,111, $113,557, and $68,821, respectively.[1]

## Classification of Injury

Understanding the anatomy and physiology of the spinal cord is important to correlating the cord damage to the clinical presentation. The spinal cord extends from the base of the brain to approximately the level of the first or second lumbar vertebra. Blood is supplied to the cord by the anterior and posterior spinal arteries. Extending from the spinal cord are the spinal nerve roots. The spinal cord is enclosed in the vertebral canal, which consists of 33 vertebrae: 7 cervical, 12 thoracic, 5 lumbar, 5 sacral (fused), and 4 coccygeal (fused). The vertebrae are held in place by ligaments, muscles, and other supporting structures.

SCIs can be classified by mechanism of injury, type of vertebral injury, level of injury, or cause. SCIs occur as a result of penetrating injury or mechanical forces. Penetrating injuries, which are most often caused by gunshot or stab wounds, damage the spinal cord and cause loss of neurologic functioning.

## Mechanism of Injury

Mechanical forces that can result in SCI include hyperflexion, hyperextension, axial loading (compression), and rotational forces (Fig. 37-1):

- **Hyperflexion**, depicted in Figure 37-1A, is caused by a sudden deceleration of the head and neck, and is often seen in patients who have sustained trauma from a head-on motor vehicle crash (MVC) or diving accident. The cervical region is most often involved, especially at the C5–C6 level.
- **Hyperextension** (Fig. 37-1B) is the most common type of injury; it can be caused by a fall, a rear-end MVC, or getting hit in the head (eg, during a boxing match). Hyperextension of the head and neck may cause contusion and ischemia of the spinal cord without vertebral column

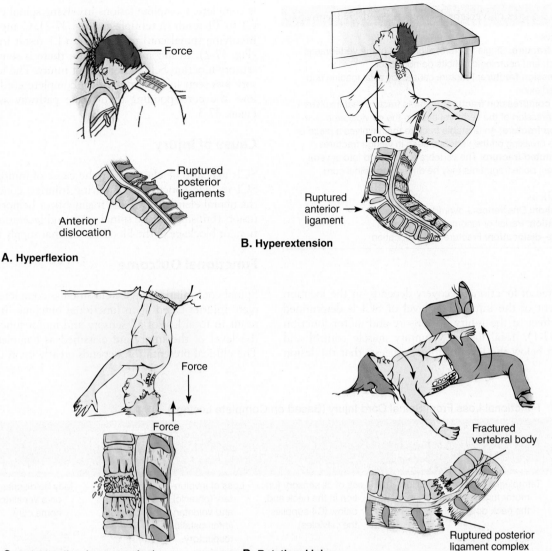

**FIGURE 37-1** Spinal cord injuries can be classified according to the mechanism of injury. **A:** With hyperflexion to the cervical spine, there may be tearing of the posterior ligamentous complex, resulting in anterior dislocation. **B:** Hyperextension injury can result in rupture of the anterior ligament. **C:** Axial loading (compression) of the spine results in fracture and subsequent spinal cord damage. **D:** When rotational force occurs, there is concurrent fracture and tearing of the posterior ligamentous complex. (Adapted from Hickey JV: Clinical Practice of Neurological and Neurosurgical Nursing, 6th ed. Philadelphia, PA: Lippincott Williams & Wilkins, 2009, pp 412–415.)

damage. Whiplash injuries are an example of a hyperextension injury.

- **Axial loading,** also known as compression (Fig. 37-1C), typically occurs when a person lands on the feet or buttocks after falling or jumping from a height, or when there is a direct blow to the head. Injury results from vertebral column compression leading to a fracture that causes damage to the spinal cord.
- **Rotational injuries** result from forces that cause extreme twisting or lateral flexion of the head and neck (Fig. 37-1D). Fracture or dislocation of vertebrae may also occur.

## Type of Vertebral Injury

Mechanical forces can result in fracture or dislocation of vertebrae, or both. If vertebral injury occurs, the type of

vertebral injury can be used to describe the person's SCI. Box 37-1 presents definitions of types of fractures and dislocations. A fracture may be considered unstable if the posterior ligaments are torn.

## Level of Injury

SCIs can also be classified according to the segment of the spinal cord that is affected:

- Upper cervical (C1–C2): Atlas fractures, atlantoaxial subluxation, odontoid fractures, and hangman's fractures
- Lower cervical (C3–C8)
- Thoracic (T1–T12)
- Lumbar (L1–L5)
- Sacral (S1–S5)

Fractures

**Simple fracture:** Single fracture; alignment of the vertebrae is intact, and neurologic deficits do not occur

**Compression fracture:** Fracture caused by axial loading and hyperflexion

**Wedge compression fracture:** A stable fracture that involves compression of the vertebral body in the cervical area

**Teardrop fracture:** An unstable fracture that involves a piece of bone breaking off the vertebra; seen in wedge fractures

**Comminuted fracture:** The vertebra is shattered into several pieces; bone fragments may be driven into spinal cord

Dislocations

**Dislocation:** One vertebra overrides another
**Subluxation:** Partial or incomplete dislocation
**Fracture–dislocation:** Fracture and dislocation

is complete. Complete lesions involving spinal cord regions C1 to T1 result in tetraplegia (Fig. 37-2). Complete lesions involving spinal cord regions T2 to L1 result in paraplegia (Fig. 37-2). In incomplete injuries, there is some motor or sensory function below the level of injury. The level of sensory loss seen in a person with a complete cord injury follows the corresponding dermatome pathway as shown in Figure 37-3.

## Cause of Injury

SCIs may also be classified by the cause of injury. Causes of SCI include concussion or jarring injuries, compression of the neural elements by bony fragments or hemorrhage, contusion (bruising) of the spinal cord, and laceration, transection, or blockage of the blood vessels that supply the cord.

## Functional Outcome

Spinal cord injuries may be classified as complete or incomplete injuries based upon functional outcome. Injuries that result in total loss of all sensory and motor function below the level of the injury are classified as complete injuries. The clinical presentation depends greatly upon the level of

The degree of functional recovery depends on the location and extent of the injury. The level of SCI is determined by the effect of the injury on sensory and motor function (Table 37-1). Total loss of voluntary muscle control and sensation below the level of injury suggests that the lesion

**TABLE 37-1** Functional Loss From Spinal Cord Injury (Based on Complete Lesions)

| Level of Spinal Injury | Motor Function | Deep Tendon Reflexes | Sensory Function | Respiratory Function | Voluntary Bowel and Bladder Function | Rehabilitative Potential |
|---|---|---|---|---|---|---|
| C1–C4 | Tetraplegia: Loss of all motor function from the neck down | All lost | Loss of all sensory function in the neck and below (C4 supplies the clavicles) | Loss of involuntary (phrenic) and voluntary (intercostals) respiratory function; ventilatory support and a tracheostomy needed | No bowel or bladder control | May be discharged home on a ventilator with home care |
| C5 | Tetraplegia: Loss of all function below the upper shoulders. Intact: Sternomastoids, cervical paraspinal muscles, and the trapezius; can control head | C5, C6 biceps | Loss of sensation below the clavicle and most portions of arms, hands, chest, abdomen, and lower extremities. Intact: Head, shoulders, deltoid, clavicle, portion of forearms (C5 supplies the lateral aspect of the arm) | Phrenic nerve intact, but not intercostal muscles | No bowel or bladder control | Use of extremity-powered devices to achieve some upper limb control. Head control facilitates wheelchair (W/C) balance. Adaptive tools, held in mouth, for typing and writing. Some adaptive tools and use of special computer technology |
| C6 | Tetraplegia: Loss of all function below the shoulders and upper arms; lacks elbow, forearm, and hand control. Intact: Deltoid, biceps, and external rotator muscles of shoulders | C5, C6 brachioradialis | Loss of everything listed for a C5 lesion, but greater arm and thumb sensation. Intact: Head, shoulders, arms, palms of hands, and thumbs (C6 supplies the forearm and thumb) | Phrenic nerve intact, but not intercostal muscles | No bowel or bladder control | Needs assistive devices to use arms (may be able to help feed, groom, and dress self). Needs a motorized W/C. Dependent for all transfers |

**TABLE 37-1** Functional Loss From Spinal Cord Injury (Based on Complete Lesions) *(continued)*

| Level of Spinal Injury | Motor Function | Deep Tendon Reflexes | Sensory Function | Respiratory Function | Voluntary Bowel and Bladder Function | Rehabilitative Potential |
|---|---|---|---|---|---|---|
| C7 | Tetraplegia: Loss of motor control to portions of the arms and hands<br>Intact: Voluntary strength in shoulder depressors, shoulder abductors, internal rotators, and radial wrist extensors | C7, C8 triceps | Loss of sensation below the clavicle and portions of arms and hands<br>Intact: Head, shoulders, most of arms and hands (C7 supplies the middle finger) | Phrenic nerve intact, but not intercostal muscles | No bowel or bladder function | Can perform some activities of daily living (ADLs)<br>Can use wrist extensor with a special splint to induce finger flexion<br>Can push a W/C with special hand grasps<br>May be able to drive a specially equipped car |
| C8 | Tetraplegia: Loss of motor control to portions of the arms and hands<br>Intact: Some voluntary control of elbow extensors, wrist, finger extension, and finger flexors | | Loss of sensation below the chest and in portions of hands<br>Intact: Sensation to face, shoulders, arms, hands, and part of chest (C8 supplies the little finger) | Phrenic nerve intact, but not intercostal muscles | No bowel or bladder function | Able to push up in the W/C<br>Improved sitting tolerance<br>Can grasp and release hands voluntarily<br>Independent in most ADLs from W/C<br>Independent in use of W/C<br>Can use hands for catheterization and rectal stimulation for bowel movements |
| T1–T6 | Paraplegia: Loss of everything below the midchest region, including the trunk muscles<br>Intact: Control of function to the shoulders, upper chest, arms, and hands | | Loss of sensation below the midchest area<br>Intact: Everything to the midchest region, including the arms and hands (T1 and T2 supply the inner aspect of the arm; T4 supplies the nipple area) | Phrenic nerve functions independently<br>Some impairment of intercostal muscles | No bowel or bladder function | Full control of upper extremities and completely independent in W/C<br>Full-time employment possible<br>Independent in managing urinary drainage and inserting suppositories<br>Able to live in a dwelling without major architectural changes |
| T6–T12 | Paraplegia: Loss of motor control below the waist<br>Intact: Shoulders, arms, hands, and long trunk muscles | | Loss of everything below the waist<br>Intact: Shoulders, chest, arms, and hands (T10 supplies the umbilicus; T12 supplies the groin area) | No interference with respiratory function | No bowel or bladder control | In addition to the previously described capabilities, there is complete abdominal and upper back control.<br>Good sitting balance (allows for greater ease of W/C operation and athletics) |
| L1–L3 | Paraplegia: Loss of most control of legs and pelvis<br>Intact: Shoulders, arms, hands, torso, hip rotation and flexion, and some leg flexion | L2–L4 (knee jerk) | Loss of sensation to the lower abdomen and legs<br>Intact: All of the above plus some sensation to the inner and anterior thigh (L3 supplies the knee) | No interference with respiratory function | No bowel or bladder control | Independent for most activities from W/C |
| L3–L4 | Paraplegia: Loss of control of portions of lower legs, ankles, and feet<br>Intact: All of the above, plus increased knee extension | | Loss of sensation to portions of the lower legs, feet, and ankles<br>Intact: All of the above, plus sensation to the upper legs | No interference with respiratory function | No bowel or bladder control | Voluntary control of hip extensors; weak abductors<br>Walking with braces possible |

*(continued)*

**TABLE 37-1** Functional Loss From Spinal Cord Injury (Based on Complete Lesions) (*continued*)

| Level of Spinal Injury | Motor Function | Deep Tendon Reflexes | Sensory Function | Respiratory Function | Voluntary Bowel and Bladder Function | Rehabilitative Potential |
|---|---|---|---|---|---|---|
| L4 to S5 | Paraplegia: Incomplete Segmental motor control L4 to S1: Abduction and internal rotation of hip, ankle dorsiflexion, and foot inversion L5 to S1: Foot eversion L4 to S2: Knee flexion S1–S2: Plantar flexion (ankle jerk) S2–S5: Bowel/bladder control | S1–S2 (ankle jerk) | Lumbar sensory nerves innervate the upper legs and portions of the lower legs L5: Medial aspect of foot S1: Lateral aspect of foot S2: Posterior aspect of calf/thigh Sacral sensory nerves innervate the lower legs, feet, and perineum | No interference with respiratory function | Bowel and bladder control possibly impaired S2–S4 segments control urinary continence S3–S5 segments control bowel continence (perianal muscles) | Can walk with braces or may use W/C Can be relatively independent |

From Hickey JV: The Clinical Practice of Neurological and Neurosurgical Nursing, 6th ed. Philadelphia, PA: Lippincott Williams & Wilkins, 2009, pp 428–429, with permission

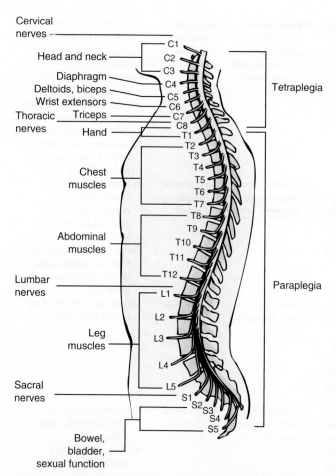

FIGURE 37-2 The level of spinal cord injury (SCI) relates to functional loss. The higher the SCI, the more motor, sensory, and autonomic functional losses are incurred. (Adapted from Hickey JV: Clinical Practice of Neurological and Neurosurgical Nursing, 6th ed. Philadelphia, PA: Lippincott Williams & Wilkins, 2009, p 411.)

injury; patients with injuries at or above C4 are particularly vulnerable to complete respiratory failure resulting from loss of innervations to both the diaphragm (C2–C4) and the intercostal muscles (T1–T4). Incomplete cord injuries often cause recognizable neurologic syndromes that are classified according to the area damaged (Fig. 37-4).

## Spinal Cord Syndromes

### Central Cord Syndrome

Damage to the spinal cord in central cord syndrome is centrally located. Hyperextension of the cervical spine often is the mechanism of injury, and the damage is greatest to the cervical tracts supplying the arms.[2] Clinically, the patient may present with paralyzed arms but with no deficit in the legs or bladder (Fig. 37-4A).

### Brown–Séquard Syndrome

The damage in Brown–Séquard syndrome is located on one side of the spinal cord. The clinical presentation is one in which the patient has either increased or decreased cutaneous sensation of pain, temperature, and touch on the same (ipsilateral) side of the spinal cord at the level of the lesion. Below the level of the lesion on the same side, there is complete motor paralysis. On the patient's opposite (contralateral) side, below the level of the lesion, there is loss of pain, temperature, and touch because the spinothalamic tracts cross to the opposite side soon after entering the cord. The posterior columns are interrupted ipsilaterally, but this does not cause a major deficit because some fibers cross to the opposite instead of running ipsilaterally. Clinically, the patient's limb with the best motor strength has the poorest sensation. Conversely, the limb with the best sensation has the poorest motor strength (Fig. 37-4B).

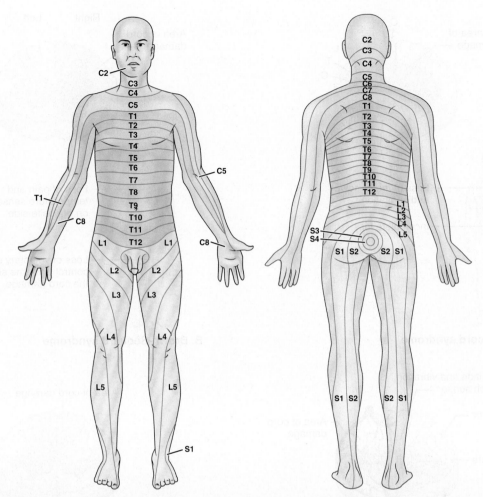

FIGURE 37-3    A person with complete SCI follows the dermatome pathways for the level of sensory loss. (From Hinkle JL, Cheever KH: Brunner & Suddarth's Textbook of Medical-Surgical Nursing, 13th ed. Philadelphia, PA: Lippincott Williams & Wilkins, 2014, p 1915.)

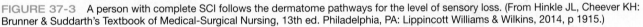

## Anterior Cord Syndrome

The area of damage in anterior cord syndrome is the anterior aspect of the spinal cord. Clinically, the patient usually has complete motor paralysis below the level of injury (corticospinal tracts) and loss of pain, temperature, and touch sensation (spinothalamic tracts), with preservation of light touch, proprioception, and position sense (Fig. 37-4C).

## Posterior Cord Syndrome

Posterior cord syndrome is usually the result of a hyperextension injury at the cervical level and is not commonly seen. Position sense, light touch, and vibratory sense are lost below the level of the injury, while motor function and pain and temperature sensation remain intact (Fig. 37-4D).

## Pathophysiology

### Primary Injury

Injury to the spinal cord that occurs at impact is referred to as the primary injury and is most often associated with damage to the vertebral column. The vertebrae may be fractured, dislocated, or compressed, leading to concussion, contusion, compression, laceration, or transaction of the spinal cord. The more mobile areas of the vertebral column (such as the cervical area) are most frequently injured.

### Secondary Injury

Equally destructive is the secondary injury or damage to the spinal cord that continues for hours to days after the initial trauma. Complex vascular, inflammatory, and chemical processes result in additional axonal damage and further neurologic deficit. Mechanisms of secondary injury include the following:

- Immune cells, which normally do not enter the spinal cord, engulf the area after an SCI. These immune cells respond as they normally do with inflammation in other parts of the body, resulting in release of regulatory chemicals, some of which are harmful to the spinal cord. Highly reactive oxidizing agents (free radicals) are produced, damaging the cell membrane and disrupting the sodium–potassium pump. Intracellular calcium increases secondary to disruption of the sodium–potassium pump, leading to release of vasoactive substances (catecholamines,

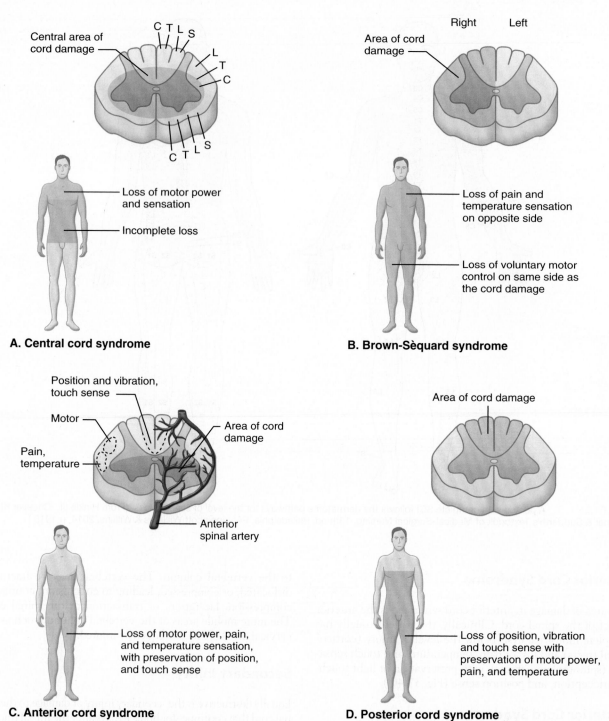

**FIGURE 37-4** Selected syndromes related to SCI. C, cervical; L, lumbar; S, sacral; T, thoracic. (Adapted from Hickey JV: Clinical Practice of Neurological and Neurosurgical Nursing, 6th ed. Philadelphia, PA: Lippincott Williams & Wilkins, 2009, pp 424–425)

histamine, and prostaglandins). This series of events ultimately leads to decreased blood flow to the spinal cord, further exacerbating cord ischemia.

- Hypoperfusion of the spinal cord from microscopic hemorrhage and edema leads to cord ischemia. Ischemic areas develop at the injury site, as well as one or two segments above and below the level of injury.
- The release of catecholamines and vasoactive substances (norepinephrine, serotonin, dopamine, and histamine)

contributes to decreased circulation and impaired cellular perfusion of the spinal cord.

- The release of excess neurotransmitters leads to overexcitation of the nerve cells. Excitotoxicity allows high levels of calcium to enter the cells, causing further oxidative damage and damage to mitochondria. Excitotoxicity is thought to damage oligodendrocytes (the cells that produce myelin), leading to demyelinated axons that are unable to conduct impulses.

# Autonomic Nervous System Dysfunction

## Spinal Shock

Spinal shock is a condition that occurs immediately or within several hours of an SCI; it is caused by the sudden cessation of impulses from the higher brain centers (Fig. 37-5). Because of a decrease in sympathetic innervation to the vascular system, massive vasodilation occurs, which initiates a series of events including decreases in preload and stroke volume. The loss of sympathetic nervous system function, accompanied by unopposed parasympathetic nervous system stimulation to the heart, leads to a decrease in heart rate, and also further decreases stroke volume. The vasodilation also leads to a decrease in afterload. Because of the changes in innervation, the patient develops hypotension and bradycardia.

Spinal shock is a unique shock state, as there is not the reflex tachycardia that usually accompanies the decrease in blood pressure. Characteristics include the loss of motor, sensory, reflex, and autonomic function below the level of the injury, with resultant flaccid paralysis, and loss of bowel and bladder function (Box 37-2). Additionally, the body's ability to control temperature is lost, and the patient's temperature tends to equilibrate with that of the external environment (poikilothermia).

If the SCI produces an incomplete transection, the suppression of function below the level of injury is temporary, lasting a few days to weeks or months. The duration of spinal shock is variable, depending on the severity of the insult and the presence of other complications. The return of perianal reflex activity signals the end of the period of spinal shock. Reflexes associated with the area surrounding the injured

- Flaccid paralysis below the level of injury
- Absence of cutaneous and proprioceptive sensation
- Hypotension and bradycardia
- Absence of reflex activity below the level of injury; may cause urinary retention, bowel paralysis, and ileus
- Loss of temperature control (Vasodilation and inability to shiver make it difficult for the patient to conserve heat in a cool environment, and the inability to perspire prevents normal cooling in a hot environment.)

cord return last. The skeletal muscles become spastic, and there is increased muscle tone and exaggerated flexor muscle movement.

## Neurogenic Shock

Neurogenic shock, a form of distributive shock, is a condition seen in patients with severe cervical and upper thoracic injuries. It is caused by the loss of sympathetic input to the systemic vasculature of the heart and subsequent decreased peripheral vascular resistance. Signs and symptoms include hypotension, severe bradycardia, and loss of the ability to sweat below the level of injury. The same clinical findings pertaining to disruption of the sympathetic transmissions in spinal shock occur in neurogenic shock.

## Orthostatic Hypotension

Orthostatic hypotension may occur in a patient with an SCI because the patient is unable to compensate for changes in

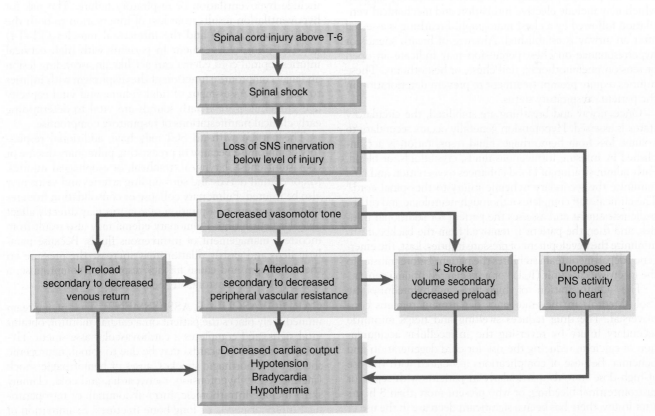

**FIGURE 37-5** Mechanisms involved in spinal shock. PNS, parasympathetic nervous system; SNS, sympathetic nervous system.

position. The vasoconstriction message from the medulla cannot reach the blood vessels because of the cord injury.

## Initial Assessment and Management

### Prehospital Management

An SCI should be suspected at the scene of an accident when the patient has decreased or absent movement or sensation. An unconscious patient or one with a head injury is treated as though an SCI has occurred until cord injury is ruled out. Because elapsed time from injury significantly affects prognosis, the patient with an SCI is transported as safely and rapidly as possible to a specialized trauma center or a hospital with adequate diagnostic and treatment facilities to handle such trauma. A primary survey performed at the scene of an accident includes a rapid assessment of airway, breathing, and circulation (ABCs). Airway patency is assessed, and the cervical spine is immobilized and stabilized. It is important to remember that a cervical collar increases the level of stability but does not provide complete immobilization, especially in the case of complete ligamentous disruption, in which the collar has a minimal immobilization effect on spinal stability.[3]

### In-Hospital Management

After the patient has been admitted to the emergency department, assessment of the patient's airway is a priority. Facial, mandibular, or laryngeal injuries, as well as broken teeth or a swollen tongue, may be a cause of airway obstruction. Based on assessment findings, the emergency department staff promptly initiates appropriate ventilatory support, which may include elective intubation and mechanical ventilation followed by a chest radiograph. Breathing is assessed after an airway is established. Absence of breath sounds or hyperresonance on chest percussion may indicate an open or tension pneumothorax, flail chest, or hemothorax. These injuries require prompt treatment to prevent deterioration in the patient's respiratory status.

Once airway and breathing are stabilized, the circulatory status is assessed. Hypotension generally occurs secondary to volume loss from hemorrhage. Fluid resuscitation is accomplished by infusing intravenous fluids, crystalloids, or blood. Early administration of blood enhances oxygenation and may minimize the secondary ischemic injury to the spinal cord.[4] The clinical staff completes a thorough neurologic and orthopedic assessment and assesses the patient for additional injuries, and then the patient is removed from the backboard to minimize the development of pressure injuries. Last, the emergency department team stabilizes the patient before transfer to the intensive care unit (ICU) or a specialized trauma center.

The administration of high-dose methylprednisolone (Solu-Medrol) in the emergency department remains controversial. The drug reduces swelling and helps minimize secondary injury by reversing the intracellular accumulation of calcium, reducing the risk for cord degeneration and ischemia. Because of complications associated with the use of high dose steroids, particularly in patients with sepsis or gastrointestinal bleeding, or who present more than 8 hours after injury, there has been a significant decrease in the use of methylprednisolone in these situations. Steroid use has also been associated with severe pneumonia and sepsis. The physician determines whether to prescribe methylprednisolone based on assessment of the patient, past medical history, and diagnostic testing.[5]

Therapeutic hypothermia, another modality used in the emergent treatment of SCI, gained national attention with the recovery of a prominent National Football League player who sustained an injury during a game. Therapeutic hypothermia was implemented for SCI prior to the initial findings regarding steroids in the early 2000s, and it is again being investigated for its therapeutic use in the management of acute SCIs.[6] The increased use of this modality may also be due to the neuroprotective effects observed in patients treated with therapeutic hypothermia after cardiac arrest. Therapeutic hypothermia involves the reduction of core body temperature, which may be achieved centrally through intravascular or regional (dural) cooling. The underlying theory concerning its effectiveness is related to the reduction of nervous system metabolism, which is thought to decrease the detrimental effects of secondary injury. While the evidence supporting the use of therapeutic hypothermia is not high-level evidence (most findings were based upon qualitative studies, descriptive studies, or randomized controlled studies with inconsistent results), there is ongoing investigational use of this modality because of its potential promise as well as to its relative safety.[7]

### Physical Examination

**RESPIRATORY ASSESSMENT.** The nurse assesses and records the patient's respiratory rate and arterial oxygen saturation (by pulse oximetry). Clinical manifestations other than those associated with concomitant injuries may include hypoventilation or respiratory failure. The risk for hypoventilation results from loss of innervation to both the diaphragm (C2–C4) and the intercostal muscles (T1–T4) and is a priority assessment in patients with high cervical injuries. Spinal cord edema can act like an ascending lesion and may compromise function of the diaphragm with injuries to C5 or C6. Assessment of tidal volume and vital capacity and auscultation of breath sounds are vital to determining early clinical manifestations of respiratory compromise.

The patient with an SCI may have additional respiratory compromise because of preexisting pulmonary disease or coexistent chest, laryngeal, tracheal, or esophageal injuries. Major cranial nerves and surrounding arteries and veins may also be injured. Pulmonary collapse or consolidation from retained secretions or aspiration of vomitus may directly affect alveolar ventilation. Pulmonary edema may also result from incorrect management of intravenous fluids. Because paralytic ileus and gastric dilation may increase the pressure on the diaphragm and cause further respiratory compromise, a nasogastric tube for stomach decompression is placed.

**CARDIOVASCULAR ASSESSMENT.** The trauma team immediately places the patient on a cardiac monitor, obtains vital signs, and completes a cardiovascular assessment. Hypotension and bradycardia may be due to spinal, neurogenic shock, or hemorrhagic shock. Causes of hemorrhagic shock (manifested by hypotension, tachycardia, and cold, clammy skin) include intrathoracic, intra-abdominal, or retroperitoneal injury or pelvic or long bone fractures. Examination of the patient determines whether other injuries are present.

The rate of intravenous infusion is adjusted based on the patient's presenting signs and symptoms and past medical history. Insertion of an indwelling Foley catheter allows for accurate monitoring of the fluid status. Chest injury often accompanies thoracic spinal cord trauma, and it is important to examine the chest, head, and abdomen for evidence of concomitant injuries. If spinal or neurogenic shock is suspected, the patient will demonstrate bradycardia, in contrast to the tachycardia associated with hypovolemia, due to loss of autonomic innervation.

**NEUROLOGIC ASSESSMENT.** Frequent assessment of neurologic status determines the extent of the SCI and allows for early recognition of changes in level of consciousness that may occur secondary to traumatic brain injury. The trauma team uses the Glasgow Coma Scale (GCS) or other standardized tools to determine patient's level of consciousness. Most SCI centers use a specialized flow sheet, such as the Standard Neurological Classification of Spinal Cord Injury flow sheet, to assess and document the patient's level of functioning (Fig. 37-6). Cranial nerve testing is necessary, particularly if the cause of the injury was penetrating trauma or involved a head injury. For a further discussion of the care of patients with a head injury, see Chapter 36.

During the early assessment of the patient, a digital rectal examination is important to determine whether the injury is incomplete or complete. The lesion is incomplete if the patient can feel the palpating finger or can contract the perianal muscles around the finger voluntarily. Sensation may be present in the absence of voluntary motor activity. Sensation seldom is absent when voluntary perianal muscle contraction is present. In either case, the prognosis for further motor and sensory return is good. Preservation of sacral function may be the only finding that indicates an incomplete lesion, and significant neurologic recovery may occur in the patient with an incomplete cord injury. Rectal tone by itself, without the presence of voluntary perianal muscle contraction or rectal sensation, is not evidence of an incomplete cord injury.

**BOWEL AND BLADDER ASSESSMENT.** Incontinence of urine and possibly feces may have occurred at the scene of the accident. To prevent the bladder from becoming distended secondary to an atonic bladder, insertion of an indwelling urinary catheter is indicated. There may be an imbalance between parasympathetic and sympathetic innervation to the bowel and therefore a loss of voluntary control.

### Diagnostic Studies

Once the patient is stabilized, definitive diagnostic tests may be completed safely. The diagnostic workup consists of radiographs of the spine, chest, and other structures as clinically indicated. A computed tomography (CT) scan provides additional information concerning bony structures and fractures. Soft tissue injury is more easily diagnosed with magnetic resonance imaging (MRI). Typical laboratory tests ordered include a complete blood count, electrolytes, glucose, blood urea nitrogen, creatinine, blood type and crossmatch, arterial blood gases, and coagulation studies.

Although rare, the incidence of missed spinal fractures is usually less than 2% with CT.[8] Consequences of a missed injury include chronic pain, deformity, and a delayed injury to the spinal cord or adjacent nerve root. The factors most associated with a missed injury are high-energy trauma, older age, closed head injury, and insufficient imaging. Ideally, flexion–extension views or an MRI is necessary in patients with altered mental status and in those who complain of pain, even when plain radiographs and CT are negative.

When the patient is in the critical care or acute care environment, a physician often orders a somatosensory evoked potential test (see Chapter 33). This test measures the ability of the spinal cord to transmit impulses along the neural pathways to the higher centers in the brain, and is used in determining treatment. In this test, a peripheral nerve in the arm or leg below the level of injury is stimulated, and the neurologic response (evoked potential) is recorded. If the injury is complete, there is no response. In incomplete injuries, varying responses occur.

## Ongoing Assessment and Management

Based on the assessment data, the interdisciplinary team develops an individual treatment plan (Box 37-3); management is based on the type and severity of injury. Collaboration with all health care disciplines is necessary to enable the patient to achieve the fullest potential after injury. The initial goals are to realign or stabilize the spine to prevent further neurologic deterioration, to prevent complications, and to initiate prompt interventions to treat any complications that do occur.

## Realignment and Stabilization of the Spine

The trauma team carefully evaluates the patient to determine the most effective treatment based on the type and cause of injury. The surgeon must balance the risks of surgery against the possible benefits associated with eventual patient outcome.

### Medical Management

Regardless of the treatment approach, medical management of the patient is an important cornerstone of initial treatment.[9] Closed reduction of a cervical fracture often involves skeletal traction. Cervical traction is used when the fracture is unstable or if subluxation has occurred. Gardner–Wells, Vinke, or Crutchfield tongs are common forms of cervical traction; however, because of the complications that accompany prolonged immobility, long-term traction with tongs is seldom used, especially since the advent of the halo vest (Fig. 37-7).

A halo device, Miami J, or Aspen collar is used for cervical immobilization. Immobilization devices for cervical and thoracic injuries may involve the use of a metal and plastic (Minerva) brace. Thoracolumbar–sacral orthosis may be accomplished using a fiberglass and plastic canvas corset or Jewett brace. Each of these devices is fitted to the patient to provide support and stabilization of the spine. Surgical stabilization may also be necessary. Bed rest is the recommended treatment for sacral and coccygeal injuries.

### Surgical Management

The goal of surgical management is to stabilize and support the spine. Emergency surgery may be necessary to remove bone fragments, a hematoma, or a penetrating object, such as

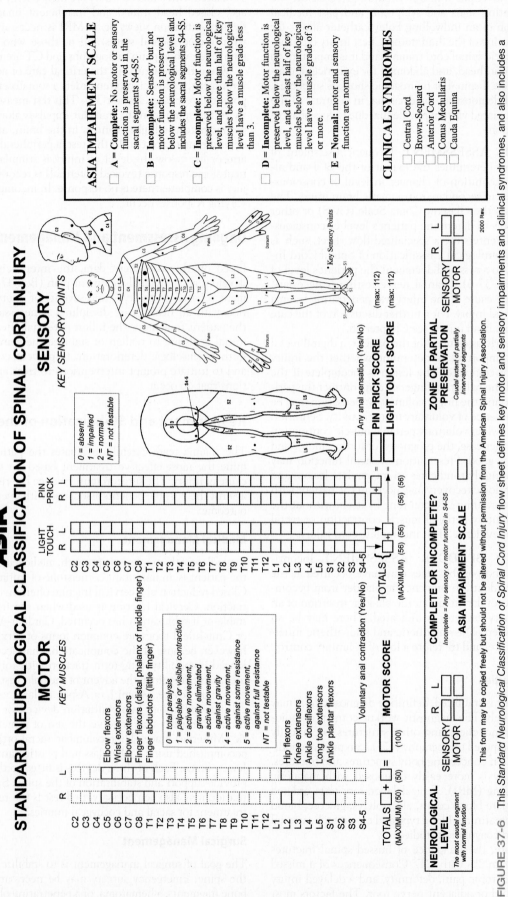

**FIGURE 37-6** This *Standard Neurological Classification of Spinal Cord Injury* flow sheet defines key motor and sensory impairments and clinical syndromes, and also includes a functional assessment scale. Motor movement of the major muscle groups is scored on a scale of 0 to 5, with 0 indicating total paralysis and 5 indicating active movement against full resistance or normal movement. Sensation testing is done starting at the area of absent or decreased sensation and proceeding to the area of normal sensation, following the sensory distribution of the skin dermatomes. Each spinal cord segment is tested for sensation and is scored as 0 for absent, 1 for impaired, or 2 for normal. (Courtesy of the American Spinal Injury Association.)

**QSEN  BOX 37-3**  *COLLABORATIVE CARE GUIDE for the Patient With Spinal Cord Injury*

| Outcomes | Interventions |
|---|---|
| **Impaired Gas Exchange** **Ineffective Breathing Pattern** | |
| Arterial blood gas values will be within normal limits. No evidence of atelectasis is demonstrated. | • Assess need for mechanical ventilation. • Provide routine pulmonary toilet, including: Airway suctioning Chest percussion, couth and deep breathing Incentive spirometer, nebulizer treatment • Turn frequently. • Mobilize out of bed to chair. • Apply abdominal binder when out of bed. • Consult pulmonologist as needed. • Obtain pulmonary function tests. |
| **Decreased Peripheral Tissue Perfusion** **Risk for Shock** | |
| There will be no evidence of neurogenic (spinal) shock (T10 injuries and higher). Blood pressure (BP) will be adequate to maintain vital organ function. There will be no development of deep venous thrombosis (DVT) or pulmonary embolism. There will be no evidence of orthostatic hypotension. | • Monitor for bradycardia, vasodilation, and hypotension. • Assess for dysrhythmias. • Prepare to administer intravascular volume, vasopressors, and positive chronotropic agents. • Begin DVT prophylaxis on admission (eg, external compression device, low-dose heparin). • Measure calf and thigh circumference daily and at same location; report increase. • Apply elastic bandage/wraps to lower extremities before mobilizing out of bed. • Monitor for orthostatic hypotension when raising head of bed and getting out of bed. • Consult cardiology department as needed. |
| **Risk for Ineffective Cerebral Tissue Perfusion** **Risk for Acute Confusion** **Risk for Autonomic Dysreflexia** | |
| There will be no evidence of deterioration in neurologic status. | • Perform neurologic check and spinal cord function checks every 2–4 h. • Monitor for deterioration in neurologic status and report to the physician or nurse practitioner. • Monitor for and prevent complications. • Provide patient and family education concerning injury, effects of injury, and rehabilitation. |
| **Electrolyte Imbalance** **Risk for Imbalanced Fluid Volume** | |
| Serum electrolytes will be within normal limits. Fluid balance will be maintained as evidenced by stable weight, absence of edema, normal skin turgor. | • Monitor laboratory studies as indicated by patient condition. • Assess for dehydration. • Administer mineral/electrolyte replacement as ordered. • Monitor gastrointestinal and insensible fluid loss. • Make accurate daily fluid intake and output measurements. • Weigh weekly. • Monitor results of laboratory studies, particularly albumin and electrolyte levels. |
| **Impaired Physical Mobility** **Risk for Activity Intolerance** **Impaired Tissue Integrity** | |
| Joint range of motion will be maintained and contractures prevented. Skin integrity will be maintained under or around stabilization devices (eg, cervical collar, Yale brace, halo vest). | • Position in correct alignment. • Consult with wound care specialist to determine correct type of bed. • Begin range-of-motion exercises early after admission. • Use high-top tennis shoes, moon boots, or extremity splints routinely. • Consult with physical and occupational therapists. • Maintain splint, brace, and adaptive device schedule; check for pressure ulcers every 4 h or more often if indicated. • Monitor skin or pin sites of stabilization devices. • Use meticulous skin care/pin care under or around stabilization devices. |
| **Impaired Tissue Integrity** | |
| Skin will remain intact. | • Consult with wound care specialist to determine correct type of bed. • Reposition at least every 2 h while patient is in bed. • Position patient to prevent pressure on bony prominences. • Use upright, straight-backed chair when patient is out of bed (not a reclining chair). Use felt pad on chair seat. • Reposition/shift weight every hour when patient is sitting upright. • Use Braden scale to monitor risk for skin breakdown. |

*(continued)*

**QSEN BOX 37-3**  **COLLABORATIVE CARE GUIDE** *for the Patient With Spinal Cord Injury (continued)*

| Outcomes | Interventions |
|---|---|
| **Imbalanced Nutrition** | |
| Protein, carbohydrate, fat, and calorie intake will meet minimal daily requirements. | • Consult dietitian.<br>• Encourage fluids, high-fiber diet.<br>• Monitor fluid intake and output, calorie count.<br>• Administer parenteral and enteral nutrition as appropriate.<br>• Assist with feeding/feed as needed. |
| **Impaired Comfort** | |
| Pain will be to verbalize a score less than "4" on visual analog scale. | • Assess and differentiate pain from anxiety or stress response.<br>• Administer appropriate analgesic or sedative to relieve pain and monitor patient response.<br>• Use nonpharmacologic pain relief techniques (eg, distraction, music, relaxation therapies). |
| **Ineffective Coping**<br>**Disturbed Body Image**<br>**Impaired Individual Resilience** | |
| Patient will adapt to loss of motor and sensory function.<br>Therapeutic strategies will be used to cope with anxiety and chronic pain syndrome.<br>Integration will be made into prior social role. | • Provide emotional support by:<br>Encouraging ventilation of sadness, fears, and the like.<br>Arranging for social services, clergy, neuropsychologist, or support groups to see patient.<br>• Provide information and counseling regarding:<br>Personal resources<br>Nonpharmacologic pain management techniques<br>Stress management strategies<br>Appropriate use of prescribed pharmacologic agents<br>• Provide patient/family counseling regarding:<br>Stages of grief<br>Sexual function and management techniques<br>Social services and community resources |
| **Teaching/Discharge Planning** | |
| Patient will adapt to loss of bowel/bladder control.<br>Patient will participate in bowel and bladder program.<br>Complications of immobility will be prevented.<br>Patient will be placed in appropriate post-acute care setting. | • Teach patient/family:<br>Bowel program and training<br>Dietary habits to maintain bowel function<br>Bladder training/intermittent catheterization<br>Prevention of and signs/symptoms of autonomic dysreflexia<br>• Teach patient/family:<br>Positioning to prevent skin breakdown<br>Physical therapy exercises<br>Pulmonary toilet<br>• Consult rehabilitation/discharge planner/social services early after admission to initiate placement arrangements. |

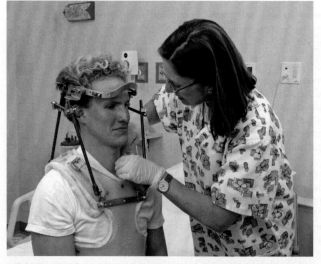

**FIGURE 37-7**  A lightweight fleece-lined vest with a halo may be used to stabilize the cervical vertebrae. Note that the vest comes in various sizes and does not need to be removed for magnetic resonance imaging studies. (Courtesy of Bremer Medical, Inc., Dawin Road, Jacksonville, FL.)

a bullet. If the patient's motor status continues to decline, a laminectomy (removal of a portion of the vertebral column) may be performed to allow for swelling of the spinal cord secondary to edema. Rod placement, laminectomy and fusion, and anterior fusion are types of surgical stabilization. Bone for fusion usually comes from the iliac crest, tibia, or ribs, or may be retrieved through a tissue bank. See Evidence-Based Practice Highlight 37-1 for information about the timing of decompression surgery.

Postoperatively, the nurse monitors the patient's neurologic status at least every hour for the first 24 hours and then every 4 hours. Any indication of deterioration in neurologic status is reported immediately to the physician. A major complication of surgery is postoperative infection. This is especially true in older patients and in those with preexisting comorbidities or with open wounds, injuries to the thoracolumbar spine, or complete injuries.[11] The causative organisms are typically gram-positive organisms, although other concurrent organisms may include *Enterococcus faecalis, Enterobacter cloacae, Pseudomonas* species, *Klebsiella* species, and *Escherichia coli.*

**QSEN**

**EVIDENCE-BASED PRACTICE HIGHLIGHT 37-1**
## Timing of Surgery for Traumatic Acute Spinal Cord Injury

In a study of 1410 patients with acute traumatic spinal cord injury, motor recovery and length of stay were evaluated in relation to time from injury to surgical intervention. Patients with incomplete injuries from C2 to L2 who underwent surgery within 24 hours demonstrated greater motor improvement, than those who had surgery after 24 hours. Patients with complete injuries

did not demonstrate the improvements. Earlier surgical intervention also correlated to shorter length of stays.[10]

Adapted from Dvorak MF, Noonan VK, Fallah N, et al. The influence of time from injury to surgery on motor recovery and length of hospital stay in acute traumatic spinal cord injury: An observational Canadian cohort study. J Neurotrauma 32(9): 645–654, 2015

## Prevention of Respiratory Problems

The patient with an SCI, especially injury above T6, is at risk for respiratory problems, such as ineffective airway clearance, ineffective breathing patterns, and impaired gas exchange. The degree of respiratory compromise is determined primarily by the level of the injury, although not entirely. For example, a 28-year-old patient with C5 tetraplegia with no lung disease may have better ventilation than a 65-year-old patient with C8 tetraplegia with a long history of smoking and chronic obstructive pulmonary disease.

Normally, ventilation is accomplished through a complex interaction between muscles of the chest, the abdominal wall, and the diaphragm. An SCI above T6 results in paralysis of the inspiratory and expiratory muscles. Dysfunction of the intercostal and accessory muscles decreases ventilation and predisposes the patient to atelectasis. Dysfunction of the abdominal muscles and expiratory intercostal muscles diminishes the patient's ability to generate a cough to clear secretions. The intercostal muscles also normally provide support to the lateral chest wall. When the intercostals are impaired, this part of the chest wall collapses during inspiration as the abdomen expands. This easily discernible breathing pattern results in ineffective ventilation.

Respiratory complications are the leading cause of death in the acute and chronic phases of SCI, especially among tetraplegic patients. The nurse and respiratory therapist auscultate breath sounds and measure respiratory parameters (eg, tidal volume and vital capacity) frequently. Respiratory failure is anticipated if the patient's vital capacity is less than 15 to 20 mL/kg and the respiratory rate is greater than 30 breaths/min. Other interventions include measuring oxygenation via pulse oximetry. If the value is less than 85 mm Hg or if the arterial carbon dioxide tension ($PaCO_2$) is above 45 mm Hg, intubation may be required. Other interventions include providing oxygen per nasal cannula and ensuring that the patient is well hydrated.

Kinetic therapy involves placing the patient on a special bed that rotates a minimum of 40 degrees on a continuous basis. This stabilizes the spine, and the continuous slow rotation prevents pulmonary complications.

The nurse encourages the patient to take deep breaths and to use an incentive spirometer every 2 hours, or more frequently if tolerated. For example, if the patient has a TV or radio in the room, every time there is a commercial, the patient can take four to five deep breaths or use the incentive spirometer independently or with the assistance of the nurse or a family member. Assisting the patient with the

quad coughing technique may help clear airways more effectively despite weakness or loss of the respiratory muscles that produce the automatic cough reflex. The quad coughing technique involves compressing the sides of the patient's chest (if the patient is on his or her side or abdomen) or the diaphragm (if the patient is supine) during exhalation. This technique is often most helpful after postural drainage or vibration of the chest.

Suctioning may be necessary if the patient's airway cannot be cleared effectively with other techniques. Nurses should remember that suctioning (or nasogastric tube insertion) might trigger an abnormal vasovagal response, resulting in bradycardia. Suctioning equipment should always be available at the bedside of the patient with high thoracic or cervical spinal cord injury.

When turning a patient to the prone position on a Stryker frame, the nurse needs to remain at the bedside for the first few turns to evaluate the patient's respiratory tolerance of the turn. Patients with high-level tetraplegia can experience respiratory arrest in the prone position because movement of the diaphragm is compromised. When the patient is in the prone position, bradycardia is also common.

## Restoration of Hemodynamic Stability

The management of arterial oxygenation and blood pressure (BP) support are critical in optimizing the potential for neurologic recovery. Continuous hemodynamic monitoring is essential to measure cardiac output and systemic perfusion. Insertion of a pulmonary artery catheter and central venous line may be necessary if this was not done in the emergency department. It is important to maintain mean arterial pressure between 85 and 90 mm Hg with the systolic BP above 90 mm Hg for the first week after injury, to promote perfusion of vital organs, including the spinal cord. The patient is at risk for cardiovascular compromise because of disruption in the autonomic nervous system. Bradycardia, hypotension, and dysrhythmias may occur. Hypotension and tachycardia may indicate hemorrhage from intra-abdominal bleeding or bleeding around fracture sites. Sequential compression devices, antiembolism stockings, or an abdominal binder may be used to promote venous return.

Left ventricular dysfunction may occur secondary to release of β-endorphins. Cardiac enzymes should be obtained if there are electrocardiographic changes. Dysrhythmias and heart block may occur. It is necessary to address adequate tissue perfusion to the spinal cord and other vital organs, such as the kidneys. Careful intravenous fluid replacement provides hydration without fluid overload. Vasopressors may not be necessary to maintain BP during spinal shock, but when the BP is not high enough to sustain vital organ perfusion, often a dopamine infusion is initiated. Bradycardia also may not require treatment, but if necessary, atropine may be used to speed up the heart rate. A transcutaneous or transvenous pacemaker may be essential if the patient remains bradycardic despite atropine.

## Neurologic Management

While in the ICU, the patient requires neurologic assessment every hour until stable, then every 4 hours. The patient's motor and sensory states warrant particular attention. If there is any deterioration in the patient's condition, the frequency of assessment increases, and the nurse notifies the physician or nurse practitioner.

Depending on the patient's motor function, an adapted nurse call system may be necessary. Useful devices include low-pressure, voice-controlled, and sip-and-puff straw-like call systems. Other communication systems can be developed in conjunction with the speech language pathologist for the patient on a mechanical ventilator.

## Pain Management

It is not unusual for the patient to complain of pain, frequently severe pain. The source of the pain may be neuropathic, musculoskeletal, central, or visceral. Abnormal sensation may occur at the level of the lesion in injuries causing diverse nerve root damage, such as occurs with gunshot or knife wounds. Pain resulting from either the SCI, surgery, or both is treated aggressively following institutional protocol and within the pain management standards of the institution.

## Medication Administration

Medications used in treating the patient with SCI include drugs:

- to minimize injury
- for cardiovascular stabilization
- for paralytic ileus and stress ulcers
- for autonomic hyperreflexia
- for skeletal muscle spasm

Nurses administering medications to patients with spinal cord injuries must consider several special considerations. Subcutaneous and intramuscular injections are not absorbed well because of the lack of muscle tone. Sterile abscesses may result, causing autonomic dysreflexia or an increase in spasms. Injection sites are the deltoid area, the anterior thigh, and the abdominal area. Rotation of injection sites is necessary, and the volume injected should not exceed 1 mL at any one site.

Nurses often start peripheral intravenous lines, but the intravenous site of choice is the subclavian vein. In this area of high blood flow, there is less chance of thrombosis secondary to vasomotor paralysis, especially during spinal shock. For this reason, the veins of the lower extremities should never be used for intravenous administration in patients with SCI.

## Thermoregulation

Ineffective thermoregulation is a common problem in patients with spinal cord injuries above the thoracolumbar area. Interruption of the sympathetic nervous system prevents the thalamic thermoregulatory mechanisms. As a result, the patient fails to sweat to eliminate body heat, and there is an absence of vasoconstriction, resulting in an inability to shiver to increase body heat when cold. The degree of thermal control and dysfunction is directly proportional to the extent of body area with loss of thermal regulation. Hence, a tetraplegic patient has more difficulty with thermoregulation than a paraplegic patient.

Hypothermia is usually managed by using warmed blankets. The room temperature is adjusted to maintain patient comfort. Electric heating blankets or hot water bottles may present a danger for body parts with no sensation, increasing the risk of thermal injury. An attempt is made to stabilize the patient's temperature above 96.5°F (35.8°C). Ideally, the patient is placed in a private room so that the room temperature does not adversely affect the other patient in the room. Over the long term, thermal control can be facilitated by use of clothing appropriate for the weather conditions.

## Nutrition

The possibility of inadequate nutrition is of significant concern during the acute phase of injury and must not go unnoticed while the focus is on hemodynamic stability. Because of protein catabolism and significant loss of lean muscle mass due to atrophy, huge nitrogen loss occurs, resulting in a negative nitrogen balance and weight loss.[12] The negative nitrogen balance contributes to skin breakdown, poor wound healing, and lack of energy for rehabilitative efforts. For these reasons, initiation of enteral feeding with 72 hours of injury is recommended to prevent further nutritional compromise.[12] Along with other required blood work, a serum albumin test is necessary. A value less than 3.5 g/dL or total lymphocyte count less than 1,500 to 2,000/mm² is indicative of clinical malnutrition. A nutritional consult should be initiated upon admission. Caloric requirements are calculated to ensure adequate, but not excessive, nutritional support. If the patient must remain nothing by mouth (NPO) for more than a few days, total parenteral nutrition should be initiated.

Patients with spinal cord injuries often have increased energy needs secondary to metabolic stress response. This can lead to a severe catabolic state and malnutrition. It is not unusual to see a significant weight loss within the first few days of injury. Total parental nutrition or enteral feedings are instituted until the patient is able to start on an oral diet. The patient's intake and output are strictly monitored.

Ensuring adequate nutrition is a collaborative problem involving the patient, family, dietitian, occupational therapist (OT), and nurse. The dietitian meets with the patient and family to identify the foods the patient enjoys and develops a menu that incorporates patient preference into the required dietary plan. Family members learn what foods they can bring from home to include in the patient's prescribed diet. The OT assesses the patient's need for assistive devices to use during mealtimes and teaches the patient and family how to use the adapted silverware. The nurse reinforces the information provided by the dietitian and OT. The nurse may teach family and friends how to assist the patient with meals and about the importance of allowing the patient as much independence as possible at mealtime. It is necessary to encourage fluid and a high-roughage diet, unless contraindicated. Before meals, the nurse assists the patient with mouth care and ensures that the patient has not been incontinent.

## Mobilization and Skin Care

Rehabilitation begins in the critical care unit and is a collaborative effort involving the patient, physician, physical therapist (PT), OT, nurse, and the patient's family. Initially, the nurse assists the patient with range-of-motion exercises. When the patient is stable, family members may be taught to assist the patient with these exercises. Based on their assessment findings, the PT and OT develop an individualized treatment plan to begin mobilization of the patient.

Positioning is not simply based on the usual every-2-hour turn schedule. Development of proper positioning protocols occurs in conjunction with the physical and OT to maximize range of motion and prevent joint contractures. When turning the patient, the nurse places a pillow under the patient's head but not under the forearms. When the patient is on his or her side, most of the upper body weight should be over the scapula that rests on the bed. Flexing of the hips and knees allows the patient to remain on the side with minimal support. The nurse places pillows and foam cushions between the knees and against the back.

Pressure is a common cause of structural damage to a muscle and its peripheral nerve supply. Preventing skin breakdown is a priority for the nurse in the critical care unit. There is a definite time–pressure relationship in the development of pressure ulcers. Microscopic tissue changes secondary to local ischemia occur in less than 30 minutes. Pressure interferes with arteriolar and capillary blood flow. When the pressure is prolonged, there is definite damage to superficial circulation and tissue. The damage may be associated with congestion and induration of the area or blistering and loss of the superficial epidermal layers of the skin. As the pressure continues, the deeper skin layers are lost, leading to necrosis and ulceration. Serous drainage from such ulceration can constitute a continuous protein loss of as much as 50 g/d. Prolongation of the pressure results in deep penetrating necrosis of the skin, subcutaneous tissue, fascia, and muscle. The destruction may progress to gangrene of the underlying bony structure. Pressure necrosis can begin from within the tissue over a bony prominence, where the body weight is greatest per square inch.

A turn schedule for the patient is important, even if the patient has not had stabilizing surgery. It may take three staff members to accomplish this safely, particularly in the patient with a cervical injury. One person stabilizes the neck, and the other two flex the hips, knees, and ankles and hold the feet flat on the bed surface while turning the patient's trunk. To maintain alignment, the nurse uses foam wedges, pillows, or air-filled rolls. Turning occurs a minimum of every 2 hours. Use of an air or egg-crate mattress does not preclude the need to turn. The nurse checks the condition of the skin before and after the position change, paying particular attention to the patient's earlobes, back of head, elbows, inner aspects of the knees, heels, and sacral area. The posterior thigh and ischial tuberosities are prone to skin breakdown from prolonged lying on the back with the head of bed elevated or when sitting in a chair. The nurse documents any change in skin integrity, notifies the wound care specialist, and implements a plan of care. Numerous kinetic beds and air beds are available for patient comfort, preventing skin breakdown and treating complications of immobility.[13]

Together with the PT and the OT, the nurse develops a plan to prevent foot drop. Initially, the heels are placed in "bunny boots." Frequently, high-top sneakers or basketball shoes are worn. It is important to ensure that the boots or shoes are the correct size, to check for signs of skin breakdown, and to ensure that the patient's feet are dry. It is necessary to develop an "on and off" schedule with the PT. When the boots or shoes are off, the nurse pays careful attention to foot positioning and assesses for pressure ulcers.

The OT determines the need for splints or braces for the patient's wrists and hands. The nurse must assess the patient's skin frequently to identify pressure areas early. If necessary, the splints are modified to prevent skin breakdown.

## Urinary Management

Acute tubular necrosis may occur within 48 hours of injury as a result of hypotension. An indwelling urinary catheter is necessary to allow for hourly measurement of urinary output during this phase, with the goal of keeping it at least 30 mL/h. The nurse closely monitors fluid and electrolyte balance. Removal of the indwelling catheter as soon as spinal shock has resolved reduces the risk for infection.

The long-range objective of bladder management, regardless of the level of the injury, is to achieve a means whereby the bladder consistently empties, the urine is sterile, and the patient remains continent. The ultimate goal is to have the patient catheter free, with consistent low residual urine checks, no urinary tract infection, and no evidence of damage to the upper urinary tract structures.

One method of bladder management involves intermittent catheterization, and it may begin in the early recovery phase after spinal shock is resolved. The purpose of this program is to exercise the detrusor muscle, again with the goal of keeping the patient catheter free. The advantage of this method is that no irritant remains in the bladder; consequently, the risk for urinary tract infection, periurethral abscess, and epididymitis is reduced.

## Bowel Management

Before the initiation of a bowel program, it is necessary to perform a systematic, comprehensive evaluation of the type of cord injury, bowel function, impairment, and possible problems. This includes an abdominal assessment, a rectal examination, and evaluation of anal sphincter tone. In addition, the anocutaneous reflex (contraction of the anal sphincter secondary to cutaneous stimulation) and bulbocavernosus reflex (also referred to as the penile reflex; compression or tapping on the dorsum of the glans penis, which leads to contraction of the bulbocavernosus muscle at the tip of the penis) require assessment to determine whether the patient has upper motor neuron or lower motor neuron dysfunction. Equally important, a bowel program must consider the ability of the patient and care givers to carry out the planned interventions at discharge.

Simple steps can prevent constipation and begin progress toward bowel continence. It is necessary to maintain appropriate intake, either through intravenous or oral fluids and diet. The nurse records bowel movements in an area that is easily accessible for review and administers stool softeners daily. Development of a consistent schedule for the bowel program is warranted. The timing of the program is usually after meals to coincide with peristalsis that occurs after meals to move food through the gastrointestinal tract. Rectal stimulation may be necessary to trigger defecation.

## Psychological Support

As soon as the patient is medically stable, the nurse begins to focus on the psychosocial issues that are of concern to the patient and family. Questions often asked of the nurse include the following: "Am I going to die?" "Will I walk or use my arms again?" "What is going to happen to me?" There are no easy answers to these questions, and it can be difficult for patients and family members to accept this uncertainty. Most patients are accustomed to receiving treatment for illnesses or conditions that have a predictable course of treatment and outcome. For example, antibiotics are prescribed for 10 days and the infection clears up, or surgery is performed and the patient is discharged home and able to return to our normal activities within an expected timeframe.

Answer questions to the best of your knowledge. Never predict the future, tell stories about patients who made a complete recovery, or ignore a question or a concern. Listen to the patient and the family. Let the patient and family talk about their fears and anxieties. Detailed patient education in a critical care unit is not generally appropriate. However, providing information the patient and family need to know while they are being cared for in the critical care unit is important. Focus on the patient care issues that present each day and on the patient's abilities. Do not minimize the patient's disabilities. Refer questions to other members of the health care team as appropriate. If indicated, ask for an order for a psychiatric consult.

Incorporate the use of technology to help the patient stay connected with family and friends. For example, place a "hands free" telephone in the room. Use a laptop computer and web cam if wireless internet is available. Explore other enhancements that may be on the patient's personal laptop that will enable continued support with others and provide a means for helping pass the long days in the critical care unit.

Psychological transition from the loss of previous physical abilities to the current state is unique to each person. Feelings of grief, loss, anger, and frustration are common. Certain emotions are characteristic after an SCI, whatever names are given to the stages of grief (Box 37-4). The rate at which a person works through this process varies, and no stage is static. A person can move back and forth between stages. The emotions felt and displayed by someone with an SCI are no different from the emotions felt by everyone at one time or another, and recognition of that fact may help promote empathy with the patient.

All staff members should have an understanding of the types of feelings and reactions the patient with an SCI may exhibit. They can share this process of recovery with family members in helping them to support the injured person and participate in recovery. It is necessary to provide psychological support for family members, who no doubt have many concerns, such as finances, role changes, and long-term prognosis. It is important to be supportive of them and help them and the patient with coping strategies.

## Addressing Concerns About Sexuality

After an SCI, patients have concerns about their ability to function sexually, although they may not verbalize this issue immediately. Critical care nurses may not deal with this problem specifically, but it is important to have some knowledge of the functional potential of the patient to begin to manage the patient's fears and concerns in this area. By avoiding discussion of this important issue, professionals validate the patient's fear that there can be no sex after an SCI, which is certainly not true.

### Male Sexuality

Many men with an SCI believe that their total sexuality is tied to erection and ejaculation. There are three general types of erection in men: psychogenic, reflexogenic, and spontaneous. A psychogenic erection can result from sexual thoughts. The area of the cord responsible for this type of erection is between T11 and L2. Therefore, if the lesion is above this level, the message from the brain cannot get through the damaged area.

Reflexogenic erections are a direct result of stimulation to the penis. Some patients may get this type of erection when their catheter is changed or the pubic hairs are pulled. The length of time the erection can be maintained is variable; therefore, its usefulness for sexual activity is variable. Reflexogenic erections are better with higher cervical and thoracic lesions. Damage to lumbar and sacral regions may destroy the reflex arc.

The third type of erection is spontaneous. This may occur when the bladder is full, and it comes from some internal stimulation. How long the spontaneous erection lasts will determine its usefulness for sexual activity. The ability to achieve a reflexogenic or spontaneous erection comes from nerves in the S2, S3, and S4 segments of the spinal cord.

### Female Sexuality

Women, like men, are concerned with sexual function after SCI; however, there are few physiologic changes in women related to sexual function after an SCI. The primary issues relate to decreased vaginal lubrication, as this is both a mental and physiologic reflex, decreased sensation, and changes in orgasm. Women with SCI may notice that it takes longer to achieve orgasm and that it feels differently than before injury. To enhance sexual satisfaction, water-based lubricants and vibrators can be used.[14]

In 50% of women with an SCI, the menstrual pattern is interrupted for approximately 6 months after injury but then is reestablished. Women are able to become pregnant and seem to have no increase in rate of miscarriage. There are potential complications for the pregnant woman, such as urinary tract infection, pressure sores, and anemia, but with careful medical attention, complications usually can be avoided or minimized.

| BOX 37-4 | Stages of Grief in a Patient With a Spinal Cord Injury |
|---|---|
| **Stage and Description** | **Implications for the Nurse** |
| 1. **Shock and disbelief:** During this phase, the patient does not request an explanation of what has happened. The patient is overwhelmed by the injury. There may be more concern with whether he or she will live than with whether he or she will walk again. This period may result in extreme dependence on the staff members. | The nurse may feel that the patient does not understand the ramifications of the injury. The nurse may identify with the feelings of being overwhelmed because he or she is often overwhelmed with the acute medical management of this catastrophic illness. |
| 2. **Denial:** The process of denial is an escape mechanism. Usually, the whole disability is not denied, but particular aspects of it are. For instance, the patient may say he or she cannot walk now but will be able to in 6 months. Bargaining, instead of being a separate stage, can be considered a form of denial. Bargains with God may be in the form of offering Him the legs if He will just return function of the arms. | The nurse often finds it difficult to deal with patients in this stage. A helpful approach is to focus on the present problems. This is not the stage to discuss long-term changes, such as ordering a wheelchair or making modifications to the home. More appropriate matters to deal with would be skin care and range-of-motion exercises. |
| 3. **Reaction:** During this stage, instead of denying the impact of the injury, the patient expresses this impact. There may be severe depression and loss of motivation and involvement. Previous hobbies or interests lose their meaning. There is great helplessness during this period, and there may be suicidal statements. | The nurse can help at this stage by listening to the patient as feelings are verbalized. The nurse should avoid setting up failure situations, which could happen if he or she pushes the patient too fast. It is important to note that both the sudden absence of muscular activity and sensations in the patient with an SCI and the mental state of helplessness appear to alter central nervous system metabolism. Depression coincides with a fall in a brain metabolite excreted in the urine as tryptamine. Thus, it is important for the nurse to understand that depression in some patients with SCI might have a metabolic basis and that a trial of pharmacologic therapy might be beneficial. |
| 4. **Mobilization:** Problem-solving behavior is seen during this stage. The patient is looking toward the future and wants to learn about self-care. In fact, the patient may become very possessive of the therapist or nurse and resent the time spent with other patients. This is a time of sharing and planning between patient and staff. | |
| 5. **Coping:** Some authorities think that patients do not accept the disability *per se* but instead learn to cope with it. Disability still is an inconvenience, but it is no longer the center of the patient's life. Life is again meaningful to the patient, and the patient is again involved with others. | |

Labor may be painless, or the woman may experience other signs that indicate labor is occurring (eg, abdominal or leg spasms, back pain, difficulty breathing). Autonomic dysreflexia is a complication of labor in women with injuries above T4 to T6 and should be anticipated so that it can be controlled. Women may breastfeed if they wish.

## Complications

### Autonomic Dysreflexia

Autonomic dysreflexia, or hyperreflexia, is a syndrome that sometimes occurs after the acute phase in patients with a spinal cord lesion at T7 or above. Autonomic dysreflexia constitutes a medical emergency. The syndrome presents quickly and can precipitate a seizure or stroke. Death can occur if the cause is not relieved.

Triggering conditions include bladder or intestinal distention, spasticity, pressure ulcers, or stimulation of the skin below the level of the injury. In men, ejaculation can initiate the reflex, and in pregnant women, strong uterine contractions can elicit it. Box 37-5 lists potential precipitating factors.

| BOX 37-5 | Precipitating Factors in Autonomic Dysreflexia |
|---|---|

- Bladder distention or urinary tract infection
- Bladder or kidney stones
- Distended bowel
- Pressure areas or decubitus ulcers
- Thrombophlebitis
- Acute abdominal problems (eg, ulcers, gastritis)
- Pulmonary emboli
- Menstruation
- Second stage of labor
- Constrictive clothing
- Heterotopic bone
- Pain
- Sexual activity; ejaculation by a man
- Manipulation or instrumentation of bladder or bowel
- Spasticity
- Exposure to hot or cold stimuli

These stimuli produce a sympathetic discharge that causes a reflex vasoconstriction of the blood vessels in the skin and splanchnic bed below the level of the injury. The vasoconstriction produces extreme hypertension and a throbbing headache. Vasoconstriction of the splanchnic bed distends

## Signs and Symptoms of Autonomic Dysreflexia

- Paroxysmal hypertension
- Pounding headache
- Blurred vision
- Bradycardia
- Profuse sweating above the level of the injury
- Flushing or splotching of the face and neck
- Piloerection
- Nasal congestion
- Nausea
- Pupil dilation

the baroreceptors in the carotid sinus and aortic arch. These baroreceptors in turn stimulate the vagus nerve, producing a bradycardia, in an attempt to lower the BP. The body also attempts to reduce the hypertension by superficial vasodilation of vessels above the SCI. As a result, there is flushing, blurred vision, and nasal congestion. Because the SCI interrupts transmission of the vasodilation message below the level of the injury, the vasoconstriction continues below the level of the injury until the stimulus is identified and interrupted. The vasoconstriction results in pallor below the injury, whereas flushing occurs above the injury. Box 37-6 summarizes the signs and symptoms of autonomic dysreflexia.

There are several things the nurse can implement quickly to relieve the patient with autonomic dysreflexia, including elevating the head of the patient's bed and frequently assessing BP. In addition, the nurse quickly checks the bladder drainage system for kinks in the tubing. The urine collection bag should not be overly full. Some protocols for checking the patency of the urinary drainage system include irrigating the catheter with 10 to 30 mL of irrigating solution. Absolutely no more than that amount is used because the addition of the fluid may aggravate the massive sympathetic outflow already present. If the symptoms persist, the catheter is changed so that the bladder can empty. Foley catheter placement may be necessary for patients on a bladder management program and those who have not voided in the past 4 to 6 hours.

If the urinary system does not appear to be the cause of the stimulus, it is necessary to check the patient for bowel impaction. Removal of the impaction should not occur until the symptoms subside. Rectal application of dibucaine or lidocaine ointment anesthetizes the area until symptoms subside. If the patient's BP does not return to normal, sublingual nifedipine (Procardia) may be effective. A sympathetic ganglionic blocking agent, such as atropine sulfate, guanethidine monosulfate (Ismelin), reserpine, or methyldopa (Aldomet), may be useful. Hydralazine (Apresoline) and diazoxide (Hyperstat) also may help. Box 37-7 presents nursing intervention guidelines for managing autonomic dysreflexia.

## Pulmonary Complications

Pulmonary complications are the most common cause of death in people with SCI, in both the acute and chronic phases. These pulmonary complications are especially prevalent in people injured above T10. If there is concomitant chest trauma or preexisting pulmonary disease, a history of smoking, or older age, there is higher risk for these complications.

BOX 37-7 | **Nursing Interventions**

For Managing Autonomic Dysreflexia
1. Elevate the head of bed.
2. Apply BP cuff, and check BP every 1 to 2 minutes.
   - If BP is above 180/90 mm Hg, proceed to step 5.
   - If BP is below 180/90 mm Hg, proceed as follows.
3. Quickly insert bladder catheter or check bladder drainage system in place to detect possible obstruction.
   - Check to make sure plug or clamp is not in catheter or on tubing.
   - Check for kinks in catheter or drainage tubing.
   - Check inlet to leg bag to make sure it is not corroded.
   - Check to make sure leg bag is not overfull.
   - If none of these are evident, proceed to step 4.
4. Determine whether catheter is plugged by irrigating the bladder slowly with no more than 30 mL of irrigation solution. Use of more solution may increase the massive sympathetic outflow already present. If symptoms have not subsided, proceed to step 5.
5. Change the catheter and empty the bladder.
6. When you are sure the bladder is empty and if BP is:
   - Above 180/90 mm Hg, call physician immediately.
   - Below 180/90 mm Hg, proceed as follows: Give sublingual nifedipine (Procardia) if protocol calls for it. Give atropine according to physician's order. If BP rises or fails to subside, call physician immediately. Guanethidine monosulfate (Ismelin), hydralazine (Apresoline), or inhaled amyl nitrate may then be ordered by the physician. Dibenzyline may be used for chronic dysreflexia.
7. Ideally, this procedure requires three people: one to check the BP, one to check the drainage system, and one to notify the physician.

If bladder overdistention does not seem to be the cause of the dysreflexia:
- Check for bowel impaction. Do not attempt to remove it, if present. Apply Nupercainal ointment or Xylocaine jelly to the rectum and anal area. As the area is anesthetized, the BP should fall. After the BP is again stable, using a generous amount of anesthetizing ointment or jelly, manually remove impaction.
- Change the patient's position. Pressure areas may be the source of dysreflexia.

### Atelectasis and Pneumonia

Atelectasis is possible in any immobilized patient. Early mobilization, ensuring the airways are clear of secretions, and bronchial hygiene may be useful in minimizing or preventing atelectasis. Pneumonia may also result from hypoventilation and an inability to keep the airways clear. Adequate hydration helps keep secretions liquefied for ease of removal, and bronchoscopy may be necessary to remove mucous plugs. Supplemental oxygen administration is used to treat hypoxia. Ventilator-dependent patients need vigorous pulmonary care (see Chapter 25).

### Deep Venous Thrombosis and Pulmonary Embolus

The Virchow triad for venous thrombosis—venous stasis, vein injury, and hypercoagulability—is found in the patient with an SCI. As a result, the patient is at increased risk for deep venous thrombosis (DVT) and pulmonary embolus. In addition to swelling and pain, obstruction to venous return can lead to compartment syndrome and limb ischemia. Although it is infrequent, hypovolemic shock can occur if enough blood and interstitial fluid pool in the extremity.[15]

If the thrombus breaks off, pulmonary emboli can obstruct venous return and lead to cardiovascular collapse and death. Patients particularly at risk for a fat embolus include those with long bone fractures; signs of chest or neck petechiae and low-grade fever may be early indications of this complication.

Leg veins should not be used as sites from which to draw blood or place intravenous catheters because of the risk that the trauma to the vessel wall will enhance platelet aggregation and clot formation. It is important to encourage smokers to quit because nicotine causes vasoconstriction, thereby slowing blood flow through the periphery.

There is some controversy about the effectiveness of serial leg measurements in monitoring for DVT. A standard measurement protocol is necessary, and all staff should follow it. For example, use a special measuring tape rather than a sewing tape, mark the area where the tape is placed, and use running averages.

Treatment of DVT and pulmonary embolus may include heparin infusion, insertion of an intravenous vena cava filter, or dissolving the clot with thrombolytic agents. Measures to prevent DVT may include the administration of low–molecular-weight heparin and the use of antiembolism stockings. Other modalities include sequential compression devices, passive range-of-motion exercises, and early mobilization. In addition, a kinetic bed can be useful; this device works by keeping the patient in continuous motion.

## Paralytic Ileus and Stress Ulcers

Early medical management of paralytic ileus and stress ulcers includes implementing NPO status, particularly for cervical spinal cord–injured patients. Nasogastric tube placement with intermittent suction is useful in treating the paralytic ileus that frequently accompanies SCI. Nasogastric tube placement also decreases the risk of aspiration and reduces abdominal distention. As soon as bowel sounds are present, safe stimulation of peristalsis may be facilitated with stool softeners, mild laxatives, or suppositories. It is important to avoid enemas, other than the oil-retention type, because the risk for intestinal perforation is high.

Patients with cervical injuries are more likely to experience gastrointestinal bleeding as a result of stress ulcers. Medical treatment includes histamine-2 ($H_2$) receptor blockers, proton pump inhibitors, antacids, or a combination of the three. Early initiation of enteral feedings also contributes to minimizing the risk of stress ulcers.

## Heterotopic Ossification

Calcification around a joint, especially the hip joint, may occur within 12 weeks of injury. Clinical manifestations include limited range of motion, swelling of the affected joint, and an elevated alkaline phosphatase level. Pain may or may not be present. The treatment goal is to prevent further damage and progression. Additional treatment includes irradiation, nonsteroidal anti-inflammatory drugs, and disodium etidronate.

## Spasticity

Spasticity develops after recovery from the period of spinal shock and affects the flexor muscles of the arms and the extensor muscles of the legs. An interdisciplinary approach is the hallmark of effective treatment. A physical therapy consult is warranted to develop an exercise, stretching, and positioning program for the patient. A variety of medications such as baclofen, dantrolene sodium, diazepam, and clonidine may be useful.

## Patient Teaching and Discharge Planning

The nurse plays an integral role in working with the patient and family in finding a rehabilitation program that has a program specific for spinal cord–injured patients. Usually, the patient is discharged to a rehabilitation setting to learn the skills needed for activities of daily living and, when possible, independent living. The nurse helps the family find a rehabilitation program specifically for patients with SCI. When searching for an appropriate rehabilitation program, the family should obtain answers to the following questions:

- How many patients with SCI are treated in the program each year?
- What is the average age of the patients in the program?
- Does the treatment plan identify both long-term and short-term goals?
- Will the patient be assigned an experienced case manager to coordinate the transition between the rehabilitation center and home?
- How much time is spent teaching the patient and family about sexuality, bowel and bladder care, and other activities of daily living?

The family should also ask whether the staff has specialized training in SCI. Rehabilitation therapies should be available for a minimum of 3 hours per day. There should be activities or programs for the patients on weekends and in the evenings. Most importantly, the facility should have 24-hour staffing with registered nurses and respiratory therapists. Box 37-8 offers a teaching guide for a person living with an SCI.

**BOX 37-8** *TEACHING GUIDE* *Living With a Spinal Cord Injury*

## Respiratory Management
- Cough and deep-breathe routinely.
- Drink plenty of fluids, unless contraindicated.
- Use postural drainage or chest physiotherapy.
- Because you are at risk for pneumonia, be careful around anyone with a cold and get an annual influenza vaccination.

## Nutritional Management
- Eat a well-balanced diet that includes protein (lean meat, dairy foods, legumes), fresh fruits, vegetables, and liquids.
- Maintain ideal body weight.

## Skin Management
- You and your helper should check your skin twice a day. Look for redness, bruises or scrapes, blisters, and rashes. Pay particular attention to bony areas. Check your groin for rashes and reddened areas.
- Keep your skin clean and dry, especially in areas where skin touches skin (eg, between the toes, underneath the breasts). Do not use antimicrobial or harsh soaps. Apply moisturizing lotion. Avoid lotions or creams that dry the skin.
- Check your feet whenever you wear new shoes. Check for ingrown toenails. Keep your nails trimmed and filed smooth and have calluses treated by a podiatrist.
- Use the wheelchair and cushion prescribed by your PT.
- Change positions frequently to relieve pressure on bony areas.
- Be sure you are not sitting or lying on anything. Avoid putting objects in your pockets.
- Check to be sure braces, leg bags, and other adaptive equipment are not too tight.
- When in bed, use padding over bony areas. Use a firm mattress. If possible, sleep on your stomach.
- Notify your health care provider of any skin breakdown.

## Urinary Tract Management
- Follow the bladder program developed by the rehabilitation team.
- Drink plenty of fluids unless contraindicated.
- If you have a Foley catheter, keep it free of kinks and change it as directed by your health care provider.
- Watch for signs and symptoms of urinary tract infection (eg, cloudy urine with a foul odor, sediment in the urine).

## Bowel Management
- Follow the bowel program developed by your rehabilitation team. Avoid the regular use of laxatives. Schedule sufficient time to complete the required activities. Notify your health care provider if you have not had a bowel movement in 3 or 4 days.
- Drink plenty of fluids, unless contraindicated.
- Monitor your diet to see what foods cause constipation and diarrhea.
- Prevent constipation through diet and fluid intake and medications as needed.
- Avoid foods that cause gas, such as beans, corn, and apples.
- Be aware of the potential for the development of autonomic dysreflexia during your bowel program.

## Home Environment Management
- Arrange for representatives from physical and occupational therapy to evaluate the patient's home for the following:
  Wheelchair accessibility
  Clearance for maneuvering a wheelchair within the home
  Necessary adaptations to the bedroom, bathroom, and kitchen
  Smoke and fire alarms
- Obtain needed equipment for home care, depending on patient's level of injury. Be sure the equipment is delivered before the patient leaves the rehabilitation facility. Also be sure that the

patient and his or her family members know how to operate the equipment.
- Make arrangements for home health care, physical therapy, occupational therapy, and job training or vocational rehabilitation, as necessary.
- Notify the electric company if there will be lifesaving equipment in the home, such as a respirator.
- Carry out patient and family education
- Locate community support groups.

## Complications

### Autonomic Dysreflexia
- This complication occurs in patients with injury at T5 or above.
- The most common cause is overfilling of the bladder. Other causes include constipation or gas, skin irritations, pressure sores, wounds, and ingrown toenails.
- Autonomic dysreflexia can be a life-threatening emergency. You or a helper must take immediate action to correct this problem.
- Signs and symptoms include a severe headache, nasal congestion, goose pimples, and restlessness.
- Be sure your head is up. If you are sitting in a chair, stay there; if you are in bed, get your head elevated.
- If you have an indwelling catheter:
  Check for kinks along the tubing.
  Empty the Foley bag; if there is no drainage, the Foley may be obstructed—change the Foley.
  Check the catheter and drainage bag for deposits.
  Check urine for color.
- If you are on intermittent catheterization, catheterize yourself.
- If the problem is related to the bowel, perform a digital stimulation and empty the bowel.
- If it is not related to a bladder or bowel problem, check for a pressure sore, ingrown toenail, or possible bone fracture.
- If none of the above actions relieve the signs and symptoms, get emergency medical treatment.

### Deep Venous Thrombosis
- Prevention is important.
- Signs and symptoms include leg swelling, chest pain, and cough.
- Call your health care provider immediately if signs or symptoms develop.

### Hypothermia and Hyperthermia
- To prevent hyperthermia:
  Drink lots of fluids.
  Dress according to the temperature you will be in.
  Watch for signs and symptoms of hyperthermia.
  Use sun block.
- To prevent hypothermia:
  - Dress appropriately for the weather.
  - Watch for signs and symptoms of hypothermia and frostbite.

### Heterotopic Ossification
- Check for development of abnormal bone in soft tissue, usually around the hip or knee.
- Signs and symptoms include a change in range of motion, decreased ability to perform activities of daily living, swelling, warmth, redness over the hip or knee, spasticity, and fever.
- Notify your health care provider immediately if any of these signs or symptoms develop.

### Pain
- Prevention of other problems such as pressure ulcers, stress ulcers, and infections is important.
- Maintain your activity program, range-of-motion exercises, and a healthy diet.

**BOX 37-8**  *TEACHING GUIDE*  *Living With a Spinal Cord Injury (continued)*

- Notify your health care provider of the type of pain you are experiencing.
- Medications and stress reduction techniques may be used.

### Orthostatic Hypotension
- Know that this is a drop in BP when you first sit up.
- Wear elastic hose or an abdominal support.
- Sit up slowly.
- If you experience orthostatic hypotension while you are sitting up, ask someone to tilt your wheelchair back until your head is parallel to the floor.
- Be sure to drink plenty of fluids.

### Spasticity
- Prevention is crucial. Watch for and immediately treat skin problems such as an ingrown toenail. Prevent pressure ulcers. Maintain your bowel and bladder program.
- Notify your health care provider if spasticity develops.

## Clinical Applicability Challenges

### CASE STUDY

S.W. is a 32-year-old accountant who was admitted to the neurotrauma critical care unit 3 days ago after suffering a stab wound during an attempted robbery. When paramedics arrived at the scene, S.W. was unconscious and breathing was shallow and labored; she was lying on her left side. The knife wound entrance was between the shoulder blades, and there was moderate bleeding at the site; the weapon was not at the scene. After stabilization by the paramedics, she was intubated in the field and placed on a spinal board. Two peripheral IV lines were placed with normal saline infusing. Pulse rate was 100 and BP was 100/60. Other than the stab wound and a small abrasion on the forehead, there were no other obvious injuries.

Upon arrival to the emergency department, S.W. was able to open her eyes and follow simple commands, such as holding up two fingers upon request; however, there was no voluntary movement of the legs or feet. The emergency room staff explained where she was and the immediate plans for treatment. S.W. tried to talk around the endotracheal tube, and the staff explained the reason for the ET tube. She was able to shrug her shoulders and had intact sensation to about the nipple line. When tested, she had no perianal reflex activity, suggesting that she was in spinal shock. Radiographic evaluation and CT scan demonstrated complete cord transection at the T3–T4 level with moderate spinal cord edema. There were no findings of head trauma on the CT scan. A loading dose of methylprednisolone (Solu-Medrol) was administered, followed by a continuous IV infusion for 23 hours.

S.W. was admitted to the neuroscience critical care unit, and after cleaning and debridement around the knife entrance wound, was stabilized on bedrest and placed in a plastic canvas corset. During the first 24 hours after admission, BP control was problematic as S.W. demonstrated signs of neurogenic shock, including decreased BP with bradycardia. In addition to IV fluids, she was also started on a continuous infusion of dopamine at 3 mcg/kg/min to maintain a mean arterial pressure of 85 to 90 mm Hg.

Currently, 2 days after the injury, S.W. is alert and oriented to person and place, and has been extubated because of improving respiratory status. Owing to continued weak inspiratory effort, she remains intubated. She also requires extensive respiratory care, including chest percussion and turning every 2 hours. Physical assessment reveals flaccid paralysis below the level of the injury. She is able to shrug her shoulders and discriminate between sharp and dull sensations at the corresponding level of her injury. She has one peripheral IV line with normal saline solution infusing at 75 mL/h. She also has a nasogastric tube connected to low intermittent suction; a Foley catheter draining clear, yellow urine; and sequential pressure devices on both legs.

Nursing interventions include monitoring vital signs every 1 to 2 hours with complete motor and sensory evaluations every 4 hours. The nurses caring for S.W. continue vigilant monitoring of her respiratory status. She is repositioned (turned) every 2 hours, and the outputs of her Foley catheter are measured and recorded every 4 hours. Every effort is made to prevent complications of immobility, both in the critical care and acute care units. After consulting physical and occupational therapy, S.W.'s health care team initiates a treatment plan. Once she is past the acute phase of her injury, plans will be made to transfer her to a rehabilitation facility for further recovery and adaptation to her injury.

1. Correlate S.W.'s clinical presentation to her T3–T4 level of injury.
2. When S.W. questions, via word board, whether she will require mechanical ventilation for the rest of her life, what is the nurse's best response?
3. How should the nurse respond to S.W.'s questions about the possibility of getting pregnant and having children in the future?

## WANT TO KNOW MORE?

A wide variety of resources to enhance your learning and understanding of this chapter are available on thePoint.

You will find:

- References
- Selected readings
- NCLEX-style review questions
- Internet resources
- And more!

# PART 9

# Gastrointestinal System

## 38

# Anatomy and Physiology of the Gastrointestinal System

ALLISON STEELE YORK AND VALERIE K. SABOL

### LEARNING OBJECTIVES

*Based on the content in this chapter, the reader should be able to:*

1. Describe the processes of ingestion, motility, digestion, absorption, and elimination.
2. Define the functions of the major structures of the gastrointestinal system.
3. Explain digestion and absorption of carbohydrates, proteins, fats, vitamins, and minerals.
4. Describe bile production, secretion, and excretion.
5. Discuss the processes involved in emesis and defecation.

The gastrointestinal system consists of the gastrointestinal tract and the accessory glandular organs that empty their contents into the gastrointestinal tract. The major structures of the gastrointestinal tract are the mouth, pharynx, esophagus, stomach, small intestine (duodenum, jejunum, ileum), and large intestine (colon, rectum, anus). The accessory glandular organs include the salivary glands, liver, gallbladder, and pancreas.

The primary physiologic functions of the gastrointestinal system are to take in nutrients for cell maintenance and growth and to eliminate waste. Cell maintenance and growth are accomplished through the processes of ingestion (taking in food), motility (mixing and propelling food through the gastrointestinal tract), digestion (breaking down food), and absorption (movement of food particles into the bloodstream). Elimination is the process by which waste is eliminated from the body.

Gastrointestinal function is regulated and coordinated by the autonomic nervous system (ANS) and a variety of peptides, which are further classified as endocrines (hormones), paracrines, and neurocrines. Endocrines are released in the general circulation and reach all tissues. Endocrine cells release paracrines, which target specific tissues. Neurocrines, or neurotransmitters, diffuse across a synaptic gap and can stimulate or inhibit the release of endocrines and paracrines.

## Structure of the Gastrointestinal System

### Macroscopic Anatomy of the Gastrointestinal System

The gastrointestinal system is composed of the gastrointestinal tract (also called the alimentary canal), that begins at the mouth and ends at the anus (Fig. 38-1). The accessory glands (eg, salivary glands) and organs (eg, liver and pancreas) release secretory products into the gastrointestinal tract.

The oral cavity opens into the pharynx, a structure that allows the passage of nutrients and air. The anterior pharynx, divided into the oropharynx and nasopharynx, connects the oral and nasal cavities. The posteroinferior end of the pharynx (at about the level of the sixth cervical vertebra) connects to the esophagus and larynx. The epiglottis, a thin cartilaginous flap covered by soft tissue, reflexively covers the larynx during swallowing and prevents the passage of food and water into the trachea.

The esophagus connects the pharynx to the stomach at the cardiac orifice (Fig. 38-2). Its main function is to deliver food to the stomach. Two muscular rings, the upper and lower esophageal sphincters, border the esophagus. The upper esophageal sphincter (UES) prevents aspiration and

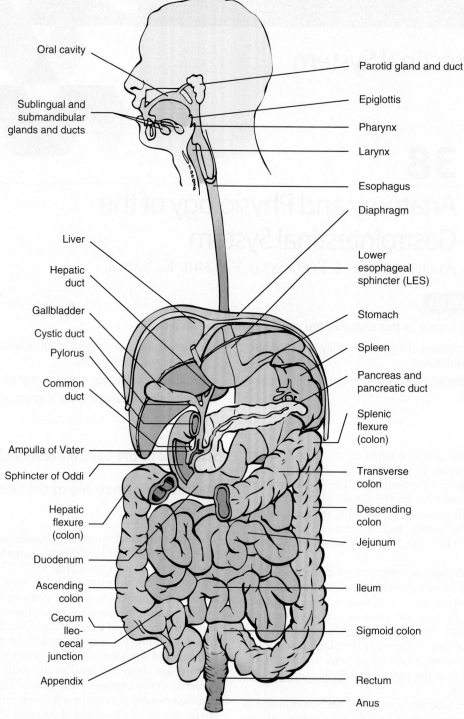

Oral cavity

Parotid gland and duct

Epiglottis

Sublingual and submandibular glands and ducts

Pharynx

Larynx

Esophagus

Diaphragm

Liver

Lower esophageal sphincter (LES)

Hepatic duct

Stomach

Gallbladder

Spleen

Cystic duct

Pancreas and pancreatic duct

Pylorus

Common duct

Splenic flexure (colon)

Ampulla of Vater

Transverse colon

Sphincter of Oddi

Hepatic flexure (colon)

Descending colon

Jejunum

Duodenum

Ascending colon

Ileum

Cecum Ileo-cecal junction

Sigmoid colon

Appendix

Rectum

Anus

**FIGURE 38-1** The gastrointestinal tract.

swallowing of excessive air. The lower esophageal sphincter (LES), a muscular ring at the gastroesophageal junction, prevents reflux of gastric contents into the esophagus. The esophageal lumen, a central hollow tube through which food passes, is surrounded by four layers of tissue (see Microscopic Anatomy of the Gastrointestinal System section for more details). From the lumen outward, these layers are the mucosa, submucosa, muscularis propria, and serosa (Fig. 38-3).

The stomach is a flask-shaped organ that lies in the upper abdomen below the diaphragm (Fig. 38-4). The main function of the stomach is storage; it acts as a reservoir for chewed food. The stomach also mixes ingested food with gastric secretions to form a semisolid liquid called chyme and regulates the release of chyme into the duodenum at a controlled rate. The esophagus joins the stomach at the cardia of the stomach. The cells of the cardia secrete mucus that helps protect the esophagus from the acidic secretions of the stomach. The dome-shaped fundus, located to the left of the cardia, acts as a reservoir. The body and the fundus have coarse folds called rugae that allow for expansion of the stomach.

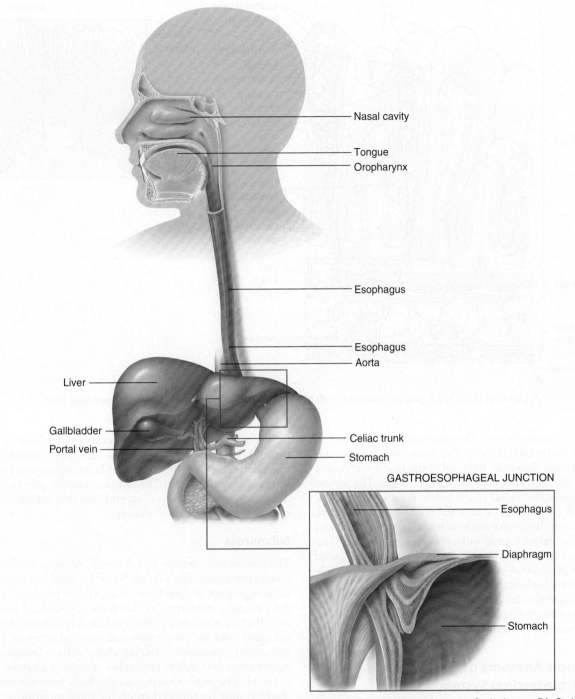

Nasal cavity

Tongue
Oropharynx

Esophagus

Esophagus
Aorta

Liver

Gallbladder
Portal vein

Celiac trunk
Stomach

**GASTROESOPHAGEAL JUNCTION**

Esophagus

Diaphragm

Stomach

**FIGURE 38-2** Gastroesophageal junction. (From Anatomical Chart Company: Atlas of Human Anatomy. Springhouse, PA: Springhouse, 2001, p 203.)

Gastric pits, which contain the acid-secreting cells of the stomach, are located mainly in the body of the stomach. The antrum, the most distal area of the stomach, is the site of G cells, which secrete gastrin. The antrum narrows into the pyloric channel, or pylorus, ending in the gastroduodenal junction at the pyloric sphincter. The pyloric sphincter, a muscular structure between the stomach and the duodenum, minimizes intestinal reflux.

Most digestion and absorption take place in the small intestine. The duodenum, the first 25 to 30 cm (10 to 12 inch) of the small intestine, begins at the pylorus. The common

bile duct opens into the duodenum at the duodenal papilla through the ampulla of Vater. The next 2.6 m (8.5 ft) of the small intestine is the jejunum. The ileum, the last 1.1 m (3.6 ft) of the small intestine, connects to the colon (cecum) at the ileocecal valve. The ileocecal valve prevents reflux of colonic contents into the ileum.

Traditionally, the colon is considered to have six sections. The *cecum* is the most proximal section and is the location of the ileocecal valve. The *vermiform appendix*, a blind-ended 2.5- to 20-cm (1- to 8-inch) tube, protrudes posteriorly from the cecum. The *ascending colon* extends superiorly from the

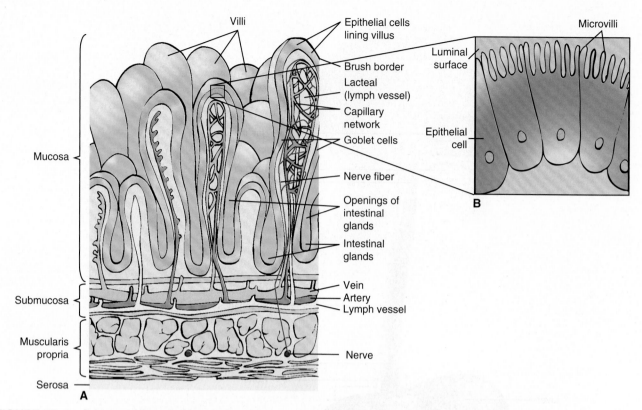

**FIGURE 38-3** **A:** Layers of tissue in the gastrointestinal tract. **B:** Microvilli on the luminal surface of intestinal epithelial cells.

cecum to the hepatic flexure. The *transverse colon* lies between the hepatic and splenic flexures. The *descending* colon extends from the splenic flexure to the level of the iliac crest. At the iliac crest, the colon becomes the sigmoid colon. The *sigmoid colon* continues downward to the pelvic floor as the rectum. The last 2.5 cm (1 inch) or so of the rectum, the anal canal, passes between the levator ani muscles of the pelvic floor and opens to the exterior body surface as the anal orifice. Two sphincters, which work to provide fecal continence, guard this orifice: an internal sphincter composed of smooth muscle and an external sphincter composed of skeletal muscle. The colon, although not necessary for life, is responsible for the reabsorption of electrolytes and fluid, thus allowing the body to maintain fluid and electrolyte balance with less fluid intake.

## Microscopic Anatomy of the Gastrointestinal System

The microscopic structure of the gastrointestinal tract varies depending on location but possesses common features that are independent of the location.

### Mucosa

The mucosa is composed of three layers: the epithelium, the lamina propria, and the muscularis mucosae. A single layer of epithelial cells lines the mucosa. The tight junctions between the epithelial cells act as a barrier to bacteria and other large molecules. In the small intestine, this layer is more convoluted and possesses finger-like projections called villi (see Fig. 38-3). Such structural modifications dramatically increase the surface area of the small intestine, thereby facilitating absorption. The lamina propria, a layer of connective tissue, contains capillaries and lymph vessels. The muscularis mucosae, the innermost layer, is composed of two layers of smooth muscle. The mucosa contains cells that produce gastrointestinal secretions and cells that are sensitive to chemical and mechanical stimuli.

### Submucosa

The submucosa contains blood vessels, nerve networks, and connective tissue. The submucosa of the small intestine contains aggregates of lymphatic tissue (Peyer patches), which are especially numerous in the ileum. Specialized mucosal cells that lie superiorly to the patches of lymphatic tissue in the small intestine absorb viral and bacterial antigens. These specialized cells sensitize the lymphatic cells to antigens and manufacture and secrete antibodies of immunoglobulin class A (IgA). The antibodies protect the body from the antigen the next time (or times) it enters the small intestine.

### Muscularis Propria

The muscularis propria consists of two layers of smooth muscle, an inner circular muscle layer and an outer longitudinal layer. The two smooth muscle layers function in the two major types of gastrointestinal motility: propulsive motion and mixing movements. The stomach has an additional layer of smooth muscle to facilitate its food-mixing movements.

### Serosa

The serosa, or adventitia, is the outermost layer of the gastrointestinal tract. The serosa is continuous with the mesentery and forms part of the visceral peritoneum.

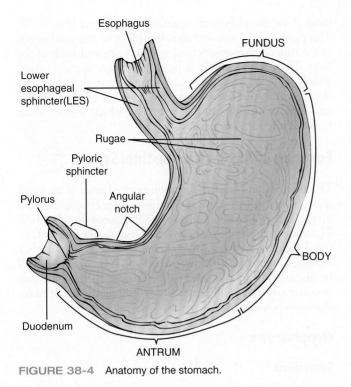

Esophagus

FUNDUS

Lower
esophageal
sphincter(LES)

Rugae

Pyloric
sphincter

Pylorus

Angular
notch

BODY

Duodenum

ANTRUM

**FIGURE 38-4** Anatomy of the stomach.

## Innervation

The gastrointestinal tract is innervated by the ANS. The ANS can be divided into the extrinsic nervous system and the intrinsic (enteric) nervous system.

### Extrinsic Nervous System

The extrinsic nervous system is further divided into parasympathetic and sympathetic branches. Parasympathetic stimulation increases gastrointestinal activity through sensory and motor fibers to promote motility, relax sphincters, and promote secretion. Activation of the sympathetic nerves usually inhibits the motor and secretory activities of the gastrointestinal system.

### Parasympathetic Branch

The parasympathetic innervation of the gastrointestinal tract is primarily through the vagus and pelvic nerves. The vagal nerve (cranial nerve X) innervates the esophagus, stomach, pancreas, gallbladder, small intestine, cecum, and proximal colon. Vagal efferents synapse onto neurons in the myenteric plexus, or Auerbach plexus. Postganglionic fibers then synapse with secretory and smooth muscle cells.

Vagal afferent (sensory) fibers originate in the esophagus, stomach, small intestine, and possibly the large intestine. Afferent fibers relay information about pain and distention to the brain and spinal cord.

The pelvic nerve, issuing from spinal routes S2 to S4, carries parasympathetic afferent and efferent fibers to innervate the rectum and descending colon.

### Sympathetic Branch

Sympathetic efferent fibers exit the spinal cord and synapse on ganglia near the spinal cord. Then, long postganglionic fibers travel to the gut and synapse on blood vessels, myenteric plexus ganglia, and secretory cells. The esophagus receives dense sympathetic innervation. Sympathetic fibers to the stomach and duodenum exit T6 to T9, synapse in the celiac ganglion, and then travel along the celiac artery. Sympathetic fibers exiting at T9 and T10 synapse in the superior mesenteric ganglion and then travel with the celiac artery to the large and small intestine. Fibers terminate on enteric neurons and blood vessels; a few fibers innervate the muscle layers.

### Intrinsic (Enteric) Nervous System

The intrinsic, more commonly known enteric nervous system (ENS), coordinates gastrointestinal motility and secretion. The ENS is grouped into several nerve plexuses, with the myenteric and submucosal plexuses being the most prominent. The nerves in these plexuses receive input from receptors in the gastrointestinal tract and from the ENS. When integrated into the intrinsic system, this input helps coordinate function. Peripheral fibers innervate the voluntary muscles responsible for chewing, swallowing, and defecating.

The ENS is a complex network embedded in the wall of the gastrointestinal tract from the pharynx to the anus. It includes enteric neurons and the processes of afferent and efferent extrinsic neurons. There are two main ganglionic plexuses containing the cell bodies of enteric neurons: an outer and inner plexus. The outer and inner plexus are responsible for controlling gastrointestinal movement and gastrointestinal secretion/blood flow, respectively. There are two main ganglionic plexuses containing the cell bodies of enteric neurons. The outer plexus, the myenteric, or Auerbach plexus, lies between the longitudinal and circular muscle layers. The inner plexus, the submucosal plexus, or Meissner plexus lies between the circular muscle and the mucosa. The myenteric plexus mainly controls gastrointestinal movement, and the submusocal plexus mainly controls gastrointestinal secretion and blood flow.

The ENS can function on its own, independent of the extrinsic nerves, although stimulation by the parasympathetic or sympathetic nerves can further activate or stimulate its function.

Nerves in the ENS are characterized by both their function and by the neurotransmitters they contain. These include acetylcholine, norepinephrine, serotonin, and dopamine. In addition, many gastrointestinal hormones have been identified in the nerves of the ENS where they act as neurotransmitters, and in the brain where they influence autonomic outflow. These include substance P, vasoactive intestinal polypeptide, gastric inhibitory peptide (GIP), and opioid peptides. There is evidence that these neuropeptides participate in the control of all gastrointestinal functions (secretion, motility, and absorption).

## Circulation

Blood supply to the gastrointestinal tract and spleen is called the splanchnic circulation. The gastrointestinal system receives about one-fourth of the resting cardiac output, more than any other organ system. When circulation is impaired (as in shock), perfusion to the splanchnic bed is shunted to the systemic circulation. Because splanchnic organs normally extract only about 20% of the oxygen from the perfusing blood, splanchnic perfusion can be reduced without compromising the organs. However, a severe reduction in splanchnic perfusion can damage the mucosal lining of the gut.

The esophageal artery branches from the thoracic aorta and perfuses the esophagus. Three branches of the abdominal aortic artery perfuse the gastrointestinal organs:

- The celiac axis (consisting of the left gastric artery, the common hepatic artery, and the splenic artery) perfuses the lower esophagus, stomach, duodenum, gallbladder, and liver.
- The superior mesenteric artery perfuses the small intestine to transverse colon.
- The inferior mesenteric artery perfuses the descending colon, sigmoid colon, and rectum.

The areas of perfusion overlap, providing some protection against ischemia.

Venous drainage of the stomach and small and large intestines is primarily through the portal vein to the liver. The blood supply from the lower rectum and the lower esophagus bypasses the portal system. Blood from the rectum drains into the inferior vena cava through the rectal veins, which empty into the external iliac vein. Blood from the esophagus drains through the hemiazygos and azygos veins into the inferior vena cava.

The blood supply of the liver is unique. The liver receives its blood supply from both venous and arterial sources. The venous blood is supplied by the portal vein, which drains most of the blood from the gastrointestinal tract (Fig. 38-5). The portal vein forms behind the spleen at the confluence of the superior mesenteric and splenic veins and leads to the liver. The arterial supply is by the common hepatic artery, which branches from the celiac trunk near the aorta and then perfuses the liver. Both sets of vessels form capillaries and then drain into the hepatic vein, which in turn feeds into the inferior vena cava.

## Function of the Gastrointestinal System

The main function of the gastrointestinal tract is to break down nutrients into a form of usable energy. Food is ingested in the form of macromolecules that cannot be absorbed. These macromolecules are converted into usable forms of energy by mixing with digestive enzymes and secretions as they move through the gastrointestinal tract. These processes will be discussed in relationship to the various parts of the gastrointestinal tract and the secretions and motility that make digestion possible.

### Oropharynx

#### Secretions

The salivary glands of the oropharynx produce saliva. Saliva is composed of mucus (a lubricant that facilitates

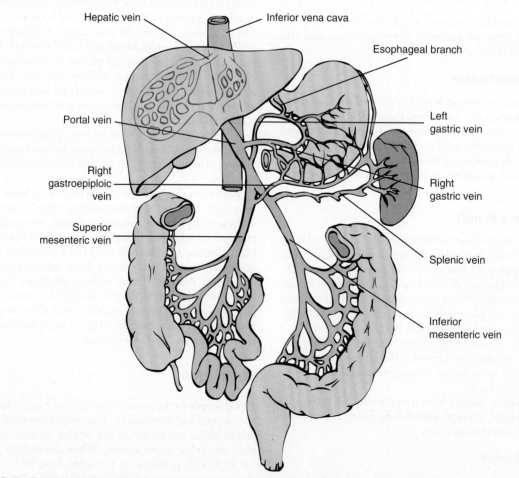

**FIGURE 38-5** Portal circulation. Blood from the gastrointestinal tract, spleen, and pancreas travels to the liver by way of the portal vein before moving into the inferior vena cava for return to the heart.

swallowing), lingual lipase (a fat-digesting enzyme secreted by tongue glands), salivary amylase (an enzyme that breaks down starch), and class A (IgA) antibodies (which provide a first line of defense against bacteria, viruses, and bacteriostatic and carcinogenic chemicals; Table 38-1). A moist oral cavity also facilitates speech. The pH of saliva is 7; saliva contains bicarbonate, which allows it to neutralize acid substances that enter the oral cavity, including regurgitated gastric acid. Lingual lipase digests about 30% of the dietary fat in the stomach. The salivary glands secrete about one-half of the digestive amylase used in digestion; the rest is secreted by the pancreas.

Saliva production is elicited by multiple stimuli, including the sight, smell, or thought of food, and by the pleasant taste or smooth texture of food in the mouth. Rough, bad-tasting, unpleasant-smelling foods reduce salivary gland secretions. Parasympathetic stimulation, or the administration of drugs that mimic stimulation (cholinergics) or enhance it (neostigmine), promotes copious secretion of watery saliva. Sympathetic stimulation or sympathomimetic drug administration produces a scanty output of thick saliva. Cholinergic blockers (eg, atropine) also inhibit salivation.

## Motility

In the mouth, chewing mechanically breaks down food into smaller particles. This produces a bolus of food held together and lubricated by saliva that can then be propelled into the

**TABLE 38-1** Major Gastrointestinal Secretions

| Location | Daily Volume | Composition (and Action) |
|---|---|---|
| Mouth | 1,000–2,000 mL | Amylase (carbohydrate digestion) |
| | | Lipase (fat digestion) |
| | | Immunoglobulins |
| | | Mucus |
| | | Water, electrolytes |
| Esophagus | 300–800 mL | Mucus |
| Stomach | 2,000 mL | Intrinsic factor (vitamin $B_{12}$ absorption) |
| | | Hydrochloric acid (activates pepsinogen) |
| | | Pepsinogen (protein digestion) |
| | | Mucus |
| | | Water, electrolytes |
| | | Gastrin (stimulates hydrochloric acid release; trophic effects on mucosa, especially in stomach) |
| Pancreas | 1,200–1,800 mL | Enzymes |
| | | • Amylase (carbohydrate digestion) |
| | | • Trypsinogen (protein digestion) |
| | | • Chymotrypsin (protein digestion) |
| | | • Elastase (protein digestion) |
| | | • Carboxypeptidase (protein digestion) |
| | | • Lipase (fat digestion) |
| | | • Colipase (fat digestion) |
| | | • Esterase (cholesterol digestion) |
| | | • Phospholipase (phospholipid digestion) |
| | | • Nucleases (RNA and DNA digestion) |
| | | Bicarbonate (protects luminal wall by neutralizing acid) |
| | | Water, electrolytes |
| Liver | 500–1,000 mL | Bile salts (emulsify fats) |
| | | Bilirubin (excretory end product of hemoglobin breakdown) |
| | | Water, electrolytes |
| Small intestine | 3,000–4,000 mL | Enzymes |
| | | • Enterokinase (activates trypsinogen) |
| | | • Lipase (fat digestion) |
| | | • Enteropeptidase (protein digestion) |
| | | • Peptidase (protein digestion) |
| | | • Nucleases (RNA and DNA digestion) |
| | | • Maltase (carbohydrate digestion) |
| | | • Lactase (carbohydrate digestion) |
| | | • Sucrase (carbohydrate digestion) |
| | | Mucus |
| | | Bicarbonate |
| | | Water, electrolytes |
| | | CCK into blood (stimulates pancreatic secretion and gallbladder contraction) |
| | | Glucose-dependent insulinotropic peptide into blood (stimulates insulin release and gastric motility, secretion) |
| | | Gastrin (stimulates gastric acid secretion) |
| Large intestine | Variable | Mucus |

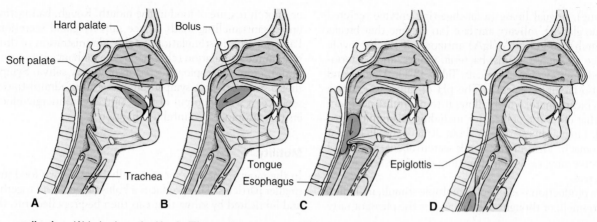

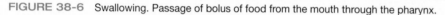

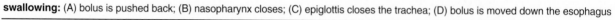

**swallowing:** (A) bolus is pushed back; (B) nasopharynx closes; (C) epiglottis closes the trachea; (D) bolus is moved down the esophagus

**FIGURE 38-6** Swallowing. Passage of bolus of food from the mouth through the pharynx.

stomach by the process of swallowing. Swallowing is a complex process that has several phases (Fig. 38-6). During the oral phase, the tongue propels the food or fluid bolus to the posterior pharynx. This is a voluntary process. During the involuntary pharyngeal phase, the presence of food or fluid in the pharynx stimulates pharyngeal sensory receptors that initiate impulses through cranial nerve V (the trigeminal nerve) to the swallowing center in the medulla. Sensory impulses reflexively trigger the outflow of impulses down motor fibers in cranial nerve IX (the glossopharyngeal nerve) and cranial nerve X (the vagus nerve) to pharyngeal and laryngeal structures. This causes the following coordinated events, which propel the solid or fluid substance into the esophagus:

1. The soft palate elevates and retracts, sealing off the nasopharynx to prevent regurgitation.
2. The vocal cords close, and the epiglottis closes over the larynx to prevent aspiration.
3. The UES relaxes.
4. The larynx pulls up and increases the opening of the esophagus and UES.
5. The pharyngeal muscles contract, propelling food or fluid into the opened esophagus.

During this phase, respiration is reflexively inhibited. Damage to sensory or motor fibers (in cranial nerves V, IX, or X) or to the swallowing center in the brainstem weakens or eliminates the ability to swallow or causes poorly coordinated swallowing, wherein food or fluid enters the nasopharynx or larynx, or both.

## Esophagus

### Secretions

Esophageal mucosal cells secrete mucus (see Table 38-1, p. xxx). The mucus protects the esophageal lining from damage by gastric secretions or food and acts as a lubricant to facilitate the passage of food.

### Motility

The esophageal phase of swallowing begins once food or fluid enters the esophagus (Fig. 38-7). Swallowing-induced

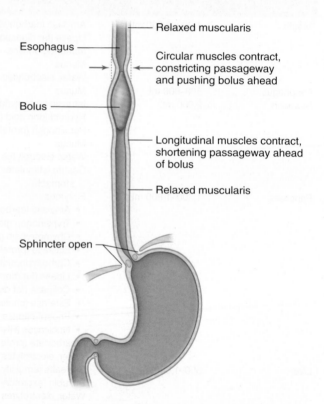

**FIGURE 38-7** Movement of a bolus of food through the esophagus by a peristaltic contraction.

contractions of the esophagus are called primary peristalsis. The wave of peristalsis causes the LES to relax, thereby allowing food to enter the stomach. If primary peristalsis cannot clear the esophagus, food or fluid distends the esophagus. This distention stimulates stretch receptors that reflexively promote relaxation of the esophageal muscles ahead of the area of distention as well as contraction of the esophageal muscles in and behind it. This propels the food or fluid ahead into the newly relaxed area, which then becomes distended. This is called secondary peristalsis. The peristalsis reflex repeatedly recurs until the food or fluid arrives at the LES.

The tone of the LES can be altered by a variety of agents (Table 38-2). Some people suffer from a hypertrophic LES,

**TABLE 38-2** Factors Influencing Lower Esophageal Sphincter Tone

| Increased Tone | Decreased Tone |
|---|---|
| Food substances: | Food substances: |
| Protein | Fats |
| Drugs: | Coffee |
| Metoclopramide | Chocolate |
| Some prostaglandins (F₂) | Alcohol |
| | Peppermint |
| | Citrus juices |
| | Tomato products |
| | Carbonated beverages |
| | CCK |
| | Progesterone (as in pregnancy) |
| | Somatostatin |
| | Dopamine |
| | Some prostaglandins (E₂, A₂) |
| | Cigarette smoking |

which impedes esophageal emptying (and can lead to overdistention of the lower esophagus), whereas others have an incompetent LES, which results in repeated episodes of gastric reflux (which can lead to lower esophageal strictures).

## Stomach

### Secretions

The major secretions of the stomach are hydrochloric acid, intrinsic factor, pepsinogen, gastrin, and mucus (see Table 38-1). Hydrochloric acid converts pepsinogen, which is secreted by the chief cells of the stomach, to pepsin, a proteolytic enzyme. The hydrochloric acid provides an ideal pH for the activity of pepsin; together, hydrochloric acid and pepsin begin the digestion of protein. The chemical action of hydrochloric acid also breaks down food molecules and helps protect the gastrointestinal tract from bacterial invasion. Intrinsic factor is necessary for the absorption of vitamin $B_{12}$ in the small intestine.

G cells, located in the gastric antrum, secrete the hormone gastrin, which promotes the secretion by the chief and parietal cells and promotes the growth of the gastric mucosa (Table 38-3). Overproduction of gastrin, a condition known as Zollinger–Ellison syndrome, results in gastric hypersecretion and peptic ulceration.

Gastric mucosal cells continuously secrete a thin coat of mucus. Mucus, a lubricant, works together with bicarbonate to neutralize acid, protecting the stomach wall from damage. This barrier can be disrupted by a variety of agents, including bile salts, alcohol, aspirin, nonsteroidal anti-inflammatory drugs, and infection with *Helicobacter pylori*.

### Factors Affecting Gastric Secretions

The gastric parietal cells contain receptors for acetylcholine, histamine, and gastrin. Stimulation of these receptors prompts the parietal cells to secrete hydrochloric acid. Hydrochloric acid secretion is inhibited by chemicals that block the histamine receptors (eg, $H_2$-receptor antagonists) or the acetylcholine receptors (eg, atropine). Proton pump inhibitors inhibit the $H^+/K^+$-adenosine triphosphatase (ATPase) enzyme pathway, the final common step in the acid secretory

pathway. Some prostaglandins also inhibit hydrochloric acid secretion. Factors that stimulate gastric secretions include alcohol, caffeine, and hypoglycemia.

### Control of Gastric Secretions

Gastric secretions are regulated in three phases: the cephalic phase, the gastric phase, and the intestinal phase (Table 38-4). These phases are controlled by neural and hormonal mechanisms.

In the cephalic phase, the sight, smell, taste, or thought of food stimulates brainstem centers, reflexively prompting parasympathetic (vagal) stimulation of salivation, pancreatic secretion, bile release, and gastric secretions of pepsinogen and hydrochloric acid by the chief and parietal cells, respectively. Sympathetic stimulation can alter the cephalic phase response. This is the mechanism by which emotions can influence gastrointestinal secretions. Fear, anger, and depression decrease secretions.

During the gastric phase, distention of the stomach by food stimulates stretch receptors in the stomach wall. Chemicals, mainly proteins, stimulate chemoreceptors in the mucosa. The stretch receptors and chemoreceptors in turn activate neurons in the submucosal plexus, which then stimulate neurons in the myenteric plexus, which in turn stimulate secretion by the parietal and chief cells. Proteins in the chyme also directly promote gastrin secretion by G cells; the gastrin provides an additional stimulus for parietal and chief cell secretion.

A combination of events eventually brings the gastric phase to a halt: the stretch receptors and chemoreceptors in the wall of the stomach become refractory to stimulation, the acidity of the chyme inhibits further gastrin secretion, and GIP decreases hydrochloric acid secretion and gastric motility.

The intestinal phase begins after chyme reaches the duodenum. The acidity of the chyme stimulates duodenal mucosal cells to release secretin into the bloodstream; proteins and fat trigger the release of cholecystokinin (CCK) into the blood from similar cells, and glucose and fat stimulate the secretion of GIP. Secretin and CCK cause pancreatic secretion and release of gallbladder contents into the duodenum. GIP stimulates the release of insulin from the islets of Langerhans and decreases gastric motility and secretions (see Table 38-3). Stretch receptors in the duodenum trigger peristalsis so that chyme is degraded, mixed with enzymes and diluents, and moved past the highly absorbent small intestinal lumen. If the chyme is less acidic, gastrin is released. Under neural control, motilin is another hormone that is cyclically released during fasting. Motilin stimulates stomach and small intestine motility.

### Motility

The passage of food from the esophagus into the stomach reflexively initiates receptive relaxation. After the stomach has filled with food, peristaltic contractions mix the food and propel gastric contents toward the pylorus, where small amounts enter the duodenum. The pyloric sphincter plays a minor role in gastric emptying; its main function is to prevent duodenal reflux. The bile acids in the chyme that reenters the stomach through duodenal reflux damage the chemical barrier that coats the surfaces of gastric mucosal

**TABLE 38-3** Hormones Controlling Secretion and Motility

| Hormone | Source | Stimulation of Release | Major Function |
|---------|--------|------------------------|----------------|
| Gastrin | Stomach, small intestine | Gastric distention, presence of partially digested protein near pylorus | Stimulates<br>• Gastric acid secretion<br>• Gastric intrinsic factor secretion<br>• Gastric motility<br>• Intestinal motility<br>• Mucosal growth<br>• Pancreatic growth<br>• Pancreatic insulin release<br>• Lower esophageal tone |
| Secretin | Small intestine | Acid entering small intestine | Stimulates<br>• Pancreatic bicarbonate secretion<br>• Pancreatic enzyme secretion<br>• Pancreatic growth<br>• Gastric pepsin secretion<br>• Bile bicarbonate secretion<br>• Gallbladder contraction<br>Inhibits<br>• Gastric emptying<br>• Gastric motility<br>• Intestinal motility |
| CCK | Small intestine | Fatty acids and amino acids in small intestine | Stimulates<br>• Gastric acid secretion<br>• Gastric motility<br>• Intestinal motility<br>• Colonic motility<br>• Gallbladder contraction and sphincter of Oddi relaxation (thus increasing bile flow into small intestine)<br>• Pancreatic bicarbonate secretion<br>• Pancreatic enzyme release<br>• Pancreatic growth<br>Inhibits<br>• Lower esophageal tone<br>• Gastric emptying |
| GIP | Small intestine | Fatty acids and lipids in small intestine | Stimulates<br>• Insulin release<br>• Intestinal motility<br>Inhibits<br>• Gastric acid secretion<br>• Gastric emptying<br>• Gastric motility |
| Motilin | Small intestine | Acid and fat in small intestine | Stimulates<br>• Gastric motility<br>• Intestinal motility |

cells. Gastric emptying can be retarded by vagotomy; by the presence of fats, proteins, or hydrochloric acid in the duodenal chyme; by duodenal distention; and by intestinal hormones.

Emesis, or vomiting, is the regurgitation of food from the stomach through the mouth. During vomiting, the abdominal muscles and diaphragm contract, and the LES relaxes, allowing reflux of gastric content into the esophagus and propulsion of gastric contents out of the mouth. In addition, irritation of the small intestine can cause reverse peristalsis. These movements move chyme toward the pyloric valve. If strong enough to force open the pylorus, intestinal contents may be vomited. When yellow bile from the duodenum is exposed to acid in the stomach, the interaction turns the vomitus green. Occasionally, vomiting of intestinal contents can be so rapid that the vomitus contains yellow bile. When blood is exposed to acid in the stomach, the exposure results in a brownish-black "coffee-ground" emesis. If the rapidity of vomiting does not allow sufficient time for this interaction

between acid and blood to occur, blood in the vomitus has its normal red color (hematemesis).

## Pancreas

The pancreas is composed of both exocrine and endocrine tissue. Endocrine tissue scattered throughout the pancreas, secrete insulin, glucagon, and pancreatic polypeptide hormones, which aid in the digestive process. The exocrine pancreas is composed of acinar cells which empty secretions into an internal pancreatic ductal system (Fig. 38-8). Because of the anatomical arrangements between the common bile duct and the duct of Wirsung, a gallstone that obstructs the ampulla of Vater can obstruct the normal flow of bile and pancreatic secretions. (Such obstruction, although rare, can lead to a stasis of pancreatic secretion, resulting in acute pancreatitis.)

The exocrine acinar cells secrete both a watery alkaline bicarbonate solution and enzymes (see Table 38-1). The large

| TABLE 38-4 | Phases of Gastric Secretion | |
|---|---|---|
| **Phase** | **Stimulus to Secretion** | **Effect** |
| Cephalic (neuronal) | Sight, smell, taste of food initiates central nervous system impulse mediated by vagus nerve | Gastric effects: Hydrochloric acid (from parietal cells) Pepsinogen (from chief cells) Mucus secretion Other effects: Salivation Pancreatic secretion Bile release |
| Gastric (neuronal and hormonal) | Food in antrum initiates central nervous system impulse mediated by vagus nerve | Gastrin release Hydrochloric acid release Pepsinogen release |
| Intestinal (hormonal) | Chyme in small intestine | pH of chyme <2: release of secretin, gastric inhibitory polypeptide, CCK (decreases gastric acid secretion) pH of chyme >3: release of gastrin (increases gastric acid secretion) |

amount of water secreted by the pancreas is instrumental in diluting chyme before absorption. In addition, the bicarbonate neutralizes the highly acidic chyme from the stomach. The pancreatic enzymes digest proteins (trypsin, chymotrypsin, elastase, and carboxypeptidase), fats (lipase, colipase, and esterase), phospholipase and nucleic acids (nucleases), and starch (amylase).

Pancreatic enzymes are secreted from the pancreas in their inactive forms. Trypsin inhibitor prevents the premature activation of trypsinogen into its active form, trypsin. Once the pancreatic secretions arrive in the duodenum, trypsinogen is activated by an intestinal mucosal enzyme, enterokinase, into its active form, trypsin. Trypsin then activates the other pancreatic enzymes.

## Gallbladder

In the duodenum, chyme mixed with pancreatic secretions is watery. The fat in chyme is not water soluble and requires a solvent enzyme mixture from the liver to render it absorbable by intestinal cells. Hepatocytes, among many other metabolic functions, make bile. Bile is a mixture of bile salts, cholesterol, bilirubin, and acids suspended in water. This solution emulsifies the fat in chyme, breaking the fat into small globules that can be absorbed across the intestinal lumen. The action of bile ionizes fat-soluble vitamins into absorbable forms. Bile also suspends cholesterol, triglycerides, and multiple-density lipoproteins in the bloodstream, thus preventing precipitation and deposition of these molecules in the vasculature until they can be catabolized.

Bile is stored and concentrated in the gallbladder. Gallbladder secretion is greatest during the intestinal phase of digestion. This activity is stimulated by CCK, which is secreted by the intestinal mucosa when fatty acids or amino acids are present. CCK causes gallbladder contraction and relaxation of the sphincter of Oddi, allowing the release of bile into the duodenum to mix with chyme.

## Small Intestine

### Secretions

In the duodenum, chyme mixes with pancreatic digestive enzymes, alkaline substances, water, mucus, and bile. When the mucosa of the small intestine is exposed to acid in the chyme, secretin is released. Secretin stimulates bicarbonate release by cells that line the bile ducts. The intestinal enzymes secretin, CCK, and enterokinase are added to this mixture, along with mucus, bicarbonate, and water. These intestinal secretions help maintain the liquidity of chyme and can dilute noxious agents.

### Motility

The small intestine has two types of characteristic movements, propulsive and mixing. Propulsive movements propel food forward, allowing for digestion and absorption. This peristalsis is stimulated by distention. During mixing movement, localized concentric contractions of the intestinal wall called segmentation promote mixing of food particles. Repetition of this process continually kneads the chyme, which increases the exposure of the molecules to the absorptive surfaces of the intestinal mucosa.

Emptying of the small intestine into the colon occurs in the same way as gastric emptying. Peristaltic waves build pressure in the ileum behind the ileocecal valve and push the chyme through the valve into the colon.

### Absorption

The major functions of the small intestine are absorption and digestion, which are facilitated by secretions from the pancreas, liver, and gallbladder. The mucosal layer of the small intestine has many folds (valvulae conniventes) covered with numerous finger-like projections (villi) and microvilli, which dramatically increase the absorptive surface area of the small intestine.

**CARBOHYDRATES.** The three major sources of carbohydrates in the human diet are sucrose, lactose, and starch. The breakdown of carbohydrates begins in the mouth when food mixes with salivary amylase during chewing. The digestion continues in the duodenum. Conversion to simple sugars continues in the small intestine by intestinal enzymes. Both active and passive transport are used to absorb sugars across the intestinal lumen into the bloodstream.

**PROTEINS.** Protein degradation is initiated in the stomach through the actions of hydrochloric acid and pepsin.

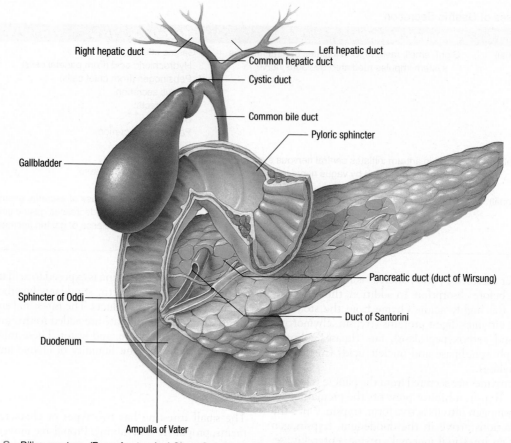

Right hepatic duct
Left hepatic duct
Common hepatic duct
Cystic duct
Common bile duct
Pyloric sphincter
Gallbladder
Pancreatic duct (duct of Wirsung)
Sphincter of Oddi
Duct of Santorini
Duodenum
Ampulla of Vater

**FIGURE 38-8** Biliary system. (From Anatomical Chart Company: Atlas of Human Anatomy. Springhouse, PA: Springhouse, 2001, p 217)

However, in the absence of pepsin and hydrochloric acid, the small intestine is capable of fully digesting all available protein. Most digestion occurs in the duodenum and jejunum by proteolytic pancreatic enzymes. Polypeptides in the small intestine are degraded into peptide fragments and amino acids by trypsin, chymotrypsin, and carboxypeptidase. Amino acids are absorbed into the blood by active and passive diffusion.

**FATS.** Triglycerides, lipids, and phospholipids are first degraded in the small intestine. Bile salts, in a process called emulsification, facilitate the creation of small droplets of fats from larger globules. Pancreatic enzymes then degrade the fats into fatty acid chains and monoglycerides. These smaller molecules form into even smaller globules, called micelles. Fatty acids and monosaccharides are transported across the intestinal mucosa from a micelle passively, leaving bile behind.

In the submucosa, free fatty acids are passed into the blood directly, if small enough. If too large for direct passive diffusion, the free fatty acid is reorganized into a triglyceride, coupled with lipoproteins and cholesterol, and passed into the lymph fluid as chylomicron.

The bile left behind in the intestine after absorption of fats from a micelle is reabsorbed in the ileum. If bile salts enter the colon, they decrease the reabsorption of sodium and water, thereby increasing the liquidity of the undigested food residues in the colon. Most fat is absorbed by the time chyme reaches the middle of the jejunum.

**VITAMINS, MINERALS, AND WATER.** Most vitamins, whether fat or water soluble, diffuse across the intestinal mucosa and submucosa into the blood. Fat-soluble vitamin $B_{12}$ couples with intrinsic factor, forming a larger molecule. In this form, vitamin $B_{12}$ is absorbed in the ileum.

Minerals and electrolytes vary in their absorption. Sodium and iron require active transport, whereas other minerals and electrolytes diffuse passively. Iron is primarily absorbed in the duodenum.

Water is absorbed passively throughout the stomach and small and large intestines. The gastrointestinal tract is highly permeable, in both directions, to water. If a hypertonic solution enters the duodenum, osmosis occurs within the lumen. The converse is also true: a hypotonic chyme in the stomach and duodenum causes extremely rapid movement of water into the bloodstream.

## Large Intestine

### Secretion

The goblet cells of the colonic mucosa secrete mucus, which lubricates the passage of chyme (see Table 38-1). The production of mucus is stimulated by irritation and by cholinergic activation.

### Motility

Colonic movements include mixing and peristaltic movements. These operate as described for the small intestine.

A third movement, unique to the colon, is mass movement. This consists of simultaneous contractions of colonic smooth muscle over large portions of the descending and sigmoid portions of the colon. Mass movement rapidly moves the undigested food residue (feces) from these areas into the rectum.

Humans cannot digest the cellulose, hemicellulose, or lignin in plant tissues. These plant materials form a large portion of the undigested food residue. They are usually termed vegetable fiber or dietary bulk. These fibers attract and hold water, creating a larger, softer stool. Low quantities of bulk result in a relatively inactive colon, leading to bowel movements that are relatively infrequent and feces that are relatively small, dry, and difficult to pass. Epidemiologic reports suggest that high-fiber diets are associated with a decreased incidence of diverticulitis and colon cancer.

Filling of the rectum triggers the defecation reflex by stimulating stretch receptors in the rectal wall. Stimulation of the stretch receptors causes sensory (afferent) nerve fibers to transmit impulses to the lower spinal cord. Because of anatomical arrangements of neurons in this part of the cord, these afferent impulses reflexively cause nerve impulses to travel out of the cord along parasympathetic motor fibers that innervate the smooth muscles of the descending and sigmoid colon, the rectum, and the internal anal sphincter. The afferent impulses also reflexively cause nerve impulses to be sent out of the cord along somatic motor neurons that innervate the skeletal muscle of the external anal sphincter. The total effect of these events is to produce coordinated expulsive contractions of the colon and rectum, relaxation (opening) of the sphincters, and expulsion of feces from the anus.

The urge to defecate begins after the pressure within the rectum reaches 18 mm Hg. After intrarectal pressure reaches 55 mm Hg, reflex bowel evacuation occurs. This defecation reflex is inhibited in a continent person by descending neuronal impulses from higher brain centers that inhibit the actions of the somatic motor neurons that innervate the external sphincter. Such inhibition keeps the external anal sphincter closed, thereby averting inappropriate defecation. After a few minutes, the defecation reflex subsides, but it usually becomes active again a few hours later. Defecation is a spinal cord reflex that does not require intact pathways between the sacral cord and the brain. In the early posttraumatic phase of spinal shock, the reflex does not work. After cord shock is ended, reflex defecation occurs once again, but voluntary inhibition is not possible (neurogenic bowel).

## Absorption

In the large intestine, most of the water and potassium are absorbed from the chyme. This produces a semisolid residue of undigested food (feces) that can be eliminated from the body. Diarrhea can reduce the transit time for chyme, thereby limiting such potassium and water reabsorption. This can result in hypokalemia and dehydration. Diarrhea can be caused by materials that hold water in the chyme (eg, magnesium sulfate), resulting in semiliquid stool.

At birth the colon is sterile, but large colonic bacterial populations become established soon afterward. Some of these organisms produce vitamin K and a number of B vitamins. Other bacteria produce ammonia, which is absorbed. Normally, ammonia is removed from the blood once it reaches the liver. However, in people with seriously impaired liver function or with collateral circulatory routes that bypass the liver (usually the result of portal hypertension), ammonia can remain in the circulation and lead to hepatic encephalopathy.

## Liver

The liver lies in the right upper quadrant of the abdomen and is divided into functional units called lobules. Each lobule consists of sheets of hepatocytes organized around a core cluster of vessels called the portal triad (Fig. 38-9). The portal triad includes the two sets of afferent vessels (portal vein and hepatic artery) and a small bile duct.

Rows of hepatocytes radiate from a central venule like spokes of a wheel. Branches of the hepatic artery and the hepatic portal vein lie at the periphery of the wheel. Kupffer cells, specialized white cells of the reticuloendothelial system, phagocytize bacteria, debris, and other foreign matter in the sinus blood. The sinuses drain into the central venule, which in turn carries blood to the hepatic vein.

Blind-ended bile canaliculi carry newly secreted bile to larger ducts located at the periphery. These smaller ducts eventually drain into the common bile duct. Bile that is leaving the liver is concentrated and stored in the gallbladder. Fluid and electrolyte reabsorption in the gallbladder can increase the concentration of bile salts, cholesterol, and bilirubin 12-fold.

The gallbladder has a maximum capacity of 50 mL and can hold a 24-hour output of bile (600 mL) from the liver. The intestinal hormone CCK (secreted by the duodenal mucosa) and vagus nerve activity stimulate gallbladder contraction as a part of food digestion, particularly lipids. CCK and local reflexes initiated by duodenal peristalsis open the sphincter of Oddi. These events permit an outflow of bile down the common bile duct into the duodenum.

The common bile duct and the main duct from the pancreas usually unite just before the duct enters the lumen of the duodenum. There is often a dilation of the tube after this junction (the ampulla of Vater). The opening of the common bile duct in the duodenum is about 8 to 10 cm from the pylorus.

The liver cells perform many vital functions, as described in the sections that follow and summarized in Table 38-5.

### Carbohydrate Metabolism

The liver participates in carbohydrate metabolism. The liver and skeletal muscle are the two primary sites of glycogen storage. Serum glucose levels are maintained by hepatic glycostatic function, involving two mechanisms. When plasma glucose levels are high, hepatocytes remove glucose from the plasma. Some of this glucose is then stored in the liver as glycogen. If plasma glucose levels decline, hepatocytes convert the glycogen back into glucose through a process called glycogenolysis, and the glucose is released into the bloodstream. Although many body tissues have the requisite cellular enzymes for glycogenolysis, hepatocytes are one of the few cell types that can release this intracellular glucose into the bloodstream. Hepatocytes do not simply respond directly to plasma glucose. These glycostatic functions are mediated by several hormones; some (eg, insulin) promote hepatic glucose uptake, and others (eg, glucagon, growth hormone, and epinephrine) stimulate glycogenolysis and the release of glucose from liver cells.

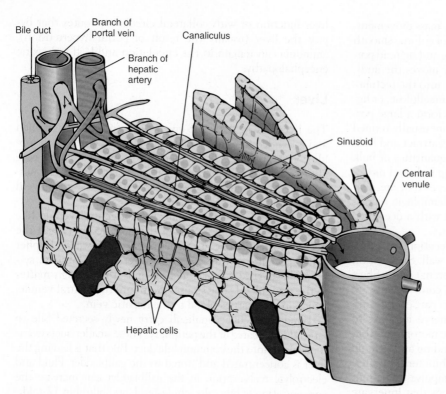

Bile duct
Branch of portal vein
Canaliculus
Branch of hepatic artery
Sinusoid
Central venule
Hepatic cells

**FIGURE 38-9**   A section of the liver lobule showing the location of the hepatic veins, hepatic cells, liver sinusoids, and branches of the portal vein and hepatic artery.

**TABLE 38-5   Hepatic Function**

| General Category | Specific Description |
|---|---|
| Carbohydrate metabolism | Glycogenesis (conversion of glucose to glycogen) |
| | Glycogenolysis (breakdown of glycogen to glucose) |
| | Gluconeogenesis (formation of glucose from amino acids or fatty acids) |
| Protein metabolism | Synthesis of nonessential amino acids |
| | Synthesis of plasma proteins (albumin, prealbumin, transferrin, clotting factors, complement factors; not γ-globulin or immunoglobulins) |
| | Urea formation from $NH_3$ ($NH_3$ formed by deamination of amino acids in liver and by action of colonic bacteria on proteins) |
| Lipid and lipoprotein metabolism | Synthesis of lipoproteins |
| | Breakdown of triglycerides into fatty acids and glycerol |
| | Formation of ketone bodies |
| | Synthesis of fatty acids from amino acids and glucose |
| | Synthesis and breakdown of cholesterol |
| Bile acid synthesis and excretion | Bile formation (containing bile salts, bile pigments [bilirubin, biliverdin]), cholesterol |
| | Bile excretion |
| Storage | Glucose (as glycogen) |
| | Vitamins (A, D, E, K, $B_1$, $B_2$, $B_{12}$, folic acid) |
| | Fatty acids |
| | Minerals (Fe, Cu) |
| | Amino acids (as albumin, β-globulins) |
| Biotransformation, detoxification, excretion of endogenous and exogenous compounds | Inactivation of drugs and excretion of the breakdown products |
| | Clearance of procoagulants, activated clotting factors, byproducts of coagulation |
| Removal of pathogens | Clearance of microorganisms by macrophages |
| Steroid catabolism | Conjugation and excretion of gonadal steroids |
| | Conjugation and excretion of adrenal steroids (cortisol, aldosterone) |

The liver does not contain enough glycogen reserves to be able to buffer plasma glucose during prolonged fasting or severe exercise. During these times, low plasma glucose levels stimulate the secretion of one or more hormones (glucagon, glucocorticoids, or thyroxine) that trigger the biochemical conversion of intracellular fatty and amino acids into glucose (gluconeogenesis), which the liver cell can then release into the bloodstream or store as glycogen. Only hepatocytes possess the enzyme that is critical for gluconeogenesis. Glycogen storage is important for other functions of liver cells.

A glycogen-rich hepatocyte conjugates bilirubin at a faster rate and is more resistant to toxins and infectious agents.

## Protein Metabolism

The liver plays an essential role in the metabolism of proteins. The amino acids that result from the breakdown of proteins are deaminated to form ammonia by the liver and then converted to urea. The liver also synthesizes plasma proteins, including albumins, globulins, fibrinogens, plasma lipoproteins, and other proteins involved in clotting. The albumins maintain normal plasma oncotic pressure. A fall in this pressure leads to edema (both systemic and pulmonary) and contributes to ascites. The globulins bind thyroid and adrenal hormones. Bound, the hormones are inactive. Decreased hepatic protein levels can lead to a clinical excess of these hormones.

## Lipid and Lipoprotein Metabolism

The liver contributes to adipose stores through the metabolism of triglycerides, fatty acids, and cholesterol. During fasting, triglycerides from adipose tissue are catabolized by the liver into fatty acids and glycerols. The free fatty acids in prolonged fasting are further catabolized into acetyl coenzyme A and then into ketone bodies. Ketone bodies provide an energy source for some (nonneuronal) tissues.

## Bile Acid Synthesis and Excretion

Hepatocytes make bile, which contains water, bile salts, cholesterol, bilirubin, gluconate, and inorganic acids. Bile salts aid digestion by emulsifying dietary fats and fostering their absorption and the absorption of fat-soluble vitamins through the intestinal mucosa. They also prevent the cholesterol in the bile from precipitating out of solution and forming calculi. More than 90% of the daily output of bile is reabsorbed for recycling by an active transport process of the ileal mucosa.

Another hepatic function is elimination of bilirubin from the body. Old or defective erythrocytes are phagocytosed by large reticuloendothelial cells that line the large veins and the sinuses of the liver and spleen. These phagocytes degrade the hemoglobin of these cells into biliverdin, iron, and globulin molecules. The last two components are recycled by the body and used for future erythropoiesis. The biliverdin is almost immediately converted to free bilirubin. Because free bilirubin is an insoluble compound, it is transported bound to plasma albumin molecules. The hepatocytes convert this insoluble bilirubin into a soluble (and thus excretable) form by conjugating it with glucuronic acid to form bilirubin gluconate. This soluble form of bilirubin is then added to the bile and is eliminated from the body by the feces. Bilirubin gluconate gives the bile its normal golden yellow color. Organisms in the intestine convert most of the bilirubin gluconate into a darker brown compound, urobilinogen, which gives the feces its natural brown color. Because it is soluble in water, urobilinogen can also be absorbed from the colon back into the bloodstream and can be excreted by the kidneys. Excess plasma levels of either conjugated (direct) or unconjugated (indirect) bilirubin produce jaundice. Excess unconjugated bilirubin can cross the immature or damaged blood–brain barrier and bind with the basal ganglia, resulting in kernicterus.

## Storage

Fat-soluble vitamins and many minerals are stored in the liver. These vitamins and minerals are released under the influence of hormones and serum concentrations of inorganic elements.

## Biotransformation

Hepatocytes possess a mixed-function oxidase (MFO) system of enzymes that degrade certain drugs, including alcohol, benzodiazepines, tranquilizers, phenobarbital, phenytoin, and sodium warfarin, among others. This system operates in addition to other intracellular systems that also degrade some of these drugs. Its clinical significance lies in the nature of the drugs that this system catabolizes and in the fact that MFO system activity can be either inhibited or augmented (induced) by these same drugs, depending on when they are taken.

Administration of two MFO system–catabolized drugs within a few hours of one another or together causes each agent to act competitively, slowing down the degradation of the other. For example, simultaneous ingestion of diazepam (Valium) and alcohol can result in slower degradation of each drug. The outcome is higher blood levels of both chemicals for a longer time after administration.

The repeated administration of one MFO system–catabolized drug for several days causes the MFO system to enlarge physically and to possess more enzymes. This is called induction. Once induced, the MFO system degrades drugs more rapidly (including the drug that initiated the induction). If administration of a second MFO system–catabolized drug is begun after MFO system induction, a larger dose of this drug is required to produce a given effect. For example, induction of the MFO system by diazepam increases the dosage of warfarin needed to produce a given therapeutic effect. Other drugs are degraded by various hepatic systems.

## Steroid Catabolism

The liver cells degrade steroid hormones, thereby preventing excess serum levels of estrogen, testosterone, progesterone, aldosterone, and glucocorticosteroids.

# Clinical Applicability Challenges

## SHORT ANSWER QUESTIONS

1. Mr. K is a 27-year-old with suspected food poisoning. What processes are involved in vomiting?
2. Mrs. D. complains of a bitter aftertaste in her mouth after meals. Other associated symptoms are suggestive of gastroesophageal reflux. Briefly describe the role of bile in the digestive process.
3. Mr. Z is a 53-year-old male who is being prepared for liver surgery. Briefly describe how the blood supply in the liver is unique.

### WANT TO KNOW MORE?

A wide variety of resources to enhance your learning and understanding of this chapter are available on thePoint.

You will find:

- References
- Selected readings
- NCLEX-style review questions
- Internet resources
- And more!

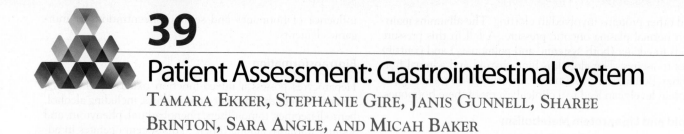

# 39

# Patient Assessment: Gastrointestinal System

TAMARA EKKER, STEPHANIE GIRE, JANIS GUNNELL, SHAREE BRINTON, SARA ANGLE, AND MICAH BAKER

## LEARNING OBJECTIVES

### Based on the content in this chapter, the reader should be able to:

1. Explain the nursing role in assessing gastrointestinal (GI) status in the critical care patient.

2. Discuss important health history components that provide information about GI system status.

3. Describe a systematic approach for conducting a complete GI physical examination.

4. Discuss the importance of pain patterns in an abdominal assessment.

5. Differentiate between normal and abnormal findings detected on physical assessment of the GI system.

6. Identify the data used to make judgments about nutrition and metabolism in a critical care patient.

7. Discuss appropriate studies and procedures used to diagnose GI disorders and the nursing implications.

The gastrointestinal (GI) system is a 30 ft (9 m) long tube with glands and accessory organs (salivary glands, liver, gallbladder, and pancreas). The GI tract begins at the mouth; extends through the pharynx, esophagus, stomach, small intestine, colon, and rectum; and ends at the anus. It is an unsterile system filled with bacteria and other flora. These organisms can cause superinfection if they develop resistance from antibiotic therapy, and they can infect other systems when an organ of the GI tract ruptures. A malfunction along the GI tract can produce a variety of metabolic effects.

Assessment of the GI system in a critically ill patient allows for early identification of GI disorders and serves as a foundation for developing a holistic plan of care for the patient. Ongoing assessment of the GI system in the critical care patient may help identify new complications. In an intensive care environment, the dynamic nature of the patient's condition may dictate a more focused patient assessment.

When a patient is critically ill, the nurse must determine whether GI assessment findings relate to the current clinical problem or a new complication. The nurse compares presenting GI signs and symptoms, and works to determine whether they are isolated entities or related to another underlying problem. Is the bright red blood in the stool a result of GI bleeding, or is it from external bleeding hemorrhoids? Is the abdominal pain due to recent bowel surgery or to a distended stomach? The nurse must be aware of the patient's changing metabolic state and nutritional status, because this information may directly affect other health outcomes.[1]

## History

An assessment of the GI system begins with a thorough and accurate history. The patient's history provides information that can lay the foundation and set the direction for the rest of the assessment. The history is the major subjective data source about a patient's health status, and provides insight into actual or potential health problems. The patient's history guides the physical assessment. The history organizes pertinent physiologic, psychological, cultural, and psychosocial information as it relates to the patient's current health status, and accounts for factors such as lifestyle, family relationships, and cultural influences.[2] Box 39-1 lists elements of a comprehensive GI health history.

The nurse focuses the history on the patient's chief complaint, precipitating events, current symptoms, medical history, and family history. Fixed information, which is obtained in the initial interview, includes data about personal health, preexisting GI conditions, previous GI or abdominal surgeries or injuries, and hospitalizations. The critical care nurse must also consider the present nutritional status of the patient, the projected length of illness, and the impact of the patient's condition on future nutritional needs or adjustments.

The GI assessment may change over the course of the illness. The data gathered during the initial history may have focused on the pressing issues facing the patient at that time, but these issues can change over the course of an admission. The critical care nurse must be vigilant, and must maintain data and incorporate additional information to provide individualized and holistic nursing care as the status of the patient evolves.[2]

Pain is often the chief complaint of patients with abdominal disorders. A thorough assessment of pain must include details about the NOPQRST assessment parameters described in Box 17-1 (see Chapter 17). To help understand the potential origin, location, and radiation of the pain, the nurse mentally divides the abdomen into regions using the quadrant method (Fig. 39-1).

With many GI problems the pain is referred; this makes diagnosis difficult. Referred pain is pain felt at a site different from that of the involved organ. Referred pain occurs because nerves that supply an organ also supply the body surface. Figure 39-2 identifies common sites of referred abdominal pain.

## BOX 39-1 Health History for Gastrointestinal Assessment

**Chief Complaint**
- Patient's description of the problem

**History of the Present Illness**
Complete analysis of the following signs and symptoms (using the NOPQRST format; see Box 17-1 in Chapter 17):
- Abdominal pain
- Anorexia
- Indigestion (heartburn)
- Dysphagia
- Eructation (burping)
- Nausea
- Vomiting
- Hematemesis
- Fever and chills
- Jaundice
- Pruritus (itching)
- Diarrhea
- Constipation
- Flatulence
- Bleeding
- Hemorrhoids
- Melena
- Change in appetite
- Recent weight gain or weight loss
- Mouth lesions
- Anal discomfort
- Fecal incontinence
- Change in abdominal girth

**Past Health History**
- Relevant childhood illnesses and immunizations: hepatitis, influenza, pneumococcal, meningococcal
- Past acute and chronic medical problems: treatments and hospitalizations—diabetes, cancer, inflammatory bowel disease (Crohn disease, ulcerative colitis, irritable bowel syndrome, diverticulitis), peptic ulcer, gallstones, polyps, pancreatitis, hepatitis or cirrhosis of the liver, previous GI bleeding, cancers or tumors of the GI tract, spinal cord injury; for women, episiotomy or fourth-degree laceration during delivery
- Risk factors: age, heredity, gender, race, tobacco use, physical inactivity, obesity, diabetes mellitus, tattoos, exposure to infectious diseases—hepatitis and influenza

- Past surgeries: previous GI surgeries (mouth, pharyngeal, esophageal, stomach, small intestine, colon, gallbladder, liver, pancreas), abdominal surgeries, or trauma
- Past diagnostic tests and interventions: upper endoscopy, colonoscopy, upper GI, barium enema, rectal manometry
- Medications (prescription drugs, over-the-counter drugs, vitamins, herbs, and supplements): aspirin, steroids, anticoagulants, nonsteroidal anti-inflammatory drugs, laxatives, stool softeners
- Allergies and reactions to medications, foods, contrast dye, latex, or other materials
- Transfusions, including type and date

**Family History**
- Health status or cause of death of parents and siblings: inflammatory bowel disease, malabsorption syndrome, cystic fibrosis, celiac disease, gallbladder disease, any cancers of the GI tract

**Personal and Social History**
- Tobacco, alcohol, and substance use
- Environment: water source
- Diet: food intolerances, taste sensations, coffee intake, special diet
- Dental status: patterns of dental care, caries, presence of dentures, braces, bridges, crowns
- Bowel habits
- Sleep patterns
- Exercise
- Cultural, spiritual, and/or religious beliefs
- Sources of stress, coping patterns, social support systems
- Travel: especially overseas

**Review of Other Systems**
- HEENT: visual changes, headaches, tinnitus, vertigo, epistaxis, sore throat, mouth lesions, swollen glands, lymphadenopathy
- Respiratory: shortness of breath, dyspnea, cough, sputum, lung disease, recurrent infections
- Cardiovascular: chest pain, palpitations, orthopnea, edema, hypertension, heart failure, dysrhythmia, angina, valvular disease
- Genitourinary: incontinence, erectile dysfunction, dysuria, frequency, nocturia
- Musculoskeletal: pain, weakness, varicose veins, sensory changes
- Neurologic: transient ischemic attacks, stroke, change in level of consciousness, syncope, seizures, cerebrovascular disease

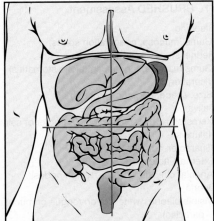

**Right upper quadrant (RUQ)**

Liver and gallbladder
Pylorus
Duodenum
Head of pancreas
Hepatic flexure of colon
Portions of ascending and transverse colon

**Left upper quadrant (LUQ)**

Left liver lobe
Stomach
Body and tail of pancreas
Splenic flexure of colon
Portions of transverse and descending colon

**Right lower quadrant (RLQ)**

Cecum and appendix
Portion of ascending colon
Portions of ileum and jejunum

**Left lower quadrant (LLQ)**

Sigmoid colon
Portion of descending colon
Portions of jejunum and ileum

**FIGURE 39-1** To aid accurate abdominal assessment and documentation of findings, the nurse can mentally divide the patient's abdomen into regions using the quadrant method.

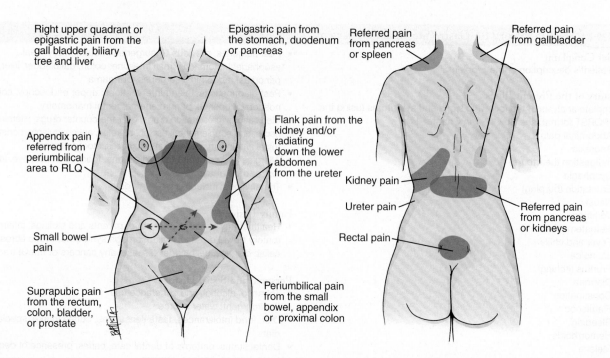

**FIGURE 39-2** Mechanisms and sources of abdominal pain. Abdominal pain may be described as visceral, parietal, or referred. (From Weber J, Kelley J: Health Assessment in Nursing, 5th ed. Philadelphia, PA: Wolters Kluwer Health, 2013, p 481.)

## Physical Examination

A focused examination of the GI system includes evaluation of the oral cavity and throat, abdomen, and rectum. Assessment of the abdomen includes assessment of the liver, gallbladder, and pancreas.[2]

## Oral Cavity and Throat

Shortly after birth, a biofilm of bacteria forms in the mouth. These biofilms train the immune system to recognize pathologic agents and help prevent pathogenic colonization.[3] A thorough assessment of the oral cavity and throat can provide information not only about the patient's GI system, but also about the likelihood of potential infections, the patient's nutritional and hydration status, and problems in the pulmonary, immune, and cardiovascular systems.

Examination of the oral cavity includes inspection and palpation using a good light source, a tongue depressor, an examining glove, and a mask. The nurse should explain the procedure to the patient. The patient assumes a comfortable position that facilitates examination; sitting upright is the best position for this part of the examination.

The BRUSHED model is an assessment tool developed by Hayes and Jones to assist nurses in completing a thorough oral cavity assessment (Table 39-1). Using the BRUSHED model, the nurse assesses the oral cavity for **B**leeding, including cracked lips or tongue, gums, the mucous membrane, and the patient's coagulation status. The nurse looks for **R**edness in and around the mouth, and notes any **U**lceration, including the size, shape, and condition of the wounds, and whether ulcers show signs of infection or appear herpetic. The nurse evaluates the patient's **S**aliva, its quantity and characteristics. The patient's breath is also assessed, and

any **H**alitosis (fecal, acidotic, fruity, or smells of infection) is noted. **E**xternal factors, such as the jaw mobility, crepitus, the lips, symmetry of neck and jaw, any swelling, and lymph nodes under the jaw and down the neck, must be examined; in addition, the nurse looks at the effects of endotracheal (ET) or GI tubes, ET tapes, and so forth. Finally, the nurse looks for **D**ebris, or any unusual particles or masses in the mouth, such as plaque, film on the tongue or mucosa, masses, or any foreign particles.[4]

Table 39-2 reviews oral assessment, normal and abnormal findings, and possible causes of abnormal findings.

Examination of the oral cavity in an intubated patient is very important, even though the tube may hinder vision during the assessment. The condition of the mouth of a critically ill patient can change rapidly, and the nurse must conduct

**TABLE 39-1  BRUSHED Assessment**

| | |
|---|---|
| B | Bleeding (Gums, mucosa, coagulation status) |
| R | Redness (Gums margins, tongue, antibiotic stomatitis) |
| U | Ulceration (Size, shape, herpetic, infected) |
| S | Saliva (Xerostomia, hypersalivation, character of saliva) |
| H | Halitosis (Character, acidotic, infected) |
| E | External Factors (Angular cheilitis, ET tape, lymph nodes) |
| D | Debris (Visible plaque, white film on tongue or mucosa, foreign particles) |

From Fouché N: Word of mouth goes a long way for critically ill patients. South Afr J Crit Care 25(2):34–35, 2009.

**TABLE 39-2  Oral Assessment**

| Structure | Normal | Abnormal Findings | Possible Cause |
|---|---|---|---|
| Lips | Smooth, pink, and moist | Dry or cracked | Febrile illness |
| | | Asymmetrical, cracked, fissured, or bleeding | Cheilitis |
| | | Cyanotic | Cold or hypoxia |
| | | Cracks at corner of lips | Possible vitamin B deficiency or poor hygiene |
| Tongue | Pink, moist with papillae present | Coated or loss of papilla and a shiny appearance (with or without redness); blistered or cracked; altered taste | Infection |
| | | Deviation to one side | Cranial nerve XII (hypoglossal nerve) problem |
| | | Nodules or ulcers on base of tongue | Cancerous lesion |
| Saliva | Watery | Thick, ropy, or absent | |
| Mucous membranes | Pink and moist | Reddened without ulcerations | Infection |
| | | Ulcerations with or without bleeding | Poor nutrition |
| | | Inflammation | Ill-fitting dentures |
| | | Leukoplakia on buccal membrane | Precancerous lesion |
| | | Cyanosis | Hypoxia |
| | | Pale mucosa | Anemia |
| | | Small areas of white scar tissue | Chronic irritation from friction of irregular tooth surfaces or biting when chewing |
| | | Inflamed or painful Stensen duct opening | Parotid gland infection |
| Gingiva | Pink, stippled, and firm | Edematous with or without redness; spontaneous bleeding or bleeding with pressure; soreness | Gingivitis |
| Teeth or dentures | Clean without debris | Plaque or debris in between teeth; plaque or debris along gum line or denture-bearing area | |
| | | Toothache, tooth abscess | |
| | | Misfit of dental appliances | |
| | | Absent or broken teeth, cavities | |
| | | Malocclusion, worn or flattened tooth edges | Bruxism |
| Voice | Normal | Deeper or raspy; difficulty talking or painful to talk | Vocal cord paralysis; recent extubation |
| Throat/swallowing | Normal | Some pain on swallowing or unable to swallow; sore throat | Infection; recent extubation; Cancerous lesion |
| Glands | Nonpalpable | Inflammation and lumps | Stones or cysts |

a periodic assessment to initiate treatment and intervene to prevent complications. It is necessary to assess the presence of any secretions, oral odor, or changes in odors coming from the oral cavity promptly. Studies have indicated that microbial colonization of the oropharynx and dental plaque are associated with pneumonia in patients who are receiving mechanical ventilation.[5]

The patient with a nasogastric, orogastric, or long tube for intestinal decompression warrants close observation because these tubes prevent the lower esophageal sphincter from closing completely. Gastric reflux or even reflux into the oropharynx may occur, which can cause erosive damage to the esophagus as well as a noxious odor in the mouth. Delayed gastric emptying may also exacerbate the reflux.

## Abdomen

The patient's comfort should be preserved as the nurse performs the abdominal examination. The patient should empty his or her bladder before the examination if possible, or this may be facilitated by an indwelling urinary catheter. A supine position with arms down and knees slightly bent is preferred, because this position relieves tension on the abdominal wall and is most comfortable for the patient. Draping exposes the abdomen while protecting the patient's modesty. This is the ideal situation for performing an abdominal examination, but it may not always be possible in a critically ill patient. The nurse must assess the circumstances and prioritize for the individual patient. If the patient is experiencing any or pain, reevaluation of the need for an examination may be warranted. Likewise, if the procedure increases discomfort or intensity of pain, the examiner should adapt and use assessment tools that preserve the patient's comfort as much as possible. The order of the abdominal examination is inspection, auscultation, percussion, and palpation. Auscultation precedes percussion and palpation because the latter can alter the frequency and quality of bowel sounds. Likewise, if the painful area is palpated first, the patient may tense the abdominal muscles, making assessment difficult or impossible.[6]

The abdomen is usually divided into four quadrants by imaginary lines crossing at the umbilicus: right upper, right lower, left upper, and left lower quadrants. Refer to Figure 39-1 for the abdominal organs and their relationship to the four quadrants. Table 39-3 presents abnormal abdominal findings and their possible causes.

**TABLE 39-3** **Abnormal Abdominal Findings**

| Finding | Characteristic | Possible Cause |
|---|---|---|
| Abdominal contour | Concave (scaphoid) | Malnutrition |
| | Distention | Tumor; excessive fluid (ascites, perforation); gas accumulation; severe malnutrition |
| Skin abnormalities | Bulging around old scar | Incisional hernia |
| | Striae | Obesity; pregnancy; abdominal tumor; Cushing syndrome (purple striae) |
| | Pink or blue | Recently developed striae |
| | White or silver | Older striae |
| | Tense, glistening | Ascites |
| | Dilated, tortuous veins | Inferior vena cava obstruction |
| Umbilicus | Everted | Increased intra-abdominal pressure |
| | Bluish ecchymosis surrounding umbilicus (Cullen sign) | Intra-abdominal bleeding; pancreatitis; ectopic pregnancy |
| | Palpable nodule bulging (Sister Mary Joseph nodule) | May indicate metastasis from pelvic or gastrointestinal (GI) cancer |
| Peristaltic wave | Strong | Intestinal obstruction |
| Abdominal aortic pulsations | Obvious and pronounced | Increased intra-abdominal pressure (from tumor or ascites) |
| Murphy sign | Sharp pain that stops respiration when palpating under liver border | Cholecystitis |
| Gray Turner sign | Flank ecchymosis | Intra-abdominal bleeding; hemorrhagic pancreatitis |
| Blumberg sign | Rebound tenderness | Peritoneal irritation; inflamed or perforated appendix |
| Iliopsoas muscle | Right lower quadrant pain when right leg elevated against tension | Inflamed or perforated appendix from inflamed psoas muscle |
| Obturator muscle | Abdominal pain when right leg rotated at hip (internal or external rotation) | Inflamed or perforated appendix |

## Inspection

The nurse begins by inspecting for symmetry of the abdomen, visible masses, and vascular pulsations. Size, shape, and movements from respirations and peristalsis should be noted. Then the nurse inspects the abdomen for tense, shiny skin, any areas of discoloration, rashes, striae (lines resulting from rapid or prolonged skin stretching), ecchymoses, petechiae (small red or purple spots caused by hemorrhage), lesions, scars, and prominent or dilated veins. It is necessary to inspect the umbilicus for position, contour, and color. Pulsation of the aorta is normally apparent in the epigastric area. In a thin person, the femoral pulses may be visible. When ascites or abdominal bleeding is suspected, the nurse should routinely measure the abdominal girth.

## Auscultation

Auscultation provides information on bowel motility and the vessels and organs that lie beneath the abdominal wall. The nurse applies light pressure on the diaphragm of the stethoscope when auscultating the four quadrants of the abdomen. The nurse starts below and to the right of the umbilicus and proceeds in a methodical direction through all four quadrants. To prevent contraction of the abdominal muscles that can obscure sounds, the nurse lifts the stethoscope completely off the abdominal wall when changing its location. Normally, air and fluid moving through the bowel by peristalsis create a soft, bubbling sound with no regular pattern, often with soft clicks and gurgles interspersed, approximately every 5 to 15 seconds. Colonic sounds are low-pitched with a rumbling feature. A hungry patient may exhibit a "growling stomach" resulting from hyperperistalsis, called borborygmi. High-pitched, rapid, loud, and gurgling bowel sounds indicate a

hyperactive bowel, and may occur in a hungry patient. High-pitched tinkling and rushes of high-pitched sounds with abdominal cramping usually indicate obstruction. Bowel sounds that occur once every minute or less frequently indicate a hypoactive bowel, which usually occurs after bowel surgery or when feces fill the colon.[2] Absent bowel sounds may be associated with peritonitis or paralytic ileus.

Edema of the abdominal wall can be detected when an imprint of the diaphragm remains after light auscultation. The nurse uses the bell of the stethoscope to listen for vascular sounds over the abdominal aorta and the renal and femoral arteries. Figure 39-3 illustrates auscultation sites of the abdomen for vascular sounds. If the nurse hears a bruit (a continuous purring, blowing, or humming sound), percussion and palpation are not performed. If a bruit is a new finding, the physician must be notified.

Table 39-4 describes abnormal abdominal sounds.

## Percussion

The nurse percusses the abdomen lightly in all four quadrants, listening for the location and distribution of tympany and dullness (Fig. 39-4A). The percussion may proceed clockwise or up and down over the abdomen (see Fig. 39-4B, C). The nurse percusses areas where the patient is not experiencing pain before examining painful areas.

Abdominal percussion helps identify air, gas, and fluid in the abdomen and helps determine the size and location of abdominal organs. The percussion sound depends on the density of the underlying structure. The sound is dull over solid organs (eg, liver), a stool-filled colon, abdominal masses, or pleural effusions. The sound is tympanic over air, such as in the gastric bubble or air-filled intestine.

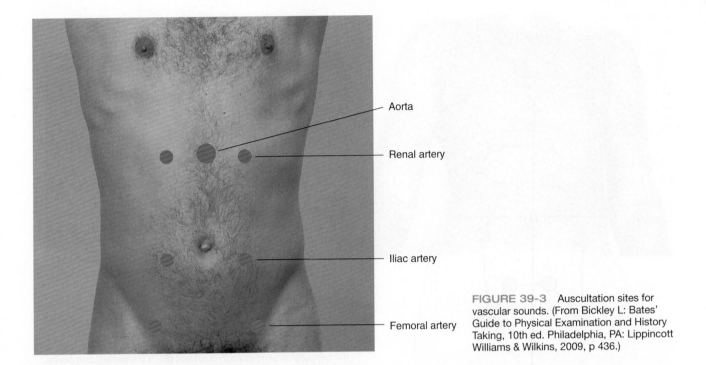

Aorta

Renal artery

Iliac artery

Femoral artery

**FIGURE 39-3** Auscultation sites for vascular sounds. (From Bickley L: Bates' Guide to Physical Examination and History Taking, 10th ed. Philadelphia, PA: Lippincott Williams & Wilkins, 2009, p 436.)

**TABLE 39-4** Abnormal Abdominal Sounds

| Description | Location | Possible Cause |
|---|---|---|
| **Bowel Sounds** | | |
| Hypoactive sounds unrelated to hunger | All four quadrants | Diarrhea or early intestinal obstruction |
| Hypoactive, then absent, sounds | All four quadrants | Paralytic ileus or peritonitis |
| High-pitched "tinkling" sounds | All four quadrants | Intestinal air and fluid under tension in a dilated bowel; early intestinal obstruction |
| High-pitched "rushing" sounds coinciding with an abdominal cramp | All four quadrants | Intestinal obstruction |
| Hyperactive sounds, long and prolonged (borborygmi) | All four quadrants | Hunger, gastroenteritis |
| Absence of sounds more than 5 min in all four quadrants | All four quadrants | Temporary loss of intestinal motility; occurs with ileus |
| **Systolic Bruits** | | |
| Vascular "blowing" sounds resembling cardiac murmurs | Abdominal aorta | Partial arterial obstruction or turbulent blood flow Dissecting abdominal aneurysm |
| | Renal artery | Renal artery stenosis |
| | Iliac artery | Hepatomegaly |
| **Venous Hum** | | |
| Continuous, medium-pitched tone created by blood flow in a large, engorged vascular organ such as the liver | Epigastric area and umbilicus | Increased collateral circulation between portal and systemic venous systems Hepatic cirrhosis |
| **Friction Rub** | | |
| Harsh, grating sound resembling two pieces of sandpaper rubbing together | Hepatic | Inflammation of the peritoneal surface of an organ Liver mass |

It may be necessary to postpone performing abdominal percussion on a critically ill patient, especially if there is abdominal guarding. Abdominal percussion or palpation is contraindicated in a patient with suspected appendicitis, abdominal aortic aneurysm, extensive abdominal surgery or trauma, polycystic kidneys or in a patient who has received an abdominal organ transplantation to prevent rupture of the organs or aorta.[2]

## Palpation

Abdominal palpation is necessary to establish the character of the abdominal wall, including the size, condition, and consistency of abdominal organs; the presence of abdominal masses; and the presence, location, and degree of abdominal pain. Abdominal palpation includes light and deep palpation. Contraindications to deep palpation are the same as those discussed for abdominal percussion.

Light palpation, which is performed first, identifies muscular resistance and areas of tenderness (Fig. 39-5). Fingertips are used to depress the abdominal wall 1 cm (0.5 inch). The nurse notes skin temperature, muscle resistance, tender areas, and masses. The femoral artery is subject to bilateral palpation. To ensure patient cooperation and relaxed muscles, the nurse always palpates a symptomatic area last.

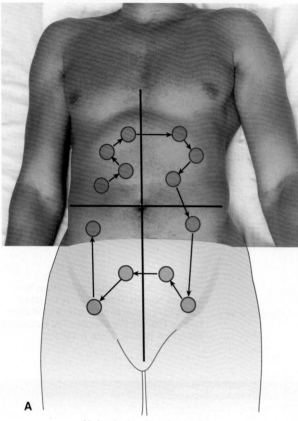

**A**

Abdominal percussion pattern

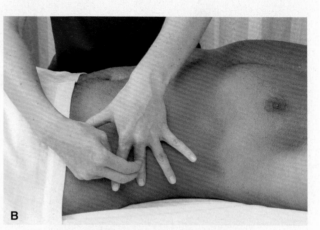

**B**

Abdominal percussion technique

**FIGURE 39-4** Percuss the abdomen systematically **(A)**, starting with the right upper quadrant and moving clockwise to the percussion sites in each quadrant **(B)**. If the patient complains of pain in a particular quadrant, adjust the percussion sequence to percuss that quadrant last. Remember when tapping to move your right finger away quickly so you do not inhibit vibrations. Abdominal percussion sequences may proceed clockwise **(B)** or up and down over the abdomen. (Adapted from Weber J, Kelley J: Health Assessment in Nursing, 5th ed. Philadelphia, PA: Wolters Kluwer Health, 2013, p 489.)

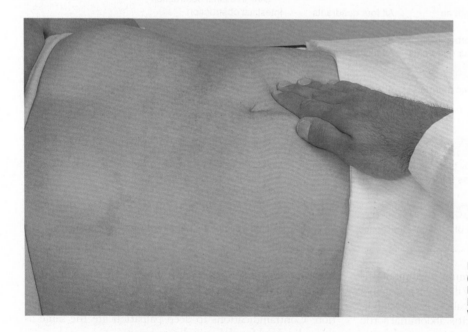

**FIGURE 39-5** Performing light palpation. (From Bickley L: Bates' Guide to Physical Examination and History Taking, 10th ed. Philadelphia, PA: Lippincott Williams & Wilkins, 2009, p 438.)

When disease is present, palpation may result in somatic or organ pain. Somatic pain is localized and reflects inflammation of the skin, fascia, or abdominal surfaces. Guarding of the abdominal muscles accompanies somatic pain. Organ pain is visceral in nature and is usually dull, diffuse, and generalized.

Deep palpation is used to locate abdominal organs (enlarged spleen, edge of the liver, pole of the right kidney; the left kidney is not usually palpable) and large masses (Fig. 39-6). The fingertips are used to depress the abdominal wall firmly to a depth of 7.5 cm (3 inches). The epigastric area is palpated for the pulse of the aorta (Fig. 39-7). If

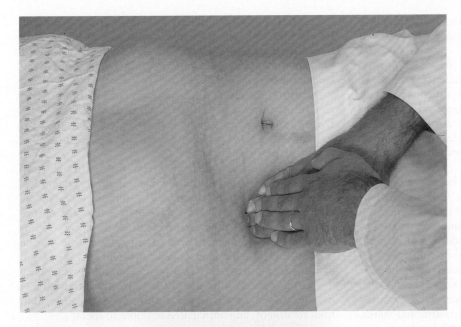

FIGURE 39-6    Two-handed deep palpation. (From Bickley L: Bates' Guide to Physical Examination and History Taking, 10th ed. Philadelphia, PA: Lippincott Williams & Wilkins, 2009, p 439.)

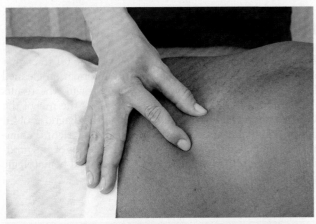

FIGURE 39-7    Palpating the aorta. (From Weber J, Kelley J: Health Assessment in Nursing, 5th ed. Philadelphia, PA: Wolters Kluwer Health, 2013, p 494.)

the nurse finds an area of tenderness with light palpation, it is necessary to check rebound tenderness by quickly withdrawing the fingertips after depression. Rebound tenderness usually indicates inflammation of the peritoneum from an abdominal process, such as organ inflammation, infection, abscess formation, or perforated bowel (release of bowel contents into the abdomen). If the nurse palpates a mass, he or she notes its location, size, shape, consistency, type of border, degree of tenderness, presence of pulsations, and degree of mobility (fixed or mobile).[2]

## Anus and Rectum

Assessment of the anus involves inspection and palpation. The skin around the anus is normally darker than the surrounding area. The nurse should inspect for inflammation, lesions, skin tags or warts, obvious fissures, and hemorrhoids. Alteration in elimination due to immobility, limited or no GI intake, opioids, or decreased intestinal peristalsis may result from a patient's disease or its treatment. Constipation may be a complication; if left untreated, it can lead to fecal

impaction or, in severe cases, bowel rupture.[2] Astute nursing assessment is critical in preventing and treating constipation or fecal impaction in any patient.

## Nutritional Assessment

Adequate nutrition of patients in the intensive care unit (ICU) improves outcomes, while malnutrition is strongly associated with increased morbidity and mortality rates among critically ill patients. GI complications are one of the main reasons why nutritional requirements for critically ill patients are not met. Nutritional support should be started in intensive care patients as early as possible. Enteral feeding should be prioritized, but it is often necessary to supplement this with parenteral feeding, as most intensive care patients are at risk of malnutrition.[7,8]

A critically ill patient's nutritional status may fall anywhere on a continuum ranging from overnutrition to malnutrition. The critical care patient may have an inadequate dietary intake because of illness or the disorder that caused the hospitalization, particularly if the disorder is GI. In addition, critically ill patients are at risk for GI problems from treatments that cause damage to the GI system and reduce the body's ability to absorb nutrients. Optimal nutrient intake provides adequate energy and can protect from complications of disease.[7]

The nurse plays an important role in evaluating the nutritional status of the patients under his or her care. Certain signs and symptoms that suggest possible nutritional deficiency are easy to note because they are specific. Conversely, fluid changes, such as edema or effusions, can mask protein and fat loss. The fact that nutritional disturbances can be subtle and are frequently nonspecific makes the need for assessment important.[8]

Nutritional assessment of the patient refers to a comprehensive evaluation of nutritional status, whereas nutritional screening is the process of identifying patients at risk for malnutrition or who are presently malnourished.[7] The detection of malnutrition in the ICU is critical to appropriately address its contribution to outcomes. Patients who are malnourished generally have longer hospitalizations and higher morbidity, mortality, and costs of care than those who are well nourished.[7]

Nurses caring for patients in the ICU are integral to the screening of patients for nutritional deficiencies or needs. Nurses assist with a formal nutritional assessment by providing information to nutrition support service and even completing screening tools for nutrition risk assessment. Serial weight measurement is perhaps the single most important indicator of nutritional status, and is the evaluation that the nurse performs most often.

An initial nutritional assessment may begin with cursory data, as dictated by the patient's condition. A registered dietitian or nutritionist or a nutritional support team may perform a more comprehensive nutritional assessment. The parameters of the nutritional assessment include anthropometric measurement, laboratory studies, physical examination, and dietary evaluation. Anthropometric measurements include height, weight, body mass index, triceps skinfold thickness, and mid-arm and arm muscle circumference.[2] Table 39-5 lists laboratory studies performed to evaluate nutritional status. Table 39-6 presents information about the physical examination and its interpretation in nutritional disorders.

The dietary evaluation may consist of a 24-hour recall to elicit all the foods and beverages consumed in the preceding 24 hours. However, this method may overestimate or underestimate a patient's usual caloric intake because the patient's recollection may not reflect long-term dietary habits. The nurse assesses the quantity and quality of food ingested by asking the patient to recall his or her normal daily intake pattern. This approach provides more information about intake patterns and tends to reflect long-term dietary habits with greater accuracy. It is also necessary to consider a patient's past or current patterns of food intake, or both, such as vegetarian or kosher dietary practices, as well as cultural background and social situation.[2] Special consideration of the geriatric patient is warranted; age-related changes in the GI system may affect dietary intake and maintenance of adequate nutrition (Box 39-2).

Nutrition screening tools are often borrowed from other care settings and have not been validated in ICU patients. Evidence supports treating patients who will be in the ICU for more than 2 days without normal oral intake as being at risk for malnutrition.[7]

The nutritional assessment directs the nutritional prescription and assists in the development of the interventions. Enteral or parenteral nutrition may be initiated if oral intake is prohibited. If the GI tract of the patient is functioning, enteral feeding is the intervention of choice. For people without a functioning GI tract, total parenteral nutrition may be the best nutritional option. (See Chapter 40 for a discussion of enteral and parenteral nutrition and refeeding syndrome.) The level of interventions is dictated by the patient's baseline nutritional state, disease status, risk for malnutrition from treatment, and anticipated response to therapy.[7]

## Laboratory Studies

Because the oral cavity is the only part of the GI tract that is visible, it is essential to combine the information gleaned from the history and physical examination with the results of laboratory and diagnostic studies to assess the rest of the GI tract. Many laboratory studies help in the diagnosis of GI and abdominal disorders in the critically ill patient. Parameters evaluated include serum electrolytes; levels of end products of metabolism, enzymes, and proteins; and hematologic parameters.

**TABLE 39-5** Laboratory Studies to Evaluate Nutritional Status

| Study | Normal Findings | Clinical and Nursing Significance |
|---|---|---|
| Hemoglobin | Males: 13–18 g/dL<br>Females: 12–16 g/dL | Main component of red blood cells (RBCs) used to transport oxygen; identifies iron-carrying capacity of the blood.<br>Helps identify anemia, protein deficiency, and excessive blood loss.<br>Elevated with dehydration, decreased in overhydration. |
| Hematocrit | Males: 40%–52%<br>Females: 36%–48% | Identifies volume of RBCs<br>Decreased value with overhydration, blood loss, poor dietary intake of iron, protein, certain vitamins |
| Albumin | 4.8 g/dL | Assesses protein levels in the body; requires functioning liver cells<br>Decreased with protein deficiency, blood loss secondary to burns, malnutrition, liver/renal disease, heart failure, major surgery, infections, cancer<br>Elevated with dehydration |
| Total protein | 6–8 g/dL | Decreased with overhydration, malnutrition, liver disease |
| Prealbumin | 15–30 mg/dL | Transport protein for thyroxine ($T_4$)<br>Short half-life makes it more sensitive than albumin to changes in protein stores<br>Decreased in malnutrition in critically ill or those with chronic disease |
| Transferrin | 200–400 mg/dL | Transport protein for iron; synthesized in the liver; shorter half-life than albumin; reflects current protein status; a more sensitive indicator of visceral protein stores<br>Elevated in pregnancy or iron deficiency<br>Decreased in acute or chronic infection, cirrhosis, renal disease, cancer |
| Total lymphocyte count | More than 2,000 mm³ | Indicator of immunocompetence<br>Mild immunocompromise: 1,200–2,000<br>Moderate immunocompromise: 800–1,199<br>Severe immunocompromise: <800<br>May indicate malnutrition when no other cause apparent; may point to infection, leukemia, or tissue necrosis |

**TABLE 39-6   Physical Assessment Interpretation in Nutritional Disorders**

| Body System or Region | Sign or Symptom | Implications |
|---|---|---|
| General | Weakness and fatigue | Anemia or electrolyte imbalance, decreased calorie intake, increased calorie use, or inadequate nutrient intake or absorption |
| | Weight loss | |
| Skin, hair, and nails | Dry, flaky skin | Vitamin A, vitamin B complex, or linoleic acid deficiency |
| | Dry skin with poor turgor | Dehydration |
| | Rough, scaly skin with bumps | Vitamin A deficiency |
| | Petechiae or ecchymoses | Vitamin C or K deficiency |
| | Sore that will not heal | Protein, vitamin C, or zinc deficiency |
| | Thinning, dry hair | Protein deficiency |
| | Spoon-shaped, brittle, or rigid nails | Iron deficiency |
| Eyes | Night blindness; corneal swelling, softening, or dryness; Bitot spots (gray triangular patches on the conjunctiva) | Vitamin A deficiency |
| | Red conjunctiva | Riboflavin deficiency |
| Throat and mouth | Cracks at the corner of mouth | Riboflavin or niacin deficiency |
| | Magenta tongue | Riboflavin deficiency |
| | Beefy, red tongue | Vitamin $B_{12}$ deficiency |
| | Soft, spongy, bleeding gums | Vitamin C deficiency |
| | Swollen neck (goiter) | Iodine deficiency |
| Cardiovascular | Edema | Protein deficiency |
| | Tachycardia, hypotension | Fluid volume deficit |
| GI | Ascites | Protein deficiency |
| Musculoskeletal | Bone pain and bow leg | Vitamin D or calcium deficiency |
| | Muscle wasting | Protein, carbohydrate, and fat deficiency |
| Neurologic | Altered mental status | Dehydration and thiamine or vitamin $B_{12}$ deficiency |
| | Paresthesia | Vitamin $B_{12}$, pyridoxine, or thiamine deficiency |

Adapted from Lee R, Neiman D: Nutritional Assessment, 5th ed. New York, NY: McGraw Hill, 2010.

**BOX 39-2   *CONSIDERATIONS for the Older Patient***

**Age-Related Changes of the GI System**

**Oral Cavity and Pharynx**
- Injury/loss or decay of teeth
- Atrophy of taste buds
- Decreased saliva production
- Reduced ptyalin and amylase in saliva

**Esophagus**
- Decreased motility and emptying
- Weakened gag reflex
- Decreased resting pressure of lower esophageal sphincter

**Stomach**
- Degeneration and atrophy of gastric mucosal surfaces with decreased production of HCl
- Decreased secretion of gastric acids and most digestive enzymes
- Decreased motility and emptying

**Small Intestine**
- Atrophy of muscle and mucosal surfaces
- Thinning of villi and epithelial cells

**Large Intestine**
- Decrease in mucous secretion
- Decrease in elasticity of rectal wall
- Decreased tone of internal anal sphincter
- Slower and duller nerve impulses in rectal area

Adapted from Smeltzer SC, Bare BG, Hinkle JL, et al (eds): Brunner & Suddarth's Textbook of Medical-Surgical Nursing, 13th ed. Philadelphia, PA: Lippincott Williams & Wilkins, 2014, p 1200.

## Liver Function Studies

The liver is responsible for many functions, the most significant being bile formation and secretion, protein and fat metabolism, detoxification of many substances, and the production of clotting factors and enzymes. Table 39-7 summarizes common laboratory studies relating to liver function.

A single laboratory test or single value from any laboratory test does not give an accurate assessment of an organ's function. A series of values from a laboratory study and combinations of studies provide a more precise picture. For example, if a patient's liver enzymes and bilirubin are elevated but the alkaline phosphatase (AP) level is normal, this usually indicates injury to the hepatocytes, such as in hepatitis and cirrhosis. If the liver enzymes are within normal range and the bilirubin and AP levels are elevated, this usually indicates an extrahepatic biliary obstruction, such as in a distal common bile duct obstruction from gallstones or pancreatic cancer.

## Pancreatic Function Studies

Table 39-8 lists serum laboratory tests that relate to pancreatic function. Amylase and lipase are digestive enzymes secreted by the pancreas. Serum amylase is found in the pancreas, parotid glands, intestine, liver, and fallopian tubes. Lipase is found primarily in the pancreas. In acute pancreatitis, serum amylase and lipase can be elevated four to six times the normal level, whereas in chronic pancreatitis, serum amylase

**TABLE 39-7** Laboratory Studies Used to Evaluate Liver Function

| Study | Normal Findings | Clinical and Nursing Significance |
|---|---|---|
| **Bile Formation and Secretion** | | |
| Serum bilirubin | | |
| Direct (conjugated)—soluble in water | <6.8 µmol/L | Elevated in biliary and liver disease; causes clinical jaundice |
| Indirect (unconjugated)—insoluble in water | 0–14 µmol/L | Abnormal in hemolysis and in functional disorders of uptake or conjugation |
| Urine bilirubin | 0 | Urine is mahogany in color; shaking the specimen results in a light-yellow foam; confirmed with Ictotest tablet or dipstick; false-positive results possible if patient is taking phenazopyridine (Pyridium). |
| Urobilinogen | <17 µmol/L | Increased in cirrhosis, biliary obstruction with biliary tract infection, hemorrhage, and hepatotoxicity; decreased in biliary obstruction without biliary tract infection, hepatocellular damage, and renal insufficiency |
| **Protein Studies** | | |
| Albumin | 35–55 g/L | Decreased in cirrhosis, chronic hepatitis |
| Globulin | 15–30 g/L | Increased in cirrhosis, chronic obstructive jaundice, viral hepatitis |
| Total serum protein | 64–83 g/L | Individual protein measurements are of greater significance than total protein measurements. |
| Transferrin | 220–400 mcg/dL | Decreased in cirrhosis, hepatitis, and malignancy; increased in severe iron deficiency anemia |
| Prothrombin time (PT) or International normalized ratio (INR) | 11.0–14.0 s 0.8–1.2 | Prolonged PT in liver disease will not return to normal with vitamin K administration, whereas prolonged PT resulting from malabsorption of fat and fat-soluble vitamins will return to normal with vitamin K administration. |
| Partial thromboplastin time PTT | 25.0–36.0 s | Increased with severe liver disease or therapy with heparin or other anticoagulants |
| Alpha-fetoprotein (AFP) | 6–20 ng/mL | Elevated in primary hepatocellular carcinoma |
| **Fat Metabolism** | | |
| Cholesterol | <200 mg/dL (adults) | Decreased in parenchymal liver disease; increased in biliary obstruction |
| High-density lipoprotein (HDL) | | |
| Men | 35–70 mg/dL | |
| Women | 35–85 mg/dL | |
| Low-density lipoprotein (LDL) | <130 mg/dL | |
| Very-low-density lipoprotein (VLDL) | 2–30 mg/dL | |
| **Liver Detoxification** | | |
| Serum alkaline phosphatase (AP) | 20–90 units/L at 30°C | Level is elevated to more than three times the normal in obstructive jaundice, intrahepatic cholestasis, liver metastasis, or granulomas; also elevated in osteoblastic diseases, Paget disease, and hyperparathyroidism |
| Ammonia | 15–56 mcg/dL | An elevation indicates hepatocyte damage (liver converts ammonia to urea) |
| **Enzyme Production** | | |
| Aspartate aminotransferase (AST) | 10–34 units/L | Any elevation indicates hepatocyte damage. |
| Alanine aminotransferase (ALT) | 7–56 units/L | Any elevation indicates hepatocyte damage. |
| Lactate dehydrogenase (LDH) | 140–280 units/L | Any elevation indicates hepatocyte damage. |
| γ-Glutamyl transferase (GGT) | 0–30 units/L at 30°C | An elevation in GGT along with an elevated AP usually indicates biliary disease; helpful in the diagnosis of chronic liver disease |

and lipase levels may be normal or very low because the pancreas may no longer be producing the enzymes.

The pancreas produces insulin and glucagon, hormones that aid in the regulation of serum glucose levels. A disruption in normal pancreatic function or the presence of a tumor may alter the production of these hormones. Frequent blood glucose monitoring is warranted in this situation. Any elevation in the serum and urine glucose levels has a cascading effect on multiple body systems, which in turn affects the patient's overall condition.[9]

## Other Laboratory Studies

Table 39-9 provides information about other selected laboratory studies that are used in the evaluation of GI disorders.

## Diagnostic Studies

The nurse caring for the critically ill patient coordinates the preparation for, and possibly the timing of, many diagnostic

**TABLE 39-8**  Laboratory Studies Used to Evaluate Pancreatic Function

| Study | Normal Findings | Clinical and Nursing Significance |
| --- | --- | --- |
| Serum amylase | 25–125 units/L | In acute pancreatitis, the serum levels peak between 4 and 8 h after onset of condition, then fall to normal within 48–72 h; low levels usually indicate pancreatic insufficiency. |
| Urine amylase | 1–7 units/h | Urine values 6–10 h behind serum values; low levels indicate pancreatic insufficiency. |
| Serum lipase | <160 units/L | Elevated only in pancreatitis, markedly in acute pancreatitis and pancreatic duct obstruction; remains elevated after amylase returns to baseline. |
| Serum glucose | 65–110 mg/dL (fasting) | Patient must fast for 12 h before specimen is obtained. |
| Serum triglycerides | <200 mg/dL | Patient must fast for 12 h before specimen is obtained; levels increased in alcoholic cirrhosis, diabetes mellitus (untreated), high-carbohydrate diet, hyperlipoproteinemia, and hypertension; levels decreased in malnutrition, vigorous exercise |
| Serum calcium | | |
| Total | 8.2–10.2 mg/dL | High total calcium levels seen in cancer of the liver, pancreas, and other organs |
| Ionized | 4.65–5.28 mg/dL | Useful in tracking the course of disorders, such as cancer and acute pancreatitis |
| Fecal fat | <7 g/24 h | Content of >6 g/24 h is suggestive of a decrease in the body's ability to absorb foods; indicative of pancreatic exocrine insufficiency as in chronic pancreatitis |

**TABLE 39-9**  Other Selected Laboratory Studies Used in the Diagnosis of GI Disorders

| Study | Normal Findings | Clinical and Nursing Significance |
| --- | --- | --- |
| **Stool Specimen** | | |
| Occult blood | None | Positive test indicates bleeding within GI tract with causes such as hemorrhoids, ulcers, or malignancy. |
| Fat | <7 g/24 h | Screening test for steatorrhea when malabsorption syndrome or pancreatic insufficiency is suspected |
| Ova and parasites | None | Positive test suggests infection. |
| Pus | None | Increased amount of pus may indicate ulcerative colitis, abscess, or anal or rectal fissure. |
| Pathogens | None | Common pathogens are *Salmonella typhi* (typhoid fever), *Shigella* (dysentery), *Vibrio cholerae* (cholera), *Yersinia* (enterocolitis), *Escherichia coli* and *Aeromonas* (gastroenteritis), *Staphylococcus aureus*, *Clostridium botulinum*, and *Clostridium perfringens* (food poisoning). |
| Urea breath test | Negative | Detects the presence of *Helicobacter pylori* |
| Hydrogen breath test | Negative | Determines the amount of hydrogen expelled in the breath after it is produced in the colon and absorbed into the blood; aids in the diagnosis of bacterial overgrowth in the intestine and short bowel syndrome |

tests. The nurse prepares the patient and family members for the test by providing a thorough explanation of how the test is performed and what information the test is expected to yield. In addition, the nurse explains the need for informed consent to perform the test, and answers any questions the patient or family members may have about the test. Table 39-10 summarizes the diagnostic studies for evaluating the GI tract, which can be divided into two categories, noninvasive and invasive.

## Radiologic and Imaging Studies

Body tissue has different densities that produce different shades of black and white on an x-ray. Bone tissue is high in density and appears white; air appears black; and soft tissue appears in shades of gray. The stomach and intestines usually contain some air and appear darker. Solid organs, such as the pancreas, spleen, kidneys, or liver, appear grayer.[10]

## Endoscopic Studies

The use of an endoscope is an important adjunct to radiographic studies because it allows direct observation of portions of the intestinal tract. A flexible fiberoptic endoscope is an instrument with a light and a lens at the end of a movable tip that can be manipulated through the intestinal tract by the operator. It also includes an instrument channel that allows for biopsy of lesions, such as tumors, ulcers, or areas of inflammation. Fluids can be aspirated from the lumen of the intestinal tract, and air can be insufflated to distend the intestinal tract for better observation. Cytology brushes and electrocautery snares can be passed through the scope. Special studies of the common bile duct and the pancreatic duct by endoscopic retrograde cholangiopancreatography use a side-viewing upper intestinal endoscope. Endoscopic ultrasonography with fine-needle aspiration is another procedure that uses an endoscope, in this case with an ultrasound probe and a biopsy needle at the end. The endoscope is inserted through an orifice, and the ultrasound probe is used to bounce high-energy sound waves off internal organs and tissues, which creates a picture on a monitor. This allows the operator to place the needle to obtain cells from a mass or lymph nodes for biopsy.[10]

Table 39-11 describes endoscopic procedures used to evaluate the GI tract.

## Other Diagnostic Studies

In addition to radiologic and imaging studies and endoscopic procedures, other studies are specifically designed to aid in the diagnosis of GI disorders. Table 39-12 provides information about other selected diagnostic studies used to diagnose specific GI disorders.

**TABLE 39-10** Diagnostic Studies Used to Evaluate the GI Tract

| Study | Description | Indications |
|---|---|---|
| Abdominal film "flat plate of the abdomen, KUB" | Noninvasive<br>Radiology test used to visualize a single flat plane; shows organ size, position, intactness, and normal gas patterns in the stomach, small intestine, and colon | Aids in diagnosis of intestinal obstruction, organ rupture, masses, foreign bodies, abnormal fluid, or air, ("stones, bones, gas, masses") |
| Upper GI studies (barium swallow) | Noninvasive<br>Preparation: NPO<br>With oral contrast<br>Radiology test used to visualize the esophagus, stomach, and duodenum; barium enhances image; double-contrast study administers barium first followed by a radiolucent substance, such as air, to help coat bowel mucosa for better visualization of any type of lesion | Aids in diagnosis of hiatal hernia, ulcers, tumors, foreign bodies, bowel obstruction |
| Upper GI series with small bowel follow-through | Noninvasive<br>Preparation: NPO<br>With oral contrast<br>Radiology test used to visualize the jejunum, ileum, and cecum. | Aids in the diagnosis of tumors, Crohn disease, Meckel diverticulum. |
| Enteroclysis | Invasive<br>With contrast<br>Preparation: NPO<br>Radiology test used to visualize entire small intestine; continuous infusion (through a duodenal tube) of air in a barium sulfate suspension along with methylcellulose fills the intestinal loops. The time it takes the contrast to move through the jejunum and ileum is timed and recorded. | Aids in diagnosis of partial bowel obstruction or diverticula. |
| Barium enema | Noninvasive<br>Preparation: Bowel prep prior to procedure; NPO/clear liquids<br>Radiology test used to visualize the colon; barium enhances image; air may be introduced after the barium to provide a double-contrast study. | Aids in diagnosis of polyps, tumors, fistulas, obstruction, diverticula, and stenosis |
| Gastric lavage | Invasive<br>Without contrast<br>Aspirations of stomach contents and washing out of the stomach by a large gastric tube | Aids in diagnosis of upper GI bleeding<br>Used to arrest hemorrhage and prepare for further tests. |
| Paracentesis | Invasive<br>Without contrast<br>Aspiration of peritoneal fluid | Laboratory studies amylase and lipase<br>Cytologic studies to detect tumors<br>Comfort measure to alleviate accumulations of ascetic fluid |
| Fast exam: Focused Assessment with Sonography in Trauma | Noninvasive<br>Ultrasound waves used to detect "free fluid" or what is most often blood in the abdominal cavity; now being used also to detect fluid in the chest cavity | Becoming the gold standard for a quick noninvasive assessment for hypotensive trauma patients<br>Most often used in the Emergency Department |
| Ultrasonography (sonogram) | Noninvasive<br>Without contrast<br>Preparation: NPO/clear liquids<br>Use of high-frequency sound waves over an abdominal organ to obtain an image of the structure | Aids in diagnosis of masses, dilated bile ducts, gallstones, and ascites<br>Gastroparesis |
| Hepatobiliary scan | Noninvasive<br>With contrast<br>Preparation: NPO<br>Intravenously injected radioisotope is primarily taken up by the liver and then secreted into the bile, allowing visualization of the biliary system, gallbladder, and duodenum (size, function, vascularity, and blood flow). | Aids in the diagnosis of GI bleeding |

**TABLE 39-10** Diagnostic Studies Used to Evaluate the GI Tract (*continued*)

| Study | Description | Indications |
|---|---|---|
| Tagged red blood cell scan (technetium-labeled red blood cell scintigraphy) | Noninvasive<br>Preparation: None<br>With contrast<br>Red blood cells are labeled with technetium and injected intravenously; images are obtained with a gamma camera that can identify areas of increased radioactivity as a site of slow or intermittent GI hemorrhage. | Aids in the diagnosis of GI bleeding |
| Computed tomography (CT scan) | Noninvasive<br>Preparation: NPO<br>With and without contrast<br>A radiologic procedure that uses narrow x-ray beams to produce cross-sectional images of organs and tissues. Three-dimensional imaging. | Visualizing the abdomen, retroperitoneal structures, tumors, cysts, or collections of fluid, air in a cavity, bleeding, or pulmonary embolism |
| Magnetic resonance imaging (MRI) | Noninvasive<br>With or without contrast<br>Preparation: No metal in patient for safety purposes. Preprocedure checklist must be completed.<br>Uses radiofrequency waves emitted from a powerful electromagnetic field to obtain tissue level deep scans | Useful in evaluating abdominal soft tissue and blood vessels, abscesses, fistulas, tumors, and sources of bleeding |
| Magnetic resonance cholangiopancreatography (MRCP) | Noninvasive<br>Without contrast<br>Preparation: No metal in patient for safety purposes. Preprocedure checklist must be completed.<br>Similar to MRI; ideal for patient with allergies to contrast | Aids in the diagnosis of disorders affecting the pancreatic ducts and biliary tree |
| Percutaneous transhepatic cholangiography (PTC) | Invasive<br>With contrast<br>Preparation: NPO<br>Uses fluoroscopy; the intrahepatic and extrahepatic biliary ducts are injected with contrast medium into biliary tree using a percutaneous needle injection. | Helps to distinguish obstructive jaundice caused by liver disease from jaundice caused by biliary obstruction (eg, from a tumor, common bile duct injury, stones within the bile ducts, or sclerosing cholangitis) |
| Percutaneous transhepatic biliary drainage (PTBD) | Invasive<br>With contrast<br>Preparation: NPO<br>A biliary catheter is placed during a PTC; the biliary catheter may be placed to the obstruction or it may bypass the obstruction to allow the free flow of bile; catheter relieves jaundice and pruritus, improves nutritional status, allows easy access into the biliary tree for further procedures, and can be used as an anatomical landmark and stent at the time of surgery. | Biliary obstruction resulting in jaundice, cholangitis, sepsis, or pain |
| Positron emission tomography (PET) | Noninvasive<br>With contrast<br>A computerized radiographic technique that uses radioactive substances to examine the metabolic activity of body structures. A PET scan can be combined with a CT scan so images can be acquired from both devices and can be taken sequentially at the same time for superimposed images. | Useful for precisely locating a tumor. Provides metabolic activity revealed by the PET scan along with the anatomic information provided by the CT scan. |
| Angiography | Invasive<br>With contrast<br>Preparation: NPO<br>Study of selected arteries and veins to see defects in the walls of the vessels; also used to evaluate blood flow through the vessels. | Usually done when initial, noninvasive procedures are insufficient in revealing the cause of a suspected vascular defect |

**TABLE 39-11 Endoscopic Studies Used to Evaluate the GI Tract**

| Study | Description | Indications |
|---|---|---|
| Esophagogastroduodenoscopy (EGD) | Invasive<br>Without contrast<br>Preparation: NPO<br>Endoscope passed through the mouth and advanced to visualize the esophagus, stomach, and duodenum; any abnormalities can be photographed and biopsied, bleeding areas may be cauterized, and varices may be injected with sclerosing agents. | Helps to diagnose acute or chronic upper GI bleeding, esophageal or gastric varices, polyps, tumors, ulcers, esophagitis, gastritis, esophageal stenosis, and gastroesophageal reflux |
| Colonoscopy | Invasive<br>Without contrast<br>Preparation: Bowel cleansing<br>A flexible fiberoptic endoscope is passed through the rectum and advanced into the large intestine for visualization of any abnormalities. These are photographed and biopsied; polyps can be removed and bleeding areas can be cauterized. | Helps to diagnose bleeding, diverticulosis, polyps, stricture, tumor, or inflammatory bowel disease (eg, Crohn disease or ulcerative colitis) |
| Proctoscopy (anoscopy) | Invasive<br>Without contrast<br>Rigid scope is passed through the rectum to visualize the mucosal surface of the anus and rectum. | Helps to diagnose polyps, bleeding, tumors, and other defects |
| Sigmoidoscopy | Invasive<br>Without contrast<br>Preparation: Enema<br>Flexible fiberoptic endoscope is passed through the rectum and advanced to visualize the rectum, sigmoid colon, and proximal colon; any lesions can be biopsied. | Helps to diagnose polyps, bleeding, tumors, and other defects |
| Endoscopic retrograde cholangiopancreatography (ERCP) | Invasive<br>With contrast<br>Preparation: NPO<br>Flexible fiberoptic endoscope is inserted into the esophagus, passed through the stomach and into the duodenum to visualize the common bile duct, hepatic bile ducts, and pancreatic ducts. The common bile duct and pancreatic duct are cannulated, and contrast medium is injected into the ducts, permitting visualization and radiographic evaluation. | Can detect extrahepatic biliary obstruction (eg, from stones, tumors of the bile duct, strictures or injuries to the bile duct), intrahepatic biliary obstruction caused by stones or tumor, and pancreatic disease, such as chronic pancreatitis, pseudocysts, and tumors |
| Endoscopic ultrasonography | Invasive<br>Without contrast<br>Preparation: NPO<br>Using endoscopy and ultrasonography, the GI tract is visualized. An ultrasonic transducer built into the distal end of the endoscope allows for high-quality resolution of the walls of the GI tract. | Useful in evaluating and staging tumors of the GI tract. |

**TABLE 39-12 Other Selected Diagnostic Studies Used in Diagnosing GI Disorders**

| Study | Description | Normal Findings |
|---|---|---|
| Gastric emptying studies | Liquid and solid components of a meal are tagged with a radionuclide marker. After ingesting the meal, the rate of passage of the radioactive substance out of the stomach is measured by a scintiscanner. Useful in diagnosing gastric motility disorders. | Normal transit |
| Gastric analysis | Analysis of gastric juice yields information about the secretory activity of the gastric mucosa and the presence or degree of gastric retention, which is useful to help diagnose patients with pyloric or duodenal obstruction. | Normal contents |
| Gastric acid stimulation | Usually performed in conjunction with gastric analysis. Histamine or pentagastrin is given subcutaneously to stimulate gastric secretions. Gastric specimens are collected at intervals for analysis. Helps to determine the presence or absence of malignant cells. | 11–20 mEq/h after stimulation |

**TABLE 39-12** Other Selected Diagnostic Studies Used in Diagnosing GI Disorders (*continued*)

| Study | Description | Normal Findings |
|---|---|---|
| Manometry | Measurement of pressures using a water-filled catheter connected to a transducer passed into the esophagus, stomach, colon, or rectum to evaluate contractility; useful in detecting motility disorders of the esophagus and lower esophageal sphincter; gastroduodenal, small intestine, and colonic manometry are used to evaluate delayed gastric emptying and gastric and intestinal motility disorders such as irritable bowel syndrome or atonic colon; anorectal manometry measures the resting tone of the internal anal sphincter and the contractility of the external anal sphincter, which are helpful in evaluation of chronic constipation or fecal incontinence. | Values differ at various levels of the intestine |
| Gastric tonometry | Monitoring modality used to determine the perfusion status of the gastric mucosa using measurements of local $PCO_2$. The $CO_2$ diffuses from the mucosa of the stomach into the lumen of the stomach and then into the silicone balloon of the tonometer. The $PCO_2$ within the balloon serves as a proxy measure for gastric mucosal $CO_2$ ($PgCO_2$). In a normally perfused gastric mucosa, $PgCO_2$ is nearly equivalent to the $PaCO_2$. With hypoperfusion, the $PgCO_2$ increases and the gap between the $PgCO_2$ and the $PaCO_2$ increases. The gap is a very sensitive indicator of gastric hypoperfusion. | The $PgCO_2$ and the $PaCO_2$ are nearly equal. |

# Clinical Applicability Challenges

## CASE STUDY

Mr. W. was seen in the GI Clinic earlier today for increased abdominal girth. He is now being admitted to the ICU for hypotension (BP 98/62, HR 110). Mr. W.'s vital signs are stable at BP 102/64, HR 106, RR 18, SpO$_2$ 96% of room air, and pain 3/10 in the abdomen. He is alert and cooperative. You notice during your assessment of Mr. W. that his abdomen is distended, taut, and tender to light palpation in all four quadrants. All bowel sounds are muffled. His skin has a slight yellow pallor.

Mr. W.'s serum lab values are hemoglobin 7.2, hematocrit 21.5, and albumin 3.1. Comprehensive metabolic panel and coagulation test results are bilirubin 9, ammonia 68, AST 45, ALT 67, and PTT 45. Mr. W. has a new order for an abdominal CT scan with contrast.

Your initial assessment and vital signs are complete, and Mr. W. is now attached to monitors.

1. What questions would you ask Mr. W. about his GI system?
2. What about your patient's appearance would cause you concern in relation to his GI health?
3. What are your priorities in caring for Mr. W.? What are your concerns?

## WANT TO KNOW MORE?

A wide variety of resources to enhance your learning and understanding of this chapter are available thePoint.

You will find:

- References
- Selected readings
- NCLEX-style review questions
- Internet resources
- And more!

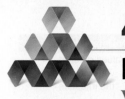

# 40

# Patient Management: Gastrointestinal System

VALERIE K. SABOL AND ALLISON STEELE YORK

## LEARNING OBJECTIVES

### Based on the content in this chapter, the reader should be able to:

1. Explain how the physiologic stressors of illness and injury alter the body's needs for energy.
2. Describe the different forms of malnutrition.
3. Discuss enteral and parenteral nutrition with regard to indications, assessment, management, and complications.
4. Discuss common medications used for patients with gastrointestinal disorders.

Health and nutrition have a symbiotic relationship. Physiologic stressors, such as illness and injury, alter the body's metabolic and energy demands. Although early identification and nutritional intervention can lessen morbidity and mortality risks in critically ill patients, the underlying disease process must be identified and corrected before the body can reverse abnormal nutrient metabolism. This chapter presents an overview of physiologic stress and its effect on metabolism, types of malnutrition, and the indications, assessment, and management of enteral and parenteral nutrition support therapies and the complications associated with these therapies.

## Malnutrition

According to the laws of thermodynamics, energy can be neither created nor destroyed. Through the processes of metabolism, people obtain energy from the foods (or organic fuels) they consume. Metabolism has two parts: anabolism and catabolism. Anabolism is a building-up and repair process that requires energy. Catabolism consists of breaking down food and body tissues to liberate energy.

Glucose is the obligatory fuel of the body, and it is the primary fuel of the brain and nervous system in particular. The nervous system cannot store or synthesize glucose as a fuel source, so it relies on glucose extraction from the bloodstream. The liver regulates glucose entry into the circulatory system because it has the ability to both store and synthesize glucose. Excess glucose is converted and stored as either glycogen or fatty acids (triglycerides). Although glucose can be converted to fatty acids for storage, there is no pathway for the conversion of fatty acids back into glucose. Instead, fatty acids are used directly as a fuel source or are converted to ketones by the liver. After prolonged starvation, the body adapts to preserve vital proteins by using ketones, rather than glucose, as energy. Ketoacidosis occurs when ketone production exceeds utilization.

The pancreatic hormones glucagon and insulin have opposing functions in metabolic processes. Glucagon stimulates glycogenolysis (glycogen breakdown) and gluconeogenesis (glucose synthesis from other sources such as proteins) and increases lipolysis (fat breakdown and mobilization). Insulin,

in contrast, helps transport glucose for storage into the cells and tissues, prevents fat breakdown, and increases protein synthesis.

Glycogenolysis is controlled by the hormone glucagon and the catecholamines epinephrine and norepinephrine, which are released from the adrenal medulla in times of stress. Once glucose and glycogen stores have been exhausted (usually within 8 to 12 hours), hepatic gluconeogenesis increases dramatically to meet metabolic demands. Hormones that stimulate gluconeogenesis include glucagon and the glucocorticoid hormone cortisol. If catabolic processes continue without the support of energy, amino acids, and essential nutrients, depletion of existing body stores compromises overall bodily health and function, and without intervention, malnutrition may develop.

The metabolic response to stress is characterized by increased release of cytokines (interleukin-1, interleukin-6, and tumor necrosis factor-$\alpha$) and increased production of counterregulatory hormones (catecholamines, cortisol, glucagon, and growth hormone).[1] These counterregulatory hormones induce catabolism and oppose the anabolic effects of insulin. This results in hypermetabolism and hypercatabolism with loss of body energy stores through proteolysis, lipolysis, and glycogenolysis. Critical illness is typically associated with catabolic stress in which patients commonly demonstrate a systemic inflammatory response.

Approximately one-third to one-half of hospitalized patients have evidence of malnutrition.[2,3] Review of data from the Healthcare Cost and Utilization Project showed that 3.2% of hospitalized patients in 2010 had a documented diagnosis of malnutrition.[4] Forty percent of patients experience considerable weight loss (more than 10 kg) during and after a stay in the intensive care unit (ICU).[5] This unintentional weight loss may deplete vital nutrient reserves, which may predispose the patient to malnutrition. Malnutrition is associated with increased morbidity and mortality, delayed wound healing, increased length of hospitalization, increased complications, immunosuppression, and organ impairment.[2,4] Malnutrition from starvation alone can usually be corrected by replacing body stores of essential nutrients. However, malnutrition resulting from critical illness and disease processes that alter metabolism is not as easily rectified.

The degree of starvation and physiologic stress determines the extent and type of malnutrition. The three major types of protein–energy malnutrition are marasmus, kwashiorkor, and protein–calorie malnutrition. Marasmus is a severe, cachectic process, whereby virtually all of the available fat stores have been exhausted from prolonged calorie deficiency. Severe muscle wasting is evident in marasmus; however, serum albumin levels may be within normal limits or only slightly reduced. Treatment requires nutrition and fluid volume replacement at slow rates to prevent the complications associated with sudden fluid shifts, electrolyte abnormalities, and cardiorespiratory failure.

In contrast to the adaptive response of relative protein sparing in marasmus, kwashiorkor and protein–calorie malnutrition are typically caused by an acute, life-threatening condition, such as surgery, trauma, or sepsis. Kwashiorkor is usually seen in children in developing countries who have had prolonged periods of protein malnutrition. Protein–calorie malnutrition is more commonly seen in developed countries and is due to depletion of fat, muscle wasting, and micronutrient deficiencies from acute and chronic illness. Typically, during periods of critical illness when the patient is relegated to NPO status (*nil per os*, nothing by mouth) for surgery, diagnostic testing, or a number of other medical complications, hypermetabolism and catabolism increase protein and energy demands. Although the critically ill patient may appear nourished, often this is due to the masking effects of generalized edema—the result of extracellular fluid shifts caused by low-protein oncotic pressures in the intravascular space. Other than edema, clinical signs of protein malnutrition include skin breakdown, poor wound healing, surgical dehiscence, or a combination of the three. Additionally, hair can easily be plucked, and hair remnants are often noted on the patient's pillowcase and sheets. Laboratory data reveal low serum albumin levels, and treatment requires aggressive repletion of protein stores. The fact that protein malnutrition is much easier to prevent than to treat reinforces the need for intense nursing vigilance over the patient's nutritional status.

Marasmus and kwashiorkor can coexist. Typically, this is seen when a patient with marasmus is exposed to an acute stressor such as surgery, trauma, or sepsis. Although each situation must be evaluated individually, aggressive protein and calorie replacement is often indicated. Regardless of the type (or types) of malnutrition, vigilant monitoring is crucial to the success of nutrition therapy.

## Nutritional Support

A nutritional assessment should be completed on all critically ill or injured patients early in their hospitalization to determine the need for nutritional support therapy. The Joint Commission requires nutrition screening within 24 hours of admission to an acute care facility. The timing of nutritional support therapy is based on evaluation of the preexisting nutritional status, the presence and extent of systemic response to inflammation, and the anticipated clinical course.[6,7] Nutritional support therapy delivered within 24 to 48 hours of admission, once patients are hemodynamically stable, is advocated.[7–9] Goals of care in nutritional support include the following: preventing and treating macronutrient and micronutrient deficiencies, maintaining fluid and electrolyte balance, maintaining immune function, preventing infection, and other complications associated with nutritional therapy, and improving patient morbidity and mortality. Meeting these goals involves a multidisciplinary approach that includes the nurse, physician, dietitian, and pharmacist. After a dietitian determines nutritional needs, a method of delivering nutritional supplementation must be selected. In patients unable to meet their nutritional needs with oral intake, nutritional supplementation may be delivered by enteral or parenteral routes. Figure 40-1 outlines the decision-making process. Considerations for elderly patients are given in Box 40-1.

## Enteral Nutrition and Delivery

Enteral nutrition refers to any form of nutrition delivered to the gastrointestinal (GI) tract. For those patients with an intact GI tract, the enteral route is the preferred method of nutritional support. A clinical rule of thumb is, "If the gut works, use it."

The GI mucosa depends on nutrient delivery and adequate blood flow to prevent atrophy, thereby maintaining the absorptive, barrier, and immunologic functions of the intestine. Enterocytes are tightly packed epithelial cells that line the intestinal lumen and function as a barrier to bacterial invasion. Gut-associated lymphoid tissue (GALT) lines the GI tract and is associated with maintenance of the immunologic function of the mucosa. GALT produces immunoglobulin A (IgA), which is secreted across the GI mucosa in response to eating. IgA coats the luminal bacteria, preventing bacterial adherence to the enterocytes. Without food, the GI mucosa atrophies, and motility is impaired. In the event of atrophy, the tissue available to absorb nutrients decreases and GALT is impaired. Preservation of the intestinal mucosal integrity is also essential to preserve its function as a barrier. With atrophy, there is a loss of the tight junctions between enterocytes, resulting in increased mucosal permeability and decreased barrier function. This decreased barrier function can allow resident GI bacteria and endotoxins to enter the systemic circulation. This process, called bacterial translocation, can trigger immune and inflammatory responses that can lead to infection, sepsis, and multisystem organ failure. In addition to its trophic effects on the GI tract, enteral nutrition is associated with enhanced utilization of nutrients, decreased infectious complications, ease and safety of delivery, and lower cost.

Enteral nutrition is considered when the patient cannot or should not eat, intake is insufficient or unreliable, the patient has a functional GI tract, and access can be safely achieved. Mechanical obstruction is the only absolute contraindication to enteral feedings. In the setting of hemodynamic compromise (ie, the patient requires significant hemodynamic support including high-dose catecholamine agents, alone or in combination with large-volume fluid or blood product administration to maintain cellular perfusion), enteral nutrition should be withheld until the patient is fully resuscitated and/or stable.[7] Accordingly, each patient situation should be evaluated individually.

Enteral nutrition can be delivered through feeding tubes placed into the stomach or the small intestine. The expected duration of nutritional support, patient's overall condition,

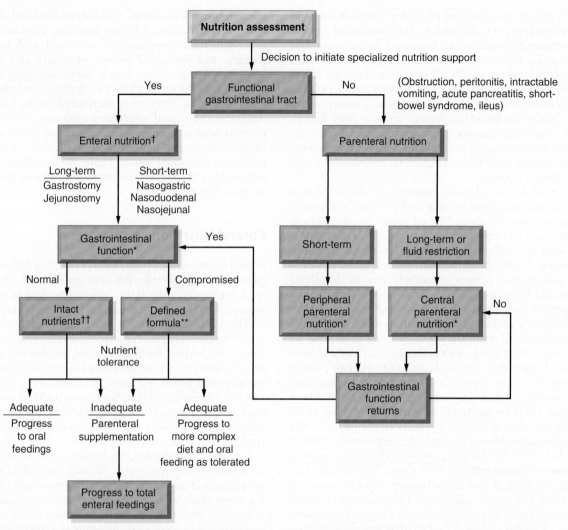

*Formulation of enteral and parenteral solutions should be made considering organ function (eg, cardiac, renal, respiratory, hepatic). **Elemental low-/high-fat content, lactose-free, fiber-rich, and modular formulas should be provided according to the patient's gastrointestinal tolerance. †Feeding may be more appropriate distal to the pylorus if the patient is at increased aspiration risk. ††Polymeric, complete formulas, or pureed diets are appropriate.

**FIGURE 40-1** Decision-making process for route of administration of specialized nutrition support. (Adapted from ASPEN Clinical Pathways and Algorithms for Delivery of Parenteral and Enteral Nutrition Support in Adults. Jacobs D (ed): Section II: Nutrition care process. J Parenter Enteral Nutr 26(1 Suppl):85A, 2002.)

risk for aspiration, function of the GI tract, and placement technique should all be considered when deciding on which type of feeding tube to place. For most patient populations, nasoenteric tubes are widely used.

## Nasoenteral Feeding and Feeding Tubes

A nasoenteric tube is indicated for short-term use in hospitalized patients, usually less than 4 to 6 weeks. Nasoenteral tubes are inserted through the nose and advanced through the esophagus into the stomach (nasogastric tube), duodenum (nasoduodenal tube), or jejunum (nasojejunal tube). The tube is identified by the distal location of its tip. Most nasoenteric tubes are soft, flexible, small-bore polyurethane or silicone tubes that are 8 to 14 French in diameter and 20 to 60 inches in length, have markers to aid measurement, and are radiopaque to allow for radiographic confirmation of placement. The shorter lengths are used for nasogastric feedings, and the longer

for nasoduodenal or nasojejunal feedings. As a general rule, the smallest-diameter tube of appropriate length is preferred because the smaller diameter has been associated with fewer complications and increased patient comfort. Small-diameter tubes may help prevent reflux and lessen the risk for aspiration because the small diameter reduces compromise of the lower esophageal sphincter. See Evidence-Based Practice Highlight 40-1 for information about the prevention of aspiration. In addition, small-diameter tubes cause less inhibition of swallowing, which is more comfortable for patients. Tubes made of polyvinyl chloride are less desirable because, over time, they can stiffen in the presence of acid, which can lead to patient discomfort and increased complications, such as tube perforation. Any nasally placed tube can cause sinusitis, erosion of the nasal septum or esophagus, otitis, vocal cord paralysis, epistaxis, or distal esophageal strictures, which may limit long-term use. Small, soft-bore tubes are less likely to cause these complications.

**BOX 40-1** CONSIDERATIONS for the Older Patient

**Nutritional Requirements**

- The risk for malnutrition increases as functional abilities decrease.
- The caloric needs of the elderly are generally less, secondary to decreased metabolism.
- Although protein requirements remain the same, it is important to monitor renal function.
- There is decreased ability to tolerate glucose loads.
- Atrophic gastritis occurs frequently in the elderly, which can result in decreased gastric acid secretion. The resultant achlorhydria or hypochlorhydria can lead to bacterial overgrowth and altered absorption of iron, vitamin $B_{12}$, folate, calcium, vitamin K, and zinc.
- Lactose intolerance increases with age; this intolerance to dairy products can contribute to osteopenia.
- Vitamin D deficiency in the elderly can be due to decreased dietary intake, decreased synthesis, or decreased exposure to sunlight.
- The elderly have less ability to regulate fluid balance, which places them at an increased risk for dehydration or overhydration.
- Encourage increased dietary fiber, fluids, and exercise to reduce the incidence of constipation.
- Decreased GI motility, exocrine function, and digestion or absorption may occur in the elderly.
- Physical changes in the jaw, including poor dentition or poorly fitting dentures, may interfere with mastication and adequate food intake.
- Swallowing may be more difficult because of decreased esophageal motility and decreased saliva production.
- Multiple medications or concomitant disease may contribute to anorexia or diminished sense of taste.

---

**QSEN**

**EVIDENCE-BASED PRACTICE HIGHLIGHT 40-1**
**Prevention of Aspiration**

**Expected Practice**

- Maintain head-of-bed elevation at an angle of 30 to 45 degrees, unless contraindicated. (Level B)
- Use sedatives as sparingly as feasible. (Level C)
- For tube-fed patients, assess placement of the feeding tube at 4-hour intervals. (Level C)
- For patients receiving gastric tube feedings, assess for GI intolerance to the feedings at 4-hour intervals. (Level C)
- For tube-fed patients, avoid bolus feedings in those at high risk for aspiration. (Level E)
- Consult with physician about obtaining a swallowing assessment before oral feedings are started for recently extubated patients who have experienced prolonged intubation. (Level C)
- Maintain endotracheal cuff pressures at an appropriate level, and ensure that secretions are cleared from above the cuff before it is deflated. (Level B)

**AACN Levels of Evidence**

**Level A** Meta-analysis of quantitative studies or metasynthesis of qualitative studies with results that consistently support a specific action, intervention, or treatment (including systematic review of randomized controlled trials)

**Level B** Well-designed, controlled studies with results that consistently support a specific action, intervention, or treatment

**Level C** Qualitative studies, descriptive or correlational studies, integrative reviews, systematic reviews, or randomized controlled trials with inconsistent results

**Level D** Peer-reviewed professional and organizational standards with the support of clinical study recommendations

**Level E** Multiple case reports, theory-based evidence from expert opinions, or peer-reviewed professional orgastandards without clinical studies to support recommendations

**Level M** Manufacturer's recommendations only

Excerpted from American Association of Critical-Care Nurses Practice Alert. The full practice alert is available online at http://aacn.org.

---

Most nasoenteric tubes have multiple ports staggered along their sides and tip, which minimize clogging and maximize flow. Many devices also have weighted tips and a stylet, which stiffens the tube to assist in placement. Another common feature of many nasoenteric tubes is a Y-port at the proximal tip, which allows for the administration of medications and irrigation without interrupting tube feeding.

**NASOGASTRIC TUBES.** Gastric feedings through a nasogastric tube are appropriate for patients who have intact gag and cough reflexes and adequate gastric emptying. Nasogastric tubes usually range from 8 to 12 French in diameter and 30 to 36 inches in length. Small-caliber nasogastric tubes are used solely for feeding, whereas large-caliber tubes can be used to decompress the stomach, monitor gastric pH, and deliver medications and feedings. Large-caliber nasogastric tubes are usually made of stiffer material and are often less comfortable for patients, possibly triggering self-extubation. These tubes are usually used to decompress and drain the stomach temporarily and are therefore typically for short-term use.

Advantages to gastric feeding include the ease of placement, the ease of checking residuals, and patient tolerability during enteral infusions. However, patients with nasogastric tubes are at the greatest risk for aspiration, especially when they are unconscious, mechanically ventilated, or otherwise unable to protect their airway. In a conscious patient, the mere physical appearance of the tube and associated discomfort may limit the clinical use of nasogastric tubes.

**NASODUODENAL TUBES AND NASOJEJUNAL TUBES.** Nasoduodenal tubes and nasojejunal tubes are thought to be better suited for long-term use than nasogastric tubes. Nasoduodenal tubes and nasojejunal tubes are advanced through the stomach, past the pylorus, and into the small intestine, usually in the third portion of the duodenum beyond the ligament of Treitz. In theory, the pyloric sphincter provides a barrier that reduces the risk for aspiration or regurgitation.

Transpyloric feeding can be given without regard to gastric emptying, providing an additional advantage over intragastric feeding. Candidates for transpyloric feedings include critically ill patients with a prior history of gastric aspiration, patients at risk for aspiration (such as ventilated patients), those with gastroparesis, those with gastric outlet obstruction, and patients with neurologic conditions who are unable to protect their airway.

A common misconception is that enteral feedings should not be started if bowel sounds are absent. Bowel sounds are an indication of GI motility, not of absorption, and the presence or absent of bowel sounds or flatus is not required before the initiation of enteral feeding.[7,9] After injury and postoperatively, bowel sounds may not be detected for 3 to 5 days owing to gastric atony. The small bowel motility is less commonly impaired than the stomach or the colon and retains its absorptive and digestive capabilities, making it possible to accept enteral feedings immediately after surgery or trauma.

Nasoduodenal tubes and nasojejunal tubes range from 8 to 16 French in diameter and 152 to 240 cm in length. The length and diameter make it more difficult to check feeding residual because the lumen is smaller and tends to collapse on itself when aspirated. In addition, clogging of medications is more common than with nasogastric tubes. The primary disadvantage associated with nasoduodenal and nasojejunal tubes relates to the difficulty in initially placing the tubing tip past the pyloric sphincter.

**PLACING NASOENTERIC TUBES.** In most ICUs, skilled nurses or physicians routinely place nasoenteric tubes. Before placing a feeding tube, institutional policy and protocol should be reviewed because nasoenteric tube placement has many potential complications. Patients with a decreased level of consciousness, poor cough or gag reflex, or an inability or unwillingness to cooperate are at increased risk for pulmonary intubation. When a patient cannot cooperate or cough when the tube enters the bronchial tree, extra precautions must be taken to ensure proper placement. Feeding tubes placed in the bronchial tree can cause pulmonary hemorrhage or pneumothorax. A cuffed endotracheal tube (ETT) does not preclude accidental pulmonary intubation. Nasoenteric tubes can also be accidentally placed in the esophagus or, in patients with basilar skull fractures, in the intracranial space.

Nasogastric tube placement is usually easier than nasoduodenal or nasojejunal tube placement. When placing a nasoenteric feeding tube in the stomach, the nurse determines the length of tube insertion by measuring the distance from the tip of the nose, to the earlobe, to the tip of the xiphoid process. Before insertion, the nurse considers using a topical anesthetic or water-soluble lubricant to assist in placement. After placing the patient's bed in a high Fowler's position, the nurse slightly flexes the patient's head (if not clinically contraindicated) and passes the lubricated tip through the nares into the nasopharynx. While advancing the tube, the nurse asks the patient to swallow repeatedly. Having the patient sip water through a straw may also assist in tube placement (if not clinically contraindicated). Rotating the tube as it is advanced may also ease advancement.

When attempting to pass the nasoenteric tube tip past the pylorus, the nurse follows the same procedure described previously and then turns the patient to the right lateral decubitus position with the head of the bed at a 30- to 45-degree angle to take advantage of gravity and peristalsis. Nasoduodenal and nasojejunal tubes depend on gastric motility to carry the tip through the pylorus, but they have a tendency to coil in the stomach. Some nasoduodenal tubes and nasojejunal tubes have weights to aid in passage through the pylorus; however, the utility of the weighted tip is dubious. Postpyloric placement with the use of bedside electromagnetic placement devices (EMPD) use real-time tracking to direct and verify accurate bedside placement of postpyloric feeding tubes.[10] An agent, such as metoclopramide or erythromycin, may be ordered before insertion because such a medication increases upper GI motility while relaxing the pylorus. Air insufflation, the process of inserting large amounts of air into the stomach, may also be helpful by distending the stomach and facilitating tube passage though the pylorus. If attempts to blindly pass a nasoduodenal or nasojejunal tube are not successful within 24 hours, endoscopic or radiologic assistance should be sought to advance the tip of the tube.

Before initiating tube feeding, proper tube placement must be confirmed by an abdominal radiograph. Feeding tubes placed surgically, by endoscopy, or under fluoroscopy do not require radiographic confirmation of placement. The external length of the tube is documented after placement is confirmed. The nurse marks the tube with tape or indelible ink at the point it enters the nares, rechecks tube placement before initiating intermittent feedings or medication administration and at least once each shift, and monitors tube placement during continuous tube feeding according to the institution's policy.

Auscultation, aspiration and inspection of aspirate, and pH testing have been used to monitor tube placement after initial placement is confirmed by an abdominal radiograph with varying degrees of accuracy. No one method is infallible, so using a combination of these methods is advised. Abdominal radiograph remains the gold standard. Injecting air into the tube and auscultation of the gastric bubble, although commonly used, is not an accurate method to verify initial tube placement. An air bubble sound can be transmitted to the epigastrium when the tube is in the esophagus. Although auscultation of insufflated air is not a reliable method to confirm initial feeding tube placement, it may still provide useful information. If no resistance is met, the tube is unlikely to be kinked, and if the patient immediately burps back air, the tip of the tube is probably in the esophagus.

Aspiration and inspection of the aspirate may help differentiate between gastric and intestinal placement, but not between intestinal and pulmonary placement. Fluid aspirated from the stomach is usually green, tan, brown, or bloody.[11] Small intestinal aspirate is usually golden yellow, clear, or bile colored and is often thicker than gastric aspirate.[11] Pulmonary fluid is usually tan, white, clear, or pale yellow and can closely mimic gastric or intestinal aspirates.[11] However, it is necessary to keep in mind that the diameter of small intestinal tubes may not allow withdrawal to check aspirate.

Measuring the pH of fluid aspirated from the feeding tube is another method of monitoring tube placement. The pH of esophageal secretions is usually 6.0 to 7.0, gastric aspirates 1.0 to 4.0, and intestinal contents 6.0 to 7.0.[11] However, the pH of gastric aspirate can be elevated with the infusion of enteral formulas, the use of acid-modifying medications, and the presence of bile reflux. The pH of both small intestinal aspirate and pulmonary fluid is usually greater than 6.0; therefore, if the pH of the aspirate is greater than 4.0, tube position cannot be determined based on pH alone.[11] For optimal results with pH testing, nothing that may alter the pH should be instilled in the tube for 60 minutes.

Capnometry and capnography detect carbon dioxide; these noninvasive monitoring techniques are used to monitor and evaluate respiratory function and ventilation. Observation of the presence or absence of a waveform is used to evaluate for accidental pulmonary placement of feeding tubes.

Suctioning and patient movement or coughing may potentially dislodge a feeding tube. If at any time tube location is in question, the nurse holds the tube feeding and requests an order for an abdominal radiograph to confirm placement. See Evidence-Based Practice Highlight 40-2 for more information.

**SECURING NASOENTERIC TUBES.** Before securing any feeding tube, the nurse cleans the skin with alcohol to remove oils and dirt and considers applying a skin protectant to maintain skin integrity. Nasoenteric tubes should be

## EVIDENCE-BASED PRACTICE HIGHLIGHT 40-2
## Verification of Feeding Tube Placement (Blindly Inserted)

### Expected Practice

- Use a variety of bedside methods to predict tube location *during* the insertion procedure:
  - Observe for signs of respiratory distress.
  - Use capnography if available.
  - Measure pH of aspirate from tube if pH strips are available.
  - Observe visual characteristics of aspirate from the tube.
  - Recognize that auscultatory (air bolus) and water bubbling methods are unreliable. (Level B)
- Obtain radiographic confirmation of correct placement of any blindly inserted tube prior to its initial use for feedings or medication administration.
  - The radiograph should visualize the entire course of the feeding tube in the GI tract and should be read by a radiologist to avoid errors in interpretation. Mark and document the tube's exit site from the nose or mouth immediately after radiographic confirmation of correct tube placement. (Level A)
- Check tube location at 4-hour intervals after feedings are started:
  - Observe for a change in length of external portion of the feeding tube (as determined by movement of the marked portion of the tube).
  - Review routine chest and abdominal x-ray reports to look for notations about tube location.
  - Observe changes in volume of aspirate from feeding tube.
  - If pH strips are available, measure pH of feeding tube aspirates if feedings are interrupted for more than a few hours.
  - Observe the appearance of feeding tube aspirates if feedings are interrupted for more than a few hours.
  - Obtain an x-ray to confirm tube position if there is doubt about the tube's location. (Level B)

### AACN Levels of Evidence

**Level A** Meta-analysis of quantitative studies or metasynthesis of qualitative studies with results that consistently support a specific action, intervention, or treatment

**Level B** Well-designed, controlled studies with results that consistently support a specific action, intervention, or treatment

**Level C** Qualitative studies, descriptive or correlational studies, integrative reviews, systematic reviews, or randomized controlled trials with inconsistent results

**Level D** Peer-reviewed professional and organizational standards with the support of clinical study recommendations

**Level E** Multiple case reports, theory-based evidence from expert opinions, or peer-reviewed professional organizational standards without clinical studies to support recommendations

**Level M** Manufacturer's recommendations only

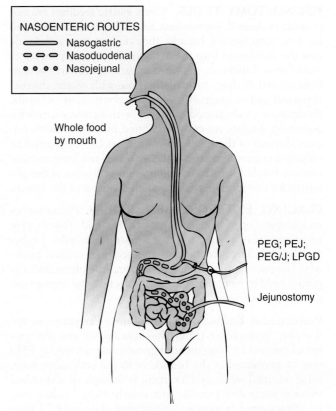

**FIGURE 40-2** Possible routes for feeding. LPGD, low-profile gastrostomy device; PEG, percutaneous endoscopic gastrostomy; PEG/J, PEG modified with a jejunal extension tube; and PEJ, percutaneous endoscopic jejunostomy.

abdomen into the stomach (gastrostomy) or jejunum (jejunostomy)[11] (Fig. 40-2). Enterostomal feeding tubes are also indicated when the nasal route is contraindicated and when the patient's swallowing is impaired or the oropharynx, larynx, or esophagus is obstructed. Enterostomal tubes are 18 to 28 French in diameter, made of silicone and polyurethane, and very durable.

**GASTROSTOMY TUBES.** Gastrostomy tubes have an internal retention bolster to prevent accidental dislodgment. Gastrostomy tubes may be used temporarily or for permanent feeding. If a gastrostomy tube is intended for permanent feedings, it may need to be replaced as the tube material deteriorates over time. Gastrostomy tubes may also be used for chronic gastric decompression. A low-profile gastrostomy device (LPGD), often referred to as a button, may be used to replace gastrostomy tubes in a mature gastrostomy tract, usually 3 to 6 months after initial placement or as an initial placement. LPGDs are anchored in the stomach and protrude through the abdomen, flush with the skin. These devices require a special extension adapter to connect with the tube-feeding bag, to check for residuals, and to use for decompression. This adapter may then be removed after use. Some LPGDs are equipped with a one-way antireflux valve to prevent leakage of gastric contents onto the skin. These devices are usually well accepted because they are durable, unlikely to irritate the skin, and difficult to dislodge. With agitated or confused adults who have a tendency to pull on their tubes, these advantages may be a benefit.

secured in a way that avoids irritation or pressure on the nares, thereby preventing necrosis. The nurse allows the tube to hang straight from the nares and secures it to the bridge of the nose or the cheek with tape (or one of the many commercially available devices). For agitated or uncooperative patients, the nurse considers soft wrist restraints or mitts to avoid accidental self-extubation (refer to your institution's policy and procedure regarding the use of restraints). It is necessary to inspect the skin and nostrils every 4 to 8 hours for signs and symptoms of irritation, erythema, or skin breakdown. Patient comfort can be maximized by providing frequent mouth care and moistening of the nares.

### Enterostomal Feeding and Feeding Tubes

If therapy is expected to last a month or more, a more permanent enterostomal device can be inserted through the

**JEJUNOSTOMY TUBES.** When gastric feedings are not possible or desired, jejunostomy tubes (J-tubes) are preferred for long-term feeding because they deliver enteral formula past the duodenum into the jejunum, decreasing pancreatic stimulation. J-tubes are indicated in patients who will benefit from jejunal feeding, particularly those with gastric disease, abnormal gastric emptying, upper GI obstruction or fistula, pancreatitis, or decreased gag reflex with significant risk for aspiration. J-tubes are contraindicated in patients with primary diseases of the small bowel (such as Crohn disease) or radiation enteritis because of the increased risk for enterocutaneous fistula formation. A limitation of J-tubes is the potential for obstruction from the small diameter of the lumen.

**PLACING ENTEROSTOMAL TUBES.** Percutaneous endoscopic, open surgical, laparoscopic, and fluoroscopic techniques may be used to place a gastrostomy tube. J-tubes may be placed by percutaneous endoscopy or surgical methods. The patient's underlying disease and the physician's expertise need to be considered when selecting the appropriate placement technique.

**Percutaneous Endoscopic Gastrostomy.** Percutaneous endoscopic gastrostomy (PEG) has rapidly become the preferred method for placement of gastrostomy devices. A PEG may be performed at the bedside or in the endoscopy suite, using minimal sedation. Placement is through an abdominal incision using direct endoscopic visualization. Feeding may be administered as soon as 2 hours after placement.[11] Other advantages of PEG include increased comfort, decreased cost, and decreased recovery time. A candidate for a PEG must have an intact oropharynx and an esophagus free from obstruction. The only absolute contraindication to PEG is the inability to bring the gastric wall into apposition with the abdomen. Prior abdominal surgeries, abdominal wall malignancy ascites, hepatomegaly, and obesity may preclude placement of a PEG.

Complications of PEG are infrequent but include wound infection related to bacterial contamination by oral flora during insertion, necrotizing fasciitis, peritonitis, and aspiration. Pneumoperitoneum, a common finding after PEG placement, is not clinically significant unless accompanied by signs and symptoms of peritonitis. Prophylactic antibiotics are usually given 30 to 60 minutes before the procedure. Correct placement is then verified by endoscopy.

In patients with severe gastroesophageal reflux disease, gastroparesis, or increased risk for aspiration related to tube feeding, a PEG can be modified with a jejunal extension tube known as a PEG/J tube. The gastric lumen of a PEG/J tube is usually used for gastric decompression, and the jejunal lumen is used for the simultaneous delivery of enteral feeding. PEG/J-tubes may decrease the risk for gastric aspiration; however, they do not necessarily provide the same protection against aspiration as jejunal tubes because the pylorus is compromised by the large catheter. The jejunal portion of a PEG/J tube may migrate back into the stomach and increase the risk for occlusion, gastric reflux, or aspiration. Both PEG and PEG/J-tubes are held in place by internal and external retention devices. The internal device rests in the stomach, which prevents migration and leakage of gastric contents. The external retention device anchors the tube to the abdomen. These tubes have a high rate of mechanical dysfunction, which limits their long-term use.

**Surgical Gastrostomy.** Surgical gastrostomy tubes are inserted through an incision in the abdominal wall with the patient receiving general anesthesia. The stomach is usually sutured to the abdominal wall to create a permanent connection between the gastric and abdominal walls. Surgical placement of a gastrostomy is usually reserved for those that fail endoscopic or radiologic placement if the surgeon wants to view the gastric anatomy clearly or as a secondary procedure during abdominal surgery. Disadvantages of surgical placement include the need for general anesthesia, increased recovery time, decreased comfort, and increased cost.

**Laparoscopic Gastrostomy.** A laparoscopically placed gastrostomy tube also requires general anesthesia or intravenous (IV) conscious sedation. Laparoscopic placement is usually reserved for patients with head, neck, or esophageal cancer. It is less invasive, is less painful, and usually involves fewer complications than a surgical gastrostomy.

**Fluoroscopic Gastrostomy.** Direct percutaneous catheter insertion of a gastrostomy tube under fluoroscopy is indicated with high-grade pharyngeal or esophageal obstruction. Disadvantages to the use of fluoroscopy to place enterostomal devices include the inability to detect mucosal disease, the potential for prolonged exposure to radiation, the necessity of transport to the fluoroscopy suite, and increased cost.

**SECURING ENTEROSTOMAL TUBES AND CARING FOR THE ENTEROSTOMY SITE.** Enterostomal tubes are secured to the abdominal wall to prevent dislodgment or migration of the tube, to avoid tension on the tubing, and to prevent the external retention device from digging into the skin. The length of the external tubing is documented to monitor for migration of the tubing.

To avoid tissue maceration, the insertion site is kept clean and dry by leaving it open to air (unless draining), and lifting or adjusting the tube is avoided for several days after the initial insertion. To avoid pulling the internal retention device taut against the gastric or intestinal mucosa, the amount of dressing between the device and the skin is limited. Any accumulated drainage may be cleaned with water. Serosanguineous drainage may be expected for 7 to 10 days after insertion. If no drainage is present, cleansing with soap and water is adequate. The skin around the insertion site and the retention device is assessed at least daily for skin breakdown, erythema, or drainage. The tissue usually heals within a month.

In-and-out play on the tubing is checked; it should be able to move one-fourth inch to prevent erosion of gastric or abdominal tissue. If the anchor is too tight, the nurse should notify the physician immediately because this may indicate "buried bumper syndrome," a situation in which the retention device is imbedded in the tissue, thereby leading to mucosal or skin erosion. If a gastrostomy tube becomes accidentally dislodged, the nurse should notify the physician immediately so that the tube can be reinserted quickly before the tract closes.

### Types and Delivery of Enteral Formulas

When selecting a tube feeding formula, nutrient requirements, the patient's clinical status, location of enteral access, GI function, cost, and duration must all be considered. Numerous tube feeding solutions are available for enteral nutrition, with many designed to assist in managing specific disease processes; however, no single formula is ideal for all patients. All contain proteins, carbohydrates, fats, vitamins, minerals, trace elements, and water. The difference lies in how these nutrients are structured and delivered. The dietary formula selected is based on the patient's ability to digest and absorb major nutrients, the total nutrient requirements, and fluid and electrolyte restrictions.

Polymeric solutions are the most commonly used formulas. These formulas are isotonic and can provide enough protein, carbohydrate, fat, vitamins, trace elements, and minerals to prevent nutritional deficiencies. They are considered nutritionally complete if given in enough volume to meet caloric needs. Standard formulas deliver 1 kcal/mL; some concentrated formulas may provide 2 kcal/mL.[12] The more concentrated formulas may be used for patients who require fluid restriction or in patients who have higher caloric requirements. All polymeric solutions contain intact proteins (most often meat, whey, milk, or soy proteins) that require normal pancreatic enzymes for digestion. Several disease-specific formulas are available.

Peptide (elemental or semielemental) formulas provide proteins as dipeptides, tripeptides, or free amino acids from hydrolysis of whey, milk, or soy proteins. Because peptides do not require pancreatic enzymes for digestion, elemental solutions are used when digestion is impaired, such as in pancreatic insufficiency, radiation enteritis, Crohn disease, or short bowel syndrome secondary to surgical resection. Elemental solutions have no proven advantage in patients with normal gut function, are usually more expensive than polymeric formulas, and have an unpleasant taste.

Modular formulas contain individual nutrient components such as protein, carbohydrates, and fat that can be mixed or added to other formulas to individualize feedings to a patient's specific nutritional needs. The involvement of a dietitian is essential in the selection of these formulas.

Attention has recently focused on the role of enteral formulas that contain additional nutrients purported to enhance immune function. These formulas, referred to collectively as immunonutrition or immune-enhancing diets, have been reported to decrease infection rates, duration of mechanical ventilation, and length of hospitalization, but they have not been shown to affect mortality.[13] Several nutrients that have attracted attention are glutamine, arginine, and omega-3 polyunsaturated fatty acids.

Glutamine is a nonessential amino acid that may become conditionally essential in critically ill adults.[12] Glutamine is an important fuel source for rapidly dividing cells, such as enterocytes, lymphocytes, and macrophages.[12] In addition, glutamine may improve immune function and reduce intestinal permeability.[12] Glutamine-enriched solutions should be considered in patients with burns and trauma.[7,9,12]

Another additive is arginine, which is also a nonessential amino acid that may become depleted in the critically ill. Arginine is a precursor of nitric oxide and is important in cell growth and proliferation, wound healing, and collagen synthesis.[12] Its role is controversial because increased nitric oxide production may increase tissue injury and trigger cardiovascular collapse in patients with sepsis or systemic inflammatory response syndrome.[7,14]

The omega-3 fatty acid is a precursor of prostaglandins, leukotrienes, and other inflammatory mediators. Use of an enteral formula with an antiinflammatory lipid profile fortified with omega-3 fatty acids or borage oil is recommended for patients with acute respiratory distress syndrome and severe acute lung injury.[7,9,14] These formulas have been shown to reduce the length of stay in the ICU, duration of mechanical ventilation, organ failure, and mortality when compared to standard formulas.[7]

When initiating enteral tube feedings, most clinicians recommend beginning with an isotonic formula at a slow rate, most often 20 to 30 mL/h, and increasing the rate incrementally every 8 to 12 hours until the goal rate is achieved. Dilution of formula may help tolerance but is not recommended because this may increase the time needed to meet the nutritional requirements.

Enteral feedings can be administered by bolus, gravity infusion, intermittent infusion, continuous infusion, or cyclic infusion. The tube tip location and tolerance generally dictate formula delivery. Gastric feedings are appropriate for patients who have intact gag and cough reflexes and adequate gastric emptying.

**BOLUS FEEDINGS.** Bolus feedings, considered the most natural method physiologically, are delivered by gravity by a large syringe in volumes as high as 400 mL over 5 to 15 minutes, three to five times a day.[11] The stomach is the preferred site for bolus feedings. The stomach and pyloric sphincter regulate the outflow of feeding from the stomach. Bolus feedings allow for increased patient mobility because the patient is free from a mechanical device between feedings. Bolus feedings are usually initiated with 60 to 120 mL of full-strength formula every 8 to 12 hours until the goal is reached.[11] Unfortunately, as a result of high residuals, bolus feedings are usually not well tolerated and are often accompanied by nausea, bloating, cramping, diarrhea, or aspiration.

**INTERMITTENT FEEDINGS.** Intermittent feedings of 300 to 400 mL are administered by slow gravity drip four to six times a day over a period of 30 to 60 minutes. The stomach is the preferred site for intermittent infusion because of its capacity. Intermittent feedings are associated with a decreased risk for osmotic diarrhea. Advantages of intermittent feedings include freedom from dependence on a mechanical device and a power source, which can decrease cost and increase patient mobility.

**CONTINUOUS FEEDINGS.** If the tip of the nasoenteric tube is in the duodenum or jejunum, tube feedings must be delivered by infusion. Continuous infusions are administered over 24 hours with the aid of a feeding pump to ensure a constant flow rate. Continuous pump feedings are the preferred method for intestinal feeding because delivery that is too rapid may lead to "dumping syndrome," characterized by osmotic diarrhea, abdominal distention, cramps, hyperperistalsis, light-headedness, diaphoresis, and palpitations. When the tube is placed in the third portion of the duodenum, past the ligament of Treitz, continuous pump feedings are associated with decreased risk for aspiration. Initiate continuous feedings of full-strength formula at 10 to 40 mL/h advancing by 10 to 20 mL increments every 8 to 12 hours until goal is reached.[11] If the feeding is advanced slowly, the small bowel can usually tolerate feedings at a rate of 150 mL/h. The continuous method is best suited to the critically ill patient because it allows more time for nutrients to be absorbed in the intestine. Continuous infusion is often used in the ICU because there is decreased incidence of gastric distention and potential for aspiration. Continuous infusion tube feeding may also act prophylactically to prevent stress ulcers and metabolic complications. As with intermittent feedings, disadvantages include the dependence on a mechanical device and a power source.

CYCLIC FEEDINGS. Cyclic feedings are continuous feedings that deliver the total daily nutritional requirements in a shorter time frame, typically over 8 to 12 hours, to allow the patient freedom from 24-hour continuous feedings. Cyclic feedings of high density and high volume are typically given at night to allow hunger to develop during the day, but they may be given during the day if a patient has difficulty with regurgitation while lying supine. This schedule may assist the patient in progressing from enteral to oral consumption.

The ultimate goal is for patients to resume adequate oral intake. Enteral feeding may be discontinued when patients can drink enough liquid to maintain hydration and can eat two-thirds of their nutritional requirements.

### Complications of Enteral Nutrition

Although enteral nutrition is in general associated with fewer complications than parenteral nutrition, complications may still occur. These complications generally fall into GI, mechanical, metabolic, and infectious categories. Many of these complications can be prevented or treated by closely observing residuals and watching for signs and symptoms of gastric intolerance.

GASTROINTESTINAL COMPLICATIONS. The patient's tolerance to enteral feeding depends on the rate of flow and the osmolality of the formula. Signs and symptoms of GI intolerance to enteral feeding include diarrhea, nausea, vomiting, abdominal discomfort, distention, and high residual returns. Food normally passes through the stomach at a rate of 2 to 10 mL/min; however, gastric emptying is delayed or absent in many critically ill patients. Unlike the stomach, the small intestine cannot act as a reservoir. If large residuals are withdrawn through a nasoduodenal tube or nasojejunal tube, the tube may have moved back into the stomach, and placement should be confirmed with an abdominal radiograph.

**High Residuals.** The monitoring of gastric residual volumes (GRVs) is a routine practice based on the assumption that GRVs are useful in predicting the risk for aspiration and pneumonia. However, studies have not shown a consistent relationship between GRV and aspiration; high GRVs do not indicate aspiration, and low GRVs do not preclude aspiration.[15] Additionally, there is no consensus among experts about what constitutes a high GRV, with reports varying from 100 to 500 mL. High GRVs have been thought to result from impaired gastric emptying caused by intolerance to enteral feedings; GRV is an imprecise measure of gastric emptying and may not take into account the volume of gastric and salivary secretions. In addition, it is difficult to determine whether gastric contents have been completely removed. Many clinicians stop tube feeding inappropriately, based on a single GRV of less than 400 to 500 mL. Although a GRV between 250 and 500 mL should raise suspicion of intolerance and cause the implementation of measures to reduce

the risk of aspiration. One high value does not mean feeding failure, and automatic cessation of feeding can delay the patient's ability to meet his or her nutritional goals.[7,9] Tube feedings should not be stopped for GRVs less than 500 mL in the absence of other signs of intolerance.[7] The nurse must be sure to evaluate the clinical status of the patient before stopping tube feeding solely on the basis of one high GRV; the key is to monitor trends.[9,16] Residuals should be checked every 4 hours during the first 48 hours of gastric feeding, every 4 hours during continuous feedings and before initiating intermittent feedings.[1,11,15]

Tube feeding should be withheld if a patient demonstrates overt signs of regurgitation, vomiting, or aspiration. A common intervention involves holding the feeding for 1 to 2 hours and rechecking GRV every 1 to 2 hours until the GRV is less than 200 to 250 mL from a nasogastric tube or less than 100 mL from a gastrostomy tube, at which point feedings can be resumed. If GRV is greater than 250 mL after two measurements, providing a promotility agent should be considered.[1,11] This allows time for normal gastric emptying and reduces the risk for aspiration. It is necessary to remember that high infusion rates result in higher GRVs and to be aware of the institution's policy and protocol regarding high GRVs.

**Nausea, Vomiting, and Bloating.** Nausea, vomiting, and bloating are commonly associated with enteral feedings. Medications, rapid infusion rate, or improper tube placement may cause both nausea and vomiting. Nausea, vomiting, and bloating are most likely to occur when gastric emptying is delayed. The nurse carefully assesses medications that may contribute to these symptoms, and the medications should be eliminated, if possible. A change of formula, reduction in delivery rate, or addition of a prokinetic medication may also help.

**Diarrhea.** Diarrhea is the most common complication of enteral feedings; however, it is important to consider other etiologies before assuming that enteral feedings are the cause of diarrhea. Diarrhea in a patient receiving enteral feeding may result from the use of antibiotics or other diarrhea-inducing medications; altered bacterial flora; formula composition; intolerance to lactose, fat, or osmolality; a rate of infusion that is too high; hypoalbuminemia; or enteral formula contamination.

The liquid form of many medications may contain hypertonic sorbitol, which can have laxative effects. Antibiotics, antacids, magnesium, and prokinetic medications can also contribute to diarrhea. Antibiotics can contribute to diarrhea by causing overgrowth of *Clostridium difficile*. To assess for *C. difficile* infection, a stool sample is assessed for *C. difficile* toxin. Treatment options include antibiotic therapy with oral metronidazole, vancomycin, or cholestyramine (a bile acid sequestrant that binds the toxin). A patient who has received antibiotics should not receive antidiarrheals until *C. difficile* infection has been ruled out because diarrhea helps eliminate the toxin from the intestinal mucosa.

Bacterial overgrowth may cause diarrhea. Reduced gastric and small bowel motility may lead to small intestinal overgrowth, which can alter intestinal microflora. Acid suppression may also permit bacterial overgrowth because bacteria can colonize the GI tract when the gastric pH is greater than 6.0.

The infusion of enteral feedings too rapidly may cause diarrhea. Intolerance of lactose, fat, or osmolality may also lead to diarrhea. Reducing the infusion rate, changing to a peptide-based formula that is easier to digest, and giving an absorbing product, such as psyllium fiber (Metamucil), may help. The use of a fiber-containing formula may be helpful in bulking stools and correction of the diarrhea.

The composition of enteral formulas makes them an ideal medium for bacterial growth, which may result in diarrhea. Many organisms have been associated with enteral feedings, including coagulase-negative staphylococci, C. difficile, and Gram-negative bacilli, such as Serratia, Klebsiella, Enterobacter, Proteus, and Pseudomonas species. Bacterial contamination from the surface of the formula container, or even water added when the preparations are mixed or poured, may lead to diarrhea. Contamination of enteral feedings may also occur as a result of retrograde movement of bacteria from the patient's own GI tract. In addition, the aspiration of gastric residuals and the removal of guide wires from the feeding tube may contribute to contamination.

Contamination of the feeding administration set may also cause diarrhea. Breaks in the system should be minimized, and the use of a closed, prefilled, ready-to-hang solution should be considered to minimize contamination from pathogens. To prevent bacterial contamination, formulas that are reconstituted in advance should be immediately refrigerated and discarded within 24 hours if not used.[11] Formulas that are exposed to room temperature for longer than 4 hours should be discarded.[11] Sterile, premixed formulas should hang no longer than 8 hours.[11] The nurse checks the expiration date of the formula and discards the formula if it has expired. Closed system administration sets should be changed every 24 to 48 hours, and open system administration sets should be changed every 24 hours.[11] All practitioners should use good hand washing technique when handling equipment and wear gloves when handling feeding systems.

In patients receiving enteral feedings, a hyperosmotic formula may also contribute to diarrhea. If diarrhea decreases when the feedings are withheld, the formula may be the cause. After consultation with the dietitian, the nurse may consider changing the formula. Also, the nurse collects a stool sample to evaluate for an osmotic gap; this may help identify osmotic diarrhea.

Hypoalbuminemia may predispose patients to diarrhea by decreasing the osmotic pressure gradient. This decrease may lead to bowel edema and malabsorption. Any formula that is not absorbed may contribute to the diarrhea. Prealbumin level is monitored because it is a more reliable indicator of current nutritional status than serum albumin.

**Constipation.** Constipation associated with enteral feedings may be related to poor hydration, lack of fiber, bed rest, impaction, obstruction, and narcotics. Adequate hydration is ensured, and adding a stool softener should be considered along with minimizing narcotic administration, encouraging ambulation, and considering the addition of fiber to relieve constipation.

**MECHANICAL COMPLICATIONS.** Mechanical complications occur when the feeding tube becomes dislodged, occluded, or malpositioned.

**Tube Dislodgment.** Tube dislodgment by patients or staff accounts for most tube removals. Soft restraints or hand mitts should be considered for agitated patients to prevent accidental self-extubation (refer to your institution's policy regarding the use of restraints).

**Tube Clogging.** Precipitation of medications, clogging of pill fragments, or coagulation of formula may cause obstruction of any feeding tube, delaying the administration of nutrients and medications. To avoid clogging, the nurse flushes enteral feeding tubes every 4 hours during continuous feedings, before and after medication administration, after checking residuals, and when turning off feedings.[11] For flushing nasoenteric tubes, the nurse always uses a large 30- to 60-mL syringe to avoid rupturing the tube with excessive pressure and irrigates with 15 to 30 mL of sterile water.[11,17] The nurse frequently checks the enteral solution container for precipitation. Crushed tablets may leave a residue that blocks the tube. To prevent clogging, the nurse administers liquid medications when available. Flushing the tube before and after each medication, administration also helps avoid incompatibilities between medications and feedings and reduces the incidence of clogging. Medication should not be directly added to enteral formulas.[11,17]

An obstruction may exist if the formula does not flow by gravity, flushing an aspirate from the tube is not possible, or the occlusion alarm of the feeding pump sounds repeatedly. If an occlusion is suspected, the nurse uses a large piston syringe to flush the tube with warm water, using a gentle push–pull motion. Although many solutions have been proposed to assist in clearing an obstructed feeding tube, they offer no demonstrable benefit over tap water. A stylet should never be used to unclog a tube because of the risk for rupturing the feeding tube and perforating the esophagus, stomach, or small intestine. Recent studies show that pancreatic enzymes have been effective in unclogging a tube when water is unsuccessful, as long as the enzymes are activated before instillation.[11]

**METABOLIC COMPLICATIONS.** Multiple metabolic complications can accompany enteral nutrition. Fluid and electrolyte imbalance may occur because of fluid excess, fluid depletion by GI or renal losses, wound drainage, diuresis, fever, or inadequate free water intake. If dehydration is due to inadequate fluid intake, the nurse may need to give the patient extra fluid by bolus or by automatic flush using specialized feeding pumps. The average patient with good renal function needs 30 to 35 mL/kg of free water per day, if not medically contraindicated. Conversely, if cardiac or hepatic function is impaired, overhydration from enteral feedings may occur. The determination of the patient's baseline fluid requirements and accurate measurement of intake and output can help maintain fluid balance. The nurse should keep in mind that many of the patients seen in the ICU may be unable to convey feelings of thirst, secondary to intubation, or diminished levels of consciousness.

Hyperglycemia may occur if patients are being overfed, during hypermetabolic states, and as a result of steroid medications. Blood glucose is monitored during enteral therapy; a decrease in formula rate or concentration may help if hyperglycemia occurs. Bolus feeding may exacerbate hyperglycemia in patients with diabetes. If feedings are abruptly stopped, hypoglycemia is assessed, especially in patients receiving insulin.

**INFECTIOUS COMPLICATIONS.** Aspiration of enteral feeding resulting in hypoxia or pneumonia is a dreaded complication of enteral feeding. The incidence of aspiration of enteral formulas is as high as 50% to 75% in patients with ETTs. Loss of consciousness, mechanical ventilation, and many medications used in critically ill patients increase the risk for aspiration. To reduce this risk, the head of the bed should be maintained at a 30- to 45-degree angle.[7,11] If head of the bed elevation is medically contraindicated, a reverse Trendelenburg position is used unless medically contraindicated.[11] Intermittent or continuous feedings are used rather than rapid boluses because they allow the restoration of gastric pH, which can minimize gastric colonization. GRV is checked frequently, and signs of feeding intolerance are assessed. Feedings are discontinued at least 30 minutes before any procedure for which the patient must lie flat. If a procedure necessitates that the head of the bed be lowered, tube feedings may be withheld. The patient is returned to an elevated position, and the feedings are restarted promptly when the procedure is completed.[11] If a patient is intubated, secretions above the tube's cuff should be cleared before deflating the tube.

Pulmonary aspiration, although often subclinical, may be signaled by a low-grade fever, coughing, shortness of breath, rhonchi during or after enteral feeding infusions, and presence of a "sweet" formula odor emanating from tracheal or oral secretions during suctioning. The addition of Food, Drug, and Cosmetic (FD&C) blue dye No. 1 to enteral feeding formula to help visually identify aspirated feeding formula was a common practice for years. However, in 2003, the U.S. Food and Drug Administration (FDA)[18] issued an FDA Public Health Advisory after several reports of toxicity, including bacterial colonization, diarrhea, systemic absorption, and death. As a result, No. 1 dye should not be used in enteral feedings. It is necessary that each nurse check his or her institution's policy and protocol regarding blue dye and its administration.

Checking tracheal suction fluid with a glucose strip and glucometer has been used to test for formula aspiration. Tracheobronchial secretions usually contain less than 5 mg/dL of glucose, so a reading greater than 20 to 25 mg/dL suggests aspiration, although there is some controversy concerning this procedure.

## Parenteral (Intravenous) Nutrition

Parenteral nutrition is indicated when oral or enteral nutrition is not possible or when absorption or function of the GI tract is not sufficient (or is unreliable) to meet the nutritional needs of the patient. Before the inception of parenteral nutrition in the early 1960s, bowel rest was thought to be the cornerstone of treatment for many GI disorders. Today, except in cases of severe hemorrhagic pancreatitis, necrotizing enterocolitis, prolonged ileus, and distal bowel obstruction, some enteral nutrition is recommended to maintain gut integrity and function.[19] If a patient was healthy prior to critical illness with no evidence of protein–calorie malnutrition, use of parenteral nutrition should be reserved and initiated after the first 7 days of hospitalization.[7,9]

There are two types of parenteral (IV) nutrition: central and peripheral. Central parenteral nutrition, also known as total parenteral nutrition (TPN), is infused through a large central vein (Fig. 40-3). TPN has sometimes been referred to as "hyperalimentation" or "hyperal." These are not preferred terms because they imply that parenteral nutrition gives more nutrients than the patient may actually require. If TPN is expected to be needed for more than a few weeks, a more permanent device such a subcutaneously tunneled Hickman catheter or Port-A-Cath can be placed. Another central venous access device that can be used for long-term nutritional support is the peripherally inserted central catheter (PICC). A PICC is inserted peripherally into the basilic vein and advanced so that the tip of the catheter rests in the superior vena cava. Peripheral parenteral nutrition (PPN), unlike TPN, is infused into smaller, peripheral veins (eg, basilic vein) and is often used for short-term nutritional support (eg, 7 to 10 days) or as a supplement during transitional phases to enteral or oral nutrition (see Fig. 40-3). Because of the risks for phlebitis, concentrations of PPN formulas must not exceed 900 mOsm/L.[20] TPN differs from standard IV fluids in that all daily required nutrients are delivered to the patient in the form of macronutrients (carbohydrates, proteins, and

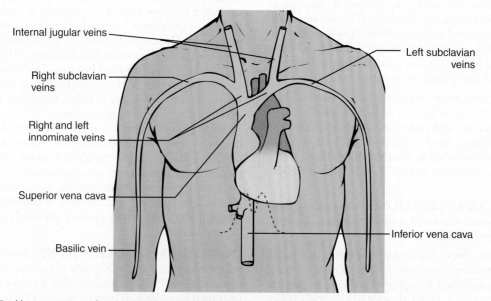

**FIGURE 40-3** Venous anatomy for parenteral nutrition routes.

fats) and micronutrients (electrolytes, vitamins, and trace minerals). Typically, the solution is infused at a constant rate over a 24-hour period to achieve maximal assimilation of the nutrients and to prevent hyperglycemia (or hypoglycemia). The aim of treatment is a continuous infusion that meets the caloric and nutritional requirements of the patient.

Critically ill patients often have issues with reliable IV access. TPN must be infused separately from other IV fluids, medications, and blood products because of the high risk for formula contamination and precipitation. Fortunately, the introduction of multiple-lumen catheters has greatly facilitated the care of patients who require multiple IV therapies by providing separate infusion ports and corresponding distal exit sites staggered along the catheter tubing. This separation prevents direct mixing of solutions before high-blood-volume dilution of the central veins. One port must be dedicated to exclusive use of TPN, whereas the remaining ports can be used for administering IV fluids and obtaining blood samples. When the central line is a single lumen, this lumen should be used exclusively for the infusion of TPN.

## Composition of Parenteral Nutrition Formulas

TPN formulas typically contain three primary macronutrients: carbohydrates, lipids (fats), and amino acids (protein). This combination is called a mixed fuel source. When all three fuel sources are combined in one TPN bag, it is often referred to as a "3-in-1" admixture. To maintain strict sterility, the desired proportions of these nutrients are prepared under a laminar flow hood by a pharmacist. Because of differences in pharmacy equipment used to mix TPN, some facilities infuse lipids separately, usually in a glass bottle. Medications are not to be added to a TPN bag after it has been prepared by the pharmacist because of the risk for contamination or precipitation of its contents. The current trend in TPN formulation is based on the specific needs of each patient; standard formulas are no longer widely prescribed.

**CARBOHYDRATES.** The primary source of energy in the body is carbohydrates (eg, dextrose). This macronutrient usually provides 40% to 60% of daily caloric requirements and is essential to central nervous system function. The most common and preferred source of carbohydrates is dextrose (D-glucose) because it is readily metabolized, stimulates the secretion of insulin, and is usually well tolerated in large quantities. Dextrose provides 3.4 kcal/g in IV form and contributes to most of the osmolality (or concentration) of the TPN solution. Initial TPN concentrations of dextrose may range from 50% to 70%, but final concentrations are diluted to approximately 25% to 30% after the addition of amino acids, lipid emulsions, and water.

Despite dilution, this concentration remains very high and requires delivery through a central venous catheter so that the higher blood volumes in the larger central veins are able to further dilute and disperse the solution. The superior vena cava is an excellent site for such delivery. Passage of a central venous catheter, by way of the subclavian vein into the superior vena cava, is the route of choice because it allows the patient the greatest freedom of movement without disturbing the insertion site. Jugular veins can also be used but may make it more difficult to keep dressings sterile, and these are not as comfortable for the patient because of limitations

in neck movement. Regardless of the site, strict adherence to insertion and infection protocols must be followed, and radiologic verification of catheter tip placement is necessary before initial infusion. (Refer to your institution's central line care and infection control policies and procedures.)

The amount of dextrose prescribed in TPN is based on metabolic needs, which, once met, allows utilization of amino acids for protein synthesis rather than solely as an energy source. Adults require a minimum of 100 g/d of dextrose to perform vital metabolic activities; however, the maximal dose of dextrose varies based on an individual's needs, medical condition, and glucose tolerance. Recommendations suggest that dextrose must not exceed 7 g/kg/d.[21] One of the most common metabolic side effects of excessive dextrose concentrations is hyperglycemia, which often requires the use of insulin. Relatively tight blood glucose control is recommended to prevent complications associated with hyperglycemia. A protocol for moderately strict control of serum glucose between a range of 100 and 150 mg/dL may be appropriate.[7,9] In addition, excessive dextrose administration may put certain patients, such as those with pulmonary compromise, at risk for carbon dioxide retention and subsequent respiratory acidosis. Because one of the end products of dextrose metabolism is carbon dioxide, elevated levels may increase minute ventilation and hence the work of breathing. Overfeeding carbohydrates may make ventilator weaning difficult, if not impossible.

**LIPIDS.** Parenteral IV lipids, or fat emulsions, primarily contain long-chain linoleic and α-linolenic acids (essential fatty acids) from safflower and soybean vegetable oils. Lipid solutions also contain egg yolk phospholipids as emulsifiers, so it is important to check for a food allergy history before administration. Lipids provide a concentrated source of calories, 9 kcal/g, and they are important in maintaining connective tissue integrity and preventing fatty acid deficiency. Symptoms of fatty acid deficiency include rough, dry, scaly skin; nasolabial seborrhea; dull or dry hair, soft or brittle nails, poor wound healing, and diarrhea. Accordingly, patients should receive 2% to 4% of their daily energy requirements as linoleic acid and 0.25% to 0.5% of their daily energy requirements from α-linolenic acid.[21] The usual prescriptive dose of lipid emulsion infusion is approximately 1.0 to 1.3 g/kg/d (not to exceed 2.5 g/kg/d) to supply up to 30% of the patient's caloric intake. Weekly administration of a 20% lipid emulsion (500 mL), however, is sufficient to prevent essential fatty acid deficiency in adults.[19,21]

Lipid emulsions are isotonic, and concentrations are available in 10%, 20%, and 30% solutions, providing 1.1, 2.0, and 2.9 kcal/mL, respectively.[20] The benefit of higher concentrations is that they provide a greater concentration of calories in less total fluid volume, an important consideration for many patients. In situations in which hyperglycemia has become problematic, dextrose solution concentrations and volumes may be reduced, and unless contraindicated, lipids concentrations and volumes can be increased. Lipids typically provide 15% to 30% of daily caloric intake; if delivery of lipids is higher than 30% of total caloric intake, vigilant monitoring for metabolic side effects is especially important. Baseline and weekly triglyceride trends monitor lipid tolerance. Elevated triglyceride levels exceeding 400 mg/dL suggest impaired lipid clearance and an increased risk for pancreatitis, so it is recommended that lipid emulsions be withheld until triglyceride levels return to normal.[22] Lipid concentrations may need to be adjusted for patients who may also be receiving additional lipids from sources other than TPN (eg, continuous infusion of propofol, a sedative delivered as a lipid emulsion). Lipid emulsions provide an excellent medium for bacterial growth, so increased manipulation and prolonged hang times are avoided. Adverse reactions to lipids include, but are not limited to, fever, chills, chest or back tightness, dyspnea, tachycardia, headache, nausea, and vomiting. If such reactions occur, the nurse stops the infusion immediately and reports the reaction to the physician and pharmacist. Long-term reactions to lipids include concerns over immune system suppression.[20] Before infusion, the nurse inspects lipid-containing TPN solutions for separation of the lipid solution, also known as cracking and coalescence. This loss of emulsion can be identified by yellow-brown marbling of the entire solution or as layering of oil at the surface of the TPN container. Such solutions are not safe for infusion and should be returned to the pharmacy for replacement.

**AMINO ACIDS.** All tissues require protein to maintain structure and facilitate wound healing. If protein intake is inadequate, the body becomes catabolic, seeking protein from skeletal muscle and vital organs. In TPN, protein is provided as a mixture of essential and nonessential crystalline amino acids, which are available in concentrations ranging from 5% to 15%. These concentrations supply approximately 15% to 20% of daily caloric needs. One gram of amino acids is equivalent to 1 g of protein, which provides 4 kcal/g. Adult amino acid requirements can range widely from 0.8 to 2.5 g/kg/d, and those patients with burns, wounds, draining fistulas, renal failure, or hepatic failure may need frequent adjustments in the amount of amino acids they receive.[19] For patients with renal disease, solutions with a higher concentration of essential amino acids are available. For patients with hepatic failure or hypercatabolic conditions, formulas with branched-chain amino acids may be used. These formulas spare the breakdown of other muscle proteins to use as energy, possibly reducing the incidence of hepatic encephalopathy.

**MICRONUTRIENTS.** Vitamins, trace minerals, and electrolytes are considered micronutrients. Unfortunately, the U.S. Recommended Dietary Allowance requirements do not apply to parenteral nutrition for several reasons. First, the liver and GI tract absorptive processes are bypassed, resulting in elimination of these micronutrients through the urine without their being utilized. Second, many diseases alter the gut's ability to absorb fat-soluble vitamins and vitamin $B_{12}$. Finally, many nutrients adhere to the plastic tubing and IV solution bags or are destroyed by exposure to light and oxygen (especially vitamin A) before reaching the bloodstream.

With these factors in mind, standard aqueous multivitamin preparations have been created and provide higher levels of thiamine, pyridoxine, ascorbic acid, and folic acid.[22] Unfortunately, hypermetabolic conditions of critical illness can exacerbate deficiencies that require additional monitoring and potential supplementation; individual vitamin products are available for supplements as needed. Until recently, vitamin K was the only vitamin not included in the multivitamin preparation; it is provided by adding up to 10 mg/wk of the vitamin to the TPN solution (unless contraindicated by

anticoagulation treatment). Because some parenteral formulas may now contain vitamin K, weekly supplementation is no longer necessary, but it is important to continue to monitor coagulation studies, especially if the patient is receiving anticoagulation treatment. Unlike patients who require additional nutrients, patients with liver or kidney disease may need to receive lower doses of certain vitamins.

Trace mineral elements are required to maintain biochemical homeostasis. They come in a variety of commercial mixtures but typically include chromium, copper, manganese, selenium, and zinc. Parenteral iron is not added to TPN solutions because of stability issues and the potential for adverse effects, and it may need to be supplemented in long-term therapy.

Most electrolyte standard mixtures contain sodium, potassium, calcium, magnesium, phosphorus, chloride, and acetate. Sodium bicarbonate is not added to TPN as precipitation with the other electrolytes may occur. Instead, acetate is used because it can be converted by the liver to bicarbonate. Depending on the patient's underlying disease process and physical assessment findings, specific electrolyte concentrations can be adjusted daily in the TPN solution. If an electrolyte deficiency is detected after the TPN solution has been prepared, or while infusing, additional IV supplements can be given separately by IV piggyback administration. Electrolyte supplements should never be added to the TPN bag after the pharmacist has formulated it because this would compromise the sterility of the solution and may cause the solution to precipitate.

**MEDICATIONS.** While preparing the TPN solution, the pharmacist can add medications, many of which are often necessitated by the TPN therapy itself. For instance, although insulin drips are now the current trend in managing hyperglycemia, insulin can be added to the TPN solution. Additionally, heparin can be added to reduce fibrin buildup along the catheter tip. The clinician ordering the medications consults with the pharmacist to ensure compatibility.

### Complications of Parenteral Nutrition

Complications can be divided into three main categories: metabolic, infectious, and mechanical.

**METABOLIC COMPLICATIONS.** TPN has been recognized as a cause of severe morbidity and life-threatening complications.[19] This is often related to the infusion amount and flow rate. Specific complications include hepatic steatosis (fatty liver), intrahepatic and extrahepatic cholestasis (suppression of bile flow), and cholelithiasis (formation of gallstones). Although the exact mechanisms of these hepatic disorders are not completely understood, it has been observed that cholestasis is less likely to occur if some form of enteral feeding is maintained.[23] GI atrophy, and all of its associated complications, may occur from disuse. If not contraindicated, oral or enteral feedings should be initiated as soon as possible.

It is important to understand that many metabolic complications stem from the patient's underlying disease processes or from imprudent formula administration. Some metabolic disturbances can be prevented by checking each bag of parenteral nutrition solution for transcription accuracy, monitoring the IV pump for infusion accuracy, and monitoring the patient's response to therapy. Virtually any metabolic disturbance can occur during parenteral nutrition infusion: the most common metabolic complications include hyperglycemia, hypoglycemia, hypophosphatemia, hypokalemia, hypomagnesemia, and hypocalcemia. These metabolic disturbances, coupled with rapid fluid shifts and imbalances, may lead to a disorder called refeeding syndrome, which is discussed later.

**Hyperglycemia.** Hyperglycemia, or a blood glucose elevated over 220 mg/dL, can occur if the pancreas does not respond to the increased glucose load. Although hyperglycemia can be caused by either enteral or parenteral feedings, it is more commonly seen in patients receiving parenteral nutrition. Even slightly elevated blood glucose levels can impair the function of lymphocytes, leading to immunosuppression and increased risk for infection. Elevated glucose concentrations have been shown to reduce neutrophil chemotaxis and phagocytosis and may be an independent risk factor for short-term infections.[6] If the renal threshold for glucose reabsorption is exceeded, osmotic diuresis results in subsequent dehydration and electrolyte imbalances. Glycemic control can be achieved by increasing the amount of insulin in the TPN solution, by maintaining a continuous insulin drip during TPN administration, or by administering sliding-scale insulin subcutaneously at regular intervals. Once TPN is discontinued, insulin requirements become notably less or nonexistent. If new TPN solution is temporarily unavailable, administration of 10% dextrose in water ($D_{10}W$) is recommended to prevent rebound hypoglycemia. In addition, if a solution is "behind schedule," the infusion rate should not be increased to make up time because this may cause sudden metabolic fluctuations and fluid overload.

**Refeeding Syndrome.** Refeeding syndrome is one of the most critical complications that occur with the initiation of TPN. This condition is characterized by rapid shifts in electrolytes (phosphorus, potassium, magnesium, and calcium), glucose, and volume status within hours to days of nutrition implementation. Parenterally delivered glucose loads stimulate insulin release, which in turn stimulates intracellular uptake of phosphorus, glucose, and other electrolytes for anabolic processes. Despite relatively normal serum phosphorus levels on standard laboratory reports, intracellular stores are markedly depleted in malnourished catabolic patients; severe hypophosphatemia (less than 1 mg/dL) can lead to neuromuscular, respiratory, and cardiac dysfunction. Low serum levels of potassium, magnesium, and calcium can precipitate cardiac dysrhythmias. The increased intravascular fluid volumes associated with parenteral nutrition can strain the viscerally depleted heart and possibly induce heart failure and myocardial damage. Risk factors for refeeding syndrome include marasmus, chronic alcoholism, anorexia nervosa, rapid refeeding, and excessive dextrose infusion.

Prevention of refeeding syndrome includes repletion of phosphorus, potassium, magnesium, and calcium before TPN initiation, limiting initial dextrose dosing, and titrating total volume and rate to evaluate for fluid overload and potential cardiac decompensation. Daily monitoring of phosphorous, potassium, and magnesium is recommended.[24] Weight-based phosphorus repletion algorithms (eg, 0.32 to 1.0 mmol/kg) have been shown to be highly efficacious in correcting hypophosphatemia during nutrition support therapy.[24] It is of paramount importance that the critical care nurse takes accurate intake and output measurements and daily weights because adequate parenteral nutrition often means giving 1.5 to 3 L of fluid/d in addition to other therapies. Progressive weight gain could be an early indicator of poor fluid tolerance.

**INFECTIOUS COMPLICATIONS.** Both the solution and the indwelling catheter are prime sites for infection because of the high glucose content. Any break in the system is a nidus for infection that can progress to a systemic infection if left unchecked. After initial preparation by a pharmacist, the access hubs on the bag of TPN are often covered with tape as a reminder that no additional solutions or medications are to be added.

At the bedside, the nurse changes the TPN solution bag and tubing according to institution policy, usually every 24 hours. He or she redresses the catheter insertion site per institution policy as well, usually every 24 to 72 hours, using either a sterile transparent or gauze dressing. Frequent dressing changes, however, have been shown to increase bacterial colonization. Fortunately, transparent dressings allow for easier observation of the catheter entrance site; visible inflammation indicates significant bacterial colonization and the need for prompt catheter removal.[25] It is important to check institutional policies and procedures regarding central and peripheral line dressing changes.

At the time of the dressing change, the nurse examines the site for signs of leakage, erythema, and/or inflammation, and then cleanses the site with an antibacterial solution to remove pathogenic organisms. Researchers have shown that chlorhexidine solution is a more effective local antiseptic than povidone–iodine solutions.[26,27] The use of impregnated chlorhexidine/silver sulfadiazine or minocycline/rifampin catheters could reduce the incidence of central venous catheter–related infections.[28] The presence of a tracheostomy or other open draining wounds near the IV insertion site requires special precautions to prevent site contamination.

Potential for infection can be minimized by meticulous catheter care. In critically ill patients, catheter-related infections range from local inflammation to systemic bloodstream infection and sepsis. Central venous catheters are a leading source of nosocomial bloodstream infection with an estimated 10% mortality.[25] If fever, rigors, or chills coincide with parenteral infusion, catheter-related sepsis should be suspected; slowing or stopping the infusion may cause fever to abate. Treatment of an infection may involve local topical antibiotics, systemic antibiotics, and, in many cases, catheter removal. If catheter sepsis is suspected, the catheter tip is usually cultured to identify the offending organism to ensure appropriate antibiotic coverage.

**MECHANICAL COMPLICATIONS.** Mechanical complications include those associated with central venous catheter insertion, such as trauma to the vessel, pneumothorax, catheter occlusion, thrombosis, and venous air embolism. After insertion of a central catheter, a chest radiograph is the standard method of confirming correct placement. If there is a clinical suspicion of catheter tip migration or other potential complications, further diagnostic testing is indicated.

Trauma to vessels and pneumothorax are complications that may warrant surgical intervention, insertion of a chest tube or tubes, or both. Catheter occlusion can simply be a result of the catheter tip lodging against the vessel wall or being physiologically "pinched" between the clavicle and first rib. Occlusion can also occur from fibrin buildup, blood or lipid deposition, drug precipitates, and catheter breakage. Another type of occlusion, "withdrawal occlusion," is an occlusion that allows infusion of a solution but prevents blood withdrawal. The addition of 6,000 units of heparin in the daily parenteral formula in hospitalized patients with temporary catheters reduces the risk of fibrin sheath formation and catheter infection.[4] Thrombosis formation in the lumen of the vessel often results from mechanical irritation (such as from traumatic catheter insertion), a small lumen, an extended duration of catheter use, the catheter material, or malpositioning. Nurses need to be aware that patients may have a thrombosis and may be asymptomatic, yet complain of vague head and eye swelling on the affected side. Vigilant assessments during parenteral nutrition administration are recommended. Treatment includes catheter removal, systemic anticoagulation, and thrombolytic therapy.

A venous air embolism is another serious complication; rapid introduction of air into the venous circulation can be fatal.[29] In a review of all patients in the literature with a cerebral air embolism associated with central venous catheters from 1975 to 1988, 54% occurred secondary to disconnection of the catheter, 31% occurred during removal of the catheter, and 15% occurred during insertion.[29] Any disruption of the closed catheter system (usually during line connection changes, when hanging a new bag of TPN, or in an accidental tubing disconnection) can increase the risk for an air embolism. If such an incident occurs, the patient will most likely experience acute, centrally located chest pain, dyspnea, and hypotension. Immediate nursing interventions include clamping the tubing of the catheter or occluding the catheter hub, attempting to aspirate air directly from the venous line (ie, for patients who have central venous access properly placed in the right atrium, attempts may be made to aspirate air bubbles from the distal port), administering 100% oxygen via a facemask, and positioning the patient head down on the left side (Durant's maneuver).[29] This position allows air to rise to the level of the right ventricle, away from the pulmonary vasculature. Prevention of an air embolism can be facilitated by having the patient perform the Valsalva maneuver or simply hum audibly during line changes. In ventilator-dependent patients, positive intrathoracic pressure can be created by initiating mechanical lung inflations or "breaths." Finally, use of sterile occlusive dressings (eg, petrolatum gauze) over the catheter entrance site is an effective measure in preventing air from entering the track after the catheter has been removed.

### Tapering Parenteral Nutrition

Tapering (gradually reducing) TPN is often initiated for those patients who are able to resume safely (and tolerate) approximately 50% to 75% of their nutritional needs by enteral or oral nutrition. In such instances, a calorie count is essential to be certain that the patient's nutritional needs are being met. If the parenteral nutrition needs to be interrupted or is to be discontinued, the infusion rate is decreased by half for 30 to 60 minutes. This allows for a plasma glucose response and prevention of rebound hypoglycemia.[30] Checking blood glucose levels for 30 to 60 minutes after discontinuation helps the nurse identify and manage immediate glucose abnormalities.

In situations in which poor prognosis does not warrant aggressive nutritional support, emotional and ethical dilemmas may surface for many nurses because feeding and hydration have long been basic tenets of nursing care. Although many institutions may have protocols in place regarding parenteral nutrition, treatment decisions and plans of care should be discussed on an individual basis. Frequent, ongoing discussions between the patient, family, and the health care team are imperative to providing the best possible care to each patient.

## Role of the Nurse in Nutritional Support

Nurses are responsible for obtaining initial "dry weight" and weekly weight measurements, vital signs, intake and output measurements, and laboratory data and for providing enteral tube and IV catheter care throughout the duration of nutrition support therapies. Many complications, whether from enteral or parenteral nutrition, can be prevented by vigilant observation and care. If the patient is awake and alert, the patient's subjective assessment of tolerance can be very informative. The nurse obtains more objective signs of feeding tolerance through abdominal examinations, which assess bowel sounds and changes in abdominal girth. Also, the nurse monitors and records volume and frequency of both urine and stool.

The nurse must also monitor for clinical signs of dehydration (thirst, dry mucous membranes, tachycardia, and poor skin turgor) and fluid excess (peripheral edema and adventitious lung sounds). Early detection and subsequent interventions may prevent the occurrence of excessive fluid shifts and cardiac compromise. This is of special concern if the patient is severely malnourished, which may precipitate refeeding syndrome and other untoward complications. Meticulous feeding tube and IV catheter care are critical to preventing local and systemic forms of infection.

Care also includes providing information and emotional support to the patient and family. Examples include explaining the procedure, what to expect, risks, and expected outcomes (Box 40-2).

## Pharmacologic Management of Gastrointestinal Disorders

Pharmacologic agents from several drug classes are used to manage patients with gastrointestinal disorders. Antacids help neutralize gastric acid and some also reduce pepsin while others bind phosphates in the GI tract. Histamine type 2 receptor antagonists inhibit histamine at the receptor sites on gastric parietal cells, which inhibits gastric acid secretion. Proton pump inhibitors are used to suppress gastric acid secretion. Laxatives work by either increasing water absorption into the intestinal lumen or by increasing peristalsis. Antiemetics act by inhibiting the chemoreceptor trigger zone, which inhibits the vomiting center or block serotonin receptors in the chemoreceptor trigger zone and GI tract.

| BOX 40-2 | *TEACHING GUIDE* | *Living With Nutritional Support* |

**General Care: Enteral Nutrition**
- Administer enteral formulas as prescribed.
- Know potential complications and appropriate treatments.
- Avoid activities that may result in high impact or stress at the insertion site and report any activity that may have damaged the enteral access site.
- Return to previous activities (eg, work, leisure, sexual activity) after obtaining physician consent.

**General Care: Parenteral Nutrition**
- Administer parenteral formulas as prescribed.
- Monitor blood glucose levels closely to help determine tolerance for parenteral solutions.
- Know the potential complications and appropriate treatments.
- Avoid activities that may result in high impact or stress at the insertion site and report any activity that may have damaged the parenteral access site.
- Return to previous activities (eg, work, leisure, sexual activity) after obtaining physician consent.

**Signs of Infections**
- Understand the rationale for aseptic technique.
- Notify the nurse of symptoms of fever, localized warmth, redness, pain, or drainage at the feeding tube or IV insertion site.

**Medications**
- Follow instructions regarding medications.
- Know the names of medications and the dose, frequency of administration, side effects, and use of each medication.
- Know the proper technique of administering medications through the feeding tube and proper flushing technique.
- Never add medications to TPN solutions—they should be added by the supplier because of risk for contamination or precipitation of the formula.

**Safety Measures**
- Inform other health care providers about enteral or parenteral access devices and notify them about any medications that the patient may be taking.

**Follow-Up Care**
- Report any problems to the home care nurse.
- Adhere to schedule for follow-up visits with patient's physician or clinic.
- Ensure that patient/caregiver learning includes determining procedures and risks, identifying patient and equipment problems early, troubleshooting, and following up with the health care provider.
- Refer to and communicate with home care services.
- Provide written instructions for patient.
- If possible, do not change the amount or rate of nutrition support on the day of discharge to home.

## Clinical Applicability Challenges

### CASE STUDY

Mrs. R., a 71-year-old morbidly obese woman with poorly controlled Type II diabetes, hypertension, and hypercholesterolemia presents with symptomatic hypoglycemia 1 month after placement of her gastrostomy feeding tube. The feeding tube was placed after a stroke that left her with mild right-sided hemiplegia and dysphagia. Upon questioning, you discover that Mrs. R. was experiencing "high" GRVs of approximately 150 mL before the next scheduled administration of her tube feeding. Although Mrs. R. continued to administer her medications as scheduled (to include her subcutaneous insulin), she had held her scheduled tube feeding. She also indicated that she

was trying to "lose weight and increase her physical activity," so she felt that holding a few doses of her tube feedings would help "speed up" her weight loss.

1. Why might Mrs. R. have residual volume in her stomach?
2. What interventions (medication- and nonmedication-related) could be considered for Mrs. R.?
3. What teaching or education would be required for Mrs. R. so that she does not experience hypoglycemia again? What other related teaching or education is required?

### WANT TO KNOW MORE?

A wide variety of resources to enhance your learning and understanding of this chapter are available on thePoint.

You will find:
- References
- Selected readings
- NCLEX-style review questions
- Internet resources
- And more!

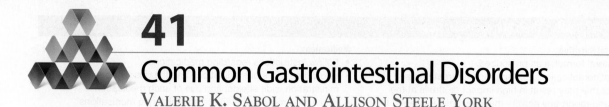

# 41

# Common Gastrointestinal Disorders

VALERIE K. SABOL AND ALLISON STEELE YORK

## LEARNING OBJECTIVES

**Based on the content in this chapter, the reader should be able to:**

1. Examine the pathophysiologic concepts that help define acute gastrointestinal bleeding (GIB), intestinal obstruction and ileus, acute pancreatitis (AP), hepatitis, complications of liver disease, and obesity.

2. Compare and contrast the pertinent history, physical examination, and diagnostic study findings for acute GIB, intestinal obstruction and ileus, AP, hepatitis, complications of liver disease, and obesity.

3. Discuss laboratory studies that are useful in the diagnosis and management of acute GIB, intestinal obstruction and ileus, AP, hepatitis, complications of liver disease, and obesity.

4. Analyze the similarities and differences in caring for patients with acute GIB, intestinal obstruction and ileus, hepatitis, complications of liver disease, and obesity.

5. Explore the nursing role in assessing, managing, and evaluating a plan of care for patients with acute GIB, intestinal obstruction and ileus, AP, hepatitis, complications of liver disease, and obesity.

The critical care nurse will inevitably provide care for patients with common yet serious disorders of the gastrointestinal (GI) tract. Some of these disorders include gastrointestinal bleeding (GIB), intestinal obstructions, and complex inflammations, such as pancreatitis and hepatitis. In addition, the critical care nurse will often have to manage patients who are obese, both postoperatively after bariatric surgery and as a general comorbidity.

## Acute Gastrointestinal Bleeding

Acute GIB is a common, and potentially lethal, medical emergency seen in people admitted to the intensive care unit (ICU). The incidence of upper GIB is 50 to 150 per 100,000 admissions per year.[1,2] The mortality rate associated with acute GIB has remained constant over the past half century despite advances in diagnosis and treatment. This constant mortality rate may result from the prevalence of comorbid disease in older adults and the widespread use of nonsteroidal anti-inflammatory drugs (NSAIDs). The cause of death is rarely from exsanguination but rather from the exacerbation of other medical illnesses. Prompt recognition and treatment of patients experiencing acute GIB requires a team approach.

Acute GIB is differentiated into upper and lower GIB. The ligament of Treitz at the junction of the duodenum and jejunum is the anatomic division between the upper and lower GI tracts. Upper GIB occurs from a source in the esophagus, stomach, or duodenum. Lower GIB occurs from a source in the jejunum, ileum, colon, or rectum. GIB from a lower GI source is less common than upper GIB.

### Upper Gastrointestinal Bleeding

#### Etiology

The possible causes of acute upper GIB are listed in Box 41-1. A complete discussion of this list is beyond the scope of this chapter. The most commonly seen causes of acute GIB in the ICU are discussed in the following sections. See Spotlight on Genetics 41-1 for a discussion of Crohn disease.

---

**BOX 41-1** | **Common Causes of Acute Gastrointestinal Bleeding (GIB)**

**Upper Gastrointestinal Bleeding**

*Esophageal Source*
- Varices
- Esophagitis
- Ulcers
- Tumors
- Mallory–Weiss tears

*Gastric Source*
- Peptic ulcers
- Gastritis
- Tumors
- Angiodysplasia
- Dieulafoy lesions

*Duodenal Source*
- Peptic ulcers
- Angiodysplasia
- Crohn disease
- Meckel diverticulum

**Lower Gastrointestinal Bleeding**
- Malignant tumors
- Polyps
- Ulcerative colitis
- Crohn disease
- Ischemic colitis
- Infectious colitis
- Angiodysplasia
- Diverticulosis
- Hemorrhoids
- Massive upper gastrointestinal hemorrhage

---

## GI SYSTEM—CROHN DISEASE

- Crohn disease is a complex, chronic disorder that primarily affects the digestive system. This condition typically involves abnormal inflammation of the intestinal walls, particularly in the lower part of the small intestine and portions of the large intestine and is most common in western Europe and North America, where it affects 100 to 150 in 100,000 people.
- The *IL23R* gene is associated with Crohn disease, and a variety of genetic and environmental factors likely play a role in causing Crohn disease. Although researchers are studying risk factors that may contribute to this complex disorder, many of these factors remain unknown.
- Crohn disease may result from a combination of certain genetic variations, changes in the immune system, and the presence of bacteria in the digestive tract. Recent studies have identified variations in specific genes, including *ATG16L1*, *IL23R*, *IRGM*, and *NOD2*, that influence the risk of developing Crohn disease. These genes provide instructions for making proteins that are involved in immune system function. Variations in any of these genes may disrupt the ability of cells in the intestine to respond normally to bacteria. An abnormal immune response to bacteria in the intestinal walls may lead to chronic inflammation and the digestive problems characteristic of Crohn disease.
- Sequence analysis of the entire coding region or targeted mutation analysis is available in the diagnosis of Crohn disease.

Data from Genetic Home Reference. Retrieved August 10, 2015, from http://ghr.nlm.nih.gov; and Palmieri O, Creanza TM, Bossa F, et al: Genome-wide pathway analysis using gene expression data of colonic mucosa in patients with inflammatory bowel disease. Inflamm Bowel Dis 21(6):1260–1268, 2015.

**PEPTIC ULCER DISEASE.** Peptic ulcer disease, which includes both gastric and duodenal ulcers, accounts for approximately 40% to 60% of acute upper GIB.[1–3] The epithelial cells of the gastroduodenal mucosa are protected from the potentially damaging effects of gastric secretions, medications, alcohol, and bacteria by several protective mechanisms. These cells secrete mucins, phospholipids, and bicarbonate, which create a pH gradient between the acidic gastric lumen and the cell surface. Prostaglandins enhance this mucosal protection by increasing mucosal secretion, increasing bicarbonate production, maintaining mucosal blood flow, and enhancing the resistance of gastroduodenal cells to injury. In addition, the tight junctions of the epithelial cells resist diffusion. When these protective factors are overwhelmed by aggressive factors, the integrity of the gastric or duodenal mucosa is interrupted, which can result in peptic ulcer disease. Bleeding from peptic ulcer disease occurs when the ulcer erodes into the wall of a blood vessel.

The primary risk factor for peptic ulcer disease is infection with the bacterium *Helicobacter pylori*. *H. pylori* infection has been associated with 90% of duodenal ulcers and 75% of gastric ulcers. *H. pylori* is a gram-negative, spiral, flagellated rod that colonizes the mucous layer overlying the gastric epithelium. The flagellum of *H. pylori* facilitates the bacterium's ability to move and adhere to the mucous layer. *H. pylori* produces urease, which converts urea to ammonia and carbon dioxide. The ammonia buffers the acid surrounding the bacterium, creating a more hospitable environment that allows the bacterium to thrive in the acidic stomach. *H. pylori* infection predisposes the mucosa to damage by disrupting the mucous layer, liberating enzymes and toxins, and adhering to the epithelium. Inflammation is furthered by a host immune response. This chronic inflammation usually results in an asymptomatic chronic gastritis. However, in some instances, ulceration develops.

In the absence of *H. pylori* infection, the ingestion of aspirin or NSAIDs accounts for most cases of peptic ulcer disease. Aspirin and NSAIDs may directly injure the mucosal layer by enhancing mucosal permeability and allowing back-diffusion of acid. Systemic effects of chronic aspirin or NSAID use include inhibition of prostaglandin synthesis by the gastroduodenal mucosa, which decreases production of mucus and bicarbonate and also decreases mucosal blood flow. This alteration in mucosal cytoprotection may lead to the development of an ulcer. Upper GIB related to NSAIDs is more common in older patients. Cigarette smoking may also predispose individuals to peptic ulcer disease, and it is linked to prolonged healing rates and high ulcer recurrence.

**STRESS-RELATED EROSIVE SYNDROME.** Stress-related erosive syndrome, also called erosive gastritis, stress ulceration, and hemorrhagic gastritis, is a common cause of acute GIB in critically ill patients. Stress ulcers are different from the ulcers of peptic ulcer disease; they tend to be more numerous, shallower, and more diffuse. These ulcers may develop in the stomach, duodenum, and esophagus within hours of injury. They are usually shallow and cause oozing from superficial capillaries but may erode into the submucosa and cause massive hemorrhage.

The risk of developing a stress ulcer depends on the severity and type of illness (Box 41-2). The common feature of the risk factors is physiologic stress. Decreased perfusion of the stomach mucosa is probably the main mechanism of ulcer development. This decreased perfusion contributes to impaired secretion of mucus, low mucosal pH, poor mucosal cell regeneration, and decreased tolerance to acidic gastric secretions.

**ESOPHAGEAL VARICES.** Portal hypertension usually develops as a result of cirrhosis, from increased resistance in the portal venous system caused by disruption of the normal liver lobular structure. This resistance impedes blood flow into, through, and out of the liver. In response to portal

**QSEN BOX 41-2** *PATIENT SAFETY*

### Risk Factors for Stress-Related Erosive Syndrome
- Hypotension or shock
- Coagulopathy
- Respiratory failure requiring mechanical ventilation
- Sepsis
- Hepatic failure
- Renal failure
- Multiple or severe trauma
- Burns over 35% of the total body surface area
- Post–organ transplantation status
- Head or spinal cord injury
- History of peptic ulcer disease or upper GIB
- Prolonged stay in intensive care unit

hypertension, collateral veins develop to bypass the increased portal resistance in an attempt to return blood to systemic circulation. As pressure rises in these veins, they become tortuous and distended, forming varicose veins or varices.

Esophageal varices account for 5% to 20% of acute upper GIB.[1,3] Varices are present in 50% of patients with cirrhosis, and approximately 30% will experience variceal bleeding within the first year of diagnosis.[4] Varices may develop in the esophagus, stomach, duodenum, colon, rectum, or anus. The most clinically significant site of varices is the gastroesophageal junction because of the propensity of varices in this area to rupture, resulting in massive GI hemorrhage. The mortality rate associated with variceal bleeding is 15% with rebleeding up to 33%.[5]

**MALLORY–WEISS TEARS.** Mallory–Weiss tears account for 8% to 15% of acute upper GIB.[2,3] These lacerations occur in the distal esophagus, at the gastroesophageal junction, and in the cardia of the stomach. Bleeding from Mallory–Weiss tears occurs when the tear involves the underlying venous or arterial bed. Mallory–Weiss tears are strongly associated with heavy alcohol use or recent binge drinking and a prior history of forceful vomiting or retching, or violent coughing. Patients with portal hypertension have an increased risk for bleeding from Mallory–Weiss tears.

**DIEULAFOY LESIONS.** Dieulafoy lesions are vascular malformations of unusually large submucosal arteries that lie in close contact with the mucosal surface. They can be found anywhere in the GI tract but most often occur in the proximal stomach. Because of the large size of the artery, bleeding from a Dieulafoy lesion may be massive and recurrent. When bleeding ceases, a Dieulafoy lesion can be difficult to identify because there is no associated ulcer, and it is likely to be the origin of many upper GIBs of unknown cause.

### Clinical Presentation

Regardless of the cause, patients with acute upper GIB have a clinical presentation consistent with the amount of blood loss. A patient's response to blood loss depends on the amount and rate of blood loss, age, degree of compensation, comorbidities, and rapidity of treatment. Patients with minimal loss may present with anemia and no further symptoms, whereas patients with rapid and severe loss may present with signs and symptoms of shock. If blood loss is moderate, the sympathetic nervous system responds with a release of the catecholamines epinephrine and norepinephrine, which initially cause an increase in heart rate and peripheral vascular vasoconstriction in an attempt to maintain an adequate blood pressure. Orthostatic changes (a decrease in blood pressure greater than 10 mm Hg with a corresponding heart rate increase of 20 beats/min in the sitting or standing position) imply volume depletion of 15% or more.

With severe blood loss, signs and symptoms of shock appear. The release of catecholamines triggers the blood vessels in the skin, lungs, intestines, liver, and kidneys to constrict, thereby increasing the volume of blood flow to the brain and heart. Because of the decreased flow of blood in the skin, the patient's skin is cool to the touch. With decreased blood flow to the lungs, hyperventilation occurs to maintain adequate gas exchange.

The classic hallmarks of GIB are hematemesis, hematochezia, and melena. Patients with upper GIB usually present with hematemesis, the vomiting of fresh, unaltered blood or "coffee-ground" material; melena, the passage of foul-smelling, black, tarry, sticky stool; or both. A patient who presents with hematemesis is usually bleeding from a source above the ligament of Treitz. Reverse peristalsis is seldom sufficient to cause hematemesis if the bleeding point is below this area. The classic coffee-ground emesis associated with upper GIB results from the partial decomposition of the blood from contact with gastric secretions. Gastric acid converts bright red hemoglobin to brown hematin, accounting for the coffee-ground appearance of the drainage. Maroon or bright red blood results from profuse bleeding and little contact with gastric juices.

Melena is black from the breakdown of the blood in transit and suggests a long transit time through the GI tract. Melena is indicative of upper GIB in most cases. It may take several days after bleeding cessation for melenic stools to clear. After upper GIB, Hemoccult stool test results may remain positive for 1 to 2 weeks. Melena should not be confused with greenish stool that results from iron ingestion or black stool caused by the ingestion of bismuth subsalicylate (Pepto-Bismol).

Hematochezia, the passage of maroon or bright red blood that may be mixed with stool, usually indicates bleeding from a lower GI source. Uncommonly, hematochezia can occur in the setting of massive, rapid hemorrhage from the upper GI tract, where the large amount of blood acts as a cathartic, resulting in rapid transit through the GI tract.

Occult GIB refers to small amounts of blood loss, which is not apparent to the patient. Obscure GIB refers to obvious bleeding with no easily identifiable source on routine examination.

### Assessment

**HISTORY.** A prompt, careful, focused history may suggest the underlying cause of GIB. A history of epigastric pain or dyspepsia or a medical history of peptic ulcer disease is suggestive of peptic ulcer disease. A medical history of GIB should be elicited because most upper GI bleeds rebleed from the same site. Heavy alcohol use increases the likelihood of cirrhosis and bleeding from esophageal varices. Patients with a history of tobacco use have a greater risk for duodenal ulcers. Underlying medical conditions may suggest an underlying cause; patients with renal failure frequently bleed from arteriovenous malformations. Vomiting, coughing, or retching before bleeding suggests a Mallory–Weiss tear. Prior use of NSAIDs or aspirin increases the risk for gastroduodenal ulcers and the likelihood of bleeding from these ulcers.

**PHYSICAL EXAMINATION.** The physical examination is directed initially to the assessment of hemodynamic stability with ongoing assessment of vital signs. Tachycardia and orthostatic hypotension indicate dehydration secondary to blood loss or vomiting. Orthostatic hypotension, syncope, lightheadedness, and tachycardia are suggestive of a greater than 15% blood volume loss and are predictive of a poor outcome. If 40% of blood volume is lost, hypotension and hypovolemia occur, with decreased perfusion of the brain and heart. Therefore, assessing for signs and symptoms of poor tissue perfusion, such as angina, cyanosis, and altered mental status, is important. A baseline electrocardiogram is critical in patients with known cardiac disease because blood loss may precipitate cardiac ischemia. A loss of circulating blood volume may also result in decreased cerebral perfusion. The nurse should be alert to signs of agitation or confusion, which may signal cerebral hypoperfusion. The abdomen is assessed for bowel sounds; abdominal tenderness; the presence of guarding, rigidity, or abdominal masses; and the stigmata of liver disease. Splenomegaly, ascites, and caput medusae suggest liver disease. A tender, board-like abdomen is suggestive of peritonitis, possibly as a result of perforation. A rectal examination is essential to assess for hematochezia and melena.

**LABORATORY STUDIES.** Laboratory studies can help determine the extent of bleeding and can often provide a clue to the etiology. Common laboratory abnormalities for the patient with acute GIB are listed in Box 41-3. The initial hematocrit and hemoglobin may not accurately reflect initial blood loss because plasma volume is lost in the same proportion as red blood cells (RBCs). Within 24 to 48 hours of the initial bleeding, redistribution of plasma from the extravascular to the intravascular space results in a decreased hematocrit. Fluids administered during resuscitation contribute to the hemodilution. Leukocytosis and hyperglycemia may reflect the body's response to stress. Hypokalemia and hypernatremia may result from loss through emesis. An elevated blood urea nitrogen (BUN) level reflects a large protein load from the breakdown of blood. A high BUN/creatinine ratio suggests an upper GI source of bleeding.[2] Coagulopathy with a prolonged prothrombin time (PT) can indicate liver disease or concurrent long-term anticoagulant therapy. Thrombocytopenia may be present in patients with cirrhosis and portal hypertension with splenomegaly. If large amounts of blood are lost, metabolic acidosis occurs as a result of anaerobic metabolism. Severe blood loss can result in hypoxemia because of decreased circulating hemoglobin with impairment of oxygen transport to cells.

### Management

**RESUSCITATION.** The initial management of any patient with acute upper GIB is directed at fluid resuscitation to reverse the effects of blood loss. Supplemental oxygen is provided to any patient with acute GIB to promote oxygen saturation and transport as well as to prevent ischemia and dysrhythmias. Intubation may be required for actively bleeding patients at high risk for aspiration, those with a diminished mental status, and those in respiratory distress. Patients with acute upper GIB should be given nothing by mouth (NPO) because urgent endoscopy or surgery may be

---

**BOX 41-3** Typical Laboratory Abnormalities in a Patient With Acute Gastrointestinal Bleeding

- Decreased hemoglobin and hematocrit
- Mild leukocytosis and hyperglycemia
- Elevated blood urea nitrogen (BUN) level
- Hypernatremia
- Hypokalemia
- Prolonged prothrombin time (PT)/partial thromboplastin time (PTT)
- Thrombocytopenia
- Hypoxemia

---

required. A Foley catheter is inserted to monitor urine output as an indication of the adequacy of fluid resuscitation. All patients with hemodynamic instability, a drop in hematocrit, transfusion requirements greater than 2 units of packed red blood cells (PRBCs), or active bleeding may warrant an ICU admission.

**Volume Resuscitation.** Patients with acute GIB require immediate intravenous (IV) access with at least two large-bore (14- to 16-gauge) IV catheters or central access. A type and cross-match should be sent early in the course of the bleeding because blood losses of greater than 1,500 mL require blood replacement in addition to fluids. While awaiting cross-matched blood, lactated Ringer or normal saline solution is infused to restore circulating volume and to prevent the progression to hypovolemic shock. PRBCs should be transfused for a hemoglobin of 7 g/dL or less to reestablish the oxygen-carrying capacity of the blood.[1,2,5] Other blood products, such as platelets and clotting factors, are ordered according to results of laboratory tests and the patient's underlying condition. Calcium replacement may be necessary if large numbers of banked RBCs are transfused because the citrate in banked blood products can bind calcium and lead to hypocalcemia. A pulmonary artery catheter or central venous catheter may be useful to help avoid overresuscitation in patients with underlying renal or cardiac disease. In patients with a coagulopathy, vitamin K can be given in the form of phytonadione (Aqua MEPHYTON), 10 mg intramuscularly or very slowly IV, in an attempt to restore the PT to normal. For patients receiving anticoagulants, correction of coagulopathy is recommended but should not delay endoscopy. Fresh frozen plasma is ordered to correct the abnormality if rapid correction of the abnormality is warranted.

Vasoactive drugs may be used until fluid balance is restored to maintain blood pressure and perfusion to vital body organs. Dopamine, epinephrine, or norepinephrine may be ordered to stabilize the patient until definitive treatment can be undertaken.

**Nasogastric Intubation.** A large-bore nasogastric tube is placed in all patients with GIB to aspirate and lavage gastric contents. A nasogastric tube documents the presence and activity of bleeding. The color of gastric aspirate is prognostically significant. Coffee-ground or black nasogastric drainage with melenic stools indicates a slow bleed, whereas bright red nasogastric drainage and bright red blood in the stools signify a rapidly bleeding upper GI source.

A nasogastric tube is also useful for decompression and lavage. Lavage helps clear blood from the stomach, which allows better visualization to identify the source of bleeding during endoscopy. Iced lavage should be avoided because it is uncomfortable, fails to control bleeding, can significantly decrease core body temperature, and can trigger cardiac dysrhythmias. Lavage should be performed with tap water or saline. A total of 250 to 500 mL is instilled through the nasogastric tube and then removed with a syringe or by intermittent wall suction until gastric secretions are clear. Nasogastric tubes are usually removed after lavage of stomach contents unless the patient is actively bleeding or is experiencing severe nausea and vomiting because a nasogastric tube may injure the gastric mucosa and contribute to bleeding.

**Acid-Suppressive Therapy.** Acid impairs platelet aggregation and clot formation and promotes fibrinolysis.[1] Patients with acute upper GIB should be treated with acid-suppressive therapy to decrease the risk for recurrent bleeding, particularly from peptic ulcers. High-dose proton pump inhibitors (PPIs) (omeprazole, lansoprazole, esomeprazole, pantoprazole, rabeprazole) should be used to maintain a gastric pH greater than 6.0. PPI therapy should be maintained for at least 72 hours after hemostasis has been achieved to prevent lysis of clots.[3] PPI therapy can be given either IV or PO. In the United States, both pantoprazole and esomeprazole are available for IV infusion.

Acid-suppressive therapy with histamine (H$_2$)-antagonistic drugs (H2RAs) (cimetidine, ranitidine, famotidine, nizatidine) is not recommended for patients with acute nonvariceal bleeding. H2RAs may be used as prophylactic therapy in patients at high risk for stress-related erosive syndrome, but their use is limited by the rapid development of tolerance.

Antacids may also be ordered, but their use is limited because of frequent dosing requirements and potential side effects. Antacids act as a direct alkaline buffer and are administered to control gastric pH. Sucralfate, a basic aluminum salt of sucrose octasulfate, acts locally as a cytoprotective drug and can be ordered for stress-related erosive syndrome prophylaxis.

**Pharmacotherapy for Decreasing Portal Hypertension.** Even before a bleeding source is identified, decreasing portal pressure with vasopressin or octreotide should be considered for patients in whom variceal hemorrhage is suspected. Vasopressin (Pitressin) decreases portal hypertension by constriction of the splanchnic arteries, which reduces portal blood flow. Vasopressin should be administered through a central line. Complications of vasopressin therapy can limit its use. Vasopressin reduces coronary blood flow and increases blood pressure, which increases oxygen demand, and causes coronary artery constriction, which can potentially result in multiple cardiac dysrhythmias. Because vasopressin also reduces blood flow to the mesenteric circulation, bowel ischemia can develop. To minimize these potential side effects, vasopressin should be given concurrently with IV, sublingual, or topical nitroglycerin, which reduces its systemic effects.

Somatostatin is a natural polypeptide that lowers portal venous pressure by vasoconstriction of splanchnic circulation. Somatostatin causes selective vasoconstriction of the splanchnic circulation and is associated with fewer systemic side effects than vasopressin. IV infusion is necessary because of its short half-life.

Octreotide (Sandostatin), a synthetic analog of somatostatin with similar hemodynamic properties but a longer half-life, is available in the United States. Octreotide causes a decrease in splanchnic blood flow with a resultant decrease in intravariceal pressure, decreases secretion of gastric acid and pepsin, and stimulates mucous production. Octreotide is usually given as a 50 to 100 mcg IV bolus followed by 50 mcg/h for 3 to 5 days. The effects of octreotide are similar to vasopressin with concurrent nitroglycerin infusion without the impact on hemodynamics or cardiac output.

**DEFINITIVE DIAGNOSIS.** After patients with acute upper GIB are resuscitated, endoscopy is considered. Endoscopy can be performed urgently at the bedside and is the procedure of choice for the diagnosis and treatment of acute upper GIB. Endoscopy within 12 to 24 hours of the initial bleeding has the best results. Early endoscopy is essential in acute GIB because the treatment is directed by the cause. Endoscopy

allows the identification of the bleeding site the majority of the time because direct mucosal inspection is possible. The patient's hemodynamic status and endoscopic appearance provide prognostic value. The presence of active bleeding, a nonbleeding visible vessel, nonbleeding and oozing ulcer indicate a high risk for of rebleeding with medical therapy alone.[3] Vital signs must be monitored closely during endoscopy. The left lateral decubitus position decreases the risk for aspiration from active bleeding.

When diagnostic endoscopy is unsuccessful because of massive hemorrhage, angiography can be used to define the site of bleeding or abnormal vasculature. Angiography can detect bleeding rates as low as 0.5 to 1.0 mL/min.[6] Angiography is insensitive in the detection of venous bleeding.

Barium studies, such as an upper GI series, are of no value in acute upper GIB. These studies lack therapeutic capability and preclude endoscopy and angiography because of retained barium. Barium studies are also often inconclusive if there are clots or superficial bleeding in the stomach.

**THERAPEUTIC INTERVENTION.** In addition to its use in diagnosis, endoscopy is the procedure of choice for treating a GIB. If this fails to meet the needs of the patient, then additional therapeutic options are available.

**Endoscopy.** In the majority of cases, endoscopic therapy results in hemostasis, although 25% of high-risk sites may rebleed.[3] Multiple therapeutic options are available, including injection sclerotherapy, thermal coagulation, the placement of hemostatic clips, and endoscopic variceal ligation (EVL). The optimal technique depends on multiple variables, including the type and appearance of the lesion and the experience of the endoscopist.

The primary methods of endoscopic control of upper GI hemorrhage from peptic ulcers include injection therapy and thermal methods. Injection therapy consists of the injection of an agent such as epinephrine around and into the bleeding vessel. Thermal methods include heater probe and bipolar electrocoagulation (where a probe is applied with pressure to heat and seal the bleeding vessel). Hemostatic clips, called endoclips, have also been used successfully to ligate bleeding blood vessels within a lesion.

EVL is the treatment of choice for variceal bleeding. In EVL, a rubber band is placed endoscopically around the base of each varix. This causes coagulative necrosis and sloughing of thrombosed varices. EVL can control acute variceal bleeding in most case although there is a 60% change of rebleeding in the first year.[5] An alternative to EVL is sclerotherapy. Injection sclerotherapy involves injecting the varices with a sclerosing agent to stop the bleeding. These agents cause local tamponade and vasoconstriction, causing necrosis and eventual sclerosis of the bleeding vessel. Acute hemostasis rates are similar to those with EVL, but sclerotherapy is associated with a higher complication rate.

**Angiography.** Most cases of GIB resolve spontaneously or can be controlled during endoscopy. However, those patients with persistent bleeding may require angiography to control the source of bleeding. During angiography, arterial GIB can be controlled by the infusion of intra-arterial vasopressin or by the embolization of the artery by an interventional radiologist. If therapeutic endoscopy fails, this is a useful therapeutic option, particularly in those who are critically ill and poor surgical candidates.

Intra-arterial vasopressin causes a generalized vasoconstriction that produces a rapid reduction in local blood flow. Patients should be monitored closely for dysrhythmias and fluid retention with resultant hyponatremia. Repeat angiography is performed after the initial infusion, and the dose can then be titrated as needed. Once bleeding is controlled, this infusion may be continued in the ICU for 24 to 36 hours and then tapered over 24 hours. Patients should have cardiac monitoring during vasopressin therapy to watch for cardiac dysrhythmias. Nitroglycerin patches or drips may be used to counteract any ischemic changes.

Embolization of a bleeding vessel consists of occluding the vessel with material that can be either temporary or permanent. Biodegradable long-acting gelatin sponges are commonly used. These sponges cause hemostasis on contact when injected into the vessel. Steel coils, balloons, and silk thread can be used to block an artery mechanically, resulting in permanent occlusion. Uncommon complications include bowel ischemia, secondary duodenal stenosis, and gastric, hepatic, or splenic infarction.

**Balloon Tamponade.** Variceal bleeding unresponsive to endoscopic therapy can be temporarily controlled with balloon tamponade. Most esophagogastric tubes have two balloons, one for the stomach and one for the esophagus, and a distal port for gastric drainage. The Sengstaken–Blakemore tube is the most widely used (Fig. 41-1).

With the use of balloon tamponade, pressure is exerted on the cardia of the stomach and against the bleeding varices. The tube is inserted to at least 50 cm to ensure gastric intubation. The gastric balloon is then slowly inflated with 250 to 300 mL of air, and gentle traction is applied until the gastric balloon fits snugly against the cardia of the stomach. Position is then confirmed by radiography. Traction is then placed on the tube where it enters the patient by means of a piece of sponge rubber, as shown in Figure 41-1, or by traction fixed to a head helmet device or the foot of the bed. If chest pain occurs, the gastric balloon must be deflated immediately because it may have shifted into the esophagus.

If bleeding continues, the esophageal balloon is inflated to a pressure of 25 to 39 mm Hg and maintained at this pressure for 24 to 48 hours. Although pressure for longer than 24 hours may be needed to control bleeding, it can cause edema, esophagitis, ulcerations, or perforation of the esophagus. After bleeding is controlled, the balloon is maintained and inflated for no longer than 12 to 24 hours to decrease the risk for gastric ischemia and necrosis. Unfortunately, rebleeding often occurs after balloon deflation unless additional therapeutic measures are taken.

A nasogastric tube should be placed in patients with a Sengstaken–Blakemore tube to aspirate oral and nasopharyngeal secretions that collect above the esophageal balloon, preventing aspiration of these secretions into the lungs. The Minnesota esophagogastric tamponade tube (see Fig. 41-1) has a suction port above the esophageal balloon in addition to the usual ports (two balloons, one gastric suction) of the Sengstaken–Blakemore tube. Nursing interventions for the patient with an esophageal tamponade tube are given in Box 41-4.

**Transjugular Intrahepatic Portosystemic Shunt.** A transjugular intrahepatic portosystemic shunt (TIPS) is a

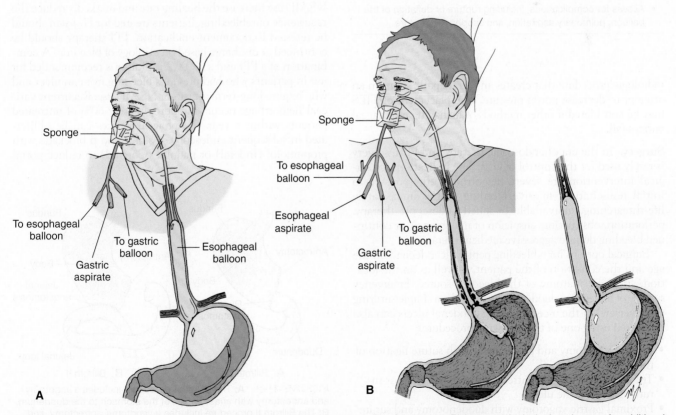

**FIGURE 41-1** Comparison of two types of esophageal tamponade tubes. **A:** The Sengstaken–Blakemore tube is the best known. An additional tube must be placed in the proximal esophagus. **B:** The Minnesota esophagogastric tamponade tube includes an esophageal aspirate lumen.

**Nursing Interventions**

**For the Patient With an Esophagogastric Balloon Tamponade Tube**

- Explain the purpose of the tube and the procedure to the patient.
- Lubricate and chill the tube as directed by the manufacturer.
- Identify and label the lumens of the tube.
- Check the patency of each lumen before insertion of the tube.
- Lavage the patient's stomach before insertion of the tube.
- Monitor the patient while the physician inserts the tube.
- Elevate the head of the bed to 30 degrees to prevent reflux.
- When a Sengstaken–Blakemore tube is in place, perform oropharyngeal suction frequently to prevent aspiration, *or* place a second nasogastric tube, if ordered, above the esophageal balloon to control secretions and prevent aspiration.
- Suction the esophageal port when a Minnesota tube is used.
- Maintain balloon pressure and traction.
- Maintain balloon position.
- Clean and lubricate the patient's nostrils frequently to prevent tube-caused pressure areas.
- Irrigate the nasogastric port every 2 hours to ensure patency and to keep the stomach empty.
- Teach the patient to avoid coughing or straining, which increases intra-abdominal pressure and predisposes to further bleeding.
- Have a second nasogastric tube, suction, and scissors available at the bedside.
- If the gastric balloon ruptures, the tube can rise into the nasopharynx, obstructing the airway. If this occurs, cut the tube immediately to deflate the balloon rapidly.
- Cut and remove the tube whenever there is a question of respiratory insufficiency or aspiration.
- Restrain the patient's arms if the patient is at risk for pulling out the tube. Agitation, confusion, and restlessness are risk factors.
- Assess for complications, including rupture or deflation of the balloon, pulmonary aspiration, and esophageal rupture.

radiologic procedure that creates an intrahepatic shunt in an attempt to decrease portal pressure. The placement of TIPS may be considered if other methods of managing esophageal varices fail.

**Surgery.** In the era of endoscopic therapy and PPIs, surgery is rarely used for the control of GIB. The indications for surgical intervention are severe hemorrhage unresponsive to initial resuscitation, massive bleeding that is immediately life-threatening, unavailable or failed endoscopic therapy, perforation, obstruction, suspicion of malignancy, or continued bleeding despite aggressive medical therapies.

Surgical options for a bleeding peptic ulcer depend on the age and the condition of the patient, as well as on the location, size, and anatomy of the bleeding source. Emergency surgery of a bleeding duodenal ulcer may be a simple suturing (eg, oversew) of the ulcer. Bleeding duodenal ulcers can also be treated using one of the following procedures:

- Truncal vagotomy and pyloroplasty with suture ligation of the ulcer
- Truncal vagotomy and antrectomy with resection or suture ligation of the ulcer
- Proximal gastric vagotomy with duodenotomy and suture ligation of the ulcer

Bleeding gastric ulcers are commonly treated with one of the following procedures:

- Truncal vagotomy and pyloroplasty with wedge resection of the ulcer
- Antrectomy with wedge excision of the proximal ulcer
- Distal gastrectomy with or without truncal vagotomy
- Wedge resection of the ulcer

A vagotomy involves severing the vagus nerve, which innervates the gastric cells. This results in decreased gastric acid secretion. A truncal (gastric) vagotomy selectively cuts the vagus distribution to the stomach. A pyloroplasty is necessary in conjunction with the vagotomy because denervation of the vagus nerve affects gastric motility. A pyloroplasty allows for continued gastric emptying. An antrectomy removes acid-producing cells in the stomach. A Billroth I procedure includes a vagotomy and antrectomy with anastomosis of the stomach to the duodenum (Fig. 41-2A). A Billroth II procedure involves a vagotomy, resection of the antrum, and anastomosis of the stomach to the jejunum (Fig. 41-2B). A gastric perforation can be surgically treated by simple closure or use of a patch to cover the mucosal hole.

Surgical decompression of portal hypertension can be used in patients with esophageal or gastric varices that are unresponsive to medical and endoscopic therapy. In this surgery, a portosystemic shunt is created, connecting the portal vein and the inferior vena cava to divert blood flow into the vena cava to decrease pressure.

**Medical Management.** Once bleeding is controlled, management focuses on treating the underlying cause of the acute upper GIB and preventing rebleeding. For patients with peptic ulcer disease, eradication of *H. pylori* and elimination of NSAID use increase the healing rate and markedly reduce the recurrence of rebleeding. Patients treated for *H. pylori* should be retested to document eradication. PPI therapy should be continued at discharge based on etiology of bleeding. A combination of a PPI and a COX-2 inhibitor is recommended for use in patients who had previous bleeding from an ulcer and who require long-term aspirin or NSAID use. Recurrent variceal hemorrhage occurs in approximately 60% of untreated patients within a year.[5] Esophageal varices can be obliterated in subsequent endoscopy sessions, and β blockade with propranolol (Inderal) or nadolol (Corgard) to reduce portal

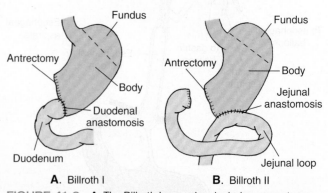

**A. Billroth I**          **B. Billroth II**

**FIGURE 41-2** **A:** The Billroth I procedure includes a vagotomy and antrectomy with anastomosis of the stomach to the duodenum. **B:** The Billroth II procedure includes a vagotomy, antrectomy, and anastomosis of the stomach to the jejunum.

pressure should be instituted to decrease the rebleeding rate. The dose should be titrated to achieve a 25% decrease in resting heart rate or a heart rate of about 55 beats/min as the desired end point.[5] The addition of isosorbide mononitrate may further decrease the risk for rebleeding. The use of prophylactic antibiotics in patients with acute bleeding varices has been shown to decrease the risk of rebleeding. Cessation of alcohol ingestion is imperative. See Box 41-5 for nursing interventions in the care of the patient with acute GIB.

## Lower Gastrointestinal Bleeding

### Etiology

Common causes of lower GIB are listed in Box 41-1. Most cases of acute lower GIB that require ICU admission result from diverticulosis or anorectal disease. Other causes include ischemia, angiodysplasia, neoplasm, colitis, inflammatory bowel disease, and hemorrhoids.

---

**BOX 41-5** | **Nursing Interventions**

For the Patient With Acute Gastrointestinal Bleeding
- Maintain a patent airway, elevate the head of the bed, and have suction available at the bedside to prevent aspiration of emesis or blood.
- Administer oxygen therapy to treat hypoxia that may result from decreased hemoglobin levels.
- Monitor pulse oximetry values.
- Assess and document signs and symptoms of shock, such as restlessness; diminished peripheral pulses; or cool, pale, or moist skin. Assess and document vital signs, urinary output, hemodynamic values, and oxygen saturation (SaO$_2$).
- Assess and document electrocardiographic monitoring and heart, lung, and bowel sounds.
- Assist with the placement of a central venous pressure (CVP) catheter or a pulmonary artery catheter.
- Monitor and document CVP, pulmonary artery pressure, pulmonary artery occlusion pressure, cardiac output, and systemic vascular resistance.
- Maintain IV access and administer IV fluids and blood products as ordered.
- Insert a nasogastric tube and lavage as ordered.
- Monitor gastric pH; consult with physician about specific pH range and antacid administration.
- Administer antisecretory medications as ordered to reduce gastric acid secretion.
- Administer vasopressin or octreotide as ordered.
- Maintain accurate intake and output every 1 to 2 hours and PRN.
- Record urine, nasogastric drainage, and emesis.
- Monitor electrolytes, which may be lost with fluids or altered due to fluid shifts, and report abnormal values.
- Monitor hemoglobin, hematocrit, red blood cell (RBC) count, PT, PTT, and BUN level and report abnormal values.
- Provide mouth care as needed.
- Explain all procedures to the patient.
- Prepare the patient for diagnostic procedures and therapeutic interventions.
- Monitor the patient for potential complications of endoscopy or colonoscopy, which include perforation, sepsis, pulmonary aspiration, and induced bleeding.
- Teach the patient the importance of seeking medical intervention if signs or symptoms of bleeding recur.
- Encourage smoking cessation and avoidance of alcohol.

---

**DIVERTICULOSIS.** Diverticula are sac-like protrusions in the colon wall that usually develop at the point where arteries penetrate the colon wall. These vessels are separated from the bowel lumen only by the mucosa and are subsequently prone to injury. Diverticular bleeding accounts for 30% to 50% of all cases of acute lower GIB, with greater incidence in the elderly.[6-9] Most patients with diverticular bleeding will stop bleeding spontaneously, but in 5% of the cases, bleeding can be massive.[9] Risk factors for diverticular bleeding include a diet low in fiber, aspirin and NSAID use, advanced age, and constipation.

**ANGIODYSPLASIA.** Angiodysplasia, also called arteriovenous malformation or angioma, is the term used to describe dilated, tortuous submucosal veins, small arteriovenous communications, or enlarged arteries. The walls of the vessels lack smooth muscle and are composed of endothelial cells. The incidence of angiodysplasia increases with age, owing to degeneration of the vessel walls; most cases occur in people older than 50 years, and two-thirds occur in those older than 70 years.

Angiodysplasia can occur anywhere in the colon, although it most often occurs in the cecum or ascending colon. As opposed to bleeding from diverticula, bleeding from angiodysplasia may be venous or arteriovenous in nature and is therefore usually less severe than bleeding from diverticular disease, which is arterial. Angiodysplasia is a common cause of lower GIB in patients with renal disease.

### Clinical Presentation

Acute lower GIB is defined by the presence of hemodynamic instability and the passage of hematochezia. Patients with diverticular bleeding usually describe the sudden onset of painless maroon or bright red hematochezia, although rarely, melena can occur. Diverticular bleeding is often painless, although patients may complain of cramping (which results from colonic spasm secondary to intraluminal exposure to blood). Blood loss from angiodysplasia usually presents as painless hematochezia.

If lower GIB is chronic, patients may present with iron-deficiency anemia and symptoms related to the anemia, such as weakness, fatigue, or dyspnea on exertion. Massive bleeding from hemorrhoids is rare but can occur in patients with rectal varices from portal hypertension.

### Assessment

**HISTORY.** Relevant findings in the medical history include abdominal surgery; a previous bleeding episode; peptic ulcer disease; inflammatory bowel disease; radiation to the abdomen or pelvis; or cardiopulmonary, renal, or liver disease. Knowledge of the patient's current medications and the existence of any allergies can also assist in diagnosis. A history of associated symptoms, including abdominal pain, fever, rectal urgency, tenesmus, weight loss, or a change in bowel habits or stool, should be elicited. The color and consistency of stool should be determined; in brisk bleeding, frequent red or maroon stools are more likely, and brown or infrequent stools are unlikely. The age of the patient may give a clue to diagnosis, because the risk for bleeding from diverticula and angiodysplasia increases with age.

**PHYSICAL EXAMINATION.** Often the physical examination findings are unremarkable. Vital signs are closely monitored to assess for hemodynamic instability. A palpable mass may reveal a neoplasm. A rectal examination is essential to assess for hematochezia and melena and exclude the possibility of bleeding hemorrhoids, which can occasionally present as a hemorrhage.

**LABORATORY STUDIES.** The initial laboratory studies include a complete blood count, serum electrolytes, BUN and creatinine levels, and PT and partial thromboplastin time (PTT). As in acute upper GIB, type and cross-match are mandatory before RBC transfusion.

### Management

**RESUSCITATION.** The management of acute lower GIB requires aggressive fluid resuscitation, as described for acute upper GIB. Patients with hematochezia should have a nasogastric tube inserted to exclude an upper GI source of bleeding because 10% of suspected lower GIB occurs from upper GI sources.[6,7] The presence of bloody aspirate confirms an upper GI source of bleeding. However, the absence of blood does not exclude an upper GI source because bleeding from a site in the duodenum may not reflux into the stomach. Nasogastric aspirate that reveals bile without blood is unlikely in bleeding from an upper GI source. Once it is determined that bleeding is coming from a lower GI source, colonoscopy is the procedure of choice for both diagnosis and treatment.

**DEFINITIVE DIAGNOSIS.** Colonoscopy is the test of choice for the evaluation of lower GIB. It has a diagnostic accuracy of up to 95% in affected patients. Other advantages of colonoscopy are the ability to locate the source of the bleeding precisely, the ability to perform biopsies, and the potential for therapeutic intervention. Before colonoscopy in the acute care setting, the colon needs to be cleansed with 4 L of polyethylene glycol solution given orally or by nasogastric tube until the waste is clear. For those patients in whom bleeding has stopped, it is reasonable to perform colonoscopy on an elective rather than emergent basis. If a source of bleeding is identified during colonoscopy, therapeutic options include thermal coagulation or injection with epinephrine or other sclerosants, as discussed previously.

**Endoscopy.** Upper endoscopy should be performed if colonoscopy is unable to distinguish a lower GI source.

**Radionucleotide Imaging.** When colonoscopy fails to identify a bleeding source, radionucleotide scanning can detect bleeding that occurs at rates as low as 0.04 mL/min.[6] This is more sensitive than angiography but less specific than either colonoscopy or a positive angiogram. The two types of scanning available are the technetium ($^{99m}$Tc)–sulfur colloid and $^{99m}$Tc pertechnetate–labeled autologous RBCs. Unfortunately, both of these techniques provide poor localization because of the peristaltic action of the bowel. However, these scans may be useful before angiography because a positive scan can aid in localizing the bleeding.

**Angiography.** Angiography is reserved for patients with massive, ongoing bleeding when endoscopy is not an acceptable option or with recurrent or persistent bleeding from a source not identified on colonoscopy. Angiography requires the active blood loss of 0.5 to 1.0 mL/min to localize a bleeding site because the contrast in the arterial system is present for only a short time.[6] A positive angiogram is associated with a high likelihood for surgical intervention. When an active source is identified, arteriographic intervention with intra-arterial vasopressin or embolization may be used. However, embolization with gelatin sponges, microcoils, or polyvinyl alcohol particles is replacing vasopressin because of the high incidence of complication and rebleeding after stopping the infusion. The nurse must be aware of the potential complications associated with arteriography, which include allergy to contrast medium, contrast-induced renal failure, bleeding from the arterial puncture site, and even embolism from thrombus.

**SURGICAL INTERVENTION.** Surgical management of lower GIB is indicated for massive or recurrent bleeding and in those patients with high transfusion requirements. An exploratory laparotomy to identify the source of the bleeding is often performed. A segmental bowel resection with a primary anastomosis is often necessary for definitive treatment of lower GIB. In patients who are unstable, a stoma and mucous fistula may be created. In those patients with severe lower GIB without a localized source, a blind total colectomy may be the operative choice. Surgical management of diverticular bleeding is indicated if bleeding is not controlled with endoscopic or angiographic means or in patients with recurrent bleeding from the same segment.

## Intestinal Obstruction and Ileus

Intestinal obstruction occurs when the passage of intestinal contents through the lumen is impaired. This can result from either mechanical (anatomical) or nonmechanical causes. Intestinal obstruction is classified as either partial or complete, depending on the degree of obstruction. In a simple obstruction there is no ischemia, whereas in cases of strangulated obstruction, ischemia is present. A closed-loop obstruction describes a mechanical obstruction with a proximal and distal occlusion of the affected intestinal segment.

Bowel obstruction can occur in both the small and large bowel. The small bowel is most commonly affected, with the ileum as the most common site of obstruction. In large bowel obstruction, the sigmoid colon is the most common site of obstruction. The location of the obstruction, the degree of obstruction, and the presence of ischemia are important distinctions because treatment varies. Prompt recognition of bowel obstruction is important for the nurse because intestinal obstruction can progress to bowel strangulation, infarction, and perforation and result in potentially life-threatening peritoneal and systemic infection. The mortality rate associated with a strangulated obstruction is high.

The causes of mechanical obstruction are varied and classified as extrinsic, intrinsic, and intraluminal (Box 41-6). Extrinsic lesions occur outside of the bowel. Examples of extrinsic lesions are adhesions, hernias, volvulus (twisting of a segment of the bowel on itself), and masses. Intrinsic lesions extend into the bowel wall. Diverticulitis, neoplasms, and radiation enteritis are examples of intrinsic lesions. Intraluminal causes of obstruction can result from the ingestion of foreign bodies, intussusception, and neoplasms.

**Causes of Mechanical Obstruction**

**Extrinsic Lesions**
Adhesions and congenital bands
Hernias
    External hernias
    Internal hernias
    Diaphragmatic hernias
    Pelvic hernias
Volvulus
    Gastric
    Midgut
    Cecal
    Sigmoid
Extrinsic masses
    Benign or malignant tumors
    Abscesses
    Aneurysms
    Hematomas
    Endometriosis

**Intrinsic Lesions**
Benign and malignant neoplasms
    Adenocarcinomas
    Lymphomas, lymphosarcomas
    Carcinoid tumors
Inflammatory conditions
    Tuberculous enteritis, Crohn disease
    Strictures secondary to potassium chloride, nonsteroidal
        anti-inflammatory drugs, and ischemia
    Radiation injury, caustic ingestants
    Eosinophilic gastroenteritis, ameboma
    Diverticulitis, pelvic inflammatory disease
Intussusception
Congenital defects
    Hypertrophic pyloric stenosis, annular pancreas
    Intestinal atresia/agenesis
    Malrotation/volvulus
    Intestinal duplication, mesenteric cysts
    Meckel diverticulum
    Hirschsprung disease
Hematoma
    Abdominal trauma
    Thrombocytopenia
    Henoch–Schönlein purpura

**Intraluminal Causes**
Meconium ileus
Barium impaction
Fecal impaction
Gallstone ileus
Gastric bezoars
Foreign bodies

From Yamada T, Alpers DH, Laine L, et al (eds): Textbook of Gastroenterology, 4th ed. Philadelphia, PA: Lippincott Williams & Wilkins, 2003, p 834.

## Small Bowel Obstruction

### Etiology

Adhesions are the most common cause of small bowel obstruction (SBO) in adults, accounting for 75% of obstructions.[10] Adhesions most commonly occur after laparotomy for colectomy, appendectomy, or gynecologic procedures. Adhesions can also develop after abdominal radiation, ischemia, or infection, or as the result of foreign bodies. Adhesions may develop only days after surgery and as late as 10 to 20 years later. Adhesive bands can form and contract and, in time, may entrap a loop of bowel.

Hernias are the second most common cause of SBO. SBO secondary to hernia carries a high risk for complete obstruction and strangulation. The herniation of a portion of the bowel after laparotomy is called a Richter hernia. The occurrence of SBO in the absence of previous laparotomy should suggest hernia as the cause.

Primary neoplasms of the small bowel are uncommon. Luminal compression of the small bowel or local invasion by gastric, pancreatic, colonic, and gynecologic cancers can cause extrinsic compression, which accounts for most cases of SBO that result from malignancy. Intraluminal strictures that result from Crohn disease, radiation therapy, ischemia, and certain drugs, such as enteric-coated potassium chloride or NSAIDs, are other possible causes of SBO.

### Pathophysiology

In SBO, large amounts of fluid and swallowed air accumulate in the intestinal lumen proximal to the obstruction, causing distention (Fig. 41-3). Fluid accumulates from oral intake; swallowed saliva; and gastric, biliary, and pancreatic juices. Swallowed air has a high nitrogen content and is poorly absorbed from the lumen.

As the obstruction continues, the bowel wall and lumen become edematous and distended. Increased intraluminal pressure leads to increased capillary permeability and movement of fluid and electrolytes into the abdominal cavity. This extravasation of fluid and electrolytes into the peritoneal cavity, combined with fluid lost through vomiting, can lead to hypovolemia, hypokalemia, and hyponatremia. Peristalsis decreases, and the normal functions of the intestine decrease or halt. In the absence of normal intestinal motility, bacterial overgrowth occurs. If oral intake continues, bacterial fermentation can contribute to gas accumulation. Within hours of acute obstruction, the contents of the lumen proximal to obstruction become malodorous and feculent because of this bacterial overgrowth.

### Clinical Presentation

The severity of symptoms is related to the site and degree of obstruction, duration, and the presence and severity of ischemia (Table 41-1). Patients with SBO usually complain of the acute onset of intermittent, crampy, periumbilical pain. Bursts of peristalsis above the obstruction cause pain. The pain is often more severe the more proximal the obstruction. Patients with an incomplete obstruction often describe crampy abdominal pain after meals. The pain in incomplete obstruction may be exacerbated by the ingestion of high-fiber meals. Patients with a closed-loop obstruction may describe pain out of proportion to physical findings.

In patients with proximal SBO, vomiting occurs frequently and early in the course of obstruction. The emesis is usually bilious, and vomiting often relieves the pain by deflating the distended bowel. Minimal abdominal distention usually accompanies proximal SBO.

In distal SBO, moderate abdominal distention and intermittent or constant pain are often present. Vomiting is intermittent. In ileal SBO, the emesis may be feculent secondary to bacterial overgrowth.

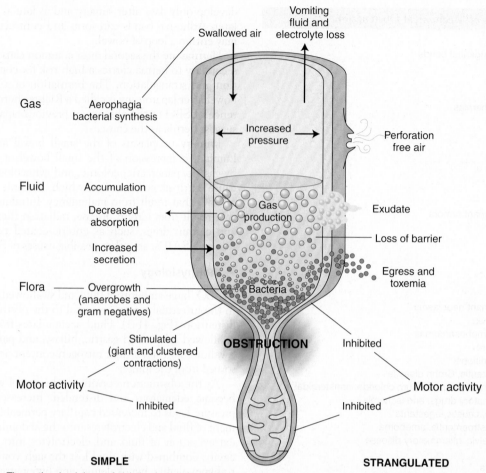

**FIGURE 41-3** The pathophysiology of simple obstruction (**left**) and strangulated obstruction (**right**) in the small intestine. (From Yamada T, Alpers DH, Laine L, et al (eds): Textbook of Gastroenterology, 4th ed. Philadelphia, PA: Lippincott Williams & Wilkins, 2003, p 830.)

**TABLE 41-1**   Clinical Features of Ileus and Obstruction Dependent on Anatomic Site

| | | Site of Obstruction | | | |
|---|---|---|---|---|---|
| Feature | Ileus | Gastric Outlet | Distal Duodenum | Jejunoileal | Colon |
| Pain | Mild | Mild | Mild | Moderate | Severe |
| Distention | Moderate to severe | Mild | Mild | Moderate | Severe |
| Emesis | | | | | |
|   Amount/frequency | Small, infrequent | Copious, frequent | Copious, frequent | Smaller/less frequent | Uncommon |
|   Nature | Sour, bilious | Clear, sour, HCl, KCl | Bile-stained, bitter, NaCl, NaHCO₃ | Malodorous, feculent | Variable |
| Acid–base imbalance | Variable | Metabolic alkalosis | Metabolic acidosis | Dehydration, hypotension | Usually not severe |

HCl, hydrogen chloride; KCl, potassium chloride; NaHCO$_3$, sodium bicarbonate; NaCl, sodium chloride.
From Yamada T, Alpers DH, Laine L, et al (eds): Textbook of Gastroenterology, 4th ed. Philadelphia, PA: Lippincott Williams & Wilkins, 2003, p 833.

In strangulated SBO, the pain is more localized and may be steady and severe. When vomiting is protracted, dehydration and hypovolemia may occur.

Fever may be present secondary to an inflammatory process or in response to bowel ischemia or perforation. Constipation is also a common complaint, although patients may continue to pass gas and stool as the bowel distal to the obstruction empties. Obstipation is an important indicator of complete obstruction, but patients with a complete bowel obstruction evacuate the contents distal to the obstruction.

Depending on the duration and severity of the obstruction, hemodynamic instability may develop as the result of massive fluid trapping in the lumen with leakage into the peritoneum.

### Assessment

**HISTORY.** A careful history provides clues to etiology. A medical history of previous abdominal surgery or trauma increases the risk for adhesions. Other pertinent medical history findings include inflammatory bowel disease, diverticulitis, abdominal or pelvic radiation, peptic ulcer disease, pancreatitis, and previous obstruction or cancer. Correlation to menses suggests endometriosis. A complete medication history is also essential. Patients with a psychiatric history should be questioned about ingestion of foreign objects.

**PHYSICAL EXAMINATION.** Patients with SBO often appear acutely ill. Inspection of the abdomen often reveals visible peristalsis and distention. Patients with a proximal SBO may have epigastric or periumbilical tenderness, whereas those with distal SBO often have more diffuse tenderness. Bowel sounds are usually hyperactive in the early course of the obstruction, then high-pitched and tinkling with loud rushes as peristaltic waves attempt to push intestinal contents past the obstruction. Bowel sounds decrease as the obstruction progresses and the bowel fatigues. Tachycardia, orthostatic hypotension, poor skin turgor, or dry mucous membranes may indicate dehydration. A palpable mass may represent a neoplasm or volvulus.

It is necessary to perform a rectal examination to assess for blood, fecal impaction, or mass. Inspection may reveal scars and external hernias. Hepatomegaly, liver masses, and palpable periumbilical, inguinal, or supraclavicular lymphadenopathy suggest malignancy. Abdominal tenderness and palpable masses may suggest abscess. Fever, rigors, and declining clinical status suggest bowel strangulation. Borborygmi, rumbling, gurgling, and tinkling noises produced by hyperactive intestinal peristalsis are often audible and may correlate with abdominal cramping. If rebound tenderness is present, observe for signs and symptoms of shock because perforation is a possibility. Percussion of the abdomen may reveal resonance or tympany from fluid trapped in the intestine. Shifting dullness to percussion indicates ascites. Palpate for inguinal, femoral, and umbilical hernias. A tender mass at the site of a hernia suggests the etiology. Tachycardia, tachypnea, altered mental status, oliguria, and hypotension may all be present in hypovolemia.

**LABORATORY STUDIES.** There is no single laboratory value that is diagnostic for SBO. A mild leukocytosis is present with simple obstructions, whereas significant leukocytosis suggests strangulation. In proximal obstruction, potassium, sodium, hydrogen, and chloride may be lost in emesis, resulting in metabolic alkalosis. BUN, creatinine, sodium, and osmolality levels reflect the fluid and electrolyte shifts that occur as fluid leaks out of the intestine and electrolytes are either reabsorbed or lost. As dehydration increases, the hemoglobin and hematocrit levels are elevated, reflecting hemoconcentration. In ischemia or strangulation, amylase, lipase, alkaline phosphatase, creatine phosphokinase, aspartate aminotransferase (AST), alanine aminotransferase (ALT), and lactate dehydrogenase levels may rise. Often, heme-positive stools are present in ischemia or carcinoma. Metabolic acidosis suggests severe hypoxemia from hypoperfusion, and metabolic acidosis refractory to fluid resuscitation suggests strangulation.

**IMAGING STUDIES.** Various imaging studies are available to confirm diagnoses.

**Radiography.** When SBO is suspected, abdominal radiographs with the patient in upright, flat, and side-lying positions can confirm the diagnosis of obstruction, localize the site of obstruction, and assist in determining the degree of obstruction. Pneumoperitoneum seen in upright films suggests intestinal perforation. Normally, there is little air in the small bowel. In complete SBO, gas and fluid accumulate proximal to the obstruction. Multiple air–fluid levels may be visible, with a stepladder pattern that demonstrates multiple loops of bowel with different air levels. Distal to the obstruction, the bowel lumen empties and collapses within 12 to 24 hours. Successive films may also confirm the diagnosis, but distinguishing between a small and large bowel obstruction or ileus is difficult.

Barium studies may be helpful in the diagnosis of obstruction if plain films are nondiagnostic. Contrast-enhanced studies can differentiate between a complete or partial obstruction. Barium is the agent of choice if SBO is suspected because it provides a better contrast than water-soluble material. In SBO, the large amount of water present proximal to the obstruction dilutes water-soluble contrast. However, if there is any question about bowel perforation, barium should be avoided because free barium in the peritoneum can cause significant inflammation. If colonic obstruction is suspected, a limited barium enema is used for diagnosis before barium is given by mouth.

**Computed Tomography.** Abdominal computed tomography (CT) can help identify obstructive lesions, neoplasms, hernias, and signs of ischemia. Abdominal CT with oral or IV contrast medium can help differentiate mechanical obstruction from pseudo-obstruction. Oral contrast seen in the colon on CT 12 hours after ingestion indicates incomplete SBO, whereas nonvisualization of oral contrast in the colon within 12 hours indicates complete SBO. The CT diagnosis of a complete SBO requires a transition zone between dilated and collapsed loops of bowel, suggesting the point of obstruction. CT is less sensitive in the diagnosis of a partial SBO. CT can also assess the entire abdomen, which can suggest alternative diagnoses and identify any complications associated with obstruction. CT is also accurate in determining the presence of strangulation or a closed-loop obstruction.

**Endoscopy.** Direct visualization with endoscopy may confirm the obstruction in the colon or proximal small bowel and aid in determining the type of obstruction.

## Management

**MEDICAL MANAGEMENT.** When possible, obstructions, especially incomplete obstructions, are treated medically rather than surgically. Oral food and fluid are withheld (ie, the patient is put on NPO status), and a nasogastric tube is placed to decompress the stomach or duodenum. Fluid and electrolytes are aggressively supplied IV with lactated Ringer or saline solution. When possible, the underlying causes are treated. Total parenteral nutrition (TPN) may be required to provide nutritional support. A Foley catheter is inserted to allow continual assessment of the fluid replacement. In patients with renal or cardiac disease, a central venous pressure (CVP) or pulmonary artery catheter may guide fluid replacement.

About 80% of SBO resolve spontaneously, and if patients continue to pass gas and stool, supportive management is continued.[11] If patients show no improvement within 3 to 5 days, or if fever or rebound tenderness occurs, a surgical evaluation is indicated.[11] All patients with intestinal obstruction should be watched closely for signs and symptoms that reflect sepsis, perforation, ischemia, necrosis, or gangrene. Broad-spectrum antibiotics are started immediately when strangulation or sepsis is suspected. The mortality rate associated with bowel ischemia resulting from obstruction is high.

**SURGICAL MANAGEMENT.** Acute complete SBO is a surgical emergency. Acute complete SBO is suspected when the patient fails to pass gas, and stool and gas are not evident in the distal intestine on radiography. An acute complete SBO is accompanied by the risk for bowel strangulation. Patients with strangulated bowel, volvulus, and incarceration of bowel loop in a hernia or a closed-loop obstruction require immediate surgery. In addition, those patients who fail conservative therapy or experience a decline in clinical status warrant surgical intervention.

Surgical procedures include laparoscopic lysis of adhesions, reduction of volvulus, resection of the involved and surrounding area of bowel with impaired blood supply, bowel decompression, and possible ostomy. These patients may require a second surgery to assess bowel viability.

## Colonic Obstruction

### Etiology

Carcinoma, sigmoid diverticulitis, and volvulus are the three most common causes of colonic obstruction and together account for the majority of colonic obstructions. Malignancy is the most common cause of colonic obstruction in the United States, accounting for approximately 60% of cases.[12] Patients with colorectal cancer present with a colonic obstruction between 10% and 30% of the time.[13] Malignancy that causes colon obstruction occurs most commonly in the sigmoid colon. Extrinsic compression or colonic invasion from pelvic tumors may also cause a colon obstruction. Diverticulitis can cause strictures in the colon that can lead to mechanical obstruction, resulting in approximately 10% of cases of colonic obstruction.[8] Volvulus, which occurs most commonly in the sigmoid colon and the cecum, causes 10% to 15% of colonic obstructions in the United States.[8,12] A closed-loop obstruction is usually produced with volvulus and carries a high incidence of strangulation. Other causes of colon obstruction include anastomotic or inflammatory strictures.

### Pathophysiology

When the ileocecal valve is competent, a closed-loop obstruction can occur because the cecum does not allow decompression of fluid and gas into the small bowel. As fluid and gas accumulate, the intraluminal pressure increases, and the colonic wall can become ischemic if this pressure exceeds the capillary pressure. In some cases, the cecum may become so severely distended that it inhibits intramural blood flow, which can result in necrosis and gangrene. In colonic obstruction, the normal colonic flora produces methane and ammonia, which contribute to the distention. Dehydration results when secretions are sequestered in the colon.

Patients with colonic obstruction have changes in intestinal flora and translocation of bacteria in mesenteric lymph nodes. This is the most likely cause of septic complications of colonic obstruction.

### Clinical Presentation

The clinical presentation of patients with colonic obstruction depends on the degree of obstruction, the cause, the presence of comorbidity, the presence of closed-loop obstruction, and the competency of the ileocecal valve. Patients with colonic obstruction typically present with abdominal pain, distention, and progressive obstipation. The pain may be colicky or severe and unremitting if peritonitis is present. Severe, constant pain suggests gangrenous bowel. If vomiting occurs, it tends to be late in the course of obstruction, especially in patients with a competent ileocecal valve. Patients with volvulus may present with a sudden onset of marked abdominal distention. Patients with obstruction from colon cancer may describe a gradual development of symptoms like altered bowel habits or a change in stool caliber. Dehydration results when secretions become sequestered in the colon. Patients with a competent ileocecal valve may have greater distention, which increases the risk for ischemia and perforation because an incompetent ileocecal valve allows decompression into the small intestine. Most patients with colonic obstruction complain of constipation; however, diarrhea may be present if stool is leaking past an obstruction. Patients may complain of dyspnea if diaphragmatic excursion is compromised by abdominal distention.

### Assessment

**HISTORY.** A history of altered bowel movements, blood in the stool, or iron-deficiency anemia is suggestive of carcinoma, as are weight loss and anorexia. Diverticulitis typically presents with left lower quadrant pain and associated fever. There may be a change in bowel habits as well. Bleeding is not usually associated with diverticulitis. A history of laxative use and constipation is common in patients with volvulus.

**PHYSICAL EXAMINATION.** Abdominal distention is common, and tympany is present with percussion. Signs of dehydration including tachycardia, hypotension, poor skin turgor, and dry mucous membranes may be seen. Bowel sounds are usually hyperactive initially but become progressively hypoactive. Abdominal masses and signs of peritoneal irritation may be elicited. The abdomen may be diffusely tender. Guarding or rebound tenderness suggests peritonitis. Ascites and hepatomegaly may be present in patients with colon cancer with liver metastasis. A rectal examination may be helpful in identifying rectal cancer. High fever and tachycardia, regardless of rehydration or the presence of peritoneal signs, suggest strangulation and warrant urgent surgical evaluation.

**LABORATORY STUDIES.** Iron-deficiency anemia may be present if obstruction results from neoplasm. Marked leukocytosis suggests diverticulitis, ischemia, or perforation.

**IMAGING STUDIES.** Plain abdominal films in the supine and upright positions identify the site of obstruction and determine the degree of obstruction. Obstruction in patients with a competent ileocecal valve causes dilation confined to the colon. Small bowel distention may be visible on abdominal films in patients with acute colonic obstruction and in patients with intact ileocecal valves. Abdominal films may also suggest volvulus.

If a contrast enema is given, water-soluble contrast medium rather than barium may be considered. Barium should never be given orally unless a barium enema, CT scan, or colonoscopy has ruled out colonic obstruction. Oral barium accumulates proximal to the colonic obstruction, and water will continually be extracted, possibly causing a barium impaction. In patients with suspected volvulus, a water-soluble contrast enema may demonstrate a point of torsion.

CT may be valuable in distinguishing between an anatomic obstruction and a pseudo-obstruction. CT can also diagnose other causes of colonic obstruction, such as inflammation as a result of colitis or diverticulitis and perforation as a result of colorectal cancer.

## Management

### MEDICAL MANAGEMENT.
The medical management of the patient with acute colonic obstruction is similar to that of the patient with SBO. Medical management focuses on fluid and electrolyte replacement. Oral intake is limited, or the patient is placed on NPO status. Nasogastric suction may assist in decompression of abdominal distention. A rectal tube may decompress the distal colon but has little effect on the proximal colon. Colonic decompression in the setting of a volvulus can be attempted by colonoscopy.

### SURGICAL MANAGEMENT.
Colonic obstruction usually requires surgery. The goals of surgery are to decompress the colon and to treat the obstructive lesion. Surgical management of the colonic obstruction is warranted if the patient fails to improve with medical management, the patient's clinical status deteriorates, or the patient has a complete colonic obstruction with a competent ileocecal valve. For obstruction of the left colon, operative decompression followed by primary anastomosis after intraoperative lavage is the treatment of choice. For obstruction in the transverse and right colon, primary resection and anastomosis can also be performed safely. Primary anastomosis should be avoided in a patient with an unprepared colon.

### ENDOSCOPIC THERAPY.
Stents that are placed endoscopically can be used as a temporary measure before surgical resection of obstruction from malignancy or as a palliative measure in nonoperative colorectal cancer. Endoscopic laser therapy, argon plasma coagulation, and snare polypectomy may be used to debulk obstructing tumors in patients unwilling or unable to have surgery.

## Ileus

Ileus, often called paralytic ileus or adynamic ileus, is the failure of intestinal contents to pass because of decreased peristalsis activity in the absence of mechanical obstruction. Ileus can have intra-abdominal or extra-abdominal causes (Box 41-7), many of which are likely to be seen in the ICU setting. Acute colonic pseudo-obstruction (ACPO), also called acute colonic ileus and Ogilvie syndrome, is a variant of ileus characterized by massive colonic dilation in the absence of mechanical obstruction.

### Etiology

Postoperative ileus (a transient inhibition of normal GI motility that usually lasts for 3 to 5 days after surgery) is the

---

### BOX 41-7 Causes of Adynamic Ileus and Acute Colonic Pseudo-Obstruction

| Intra-Abdominal Causes | Extra-Abdominal Causes |
| --- | --- |
| **Reflex Inhibition** | **Reflex Inhibition** |
| Laparotomy | Craniotomy |
| Abdominal trauma | Spine or pelvic fractures |
| Renal transplantation | Myocardial infarction |
| | Coronary bypass |
| **Inflammatory Conditions** | Open heart surgery |
| Perforated viscus or penetrating wounds | Pneumonia, pulmonary embolus |
| Bile peritonitis | Burns |
| Chemical peritonitis | Black widow spider bites |
| Intraperitoneal hemorrhage | |
| Toxic megacolon | **Drug-Induced** |
| Familial Mediterranean fever | Anticholinergic/ganglionic antagonists |
| Acute pancreatitis | Opiates |
| Acute cholecystitis | Chemotherapeutic agents |
| Celiac disease | Tricyclic antidepressants |
| Inflammatory bowel disease | Phenothiazines |
| **Acute Irradiation Injury** | |
| Abdominal irradiation | **Metabolic Abnormalities** |
| | Septicemia |
| **Infectious Processes** | Electrolyte imbalance |
| Bacterial peritonitis | Heavy metal poisoning (lead, mercury) |
| Appendicitis | Porphyria |
| Diverticulitis | Uremia |
| Herpes zoster virus | Diabetic ketoacidosis |
| Anorectal herpes simplex virus | Sickle cell disease |
| | Pulmonary failure |
| **Ischemic Processes** | |
| Arterial insufficiency | |
| Venous thrombosis | |
| Mesenteric arteritis | |
| Strangulation obstruction | |
| **Retroperitoneal Processes** | |
| Ureteropelvic stones | |
| Pyelonephritis | |
| Retroperitoneal hemorrhage | |
| Pheochromocytoma | |
| Malignancy (Ogilvie syndrome) | |

From Yamada T, Alpers DH, Laine L, et al (eds): Textbook of Gastroenterology, 4th ed. Philadelphia, PA: Lippincott Williams & Wilkins, 2003, p 836.

---

most common cause of a delayed discharge after surgery, abdominal or otherwise. An underlying disease is present in the majority of ileus. Causes of ileus include metabolic abnormalities (electrolyte disturbances, diabetic ketoacidosis, uremia, heavy metal poisoning), drugs (narcotics, catecholamines, antihistamines, calcium channel blockers, adrenocorticotropic hormones, anticholinergics), and local or systemic inflammation (sepsis, peritonitis, ischemia, pancreatitis). Ileus may also be present after spinal cord injury. Blood-borne toxins, abnormalities in acid–base balance, electrolyte disturbances, and decreased oxygen supply are all possible causes of ileus.

### Pathophysiology

Although the etiology of ileus can be defined, the pathophysiology of ileus is poorly understood. Postoperative ileus has been widely studied, and multiple mechanisms are thought to play a role, including sympathetic neural reflexes that inhibit normal bowel motility, local and systemic inflammatory mediators that result in bowel edema, and changes in neural and hormonal transmitters. The effects of anesthesia, combined with inflammation or ischemia in the operative area, may also interfere with nerve conduction. Opioid narcotics may also contribute to postoperative ileus because they decrease propulsive motility of the intestine. In ileus, peristalsis ceases or is decreased, and distention of the intestine occurs as gas, fluid, and electrolytes accumulate in a process similar to that seen in mechanical obstruction.

### Clinical Presentation

Patients with ileus may complain of diffuse abdominal discomfort and distention (see Table 41-1). ACPO is more common in men and patients 60 years of age and older. Nausea and vomiting are often predominant in patients with postoperative ileus. Vomiting is frequent, and the emesis usually contains gastric contents and bile. The vomiting of feculent material is rare. The pain is usually less intense than in small bowel or colonic obstruction. The patient with ileus also complains of constipation and usually denies the passage of flatus. Other common symptoms are nausea, anorexia, hiccups, and bloating.

### Assessment

**HISTORY.** A history of thyroid or parathyroid disease, heavy metal exposure, diabetes mellitus, and scleroderma should be elicited to identify underlying causes.

**PHYSICAL EXAMINATION.** Abdominal distention is often prominent in ileus. Auscultation of the abdomen usually reveals infrequent or absent bowel sounds. The abdomen is usually resonant to percussion secondary to air in the dilated loops of intestine. Abdominal distention may cause labored breathing. Abdominal girth is assessed at frequent intervals. Peritoneal signs may indicate impending perforation. Tachycardia, orthostatic hypotension, poor skin turgor, or dry mucous membranes may indicate dehydration.

**LABORATORY STUDIES.** Electrolyte abnormalities commonly associated with ileus are similar to those seen in patients with mechanical obstruction.

**IMAGING STUDIES.** Abdominal radiography that shows massive colonic dilation confirms the diagnosis of ileus. In ileus, gas and fluid accumulate in loops of mildly dilated bowel proximal or adjacent to the site of an acute inflammatory process, such as appendicitis or pancreatitis. These loops are involved in localized ileus and are called sentinel loops. In ACPO, the entire colon becomes dilated, with the cecal diameter the greatest. Chest radiography may help identify pneumonia or other causes of ileus. Contrast-enhanced enema studies can be used to differentiate complete obstruction from partial obstruction and ileus. CT of the abdomen may identify causes that can contribute to ileus. Ultrasonography has no role in the diagnosis of ileus because the dilated loops of bowel prevent imaging.

### Management

Treatment of ileus focuses on management of underlying causes. Because ileus may present in much the same way

as mechanical obstruction, exclusion of mechanical causes is necessary. Treatment usually consists of supportive care. Patients with ileus have traditionally been placed on NPO status, although recent studies suggest that early feeding is safe. Fluid and electrolyte replacement is directed by clinical status and laboratory values as needed. Nasogastric suction limits the collection of swallowed air that can contribute to abdominal distention. Medications that can adversely affect colonic motility including narcotics and anticholinergics should be discontinued when possible. Laxative use should be avoided because these agents can provide a substrate for bacterial fermentation, which results in further gas accumulation. In addition, patients should be mobilized and encouraged to get out of bed if they are ambulatory.

If patients show no improvement in 3 to 5 days, a further search for underlying causes is initiated. Neostigmine has been effective in treating colonic ileus not responsive to conservative therapy. Neostigmine is a parasympathomimetic that can correct the autonomic imbalance thought to contribute to ileus. Neostigmine can cause bradycardia and dysrhythmias, so careful cardiac monitoring is required. Prokinetic medications, such as metoclopramide (Reglan) and erythromycin, have not been found to be effective in treating ileus.

Therapeutic interventions for decompressing the colon include colonoscopy, open or percutaneous cecostomy, and a decompression colostomy. Colonoscopy is the procedure of choice for decompression in patients who do not respond to conservative or medical therapy.

Surgery is indicated for patients who fail conservative management or in patients who develop a perforation or evidence of ischemia.

## Acute Pancreatitis

Acute pancreatitis (AP) is an acute inflammation of the pancreas that can also involve surrounding tissues, remote organs, or both. There are approximately 300,000 hospital admissions a year in the United States caused by AP.[14] AP refers to an acute attack in a previously healthy individual, with resolution of symptoms after the attack. Chronic pancreatitis refers to repeated attacks with continued symptoms. AP can be mild, moderate, or severe. Mild AP is not associated with organ dysfunction or complications, and recovery is usually uneventful, within a week. Moderately severe AP is defined by the presence of transient organ failure, local complications or exacerbation of comorbid disease; in severe AP, there is persistent organ failure that last for more than 48 hours.[15] Approximately 20% of patients with AP develop severe AP, also called necrotic or hemorrhagic pancreatitis.[16] In severe AP, there is extensive fat necrosis in and around the pancreas, pancreatic cellular necrosis, and hemorrhage in the pancreas. The incidence of AP varies among populations based on the prevalence of precipitating factors, such as alcohol use and gallstone disease.

### Etiology

There are multiple causes of AP (Box 41-8). Gallstones and excessive alcohol use together account for the majority of cases.

Gallstones are responsible for 40% of cases.[16] Gallstones and biliary sludge may become lodged as they pass through

**Major Causes of Acute Pancreatitis**

- Biliary disease: gallstones or microlithiasis, common bile duct obstruction, biliary sludge
- Pancreas divisum
- Alcohol abuse
- Drugs: thiazide diuretics, furosemide, procainamide, tetracycline, sulfonamides, azathioprine, 6-mercaptopurine, angiotensin-converting enzyme inhibitors, valproic acid
- Hypertriglyceridemia
- Hypercalcemia
- Idiopathic
- Miscellaneous (postoperative, ectopic pregnancy, ovarian cyst, total parenteral nutrition)
- Abdominal trauma
- Endoscopic retrograde cholangiopancreatography
- Infectious processes

biliary system, blocking pancreatic secretions from emptying into the duodenum. Reflux of bile into the pancreatic duct resulting from this obstruction is thought to be the inciting factor. Gallstone pancreatitis is more common in women.

Alcoholism is the second leading cause of pancreatitis and accounts for 35% of the cases of AP.[16] The exact mechanism by which alcohol induces AP is unknown. Alcohol may also have a direct toxic effect and increase the sensitivity of the pancreas to injury by environmental or genetic factors. Another theory is that alcohol causes sphincter of Oddi spasm, which causes pancreatic enzymes to back up into the pancreas. Alcoholic pancreatitis is more common in men. AP is rarely the result of binge drinking unless the pancreas is already damaged by chronic alcohol use. Drinking five to eight alcoholic beverages a day for more than 5 years is a risk factor for the pancreatitis.[14]

Metabolic causes of AP include hypercalcemia and hypertriglyceridemia. Many drugs, including diuretics, sulfonamides, metronidazole, aminosalicylates, and estrogen, can precipitate AP as a result of toxic metabolites or a drug reaction. Idiopathic pancreatitis is associated with pregnancy, the administration of TPN, or major surgery. Pancreatitis has also occurred after blunt or penetrating abdominal trauma or after endoscopic manipulation of the ampulla of Vater. Other possible precipitating factors include infectious processes, such as mumps, staphylococcal infection, scarlet fever, and viral infections, as well as the congenital variant of pancreas divisum. Pancreatitis may occur as an isolated event, or the patient may suffer repeated attacks.

## Pathophysiology

The acinar cells of the pancreas synthesize and secrete digestive enzymes to assist in the breakdown of starch, fat, and proteins. Under normal circumstances, these enzymes remain inactive until they enter the duodenum. As pancreatic juice enters the duodenum, trypsinogen is activated by enterokinase into its active form, trypsin.

In AP, pancreatic enzymes become prematurely activated in the pancreas. This premature activation results in autodigestion of the pancreas and the peripancreatic tissue. The exact mechanism by which pancreatic enzymes become activated and initiate autodigestion is not fully understood. However, the activation of trypsinogen is thought to be the critical event that promotes the activation of other injurious enzymes, including elastase, kinases, and phospholipase A. Elastase can cause dissolution of elastic fibers in blood vessels, which can lead to hemorrhage. Activated kinins cause systemic vasodilation and increased vascular permeability, which promotes edema. Phospholipase A causes necrosis of the pancreas and the surrounding fatty tissue.

Pancreatic enzymes, vasoactive substances, hormones, and cytokines released from the injured pancreas cause a cascade of events that can lead to edema, vascular damage, hemorrhage, and necrosis. Systemic effects mediated by the immune system can lead to a systemic inflammatory response syndrome (SIRS), which can result in distant organ damage and multisystem organ failure. This immune response is independent of the event that causes AP but is responsible for the majority of the morbidity and mortality associated with it.

## Clinical Presentation

The diagnosis of AP requires the presence of two of the three following features: abdominal pain consistent with pancreatitis, serum lipase at least three times or greater the upper limit of normal, and characteristic findings on CT, MRI, or US.[15] The severity of the pain correlates to the degree of pancreatic involvement. The pain is usually deep and boring, midepigastric or periumbilical, with radiation to the back, but it may radiate to the spine, flank, or left shoulder. The pain usually begins abruptly and increases in intensity over several hours. It is usually steady, but can be exacerbated by intake. Pain associated with gallstone pancreatitis may be more localized to the right upper quadrant, more colicky, and more variable in intensity. The pain is usually exacerbated when the patient lies supine and is usually relieved when the patient sits and leans forward or lies in a fetal position. Patients are often restless and agitated. Nausea and vomiting without pain relief is common. Tachycardia, abdominal distention, and hypotension are other common symptoms. A low-grade fever may or may not be present. A persistent fever may indicate complications, such as peritonitis, cholecystitis, or intra-abdominal abscess.

The diagnosis of AP is often challenging because AP can mimic many other conditions. The differential diagnosis includes gastritis, perforated duodenal or gastric ulcers, acute SBO, ruptured ectopic pregnancy, sickle cell crisis, acute cholecystitis, mesenteric artery occlusion, and ruptured aortic aneurysm. Diagnosis is made on the basis of the patient's clinical presentation, history, physical examination findings, and the results of laboratory and radiographic studies (Box 41-9).

## Assessment

**HISTORY.** A careful history can provide important clues to diagnosis. A history of biliary tract disease, alcohol intake, diabetes, and medication use should be elicited to identify precipitating causes. A family history of AP may suggest hereditary causes. The patient may report anorexia, weight loss, nausea, vomiting, or abdominal distention. Assessment of the location, duration, quality, quantity, and precipitating factors of pain is important to help identify potential causes.

**PHYSICAL EXAMINATION.** Diffuse abdominal tenderness and guarding may be present during abdominal

**Physical Examination Findings**
- Abdominal pain
- Low-grade fever
- ± Jaundice
- Abdominal guarding or distention
- Paralytic ileus
- Grey Turner sign
- Cullen sign
- Nausea or vomiting without relief

**Laboratory Findings**
- Elevated serum and urine amylase
- Elevated serum lipase
- Elevated white blood cell (WBC) count
- Hypokalemia
- Hypocalcemia
- Elevated bilirubin, aspartate aminotransferase (AST), and PT (with liver disease)
- Elevated alkaline phosphatase level (with biliary disease)
- Hypertriglyceridemia
- Hyperglycemia
- Hypoxemia

palpation. The upper abdomen may be distended and tympanic to percussion. Bowel sounds may be hypoactive or absent, owing to decreased intestinal mobility or paralytic ileus. Jaundice may be present in gallstone disease or from obstruction of the biliary tree from pancreatic edema. Ascites or palpable abdominal masses may be present. Patients with severe acute hemorrhagic pancreatitis may have signs of dehydration and hypovolemic shock. These signs may worsen when fluid is lost into the bowel lumen because of a paralytic ileus. The presence of a bluish discoloration of the lower abdominal flanks (Grey Turner sign) or around the umbilical area (Cullen sign) indicates hemorrhagic pancreatitis and an accumulation of blood in these areas. These findings are rare, but if they occur, the findings usually do not appear until 48 hours or more after onset of symptoms.

**LABORATORY STUDIES.** No single laboratory study is diagnostic of AP; however, elevations of serum amylase and lipase enzymes are often seen in AP (see Chapter 39, Table 39-7). These enzymes are released as the pancreatic cells and ducts are destroyed. Serum amylase levels rise within 2 to 12 hours of the onset of symptoms and gradually return to baseline within 3 to 5 days in AP. In mild pancreatitis, amylase levels can be close to normal. If a few days have elapsed since symptoms began, amylase values can also be normal even with an active inflammatory process in the pancreas. The sensitivity of serum amylase is limited in patients with hypertriglyceridemia and in patients with an acute chronic alcoholic pancreatitis. The specificity of serum amylase is decreased in biliary tract disease, tumors, salivary gland lesions, cerebral trauma, gynecologic disorders, and renal failure. However, serum amylase levels that are more than three times the upper limits of normal are highly specific for pancreatitis.[15]

Compared with serum amylase levels, serum lipase levels rise later and remain elevated. Serum lipase levels usually rise within 4 to 8 hours of the onset of symptoms, peak at 24 hours, and return to normal after 8 to 14 days. Because the serum lipase level stays elevated longer, it is a useful test in diagnosis if there is a delay in examination. Like amylase, serum lipase levels may be elevated in patients who have intra-abdominal inflammation or renal insufficiency.

Elevations of isoenzymes, urinary amylase, and the amylase values of pleural fluid and paracentesis drainage support the presence of AP. Leukocytosis, hypokalemia, hypocalcemia, and hypertriglyceridemia may be present but are not specific to AP. Leukocytosis frequently results from infection, stress, or dehydration. Persistent vomiting may result in hypokalemia. Hypocalcemia may indicate the presence of pancreatic fat necrosis because calcium binds with fatty acids during tissue necrosis. In addition, trypsin inactivates parathyroid hormone, which is needed for calcium absorption. Hyperglycemia may result from decreased insulin release from damaged β cells, increased glucagon release, and the stress response. Hemoconcentration may occur as fluid is lost into the peritoneal space. Elevations in serum bilirubin, AST, and PT are common in the presence of concurrent liver disease. A greater than threefold elevation in ALT suggests biliary pancreatitis. Alkaline phosphatase is elevated with biliary tract disease. Triglyceride levels associated with AP are usually greater than 1,000 mg/dL.[14]

**IMAGING STUDIES.** Radiographs of the chest and abdomen are useful to exclude other causes of abdominal pain, including intestinal ileus, perforation, pericardial effusion, and pulmonary disease.

Abdominal ultrasonography is of limited use in visualization of the pancreas because of intestinal gas and adipose tissue. Abdominal ultrasonography is used to evaluate the biliary tree for gallstones, sludge, or ductal dilation as the etiology of pancreatitis. CT is the best imaging study to confirm the diagnosis and determine the severity of AP. CT can visualize the size of the pancreas and identify the presence of peripancreatic fluid, pancreatic pseudocysts, and abscesses. Dynamic CT done with contrast can help identify areas of necrosis in the pancreas. CT findings of extensive necrosis have correlated with a high risk for pancreatitis-related infection and death. Sequential CT allows for assessment of progressive disease or resolution. CT can also demonstrate fluid collection and areas of necrosis and can be used to guide percutaneous needle aspiration for culture.

Magnetic resonance cholangiopancreatography may have a sensitivity of more than 90% for bile duct stones. It can be used in patients who are pregnant and those who have allergies to the contrast used in CT or those with renal disease. Endoscopic retrograde cholangiopancreatography plays a role in locating and removing stones in the common bile duct if gallstone pancreatitis is present.

**TOOLS FOR PREDICTING SEVERITY.** AP is self-limiting and mild in 75% of patients, resolving spontaneously within 5 to 7 days.[17] These patients usually require conservative care. However, in 10% to 20% of patients with AP, increased intrapancreatic and extrapancreatic inflammation results in a systemic inflammatory response. Although the mortality rate for severe AP is 10%, this value rises to 30% or more when there are complications.[17] Multiple assessment tools have been developed in attempts to identify patients who are likely to develop severe AP so that aggressive treatment and surveillance can decrease complications and mortality.

---

**BOX 41-10** Ranson Criteria for Acute Pancreatitis

Evaluate on admission or on diagnosis:
- Age more than 55 years
- Leukocyte count more than 16,000/mL
- Serum glucose more than 200 mg/dL
- Serum lactate dehydrogenase more than 350 IU/mL
- Serum AST more than 250 IU/dL

Evaluate during initial 48 hours:
- Fall in hematocrit more than 10%
- BUN level rise more than 5 mg/dL
- Serum calcium less than 8 mg/dL
- Base deficit more than 4 mEq/L
- Estimated fluid sequestration more than 6 L
- Arterial $PaO_2$ less than 60 mm Hg

---

**BOX 41-11** Major Complications of Acute Pancreatitis

Local
- Pancreatic necrosis
- Pancreatic pseudocyst
- Pancreatic abscess

Pulmonary
- Atelectasis
- Acute respiratory distress syndrome
- Pleural effusions

Cardiovascular
- Hypotensive shock
- Septic shock
- Hemorrhagic shock

Renal
- Acute renal failure

Hematologic
- Disseminated intravascular coagulation (DIC)

Metabolic
- Hyperglycemia
- Hypertriglyceridemia
- Hypocalcemia
- Metabolic acidosis

Gastrointestinal
- Gastrointestinal bleed

---

Ranson criteria have been widely used to assess the severity of AP (Box 41-10). Ranson criteria consist of multiple clinical criteria used to identify those patients at risk for increased morbidity and mortality. The criteria assessed at admission indicate the severity of the acute inflammatory response, and the criteria assessed at 48 hours evaluate systemic effects. Three or more signs identified at the time of admission or during the initial 48 hours are predictive of severe AP. Ranson criteria have a greater than 90% accuracy rate and are useful clinically in identifying high-risk patients.[17] The primary disadvantage to Ranson criteria is the 48-hour delay before the assessment is completed.

Extravasation and third spacing seen in severe AP can cause significant intravascular volume depletion. This depletion can lead to decreased perfusion of the pancreas and cause pancreatic necrosis. Some experts have proposed that hemoconcentration, as detected by an elevated serum hematocrit, is a reliable predictor of necrotizing pancreatitis; however, there is no consensus.

The presence of peripancreatic inflammation, peripancreatic fluid collection, and extent of pancreatic necrosis found on CT have been shown to predict severity of AP. The CT severity index uses CT findings to grade pancreatic severity.

The use of serum markers to prognosticate severity has been tested. The most promising has been quantification of C-reactive protein (CRP). CRP rises in relation to severity, is inexpensive, and readily available. Unfortunately, CRP does not become significantly elevated until 48 hours after inflammation, which limits its use in diagnosis of AP.

## Complications

The local and systemic complications of AP are summarized in Box 41-11.

**LOCAL COMPLICATIONS.** The local effects of pancreatitis include inflammation of the peritoneum around the pancreas and fluid accumulation in the peritoneal cavity. These changes can lead to pancreatic pseudocyst, pancreatic abscess, and acute GI hemorrhage.

Pancreatic pseudocysts occur in up to 15% of all cases of AP. A pseudocyst is a collection of inflammatory debris and pancreatic secretions, enclosed by lined epithelial tissue and free of solid debris, that must be present for 4 weeks or more. The pseudocyst can rupture and hemorrhage or become infected, causing bacterial translocation and sepsis. A pseudocyst is suspected in any patient who has persistent

abdominal pain with nausea and vomiting, a prolonged fever, and elevated serum amylase. Surgery may also be indicated for pseudocysts; however, it is usually delayed because most pseudocysts resolve spontaneously. Surgical treatment of the pseudocyst can be done through internal or external drainage or needle aspiration. Acute surgical intervention may be required if the pseudocyst becomes infected or perforates.

A pancreatic abscess is a walled-off collection of purulent material in or around the pancreas that usually occurs 6 weeks or more after the onset of AP. Signs and symptoms of an abdominal abscess or infected pancreatic necrosis include increased white blood cell count, fever, abdominal pain, and vomiting. Pancreatic infection from an abscess, pseudocyst, or necrotic tissue may be present whenever a patient has a temperature greater than 39°C (102.2°F), tachycardia, or leukocytosis or shows other signs of clinical deterioration. Often, infections after the onset of pancreatitis, if untreated, are fatal. Broad-spectrum antibiotics are given to those patients with suspected infection.

GI complications of AP include GIB and bacterial translocation. GIB, the most common GI complication of AP, includes bleeding from peptic ulcers, hemorrhagic gastroduodenitis, stress ulcers, and Mallory–Weiss syndrome. Decreased peristalsis can lead to bacterial translocation.

**PULMONARY COMPLICATIONS.** Enzymes and inflammatory cytokines that reach the pulmonary circulation are thought to cause the many pulmonary complications associated with AP. Leukocytes that reach the pulmonary microcirculation migrate into the interstitium, which results in endothelial permeability and tissue edema. This causes lung congestion and alveolar collapse, and it can lead to adult respiratory distress syndrome. Arterial hypoxemia can occur in patients with mild disease without clinical or radiographic findings to support the pulmonary dysfunction. Arterial blood gas results and pulse oximetry should be followed closely for the first few days to detect this complication. Treatment of hypoxemia includes vigorous pulmonary care (eg, deep breathing and coughing) and frequent position changes. Oxygen therapy can also be used to improve overall oxygenation status. Careful fluid administration is also necessary to prevent fluid overload and pulmonary congestion. Patients with acute respiratory compromise may require mechanical ventilatory support. Abdominal distention and diminished diaphragmatic excursion may also contribute to atelectasis seen in AP.

**CARDIOVASCULAR COMPLICATIONS.** Hemodynamically significant fluid sequestration is characteristic of fulminant pancreatitis. Another major systemic effect of enzyme release into the circulatory system is peripheral vasodilation, which in turn can cause hypotension and shock.

Decreased perfusion to the pancreas itself can result in the release of myocardial depressant factor (MDF). MDF decreases heart contractility and affects cardiac output. Perfusion of all body organs can then become compromised. Early and aggressive fluid resuscitation is thought to prevent the release of MDF. Trypsin activation causes abnormalities in blood coagulation and clot lysis. This promotes the development of disseminated intravascular coagulation (DIC) with its associated bleeding (see Chapter 49).

**RENAL COMPLICATIONS.** Acute renal failure is thought to be a consequence of hypovolemia and decreased renal perfusion. Death during the first 2 weeks of AP usually results from pulmonary or renal complications.

**METABOLIC COMPLICATIONS.** Metabolic complications of AP include hypocalcemia and hyperlipidemia, which are thought to be related to areas of fat necrosis around the inflamed pancreas. Hyperglycemia may occur as a result of damage to the cells of the islets of Langerhans; metabolic acidosis can result from hypoperfusion and activation of anaerobic metabolism.

### Management

**MEDICAL MANAGEMENT.** Conventional care of the patient with AP focuses on fluid and electrolyte replacement to maintain or replenish vascular volume and electrolyte balance, pain management, resting the pancreas in an effort to prevent the release of pancreatic secretions, and maintaining the patient's nutritional status. Close observation and clinical judgment are the basis for therapy and management.

**FLUID AND ELECTROLYTE REPLACEMENT.** Most patients with AP require the infusion of IV fluids to replace fluid lost through third spacing into the retroperitoneal space or peritoneal cavity, and intravascular volume depletion as a result of inflammatory mediators and local inflammation caused by pancreatic enzyme exudates. Patients with severe AP may need up to 5 to 10 L of fluid replacement within 24 hours during their initial days of hospitalization. The goal is to administer enough fluid to obtain a circulating volume sufficient to maintain organ and tissue perfusion and prevent end-stage shock. Hypovolemia and shock are major causes

of death early in the disease process when aggressive fluid resuscitation fails to reverse the shock process.

Colloid and crystalloid solutions, such as albumin and lactated Ringer solution, are used for volume replacement. Patients with acute hemorrhagic pancreatitis may also need PRBCs to restore blood volume. Fluid replacement is evaluated by monitoring intake and output and daily weights. Patients with more severe disease may require hemodynamic monitoring with measurement of pulmonary artery occlusion pressure or CVP. Patients with severe disease whose hypotension fails to respond to fluid therapy may need medications to support blood pressure. The drug of choice is dopamine at low doses to maintain renal perfusion while supporting blood pressure.

Urinary output is a sensitive measure of the adequacy of fluid replacement, and it should be maintained at greater than 30 mL/h or 0.6 mL/kg/h. Blood pressure and heart rate are also sensitive measures of volume status.

Patients with severe hypocalcemia are placed on seizure precautions with respiratory support equipment on hand. The nurse is responsible for monitoring calcium levels, administering replacement solutions, and evaluating the patient's response to any calcium supplementation. Calcium replacements should be infused through a central line because peripheral infiltration can cause tissue necrosis. The patient also needs to be monitored for calcium toxicity; symptoms include lethargy, nausea, shortening of the QT interval, and decreased excitability of nerves and muscles. Hypomagnesemia may also be present, so magnesium may need to be replaced as well. Serum magnesium levels usually need to be corrected before calcium levels can return to normal. Potassium may need to be replaced early in the treatment regimen because it is lost through vomiting and sequestration of potassium-rich pancreatic juices.

Hyperglycemia is related to impaired secretion of insulin, an increased release of glucagon, or increased stress response. In some cases, hyperglycemia can be associated with dehydration or other electrolyte imbalances. Sliding-scale regular insulin may be ordered; it needs to be administered very cautiously because glucagon levels are only transiently elevated in AP. Successful fluid replacement is marked by return of alert mental status, urine output, cardiac output, stable hemodynamic values, and a normal serum lactate level.

**PAIN MANAGEMENT.** Pain control is a nursing priority for patients with AP, not only because of the extreme discomfort but also because pain increases pancreatic enzyme secretion. Pain is related to the degree of pancreatic inflammation, can be severe and constant, and can last for many days.

Adequate pain control with the use of IV narcotics, preferably delivered by patient-controlled analgesia, is essential in the treatment of AP. Meperidine (Demerol) has traditionally been the analgesic of choice because of the potential for sphincter of Oddi spasm that can accompany opioid use. However, meperidine is not always effective, and other analgesics (including opioids) should not be withheld. Fentanyl citrate (Sublimaze) and hydromorphone (Dilaudid) have been used successfully to control the pain of AP.

Analgesia should be routinely administered at least every 3 to 4 hours to prevent uncontrollable abdominal pain. Use of a pain rating scale is recommended for evaluating the patient's response to medication. Be alert to the patient's respiratory status because narcotics can induce respiratory depression. A nasogastric tube attached to low intermittent suction can help ease pain considerably, although the use of a nasogastric tube is controversial in patients without vomiting. Patient positioning can also relieve some of the discomfort.

**RESTING THE PANCREAS.** In some patients with AP, nasogastric suction is used to decompress the stomach and decrease stimulation of secretin. Secretin, which stimulates production of pancreatic secretions, is released in response to acid in the duodenum. Nausea, vomiting, and abdominal pain may decrease when a nasogastric tube is placed and connected to suction early in treatment. A nasogastric tube is also necessary in patients with severe gastric distention or a paralytic ileus. Patients with AP should be placed on NPO status until the abdominal pain subsides and serum amylase levels have returned to normal. Starting oral intake sooner can cause the abdominal pain to return and can induce further inflammation of the pancreas by stimulating the autodigestive disease process.

**NUTRITIONAL SUPPORT.** For those patients with AP who are on prolonged NPO status with nasogastric suction because of paralytic ileus, persistent abdominal pain, or pancreatic complications, nutritional support is recommended. TPN has been traditionally used because it was believed that stimulation of the pancreas by solid or liquid nutrients caused pancreatic stimulation and adversely affected the course of AP. Oral or enteral nutrition within 48 to 72 hours of admission is recommended.[18] In addition, enteral nutrition may reduce infectious complications by maintaining intestinal barrier function and avoiding some of the complications of parental nutrition. Lipid administration is avoided to prevent increasing triglyceride levels, which can exacerbate the inflammatory process. In the patient with mild AP, oral fluids can usually be restarted within 3 to 7 days, with solid food introduced slowly and as tolerated. Supplementation with TPN is appropriate if oral and enteral nutrition cannot provide enough calories to prevent catabolism.

Prolonged NPO status is often difficult for patients. Frequent mouth care and proper positioning of the nasogastric tube are important to maintain skin integrity and maximize patient comfort. Bed rest is prescribed to decrease the patient's basal metabolic rate; this, in turn, decreases the stimulation of pancreatic secretions.

**SURGICAL MANAGEMENT.** Surgery for AP is indicated if massive pancreatic necrosis is present in a patient with a worsening clinical status. A pancreatic resection for acute necrotizing pancreatitis can be performed to prevent systemic complications of the disease process. In this procedure, dead or infected pancreatic tissue is surgically removed. In some cases, the entire pancreas is removed. Broad-spectrum antibiotics are given to patients who require surgical débridement of necrotic tissue.

## Hepatitis

### Etiology

Diffuse inflammation of the liver, otherwise known as hepatitis, is commonly a consequence of a viral infection, but can be secondary to bacterial, fungal, or parasitic infection; a result

---

| BOX 41-12 | Selected Causes of Hepatic Inflammation |
|---|---|

**Infectious Diseases**
- Viral hepatitis (A, B, C, D, E)
- Epstein–Barr virus
- Cytomegalovirus
- Herpes simplex virus
- Coxsackievirus B
- Toxoplasmosis
- Adenovirus
- Varicella-zoster virus

**Drugs and Toxins**
- Alcohol
- Acetaminophen
- Isoniazid
- Salicylates
- Anticonvulsants
- Antimicrobials
- HMG-CoA reductase inhibitors
- α-Methyldopa
- Amiodarone
- Estrogens
- *Amanita phalloides* mushrooms
- Ecstasy (methylenedioxymethamphetamine)
- Herbal medicines (ginseng, comfrey tea, pennyroyal oil, *Teucrium polium*)

**Autoimmune Diseases**
- Autoimmune hepatitis
- Primary biliary cirrhosis
- Primary sclerosing cholangitis

**Congenital Diseases**
- Hemochromatosis (iron overload)
- Wilson disease (copper deposition)
- $\alpha_1$-Antitrypsin deficiency

**Miscellaneous Causes**
- Nonalcoholic fatty liver
- Fatty liver of pregnancy
- Severe right-sided congestive heart failure
- Budd–Chiari syndrome (vascular obstruction)

---

of toxic exposure; a side effect of a prescribed medication; or a consequence of an immunologic disorder (Box 41-12). Acute hepatitis lasts less than 6 months; it either resolves completely with return of normal liver function or progresses to chronic hepatitis, then cirrhosis, and possibly liver failure. Chronic hepatitis is an inflammatory process that lasts longer than 6 months and may also progress to cirrhosis and possibly liver failure.

**NONINFECTIOUS HEPATITIS.** Noninfectious hepatitis can be caused by excessive alcohol consumption, autoimmune disorders, metabolic or vascular disorders (including right-sided heart failure), acute biliary obstruction, and many individual drugs and drug classes (depending on the amount ingested and length of exposure). Examples include but are not limited to acetaminophen (both intentional and unintentional overdosing), isoniazid, HMG-CoA reductase inhibitors, anticonvulsants, antimicrobials, α-methyldopa, amiodarone, and estrogens. Although only a minority of chronic alcohol abusers develop the syndrome of alcoholic hepatitis, severe cases carry a significant mortality rate, particularly in the elderly.

Other liver toxins include poisonous mushrooms (*Amanita phalloides*), ecstasy (methylenedioxymethamphetamine), and some herbal medicines (ginseng, comfrey tea, pennyroyal oil, and *Teucrium polium*). Autoimmune hepatitis, a condition in which the patient's own immune system attacks the liver, causes inflammation and hepatocyte injury or death. Autoimmune hepatitis can be mistaken for an acute viral hepatitis if the patient presents with severe symptoms.

**INFECTIOUS HEPATITIS.** Viral hepatitis is a highly contagious inflammatory condition. Just like noninfectious hepatitis, infectious hepatitis can be acute, or it can be chronic if infection lasts longer than 6 months. Viral infections of the liver parenchyma have been classified according to their specific infecting agent and corresponding serology markers. Hepatitis A, B, C, D, and E are summarized in Table 41-2. Other viral causes of hepatitis include herpes simplex virus, Epstein–Barr virus, cytomegalovirus, adenovirus, coxsackievirus B, and varicella-zoster virus. Typically, patients with viral hepatitis present with nonspecific, flu-like symptoms, such as malaise, nausea, vomiting, diarrhea, loss of appetite, midepigastric abdominal discomfort, and low-grade fever. In patients with hepatitis B virus (HBV), symptoms may be more severe.

**Hepatitis A.** In the United States, the Centers for Disease Control and Prevention (CDC) have reported a significant decline in the incidence of acute hepatitis A virus (HAV) since the vaccine first became available in 1995.[19] However, sporadic outbreaks continue to be reported due to consumption of contaminated food or direct person-to-person contact.[19] HAV is caused by an RNA enterovirus transmitted through the oral–fecal route, predominantly by ingestion of contaminated water or raw or partially cooked shellfish. In most patients, symptoms of HAV infection are either relatively mild or nonexistent, although older patients are at greater risk for more severe symptoms. The incubation period ranges from 15 to 45 days after exposure. HAV infection causes only acute liver disease; recovery is usually complete and does not lead to chronic hepatitis or cirrhosis. Blood tests usually reveal elevations in the aminotransferases (ALT and AST), bilirubin concentrations, and alkaline phosphatase level. In severe cases, the PT may be prolonged. Diagnosis can be made with serology antibody testing. Anti-HAV immunoglobulin G (IgG) antibodies provide immunity and can be found in people who have had a previous HAV infection, but these are not helpful in diagnosing an acute infection. Instead, a positive anti-HAV IgM serology marker indicates HAV infection within the preceding 6 months. HAV infection does not induce a carrier state.

Early in the course of the disease, there is an incubation period during which the patient is asymptomatic but highly contagious, particularly with high HAV levels in the stool. After symptoms are apparent, the hepatitis infection can be misdiagnosed because many of the symptoms are similar to those of the flu. Some patients seek medical attention because they become jaundiced. The two most common physical examination findings are jaundice and hepatomegaly. Acute symptoms can progress or disappear once jaundice is present. By the time symptoms occur, the virus is no longer shed in the stool, and the patient is usually not infectious. Recovery is signaled by liver function test (LFT) results returning to normal.

After exposure to HAV, passive immunization can be achieved through the use of immune serum globulin. Most preparations of immune serum globulin contain adequate quantities of anti-HAV and should be given within 2 weeks of exposure. The immune serum globulin may not entirely abort an infection, but it significantly ameliorates the symptoms. It is usually given to intimate contacts of patients with HAV. There are also two US Food and Drug Administration (FDA)–approved vaccines: Havrix and Vaqta. A combination vaccine, Twinrix, contains both HAV and HBV virus antigens. All of these vaccines are inactivated. Vaccination is encouraged for all high-risk groups, all children aged 12 to 23 months, and children/adolescents aged 2 to 18 years who live in communities where there is a high disease incidence.[19]

**Hepatitis B.** HBV is a DNA virus of the Hepadnaviridae family that replicates by reverse transcription. Infection causes both acute and chronic hepatitis, and the incubation period is 30 to 180 days, with the average at 12 weeks. HBV is

| TABLE 41-2 | Summary of Types of Hepatitis | | | | |
| --- | --- | --- | --- | --- | --- |
| | **Hepatitis A** | **Hepatitis B** | **Hepatitis C** | **Hepatitis D** | **Hepatitis E** |
| Incubation (days) | 15–45 | 30–180 | 15–160 | 30–180 | 14–60 |
| Onset | Acute | Insidious | Insidious | Acute or insidious | Acute |
| Transmission | Fecal/oral | Blood | Blood | Blood | Fecal/oral |
| | Contaminated food, water | Sexual Perinatal Percutaneous | May be sexual | Sexual (comorbid infection with HBV) | Contaminated food, water |
| Severity | Mild | Often severe | Moderate | May be very severe | Virulent, especially in pregnant women |
| Prognosis | Generally good | Worse with age, debility | Moderate | Fair, worse with chronic disease | Good, unless pregnant |
| Diagnosis | | | | | |
| Acute | Anti-HAV IgM | HBsAG Anti-HBc (IgM) HBeAg | HCV ELISA Anti-HCV RIBA HCV RNA | HDV Ag | Clinical |
| Chronic | — | Anti-HBc (IgG) | Anti-HCV | Anti-HDV | — |
| Prophylaxis (adults) | Immune globulin | Hepatitis B vaccine Immune globulin | Immune globulin | None available | None available |
| Carrier | No | Yes | Yes | Yes | No |

spread by contact with blood or blood products. The antigen has been identified in body secretions, such as semen, mucus, and saliva; sexual exposure to a person with HBV is the most common mode of transmission. It appears that a break in the skin or the mucous membrane is necessary for the transmission to occur. HBV is also transmitted parenterally through blood transfusions, occupational needlestick injuries, and the use of contaminated needles (eg, illicit drug use). Maternal perinatal transmission can also occur.

The diagnostic criteria of HBV include serologic markers, biochemical markers of liver disease (including elevated liver enzyme levels), and histologic changes in the liver. Incorrect interpretation of HBV serologic markers is common. Familiarity with the serology testing is important for the nurse who is assisting in the diagnostic evaluation of a suspected case of viral hepatitis to prevent inappropriate laboratory testing and patient discomfort. Hepatitis B surface antigen (HBsAg) is a protein that coats the outer surface of the HBV and is produced in great excess during viral replication. HBsAg is the single most important test to detect infection with HBV; a positive result indicates that a patient is infected with HBV and is also infectious to others. If the presence of HBsAg is associated with an acute illness (less than 6 months) and a marked rise in the aminotransferases as well as the presence of hepatitis B core IgM antibody (IgM anti-HBc), the patient has acute HBV infection. If HBsAg disappears from the blood within 6 months, there is resolution of infection, and the patient does not advance to chronic disease. If HBsAg disappears from the blood within 6 months, this indicates resolution of infection and the patient does not advance to chronic disease. In patients with acute HBV infection who eradicate the virus by developing antibodies against hepatitis B surface antigen (anti-HBsAg), said antibodies will be detected through a positive hepatitis B surface antibody (anti-HBs) result. In some laboratories, these results may be reported as hepatitis B surface antibody (HBsAb) instead of anti-HBs. Regardless of the nomenclature, these individuals are protected against future HBV infection. A person who is successfully vaccinated against HBV with the HBV vaccine will also be anti-HBs (or HBsAb) positive. One additional marker in HBV testing includes the total hepatitis B core antibody (anti-HBc), which appears at the onset of symptoms and persists for life; a positive result indicates previous or chronic infection in an undefined time frame. In chronically infected patients, serum testing will reveal: HbsAg (positive), anti-HBc (positive), IgM anti-HBc (negative), and anti-HBs (negative).[20]

Clinical signs and symptoms of HBV infection during the acute phase are the same as those of HAV infection. Arthralgia, high fever, and rash are hallmark signs of an acute HBV infection. Acute HBV infection resolves in most adults; however, it can become chronic, particularly in those individuals with immune deficiencies. Those individuals who develop chronic HBV infection will continue to have high levels of HBsAg and can be infectious to others; individuals with a high viral load will also have an increased risk of chronic liver disease (eg, cirrhosis) and hepatocellular carcinoma. Cirrhosis should be suspected if the patient develops hypersplenism, hypoalbuminemia (in the absence of nephropathy), thrombocytopenia, and prolongation of serum PT. Although less than 1% of cases of those infected with HBV will progress to fulminant liver failure (typically occurs

within 4 weeks of the onset of symptoms), it is associated with encephalopathy, multiorgan failure, and a mortality rate of 75% if not treated with liver transplantation.[20]

HBV exposure is associated with high risk. After accidental exposure, such as an inadvertent needlestick, passive immunoprophylaxis can be achieved by using high anti-HBs titer hepatitis B immune globulin (HBIG). This is a pooled serum containing high titers of the anti-HBIG. It is recommended that HBIG be given within 48 hours of postexposure as inoculations to high-risk patients, to close contacts of patients with active HBV (within 2 weeks after sexual or personal contact with infected body fluids), and to those traveling to endemic areas who do not have time to go through the normal three-dose vaccination series.[20] The following medications are currently approved by the FDA for treating chronic HBV infection and include standard interferon alpha (INF-$\alpha$ 2b), pegylated interferon alpha (INF-$\alpha$ 2a), and oral antiviral agents (ie, lamivudine, adefovir, entecavir, telbivudine, and tenofovir).[20]

Fortunately, vaccines exist for active immunization against HBV (ie, Recombivax-HB or Engerix-B). Vaccination, administered prophylactically over a 6-month period, provides active immunization against HBV. It is highly recommended for health care personnel at risk for infection with HBV. It is also recommended for people who have had intimate contacts with people already infected with HBV. Precautions to protect against exposure to blood-borne pathogens must be followed. In the United States, children are universally vaccinated against HBV. Other combination vaccine preparations include Twinrix (HBV and HAV) and Pediarix (HBV, diphtheria, tetanus, acellular pertussis, and inactivated polio virus).[20]

**Hepatitis C.** Hepatitis C virus (HCV) has surpassed alcoholism to become the leading cause of liver cirrhosis and end-stage liver disease requiring liver transplantation in the United States.[21] As diagnostic tests improved, HCV, formerly called non-A, non-B hepatitis, was identified in 1989. It is a single-stranded RNA virus related to the Flaviviridae family. There are at least 6 known genotypes and more than 50 subtypes of HVC; all have different treatment options, duration of therapy and outcomes.[21] These differences highlight not only the importance of genotyping (ie, to determine the best treatment pathway) but also the challenges associated with vaccine development. Currently, no vaccine is available to prevent HCV and immune globulin does not afford protection to people who have been exposed.

HCV, a blood-borne virus, can cause both acute and chronic hepatitis. Of those people who develop acute HCV, chronicity can occur in as many as 75% to 85%, and 5% to 20% reportedly develop cirrhosis over approximately 20 to 30 years.[21] Of those individuals who develop cirrhosis, 1% to 5% will die from complications of cirrhosis or hepatocellular carcinoma.[21] Before 1992, when testing for HCV was mandated, many people acquired HCV through blood transfusions. The main risk factors in the United States include shared contaminated needles from illicit drug use and occupational needlestick exposure. There are indications that the virus might also be transmitted through perinatal, sexual, and household contacts (eg, sharing of razors and toothbrushes), although these modes of transmission are not as common. It has also been suggested that acupuncture, body piercing, tattooing, and even commercial barbering carry a risk for HCV transmission. Incubation of HCV is 15 to 160 days, with an average of 7 weeks. Within 6 months of infection, patients may produce anti–hepatitis C antibodies, but these do not confer immunity.

Although most patients with newly acquired HCV infection are asymptomatic (70% to 85%), up to 85% will continue on to chronic infection.[21] Although the majority may be asymptomatic, liver enzymes like alanine aminotransferase (ALT) may be elevated to greater than 200 IU/L. Those who clear the virus on their own are categorized as having resolved the HCV infection. The most commonly reported symptoms of HCV infection include fever, fatigue, dark urine, clay-colored stool, abdominal pain, anorexia, joint pain, and jaundice. HCV antibodies usually do not appear until several months after exposure but will always be present in the later stages of the disease. Diagnostic evaluation for HCV infection (ie, HCV antibody) includes either an HCV enzyme-linked immunosorbent assay (EIA), an enhanced chemiluminescence immunoassay (CIA), or a more anti-HCV specific assay (ie, recombinant immunoblot assay, RIBA). An HCV RNA test is ordered when anti-HCV is reactive (ie, antibody positive) and there remains a high index of suspicion for HCV infection. HCV RNA tests for the presence of the virus RNA in the blood (rather than antibodies against the virus); if detected, the patient has current HCV infection. If HCV RNA is not detected, there is no current HCV infection. However, it is important to differentiate a resolved HCV infection from a false positive HCV antibody test (ie, another HCV antibody assay test can be repeated).[21] Approximately 40% of those infected with HCV will have detectable antibody in their serum (positive anti-HCV) at 10 to 11 weeks postexposure; almost all infected persons will have a positive anti-HCV test 6 months postinfection. Since the discovery of HCV protease inhibitor therapies in 2011, evolution of additional drug therapies and improved patient outcomes are particularly impressive. The goal of HCV treatment is to reduce all-cause mortality and liver-related health adverse consequence, including end-stage liver disease and hepatocellular carcinoma, through the achievement of virologic cure as evidenced by a sustained virologic response (or SVR) at least 12 weeks after the completion of therapy.[22] Accordingly, the American Association for the Study of Liver Diseases and the Infectious Diseases Society of America recommend early treatment of chronic HCV infection before the development of liver disease and other complications to improve overall survival rates because recent studies demonstrate that new treatments cure more than 99% of patients who were followed for 5 years.[23,24]

Until recently, the mainstay of treatment for HCV infection has been pegylated interferon-α 2a or 2b plus ribavirin with or without first generation protease inhibitors (boceprevir and telaprevir) for HCV genotype 1, the most common genotype found in the United States. Individuals with genotypes 2 and 3 are almost three times as likely as individuals with genotype 1 to respond to α interferon or the combination of α interferon and ribavirin. For genotypes 2 and 3, a 24-week course of combination therapy is considered adequate whereas for genotype 1, a 48-week course is recommended.[21] It is important to note that once the genotype is identified, it does not need to be tested again (ie, genotypes will not change). A new class of potent direct-acting antiviral agents (DAA) has been included in treatment guidelines. Between 2013 and 2014, the FDA-approved two new potent DAAs, sofosbuvir and simeprevir, and a nonstructural 5A protein (NS5A) inhibitor, ledipasivir, to be used in various combination therapies (with or without interferon; with or without ribavirin) to treat chronic HCV infection with compensated liver disease, cirrhosis, HIV coinfection, and hepatocellular carcinoma awaiting liver transplant.[21] Although these new medications have once to twice daily oral administration frequency and reduced side effects (compared to interferon and ribavirin), duration of therapy (8 weeks minimum) can play a significant role in treatment adherence.

**Hepatitis D.** Hepatitis D (delta virus or HDV) is an incomplete RNA virus that depends on HBV envelope proteins to reproduce. It cannot exist or be spread in the absence of HBV. It is spread through percutaneous or mucosal contact with infectious blood. HDV infection may occur as a superinfection in the patient who has chronic HBV, or it may occur simultaneously with an acute HBV infection. Although uncommon in the United States, HDV can progress to fulminant hepatitis and chronic disease. Early in the disease, the hepatitis D antigen (HDV Ag) is present in the blood. Later in the disease, antibodies to the HDV are present (anti-HDV).

Because this disease coexists with HBV, patients with HDV have symptoms similar to those of acute or chronic HBV, but symptoms may be more pronounced. Quantitative real-time polymerase chain reaction (PCR) assays for HDV RNA are monitored at 3 and 6 months. Current treatment options are limited, but include standard INF, and recent research suggests that pegylated INF-α 2b may improve SVR. The addition of ribavirin has not been shown to provide any additional benefit.[25] There is no HDV vaccine, but vaccination against HBV may prevent HDV infection.[25]

**Hepatitis E.** Hepatitis E virus (HEV) is a single-stranded RNA virus similar to HAV. Although rare and sporadic in industrialized countries, it is the most common epidemic, water-borne form of hepatitis in developing countries.[26] It is transmitted by the oral–fecal route from contaminated water and food (individuals living in refugee camps or overcrowded temporary housing after natural disasters are at increased risk). Foodborne infection could occur from consumption of uncooked/undercooked meat/meat organs of infected animals (pork, boar, and deer meat).[26] Four different viral genotypes have been identified, each displaying different clinical characteristics. HEV genotype 1 is typically found in Asia and Africa; genotype 2 in Mexico or West Africa; and genotype 4 in Taiwan and China. HEV genotype 3 is often found in isolated cases in developed countries.[26] Symptoms typically present 15 to 60 days after exposure and can include fever, anorexia, nausea, vomiting, abdominal pain, hepatomegaly, and jaundice. Serum aminotransferase levels will be significantly elevated, but the infection is typically self-limited. For reasons that are still unclear, pregnant women have a more severe illness, with a mortality rate of 10% to 30% for women in their third trimester.[26] Because the incidence of HEV infection is rare in the United States, the nurse should pay careful attention if a patient presenting with symptoms of hepatitis has recently traveled or lived in endemic areas. There is no FDA-approved vaccine available for use in the United States; however, there is a recombinant vaccine that has recently been approved for use in China.[26] Unfortunately, previous HEV infection is not necessarily protective.

## Pathophysiology

To improve patient outcomes, nurses must have a solid knowledge base regarding the underlying pathophysiology, assessment, and management of acute and chronic liver disease. Hepatocytes, the functional cells of the liver, perform many essential functions, including the metabolism of nutrients (eg, glucose, proteins, lipids, vitamins) and the detoxification of medications, alcohol, ammonia, toxins, and hormones. In addition, hepatocytes are responsible for synthesis of clotting factors, conjugation and secretion of bilirubin, and synthesis of bile salts. Abnormal liver function is usually not apparent unless a significant acute insult occurs or chronic liver disease is fairly advanced. Liver failure occurs when there is a loss of 60% of the hepatocytes, and symptoms are usually detectable after 75% or more of the hepatocytes are injured or killed. LFT and evaluation begin with a complete history and physical examination. Interpretation of liver serum enzymes, synthetic function, and cholestasis (or excretory function) tests are important for the nurse to understand and are discussed later in this chapter.

Acute liver disease, typically caused by viral or chemical insults, occurs suddenly and resolves, becomes chronic, or results in a patient's death. Chronic liver disease leading to cirrhosis, typically more insidious in nature, is the 12th leading cause of death in the United States.[27] Disease processes in the liver can affect the hepatocytes, the blood vessels, and the Kupffer cells, which are responsible for uptake and subsequent degradation of foreign and potentially harmful substances in the body. If the injury is mild and reversible, hepatocytes may regenerate, and liver function may return to normal. However, if the injury is more severe or sustained, regeneration may be incomplete, or the healing process may cause fibrosis. Fibrotic changes alter the liver architecture and can lead to cirrhosis and impediment of blood flow through the liver. An acute insult to the liver can progress to fulminant liver failure, which is defined as hepatic encephalopathy (HE) occurring within 8 weeks of jaundice. HE is a state of abnormal mental functioning as a result of the inability of the liver to remove ammonia and other toxins from the blood. If liver function does not return and liver transplantation is unavailable, fulminant liver failure can progress to cerebral edema, coma, and death from brain herniation.

## Assessment

**HISTORY.** Questions regarding the patient's alcohol consumption and illicit drug use, use of prescription and over-the-counter medications, use of herbal supplements, surgical and transfusion history, occupational or travel exposure history, and sexual history may be helpful in determining the diagnosis, nursing plan of care, and teaching needs of the patient. In chronic hepatitis, most patients are asymptomatic except for mildly elevated liver enzymes. Constitutional symptoms vary widely but typically include malaise, fatigue, low-grade fever, nausea, vomiting, and sometimes diarrhea.

**PHYSICAL EXAMINATION.** When cirrhosis and portal hypertension resulting from chronic hepatitis are present, jaundice (yellow staining of the skin and mucous membranes as a result of bilirubin pigments) may be noted. Hepatomegaly (enlargement of the liver) may result in right upper quadrant tenderness and is a result of portal hypertension or congestion in the liver from altered blood flow resulting from cirrhosis. The liver edge is often firm and nodular. In advanced cirrhosis, although the left lobe may be enlarged, overall liver size is often decreased and difficult to palpate. Dullness of percussion over the liver span can provide serial observations of resolution of hepatitis or progression of cirrhosis. Splenomegaly as a result of portal hypertension and sequestration of fluid in the spleen may result in left upper quadrant tenderness. Muscle wasting and abdominal ascites may develop as a result of malnutrition, portal hypertension, and hypoalbuminemia from the liver's impaired ability to synthesize proteins. Peripheral edema may result from hypoalbuminemia, sodium retention, and ascites obstructing blood return from the lower extremities. Vitamin deficiencies may result in glossitis of the tongue and cheilosis of the lips. Bruising and bleeding tendencies may develop as a result of impaired production of clotting factors and sequestration of platelets in the spleen. Other manifestations include telangiectasis or spider nevi (usually of the upper half of the body). These lesions consist of a pulsating arteriole from which smaller vessels radiate. Palmar erythema, or redness of the palms, is a result of increased blood flow from hyperdynamic cardiac dysfunction associated with hepatitis (with ascites). In men, there may be a loss of body hair, testicular atrophy, and gynecomastia. These changes are thought to be related to altered hormone metabolism and estrogen excess in the liver.

Physical examination may also reveal abdominal wall vein dilation around the umbilicus, known as caput medusae. This is the result of portal hypertension and congestion and collateral vessel development. This congestion may be auscultated as an arterial bruit (systolic phase) or a venous hum (both systolic and diastolic phases) over the liver and epigastrium. Encephalopathy, ascites, and peripheral edema, reflective of advanced disease, may be present. Other observable assessment findings include frothy, dark amber urine and clay-colored stools as a result of alterations in bilirubin excretion. Common signs and symptoms of noninfectious and infectious hepatitis are summarized in Table 41-3. Patients with signs and symptoms of hepatic decompensation (eg, portal hypertension, ascites, encephalopathy, and coagulopathy) should be hospitalized, evaluated, and treated more expeditiously than those patients who demonstrate adequate hepatic compensation and stability.

## LABORATORY STUDIES.

**Tests for Evaluating Hepatocellular Injury.** The clinical significance of any liver chemistry must be evaluated in the context of the patient's history and clinical situation. LFT is a commonly used but inaccurate term. Some laboratory tests do measure liver synthetic function, and these include albumin, PT, and total bilirubin. However, other laboratory tests are markers of hepatocellular injury and include AST, previously known as serum glutamic oxaloacetic transaminase, and ALT, previously known as serum glutamic pyruvic transaminase. See Chapter 39, Table 39-6.

ALT and AST are enzymes present inside the hepatocytes. When hepatocytes are injured or die, they release AST and ALT into the serum. Therefore, the presence of these enzymes in the blood signals the presence of hepatocyte injury. However, AST and ALT lack sensitivity (for a particular

| TABLE 41-3    Common Signs and Symptoms of Hepatitis | |
|---|---|
| **Signs and Symptoms** | **Cause** |
| **Constitutional** | |
| Fever, chills | Immune response to viral infection |
| Generalized weakness, malnutrition | Inability to metabolize nutrients |
| **Gastrointestinal** | |
| Right upper quadrant pain | Hepatomegaly |
| Left upper quadrant pain | Splenomegaly |
| Loss of appetite | Ascites, fatigue |
| Abdominal distention | Ascites |
| Nausea, vomiting/hematemesis | Portal hypertension |
| Clay-colored feces | Inability to excrete conjugated bilirubin |
| Diarrhea | Impaired fat metabolism |
| Melena, hematochezia | Portal hypertension |
| **Pulmonary** | |
| Shortness of breath | Ascites, decreased lung and diaphragmatic expansion |
| Increased work of breathing | |
| Decreased oxygen saturation | |
| Decreased partial pressure of oxygen | |
| **Cardiac** | |
| Increased heart rate | Hypotension, sequestration of fluid in the liver and spleen, third spacing in the periph- |
| Decreased blood pressure | eral extremities from decreased protein metabolism/low albumin levels |
| Dysrhythmias | Electrolyte disturbances |
| Peripheral edema | Impaired protein metabolism |
| **Neurologic** | |
| Headache | Impaired metabolism of ammonia and other circulating toxins |
| Depression/irritability | |
| Asterixis | |
| **Genitourinary** | |
| Decreased urinary output | Decreased circulating volume and impaired glomerular filtration rate |
| Frothy, dark amber urine | Excretion of conjugated bilirubin (water-soluble bile) |
| **Integumentary** | |
| Jaundice | Impaired excretion of bile |
| Pruritus, dry skin | Impaired excretion of bile |
| Bruising, ecchymosis | Impaired ability to synthesize clotting factors |
| Spider nevi, caput medusae | Portal hypertension |
| Palmar erythema | Portal hypertension |
| Hair loss | Impaired metabolism of circulating hormones |
| **Endocrine** | |
| Hypoglycemia | Impaired glucose metabolism and storage |
| Increased weight | Ascites, third spacing of fluid |
| Gynecomastia, testicular atrophy (in men) | Inability to metabolize hormones (eg, estrogens) |
| **Immune** | |
| Infection, spontaneous bacterial peritonitis | Impaired Kupffer cell function, splenomegaly |

diagnosis) in evaluating chronic liver injury for two reasons. First, AST and ALT are also found (to a lesser degree) in the skeletal muscle, and as such, elevations may be related to a skeletal muscle injury or overexertion. This is particularly true for AST because ALT is almost exclusively present in hepatocytes and is the most specific test for hepatocellular damage. Second, it is thought that dying hepatocytes synthesize less AST and ALT enzymes than healthy ones. Therefore, despite inflammation detected on a liver biopsy, patients with chronic hepatitis may have relatively normal levels of AST and ALT.

Despite these difficulties in laboratory interpretation, elevations of AST and ALT are often helpful in evaluating acute liver injury, response to treatment, and monitoring those at risk for liver disease because of medical interventions. Elevations of these enzymes suggest hepatocyte death, and the degree of elevation roughly approximates the amount of liver cell death. AST and ALT elevate at relatively equal levels, but an exception occurs in alcoholic hepatitis, in which AST levels tend to be higher than ALT levels. Although the AST/ALT ratio is not diagnostic, a ratio greater than 2:1 suggests alcohol-induced injury. This is thought to be due to the depletion of vitamin $B_6$ (pyridoxine) in patients with chronic alcoholism; ALT synthesis is more strongly inhibited by pyridoxine deficiency than AST synthesis. In chronic hepatitis, AST and ALT levels are usually less than 10 times normal. However, in acute viral, toxin-induced, or ischemic hepatitis, these elevations may be greater than 1,000 units/L. In addition, alcoholic hepatitis causes smaller elevations (less than 300 units/L). Unfortunately, AST and ALT levels have low prognostic value.

**Tests for Evaluating Liver Synthetic Function.** As mentioned earlier, albumin, total protein, and PT are measures of actual liver synthetic function. Because proteins are synthesized by the liver, albumin and other proteins are an index of liver function. Albumin is the predominant protein in the serum; patients with advanced liver disease and cirrhosis tend to have low serum concentrations (hypoalbuminemia). Because albumin is responsible for colloid osmotic pressure, low concentrations lead to leakage of intravascular fluids into interstitial spaces and peripheral edema. Because albumin levels are also influenced by poor nutrition and renal disease, care must be taken when interpreting laboratory test results.

The PT is a measure of the liver's capacity to synthesize clotting factors. The liver synthesizes blood clotting factors II, V, VII, IX, and X. An elevation in PT values is not seen until more than 80% of hepatocyte function is lost. However, because of the short half-life of factor VII, a PT is helpful in evaluating acute liver failure. Evaluation for vitamin K deficiency is performed because malabsorption or poor nutritional intake must be excluded in a patient who is hypoprothrombinemic. Failure of improvement in a PT level after vitamin K supplementation (5 to 10 mg orally for 3 days) may indicate intrinsic liver disease.

**Tests for Evaluating Cholestasis (Excretory Function).** Tests for cholestasis (lack of bile flow) help determine what is happening in the bile ducts. Obstruction of bile flow may be extrahepatic (eg, gallstones, postsurgical stricture, or malignancy) or intrahepatic (eg, poor hepatocyte function or damage to the small septal or intralobular bile ducts). Present in the biliary epithelium, elevated alkaline phosphatase and $\gamma$-glutamyltransferase levels reflect damage to the bile ducts or obstruction of bile flow.

An elevated serum bilirubin level is roughly proportional to the amount of liver dysfunction or disease severity. Bilirubin is the major source of hemoglobin metabolism from the destruction of adult RBCs. The unconjugated (indirect) form of bilirubin is not water soluble and is bound to albumin as a means of transport to the liver for conjugation and subsequent excretion in the bile. In the hepatocytes, unconjugated bilirubin is combined with glucuronic acid to make it water soluble (or conjugated) for excretion into the bile and feces. Cholestasis causes reflux of conjugated bilirubin into the blood (a condition called conjugated hyperbilirubinemia), so the conjugated bilirubin is instead excreted through the kidneys. The urine becomes frothy and very dark amber in color from bilirubin pigments. The nurse may be asked to perform a dipstick test on the urine for bilirubin to confirm this clinical suspicion. Unconjugated hyperbilirubinemia results from a poor nutritional state (eg, decreased albumin available for transport of bilirubin to the liver) or hepatocyte dysfunction in the conjugation process. Jaundice is usually present when the serum bilirubin level is greater than 2.5 mg/dL.

## Management

The primary treatment of acute hepatitis of any type is primarily supportive. Measures include providing rest and adequate nutrition and preventing further liver injury by avoiding hepatotoxic medications and substances. Hospitalization is rarely required but is needed in cases of disease complicated by hemodynamic instability, failure to maintain adequate nutrition and fluid intake, encephalopathy, blood coagulopathies, and renal failure.

In situations of hemodynamic instability, monitoring of blood pressure, heart rate, cardiac dysrhythmias, and urine output is essential. IV fluids will most likely be needed. It is important to avoid lactated Ringer solutions because of the inability of the impaired liver to metabolize lactate, which could induce or exacerbate a metabolic acidosis. Frequent monitoring of hepatic enzymes and synthetic function is requested to evaluate disease progression and response to treatment interventions. Electrolyte, nutrient, and vitamin abnormalities from disease progression, malnutrition, and nausea and vomiting require repletion. The nurse may have to assist in invasive treatments or procedures, such as placement of a Sengstaken–Blakemore tube for control of bleeding esophageal varices, paracentesis for ascites, and liver biopsy. In the event of fluid volume overload, diuretics, albumin, and protein supplements may be prescribed. Accurate intake and output, daily weight, and abdominal girth measurements may alert the nurse to significant volume shifts and potential hemodynamic or respiratory issues.

Maintaining adequate nutrition is a priority. Small, frequent meals and antiemetics are administered as needed. A high-calorie, low-protein diet is recommended to prevent complications associated with impaired protein and ammonia metabolism associated with acute HE. However, a low-protein diet is used only in the short term because seriously ill patients actually have increased protein requirements to build and maintain muscle mass and to assist in healing and repair. Parenteral nutrition is needed only if oral intake is impaired by intractable nausea and vomiting. Patients with severe fatigue require frequent rest and spacing of activities.

Because of the risk for coagulopathy, the nurse must monitor for bleeding gums, epistaxis, ecchymosis, petechiae, hematemesis, hematuria, and melena. Vitamin K may be prescribed to help reduce the effects of bleeding tendencies, and a PT may be ordered to monitor the efficacy of treatment.

Avoidance of alcohol, narcotics, barbiturates, and medications that are metabolized by the liver is recommended. Careful observation and documentation of patient responses (eg, mental status, level of consciousness) to medications and treatment regimens is recommended. Because of the liver's inability to metabolize or detoxify many foods, drugs, and toxins, the nurse may be asked to administer frequent medications, such as lactulose, neomycin sulfate, and metronidazole, to treat HE. Lactulose is a laxative that acidifies the colon to prevent the absorption of ammonia. The dose of lactulose is titrated so that the patient has two to three soft stools per day without diarrhea. Neomycin and metronidazole act as antibiotics to clear the colon of bacteria that produce ammonia.

If severe pruritus from jaundice is present, a bile salt sequestering agent (eg, cholestyramine), a topical emollient, or both can be used to help alleviate this symptom. Mittens may need to be used to prevent excessive scratching and subsequent skin breakdown in a confused patient.

Patient teaching for the patient with hepatitis includes measures to prevent infection and transmission, dietary limitations and alcohol avoidance, and the necessity for follow-up care. The patient is advised to monitor activity tolerance and fatigue. If signs and symptoms persist and liver enzymes remain elevated for greater than 6 months, the patient will progress to chronic disease. This is more common in HBV and HCV infection and is confirmed by liver biopsy.

## Complications of Liver Disease

Complications of advanced liver disease include cirrhosis, HE, hepatorenal syndrome (HRS), spontaneous bacterial peritonitis (SBP), and hepatocellular carcinoma.

## Cirrhosis

### Etiology

As noted earlier, chronic HCV infection and alcohol abuse are the most common causes of liver cirrhosis. However, cirrhosis of the liver can result from a number of other diseases, which include but are not limited to nonalcoholic steatohepatitis, hereditary hemochromatosis, Wilson disease, and $\alpha_1$-antitrypsin deficiency.

### Pathophysiology

Cirrhosis, which develops over time, can cause severe alterations in the structural architecture of the liver and function of the hepatocytes. These changes are characterized by inflammation and liver cell necrosis, which can be focal or diffuse. Necrosis is followed by regeneration of liver tissue but not in a normal fashion. Fibrous tissue and regenerative nodules develop over time, which distorts the normal architecture of the liver lobule and alters blood flow. These fibrotic changes are irreversible, resulting in chronic liver dysfunction and eventual liver failure. Fatty deposits in the parenchymal cells may be seen initially. The cause of the fatty changes is unclear, but it may be a response to alterations in enzymatic function responsible for normal fat metabolism. Eventually, all of the liver's metabolic processes are altered.

Inflammation, fibrotic changes, and increased intrahepatic vascular resistance cause compression of the liver lobule, leading to increased resistance or obstruction of normal blood flow through the liver, which is normally a low-pressure system. This portal hypertension results in significant venous congestion and dilation (Fig. 41-4). Subsequently, nutrient-rich blood from the GI tract is shunted away from the liver, the first site of metabolism for many nutrients, drugs, and toxins. Pressure builds up in the systemic venous circulation, causing congestion where the portal and systemic venous systems connect: the esophagus, stomach, and rectum. These vascular changes result in varicose veins, or varices.

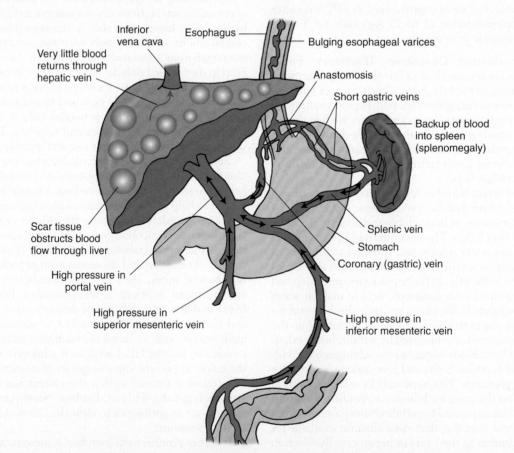

**FIGURE 41-4** Esophageal varices develop from increased portal pressure. In an attempt to return blood to the systemic circulation, collateral veins develop to bypass increased portal resistance. These collateral vessels become tortuous and distended and are called varices.

Esophageal varices and gastric varices are of particular concern in the care of these patients because they are extremely friable. Rupture from these varices can result in massive internal bleeding that may be life-threatening. Portal hypertension also promotes increased collateral circulation and allows blood to flow from the intestines directly to the vena cava. This congestion is often seen as a collection of prominent vessels on the surface of the abdomen and is known as caput medusae. Splenomegaly results from the sequestration of trapped blood from portal hypertension. Of particular concern is the trapping of platelets, which can be seen clinically by bleeding tendencies and a thrombocytopenia on laboratory evaluation. Frank hematemesis or bleeding from esophageal and gastric varices can cause melena. Hemorrhoidal varices, or hemorrhoids, can also result from portal hypertension. Finally, portal hypertension may result in abdominal fluid accumulation, known as ascites. As liver disease progresses and cirrhosis develops, mild to moderate high-output cardiac dysfunction may occur. This hyperdynamic dysfunction is characterized by splanchnic and systemic vasodilation, an afterload effect that decreases cardiac work and elevates cardiac output. Clinically, it is seen as hypotension, tachycardia, and cardiac flow murmurs. As hepatic cirrhosis progresses, these clinical findings become more pronounced. Figure 41-5 illustrates clinical effects of cirrhosis.

## Assessment

In some patients, cirrhosis may be subclinical. However, history and physical examination findings may reveal clues to altered liver function. For example, altered carbohydrate metabolism can result in unstable blood glucose levels. Altered fat metabolism can cause fatigue and decreased activity tolerance. Altered protein metabolism results in a decreased synthesis of albumin. Albumin is necessary for colloid osmotic pressure, which holds fluid in the intravascular space. A decrease leads to interstitial tissue edema and decreased plasma volume. Globulin, another protein, is essential for normal blood clotting. This, coupled with a decreased synthesis of many blood clotting factors and decreased metabolism of vitamins and iron, predisposes the patient to hematologic complications that range from bruising to hemorrhage. A low-grade DIC also may develop. Portal hypertension, ascites, and lower extremity edema cause hypotension. Initially, the patient may have flushed skin and bounding pulses from the vasodilation in the portal venous system, which leads to a hyperdynamic state with peripheral circulation vasodilation and hypotension. Table 41-4 summarizes laboratory findings in patients with cirrhosis and impending liver failure.

## Management

Management goals include preventing additional stress on liver function and early recognition and treatment of complications. Liver functions under stress include nutritional metabolism, clearing medication and metabolic waste products, and formation of clotting factors. Interventions include monitoring nutritional markers and providing nutrition; monitoring fluid balance, urinary output, electrolyte and chemistry studies, drug type, and dose requirements; monitoring bleeding times, platelet function, and hematocrit; and detecting signs of bleeding (Box 41-13). Bowel cleansing regimens may be ordered. The early recognition of complications includes

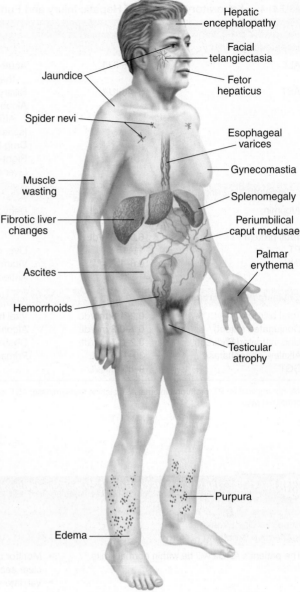

**FIGURE 41-5** Clinical effects of cirrhosis of the liver. (From Porth CM: Pathophysiology: Concepts of Altered Health States, 8th ed. Philadelphia, PA: Wolters Kluwer Health/Lippincott Williams & Wilkins, 2009, p 968.)

detecting signs of impending liver failure: changes in neurologic and mental status, increasing ascites, and HRS.

The critically ill patient in liver failure is often in some state of unconsciousness, with jaundiced skin and sclera. Coagulation times are prolonged, so bleeding is apt to occur from many sources. There is a risk for sores and skin breakdown because of the patient's debilitated state.

Maintaining fluid and electrolyte balance requires ongoing nursing assessment. Imbalance can result from replacement therapy, malnutrition, gastric suction, diuretics, vomiting, diaphoresis, ascites, diarrhea, inadequate fluid intake, and elevated aldosterone levels. The patient may complain of headache, weakness, numbness and tingling of extremities, muscle twitching, thirst, nausea, or muscle cramps and may become confused. The nurse is asked to monitor weight and

**TABLE 41-4** Laboratory Studies for Hepatic Injury and Function

| Parameter | Normal | Increased | Decreased |
|---|---|---|---|
| **Hepatocellular Injury** | | | |
| ALT | 5–35 IU/L | Acute viral hepatitis (ALT more than AST) | Vitamin B deficiency |
| AST | 5–40 IU/L | Biliary tract obstruction | |
| | | Alcoholic hepatitis (AST more than ALT) | |
| | | Ischemia or hypoxia ("shock liver") | |
| | | Drug toxicity | |
| | | Right-sided heart failure | |
| | | Liver cancer | |
| **Liver Synthetic Function** | | | |
| Albumin | 3.4–4.7 g/dL | Dehydration, shock | Chronic liver disease, malnutrition, malabsorption |
| Total protein | 6.0–8.0 g/dL | | |
| PT | 11–15 s | Liver disease | N/A |
| INR | 0.8–1.2 s | Vitamin K deficiency | |
| | | Anticoagulants | |
| **Cholestasis or Excretory Function** | | | |
| Total bilirubin | 0.2–1.3 mg/dL | Viral hepatitis | N/A |
| Conjugated (direct) | 0.1–0.3 mg/dL | Alcoholic hepatitis | |
| Unconjugated (indirect) | 0.2–0.7 mg/dL | Obstructive jaundice | |
| Alkaline phosphatase | 30–115 IU/L | Primary biliary cirrhosis | |
| GGT | 9–85 units/L | | |

N/A, not applicable; PT, prothrombin time; ALT, alanine transaminase; AST, aspartate aminotransferase; GTT, gamma-glutamyl transpeptidase; INR, international normalized ratio.

---

**QSEN BOX 41-13** *COLLABORATIVE CARE GUIDE for the Patient With Cirrhosis and Impending Liver Failure*

| Outcomes | Interventions |
|---|---|
| **Impaired Gas Exchange** **Ineffective Breathing Pattern** | |
| The patient's ABGs will be within normal limits. | • Monitor pulse oximetry and ABG values, respiratory rate and pattern, and ability to clear secretions. |
| | • Validate significant changes in pulse oximetry with co-oximetry arterial saturation measurement. |
| The patient has no evidence of pulmonary edema or atelectasis. | • Assist patient to turn, cough, deep breathe, and use incentive spirometer every 2 h. |
| Breath sounds are clear bilaterally. | • Provide chest percussion with postural drainage if indicated every 4 h. |
| | • Monitor effect of ascites on respiratory effort and lung compliance. |
| | • Position patient on side and with head of bed elevated to improve diaphragmatic movement. |
| **Decreased Cardiac and Tissue Perfusion** **Risk for Bleeding** **Risk for Ineffective Gastrointestinal Perfusion** | |
| Patient will achieve or maintain stable blood pressure and oxygen delivery. | • Monitor vital signs, including cardiac output, systemic vascular resistance, oxygen delivery, and oxygen consumption. |
| Serum lactate will be within normal limits. | • Monitor lactate daily until it is within normal limits. |
| | • Administer RBCs, positive inotropic agents, colloid infusion as ordered to increase oxygen delivery. |
| Patient will not experience bleeding related to coagulopathies, varices, hepatorenal syndrome. | • Monitor PT, PTT, complete blood count daily. |
| | • Assess for signs of bleeding (eg, blood in gastric contents, stools, or urine); observe for petechiae, bruising. |
| | • Administer blood products as indicated. |
| | • Assist with insertion and manage the esophageal tamponade balloon tube. |
| | • Perform gastric lavage as needed. |

**QSEN BOX 41-13** *COLLABORATIVE CARE GUIDE for the Patient With Cirrhosis and Impending Liver Failure (continued)*

| Outcomes | Interventions |
|---|---|
| **Electrolyte Imbalance** **Risk for Imbalanced Fluid Volume** | |
| Patient is euvolemic. Patient will not gain weight due to fluid retention. | • Daily weights • Monitor intake and output. • Monitor electrolyte values. • Measure abdominal girth daily at the same location on the abdomen. • Monitor signs of volume overload: Cardiac gallop Pulmonary crackles Shortness of breath Jugular vein distention Peripheral edema • Administer diuretics as ordered. |
| **Risk for Injury** **Impaired Physical Mobility** **Risk for Activity Intolerance** **Risk for Infection** | |
| Patient is alert and oriented. Ammonia level is within normal limits. Patient achieves or maintains ability to conduct activities of daily living and mobilize self. No evidence of infection, WBC within normal limits. | • Assess serum ammonia level. • Administer lactulose as ordered. • Monitor level of consciousness, orientation, thought processing. • Assess asterixis. • Take precautions to prevent falls. • Consult physical therapist. • Conduct range-of-motion and strengthening exercises. • Monitor SIRS criteria: increased WBC, increased temperature, tachypnea, tachycardia. • Use aseptic technique during procedures and monitor others. • Maintain invasive catheter tube sterility. • Change invasive catheters, culture blood, line tips, or fluids, provide site care, etc., according to hospital protocol. |
| **Impaired Skin Integrity** | |
| Skin will remain intact. | • Assess skin every 8 h and each time patient is repositioned. • Turn patient every 2 h. Assist or teach patient to shift weight or reposition. • Consider pressure relief/reduction mattress. |
| **Imbalanced Nutrition** | |
| Caloric and nutrient intake meets metabolic requirements per calculation (eg, basal energy expenditure). Evidence of metabolic dysfunction is minimal. | • Provide nutrition by oral, enteral, or parenteral feeding. • Adhere to sodium, protein, fat, or fluid restrictions as necessary. • Consult dietitian or nutritional support service to evaluate nutritional needs and restrictions. • Provide small, frequent feedings. • Monitor albumin, prealbumin, transferrin, BUN, cholesterol, triglycerides, bilirubin, aspartate transaminase, alanine transaminase. • Administer cleansing enemas and cathartics if ordered. |
| **Impaired Comfort** | |
| Patient will have minimal pain. Patient will have minimal pruritus. | • Assess pain and discomfort from ascites, bleeding, pruritus. • Administer analgesics cautiously and monitor patient response. • Bathe with cool water, blot dry. • Lubricate skin. • Administer antipruritic medication; apply to skin PRN as ordered. |
| **Ineffective Coping** **Anxiety** | |
| Patient demonstrates decreased anxiety. | • Assess patient's response to illness. Provide time to listen. • Assess effect of critical care environment on the patient. • Minimize sensory overload. • Provide adequate time for uninterrupted sleep. • Encourage flexible visiting hours for family. • Plan for consistent care giver. |

*(continued)*

**QSEN** **BOX 41-13** *COLLABORATIVE CARE GUIDE for the Patient With Cirrhosis and Impending Liver Failure (continued)*

| Outcomes | Interventions |
|---|---|
| **Teaching/Discharge Planning** | |
| Patient/significant others understand procedures and tests needed for treatment of hepatic dysfunction. | • Prepare patient/significant others for procedures such as paracentesis or laboratory studies.<br>• Teach patient and family information regarding sodium, protein, and fluid restrictions. Give written instructions. |
| Patient/significant others are prepared for home care. | • Teach signs and symptoms of progressing hepatic failure (eg, change in mentation, skin coloration, ascites).<br>• Teach signs and symptoms of occult bleeding and respiratory infection.<br>• Teach home medication regimen.<br>• Teach comfort measures. |

CVP trends to help determine fluid retention and vascular loading. Other assessment clues to monitor include any increase or decrease in urinary output, cardiac dysrhythmias, changes in mental status or level of consciousness, prolonged vomiting or frequent liquid stools, muscle tremors, spasms, edema, or poor skin turgor.

Impaired handling of salt and water by the kidney and other abnormalities in fluid homeostasis predispose the patient to ascites, an accumulation of fluid in the peritoneum. This complication can be problematic because it can restrict movement of the diaphragm, impairing the patient's breathing pattern. Therefore, monitoring respiratory status by the nurse is crucial. Ascites is managed through bed rest, a low-sodium diet of no more than 2,000 mg/d, fluid restriction, and diuretic therapy.[28] It has been demonstrated that ascites absorption has an upper limit of 700 to 900 mL/d during diuresis therapy. If diuresis exceeds this limit, it may be at the expense of the intravascular volume and may potentiate hemodynamic instability. Diuresis with spironolactone, an aldosterone antagonist, is first-line diuretic therapy for ascites, although combination therapy with furosemide is more effective.[28] Monitoring for electrolyte imbalance, particularly hypokalemia, is essential. In addition to strict intake and output balance and daily weights, abdominal girth should be measured daily.

Paracentesis is also used to treat ascites in patients unresponsive to salt restriction and maximal diuretic therapy.[28] In this procedure, ascitic fluid is withdrawn from the abdomen through percutaneous needle aspiration. As much as 4 to 6 L/d of ascitic fluid can be withdrawn, and close monitoring of vital signs is important during this procedure because a sudden loss of intravascular pressure may precipitate hypotension, decreased renal perfusion, and tachycardia. Volume expanders are recommended if 5 L or more of ascitic fluid are withdrawn during a single paracentesis procedure (eg, replacement of 5 to 10 g of albumin per liter of removed ascites fluid).[28] As with any invasive procedure, there is an increased risk for infection, particularly with repeated large-volume paracentesis procedures (eg, refractory ascites). Refractory ascites results from continued deterioration of liver function and increased portal pressure, increased circulating vasoconstrictors, and decrease in renal blood flow. Refractory ascites marks a sentinel deterioration in the patient's disease trajectory. Refractory ascites requires repeated paracentesis, with decreasing intervals of time between procedures. Unfortunately, paracentesis does not improve the overall poor prognosis, and all patients with refractory ascites should be referred for consideration for a liver transplantation.

A venous–peritoneal (VP) shunt is used to relieve ascites that is resistant to other therapies. The LeVeen shunt (Fig. 41-6) is inserted by placing the distal end of a tube in the abdominal cavity and tunneling the other end into a central vein (eg, the superior vena cava). This perforated intra-abdominal tube allows for ascitic fluid to flow into the central vein. Complications related to placement and use include sepsis, peritonitis, DIC, thrombi formation, and variceal hemorrhage. It is not recommended for patients with infected ascites, encephalopathy, or renal failure. Although the VP shunt controls ascites better than paracentesis, occlusion rates within the first year of placement are high. Because of the aforementioned complications, these shunts are rarely placed in current hepatology practice.

A nonsurgical approach to managing ascites and acute variceal hemorrhage is the TIPS, illustrated in Figure 41-7. The purpose of a TIPS is to decompress the portal venous system and therefore prevent rebleeding from varices or stop or reduce the formation of ascites.[28] TIPS has been associated

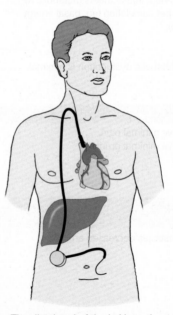

**FIGURE 41-6**  The distal end of the LeVeen shunt is tunneled into a central vein. The shunt allows ascites fluid to drain from the abdominal cavity.

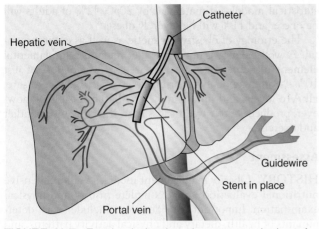

**FIGURE 41-7** Transjugular intrahepatic portosystemic shunt. A stent is inserted through a catheter to the portal vein to divert blood flow and reduce portal hypertension. (Hinkle JL, Cheever KH: Brunner and Suddarth's Textbook of Medical-Surgical Nursing, 13th ed. Philadelphia, PA: Lippincott Williams & Wilkins, 2014, p 1348.)

with improved survival rates, improved renal function via improved flow, and it has even allowed some patients to stop hemodialysis. Absolute contraindications to a TIPS procedure include congestive heart failure, severe tricuspid regurgitation, multiple hepatic cysts, uncontrolled systemic infection or sepsis, unrelieved biliary obstruction, and severe pulmonary hypertension (mean pressures more than 45 mm Hg; these patients are not candidates for liver transplantation). Using an angiographic catheter, a guide wire with a dilating balloon is inserted into the internal jugular vein and is advanced through the liver parenchyma to connect the portal vein, where most of the blood flowing to the liver enters, to the hepatic vein, which empties blood into the inferior vena cava. A stent is then placed to create a conduit between the hepatic and portal vein, which decreases portal pressure. Complications include shunt occlusion, shunt stenosis, and HE. HE increases after a TIPS procedure because this portacaval shunt diverts portal blood flow away from the liver parenchyma. Although TIPS is fairly successful in treating ascites, recent meta-analyses concluded that it can also be associated with the development of increased encephalopathy.

## Hepatic Encephalopathy

Patients with severe liver disease can progress to HE, a reversible decrease in neurologic function caused by liver disease. In general, clinical manifestations of HE can be subtle, with changes in memory, personality, concentration, and reaction times. HE can progress to more apparent neurologic cognitive changes, irritability or agitation, reversal of day and night schedules, somnolence, and eventually terminal coma if left untreated. These changes can be graded by clinical manifestations: Grade 1 includes changes in behavior, mild confusion, slurred speech and/or disordered sleep; Grade 2 includes lethargy and/or moderate confusion; Grade 3 includes marked confusion (stupor), incoherent speech, sleeping but arousable; and Grade 4 presents as coma, unresponsive to pain. Treatment will vary depending on HE grade severity.

The cause of the HE is thought to be related to the accumulation of toxic agents absorbed from the intestinal tract. These substances accumulate because the liver has lost the ability to metabolize and detoxify these substances. Elevated serum ammonia, a byproduct of protein and amino acid metabolism, is one of the suspected neurotoxins. Normally, ammonia is metabolized into urea before entering the systemic circulation, and the urea is then excreted. If the liver is unable to perform this detoxification or if a good portion of the portal blood is shunted around the liver from portal hypertension, the circulating level of ammonia rises. If ammonia and the other toxic agents can be reduced through effective therapy, the encephalopathy gradually clears. Although arterial ammonia levels are more reliable than venous samples, they are often more difficult to obtain and more painful for the patient. In addition, symptoms of HE may lag behind ammonia level elevations, and improvements in HE symptoms may occur before any improvement in ammonia levels.

Treatment is generally targeted toward interventions that lower ammonia production and absorption with medications such as lactulose and/or rifaximin. Lactulose is used to facilitate bowel movements and clearance of nitrogenous products and it also decreases the colonic pH to prevent the absorption of ammonia. Antibiotics like neomycin or metronidazole may be given to clear the gut of bacteria that promote nitrogenous production. In addition, restricting dietary protein intake is no longer recommended for the majority of patients because patients with cirrhosis are often malnourished. In patients with portal hypertension (as a result of cirrhosis), bleeding from esophageal varices or other sites in the GI tract introduces a significant nitrogenous load into the GI tract. Breakdown of RBCs from bacterial deamination produces additional ammonia, makes a portosystemic shunt an important treatment option (ie, reduce portal hypertension/risk of bleeding). Bypassing the liver with a portosystemic shunt, however, may result in decreased clearance and increased accumulation of toxins, allowing opportunity for HE to rapidly develop. Nursing measures to monitor for changes in mental status and provide a safe environment are a priority.

## Hepatorenal Syndrome

HRS is the most frequently fatal complication of cirrhosis. It is defined as the development of renal failure in patients with severe liver disease (acute or chronic) in the absence of any other identifiable cause of renal pathology.[29] HRS has been defined as type 1 and type 2. The onset of type 1 is rapid, with a creatinine value of more than 2.5 mg/dL or a 50% reduction in initial 24-hour creatinine clearance and a decrease in glomerular filtration rate to less than 20 mL/min within 2 weeks. Type 1 is often observed in acute liver failure or alcoholic hepatitis, or following acute decompensation of a patient with a history of cirrhosis. Patients often appear jaundiced and have a significant coagulopathy. Survival time in patients with type 1 HRS is 2 weeks.[30] Mortality from type 1 HRS usually results from a combination of liver and renal failure or variceal bleeding. Type 2 HRS usually occurs in patients with diuretic-resistant ascites. Onset is more insidious, with deterioration in renal failure over months, but it is also associated with a poor prognosis with a median survival of 6 months.[30] In both type 1 and 2 HRS, failure of the kidneys is the result of the extreme systemic vasodilation (from the portal hypertension of liver failure), which decreases the effective circulating blood volume. This leads to a compensatory increase in cardiac output and maximal renal vasoconstriction, which reduces renal perfusion and subsequent renal failure.

Ascites, jaundice, hypotension, and oliguria are clinical findings in HRS; laboratory findings typically include azotemia, elevated serum creatinine, urine sodium less than 10 mEq/L, and hyponatremia. Management goals include therapies to support liver and kidney functions. Historically, liver transplantation had been the treatment of choice. However, because elevated pretransplantation serum creatinine levels have been demonstrated as a poor posttransplantation prognostic factor, it is now being suggested that both a liver and kidney transplantation would improve patient survival.

## Spontaneous Bacterial Peritonitis

Patients with liver disease may be more susceptible to infection because the hepatic Kupffer cells, which are responsible for uptake and subsequent degradation of foreign and potentially harmful substances in the body, do not function as efficiently. SBP is an ascitic fluid infection without an identifiable intra-abdominal source (ie, absence of recognizable intestinal perforation). Ascitic fluid contains low concentrations of albumin, which is thought to normally provide some protection against bacteria. Subsequent leakage of bacteria through the abdominal wall or from invasive procedures (eg, endoscopy, nasogastric tube, IV line, or indwelling bladder catheter placement) is thought to precipitate SBP.

Patients with SBP may complain of fever, chills, generalized abdominal pain, or tenderness with palpation (but rarely with rebound tenderness). However, symptoms may be minimal, with only subtle worsening of jaundice or encephalopathic trends.

SBP leads to renal impairment in approximately 30% to 40% of patients with cirrhosis and is a strong predictor of death during hospitalization.[31] *Escherichia coli*, *Klebsiella* sp., *Enterobacter* sp., and *Staphylococcus aureus* are the most common causative organisms.[31] Early recognition of SBP symptoms in advanced cirrhosis (ie, fever, abdominal pain/tenderness, and altered mental status) is important before shock ensues. Since patients with advanced cirrhosis are often mildly hypothermic, a temperature of 37.8°C (100°F) should be clinically suspect (ie, similar to managing a patient with neutropenia). If SBP is suspected, the ascitic fluid should be evaluated for cell count, differential, and culture. Treatment with broad-spectrum antibiotic coverage is recommended until the results of these tests are returned. In addition, SBP must be differentiated from peritonitis secondary to an abscess or perforation because the latter needs immediate surgical treatment.

## Obesity

### Etiology

Obesity rates in the United States are on an upward trajectory. Currently, over two-thirds of Americans are overweight (defined as body mass index [BMI] between 25 and 30 kg/m²) or obese (defined as BMI greater than 30 kg/m²).[32] Recent statistical models estimate that by 2030, 42% of adults will be obese, and 11% will be severely obese.[33]

The etiology of obesity is genetic as well as environmental. A well-balanced, nutritious diet remains a fundamental element in achieving a healthy weight; weight loss of just 10% is often enough to bring down high blood pressure, HbA1c levels, and lipid parameters. Bariatric surgery, however, produces better weight loss than the conventional diet and exercise.

### Assessment

**HISTORY.** Obesity management includes a comprehensive nutritional evaluation and a complete history and physical examination. Important considerations include social determinants of health, dietary and physical activity patterns, and medication review for medications that may promote weight gain. There are many comorbidities associated with obesity, including but not limited to diabetes, hypertension, obstructive sleep apnea, and osteoarthritis.

**PHYSICAL EXAMINATION.** The Quetelet index, better known as the body mass index (BMI), is a quick and simple way to assess body adiposity in relation to height and weight, independent of body frame size. However, BMI may overestimate or underestimate body fat in certain individuals; it does not address differences in gender or ethnicity; and it does not measure overall fat or lean tissue (muscle) content. Standardized nomograms or online calculators easily determine BMI; obesity can be classified into three progressive grades that reflect increased risk of developing disease.

**LABORATORY STUDIES.** No single laboratory study is diagnostic of obesity. Bariatric surgery requires regular monitoring of basic metabolic profiles (ie, complete blood count, electrolytes, renal function, liver function, PT, and PTT); the critical care nurse should be familiar with hospital-specific protocols.

### Management

In June 2013, the American Medical Association[34] adopted a policy that recognized obesity as a disease requiring a range of medical interventions to advance obesity treatment and prevention.[34] This policy comes after decades of various weight-loss-targeted (or bariatric) surgeries with variable outcomes and health insurance coverage.

The jejunoileal bypass (JIB), first performed in 1954, was the first bariatric surgery ever performed. Because of a high incidence of complications (ie, diarrhea, liver cirrhosis, nephrolithiasis, and renal failure), this technique was eventually banned in the 1990s. The first Roux-en-Y gastric bypass (RYGB) was performed in 1977, and the first laparoscopic gastric bypass (LRYGB) was performed in 1994.[35]

Most bariatric surgeries worldwide are now performed laparoscopically. A very low calorie diet (VLCD) is often prescribed preoperatively to help decrease the size of the liver to improve technical accuracy, as well as to reduce comorbidities that are often associated with obesity by improving serum glucose and blood pressure parameters. In addition to weight loss, long-term benefits of bariatric surgery include improved metabolic control of comorbidities like diabetes mellitus and hypertension.

The goal of bariatric operations is restriction of food intake, restriction of food absorption, or both to promote weight loss. The most common types of bariatric surgeries performed worldwide include the laparoscopic adjustable gastric band (LAGB), the RYGB, and the sleeve gastrectomy (SG). The LAGB is the least invasive: an adjustable band is placed around a portion of the stomach and works in a restrictive manner (ie, it allows an individual to feel full after consuming a smaller portion of food). The RYGB is considerably more invasive: the stomach is reduced to the size of a small pouch and surgically attached to the lower part of the small intestine. The RYGB works by restricting both food intake and food absorption (ie, smaller portions are consumed and most of the stomach and the duodenum are bypassed). The SG involves the longitudinal excision and removal of almost 85% of the stomach; the remaining stomach resembles a tube or a sleeve.

Following laparoscopic RYGB and SG procedures, a gastrografin leak test is typically performed on the first postoperative day to ensure that there is no anastomotic surgical leak. If no leak has been identified, sips of a clear liquid diet may be initiated. The critical care nurse needs to be particularly vigilant in anticipating potential postoperative complications. For example, patients who are obese typically present with a restrictive ventilation pattern, putting them at increased risk for postoperative pulmonary complications like hypoventilation, hypoxemia, and prolonged mechanical ventilation. Extreme obesity (BMI of 40 kg/m$^2$ or higher) has been associated with an increased risk of prolonged mechanical ventilation in the acutely ill patients.[36] Additionally, increased abdominal pressure from the increased weight of adipose tissue on the chest and abdomen increases the risk of aspiration. Preventive strategies include reverse Trendelenburg positioning and positive end-expiratory pressure (PEEP) during mechanical ventilation, which may improve work of breathing, oxygenation, and early extubation. Other immediate postoperative complications include bleeding, leaking at the surgical anastomotic site, infection, and thromboembolism. Unit-based postoperative care protocols are frequently employed (ie, pain management, hemodynamic monitoring, intravenous fluids, pulmonary hygiene, and early mobility).

Long-term complications of bariatric surgery potentially include incisional herniation, cholelithiasis (gallstones), and renal stone formation. Because of alteration of the stomach's anatomy, insertion of a nasogastric tube places the patient at risk for mucosal perforation, and tube advancement should be done with caution (ie, avoid advancing the tube against resistance). Fluoroscopic guidance during insertion, which allows visualization of the tip of the tube, is a strategy that could decrease the risk of perforation. Other strategies to prevent accidental perforation include using soft, flexible tubes made of polyurethane or silicone (rather than polyvinylchloride [PVC]).[37]

## Clinical Applicability Challenges

---

**CASE STUDY**

J.S. is a 45-year-old man who was admitted with complaints of progressively severe, constant right upper quadrant abdominal pain, nausea, and vomiting for the past 24 hours. He was at a party the previous weekend, where he consumed large quantities of alcohol at a family reunion, but reports that he does not drink alcohol regularly. He takes a multivitamin daily and is not on any prescription medication.

On physical exam, he is noted to be in acute distress with facial grimacing and clutching his abdomen. Vitals signs reveal a temperature of 100.4°F (38°C); blood pressure of 102/58 mm Hg; pulse at 101 beats/min; and respirations at 16/min. Laboratory data reveal a white blood cell count of 11,000 cells/mm$^3$, hematocrit 45%, serum creatinine 1.4 mg/dL, total serum bilirubin 3.4 mg/dL, and serum amylase of 650 U/L. AST and ALT levels are both elevated. An abdominal ultrasound reveals a stone in the common bile duct. Treatment includes NPO status, placement of a nasogastric tube (placed on low suction), initiation of IV fluids, and analgesics for pain control. J.S. is diagnosed with acute biliary pancreatitis and is scheduled for an endoscopic retrograde cholangiopancreatography (ERCP) procedure to remove the gallstone in his common biliary duct.

1. What signs and symptoms are typical in AP, and what is the pathophysiologic mechanism?
2. What clinical and laboratory indices are used to assess prognosis in AP?
3. What is the treatment for AP?

---

**WANT TO KNOW MORE?**

A wide variety of resources to enhance your learning and understanding of this chapter are available on thePoint.

You will find:

- References
- Selected readings
- NCLEX-style review questions
- Internet resources
- And more!

## 42

# Anatomy and Physiology of the Endocrine System

JANE KAPUSTIN AND AMEERA CHAKRAVARTHY

**LEARNING OBJECTIVES**

*Based on the content in this chapter, the reader should be able to:*

1. Describe the production, action, and regulation of antidiuretic hormone, growth hormone, and the thyroid hormones.

2. Discuss how activated vitamin D, parathyroid hormone, and calcitonin each influence calcium concentrations in the blood.

3. Describe the eight underlying mechanisms of the pathogenesis of type 2 diabetes mellitus.

4. Compare and contrast the pathophysiology of types 1 and 2 diabetes.

5. Describe the roles of counter-regulatory hormones, gut hormones, and glucagon on the regulation of blood glucose.

6. Explain how glucocorticoids are secreted.

7. Discuss the significant effects of glucocorticoid medications.

8. Summarize the renin–angiotensin mechanism for regulating mineralocorticoid secretion.

Communication between systems in the body is accomplished in three ways. One method of communication is the nervous system. A second method is the cellular secretion of chemicals that are released into the interstitial fluid. Examples of this method of communication include the chemicals that trigger a local inflammatory response, such as histamine, complement, and prostaglandins. The third method of communication is the cellular secretion of chemicals that are circulated through the bloodstream. This communication is known more commonly as the endocrine system (Fig. 42-1, Table 42-1). The secretions of endocrine cells are termed hormones. Hormones are molecules synthesized and secreted by specialized cells and released into blood vessels to exert biochemical effects on target cells distant from the site of origin. They control metabolism, transport of substances across the cell membrane, fluid and electrolyte balance, growth and development, adaptation, and reproduction.

Hormone action is specific and depends on linkage with a specialized hormone receptor on the target cell. This hormone–receptor complex is responsible for a series of biologic responses. Hormones are either stimulatory or inhibitory. Either their actions are very organ specific, such as prolactin (which only affects the mammary glands), or their effects are generalized, such as insulin (which affects most cellular functions of the body).

Hormone production is maintained by a feedback loop mechanism involving the hypothalamic–pituitary axis system (Fig. 42-2). Release of a specific hormone is made possible when the circulating level of that hormone is low (positive feedback). Conversely, when the circulating level of a hormone is high, the release of more hormones is inhibited (negative feedback) until a lower level is reached. This system is regulated by specialized sensors in the hypothalamus that continuously monitor hormone assays to maintain self-regulated homeostasis. Theoretically, when functioning properly, this system prevents the overproduction of hormones.

The effects of aging can influence the endocrine system as well (Box 42-1). As humans age, target organ sensitivity decreases. The target organs demonstrate the effects of aging by either increasing in pigmentation or shrinking in size. This, in effect, decreases hormone receptor binding. This phenomenon explains why older patients, women in particular, are at higher risk for development of hypothyroidism: aging can decrease production of triiodothyronine ($T_3$) and thyroxine ($T_4$) and can lead to thyroid gland atrophy.

Endocrine dysfunction can be identified as belonging to one of five major categories:

- Subnormal hormone production as a result of gland destruction or malformation
- Hormone excess
- Production of abnormal hormone resulting from gene mutation

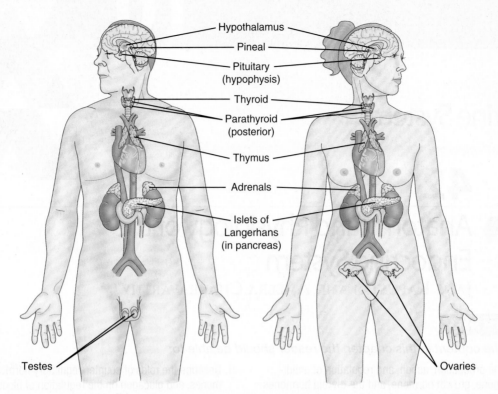

FIGURE 42-1   The endocrine system. (From Hinkle JL, Cheever KH: Brunner & Suddarth's Textbook of Medical–Surgical Nursing, 13th ed. Philadelphia, PA: Lippincott Williams & Wilkins, p 1464, 2014.)

### TABLE 42-1   Endocrine System in Summary

| Endocrine Gland and Hormone | Principal Site of Action | Principal Processes Affected |
|---|---|---|
| **Pituitary Gland** | | |
| *Anterior Lobe* | | |
| GH, somatotropin | General | Growth of bones, muscles, and other organs |
| TSH | Thyroid | Growth and secretory activity of thyroid gland |
| ACTH | Adrenal cortex | Growth and secretory activity of adrenal cortex |
| FSH | Ovaries | Development of follicles and secretion of estrogen |
| | Testes | Development of seminiferous tubules, spermatogenesis |
| LH or interstitial cell–stimulating hormone | Ovaries | Ovulation, formation of corpus luteum, secretion of progesterone |
| Prolactin (LTH) | Testes | Secretion of testosterone |
| MSH | Mammary glands and ovaries | Secretion of milk; maintenance of corpus luteum |
| β-Lipotropin | Skin | Pigmentation |
| *Posterior Lobe* | | |
| ADH (vasopressin) | Kidney | Reabsorption of water; water balance |
| | Arterioles | Blood pressure |
| Oxytocin | Uterus | Contraction |
| | Breast | Expression of milk |
| **Pineal Gland** | | |
| Melatonin | Gonads | Sexual maturation |
| **Thyroid Gland** | | |
| Thyroxine ($T_4$) and triiodothyronine ($T_3$) | General | Metabolic rate; growth and development; intermediate metabolism |
| Calcitonin | Bone | Inhibits bone resorption; lowers blood level of calcium |
| **Parathyroid Glands** | | |
| PTH | Bone, kidney, intestine | Promotes bone resorption; increases absorption of calcium; raises blood calcium level |

| TABLE 42-1 | Endocrine System in Summary *(continued)* | |
|---|---|---|
| **Endocrine Gland and Hormone** | **Principal Site of Action** | **Principal Processes Affected** |
| **Adrenal Glands** | | |
| *Cortex* | | |
| Mineralocorticoids (eg, aldosterone) | Kidney | Reabsorption of sodium; elimination of potassium |
| Glucocorticoids (eg, cortisol) | General | Metabolism of carbohydrate, protein, and fat; response to stress; anti-inflammatory |
| Sex hormones | General | Preadolescent growth spurt |
| *Medulla* | | |
| Epinephrine | Cardiac muscle, smooth muscle, glands | Emergency functions: same as stimulation of sympathetic nervous system |
| Norepinephrine | Organs innervated by sympathetic nervous system | Chemical transmitter substance; increases peripheral resistance |
| **Islet Cells of Pancreas** | | |
| Insulin | General | Lowers blood glucose; utilization and storage of carbohydrate; decreases gluconeogenesis |
| Glucagon | Liver | Raises blood glucose; glycogenolysis |
| Somatostatin | General | Lowers blood glucose by interfering with release of GH and glucagon |
| **Testes** | | |
| Testosterone | General | Development of secondary sex characteristics |
| | Reproductive organs | Development and maintenance; normal function |
| **Ovaries** | | |
| Estrogens | General | Development of secondary sex characteristics |
| | Mammary glands | Development of duct system |
| | Reproductive organs | Maturation and normal cyclic function |
| Progesterone | Mammary glands | Development of secretory tissue |
| | Uterus | Preparation for implantation; maintenance of pregnancy |
| **Gastrointestinal Tract** | | |
| Gastrin | Stomach | Production of gastric juice |
| Enterogastrone | Stomach | Inhibits secretion and motility |
| Secretin | Liver and pancreas | Production of bile; production of watery pancreatic juice (rich in $NaHCO_3$) |
| Pancreozymin | Pancreas | Production of pancreatic juice, rich in enzymes |
| CCK | Gallbladder | Contraction and emptying |

- Hormone receptor disorders resulting from autoimmune processes
- Disorders of hormone transport or metabolism, resulting in increased levels of "free" hormones in the blood

## The Hypothalamus and Pituitary Gland

The key to understanding the physiology of the hormones of the pituitary gland lies in visualizing the anatomy of the gland and its blood supply. The hypothalamus and pituitary share two connecting pathways: a rich vascular network, which connects the hypothalamus with the anterior pituitary, and nerve fibers, which link the hypothalamus with the posterior pituitary. Together, these two glands form a unit that controls the thyroid gland, the adrenal glands, and the gonads, and exerts control over the growth and metabolism of the organism.

Because of the control the pituitary gland exerts over all body functions, it is often referred to as the master gland. It has two distinct regions: the anterior (front) lobe and the posterior (back) lobe. Despite being well protected, the pituitary is still susceptible to injury as a result of head or facial trauma, edema, or surgical complications. Because it is so vascular, the pituitary is extremely vulnerable to injury from ischemia and infarction.

The hypothalamus is a small area at the base of the brain connected to the posterior pituitary (also known as the neurohypophysis) by the pituitary stalk. This stalk is a direct outgrowth of the neuroectoderm of the base of the brain that drops during development of the gland into the bony sella turcica. This is in direct contrast to the anterior pituitary (adenohypophysis), which arises from the buccal endothelium and develops separately in the same bony structure. Because the hypothalamus controls the releasing or inhibiting hormones that influence the pituitary, it assumes the function of the coordinating center of the brain for endocrine, behavioral, and autonomic nervous system function. The hypothalamus is responsible for communicating emotion, pain, body temperature, and other neural input to the endocrine system.

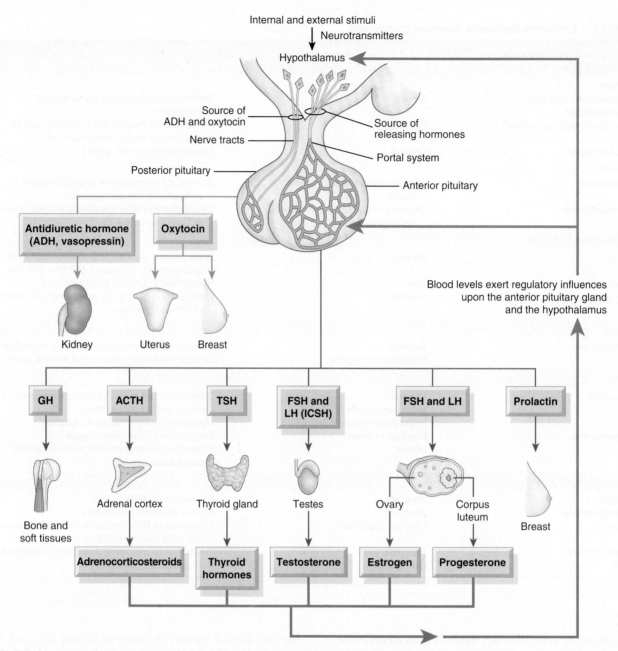

**FIGURE 42-2** The feedback loop mechanism that controls hormone production. Sensors in the hypothalamus monitor hormone levels and initiate or suppress production accordingly. (From Hinkle JL, Cheever KH: Brunner & Suddarth's Textbook of Medical–Surgical Nursing, 13th ed. Philadelphia, PA: Lippincott Williams & Wilkins, p 1467, 2014.)

The anterior pituitary hormones are controlled by releasing factors that are secreted from the hypothalamus. Both growth hormone (GH, somatotropin) and prolactin are dually controlled by a stimulatory and an inhibitory

**BOX 42-1** **CONSIDERATIONS for the Older Patient**

**Physiologic Changes in the Endocrine System That Occur With Aging**
a. Production of thyroid hormone, cortisol, and aldosterone decreases with age.
b. Levels of somatostatin, triiodothyronine ($T_3$), thyroxine ($T_4$), TSH, aldosterone, renin, calcitonin, and vasopressin decrease with age, as does glucose tolerance.
c. Levels of norepinephrine, PTH, ANP, insulin, and glucagon increase with age.

hypophysiotropic hormone. In addition to controlling the pituitary gland through releasing factors, the hypothalamus controls other endocrine roles through releasing factors that control appetite, thirst, emotions, sleep–wake cycles, and cognition.

Such hypothalamic regulation of pituitary functioning can be disrupted by hypothalamic lesions. This can lead to oversecretion or undersecretion of one or more hormones released from the anterior or posterior pituitary. The hypothalamus also receives input from various higher and lower brain centers. These neural connections, together with the influence of the hypothalamus on the pituitary, provide the biologic basis for the construction of conceptual models that describe how stress, emotions, environmental stimuli, and perceptions affect endocrine functions.

## Posterior Pituitary (Neurohypophysis) Hormones

The two major hormones of the posterior pituitary gland are antidiuretic hormone (ADH, vasopressin) and oxytocin (see Table 42-1). Because oxytocin does not have a role in critical care, it is not discussed here.

The two major actions of ADH are to concentrate the urine (by permitting only water reabsorption from the hypotonic tubular fluid in the distal nephron) and to constrict smooth muscles in the arterial wall. ADH binds to specific receptors in the distal renal tubules to increase their permeability to water. This results in increased water reabsorption but without electrolyte reabsorption. This reabsorbed water increases the volume and decreases the osmolality of the extracellular fluid (ECF). At the same time, it decreases the volume and increases the concentration of the urine excreted. Without ADH, the distal convoluted tubule would be impermeable to water. In the presence of ADH, the tubule and collecting duct are permeable to water, which diffuses from the hypotonic tubular fluid to the hypertonic tissue surrounding the tubules. This concentrates the tubular fluid and ultimately the urine.

The term *vasopressin* originated from the observation that large, supraphysiologic dosages of ADH act on arteriole smooth muscle to elevate blood pressure. Although this pressor action of ADH does not appear to play a role in the normal homeostasis of blood pressure, it does counteract a fall in blood pressure that results from hemorrhagic or other drastic hypovolemic states and can be used pharmacologically for that purpose.

There are three major stimuli for the regulation of ADH secretion. The first is plasma osmolality, which is monitored by osmoreceptors in the anterior hypothalamus. An increase above the normal osmolality of plasma (290 mOsm/kg) results in neural stimuli from these receptors to the ADH-secreting cells, increasing ADH secretion. This increases water retention, thereby diluting the ECF and lowering the plasma osmolality back to normal. Similarly, a fall in plasma osmolality triggers a decrease or cessation in ADH secretion. This allows more water excretion, thereby raising the ECF osmolality. ADH secretion can be altered by changes in osmolality of less than 1%. This osmoreceptor-mediated reflex arc functions to maintain osmotic homeostasis of the ECF.

The second stimulus consists of changes in ECF volume. Stretch receptors in the low-pressure portion of the cardiovascular system (eg, the vena cava, the right atrium of the heart, and the pulmonary vessels) monitor blood volume. Stimuli from these receptors are conducted by afferent fibers to the hypothalamus (by way of the brainstem). A decrease in blood volume stimulates ADH secretion. The resultant increase in water retention elevates the blood volume. An increase in blood volume stops ADH secretion. This halts water retention, thereby restoring the normal volume of the ECF compartment. This mechanism alters ADH secretion in response to changes in body position. Movement from the recumbent to the upright position causes a temporary decrease in the stimulation of volume receptors because blood pools in the legs. This results in an increase in ADH secretion. Recumbency increases venous return from the legs. The increased volume triggers a decrease in ADH secretion, thereby increasing the volume of urine excreted.

**BOX 42-2 Drugs That Influence Antidiuretic Hormone Secretion**

**Drugs That Stimulate ADH Secretion**
  i. Diuretics
  ii. Barbiturates
  iii. Glucocorticoids
  iv. Tricyclic antidepressants
  v. Carbamazepine
  vi. Chlorpropamide
  vii. Anesthetics
  viii. Acetaminophen

**Drugs That Inhibit ADH Secretion**
  i. Alcohol
  ii. Phenytoin
  iii. Narcotics
  iv. Lithium
  v. Demeclocycline
  vi. Norepinephrine
  vii. Chlorpromazine

The third stimulus, changes in arterial blood pressure, also can regulate ADH secretion. The hypothalamus receives information from pressure receptors located in the carotid sinuses and aorta. A fall in arterial pressure increases ADH secretion. The water retention thereby produced increases the plasma volume and pressure. A rise in arterial pressure produces the opposite effect. This mechanism is most important in compensating for large changes in arterial blood pressure (eg, impending or actual shock).

Various other stimuli have been shown to influence ADH secretion. Increased ADH secretion can be prompted by angiotensin II, pain, increased serum osmolality, hypovolemia, nausea and emesis, hypoglycemia, stress, acute infections, malignancies, nonmalignant pulmonary conditions, and trauma to the hypothalamic–hypophyseal system. Secretion of ADH is inhibited by decreased serum osmolality, hypervolemia, water intoxication, cold, trauma to the hypothalamic–hypophyseal system, carbon dioxide inhalation, and alcohol ingestion. Many drugs affect ADH secretion (Box 42-2).

## Anterior Pituitary (Adenohypophysis) Hormones

This anterior lobe of the pituitary gland contains five morphologically different types of cells that secrete polypeptide hormones:

- Somatotrophs, which secrete GH (somatotropin)
- Mammotrophs, which secrete prolactin (luteotropic hormone or LTH)
- Thyrotrophs, which secrete thyroid-stimulating hormone (TSH)
- Corticotrophs, which secrete adrenocorticotropic hormone (ACTH), β-lipotropin, β-endorphin, and melanocyte-stimulating hormone (MSH)
- Gonadotrophs, which secrete luteinizing hormone (LH) and follicle-stimulating hormone (FSH).

Each type of cell is separately regulated by hypophysiotropic hormones (Fig. 42-3).

LTH, LH, and FSH are not significant in the critical care arena and are not discussed in this chapter. TSH, which

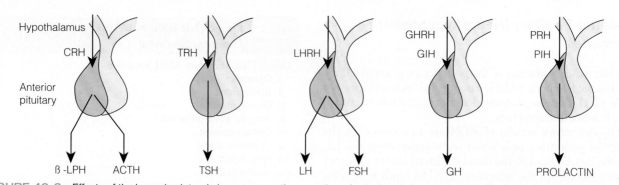

**FIGURE 42-3** Effects of the hypophysiotropic hormones on the secretion of anterior pituitary hormones. The hypophysiotropic hormones are CRH, TRH, luteinizing hormone–releasing hormone (LHRH), growth hormone–releasing hormone (GHRH), growth-inhibiting hormone (GIH), prolactin-inhibiting hormone (PIH); and prolactin-releasing hormone (PRH). CRH prompts the release of β-lipotropin (β-LPH) and ACTH. TRH prompts the release of TSH. LHRH prompts the release of LH and FSH. GHRH and GIH promote and inhibit the secretion of GH, respectively. PRH and PIH promote and inhibit the secretion of prolactin, respectively.

stimulates cells of the thyroid gland to produce and secrete the two thyroid hormones, is discussed later in this chapter, and GH is described in the following paragraph.

The production and secretion of GH occur in the anterior pituitary in response to GH-releasing hormone produced in the hypothalamus. Growth-inhibiting hormone inhibits the secretion of GH. GH acts both directly on target cells and indirectly by stimulating the liver and other as-yet-unidentified tissues to secrete various growth factors termed somatomedins. These growth factors are structurally similar to insulin. Direct actions of GH include increasing the breakdown of fats (lipolysis) in adipose cells and releasing the fatty acids produced by lipolysis into the bloodstream (this is termed its ketogenic effect); increasing hepatic glycolysis and thereby increasing plasma glucose levels; increasing the sensitivity of insulin-producing cells to certain

stimuli; increasing the cellular uptake of amino acids; and stimulating erythropoiesis.

## The Thyroid and Parathyroid Glands

The thyroid gland is a richly vascularized structure. The lobes lie lateral to the trachea just beneath the larynx and are connected by a bridge of thyroid tissue, the isthmus that runs across the anterior surface of the trachea (Fig. 42-4). The follicles produce, store, and secrete the two major thyroid hormones: $T_3$ and $T_4$. Parafollicular cells (C cells), which produce the hormone calcitonin, are scattered between the follicles of the thyroid gland.

Each lobe of the thyroid gland typically contains two parathyroid glands: one in its superior pole and one in its inferior

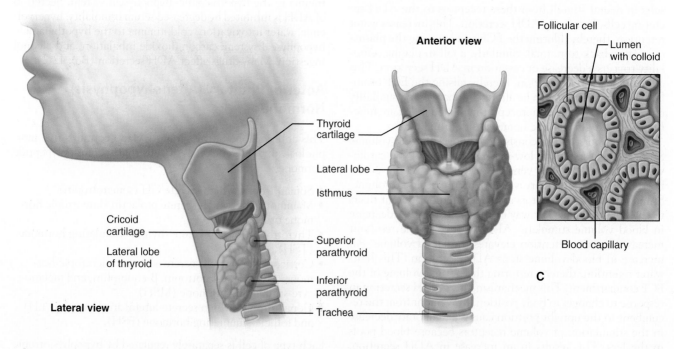

**FIGURE 42-4** **A–C:** The thyroid gland. (Adapted from Porth CM: Pathophysiology: Concepts of Altered Health States, 9th ed. Philadelphia, PA: Lippincott Williams & Wilkins, 2013.)

pole. The parathyroid glands produce parathyroid hormone (PTH) that is active with maintaining calcium balance.

## Thyroid Hormones

The follicular cells absorb tyrosine (an amino acid) and iodide from the plasma and secrete them into the central colloid portion of the follicle, where they are used in the synthesis of $T_3$ and $T_4$. Because of the role of iodine in the manufacture of thyroid hormones, storage and release of small amounts of radioactive iodine by the thyroid can be used to measure the activity of this gland. Because the thyroid gland is virtually the only tissue of the body that absorbs and stores iodine, larger amounts of radioactive iodine can be used to destroy portions of the thyroid gland as a treatment for hyperthyroidism.

$T_3$ and $T_4$ are stored in the colloid until they are needed. When they are to be secreted, the follicular cells transport them from the colloid to the plasma. The plasma proteins involved in transporting $T_3$ and $T_4$ are manufactured in the liver. Consequently, liver damage that decreases the plasma levels of these proteins can produce a condition resembling thyroid hormone excess (ie, hyperthyroidism). Plasma levels of these proteins can also be depressed by glucocorticoids, androgens, and L-asparaginase (an antineoplastic drug). They are elevated during pregnancy, and by estrogens, opiates, clofibrate, and major tranquilizers. Thyroid hormones are deiodinated and catabolized by the liver, kidneys, and various other tissues.

The actions of thyroid hormones are widespread and apparently arise from their stimulation of the basal metabolic rate of most tissues (excluding tissues of the brain, anterior pituitary, spleen, lymph nodes, testes, and lung). Thyroid hormone increases the number of $\beta_1$- and $\beta_2$-adrenergic receptors in various tissues and the affinity of these receptors for catecholamines; thus, an increased heart rate and sweating often occur in hyperthyroidism. Thyroid hormones increase the catabolism of skeletal muscle proteins to such a degree that pronounced muscle weakness results from prolonged hyperthyroidism (thyrotoxic myopathy). Thyroid hormones increase the rate of carbohydrate absorption from the small intestine and decrease circulating levels of cholesterol.

Thyroid hormones are essential for the normal growth and development of many body systems, notably the skeletal and nervous systems. These hormones stimulate the secretion of GH and potentiate its effect on various tissues. Thyroid hormones are also necessary for normal levels of neuronal functioning. Thyroid insufficiency leads to slowed reflexes, slowed mentation, and decreased level of consciousness (through decreased levels of reticular activating system activity). Hyperthyroidism lowers synaptic thresholds in the central nervous system (CNS), causing hyperreflexia and a fine muscle tremor. The pervasive effects of thyroid hormones on the nervous system are best illustrated by cretinism, a condition resulting from congenital thyroid insufficiency.

The secretion of $T_3$ and $T_4$ by the thyroid gland is primarily regulated by the secretion of TSH from the anterior pituitary. In turn, TSH secretion is regulated by a hypothalamic neurosecretory material termed thyrotropin-releasing hormone (TRH). After receiving stimuli from TRH from the hypothalamus, the thyroid secretes TSH to stimulate the manufacture and secretion of $T_3$ and $T_4$. A negative feedback regulatory loop exists whereby increased levels of free (unbound) $T_3$ and $T_4$ suppress TSH secretion. Decreased plasma TSH results in decreased thyroid function, which causes a fall in free plasma $T_3$ and $T_4$. Low $T_3$ and $T_4$ levels stimulate TSH secretion. If a TSH-induced increase in thyroid activity does not raise the plasma levels of free $T_3$ and $T_4$, the continued high levels of TSH eventually cause an increase in the size of the thyroid gland (nontoxic goiter). In this case, an enlarged thyroid is not associated with overproduction of hormone. This feedback loop maintains homeostasis of the daily secretion of TSH and thyroid hormones.

## Calcitonin and Parathyroid Hormone

Calcitonin, which is secreted by the parafollicular cells of the thyroid gland, and PTH, which is produced and secreted by the parathyroid glands, exert a major influence on calcium metabolism in conjunction with 1,25-dihydroxycholecalciferol, which is produced by the action of the liver and the kidneys on vitamin D. Ultraviolet light changes 7-dehydrocholesterol provitamins in the skin to a group of compounds, collectively called vitamin D. One of these, $D_3$, can also be obtained from vitamin D–enriched and other foods. The liver converts $D_3$ to 25-hydroxycholecalciferol, which is then altered by kidney cells to a more active form, 1,25-dihydroxycholecalciferol. (The hypocalcemia seen in chronic renal disease results from an activated vitamin D deficiency.) Activated vitamin D acts on intracellular enzymes of the intestinal mucosal cells to increase calcium absorption. To a lesser extent, it also increases the active transport of calcium out of osteoblasts into the bloodstream. Both of these actions elevate plasma calcium levels. In vitamin deficiency states, the effect of decreased intestinal absorption outweighs any decrease in the mobilization of calcium from bone to produce an overall hypocalcia and poor mineralization of bone.

Vitamin D is synthesized in the skin, absorbed in the small intestine, and transported into the plasma bound to vitamin D–binding proteins. The metabolism of vitamin D is strictly regulated by phosphate concentration in the kidney and by PTH. Thus, the effect of a decrease in dietary phosphate or serum phosphate is to increase levels of 1,25-dihydroxycholecalciferol.

### Parathyroid Hormone

PTH is a polypeptide produced and secreted by the chief cells of the parathyroid glands. This hormone is stored in secretory granules and released in response to a decrease in ionized calcium concentrations. It is cleaved into active form in the kidneys and liver. Plasma calcium and phosphate levels operate in a negative feedback loop to influence the activity of the renal enzyme system, which catalyzes the conversion of metabolically inactive vitamin D to the metabolically active form. High plasma calcium levels decrease this activation process, whereas low levels increase it. The formation of activated vitamin D is also facilitated by PTH and decreased by metabolic acidosis and hypoinsulinemia (diabetes mellitus).

PTH is transported free (unbound) in the plasma and is metabolically degraded by cells in the liver. A decrease in calcium concentration increases PTH secretion. PTH acts on two target tissues: bone cells and kidney tubules. In bone, it stimulates osteoclast activity and inhibits osteoblast activity. This results in bone reabsorption with consequent mobilization of calcium and phosphate from the bony matrix into the bloodstream. In the kidney, PTH increases the reabsorption of calcium by distal tubule cells and decreases the reabsorption of phosphate by proximal tubule cells. The effect of these multiple actions is elevation of plasma calcium levels and lowering of plasma phosphate levels.

Plasma calcium levels alter PTH secretion through a negative feedback loop. Secretion is inhibited by high plasma calcium levels and stimulated by low blood levels of calcium. The activated vitamin D deficiency–induced hypocalcemia, which occurs in chronic renal failure, typically produces a secondary hyperparathyroidism. Secretion of PTH by the parathyroid gland is also stimulated by hypomagnesemia, adrenergic agonists, and prostaglandins.

### Calcitonin

This polypeptide hormone is produced by the parafollicular cells (C cells) of the thyroid gland. It can also be secreted by nonthyroidal tissue (eg, tissue of the lung, intestine, pituitary, and bladder). Calcitonin is transported unbound in the plasma. It has a half-life of 5 minutes and is predominantly metabolized in the kidney. Calcitonin lowers plasma calcium and phosphate levels by inhibiting osteoclastic bone reabsorption and increasing urinary phosphate and calcium excretion. Calcitonin levels are elevated during pregnancy and lactation, suggesting that calcitonin may help to protect the mother's skeleton from excess calcium loss during these periods of calcium drain.

Calcitonin does not function in the normal daily homeostasis of plasma calcium levels. It appears to serve more of an emergency function in that it is secreted only if the plasma calcium level exceeds 9.3 mg/dL. At high blood calcium levels, calcitonin secretion is stimulated by increased levels of plasma calcium. Calcitonin is also released by the action of gastrin, glucagon, and secretion of gastrointestinal hormones.

Table 42-2 summarizes the hormones secreted by the thyroid and parathyroid glands.

## The Endocrine Pancreas

The pancreas has both endocrine and exocrine functions, which are under the control of different groups of cells. The organ is made up of two tissue types: the acini, the exocrine portion, and the islets of Langerhans, the endocrine portion. The acini secrete digestive enzymes into the duodenum, whereas the islets of Langerhans secrete hormones into the blood.

The islets of Langerhans secrete the peptide hormones involved in blood glucose regulation. The name "islets of Langerhans" refers to the more than 1 million ovoid islands (clusters) of cells that are scattered throughout the pancreas, predominantly in the tail. Because of this distribution of islet cells, acute attacks of pancreatitis, which usually spare the tail, tend to spare the islets. Episodes of chronic recurrent pancreatitis typically involve the entire pancreas. Consequently, chronic episodes can cause islet cell destruction and diabetes mellitus.

Each cell cluster is richly supplied with capillaries, into which its hormones are secreted. The islets are composed of four types of cells: α cells, which secrete glucagon; β cells, which secrete insulin; δ cells, which secrete somatostatin; and F cells, which secrete pancreatic polypeptide. The hormones secreted by the pancreas are summarized in Table 42-3.

## Insulin

Insulin, an anabolic hormone, is regulated by a number of stimulatory and inhibitory factors. It is responsible for the control of blood glucose concentrations and storage of carbohydrate, proteins, and fats. Insulin facilitates the use of glucose as the main source of energy for most body tissues. Insulin is the only hormone with the ability to directly lower the blood glucose level. Also, insulin facilitates an increase in the cellular transport of glucose, amino acids, and fatty acids across cell membranes and modulates intracellular metabolic synthesis of nucleic acids. Cell membranes require a glucose transporter to carry glucose into the cell at a faster rate than diffusion. GLUT-4 is the glucose transporter for skeletal muscle and adipose tissue, and GLUT-2 carries glucose into β cells and liver tissue.

The precursor of insulin, proinsulin, is manufactured in the β cells of the islets of Langerhans. Proinsulin can be found in the plasma as a result of certain islet tumors (insulinoma) or overstimulation of the β cells. Connecting peptide

**TABLE 42-2** Hormones of the Thyroid and Parathyroid Glands and Their Actions

| Gland | Hormone | Action |
|---|---|---|
| Thyroid gland | Thyroxine (T₄) | Controls basic metabolic rate |
| | Triiodothyronine (T₃) | Induces growth and development |
| | | Inhibits bone resorption |
| | Calcitonin | Inhibits calcium reabsorption in gastrointestinal tract |
| | | Increases calcium excretion from kidney |
| Parathyroid gland | PTH | Promotes bone resorption |
| | | Increases calcium reabsorption |
| | | Increases calcium blood levels |

**TABLE 42-3** Hormones of the Pancreas and Their Actions

| Hormone | Cell | Stimulant | Response |
|---|---|---|---|
| Insulin | β | Glucose | Decreased glucose level |
| | | | Increased fat storage |
| | | | Increased protein synthesis |
| | | | Increased glucogenesis |
| Glucagon | α | Decreased glucose level, exercise | Increased glucose level |
| | | | Increased gluconeogenesis |
| | | | Increased glycogenolysis |
| Somatostatin | δ | Hyperglycemia | Increased glucose |
| | | | Increased glycogen |
| Pancreatic polypeptide | F | Acute hypoglycemia | Increased gallbladder contraction |
| | | | Increased pancreatic enzymes |

---

**BOX 42-3** | **Major Actions of Insulin on Adipose and Muscle Cells**

**Muscle Cells**
Increased glucose entry
Increased K$^+$ uptake
Increased glycogen synthesis
Increased amino acid entry
Increased protein synthesis
Decreased protein catabolism
Increased ketone entry into cells

**Adipose Cells**
Increased glucose entry
Increased K$^+$ uptake
Increased fatty acid entry and synthesis
Increased fat deposition
Increased conversion of glucose to fatty acids
Inhibition of lipolysis

---

**BOX 42.4** | **Factors Affecting Insulin Secretion**

**Stimulators**
Glucose
Mannose
Amino acids (leucine, arginine, others)
Intestinal hormones (gastric inhibitory peptide, gastrin, secretin, CCK, glucagon, others)
β-Keto acids
Acetylcholine
Glucagon
Cyclic adenosine monophosphate (AMP) and various cyclic AMP–generating substances
β-Adrenergic-stimulating agents
Theophylline
Sulfonylureas

**Inhibitors**
Somatostatin
2-Deoxyglucose
Mannoheptulose
α-Adrenergic-stimulating agents (norepinephrine, epinephrine)
β-Adrenergic-blocking agents (propranolol)
Diazoxide
Thiazide diuretics
Phenytoin
Alloxan
Microtubule inhibitors
Insulin

---

(C-peptide) is a biologically inactive chain and is secreted into the bloodstream along with insulin. Because there is a 1:1 ratio between C-peptide and insulin, plasma C-peptide levels can be used to measure endogenous insulin secretion or degree of β-cell activity. Clinically, C-peptide levels can assist with distinguishing between types 1 and 2 diabetes (C-peptide is low in type 1 diabetes, reflecting autodestruction of β cells and no further production of insulin).[1]

The actions of insulin are summarized in Box 42-3. In general, insulin enables glucose to be readily available for aerobic oxidation in muscle, adipose, and connective tissue cells. Facilitation of the preferential use of glucose as cellular fuel means that the cells do not need to oxidize fatty or amino acids. Instead, these can be conserved. Protein synthesis and fat storage are increased in liver, muscle, and adipose tissue. Breakdown of fats and proteins is decreased. Hepatic gluconeogenesis also is decreased or halted, and glycogen synthesis is increased.

Insulin acts only on a few types of tissues. However, the membranes of nearly all types of body cells possess insulin receptors. Binding of insulin to the insulin receptors initiates the physiologic action of insulin on the cell. About 80% of all circulating insulin is catabolized by liver and kidney cells.

Insulin secretion is influenced by a variety of factors as listed in Box 42-4. Monosaccharides are the primary regulatory mechanism for insulin secretion. Elevated plasma levels of glucose act in a negative feedback loop to increase the secretion of insulin. Lower levels of glucose decrease insulin output. Glucagon, β-adrenergic agonists, and theophylline increase insulin secretion. β-Cells are also stimulated to secrete insulin by tolbutamide and other sulfonylurea derivatives; acetylcholine; impulses from vagal nerve branches to the islets; selected amino acids, such as arginine; and β-ketoacids. The mechanisms of action of these stimuli are as yet unclear. Insulin production is inhibited by α-adrenergic agonists, β-adrenergic blocking agents, diazoxide (Proglycem), thiazide diuretics, phenytoin (Dilantin), alloxan, agents that prevent glucose metabolism (eg, 2-deoxyglucose and mannoheptulose), somatostatin, and insulin itself.

Chronic stimulation of β cells, such as by a high-carbohydrate diet for several weeks, can cause a limited amount of hypertrophy and subsequent increase in the insulin-producing capacity. However, overstimulation produces β-cell exhaustion. Stimulation of these exhausted cells produces β-cell death and depletes the β-cell reserve. β-Cell activity is also decreased by the administration of exogenous insulin. Such decreased activity enables the cells to rest and results in temporary hyperproduction after the withdrawal of exogenous insulin.

## Insulin Resistance

Insulin resistance, characteristic of type 2 diabetes, is one of the main defects seen with the development of hyperglycemia, hyperinsulinemia, and consequent β-cell loss. Insulin resistance is a physiologic condition in which a person needs more insulin to lower serum glucose effectively than would normally be required. To compensate for insulin resistance, the pancreas initially secretes more insulin in an attempt to maintain normal glucose levels. The degree of obesity directly affects the resistance to insulin in most patients with type 2 diabetes. One principal mechanism may be a defect in insulin receptor function because of a genetic mutation of the insulin receptor gene. The quantity and activity of insulin receptors also can be regulated by various factors. Increased amounts of insulin, obesity, acromegaly, excess glucocorticoids, and human immunodeficiency virus therapies can exacerbate insulin resistance by decreasing the receptors' number or activity, or both. Exercise and decreased circulating levels of insulin increase the activity of insulin receptors[2]; therefore, leading a sedentary lifestyle may contribute to insulin resistance.

Aside from type 2 diabetes, insulin resistance plays a role in other metabolic abnormalities including obesity, high levels of triglycerides, low levels of high-density lipoproteins, hypertension, and systemic inflammation, macrovascular disease, and abnormal fibrinolysis. These signs and symptoms are called metabolic syndrome, and obesity along with sedentary lifestyle are major factors that can lead to the development of type 2 diabetes.

There are eight conditions (termed the *Ominous Octet*) that play a role in the pathogenesis of type 2 diabetes mellitus: insulin resistance, β-cell dysfunction, excess hepatic glucose production, decreased incretin effect, increased lipolysis, increased glucagon secretion, increased renal glucose reabsorption, and neurotransmitter dysfunction. When type 2 diabetes mellitus is diagnosed, approximately 50% to 80% of β-cell function is already lost.[3]

Several theories explain the development of β-cell dysfunction:

- Cell exhaustion results when the pancreas must keep up with the higher demands for insulin. Some functional and morphologic changes occur to compensate for the increased demand, but eventually β-cell exhaustion occurs.
- Chronic hyperglycemia leads to the development of glucotoxicity—direct toxicity to the β cells.
- Chronic exposure of β cells to excess free fatty acids damages them, leading to lipotoxicity.
- Apoptosis, or programmed cell death, occurs secondary to chronic glucotoxicity and lipotoxicity. This leads to progressive β–islet cell loss.
- Abnormal deposition of amyloid matter leads to islet cell destruction.[4]

Insulin resistance interferes with normal cellular interactions between insulin, skeletal muscles, and adipose tissues. Insulin binds with cell-surface receptors, causing a cascade of intracellular signals; this results in the translocation of glucose transporter cells to cell surfaces and allows entry of glucose into the cell. In addition, insulin may bind normally to receptors but has to work with disrupted signals, resulting in insufficient translocation of glucose transporter molecules. This ultimately leads to excess glucose accumulation.[2]

Insulin resistance triggers β cells to produce more insulin as a compensatory mechanism. Hyperinsulinemia initially meets the additional needs created by excess glucose. However, when β-cell function fails to satisfy these demands, hyperglycemia and type 2 diabetes mellitus ensue.[4] Data from a landmark trial, the United Kingdom Prospective Diabetes Study, suggest that the process of declining β-cell function occurs for approximately 10 years before the diagnosis of type 2 diabetes is made.[5]

## Glucagon

Glucagon is manufactured and secreted by the α cells of the islets of Langerhans and is stimulated by pure protein meal ingestion that produces an aminoacidemia. Glucagon influences enzyme systems in liver, fat, and muscle cells and is degraded mainly by the liver.

The major function of glucagon is to elevate blood glucose levels and then to enable this plasma glucose to enter and be used by the cells of the body (eg, the muscle cells) by stimulating the secretion of insulin. In this manner, glucagon prevents hypoglycemia between meals, during exercise, during the first few days of fasting, and after a high-protein meal. Dietary protein stimulates an increase in plasma insulin, which causes a rapid cellular uptake of absorbed dietary carbohydrates.

To elevate blood glucose levels, glucagon stimulates liver cells to perform glycogenolysis and gluconeogenesis. This increases the glucose concentration in liver cells, and because these cells can dephosphorylate intracellular glucose, this glucose can be released from the liver into the bloodstream. The fatty acids and amino acids needed for gluconeogenesis are supplied by the glucagon-stimulated breakdown of fats in adipose cells and the release of fatty acids into the bloodstream. If the supply of fatty acids is insufficient, glucagon also stimulates the breakdown of proteins into amino acids in muscle cells and the release of amino acids into the plasma. These fatty acids and amino acids are then taken up by hepatocytes and used as raw materials in gluconeogenesis. Glucagon also elevates plasma ketone levels by increasing hepatic ketone production, and promotes the secretion of somatostatin and GH.

Although glucagon opposes the effects of insulin on blood glucose levels, it also stimulates the secretion of insulin. This apparent contradiction is actually a logical second step in the biologic function of this hormone. It enables the increased plasma glucose to enter and be used by various tissues. An elevated plasma glucose level stimulates insulin secretion, but this takes a while. The direct action of glucagon on β cells is simply faster.

As is the case with β cells, α cells are stimulated by β-adrenergic agonists, theophylline, elevated plasma levels of dietary amino acids (primarily those used in gluconeogenesis), and vagal (cholinergic) stimulation. Glucagon secretion is also prompted by glucocorticoids (eg, cortisol), catecholamines, GH, cholecystokinin (CCK), and gastrin. Exercise, physical stress, and infections also increase α-cell activity. Whereas the effects of exercise on glucagon secretion appear to be mediated by increased β-adrenergic activity, stress and infection probably operate by increasing plasma glucocorticoid levels. Dietary amino acids are believed to enhance glucagon secretion by their effects on CCK or gastrin, or both, because intravenous amino acids exert little or no effect on α cells.

Elevated plasma glucose levels enact a negative feedback loop to retard or halt the output of glucagon; however, plasma insulin must be present for this mechanism to operate. Like β-cell secretion, α-cell secretion is inhibited by adrenergic agonists, phenytoin, and somatostatin. Fatty acids and ketone bodies in the plasma can inhibit glucagon secretion, but this inhibition must be weak because plasma glucagon levels can be quite elevated during diabetic ketoacidosis.

In addition to glucagon, other hormones—cortisol, epinephrine, and GH—have great influence on the regulation of glucose and insulin. These counter-regulatory hormones have a synergistic effect on glucose production as a mechanism to protect the body during stress. They act to inhibit insulin while increasing glucagon, producing an insulin-resistant state, and increasing overall serum glucose levels to produce sufficient energy levels during "fight-or-flight" responses. These hormones elevate serum glucose levels to protect against hypoglycemia and to prepare the body for stress. However, they can also further aggravate a state of hyperglycemia and can lead to dangerous levels of glucose, as seen in diabetic emergencies.[6]

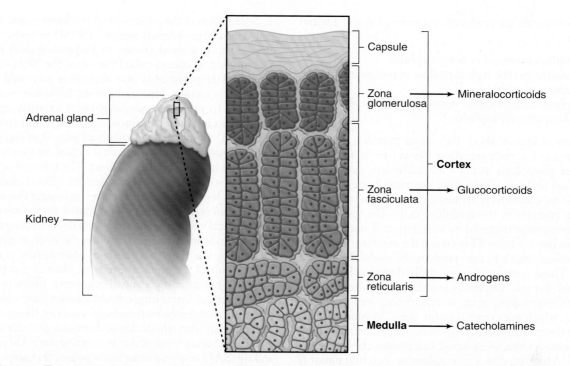

**FIGURE 42-5**   The adrenal gland has a cortex and a medulla. (Adapted from Seifter J, Ratner A, Sloane D: Concepts in Medical Physiology. Philadelphia, PA: Lippincott Williams & Wilkins, p 541, 2005)

Another group of hormones, incretins, are released by the gut in response to nutrient ingestion. One hormone, glucagon-like peptide-1, is a potent insulin secretagogue released from the L cells in the distal small bowel that will assist with assimilating nutrients. It inhibits glucagon secretion, delays gastric emptying, and reduces appetite and food intake. When used pharmacologically, incretins can lower blood glucose substantially.[6–8]

## Somatostatin

Somatostatin is produced not only by the δ cells of the pancreas but also by the hypothalamus, where it functions as an inhibitor of anterior pituitary GH secretion; neurons of the CNS, where it probably functions as a synaptic neurotransmitter agent; and δ cells in the gastric mucosa, where it inhibits the secretion of gastrin and other lesser known gastrointestinal hormones. Islet cell somatostatin is secreted into the bloodstream and therefore functions as a hormone. Little is known of the metabolism of somatostatin because it is so tightly bound with the actions of GH.

Somatostatin inhibits the release of insulin and glucagon from the pancreas. Pancreatic somatostatin inhibits the activity of all other islet cells. The biologic significance of this action is not yet known. The only clinical data of relevance concern δ-cell tumors. These produce a clinical picture that resembles diabetes mellitus but that is reversible with tumor ablation. The secretion of somatostatin from islet cells is increased by glucose, certain amino acids, and CCK. Factors that inhibit islet somatostatin secretion are unknown.

## Pancreatic Polypeptide

Not much is known about this islet hormone in humans. It is produced by the endocrine cells and its secretion is enhanced by dietary protein, exercise, acute hypoglycemia, and fasting. Somatostatin and elevated plasma glucose levels decrease the secretion of this polypeptide. It appears to have a role in smooth muscle relaxation of the gallbladder.

## The Adrenal Glands

The adrenal glands lie at the superior pole of each kidney retroperitoneally. Each gland is composed of an inner core, the medulla, surrounded by an outer layer, the cortex (Fig. 42-5). The hormones produced by the adrenal glands are summarized in Table 42-4.

## Medullary Hormones

The adrenal medulla is basically a modified sympathetic ganglion. Because the adrenal medulla secretes chemicals directly into the bloodstream, it may be appropriately viewed as an endocrine extension of the autonomic nervous system.

**TABLE 42-4**   Hormones of the Adrenal Gland and Their Actions

| Gland | Hormone | Action |
|---|---|---|
| Adrenal gland cortex | Mineralocorticoids | Reabsorption of sodium |
|  |  | Elimination of potassium |
|  | Glucocorticoids | Responds to stress |
|  |  | Decreases inflammation |
|  |  | Alters metabolism of protein and fat |
| Medulla | Epinephrine | Stimulates sympathetic system |
|  | Norepinephrine | Increases peripheral resistance |

Four chemicals are produced and secreted in the adrenal medulla:

- Dopamine, a precursor of norepinephrine
- Norepinephrine, the typical product of postganglionic sympathetic neurons
- Epinephrine, a methylated version of norepinephrine
- Opioid peptides (enkephalins).

Not much is known about the opioid peptides. The specific stimulus for their secretion has yet to be identified, and their physiologic actions are unknown, as are their metabolism and fate. Dopamine, norepinephrine, and epinephrine are collectively termed catecholamines. They are stored in granules in the medullary cells. The secretion of these chemicals is triggered by stimulation of neurons that innervate the medulla. This causes the neurons to release acetylcholine, which in turn prompts the medullary cells to secrete. These compounds are rapidly degraded by plasma renal and hepatic catechol-O-methyltransferase enzymes into vanillylmandelic acid, metanephrine, and normetanephrine, which are excreted in the urine. Measuring urine levels of these compounds is significant if an adrenal tumor, pheochromocytoma, is suspected. In this case, the levels will be high, indicating that a catecholamine secreting tumor is likely.

Predictably, the epinephrine and norepinephrine secreted by the adrenal medulla mimic the effects of a mass discharge from sympathetic neurons. However, apart from this, they produce several metabolic actions. First, they elevate blood glucose levels by activating an enzyme, phosphorylase, which promotes hepatic glycogenolysis. Because liver cells possess the enzyme glucose-6-phosphatase, the glucose produced by this glycogen breakdown is able to diffuse out of hepatocytes and into the bloodstream. These hormones also induce muscle cells to participate in elevating blood glucose levels, although this process is less direct. These hormones can also elevate plasma glucose levels by stimulating the secretion of glucagon and can increase the uptake of glucose into body tissues by stimulating the secretion of insulin. Epinephrine and norepinephrine can also produce the opposite effects by stimulating $\alpha$-adrenergic receptors on islet cells. Because of differential effects of both hormones on $\alpha$- and $\beta$-adrenergic receptors, the result is that epinephrine elevates plasma glucose levels much more than does norepinephrine.

A second metabolic effect of catecholamines is promotion of lipolysis in adipose tissue. This elevates plasma-free fatty acid levels and provides an alternative energy source for many body cells. Circulating catecholamines also increase alertness by stimulating the reticular activating system. Last, these hormones produce an increase in the metabolic rate of the body and a cutaneous vasoconstriction, both of which result in an elevation in body temperature. However, the accelerated metabolism requires the presence of the thyroid and adrenal cortex hormones.

Although the physiologic action of adrenal medullary dopamine is unknown, exogenous dopamine is useful in combating certain shocks because it has a positive inotropic effect on the heart (by way of $\beta$ receptors) and produces renal vasodilation and peripheral vasoconstriction. The overall effect of moderate dosages is elevation of systolic blood pressure (without an appreciable increase in diastolic blood pressure) together with retention or restoration of renal output.

Stimulation of the adrenal medulla glands is part of a general sympathetic–adrenal medulla (SAM) response to exercise and to perceived threats to biopsychological integrity and survival. (Cannon called the latter the "fight-or-flight" response.) Hypoglycemia also stimulates increased adrenal medullary secretion. The results of the SAM response enable the body to perform vigorous physical exertion optimally. The heart rate and blood pressure are increased (increasing perfusion), and blood flow is shunted away from the skin and gastrointestinal tract to more vital organs for exertion, such as skeletal muscles, brain, and heart. The reticular activating system is stimulated, fostering alertness. Blood glucose and fatty acid levels are raised, thereby increasing the available energy sources for cells. Pupils are dilated, increasing the field of peripheral vision and the amount of light entering the eyes. Sweat glands are stimulated, cooling the body in advance of and during the time that the body temperature is elevated as the result of the physical exertion. Most of this SAM response is mediated by sympathetic nerve fibers to various body structures; circulating catecholamines play only a minor role. Furthermore, many tissue responses (eg, those of muscle cells) to such sympathetic demands require glucocorticoids to enable the tissues to meet the demands of the SAM response, and the SAM response often accompanies the stress-induced secretion of adrenal steroids discovered by Selye. (This and the endocrine response to physical and psychological stress are discussed in the section on cortical hormones.)

## Cortical Hormones

The adrenal cortex is composed of three histologically different layers (see Fig. 42-5).

Its exterior is covered by a capsule. The outermost layer, the zona glomerulosa, produces and secretes primarily mineralocorticoids, such as aldosterone. The inner two layers, the zona fasciculata and zona reticularis, manufacture and secrete glucocorticoids (cortisol and corticosterone) and adrenal androgens and estrogens. If these inner cortical layers are destroyed, they can be regenerated from zona glomerulosa cells.

Figure 42-6 depicts the metabolic pathways for synthesis of all adrenocortical hormones. Each of these metabolic steps is governed by a specific enzyme. Genetic deficiencies in one or more of these enzymes produce syndromes involving the underproduction or overproduction of various cortical hormones. Drugs that inhibit specific enzymes are used clinically to assess cortical function. One such drug is metyrapone, which inhibits cortisol synthesis.

After secretion, plasma cortisol and, to a lesser extent, corticosterones are bound to a plasma globulin called corticosteroid-binding globulin (CBG), or transcortin. Only the unbound hormones are physiologically active. The bound glucocorticoids serve as a hormone reservoir that is used to replace degraded unbound hormones. CBG is manufactured by liver cells. Therefore, decreased hepatic function (eg, cirrhosis) can lead to subnormal quantities of plasma CBG, resulting in excess quantities of circulating unbound, active glucocorticoids, leading to hyperdynamic circulation. Only a small amount of aldosterone is bound to plasma proteins. Adrenal steroids are degraded by the liver. Depressed hepatic function can retard the degradation of adrenal steroids, thereby producing a clinical picture of hormone excess. The soluble degraded steroid metabolites are excreted by the kidneys.

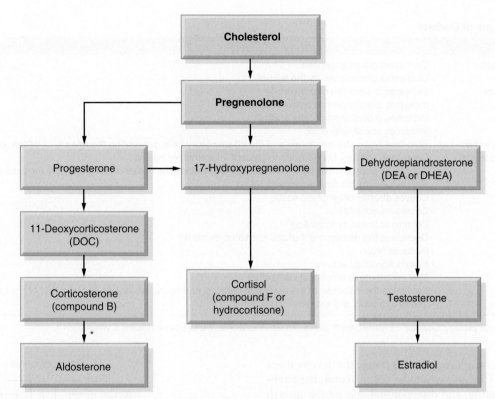

**FIGURE 42.6** Biosynthetic pathways for adrenal cortical hormones. Only cells of the zona glomerulosa can convert corticosterone to aldosterone (*asterisk*). All the other pathways can be carried out by cells in all three layers of the adrenal cortex.

## Glucocorticoids

As the name glucocorticoid suggests, cortisol and corticosterone influence glucose metabolism. They elevate plasma glucose levels by promoting hepatic gluconeogenesis and glycogenolysis. To facilitate gluconeogenesis, these hormones cause the breakdown of fat and proteins and the release of fatty and amino acids into the bloodstream, which carries them to the liver. Excessive gluconeogenesis can lead to severe hyperglycemia often seen in diabetic patients receiving glucocorticoids.

Glucocorticoids enable tissues to respond to glucagon and catecholamines; they also prevent rapid fatigue of skeletal muscle. Cortisol and corticosterone also act on the kidneys to permit the excretion of a normal water load in one of three ways: glucocorticoids make distal or collecting tubules more permeable to the reabsorption of water independently of sodium reabsorption, they increase the glomerular filtration rate (GFR), or they reduce the output of ADH.

The effects of glucocorticoids on plasma components are mixed. They decrease the number of plasma eosinophils and basophils but increase the number of circulating neutrophils, platelets, and erythrocytes. By suppressing production and increasing destruction, glucocorticoids decrease the number of lymphocytes. They also decrease the size of lymph nodes. A major function of lymphocytes is to provide either humoral immunity (with antibodies) or cell-mediated immunity. Stress-induced elevations in glucocorticoid secretion and the resulting decrease in lymphocytes may explain the decrease in immunocompetence that often occurs in people who are under psychological or physical stress.

Other effects of physiologic levels of glucocorticoids include decreasing olfactory and gustatory sensitivity. People with adrenal insufficiency can detect various chemicals (eg, sugar, salt, urea, and potassium chloride) by either taste or smell with a sensitivity that is 40 to 120 times greater than normal.

The effects of pharmacologic dosages of glucocorticoids are considered separately from those of normal physiologic levels. In pharmacologic dosages, glucocorticoids possess immunosuppressive, anti-inflammatory, and antihistaminic activity. Glucocorticoids suppress the immune system by inhibiting the production of interleukin-2 by $T_4$ (helper) lymphocytes. Decreases in interleukin-2 reduce the proliferation of $T_8$ (suppressor, cytotoxic) T cells and B lymphocytes. Glucocorticoids act in several ways to suppress the inflammatory response, including the influx of phagocytes and the activation of complement and kinins.

Conversely, glucocorticoids can be of great benefit in the treatment of certain noninfective inflammatory conditions (eg, rheumatoid arthritis and systemic lupus erythematosus). Glucocorticoids can also be beneficial in treating certain allergies (eg, asthma, hives, and minimal-change glomerular disease) because they prevent the release of histamines from mast cells. Their use as immunosuppressives enables patients to receive organ transplants. In any case, the potentially deleterious side effects of glucocorticoids usually require that they be used only after other treatments (eg, nonsteroidal anti-inflammatory drugs [NSAIDs] or antihistamines) have failed or if the benefits clearly outweigh the risks (eg, in renal disease or with organ transplants). In addition to

**TABLE 42-5** Actions of Cortisol

| Major Influence | Effect on Body |
| --- | --- |
| Glucose metabolism | Stimulates gluconeogenesis |
| | Decreases glucose use by the tissues |
| Protein metabolism | Increases breakdown of proteins |
| | Increases plasma protein levels |
| Fat metabolism | Increases mobilization of fatty acids |
| | Increases use of fatty acids |
| Anti-inflammatory action (pharmacologic levels) | Stabilizes lysosomal membranes of the inflammatory cells, preventing the release of inflammatory mediators |
| | Decreases capillary permeability to prevent inflammatory edema |
| | Depresses phagocytosis by white blood cells to reduce the release of inflammatory mediators |
| | Suppresses the immune response |
| | Causes atrophy of lymphoid tissue |
| | Decreases eosinophils |
| | Decreases antibody formation |
| | Decreases the development of cell-mediated immunity |
| | Reduces fever |
| | Inhibits fibroblast activity |
| Psychic effect | May contribute to emotional instability |
| Permissive effect | Facilitates the response of the tissues to humoral and neural influences, such as that of the catecholamines, during trauma and extreme stress |

From Porth CM: Pathophysiology: Concepts of Altered Health States, 9th ed. Philadelphia, PA: Lippincott Williams & Wilkins, 2013.

immunosuppression, glucocorticoids trigger the development of all or part of Cushing syndrome (eg, diabetes, hypertension, protein wasting, and osteoporosis) and inhibit growth in infants and children. The pharmacologic and physiologic actions of glucocorticoids are summarized in Table 42-5.

Regulation of glucocorticoid secretion is outlined in Figure 42-7. The secretion of glucocorticoids is triggered by the release of corticotropin-releasing hormone (CRH), a neurosecretory material released by the hypothalamus. CRH stimulates the cells of the anterior pituitary to secrete ACTH. Without the stimulus of ACTH, the cells of the zona fasciculata and zona reticularis do not secrete glucocorticoids. Elevated plasma glucocorticoid levels function in a negative feedback loop to decrease or halt the secretion of CRH and thereby indirectly inhibit the secretion of ACTH as well.

There is a diurnal rhythm to the secretion of CRH that causes a similar rhythm in the output of ACTH and glucocorticoids. The result is that maximal glucocorticoid secretion occurs between 6:00 AM and 8:00 AM in people sleeping from midnight to 8:00 AM in a 24-hour day. Tumors that secrete CRH, ACTH, or glucocorticoids do not demonstrate such a rhythm, a fact that is useful in their diagnosis. The biologic clock that regulates this and other diurnal, or circadian, rhythms is located in the hypothalamus, just above the area where the optic nerves cross (optic chiasma).

The beneficial functions of normal levels of glucocorticoids in enabling tissues to respond to glucagon and catecholamines are more than adequate to meet the needs of the SAM mechanism for a short time. If these needs continue, additional stress-induced glucocorticoid secretion is required. Eventually, if the stress continues unameliorated, exhaustion of the adrenal cortex occurs, glucocorticoid levels drop, tissues are no longer able to meet the demands of the SAM mechanism, muscle fatigue occurs, readily available cell energy sources (eg, plasma glucose and fatty acid) are depleted, and vascular collapse and death result.

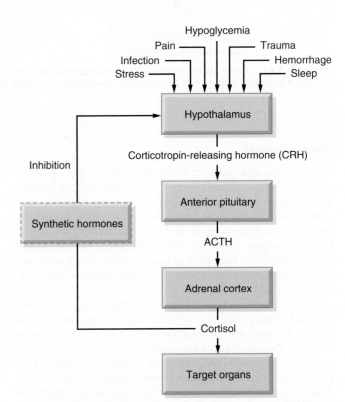

FIGURE 42-7 The hypothalamic–pituitary–adrenal (HPA) feedback system that regulates glucocorticoid (cortisol) levels. Cortisol release is regulated by ACTH. Stress exerts its effects on cortisol release through the HPA system and CRH, which controls the release of ACTH from the anterior pituitary gland. Increased cortisol levels incite negative feedback inhibition of ACTH release. Pharmacologic doses of synthetic steroids inhibit ACTH release by way of the hypothalamic CRH.

## Mineralocorticoids

Aldosterone and glucocorticoids that have some mineralocorticoid function (eg, 11-deoxycorticosterone) increase sodium reabsorption by the cells of the collecting ducts and distal tubules of the nephrons. Because of the cation exchange system in the distal tubule cells, such sodium reabsorption can increase potassium secretion and thereby foster potential hypokalemia. The reabsorption of sodium osmotically causes water reabsorption. This expands the volume of ECF. The increase in blood volume causes an elevation in blood pressure. However, edema does not usually result. Above a certain level of aldosterone-induced sodium reabsorption, the expansion of the ECF compartment can trigger secretion of natriuretic hormone or decreased sodium reabsorption in the proximal tubule. Either of these effects opposes the action of aldosterone and sodium excretion.

The primary mechanism for regulating aldosterone secretion is the renin–angiotensin system (Fig. 42-8). Pituitary ACTH does not stimulate zona glomerulosa cells under normal conditions. Cells of the juxtaglomerular apparatus are wedged between the renal afferent arteriole as it enters the

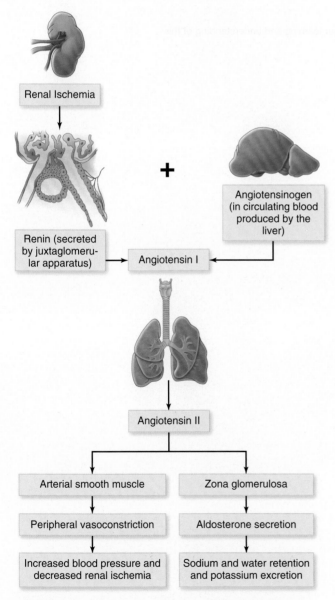

**FIGURE 42.8** The renin–angiotensin system induces aldosterone secretion and vasoconstriction, which in turn elevates the systemic blood pressure.

glomerulus and the distal tubule as it passes by this area. The juxtaglomerular apparatus contains baroreceptor cells that monitor the afferent arteriole blood pressure and other cells that monitor the sodium and chloride concentration in the urine in the distal tubule (the lower the concentration, the slower the formation of filtrate, if all other factors are equal). A decrease either in the blood pressure or in the concentration of electrolytes stimulates the juxtaglomerular apparatus to secrete the glycoprotein hormone, renin. The major classes of stimuli that trigger renin secretion are decreased renal perfusion (eg, cardiac failure, dehydration, and hemorrhage) and low ECF salt concentrations (eg, from excessive use of diuretics).

Renin converts a circulating plasma globulin into angiotensin I. As the blood passes through the lungs (and to a lesser extent in other parts of the circulatory system), angiotensin I is converted to angiotensin II. This physiologically active chemical acts on the zona glomerulosa to promote aldosterone secretion, which leads to retention of salt and water, and contraction of vascular smooth muscle, thereby stimulating profound vasoconstriction. The result of both actions of angiotensin II is elevation of systemic blood pressure, which, among other things, improves renal perfusion.

The juxtaglomerular apparatus contains $\beta_1$ receptors and can be stimulated by sympathetic fibers. Prostaglandins also stimulate the juxtaglomerular apparatus. Sympathetic stimulation through $\beta_1$ receptors, renal artery hypotension, and decreased sodium delivery to distal tubules stimulate the secretion of renin. Therefore, the secretion of renin can be pharmacologically decreased by $\beta$-blockers (eg, propranolol or atenolol). Prostaglandin inhibitors (aspirin and NSAIDs) can exert a similar action. Angiotensin-converting enzyme (ACE) inhibitors (eg, lisinopril) prevent the conversion of angiotensin I to angiotensin II. These effects have made ACE inhibitors and $\beta$-blockers useful as antihypertensive agents.

Aldosterone secretion is also stimulated by an increase in plasma potassium levels, but not by increased sodium levels. Another regulating factor for aldosterone secretion is posture. An upright body position increases aldosterone levels by increasing production and decreasing degradation. How this works is unclear, but because of this, aldosterone levels of bedridden patients are slightly subnormal. There is also a poorly understood diurnal rhythm of aldosterone secretion, with highest levels occurring in the early morning hours just before the person awakens.

## Atrial Natriuretic Peptide (Natriuretic Hormone)

Atrial natriuretic peptide (ANP) is manufactured by cells in the walls of the atria of the heart. The main stimulus for ANP secretion is atrial stretch. ANP increases renal excretion of salt and water. Some evidence suggests that ANP acts by increasing glomerular filtration. Other evidence indicates that ANP inhibits the membrane active transport mechanism responsible for the reabsorption of sodium by renal tubule cells. Decreased sodium reabsorption decreases the movement of water from the urine in the nephron back into the blood of the peritubular capillaries, thereby increasing the elimination of water and salt from the body. ANP also inhibits the secretion of renin by the juxtaglomerular apparatus, thereby lowering plasma angiotensin levels. In addition,

ANP inhibits the membrane active transport mechanism responsible for pumping sodium out of vascular smooth muscle cells. The consequent rise in intracellular sodium inhibits the entry of calcium ions, thereby lowering the intracellular concentration of calcium ions. The decrease in the intracellular free calcium promotes vasodilation and a lowering of the systemic blood pressure.

ANP is secreted in response to an increase in ECF volume caused by the ingestion of salt and water. The exact stimulus appears to be a stretch of the muscle fibers in the atrial walls, which results from the increased venous return that is caused by the rise in ECF volume. As the natriuresis causes the ECF volume to fall back to normal, the secretion of ANP stops. The capability of ANP to increase the GFR, together with its direct effects on the collecting tubules, results in a profound natriuresis and diuresis.

The metabolic fate of ANP is unknown, but circulating levels of this hormone are elevated in patients with congestive heart failure, cirrhosis, or renal insufficiency and are low in those with nephrotic syndrome or volume depletion. These results suggest liver and kidney regulation.

## Clinical Applicability Challenges

### SHORT ANSWER QUESTIONS

1. Discuss the impact critical illness might have on the three major stimuli for the regulation of ADH secretion.
2. Describe the conditions that can influence the negative feedback loop for thyroid hormone secretion.
3. Describe the significance of and the specific metabolic defects of the Ominous Octet.

---

### WANT TO KNOW MORE?

A wide variety of resources to enhance your learning and understanding of this chapter are available on thePoint.

You will find:

- References
- Selected readings
- NCLEX-style review questions
- Internet resources
- And more!

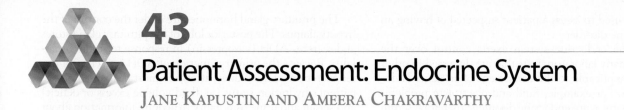

# 43

# Patient Assessment: Endocrine System

JANE KAPUSTIN AND AMEERA CHAKRAVARTHY

## LEARNING OBJECTIVES

*Based on the content in this chapter, the reader should be able to:*

1. Examine the relationship between dysfunction of the hypothalamus and the pituitary gland and the signs and symptoms of the resultant disorder.

2. Analyze differences between the signs and symptoms of hypothyroidism and hyperthyroidism.

3. Identify the parathyroid hormone's role in regulating serum calcium and phosphorus.

4. Describe the pathogenesis of the signs and symptoms associated with hyperglycemic emergencies.

5. Compare normal with abnormal history and physical findings for adrenal gland disturbance.

6. Explain appropriate diagnostic and laboratory tests used to diagnose acute endocrine disorders.

Endocrine disorders can affect all body systems and are usually caused by the overproduction or underproduction of hormones. This chapter presents an overview of the history, physical examination, and diagnostic studies that help diagnose thyroid crisis, myxedema coma, adrenal crisis, syndrome of inappropriate antidiuretic hormone (SIADH), diabetes insipidus, diabetic ketoacidosis (DKA), hyperglycemic hyperosmolar state (HHS), and hypoglycemia. It builds on the content presented in Chapter 42, which explored the far-reaching effects of the endocrine system on body functions. This chapter also provides a foundation for understanding specific disorders and their management, as described in Chapter 44.

Because the endocrine system affects so many areas of the body, assessment must include a variety of signs and symptoms. General manifestations of disorders are evident through vital signs, energy level, fluid and electrolyte imbalances, and ability to carry out activities of daily living. Other parameters to be assessed include heat or cold intolerance, changes in weight, fat redistribution, changes in sexual functioning, and altered sleep patterns. Box 43-1 summarizes

---

**BOX 43-1**  **HEALTH HISTORY for Endocrine Assessment**

**Chief Complaint**
Patient's description of the problem

**History of the Present Illness**
*Hypothalamus and pituitary disorders*: excessive or inadequate urinary output, excessive thirst, poor skin turgor, cognitive changes, dehydration, or water intoxication
*Thyroid disorders*: cold or heat intolerance; edema; cognitive changes, such as slowed mentation, agitation, memory impairment, and stupor; tremulousness; insomnia; fatigue; tachycardia, atrial fibrillation; bradycardia; hypoventilation; constipation; diarrhea; menstrual cycle irregularities; skin problems; husky voice; diplopia, exophthalmos; eye pain, change in vision; depression; hematuria
*Parathyroid disorders*: apathy, fatigue, weakness, tetany, joint pain
*Diabetes mellitus*: weight gain or loss, excessive urination, excessive thirst, excessive appetite, blurred vision, dental caries, poor wound healing, chronic vaginitis, neuropathy, nocturia, dehydration, cognitive changes
*Adrenal disorders*: nausea, vomiting; striae; central obesity with peripheral wasting; moon facies; hirsutism; petechiae, easy bruising; dehydration; fatigue, lethargy

**Past Health History**
*Relevant childhood illnesses and immunizations*: history of adenoid or neck/chest radiation, mental retardation, iodine deficiency
*Past acute and chronic medical problems*: diabetic emergencies, hypertension, high cholesterol, tachydysrhythmias, congestive

heart failure, myocardial infarction, Graves disease, Hashimoto thyroiditis, head injury, cerebral vascular accident, pancreatitis, unexplained infections
*Risk factors*: age, heredity, gender, race, tobacco use, alcohol use, elevated cholesterol, obesity, sedentary lifestyle, growth spurt cycles, pregnancy, gestational diabetes, delivery of an infant weighing more than 9 lb, anemia
*Past surgeries*: neurosurgical procedures, thyroidectomy, parathyroidectomy, adrenalectomy
*Medications*: amiodarone, phenytoin, carbamazepine, chlorpropamide, corticosteroids, opioids, lithium, aspirin, iodides, heparin, levothyroxine (Synthroid), neoplastic drugs, estrogen, methadone, androgens, β-blockers, nonsteroidal anti-inflammatory drugs, potassium, diuretics
*Allergies* and reactions to medication, foods, contrast dye, latex, or other materials
Transfusion history
*Family history*: thyroid disease, diabetes, lipid disorders, cerebral aneurysms, cancers, autoimmune disorders
*Personal and social history*: tobacco, alcohol, substance abuse; occupation; living environment; diet, exercise; sleep patterns; cultural beliefs; spiritual/religious beliefs; leisure activities

**Review of Other Systems**
*HEENT*: headaches, dizziness, weakness, visual changes
*Lymphatics:* edema, lymphadenopathy
*Genitourinary*: sexual dysfunction, infertility, abnormal vaginal bleeding

the approach used to assess a patient suspected of having an acute endocrine disorder.

Because the endocrine system exerts control over the entire body, many laboratory tests that are discussed in other chapters are applicable to the assessment of an acute endocrine disorder. For example, fluid and electrolyte problems accompany many acute endocrine disorders; therefore, serum sodium, potassium, magnesium, and osmolality are assessed. Blood urea nitrogen (BUN) and creatinine levels may also help assess renal involvement (see Chapter 29). Arterial blood gases, bicarbonate levels, and anion gap calculation may be necessary to diagnose acidosis. Laboratory studies specific to endocrine gland dysfunction are described in the following sections and summarized in Table 43-1.

Similarly, in the evaluation of endocrine disorders, it is often necessary to evaluate body systems other than the endocrine system using diagnostic studies. For example, electrocardiography and cardiac monitoring may be needed to diagnose cardiac problems, whereas a chest radiograph may be necessary to detect pulmonary problems, such as the pleural effusion that can occur in myxedema coma. Computed tomography (CT), magnetic resonance imaging (MRI), and ultrasound may be used to localize tumors.

## The Hypothalamus and the Pituitary Gland

Some hormones of the hypothalamus and the pituitary gland have a profound impact on the critically ill patient and are described in detail in this section. They include antidiuretic hormone (ADH), adrenocorticotropic hormone (ACTH), and thyroid-stimulating hormone (TSH). Those hormones that are mainly responsible for normal physiological functioning of the reproductive system—oxytocin, follicle-stimulating hormone, luteinizing hormone, growth hormone, melanophore-stimulating hormone—are not significant in the care of the critically ill adult and therefore are not covered in this section.

The pituitary gland hormones are under the control of the hypothalamus. The posterior lobe of the pituitary gland stores and secretes ADH (vasopressin) in response to serum osmolality. Because the primary function of ADH is to control water excretion by the kidney, attention must be focused on the patient's hydration status (ie, fluid volume excess or deficit) and serum and urine osmolality to acquire information about the general functioning of this part of the pituitary.

## History and Physical Examination

The nurse obtains important information about the nature of endocrine disorders by conducting a thorough history. Because disorders of the pituitary that could result in critical care admission affect fluid and electrolyte balance, the nurse inquires about general hydration status. Specific parameters are included in the endocrine health history (see Box 43-1).

Physical examination of the patient includes assessment of hydration status. Skin turgor, buccal membrane moisture, vital signs, and weight are assessed. A patient with hypovolemia (as seen in diabetes insipidus) would experience weight loss from excretion of large volumes of dilute urine. Eventually, the patient would experience tachycardia, hypotension, poor skin turgor, dry buccal membranes, and cognitive changes associated with dehydration and hypernatremia. Conversely, a patient with hypervolemia (as seen in SIADH) would display signs of water intoxication, such as edema, scant urinary output, weight gain (1 L of fluid equals 2.2 lb of weight), hypertension, moist buccal membranes, good skin turgor, and cognitive changes associated with hyponatremia.

For patients experiencing fluid balance alterations, the nurse needs to maintain strict measuring of intake and output. Urine specific gravity is measured routinely, noting the nature of the urine (color, concentration, and volume). In addition, critically ill patients with fluid imbalance often have advanced monitoring techniques in place, such as

| TABLE 43-1 | Sampling of Laboratory Studies Used to Assess Acute Endocrine Disorders | |
|---|---|---|
| **Test** | **Normal Adult Values** | **Abnormal Values** |
| Total T$_4$ | 4–12 mcg/dL | High in hyperthyroidism |
| | | Low in hypothyroidism |
| Free T$_4$ | 0.8–2.7 ng/mL | High in hyperthyroidism |
| | | Low in hypothyroidism |
| Free T$_4$ index | 4.6–12 ng/mL | High in hyperthyroidism |
| | | Low in hypothyroidism |
| Free T$_3$ | 260–480 pg/dL | Low in hypothyroidism |
| TSH | 260–480 pg/dL | High in hypothyroidism (primary) |
| | | Low in hypofunction of anterior pituitary (secondary hypothyroidism) |
| Cortisol | 8 AM 5–23 mcg/dL | High in Cushing disease (increased ACTH secretion by pituitary) |
| | 4 PM 3–16 mcg/dL | High in stress, trauma, and surgery |
| | | Low in hyposecretion of ACTH by pituitary and adrenal insufficiency |
| Cortisol stimulation | Should increase to 18 mcg/dL | Low or absent in adrenal insufficiency and hypopituitarism |
| Urine vanillylmandelic acid (VMA) and catecholamines | VMA up to 2–7 mg/24 h | High in pheochromocytoma |
| | Catecholamines: 270 mcg/24 h | High in hypothyroidism and diabetic acidosis |
| Urine specific gravity | 1.010–1.025 with normal hydration and volume | Low in diabetes insipidus |
| | | High in diabetes mellitus with dehydration |
| | | High in SIADH |
| Urine ketones | Negative | Positive in DKA |

T$_3$, triiodothyronine; T$_4$, thyroxine.

**TABLE 43-2**  Comparison of Laboratory Values in Diabetes Insipidus and Syndrome of Inappropriate Antidiuretic Hormone

| Laboratory Test | Diabetes Insipidus | SIADH |
| --- | --- | --- |
| ADH | Decreased | Increased |
| Serum osmolality | Increased | Decreased |
| Sodium | Increased | Decreased |
| Urinary output | Increased | Decreased |
| Urine specific gravity | Decreased | Increased |
| Urine osmolality | Decreased | Increased |

central venous pressure or hemodynamic monitoring with a pulmonary artery catheter. Vigilant monitoring of the patient's fluid status must be maintained.

## Laboratory Studies

### Serum Antidiuretic Hormone

The normal serum ADH level is 1 to 13.3 pg/mL. This radioimmunoassay level distinguishes between central diabetes insipidus and SIADH. Elevated serum ADH compared with low serum osmolality and elevated urine osmolality confirms the diagnosis of SIADH. Conversely, reduced levels of ADH with a correspondingly high serum osmolality, hypernatremia, and reduced urine concentration indicate central diabetes insipidus. Table 43-2 compares and contrasts laboratory values for diabetes insipidus and SIADH.

### Urine Specific Gravity

Specific gravity reflects the kidneys' ability to dilute and concentrate urine. The range depends on hydration, urine volume, and the amount of solids in the urine. The specific gravity can be measured by using a multiple-test dipstick that has a reagent for specific gravity or by using a refractometer. Low specific gravity (1.001 to 1.010) is seen in diabetes insipidus and is accompanied by copious, dilute urine. Increased specific gravity (1.025 to 1.030) is seen in diabetes mellitus with dehydration; the urine in general is more concentrated with smaller volumes.

### Serum Osmolality

Serum osmolality ranges from 270 to 300 mOsm/kg and measures the concentration of diluted particles in the bloodstream. Elevated serum osmolality (hemoconcentration) stimulates the release of ADH, which enhances the reabsorption of fluid and sodium at the nephron level. Through this process, extracellular fluid (ECF) volume is restored, and the plasma becomes less concentrated.

Conversely, hemodilution or decreased serum osmolality inhibits ADH, causing excess fluid to be eliminated by the kidneys to maintain homeostasis. Concentration of the plasma is restored.

### Urine Osmolality

This test is a more exact measure of urine concentration. It is also a more useful test when performed in conjunction with serum osmolality. It can be used to diagnose kidney function, diabetes insipidus, and psychogenic water drinking. The urine osmolality is increased in Addison disease, SIADH, dehydration, and renal disease. It is decreased in diabetes insipidus and psychogenic water drinking. The normal range is 300 to 900 mOsm/kg/24 h and 50 to 1,200 mOsm/kg in a random sample.

### Water Deprivation Test

Water restriction is a useful test, because healthy people respond with a rapid decrease in urine volume when water intake is withheld. However, people with diabetes insipidus have no decrease in urine volume in response to severe water restriction. This signifies that the normal mechanism of ADH release in the face of water restriction and dehydration is dysfunctional. However, this test is rarely performed in a critical care unit because the patient is too ill and fragile to withstand the rigors of severe dehydration. The preferred test is measurement of serum ADH to diagnose diabetes insipidus.

### Antidiuretic Hormone Administration

One final laboratory test used to diagnose diabetes insipidus is ADH administration. Exogenous ADH (vasopressin or Pitressin) given subcutaneously to the person suspected of having diabetes insipidus causes a temporary increase in urine osmolality. For a brief time, the person displays the appropriate response to ADH by conserving water at the kidney level, and urine output slows down in an attempt to restore ECF. This test also helps distinguish between the two types of diabetes insipidus: nephrogenic and central. In nephrogenic diabetes insipidus, the person does not demonstrate a reaction to exogenous ADH because the kidney receptors in the collecting duct are unresponsive to ADH. People with central diabetes insipidus respond readily to the exogenous ADH.

## Diagnostic Studies

Diagnostic imaging studies are frequently used for patients suspected of having pituitary or hypothalamic disorders. CT and MRI are essential in diagnosing primary diseases affecting this area of the brain. Examples of disorders that affect the pituitary–hypothalamic axis are brain tumors, aneurysms, edema from surgical exploration or traumatic injuries, and necrotic lesions. Imaging techniques are used to view the sella turcica and the surrounding structures, including the pituitary within the bony encasement of the middle cranial fossa. Angiography assists with precise viewing of the vascular supply in the area.

The critically ill patient requires monitoring at all times during these procedures. Quite often, the patient requires sedation to eliminate all patient motion in an effort to ensure clear images. CT is often used with contrast media to highlight specific areas of the brain, and the patient needs to be monitored for adverse allergic reactions if sensitive to iodine, which may be contained in the contrast agent. Institutional policies and procedures need to be followed during diagnostic testing.

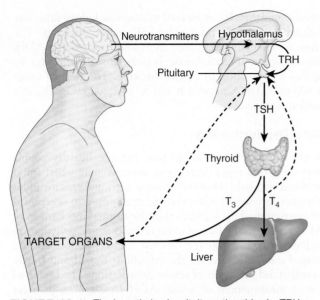

**FIGURE 43-1**   The hypothalamic–pituitary–thyroid axis. TRH from the hypothalamus stimulates the pituitary gland to secrete TSH. TSH stimulates the thyroid to produce thyroid hormone ($T_3$ and $T_4$). High circulating levels of $T_3$ and $T_4$ inhibit further TSH secretion and thyroid hormone production through a negative feedback mechanism (*dashed lines*). (From Hinkle JL, Cheever KH: Brunner & Suddarth's Textbook of Medical–Surgical Nursing, 13th ed. Philadelphia, PA: Lippincott Williams & Wilkins, 2014, p 1471.)

## The Thyroid Gland

The thyroid hormones are regulated by the hypothalamus and the pituitary gland in a negative feedback system as previously described. Low levels of triiodothyronine ($T_3$) and thyroxine ($T_4$) cause the hypothalamus to secrete thyrotropin-releasing hormone (TRH), which then stimulates the anterior pituitary gland to release TSH. TSH stimulates the production and release of the thyroid hormones (Fig. 43-1).

Increased thyroid hormone production results in hyperthyroidism, which can lead to an extreme form of thyrotoxicosis. This is a rare, life-threatening illness necessitating critical care admission for management of the patient. Conversely, hypothyroidism can occur, resulting in a severe hypometabolic state. If hypothyroidism is untreated, myxedema coma can develop in the patient, which is most likely to be managed and treated in a critical care unit.

## History and Physical Examination

Thyroid hormones affect nearly every cell and tissue in the body. Therefore, manifestations of these disorders are widespread. The typical course of disease progression is insidious, and the nurse needs to take a detailed history to uncover signs and symptoms of either hypothyroidism or hyperthyroidism. History taking focuses on the variety of expected signs and symptoms associated with hypothyroidism and hyperthyroidism. Table 43-3 compares and contrasts the two disorder. Box 43-2 explores the incidence of thyroid disorders in the older patient.

Because of their deep, protected locations in the body, the endocrine glands are in general inaccessible to palpation, percussion, and auscultation. The exception is the thyroid gland, which can be examined physically when it is enlarged. Assessment begins with inspection of the anterior neck area for enlargement, nodules, and symmetry of the gland. The patient is then asked to swallow while the nurse observes the thyroid rising. Next, the thyroid is palpated for size, shape, symmetry, and presence of tenderness (Fig. 43-2). See Box 43-3 for a more detailed description of the steps for palpating the thyroid gland. Thyromegaly (goiter) or thyroid nodules can be detected by palpation. Both lobes of the gland and the isthmus are palpated. Occasionally, a thyroid bruit can be detected by listening over the gland with the bell of the stethoscope. A bruit is caused by excessive or turbulent blood flow associated with hyperthyroidism and the resultant hypermetabolic state.

**TABLE 43-3**   Manifestations of Hypothyroid and Hyperthyroid States

| Hyperthyroidism | Hypothyroidism |
|---|---|
| *Symptoms of Thyroid Dysfunction* | |
| Nervousness | Fatigue, lethargy |
| Weight loss despite an increased appetite | Modest weight gain with anorexia |
| Excessive sweating and heat intolerance | Cold intolerance |
| Palpitations | Swelling of face, hands, and legs |
| Frequent bowel movements | Constipation |
| Muscular weakness of the proximal type and tremor | Weakness, muscle cramps, arthralgias, paresthesias, impaired memory and hearing |
| *Signs of Thyroid Dysfunction* | |
| Tachycardia or atrial fibrillation | Bradycardia and, in late stages, hypothermia |
| Increased systolic and decreased diastolic blood pressures | Decreased systolic and increased diastolic blood pressures |
| Hyperdynamic cardiac pulsations with an accentuated $S_1$ sound | Dry, coarse skin, and intensity of heart sounds sometimes decreased |
| Warm, smooth, moist skin | Dry, coarse, cool skin, sometimes yellowish from carotene, with non-pitting edema and loss of hair |
| Tremor and proximal muscle weakness | Impaired memory, mixed hearing loss, somnolence, peripheral neuropathy, carpal tunnel syndrome |
| With Graves disease, eye signs such as stare, lid lag, and exophthalmos | Periorbital puffiness |

*CONSIDERATIONS for the Older Patient*

### Endocrine Disorders

- Expect a higher prevalence of hypothyroidism in the elderly population. Often, the older patient presents with atypical initial symptoms such as depression, apathy, and immobilization.
- Hyperthyroidism in the elderly is much less common; however, the older patient may present with a subclinical picture. Common complaints such as weight loss, fatigue, palpitations and tachycardia, mental confusion, and anxiety are typically attributed to "old age," thus making the disorder harder to detect. Worsening heart failure or unstable angina may result, and often the elderly patient presents with new-onset atrial fibrillation. For these reasons, the highly sensitive TSH test should be considered for the older patient with cardiovascular and neurological manifestations.
- The older adult experiences increased insulin resistance and hyperinsulinemia, and is, therefore, at higher risk for developing type 2 diabetes.
- HHS affects the frail elderly population, with the acutely ill older patient at higher risk. Be suspicious of the older patient with diabetes and the new onset of acute illness, such as myocardial infarction, pancreatitis, pneumonia, or other serious infections or illnesses.
- Another expected result of aging is the decrease in secretion of aldosterone and cortisol. This can result in a diminished response to acute illness or trauma. The older patient may have a decreased ability to maintain appropriate fluid and electrolyte balance. In general, older adults display diminished responses to stressors, such as critical illness or trauma.

Other assessment parameters include noting vital sign changes, skin changes (including edema), neurological changes, and weight changes associated with either disorder. Hypothyroidism is frequently associated with hypotension, bradycardia, hypoventilation, and subnormal temperature. The patient often has dry, flaky skin; edema over the pretibial area; and a deep or husky voice. The patient displays slowed cognitive functioning with slower-than-normal verbal responses, slowed rapid alternating movements, and decreased deep tendon reflexes.

Patients with hyperthyroidism have more neurological manifestations, such as tremor, nervousness, insomnia and

**Steps for Palpating the Thyroid Gland**

- Ask the patient to flex the neck slightly forward to relax the sternomastoid muscles.
- Place the fingers of both hands on the patient's neck so that your index fingers are just below the cricoid cartilage.
- Ask the patient to sip and swallow water as before. Feel for the thyroid isthmus rising up under your finger pads. It is often but not always palpable.
- Displace the trachea to the right with the fingers of the left hand; with the right-hand fingers, palpate laterally for the right lobe of the thyroid in the space between the displaced trachea and the relaxed sternomastoid. Find the lateral margin. In similar fashion, examine the left lobe.
- The lobes are somewhat harder to feel than the isthmus, so practice is needed.
- The anterior surface of a lateral lobe is approximately the size of the distal phalanx of the thumb and feels somewhat rubbery.
- Note the *size*, *shape*, and *consistency* of the gland and identify any *nodules* or *tenderness*.

  If the thyroid gland is enlarged, listen over the lateral lobes with a stethoscope to detect a *bruit*, a sound similar to a cardiac murmur but of noncardiac origin.

From Bickley LS: Bates' Guide to Physical Examination and History Taking, 10th ed. Philadelphia, PA: Wolters Kluwer/Lippincott Williams & Wilkins, 2009, p. 242.

restless movements, and hyperactive reflexes. Characteristic vital signs are hypertension, tachycardia, tachypnea, and hyperthermia. The patient may have a goiter with detectable bruit. Also, the patient may have exophthalmos or proptosis of the eyes. The eyes may unilaterally or bilaterally protrude from the eye sockets, rendering the patient unable to close one or both eyes (Fig. 43-3).

## Laboratory Studies

### Thyroid-Stimulating Hormone Test (Thyrotropin Assay)

The TSH test is a highly sensitive test used to diagnose hypothyroidism and hyperthyroidism. The third-generation immunometric assay tests of TSH are 100 times more sensitive than the earlier methods for measuring TSH, and this test is the preferred method for diagnosing and monitoring

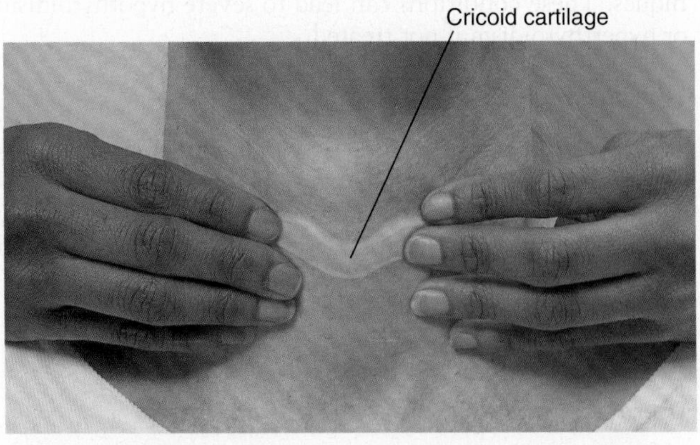

Cricoid cartilage

**FIGURE 43-2**   The thyroid is examined from behind, with the patient in a sitting position, avoiding hyperextension of the neck. (From Bickley LS: Bates' Guide to Physical Examination and History Taking, 10th ed. Philadelphia, PA: Wolters Kluwer/Lippincott Williams & Wilkins, 2009, p 242.)

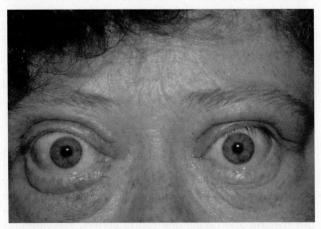

**FIGURE 43-3**   A woman with Graves disease (hyperthyroidism). Note the exophthalmos. (From Goodheart HP: Goodheart's Photoguide to Common Skin Disorders: Diagnosis and Management, 2nd ed. Philadelphia, PA: Lippincott Williams & Wilkins, 2003, p 391.)

**Tests That Assess Thyroid Function**
- Radioactive iodine uptake

**Tests That Assess the Hypothalamic–Pituitary Axis**
- Sensitive TSH
- TSH-releasing hormone stimulation test

**Tests That Assess Thyroid Hormone Binding Peripherally**
- Total $T_4$ and total $T_3$
- Free $T_4$ and free $T_3$
- In vitro uptake tests ($T_3$ resin uptake)
- Thyroid hormone–binding ratios (free $T_4$ index)
- $T_4$-binding globulin

**Diagnostic Studies**
- Iodine-131, technetium-99m scans
- Ultrasonography
- CT
- MRI
- Computerized rectilinear thyroid

**Miscellaneous Tests**
- Thyroid antibodies (thyroid peroxidase, thyroid-stimulating immunoglobulin)
- Thyroglobulin
- Calcitonin
- Basal metabolic rate

progression of thyroid disease. Box 43-4 provides a review of common thyroid tests. Table 43-4 lists medications that may interfere with thyroid tests.

The TSH test measures circulating TSH from the anterior pituitary. TSH stimulates the release and distribution of the $T_3$ and $T_4$ stored in large amounts in the thyroid gland. Measuring TSH helps determine whether the hypothyroidism is primary (ie, caused by dysfunction of the thyroid gland) or secondary (ie, caused by hypofunction of the anterior pituitary gland). A high TSH level helps diagnose primary hypothyroidism. Measuring the TSH level also helps guide medication titrations for patients requiring exogenous thyroid hormone. However, the levels of TSH and free $T_4$ are highly influenced by stress in critically ill patients because of problems with protein levels that are often seen in critical care. Malnutrition, hepatic dysfunction, pregnancy, and drugs affect the TSH and free $T_4$ levels, and actual thyroid disease is not present. This is termed euthyroid sick syndrome.[1] Therefore, the results of the TSH test need to be analyzed carefully in the critically ill patient. The normal adult value for TSH is 0.4 to 5.4 mIU/L.

## Total Thyroxine

The total $T_4$ test measures both the free $T_4$ and the portion carried by thyroxine-binding globulin (TBG). $T_4$ is increased in hyperthyroidism and decreased in hypothyroidism. Any factor that affects protein binding affects the results of the total $T_4$; these factors include pregnancy, estrogen or androgen therapy, and taking oral contraceptives, salicylates, or phenytoin. Normal values depend on the laboratory method used. The normal value is 9.8 to 22.6 mcg/dL in infants; childhood norms are up to 5.6 to 16.6 mcg/dL. Normal adult

values range from 4.6 to 12 mcg/dL and are higher during pregnancy. Older adults have lower values because plasma proteins decrease as people age.

## Free Thyroxine and Free Thyroxine Index

Free $T_4$ and free $T_4$ index measure the free part of $T_4$, the part that is not bound to protein. Free $T_4$ is the metabolically active form of the hormone that can be used by tissues. It makes up a small part of the total $T_4$. The free $T_4$ test is more useful than the total $T_4$ test in diagnosing hypofunction and hyperfunction of the thyroid gland because it helps diagnose thyroid function when TBG levels are abnormal. This test can also evaluate thyroid replacement therapy. Radioisotopes can interfere with test results, and heparin can give false high readings. This test can be performed by direct assay or by indirect measurement. The direct assay normal value is 0.8 to 2.7 ng/mL, whereas the free $T_4$ index is 4.6 to 12 ng/mL.

## Free Triiodothyronine

Free $T_3$ measures the circulating $T_3$ that exists in the free state in the blood, unbound to protein. This is one measure to evaluate thyroid function. $T_3$ is about five times more potent than $T_4$ and is more metabolically active. Decreased values indicate hypothyroidism. Radioisotopes also affect results. Normal adult values are 260 to 480 pg/dL.

## Triiodothyronine Resin Uptake Test

The $T_3$ resin uptake test is an indirect measure of TBG available to bind $T_3$ and $T_4$. It is increased with thyrotoxicosis.

## Calcitonin

Calcitonin, or thyrocalcitonin, is a hormone secreted by the thyroid. It is secreted in response to high levels of calcium and reduces the calcium level by increasing its deposition in bone.

## Thyroid Antibodies

Several autoimmune thyroid diseases produce detectable antibodies. Specifically, Graves disease, Hashimoto thyroiditis, and chronic autoimmune thyroid disease cause elevations in antithyroid antibodies, detectable by immunoassay techniques. These conditions can lead to severe hypothyroidism or hyperthyroidism if not treated.

## Thyroglobulin

Thyroglobulin can be measured by radioimmunoassay and is elevated in most thyroid disorders. This test has limited diagnostic value because it is nonspecific. It is used clinically to follow the progression of disease in a patient being treated for thyroid cancer.

# Diagnostic Studies

## Thyroid Scan and Radioactive Iodine Uptake

The radioactive iodine uptake test measures the rate of iodine uptake by the thyroid gland after the administration of iodine-123 tracer (by capsule, solution, or intravenous injection). A scintillation counter then measures gamma rays

| TABLE 43-4 | Medications That May Interfere With Thyroid Tests | |
|---|---|---|
| **Substance Determined** | **Drugs Causing Increased Values or False-Positive Values** | **Drugs Causing Decreased Values or False-Negative Values** |
| Calcitonin (plasma) | Estrogen/progestin, calcium, cholecystokinin, epinephrine, glucagon | Octreotide, phenytoin |
| T$_4$ free (serum) | Amiodarone, aspirin, carbamazepine, danazol, furosemide, levothyroxine, phenytoin, probenecid, propranolol, oral contraceptives, radiographic agents, tamoxifen, T$_4$, valproic acid | Amiodarone, anabolic steroids, anticonvulsants (eg, carbamazepine), asparaginase, clofibrate, corticosteroids, furosemide, isotretinoin, levothyroxine, methadone, methimazole, octreotide, phenobarbital, phenytoin, ranitidine |
| Free T$_3$ (serum) | Amiodarone, aspirin, carbamazepine, fenoprofen, levothyroxine, phenytoin, ranitidine, T$_4$ | Amiodarone, carbamazepine, corticosteroids, methimazole, phenytoin, propranolol, radiographic agents, somatostatin |
| Free T$_4$ index (serum) | Amiodarone, amphetamine, furosemide, levothyroxine, oral contraceptives, phenobarbital, propranolol | Aspirin, carbamazepine, clomiphene, corticosteroids, co-trimoxazole, ferrous sulfate, iodides, isotretinoin, lovastatin, methimazole, phenobarbital, phenytoin, primidone, radioactive iodine |
| Thyroglobulin (serum) | Amiodarone | Carbamazepine, neomycin, T$_4$ |
| TSH (serum) | Aminoglutethimide, amphetamine, atenolol, calcitonin, carbamazepine, chlorpromazine, clomiphene, estrogen, ethionamide, ferrous sulfates, furosemide, iodides, lithium, lovastatin, mercaptopurine, metoprolol, morphine, nitroprusside, phenytoin, potassium iodide, prazosin, prednisone, propranolol, radiographic agents, rifampin, sulfonamides, TRH | Amiodarone, anabolic steroids, antithyroid drugs, aspirin, carbamazepine, clofibrate, corticosteroids, danazol, dobutamine, dopamine, fenoldopam, growth hormone-releasing hormone, hydrocortisone, interferon, levodopa, levothyroxine, nifedipine, octreotide, phenytoin, pimozide, pyridoxine, somatostatin, T$_4$, troleandomycin |
| TBG (serum) | Carbamazepine, clofibrate, diethylstilbestrol, estrogens, mestranol, oral contraceptives, perphenazine, phenothiazines, progesterone, tamoxifen, thyroid agents, warfarin | Anabolic steroids, asparaginase, aspirin, chlorpropamide, colestipol, corticosteroids, cortisone, cytostatic therapy, phenytoin, propranolol, sulfonamides |
| T$_3$ total (serum) | Amiodarone, amphetamine, clofibrate, estrogens, fenoprofen, fluorouracil, insulin, levothyroxine, mestranol, methadone, opiates, phenothiazines, phenytoin, propylthiouracil, prostaglandins, ranitidine, rifampin, somatotropin, tamoxifen, terbutaline, TRH, valproic acid | Amiodarone, anabolic steroids, androgens, anticonvulsants (eg, phenytoin), asparaginase, aspirin, atenolol, cholestyramine, cimetidine, clomiphene, clomipramine, colestipol, corticosteroids, co-trimoxazole, furosemide, interferon, iodides, isotretinoin, lithium, methimazole, metoprolol, neomycin, netilmicin, oral contraceptives, penicillamine, phenobarbital, phenytoin, potassium iodide, propranolol, propylthiouracil, radiographic agents, reserpine, salicylates (eg, aspirin), somatostatin, sulfonylureas |
| T$_3$ uptake (blood) | Anabolic steroids, androgens, aspirin, colestipol, corticosteroids, cytostatic therapy, dicoumarol, heparin, phenytoin, propranolol, salicylates, sulfonamides, thyroid agents, warfarin | Antiovulatory drugs, antithyroid drugs, carbamazepine, clofibrate, diethylstilbestrol, estrogens, heparin, heroin, mestranol, methadone, oral contraceptives, perphenazine, phenothiazines, progesterones, tamoxifen, thiazide diuretics (eg, hydrochlorothiazide), thyroid agents, warfarin |

From Fischbach FT, Dunning MB: A Manual of Laboratory and Diagnostic Tests, 8th ed. Philadelphia, PA: Lippincott Williams & Wilkins, 2009, pp 1253–1254.

released from the breakdown of the tracer in the thyroid, producing a visual representation of the radioactivity in the thyroid gland, neck, and mediastinum. Scan time is about 20 minutes. Normally, the radioactive iodine is evenly distributed in the thyroid gland, and the scan shows a normal size, position, and shape.

The thyroid scan may be performed in conjunction with a radioactive iodine uptake study. After the patient takes the radioactive iodine, a count is made over the thyroid gland with a scintillation counter at specific times. These nuclear tests can indicate areas of increased and decreased function and provide data to diagnose hyperthyroidism, hypothyroidism, nodules, ectopic thyroid tissue, and cancer of the thyroid.

### Fine-Needle Biopsy

Fine-needle biopsy is the diagnostic tool of choice for detecting malignancy for a thyroid nodule. It is often the initial test for evaluation of any thyroid mass. The test is safe, quick, and accurate, and results are usually available within hours to several days.

### Ultrasound

Ultrasound of the thyroid gland uses high-frequency sound waves to produce an image of the gland. Ultrasound is an easy, noninvasive procedure that has no radiation risks and can be performed at the bedside. The test produces good images of structures and can detect masses, nodules, cysts, and enlargements of the gland.

# The Parathyroid Gland

The parathyroid gland produces parathyroid hormone (PTH), which maintains blood calcium and phosphorus levels, neuromuscular activity, blood clotting function, and cell membrane permeability. The four parathyroid glands are located just posterior to the thyroid gland and are sometimes damaged during thyroid surgery.

The output of PTH is regulated by the serum level of calcium under a negative feedback system. Overproduction of PTH results in hyperparathyroidism and is characterized by bone decalcification and the development of renal stones containing calcium.

Hypocalcemia, as a result of hypoparathyroidism, manifests neurologically as tetany (general muscular hypertonia, tremor, and spasmodic movements) when calcium levels dip below 5 to 6 mg/dL. The patient may complain of numbness, tingling, and cramps in the extremities. As the hypocalcemia worsens, the patient experiences bronchospasm, laryngeal spasm, carpopedal spasm (flexion of the elbows and wrists with extension of the carpophalangeal joints), dysphagia, photophobia, cardiac dysrhythmias, and seizures.

## History and Physical Examination

The nurse establishes a history of electrolyte imbalance, specifically related to calcium and phosphorus. Additional information includes a history of a variety of other symptoms listed in the endocrine health assessment (see Box 43-1). The patient may present with kidney stone symptoms, such as severe flank pain, groin pain, frequent urination, hematuria, and nausea and vomiting. The patient may experience joint and bone pains and may sustain pathological fractures, especially of the spine. The nurse remains vigilant for signs of tetany and related complications.

Tetany can be assessed by evaluating the patient for Trousseau sign or Chvostek sign (Fig. 43-4). Trousseau sign is positive when carpopedal spasm is induced by occluding the blood flow to the arm for 3 minutes with the use of a blood pressure cuff. If tapping over the facial nerve just in front of the parotid gland causes twitching of the mouth or eye, the patient has a positive Chvostek sign.

## Laboratory Studies

Normal calcium levels range from 8.6 to 10.3 mg/dL. Most (99%) of body calcium is in the bone, and the remaining 1%

is in the ECF. Nearly 50% of serum calcium is ionized or free, whereas the remainder is bound to albumin.

Marked serum calcium elevations (levels greater than 10.3 mg/dL) are the most obvious manifestation of hyperparathyroidism. Common causes include primary hyperparathyroidism, malignancy, sarcoidosis, vitamin D toxicity, hyperthyroidism, and some medications, such as thiazide diuretics and lithium.

Low serum calcium levels are the marker for hypoparathyroidism. Tetany develops at calcium levels of 5 to 6 mg/dL or lower. Common causes of hypocalcemia include hypoalbuminemia, renal failure, hypoparathyroidism, acute pancreatitis, tumor lysis syndrome, severe hypomagnesemia, and multiple citrated blood transfusions.

# The Endocrine Pancreas

Diabetes is a disorder of the endocrine pancreas characterized by chronic hyperglycemia; it results in major shifts of fluids and electrolytes as well as in blood glucose levels. The risk of developing diabetes increases with age. The two main types of diabetes are type 1 and type 2, and both forms of diabetes can lead to serious illnesses requiring critical care.

## History and Physical Examination

A complete history is multisystem focused, because glucose dysfunction affects every system of the body. A good family history is obtained to document the role of familial patterns often seen in type 2 diabetes. The characteristics of patients at risk for developing type 2 diabetes are reviewed in Box 43-5.

For the patient with known diabetes who enters the critical care arena, the nurse focuses on gathering information about the extent of the disease and its duration, the onset of complications, the medications taken for the disease, and other past medical and surgical history. Chronic complications, such as neuropathy, retinopathy, and nephropathy, are explored, as well as the coexistence of related medical conditions such as hypertension, hyperlipidemia, obesity, and peripheral vascular disease. Refer to Box 43-1 for a health history review of the endocrine system.

Physical examination focuses on the severe fluid and electrolyte and neurological dysfunction seen with acute diabetes complications such as DKA, HHS, and hypoglycemia. Observation of fluid status and hydration is essential. Skin

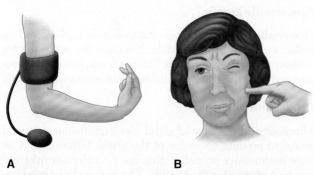

**A**          **B**

FIGURE 43-4  Tetany is caused by tonic spasm of the intrinsic hand muscles. Evaluate the patient for Trousseau sign (**A**) or Chvostek sign (**B**).

**QSEN  BOX 43-5**   *PATIENT SAFETY*

**Risk Factors Associated With Developing Type 2 Diabetes**
- Family history of diabetes (parents, grandparents, siblings)
- Obesity (body mass index >27 kg/m$^2$)
- Race and ethnicity (African American, Native American, Hispanic American, Asian American, Pacific Islander)
- Age greater than 45 years
- History of IFG or IGT
- Hypertension
- High-density lipoprotein cholesterol less than 35 mg/dL
- Triglyceride level greater than 250 mg/dL
- History of gestational diabetes, the delivery of a baby greater than 9 lb, or both

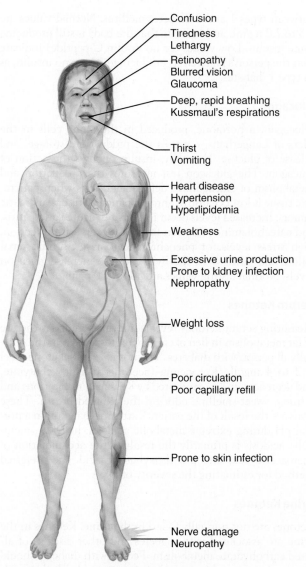

- Confusion
- Tiredness
- Lethargy
- Retinopathy
- Blurred vision
- Glaucoma
- Deep, rapid breathing
- Kussmaul's respirations
- Thirst
- Vomiting
- Heart disease
- Hypertension
- Hyperlipidemia
- Weakness
- Excessive urine production
- Prone to kidney infection
- Nephropathy
- Weight loss
- Poor circulation
- Poor capillary refill
- Prone to skin infection
- Nerve damage
- Neuropathy

**FIGURE 43-5** Clinical features of diabetes mellitus.

presence of a fruity odor on the breath (associated with ketonemia) should be noted. In addition, the patient may display Kussmaul respirations as an attempt to rapidly exhale excess carbon dioxide. This respiratory pattern is characterized by deep, rapid breathing. Figure 43-5 summarizes the physical features seen in the patient with diabetes mellitus. Table 43-5 compares DKA and HHS.

## Laboratory Studies

### Fasting Blood Glucose Level and Fingerstick Glucose Analysis

The fasting blood glucose level provides a foundation for managing diabetes mellitus. Very high blood glucose levels can occur in DKA and HHS. In addition, elevated glucose levels can occur in Cushing syndrome, high-stress states, pancreatitis, and chronic renal and liver disease. Hypoglycemia can occur in Addison disease, pancreatic tumors, starvation, and hypopituitary problems. The normal value for fasting glucose in adults is 65 to 110 mg/dL. Two-hour postprandial blood glucose testing helps further evaluate carbohydrate metabolism, and the normal value is 65 to 126 mg/dL.

In addition, the ADA recognizes an intermediate group of people who have glucose levels less than 126 mg/dL but too high to be considered normal. If their fasting glucose is greater than 100 mg/dL but less than 126 mg/dL, they have the abnormality known as impaired fasting glucose (IFG). If the oral glucose tolerance test (GTT) is performed to diagnose glucose abnormalities, the 2-hour post-load level of less than 140 mg/dL is considered normal, a level of 140 to 199 mg/dL is considered impaired glucose tolerance (IGT), and a level greater than 200 mg/dL is provisionally diagnostic of diabetes.[2] Patients with IFG or IGT are now diagnosed with "prediabetes"; they are at high risk for developing diabetes as well as cardiovascular disease. IFG and IGT are associated with metabolic syndrome, which is manifested by increased abdominal obesity, high triglyceride levels, low high-density lipoprotein cholesterol levels, and hypertension.[3]

Numerous drugs can interfere with glucose regulation, including corticosteroids, diuretics, lithium, phenytoin, β-blockers, and estrogen. Hypoglycemic reactions can result from sulfonylureas, insulin, alcohol, β-blockers, angiotensin-converting enzyme inhibitors, and aspirin.

turgor, buccal membranes, weight, urine specific gravity, and vital signs are assessed. The nurse monitors the patient's neurological status frequently as well as central venous pressures, and used other advanced monitoring if available. The

| TABLE 43-5 | Comparison of Diabetic Ketoacidosis and Hyperglycemic Hyperosmolar Syndrome | |
| --- | --- | --- |
| **Characteristics** | **DKA** | **HHS** |
| Patients most commonly affected | Can occur in type 1 or type 2 diabetes; more common in type 1 diabetes | Can occur in type 1 or type 2 diabetes; more common in type 2 diabetes, especially older patients with type 2 diabetes |
| Precipitating event | Omission of insulin; physiologic stress (infection, surgery, CVA, MI) | Physiologic stress (infection, surgery, CVA, MI) |
| Onset | Rapid (<24 h) | Slower (over several days) |
| Blood glucose levels | Usually >250 mg/dL (>13.9 mmol/L) | Usually >600 mg/dL (>33.3 mmol/L) |
| Arterial pH level | <7.3 | Normal |
| Serum and urine ketones | Present | Absent |
| Serum osmolality | 300–350 mOsm/L | >350 mOsm/L |
| Plasma bicarbonate level | <15 mEq/L | Normal |
| BUN and creatinine levels | Elevated | Elevated |
| Mortality rate | 1%–5% | 10%–20% |

CVA, cerebrovascular accident; MI, myocardial infarction.
Adapted from Reynolds, IG: How to recognize and intervene for hyperosmolar hyperglycemic syndrome. Am Nurs Today 7(7), 12–15, 2012.

Fingerstick glucose testing can be used at the bedside for immediate feedback regarding the patient's glucose status. In addition, patients can be taught to use fingerstick devices at home to monitor their glucose levels and responses to medication. Standardization of the equipment must be ensured when these devices are used for patient monitoring.

In general, point-of-service testing such as this may not be appropriate for the critically ill patient because fingerstick testing requires adequate tissue perfusion for accuracy, and many critically ill patients do not have this required level of perfusion. Testing glucose from more direct sources of blood (ie, veins, venous lines, central lines, arterial lines) may enhance accuracy.

### Glycosylated Hemoglobin

Glycosylated hemoglobin ($HbA_{1c}$) testing offers information about the average amount of serum glucose that is bound to hemoglobin for the 100- to 120-day life span of erythrocytes. This information is now used to diagnose diabetes[4] and to assess data trends for a person who has been previously diagnosed with diabetes. The percentage result (normal: 4% to 7%) reflects an average of 3 months and enhances accuracy because it controls for many variables such as stress, exercise, fasting state, interfering medications, and recent changes in patient compliance. In comparison with the highly variable "snapshot view" that is provided by a fasting glucose level, $HbA_{1c}$ testing provides insight into the patient's overall status over the previous months.[5]

### Fructosamine

Serum fructosamine level measures glycosylation of serum protein albumin. Albumin has a half-life of approximately 2 weeks, as opposed to the half-life of hemoglobin. It is a useful index that reflects chronic glycemic control in patients with diabetes for whom $HbA_{1C}$ may be inaccurate, such as those with anemia or hemoglobin abnormalities (eg, sickle cell disease).[6]

### Insulin

An insulin test helps measure abnormal carbohydrate metabolism by measuring the amount of circulating serum insulin in the fasting state. Insulin is released in response to serum glucose levels. When glucose is elevated, insulin levels should increase as well. Abnormally high levels of insulin may help diagnose insulinoma, a tumor of the islets of Langerhans. The normal adult value is 6 to 24 mcU/mL.

A low insulin level helps diagnose diabetes mellitus, especially in the presence of an abnormal GTT. A fasting blood sample is tested. If the insulin test is performed in conjunction with a GTT, blood samples are drawn at that time. Oral contraceptives and recent administration of radioisotopes interfere with results.

### C-Peptide Level

C-peptide is a single chain of amino acids connecting A and B chains of insulin in the proinsulin molecule. It has no known physiological function, but because it persists in higher concentrations than insulin, it may be a more accurate reflection of insulin levels. It provides a useful monitor of average β-cell insulin secretion and can be used to distinguish between types 1 and 2 diabetes mellitus. Normal values are 0.5 to 2.0 ng/mL and indicate that the body is still producing some insulin. Low values (or no insulin C-peptide) indicate that the person's pancreas is producing little or no insulin, as in type 1 diabetes.[7]

### Glucagon

Glucagon, a hormone, produced in the alpha cells in the islets of Langerhans, controls the production, storage, and release of glucose. Normally, insulin opposes the action of glucagon. The glucagon test measures the production and metabolism of glucagon. A deficiency occurs when pancreatic tissue is lost because of chronic pancreatitis or pancreatic tumors. Increased levels occur in diabetes, acute pancreatitis, and catecholamine secretion (such as occurs with infection, high stress levels, or pheochromocytoma). Chronic renal failure and cirrhosis of the liver can also increase glucagon levels. Normal fasting values are 50 to 200 pg/mL.

### Serum Ketones

Measuring serum ketones reveals information about the use of fat metabolism in lieu of carbohydrates as seen in the critically ill person with diabetes. The normal serum ketone level is 2 to 4 mg/dL. Ketonemia (acetone, β-hydroxybutyrate, and acetoacetate) is manifested by Kussmaul respirations and a fruity, sweet-smelling odor on the exhaled breath. These signs are the result of the patient's attempt to maintain a normal pH during extreme metabolic acidosis. In DKA, metabolic acidosis is primarily the result of the accumulation of acetoacetic acid and β-hydroxybutyric acid, the preferred method for estimating the severity of DKA.[8]

### Urine Ketones

Ketones are not normally found in the urine. Ketones in the urine are associated with diabetes and other diseases of altered carbohydrate metabolism. People with diabetes should test for ketones whenever their urine or blood glucose is high. Because ketones appear in the urine before they can be detected in the blood, this test is often used in the emergency department when screening for acidosis. The test is performed by dipping a ketone reagent strip in a fresh urine sample. The presence of ketones in the urine results from lipolysis or fat breakdown in the absence of adequate insulin.

## The Adrenal Gland

The adrenal gland is anatomically and functionally divided into two distinct parts—the outer cortex and the inner medulla (see Chapter 42, Fig. 42-6). The two regions secrete different hormones. The cortex produces mineralocorticoids (eg, aldosterone), glucocorticoids (eg, cortisol), and androgens. The medulla secretes catecholamines such as epinephrine, norepinephrine, and dopamine. Disorders of the adrenal gland have widespread effects on the human body because these hormones regulate major body functions, such as fluid and electrolyte balance, sympathetic nervous system responses, inflammation, and metabolism.

The secretion of hormones by the adrenal gland is regulated in a negative feedback system through the hypothalamic–pituitary axis. The hypothalamus releases corticotropin-releasing hormone, which in turn stimulates the release of ACTH from the anterior pituitary. ACTH then stimulates the adrenal cortex to secrete cortisol.

## History and Physical Examination

Refer to Box 43-1 for a review of relevant health history questions related to adrenal disorders. Clinical manifestations of adrenal gland dysfunction depend on the nature of the lesion and which hormone is adversely affected. Adrenal medulla lesions may affect the release of catecholamines and cause sudden, severe headache, diaphoresis, palpitations, and other symptoms associated with paroxysmal hypertension. One such lesion is pheochromocytoma, a benign adrenal medulla tumor that mediates this severe outpouring of catecholamines.

Another common pathology affecting the adrenal gland is a pituitary tumor that leads to hypersecretion of ACTH. The resulting disease, Cushing syndrome, manifests as central obesity, unusual fat deposits, thin extremities, fragile skin, skin discoloration (striae), sleep disturbances, and catabolism (Fig. 43-6). The same clinical picture can result from chronic exogenous steroid use.[9]

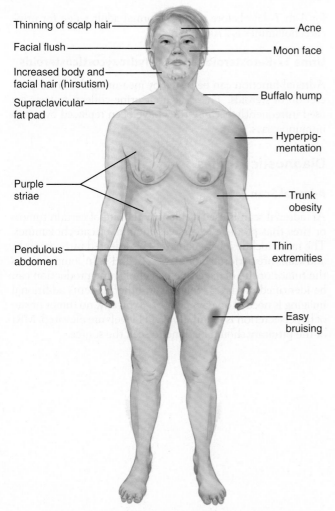

Thinning of scalp hair

Facial flush

Increased body and facial hair (hirsutism)

Supraclavicular fat pad

Purple striae

Pendulous abdomen

Acne

Moon face

Buffalo hump

Hyperpigmentation

Trunk obesity

Thin extremities

Easy bruising

**FIGURE 43-6**  Clinical manifestations of Cushing syndrome.

Adrenal insufficiency from autoimmune Addison disease can lead to an adrenal crisis. The patient lacks adequate stimulation of the adrenal gland, or the adrenal gland is rendered ineffective and stops secreting adequate levels of hormone. Consequently, the patient becomes lethargic, dehydrated, and unable to mount any stress response to handle acute illness or trauma.

The critically ill patient often suffers from mild forms of adrenal insufficiency because the patient's normal stores of hormones are used quickly in response to the illness. Many require exogenous steroids to assist with recovery. A summary of the clinical manifestations of adrenal cortical insufficiency and glucocorticoid excess is given in Table 43-6.

## Laboratory Studies

### Cortisol (Hydrocortisone)

The cortisol test evaluates the ability of the adrenal cortex to produce the glucocorticoid hormone cortisol. Cortisol is elevated in adrenal hyperfunction and decreased in adrenal hypofunction. Adrenal hyperfunction may be caused by excess secretion of ACTH by the pituitary gland (Cushing syndrome), high stress, trauma, and surgery. Adrenal hypofunction may be the result of anterior pituitary hyposecretion, hepatitis, and cirrhosis.

Cortisol secretion is diurnal; it is normally higher in the early morning (6:00 AM to 8:00 AM) and lower in the evening (4:00 PM to 6:00 PM). This variation is lost in patients with adrenal hyperfunction and in people under stress. Serum samples are drawn between 6:00 AM and 8:00 AM and between 4:00 PM and 6:00 PM. Normal 8:00 AM values are 5 to 23 fg/dL or 138 to 635 mmol/L. Normal 4:00 PM values are 3 to 16 fg/dL or 83 to 441 mmol/L.

### Cortisol (Dexamethasone) Suppression

The cortisol suppression test is the test of choice to diagnose Cushing syndrome.[10] Before this test is started, medications are discontinued for 24 to 48 hours—in particular, estrogens, phenytoin, and cortisol-related preparations. Also, radioisotopes should not be given within 1 week of this test.

For this test, a low dose of dexamethasone (chemically similar to cortisol) is given at bedtime. Blood samples are taken the next day at 8:00 AM and 4:00 PM. When healthy people receive a low dose of dexamethasone, ACTH production is suppressed, but people with adrenal hyperfunction and some with endogenous depression continue to produce ACTH and do not have a diurnal variation of cortisol.

### Cortisol Stimulation

Cortisol stimulation is the preferred test to diagnose Addison disease. The cortisol stimulation test measures the response of the adrenal glands to an injection of cosyntropin (Cortrosyn, a synthetic ACTH preparation). Blood is drawn for a fasting 8:00 AM cortisol level before cosyntropin is administered, and then blood samples are taken 30 and 60 minutes after it is administered. The adrenal glands normally respond to the cosyntropin by synthesizing and secreting adrenocorticoids. The plasma cortisol level should increase to at least 18 fg/dL. The response to cosyntropin is decreased or absent in people

TABLE 43-6    Manifestations of Adrenal Cortical Insufficiency and Excess

| Parameter | Adrenal Cortical Insufficiency | Glucocorticoid Excess |
|---|---|---|
| Electrolytes | Hyponatremia* <br> Hyperkalemia* | Hypokalemia |
| Fluids | Dehydration* (eg, elevated BUN) | Edema |
| Blood pressure | Hypotension <br> Shock* <br> Orthostatic hypotension | Hypertension |
| Musculoskeletal | Muscle weakness* <br> Fatigue* | Muscle wasting <br> Fatigue |
| Hair and skin | Skin pigmentation | Easy bruising <br> Hirsutism, acne, and striae (abdomen and thighs) |
| Inflammatory response | Low resistance to trauma, infection, and stress | Decrease in eosinophils, lymphocytopenia |
| Gastrointestinal | Nausea, vomiting* <br> Abdominal pain* | Possible gastrointestinal bleeding |
| Glucose metabolism | Hypoglycemia* | IGT <br> Glycosuria <br> Elevated blood glucose |
| Emotional | Depression and irritability | Emotional lability to psychosis |
| Other | Menstrual irregularity <br> Decreased axillary and pubic hair in women | Oligomenorrhea <br> Impotence in the male <br> Centripetal obesity (moon face and buffalo hump) |

*Occurs with acute adrenal insufficiency.
Adapted from Porth CM: Porth's Pathophysiology: Concepts of Altered Health States, 9th ed. Philadelphia, PA: Wolters Kluwer/Lippincott Williams & Wilkins, 2014.

with adrenal insufficiency or hypopituitarism. Long-term steroid therapy affects results. This test may be contraindicated in the presence of infections, inflammatory diseases, and cardiac disease.

### Urine and Plasma Catecholamine Levels

Urine vanillylmandelic acid, a metabolite of catecholamines, is rarely used diagnostically today. It is preferred to measure free and fractionated plasma metanephrines, fractionated and total urine metanephrines, and plasma normetanephrines, because they yield higher sensitivity levels for pheochromocytoma. Since metanephrines have high concentration in the urine and are easy to detect, a 24-hour urine test is performed when a person is suspected of having hypertension due to pheochromocytoma. Elevated levels of catecholamines can be found in patients with hypothyroidism, DKA, neuroblastomas, and ganglioneuromas.

Urine should not be collected when the patient is fasting. Test results are also affected by many drugs and foods, such as tea, coffee, vanilla, and fruit juice. Therefore, some laboratories restrict certain foods for 2 days before testing and on the day of testing. Certain drugs may also be discontinued

for 4 to 7 days before testing. Normal adult value for urine catecholamines is 270 fg/24 h.

### Urine 17-Ketosteroids and 17-Hydroxycorticosteroids

Adrenal function can be tested by measuring the urinary excretion of steroids. These 24-hour urine collection tests are used infrequently because they have been replaced by serum immunoassays.

## Diagnostic Studies

### Adrenal Scan

An adrenal scan is used to identify the site of certain tumors or sites that produce excessive amounts of catecholamines. The radionuclide iobenguane ($^{131}$I) is injected intravenously, and scans are performed on days 2, 3, and 4. In some patients the tumor or site of excessive catecholamine production can be identified on day 2, whereas in other patients additional imaging is needed on days 6 and 7. Typically, no tumor or site of hypersecretion is found. If ACTH levels are elevated, MRI of the pituitary should be done to seek the source.

# Clinical Applicability Challenges

**CASE STUDY**

Mrs. T., a 53-year-old Hispanic woman with a medical history of obesity, diabetes, dyslipidemia, and reactive airway disease, presented to an emergency department with a 5-day history of weakness, fever, productive cough, nausea, and vomiting. She reports that 2 years before this presentation, her diabetes had been managed with diet alone. In the past year, glipizide (Glucotrol) and metformin (Glucophage) were added by her primary care provider because of worsening glycemic control.

On examination, Mrs. T.'s temperature is 101.1°F, blood pressure 98/64 mm Hg, pulse 136/min, and respirations 36/min. The patient is drowsy but rational. Her head and neck exam reveal poor dentition and periodontal disease. Lung sounds are clear, but no lung sounds are audible in the right lower lobe. Heart sounds are normal.

The abdominal exam reveals mild epigastric tenderness to deep palpation but no rebound tenderness or guarding. Extremities are well perfused with symmetric pulses.

Laboratory results are remarkable for a room air arterial blood gas with pH of 7.14, $pCO_2$ of 17 mm Hg, $PaO_2$ 92, and bicarbonate of 5.6 mEq/L. Urinalysis reveals 4+ glucose and 2+ ketones. Chemistry panel reveals a glucose of 420 mg/dL, BUN 16 mg/dL, creatinine 1.3 mg/dL, sodium 139 mEq/L, chloride 112 mEq/L, $CO_2$ 11.2 mmol/L, and potassium 5.0 mEq/L. Chest x-ray reveals a small infiltrate in the right lower lobe.

1. Is Mrs. T. experiencing DKA?
2. What type of diabetes does Mrs. T. have?
3. What is the etiology of DKA in Mrs. T.?

**WANT TO KNOW MORE?**

A wide variety of resources to enhance your learning and understanding of this chapter are available on *the*Point.

You will find:

- References
- Selected readings
- NCLEX-style review questions
- Internet resources
- And more!

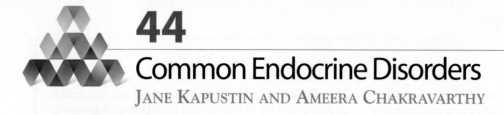

# 44

# Common Endocrine Disorders

JANE KAPUSTIN AND AMEERA CHAKRAVARTHY

## LEARNING OBJECTIVES

*Based on the content in this chapter, the reader should be able to:*

1. Review the underlying pathophysiologic mechanisms that help explain thyrotoxic crises, myxedema coma, adrenal crises, pheochromocytoma, syndrome of inappropriate antidiuretic hormone secretion, diabetes insipidus, diabetic ketoacidosis, hyperosmolar hyperglycemic state, and hypoglycemia.

2. Discuss key precipitating factors, history, and clinical manifestations of endocrine disorders.

3. Discuss at least five laboratory studies that are useful in diagnosing acute endocrine disorders.

4. Describe the similarities and differences in caring for patients with hypo- or hyperfunctioning endocrine disorders.

5. Explore the nursing role in assessing, managing, and evaluating a plan of care for acutely ill patients with endocrine disorders.

Endocrine disorders have multisystem effects and should be considered in the assessment and management of all critically ill patients. Acute illness may lead to hypofunction and, less commonly, hyperfunction of the neuroendocrine system. In addition, some patients present with a known endocrine disorder, whereas other patients may have a preexisting endocrine disorder that is only recognized when they experience an acute illness.

## Hypothalamic–Pituitary–Adrenal Function During Critical Illness

Severe illness and stress activate the hypothalamic–pituitary–adrenal (HPA) axis, resulting in the release of cortisol from the adrenal cortex. This mechanism is key to initiating positive adaptation to severe stressors and for general cellular and organ homeostasis. The nervous and endocrine systems are both influenced by responses to stress, and the actions of these systems are intertwined and interdependent. For example, the neurosensory pathways and chemical mediators in the vascular system will detect a potential stressor, and the endocrine and immune systems will be stimulated to provide both an interaction and reaction to deal effectively with it. Table 44-1 defines the hormones that are intricately involved in the response to stress. The stress response is first activated at the level of the central nervous system (CNS). Communication occurs along the many neuronal pathways in the cerebral cortex, limbic system, thalamus, hypothalamus, pituitary gland, and reticular activating system (Fig. 44-1). One area of the brainstem, the locus ceruleus, is responsible for the autonomic nervous system release of norepinephrine, one of the most basic survival responses to stress. This release causes a chain of events that prepares humans for mounting an appropriate reaction to the stressor. In turn, corticotropin-releasing factor induces the secretion of the adrenocorticotropic hormone (ACTH), which triggers the synthesis and release of cortisol from the adrenal gland.[1]

Acute and chronic stressful events can initiate a significant physiologic response in an effort to maintain homeostasis. The "fight-or-flight" response is the initial reaction to a severe stressor, and release of norepinephrine and epinephrine follows. Activation of the HPA axis occurs in response to stress and critical illness, resulting in secretion of cortisol, the primary glucocorticoid hormone. Cellular actions of cortisol include stimulation of gluconeogenesis, anti-inflammatory effects of the immune system, maintenance of vascular tone and endothelial integrity, increased sensitivity to pressors, reduction of nitric oxide–mediated vasodilation, and modulation of angiotensinogen synthesis. This hormone plays an important role in surviving major stressful events. Cortisol stimulates the HPA axis during acute and chronic events, such as surgery, sepsis, trauma, burns, and other severe critical illnesses. Typically, elevated cortisol levels are detected initially in the critically ill patient; however, if the stressor is prolonged, cortisol levels become depleted. Refer to Table 44-1 and to Chapter 42 for a review of the hormones activated in the neuroendocrine response to stress.

This chapter presents an overview of acute endocrine disorders, including pathophysiology, patient assessment and management, and complications. Thyroid dysfunctions, adrenal gland dysfunctions, antidiuretic hormone (ADH) dysfunctions, and emergencies in patients with diabetes are reviewed. The accompanying box, Spotlight on Genetics 44-1, discusses maturity-onset diabetes of the young (MODY).

## Thyroid Dysfunction

Thyroid dysfunction is a common clinical problem in the United States. Women are 5 to 10 times more likely than men to present with thyroid disease. The most common thyroid conditions are hyperthyroidism, hypothyroidism, and thyroid nodule. Clinical presentations may be quite subtle; therefore, patients with endocrine manifestations must be regarded with a high index of suspicion. Figure 44-2 compares the signs and symptoms of hyperthyroidism and hypothyroidism.

| TABLE 44-1 | Hormones Involved in the Neuroendocrine Response to Stress | |
| --- | --- | --- |
| **Hormones Associated With the Stress Response** | **Source of the Hormone** | **Physiologic Effects** |
| Catecholamines (norepinephrine, epinephrine) | Locus ceruleus, adrenal medulla | Produces a decrease in insulin release and an increase in glucagon release resulting in increased glycogenolysis, gluconeogenesis, lipolysis, proteolysis, and decreased glucose uptake by the peripheral tissues; an increase in heart rate, cardiac contractility, and vascular smooth muscle contraction; and relaxation of bronchial smooth muscle |
| Corticotropin-releasing factor | Hypothalamus | Stimulates ACTH release from anterior pituitary and increased activity of neurons in locus ceruleus |
| ACTH | Anterior pituitary | Stimulates the synthesis and release of cortisol |
| Glucocorticoid hormones (eg, cortisol) | Adrenal cortex | Potentiates the actions of epinephrine and glucagon; inhibits the release and/or actions of the reproductive hormones and TSH; and produces a decrease in immune cells and inflammatory mediators |
| Mineralocorticoid hormones (eg, aldosterone) | Adrenal cortex | Increases sodium absorption by the kidney |
| ADH (vasopressin) | Hypothalamus, posterior pituitary | Increases water absorption by the kidney; produces vasoconstriction of blood vessels; and stimulates the release of ACTH |

From Porth CM: Porth's Pathophysiology: Concepts of Altered Health States, 8th ed. Philadelphia, PA: Wolters Kluwer Health, 2009, p.202.

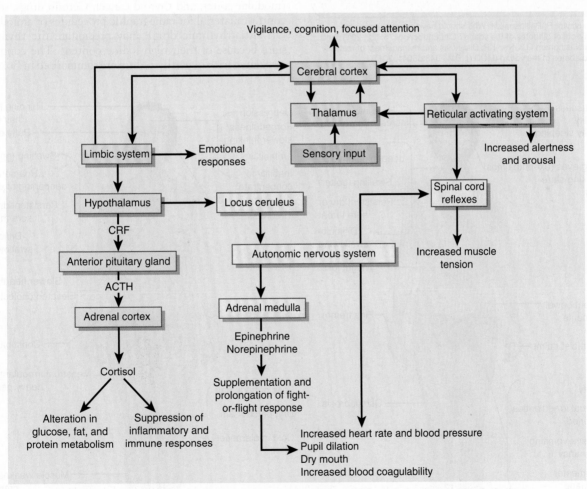

**FIGURE 44-1**  Neuroendocrine pathways and physiologic responses to stress. CRF, corticotropin-releasing factor.

(From Grossman S, Porth CM: Porth's Pathophysiology: Concepts of Altered Health States, 8th ed. Philadelphia, PA: Wolters Kluwer Health, 2009, p 203.)

**MATURITY-ONSET DIABETES OF THE YOUNG**

- MODY affects 1% to 2% of people with diabetes but may go unrecognized. It is important to detect since it is treated differently than other types of diabetes.
- It is a monogenic disorder with autosomal dominance inheritance, so children of an affected parent will have 50% chance of inheriting the gene and getting MODY.
- Each different mutated gene causes a slightly different type of diabetes.
  - There are six types of MODY identified.
  - Most common forms: *HNF1α*-MODY (MODY3) and *GCK*-MODY (MODY2), due to mutations in the *HNF1A* and *GCK* genes, respectively.
- MODY is typically diagnosed in late childhood, adolescence. or early adulthood.
- Some forms of MODY are treated with oral medication (sulfonylurea) and some respond best to insulin therapy. Genetic testing, therefore, is necessary to determine the type of optimal treatment.

Data from Naylor R, Philipson LH: Who should have genetic testing for maturity-onset diabetes of the young? Clin Endocrinol 75:422, 2011; and Thanabalasingham G, Owen KR: Diagnosis and management of maturity onset diabetes of the young (MODY). BMJ 343:d6044, 2011.

## Thyrotoxic Crisis

Thyrotoxic crisis is a severe form of hyperthyroidism often associated with physiologic or psychological stress. When the thyroid state worsens critically, it is called thyrotoxic crisis. The condition may develop spontaneously, but it occurs most frequently in people who have undiagnosed or partially treated severe hyperthyroidism. Rapid deterioration and death can occur if the condition is untreated. Patients in thyrotoxic crisis must be admitted to the intensive care unit for supportive measures, antithyroid medications, steroids, and continuous nursing care. Consultation with an endocrinologist and cardiologist is essential. Even in the patient without preexisting coronary artery disease, untreated thyrotoxic crisis can cause angina pectoris and myocardial infarction, heart failure, cardiovascular collapse, coma, and death.

By definition, hyperthyroidism is a condition in which the actions of the thyroid hormones result in greater-than-normal responses. Specific diseases that can cause hyperthyroidism include Graves disease, exogenous administration of levothyroxine, thyroiditis, toxic nodular goiter, toxic multinodular goiter, and thyroid cancer. Certain drugs, such as contrast material for radiographic procedures or amiodarone (an antiarrhythmic drug), may precipitate the thyrotoxic state because of their high iodine content. The conditions associated with hyperthyroidism are summarized in Box 44-1.

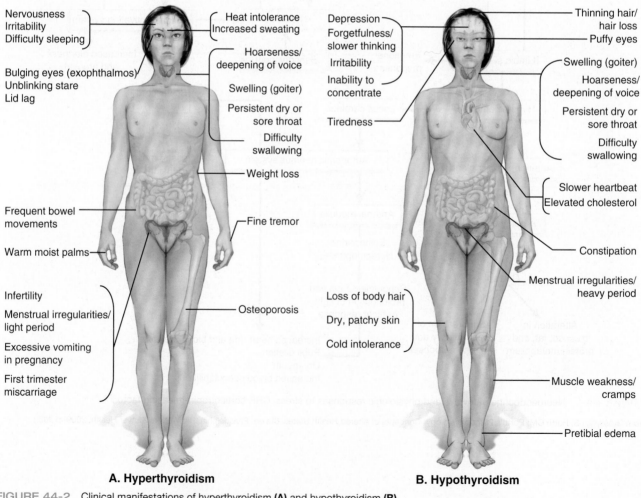

**A. Hyperthyroidism**

Nervousness
Irritability
Difficulty sleeping

Heat intolerance
Increased sweating

Bulging eyes (exophthalmos)
Unblinking stare
Lid lag

Hoarseness/
deepening of voice

Swelling (goiter)

Persistent dry or
sore throat

Difficulty
swallowing

Weight loss

Frequent bowel
movements

Fine tremor

Warm moist palms

Infertility

Menstrual irregularities/
light period

Osteoporosis

Excessive vomiting
in pregnancy

First trimester
miscarriage

**B. Hypothyroidism**

Depression
Forgetfulness/
slower thinking

Irritability

Inability to
concentrate

Tiredness

Thinning hair/
hair loss

Puffy eyes

Swelling (goiter)

Hoarseness/
deepening of voice

Persistent dry or
sore throat

Difficulty
swallowing

Slower heartbeat
Elevated cholesterol

Constipation

Menstrual irregularities/
heavy period

Loss of body hair

Dry, patchy skin

Cold intolerance

Muscle weakness/
cramps

Pretibial edema

**FIGURE 44-2** Clinical manifestations of hyperthyroidism **(A)** and hypothyroidism **(B)**.

## Pathophysiology

The cause of thyrotoxic crisis, often referred to as thyroid storm, is poorly understood. Physiologic mechanisms that are thought to induce thyrotoxic crises include the sudden release of large quantities of thyroid hormone, low tissue tolerance to triiodothyronine ($T_3$) and thyroxine ($T_4$), adrenergic hyperactivity, and excessive lipolysis and fatty acid production. The abrupt release of large quantities of thyroid hormone is thought to produce the hypermetabolic manifestations seen during thyrotoxic crises. The many different endocrine, reproductive, gastrointestinal, integumentary, and ocular manifestations are caused by increased circulating levels of thyroid hormone and by stimulation of the sympathetic nervous system.

Adrenergic hyperactivity is considered a possible link to thyrotoxic crisis. Although thyroid hormone and catecholamines potentiate each other, catecholamine levels during thyrotoxic crisis are usually within the normal range. It is uncertain whether the effects of hypersecretion of thyroid hormone or increased catecholamine levels cause heightened sensitivity and thyroid overfunction. Thyroid–catecholamine interactions result in an increased rate of chemical reactions, increased nutrient and oxygen consumption, increased heat production, alterations in fluid and electrolyte balance, and a catabolic state.

Another mechanism that may contribute to thyrotoxic crisis is excessive lipolysis and fatty acid production. With excessive lipolysis, increased fatty acids are oxidized and produce an overabundance of thermal energy that is difficult to dissipate through vasodilation.

## Assessment

**HISTORY AND PHYSICAL EXAMINATION.** Accurate identification of the precipitating factor for thyrotoxic crisis allows for proper treatment to be initiated. Precipitating factors for people with recognized and unrecognized existing thyroid disease are listed in Box 44-2. Hyperthyroidism's most common form, Graves disease, is an autoimmune

condition caused by thyroid-stimulating immunoglobulins. It is not always apparent that the patient is suffering from this particular disease; therefore, subtle clues need to be explored, such as the patient's exposure to iodine, prior or current use of thyroid hormone, anterior neck pain, thyroid enlargement, exophthalmos (ie, protrusion of one or both eyes) or other eye symptoms, pregnancy, a history of goiter, and a family history of thyroid disease.

Signs and symptoms of hyperthyroidism affect all body systems and include sweating, heat intolerance, nervousness, tremors, palpitations, tachycardia, hyperkinesis, and increased bowel sounds. Extremes of these manifestations—specifically, a temperature greater than 104F (40°C) in the absence of an infection, tachycardia, and CNS dysfunction—may be present in hyperthyroidism. CNS abnormalities include agitation, restlessness, delirium, seizures, or coma. Signs of thyroid emergencies are listed in Box 44-3.

As discussed in Box 44-4, older patients may not have the classic signs and symptoms of thyrotoxic crisis, causing this condition to be overlooked; however, they frequently have suggestive signs and symptoms. In these circumstances, the nurse asks older patients if they have heart disease and what medications they take. This can be important in determining whether there is underlying thyroid disease, because β-blocker medication may mask cardiovascular clues.

## OSEN BOX 44-3    *PATIENT SAFETY*

### Possible Indications of Thyroid Emergencies

| Thyroid Storm | Myxedema Coma |
|---|---|
| Tachycardia | Bradycardia |
| Hyperthermia | Hypothermia |
| Tachypnea | Hypoventilation |
| Diaphoresis | |
| Hypercalcemia | Hyponatremia |
| Hyperglycemia | Hypoglycemia |
| Metabolic acidosis | Respiratory and metabolic acidosis |
| Diarrhea | |
| Cardiovascular collapse | Cardiovascular collapse |
|    Cardiogenic shock |    Decreased vascular tone |
|    Hypovolemia | |
|    Cardiac dysrhythmias | |
| Irritability | |
| Depressed LOC | Depressed LOC |
| Emotional lability | Seizures, coma |
| Psychosis | |
| Tremors, restlessness | Hyporeflexia |
| Weight loss | Weight gain |

## BOX 44-4    *CONSIDERATIONS for the Older Patient*

**Hyperthyroidism**

Elderly patients with hyperthyroidism often present with atypical signs and symptoms of the disorder. Apathetic hyperthyroidism, as seen in the older patient, manifests with a single symptom such as depression, atrial fibrillation, heart failure, or muscle weakness. Thus, the elderly patient may present with palpitations, shortness of breath, tremor, and nervousness, but many other symptoms, as seen in younger patients, are masked. Much time can transpire until the patient deteriorates into full-blown thyroid storm.

**LABORATORY STUDIES.** Laboratory studies may show elevated total $T_4$, free $T_3$, and free $T_4$ levels. The thyroid-stimulating hormone (TSH) level is extremely low (usually less than 0.1 mcg/mL) in hyperthyroidism. TSH is suppressed because the levels of circulating hormones, $T_3$ and $T_4$, are elevated. Recall that TSH is secreted when thyroid hormone levels are low.

Serum electrolytes, liver function tests, and complete blood counts, although not diagnostic, may help uncover abnormalities that require treatment. They may also help identify the precipitating cause. Electrolyte imbalances from dehydration, excessive bone resorption, and increased insulin degradation often occur. The serum calcium level is often elevated, whereas potassium and magnesium levels are decreased, and liver function test values are increased. Hyperglycemia resulting from insulin resistance and breakdown of stored glucose often occurs.

**DIAGNOSTIC STUDIES.** Diagnostic tests include the radioactive iodine uptake test; iodine update is usually increased. Electrocardiography (ECG) and cardiac monitoring may show atrial fibrillation, supraventricular tachycardia, sinus bradycardia, heart block, conduction disturbances, and ventricular dysrhythmias, all reflective of the hypermetabolic state and the synergized catecholamines.

## Management

Management goals for thyrotoxic crises are fourfold: (1) treating the precipitating factor or factors, (2) controlling excessive thyroid hormone release, (3) inhibiting the thyroid hormone biosynthesis, and (4) treating the peripheral effects of thyroid hormone.[1]

Antithyroid drugs are used to control thyroid release or biosynthesis. Propylthiouracil (PTU) is the preferred agent during pregnancy, although it can only be given orally. PTU is preferred because it blocks the conversion of $T_4$ to $T_3$ in peripheral tissues and binds iodine to prevent synthesis of the hormone. If the oral route is not possible, methimazole can be given rectally. PTU has been associated with severe hepatic side effects; close monitoring is warranted to avoid irreversible damage.

Iodine solutions, such as sodium iodide IV, or potassium iodide or Lugol's solution orally, are given to block the release of thyroid hormone. These agents should not be given until 1 hour after the administration of antithyroid medications. Lithium is the choice for patients who are iodine sensitive. Glucocorticoids may be ordered because they also inhibit thyroid hormone release.

Emergency removal of excess circulating hormone replacement therapy can be accomplished by instituting plasmapheresis, dialysis, or hemoperfusion adsorption. Cholestyramine may be used to assist with oral absorption of excess hormone.

Blocking the catecholamine effects that may result in cardiovascular decompensation secondary to decreased stroke volume and reduced cardiac output may be instituted. β-Blockers, specifically propranolol, are used to treat the symptoms of the hyperthyroidism rather than the primary thyroid disease. This therapy may be ordered to restore cardiac function by decreasing the catecholamine-mediated symptoms. The response to β-blockers is carefully monitored because intrinsic cardiac disease may worsen as a result of the negative inotropic effects.[2] Digoxin, diltiazem (Cardizem), diuretics, or a combination of these agents may also be used to treat heart failure or supraventricular tachydysrhythmias. Oxygen is delivered to address the additional metabolic requirements. The goal of therapy is to decrease myocardial oxygen consumption, decrease the heart rate (ideally to below 100 beats/minute), and increase cardiac output.

Corticosteroids may be used to help treat coexisting adrenal insufficiency and thyroid storm. Intravenous (IV) dexamethasone or hydrocortisone can be given to assist with blunting excess thyroid hormone release in this emergency state.

Management also focuses on monitoring multisystem effects from the hypermetabolism of thyrotoxic crisis and the response to treatment. Cardiovascular function, fluid and electrolyte balance, and neurologic status require close attention. It is necessary to assess blood pressure, heart rate and rhythm, respiratory rate, and extra heart sounds every hour.

The nurse evaluates fluid status and laboratory values. Hourly monitoring of body temperature is warranted because the patient is at risk for hyperthermia. Antipyretic agents, particularly acetaminophen, are recommended for fever control; aspirin is not appropriate because it increases free $T_3$ and $T_4$ levels. Tepid baths or a cooling blanket may be necessary. It is important to avoid cooling to the point of shivering and piloerection, because this may have a rebound effect of raising body temperature. IV fluids are necessary to replace the fluids lost from excessive hyperthermia, tachypnea, diaphoresis, and diarrhea that often accompany thyrotoxic crisis.

The nurse assesses neurologic status at least hourly, and initiates seizure precautions and safety measures to prevent injury. If the patient's level of consciousness (LOC) decreases, it is important to assess airway patency and safety issues. Maintaining a calm environment is necessary to help manage the extreme agitation and restlessness seen in the patient with thyrotoxic crisis.

Energy and nutritional needs are heightened because of the hypermetabolism. Interventions include administering glucose-containing solutions, nutritional support, vitamin supplementation, and sedation if needed. The nurse monitors the patient's glycemic status, because the administration of corticosteroids and excess glucose-rich nutrients may lead to hyperglycemia in some patients.

Effective therapy can be expected to result in clinical improvement within 24 to 48 hours. The nurse monitors the patient's mental status carefully, and also checks for stabilization of vital signs and normalization of body temperature. Patient follow-up to prevent another episode is necessary and may involve lifelong medication or suppressive therapy with thyroid ablation.

## Myxedema Coma

Hypothyroidism is a common disorder with a broad clinical spectrum: patients may be asymptomatic, or they may be severely ill with myxedema coma. Hypothyroidism is more common among women, and the incidence increases with age. Approximately 10% to 15% of elderly patients have elevated TSH associated with hypothyroidism, and routine screening of high-risk populations is often done in primary care settings.[3]

Myxedema coma is a rare, life-threatening emergency brought on by extreme hypothyroidism. It is usually seen in older patients during winter months after certain precipitating factors, such as stress, exposure to extreme cold temperatures, or trauma. In addition to coma, complications of myxedema coma include pericardial and pleural effusions, megacolon with paralytic ileus, and seizures. Death can result if severe hypoxia and hypercapnia are not reversed.

### Pathophysiology

Deficient production of thyroid hormone results in the clinical state termed hypothyroidism. Hypothyroidism, a chronic disease, is 10 times more common in women than in men. It occurs in all age groups but most commonly in those older than 50 years. It is more common than hyperthyroidism.

Hypothyroidism can be primary or secondary. Primary causes include congenital defects, loss of thyroid tissue after treatment for hyperthyroidism, defective hormone synthesis from an autoimmune process, and antithyroid drug administration or iodine deficiency. Secondary causes include peripheral resistance to thyroid hormone, pituitary infarction, and hypothalamic disorders. Transient hypothyroidism can occur after withdrawal of prolonged $T_4$ or $T_3$ treatment. The common causes of hypothyroidism are summarized in Box 44-5.

---

> **BOX 44-5** **Causes of Hypothyroidism**
>
> - Destruction of the thyroid gland (eg, surgery, radioactive iodine, external radiation to the neck)
> - Infiltrative disease (eg, sarcoidosis, amyloidosis, lymphoma)
> - Autoimmune disease (eg, Hashimoto's disease, post-Graves disease)
> - Thyroiditis (eg, viral, silent, postpartum)
> - Drug induced (eg, iodides, lithium, amiodarone)
> - Hereditary hypothyroidism
> - Thyrotropin-releasing hormone deficiency
> - TSH deficiency

---

Hypothyroidism usually affects all body systems. A low basal metabolic rate and decreased energy metabolism and heat production are characteristic. The patient with chronic hypothyroidism may have myxedema, an alteration in the composition of the dermis and other tissues. The connective fibers are separated by an increased amount of protein and mucopolysaccharides; this binds water, producing nonpitting, boggy edema, especially around the eyes, hands, and feet; it is also responsible for thickening of the tongue and the laryngeal and pharyngeal mucous membranes, resulting in slurred speech and hoarseness.

### Assessment

**HISTORY AND PHYSICAL EXAMINATION.** Signs and symptoms of hypothyroidism include fatigue, weakness, decreased bowel sounds, decreased appetite, weight gain, and ECG changes. Myxedema coma is a rare manifestation of hypothyroidism, characterized by severe depression of the sensorium, hypothermia, hypoventilation, hypoxemia, hyponatremia, hypoglycemia, hyporeflexia, hypotension, and bradycardia. Patients with myxedema coma do not shiver, although body temperatures below 80 F (26.6°C) have been reported. The diagnosis of myxedema coma depends on recognizing the clinical symptoms and identifying the underlying precipitating factor. The most common precipitating factor is pulmonary infection; other factors include trauma, stress, infections, drugs (eg, narcotics or barbiturates), surgery, and metabolic disturbances (see Box 44-3).

**LABORATORY STUDIES.** A decrease in $T_4$ and free $T_4$ levels is most common; sodium is usually decreased, and potassium is increased. TSH is markedly elevated in severe hypothyroidism. Arterial blood gas (ABG) findings usually show a severe hypercapnia with decreased arterial oxygen tension ($PaO_2$) and increased arterial carbon dioxide tension ($PaCO_2$).

**DIAGNOSTIC STUDIES.** A chest radiograph detects pleural effusion. ECG changes include bradycardia, a prolonged PR interval, and decreased amplitude of the P wave and QRS complex. Heart block may develop.

### Management

The most serious complication of hypothyroidism is progression to myxedema coma and death, if the condition is untreated. A multisystem approach must be used in treating this emergency. Mechanical ventilation is used to control hypoventilation, hypercapnia, and respiratory arrest.

IV hypertonic normal saline and glucose solutions correct the dilutional hyponatremia and hypoglycemia. Fluid administration plus vasopressor therapy may be necessary to correct hypotension.

Pharmacologic therapy includes the administration of thyroid hormone and corticosteroids. Hormone replacement should occur slowly, with continuous monitoring of the patient during treatment to avoid sudden increased metabolic demand and resultant myocardial infarction. Methodical fluid replacement and rewarming of the patient also help to avoid complications.

Additional interventions include treating abdominal distention and fecal impaction and managing hypothermia by gradually rewarming the patient using blankets and socks. Mechanical devices are not used. The nurse monitors the patient for neurologic status and changes in LOC, and implements seizure precautions. Care of the comatose patient includes preventing complications related to aspiration, immobility, skin breakdown, and infection. Monitoring of cardiovascular and respiratory function is necessary. Fluid administration must also be monitored because of a risk for fluid overload. An important aspect of care is to detect early signs of complications. As the patient recovers, interventions focus on patient self-care and education.

Patient follow-up includes a thorough investigation of how the severe hypothyroidism occurred and how it can best be avoided in the future. Patient teaching, family follow-up, medical alert activation, and involvement of community supports may be necessary for this complex patient.

# Adrenal Gland Dysfunction

## Adrenal Crisis

### Pathophysiology

Adrenal insufficiency, also known as hypoadrenalism or hypocorticism, is a rare but life-threatening dysfunction of the adrenal cortex. Adrenal hormone insufficiency may be either primary (ie, directly involving the adrenal gland) or secondary (ie, due to hypothalamic–pituitary disease).

Primary adrenal insufficiency is termed Addison disease. The most common cause of primary hypoadrenalism in the industrialized West is autoimmune adrenalitis. Autoimmune antibody formation leads to the gradual destruction of the adrenal gland, resulting in adrenal insufficiency. The second leading cause of primary adrenal insufficiency is destruction of the gland secondary to *Mycobacterium tuberculosis* infection. Worldwide, tuberculosis remains the most common cause of primary adrenal insufficiency. Other causes include bilateral hemorrhage of the glands secondary to bacterial infection with sepsis and shock, metastatic malignancies, acquired immunodeficiency syndrome (AIDS), fungal infections, surgical adrenalectomy, and sarcoidosis.

The most common cause of secondary adrenal insufficiency is iatrogenic, resulting from abrupt withdrawal of exogenous ACTH or as a complication of cortisol therapy. Suppressed ACTH secretion as a result of exogenous cortisol therapy disrupts the body's natural feedback loop that controls cortisol secretion, rendering the patient in an acute state of adrenal insufficiency. Other causes of secondary adrenal insufficiency include metastatic carcinomas of the lung or breast, pituitary infarction, surgery or irradiation, and CNS disturbances, such as basilar skull fractures or infections.

Acute adrenal insufficiency, or adrenal crisis, occurs when there is a change in the chronic condition or massive adrenal hemorrhage. In addition to the chronic disease, severe infection, septic shock, trauma, a surgical procedure, or some extra stress occurs, precipitating acute adrenal crisis in the patient. The patient is therefore unable to meet the requirements for normal metabolic function or increased metabolic needs as necessary for stress or illness. Any stressed, critically ill patient can develop adrenal insufficiency as a result of suddenly imposed extraneous stressors. As the patient struggles to survive, he or she quickly depletes cortisol stores and may require exogenous replacement.[4]

### Assessment

**HISTORY AND PHYSICAL EXAMINATION.** Symptoms of adrenal insufficiency are the same for primary and secondary disease. Because adrenal insufficiency affects both glucocorticoids and mineralocorticoids, many body functions are affected, including glucose metabolism, fluid and electrolyte balance, cognitive state, and cardiopulmonary status. Weakness, fatigue, anorexia, nausea, vomiting, diarrhea, and abdominal pain may be initial clues to adrenal crisis. These findings are nonspecific until linked with the history of a chronic condition requiring past or present corticosteroid use.[5] Specifically, use of more than 20 mg of hydrocortisone or its equivalent, taken for longer than 7 to 10 days, has the potential for suppressing the HPA axis.

Hyperpigmentation on areas of the elbows, knees, hands, or buccal mucosa is seen in primary adrenal insufficiency. The presence of hyperpigmentation, secondary to the deposition of melanin in the skin, strengthens the clinical picture of adrenal crisis. The most common physical changes include signs of severe dehydration, such as weight loss and orthostatic hypotension. Dehydration occurs secondary to the nephrons' insufficient ability to reabsorb sodium and water. Signs and symptoms of an impending adrenal crisis are summarized in Box 44-6.

**LABORATORY STUDIES.** Laboratory values in acute conditions of glucocorticoid and mineralocorticoid deficiency show hyponatremia, hyperkalemia, decreased serum bicarbonate levels, and elevated blood urea nitrogen (BUN). Metabolic acidosis may occur because of dehydration. Hypoglycemia is usually present. Other abnormal laboratory findings include anemia and lymphocytosis with eosinophilia. In primary adrenal insufficiency, the patient presents with chronically elevated ACTH levels. ACTH levels are normal or decreased in the patient with secondary adrenal insufficiency.

Serum cortisol levels and cortisol stimulation (ACTH stimulation) tests are also used to confirm the diagnosis. Cortisol levels below 15 mcg/dL are indicative of adrenal dysfunction. In primary adrenal insufficiency, repeated injections of ACTH (or Cortrosyn) do not cause a rise in cortisol levels because the adrenal gland is dysfunctional. In secondary adrenal insufficiency, ACTH injections cause a normal but delayed response.

**DIAGNOSTIC STUDIES.** A computed tomography (CT) scan of the adrenal glands and the head may be done to detect tumors or other pathology of the adrenal and pituitary gland.

## Indications of Impending Adrenal Crisis

**Aldosterone Deficiency**
- Hyperkalemia
- Hyponatremia
- Hypovolemia
- Elevated (BUN)

**Cortisol Deficiency**
- Hypoglycemia
- Decreased gastric motility
- Decreased vascular tone
- Hypercalcemia

**Generalized Signs and Symptoms**
- Anorexia
- Nausea and vomiting
- Abdominal cramping
- Diarrhea
- Tachycardia
- Orthostatic hypotension
- Headache, lethargy
- Fatigue, weakness
- Hyperkalemic electrocardiographic changes
- Hyperpigmentation

## Management

The immediate goal of therapy is to administer the needed hormones and restore fluid and electrolyte balance. Fluid resuscitation is also started immediately with normal saline and 5% dextrose solutions. The rate of fluid and electrolyte replacement is dictated by the degree of volume depletion, serum electrolyte levels, and clinical response to therapy. Associated medical or surgical problems may indicate the need for invasive blood pressure and hemodynamic monitoring.

Another management goal is to prevent complications by monitoring signs and symptoms of electrolyte imbalance (hyponatremia and hypercalcemia) and respiratory and cardiovascular function. The nurse looks for changes in blood pressure, heart rate and rhythm, skin color and temperature, capillary refill time, and central venous pressure (CVP), as well as orthostatic hypotension, bradycardia, and dysrhythmias. The nurse also monitors neuromuscular signs, such as weakness, twitching, hyperreflexia, and paresthesia.

Emotional support, a simple explanation, and a quiet environment are effective in assisting the patient emotionally through the physiologic crisis. Once the acute crisis is over, patient education is a goal of care. Patient education is necessary because the ultimate prognosis depends on the patient's ability to understand and follow through with self-care. Self-care includes knowing the medication regimen, recognizing stress factors and knowing their effect on the disease, and being aware of signs of impending crisis; wearing a medical identification tag or bracelet, or carrying a wallet card; and taking medication as prescribed.

## Pheochromocytoma

Pheochromocytoma is a rare catecholamine-secreting tumor that arises from chromaffin cells in the adrenal gland. Because of excessive catecholamine secretion, pheochromocytoma may precipitate life-threatening hypertension or cardiac dysrhythmias when norepinephrine or epinephrine is released in larger quantities. The trigger for the release of catecholamines is unknown, but the high levels can lead to severe hypertension, atrial fibrillation, ventricular fibrillation, myocardial infarction, or cerebral infarction.

Pheochromocytomas can occur in people of all ages and ethnicities; the peak incidence is between the third and fifth decades of life. The classic symptomatic triad consists of headaches, palpitation, and sweating. When associated with severe, paroxysmal hypertension, the triad is found to be over 90% sensitive and specific for pheochromocytoma. Typically, the symptoms worsen with time and become more severe as the tumor grows.

Diagnosis is based on the suspicion of pheochromocytoma for the patient who presents with paroxysmal hypertension and other associated symptoms. Choice laboratory studies include measurement of fractionated plasma and urine metanephrines and normetanephrines. Vanillylmandelic acid is rarely measured because of its limited ability to detect a true positive result (low sensitivity). Diagnosis is confirmed with imaging studies such as abdominal magnetic resonance imaging or CT. Medical care includes surgical resection of the tumor and careful control of the hypertension. Medications that are required preoperatively to control blood pressure and to prevent hypertensive crisis include α-blockers and β-blockers. Usually, the hypertension is no longer a problem postoperatively.

# Antidiuretic Hormone Dysfunction

Two disorders involve ADH dysfunction. One, syndrome of inappropriate antidiuretic hormone secretion (SIADH), is an excess of ADH. The second, diabetes insipidus, involves a deficiency of ADH. Both of these disorders can produce severe fluid and electrolyte imbalances and adverse neurologic changes. Recall that ADH is synthesized in the hypothalamus and stored in the posterior pituitary. It is released when stimulated by specific conditions and causes the renal tubules to reabsorb more water and sodium.

## Syndrome of Inappropriate Antidiuretic Hormone Secretion

### Pathophysiology

In SIADH, there may be either increased secretion or increased production of ADH. The increase in ADH occurs despite normal initial osmolality. As a result, increased ADH production causes an increase in total body water. SIADH is considered whenever the patient experiences hypotonic hyponatremia with elevated urine osmolality, the hallmark of the disorder. In SIADH, no edema or hypovolemia is associated with the hyponatremia.

The secretion of ADH is considered "inappropriate" in that it continues despite the decreased osmolality of the plasma. The normal feedback system regulating the release and inhibition of ADH fails, and ADH secretion continues. The circulating ADH acts on the renal tubules, causing reabsorption of water that is inconsistent with the body's needs. Other reasons for the continued secretion of ADH are also

## BOX 44-7 Common Causes of Syndrome of Inappropriate Antidiuretic Hormone Secretion

**Malignancies**
- Bronchogenic carcinoma
- Pancreatic adenocarcinoma
- Prostate or thymus cancer
- Leukemia

**CNS Causes**
- Head injury
- Hemorrhage (subdural hematoma, subarachnoid hemorrhage)
- Brain abscess
- Infection, abscess, meningitis
- Hydrocephalus

**Pulmonary Causes**
- Mechanical ventilation
- Chronic obstructive pulmonary disease
- Respiratory failure
- Lung abscess, infection, pneumonia

**Medications**
- Nicotine
- Opiates, morphine
- Chlorpropamide, hypoglycemics, insulin
- Antineoplastics
- Tricyclic antidepressants, SSRIs
- Anesthetics
- Clofibrate
- Diuretics

**Other Causes**
- Human immunodeficiency virus, AIDS
- Senile atrophy
- Pain
- Fear
- Myocardial infraction
- Idiopathic

lacking. There is no hypokalemia and edema; cardiac, renal, and adrenal functions are normal; and there is normal or expanded plasma and extracellular fluid (ECF) volumes.

Occasionally, the cause of SIADH is a pituitary tumor, but more commonly it occurs as the result of a bronchogenic (oat cell) or pancreatic carcinoma. These tumors actually secrete ADH but are independent of normal physiologic controls. Other possible causes of SIADH include head injuries; other endocrine disorders; pulmonary diseases, such as pneumonia and lung abscesses; CNS infections or tumors; and drugs. Box 44-7 outlines the most common causes of SIADH.

### Assessment

**HISTORY AND PHYSICAL EXAMINATION.** SIADH is characterized by water retention and eventually water intoxication secondary to sustained ADH effect. The hyponatremia in SIADH has two components, an early dilutional component caused by increased intravascular water, and a later, clinically undetectable component, caused by the increased urinary sodium excretion.

The signs and symptoms produced by SIADH are predominantly neurologic and gastrointestinal. The most common signs and symptoms are personality changes, headache,

decreased mentation, lethargy, abdominal cramps, nausea, vomiting, diarrhea, anorexia, decreased tendon reflexes, disorientation, confusion, and finally, seizures and coma. Many patients remain asymptomatic until the sodium level drops well below 125 mEq/L. Subtle neurologic findings such as altered mental state, slight confusion, anorexia, inability to concentrate, and complaints of weakness may be the earliest indication of impending problems.

Hyponatremia is the clinical focus and probable cause of hospital admission. When the serum sodium falls to less than 120 to 125 mEq/L, more pronounced symptoms associated with cerebral edema, such as headache, nausea and vomiting, restlessness, muscular irritability, and seizures, often result. When the condition develops acutely (ie, within 24 hours), a mortality rate of 50% has been reported. Children and the elderly are more susceptible to hyponatremia because of their lower body water content.

Physical evidence of hyponatremia includes dyspnea, jugular venous distention, restlessness, hypothermia, weight gain, mild to no edema, reduced and concentrated urine, anorexia, abdominal cramps, and disorientation. Often, the nurse is the first to identify these early, subtle signs.

**LABORATORY STUDIES.** The main laboratory abnormalities in SIADH are a plasma hyponatremia and hypo-osmolality. The urine is simultaneously hyperosmolar, and there is a high excretion of urinary sodium. The urine specific gravity is high (concentrated), usually greater than 1.025, and the overall urinary output is lower (less than 30 mL/hour). Other laboratory findings include low BUN, creatinine, and uric acid levels; hypocalcemia and hypokalemia; and decreased hemoglobin and hematocrit values. The diagnosis can be confirmed by radioimmunoassay of plasma ADH, which is inappropriately elevated relative to plasma osmolality. Table 44-2 presents a comparison of laboratory values in SIADH and diabetes insipidus.

### Management

There are three goals in SIADH management: (1) treating the underlying disease, (2) alleviating excessive water retention, and (3) providing the comprehensive care needed when the patient has a depressed LOC.

Treatment of the underlying cause of SIADH may or may not be possible, depending on the pathologic process. Surgical resection, radiation, or chemotherapy may alleviate some of the water retention caused by some cancers. No drug completely inhibits the release of ADH from the pituitary gland or a tumor. When the cause of the SIADH is unknown, the treatment consists of fluid restriction.

The first step in managing SIADH is to restrict fluid intake. In mild cases, fluid restriction is sufficient. It slows renal blood flow and glomerular filtration, enhancing proximal tubular reabsorption of salt and water; increases aldosterone secretion; and enhances distal tubule sodium reabsorption. As a general guideline, water intake should not exceed urinary output until the serum sodium concentration normalizes and symptoms abate. Fluid restriction is usually successful for the patient with sodium levels between 125 and 135 mEq/L.

In severely symptomatic patients with acute hyponatremia, administration of 3% hypertonic saline solution and furosemide is used to correct hyponatremia in an emergency situation. Infusion of hypertonic saline solution at 0.1 mg/kg/minute prevents rapid volume overload and pulmonary edema. Usually, 300 to 500 mL given IV over 4 to 6 hours is appropriate.

**TABLE 44-2    Laboratory Values: Syndrome of Inappropriate Antidiuretic Hormone Secretion and Diabetes Insipidus**

| Value | Normal | SIADH | Diabetes Insipidus |
|---|---|---|---|
| Serum ADH | 1–5 pg/mL | Increased | Decreased |
| Serum osmolality | 285–300 mOsm/kg | <285 mOsm/kg | >300 mOsm/kg |
| Serum sodium | 133–145 mEq/L | <33 mEq/L | >145 mEq/L |
| Urine osmolality | 300–1,400 mOsm/kg | >300 mOsm/kg | <300 mOsm/kg |
| Urine specific gravity | 1.005–1.030 | >1.030 | <1.005 |
| Urine output | 1.0–1.5 L/24 h | Below normal | 30–40 L/24 h |
| Fluid intake | 1.0–1.5 L/24 h | Goal: <600–800 mL/24 h (restricted fluid intake) | >50 L/24 h |

One major complication to avoid is central pontine myelinolysis. This may occur when correction of hyponatremia by hypertonic saline infusion is too rapid. Rapid correction of hyponatremia may lead to brain dehydration, cerebral bleeding, demyelination, neurologic injury, or death. Initial signs and symptoms include seizures, movement disorders, akinetic mutism, quadriparesis, and unresponsiveness. The best plan is to replace sodium at a rate no faster than 1 to 2 mEq/L/hour to avoid the syndrome.

Other medications effectively interfere with the ADH–renal tubule interaction. Conivaptan (Vaprisol) is an inhibitor of ADH that can be administered IV for hospitalized patients with euvolemic hyponatremia. It blocks vasopressin receptors in the renal collecting ducts to decrease water reabsorption. Demeclocycline, an antibiotic, has been effective because it interferes with the normal ADH effect in kidney tubules. Other medications that block the effects of ADH at the tubules include phenytoin (Dilantin), lithium, and fludrocortisone (Florinef).

The nurse monitors fluid and electrolyte balance, especially the serum sodium level. In addition, it is necessary to evaluate intake and output, including hourly urine amounts, and observe for signs of fluid overload. Output should exceed intake. Adequate intake of dietary protein and salt need to be encouraged.

The nurse evaluates the patient's neurologic status. Rapid changes in sodium levels can result in neurologic deterioration. When the serum sodium is less than 125 mEq/L, there is a significant risk for neurologic symptoms, including disorientation and decreasing consciousness. Seizure precautions may be necessary. Complications of SIADH include neurologic deterioration leading to seizures, coma, and death.

Patients may find it difficult to limit their fluid intake. Mealtimes may also be difficult because menus are aimed at meeting nutritional needs without increasing fluid intake. Providing good oral care and offering substitutions for fluids (eg, Toothettes, lemon-glycerin swabs) may be helpful for the persistently thirsty patient. Providing information and emotional support and acknowledging the deprivation may help patients through this period.

## Diabetes Insipidus

### Pathophysiology

Diabetes insipidus is a disease characterized by water imbalance resulting from inadequate ADH or resistance to ADH, leading to water diuresis and dehydration. Polyuria is the hallmark of the disorder: the kidneys can excrete great quantities of dilute urine, at times up to 20 L/d. Normally, the posterior pituitary releases ADH, which then acts on the distal renal tubules to promote reabsorption of water. When there is an absence of or deficit in ADH, the kidneys lose their ability to reabsorb water and control fluid output (see Chapter 42).

Diabetes insipidus may manifest in two forms: central and nephrogenic. Central diabetes insipidus is the more common condition that results in ADH deficiency; it responds favorably to exogenous vasopressin administration. This type of diabetes insipidus is the disease most often encountered in the critical care environment. Nephrogenic diabetes insipidus is a rare genetic disorder that results from the failure of the kidney to respond to ADH. Only central diabetes insipidus is discussed in this chapter.

Diabetes insipidus can be transient, temporary, partial, or permanent, depending on the initial cause and circumstances surrounding the patient illness or injury. The osmolality sensors of the hypothalamus control ADH release from the posterior pituitary. As the osmolality increases, the osmoreceptors are stimulated, releasing more ADH. In the kidneys, ADH causes more water and sodium to be absorbed, restoring adequate fluid balance. In the absence of ADH, the renal tubules and collecting ducts are impermeable to water; consequently, large volumes of dilute urine are excreted. Serum osmolality and sodium rise, and the patient continues to become progressively more dehydrated. The thirst sensation may or may not be affected, depending on the patient's LOC. For patients with an impaired thirst mechanism, dehydration and hypovolemic shock will result more quickly if the condition is not corrected.

Diabetes insipidus can develop after any event that causes edema or direct damage to the neurohypophysis. After surgery, diabetes insipidus may occur when regions of the brain around the hypothalamus and pituitary are affected. It can occur after head injuries, gunshot wounds, and lesions that disrupt blood supply to the area. Damage to the sphenoid bone, maxillofacial injuries, hypothalamic tumors, and nasopharyngeal tumors that invade the base of the skull may also lead to the development of diabetes insipidus. Direct trauma or ischemic events involving the hypothalamus, such as hemorrhage, infection, or neoplasm, may result in diabetes insipidus. Also, diseases or drugs that affect the renal collecting tubules may lead to diabetes insipidus. There is also a psychogenic polydipsia, in which excessive water is consumed, resulting in excess output.

After trauma or surgery, diabetes insipidus can be transient until initial edema subsides. The neurohypophysis is very sensitive to extraneous pressure; consequently, these structures may be unable to produce, secrete, or release ADH

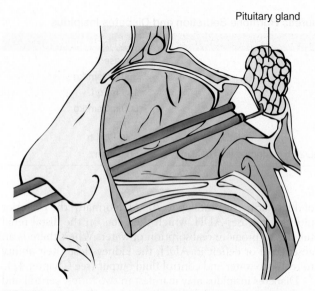

Pituitary gland

FIGURE 44-3 The transsphenoidal approach to a pituitary tumor can lead to transient diabetes insipidus. The neurohypophysis is very sensitive to extraneous pressure; consequently, these structures may be unable to produce, secrete, or release ADH as needed. The resultant diabetes insipidus resolves as the edema (from the surgery) resolves.

as needed. The patient displays temporary signs of diabetes insipidus. As the edema abates, ADH secretion resumes its normal course, and the diabetes insipidus is eventually corrected. In some cases of severe trauma or hemorrhage, the structures may be completely damaged, and the patient may permanently develop diabetes insipidus.

The classic example of the transient type of disorder is illustrated by the patient undergoing a transsphenoidal approach for a hypophysectomy to remove a pituitary tumor. In most cases, the patient experiences temporary problems related to an inability to synthesize, store, or release ADH due to edema of the hypothalamus and pituitary. This patient requires close monitoring for the development of diabetes insipidus and may need treatment. Figure 44-3 illustrates a transsphenoidal approach to a pituitary tumor.

### Assessment

Polyuria, polydipsia, and dehydration are the hallmarks of diabetes insipidus. Patients can excrete from 3 to 20 L of urine/d. When patients are alert, they experience excessive thirst and excessive urinary output. They try to increase their fluid intake, but this can cause exhaustion and eventually result in dehydration. On the other hand, when people are not alert enough to detect thirst and increase their fluid intake, they can quickly become hypovolemic because of the fluid loss. If left untreated, this can lead to death.

Signs of dehydration include dry skin, dry mucous membranes, confusion, sunken eyeballs, constipation, poor skin turgor, lethargy, muscle weakness, muscle pain, and pallor. Vital signs are adversely affected, with severe tachycardia, hypotension, low CVP, and a possible rise in body temperature. Weight loss may be apparent.

Recognizing diabetes insipidus may be more difficult when patients are recovering from surgery because steroids and cerebral dehydrating agents used before and during surgery promote diuresis for the first postoperative day or so. If awake,

the patient complains of progressive thirst if diabetes insipidus is present. Urine output increases and persists regardless of the amount of fluid intake. Urine specific gravity falls or remains at about 1.001 to 1.005. Urine is copious, clear, and almost colorless. Plasma osmolality increases, often to levels greater than 300 mOsm/kg. Urine osmolality decreases to 50 to 100 mOsm/kg. The urine sodium concentration is below normal, whereas the serum sodium concentration is elevated (see Chapter 43, Table 43-2). The water deprivation test is also helpful to diagnose diabetes insipidus. These tests, combined with the constellation of signs and symptoms, lead to the diagnosis. Table 44-2 presents laboratory values for patients with diabetes insipidus.

### Management

The objective of therapy is to prevent dehydration and electrolyte imbalance, while treating the underlying cause and preventing complications. Hypotonic IV solutions, such as 0.45% sodium chloride solution, are administered to match the urine output. The volume of replacement fluids depends on the degree of dehydration and the amount needed to reverse hypovolemic shock.

A variety of replacement ADH (vasopressin) therapies are available. Desmopressin acetate is synthetic ADH that can be administered IV, orally, or as a nasal spray. Aqueous vasopressin (Pitressin) may be given as an IV bolus, continuous infusion, or subcutaneously. The medications can be used for temporary or permanent ADH replacement. Permanent hormone replacement requires additional patient and family education. The patient should also obtain medical identification to carry at all times. Medications administered for the treatment of diabetes insipidus include desmopressin, aqueous pitressin, lysine vasopressin nasal spray, chlorpropamide (Diabinese), and clofibrate.

Management also focuses on monitoring fluid and electrolyte balance. The nurse detects fluid excesses or deficits by evaluating hourly intake and output, serum and urine electrolytes and osmolality results, and urine specific gravity. Also noted are changes in blood pressure, pulse, and respirations, as well as the onset of pulmonary crackles, neck vein distention, peripheral edema, and increasing CVP and pulmonary artery occlusion pressure (PAOP, also known as pulmonary artery wedge pressure). The nurse observes skin turgor and mucous membranes, and changes in alertness and cognition. Drowsiness, confusion, and headache may indicate water intoxication. Body weight is another indicator of fluid status.

### Complications

Major complications of diabetes insipidus are cardiovascular collapse and tissue hypoxia. Seizures and encephalopathy can also result from fluid and electrolyte imbalance. Prognosis is excellent as long as the patient receives prompt and aggressive treatment.

## Emergencies for Patients With Diabetes Mellitus

Diabetes mellitus is a complex and chronic metabolic disorder characterized by hyperglycemia and defects in insulin secretion. Figure 44-4 illustrates how chronic hyperglycemia

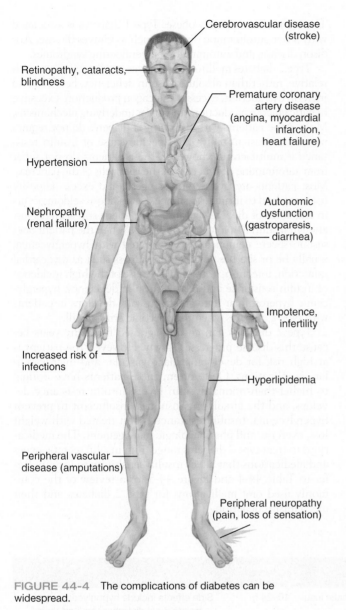

Cerebrovascular disease (stroke)

Retinopathy, cataracts, blindness

Premature coronary artery disease (angina, myocardial infarction, heart failure)

Hypertension

Autonomic dysfunction (gastroparesis, diarrhea)

Nephropathy (renal failure)

Impotence, infertility

Increased risk of infections

Hyperlipidemia

Peripheral vascular disease (amputations)

Peripheral neuropathy (pain, loss of sensation)

**FIGURE 44-4** The complications of diabetes can be widespread.

disease are the primary causes of morbidity and mortality in people affected with diabetes.

The incidence of diabetes in the United States has risen dramatically, and diabetes morbidity and mortality are also increasing. Diabetes is one of the most common diseases in the United States, with an estimated 29.1 million adults afflicted, representing 9.3% of the population.[6] Prevalence rates approach 50% in certain population subgroups (Native American, Hispanic American, African American). This rate is strongly related to the epidemic of obesity and the socioeconomic inequalities that plague the United States.

The pathogenic processes associated with diabetes mellitus range from autoimmune destruction of the islet beta cells of the pancreas (type 1 diabetes mellitus) to insulin resistance (type 2 diabetes mellitus). The derangements of carbohydrate, protein, and fat metabolism all result from deficient action of insulin on target tissues. The main effect is hyperglycemia. Hyperglycemia is manifested as polyuria, polydipsia, polyphagia, weight loss, and blurred vision. Acute, critical illnesses associated with diabetes are hyperglycemia with ketoacidosis and nonketotic hyperosmolar state.

Often, almost half of patients with type 2 diabetes mellitus are not diagnosed until complications have already developed, and many suffer acute syndromes requiring emergency department evaluation, intensive care management, or both. The critical care nurse must be vigilant in identifying high-risk patients.

Most patients with diabetes can be classified into two main groups: those with type 1 diabetes mellitus and those with type 2 diabetes mellitus (Table 44-3). The cause of type 1 diabetes is an absolute deficiency of insulin secretion. This insulin secretion impairment results from autoimmune destruction of the beta cells of the pancreas. Markers of immune destruction include islet cell autoantibodies (ICAs), glutamic acid decarboxylase antibodies, islet cell antibodies (ICA512-1A-2), and insulin antibodies. The best predictor for future development of type 1 diabetes is the expression of multiple autoantibodies.[7] The rate of islet cell destruction is variable, and it occurs more rapidly in younger patients and more slowly in older patients. Some children and adolescents present with ketoacidosis as the first manifestation of the disease. As the islet cell destruction occurs, the patient is rendered insulin dependent for survival.

Type 1 diabetes is primarily a disease of the young, with a peak incidence at ages 10 to 12 years for females and 12 to 14 years for males. Although onset occurs mainly during childhood or at puberty, and most patients receive a diagnosis

is associated with long-term organ dysfunction, particularly of the eyes, kidneys, nerves, heart, and blood vessels. These long-term microvascular and macrovascular complications of retinopathy, neuropathy, nephropathy, and cardiovascular

| TABLE 44-3 | Comparison of Type I and Type 2 Diabetes Mellitus | |
|---|---|---|
| | **Type 1 Diabetes** | **Type 2 Diabetes** |
| Etiology | Autoimmune destruction of islet cells | Insulin resistance |
| Incidence | 5%–10% | 90%–95% |
| Age of onset | Usually before 35 y | Usually after 35 y |
| Speed of onset | Usually rapid | Usually gradual |
| Nutritional state | Usually thin | Usually overweight, obese |
| Endogenous insulin | Absent | Low or high, rarely absent |
| Symptoms | Polyuria, polydipsia, polyphagia, weight loss | Same, plus blurred vision, fatigue |
| Ketosis | Frequently present with poor control | Infrequent |
| Treatment goal | Exogenous insulin management | Weight loss, exercise, improved insulin resistance |
| Treatment | Exogenous insulin, diet control, exercise, weight maintenance | Oral and injectable (non-insulin) agents, diet control, exercise, weight loss, can progress to insulin |

## TYPE 1 DIABETES

- Type 1 diabetes occurs in 10 to 20 per 100,000 people per year in the United States. Type 1 diabetes accounts for 5% to 10% of cases of diabetes worldwide and during the past 20 years has been increasing 2% to 5% each year, worldwide.
- The risk of developing type 1 diabetes is increased by certain variants of the *HLA-DQA1*, *HLA-DQB1*, and *HLA-DRB1* genes. The *HLA-DQA1*, *HLA-DQB1*, *and HLA-DRB1* genes belong to a family of genes called the human leukocyte antigen (HLA) complex. The HLA complex helps the immune system distinguish the body's own proteins from proteins made by foreign invaders such as viruses and bacteria.
- Type 1 diabetes is generally considered an autoimmune disorder usually due to the numerous variants found *HLA-DQA1*, *HLA-DQB1*, and *HLA-DRB1* genes. For unknown reason the HLA complex damages the insulin-producing beta cell sounds in the pancreas.
- Genetic testing is available to identify risk of developing Type-1 diabetes.

Data from Genetic Home Reference http://ghr.nlm.nih.gov—Accessed August 10, 2015; and Morahan G: Insights into type 1 diabetes provided by genetic analyses. Curr Opin Endocrinol Diabetes Obes 19(4):263–270, 2012.

before age 20 years, the disease can occur at any age. Type 1 diabetes accounts for approximately 5% to 10% of all cases of diabetes. A genetic predisposition for type 1 diabetes may exist: it appears that genetically predisposed patients contract the disorder after an environmental factor (viruses, congenital rubella, enteroviruses) triggers the autoimmune destruction of the islet cells, leading to insulin deficiency.[7,8] (See the accompanying box, Spotlight on Genetics 44-2: Type 1 Diabetes.)

These patients are rarely obese. Type 1 diabetes is associated with other autoimmune diseases, such as Graves disease, Addison disease, and autoimmune polyendocrine syndromes.

Type 2 diabetes mellitus manifests as insulin resistance with relative, rather than absolute, insulin deficiency, beta cell and incretin dysfunction, excessive glucagon production, excessive hepatic glucose production, and other underlying mechanisms. Most of the patients with this form of diabetes do not require insulin, at least initially. The specific cause of insulin resistance is multifactorial; however, these patients do not suffer from autoimmune destruction of the islet cells of the pancreas. Most patients are overweight or obese, and excess adiposity itself can lead to insulin resistance. Ketoacidosis seldom occurs in this form of diabetes because the patient still secretes just enough insulin to avoid critical illness. When the patient does sustain severe complications associated with hyperglycemia, usually he or she has concomitant illness such as myocardial infarction, infection, or trauma. Because of the high incidence of insulin resistance and relative insulin deficiency, hyperglycemic hyperosmolar state (HHS) usually develops in patients with type 2 diabetes when they become critically ill.

Type 2 diabetes can go undiagnosed for many years because this disease progresses slowly. However, the patient is at high risk for developing macrovascular and microvascular complications. Quite often, these patients have normal to higher-than-normal insulin levels; insulin resistance develops, and the circulating insulin is insufficient to prevent hyperglycemia. Insulin resistance is best treated with weight loss, exercise, and pharmacologic management. The medications to treat type 2 diabetes range from insulin secretagogues and medications that affect insulin sensitivity to insulin. Refer to Table 44-4 and Figure 44-5 for a review of the commonly used oral medications for type 2 diabetes and their mechanisms of action.

**TABLE 44-4    Oral Drugs Used to Treat Diabetes Mellitus**

| Drug | Example | Action | Duration of Action | Nursing Considerations |
|---|---|---|---|---|
| Second-generation sulfonylureas | Glyburide, glucotrol, Micronase, Amaryl | Stimulates pancreatic insulin secretion | 10–24 h | Side effects include hypoglycemia, gastrointestinal disturbances, and rash<br>Safer in elderly patients |
| Biguanides | Metformin (Glucophage) | Reduces hepatic glucose production, increases insulin sensitivity | 8 h | Lactic acidosis is a serious side effect (stop when using contrast medium for x-rays); other side effects include gastrointestinal disturbances (eg, flatulence, diarrhea, nausea)<br>Use with caution in PATIENTS with renal disease<br>Improves insulin resistance<br>Promotes weight loss |
| Thiazolidinediones | Actos | Enhances insulin's effects at receptor sites | 12–24 h | Will not increase level of circulating insulin<br>Side effects include edema, weight gain, and anemia<br>Monitor liver function tests<br>Improves lipid profile<br>Contraindicated with Class 3 and 4 heart failure |
| α-Glucosidase inhibitors | Precose, Miglitol | Inhibits metabolism of carbohydrates in intestines | 8 h | Take with meals<br>Side effects include gastrointestinal symptoms (eg, flatulence, abdominal pain, diarrhea, nausea)<br>Use with caution in patients with renal disease |

**TABLE 44-4**    Oral Drugs Used to Treat Diabetes Mellitus (*continued*)

| Drug | Example | Action | Duration of Action | Nursing Considerations |
|---|---|---|---|---|
| Meglitinides | Prandin | Stimulates β-cell insulin release | | Side effects include hypoglycemia, upper respiratory infection, headache, and diarrhea<br>Use with caution in patients with hepatic or renal disease |
| Amino acid derivatives (insulin secretagogue) | Starlix | Stimulates β-cell insulin release | | Side effects include hypoglycemia, gastrointestinal disturbances (eg, nausea), upper respiratory tract symptoms, and dizziness<br>Use with caution in patients with hepatic disease |
| Incretion mimetics | | | | |
|   Glucagon-like peptide-1 (GLP-1) receptor agonists | | Decreases postprandial glucose rise, promotes insulin secretion, and slows gastric emptying, promotes satiety | 8–12 h | Given subcutaneously<br>May produce weight loss<br>Caution with renal dysfunction<br>Risk of pancreatitis, risk of thyroid C-cell cancer |
|   Exenatide | Byetta<br>Bydureon (weekly injected exenatide) | | 8–12 h<br>weekly | |
|   Dulaglutide | Trulicity | | Weekly | |
|   Albiglutide | Tanzeum | | Weekly | |
|   Liraglutide | Victoza | | 24 h | |
| Amylin analogue | Symlin | As above | | |
| Dipeptidyl peptidase-4 inhibitors | | Increases availability of GLP-1 above actions | 12–24 h | Given orally<br>May produce weight loss but usually weight neutral; caution with renal disease, risk of pancreatitis |
|   Linagliptin | Tradjenta | | | |
|   Sitagliptin | Januvia | | | |
|   Saxagliptin | Onglyza | | | |
|   Alogliptin | Nesina | | | |
| Sodium glucose co-transporter-2 inhibitors | | Increases glucosuria to lower glucose levels | 12–24 h | Requires adequate renal function<br>May help with weight reduction<br>Risk of genital mycotic infections, UTI and postural hypotension |
|   Canagliflozin | Invokana | | | |
|   Dapagliflozin | Farxiga | | | |
|   Empagliflozin | Jardiance | | | |
| Combination therapy | | | | |
|   Glyburide and metformin | Glucovance | As above with each drug | As above with each drug | As above with each drug |
|   Metformin and glipizide | Metaglip | As above with each drug | As above with each drug | As above with each drug |
|   Repaglinide and metformin | PrandiMet | As above with each drug | As above with each drug | As above with each drug |
|   Sitagliptin and metformin | Janumet | As above with each drug | As above with each drug | As above with each drug |
|   Alogliptin and metformin | Kazano | | | |
|   Linagliptin and metformin | Jentadueto | | | |
|   Saxagliptin and metformin | Kombiglyze XR | | | |
|   Pioglitazone and metformin | Actoplus MET | As above with each drug | As above with each drug | As above with each drug |
|   Pioglitazone and glimepiride | Duetact | As above with each drug | As above with each drug | As above with each drug |
|   Rosiglitazone and glimepiride | Avandaryl | As above with each drug | As above with each drug | As above with each drug |
|   Canagliflozin and metformin | Invokamet | As above with each drug | As above | As above |
|   Dapagliflozin and metformin | Xigduo | As above with each drug | As above | As above |

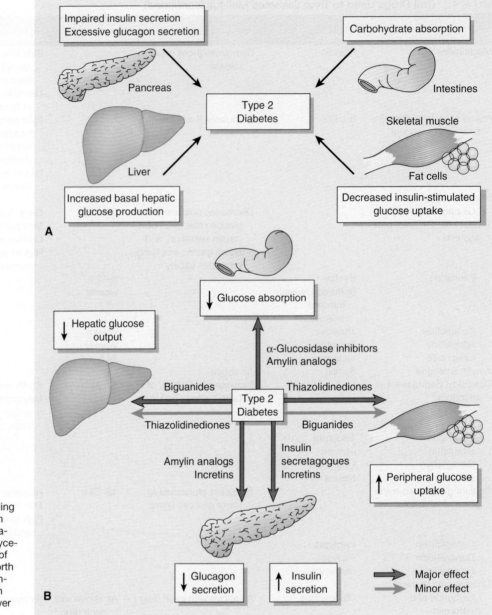

**FIGURE 44-5** **A:** Factors leading to elevated blood glucose levels in type 2 diabetes mellitus. **B:** Mechanisms of action of the oral hypoglycemic agents used in the treatment of type 2 diabetes mellitus. (From Porth CM: Porth's Pathophysiology: Concepts of Altered Health States, 8th ed. Philadelphia, PA: Wolters Kluwer Health, 2009, p 1063.)

Many people with diabetes require insulin as their disease progresses. The risk of developing type 2 diabetes increases with age, obesity, sedentary lifestyle, and family history of type 2 diabetes. Its incidence varies with ethnicity but is increasingly more common in African Americans, Hispanics, Native Americans, South Pacific Islanders, and Asian Americans. Epidemiologic and genetic studies suggest a strong genetic basis for developing type 2 diabetes; however, candidate genes that account for the majority of cases have not been identified. Type 2 diabetes is a multifactorial disorder with genetic and environmental implications.

Results from two landmark trials involving people with types 1 and 2 diabetes mellitus—the Diabetes Control and Complications Trial (DCCT)[9] and the United Kingdom Prospective Diabetes Study (UKPDS)[10]—have profoundly affected the current management of diabetes. These two trials demonstrated that very tight glycemic control is necessary to avoid the costly and life-threatening complications resulting from poorly controlled diabetes. This approach extends to the management of diabetic emergencies in the critical care arena as well; another landmark trial conducted in 2001 demonstrated significant improvement in patient outcomes when glycemic control was maintained at 80 to 110 mg/dL. The evidence that was produced by these trials significantly changed the management of diabetes among the critically ill, and instituted the practice of continuous IV insulin infusions to control the patient's glucose at all times. The critical care nurse needs to monitor the patient very closely to avoid serious complications associated with insulin infusions.

New evidence now exists that questions the need for very strict glycemic control in the hospital setting. In 2008, the Action to Control Cardiovascular Risk in Diabetes Trial,[11] aiming to lower Hb A₁C levels below 6% to study effects on cardiovascular risk, was discontinued prematurely after participants in the intensive therapy group experienced higher mortality rates. The Normoglycemia in Intensive Care Evaluation–Survival Using Glucose Algorithm Regulation (NICE-SUGAR) trial,[12] a large randomized prospective study that assessed the effects of intense glucose lowering on critically ill adults (80 to 108 mg/dL), demonstrated that study participants experienced unacceptably severe hypoglycemic episodes of less than 40 mg/dL and an associated higher risk of mortality than among the control group. The two trials' results have led to revisions in the standards of care that now sanction more moderate glycemic control in critically ill patients.

## Diabetic Ketoacidosis

### Pathophysiology

Diabetic ketoacidosis (DKA) is a critical illness that manifests with severe hyperglycemia, metabolic acidosis, and fluid and electrolyte imbalances. DKA results from severe insulin deficiency that leads to the disordered metabolism of proteins, carbohydrates, and fats. The concomitant elevation of counter-regulatory hormones such as growth hormone (GH), cortisol, epinephrine, and glucagon exacerbates the condition, leading to further hyperglycemia and hyperosmolality, ketoacidosis, and volume depletion. Figure 44-6 outlines these mechanisms and their interrelationships.

DKA continues to be an important cause of morbidity and mortality among people with diabetes. DKA is responsible for more than 100,000 hospital admissions per year in the United States. Most patients with DKA have type 1 diabetes mellitus; however, it is possible for patients with type 2 diabetes to manifest DKA during catabolic stress associated with severe critical illness. DKA is associated with less than 2% mortality rate overall, but it is a common cause of death due to cerebral edema among children and adolescents with type 1 diabetes mellitus.[13] Treatment can cost more than one of every four health care dollars spent on direct medical care for adults with type 1 diabetes mellitus, resulting in up to 2.4 billion US dollars annually.[14] Death is rarely a direct result of the metabolic acidosis or hyperglycemia; instead, death is more often related to the underlying illness that precipitated the metabolic decompensation. Therefore, successful treatment requires prompt attention to the precipitating causes of the hyperglycemic event.

Three major physiologic disturbances exist in DKA: (1) hyperosmolality from hyperglycemia, (2) metabolic acidosis from accumulation of ketoacids, and (3) volume depletion from osmotic diuresis. Each of these three disturbances may be more or less severe in any patient. Furthermore, interactions among these disturbances may occur, aggravating (or possibly partially compensating for) one another.

**HYPERGLYCEMIA AND HYPEROSMOLALITY.** The first major consequence of DKA is hyperosmolality resulting

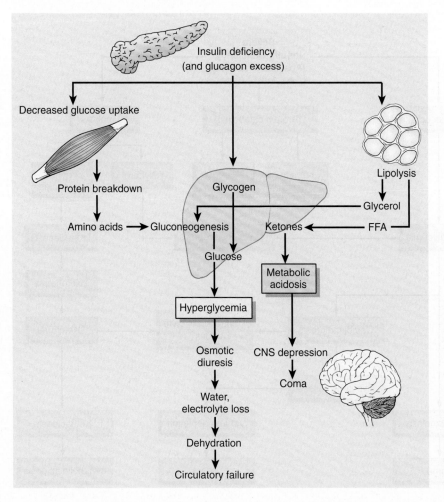

**FIGURE 44-6** Mechanisms of DKA. DKA is associated with very low insulin levels and extremely high levels of glucagon, catecholamines, and other counter-regulatory hormones. Increased levels of glucagon and catecholamines lead to mobilization of substrates for gluconeogenesis and ketogenesis by the liver. Gluconeogenesis in excess of that needed to supply glucose to the brain and other glucose-dependent tissues produces a rise in blood glucose levels. Mobilization of FfAs from triglyceride stores in adipose tissue leads to accelerated ketone production and ketosis. (From Porth CM: Porth's Pathophysiology: Concepts of Altered Health States, 8th ed. Philadelphia, PA: Wolters Kluwer Health, 2009, p 1068.)

from hyperglycemia. The hyperglycemia seen in DKA is the result of insulin deficiency, gluconeogenesis (excessive hepatic glucose production), and glycogenolysis (excessive renal glucose production), and reduced glucose utilization in peripheral tissues. With insulin deficiency, the plasma glucose level rises. As illustrated in Figure 44-7, the concomitant effects of the counter-regulatory hormones, particularly cortisol and catecholamines, further aggravate hyperglycemia by enhancing gluconeogenesis, insulin resistance, and lipolysis. This leads to hepatic fatty acid oxidation to ketone bodies (β-hydroxybutyrate and acetoacetate), ketonemia, and metabolic acidosis.

The central mechanism that protects against hyperosmolality is excretion of glucose by the kidneys. Glucose is filtered at the kidney glomerulus. With normal circulating blood volume and a normal glucose load, all this glucose is reabsorbed into the bloodstream. However, when the blood glucose level exceeds the normal threshold of about 180 mg/dL, glucose begins to escape into the urine because the reabsorption capacity of the tubules is exceeded. As the glucose load to be filtered increases, glucose is lost rapidly in the urine. Eventually, nearly all of the additional glucose put into the circulation is lost into the urine. The renal "escape valve" serves as a protective device to prevent extreme accumulation of glucose in blood. Indeed, in people with diabetes whose circulating blood volume is well maintained, it is extremely unusual to find blood glucose levels in excess

of 500 mg/dL because of the intense glucose diuresis. Conversely, any patient whose blood glucose level is higher than this level has a severely reduced circulating blood volume, renal damage, or both.

Glycosuria is largely responsible for volume depletion. Additionally, high ketone levels cause osmotic diuresis that leads to hypovolemia and decreased glomerular filtration rate. A vicious cycle occurs in a patient whose diabetes is badly out of control and who cannot take in enough sodium and water to compensate for urinary losses. Hyperglycemia leads to volume depletion, which in turn reduces urinary glucose losses and permits the blood glucose level to rise even higher.

This hyperosmolality of body fluids and dehydration probably accounts for the lethargy, stupor, and, ultimately, coma that occur as DKA worsens. Diabetic patients who have ketoacidosis without hyperosmolality are less likely to have changes in consciousness.

**KETOSIS AND ACIDOSIS.** The second major consequence of severe insulin deficiency is uncontrolled ketogenesis (see Fig. 44-7). The combination of insulin deficiency and enhanced effects of the counter-regulatory hormones causes the activation of lipase in adipose tissue. Lipase causes the breakdown of triglycerides into glycerol and free fatty acids (FfAs); massive amounts of FfAs are released as precursors of ketoacids. In the liver, they are oxidized to ketone bodies.

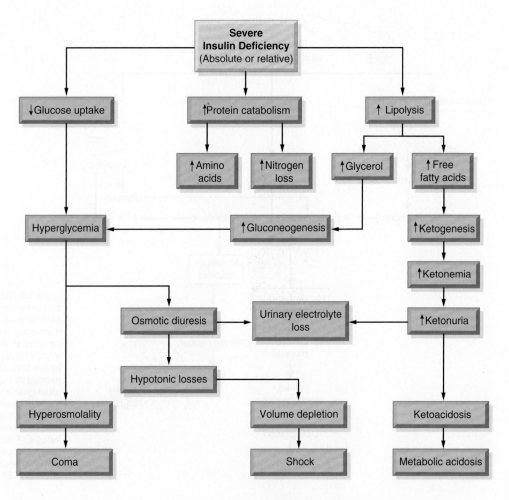

**FIGURE 44-7**  The metabolic consequences of severe insulin deficiency and the interrelations of these consequences lead to DKA.

As ketoacids enter the ECF, the hydrogen ion is stripped from the molecule and neutralized by combining with the bicarbonate ion buffer, thereby protecting the pH of the ECF and leaving behind ketoacid anion residues. The resulting carbonic acid breaks down into water and carbon dioxide gas, which is exhaled. As ketoacid anions accumulate, they progressively displace bicarbonate from the ECF. The usual laboratory determination of electrolytes does not measure ketoacid concentration directly. However, an excess of total measured cations (sodium plus potassium) over total measured anions (chloride plus bicarbonate) provides a clue to the presence of these so-called unmeasured anions. This excess, referred to as the anion gap, can serve as an indirect measure of the quantity of ketoacids present.

The following formula is used to calculate the anion gap:

$$(sodium) - (chloride + HCO_3)$$

The normal value is less than 15 mEq/L. An abnormal result indicates metabolic acidosis. For example, if sodium = 144 mEq/L, chloride = 92 mEq/L, and bicarbonate = 26 mEq/L, then the anion gap is 26 mEq/L, a value that indicates severe metabolic acidosis. As the ketoacids continue to accumulate, the serum bicarbonate falls and the anion gap increases. If this continues, the pH falls, and the acidosis becomes life-threatening.

Another cause of metabolic acidosis in DKA is the formation of lactic acidosis resulting from poor tissue perfusion and hypovolemia. This further exacerbates the anion gap, decreasing the serum bicarbonate level. Neutrality of body fluids is protected primarily by the bicarbonate buffering system, which determines the pH at all times by the ratio of bicarbonate anion to carbon dioxide in plasma. If bicarbonate anion is lost because of its displacement by ketoacid anions, excess carbon dioxide gas must be driven off at the level of the lung by hyperventilation. This process keeps the ratio at or close to its usual value of 20:1 and maintains the pH close to its physiologic value of 7.4. Hyperventilation, which is gradual at first and then rapidly becomes more vigorous and more obvious as the arterial pH drops below 7.2, is a characteristic physical finding in DKA. This dramatic increase in ventilation, which occurs more by an increase in the depth than in the frequency of breathing, is known as Kussmaul respirations. It is associated with the classic "fruity" odor of the breath in DKA. The presence of clearcut Kussmaul respirations is a signal that the ECF pH is at or below 7.2, a relatively severe degree of acidosis.

**VOLUME DEPLETION.** Ketoacids are excreted in the urine largely as sodium, potassium, and ammonium salts. This contributes to the third pathophysiologic problem of DKA: volume depletion and fluid and electrolyte loss as a result of osmotic diuresis. The fluid loss associated with DKA is approximately 6 L.

Although loss of glucose through the kidneys helps protect against the ravages of extreme hyperosmolality, the diabetic patient who develops ketoacidosis pays a price for this glycosuria. Glucose remaining in the glomerular filtrate, after the renal tubules have reabsorbed all they can, forces water to remain in the tubules. This glucose-rich filtrate then flows out of the body, carrying with it water, sodium, potassium, ammonium, phosphate, and other salts. This rapid urine flow and obligate loss of water and electrolytes is known as an osmotic diuresis. Salts of ketone bodies and the urea resulting from rapid protein breakdown and accelerated gluconeogenesis also contribute to the solute load in the renal tubule, further aggravating the diuresis. The average amounts of salts and water lost to the body through osmotic diuresis during the development of DKA have been measured. Overall water loss in a 70 kg adult patient with DKA can be 5 to 8 L, or 15% of total-body water.

The fluid lost to the body is slightly hypotonic: it contains a slight excess of water compared with the volume of salts. This is expected from an osmotic diuresis due to glucose and urea. The fluid losses result from the combination of many different factors, including the intensity and duration of the hyperglycemia and osmotic diuresis; the amount of water and electrolyte replaced orally during this time; the presence of other fluid and electrolyte losses, such as vomiting, diarrhea, or sweating; and the integrity of renal function.

Sodium and water make up the central structure of the ECF, including the vascular volume. When large quantities of sodium and water are lost in the urine, the body perceives it as a serious threat to the maintenance of the circulation. A variety of compensatory mechanisms are called into play to prevent vascular collapse and shock. For example, an increase in pulse rate usually occurs, which helps maintain cardiac output in the face of shrinking intravascular volume.

At least as important, however, is a protective shift in body fluid brought about by the hyperglycemia. Because free glucose is limited almost entirely to the extracellular water, an osmotic pressure gradient is set up across the cell membrane, between the extracellular compartment and the interior of the cells. Therefore, the higher the blood glucose, the more water is drawn out of cells and into the extracellular space. As sodium and water are lost into the urine, shrinking the ECF, they are "replaced" (at least as to their osmotic effect) by glucose entering from the liver and by water entering from all cells; this re-expands the ECF.

Although hyperosmolality produces damaging CNS effects and osmotic diuresis, it provides a temporary mechanism for preventing vascular collapse. Despite these compensatory mechanisms, circulatory volume falls as DKA progresses. This leads to decreased glomerular filtration, decreased tissue perfusion, metabolic acidosis, and shock.

As the vascular volume falls, glomerular filtration also falls. This decreasing renal function leads to increasing blood levels of glucose, potassium, urea nitrogen, and creatinine. The excretion of potassium by the kidney occurs through the exchange of potassium for sodium. Therefore, adequate sodium must be present at the exchange site in the kidney for the rate of potassium excretion to keep pace with the need for excretion. If renal perfusion falls, enough sodium may not be available for this exchange. As a result, despite a total-body depletion of potassium, the serum potassium level may rise above normal, even to dangerously high levels.

A second major consequence of diminished vascular volume is a generalized decrease in tissue perfusion. Well before the drop in volume has reached the point at which blood pressure actually falls and frank shock occurs, blood is shunted away from many tissues, and the perfusion of nearly all tissues suffers. The resulting decrease in oxygen causes those tissues to shift to some degree of anaerobic glucose metabolism. This results in the increased production of lactic acid. The release of lactic acid into the circulation lowers the bicarbonate further, aggravating the already existing metabolic acidosis. Therefore, in patients with DKA, combined lactic acidosis and ketoacidosis is a common finding.

The loss of phosphate in the urine worsens tissue hypoxia. As body phosphate stores are depleted, circulating plasma phosphate levels fall quite low, depriving the red blood cells of organic phosphate compounds. Under these circumstances, the red blood cells become depleted of certain key phosphate derivatives, increasing the tightness of oxygen binding to the hemoglobin in these cells. Therefore, less oxygen is given up, and tissue hypoxia worsens.

Finally, if vascular volume falls low enough, compensation mechanisms fail, blood pressure drops, and true shock supervenes, changing the situation. A rapidly worsening cycle of acidosis, tissue damage, and deepening shock may then occur, leading ultimately to irreversible vascular collapse and death. The complete syndrome of DKA is characterized by major contributions from all three major pathophysiologic disruptions, each of which is primarily responsible for one of the major clinical features: coma, shock, and metabolic acidosis. There is evidence to suggest that hyperglycemia crisis is associated with severe inflammatory state due to the elevation of proinflammatory cytokines, C-reactive protein, reactive oxygen species, and lipid peroxidation as well as plasminogen activator inhibitor-1. This partially explains the hypercoagulable state associated with hyperglycemic crisis.[15]

## Causes

The most common cause of DKA is infection, occurring in 30% to 50% of cases. Urinary tract infection (UTI) and pneumonia account for the majority of infections.[8] Other precipitating factors include inadequate insulin therapy, insulin noncompliance, severe illness (cerebrovascular accident [CVA], myocardial infarction, pancreatitis), alcohol or drug abuse, trauma, and certain medications (eg, antipsychotics, steroids). In addition, many people with type 1 diabetes present with DKA on initial diagnosis. Also, many patients with type 1 diabetes suddenly discontinue their insulin and deteriorate; reasons for insulin omission in younger patients include fear of weight gain, fear of hypoglycemia, rebellion against authority, and the stress of chronic disease. In one study of 341 females with type 1 diabetes, psychological problems complicated by disorders were a contributing factor in 20% of cases.[13] Other reasons given for sudden discontinuation of insulin or oral medications include lack of knowledge and poor compliance related to lack of financial resources. Noncompliance with therapy has been implicated as a major precipitating cause of DKA in urban African American and medically indigent patients.[8]

## Assessment

Initial laboratory analysis should include an immediate glucose level using a venous sample and glucose meter measurement at the bedside to confirm the diagnosis. While these preliminary data are collected, the nurse inserts an IV line and starts volume replacement. A more considered assessment follows, which begins with details of the history and physical examination, a search for precipitating causes, and more complete laboratory tests. Physical examination and laboratory findings in DKA are summarized in Box 44-8.

---

**BOX 44-8** Signs of Diabetic Ketoacidosis (DKA)

- Hyperventilation
- Kussmaul's respirations and "fruity" breath
- Lethargy, stupor, coma
- Hyperglycemia
- Glycosuria
- Volume depletion
- Hyperosmolality
- Increased anion gap (>7 mEq/L)
- Decreased bicarbonate (<10 mEq/L)
- Decreased pH (<7.4)

---

**HISTORY AND PHYSICAL EXAMINATION.** If ketoacidosis is strongly suspected, an effort is made to establish the diagnosis quickly so that life-preserving therapy can be started. Initial data collection includes an abbreviated history from the family or friends of an unconscious patient, a search for a diabetic identification card, and rapid assessment for clinical clues of volume depletion. After asking about the diabetic regimen, medications, and recent changes in health, the clinician should perform a review of systems. Questions concern appetite, weight change, food and fluid intake, thirst, abdominal bloating and discomfort, bowel function, and urinary frequency and amount. During the interview, the clinician should observe the patient's cognition and responsiveness.

DKA develops rapidly, and patients may display polydipsia, polyuria, and weight loss several days before ketoacidosis is established. Frequently, abdominal pain and vomiting are presenting symptoms. Approximately 40% to 75% of patients experience abdominal pain that mimics an acute abdomen; the severity of abdominal pain often correlates with more severe metabolic acidosis. Other possible findings include thirst, frequent urination, poor appetite, nausea and vomiting, fatigue, weakness, and drowsiness. The patient may also have symptoms related to UTI, upper respiratory infection, and chest symptoms, because infection is often a precipitating factor.

The physical examination includes blood pressure, heart and respiratory rate, breathing pattern, heart sounds and rhythm, breath sounds, capillary refill, skin color and warmth of extremities, temperature, signs of hydration (eg, skin turgor, mucus pool under tongue), deep tendon reflexes, LOC, and an abdominal examination. Possible findings include hyperventilation, Kussmaul respirations and fruity breath, dehydration, abdominal distention, dry mucous membranes, flushed skin, poor skin turgor and perfusion, hypotension, tachycardia, and varying degrees of responsiveness from lethargy to coma. Even though infection is often concurrent, the patient may be normothermic due to vasodilation. Severe hyperthermia is a poor prognostic sign.

**LABORATORY STUDIES.** Laboratory studies include blood glucose, chemistries, CBC with differential, osmolality, anion gap, pH, ABGs, urine acetone, and glucose. Possible findings include hyperosmolality, increased anion gap (greater than 7 mEq/L), decreased bicarbonate (less than 10 mEq/L), and decreased pH (less than 7.4). The serum glucose may range from 250 to 800 mg/dL or higher. Sodium, potassium, creatinine, and BUN levels are all elevated. Magnesium and phosphate may also be high. Patients with DKA often present with leukocytosis and the presence of greater than 10% neutrophil bands. The key diagnostic feature of DKA is the presence of serum ketones per the nitroprusside test or by direct measurement of β-hydroxybutyrate.[8,15]

**DIAGNOSTIC STUDIES.** Tissue cultures of the throat, urine, or blood may also be performed to determine the presence of infection, especially if bandemia is present. A chest radiograph should be obtained to rule out acute infection, and an ECG should be obtained.

### Management

The severity of DKA can be categorized as mild, moderate, or severe depending on the level of metabolic acidosis and altered mental state. Treatment goals for the patient with DKA include the following:

- Improve circulatory volume and tissue perfusion
- Correct electrolyte imbalances
- Decrease serum glucose concentration
- Correct ketoacidosis
- Determine precipitating events.

Treatment protocols for the adult with DKA are given in Figure 44-8, and a Collaborative Care Guide is given in Box 44-9.

**FLUID REPLACEMENT.** The immediate threat to life in a critically ill ketoacidotic patient is volume depletion. After establishing an IV line, the nurse rapidly infuses 0.9% (normal) saline solution. The goal is to reverse the severity of the extracellular volume depletion and restore renal perfusion as soon as possible. The first liter may be infused in 1 hour in patients with normal cardiac function; on average, the rate will be equal to 15 to 20 mL/kg body weight per hour. This replaces only a fraction of the extracellular loss in the average patient, which can range from 6 to 10 L.

Fluid replacement continues at roughly 1 L/hour until the heart rate, blood pressure, and urine flow indicate that hemodynamic stability is attained. Hypotonic solutions, such as 0.45% (half normal) saline solution, can be administered at a rate of 150 to 250 mL/hour after the intravascular volume has been restored, or if the serum sodium level is greater than 155 mg/dL. Other plasma expanders, such as albumin and plasma concentrates, may be necessary if low blood pressure and other clinical signs of vascular collapse do not respond to saline solution alone.

Rapid infusion of saline solution in DKA has possible complications. It can dilute plasma proteins and lower the osmotic pressure of the plasma. This allows fluid to leak out of the vascular space through the capillary walls and contributes to the development of pulmonary edema or cerebral edema, particularly in children and older adults. Therefore, patients must be observed carefully during the first 24 to 36 hours for signs of pulmonary or cerebral edema.

Volume losses continue throughout the first hours of treatment until the glycosuria and osmotic diuresis are controlled. The next step of fluid replacement can be based on an estimate of the patient's total-body fluid loss. About 80% of the fall in blood glucose level during treatment of DKA is due to glucose loss into the urine, rather than the result of insulin-induced changes in glucose production and

consumption. Therefore, in the earliest phases of treatment, insulin therapy complements fluid and electrolyte replacement. Lowering of glucose levels will occur more rapidly (as long as 6 hours) than correction of ketoacidosis (as long as 12 hours).

**INSULIN THERAPY.** Insulin therapy is the cornerstone of managing ketoacidosis for several reasons. It decreases the production of ketones by shutting off the supply of FFAs emerging from adipose tissue. It inhibits hepatic gluconeogenesis, thereby preventing further glucose from being added to the ECF. Simultaneously, hepatic ketogenesis is further reduced. Insulin also restores cellular protein synthesis. This effect occurs more slowly and permits the restoration of normal potassium, magnesium, and phosphate stores in tissues. Insulin also increases peripheral glucose utilization.

Careful glycemic control is the goal for managing patients with diabetes in the acute care setting. However, the blood glucose level should not fall too fast or too far. Sudden and rapid lowering of the blood glucose with insulin allows water to move very rapidly back into the cells and this can potentially lead to vascular collapse. Instead, early volume replacement should include sodium and water either before or along with insulin therapy.

It is necessary to give low-dose regular insulin by continuous IV infusion rather than by IV bolus or subcutaneous doses for more severe DKA or HHS cases. Subcutaneous insulin injections given every 1 to 2 hours are an alternative to IV insulin for mild or moderate DKA, and usually rapid-acting analog insulin (lispro, aspart, or glulisine) is used.[12] Box 44-10 summarizes guidelines for insulin administration.

Initially, insulin administration involves giving an IV bolus of regular insulin at 0.15 units/kg body weight followed by a continuous infusion of regular insulin at a dose of 0.1 units/kg/hour (5 to 10 units/hour). This produces a steady decline in glucose concentrations at a rate of 65 to 125 mg/hour. An hourly insulin infusion of 0.14 units/kg/hour without initial bolus is sufficient to lower glucose and suppress hepatic ketone body production.

When the plasma glucose reaches 200 to 250 mg/dL, it is necessary to decrease the insulin infusion to 0.5 units/kg/hour and add dextrose (5% or 10%) to the IV fluids. To prevent cerebral edema that may occur when the blood–brain barrier is affected by extreme fluid shifts, avoidance of hypoglycemia is warranted at this point. It is vital to start subcutaneous basal insulin 1 to 2 hours *before* IV insulin is stopped.[8,15] See Table 44-5 on page 885 for commonly used insulins.

**POTASSIUM AND PHOSPHATE REPLACEMENT.** The initial plasma potassium in patients with DKA can range from very low to very high; therefore, potassium is not given until the laboratory report is available. Beginning IV potassium therapy in the presence of unrecognized hyperkalemia and inadequate renal mechanisms for handling potassium loads can be fatal. Although the ECG can provide clues to the presence of high or low potassium levels, potassium therapy should not be based on the ECG alone.

If the initial serum potassium level is low, IV potassium is usually started right away. This is particularly important because both insulin and saline solutions drive the potassium even lower, possibly to dangerously low levels at which skeletal muscle paralysis and cardiac arrest may occur. If the initial

Complete initial evaluation. Check capillary glucose and serum/urine ketones to confirm hyperglycemia and ketonemia/ketonuria. Obtain blood for metabolic profile. Start IV fluids: 1.0 L of 0.9% NaCl per hour.[†]

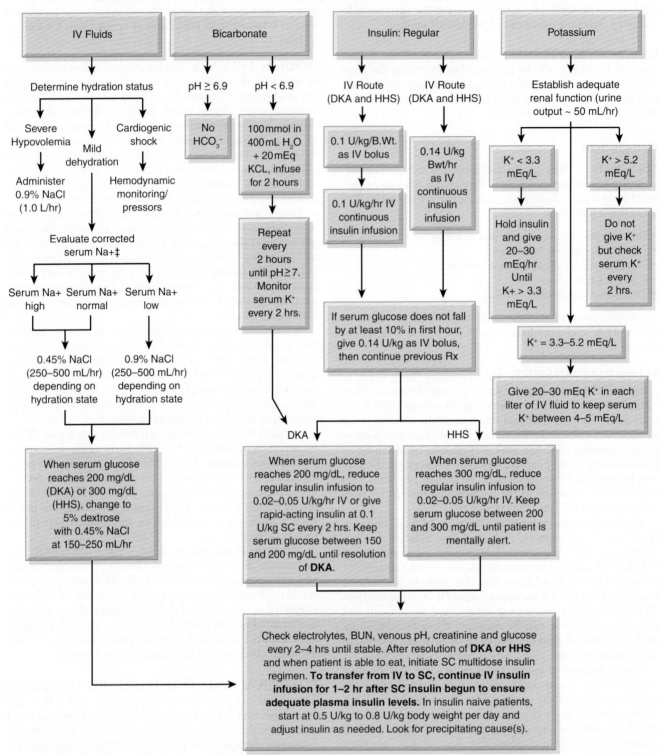

**FIGURE 44-8** Protocol for management of adult patients with DKA or HHS. DKA diagnostic criteria: blood glucose 250 mg/dL, arterial pH 7.3, bicarbonate 15 mEq/L, and moderate ketonuria or ketonemia. HHS criteria: serum glucose greater than 600 mg/dL, arterial pH greater than 7.3, serum bicarbonate greater than 15 mEq/L, and minimal ketonuria and ketonemia.

[†]15 to 20 mL/kg/h; [‡]serum Na should be corrected for hyperglycemia (for each 100 mg/dL glucose, add 1.6 mEq to sodium value for corrected serum value). Bwt, body weight; SC, subcutaneous. (From Kitabchi AE, Umpierrez GE, Miles JM, et al: Hyperglycemic crises in adult patients with diabetes. Diabetes Care 32[7]:1335–1343, 2009.)

**QSEN BOX 44-9** *COLLABORATIVE CARE GUIDE for the Patient With DKA*

| Outcomes | Interventions |
|---|---|
| **Impaired gas exchange**<br>**Ineffective breathing pattern** | |
| Arterial blood gases are maintained within normal limits<br><br>No evidence of acute respiratory failure | • Provide chest physiotherapy, turn, deep breath, cough, incentive spirometer every 4 h and PRN<br>• Continuously monitor patient's respiratory rate, depth, and pattern. Observe for Kussmaul's respiration, rapid and shallow breathing, and other signs of respiratory distress<br>• Monitor arterial blood gases, pulse oximetry, and, if intubated, end-tidal $CO_2$<br>• Provide supplemental oxygen<br>• Prepare for intubation and mechanical ventilation (see Box 25-16) |
| The patient's lungs are clear<br>There is no evidence of atelectasis or pneumonia | • Auscultate breath sounds every 2 h and PRN<br>• Take daily chest x-ray<br>• Provide chest physiotherapy every 4 h<br>• Mobilize out of bed as soon as patient is stabilized |
| **Decreased cardiac perfusion** | |
| Blood pressure and heart rate are within normal limits<br>If pulmonary artery catheter is in place, hemodynamic parameters are within normal limits | • Monitor vital signs hourly and PRN<br>• Assess for dehydration/hypovolemia: tachycardia, decreased CVP and PAOP<br>• Assess for hypervolemia: neck vein distention, pulmonary crackles and edema, increased CVP and PAOP<br>• Administer vasopressor agents if hypotension is related to vasodilation |
| Patient is free of dysrhythmias | • Monitor ECG continuously<br>• Evaluate and treat the cause of dysrhythmias (eg, acidosis, hypoxia, hypokalemia/hyperkalemia) |
| **Ineffective renal perfusion**<br>**Decreased fluid volume**<br>**Risk for electrolyte imbalance**<br>**Risk for unstable glucose level** | |
| Evidence of rehydration without complications:<br>• balanced intake and output<br>• normal skin turgor<br>• hemodynamic stability<br>• intact sensorium | • Infuse normal saline or lactated Ringer's solution, then 0.45% normal saline solution<br>• Monitor serum osmolality, urine output, neurologic status, and vital signs closely during rehydration. Observe for complications of DKA (eg, shock, renal failure, decreased LOC, and seizures)<br>• Assess BUN, creatinine, and urine for glucose and ketones |
| Normal serum electrolytes and acid–base balance | • Assess and replace electrolytes, Mg, and $PO_4$, as indicated<br>• Closely monitor potassium fluctuations as serum glucose is decreased and acidosis reversed<br>• Assess arterial pH and bicarbonate level every 2–4 h during rehydration and insulin administration |
| Serum glucose returns to normal range | • Monitor serum glucose every 30–60 min, then every 1–4 h after level is <300 mg/dL<br>• Administer IV insulin bolus then continuous low-dose infusion<br>• Infuse D5 half normal saline solution or D5W, after glucose level is <300 mg/dL |
| **Impaired physical mobility**<br>**Risk for injury**<br>**Risk for falls** | |
| The patient will be free of injury related to altered sensorium or seizures | • Place on seizure and falls precautions<br>• Assess neurologic status hourly, then every 2–4 h after initial rehydration phase |
| Maintain muscle tone and joint range of motion | • Provide range-of-motion exercises every 4 h<br>• Reposition in bed every 2 h<br>• Mobilize to chair when condition stable<br>• Consult physical therapist |
| **Impaired skin integrity** | |
| Skin will remain intact | • Assess risk for skin breakdown using the Braden Scale (see Fig. 51-7, p. 1164)<br>• Initially assess skin and circulation every 1–2 h for 12 h<br>• If risk for skin breakdown is low, assess skin every 8 h and each time patient is repositioned<br>• Turn patient every 2 h<br>• Consider pressure relief/reduction mattress if at risk for skin breakdown |

*(continued)*

**QSEN BOX 44-9** **COLLABORATIVE CARE GUIDE** for the Patient With DKA (continued)

| Outcomes | Interventions |
| --- | --- |
| **Imbalanced nutrition** **Electrolyte imbalance** | |
| Calorie and nutrient intake meet metabolic requirements per calculation (eg, basal energy expenditure) | • Provide parenteral feeding if patient is fasting (NPO)<br>• Provide clear, then full liquid diet, and assess patient response<br>• Progress to diabetic diet (ADA)<br>• Consult dietitian or nutritional support service regarding special nutritional needs |
| No evidence of metabolic dysfunction | • Monitor albumin, prealbumin, transferrin, cholesterol, triglycerides, glucose, and protein levels |
| **Impaired comfort** | |
| Patient will have minimal pain, <5 on pain scale | • Assess pain and discomfort. If pain present, use objective pain scale every 4 h PRN and following administration of pain medication<br>• If analgesics are needed, administer cautiously due to risk of respiratory and neurologic complications<br>• Consider nonpharmacologic pain management techniques (eg, distraction, touch) |
| The patient's nausea, vomiting, and abdominal pain or tenderness will resolve | • Maintain nasogastric tube patency<br>• Assess bowel sounds every 1–2 h<br>• Administer antiemetic as ordered<br>• Provide ice chips and frequent oral hygiene |
| **Ineffective coping** | |
| Patient demonstrates decreased anxiety | • Provide nonjudgmental atmosphere in which patient can discuss concerns and fears<br>• Provide patients who are intubated with a method to communicate<br>• Provide patients with decreased LOC with sensory input<br>• Provide for adequate rest and sleep |
| **Teaching/Discharge Planning** | |
| Patient/significant others understand the tests needed for treatment<br>Significant others understand the severity of the illness, ask appropriate questions, and anticipate potential complications | • Prepare patient/significant others for procedures such as electroencephalography, ECG, and multiple laboratory studies<br>• Explain the widespread effects of diabetes and the potential for complications of DKA such as seizures, renal failure, or vascular collapse<br>• Encourage significant others to ask questions related to complications, pathophysiology, monitoring, treatments, and so on |
| Patient/significant others are prepared for home care | • Teach patient and family information needed to manage diabetes: diabetic diet, skin care, glucose monitoring, insulin administration, signs and symptoms of hypoglycemia and hyperglycemia, and appropriate actions<br>• Discuss sick-day management and factors that can precipitate DKA<br>• Initiate contacts with diabetic support groups, social services, and home health agency |

**BOX 44-10** **Nursing Interventions**

**For Insulin Administration**
- Administer insulin IV to the patient with DKA to minimize the trauma of repeated injections
- Administer the insulin infusion through an IV infusion pump. Flush tubing well with insulin mixture before infusing to patient to prevent tubing from absorbing too much insulin.
- When the serum glucose level reaches 200 to 250 mg/dL, the IV fluids should be changed to a glucose-based solution
- Changes in blood glucose level and clinical state should indicate a clear-cut beneficial response to insulin and fluid replacement. If blood glucose level does not drop and blood pressure and urine output do not stabilize, insulin or fluid replacement may not be adequate.

potassium is normal or high, IV potassium is usually withheld until the level has begun to drop and urine flow is established. Potassium is usually replaced at concentrations of 20 to 40 mEq/L of IV fluid, depending on the serum potassium level. Failure of the potassium level to fall can occur for the following reasons:

- Persistent, uncorrected acidosis (which drives potassium out of cells and into ECF)
- Hyperosmolality
- Intrinsically impaired renal function
- Insufficient circulating volume.

Phosphate levels usually also drop during therapy, aggravating any preexisting tendency of red blood cells to bind oxygen more tightly. Therefore, many patients receive phosphate in the middle and later phases of therapy. It is usually combined with potassium replacement in the form of potassium phosphate salts added to the IV infusion. Patients who are receiving IV phosphate therapy should be watched carefully for signs of tetany: tingling around the mouth or in the hands, neuromuscular irritability, carpopedal spasm, or even seizures. Tetany can occur because phosphate lowers the level of circulating calcium.

**TABLE 44-5** Types of Insulin

| Preparation | Brand | Onset (h) | Peak (h) | Duration (h) | Nursing Points |
|---|---|---|---|---|---|
| **Very Rapid Acting** | | | | | |
| Insulin analog | Humalog (Lispro) NovoLog (Aspart) Glulisine (Apidra) | <0.25 | 0.5–1.5 | 3–5 | Must take with food (shorter acting than regular) |
| **Short Acting** | | | | | |
| Regular (R) | Humulin R Novolin R Velosulin BR Afrezza | 0.5–1 | 2–3 | 5–8 | Only form available for IV continuous infusion Powder, given by hand-held inhaler device |
| **Intermediate Acting** | | | | | |
| NPH | Humulin N | 1–4 | 4–12 | 10–16 | Should look uniformly cloudy |
| Insulin Regular (R) | Novolin N | 0.5–1.0 | 1.7–4 | 6–8 | |
| Regular | Humulin R U-500 | 0.5 | 1.75–4 | 24 | Five times the concentration of insulin; for patients on high doses of insulin |
| **Long Acting** | | | | | |
| Insulin glargine | Lantus | 1–2 | None | 24 | Cannot be mixed with any other insulin |
| Insulin glargine 300 | Toujeo | 6 | None | 24 + | |
| Insulin detemir | Levemir | 0.8–2 | 3–9 | Up to 24 | |
| **Combination** | | | | | |
| NPH and R (70/30) | 70/30 (70% NPH, 30% regular) 50/50 (50% NPH, 50% regular) | 0.5–3 | Dual | 12–14 | Mixture of long- and short-acting insulins |
| Humalog Mix (75/25) | 75% insulin lispro protamine 25% insulin lispro (Humalog mix 75/25) | 0.1–0.25 | Dual | 10–16 h | |
| Humalog Mix (50/50) | 50% insulin lispro protamine 50% insulin lispro | 0.1–0.25 | Dual | 10–16 h | |
| NovoLog Mix (70/30) | 70% insulin aspart protamine 30% insulin aspart | 0.1–0.25 | Dual | 10–16 | |

**BICARBONATE REPLACEMENT.** Patients with mild or moderate ketoacidosis who are treated with salt, water, and insulin eventually excrete and metabolize the ketone bodies remaining in ECF. As this process continues, more bicarbonate anions are reabsorbed from the renal tubules, and the bicarbonate deficit is slowly repaired. Sometimes the large amounts of chloride administered along with the sodium in IV saline solution can produce a transient hyperchloremia; this delays the full return of the bicarbonate level to normal for several days.

Bicarbonate replacement in patients with DKA remains controversial because evidence-based research has failed to demonstrate benefit in patients with an arterial pH between 6.9 and 7.1.[8] However, the American Diabetes Association recommends bicarbonate replacement with severe acidosis as indicated by an arterial pH of 6.9 or less. It is also necessary to give bicarbonate when there is cardiac decompensation. The bicarbonate deficit can be calculated and replaced IV over several hours to raise the level at least to the 10 to 12 mEq/L range. Sodium bicarbonate should be administered by slow IV infusion over several hours. It is administered as a bolus injection only in the case of cardiac arrest. Sodium bicarbonate administration can cause a rapid reduction in plasma potassium concentration and sodium overload.

**REESTABLISHING METABOLIC FUNCTION.** Gastric motility is greatly impaired in DKA. Gastric distention with dark, hemopositive fluid and vomiting is common. Abdominal pain, tenderness, and a paralytic ileus may also be due to DKA. The patient may need a nasogastric tube to decompress the stomach; this increases comfort and decreases the risk for aspiration. Patients should not eat or drink in this phase of illness. Ice chips may decrease thirst. Later, when distention lessens and motility returns, oral intake begins in order to provide the complex nutritional requirements for recovery.

Metabolic abnormalities should not be corrected too rapidly, especially in patients in whom DKA has been developing for a long time. The key risks during this phase are worsening stupor or coma, hypotension, and hyperkalemia. Osmotic or pH disequilibrium may occur when blood glucose or bicarbonate has been corrected too rapidly. The patient's mental state may worsen even though the blood chemistries are improving. Rapid reduction of blood glucose without sufficient sodium and water replacement may be responsible for hypotension; however, sepsis, myocardial infarction, and other causes of shock may also cause hypotension. Hyperkalemia usually results from premature potassium infusion, persistent acidosis, and insufficient volume replacement;

---

**BOX 44-11** | *TEACHING GUIDE*   *Self-Management After Ketoacidosis*

- A person with diabetes, as any other person, must have insulin, even if no food is being taken in.
- The amount of insulin required when the person with diabetes is not eating is about half the total needed when eating.
- The amount of insulin required when a person with diabetes is fasting must be spread out as an insulin "trickle" rather than as an insulin "burst."
- Illness generally increases the need for insulin so that even if the person with diabetes is not eating, he or she may actually require more than 50% of the usual daily dose.
- Always keep enough insulin on hand for daily injections.
- Know how to reach a health care provider for timely phone advice.
- When you are ill, adjustments for managing your diabetes may need to be made.

---

however, there may be an early occlusion of the arterial supply to a limb that can cause large amounts of potassium to leak into the circulation. Therefore, limbs are monitored for asymmetrical pallor, coolness, and rubor.

Although patients begin to improve during the initial phase of treatment, recovery may take place over several days. Reversal of most metabolic abnormalities and replenishment of body stores of many nutrients (eg, magnesium, protein, and phosphate) occur during this time. Once recovery is well underway, it is time to help the patient and family understand how to prevent a recurrence.

### Patient Education

Many cases of DKA are preventable with good education. Patients and families who are well informed about diabetes may be more likely to recognize early signs of complications, minimize their development, and seek help if they begin to occur. Although people usually understand the need for insulin injections when they are hungry and eating normally, they may not understand why they need their insulin when they are ill, have no appetite, are not eating, or are vomiting. Box 44-11 outlines appropriate teaching points after an episode of DKA.

## Hyperosmolar Hyperglycemic State

Sometimes a marked hyperglycemia and hyperosmolality without ketoacidosis develop in patients with diabetes; this is characteristic of HHS. Usually, patients with HHS are middle-aged or older (55 to 70 years), have undiagnosed type 2 diabetes, and are frequently residents of nursing homes. HHS is the initial manifestation in 7% to 17% of patients.[15]

HHS has a higher mortality rate than any other complication of diabetes, reflecting the higher morbidity associated with patients affected by this type of diabetic emergency. Often, these elderly, obese patients suffer from other severe medical conditions, such as congestive heart failure or kidney disease. Extremely high levels of glucose, coupled with severe dehydration in a vulnerable, elderly patient with other medical illnesses, explain the higher mortality rate associated with this diabetic complication. HHS is compared with DKA in Table 44-6.

### Pathophysiology

It is not known specifically why some people with diabetes develop HHS rather than DKA, although it is speculated that these patients may have just enough insulin to prevent ketosis. Pathophysiologically, the mechanisms of disease are the same as for DKA. A reduction in circulating insulin, coupled with the effects of counter-regulatory hormones such as cortisol and epinephrine, leads to the development of hyperglycemia and the extreme hyperosmolar state. Usually, the patient has coexisting impaired renal excretion of glucose and antecedent renal insufficiency or prerenal azotemia. Because basal insulin levels are unaffected, excessive ketone production does not occur. The acidosis that these patients develop is attributed to lactic acidosis from poor tissue perfusion instead of ketoacidosis.

HHS develops slowly over days to weeks, and patients often experience polydipsia, polyuria, and progressive decline in LOC. Marked dehydration occurs if the patient is unable to maintain an adequate fluid intake. The typical fluid loss associated with HHS is 9 L. As dehydration worsens,

---

**TABLE 44-6**   Comparing Signs and Symptoms of Diabetic Ketoacidosis (DKA) and Hyperglycemic Hyperosmolar State (HHS)

| Characteristics | DKA | HHS |
|---|---|---|
| Onset | Gradual or sudden, usually <2 d | Gradual, usually >5 d |
| Previous history of diabetes mellitus | 85% (15% have new onset) | 60% |
| Type of diabetes mellitus | Type 1, rarely Type 2 | Type 2 |
| Age of patient | Usually younger than 40 y | Usually older than 60 y |
| Mortality risk | 1%–15% | 20%–40% |
| Drug history | Insulin | Steroids, thiazides, oral agents |
| Physical signs | Polydipsia, polyuria, dehydration, Kussmaul's respirations, mental status changes, "fruity breath," febrile at times, ketoacidosis, nausea and vomiting | Dehydration; obtundation; hypothermia; toxic appearance; Kussmaul's respirations absent; nonketotic |
| Glucose level | Mean, 600 mg/dL   Range, 250–1,200 mg/dL | Mean, 1,100 mg/dL   Range, 400–4,000 mg/dL |
| Ketones | Present | Absent |
| Osmolarity | Mean, 320 mOsm/L | Mean, 400 mOsm/L |
| Arterial pH | Mean, 7.07 | Mean, 7.26 |
| Bicarbonate | Markedly low (<10 mEq/L) | Normal or >15 mEq/L |
| Anion gap | >12 mEq/L | <12 mEq/L, variable |

Adapted from Kitabchi AE, Umpierrez GE, Miles JM, et al: Hyperglycemic crises in adult patients with diabetes. Diabetes Care 32(7):1335–1343, 2009.

the patient develops increasing serum glucose concentrations and serum osmolality. The life-threatening cycle of hyperglycemia, hyperosmolality, osmotic diuresis, and profound dehydration triggers the sympathetic nervous system fight-or-flight response. The counter-regulatory hormones epinephrine and cortisol stimulate gluconeogenesis and increase hepatic glucose production. Dehydration worsens and leads to CNS dysfunction. Confusion and lethargy ensue quickly. Hemoconcentration of the blood increases the risk for clot formation, thromboemboli, and infarctions in major organs.

### Causes

Infection is a major cause of HHS, occurring in 30% to 60% of patients. UTIs and pneumonia are the most common associated infections. In some cases, acute illness such as CVA, myocardial infarction, or pancreatitis provokes the release of counter-regulatory hormones, resulting in hyperglycemia. HHS may also occur secondary to extreme stress associated with severe medical illness, such as stroke, myocardial infarction, pancreatitis, trauma, sepsis, burns, or pneumonia. Often, HHS results from excessive exposure or carbohydrate intake, such as dietary supplements, total enteral support with tube feedings, or peritoneal dialysis. Elderly people are at particularly high risk, especially those who have impaired cognition and who are in long-term chronic care facilities. Drugs such as corticosteroids, thiazide diuretics, sedatives, and sympathomimetics affect carbohydrate metabolism adversely and may lead to glucose impairment.

### Assessment

**HISTORY AND PHYSICAL EXAMINATION.** The nurse assesses the patient for precipitating or associated events. This syndrome can be iatrogenic (eg, induced by certain medications such as steroids, hemodialysis against hyperosmolar glucose solutions, or prolonged IV hypertonic glucose infusions such as those given for total parenteral nutrition). It can also be precipitated by serious medical illnesses such as pneumonia or pancreatitis.

Often family members or long-term-care personnel report that the patient has become a bit drowsy, taken in less food and fluid over several days, and slept more until he or she became difficult to awaken. The patient often arrives at the hospital with serious volume depletion and in a stupor or coma. The signs and symptoms of HHS are given in Table 44-6. The clinical manifestations may take days to weeks to develop, and the patient often displays weakness, polyuria, polydipsia, and impaired mental state ranging from confusion to coma. Dehydration is manifested by tachycardia, hypotension, low cardiac output, poor skin turgor, rapid respirations without Kussmaul breathing, and warm, flushed skin. The presence of hypothermia is a poor prognostic sign in HHS.

**LABORATORY STUDIES.** Laboratory values for HHS are similar for those with DKA with four main exceptions:

1. The hyperglycemia in HHS is, by definition, a blood glucose level greater than 600 mg/dL; this is a significantly higher level than in DKA. Glucose can be in excess of 2,000 mg/dL.

2. Plasma osmolality is higher than in DKA and is reflective of more severe dehydration. In addition to extracellular sodium and water losses, a large additional "free water" deficit exists, probably because patients do not become thirsty, causing them to take in decreasing amounts of fluid. As a result, patients have very high serum levels of sodium and glucose. Serum osmolality is extremely high (greater than 310 to 320 mOsm/kg).

3. Patients may have some degree of ketosis as well but are usually nonketotic. In DKA, the degree of ketosis is much more severe.

4. In HHS, acidosis is not present or is very mild. In HHS, the anion gap attributable to ketoacids is usually less than 7 mEq/L. The patient may present with azotemia, hyperkalemia, and lactic acidosis.

### Management

Therapy for HHS is directed at correcting the volume depletion, controlling hyperglycemia, and identifying and treating the underlying cause. The volume depletion is usually greater in HHS than in DKA. Rapid rehydration is more cautiously carried out because of the fragile state of the patient, who often has comorbidities. Isotonic saline or hypotonic saline solution is administered initially to correct the fluid imbalance; some patients may require as much as 9 to 12 L of fluid overall. The nurse should be vigilant for the signs of fluid overload during rehydration.

Critically ill patients require hemodynamic monitoring during fluid resuscitation, especially elderly patients with cardiac or renal disease. Careful monitoring of fluid intake, urine output, blood pressure, hemodynamic pressures, pulse, breath sounds, and neurologic status is one of the nurse's primary responsibilities. In addition, the patient requires frequent monitoring of laboratory test findings.

Patients receive low doses of insulin along with the fluid replacement. It is necessary to give low-dose insulin by continuous infusion (0.1 mg/kg/hour) because these patients are vulnerable to the sudden loss of circulating blood volume that occurs with higher doses of insulin and a rapid blood glucose reduction. As the glucose level returns close to normal (250 to 300 mg/dL), it is appropriate to stop the insulin infusion and add dextrose to the IV fluids to prevent a sudden drop in the blood glucose level. At this point, subcutaneous administration of insulin can proceed.

Investigation of the underlying cause of HHS is warranted, and treatment, if possible, is necessary. For example, management of underlying infection from pneumonia involves aggressive use of antibiotics, chest physiotherapy, turning, and coughing and deep breathing or suctioning as needed to clear the infiltrate. Removal of exogenous sources of glucose (tube feedings, peritoneal dialysis, medications) is appropriate while treating the hyperglycemic state.

Older patients who develop HHS have frequent complications and high mortality rates. They often have difficulty handling the fluid volume shifts that occur during the development and treatment of this disorder. The nurse gives fluid slowly to avoid complications associated with cerebral edema, such as seizures and an altered neurologic state. These patients are also at risk for intravascular thrombosis and focal seizures because of the hemoconcentration of the blood and the hyperosmolar state. Use of seizure precautions is necessary at all times. Treatment of acute cerebral edema usually involves infusion of osmotic diuretic such as 20% mannitol. Because these patients usually have a preexisting cardiac or renal history that predisposes them to complications, fluid resuscitation should proceed slowly and carefully.

Critical care management continues until the patient's hyperglycemic state has stabilized, his or her neurologic condition and vital signs return to normal, and the precipitating cause has resolved. Discharge criteria also include having an adequate plan in place for the patient to maintain glycemic control and avoid future hyperglycemic emergencies.

### Patient Education

As with patients who have DKA, the patient and family experiencing HHS need education. The prevention of many cases of HHS and DKA entails better access to medical care, proper education, and effective communication with a health care provider during an intercurrent illness. Many uninsured or underinsured patients stop insulin therapy for economic reasons; the nurse must assess for this possibility.

For the person with newly diagnosed diabetes, the nurse needs to provide information about the pathophysiology of the disease, the signs and symptoms of complications, and methods of treatment, including medications, diet, and exercise. Information about how to manage "sick days" and other tips to avoid acute complications such as HHS must be part of the educational plan.

The patient may need instruction on home management and glucose testing. Often the critical care staff consults with the diabetes educator as the patient's educational plan is being formulated. The main theme should focus on effective techniques to avoid emergency intervention in the future. It is necessary to make appropriate referrals to a diabetic educator, social worker, dietitian, or a combination of these because diabetes outcomes are optimized when a team approach is used.

## Hypoglycemia

Hypoglycemia is a well-recognized complication among patients with type 1 diabetes, and it is the most common diabetes-related emergency.[16] The issue of hypoglycemia is well documented in the landmark DCCT,[9] in which people with diabetes who maintained strict, intensive therapy for their diabetes experienced a threefold greater incidence of severe hypoglycemia than those patients with less strict treatment protocols. The UKPDS[10] demonstrated some increased incidence of hypoglycemia among people with type 2 diabetes, although few severe, life-threatening cases were documented in the study.

Insulin-induced hypoglycemia reactions often occur in the midst of the patient's daily life; this can be, at the very least, embarrassing, and at worst, dangerous. Mild hypoglycemia causes unpleasant symptoms and discomfort; however, severe hypoglycemia can lead to life-threatening complications such as seizures, coma, and even death if not reversed. Even though measurable recovery from hypoglycemia is rapid and complete within minutes after proper treatment, many patients remain emotionally (and possibly physiologically) shaken for hours or even days after insulin reactions. In extreme situations, prolonged or recurrent hypoglycemia,

| BOX 44-12 | Signs and Symptoms of Hypoglycemia |
|---|---|
| **Signs** | **Symptoms** |
| Hypothermia | Headache |
| Tachypnea | Personality changes |
| Tachycardia | Palpitations |
| Dysrhythmias | Blurred vision |
| Hypertension | Combativeness, confusion, coma, |
| Diaphoresis | convulsions |
| Tremulousness | |
| Hunger | |
| Nausea | |
| Belching | |

although uncommon, has the potential to cause permanent brain damage and can even be fatal.

### Pathophysiology

Minute-to-minute dependence of the brain on glucose supplied by the circulation results from the inability of the brain to burn long-chain FfAs, the lack of glucose stored as glycogen in the adult brain, and the unavailability of ketones. The brain recognizes its energy deficiency when the serum glucose level falls abruptly to about 45 mg/dL. The term *neuroglycopenia* refers to the degree of hypoglycemia sufficient to cause brain dysfunction resulting in personality changes and intellectual deterioration. The exact level at which symptoms occur varies widely from person to person, however, and it is not uncommon for levels as low as 30 to 35 mg/dL to occur (eg, during glucose tolerance tests) with no symptoms whatsoever among the long-term diabetic population. See Box 44-12 for common signs and symptoms of hypoglycemia.

Symptoms result from either the sympathetic nervous system response to hypoglycemia or the neuroglycopenic response. The hypothalamus reacts to the lower glucose levels by mounting the adrenergic response, which results in tachycardia, palpitations, tremors, and anxiety. The goal is to activate the counter-regulatory hormones (glucagon, catecholamines, cortisol, GH) to raise the glucose level and protect vital organs from hypoglycemia. This involves glycogenolysis and gluconeogenesis.

### Assessment

Occasional reactions occur in even the most stable insulin-dependent diabetic patient. As long as the reactions are mild, they can usually be tolerated without difficulty and are not cause for alarm or for changes in regimen. Frequently, the precipitating event is clear (eg, a skipped meal or an unusually strenuous bout of exercise). Box 44-13 reviews the common causes of hypoglycemia.

When hypoglycemic reactions are frequent, recurrent, or severe, it is important to identify the cause and prevent further reactions; otherwise patients may limit their functional activities and may become unwilling or unable to drive—in other words, they may overeat in an effort to prevent reactions. Usually the underlying mechanism can be discovered; if not, the patient should be admitted for work-up and further evaluation.

| BOX 44-13 | Common Causes of Hypoglycemia |
|---|---|
| Insulin shock | Severe sepsis |
| Insulinoma | Drug effects |
| Inborn errors of metabolism | • Ethanol |
| Stress | • Salicylates |
| Weight loss | • Quinine |
| Postgastrectomy | • Haloperidol |
| Alcohol excess | • Insulin |
| Glucocorticoid deficiency | • Sulfonylureas |
| Fasting hypoglycemia | • Sulfonamides |
| Profound malnutrition | • Allopurinol |
| Prolonged exercise | • Clofibrate |
| Severe liver disease | • β-Adrenergic agents |

**HISTORY AND PHYSICAL EXAMINATION.** The nurse asks about food intake and exercise, because these often contribute to hypoglycemia. Problems with insulin dosage or administration may be noted. It is necessary to investigate every detail of insulin therapy thoroughly, including insulin purchase and its appearance, species, and units; syringes, injection sites, and injection technique; and especially any recent change in any part of the regimen. The nurse explores for flaws and inconsistencies in reporting. Prescription errors, mismatched syringe and insulin units, use of new injection sites, and other errors may emerge.

The administration or withdrawal of other drugs may be the precipitating event for recurrent insulin reactions. For example, salicylates in large doses can reduce blood glucose and, in combination with insulin, can produce hypoglycemia. Also, the nurse asks about the use of glucocorticoid medications. Because these medications cause insulin resistance, insulin doses are often raised to meet the increased insulin demand. If the steroids are then tapered without reducing the insulin dose, hypoglycemic reactions can occur. Alcohol often causes hypoglycemia. Not only do patients often eat less when they have a few drinks, but also alcohol shuts off gluconeogenesis by interfering with intermediate biochemical steps in the liver. When combined with injected insulin, this frequently leads to hypoglycemia. Oral hypoglycemic agents can also produce severe and long-lasting hypoglycemia. Patients who experience such episodes tend to be older and undernourished with impaired renal or hepatic function. Nevertheless, any patient on oral agents can become hypoglycemic, especially when substances such as salicylates and alcohol potentiate the effects of the oral agents.

Another common mechanism that can cause hypoglycemia is an atypical (eg, early or late) response to insulin therapy. Once the response pattern is defined, it is possible to adjust the insulin regimen and eliminate the insulin reactions. Occasionally, when a stable, reaction-free patient begins to experience hypoglycemic episodes, the clinician should explore the likelihood of insulin sensitivity due to weight loss or the onset of azotemia.

As the blood glucose level falls below normal, the CNS responds in two distinct ways: first, with impairment of higher cerebral functions, and second, soon thereafter, with an "alarm" response in vegetative functions. Patients most commonly describe the symptoms of mild or early insulin reactions as fuzziness in the head, trouble thinking or concentrating, shakiness, light-headedness, or giddiness. These changes occur when the cerebral cortex is deprived of its main energy supply, usually when the blood glucose level has fallen to 50 mg/dL or less or is rapidly declining. The cerebral cortex is apparently the most sensitive to the loss of glucose.

Changes in personality and behavior vary with the person and may not be apparent to the individual during an insulin reaction. Changes range from silly, manic, inappropriate behavior to withdrawn, sullen, grumpy, irritable, suspicious behavior. There may be difficulties in motor function, such as trouble walking and slurred speech, and patients who are well into insulin reactions may closely resemble people who have been drinking alcohol in excess.

Some patients experience aphasia, vertigo, localized weakness, and even focal seizures with their insulin reactions. Such focal changes usually occur when there is prior damage to a specific area of the cortex, such as a head injury or CVA. Closely following the cortical changes is a series of autonomic neurologic responses. The primary response is discharge from the centers that control adrenergic autonomic impulses; this results in the release of norepinephrine throughout the body and epinephrine from the adrenals. Tachycardia, pallor, sweating, anxiety, and tremor are characteristic signs of hypoglycemia and are important early warning signs for patients who recognize a reaction. Headache can occur, and the stress response can occasionally trigger secondary sequences of symptoms, including angina or pulmonary edema in patients with fragile cardiovascular disease.

As hypoglycemia persists and worsens, consciousness is progressively impaired, leading to stupor, seizure, or coma; this is characteristic of severe hypoglycemia. The autonomic centers controlling fundamental systems, such as respiration and blood pressure, are the most resistant to hypoglycemia and continue to function even when most other cerebral functions are lost.

The more profound the hypoglycemia and the longer it lasts, the greater the chance of transient or even permanent cerebral damage after the blood glucose level is restored. There does not seem to be a clear duration threshold for such damage, but severe hypoglycemia lasting more than 15 to 30 minutes can result in some symptoms that persist for a time after glucose is given. Blood glucose measurement, before the administration of glucose if possible, verifies the diagnosis, but waiting for a glucose test result should be avoided in an emergency situation.

### Management

Treatment for insulin reactions is always glucose. If the patient can swallow, the most convenient form is a glucose- or sucrose-containing drink because it probably gets through the stomach and into the absorbing intestine in this form in the shortest possible time. If the patient is too groggy, stuporous, or uncooperative to drink, the glucose is administered in the form of an IV bolus of 25 g of 50% dextrose, given over several minutes. If this route or dosage is unavailable, 1 mg of glucagon given subcutaneously or intramuscularly reverses the symptoms by inducing a rapid breakdown and release of glucose into the bloodstream from hepatic glycogen stores.

The amount of glucose needed to reverse an insulin reaction acutely is not large. In an average-sized adult, less than 15 g (three teaspoons) of glucose can raise the blood glucose from 20 to 120 mg/dL. Glucose in almost any oral form will serve. Typical treatments for hypoglycemia include three glucose tablets, 6 oz of regular cola, 6 oz of orange juice, 4 oz of skim milk, or 6 to 8 lifesaver candies. Starch, found in crackers and cookies, is broken down to free glucose after passing through the stomach and is absorbed so rapidly that blood glucose rises virtually as fast as with free glucose or sucrose.

Patients frequently express concern about what to do if they do not respond to the initial therapy, and they fear that they might "never wake up" from a nocturnal insulin reaction. The nurse must reassure them that if the first bolus of glucose consumed does not seem to work, the sensible thing to do is to take in more. Insulin reactions are always reversible with enough glucose. The response to oral glucose, of course, takes time, perhaps 5 to 15 minutes, whereas the response to IV glucose should occur within 1 or 2 minutes at most. Failure to respond fully in the appropriate time indicates that not enough glucose has been given, that the diagnosis is incorrect, or that the hypoglycemia has been long and severe enough to produce persistent, although not necessarily permanent, cerebral dysfunction.

## Patient Education

The nurse should teach all people with diabetes to report hypoglycemic reactions to their health care provider for adjustments in their medical regimen. If they are taking insulin, they should know when to expect peak effects of the drug so that they can predict high-risk times for hypoglycemia. They should always carry a high-glucose snack with them for emergency use. The nurse should encourage them to carry medical identification at all times.

## Clinical Applicability Challenges

### CASE STUDY

S.T., a 19-year-old college student, was admitted to the hospital with symptoms of the flu: fever, nausea, vomiting, and cough for 3 days. He had been diagnosed with diabetes mellitus at 12 years of age and has been taking a maintenance insulin regimen of 24 units of longer-acting insulin glargine (Lantus) at bedtime and a sliding-scale dose of aspart (NovoLog) before meals. For the past 3 days, he omitted his insulin because he was not eating anything and still vomiting. His college roommate called 911 when S.T. could not stay awake and looked very ill.

S.T.'s vital signs are temperature 102.5 F (39.2°C); pulse 124 beats/minute; respirations 36 breaths/minute and deep; and blood pressure 82/52 mm Hg. He is lethargic but fully oriented, complaining of chills and right lower chest discomfort. Admission laboratory work reveals hematocrit 48.2%; white blood cells 36,500/mm³; glucose 560 mg/dL; sodium 140 mEq/L; potassium 5.7 mEq/L; chloride 90 mEq/L; bicarbonate 4 mEq/L; BUN 43 mg/100 mL; creatinine 2.2 mg/dL; serum ketones 4+; and urine glucose and ketones 4+. ABG values are arterial blood pH 7.06; PaO$_2$ 86 mm Hg; PaCO$_2$ 13 mm Hg; and bicarbonate 2.5 mEq/L. His chest x-ray confirms right-sided pneumonia. S.T. did not get a flu shot last fall.

Emergency department physicians diagnose S.T. with moderate to severe DKA with right lower lobe pneumonia. The initial therapy consists of several liters of normal saline solution infused intravenously and 20 units regular insulin by IV push, followed by an infusion of insulin at 5 units/hour during the first 6 hours. He is immediately started on broad-spectrum antibiotics, antipyretics. His mental status improves as he is rehydrated. The flow sheet below summarizes the biochemical changes over the first 15 hours.

**Biochemical Flow Sheet Indicating Diabetic Ketoacidosis for S**

| Time | Sugar | pH | Na | K | Cl | HCO$_3$ | BUN/ Creatinine |
|------|-------|------|-----|-----|-----|------|----------------|
| 1:00 PM | 560 | 7.06 | 138 | 5.7 | 90 | 4 | 40/2.1 |
| 3:00 PM | 490 | | 137 | 4.8 | 101 | 6 | 41/1.7 |
| 5:15 PM | 375 | 7.25 | 137 | 4.1 | 106 | 8 | 45/1.4 |
| 10:00 PM | 303 | | 139 | 4.7 | 114 | 15 | 27/1.2 |
| 4:00 AM | 204 | | 143 | 4.3 | 113 | 22 | 22/1.1 |

By the time of discharge 5 days later, S.T. is eating well, his fever is gone, and he has well-controlled blood glucose levels on his usual doses of insulin glargine and insulin aspart.

1. S.T. receives the diagnoses of ketosis and acidosis. What are the indicators of ketosis and acidosis?
2. S.T. experiences volume depletion and electrolyte imbalances. Why does this occur and what are the clues?
3. What are the main teaching points regarding future management of S.T.'s diabetes in this case?

### WANT TO KNOW MORE?

A wide variety of resources to enhance your learning and understanding of this chapter are available on thePoint.

You will find:

- References
- Selected readings
- NCLEX-style review questions
- Internet resources
- And more!

# PART 11

# Hematologic and Immune Systems

## 45

# Anatomy and Physiology of the Hematologic and Immune Systems

THOMASINE D. GUBERSKI

*Based on the content in this chapter, the reader should be able to:*

1. Describe the blood and its components and the function of each component.
2. Delineate the clotting factors and the role each plays in coagulation.
3. Describe the anatomy and physiology of the immune system.
4. Differentiate between innate and adaptive immunity including humoral and cell-mediated immunity.

Because cells for both the hematologic and the immune systems originate in bone marrow, the systems are interrelated. As a result, a change in one system can manifest itself in the other system. For example, a decrease in the number of white blood cells results in an immune system that is less able to resist infection. The anatomy and physiology of these two systems are discussed separately in this chapter, but the reader should keep in mind their close relationship.

## Hematologic System

Veins, venules, capillaries, arterioles, and arteries constitute an intricate network of conduits for the transportation of blood, which carries respiratory gases, nutrients, and waste products to and from body tissue. A delicate balance must be maintained in the vasculature to ensure both its patency and the liquid state of blood so that neither thrombosis nor hemorrhage occurs. This delicate balance is provided by the hemostatic and fibrinolytic systems working in concert.

### Blood and Its Functions

Blood is an aqueous solution of colloid and electrolytes that serves as a medium of exchange between body cells (interior environment) and the exterior, or external, environment. It has distinct characteristics, including variable color (arterial blood is bright red; venous blood is dark red), viscosity (blood is three to four times thicker than water), a pH of 7.35 to 7.4, and a volume of approximately 70 to 75 mL/kg of body weight (5 to 6 L). Plasma constitutes approximately 55% of blood volume, whereas cellular elements suspended in the

plasma constitute the remaining 45%. The vital functions of blood are as follows:

- Transport of oxygen and absorbed nutrients to cells
- Transport of carbon dioxide and other waste products to the lungs, kidneys, gastrointestinal system, and skin
- Transport of hormones from endocrine glands to target organs and tissues
- Protection of the body from life-threatening microorganisms
- Regulation of acid–base balance
- Protection from blood loss through hemostasis
- Regulation of body temperature by heat transfer.

See Chapter 16 for a more detailed discussion of circulation.

### Components of Blood

#### Plasma

Plasma, the liquid portion of the blood, contains a wide variety of organic and inorganic components (Table 45-1). The concentration of these components reflects diet, metabolic demand, hormones, and vitamins. Plasma is approximately 90% water and 10% dissolved solutes. The most prevalent solutes by weight are the plasma proteins and clotting factors. Serum is plasma that has had clotting proteins removed.

Plasma proteins play a role in transport, volume regulation, immune function, and coagulation. Most plasma proteins, including albumin and fibrinogen, are synthesized by the liver; however, the immunoglobulins (Igs) are synthesized by B lymphocytes. Albumin is essential for regulation of the colloidal osmotic pressure, which is critical for movement

**TABLE 45-1** Organic and Inorganic Components of Arterial Plasma

| Constituent | Amount/Concentration | Major Functions |
|---|---|---|
| Water | 93% of plasma weight | Medium for carrying all other constituents |
| Electrolytes | Total <1% of plasma weight | Maintain $H_2O$ in extracellular compartment; act as buffers; function in membrane excitability |
| $Na^+$ | 142 mEq/L (142 mM) | |
| $K^+$ | 4 mEq/L (4 mM) | |
| $Ca^{2+}$ | 5 mEq/L (2.5 mM) | |
| $Mg^{2+}$ | 3 mEq/L (1.5 mM) | |
| $Cl^-$ | 103 mEq/L (103 mM) | |
| $HCO_3^-$ | 27 mEq/L (27 mM) | |
| Phosphate (mostly $HPO_4^{2-}$) | 2 mEq/L (1 mM) | |
| $SO_4^{2-}$ | 1 mEq/L (0.5 mM) | |
| Proteins | 7.3 g/dL (2.5 mM) | Provide colloid osmotic pressure of plasma; act as buffers; bind other plasma constituents (eg, lipids, hormones, vitamins, minerals, and so on); clotting factors; enzymes; enzyme precursors; antibodies (immune globulins); hormones; transporters |
| Albumins | 4.5 g/dL | |
| Globulins | 2.5 g/dL | |
| Fibrinogen | 0.3 g/dL | |
| Transferrin | 250 mg/dL | |
| Ferritin | 15–300 mcg/L | |
| Gases | | |
| $CO_2$ content | 22–32 mmol/L plasma | Byproduct of oxygenation, most $CO_2$ content from $HCO_3$ and acts as a buffer |
| $O_2$ | $PaO_2$ 80 torr or greater (arterial); $PvO_2$ 30–40 torr (venous) | Oxygenation |
| $N_2$ | 0.9 mL/dL | Byproduct of protein catabolism |
| Nutrients | | Provide nutrition and substances for tissue repair |
| Glucose and other carbohydrates | 100 mg/dL (5.6 mM) | |
| Total amino acids | 40 mg/dL (2 mM) | |
| Total lipids | 500 mg/dL (7.5 mM) | |
| Cholesterol | 150–250 mg/dL (4–7 mM) | |
| Individual vitamins | 0.0001–2.5 mg/dL | |
| Individual trace elements | 0.001–0.3 mg/dL | |
| Iron | 50–150 mcg/dL | |
| Waste products | | |
| Urea (blood urea nitrogen) | 7–18 mg/dL (5.7 mM) | End product of protein catabolism |
| Creatinine (from creatine) | 1 mg/dL (0.09 mM) | End product from energy metabolism |
| Uric acid (from nucleic acids) | 5 mg/dL (0.3 mM) | End product of protein metabolism |
| Bilirubin (from heme) | 0.2–1.2 mg/dL (0.003–0.018 mM) | End product of red blood cell destruction |
| Individual hormones | 0.000001–0.05 mg/dL | Functions specific to target tissue |

From McCance KL, Heuther SE: Pathophysiology: The Biologic Basis for Disease in Adults and Children, 7th ed. St. Louis, MO: Elsevier Mosby, 2014, p 947.

of water and solutes through the microcirculation. Plasma is also a carrier molecule for normal blood components and exogenous agents, such as drugs. Igs (antibodies) are essential for defense against infectious microorganisms (see the Immune System section in this chapter for a further description). Fibrinogen is the clotting factor that forms the fibrin clot, essential to the clotting cascade.

Lipoproteins, which include the plasma lipids, triglycerides, phospholipids, cholesterol, and fatty acids, are carried through the blood as complexes with the plasma proteins. Also contained within the plasma, electrolytes (sodium, potassium, calcium, magnesium, chloride, bicarbonate, phosphate, and sulfate) maintain the pH and osmolality of the blood. Plasma nutrients, such as glucose, and gases, such as oxygen and carbon dioxide, are circulated to and from the tissues. Waste products, a final component of plasma, are carried to the appropriate organ for excretion.

## Cellular Elements

Summarized in Table 45-2 along with their functions, the cellular elements of the blood are erythrocytes (red blood cells), leukocytes (white blood cells), and platelets. All blood cell types are believed to be derived from a single stem cell known as the pluripotent stem cell, as shown in Figure 45-1. The production of blood cells (hematopoiesis) occurs in the bone marrow. Mitosis occurs, and proliferation continues until the needed number of mature daughter cells enters the circulation. Stress may trigger the release of an increased number of immature cells.

## Erythrocytes

There are approximately 5 million erythrocytes per cubic millimeter of blood. They are produced in the red bone marrow found in the sternum, ribs, skull, vertebrae, and bones of

**TABLE 45-2** Cellular Components of the Blood

| Cell | Structural Characteristics | Normal Amounts in Circulating Blood | Function | Life Span |
|---|---|---|---|---|
| Erythrocyte (red blood cell) | Non-nucleated cytoplasmic disk containing hemoglobin | 4.2–6.2 million/mm$^3$ | Gas transport to and from tissue cells and lungs | 80–120 days |
| Leukocyte (white blood cell) | Nucleated cell | 5,000–10,000/mm$^3$ | Bodily defense mechanisms | See below |
| Lymphocyte | Mononuclear immunocyte | 25%–33% of leukocyte count (leukocyte differential) | Humoral and cell-mediated immunity | Days or years, depending on type |
| Monocyte and macrophage | Large kidney-shaped mononuclear phagocyte | 3%–7% of leukocyte differential | Phagocytosis; mononuclear phagocyte system | Months or years |
| Eosinophil | Segmented polymorphonuclear granulocyte with granules stainable by eosin dyes | 1%–4% of leukocyte differential | Phagocytosis; response to parasites, control of allergic reactions | 8–12 days |
| Neutrophil | Segmented polymorphonuclear granulocyte with granules stainable by neutral staining | 57%–67% of leukocyte differential | Phagocytosis, particularly during early phase of inflammation, bacterial killing | 4 days |
| Basophil | Lobate nuclear granulocyte with granules stainable by basic dyes | 0%–0.75% of leukocyte differential | Similar to mast cell, secretes inflammatory mediators (eg, histamine, chemotactic factors for eosinophils and neutrophils), involved with allergic reactions | Few hours to days |
| Platelet | Irregularly shaped cytoplasmic fragment (not a cell) | 140,000–340,000/mm$^3$ | Hemostasis following vascular injury; normal coagulation and clot formation/retraction | 8–11 days |

From McCance KL, Heuther SE: Pathophysiology: The Biologic Basis for Disease in Adults and Children, 7th ed. St. Louis, MO: Elsevier Mosby, 2014, p 948.

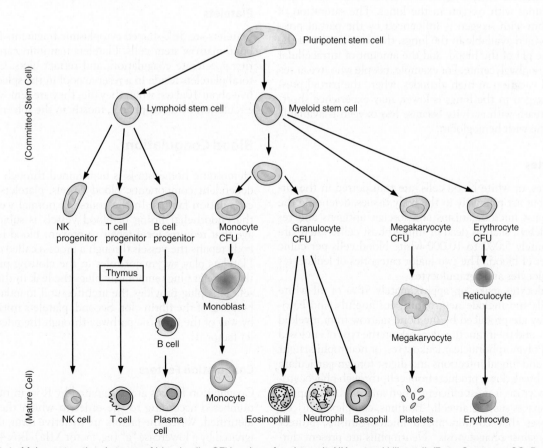

**FIGURE 45-1** Major maturational stages of blood cells. CFU, colony-forming unit; NK, natural killer cell. (From Grossman SC, Porth CM: Porth's Pathophysiology: Concepts of Altered Health States, 9th ed. Philadelphia, PA: Lippincott Williams & Wilkins, 2014, p 645.)

the hands, feet, and pelvis. Normal cell formation requires nutrients such as iron, vitamin B$_{12}$, folic acid, and pyridoxine. Reticulocytes (immature nucleated red blood cells) are released from the bone marrow.

The erythrocyte has volume ratio that is optimal for the diffusion of gases into and out of the cell. Reversible deformability allows the cell to alter its shape to squeeze through the microcirculation and then return to its normal shape.

Hemoglobin is the iron-containing substance of the erythrocyte. The normal amount of hemoglobin in the body is 12 to 18 g/dL of blood, with the lower level more common in women and the higher level more common in men. Hemoglobin is composed of a red compound called heme (which contains iron and porphyrin) and a simple protein called globin. Two thirds of this is in hemoglobin, whereas the rest is stored in the bone marrow, spleen, and liver. When red blood cells break down, hemoglobin splits into heme and globin factors. The liver stores the iron portion of heme for production of new hemoglobin, and the remainder is converted into bilirubin, which is excreted in feces and urine after conjugation by the liver. This conjugation process is important to the excretion of bilirubin, which causes jaundice when it accumulates in the tissues (see Chapter 38). Each red blood cell contains 200 to 300 million molecules of hemoglobin, which combines with oxygen to form oxyhemoglobin. Hemoglobin also combines with carbon dioxide. Thus, the blood can carry oxygen to the tissues and carbon dioxide from the tissues to the alveoli of the lungs, where it is expelled into the atmosphere. Hemoglobin can also combine preferentially with carbon monoxide, which displaces oxygen.

Respiration is a major function of erythrocytes. Hemoglobin combines with oxygen in the lungs. The saturation of hemoglobin with oxygen is influenced by the partial pressure of oxygen available in the lungs, the temperature of the blood, the pH of the blood, and the amount of intracellular 2,3-biphosophyglycerate. For example, people who live at sea level and vacation in high altitudes, where the partial pressure of oxygen in the lungs is lower, may experience shortness of breath with activity because less oxygen is available to combine with hemoglobin.

### Leukocytes

Leukocytes, or white blood cells, are transported in the circulation but act primarily in the body tissues, defending the body against microorganisms and foreign antigens and removing debris, such as dead or injured host cells. There are approximately 5,000 to 10,000 white blood cells per cubic millimeter of blood. The two major categories of leukocytes are granulocytes and agranulocytes.

Granulocytes make up approximately 70% of all white blood cells and include neutrophils, eosinophils, and basophils. They are produced by the bone marrow from myeloid stem cells, and their function depends on the type of enclosed granule. Polymorphonuclear leukocytes, or neutrophils, fight bacterial and fungal infections and digest foreign particulate matter or break down products from cells through phagocytosis. Phagocytosis is most efficient when microbes are trapped in small spaces such as alveoli.[1] Biofilms, complex multicellular masses that contain mixed microorganisms, protect bacteria against phagocytosis.[2] Neutrophils are present during the early acute phase of an inflammatory reaction. After

bacterial invasion or tissue injury, they migrate from the capillaries into the inflamed area or tissues, reaching their peak activity in 6 to 12 hours. In the inflamed area, they destroy and ingest microorganisms and other debris. They die in 1 or 2 days, releasing digestive enzymes that dissolve cellular debris and prepare the inflamed site for healing.

Eosinophils are particularly important in detoxifying foreign protein. They ingest antigen–antibody complexes, attack parasites and some viruses, and are elevated during allergic reactions.

Basophils contain cytoplasmic granules with histamine, bradykinin, and serotonin (vasoactive amines), which are thought to play a role in the symptoms of acute immunoglobulin E (IgE)-mediated systemic allergic reactions. Basophils contribute to B cell differentiation.

Agranulocytes (monocytes, macrophages, and lymphocytes) are leukocytes that do not contain lysosomal granules in their cytoplasm. Monocytes (immature macrophages) and macrophages are responsible for the phagocytosis of dead leukocytes and erythrocytes in the blood and for processing antigenic material as neutrophils start to decrease in number. Some of the circulating macrophages migrate out of the blood vessels in response to inflammation or infection, whereas others migrate to fixed sites in lymphoid tissues of the liver, spleen, lymph nodes, peritoneum, or gastrointestinal tract, where they may remain active for months or years. Lymphocytes are involved in producing antibodies and maintaining the immune response. The most important classifications are B and T lymphocytes, which are discussed later in the chapter.

### Platelets

Platelets are disk-shaped cytoplasmic fragments formed from bone marrow stem cells. Platelets maintain capillary integrity, accelerate coagulation, and retract clots. One third of total platelets reside in a reserve pool in the spleen. Platelets live about 10 days; when they die, they are removed from the circulation by macrophages, mostly in the spleen.

## Blood Coagulation

Hemostatic homeostasis is maintained through three interdependent components: blood vessels, platelets, and blood coagulation factors. In the course of normal wear and tear, the endothelial lining of blood vessels is subject to damage that requires local repair to prevent blood leakage. The body repairs the vessels through a process called coagulation. Platelets play two major roles in the clotting process. First, the platelet plug temporarily plugs the leak in the blood vessel. This plug provides the architectural foundation for the building of the fibrin clot. Second, platelets initiate clotting by way of the intrinsic pathway through the release of platelet factor III.

### Coagulation Factors

Coagulation factors are designated by Roman numerals and numbered according to the order in which they were first identified. When the factors are in active form, they are designated by a lowercase "a" (eg, factor XIIa). Box 45-1 lists the factors by Roman numeral and common name.

## Coagulation Pathways

Blood coagulation proteins, or coagulation factors, are found in the extrinsic and intrinsic pathways to coagulation. Tissue factor TFVIIa activates the coagulation pathway. There is interplay between the extrinsic and intrinsic pathways. Activation of factor VII, found in the extrinsic pathway, can activate intrinsic pathway factor XI. Likewise, several factors in the intrinsic pathway activate factor VII.

## Extrinsic Pathway

The extrinsic pathway is a series of chemical reactions that originate outside the injured structure. Critical steps are shown in Figure 45-2. Injury to tissues and blood vessels triggers coagulation and results in the release of thromboplastin into the circulation. Thromboplastin, catalyzed by factor VII proconvertin, activates factor X. In the presence of calcium ions, proaccelerin, and platelet factor III, factor Xa catalyzes the conversion of prothrombin to thrombin and fibrinogen to the fibrin clot.

The result of the interaction is fibrin formation. The intrinsic and extrinsic pathways merge into a final common pathway to clot formation. Figure 45-2 diagrams the sequence of clot formation.

Calcium plays an important role along the clotting cascade and creates a strong affinity for the factors to bind at the site of clotting.

## Intrinsic Pathway

Normally, blood coagulation factors circulate in an inactive state. After an initiating stimulus, changes in the coagulation factors occur immediately. The stimulus, damaged subendothelium, causes molecular alteration in any inactive coagulation factor, known as a proenzyme, converting it to an active form. The product of this enzymatic reaction activates the next coagulation factor in a chain-like reaction, leading to final clot formation. This chain of chemical reactions is termed the intrinsic pathway, which indicates its origin from within the tissue.

## Coagulation Inhibitors

Unchecked activation of the blood clotting factors would cause clots to form on top of the platelet plug, releasing thrombin in the process of clotting, further attracting platelets to the clot site, and causing additional clots to form at the local site of the vessel leak (Fig. 45-3). There would be

| BOX 45-1 | Coagulation Factors |
|---|---|
| I | Fibrinogen |
| II | Prothrombin (thrombin in active form–IIa) |
| III | Thromboplastin |
| IV | Calcium |
| V | Proaccelerin |
| VI | Unassigned |
| VII | Proconvertin; prothrombinogen; convertin |
| VIII | Antihemophiliac factor A (factor VIIIR–von Willebrand) |
| IX | Antihemophiliac factor B; Christmas factor; platelet cofactor II |
| X | Stuart–Prower factor; prothrombinase |
| XI | Plasma thromboplastin antecedent |
| XII | Hageman factor; glass factor |
| XIII | Fibrin-stabilizing factor; Laki–Lorand factor |

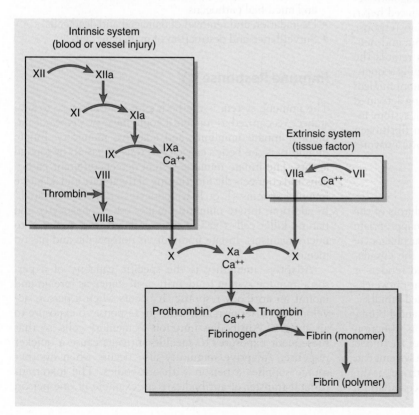

**FIGURE 45-2** The coagulation cascade. (From Grossman SC, Porth CM: Porth's Pathophysiology: Concepts of Altered Health States, 9th ed. Philadelphia, PA: Lippincott Williams & Wilkins, 2014, p 651.)

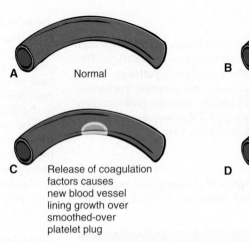

**A** Normal

**B** Vessel injury causes small vessel leak and minute platelet plug

**C** Release of coagulation factors causes new blood vessel lining growth over smoothed-over platelet plug

**D** Cumulative injury causes overgrowth of platelet plug with subsequent blood eddy currents and total vessel thrombosis

FIGURE 45-3 **A–D:** Sequence of thrombus formation in blood vessels.

total vessel occlusion if there were no mechanisms operating to maintain the blood in a fluid state and prevent uncontrolled clotting.

However, there is a well-controlled balance between clot formation and clot inhibition. Through the action of physiologic coagulation inhibitors, the blood is maintained in its fluid state, and blood vessels remain patent. These inhibitors—adequate blood flow, mast cells, antithrombin III, the mononuclear phagocyte system, and the fibrinolytic system—work by limiting reactions that promote clotting and by lysing any clots that do form, thereby preventing total occlusion of the vessels. Maintaining adequate blood flow facilitates the quick delivery of dilute-activated clotting factors to the liver, where they are cleared from circulation. Also, mast cells, which are located in most body tissues, produce heparin (which has a low anticoagulant activity compared with that of commercially produced heparin). Next, the liberation of antithrombin III in response to thrombin inactivates the circulating thrombin and neutralizes activated factors XII, XI, and X. This retards the conversion of fibrinogen to fibrin, thereby stopping sequential activation of clotting factors. Also, the mononuclear phagocyte system inhibits coagulation by clearing activated factors from the blood. Finally, the fibrinolytic system interferes with thrombin at its site of action on fibrinogen and also involves a chain reaction whereby lytic enzymes dissolve clots.

### Fibrinolytic System Inhibitors

Similar to coagulation inhibitors, there are inhibitors of the fibrinolytic system. These inhibitors prevent inappropriate lysis of needed clot formation. The mononuclear phagocyte system clears fibrin degradation products from the circulation. Also, antiplasmin binds with plasmin and renders it inactive. The level of circulating antiplasmin far outweighs plasmin concentrations, and plasmin is neutralized rapidly.

It is evident that the systems of hemostasis and fibrinolysis, in conjunction with their system inhibitors, function within a narrow margin to ensure the liquidity of the blood and patency of the vasculature. An upset in these systems can result in clinical evidence of thrombosis, hemorrhage, or the catastrophic event of disseminated intravascular coagulation.

## Immune System

The immune system is composed of the following organs: spleen, lymph nodes, thymus, bone marrow, appendix, tonsils, and adenoids; and cells: B and T lymphocytes, eosinophils, basophils, and phagocytes. The organs of the system are connected with one another and with other organs through a network of lymphatic vessels. Immune cells and foreign particles are conveyed through the vessels in lymph fluid.

Both the hematologic and immune systems originate in the bone marrow and blood carries components of the immune system throughout the body. The coagulation system helps keep microorganisms at the inflammatory site. The following are functions of a healthy immune system:

- Protection of the body from destruction by foreign agents and microbial pathogens
- Degradation and removal of damaged and dead cells
- Surveillance and destruction of malignant cells.

## Immune Response

The immune system is the body's internal response to substances recognized as foreign. People have two types of immunity: innate immunity and adaptive immunity. Innate immunity is the body's capacity to resist invasion by foreign agents. The innate immune system detects different pathogens and connects the functioning of the innate and adaptive immune systems. T & B lymphocytes are both activated.[1] In addition, innate immunity makes use of phagocytes and natural killer cells (NKCs) in its inflammatory response to microorganisms. Innate immunity is nonspecific and has no memory.

Adaptive immunity is the specific capacity of a person's immune system to identify a substance as foreign and mount an antibody response. It occurs when a person develops his or her own antibodies in response to exposure to an antigen. Antibodies function as memory cells, so that subsequent exposures to specific antigens cause a quicker response. Adaptive immunity also occurs when another source supplies a person with antibodies. The maternal-to-fetal transfer of antibodies is an example of one person supplying antibodies to another. Because it may take several days for acquired immunity to generate sufficient activity to protect a person, a major role of the innate immune system is to limit microbial replication until the specific immune response is mobilized.

Basically, the immune system protects the body, or "self," from invasion by "nonself." The concept of immune tolerance infers a nonactive immune system with self while producing immunity to foreign substances. Any foreign substance capable of eliciting a specific immune response is referred to as an antigen. Antigens can act as antigenic materials. Bacteria, viruses, fungi, parasites, and foreign tissue are all antigens. For instance, transplant rejection occurs when the body recognizes transplanted tissues or organs as foreign. Discrete, immunologically active sites on antigens enable Igs, lymphocytes, or antibodies to identify target cells, against which destructive forces are directed. Immune responses are not equally potent. The intensity of the system's response is affected by the route of invasion, the dosage of the antigen, and the antigen's degree of foreignness.

Immunologic competence refers to the immune system's capacity to identify and reject foreign materials. The system's failure to recognize antigens and mobilize effective defenses results in infection or malignancy. Failure to recognize markers of self can result in autoimmune diseases, such as multiple sclerosis, rheumatoid arthritis, or systemic lupus erythematosus. The system's "battle against imaginary enemies," such as pollen or dust, may result in allergies.

The major histocompatibility complex, essential for recognizing self from nonself, is a group of genes encoding molecules that mark a cell as self. These genes vary widely in structure from one person to another. Their presence is a major factor in transplant rejection because they determine to which antigens one responds and how strongly. More similar is better. They also allow immune cells to recognize and communicate with one another.

## Innate Immunity

Innate immunity is present in all healthy people and forms the first line of defense against illness. Previous exposure to an organism or toxin is not required for activation. Also, mechanisms of innate immunity do not distinguish among microorganisms of different species and do not alter in intensity on re-exposure. Innate immune defenses include physical, chemical, and mechanical barriers; biologic defenses; phagocytosis; inflammatory processes; and cytokines, dendritic cells, macrophages, and neutrophils.

## Physical, Chemical, and Mechanical Barriers

Physical barriers prevent harmful organisms and other substances from gaining entrance into the body or body cavities. These barriers include skin, mucous membranes, the epiglottis, respiratory tract cilia, and sphincters. Chemical barriers such as antibacterial agents, antibodies, and acid solutions create an environment hostile to many pathogens. Lysozymes in tears, lactic acid in vaginal secretions, and hydrochloric acid in gastric secretions all act as chemical barriers. Mechanical barriers help rid the body of potentially harmful substances through some action (eg, lacrimation, intestinal peristalsis, urinary flow).

## Biologic Defenses

Under normal conditions, large areas of the human body are colonized with microorganisms of low pathogenicity. The skin and mucous membranes of the oropharynx, nasopharynx, intestinal tract, and parts of the genital tract each have their own microflora, referred to as normal flora. These microorganisms influence patterns of colonization by competing with more harmful organisms for essential nutrients and by producing substances that inhibit the growth of other microorganisms. Vitamin D deficiency, a decrease in normal skin flora, or certain autoimmune diseases may increase the risk of infection in epithelial tissues.

## Phagocytes and Phagocytosis

Phagocytosis is a process by which injured cells and foreign invaders are ingested by leukocytes, specifically, neutrophils and mononuclear phagocytes (monocytes and macrophages). Neutrophils provide the "first-wave" cellular attack on invading organisms during the acute inflammatory process. The second wave of cells is primarily monocytes. Once in the tissue, monocytes swell to much larger sizes to become macrophages, which either attach to certain tissues and destroy bacteria, or wander through the tissue phagocytizing foreign matter. Macrophages in different tissues differ in appearance because of environmental variations and are known by different names (ie, Kupffer cells in the liver, alveolar macrophages in the lungs, histiocytes in the skin and subcutaneous tissue, and microglia in the brain).

## Inflammatory Responses

Inflammation is an acute physiologic nonspecific response of the body to tissue injury caused by factors such as chemicals, heat, trauma, or microbial invasion. It is the primary process through which the body repairs tissue damage and defends itself against infection. The initial inflammatory response is localized but may lead to systemic consequences such as fever, malaise, and neutrophilia. The inflammatory response contains three stages:

1. The vascular stage involves an immediate but short-term vasoconstriction, followed by vasodilation of arterioles and venules and hyperemia and swelling resulting from the secretion of histamine, prostaglandins, serotonin, and kinins.
2. The cellular exudate stage is characterized by neutrophilia, secretion of colony-stimulating factors into the interstitial fluid, and formation of exudate, a clear serous fluid with a high protein count. The functions of exudate are to transport leukocytes and antibodies to the inflammatory site, dilute toxins and irritating substances, and transport materials necessary for tissue repair. As the inflammatory process continues, the serous exudate changes to a creamy white fluid containing cellular debris.
3. The tissue repair and replacement stage, in which inflammatory material is removed and connective tissue cells proliferate. Collagen synthesis occurs, resulting in tissue replacement.

The most important result of these processes is accumulation at the site of injury of large numbers of neutrophils and macrophages, which inactivate or destroy invaders, remove debris, and begin the initial tissue repair.

## Cytokines

Cytokines are chemical messengers produced by T lymphocytes that function as immune system hormones and play a role in adaptive immunity and in mediating the inflammatory response. They enhance cell growth, promote cell activation, direct cellular traffic, stimulate macrophage function, and destroy antigens. They are also called interleukins because they serve as messengers between leukocytes. Interferons and tumor necrosis factor are also cytokines.

Cytokines can be classified as either lymphokines (secreted by lymphocytes) or monokines (secreted by monocytes or macrophages). Interferons (a type of lymphokine) provide some protection to the body against invasion by viruses until more slowly reacting specific immune responses take over. Interferons are produced when a virus infects a host cell; they affect the transcription and translation of viral genes. In addition, interferons appear to be involved in protecting the body against some forms of cancer. Specifically, these substances have been demonstrated to interfere with cellular division and proliferation of abnormal cells. They also enhance the activity of NKCs. Inflammatory cytokines cause fever in patients and also increase the synthesis of C-reactive protein (CRP), an acute-phase inflammatory marker.

## Adaptive Immunity

If a foreign agent persists despite innate immune responses, the activation of adaptive immune responses occurs. To be most effective, these responses require previous exposure to a foreign agent or organism. The cellular components of these types of responses are capable of distinguishing among microorganisms and can alter their intensity and response time significantly on re-exposure. The adaptive immune response has antigenic specificity and memory.

Two types of adaptive immune responses have been identified: cell-mediated immunity and humoral immunity. Most foreign substances stimulate both cellular and humoral immune responses; this results in an overlapping of their reactions and maximal protection against damage from the invading substances. Symptoms of some infectious diseases such as hypotension and shock are the result of massive amounts of bacterial toxins and a lack of sufficient protective antibodies.

## B and T Lymphocytes

B and T lymphocytes originate from stem cells produced in the bone marrow and mature into the competent cells responsible for cell-mediated and humoral immune responses.

As they develop, each of these "preprogrammed" B or T lymphocytes (on activation by its specific antigen) are capable of producing tremendous numbers of clones or duplicate lymphocytes. The different types of T cells that confer long-term immunity are categorized according to their function, as shown in Table 45-3.

## Lymphoid System

Secondary lymphatic tissue is located extensively in the lymph nodes. It is also found in special lymphoid tissue, such

| **TABLE 45-3** | **Types of T Cells and Their Functions** |
|---|---|
| **Cell Type** | **Function** |
| Cytotoxic T cells (T8) | Direct-attack cells capable of killing many microorganisms; predominant effector cell |
| | Virus-infected cells, cancer cells, and transplanted cells especially susceptible |
| Helper-inducer T cells (T4) | Most numerous |
| | Play pivotal role in overall regulation of immune response |
| | Often called "master conductor" |
| | Secrete lymphokines |
| Suppressor T cells (T8) | Act as negative feedback controllers of T4 cells |
| | May also limit ability of immune system to attack body tissues |
| Memory T cells | Sensitized to antigens during specific immune responses |
| | Remain stored in body |
| | Capable of initiating far more rapid response by T cells on re-exposure to same antigen |

as that of the spleen, tonsils, adenoids, appendix, bone marrow, and gastrointestinal tract. This lymphoid tissue is placed advantageously throughout the body to intercept invading organisms or toxins before they can enter the bloodstream and disseminate widely.

## Cell-Mediated Immune Response

Cell-mediated immunity provides a response to fungi, parasites, and intracellular bacteria. It also plays a major role in the rejection or acceptance of certain tissue grafts, the stimulation and regulation of antibody production, and defense against various malignant changes.

Each T cell, when activated by its specific antigen, migrates to lymphoid tissue, where it directly attacks antigens and malignant cells and regulators of both the cellular and humoral immune response.

Antigenic stimulation of T lymphocytes initiates the cell-mediated response. This step of the response may be mediated by macrophages that bind to the antigen, facilitating its recognition. The macrophages then produce cytokines, which stimulate T lymphocytes, increase B-lymphocyte proliferation, and activate phagocytes. People with impaired cell-mediated immunity are at high risk for infections with pathogens that replicate within cells such as viruses or parasites.

## Humoral Immune Response

The humoral immune response occurs in blood and tissue fluid. It begins in response to most bacteria, bacterial toxins, and the extracellular phase of viral invasion. Humoral immunity involves two types of serum proteins: Igs and complement. Vitamin D can decrease Ig production and slows differentiation of B cell precursors into plasma cells.[3]

Igs are antibody molecules made by B lymphocytes that differentiate to plasma cells and memory cells. The plasma cells then secrete antibodies that bind to antigens; the resulting antigen–antibody complexes are ingested by phagocytes. After the complexes are eliminated, the memory cells remain in circulation and in lymphoid tissue to mature into plasma cells when the antigen is encountered again. Igs are specific to antigens and are of several types:

- IgA (two types) concentrates in body fluids, such as tears, saliva, and secretions of respiratory and gastrointestinal tracts; it guards entrances to the body.
- IgM tends to remain in the bloodstream, where it is effective in killing bacteria.
- IgG (four types) is able to enter tissue spaces and works efficiently to coat microorganisms before phagocytosis occurs.
- IgD is found mostly in the membrane of B cells, where it is believed to regulate the cells' activation.
- IgE is normally present in only trace amounts; it is responsible for symptoms of allergy by activating mast cells.

Complement is a nonspecific series of 15 proteins synthesized by macrophages that circulate in an inactive form in the bloodstream. These proteins activate one another in a cascading sequence when the first complement encounters an antigen–antibody complex. The end product of the cascade kills the target cell.

Complement is activated by the antibody–antigen complex (Fig. 45-4).[2] Complement facilitates antigen–antibody interaction and enhances all aspects of the inflammatory process.

## Combined Immune Responses

The specific immune response is complex and involves the interaction of macrophages, complement proteins, and the cellular components of both the cellular and humoral systems (Fig. 45-5). All these components work together to destroy the antigen, either through complex processes involving direct attack or through modulation by chemical processes. Suppressor T cells provide feedback to the T4 helper cells to halt these defense reactions when they are no longer needed, and memory cells reactivate them on re-exposure to the antigen.

## Impaired Host Resistance

The various components of the immune system provide a complex network of mechanisms that, when intact, defend the body against foreign microorganisms and malignant cells. However, in some situations, components of the system can fail, resulting in impaired host resistance. Often the state of immunosuppression is chemically induced by drugs or medications, such as corticosteroids and cytotoxic chemotherapeutic agents. People who acquire an infection because of a deficiency in any of their host defenses are referred to as immunocompromised or immunosuppressed.

The exact effects of, and symptoms related to, defects in host defense vary according to the part of the immune system affected (Table 45-4). General features associated with compromised host resistance include recurrent infections, infections caused by usually harmless agents (opportunistic organisms), chronic infections, skin rashes, diarrhea, growth impairment, and increased susceptibility to certain cancers.

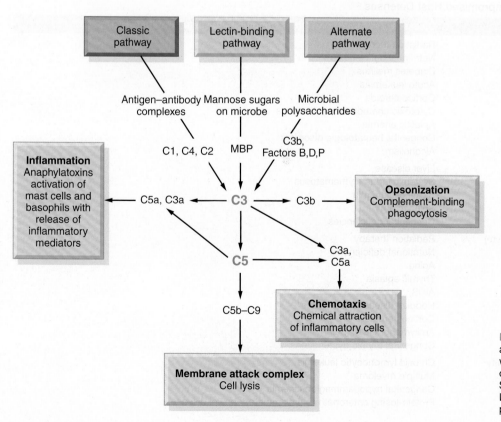

**FIGURE 45-4** Classic, lectin, and alternative complement pathways. (From Porth CM: Pathophysiology: Concepts of Altered Health States, 7th ed. Philadelphia, PA: Lippincott Williams & Wilkins, 2005, p 381.)

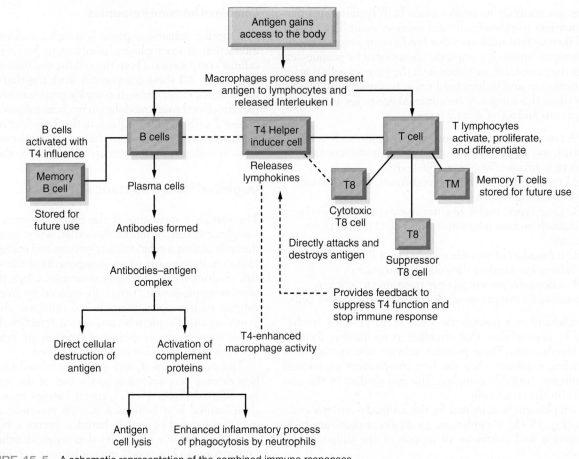

FIGURE 45-5  A schematic representation of the combined immune responses.

**TABLE 45-4  Risk Factors for Compromised Host Defenses**

| Host Defect | Diseases, Therapies, and Other Conditions Associated With Host Defects |
| --- | --- |
| Impaired phagocyte functioning | Radiation therapy<br>Nutritional deficiencies<br>Diabetes mellitus<br>Acute leukemias<br>Corticosteroids<br>Cytotoxic chemotherapeutic drugs<br>Aplastic anemia<br>Congenital hematologic disorders<br>Alcoholism |
| Complement system deficiencies | Liver disease<br>Systemic lupus erythematosus<br>Sickle cell anemia<br>Splenectomy<br>Congenital deficiencies |
| Impaired cell-mediated (T lymphocyte) immune response | Radiation therapy<br>Nutritional deficiencies<br>Aging<br>Thymic aplasia<br>AIDS<br>Hodgkin disease/lymphomas<br>Corticosteroids<br>Antilymphocyte globulin<br>Congenital thymic dysfunctions |
| Impaired humoral (antibody) immunity | Chronic lymphocytic leukemia<br>Multiple myeloma<br>Congenital hypogammaglobulinemia<br>Protein-losing enteropathies (inflammatory bowel disease) |

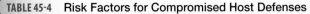

**TABLE 45-4 Risk Factors for Compromised Host Defenses**

| Host Defect | Diseases, Therapies, and Other Conditions Associated With Host Defects |
|---|---|
| Interruption of physical/mechanical/chemical barriers | Traumatic injury |
| | Decubitus ulcers/skin defect |
| | Invasive medical procedures |
| | Vascular disease |
| | Skin diseases |
| | Nutritional impairments |
| | Burns |
| | Respiratory intubation |
| | Mechanical obstruction of body drainage systems, such as lacrimal and urinary systems |
| | Decreased level of consciousness |
| Impaired mononuclear phagocyte system | Liver disease |
| | Splenectomy |

## Clinical Applicability Challenges

### SHORT ANSWER QUESTIONS

1. A patient is thought to be undergoing transplant rejection. What is the mechanism responsible?
2. What are the major differences between the functions of toll-like receptors and dendritic cells in immune functioning?
3. A patient with a staph infection develops hypotension, fever, and a rising CRP. What is happening?

---

### WANT TO KNOW MORE?

A wide variety of resources to enhance your learning and understanding of this chapter are available on thePoint.

You will find:

- References
- Selected readings
- NCLEX-style review questions
- Internet resources
- And more!

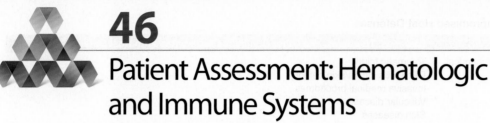

# 46

# Patient Assessment: Hematologic and Immune Systems

PATRICIA GONCE MORTON

## LEARNING OBJECTIVES

*Based on the content in this chapter, the reader should be able to:*

1. Describe areas of a patient's history and physical assessment pertinent to assessing hematologic and immune disorders.

2. Differentiate diagnostic tests used to assess hematologic and immune disorders.

3. Synthesize the results of a patient's history, physical examination, and diagnostic tests to identify hematologic and immune disorders.

4. Describe key aspects of the assessment of the immunocompromised patient.

Hematologic and immune disorders encompass numerous ailments, many of which are life threatening. In general, hematologic disorders can be classified as overproduction or underproduction of hematologic components or dysfunction of these components. Immune disorders are usually caused by underactivity or overactivity of immune system elements. Immune disorders can be inherited, or they can be acquired through disease or treatments, such as chemotherapy and transplant immunosuppression. The hematologic and immune systems are complex and closely interrelated; therefore, disorders or dysfunctions of one system often alter the effectiveness of the other.

## History

The patient history is essential when evaluating potential hematologic or immune disorders. While discussing the chief complaint, a patient may state symptoms that seem vague and unrelated, so a detailed history is critical. It is important to keep in mind the complex physiology of these systems when assessing a patient's health history (see Chapter 45). After obtaining information about the chief complaint and history of the present illness, the nurse inquires about the patient's past health history, family history, and personal and social history (Box 46-1). The patient's immunization history and occupation may provide helpful clues. A review of relevant systems concludes the history. Table 46-1 summarizes conditions and treatments that may predispose patients to hematologic and immune disorders (see Chapters 48 and 49). Box 46-2 summarizes special considerations for older patients.

## Physical Examination

A thorough physical examination is necessary to identify physical signs that may indicate a hematologic or immune system disorder. Table 46-2 on page 905 summarizes physical findings that may suggest various disorders of these systems. (Many of these disorders are further described in Chapter 49.)

The physical examination of the hematologically or immunocompromised patient focuses on four major areas: skin, liver, spleen, and lymph nodes. The entire examination must be thorough to help identify the exact source of the problem. The nurse examines the patient's skin for pallor or jaundice as well as for signs of abnormal bleeding. He or she also evaluates the patient's joints for pain, swelling, and limited range of motion, which may suggest hemarthrosis from coagulopathy or sickle cell anemia. Superficial mucocutaneous bleeding and a dependent distribution of petechiae can indicate thrombocytopenia, whereas clusters of palpable, pruritic petechiae can suggest vasculitis. Extensive superficial purpura, deep hematomas, or hemarthroses may indicate a coagulation disorder. The nurse also notes skin rashes, pruritus, and excoriations. It is necessary to assess the extremities for areas of redness, tenderness, warmth, or swelling, which can indicate thrombophlebitis. Leg and ankle ulcers may be present in patients with sickle cell anemia. The nurse assesses the lips and nail beds for cyanosis; digital clubbing may be present in patients with chronic hypoxemia. For more information on assessment of nails, see Chapter 51.

The nurse also examines the patient's eyes and mouth. Visual changes can indicate hyperviscosity from polycythemia or retinal infarcts from sickle cell anemia. It is important to assess the nares, gums, and mucous membranes of the mouth for signs of bleeding. The oral examination is a good time to ask about bleeding gums while brushing. Pallor of the oral mucosa can be a significant indicator of anemia. Tongue changes can occur in patients with an iron deficiency and megaloblastic anemias. Inspection of the throat and palpation of lymph nodes to assess for infection or malignancy is warranted. Figure 46-1 on page 906 shows the location of the lymph nodes in the neck.

Tachycardia and tachypnea may be present in patients with anemia or infection. An $S_4$ heart sound may be heard in persons with severe anemia. Dyspnea on exertion and orthostatic changes in blood pressure can be other symptoms of anemia and not just volume insufficiency. Many patients present with new-onset chest pain made worse by anemia. As the body loses oxygen-carrying capacity resulting from

## BOX 46-1   Health History for Hematologic and Immune Assessment

**Chief Complaint**
- Patient's description of the problem

**History of the Present Illness**
- Complete analysis of the following signs and symptoms (using the NOPQRST format; see Box 17-1)
- Unusual bruising or bleeding, frequent infections, fatigue/malaise, headache, dizziness/gait disturbance, pain, enlarged lymph nodes, fevers, night sweats, weakness, limb pain/limp, seizure, weight loss, abdominal pain, vomiting, heat intolerance, poor wound healing, nevi

**Past Health History**
- Relevant childhood illnesses and immunizations—mononucleosis, malabsorption, hepatitis, pernicious anemia
- Past acute and chronic medical problems, including treatments and hospitalizations—anemia, cancer, infections, autoimmune hemolytic anemia/Evans syndrome, hemochromatosis, hereditary spherocytosis, iron deficiency anemia, polycythemia, hemophilia, sickle cell disease, thalassemia, idiopathic thrombocytopenia, glucose-6-phosphate dehydrogenase (G6PD) deficiency, aplastic anemia, myelodysplastic syndrome, cirrhosis, HIV, major trauma, sepsis
- Risk factors—recent exposure to benzenes, pesticides, mustard gas, antineoplastic agents
- Past surgeries—splenectomy, cardiothoracic surgery, total gastrectomy
- Past diagnostic tests and interventions—bone marrow aspiration, radiation therapy, chemotherapy, multiple blood transfusions, administration of blood products (cryoprecipitate)
- Medications including prescription drugs, over-the-counter drugs, vitamins, herbs, and supplements—chemotherapeutic agents, antibiotics, antihypertensives, diuretics, glucocorticoids, nonsteroidal anti-inflammatory drugs, aspirin, heparin, warfarin, antiplatelet agents
- Allergies and reactions to medications, foods, dye, latex, and other materials
- Transfusions, including type and date

**Family History**
- Health status or cause of death of parents and siblings—cancer, anemia, inherited hematologic disorders

**Personal and Social History**
- Tobacco, alcohol, and substance use
- Environment: exposure to chemicals
- Diet: insufficient intake of foods rich in iron, folic acid, and vitamin $B_{12}$
- Sleep patterns—disruptive sleep patterns
- Exercise

**Review of Systems**
- HEENT: oral infections, gum bleeding, epistaxis, mouth sores, sore throat, smooth tongue texture, jaundiced sclera, conjunctival pallor, retinal hemorrhages
- Cardiac: palpitations, tachycardia, new onset chest pain
- Respiratory: recent upper or lower respiratory infections, hemoptysis
- Gastrointestinal: blood in emesis or stools, "tarry" stools, unintentional weight loss
- Musculoskeletal: weakness, bone pain, back pain, arthralgia
- Neurologic: mental status changes, pain to touch
- Genitourinary: blood in urine, urinary tract infections, heavy menstruation, vaginal bleeding

---

loss of hemoglobin, the myocardium becomes stressed and can trigger angina. It is necessary to perform thorough lung auscultation and inspection of sputum, if present, to rule out respiratory infection and hemoptysis. Symptoms of intermittent claudication (see Chapter 19) and angina pectoris (see Chapter 21) indicate problems with oxygen delivery in patients with polycythemia. Polycythemia is an unusual myeloproliferative disease in which there is excessive production of erythrocytes. The increased number of erythrocytes results in increased blood volume, increased viscosity of blood, and clogging of microcirculatory blood vessels, which leads to decreased tissue perfusion. Subsequently, patients with polycythemia commonly experience hypertension as part of the sympathetic response to decreased tissue perfusion.

Pertinent physical assessment findings of the abdominal and pelvic region include lymphadenopathy, splenomegaly, and hepatomegaly, which can indicate a number of hematologic or immune conditions. Figure 46-2 on page 906 shows the technique for palpating the spleen in the supine and side-lying positions. Figure 46-3 on page 906 shows the degrees of splenomegaly. The nurse also thoroughly assesses for urinary tract infections, vaginal infections (including those with yeast), and perirectal inflammation. In addition, the nurse checks all body secretions and fluids (stool, urine, emesis, or gastric secretions) for the presence of blood.

Neurologic abnormalities may be present in patients with hematologic conditions. Altered mental status, paresis, aphasia, dysphasia, coma, seizures, paresthesia, and visual problems may be caused by thrombotic thrombocytopenic purpura (TTP; see Chapter 49). An altered level of consciousness, papilledema, vomiting, and bradycardia with widening pulse pressure are signs of increased intracranial pressure, which may be caused by intracranial bleeding in patients with coagulopathy.

# Diagnostic Studies and Interpretation of Results

Laboratory test results are usually the most sensitive and specific determinants of hematologic and immune problems. Specialized testing may be required to ascertain whether the components are functioning properly. Because patients with severe presentations of hematologic and immune conditions may be seen in the intensive care unit (ICU), tests to differentiate the conditions and their causes are presented here.

## Tests to Evaluate Red Blood Cells

Red blood cells (RBCs) are essential for oxygenating tissues. An overproduction of RBCs results in polycythemia, which is indicated by a high hematocrit level and an increased RBC mass (see Chapter 49). Anemia is a condition marked by a decrease in the RBC mass caused by decreased production of RBCs, increased RBC destruction, a combination of these two conditions, or acute blood loss. All patients being evaluated for anemia should have a complete blood count (CBC) with RBC indices, a reticulocyte count, iron studies, and a

**TABLE 46-1** Hematologic and Immune Disorders Based on Patient History

| Patient History | Potential Disorder |
| --- | --- |
| Chronic disease (inflammation, infection) | Anemia |
| Nutritional deficiencies (iron, folate, vitamin $B_{12}$) | Anemia |
| Nutritional deficiencies (vitamin K, malabsorption) | Coagulopathy |
| Endocrine (thyroid, pituitary) dysfunction | Anemia |
| Hypersplenism | Anemia, thrombocytopenia |
| Acquired immunodeficiency syndrome | Anemia, neutropenia |
| Malignancy | Pancytopenia |
| Chemical exposure | Neutropenia, hemolytic anemia |
| Prosthetic heart valve or vascular graft | Hemolytic anemia |
| Collagen vascular disorder | TTP |
| Hypersensitivity reaction | TTP |
| Viral, bacterial, or fungal infection | TTP |
| Uremia | Coagulopathy |
| Chronic alcoholism | Coagulopathy |
| Liver disease | Coagulopathy, thrombosis |
| Vasculitis | Thrombosis |
| Atherosclerosis | Thrombosis |
| Chronic obstructive pulmonary disease | Polycythemia |
| Smoking | Polycythemia |
| Congenital cardiac disease | Polycythemia |
| **Previous Therapies/Medications** | |
| Heparin | Thrombocytopenia |
| Antibiotics | Agranulocytosis |
| Carbamazepine | Agranulocytosis |
| Alkylating agents | Leukemia, lymphoma, pancytopenia |
| Blood transfusion | Anemia |
| Aspirin, nonsteroidal anti-inflammatory drugs | Coagulopathy |
| Warfarin | Coagulopathy |
| Steroids | Leukocytosis |
| Various drugs, chemicals, and toxins (see Box 49-1) | Hemolytic anemia |
| **Family History** | |
| Sickle cell anemia | Anemia |
| Thalassemia | Anemia |
| Congenital hemolytic anemia | Anemia |
| Polycythemic disorders | Polycythemia vera |
| von Willebrand disease | Bleeding disorder |
| Hemophilia | Bleeding disorder |

peripheral smear analysis. Abnormalities in these test results indicate the need for subsequent testing.

## Complete Blood Count

The CBC provides an overall indication of bone marrow production of RBCs, white blood cells (WBCs), and platelets. It also indicates the patient's hemoglobin level, hematocrit value, RBC indices, and WBC differential. (See Chapter 17, Table 17-2 for normal hemoglobin and hematocrit values.) Patients usually extract about 25% of the oxygen from saturated hemoglobin. An increase in oxygen extraction can

**BOX 46-2** CONSIDERATIONS FOR THE OLDER PATIENT

**Risk Factors for Hematologic Disorders**
- Decreased iron intake, resulting from poor dentition (difficulty chewing meat) or a fixed income (making sources of iron such as meat or supplements unaffordable), can place the older adult at risk for iron deficiency anemia.
- Older adults may experience low-grade gastrointestinal bleeding as a result of nonsteroidal anti-inflammatory drug use for the treatment of arthritis, from hemorrhoids and polyps, or from undiagnosed colon cancer. This blood loss may also place them at risk for iron deficiency anemia.
- Poor absorption of vitamin $B_{12}$ (as a result of atrophic gastritis) places the older adult at risk for megaloblastic anemia.
- Declining immune function places the older adult at risk for leukemia, lymphoma, and multiple myeloma.
- Anticoagulation therapy (eg, to treat atrial fibrillation) can result in platelet dysfunction and places the older adult at risk for hemorrhage. This is a particularly significant risk in older adults who are disoriented or have decreased mobility.

occur in patients with extreme anemia. As the patient's extraction increases, so does his or her oxygen debt and shock state. Anemia from any cause is a major determinant in tissue hypoxia.

### Red Blood Cell Indices

RBC indices are laboratory values that describe RBC structure or function. Table 46-3 on page 907 presents RBC indices and some of the conditions that can cause abnormal laboratory results.

### Peripheral Smear

The peripheral smear can indicate disorders of the structure of RBCs. Table 46-4 on page 908 lists various abnormalities detected by examining the peripheral smear, along with further testing that may be appropriate.

Mature RBCs do not contain a nucleus. Nucleated RBCs mature in the bone marrow and are not normally present in peripheral blood. They appear in the peripheral smear after profound stimulation, such as that from acute hemorrhage, hypoxemia, hemolytic anemia, or megaloblastic anemia. If these causes are ruled out, the appearance of nucleated RBCs may be caused by infiltrative processes in the bone marrow from malignancy, myelofibrosis, or granuloma. Nucleated RBCs may also be seen in asplenic patients because the spleen normally recognizes and removes these abnormal cells.

Spherocytes and elliptocytes are abnormally shaped RBCs. They usually appear in patients with a hereditary disorder that causes RBC membrane defects. These irregular cells are trapped and destroyed in the spleen, causing hemolytic anemia. Testing for RBC osmotic fragility demonstrates that these cells are more likely to lyse than normal RBCs. Serum lactate dehydrogenase and serum bilirubin levels should be ordered if hemolysis is suspected.

The presence of Rouleaux formations (the RBCs on the peripheral smear resemble a stack of coins) can indicate multiple myeloma.[1] If clinical findings support this suspicion, serum protein electrophoresis and urine analysis for Bence Jones protein are the next steps in determining a diagnosis.

Target cells, sickled cells, and RBC cytoplasmic inclusions on the peripheral smear suggest the need for hemoglobin electrophoresis and analysis of hemoglobin F and $A_2$ levels.

**TABLE 46-2**   Findings Indicating Possible Hematologic or Immune Disorders

| Physical Findings* | Related Information From Patient History | Possible Disorder |
|---|---|---|
| Pallor, dyspnea, dizziness, tachycardia, glossitis | Fatigue<br>Headache<br>Pica (compulsive craving for clay, laundry starch, earth, or ice) | Iron deficiency anemia |
| As above, also smooth tongue, stomatitis, icterus, paresthesias, gait ataxia, mental status changes | Fatigue<br>Headache<br>Premature graying of hair | Megaloblastic anemia |
| Bleeding (ecchymosis, petechiae, epistaxis, hemorrhage), pallor, dizziness, tachycardia | Fatigue<br>Headache<br>History of frequent infections (eg, upper respiratory, cellulitis, perirectal)<br>Previous viral infection (hepatitis, infectious mononucleosis, HIV, cytomegalovirus)<br>Family history of aplastic anemia | Aplastic anemia |
| Pallor of conjunctiva, mucous membranes, palms and soles of feet; dyspnea; dizziness; tachycardia; bone pain; pain in chest or abdomen; splenomegaly; fever; leg and ankle ulcers; painless hematuria | African American descent<br>Family history of sickle cell anemia<br>Frequent infections<br>Impaired vision<br>Damage to joints<br>Chronic renal failure<br>History of stroke | Sickle cell anemia |
| Pallor, dyspnea, dizziness, jaundice, splenomegaly, cholelithiasis | Mediterranean descent, also Middle Eastern, South and Southeast Asian, and African | Thalassemia |
| Splenomegaly, hepatomegaly, facial and conjunctival plethora, hypertension, pruritus, dizziness, headache, thrombosis, thrombophlebitis | Visual disturbances<br>Epigastric distress<br>Cardiovascular insufficiency<br>Bleeding tendency<br>Numbness and burning of toes (from peripheral vascular insufficiency) | Polycythemia |
| Mouth sores, sore throat, lymphadenopathy, splenomegaly, hepatomegaly, infection (signs of infection may be minimal) | History of recurrent, severe infections<br>Fatigue<br>Recent radiation or chemotherapy treatment | Leukopenia |
| Infection, bleeding, bone pain, splenomegaly, skin and gum lesions, leukostasis if WBC count is extremely high (headache, confusion, central nervous system infarctions, acute respiratory insufficiency, pulmonary infarctions) | History of recurrent infections<br>Fatigue<br>Anorexia<br>Weight loss | Acute or chronic leukemia |
| Bone pain, pallor, weakness, fatigue | History of recurrent infections<br>Renal insufficiency<br>Hypercalcemia (thirst, lethargy, confusion, polyuria, constipation) | Multiple myeloma |
| Weight loss, fever, night sweats, painless lymphadenopathy, splenomegaly, abdominal pain | Fatigue<br>Anorexia<br>History of infections | Hodgkin disease or non-Hodgkin lymphoma |
| Superficial mucocutaneous bleeding, petechiae on dependent areas of the body, epistaxis, hemoptysis, hematemesis, hematuria, rectal bleeding, vaginal bleeding, intra-abdominal hemorrhage (diffuse abdominal pain, restlessness, anxiety, pallor, rigidity, dusky coloration of abdominal skin, tachycardia, tachypnea, and hypotension), intracranial bleeding (headache, vomiting, decreasing level of consciousness, papilledema, bradycardia) | History of viral or bacterial infection<br>Hypersplenism<br>Malignancies affecting the bone marrow<br>History of immune disorders<br>Alcoholism<br>Pregnancy | Thrombocytopenia |
| Confusion, headache, altered mental status, paresis, aphasia, dysphagia, coma, seizures | Paresthesias<br>Visual disturbances | TTP |
| Superficial purpura, mucocutaneous bleeding, hemorrhage, joint pain and swelling (from bleeding into joints), deep hematomas | History of excessive or recurrent bleeding in patient or family members<br>Alcoholism<br>Hepatitis<br>Liver disease<br>Malnutrition<br>Malabsorption syndromes (affects absorption of vitamin K from gastrointestinal tract) | Coagulation disorder |

*Findings listed may not always be present.

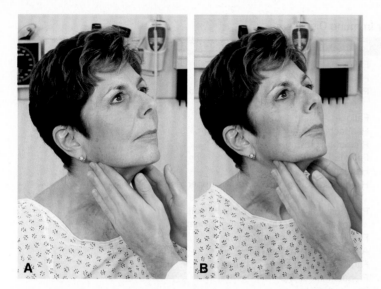

FIGURE 46-1 **A:** Palpating the tonsillar nodes. **B:** Palpating the submandibular nodes. (From Weber J, Kelley J: Health Assessment in Nursing, 5th ed. Philadelphia, PA: Wolters Kluwer Health/Lippincott Williams & Wilkins, 2014, p 287.)

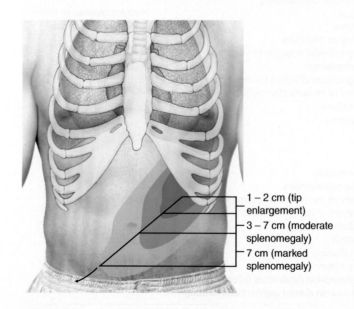

FIGURE 46-2 **A:** Palpating the spleen in the supine position. **B:** Palpating the spleen in the side-lying position. (From Weber J, Kelley J: Health Assessment in Nursing, 5th ed. Philadelphia, PA: Lippincott Williams & Wilkins, 2014, pp 495, 500.)

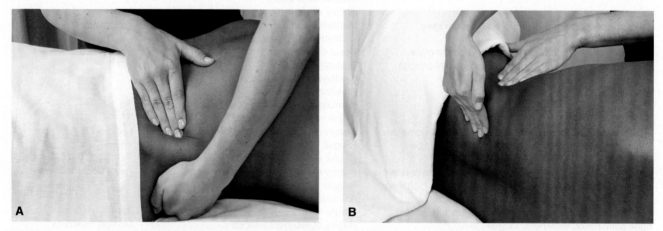

1 – 2 cm (tip enlargement)

3 – 7 cm (moderate splenomegaly)

7 cm (marked splenomegaly)

FIGURE 46-3 Degrees of splenomegaly.

The most common anemias diagnosed in this manner are β-thalassemia and sickle cell anemia.

The presence of schistocytes in a patient with a prosthetic heart valve may indicate mechanical hemolysis. Schistocytes in a patient with fever, thrombocytopenia, renal dysfunction, and neurologic abnormalities require immediate interventions for suspected TTP (see Chapter 49).

## Tests to Evaluate White Blood Cells

Because WBCs detect and destroy pathogens, an elevated WBC count usually indicates infection and tends to correlate with the severity of the infection.

### White Blood Cell Count

The WBC count measures circulating leukocytes and should always be assessed in conjunction with the WBC differential and the patient's clinical condition. The WBC differential is relative and describes the percentages of the WBC subtypes (neutrophils, eosinophils, basophils, monocytes, and

**TABLE 46-3   Red Blood Cell Indices: Laboratory Abnormalities**

| Test | Normal Value | Significance | Possible Causes for Abnormal Results |
|---|---|---|---|
| Mean corpuscular volume | 82–98 m³ | Indicates the average volume of a RBC in the blood sample.<br>Low value indicates RBCs are smaller than normal (microcytic).<br>High value indicates RBCs are larger than normal (macrocytic). | *Decreased*: Anemia (iron deficiency, sickle cell, hemolytic), α- or β-thalassemia, chronic disease, radiation therapy, endocarditis, diverticulitis, warm autoantibodies<br>*Increased*: Alcoholism, cirrhosis, folate deficiency, vitamin B₁₂ deficiency, pancreatitis, chronic lymphocytic leukemia, aplastic anemia |
| Mean corpuscular hemoglobin | 26–34 pg | Indicates the average weight of hemoglobin in each RBC. | *Decreased*: Anemia (iron deficiency, microcytic, normocytic)<br>*Increased*: Anemia (macrocytic, pernicious), cold agglutinin conditions, presence of monoclonal blood proteins, heparin sodium, heparin calcium |
| Mean corpuscular hemoglobin concentration | 31%–38% | Indicates the amount of hemoglobin in the RBC compared with its size.<br>Results expressed as hypochromic or normochromic, referring to the concentration of hemoglobin and color of RBCs. | *Decreased*: Anemia (iron deficiency, chronic, megaloblastic, microcytic, sideroblastic)<br>*Increased*: Cold agglutinins, hereditary spherocytosis, intravascular hemolysis, heparin calcium, heparin sodium |
| Red cell distribution width | 13.4%–14.6% | Measures the amount of homogeneity in the RBC width in the blood sample.<br>Much variation in RBC width indicates the red cell distribution width is elevated. RBCs of similar size indicate red cell distribution width is low. | *Decreased*: Defects in iron reutilization<br>*Increased*: Iron deficiency states |
| Reticulocyte count | 1%–2% | Indicates the amount of immature RBCs that have been recently released from the bone marrow, expressed as a percentage of the total RBCs.<br>Low reticulocyte count in presence of decreased RBCs indicates possible bone marrow dysfunction. | *Decreased*: Alcoholism, anemia (aplastic, iron deficiency, megaloblastic, pernicious), chronic infection, myxedema, radiation therapy<br>*Increased*: Hemolytic anemia, hemorrhage, leukemia, malaria, polycythemia, pregnancy, sickle cell anemia, thalassemia, TTP |
| Serum iron | Adult men 50–160 mcg/dL<br>Adult women 40–150 mcg/dL | Indicates the amount of iron in the serum.<br>Low serum iron needs to be correlated with other testing (ie, ferritin, transferrin, and total iron binding capacity) to determine if iron deficiency anemia is present. | *Decreased*: Acute blood loss, iron deficiency anemia, gastrectomy, malabsorption, malignancy, rheumatoid arthritis, uremia<br>*Increased*: Acute hepatitis, aplastic anemia, blood transfusion, hemochromatosis, lead poisoning, pernicious anemia, thalassemia, vitamin B₆ deficiency |
| Serum ferritin | Adult men 15–200 ng/mL<br>Adult women 40 y or older, 11–122 ng/mL<br>Adult women younger than 40 y, 12–263 ng/mL | Correlates well to the size of iron stores in the body. Ferritin is stored in the liver and reticuloendothelial system and released into the serum to meet the body's demand for iron. | *Decreased*: Hemodialysis, inflammatory bowel disease, iron deficiency anemia, gastrointestinal surgery, pregnancy<br>*Increased*: Anemia (chronic, hemolytic, megaloblastic, pernicious, sideroblastic), chronic infection, chronic inflammation, chronic renal disease, excess ingestion of iron, hepatic disease, liver disease, malignancy, multiple blood transfusions, rheumatoid arthritis, thalassemia |
| Total iron-binding capacity | 250–400 mg/dL | Indicates the maximum amount of iron that can be bound to transferrin.<br>Useful for differentiating anemia from chronic inflammatory disorders. | *Normal*: Chronic inflammatory disorders<br>*Increased*: Iron deficiency anemia |
| Serum transferrin | 200–400 mg/dL | Plasma protein that transports iron by binding iron to serum transferrin receptors.<br>Emerging as more sensitive indicator of iron deficiency and may replace more conventional indices (serum iron and ferritin). | *Decreased*: Cirrhosis, hemochromatosis, inflammatory states, renal disease, hemorrhage, hepatitis, hypothyroidism, microcytic anemia, pernicious anemia, thalassemia<br>*Increased*: Iron deficiency states |

Data from Chernecky CC, Berger BJ: Laboratory Tests and Diagnostic Procedures, 6th ed. St. Louis, MO: Saunders, 2013.

**TABLE 46-4** Peripheral Smear Red Blood Cell Abnormalities

| Abnormality | Potential Diagnoses | Further Testing |
|---|---|---|
| Nucleated RBCs 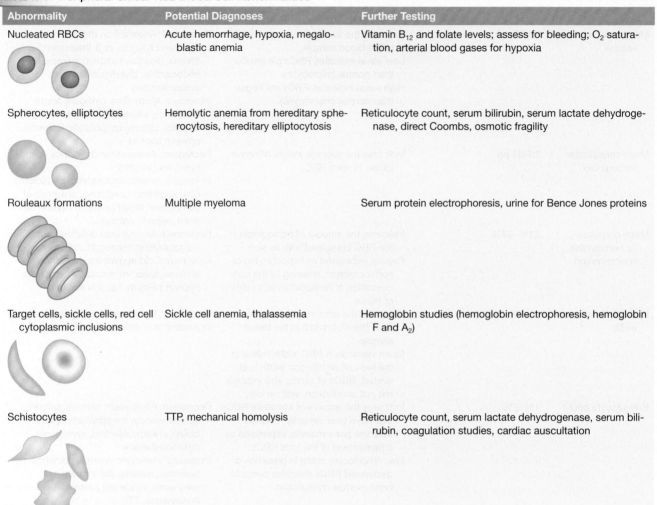 | Acute hemorrhage, hypoxia, megalo-blastic anemia | Vitamin $B_{12}$ and folate levels; assess for bleeding; $O_2$ saturation, arterial blood gases for hypoxia |
| Spherocytes, elliptocytes | Hemolytic anemia from hereditary spherocytosis, hereditary elliptocytosis | Reticulocyte count, serum bilirubin, serum lactate dehydrogenase, direct Coombs, osmotic fragility |
| Rouleaux formations | Multiple myeloma | Serum protein electrophoresis, urine for Bence Jones proteins |
| Target cells, sickle cells, red cell cytoplasmic inclusions | Sickle cell anemia, thalassemia | Hemoglobin studies (hemoglobin electrophoresis, hemoglobin F and $A_2$) |
| Schistocytes | TTP, mechanical homolysis | Reticulocyte count, serum lactate dehydrogenase, serum bilirubin, coagulation studies, cardiac auscultation |

lymphocytes). WBC subtypes can also be measured using absolute numbers. It is important to consider both the absolute and relative values of the WBC subtypes when assessing the differential. For example, 60% segmented neutrophils may seem within normal limits, but if the total WBCs are 18,000 cells/mm³, the absolute value (18,000 × 0.60) is 10,800 cells/mm³, which is well above normal. Table 46-5 indicates normal absolute and differential values for the WBC count.

Conditions other than infection that may elevate the WBC count (leukocytosis) include use of steroids, trauma, stress, leukemia, hemorrhage, tissue necrosis, and dehydration.[2–4] Table 46-5 summarizes abnormalities of WBC overproduction and potential physiologic causes. In some cases, patients with leukemia have WBC counts greater than 100,000 cells/mm³ because of excessive bone marrow production of blast cells (immature granulocytes). These patients are at risk for leukostasis, in which blasts aggregate in the capillaries of the brain and lungs. Clinical findings of leukostasis include headache, confusion, central nervous system infarcts, acute respiratory insufficiency, and pulmonary infiltrates.

A low WBC count usually indicates decreased production caused by immunosuppressive therapy or a disorder of bone marrow production due to infiltrative processes or bone marrow failure. Decreases in circulating neutrophils may be caused by decreased production from bone marrow injury, bone marrow infiltration, nutritional deficiencies, or congenital defects of the stem cells in the bone marrow. Other causes of neutropenia are splenic sequestration and destruction, immune-mediated granulocyte destruction, or overwhelming infection. Lymphocytopenia is most commonly caused by malignancy, followed by collagen vascular disease. Acquired immunodeficiency syndrome (AIDS) and AIDS-related complex are other notable causes of lymphocytopenia (see Chapter 48).

There are numerous potential abnormalities in the WBC differential. A left shift refers to an increase in the number of bands (neutrophil precursors), which usually indicates an infectious process. The presence of blasts in the peripheral blood is always an aberrant finding and suggests the presence of leukemia or a myeloproliferative disorder.

## T- and B-Lymphocyte Tests

As discussed in Chapter 45, lymphocytes are classified as T cells and B cells. T cells are important in the body's ability to

**TABLE 46-5** White Blood Cell Count and Differential: Laboratory Abnormalities

| Test | Normal Value: Relative | Normal Value: Absolute (cells/mm³) | Significance | Possible Causes of Abnormal Results |
|---|---|---|---|---|
| WBC count | | 4,500–10,000 | Measures number of WBCs | Infection, inflammation, leukemia, trauma, stress |
| Differential | All percentages for various types of WBCs must add up to 100% | | Describes the percentage of each WBC found in blood | See examples of specific cell type below |
| Granulocytes | 50%–70% | | Type of WBC categorized by presence of granules in cytoplasm | See specific granulocyte subtypes below |
| Segmented neutrophils | 50%–70% | 2,500–7,000 | Mature neutrophil with nuclei segmented into lobes | *Increased*: bacterial infection, inflammatory disorder, tissue destruction, malignancy, drug-induced hemolysis, diabetic ketoacidosis, myeloproliferative disorders, idiopathic, smoking, obesity<br>*Decreased*: compromised immune system, depressed bone marrow, heart–lung bypass, hemodialysis, overwhelming infection, tuberculosis, typhoid |
| Band neutrophils | 1%–3% | 135–500 | Immature neutrophil with nuclei that have smooth edges, unsegmented | *Increased*: acute stress, active bacterial infection<br>*Decreased*: compromised immune system |
| Eosinophils | 1%–3% | 100–300 | Also known as acidophils (acid loving); combat infections caused by parasites; play a role in allergic reactions; cause bronchoconstriction in asthma | *Increased*: parasitic infection, asthma, allergies, dermatoses (hives and eczema), adrenal insufficiency<br>*Decreased* (note: a low eosinophil count is not a cause for concern): Cushing disease; administration of glucocorticosteroids; various pharmaceuticals |
| Basophils | 0.4%–1% | 40–100 | Similar mechanism to mast cells in allergic response; triggered by immunoglobulin E binding to antigens; releases proinflammatory mediators | *Increased*: hyperlipidemia, viral infections (smallpox, chickenpox), inflammatory conditions (ulcerative colitis, chronic sinusitis, asthma), Hodgkin lymphoma, increased estrogen, hypothyroidism, myeloproliferative disorders<br>*Decreased*: stress, hyperthyroidism, pregnancy |
| Monocytes | 4%–6% | 200–600 | Monocytes become macrophages after migration into tissue; macrophages perform phagocytosis | *Increased*: viral infection, parasitic infection, myeloproliferative disorders, inflammatory bowel disease, sarcoidosis, cirrhosis, drug reactions<br>*Decreased*: administration of glucocorticoids, aplastic anemia, lymphocytic anemia |
| Lymphocytes | 25%–35% | 1,700–3,500 | Primary source of viral defense and antibody production | *Increased*: viral infections, pertussis, tuberculosis, acute lymphoblastic leukemia, cytomegalovirus infection, mononucleosis, post transfusion, splenomegaly, hyperthyroidism, connective tissue disorder<br>*Decreased*: AIDS, bone marrow suppression, aplastic anemia, steroid use, neurologic disorders (multiple sclerosis, myasthenia gravis, Guillain–Barré syndrome) |

distinguish between self and nonself. Monoclonal antibodies against specific lymphocyte surface proteins are used to identify types of circulating lymphocytes and their subset populations, which can be useful in characterizing hematologic malignancies and identifying immunologic and autoimmune diseases. A specific example of this is assessment of the CD4$^+$ subpopulation of T cells in patients with AIDS. Table 46-6 lists possible causes of lymphocytosis and lymphopenia.

When an antigen stimulates B cells, they differentiate into plasma cells and produce antibodies. Although plasma cells reside in lymphoid tissue, their antibody production can be evaluated through serum and urine protein electrophoresis. Autoimmune diseases occur when the body produces antibodies directed against its own tissues. These diseases can be organ specific (eg, Graves disease in the thyroid) or widely disseminated and involving multiple organs, such as systemic lupus erythematosus, which can attack almost every body system. Laboratory testing is aimed at the detection of serum antibodies against various tissues. C-reactive protein, antinuclear antibody, rheumatoid factor, and erythrocyte sedimentation rate are additional tests used in diagnosing autoimmune disorders.[1]

## Tests to Evaluate Disorders of Primary Hemostasis

Laboratory testing that evaluates hematologic dysfunction should be guided by the information gathered in the history and physical examination. Family history, underlying clinical conditions, and the duration and type of abnormal bleeding can indicate appropriate testing and diagnostic workup. Because hematologic and immune disorders are so pervasive in the human body, the nurse must be careful not to disregard innocuous symptoms. The patient's history must be thorough.

Primary bleeding disorders are caused by problems with platelets and small blood vessels that can result in subtle bleeding. For instance, mucocutaneous bleeding, petechiae, and superficial purpura may be early signs of impending critical illness. Decreased platelets or increased capillary fragility can cause the sudden appearance of petechiae, especially in dependent areas, such as the lower extremities.

### Platelet Count

The primary phase of hemostasis involves aggregation of platelets at the site of vessel injury. These platelets initiate the coagulation cascade, which results in the deposit of fibrin at the site of injury to stabilize the clot (secondary hemostasis). See Chapter 45, Figure 45-2, for an illustration of the processes that occur during hemostasis.

When evaluating primary hemostasis, one first obtains a platelet count from the CBC. A platelet count of less than 150,000/mm$^3$ is abnormal, but bleeding from thrombocytopenia alone usually does not happen unless the platelet count falls below 20,000/mm$^3$. However, prolonged bleeding from surgery or trauma may occur with platelet counts of 40,000 to 50,000/mm$^3$. Severe, spontaneous hemorrhage may result when platelet counts reach 5,000 to 10,000/mm$^3$. Causes of thrombocytopenia include decreased bone marrow production, splenic sequestration due to splenomegaly, or peripheral destruction of platelets by the body's own immune system. Disseminated intravascular coagulation (DIC) and TTP (see Chapter 49) are other serious disorders that involve low platelet counts. Drugs are the first suspect in thrombocytopenia (Box 46-3); once the nurse has ruled them out, she or he moves to consider other causes (Box 46-4). Finally, one must consider that some people may produce adequate numbers of platelets but ones that function abnormally.

An elevated platelet count greater than 400,000/mm$^3$ indicates increased platelet production or decreased platelet destruction. These platelets may function abnormally, causing aberrant bleeding and clotting. A cause of primary thrombocytosis is bone marrow disease. Causes of reactive thrombocytosis include chronic inflammation, infection, malnutrition, acute stress, malignancy, splenectomy, and the postoperative state.

### Peripheral Smear

A peripheral blood smear may reveal megathrombocytes (large platelets), which may be present during premature platelet destruction. Also, note that some patients' platelets clump when exposed to ethylenediamine tetraacetic acid

| TABLE 46-6 | Possible Causes of Lymphocytosis and Lymphopenia |
|---|---|
| **Finding** | **Possible Causes** |
| Lymphocytosis | Lymphatic leukemia, Epstein–Barr virus, viral infections of the upper respiratory track, cytomegalovirus, measles, mumps, chickenpox, acute HIV infection, infectious hepatitis, tuberculosis, Crohn disease |
| Lymphopenia | Aplastic anemia, Hodgkin disease, acquired immune deficiency syndrome, congestive heart failure |
| | Drugs include chemotherapeutic agents, immunosuppressive medications, radiation therapy |

Data from Fischbach FT, Dunning MB: A Manual of Laboratory and Diagnostic Tests, 9th ed. Philadelphia, PA: Wolters Kluwer: Lippincott Williams & Wilkins, 2014.

**QSEN BOX 46-3** *PATIENT SAFETY*

**Drugs That Decrease Platelet Production or Function**
The drugs listed below may cause complications, interactions, or other undesired effects.

| | |
|---|---|
| • Aspirin | • Glyburide |
| • Barbiturates | • Ibuprofen |
| • Cimetidine | • Penicillin |
| • Chemotherapeutic agents | • Phenobarbital |
| • Chloramphenicol | • Quinidine |
| • Chlorothiazide | • Streptomycin |
| • Digitalis | • Sulfonylureas |
| • Digitoxin | • Tetracycline |
| • Furosemide | |

Data from Fischbach FT, Dunning MB: A Manual of Laboratory and Diagnostic Tests, 9th ed. Philadelphia, PA: Wolters Kluwer: Lippincott Williams & Wilkins, 2014.

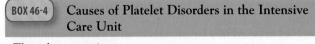

**BOX 46-4** Causes of Platelet Disorders in the Intensive Care Unit

Thrombocytopenia
Heparin (1% to 3%)
Sepsis (greater than 50%)
AIDS (40% to 60%)
DIC
TTP

Abnormal Platelet Function
Renal insufficiency
Cardiopulmonary bypass
Aspirin
Dextran
The incidence of platelet disorders is indicated in parentheses.

From Marino PL: Marino's the ICU Book, 4th ed. Philadelphia, PA: Wolters Kluwer Health/Lippincott Williams & Wilkins, 2014.

(the anticoagulant used in the "purple top" or CBC tube). Examination of the peripheral smear shows this clumping, and a repeat CBC in a heparinized "green top" blood collection tube reveals an accurate platelet count.

### Platelet Function Assay

The platelet function assay is a screening method that tests platelet function in adhesion and aggregation quality. This test is helpful in the evaluation of platelet function in patients with menorrhagia, drug-induced platelet dysfunction, and high-risk pregnancy.

### Bleeding Time

The bleeding time test assesses the length of time required for a clot to form at the site of vessel injury. A prolonged bleeding time in a patient with a normal platelet count may indicate a disorder of platelet function that requires further testing. Remember that patients can bleed to hemorrhage with a normal platelet count if the platelets are not functioning. A deficiency in factor VIIIR (von Willebrand disease) results in decreased ability of the platelets to adhere to the injured vessel wall. Uremia from renal failure, drugs (especially aspirin), foods, and spices can also cause abnormal platelet function. Box 46-3 lists some drugs known to decrease platelet production or function. Platelet aggregation studies are performed to detect inherited or acquired disorders in platelet function.

### Screening Tests for Coagulation Abnormalities

**PROTHROMBIN TIME AND ACTIVATED PARTIAL THROMBOPLASTIN TIME.** Screening for coagulation abnormalities includes evaluating the prothrombin time (PT) and the activated partial thromboplastin time (aPTT). Prolongation of either of these tests indicates coagulation factor deficiencies or inhibition.

The PT test screens for dysfunction in both the extrinsic portion that includes tissue thromboplastin and factor VII and in the common pathway that includes factors X, V, and II and fibrinogen. Prolongation of PT can result from disorders such as liver disease, vitamin K deficiency, clotting factor deficiencies, and DIC. Numerous medications, including allopurinol, aspirin, β-lactam antibiotics, chlorpropamide, digoxin, diphenhydramine, and phenytoin sodium, can also

cause a prolonged PT. PT is also used to monitor patient response to anticoagulation therapy with warfarin. The international normalized ratio (INR) provides a common standard for interpretation of PT. The INR value depends on the sensitivity ratio of the thromboplastin reagent used in the laboratory to the International Reference Preparation. Assessment of the level of anticoagulation and warfarin dosing are based on the INR ratio.

The aPTT measures how well the coagulation sequences of the intrinsic pathway (factors XII, XI, IX, VIII) and the common pathway (factors X, V, II, and fibrinogen) are functioning. An elevated aPTT could indicate disorders of any coagulation factor except VII and XIII. Clinical conditions associated with an elevated aPTT include DIC, von Willebrand disease, and liver disease. Drugs that may affect aPTT include chlorpromazine, codeine, phenothiazines, salicylates, and warfarin. The aPTT test is also used to monitor patient response to heparin therapy.

**THROMBIN TIME.** Thrombin time is a test that measures the clotting time of a sample of plasma to which thrombin has been added. Thrombin is important in converting fibrinogen to fibrin in the final phase of the coagulation cascade. Thrombin time is increased in conditions such as DIC, liver disease, clotting factor deficiencies, shock, and hematologic malignancies. Decreased thrombin time occurs with thrombocytosis.

**FIBRINOGEN LEVEL.** Fibrinogen is converted by thrombin to fibrin, which then combines with platelets to form a stable clot. Patients with DIC, severe liver disease, sepsis, TTP, or trauma have a low fibrinogen level. Elevated fibrinogen levels occur in conditions involving tissue damage and inflammation.

**FIBRIN DEGRADATION PRODUCT LEVEL.** Fibrin degradation products (FDPs) accumulate when a large amount of clotting has occurred and has then been broken down. Increased FDPs, along with an elevated PT/aPTT, decreasing platelets, and a low fibrinogen level, indicate possible DIC (see Chapter 49).

**D-DIMER.** D-Dimer is a more specific test than FDP measurement for detecting an event in which fibrin is being broken down. Its indications include ruling out and monitoring DIC, deep venous thrombosis, venous and arterial thrombotic conditions, and the monitoring of thrombolytic therapy.

### Tests to Evaluate Disorders of Secondary Hemostasis

Disorders of secondary hemostasis involve clotting factor deficiencies and are characterized by recurrent oozing of blood and hematoma formation. The onset of these symptoms may be delayed because of the initial plugging of the vessel injury; however, defective clotting mechanisms fail to provide a stable fibrin clot.

When assessing disorders of secondary hemostasis, one must determine whether the disorder is congenital or acquired. A history of excessive or recurrent bleeding in the individual or family members suggests a congenital disorder as the more likely cause. Table 46-7 describes potential complications experienced by people with congenital bleeding

**TABLE 46-7** Potential Complications in Congenital Bleeding Disorders

| Site | Potential Complication |
|---|---|
| Abdomen | Hypotension, hypovolemic shock (eg, retroperitoneal) |
| Muscle | Compartment syndrome |
| Joint | Hemarthrosis with destruction of bone and cartilage in joint capsule |
| Intracranial | Increased intracranial pressure |
| Retropharyngeal | Airway obstruction |
| Gastrointestinal | Anemia, melena |
| Urinary tract | Hematuria; clots in ureters may occur after factor administration |

Data from Stabler SP: Hemophilia. In: Wood ME (ed): Hematology/Oncology Secrets, 3rd ed. Philadelphia, PA: Hanley & Belfus, 2003.

disorders. The most common congenital bleeding disorders are von Willebrand disease, hemophilia A, and hemophilia B. PT and aPTT are ordered for patients with suspected congenital disorders, along with factor VIIIR, VIII, and IX assays. A deficiency in von Willebrand factor (VIIIR) results in the decreased ability of platelets to adhere to the injured vessel wall and a deficiency of factor VIII. A deficiency of factor VIII causes hemophilia A; a deficiency of factor IX causes hemophilia B. Table 46-8 summarizes laboratory abnormalities that indicate these congenital disorders.

An acute bleeding problem without a prior history of chronic bleeding suggests an acquired disorder. Acquired disorders of hemostasis occur with vitamin K deficiency, severe trauma, hemorrhage, massive transfusion, overwhelming infection, severe liver disease, and DIC. A deficiency of vitamin K decreases synthesis of prothrombin, factor VII, factor IX, and factor X. Liver disease impairs the absorption of vitamin K by decreased production of bile salts necessary for vitamin K absorption from the gut or through obstruction of the biliary system. Dysfunctional hepatocytes in the liver are unable to produce the vitamin K–dependent factors, as well as fibrinogen; factors V, XI, XII, and XIII; and other clotting factors. Some patients with liver disease may demonstrate thrombotic tendencies caused by decreased liver synthesis of anticoagulants, such as protein C, protein S, plasminogen, and antithrombin III.

Laboratory testing for an acquired disorder of hemostasis varies based on the suspected etiology of the disorder. In general, testing includes PT, aPTT, thrombin time, bleeding time, liver enzyme and liver function tests, fibrinogen levels, and FDPs. Table 46-9 summarizes laboratory abnormalities that indicate some of the acquired coagulation disorders.

A hypercoagulable state causes an increased tendency for thrombosis. Box 46-5 summarizes some of the risk factors for hypercoagulability. Hereditary thrombotic disease is a group of genetic abnormalities causing defects of coagulation, fibrinolysis, or their regulatory systems. Laboratory abnormalities in hereditary hypercoagulability include deficiencies of antithrombin III, protein C, protein S, plasminogen, tissue plasminogen activator, and fibrinogen; however, 65% to 70% of the causes remain unknown. Lupus anticoagulant (LA) is an autoimmune disorder in which patients have an elevated aPTT, yet thrombosis develops in 30% of the patients. LA is confirmed by the presence of anticardiolipin antibodies, positive platelet neutralization procedure, or positive dilute Russell viper venom test.

## Tests to Evaluate Hematologic and Immune Disorders

Table 46-10 lists common laboratory tests to assess immune system functioning. Diagnostic tests for human immunodeficiency virus (HIV) are listed in Chapter 48.

Bone marrow aspiration and biopsy are the most important diagnostic tests for determining bone marrow function. The biopsy provides information about the precursors of the blood's components to determine whether hematologic abnormalities are a production defect. Bone marrow examination is useful in detecting infiltrative processes, such as malignancy, which can affect blood cell production. This procedure is also performed to determine response to therapy in patients with hematologic malignancies or solid tumor infiltration of the bone marrow.

Tissue biopsy may be performed on skin lesions in which malignancy (eg, cutaneous T-cell lymphoma) or an autoimmune process (eg, pemphigus) is suspected. Lymph node biopsy is required for lymphadenopathy that does not appear to be caused by an infectious process.

Internal lymph nodes of the chest, abdomen, and pelvis can be evaluated by computed tomography (CT) scanning. A CT scan may be used to determine the presence of masses in suspected malignancy, especially lymphoma. Positron emission tomography is used in lymphoma and non-Hodgkin lymphoma to diagnose and stage cancer, evaluate response to therapy, and assess for recurrence. Liver disease, an important factor in coagulopathy, and splenomegaly may also be evaluated through a CT scan. A skeletal survey (skull, vertebrae, ribs, pelvis, arms, forearms, thighs, and lower legs) is done in patients with suspected multiple myeloma to assess for the typical "punched-out" lytic lesions that occur in this condition.

Intradermal skin testing is used to evaluate cell-mediated immunity. Various antigens are injected just below the skin's surface to check for delayed-type hypersensitivity. Commonly used antigens include mumps, *Candida* species, trichophytin, and tuberculin. If the patient fails to respond to the

**TABLE 46-8** Laboratory Abnormalities in Congenital Bleeding Disorders*

| | PT | aPTT | vWF | vWF Antigen | VIII | IX | BT† |
|---|---|---|---|---|---|---|---|
| von Willebrand disease | N | ↑ | ↓ | ↓ | ↓ | N | ↑ |
| Hemophilia A | N | ↑ | N | N | ↓ | N | ↑ |
| Hemophilia B | N | ↑ | N | N | N | ↓ | ↑ |

*Other congenital bleeding abnormalities are rare and not mentioned in this text.
†BT depends on the severity of the condition; it may be normal in mild cases.
vWF, von Willebrand factor; VIII, factor VIII; IX, factor IX; BT, bleeding time; N, normal.

## TABLE 46-9 Laboratory Abnormalities in Acquired Bleeding Disorders

| | PT | aPTT | TT | FDP | Plt |
|---|---|---|---|---|---|
| Vitamin K deficiency | × | × | | | |
| Liver disease: Acute hepatitis, early liver disease | × | | | | |
| Chronic liver disease | × | × | × | × | × |
| DIC | × | × | × | × | × |
| Massive transfusion | × | × | × | | × |

TT, thrombin time; Plt, platelets; ×, elevated laboratory result.

### QSEN BOX 46-5 *PATIENT SAFETY*

**Risk Factors for Hypercoagulability**

**Physiologic**
- Pregnancy
- Postpartum
- Venous stasis
- Age more than 40 years
- Immobilization
- Varicose veins
- Previous venous thromboembolism

**Pathologic**
- Malignancy
- Liver disease
- Disseminated intravascular coagulation
- Polycythemia
- Lupus anticoagulant
- Vascular injury
- Sepsis
- Heart failure
- Myocardial infarction
- Inherited abnormalities

**Environmental**
- Smoking
- Stress
- Heat

**Iatrogenic**
- Surgery
- Postsurgical
- Oral contraceptives
- Estrogens

injected antigens, he or she is said to have cutaneous anergy; this implies a defect in the patient's cellular immunity. Some causes of cutaneous anergy include AIDS, acute leukemia, chronic lymphocytic leukemia, carcinoma, Hodgkin disease, non-Hodgkin lymphoma, congenital immune conditions, bacterial, fungal, or viral infections, immunosuppressive medications, cirrhosis, and malnutrition.

## Assessment of the Immunocompromised Patient

Immunocompetence refers to the body's ability to protect itself against disease (see Chapter 45). Figure 46-4 illustrates areas to be assessed for immunocompetence.

It is essential that critically ill patients' immunocompetence be assessed at frequent intervals. Physical and psychological stress from overwhelming illness or trauma in the critically ill patient can depress functioning of the immune system. Invasive procedures, indwelling catheters, intravenous lines, mechanical ventilation, nutritional compromise, and the intensive care environment itself can predispose patients to infections and sepsis. As always, handwashing is the best tool available for these patients. Also, patient teaching and aseptic technique are essential to minimize exposure to infectious organisms. The nurse closely monitors potential sites of infection, changes or fluctuations in body temperature, nutritional status, and laboratory findings for indications of compromised immune function or the onset of infection.

Septic shock is a life-threatening complication that can develop rapidly in immunocompromised patients. Patient outcomes are greatly improved when septic shock is detected in its early stages and interventions are instituted promptly. Box 46-6 presents signs of early septic shock (also see Chapter 54).

### History

Reducing susceptibility to infection is key to the care of patients in the ICU, and the history can identify susceptibility and guide critical care nursing practice. The type of infection often provides the clues regarding the nature of the immune defect. For example, patients with defects in humoral immunity may have recurrent or chronic bacterial infections, such as meningitis or bacteremia. Repeated viral or fungal infections can indicate a defect in cell-mediated immunity. (See Chapter 45 for a review of humoral and cell-mediated immunity.)

### Risk Factors for Immunocompromise

Certain factors, such as chronologic age, place critically ill patients at a higher risk of immunocompromise. A patient who has a chronic disease or is already immunosuppressed may also be predisposed to further immune difficulties. Finally, certain medications and treatments can alter a patient's immunocompetence, as can his or her nutritional status and skin integrity. Nurses should be especially aware of these risk factors during their assessment of immunocompetence.

#### Age

The patient's chronologic age influences immunocompetence. Immune response may be depressed in the very young because of the underdevelopment of the thymus gland. Older patients experience a decline in immune system function, making them more susceptible to infections; thus, they should be closely assessed for alterations in their immunocompetence. Box 46-7 describes factors that contribute to the overall decline of immunocompetence in older people.

#### Chronic Disease

Many chronic diseases are associated with compromised immune functioning. Diabetes, hepatic disorders, cancer, and aplastic anemia are just a few examples of diseases in which immune deficiencies occur. Because many critically ill patients have an underlying chronic disease, the existence and severity of such diseases should be considered contributing factors to immunocompromise when these patients are assessed.

**TABLE 46-10** Common Laboratory Tests of the Immune System

| Laboratory Test | Reference Range | Use |
|---|---|---|
| C-reactive protein | Not available; levels less than 10 mg/L indicate patient no longer has clinically active inflammation; high or increasing levels are consistent with infection and/or inflammation | Evaluation of various inflammatory conditions, including rheumatoid arthritis and systemic lupus erythematosus |
| Antinuclear antibody | Low titers are negative; elevated titers demonstrate an elevated concentration of antinuclear antibodies | Screening and diagnosis of autoimmune disorders |
| Human leukocyte antigen (HLA) typing | Reported as phenotype for each of the six HLA loci tested. HLA (protein marker found on most of the body's cells) typing involves either serologic or DNA methods.<br><br>Antibody screen test is reported as the percentage of panel reactive antibodies (PRAs); percent PRA is number of wells reactive with patient's serum expressed in percent.<br><br>Cross-match is reported as compatible or incompatible. | Determination of tissue compatibility for organ transplantation; also used to determine paternity and to diagnose HLA-related disorders |
| Erythrocyte sedimentation rate (ESR) | 1–13 mm/h for males; 1–20 mm/h for females | Evaluation of inflammatory state; females tend to have a higher ESR; ESR increases with age |
| Immunoglobulins (Igs) | IgA: 160–260 mg/dL<br>IgG: 950–1,550 mg/dL<br>IgM: 50–300 mg/dL<br>IgD: 0–9 mg/dL<br>IgE: 0.002–0.2 mg/dL | Assessment of immunodeficiency state and certain cancers, including multiple myeloma and macroglobulinemia; also used to assess response to immunizations |
| Complement system | C3: 75–150 mg/dL<br>C4: 13–40 mg/dL | Diagnosis of systemic lupus erythematosus and other immunologic disorders |

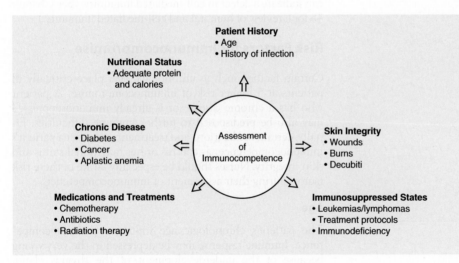

FIGURE 46-4 In addition to obtaining his or her history, assessment of the immunocompromised patient should cover six major areas.

## Immunosuppressed States

Patients with leukemia, lymphoma, multiple myeloma, and other hematologic conditions can experience impaired immunity and recurrent infections. Immunodeficiency states can be congenital or acquired. People with congenital immunodeficiencies frequently do not survive childhood. Immunodeficiency syndromes in adults may occur through a spontaneous defect in the immune system or through HIV infection (see Chapter 48).

Patients who are severely immunosuppressed have impaired responses to infectious agents and may not display the typical signs of infection. Fever and redness or pus at infection sites may be diminished because of the decreased numbers of WBCs required to promote these physical signs. Nurses should thus be extremely vigilant about monitoring for potential infection in these patients.

## Medications and Treatments

Many medications affect immunocompetence. Antibiotics such as tetracycline and chloramphenicol impair bone marrow function. Steroids display many immunologic effects, including decreased lymphocyte and antibody concentration.

BOX 46-6 | *PATIENT SAFETY*

**Signs of Early Septic Shock**
- Fever
- Chills
- Confusion
- Irritability
- Tachycardia
- Tachypnea
- Decreased peripheral pulses
- Hypotension
- Warm, dry skin

BOX 46-7 | *CONSIDERATIONS FOR THE OLDER PATIENT*

**Factors Contributing to Diminished Immunocompetence**
- Decline in immune system functioning
- Decreased nutritional intake (decreased taste, poor teeth, declining appetite)
- Chronic illnesses (diabetes, chronic obstructive pulmonary disease, renal disease)
- Increased risk for malignancy
- Possible urinary incontinence
- Prostatic hypertrophy and urinary retention
- Skin breakdown and impaired wound healing
- Decreased ability to care for self
- Impaired communication
- Decreased mobility

BOX 46-8 | **Nursing Interventions**

**For the Immunocompromised Patient***
- Provide a private room or uninfected roommate.
- Use a laminar flow or positive pressure room.
- Maintain strict handwashing with antiseptic soap.
- Use no rectal thermometers, enemas, or suppositories.
- Restrict staff and visitors with infections (or require masks).
- Provide patient with a mask when he or she goes to other departments or crowded areas.
- Permit cooked foods only.
- Allow no fresh flowers or live plants.
- Avoid sources of stagnant water (vases, water pitchers, humidifiers, denture cups).

*Precautions taken may vary according to institutional policy and the severity of immunosuppression.

*Example:*

Segs = 42%

Bands = 10%

Total WBC count = 4,100 cells/mm$^3$

$42 + 10 = 52\%$

$4,100 \times 0.52 = 2,132$ cells/mm$^3$ (ANC)

Usually, protective measures, such as those summarized in Box 46-8, are instituted for patients with an ANC of less than 1,000 cells/mm$^3$. However, all patients in the ICU are considered at risk for immunocompromise and should have the benefit of scrupulous handwashing, rigorous monitoring, and protective interventions.

**Nutritional Status**

The patient's nutritional status has a major impact on immune function. Inadequate intake of protein and calories can alter immune responses and resistance to infection by decreasing lymphocyte and antibody production as well as impairing wound healing. A multidisciplinary approach including a nutritionist can assist the nurse in assessing dietary intake and nutritional requirements for the critically ill immunocompromised person. Supplemental intravenous or enteral feedings may be necessary to prevent further deterioration of the body's nutritional status and ability to fight infection.

**Skin Integrity**

The integumentary system, including the skin and mucous membranes, provides a physical barrier to infection. Surgical or traumatic wounds, burn injuries, and pressure sores breach these physical defenses and predispose the critically ill patient to infection. Also, in a critical care setting in which intravenous and intraarterial catheters, urethral catheters, or endotracheal tubes are used, multiple portals of entry for pathogens can provide simultaneous sites for potential infection. Therefore, all wounds and portals of entry should be carefully monitored for signs and symptoms of infection.

Patients who have received organ or bone marrow transplants (see Chapter 47) often must remain on medications (eg, cyclosporine) that severely suppress the immune system. Patients placed on treatment regimens with any immunosuppressive medications are monitored for early symptoms of infection that would indicate compromise in immune functioning.

Various treatments also impair immunocompetence. Treatment protocols for patients with cancer can lead to life-threatening complications, such as infection and sepsis. Biologic therapy with interferon-α and interleukin-2 can cause leukopenia. Patients who receive multiple transfusions with RBCs can demonstrate suppressed immunity. Most chemotherapeutic agents and radiation to the pelvis, spine, ribs, sternum, skull, and metaphyses of the long bones can adversely affect the bone marrow's ability to produce WBCs. The lowest point in WBC levels, or the nadir, may not be seen until several days or weeks after the initiation of treatment. The absolute neutrophil count (ANC) is calculated in neutropenic patients to determine the degree of immunosuppression. The ANC is calculated as follows:

1. Add segmented neutrophils and band neutrophils (from the WBC differential).
2. Multiply the total WBC count by the total obtained in step 1.

# Clinical Applicability Challenges

Mrs. J., a 79-year-old woman, was admitted to the intensive care unit with a diagnosis of a lower gastrointestinal bleed. Her vital signs are heart rate 110 beats per minute, respiratory rate 26 breaths per minute, temperature 98.4°F (36.9°C), and blood pressure 88/58 mm Hg. Her red blood cell count is $3.4 \times 10^6/mm^3$, hematocrit is 32%, and hemoglobin is 10 g/100 mL. Although Mrs. J. has no cardiac history, her family tells you that she had new onset chest pain this morning.

1. Mrs. J.'s gastrointestinal bleed has most likely caused what other problem?
2. Explain why Mrs. J. has developed new onset chest pain.
3. On physical examination of the cardiovascular system, what other findings may you anticipate?

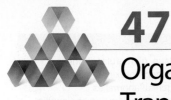

# 47

# Organ and Hematopoietic Stem Cell Transplantation

SANDRA A. MITCHELL, JO ANN HOFFMAN SIKORA,
AND ESMERALDA L. MATTHEWS

**LEARNING OBJECTIVES**

*Based on the content in this chapter, the reader should be able to:*

1. Analyze the criteria used to evaluate and prepare patients for transplantation.

2. Evaluate the principles of organ and hematopoietic stem cell compatibility and immunosuppression.

3. Discuss nursing assessment and management for patients undergoing solid organ transplantation (kidney, liver, heart, pancreas, lung) or hematopoietic stem cell transplantation (HSCT).

4. Describe the early and late-phase complications of organ and HSCT.

Transplant research began in the early 1900s, but kidney transplantation did not become a realistic treatment for chronic renal failure in humans until the early 1950s. Heart and liver transplantations followed in the 1960s and since the 1980s, have steadily increased in frequency as a treatment for end-stage organ failure. Pancreas transplantation also began in the mid-1960s with good graft survival rates being achieved in the 1980s. The number of lung transplantations is small, primarily because of a lack of medically suitable donors. Table 47-1 gives survival rates for solid organ transplantations.

During the past 40 years, hematopoietic stem cell transplantation (HSCT) has evolved from an experimental treatment for patients with advanced acute leukemia into a therapeutically effective modality that is now standard therapy for selected diseases. HSCT, which is known to be curative in several malignant and nonmalignant disorders, is a transplantation using hematopoietic stem cells at various stages of differentiation and maturation. Decreased treatment-associated mortality and improved supportive care have helped make this possible.

This chapter describes the major aspects of care for patients receiving kidney, liver, heart, pancreas, and lung transplantations and HSCT. It covers principles that apply to all types of transplantation and discusses content unique to specific types of transplants.

## Patient Selection

Many factors influence the indications and patient eligibility for transplantation. Currently, end-stage disease is the primary reason for most organ transplantations. HSCT is now used when bone marrow is defective or destroyed by a disease process or as a result of treating an underlying disease.[1] New information concerning patient outcomes, complications, surgical techniques, immunosuppressive drugs, and availability of organs and hematopoietic stem cells is also considered. Table 47-2 presents indications for transplantation.

Selecting the ideal candidate for transplantation is an intricate process. To evaluate a patient's suitability for transplantation, a comprehensive multisystem analysis is performed. This includes both physiologic and psychosocial factors that affect the patient's chance for a successful transplantation. During this evaluation phase, treatment of newly diagnosed conditions occurs, and clinicians make plans to ensure adequate nutrition, mobility, and muscle strength. The goal is to have the patient in the best possible physical condition for transplantation. When transplantations are performed earlier, rather than later in the disease process, there are fewer disabilities and a greater chance for survival.

Financial guidance is provided so that patients and families know what their insurance will cover and the nature

**TABLE 47-1** Graft and Patient 1-Year Survival Rates for Adult Solid Organ Transplants Performed in 2009–2010

| Organ | Graft Survival Rate (%) | Patient Survival Rate (%) |
|---|---|---|
| Kidney—living donor | 95 | 98 |
| Kidney—deceased donor | 89 | 94 |
| Heart | 86 | 87 |
| Lung | 82 | 83 |
| Liver—living donor | 82 | 90 |
| Liver—deceased donor | 82 | 86 |
| Pancreas | 76 | 94 |
| Kidney/pancreas | 91 (pancreas graft 89.1) | 95 |
| Intestine | 75 | 78 |

Data from the 2015 Annual Report of the U.S. Organ Procurement and Transplantation Network and the Scientific Registry of Transplant Recipients: Transplant Data. Rockville, MD: U.S. Department of Health and Human Services, Health Resources and Services Administration, Healthcare Systems Bureau, Division of Transplantation.

**TABLE 47-2** Indications for Transplantation

| Organ | Indications for Transplantation | Common Causes |
|---|---|---|
| Kidney | End-stage renal disease | Hypertension, diabetes mellitus, glomerular nephritis, urologic disorders, cancer, nephrotoxins, trauma, hemolytic disorders, congenital anomalies |
| Liver | *Adults*: irreversible liver disease, malignancy, and hepatic failure resulting in synthetic liver dysfunction<br>*Children*: biliary atresia, α-1-antitrypsin deficiency | Acute or chronic hepatitis, primary sclerosing cholangitis, primary biliary cirrhosis, hepatocellular carcinoma, Budd–Chiari syndrome, alcoholic cirrhosis |
| Heart | End-stage heart failure | Ischemic cardiomyopathy, idiopathic cardiomyopathy, valvular heart disease, congenital anomalies |
| Pancreas | Type 1 diabetes mellitus with end-stage renal disease either alone or in combination with a kidney transplant | Diabetes mellitus |
| Lung | Chronic obstructive pulmonary disease | Emphysema and bronchiectasis, idiopathic pulmonary fibrosis, emphysema due to α-1-antitrypsin deficiency, primary pulmonary hypertension |
| Heart–lung | Eisenmenger syndrome | Pulmonary hypertension with irreversible right-sided heart failure not amenable to heart transplantation alone |
| Hematopoietic stem cell | Malignant disorders | Leukemias, myelodysplastic syndrome, Hodgkin lymphoma, non-Hodgkin lymphoma, multiple myeloma, and selected solid tumors (eg, renal cell tumors, germ cell tumors, neuroblastoma, pinealoblastoma)[2] |
|  | Nonmalignant disorders | Aplastic, sickle cell, and Fanconi anemias; selected metabolic disorders; thalassemia; and immunodeficiency syndromes[2] |

and amount of their expected out-of-pocket expenses. Transplantation involves costs before, during, and after the actual transplant surgery. Such costs include laboratory tests, organ procurement, transplant surgeon and other operating personnel, in-hospital stays, transplantation to and from the hospital for surgery, check-ups, rehabilitation, and medications, which can cost up to $2,500 per month. The average cost of transplantation in 2008 ranged from $259,000 for a single kidney to over $1,200,000 for a heart-lung transplant.[3–5]

Transplantation centers may require proof of the patient's ability to cover medication expenses before accepting a patient for transplantation.

The following general criteria guide the selection of candidates for transplantation:

- Biologic rather than chronologic age is evaluated individually. Individuals eligible for transplantation may range from newborns to 70-year-olds. People older than age 55 may be at increased risk for complications.
- Acute or chronic infection is absent or has been treated. Localized liver infection may be an exception. Inflammatory diseases, such as systemic lupus erythematosus, do not rule out transplantation but should be quiescent at the time of the procedure.
- For the patient undergoing HSCT for a malignancy, care is taken to distinguish patients who can be saved by transplantation from those who may relapse or succumb to the rigors and toxicities of treatment.

Table 47-3 lists organ-specific criteria for transplantation. In general, evaluations common to all transplantation procedures include the following:

- ABO typing
- Tissue typing, HLA matching, mixed lymphocyte culture (MLC) matching
- Transfusion history
- Infectious disease screening (tuberculin skin test, human immunodeficiency virus [HIV], hepatitis B surface

antigen, hepatitis C virus, Epstein–Barr virus, cytomegalovirus [CMV], toxoplasmosis titers, herpes simplex, varicella virus, venereal disease)

- Liver function studies
- Renal function studies
- Complete blood count (CBC)
- Coagulation studies
- Gastrointestinal evaluation (depending on age and history)
- Gynecologic examination
- Electrocardiogram (ECG)
- Chest radiograph
- Dental examination to rule out infection
- Social history, review of patient motivation, ability to follow postoperative regimen, and psychiatric evaluation.

Contraindications are based on conditions and behaviors that decrease the chance of survival. For solid organ transplantation, these include serious active infection or sepsis, recent cancer (unless that is the reason for transplantation), current substance abuse, HIV infection, severe cachexia, active peptic ulcer disease, psychiatric disorders that impair the ability to give informed consent or adhere to the treatment regimen, and repeated noncompliance. Table 47-3 lists these contraindications.

## Donor Selection

After a person is determined to be a candidate for transplantation, a donor source must be selected.

## Determining Compatibility

Determination of compatibility in transplantation involves the evaluation of two major antigen systems. The primary determinant for solid organ transplantation is ABO grouping. A mismatch in compatibility may cause an immediate reaction leading to organ loss.

## Organ Transplantation

The rules of compatibility that apply to the administration of blood products also apply to solid organ transplantation: type A blood has the A antigen, type B blood has the B antigen, type AB blood has both A and B antigens, and type O blood has neither antigen.

Histocompatibility testing (tissue typing) is the identification of donor and recipient antigens and the evaluation of donor antigens against recipient antibodies. This evaluation determines the compatibility between donor and recipient, which predicts the chances of graft acceptance. In the HLA antigen system, genes of the major histocompatibility complex code for the antigens that compose a person's tissue type. These genes contain information for antigens present on the surface of the nucleated cells and serve to signal the immune system in differentiating self from nonself. The

**TABLE 47-3 Criteria, Contraindications, and Evaluations in Transplantation**

| Organ | Specific Criteria | Contraindications | Specific Evaluation |
|---|---|---|---|
| Kidney | • End-stage or near end-stage renal failure (defined as a glomerular filtration rate of less than 10 mL/min)<br>• Pre–end stage preferable for some patients (ie, children, patients with diabetes mellitus, and those for whom there is a living donor) | • Severe or uncorrectable coronary artery disease, peripheral vascular disease, or pulmonary disease<br>• Severe cardiomyopathy | • Voiding cystourethrogram to evaluate for obstruction or reflux (medical history dependent)<br>• Cardiac evaluation (age and medical history dependent) |
| Liver | • Malnutrition<br>• Severe blood clotting abnormalities<br>• Variceal bleeding<br>• Hepatic encephalopathy<br>• Severe, intractable ascites<br>• Severe, intractable pruritus | • Multiple uncorrected congenital anomalies<br>• Advanced cardiopulmonary disease<br>• Severe pulmonary hypertension | • Abdominal computed tomography (CT) scan (to detect hepatoma)<br>• Doppler ultrasound (to identify patency of portal vein)<br>• Liver disease studies and autoimmune markers, such as ceruloplasmin, carcinoembryonic antigen, alpha-fetoprotein, antimitochondrial and antinuclear antibody<br>• Endoscopic retrograde cholangiopancreatography/cholangiogram (if indicated, usually for patients with cholestasis)<br>• Liver biopsy (if indicated)<br>• Upper and lower endoscopy (if indicated) |
| Pancreas | • End-stage renal failure (combine kidney and pancreas transplant)<br>• Absence of (or corrected) coronary artery disease | • Severe or uncorrectable coronary artery disease, peripheral vascular disease, or pulmonary disease<br>• Previous major amputation<br>• Blindness (not absolute contraindication)<br>• Severe cardiomyopathy | • Thallium stress test or coronary angiogram<br>• Cardiology consult<br>• Gastric emptying study<br>• Ophthalmology evaluation<br>• Endocrine studies: glycosylated hemoglobin, serum amylase and lipase, islet cell antibody, urine, and serum peptide measurements |
| Heart | • Cardiac disease, New York Heart Association Class IV (or advanced III)<br>• Condition not amenable to other forms of medical or surgical therapy<br>• End-stage cardiac disease with less than a 25% likelihood of survival at 1 y without a transplant<br>• Patients with potentially fatal dysrhythmia not amenable to other therapies | • Fixed pulmonary hypertension with pulmonary vascular resistance: more than 6–8 Wood units (more than 480–640 dynes/s/cm$^{-5}$ or pulmonary arteriolar gradient greater than 15 mm)<br>• Recent unresolved pulmonary infarct (increased posttransplant risk for pulmonary infection)<br>• Advanced or poorly controlled diabetes mellitus | • Right heart catheterization; full cardiac catheterization if indicated<br>• Cardiopulmonary exercise testing (MVO$_2$)<br>• Pulmonary function tests, including diffusion capacity (DLCO)<br>• Cardiac rehabilitation consultation<br>• Multigated acquisition (MUGA) analysis or echocardiogram |
| Lung | • Untreatable end-stage pulmonary disease (parenchymal or vascular)<br>• Medical therapy ineffective<br>• Estimated survival (without lung transplant) less than probability of survival with lung transplant | • Significant coronary artery disease<br>• Poor nutritional status (ie, less than 10%–15% of ideal body weight)<br>• Previous cardiothoracic surgery<br>• Corticosteroid use more than 15 mg/d<br>• Ventilation dependency | • Quantitative ventilation/perfusion scan<br>• Cardiac evaluation<br>• Full pulmonary function testing, including DLCO, arterial blood gases (ABGs), lung volume<br>• 6-min walk test (rehabilitation assessment)<br>• Nutritional assessment |

*(continued)*

**TABLE 47-3** Criteria, Contraindications, and Evaluations in Transplantation (*continued*)

| Organ | Specific Criteria | Contraindications | Specific Evaluation |
|---|---|---|---|
| Hematopoietic stem cells | • *Malignant disorders*: replacement of hematopoietic and immune system destroyed by high-dose chemotherapy or radiation with new immune system that can recognize malignant cells as foreign and mount immunologic response against tumor<br>• *Nonmalignant disorders*: replacement of an immune or hematopoietic system that is either defective or has failed | • Poor or no response to conventional-dose chemotherapy for malignant disorders (exception is acute leukemia that fails to respond to induction therapy [primary induction failure]; high-dose chemotherapy and allogeneic transplant is an accepted indication)<br>• Poor performance status (using Karnofsky Performance Status scale to assess physical functioning)<br>• Advanced cardiopulmonary or renal disease (left ventricular ejection fraction less than 50%; DLCO less than 70; creatinine clearance, 60 mL/min [exception may be multiple myeloma patients])<br>• Brain metastasis<br>• Age greater than 70 y | • Disease restaging, including CT scans, nuclear medicine scans, bone marrow aspirate and biopsy, lumbar puncture, immunoglobulin levels, cytogenetics, molecular diagnostics, and measures of minimal residual disease<br>• DNA procurement for future engraftment studies<br>• ABO and Rh typing<br>• Human leukocyte antigen (HLA) typing and HLA-matched platelet transfusion support (allogeneic transplant patients only)<br>• Chest x-ray, ECG and MUGA scan, pulmonary function tests, including DLCO, 24-h urine for creatinine clearance<br>• Baseline CT scans of chest and sinuses, particularly if there are symptoms or a history of repeated infections<br>• Dental evaluation, including full mouth x-rays and cleaning<br>• Fertility preservation<br>• Autologous stem cell backup if patient is undergoing unrelated or mismatched transplantation<br>• Consultations with radiation therapy and infectious disease |

major histocompatibility complex involved in the immune response includes class I antigens (A, B) and class II (DR) antigens. Class I antigens (HLAs) are present on the surface of all nucleated cells and platelets, whereas class II antigens are found on the surface of lymphocytes. Each person has six A-, B-, and DR-locus antigens that are inherited as a haplotype (ie, a single unit), receiving one HLA haplotype from each parent. Individuals have two HLA haplotypes, one for each chromosome. Offspring then share one haplotype with each parent, and on average, there is a one in four chance that they will share both haplotypes with at least one of their siblings. There is also a one in four chance that they will share neither haplotype with their siblings. Many possible alleles occur at each locus, resulting in a large number of HLA combinations. Therefore, it is rare that unrelated people have identical antigens.

The higher the number of antigens that match, the higher the likelihood of compatibility, and the lower the risk for rejection. A six-antigen match is associated with the greatest potential for successful transplantation. HLA matching is performed for both solid organ and hematopoietic stem cell transplants. It is most important in kidney and stem cell transplantation. Transplantation requires the suppression of the normal immune response with the postoperative administration of antirejection medications to prevent graft rejection. The greater the similarity of the donor and recipient tissue type, the less likely the occurrence of rejection.

In the case of living related donors, a direct white blood cell (WBC) cross-match may be performed. The sera of the donor and the recipient are tested and evaluated for cell death. For those patients not receiving living related donation, screening is routinely performed against a pool of lymphocyte samples from multiple random donors against the sera of the recipient. The percentage of samples to which the recipient reacts is referred to as the panel reactive antibody (PRA) percentage. A high PRA is predictive of a high risk for rejection, and a prospective cross-match, such as is used in living donors, would be advised. PRA should be repeated monthly because the titer may change from time to time.

Blood transfusions are avoided if possible in patients awaiting organ transplantation because of the risk for antibody production and a resultant high PRA or positive cross-match between donor and recipient. If blood transfusions are necessary, leukocyte-filtered blood should be administered.

## Hematopoietic Stem Cell Transplantation

Selection of a donor for HSCT is based on the type and stage of the underlying disease, age, comorbidities, and availability of an appropriate HLA- and MLC-matched donor. MLC matching is performed to observe for interaction between the potential donor's cells and recipient cells. Low reactivity indicates greater compatibility.

There are many sources of hematopoietic stem cells. The types of HSCT may be differentiated in terms of the hematopoietic stem cell donor, the method used to collect the cells, and the intensity of the conditioning regimen (Box 47-1).

---

> **BOX 47-1** Types of Hematopoietic Stem Cell Transplantation
>
> Differentiated based on *donor* source for stem cells
> Autologous—self
> Syngeneic—identical twin
> Allogeneic—nonself
> - Related
> - Unrelated (National Marrow Donor Program)
> Cord blood
> - Related
> - Unrelated (cord blood bank)
> Differentiated based on *method* of collecting stem cell
> - Bone marrow harvest
> - Peripheral blood stem cell collection by apheresis
> Differentiated based on *intensity* of conditioning regimen
> - Myeloablative: high doses of chemotherapy and sometimes radiation therapy given to destroy hematopoietic and immune systems of recipient. Transplantation of new stem cells allows hematopoietic and immune reconstitution. High morbidity and mortality rates restrict this treatment to younger patients and those in good medical condition.
> - Reduced intensity: lower chemotherapy doses (those that do not fully destroy patient's own hematopoietic and immune systems) are given along with immunosuppression to facilitate engraftment of donor hematopoietic cells. Significant long-term risks for infection and chronic graft-versus-host disease (GVHD) persist.

For patients who receive hematopoietic stem cells from another person (ie, allogeneic transplant), donor selection is based on the availability of HLA- and MLC-matched donors, who may or may not be related. A related donor is usually a sibling (siblings have the greatest chance of matching on both HLA and on other minor and as yet unrecognized antigens). If more than one donor is HLA-identical to the patient, donor selection is based on sex compatibility with the patient, ABO compatibility with the patient, negative viral titers, overall health, younger donor age, minimal donor exposure to blood products, and donor nulliparity because all these factors are associated with an improved outcome of HSCT.

If the patient does not have a suitable family donor, a search for an unrelated donor may be undertaken. The National Marrow Donor Program (NMDP) is a federally funded registry that coordinates the donor search and matching process. The NMDP maintains the world's largest and most diverse registry of more than 6 million volunteer blood stem cell donors and more than 60,000 cord blood units donated by parents after their infant's birth. Umbilical cord blood is another potential stem cell source, particularly in pediatric allogeneic transplantation. The NMDP also works with the American Red Cross and with international registries to access 4 million additional donors and cord blood units around the world.

A difference in ABO blood groups between patient and donor does not interfere with donor selection; however, it does present unique clinical problems. The hematopoietic stem cell product may have to be depleted of red blood cells (RBCs) to prevent, during infusion, a hemolytic reaction caused by ABO antibodies still circulating in the patient's bloodstream. After engraftment and approximately 100 days after transplantation, the patient will seroconvert to the ABO type of the donor.

## Living Donors

Since the beginning of transplantation, there has been a dire shortage of available suitable donor organs. While the numbers of transplantation candidates continue to grow, the numbers of cadaveric organ donors remain relatively constant. In an effort to address the widening disparity between the demand and supply of adequate organs, there has been an increase in the use of living donor organs.[6] Living donors are increasingly being used in kidney, liver, pancreas, and lung transplantation. Living donors are used exclusively in HSCT.

Once identified, a potential donor has a thorough medical evaluation to determine that the organ functions normally, there is no underlying disease, and donation would not jeopardize the donor's well-being in any obvious way. After successful completion of this evaluation, a living donor transplantation may occur.

People continue to raise ethical questions about the use of living donors. Long-term studies of living donors have shown that the risks and adverse effects of donation are rare, and, in fact, some donors report beneficial psychological effects from donating. However, some question the risk of coercion in living donors, especially when the donor is the parent of a child who will die without transplantation. To ensure freely given and informed consent, there may be an assessment by a psychiatrist and involvement of a non–transplant-related physician, together with education and counseling of the donor.

### Kidney Donor

Historically, living donors have been blood relatives because tissue matching was considered more likely. However, more recently, living kidney donors have been spouses and friends, and the results have been comparable with those obtained with living blood-related donors. Although either kidney may be used for transplantation, the left is preferred because the left renal vein is longer than the right.[7]

### Liver Donor

Living donor liver transplantation involves the removal of a portion of the liver from a living adult for transplantation into a recipient. The 1-year graft survival rate in the United States is 97%.[5]

### Pancreas Donor

Transplanting part of the pancreas from a living person is rarely performed. The donor must not be at risk for diabetes mellitus.

### Lung Donor

Recently, the use of living related donors in lung transplantation has been successful. Either the lobe of one lung from one parent is transplanted into the child, or one lobe from each parent is used for a bilateral lobar transplantation. The major advantage of lobar transplantation is that it enables children to have the transplantation either at a time when they are in the best condition or when they become critically ill and a cadaveric donor is unavailable.

# Cadaveric Donors

If a cadaveric donor is needed, the recipient is placed on the national waiting list. The National Organ Transport Act was designed to improve the organ matching and placement process. The act outlawed the sale of human organs and authorized grants to establish and operate organ procurement organizations (OPOs). The United States is divided into approximately 60 areas; an OPO is responsible for recovering and transporting organs to transplantation hospitals in each area. The United Network for Organ Sharing (UNOS) is the private, nonprofit organization that administers organ waiting lists and allocates organs throughout the United States on behalf of the recipients.

Patients are placed on the UNOS national list based on blood type and listing date. The size of hearts, lungs, and livers is important for donation. The waiting time varies by organ. Patients awaiting heart transplantation are risk stratified based on condition and classified according to status. Those awaiting heart transplantation who require inotropic medications or ventricular assist devices may have a higher priority (status 1) than those waiting at home on stable oral heart failure medications (status 2). Patients awaiting lung transplantation are ranked using a new UNOS-developed lung allocation system that uses medical information specific to each patient to estimate the severity of illness and chance of success following transplantation. The UNOS score is used to prioritize recipients who are awaiting a lung transplant. A candidate with a higher lung allocation score receives higher priority for a lung offer when a compatible lung becomes available.[4,5] Patients awaiting liver transplantation are also risk stratified based on the model for end-stage liver disease (MELD) score. Status rankings 1, 2A, 2B, and 3 are used based on the severity of the disease process. A patient who is projected to live less than 7 days without transplantation is status 1, whereas a patient who is living at home with chronic liver disease is status 3.[8–10]

Despite the continued need for transplantations, the supply of donor organs remains inadequate. Currently, according to UNOS, about 122,446 patients are awaiting organ transplantation in the United States. The Scientific Registry of Transplant Recipients reported in 2012, there were 28,051 organ donors; this number includes living and deceased donors.[4,11] Lack of consent to a request for donation is the primary cause of the gap between the number of potential donors and the numbers of actual donors. The donation rate is calculated as the number of eligible donors per 100 eligible deaths. In 2011, 72.9 eligible donors per 100 eligible deaths were converted to organ donors.[4]

A major factor in the discrepancy between potential and actual donors is lack of education for potential donor families.[12] When a patient is determined to be brain dead, or support is withdrawn from a patient who is not brain dead, many hospitals alert the local OPO as a matter of policy. In some larger institutions, a nurse with advanced training in the area of organ donation and family support is trained as a donor advocate. The role of this nurse is to support the family in the grieving process while initiating the discussion of organ donation. It is important that all potential organ donors be identified. Often, potential donors are victims of trauma, cerebral aneurysm, or a variety of other circumstances. Potential donors may be precluded from donating solid organs for reasons, such as advanced age, infection, or coma, though such donors may be considered for donation of the cornea, skin, or cardiovascular tissue (such as heart valves or portions of the aorta).

## Determination of Death

With current technology, death can be determined in two ways. The absence of cardiopulmonary function is the better-known method; however, the absence of brain function (brain death) also is a common method of determining death (see Chapter 36 for neurologic criteria for determining death). Most patients who are organ donors are pronounced dead based on the absence of brain function. The critical care nurse should be familiar with the laws in his or her state related to "brain death" and with the institutional policies for the determination of death.

## Role of the Nurse

Critical care nurses are an integral part of the organ donation team. Almost all organ donors die in critical care units; therefore, the critical care nurse is a key person in identifying potential donors. Moreover, the nurse plays an important role as advocate by making certain that all efforts are made to determine and act on the patient's wishes regarding donation. Nurses also play a vital role in supporting the family psychologically, particularly when they are trying to accept the donor's death. The role of the donor coordinator has developed to allow a nurse with specialized skills to interact with the potential donor's family during the process and to provide support for the nursing staff caring for the donor. When a decision is made for organ donation, the nurse also plays an important role in supporting the donor physiologically.

The care of the potential donor, once identified, becomes the responsibility of the OPO. A nurse who is specially trained to maintain hemodynamic stability of the donor works with the bedside nurse to care for the patient. It is essential to maintain hemodynamic stability so that the vital organs are perfused adequately.

Given the massive hemodynamic shifts seen following brain death, hemodynamic management occurs in two phases. In the first phase, hemodynamic surges consequent to endogenous catecholamine mobilization produce hypotension. Short-acting agents, such as nitroprusside or esmolol, which are easily titrated and have a short duration of action, are used to control blood pressure and heart rate.

Phase 2 begins after depletion of catecholamine stores, at which time the donor experiences a dramatic fall in blood pressure. Initial intervention in phase 2 involves rapid replacement of circulating blood volume with crystalloid or colloid intravenous (IV) fluids. Aggressive fluid resuscitation in this phase must account for the relative fluid volume deficit produced by a vasodilatory state from endogenous catecholamine depletion as well as the systemic inflammatory response.[6,13] The goal of blood pressure management in phase 2 should be to sustain a mean arterial pressure of 70 mm Hg. Recommended pharmacologic therapy for vasopressor support includes dopamine or dobutamine, with target doses of less than 10 mcg/kg/min if the focus is cardiac donation. In other instances, norepinephrine may be used, with a target dose of 0.5 to 5.0 mcg/min. The administration of vasopressors and inotropes, in addition to providing cardiovascular support for the organ donor, promotes a lower incidence of kidney rejection and better long-term graft survival.[13,14] As the need for vasopressors and inotropes increases, the possibility for multiorgan recovery decreases.

Optimal pulmonary management, including suctioning for airway clearance and aspiration precautions, is necessary. Ventilator management should include close titration of fluids to minimize the risk for pulmonary edema. Positive end-expiratory pressure should be less than 5 cm $H_2O$, and peak airway pressures should be maintained at less than 30 mm Hg if possible. Ventilation with tidal volumes of 10.0 to 12.0 mL/kg may maintain minute ventilation and attenuate risk for barotrauma.[13]

It is also essential to assess urine output hourly to detect diabetes insipidus. This is common in organ donors and is caused by failure of the posterior pituitary to produce or release antidiuretic hormones. This can lead to electrolyte imbalances. It may be necessary to order aqueous vasopressin or desmopressin acetate to reduce urine output and help maintain fluid balance.

Laboratory results, such as electrolytes, CBC, liver and renal function tests, and arterial blood gases (ABGs) values, are necessary to assess organ function and determine appropriate intervention. An ECG and echocardiogram are required for heart donation. Serial chest radiographs, bronchoscopy, sputum for Gram stain and visual inspection at the time of organ procurement are required for lung donation.

### Role of the Donor Coordinator

The role of the donor coordinator developed as a result of the disparity between potential donors and the numbers of patients awaiting organ donation. The donor coordinator, usually a nurse, introduces the concept of organ donation to the family; this approach results in the highest rates of consent.[15] The donor coordinator is involved in coordinating and procuring all transplantable organs. (Kidneys are the most commonly transplanted organ; heart, lung, liver, pancreas, intestine, cornea, skin, bone, and other organs or tissue may also be donated.) In addition, the donor coordinator usually ensures that the family has the information necessary to give informed consent and provides them with access to bereavement support. The donor coordinator also serves as a resource for the health care team and as a liaison between the transplantation program and the critical care area. Cooperation between the critical care staff and the transplantation program helps ensure that the option of donation is offered to families of all potential donors.

### Preservation Time

Cells rapidly switch from aerobic to anaerobic metabolism in the absence of circulation. During anaerobic metabolism, more glucose substrate is required to generate adenosine triphosphate (ATP) than aerobic metabolism. Subsequently, the result is rapid consumption of energy substrate, depletion of intracellular energy stores, and accumulation of metabolites and lactic acid. The purpose of organ preservation is to prevent arrest these changes as quickly as possible.[6]

There is a broad range of acceptable preservation times for organs. However, the goal is to transplant organs as soon as possible. Kidneys can be stored for up to 48 hours using pulsatile perfusion preservation and for 24 to 36 hours using cold storage. Livers can be stored for up to 20 hours, pancreas

up to 12 hours, and hearts and lungs for 4 to 6 hours. To decrease cellular injury, organs are stored in a solution and kept in ice. The preservative solutions used are different for each organ and are based on the metabolic needs of the organ, with center-specific variability. The focus of preservation is to protect the organ from ischemic injury.[5,13]

## Organ Transplantation: Assessment and Management

The role of the transplant coordinator extends across the continuum of care from pre–evaluation of potential recipients through transplantation and follow-up. This person is responsible for coordinating the evaluation and teaching the recipient and family about the evaluation testing process, the listing process, and organ allocation. A major contribution is reviewing preoperative through postoperative procedures, the immunosuppressive regimen, and follow-up care. In many institutions, a nurse practitioner, who also provides medical care and follow-up for the patients, fulfills this role.

### Preoperative Phase

The immediate preoperative phase, which usually occurs within the few hours after an organ becomes available, includes comprehensive laboratory studies, chest radiograph, ECG, and, for kidney transplant recipients, dialysis within 24 hours of transplantation. Laboratory studies usually include CBC, prothrombin time (PT), partial thromboplastin time (PTT), electrolytes, blood glucose, blood urea nitrogen (BUN), creatinine, liver function tests, type and cross-match, and urinalysis.

### Surgical Procedure

#### Kidney

Typically, the kidney is placed retroperitoneally in the iliac fossa. The hypogastric or internal artery and the external iliac vein are usually used for vascular anastomosis. When it is mechanically difficult to access these vessels, as with children, it may be necessary to anastomose the renal vessels to the inferior vena cava and aorta.

Two common types of ureteral anastomoses can be performed. In the first procedure, the donor ureter is implanted into the recipient's bladder by a vertical cystotomy and a submucosal antireflux tunnel because the ureter lacks innervation and normal peristalsis. In the second type, used less frequently, the donor kidney is anastomosed at the ureteropelvic junction to the recipient ureter. An indwelling catheter is used for both types of anastomoses, and occasionally, a ureteral stent may be used. In either case, hematuria is present for several days. In the first, more common procedure, clots may be seen in the urine because of the vascular nature of the bladder. In the second, less common, procedure, the urine changes to pink within the first postoperative day because there are no sutures in the bladder.

#### Liver

The liver is transplanted orthotopically, that is, in its normal position after the native liver is removed. Four vascular anastomoses must be performed: the suprahepatic vena cava, the infrahepatic vena cava, the portal vein, and the hepatic artery (Fig. 47-1). Then the liver is reperfused, and the bile duct is anastomosed, usually to the recipient bile duct.[16] A T-tube is usually inserted. During liver transplantation, a rapid infusion system is used for administering blood and blood products, a cell saver is often used to limit the amount of banked blood required, and a pump for venovenous bypass is often used in adults to return blood to the heart. This is performed by inserting a catheter into the saphenous or femoral vein and another into the axillary vein (usually on the left side), which allows blood to circulate from the lower extremities back to the heart. Surgery usually takes between 8 and 16 hours.

### Heart

Procedures for heart transplantation include orthotopic and heterotopic approaches. Orthotopic transplantation involves replacing the damaged heart with the donor heart. With heterotopic transplantation, the patient's own heart is not removed. The donor heart is positioned so that the chambers and blood vessels of both hearts can be connected, thus allowing the donor heart to assist the damaged heart.

**ORTHOTOPIC TRANSPLANTATION.** Orthotopic heart transplantation (OHT) is the most common heart transplantation performed. The surgeon excises the recipient's heart and implants the donor heart in its place. A median sternotomy incision is made, cardiopulmonary bypass is initiated, and the recipient's heart is removed by incising the left and right atria, pulmonary artery, and aorta. The Lower and Shumway technique has been the gold standard for OHT. The atrial septum and posterior and lateral walls of the recipient's atria are left intact, including the areas of the sinoatrial node, inferior and superior venae cavae to the right atrium, and pulmonary veins to the left atrium. The remnant atria serve as anchors for the donor heart.

The donor atria are trimmed to preserve the anterior arterial walls, sinoatrial node, and internodal conduction pathways. Then anastomoses are made between the recipient and donor left and right atria, the pulmonary arteries, and the

aortas. Atrial and ventricular pacing wires are placed at the time of surgery so that temporary pacing can easily be initiated. Cardiopulmonary bypass is weaned off, and the donor heart assumes the role of providing the cardiac output (Fig. 47-2A).

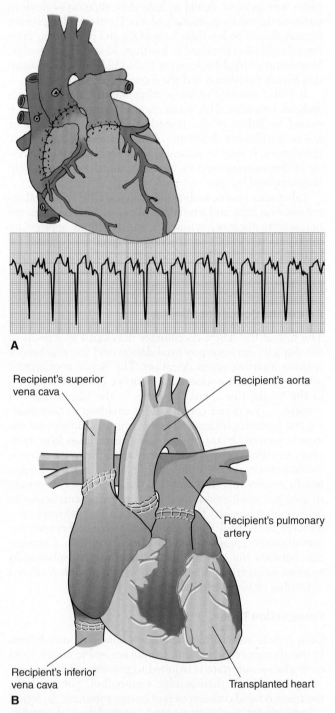

**A**

**B**

FIGURE 47-2 Orthotopic method of transplantation. **A:** Lower and Shumway technique. Both the donor and the recipient sinoatrial nodes are intact (X), resulting in the electrocardiogram (ECG) tracing. Note the double P wave at the independent rates. **B:** Bicaval technique. The anastomoses are made between the inferior and superior venae cavae rather than the atria. (**B** from Smeltzer SC, Bare BG, Hinkle JL, et al: Brunner and Suddarth's Textbook of Medical-Surgical Nursing, 12th ed. Philadelphia, PA: Lippincott Williams & Wilkins, 2010, p 811.)

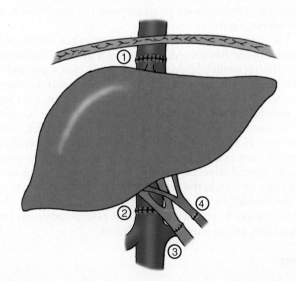

FIGURE 47-1 Diagram of vascular anastomoses in liver transplantation: (1) suprahepatic vena cava, (2) infrahepatic vena cava, (3) portal vein, and (4) hepatic artery.

An alternative to the atrial-to-atrial cuff technique is the bicaval technique (see Fig. 47-2B), which preserves atrial anatomy disrupted by the Lower and Shumway technique. The donor atria are intact, and the anastomoses are between the donor and recipient inferior and superior venae cavae rather than the atria. This avoids the loss of atrial anatomy, which has been responsible for the development of posttransplantation complications, such as mitral and tricuspid regurgitation, atrial thrombus formation, and tachydysrhythmia.[17,18]

### HETEROTOPIC TRANSPLANTATION.
Heterotopic transplantation, or piggyback procedure, is an infrequently used technique. The recipient's heart is left in place, and the donor heart is placed next to it in the right chest. The two hearts are connected in parallel by anastomoses made between the donor and recipient left and right atria, aortas, and pulmonary arteries using a synthetic tube graft. By allowing blood to flow through either or both hearts, two functional hearts work together to provide the cardiac output (Fig. 47-3).

Heterotopic transplantation may be used in patients with pulmonary hypertension in whom the donor heart alone would not have a strong enough right ventricle to pump against the increased pulmonary vascular resistance. It can also be used as a lifesaving procedure in urgent cases if the only available donor heart is too small for the size of the recipient. Limitations of heterotopic transplantation include thromboembolism from the native heart with need for anticoagulation, limited space in the chest cavity, and, in ischemic heart disease, ongoing angina and the possibility of

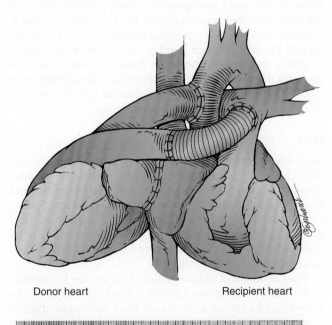

Donor heart                          Recipient heart

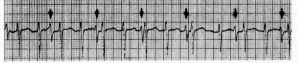

**FIGURE 47-3**  Heterotopic method of heart transplantation. The donor heart is anastomosed with a Dacron graft to the recipient's heart, resulting in this ECG tracing. Note the "extra" QRS at an independent rate. (From Smeltzer SC, Bare BG: Brunner and Suddarth's Textbook of Medical-Surgical Nursing, 10th ed. Philadelphia, PA: Lippincott Williams & Wilkins, 2004, p 775.)

ischemia-induced dysrhythmias in the native heart. The survival rates are less favorable for heterotopic transplantation than for orthotopic transplantation.

### Pancreas

Transplantation of the entire pancreas is performed most commonly. Pancreas transplantation may be performed in combination with kidney transplantation for recipients with end-stage renal disease secondary to diabetes mellitus. The pancreas and kidney may be transplanted at the same time or months apart. Clinical trials are ongoing to determine the feasibility and outcomes of islet cell transplantation for patients with type 1 diabetes not controlled with insulin. With this experimental procedure, only the insulin-producing islet cells are transplanted. The recipient still requires immunosuppressive medications to prevent rejection.

The pancreas is placed into a heterotopic position, usually the right iliac area. Techniques vary for vascular and exocrine anastomoses. The most controversial aspect of the surgical technique is the approach for draining exocrine secretions. The exocrine duct may be occluded, or exocrine secretions may drain either into the small bowel or bladder. There is no consensus about the best approach, and all have advantages and disadvantages.

### Lung

Both single- and double-lung transplantations are performed. In single-lung transplantations, the left lung mainstem bronchus is longer, which makes the procedure easier technically. The preferred lung is based on perfusion abnormalities (as determined by ventilation–perfusion scan) and functional abnormalities. Anastomoses are made at the mainstem bronchus, pulmonary artery, and cuff of atrium containing pulmonary veins. Cardiopulmonary bypass is not always necessary and depends on the patient's pulmonary artery pressure, blood pressure, and gas exchange. Incision is made at the fifth intracostal space using a posterior lateral thoracotomy for single-lung transplantations, whereas a median sternotomy incision or a clamshell incision is made for double-lung transplantations. Surgeons telescope the recipient's bronchus into the donor lung or vice versa, or perform an end-to-end anastomosis with omentopexy in which an omental flap is wrapped around the tracheal anastomosis to increase blood supply to the area.

### Postoperative Phase

Immediately after surgery, transplant recipients require care in a closely monitored area until their condition stabilizes. Kidney transplant recipients often go to a postanesthesia care unit and then directly to a transplant unit. Other organ recipients go to an intensive care unit (ICU) from the operating room.

When a patient arrives in the postanesthesia or intensive care area, the nurse makes the following assessments:

• Blood pressure, heart rate, respirations, oxygenation and ventilator settings, temperature, central venous pressure, and cardiopulmonary hemodynamics. In renal transplant recipients, it is necessary to take blood pressure on an extremity that does not have a functioning vascular access site because even momentary interference with arterial blood flow may lead to access malfunction.

- Patient's level of consciousness and degree of pain
- Number of IV and arterial lines, noting the site, type of solution, and flow rate
- Abdominal or chest dressing for drainage, noting the presence of drains and amount and type of drainage
- Presence of bladder and possible ureteral catheters and patency and urinary drainage
- Attachment of nasogastric tube to appropriate drainage system and amount and character of drainage
- Most recent hemodynamic and intraoperative laboratory results

### Kidney

Care of the kidney transplant recipient emphasizes assessing renal function and administering immunosuppressive therapy. Therefore, answers to the following questions help guide care:

- Are the patient's own kidneys present in addition to the graft, and if so, how much urine do they produce daily? This information helps determine how much urine is from the transplanted kidney.
- What are the preoperative results of laboratory tests (BUN, creatinine, hematocrit)?
- How much and what kind of IV fluid has the patient received?
- What immunosuppressive drugs were given before or during surgery? What immunosuppressive therapy should be given after surgery?

Nursing responsibilities also involve the following:

- Observing the function of the transplanted kidney
- Monitoring fluid and electrolyte balance
- Helping avoid sources of infection
- Detecting early signs of complications
- Supporting the patient and family through the recovery phase

In addition, at regular intervals, the nurse evaluates the patency and the vascular access used for dialysis. This is done by placing either fingers or a stethoscope directly over the access site and feeling or listening for a characteristically loud, pulsating noise called a *bruit*. If the patient has been maintained on peritoneal dialysis and the catheter is in place, it is essential that the catheter system is sterile and capped.

**RENAL GRAFT FUNCTION.** The amount of urine produced by the transplanted kidney varies from a large amount (200 to 1,000 mL/h) to small amounts (less than 20 mL/h). The degree of renal function is related to ischemic injury in the donor kidney, usually from either hypotensive periods in a cadaveric donor or from the time the kidney is stored outside the body (preservation time). Renal function is better when kidney preservation time is less than 24 hours. Most posttransplantation dysfunction is reversible but may take up to 4 weeks to return to normal.

Assessments of renal function include periodic BUN and creatinine levels and, in some centers, a $\beta_2$-microglobulin level. The glomerular basement membrane readily filters this low–molecular-weight globulin, which the proximal renal tubules reabsorb and metabolize almost completely.

A renal scan is a radionuclide test used to determine renal perfusion, filtration, and excretion. It is usually performed in the first 24 hours to obtain baseline data and then periodically thereafter when laboratory values or clinical changes suggest an alteration in renal function.

**URINARY DRAINAGE PROBLEMS.** When a change in urinary output occurs, such as a large volume in 1 hour and a diminished amount in the next, mechanical factors that interfere with urinary drainage should be suspected. Clotted, kinked, or compressed tubing in the urinary drainage system may be the cause of the decreased output. When the catheter is occluded by a clot, the patient may complain of pain, feel an urgency to void, or have bloody leakage around the catheter. Milking is the preferred way to dislodge clots because irrigation, even under aseptic conditions, increases the risk for infection. However, gentle irrigation with strict aseptic technique may be necessary. Small amounts of irrigant (30 mL or less) are recommended because patients commonly have small bladders. Vigorous irrigation also could cause extravasation at the ureteral anastomosis site.

**URINARY LEAKAGE.** Urinary leakage on the abdominal dressing and severe abdominal discomfort or distention may indicate retroperitoneal leakage from the ureteral anastomosis site. It is important to report decreased urinary output or severe abdominal pain in the presence of good renal function and adequate pain medication because technical and surgical complications can result in loss of graft function.

**HYPERKALEMIA.** The most frequent electrolyte disturbance in the acute postoperative phase is hyperkalemia. If the graft functions and excretes a high volume of urine, it is usually also able to excrete the excessive serum potassium created by surgical tissue damage. If the patient is oliguric or anuric after surgery, the serum potassium may increase to unacceptable levels. Interventions include administration of glucose and insulin to transport potassium into the cell and administration of oral polystyrene sulfonate.

### Liver

Immediate postoperative care focuses on hemodynamic stability, adequate oxygenation, fluid and electrolyte balance, adequate hemostasis, and graft function. An arterial line and pulmonary artery catheter are in place. The pulmonary artery catheter readings help monitor cardiac function and fluid status because high cardiac output and low systemic vascular resistance related to the effects of end-stage liver disease continue immediately after surgery.

Vasopressors and additional fluid boluses may be required in the first 24 to 36 hours. Central venous pressure should be maintained at greater than 10 cm $H_2O$ to balance the importance of good cardiac function against the risk for passive congestion of the liver. Hypotension is most often caused by intra-abdominal bleeding. An increase in abdominal girth or excess bloody drainage from Jackson–Pratt drains is indicative of a severe problem.

**OXYGENATION.** Adequate ventilation is crucial for graft perfusion and helps reduce the risk for pulmonary complications. The critical care team determines ventilator settings, and the nurse monitors the arterial ($SaO_2$) and mixed venous

($SvO_2$) oxygen saturations. Pulse oximetry may be used, but severe jaundice may interfere with saturation measurements. Postoperative pleural effusion is common owing to the presence of ascites and risk of injury to the diaphragm during surgery. A chest tube may be required for drainage.

Ventilator support is usually withdrawn when the patient is fully awake. However, if the patient is going to receive a monoclonal antibody, such as muromonab-CD3, the first dose should be given before extubation because there is a risk for pulmonary edema as a reaction to the medication.

**COAGULATION.** Abnormal clotting factors, bleeding at the site of anastomosis, and impaired graft function may all contribute to problems with hemostasis. Therefore, the nurse monitors PT, PTT, fibrinogen, and factor V level along with the amount, color, and consistency of bleeding from the incision and drainage tubes.

The patient may need infusions of platelets, RBCs, or cryoprecipitate. Blood products should be leukocyte reduced to avoid introduction of CMV, especially if the patient is negative for CMV. It is necessary to take care to avoid overcorrecting coagulation deficiencies, which could lead to vascular thrombosis of the extremities or the graft. As a result of the venovenous bypass system, there is also a risk for phlebitis or thrombosis in the femoral and axillary access site. This may be indicated by ipsilateral swelling in these extremities. Anticoagulation or an inferior vena cava filter may be necessary if deep venous thrombosis develops.

**ELECTROLYTE BALANCE.** Hyperglycemia; hyperkalemia; metabolic alkalosis; and calcium, phosphorus, and magnesium disorders may occur. Hyperglycemia is an indication that the liver is able to store glycogen and convert it to glucose. Hyperkalemia can indicate nonfunctional hepatocytes and, in turn, a nonfunctional graft. Metabolic alkalosis is related to the citrate in stored blood (metabolized to bicarbonate), hypokalemia, diuretic therapy, and the administration of large volumes of fresh frozen plasma. This usually resolves spontaneously, but hypoventilation in response to the alkalosis may slow weaning from mechanical ventilation. Calcium, phosphorus, and magnesium disturbances primarily result from the administration of fluid and blood products.

Some degree of postoperative renal dysfunction is also common due either to hepatorenal syndrome or hypotension during surgery. In addition, some immunosuppressive medications are nephrotoxic. This can affect fluid and electrolyte balance. On occasion, when dialysis is needed, continuous arteriovenous or venovenous hemofiltration is used because it interferes least with hemodynamic stability.

**LIVER FUNCTION.** Function of the transplanted liver can range from excellent to primary nonfunction. Although the cause of primary nonfunction is not known, it is believed to be related to preservation injury, and retransplantation is necessary. Liver function is initially assessed by bile production, coagulation factors, and later by liver function tests. Measuring bile production from the biliary drainage tube helps assess the excretory function of the liver and is a good early indicator of graft function. PT and the international normalized ratio (INR) provide a measure of the synthetic function of the liver. Aminotransferases (alanine aminotransferase and aspartate aminotransferase) provide information about the degree of hepatic injury related to preservation. In addition, improvement in the clearance of lactate, encephalopathy, and glucose metabolism are also assessments of liver function. All liver function test results are elevated initially and gradually decrease.

## Heart

Postoperative care of the heart transplant recipient is similar to that for any person undergoing cardiac surgery. However, there are several major differences, including changes in cardiac rhythm and function caused by denervation of the donor heart and the potential for right ventricular failure. Only the more common orthotopic transplantation is discussed here.

**REMNANT P WAVES.** In the standard atrial cuff technique, the recipient sinoatrial node and portions of the recipient atria are left intact at the time of surgery. Therefore, two P waves are usually seen on the ECG. The recipient sinoatrial node initiates an impulse that depolarizes the remnant recipient atria; however, this depolarization wave usually does not cross the atrial suture line. The donor sinoatrial node initiates the impulse that causes depolarization of the entire donor heart and elicits the QRS complex. Because the two sets of atria beat independently of each other, two different P waves may appear on the ECG. Remnant P waves may be identified by their dissociation or lack of relationship to the QRS complexes. They usually occur at a slower rate than the donor P waves, and their rate may speed up or slow down because the remnant P waves are still under autonomic nervous system influence, whereas the donor P waves are denervated. The two sets of atria may also be in different rhythms. For example, the recipient atrial remnants may be in atrial fibrillation while the donor heart is in normal sinus rhythm.

**EFFECTS OF DENERVATION.** During removal of the donor heart, the nerve supply is severed, resulting in a lack of autonomic nervous system innervation of the transplanted heart. Because of the loss of vagal influence, the resting sinus rate is higher than normal—usually between 90 and 110 beats/min—and heart rate variations caused by respiration do not occur.

Decreased donor sinoatrial node automaticity can also occur after transplantation as a result of injury to the node during procurement, transport, surgical procedure, or postoperative edema of the atrial suture line. Usually, these problems resolve within 1 to 2 weeks after transplantation, but temporary pacing may be needed to maintain an adequate heart rate. Atropine, which blocks vagal stimulation, is ineffective in treating bradydysrhythmias in the transplanted heart because there is no parasympathetic innervation. If the sinus rate is reduced, junctional rhythms can occur earlier than normal because of the loss of vagal tone.

Normal cardiovascular reflexes are also removed by denervation. In the normal heart, the body's increased metabolic demands cause direct compensatory stimulation of the heart by the sympathetic nervous system, which immediately increases heart rate, contractility, and cardiac output. Because direct sympathetic nervous system stimulation of the transplanted heart is absent, this response is mediated through release of circulating catecholamines from the adrenal medulla. Therefore, increases in heart rate, contractility, and cardiac output occur much more slowly than normal. With exercise, heart rate and cardiac output increase gradually over 3 to 5 minutes and remain elevated longer after exercise. Prolonged warm-up before and cooldown after exercise help compensate for these changes.

Orthostatic hypotension can occur because the normal, immediate reflex tachycardia, which compensates for venous pooling with position change, does not occur. When patients begin ambulating, they should be cautioned to change position gradually to prevent orthostatic hypotension.

Because of denervation, the cardiac effects of medications normally mediated by the autonomic nervous system are abnormal. Atropine, which increases heart rate by blocking parasympathetic influence, is ineffective. Isoproterenol, a positive chronotropic agent, has been widely used because it stimulates myocardial receptors directly for pharmacologic management of symptomatic bradydysrhythmias. However, isoproterenol is not widely available. Instead, dobutamine and epinephrine, along with temporary epicardial pacing, are frequently used.

Digitalis preparations are ineffective in decreasing the heart rate or increasing the atrioventricular nodal refractory period because these effects are mediated primarily by the parasympathetic nervous system. Digitalis does increase myocardial contractility by its direct action on myocardial cells. Beta-blocking drugs or calcium channel blockers (eg, verapamil) can be used to control supraventricular tachydysrhythmias in the transplanted heart; carotid sinus pressure, the Valsalva maneuver, and digitalis are ineffective.

Finally, denervation prevents transmission of pain impulses from ischemic myocardium to the brain, so the patient does not experience angina. Severe myocardial ischemia or infarction may go unnoticed. For this reason, ECG stress testing and annual coronary angiography or coronary vascular ultrasonography are usually performed.

**POTENTIAL FOR VENTRICULAR FAILURE.** Posttransplantation ventricular failure, causing decreased cardiac output, occurs for the same reasons as in other cardiac surgical procedures. In addition, a prolonged ischemia time, inotropic support of the donor, or rejection can cause myocardial depression in a transplant recipient.

Right ventricular failure is the most common cause of primary graft failure after transplantation. Reasons for right-sided heart dysfunction are not entirely clear but are related to acute changes in pulmonary vascular resistance. The newly transplanted heart is required to work against elevated pulmonary pressures secondary to long-standing heart failure in the recipient. Postoperative changes in pH or ABGs can cause pulmonary vascular spasm. Both pulmonary hypertension and spasm increase the pulmonary vascular resistance or resistance to ejection of blood by the right ventricle. The normal right ventricle of the donor heart may be unable to increase its output acutely to overcome a high preexisting pulmonary vascular resistance. Signs of acute right ventricular failure include elevated central venous pressure and jugular venous distention. Left ventricular cardiac output decreases because the right ventricle is unable to pump enough blood through the lungs.

Treatment of posttransplantation right-sided heart failure involves the use of drugs to decrease right heart afterload (dobutamine, milrinone, inhaled nitric oxide). Inhaled nitric oxide, a direct pulmonary vasodilator, may be administered through the ventilator circuit, thereby avoiding the systemic effects of the drugs that are administered IV. Conditions that increase right heart afterload (eg, hypoxia, acidosis, excessive blood transfusions) should be avoided.

## Pancreas

The critical care of a pancreas transplant recipient is comparable to the critical care of any patient who has had major abdominal surgery. The differences relate to pancreatic function, the type of surgical procedure, and secondary effects of diabetes mellitus.

Blood glucose response usually returns within the first few postoperative hours; however, an insulin drip may be required until the blood glucose level is normal. Pancreatic function is monitored by glucose levels before and after meals, by the results of glycosylated hemoglobin, and sometimes by glucose tolerance testing. Even minor abnormalities may indicate rejection or vascular thrombosis of the graft.

When a section of duodenum is used for exocrine drainage, the prevention of infection is particularly challenging. Antibiotics are usually administered until the intraoperative culture of the duodenum is reported. When the bladder is used for exocrine drainage, bicarbonate wasting in the urine may occur. The standard method for pancreatic transplantation involves drainage of exocrine secretions into the urinary bladder with venous outflow into the systemic circulation. Despite the high success rate associated with this approach, it often leads to complications, which can include urinary tract infections, reflux pancreatitis, metabolic acidosis, and hyperinsulinemia. Depending on the patient's ability to void, the catheter may be needed for several days or possibly weeks if there is long-standing neurogenic bladder dysfunction secondary to diabetes mellitus. The surgical approach remains center and surgeon specific.

It is necessary to keep a nasogastric tube in place until bowel activity returns. This may take 3 to 5 days if there is diabetic gastroparesis. If the nasogastric tube remains in place, enteral or parenteral feedings may be necessary.

## Lung

On arrival to the ICU, the lung transplant recipient is anesthetized, intubated, and mechanically ventilated. Usually, extubation occurs 24 to 36 hours after surgery when the patient's oxygenation is optimized and secretions are minimal. Extubation usually proceeds more quickly in patients with emphysema and a single-lung transplant than in patients with pulmonary hypertension, who may need a longer intubation period.

The lung transplant recipient does not have a cough reflex because of denervation. Therefore, when suctioning, the nurse avoids inserting the catheter where it can cause damage. The surgical team performs frequent bronchoscopy to ensure intact anastomoses and pulmonary toileting. A common problem in the immediate posttransplantation period is pulmonary edema due to a phenomenon known as "reperfusion" injury. As a result, it is best to maintain the patient in a relatively hypovolemic state for the first few days. Diuresis begins when the patient is hemodynamically stable.

The lungs are constantly exposed to the outside world, and therefore prevention of infection is especially important after lung transplantation. Antibiotics are given prophylactically and are determined by donor cultures, preoperative serology results, and sputum samples. Patient care measures to prevent infection include giving oral care, encouraging physical activity early in the postoperative course, and performing daily respiratory and chest physiotherapy. Continuous pulse oximetry is used to monitor oxygen saturation, and daily chest radiographs help monitor progress. Infection control measures by staff include washing hands and using aseptic suctioning technique. Staff and visitors with active infections should avoid caring for or visiting the patients.

## Hematopoietic Stem Cell Transplantation: Assessment and Management

HSCT involves replacing diseased, destroyed, or nonfunctioning hematopoietic cells with healthy progenitor cells, also called stem cells. Stem cells are primitive hematopoietic cells capable of self-renewal; they are pluripotent, meaning that they are capable of maturation into an RBC, WBC, or platelet. These stem cells may be collected directly from the bone marrow spaces by a bone marrow harvest procedure, or from the peripheral blood, by apheresis. HSCT is an important advance in restoring hematopoietic function in patients whose bone marrow has been destroyed by high-dose chemotherapy and radiation therapy (see Table 47-1).

In both autologous and allogeneic HSCT, peripheral blood stem cells have become the preferred source of hematopoietic stem cells for grafting, although for selected allogeneic HSCT recipients, bone marrow grafting may offer specific advantages over peripheral blood stem cells.

Collection of cells through apheresis is easier and less costly and may also result in a more rapid recovery of neutrophil and platelet counts. In unrelated allogeneic transplantation, the source of stem cells may be either a bone marrow harvest procedure or a peripheral blood stem cell collection. Table 47-4 presents a detailed comparison of autologous and allogeneic stem cell transplantation. Box 47-2 outlines the benefits and limitations of the various sources of stem cells for transplantation.

## Stem Cell Harvesting, Mobilization, and Collection

Stem cells are most numerous in the bone marrow spaces, and some circulate in the peripheral blood. The process of harvesting and collecting hematopoietic stem cells differs depending on whether progenitor cells will be obtained through a bone marrow harvest or collected from the peripheral bloodstream.

When stem cells are obtained from the bone marrow, the harvesting procedure is performed in the operating room with the patient anesthetized. Multiple aspirations are obtained from each posterior iliac crest using large-bore needles until a total of 2 to $3 \times 10^8$ nucleated cells per kilogram of recipient body weight is obtained. The total volume of aspirate is 1 to 2 L. The marrow is placed in a heparinized tissue culture medium and filtered for the removal of fat and bone particles, and the cells are taken directly to the recipient's room for infusion. The bone marrow harvest procedure usually takes 1 to 2 hours. Pressure dressings are applied to the aspirate sites, and the donor is usually admitted to the hospital for overnight observation. The harvest sites may be mildly uncomfortable for 2 to 7 days after the procedure.

**TABLE 47-4**  Comparison of Autologous and Allogeneic Stem Cell Transplantation

| | Autologous | Allogeneic |
|---|---|---|
| Indications | Hematologic malignancies and solid tumors<br>Possible role in treatment of autoimmune disorders<br>Future role in combination with gene therapy to treat genetic disorders and HIV infection | Hematologic malignancies, aplastic anemia, congenital bone marrow disorders, immune deficiency states, some inborn errors of metabolism |
| Source of stem cells | Stem cells collected from bone marrow or peripheral blood of the patient and then reinfused after high-dose conditioning regimen<br>Stem cells given to rescue the patient from hematologic toxicity of conditioning regimen | Marrow, peripheral blood, cord blood, family donors, unrelated donors, HLA-matched or partially matched |
| Preparative regimen | High-dose chemotherapy to eradicate malignant disease | High-dose chemotherapy and sometimes total-body radiation as intensive therapy for malignant disease and to provide immunosuppression to allow engraftment (makes "space" for incoming stem cells) |
| Posttransplantation treatment | Supportive care, transfusions, growth factors, immune manipulation | Supportive care, transfusions, growth factors, immune manipulation, prophylaxis and treatment of graft-versus-host disease (GVHD) |
| Risk for infectious complications | Lower risk; infections occur mainly in early posttransplantation period | Higher risk; sustained risk for infection for months or years |
| Major complications | Preparative regimen toxicity, disease recurrence or progression | Preparative regimen toxicity, disease recurrence or progression, GVHD, immunodeficiency |
| Treatment-related mortality rate | Usually less than 5% | 5%–30% depending on many patient-, donor-, and disease-related factors |

Adapted from Treleaven J, Barrett AJ (eds): Hematopoietic Stem Cell Transplantation in Clinical Practice. Edinburgh, UK: Elsevier Limited, 2009.

Hematopoietic stem cells may also be collected from the peripheral blood. However, because stem cells are not abundant in the peripheral blood, chemotherapy or colony-stimulating factors (CSFs) (granulocyte colony-stimulating factor [G-CSF] or granulocyte–macrophage colony-stimulating factor [GM-CSF]) must be given before collection to drive progenitor cells into the peripheral circulation. This process is termed *mobilization* or *priming*. The chemotherapy that patients receive for stem cell mobilization is also useful for tumor reduction. For related and unrelated donors, colony-stimulating factors alone are used to increase the number of stem cells in the peripheral blood. Protocols vary, but G-CSF or GM-CSF is given by a subcutaneous injection daily. Stem cell collections begin after 4 or 5 days of cytokine injections.

Hematopoietic progenitor cells are collected from the peripheral blood by a method called *leukapheresis*. A commercial cell separator machine collects the progenitor cells and returns the remainder of the plasma and cellular components to the bloodstream. This is performed either through wide-bore double-lumen central catheters or large-bore antecubital IV catheters. The procedure takes approximately 3 to 4 hours, and the number of leukapheresis procedures required is determined by the number of stem cells harvested at each session. The goal is to collect $5 \times 10^6$ CD34-positive cells per kilogram of recipient body weight. The CD34-positive antigen is an antigen expressed on the surface of early progenitor cells. With autologous hematopoietic progenitor cells, the cells are immediately cryopreserved and stored in liquid nitrogen until the recipient is ready for reinfusion. The donor may experience a transient hypocalcemia reaction with chills, fatigue, tingling in the lips and extremities, and vertigo resulting from the citrate infusion, which is used to prevent clotting of the blood during the procedure. The symptoms can be prevented or treated by taking a calcium supplement.

## Conditioning Regimen

After the progenitor cells have been obtained, the recipient begins the conditioning regimen designed to prepare him or her to receive transplanted stem cells. The goal of the conditioning regimen depends in part on whether the transplant is autologous or allogeneic and on the nature of the recipient's underlying disease. In allogeneic transplantation, the purpose of conditioning is to eradicate any malignant disease, eliminate the bone marrow to create a space for the new donor stem cells, and provide sufficient immunosuppression to allow engraftment of the transplanted stem cells. In autologous transplantation, immunosuppression is not required because the recipient of the hematopoietic stem cells is also the donor, and therefore, there is no tissue incompatibility. However, the high-dose therapy is still needed to eradicate malignant disease.

High-dose chemotherapy is based on the hypothesis that increasing the total dose or dose rate will kill more tumor cells, resulting in improved response and survival rates. Drugs with different (ie, nonoverlapping) nonhematologic dose-limiting toxicities are combined in maximal doses. Alkylating agents (cyclophosphamide, carboplatin, busulfan, thiotepa, cisplatin, melphalan, carmustine), etoposide, cytarabine, and sometimes total-body irradiation are used to destroy the bone marrow and eradicate disease. The regimen is administered over 2 to 8 days. The individual drugs that may be used in combination as part of the transplant conditioning regimen may have several adverse effects (Box 47-3).

The stem cell recipient is allowed 1 to 2 rest days to clear the chemotherapeutic agents from the system before the infusion of stem cells. Bone marrow aplasia occurs within days after the conditioning regimen is completed. The acute toxicity from the regimen can last for a few weeks or until engraftment occurs.

Reduced-intensity conditioning regimens (sometimes called nonmyeloablative) followed by allogeneic HSCT may provide improved transplantation outcomes for selected candidates. Reduced-intensity transplantation may provide a treatment option for patients who, because of advanced age or preexisting lung, kidney, or liver damage, cannot tolerate the toxicities of a traditional allogeneic transplant.[19] The theory behind a reduced-intensity transplantation is that the immune-mediated graft-versus-tumor effect provided by the new immune system, rather than the conditioning regimen itself, cures the disease. Specific regimens under investigation include fludarabine, single-dose total-body irradiation, and a combination of potent immunosuppressive medications. These regimens are not without risk, and patients undergoing reduced-intensity transplantation still experience many of the expected complications of myeloablative allogeneic transplantation. The problems encountered in the early posttransplantation period, such as infection, bleeding, and regimen-related toxicities, may be reduced compared with myeloablative transplantation, but the risk for GVHD and the long-term risks for infection continue to be important.

## Transplantation: Hematopoietic Stem Cell Infusion

In allogeneic HSCT, the stem cells are usually infused immediately after they are collected. Autologous stem cells are

**Nonhematologic Adverse Effects of High-Dose Therapy Regimens**

**Busulfan:** Interstitial pulmonary fibrosis, hepatic dysfunction (including veno-occlusive disease of the liver), acute cholecystitis, generalized seizures, mucositis, skin adverse effects (hyperpigmentation, desquamation, acral erythema), nausea and vomiting

**Carmustine (BCNU):** Hepatic, pulmonary, and central nervous system adverse effects, cardiac adverse effects (dysrhythmias and hypotension), nausea and vomiting

**Cytosine arabinoside (Ara-C):** Cerebellar toxicity, encephalopathy, seizures, conjunctivitis, skin adverse effects (rash, acral erythema), nausea and vomiting, diarrhea, renal insufficiency, liver function abnormalities, pancreatitis, noncardiogenic pulmonary edema, fever, arthralgias

**Cyclophosphamide:** Cardiac adverse effects (cardiomyopathy, congestive heart failure, hemorrhagic cardiac necrosis, pericardial effusion, ECG abnormalities), interstitial pulmonary fibrosis, hemorrhagic cystitis, elevation in liver enzymes, nausea and vomiting, metabolic adverse effects (syndrome of inappropriate antidiuretic hormone secretion)

**Carboplatinum:** Nausea and vomiting, nephrotoxicity, liver function abnormalities (including veno-occlusive disease of the liver), ototoxicity

**Cisplatinum:** Nausea and vomiting, neurotoxicity (peripheral neuropathy, ataxia, visual disturbances), ototoxicity, renal adverse effects

**Etoposide:** Hypersensitivity reactions, hypotension, liver function abnormalities and chemical hepatitis, renal dysfunction, nausea and vomiting, metabolic adverse effects (metabolic acidosis), mucositis, stomatitis, painful skin rash (on the palms, soles, and periorbital area)

**Ifosfamide:** Hemorrhagic cystitis, nausea, vomiting

**Melphalan:** Acute hypersensitivity reaction, renal adverse effects, mucositis, nausea and vomiting, hepatic toxicity (including veno-occlusive disease of the liver)

**Thiotepa:** Hyperpigmentation, acute erythroderma, dry desquamation, liver function abnormalities (including veno-occlusive disease of the liver), mucositis, esophagitis, dysuria, hypersensitivity reactions

**Total-body irradiation:** Nausea and vomiting, diarrhea, fever, parotitis, xerostomia, stomatitis, erythema, pneumonitis, veno-occlusive disease of the liver

cryopreserved with dimethylsulfoxide (DMSO) and must be thawed in a warm normal saline bath at the bedside immediately before reinfusion.

The actual infusion of stem cells is a relatively simple procedure, much like a blood transfusion. The cells are infused into a central venous catheter over 30 to 60 minutes, depending on the total volume of the product. Patients usually are premedicated with acetaminophen, hydrocortisone, and diphenhydramine, and they are prehydrated to maintain renal perfusion. Diuretics, mannitol, and antihypertensives may be required to prevent volume overload and manage hemodynamic changes during infusion. Vital signs are monitored, and oxygen and cardiac monitoring are readily available.

Complications of stem cell infusion include pulmonary edema, hemolysis, infection, and anaphylaxis; however, these are rare. A garlicky odor or taste may occur; excretion of DMSO causes this. DMSO-associated RBC hemolysis may also occur, and patients require vigorous hydration to prevent renal toxicity. An infusion reaction that may include bradycardia (rarely heart block), hypertension, and an acute

hypersensitivity reaction is another potential adverse effect of DMSO during the administration of cryopreserved autologous HSCT. During HSCT, monitoring for volume overload and for complaints suggestive of embolism, such as chest pain, dyspnea, and cough is necessary. Patients may also experience an acute hemolytic transfusion reaction if they are receiving hematopoietic stem cells from an ABO-mismatched donor.

## Engraftment

After IV infusion, the hematopoietic stem cells migrate to the bone marrow spaces, where they are attracted by chemotactic factors. Engraftment occurs when the transplanted progenitor cells begin to grow and manufacture new hematopoietic cells in the bone marrow. Engraftment is generally defined as an absolute neutrophil count greater than $0.5 \times 10^9/L$ for 3 consecutive days and a platelet count greater than $20 \times 10^9/L$ achieved without transfusion support. The rate of engraftment depends on the source of the progenitor cells, the total progenitor cell dose, the use of colony-stimulating factors, the complications the patient experiences in the pre-engraftment period, and the choice of prophylaxis against GVHD. Time to engraftment in HSCT varies according to the origin of the hematopoietic stem cells: for bone marrow–derived stem cells, 2 to 3 weeks; for peripheral blood stem cells, 11 to 16 days; and for cord blood–derived stem cells, 26 days (average; as long as 42 days).

Patients usually receive their conditioning treatment and immediate posttransplantation care in an inpatient unit. However, improved symptom management and technological advances, including the use of hematopoietic growth factors, have allowed earlier discharge from the hospital.

After the transplantation but before complete hematopoietic cell engraftment, patients experience severe pancytopenia and immunosuppression, and the resulting complications may include infection and bleeding. Patients take hematopoietic growth factors (eg, G-CSF, GM-CSF) to accelerate neutrophil recovery, thereby reducing the period of pancytopenia and the highest risk for infection. While patients have pancytopenia, until their blood counts begin to recover, they typically receive broad-spectrum antimicrobial drugs directed at bacteria, viruses, and fungi, as well as blood components, such as platelets and packed RBCs.

All blood products given to HSCT recipients require filtration to remove WBCs that may transmit CMV and irradiation to prevent transfusion-associated GVHD. Studies have determined that leukodepletion by either bedside filtration during transfusion or by prestorage leukocyte depletion of blood products is an effective method of preventing transfusion-associated CMV infection in HSCT because leukocytes transmit CMV.[20] In addition, filtered blood products may also prevent febrile transfusion reactions and delay alloimmunization.[21,22] However, use of a leukocyte depletion filter does not affect the risk for transmission of viral hepatitis.

Transfusion-associated GVHD is a rare but almost uniformly fatal complication of transfusion, resulting from the infusion of immunocompetent lymphocytes capable of proliferation into an immunocompromised recipient who is unable to destroy them.[23,24] The infused lymphocytes recognize host tissues as foreign and mount a reaction.

To prevent transfusion-associated GVHD, all cellular blood products except for stem cell grafts and donor lymphocytes given for graft-versus-tumor effect, should be irradiated with 2500 cGy prior to transfusion.[23,24] The blood component should be labeled as irradiated. It is not radioactive, and no additional precautions for handling the blood product are required. Other patients can use irradiated blood products; the irradiating process does not alter the efficacy or cellular content of the product and does not harm the recipient in any way. Patients who have undergone allogeneic or autologous HSCT should receive irradiated cellular components, both before and after stem cell transplantation.[16] Most centers recommend that allogeneic stem cell recipients receive irradiated blood products for the rest of their lives. Box 47-4 presents a collaborative care guide for the patient with allogeneic HSCT.

---

**QSEN BOX 47-4**    *COLLABORATIVE CARE GUIDE for the Allogeneic Hematopoietic Stem Cell Transplantation*

| Outcomes | Interventions |
|---|---|

**Impaired Gas Exchange**
**Ineffective Breathing Patterns**

| Outcomes | Interventions |
|---|---|
| The patient will demonstrate pulmonary hygiene techniques, including coughing, deep breathing, incentive spirometry, and daily exercise as tolerated.<br><br>The patient will demonstrate improvement in respiratory pattern and lung sounds, with subjective reduction in complaints of dyspnea, cough, pleuritic chest pain, and weakness.<br><br>The patient's risk for aspiration will be eliminated or minimized. | • Auscultate lung sounds and vital signs and pulse oximetry every 4 hours and PRN.<br>• Note skin color capillary refill and presence of central or peripheral cyanosis.<br>• Assess the quality of respirations including use of accessory muscles, nasal flaring, and grunting.<br>• Note cough and complaints of shortness of breath, orthopnea, or pleuritic pain.<br>• Determine effects of medications that may affect respiratory status, including narcotics and sedatives.<br>• Suction oropharynx or nasotrachea to remove secretions.<br>• Encourage deep-breathing and coughing exercises, and teach patient proper use of incentive spirometry.<br>• Encourage patient to maintain optimal level of activity, including walking, exercise bicycle, and working daily with physical therapist.<br>• Instruct patient on methods of preventing respiratory complications related to mucositis or aspiration, such as avoiding drinking liquids after using topical local anesthetics, keeping head of bed elevated and having oral suction in a convenient location.<br>• Implement measures to manage anemia and control bleeding, if present.<br>• Administer supplemental oxygen as indicated.<br>• Administer diuretics as ordered. |

**Decreased Cardiac Tissue Perfusion**
**Risk for Shock**
**Risk for Bleeding**
**Risk for Imbalanced Fluid Volume**

| Outcomes | Interventions |
|---|---|
| The patient will exhibit the absence or control of signs and symptoms of potential physiologic problems:<br><br>**Bleeding/hemorrhage**<br><br>**Hypotension** secondary to sepsis, hemorrhage, medication side effects, or dehydration<br><br>**Hypertension** secondary to medication side effects<br><br>**Dehydration** secondary to decreased oral fluid intake as a result of nausea, vomiting, or mucositis, or increased fluid losses through fever, diarrhea, or insensible fluid losses through the skin | • Develop a nursing plan to manage individual cardiovascular problems. Cardiovascular problems may include hypertension, orthostatic hypotension, sepsis-induced hypotension, dysrhythmias, pericarditis, superior vena cava syndrome, thrombus formation, and myocardial infarction.<br>• Replace fluid losses with packed RBCs or hydration.<br>• Use appropriate measures to decrease fluid losses secondary to fever, diarrhea, vomiting, or hemorrhage.<br>• Administer antihypertensives, diuretics, antiarrhythmics, or vasoactive drugs as ordered and monitor their effectiveness.<br>• Provide information to patient and family regarding cardiac status, and rationale for specific nursing interventions.<br>• Monitor platelet count and coagulation profile carefully, especially in patients experiencing hypertension.<br>• Instruct patient about appropriate safety measures during period of altered cardiac status. Patients who are orthostatic may become dizzy when standing. Provide assistance as needed.<br>• Although hypotension and hypertension may occur without symptoms, alert patient to these signs and symptoms, and encourage prompt reporting to the health care team. Common signs of hypertension include headache and visual disturbance. Hypotension may be associated with dizziness, visual disturbances, tachycardia, and cool or diaphoretic skin.<br>• Emphasize the importance of taking oral antihypertensive medications when scheduled. |

| Outcomes | Interventions |
|---|---|
| **Electrolyte Imbalance**<br>**Risk for Imbalanced Fluid Volume**<br>**Ineffective Renal Perfusion** | |
| The patient will exhibit the absence of or control of signs and symptoms of potential physiologic problems:<br>**Veno-occlusive disease of the liver,** as manifested by sudden weight gain, increase in bilirubin, aspartate aminotransferase, and alkaline phosphatase levels, hepatomegaly, ascites, and encephalopathy<br>**Renal insufficiency/failure,** as manifested by a decreased urine output or rising serum creatinine<br>**Dehydration** secondary to decreased oral fluid intake as a result of nausea, vomiting, or mucositis, or increased fluid losses through fever, diarrhea, or insensible fluid losses through the skin.<br>**Electrolyte disorders** secondary to steroid-induced hyperglycemia, syndrome of inappropriate antidiuretic hormone secretion, tumor lysis syndrome, or medication-induced electrolyte shifts | • Strictly monitor intake, output, and fluid balance every 4–8 hours.<br>• Check weight twice daily.<br>• Measure abdominal girth daily in patients with veno-occlusive disease.<br>• Perform pulmonary assessment, including pulse oximetry, respiratory rate, quality, and presence of adventitious breath sounds.<br>• Perform cardiac assessment, noting presence of orthostatic hypotension, extra heart sounds, or neck vein distention.<br>• Assess for peripheral and sacral edema.<br>• Monitor serum electrolytes, liver function tests, and urine specific gravity once or twice daily as ordered.<br>• Monitor for and treat steroid-induced hyperglycemia.<br>• Adjust dose or eliminate nephrotoxic drugs in patients with renal insufficiency or renal failure.<br>• Administer intravenous fluids as ordered to replace gastrointestinal losses and to supplement inability to consume sufficient oral fluids.<br>• Administer electrolyte replacements as ordered.<br>• Administer antiemetics and antidiarrheal agents as ordered.<br>• Monitor stools for volume, consistency, color, and odor.<br>• Monitor for fluid losses through sloughing of the skin. |
| **Risk for Falls**<br>**Impaired Physical Mobility**<br>**Risk for Injury**<br>**Risk for Activity Intolerance** | |
| The patient will:<br>Maintain baseline strength and endurance and minimize focal muscle weakness, fatigue, and dyspnea<br>Participate in measures to prevent a decrease in strength and endurance<br>Experience minimal complications from decreased mobility<br>Use safety measures to prevent injury | • Encourage patient to continue daily activities throughout the transplantation course. Provide rationale and explain the complications of inactivity to both patient and family.<br>• Develop an individualized plan to address factors contributing to limited mobility, including pain, nonadherence, depression, medication side effects, nausea, generalized weakness and malaise, and altered level of consciousness.<br>• Refer to physical and occupational therapy for assessment and treatment.<br>• Encourage focused exercises that provide proximal muscle strengthening in patients on corticosteroids.<br>• Encourage patient to maintain maximal independence in activities of daily living (ADLs) and self-care.<br>• Develop a schedule that allows adequate rest by coordinating all activity and treatments (ADLs, medications, health team rounds).<br>• Identify signs of impaired activity tolerance and set specific goals for improving tolerance/endurance in activities. |
| **Impaired Skin Integrity** | |
| The patient will:<br>Maintain skin integrity<br>Demonstrate techniques of skin care<br>Demonstrate basic understanding of skin GVHD<br>Exhibit control of symptoms associated with skin GVHD | • Assess skin daily for maculopapular rash, erythema, sloughing, or open lesions.<br>• Monitor skin for the development of signs of infection such as warmth, erythema, swelling, or tenderness.<br>• Apply skin emollients and other topical agents, including topical antimicrobial agents, as ordered.<br>• Consider use of antipruritic or steroid topical agents to manage symptoms of itching and inflammation.<br>• If skin breakdown occurs, consult enterostomal therapist or wound management specialist concerning nonadherent, absorptive dressings and the role of special beds/mattresses.<br>• Monitor patient for dehydration if there are increased insensible losses of fluid through the skin.<br>• Teach patient and family the importance of avoiding direct sun exposure and the importance of using sun block and protective clothing when outdoors because sun exposure can initiate a flare of GVHD of skin. |

*(continued)*

**QSEN** **BOX 47-4**    *COLLABORATIVE CARE GUIDE for the Allogeneic Hematopoietic Stem Cell Transplantation (continued)*

| Outcomes | Interventions |
| --- | --- |

### Imbalanced Nutrition
### Electrolyte Imbalance

The patient will:

Have nutritional balance maintained through diet and parenteral nutrition

Demonstrate understanding of dietary restrictions related to a specific gastrointestinal problem

Demonstrate methods for maintaining nutritional requirements as an outpatient

- Evaluate oral mucosal integrity and note presence of oral problems.
- Note subjective data, including complaints of nausea, loss of appetite, taste changes, early satiety, pain or abdominal cramping, and any precipitating factors.
- Monitor calorie counts, intake and output totals, and weights to determine adequacy of nutritional intake.
- Develop a multidisciplinary plan for nutritional management. Discuss approaches to use when experiencing taste changes; thick, viscous saliva and mucus; xerostomia; early satiety; nausea/vomiting; mucositis or esophagitis; and other troubling symptoms.
- If patient is receiving high-dose steroids, ensure increased protein intake and calcium and vitamin D supplementation. Consider restricted concentrated carbohydrate intake if hyperglycemia is present. Consider restricted sodium intake if fluid retention is especially problematic.
- Increase protein intake in patients with extensive skin or gastrointestinal GVHD.
- Consider multiple vitamin without iron (to prevent iron overload), and folic acid supplementation 1 mg orally daily.
- Maintain nutritional requirements through use of hyperalimentation as required.
- Encourage patient to try different foods as tolerated.
- Advance diet as tolerated and note response to advancement.
- Encourage small, frequent meals and a bedtime snack.
- Medicate for nausea or pain as needed.
- Encourage family members to be supportive and patient. Pressure from family or staff can produce anxiety that will have a negative effect on eating habits.

### Impaired Comfort

Patient will be able to:

Identify activities that increase or decrease pain

Relate location and characteristics of pain as well as degree of pain relief to the health care team

Participate in daily care without interference from pain or side effects of pain control measures

Achieve acceptable level of pain control

- Monitor for the potential sources of pain/discomfort in the hematopoietic stem cell transplant recipient, including:
  - Pain associated with diagnostic or therapeutic procedures
  - Neuropathic pain secondary to immunosuppressive medications
  - Mucositis/esophagitis
  - Rectal pain/hemorrhoids
  - Painful urination from hemorrhagic cystitis
  - Abdominal pain secondary to infections, severe diarrhea/enteritis, or liver distention
  - Cutaneous discomfort secondary to GVHD of skin
- Teach patient importance of reporting pain and the effectiveness of pain relief measures to health care team.
- Assess location, onset, frequency, intensity, and quality of pain. Use a 0–10 pain scale to assess patient's perception of pain and to assist in evaluating effectiveness of treatment. For patients unable to communicate, monitor changes in vital signs and observe for increased restlessness, which could indicate inadequate pain control.
- Premedicate patient before potentially painful procedures.
- Teach proper and safe use of patient-controlled analgesia if ordered.
- For patients receiving continuous infusion, consider the need for a bolus of analgesic before disconnecting patient from continuous infusion, while disconnected, and after resuming continuous infusion.
- Suggest consultation with pain management team if indicated.
- Monitor narcotic dosages and patient response carefully in patients with hepatic dysfunction secondary to veno-occlusive disease or GVHD.
- In the nonventilated patient, adjust analgesic dosages in the presence of markedly deceased respiratory rate or markedly altered level of consciousness.

| Outcomes | Interventions |
|---|---|
| **Ineffective Coping** | |
| Patient and family will be able to:<br>Identify effective and ineffective coping patterns<br>Identify personal strengths<br>Verbalize their needs<br>Actively participate in problem solving<br>Use resources and support systems to strengthen their coping skills | • Provide opportunities for patient and family to communicate with each other, as well as with psychosocial support professionals and other health care team members.<br>• Reinforce successful coping skills (ie, clearly verbalizing needs, using activities that reduce stress, and effective patient/family/team communication).<br>• Provide reassurance and review support systems, options, and resources available to support effective coping.<br>• Establish trust and congruence in goals and objectives.<br>• Provide information in a timely and specific manner.<br>• Allow patient as much choice and control as appropriate and feasible.<br>• Avoid the use of approaches that foster dependency (coercion, persuasion, manipulation).<br>• Demonstrate caring, respect, and concern for patient and family.<br>• Use positive reinforcement. |
| **Teaching/Discharge Planning** | |
| The patient and family will demonstrate knowledge of:<br>The overall process of HSCT and the expected complications and self-care requirements, including preparative regimen and side effects, infusion of peripheral stem cells and side effects, engraftment, complications, discharge criteria, follow-up care, symptoms to report, protective precautions (neutropenic and thrombocytopenic precautions), dietary restrictions, and specific psychomotor skills, including central venous catheter care, medication administration, and vital sign monitoring<br>The structure of the inpatient unit, unit routines, and the programs and resources available to make their inpatient stay more comfortable and facilitate their self-care<br>The importance of the active involvement of patient and family in the daily care and decision making throughout the HSCT process<br>On discharge, patient and family will demonstrate knowledge of:<br>Signs and symptoms that should be reported immediately to the health care team, including fever, chills, skin rash, bleeding, nausea, vomiting, diarrhea or abdominal pain, shortness of breath, cough, dyspnea, and an inability to take oral medication or consume sufficient fluids<br>Names of medication, rationale for each medication, the required schedule for administration, and potential side effects<br>Contact telephone numbers for day and after-hours care<br>Psychomotor skills necessary for administration of oral and IV medications, self-care of central venous catheter, and any other self-care skills such as administration of total parenteral nutrition and home IV hydration | • Orient patient to unit, room environment, ancillary services, and general routines. The patient and family may be initially overwhelmed by the amount of new information and may require reinforcement of information.<br>• Allow patient and family to share concerns and request additional information about the transplantation process.<br>• Encourage questions throughout the transplantation process, and provide clarification on all aspects of treatment.<br>• Explain the need for active patient and family involvement in daily care and decision making throughout the HSCT process.<br>• Teach the importance of daily hygiene, diligent oral care, daily exercise, nutrition, and other routines.<br>• Encourage patient to maintain open communication with health care team.<br>• Integrate discharge teaching while fostering patient family participation in daily care.<br>• Provide patient with written instructions on outpatient self-care guidelines, medication schedule, and other self-care activities.<br>• Refer to home health agency for continued education and support of patient at home, as indicated.<br>• Provide teaching/instruction using methods adapted to patient's learning style. Discuss with patient how he or she learns best: by doing, by listening, or by watching.<br>• Document teaching provided, areas requiring continued reinforcement and follow-up, and learning outcomes achieved in the patient's record. |

## Factors Affecting Outcomes

Astute nursing care for HSCT patients is essential to prevent treatment-related complications and death. Other factors that may affect the outcomes of HSCT include the type and stage of disease at the time of transplantation, the type of transplant (allogeneic versus autologous), the degree of human leukocyte antigen (HLA) matching in allogeneic transplants, the stem cell source, the intensity of the conditioning regimen, the ages of both the donor and the recipient, and the experience of the transplantation center. In general, the transplant-related mortality risk in allogeneic HSCT is about 20% to 30% higher than in autologous HSCT. The transplant-related mortality rate in autologous HSCT is less than 5% at most centers.

## Immunosuppressive Therapy

After transplantation, graft function requires immunosuppression. If immunosuppression is stopped, rejection takes place and the graft dies.

In solid organ transplantation, the transplanted organ is foreign to the recipient, whose immune system eventually will recognize this and mobilize to reject the transplanted organ. Therefore, immunosuppressive therapy is necessary to suppress the immune response so the transplanted organ will be accepted. In allogeneic HSCT, because the immune system is generated from donor cells, immunosuppressive therapy is used to prevent GVHD, a response in which donor T lymphocytes attack the recipient's cells. The challenge of immunosuppressive therapy is to provide the recipient with adequate immunosuppression without undue toxicity, unfavorable reactions, and excess susceptibility to opportunistic infections. Therapeutic regimens may be individualized based on the needs of a particular patient.

Immediately after transplantation, high levels of immunosuppression are required, but thereafter, doses can be reduced to a maintenance level. In solid organ transplants, immunosuppression strategies consist of induction and maintenance therapy.[25–28] The goals of these strategies are to reduce cellular rejection occurrence while minimizing immunosuppression associated complications such as infections, renal insufficiency, and neurotoxicity.

## Induction Therapy

Induction therapy consists of the administration of an immunosuppressant at the time of antigen presentation during the peri-transplant period. It is used to enhance immunosuppression to prevent clinically significant acute cellular rejection during the early post–transplant period. Other benefits include improving (prolonging) graft survival, renal protection (prevention of early nephropathy associated with calcineurins), and minimizing steroid use.[25,26,28,29]

In the absence of positive crossmatch, early allograft injury is primarily due to T-cell responses; thus, induction strategies focuses on T-cell inhibition. There are two methods of induction therapy, both of which involve the use of antibodies. The first method depletes T-cells (as well as other immune cells) with the use of monoclonal or polyclonal antibodies with reactivity against one or more lymphocyte surface antigens. The second method uses nondepleting antibodies (monoclonal chimeric antibodies) that prevent T-cell activation and subsequently lymphocyte proliferation without causing direct destruction or cytolysis of T-cells. Regardless of which induction therapy method is used, the result is a decrease in T-cells.

Depleting agents use monoclonal or polyclonal antibodies that target various antigens on the surface of T and B cells, with reactivity against one or more lymphocyte surface antigens to deplete T-cells (and B-cells) resulting in cell lysis (cytolysis). Examples of polyclonal antibodies include antilymphocyte (ALG) and antithymocyte (ATG). Examples of monoclonal antibodies include muromonab-CD3 (OKT3), which was voluntarily withdrawn from the U.S. market in 2009 because of decreased utilization, and alemtuzumab (Campath). Alemtuzumab works directly against the CD-52 antigen, which is present on the cell surface of B and T-cells as well as monocytes, macrophages, NK cells, and thymocytes. Originally, alemtuzumab was prescribed in chronic lymphocytic leukemia and lymphoma; it was introduced in renal transplant in the late 1990s. The use of T-cell depleting agents (monoclonal and polyclonal antibodies) causes cytokine-release syndrome: hemodynamic instability, fevers, rigors, and anaphylaxis. To combat the cytokine-release syndrome, patients should be premedicated with Tylenol, Benadryl, and steroids. Other side effects include leukopenia, thrombocytopenia, glomerulonephritis, pulmonary edema, aseptic meningitis, renal insufficiency, and seizure.[25,28]

The second method of induction therapy uses non–depleting T-cell antibodies, the IL-2 receptor antagonists (chimeric monoclonal antibodies). These antagonists target only activated T-cells. Examples are daclizumab (Zenapax) and basiliximab (Simulect). The IL-2 antagonists generally have minimal side effects but have been reported to cause pulmonary edema and an acute respiratory distress syndrome (ARDs)–like syndrome.[28]

## Maintenance Therapy

To suppress the immune response in both solid organ and hematopoietic stem cell transplant recipients, several drugs may be necessary. A single medication usually cannot accomplish this effectively. Therefore, immunosuppressive regimens include medications that complement each other and increase the effectiveness of the immunosuppression. The foundation of most immunosuppressant regimens for solid organ transplantation is triple, or three-drug, therapy. The combination of drugs used for organ transplantation and HSCT may differ.

Triple therapy is a combination of low-dose prednisone, azathioprine or mycophenolate mofetil (MMF), and cyclosporine A or tacrolimus. By combining three agents, the dose of each drug is lower so that patients experience fewer adverse effects than they would from one drug alone. For example, the risk for aseptic necrosis, diabetes mellitus, cataracts, and gastrointestinal complications attributed to chronic steroid therapy is greatly reduced with the combination therapy. Because the dosage of azathioprine is low, the potential for hepatotoxicity and leukopenia is decreased. Problems associated with higher doses of cyclosporine A, including lymphoma, hirsutism, hepatotoxicity, gingival hyperplasia, seizures, and gastrointestinal disturbances, occur at a lower frequency.

Quadruple, or sequential, therapy is a combination of the same three drugs that are used in triple therapy (prednisone, azathioprine or MMF, and either cyclosporine A or tacrolimus) plus antithymocyte antibody preparations or monoclonal antibody, monomurab-CD3. The calcineurin inhibitors, cyclosporine A or tacrolimus, are withheld until renal function is present. All four drugs are given for several days, after which the polyclonal or monoclonal antibody preparation is discontinued. A triple-drug regimen is then continued for maintenance therapy.

Because of the nephrotoxicity of calcineurin inhibitors and the risks of drug accumulation and resultant toxicity in the absence of renal function, not using the calcineurin inhibitors in the early posttransplantation period has advantages. Quadruple therapy permits both broad and specific immunosuppression while limiting toxicity until renal function has improved. However, it does have a disadvantage: the potential inability to use the polyclonal or monoclonal antibody preparation for treatment of rejection episodes or as "rescue" therapy.

## Rescue Therapy

High-dose corticosteroids are the mainstay of rescue therapy for episodes of organ rejection. For rejection episodes that are refractory to high-dose corticosteroids, other treatment options include antithymocyte globulin and monoclonal antibodies, including muromonab-CD3, basiliximab, or daclizumab for rejection episodes that are refractory to high-dose corticosteroids. A second course of muromonab-CD3 may be given as a rescue therapy for recurrent rejection; although repeat treatment may be associated with complications from the development of antimouse antibodies. Other rescue treatment options for steroid-resistant rejection episodes include rapamycin, mycophenolate mofetil, and azathioprine.

## Complications of Transplantation

Complications after solid organ transplantation and HSCT are usually due to graft function, problems with immunosuppression, or the adverse effects of the transplantation preconditioning regimen. Other common complications after HSCT are GVHD and infection.

### Organ Transplantation Complications

Recipients of kidney, liver, heart, pancreas, and lung transplants are at risk for a number of complications, including acute and chronic organ rejection, infection, and bleeding.

#### Organ Rejection

The early recognition and management of organ rejection and its associated problems are key priorities for the critical care nurse. The transplanted organ represents a continuous source of HLA alloantigens capable of inducing a rejection response. This immunologic response involves the recognition of HLA antigens of donor endothelial tissues cells by recipient lymphocytes or antibodies. The allograft continuously activates the immune response, resulting in lifelong overproduction of cytokines, constant cytotoxic activity, and sustained alteration in the graft vasculature. Transplantation of a vascular organ induces sensitization through direct stimulation of circulating host immune cells as they encounter donor antigens on allograft cell surfaces. Rejection leads to subsequent destruction of the antigen-bearing graft. The pathophysiologic mechanisms of graft rejection are depicted in Figure 47-4.

Both donor and host factors contribute to the immune response of rejection. The major donor factor is the expression of antigens on the donor tissue and the presence of antigen-presenting cells within the transplanted graft. The major host factor is prior sensitization against ABO and HLA antigens expressed in the graft.[30]

Because the transplanted organ is not immunologically identical to the recipient, it acts as an antigen or foreign substance and triggers the immune system to reject it. Rejection can vary in degree from mild to severe and may be irreversible. Rejection may occur at any time, but the risk is highest in the first 3 months after transplantation. It is important to maintain therapeutic levels of immunosuppression and to provide patient and family education about the importance of taking all medications as instructed and the rationale for routine laboratory monitoring of the levels of immunosuppressive drugs. The earlier and more severe the rejection episode, the worse the prognosis for graft survival. Biopsy of the transplanted organ is usually needed to diagnose rejection definitively. Four types of rejection are defined: hyperacute, accelerated, acute, and chronic, although all types do not occur in all transplanted organs.

**HYPERACUTE REJECTION.** Hyperacute rejection occurs in the operating room immediately after transplantation. It is a humoral immune response in which the recipient has preformed antibodies that immediately react against antigens of the donor organ. Vascular damage occurs, resulting in severe thrombosis and graft necrosis. In kidney and heart transplantation, hyperacute rejection always results in graft failure and the need for retransplantation. Fortunately, hyperacute rejection is uncommon and can usually be prevented by pretransplantation cross-matching.

**ACCELERATED REJECTION.** Accelerated rejection is defined only in kidney transplantation, and it occurs within 1 week after transplantation. Clinically, the patient may have anuria, increased BUN and creatinine levels, and pain at the graft site. Accelerated rejection is due either to preformed antibodies against the donor antigens in the recipient's blood or to lymphocytes in the recipient that are already sensitized to some of the donor antigens. Like hyperacute rejection, accelerated rejection is seen infrequently because of improved tissue typing and cross-matching. It is treated aggressively with immunosuppressants and usually results in loss of the transplanted kidney.

**ACUTE REJECTION.** Acute rejection occurs within the first 3 months after transplantation. This is the most common type of rejection, and most patients experience at least one episode. Acute rejection occurs when antigens on the donor organ trigger lymphocytes to mature into helper T cells. The helper T cells increase the production of cytotoxic killer T cells, which bind to the transplanted organ and damage it by secreting lysosomal enzymes and lymphokines. Acute rejection is also the type of rejection that responds best to immunosuppressive therapy.

**CHRONIC REJECTION.** The pathophysiology of chronic rejection is not completely understood. Most likely it is a combination of a cell-mediated response and a response to circulating antibodies. Second in frequency to acute rejection, chronic rejection usually occurs from 3 months to years after transplantation and is accompanied by deteriorating organ function.

**KIDNEY.** Acute rejection occurs after the first postoperative week. It is the most frequently seen form of rejection and the type that responds best to therapy. Changes in laboratory values are the earliest and most reliable indicators that graft function is deteriorating. Clinical manifestations of rejection are more subtle and may not be seen. The patient may experience any, all, or none of the following laboratory findings during an acute rejection episode:

- Increased serum creatinine, BUN, serum $\beta_2$-microglobulin levels
- Decreased creatinine clearance
- Decreased urine creatinine level
- Possibly decreased urine sodium level
- Decreased blood flow identified by renal scan

Clinical manifestations of rejection include:

- Decreased urine output
- Weight gain
- Edema

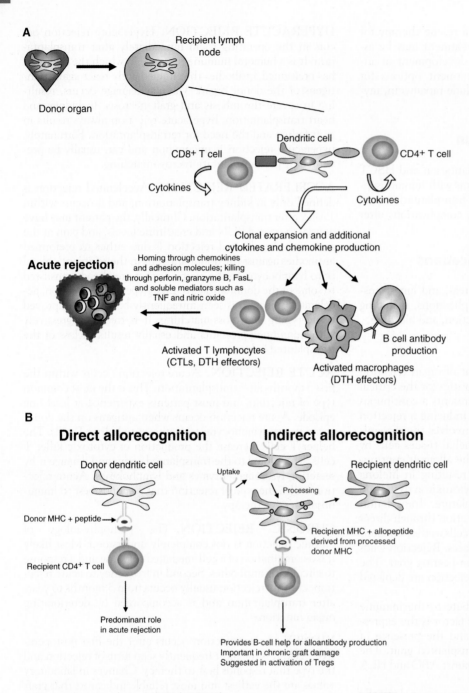

**A**

Donor organ

Recipient lymph node

CD8+ T cell

Dendritic cell

CD4+ T cell

Cytokines

Cytokines

Clonal expansion and additional cytokines and chemokine production

**Acute rejection**

Homing through chemokines and adhesion molecules; killing through perforin, granzyme B, FasL, and soluble mediators such as TNF and nitric oxide

Activated T lymphocytes (CTLs, DTH effectors)

Activated macrophages (DTH effectors)

B cell antibody production

**B**

**Direct allorecognition**

Donor dendritic cell

Donor MHC + peptide

Recipient CD4+ T cell

Predominant role in acute rejection

**Indirect allorecognition**

Uptake

Processing

Recipient dendritic cell

Recipient MHC + allopeptide derived from processed donor MHC

Provides B-cell help for alloantibody production
Important in chronic graft damage
Suggested in activation of Tregs

**FIGURE 47-4**   Mechanisms of graft rejection. **A:** Within 24 to 48 hours after engraftment, dendritic cells that normally reside within the donor organ migrate to regional recipient lymphoid tissue. In the lymph node, they stimulate alloreactive CD4+ and CD8+ T cells. Activated T cells, particularly CD4+ cells, produce cytokines (eg, interleukin-2, interleukin-4, interferon-$\gamma$), and both populations respond by proliferating and differentiating. Activated T lymphocytes can cause graft destruction by direct lysis (cytotoxic T lymphocytes, or CTLs) or by local production of cytokines, a delayed-type hypersensitivity (DTH) reaction. Cytokines also promote macrophage and eosinophil activation and recruitment, and these cells can also secrete soluble inflammatory mediators that kill their targets. Last, activated T cells provide help for alloantibody production by B cells. **B:** There are two types of allorecognition. Direct allorecognition occurs when T cells recognize intact foreign major histocompatibility complex (MHC) molecules (as depicted in part A). This is thought to be the dominant initiator of acute graft rejection. T cells may also recognize peptide fragments derived from processing of donor antigens presented on self-MHC molecules. This is termed *indirect allorecognition*, and it is believed to be important in chronic graft dysfunction, in part perhaps because of its role in providing T-cell help for alloantibody production by B cells. Indirect allorecognition is also implicated in activating regulatory T cells, which may act to limit graft damage and promote tolerance. (From Lechler RI, Sykes M, Thomson AW, et al: Organ transplantation: How much of the promise has been realized? Nat Med 11(6):605–613, 2005.)

• Temperature at least 100°F (37.8°C)
• Tenderness over the graft site, with possible swelling of the kidney
• General malaise
• Increased blood pressure

Chronic rejection is the result of repeated episodes of acute rejection in which the vessels become infarcted owing to the vasculitis, and the renal tissue becomes scarred. This gradually leads to deteriorating kidney function. The symptoms are similar to those of acute rejection except for fever and graft enlargement. Laboratory findings are similar to those of acute rejection but also include signs of chronic renal failure, such as a declining hematocrit and calcium–phosphorus imbalance. The rate of deterioration can vary from months to years. A transplant nephrectomy is not usually required unless the kidney becomes necrotic and life threatening.

**LIVER.** Acute rejection in liver transplantation is suspected when liver function tests, specifically PT/INR (most sensitive), aminotransferases, alkaline phosphatase, and total bilirubin, are increased. Clinical signs, such as decreased bile production and perigraft tenderness, may or may not occur.[31,32] Chronic rejection is believed to be due to multiple acute rejection episodes or a positive cross-match. A definitive diagnosis is made when a biopsy shows portal and bile duct inflammation and inflammatory cells, such as T lymphocytes.[31,32]

**HEART.** Although acute rejection is often asymptomatic, subtle signs and symptoms may include decreased cardiac output, atrial flutter or fibrillation, elevated WBC count, and low-grade fever. Endomyocardial biopsy is performed weekly for the first month and then less frequently to diagnose rejection. Acute rejection is a major cause of death in the first year after transplantation. Chronic rejection is the leading cause of death after the first year of cardiac transplantation. The prevalence within 5 years of transplantation is at least 60%. This cell-mediated rejection causes progressive myocardial fibrosis, leading to heart dysfunction. The lesions in allographic vasculopathy are concentric, not focal, unlike in typical atherosclerosis, and allographic vasculopathy can often be missed on standard cardiac catheterization. Angina cannot be used as a warning sign for coronary artery disease because the heart is denervated. Instead, decreased exercise tolerance during stress testing or intravascular ultrasonography is used for diagnosis.[33]

**PANCREAS.** Rejection is a major cause of graft loss in pancreas transplantation. This may be attributed to the difficulty in diagnosing rejection. Elevated blood glucose levels are a late sign and may occur too late to initiate successful treatment. When the bladder is used for exocrine drainage, urinary amylase levels reflect rejection before hyperglycemia becomes obvious. In combined kidney–pancreas transplantation, an elevated serum creatinine level may indicate rejection, although rejection can occur in one organ and not the other. Some experts state that chronic pancreas rejection may not occur in combined kidney–pancreas transplantation. The best pancreas transplant survival rate occurs when the procedure is performed simultaneously with kidney transplantation.[4,34] (see Table 47-1). Needle biopsy during cystoscopy is used for definitive diagnosis.

**LUNG.** The signs and symptoms of lung transplant rejection are difficult to distinguish from pulmonary infection. Decreased lung function (ie, forced expiratory volume), dyspnea, cough, decreased breath sounds, fever, and tachypnea may occur in both rejection and infection. Immediately after surgery, rejection may also be confused with volume overload, reperfusion injury, or ischemic injury secondary to preservation. Chest radiographs showing interstitial and perihilar edema may be signs of rejection and signal the need for biopsy. Even so, biopsies must be carefully interpreted to rule out infectious complications, such as infection with CMV or *Pneumocystis carinii*, which can have histologic findings similar to those of acute rejection.

Chronic rejection is known as obliterative bronchiolitis and occurs in approximately 15% to 25% of lung transplant recipients. Acute rejection and infection are believed to play a role in obliterative bronchiolitis. Acute rejection remains common, with 36% of lung transplant patients experiencing at least one episode of acute rejection in the first year after transplant.[35]

## Infection

Infection is the most common posttransplantation complication. Alterations in the integrity of mucosal barriers and severe neutropenia from the pretransplantation conditioning regimen produce an environment conducive to serious bacterial and fungal infection.

The causative agents are often from the patient's own flora, particularly from the gastrointestinal tract and integumentary system. Pathogens may be bacteria, fungi, viruses, and even protozoa. The latter three groups of organisms are referred to as opportunistic pathogens. Normally harmless and found in humans and in the environment, they pose serious threats to patients with compromised immune systems. They take advantage of the decreased host defenses—hence the term "opportunistic." Examples of opportunistic infections include herpes simplex and herpes zoster viruses, CMV, *Candida albicans*, *P. carinii*, *Aspergillus* species, and *Cryptococcus* species.[36]

All transplant recipients are at risk for bacterial infections from intravascular lines and urinary drainage catheters, but organ transplant recipients can also acquire postoperative wound and lung infections. Usually broad-spectrum antibiotics are given prophylactically for 48 hours after organ transplantation or until invasive lines and drains are removed. HSCT recipients receive antibiotics prophylactically for months after transplantation. Table 47-5 lists infections caused by bacteria and other organisms that commonly occur after allogeneic HSCT.

Recipients of organ transplants are at high risk for infection during the first 3 months after transplantation because they receive high dosages of immunosuppressants. Infections in the post–stem cell transplantation period usually follow a predictable pattern based on the recovery of the immune system. Therefore, recipients of HSCT are at high risk for infection during the first month, which is the pre-engraftment phase, because of neutropenia. HSCT recipients may receive colony-stimulating factors to reduce their risk for infection by accelerating WBC recovery. They remain at high risk for infection if they are receiving immunosuppressive medications to prevent or treat GVHD.

During the first month, the predominant fungal infections in recipients of HSCT are *Aspergillus* species and *Candida* species, for which amphotericin B or fluconazole may be used prophylactically. The most frequent viral infection is herpes simplex, and 80% of the patients who were seropositive before transplantation experience a reactivation of herpes simplex unless they receive acyclovir prophylactically.[35,37]

**TABLE 47-5  Infections After Allogeneic Hematopoietic Stem Cell Transplantation**

| Period of Neutropenia (Days 0–30) | Period of Acute GVHD (Days 30–100) | Period of Chronic GVHD (Days 100+) |
|---|---|---|
| Gram-negative bacteria | Gram-negative bacteria | Encapsulated bacteria |
| Gram-positive bacteria | Gram-positive bacteria | Varicella-zoster virus |
| Herpes simplex | Cytomegalovirus (CMV) | CMV |
| *Candida* species | Polyomavirus (BK virus) | *P. carinii* |
| *Aspergillus* species | Adenovirus | *Aspergillus* species |
| | Varicella-zoster virus | |
| | *Candida* species | |
| | *Aspergillus* species | |
| | *Pneumocystis carinii* | |
| | *Toxoplasma gondii* | |

Based on information from: Wingard JR, Hsu J, Hiemenz JW: Hematopoietic stem cell transplantation: An overview of infection risks and epidemiology. Hematol Oncol Clin North Am 25(1):101–116, 2011. doi:10.1016/j.hoc.2010.11.008

After the first month, the most common infection in all transplant recipients is CMV. The consequences of CMV infection include enteritis, retinitis, pneumonitis, and marrow suppression. To prevent CMV infection, patients who are CMV seronegative should receive only CMV-negative blood products. Many centers require that all blood transfusions be filtered. Current recommendations are to treat solid organ transplant recipients, who are CMV negative and who receive a CMV-positive organ, prophylactically with oral valacyclovir (Valtrex) for 3 to 6 months after transplantation.[37,38] Ganciclovir may be appropriate for patients who are CMV seropositive and who are receiving increased immunosuppression for an episode of acute organ rejection. Close monitoring of HSCT recipients for CMV reactivation, as demonstrated by a rising level of CMV antigen by polymerase chain reaction in the blood, is imperative, with early preemption. Prevention is important in heart transplant recipients because there is a connection between CMV and coronary artery disease.[36,38] CMV may affect many organ systems; therefore, signs and symptoms of hepatitis, retinitis, enteritis, pneumonitis, fever, chills, and malaise may occur.[37,38]

A small number of HSCT recipients contract severe and potentially fatal infections 3 months or more after transplantation, during the late recovery phase, because of cellular and humoral immune deficiencies. The most frequent causes of these infections are *Pneumococcus* species, *Staphylococcus aureus*, *Candida* species, and varicella-zoster virus.

If infection develops in immunosuppressed patients, the usual signs and symptoms may be absent. In these patients, even a small increase in temperature (99°F [37.2°C]) may be significant. Daily monitoring of the WBC count is necessary. After organ transplantation, the leukocyte count is usually slightly elevated because of surgery and steroid treatment. However, infection may be present if the elevation persists, a rapid elevation occurs after a decline, or there is an increase in the percentage of immature WBCs (bands) noted on the differential.

It is essential to prevent infection in transplant recipients, who are immunosuppressed and may be neutropenic. Important nursing responsibilities include maintaining protective environments, practicing consistent and thorough provider handwashing and good oral and skin hygiene, monitoring vital signs frequently, and performing head-to-toe assessments. In some centers, additional protective measures include protective isolation systems, air filtration, gut and skin decontamination, and low-microbial diets. The benefit of these interventions has been debated, and their application is institution or protocol specific.[39]

In combined kidney–pancreas transplantation, immunosuppressive drugs may be discontinued in the presence of a severe infection to mobilize the patient's immune system. Consequently, the graft may be lost to save the patient. In heart, lung, and liver transplantation, immunosuppression may be decreased but must be continued.

### Bleeding

Bleeding, oozing from the surface of the transplanted organ, or the presence of hematoma or lymphocele may occur after surgery. The heart transplant recipient is at risk for bleeding because the pericardial sac has stretched to accommodate an enlarged heart. When a smaller, healthy heart is implanted, the larger pericardial sac becomes a reservoir that can conceal postoperative bleeding. This may result in cardiac tamponade. Long-term coagulation therapy and liver congestion from pretransplantation heart failure also increase the risk for bleeding.

After liver transplantation, bleeding may occur as a result of coagulopathy because of liver dysfunction or from small vessels that continue to bleed after surgery. When the bladder drainage technique is used for exocrine drainage in pancreas transplantation, patients may have postoperative hematuria if the transplanted duodenal segment becomes ulcerated or if cystitis develops. Electrocautery using cystoscopy may be required for severe bleeding.

### Gastrointestinal Complications Related to Steroid Therapy

Chronic steroid therapy increases the risk for peptic ulceration and erosive gastritis because it increases the secretion of hydrochloric acid and pepsinogen. Massive gastrointestinal bleeding may occur not only from steroid therapy but also from stress and decreased tissue viability caused by long-term protein restriction. For these reasons, patients usually are given histamine-2 ($H_2$) receptor antagonists (eg, nizatidine or ranitidine) or proton pump inhibitors (eg, omeprazole). The degree of renal function, together with concurrent medications, dictates which class of agent is selected for gastric cytoprotection.

Other serious gastrointestinal complications include acute pancreatitis, diverticulitis, *Candida* infection, esophagitis, obstruction from bowel adhesions, and ulcerative colitis. Infection becomes an added risk if the patient has an intestinal perforation. Ischemic bowel disease has been observed in the early posttransplantation period as a result of dehydration or ischemia resulting from low cardiac output.

More than one complication may occur simultaneously. In addition, signs and symptoms of gastrointestinal bleeding or perforation may be obscured by the anti-inflammatory effects of steroids. Therefore, complaints and changes in the patient's progress require thorough and prompt assessment.

The gastrointestinal tract of the patients who have had HSCT may also suffer the effects of the total-body irradiation and chemotherapy used in the preparatory regimen. Symptoms may include mucositis, nausea, vomiting, diarrhea, cramping, dyspepsia, anorexia, taste changes, and xerostomia.

## Hematopoietic Stem Cell Transplantation Complications

### Graft Failure

The incidence of graft failure is less than 5% and is typically defined as a complete absence of engraftment or a seemingly initial hematopoiesis after transplantation, with later decreasing blood cell counts and an absence of hematopoiesis.[40] Table 47-6 describes graft failure in terms of its risk factors, possible causes, and therapeutic and preventive measures.

### Veno-Occlusive Disease of the Liver (Sinusoidal Obstructive Syndrome)

Veno-occlusive disease of the liver (also called sinusoidal obstructive syndrome) is a potentially fatal liver disease that

**TABLE 47-6** Graft Failure After Hematopoietic Stem Cell Transplantation: Risk Factors, Causes, and Preventive Measures

| | Risk Factors | Causes | Preventive/Supportive Measures |
|---|---|---|---|
| *Autologous stem cell transplants* | • Patients with acute myelocytic leukemia, patients extensively pretreated<br>• Low cell dose<br>• Purged marrow<br>• Marrow-suppressive drugs<br>• Viral infection | • Defective marrow microenvironment with stromal cell damage<br>• Collection of damaged stem cells due to extensive previous treatment<br>• Drug-induced myelosuppression<br>• Viral effects on stroma of bone marrow | • Harvest autologous stem cells early, before multiple cycles of potentially stem cell–toxic regimens have been given<br>• Maximize number of infused cells (minimum number of autologous peripheral blood stem cells that results in consistent engraftment is at least $1 \times 10^6$ CD34+ cells/kg of body weight, below which engraftment may be incomplete or there may be failure of engraftment)<br>• Avoid myelosuppressive drugs after transplantation<br>• Adjust doses of medications for renal dysfunction<br>• Treat/prevent viral infections<br>• Keep unmanipulated cells as backup in case or purged or manipulated grafts<br>• Ensure that there is no folate or vitamin B12 deficiency<br>• Administer G-CSF and rEPO as needed |
| *Allogeneic stem cell transplants* | • Diseases associated with a defective marrow microenvironment, including aplastic anemia and myelofibrosis<br>• Stem cell source from HLA-mismatched, unrelated, or cord blood donor<br>• Pretransplant transfusions, especially from a related donor<br>• T-cell depletion, low cell dose, purging<br>• Patients whose clinical condition precludes a sufficiently intensive conditioning regimen<br>• Inadequate posttransplantation immunosuppression<br>• Marrow-suppressive drugs<br>• Viral infection, including infection with CMV | • Defective marrow microenvironment with stromal cell damage<br>• Histocompatibility barriers<br>• Allosensitization by transfusions<br>• Damaged or inadequate number of stem cells infused<br>• Persistence of host hematopoiesis<br>• Persistence of immunocompetent host lymphocytes<br>• GVHD-associated damage to bone marrow microenvironment<br>• Drug-induced myelosuppression<br>• Viral effects on stroma of bone marrow | • Avoid pretransplantation transfusions, especially from relatives<br>• Select histocompatible donors<br>• Ensure that the conditioning regimen is adequately immunosuppressive<br>• Provide sufficient stem cell dose (minimum number of allogeneic peripheral blood stem cells that results in consistent engraftment is at least $2 \times 10^6$ CD34+ cells/kg of body weight, below which engraftment may be incomplete or there may be failure of engraftment)<br>• Use posttransplantation immunosuppression with cyclosporine, tacrolimus, or methotrexate<br>• Avoid all myelosuppressive drugs after transplantation<br>• Adjust doses of medications for renal dysfunction<br>• Treat/prevent viral infections<br>• Ensure that there is no folate or vitamin B12 deficiency<br>• Administer G-CSF, rEPO as needed<br>• Consider cryopreserving autologous peripheral blood stem cells preallograft for possible use in the event of graft failure and overwhelming clinical problems such as hemorrhage or life-threatening infection |

rEPO, recombinant erythropoietin; G-CSF, granulocyte colony-stimulating factor.

Data from Rees C, Beale P, Judson I: Theoretical aspects of dose intensity and dose scheduling. In: Barrett J, Treleaven J (eds): The Clinical Practice of Stem Cell Transplantation. Oxford, UK: Isis Medical Media, 1998, pp 17–29; Potter M: Graft failure. In: Treleaven J, Barrett AJ (eds): Hematopoietic Stem Cell Transplantation in Clinical Practice. Edinburgh, UK: Elsevier Limited, 2009, pp 381–385; Lowe T, Bhatia S, Somlo G: Second malignancies after allogeneic hematopoietic cell transplantation. Biol Blood Marrow Transplant 13(10):1121–1134, 2007.

occurs in 15% to 20% of recipients of HSCT. Veno-occlusive disease is a complication of the conditioning regimen, and patients who have received total body irradiation are at increased risk. Veno-occlusive disease has a mortality rate close to 50%, and may result in multisystem organ failure.[41]

Veno-occlusive disease occurs when fibrous material accumulates, resulting in obstruction of small venules in the liver. Subsequently, portal hypertension, acute liver congestion, and destruction of liver cells develop. Veno-occlusive disease also affects the kidneys; there is a decrease in renal blood flow, causing further water and sodium retention.

Clinical manifestations of veno-occlusive disease usually begin during the first 3 weeks after transplantation and are characterized by hyperbilirubinemia, rapid weight gain, ascites, right upper quadrant pain, hepatomegaly, splenomegaly, and jaundice.[42] Treatment is supportive and focuses on maintaining intravascular volume and renal perfusion while minimizing fluid accumulation.[42] This may require central venous pressure monitoring and mechanical ventilation, as well as pulmonary artery pressure monitoring if excess fluids accumulate in the lungs. Sodium restriction is warranted, and spironolactone administration is necessary to decrease extravascular accumulation. Other supportive strategies may include renal-dose dopamine infusion, avoidance of diuretics that deplete intravascular volume, and chest physiotherapy to avoid pulmonary atelectasis.[42]

Strategies for preventing veno-occlusive disease of the liver are currently undergoing investigation. These include anticoagulation with heparin; fibrinolytics, such as tissue plasminogen activator or antithrombin III concentrates, defibrotide, prostaglandin E; and ursodeoxycholic acid (Actigall).[43]

## Pulmonary Complications

Pulmonary complications develop in 30% to 60% of patients after HSCT.[36] Pulmonary complications may result from (1) infection, pulmonary edema, aspiration pneumonia, acute respiratory distress syndrome, and septic shock and (2) lung damage from total-body irradiation or pulmonary toxic chemotherapy agents.[44-47] Box 47-5 lists the pulmonary complications of HSCT.

---

**BOX 47-5** **Pulmonary Complications of Hematopoietic Stem Cell Transplantation**

**Acute (Before Day 30)**
Pulmonary edema (secondary to fluid overload, cardiac dysfunction, or allergic reaction to medications/therapy)
Oropharyngeal mucositis
Aspiration pneumonia
Pulmonary hemorrhage/diffuse alveolar hemorrhage
Bacterial or fungal pneumonia
Atelectasis
Pleural effusion
Recall radiation pneumonitis
Allergic bronchospasm
Transfusion-associated lung injury
ARDS and septic shock

**Early (Before Day 100)**
Idiopathic interstitial pneumonitis
Pulmonary embolism
Viral pneumonia (CMV, herpes simplex virus, varicella-zoster virus, respiratory syncytial virus, adenovirus, parainfluenza, influenza)
Protozoal pneumonia (*Pneumocystis carinii* pneumonia)
Fungal pneumonia
Bacterial pneumonia
Transfusion-associated lung injury
ARDS and septic shock

**Late (After Day 100)**
Idiopathic interstitial pneumonitis
Bacterial, fungal, or viral pneumonia
Bronchiolitis obliterans/GVHD of lung

ARDS, acute respiratory distress syndrome.

---

## Graft-Versus-Host Disease

GVHD, which is unique to allogeneic HSCT, results when the infused donor stem cells (graft) recognize the recipient (host) as foreign tissue. The graft then mounts an immunologic response attacking the host tissues, resulting in a T-cell–mediated reaction in the skin (rash), gastrointestinal tract (enteritis), and liver (elevated liver function test results). Figure 47-5 shows examples of the skin and gastrointestinal tract manifestations that may occur in acute GVHD.

The incidence of GVHD is 30% to 60% in cases involving histocompatible, sibling-matched allografts, with more GVHD occurring when there is greater HLA mismatch between the donor and recipient.[48,49] The mortality rate due directly or indirectly to GVHD may reach 50%.[50] Risk factors other than histoincompatibility include sex mismatching; donor parity; older age; posttransplantation infectious complications, especially viral infections; the use of donor lymphocyte infusions after transplantation; and the type of GVHD prophylaxis used.[51]

GVHD is a serious complication, but it also has a beneficial effect in controlling the patient's malignancy in that immunocompetent donor cells are able to recognize the patient's malignant cells as foreign and eliminate them. This effect was originally identified in leukemia patients and was termed *graft-versus-leukemia effect*. Leukemia relapse was seen less often in patients with GVHD than in those without GVHD. The absence of GVHD in autologous transplant recipients is suspected to play a role in the higher disease relapse rates these patients experience. Recently, researchers are applying the graft-versus-malignancy effect to prevent disease recurrence after stem cell transplantation by the infusion of donor lymphocytes.[52,53] This approach is called donor lymphocyte infusion. Research is also under way to devise strategies to induce GVHD in autologous recipients of HSCT.

**ACUTE GRAFT-VERSUS-HOST DISEASE.** Acute GVHD may occur as early as 7 to 21 days after transplantation but peaks 30 to 40 days after transplantation. Acute GVHD targets the skin, liver, and gastrointestinal system. Skin reactions, which often occur first, include an itchy maculopapular, erythematous rash on the palms, soles, ears, face, and trunk. This may resolve or progress to generalized erythroderma and desquamation. Gastrointestinal symptoms include nausea, vomiting, anorexia, abdominal cramping, and large-volume diarrhea that is green and watery. Stool may be guaiac-positive as a result of intestinal mucosa sloughing. An enlarged liver, right upper quadrant pain, jaundice, and elevated bilirubin and alkaline phosphatase levels may occur. The severity and extent of acute GVHD are evaluated using a grading system (Table 47-7).

**CHRONIC GRAFT-VERSUS-HOST DISEASE.** Chronic GVHD usually occurs in patients who have had acute GVHD, although it can occur in the absence of acute GVHD. Chronic GVHD typically occurs between 100 and 400 days after transplantation. Among patients who survived 150 days after allogeneic stem cell transplantation, researchers observed chronic GVHD in 33% to 49% of HLA-identical related transplants and in 64% of matched unrelated donor transplants.[44]

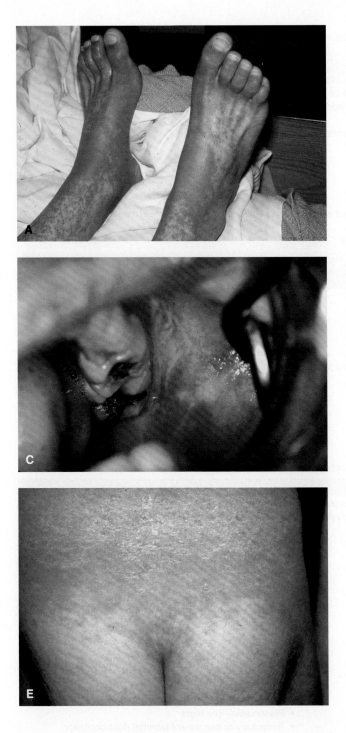

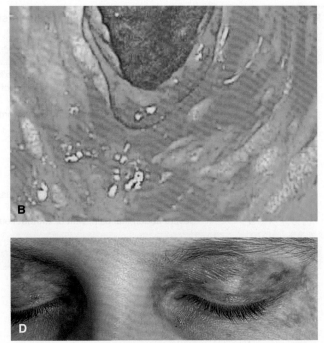

**FIGURE 47-5** Acute and chronic graft-versus-host disease (GVHD). **A:** GVHD of the skin is characterized by fine, discrete or confluent, erythematous macules and papules. Lesions may be pruritic or slightly tender with palpation. Earliest skin findings are usually seen on the face, palms and soles, and upper trunk. **B:** GVHD of the gastrointestinal tract. Images obtained during endoscopy demonstrate tissue edema, extensive erythema, and mucosal ulcerations. **C:** Oral lichen planus changes in a patient with chronic GVHD more than 130 days after allogeneic peripheral blood stem cell transplantation. Note the confluent, smooth, white papules that create a lacy pattern on the buccal mucosa. **D:** Chronic GVHD of the skin with irregularly shaped, deeply hyperpigmented macular lesions. Note the atrophy of the dermal and subcutaneous tissues with paper-thin skin giving an easily wrinkled or shiny appearance. The term *poikiloderma* is used to describe the classic features of patchy hypopigmentation and hyperpigmentation, dermal atrophy, and telangiectasias (small-diameter linear blood vessels seen on the skins surface). **E:** Lichenoid chronic GVHD of the skin of the lumbar region with flat-topped, violaceous papules; the surface is shiny and has a lacy white pattern. The eruption is confluent in some areas, and hypertrophic plaques have developed. Postinflammatory hyperpigmentation may develop. (**B**, photo courtesy of Bruce Greenwald, MD, University of Maryland Medical System, Baltimore, MD; **C**, photo courtesy of Jane Fall-Dickson, RN, PhD, AOCN, National Institutes of Health, Bethesda, MD; **D** and **E**, photos courtesy of TL Diepgen and G Yihune, Dermatology Online Atlas [http://www.dermis.net/doia].)

Risk factors for chronic GVHD include previous acute GVHD, older recipient age, and sex mismatching (female donor and male recipient).[54] The incidence of chronic GVHD may also be higher in recipients of peripheral blood stem cells than in recipients of bone marrow–derived stem cells.[55] Another significant risk factor for the development of chronic GVHD is a continuing need for corticosteroids for control of GVHD by day 100 after transplantation.[55]

Clinical manifestations of chronic GVHD, which may be clinically mild, moderate or severe, are present in the skin, liver, eyes, oral cavity, lungs, gastrointestinal system, neuromuscular system, and a variety of other body systems. Although the onset of chronic GVHD typically occurs much

later than acute GVHD, generally 100 to 400 days after transplantation, there is a growing recognition that acute and chronic GVHD are best differentiated by their features, not their onset. Features of acute GVHD, including erythematous skin rash, liver function test abnormalities, nausea, vomiting, diarrhea, and abdominal pain, may also occur after donor lymphocyte infusion. The contemporary paradigm for classifying GVHD as acute or chronic is based on the signs and symptoms of acute or chronic GVHD, rather than on the number of days after transplantation.[56] In addition, contemporary classification systems now identify an overlap syndrome in which diagnostic or distinctive features of chronic GVHD and acute GVHD appear together.[57] Table 47-8 summarizes the clinical

**TABLE 47-7** Staging and Grading System for Acute Graft-Versus-Host Disease

**Clinical Staging of Individual Organ Manifestations**

| Organ | Stage* | Description |
|---|---|---|
| Skin[†] | +1 | Maculopapular eruption over less than 25% of body area |
| | +2 | Maculopapular eruption over 25%–50% of body area |
| | +3 | Generalized erythroderma |
| | +4 | Generalized erythroderma with bullous formation and often with desquamation |
| Liver | +1 | Bilirubin 2.0–3.0 mg/dL |
| | +2 | Bilirubin 3.1–6.0 mg/dL |
| | +3 | Bilirubin 6.1–15 mg/L |
| | +4 | Bilirubin greater than 15 mg/dL |
| Gut | +1 | Diarrhea less than 500 mL/d |
| | +2 | Diarrhea 500–999 mL/d, or persistent nausea with histologic evidence of GVHD in the stomach or duodenum |
| | +3 | Diarrhea 1,500 or more mL/d |
| | +4 | Severe abdominal pain, with or without ileus |

**Overall Grade**

| Grade | Skin[‡] | Liver | Gut |
|---|---|---|---|
| I | +1 to +2 | 0 | 0 |
| II | +1 to +3 | +1 and/or | +1 |
| III | +2 to +3 | +2 to +3 and/or | +2 to +3 |
| IV | +2 to +4 | +2 to +4 and/or | +2 to +4 |

*Criteria for staging minimal degree of organ involvement required to confer that stage.
[†]Use rule of nines or burn chart to determine extent of rash.
[‡]If no skin disease is present, the overall grade is the highest single organ stage.

**TABLE 47-8** Chronic Graft-Versus-Host Disease: Clinical Manifestations and Interventions

| Organ/System | Clinical Manifestations | Interventions |
|---|---|---|
| Dermal | Dyspigmentation, xerosis (dryness), erythema, hyperkeratosis, pruritus, sclerosis, lichenification, onychodystrophy (nail ridging/nail loss), alopecia | • Systemic Immunosuppressive therapy<br>• PUVA; extracorporeal photopheresis<br>• Topical tacrolimus ointment (Protopic)<br>• Topical treatment with steroid creams, moisturizers/emollient, antibacterial ointments to prevent suprainfection; aggressive lubrication of the skin<br>• Because the sweat glands are affected, avoid overheating because heat prostration and heat stroke can occur<br>• Avoid sunlight exposure, use sunblock lotion and wear a large hat that shades the face when outdoors |
| Oral | Lichen planus, xerostomia, ulceration | • Steroid mouth rinses, oral PUVA, pilocarpine for xerostomia, fluoride gels/rinses to decrease caries<br>• Careful attention to oral hygiene; regular dental evaluations |
| Ocular | Keratitis, sicca syndrome | • Regular ophthalmologic follow-up<br>• Preservative-free tears<br>• Temporary or permanent lacrimal duct occlusion<br>• Fluid-ventilated, gas-permeable scleral lens prosthesis<br>• Consider trial of cyclosporine ophthalmic emulsion (Restasis) |
| Hepatic | Jaundice, abdominal pain | • Consider bile acid displacement therapy with ursodeoxycholic acid (Actigall) 300 mg PO three times a day |
| Pulmonary | Obstructive/restrictive pulmonary disease, shortness of breath, cough, dyspnea, wheezing, fatigue, hypoxia, pleural effusion | • Prevent and treat pulmonary infections, including *Pneumocystis carinii* and *Streptococcus pneumoniae*<br>• Aggressively investigate changes in pulmonary function because these may represent chronic GVHD of lung/bronchiolitis obliterans<br>• Encourage smoking cessation<br>• Consider treatment with montelukast and low dose azithromycin |

| Organ/System | Clinical Manifestations | Interventions |
|---|---|---|
| Gastrointestinal | Nausea, odynophagia, dysphagia, anorexia, early satiety, malabsorption, diarrhea, weight loss | • Referral to gastroenterologist; consultation with nutritionist and nutrition support<br>• Consider empirical trial of pancreatic enzyme supplementation<br>• Aggressive management of gastrointestinal symptoms such as nausea and vomiting<br>• Consider the use of cholestyramine (Questran) in the management of diarrhea<br>• Consider a trial of oral beclomethasone, budesonide, or both |
| Nutritional | Protein and calorie deficiency, malabsorption, dehydration, weight loss, muscle wasting | • Nutritional monitoring, supplementation, symptom specific interventions<br>• Trial of megestrol (Megace) or other approaches to appetite stimulation (eg, mirtazapine [Remeron] or similar antidepressants; dronabinol [Marinol]) |
| Genitourinary | Vaginal sicca, vaginal atrophy, stenosis, dyspareunia, vulvodynia | • Consider trial of mucosal application of corticosteroid ointment, cyclosporine ointment, or tacrolimus ointment<br>• Vaginal dilators<br>• Vaginal lubricants<br>• Sexual counseling |
| Immunologic | Hypogammaglobulinemia, autoimmune syndromes, development of autoantibodies | • IV immunoglobulin supplementation as indicated, and prophylactic antimicrobials (rotating antibiotics for recurrent sinopulmonary infections, PCP prophylaxis, topical antifungals)<br>• Screening for CMV and other opportunistic infections with frequent surveillance cultures and antigen detection<br>• Consider vaccination against influenza and pneumococcus |
| Musculoskeletal | Myositis fascitis, contractures, debility, muscle cramps/aches, carpal spasm | • Physical therapy for stretching and endurance<br>• Correct electrolyte imbalances<br>• Consider clonazepam, magnesium supplementation treatment for muscle cramping or myalgias |

MRI, magnetic resonance imaging; CT, computed tomography; PCP, *Pneumocystis carinii* pneumonia; PUVA, psoralen and ultraviolet A.

features, screening and evaluation, and interventions recommended for patients with chronic GVHD.[51,54,58–61]

## TREATMENT AND PROPHYLAXIS OF GRAFT-VERSUS-HOST DISEASE.

The first and most important way to limit GVHD is to find an HLA-matched donor. Despite such optimal matching of donor and recipient, further strategies to limit GVHD must be taken. The two major approaches to the prophylaxis of GVHD after HSCT are T-cell depletion of the graft and pharmacologic therapy to prevent and treat GVHD.

T cells play a major role in the recognition of self from nonself proteins, and decreasing the number of T cells in the graft before transplantation may decrease the incidence and severity of GVHD. Methods of T-cell depletion involve physical, immunologic, and pharmacologic techniques. The desired outcome is a reduction or elimination of T cells capable of initiating life-threatening GVHD. However, T cells also play a role in engraftment, and T-cell depletion carries greater risks for infection, graft failure, and disease relapse.

A variety of immunosuppressive agents, alone or in combination, have been used prophylactically for acute GVHD.[50,62–65] Immunosuppressive medications minimize the ability of the newly developing donor immune system to recognize the host or patient as foreign and limit the immune response. Immunosuppressive drugs may need to be taken for months or years after an allogeneic HSCT. Immunosuppression may involve a single drug (often tacrolimus or cyclosporine A) or a combination of drugs (methotrexate, tacrolimus, cyclosporine A, steroids, MMF, antithymocyte globulin [ATG]), sometimes in combination with T-cell depletion.[66,67,68]

For patients at higher risk for GVHD, especially those undergoing matched unrelated HSCT, more intensive strategies for GVHD prevention are necessary. Many drug–drug interactions are associated with cyclosporine A and tacrolimus. Table 47-9 lists drugs that may interact with cyclosporine A and tacrolimus. It is important to instruct patients to take their immunosuppressive medication exactly as directed and to contact their physician before starting any new medication.

Prospective, randomized trials have demonstrated that combination therapy is superior to single-drug therapy in preventing acute GVHD. However, to date, research has not shown that any one prophylactic regimen is superior in preventing acute GVHD or improving overall outcome.[62,69] The most widely used pharmacologic regimen for the prophylaxis of acute GVHD is a combination of methotrexate and either cyclosporine A or tacrolimus.[63] Other drugs included in some GVHD prophylaxis regimens are corticosteroids, ATG, daclizumab, and MMF.[65] Box 47-6 presents several sample regimens for GVHD prophylaxis.

**TABLE 47-9** Drugs That May Alter Levels of Cyclosporine and Tacrolimus

| Known Interactions | Suspected Interactions |
|---|---|
| **Increase Serum Levels** | |
| Erythromycin | $H_2$ antagonists |
| Clarithromycin | Cephalosporins |
| Itraconazole | Thiazide diuretics |
| Fluconazole | Furosemide |
| Ketoconazole | Acyclovir |
| Corticosteroids | Warfarin |
| | Calcium channel blockers (ie, diltiazem, verapamil, nicardipine) |
| | Oral contraceptives |
| | Doxycycline |
| | Metoclopramide |
| | Coadministration with grapefruit juice |
| **Decrease Serum Levels** | |
| Phenytoin or phenobarbital | Sulfinpyrazone |
| Rifampin or isoniazid | Carbamazepine |
| Sulfadiazine + trimethoprim (IV) | Anticonvulsants |
| **Cause Additive Nephrotoxicity** | |
| Amphotericin B | Nonsteroidal anti-inflammatory drug |
| Aminoglycosides | |
| Melphalan | |
| Trimethoprim-sulfamethoxazole | |
| **Alter Immunosuppressive Effects** | |
| | Propranolol |
| | Verapamil |
| | Etoposide |

Data from Evans SO: The transplant pharmacopeia. In: Treleaven J, Barrett AJ (eds): Hematopoietic Stem Cell Transplantation in Clinical Practice. Edinburgh, UK: Elsevier Limited, 2009, pp 331–342.

**BOX 47-6** Examples of Commonly Used Drug Regimens for Prophylaxis of Acute GVHD

Cyclosporine/Steroids
Cyclosporine 3 mg/kg/d IV infusion from day −2, taper 10% weekly starting day +180*
Methylprednisolone 0.25 mg/kg twice a day, days +7 to +14; 0.5 mg/kg twice a day, days +15 to +28; 0.4 mg/kg twice a day, days +29 to +42; 0.3 mg/kg twice a day, days +43 to +58; 0.25 mg/kg twice a day, days +59 to +119; and 0.1 mg/kg daily, days +120 to 180

Cyclosporine/Methotrexate/Steroids
Cyclosporine 5 mg/kg/d IV infusion from day −2, taper 20% every 2 weeks starting day +84*
Methotrexate 15 mg/m² on day +1, 10 mg/m² on days +3 and +6
Methylprednisolone 0.25 mg/kg twice a day, days +7 to +14; 0.5 mg/kg twice a day, days +15 to +28; 0.4 mg/kg twice a day, days +29 to +42; 0.3 mg/kg twice a day, days +43 to +58; 0.25 mg/kg twice a day, days +59 to +119; and 0.1 mg/kg daily, days +120 to 180

Tacrolimus/Mini-Methotrexate
Tacrolimus 0.03 mg/kg/d infusion from day −2, taper 20% every 2 weeks starting day +180*
Methotrexate 5 mg/m² on days +1, +3, +6, and +11

ATG/Cyclosporine/Methotrexate
ATG 20 mg/kg IV days −3, −2, and −1
Cyclosporine 5 mg/kg/d IV infusion from day −1, taper 10% weekly starting day +180*
Methotrexate 10 mg/m² on days +1, +3, +6, and +11

*Either tacrolimus or cyclosporine has been used with this methotrexate or steroid dose schedule.

If grade II to IV acute GVHD develops, treatment is usually required.[62] Corticosteroids are the main component of therapy, along with continuing treatment with the immunosuppressive agent used for prophylaxis (tacrolimus or cyclosporine A). Corticosteroids are the main component of therapy, along with continuation of the immunosuppressive agents used for initial prophylaxis.[58,67] High doses of methylprednisolone (1 to 20 mg/kg/d) may be used. However, these high-dose regimens are associated with fatal infections and cannot be administered for more than a few days, and the dose of methylprednisolone is rapidly tapered to 2 mg/kg/d in divided doses. Once maximal improvement is achieved, the steroid dosage is tapered over 8 to 20 weeks, based on patient response.

For patients with GVHD in whom initial therapy has failed, a variety of salvage or secondary regimens, including MMF, rituximab, montelukast, infliximab, and daclizumab, are available.[59] Once chronic GVHD develops, the usual therapy involves steroids, cyclosporine A, tacrolimus, and a variety of other immunosuppressive agents.[65] Gut rest, pain control, and antimicrobial prophylaxis coupled with hyperalimentation, if needed, are important aspects of the supportive care of patients with acute GVHD.[62] The outcome of treatment of acute GVHD is predicted by the overall grade of acute GVHD; higher overall grades are associated with poorer outcomes.[48] Response to treatment is another key determinant of outcome, and mortality is greatest in patients who do not achieve a complete response to the initial treatment strategy for acute GVHD.[48]

## Long-Term Considerations

Organ transplantation can lead to long-term survival. Increasing numbers of recipients lead healthier and longer lives. However, complications may occur long after transplantation.

Long-term care focuses on monitoring the patient's progress and adherence to the health care regimen. In solid organ transplant recipients, a major cause of graft loss in the long term is failure of patients to adhere to the medication regimen. Patients must also be monitored for the development of late complications, including infections, hypertension and cardiovascular disease, chronic rejection, and recurrence of the original disease, such as hepatitis in liver transplantation and recurrent glomerulonephritis in kidney transplantation. There is also increased incidence of posttransplantation lymphoproliferative disease in solid organ transplant recipients who are receiving long-term immunosuppression.[70,71]

Weight gain can be a significant complication after transplantation as a result of steroid use or because of general improved well-being related to the organ transplantation. Osteoporosis secondary to high steroid use is also a long-term issue for organ transplant recipients, more often for heart, liver, and stem-cell transplant recipients than for kidney transplant recipients.

The refinement and success of HSCT has resulted in a large population of patients who have achieved control of their underlying disease. However, these patients must often deal with long-term sequelae and late effects of HSCT. In addition to chronic GVHD and infectious risks, they may experience a wide range of complications (Box 47-7).[72–79] In general, autologous transplantation has fewer long-term complications, largely because no GVHD is associated with

autologous transplantation. Disease-free survival 5 years after HSCT varies substantially, depending on the age of the recipient, the underlying disease, prognostic risk factors, disease status at the time of transplantation, the type of HSCT procedure, and the extent of prior treatment. Depending on these factors, disease-free survival rates vary from 10% to 75% (Table 47-10).[2,80–85] Advances in histocompatibility matching, immunosuppression, stem-cell collection, and cryopreservation techniques, as well as the development of safer and less toxic conditioning regimens along with more effective drugs to manage posttransplantation infections, stimulate hematopoiesis, and manage graft-versus-host disease have helped increase the success of HSCT.[86,66]

---

**BOX 47-7** **Early and Late Complications of Autologous and Allogeneic Hematopoietic Stem Cell Transplantation**

**Early (Occurring Before Day 100)**
Regimen-related toxicity
- Hemorrhagic cystitis
- Veno-occlusive disease of the liver
- Pulmonary complications
- Renal complications
- Neurologic complications
Nutritional complications
Idiopathic pneumonitis
Graft failure
Infection
- Viral
- Bacterial
- Fungal
Graft-versus-host disease
Relapse

**Late (Occurring After Day +100)**
Regimen-related toxicity
- Cataracts
- Neurologic conditions (peripheral and autonomic neuropathies)
- Gonadal dysfunction
- Endocrine dysfunction
Immunodeficiency
Infection
Musculoskeletal
- Osteoporosis
- Avascular necrosis
Chronic GVHD
Relapse of malignancy
Secondary malignancy

---

**TABLE 47-10** **Disease-Free Survival 5 Years After Hematopoietic Stem Cell Transplantation**

| Disease and Stage | Allogeneic (% Survival) | Autologous (% Survival) |
|---|---|---|
| **Acute Myeloid Leukemia** | | |
| First remission | 45–70 | 40 |
| First relapse, second or later remission | 23–45 | 20–30 |
| Refractory, multiply relapsed | 10–15 | <less than 10 |
| **Acute Lymphocytic Leukemia** | | |
| First or second remission | 30–60 | 40 |
| Relapse | 10 | — |
| **Chronic Myelogenous Leukemia** | | |
| Chronic phase | 50–70 | — |
| Accelerated or blastic phase | 10–30 | — |
| **Aplastic Anemia** | | |
| Untranfused | 80–90 | — |
| Transfused | 50–70 | — |
| Myelodysplastic syndrome | 10–25 | — |
| Hodgkin lymphoma | — | 50–80 |
| Non-Hodgkin lymphoma | 40–50 | 30–60 |
| Multiple myeloma | 20–40 | <less than 10* |

*15%–25% with tandem autologous transplantation.

Data from Arnaout K, Patel N, Jain M, et al: Complications of allogeneic hematopoietic stem cell transplantation. Cancer Invest 32(7):349–362, 2014; Gyurkocza B, Rezvani A, Storb RF: Allogeneic hematopoietic cell transplantation: The state of the art. Expert Rev Hematol 3(3):285–299, 2010; and Barrett JA, Chao NJA, Bishop MR: Are More Patients Being Cured with Allogeneic Stem Cell Transplantation? American Society of Clinical Oncology, 2006 Educational Book. Alexandria, VA: American Society of Clinical Oncology, 2006.

# Clinical Applicability Challenges

## CASE STUDY

Mrs. G.S. was a 52-year-old woman with usual interstitial pneumonia (UIP) and pulmonary hypertension. She began experiencing progressive dyspnea over the last 2 years, which worsened last summer. She was able to walk on a flat surface for approximately 5 minutes, got short of breath when walking a slight incline, and complained of minimal cough. She was on home oxygen (3–5 L) via a nasal cannula.

Mrs. G.S.'s past medical history consisted of anxiety, hypertension, hyperlipidemia, and mitral valve prolapse with endocarditis. She had a mitral valve replacement (tissue valve) in 2007. She was married, was a retired teacher, had a 5 pack year history of tobacco use (she had quit 15 years ago), drank wine occasionally, and had never used recreational drugs.

A chest radiograph revealed extensive bilateral lung opacity consistent with infiltrates or edema of multiple etiologies. No pneumothorax and no pleural effusions were evident. Her heart was mildly enlarged and a sternotomy with valve replacement was visible. A chest CT scan showed mild-to-moderate diffuse interstitial fibrotic change especially involving the lung periphery, greater in the lower lobes and nearly entirely involving the left lower lobes, with bronchiectasis and cystic bullous changes in the anterior left upper lobe. A ventilation/perfusion (V/Q) scan showed right ventilation 71.2%, perfusion 83%, and left ventilation 28.4%, perfusion 17%. Her pulmonary function test revealed an FVC 2.77, FEV1 2.32, DLCO 5.8. Her 6-minute walk test was 1,200 ft on 3L NC and ABG 7.43/42/49/81%. A transthoracic echocardiogram showed an EF 50% to 60%, mild MR, mild MS, moderate TR, mild AR, and moderate to severe pulmonary hypertension. Her right cardiac catheterization results were as follows: RA 2, PAS 72, PAD 25, PAM 43, PCW 16, PVR 42, Fick CO 6.4, Fick CI 2.32. A left cardiac catheterization revealed no significant AS or MS, and no significant coronary artery disease.

Mrs. G.S. was seen by a pulmonologist, who has been managing her interstitial lung disease. A cardiothoracic surgeon has also evaluated her and she had been listed as a lung transplant candidate.

When a suitable donor lung became available, Mrs. G.S. was admitted and underwent a left orthotopic lung transplantation. The operative procedure was uneventful. She was on epinephrine drip at 0.05 mcg/kg/min and vasopressin drip at 0.04 units/min. She remained intubated from the operative procedure and was transferred to the cardiac surgery intensive care unit (CSICU). Mrs. G.S. was extubated on postoperative day 1. She had no bleeding complications in the CSICU. Weaning from the vasopressin and epinephrine drips occurred within the first 24 hours. She received induction therapy with alemtuzumab (Campath) 30 mg IV infused over 2 hours. She was premedicated prior to the induction therapy with 650 mg acetaminophen (Tylenol), 50 mg IV diphenhydramine (Benadryl), and 500 mg IV methylprednisolone.

Twenty-four hours after the induction therapy, tacrolimus (Prograf) was initiated at low doses, with close attention to urinary output and renal indices, as well as oral steroids for immunosuppression. Mycophenolate mofetil (CellCept) was not initiated immediately secondary to the alemtuzumab induction. Blood urea nitrogen and creatinine values remained within normal limits, and the tacrolimus was increased with a goal level of 6 to 8 ng/mL. Mrs. G.S. was also started on voriconazole 200 mg twice a day, valganciclovir (Valcyte) 900 mg daily, azithromycin 250 mg every Monday, Wednesday, Friday, and sulfamethoxazole/trimethoprim (Bactrim DS) one tablet every Monday, Wednesday, Friday. Because of cytomegalovirus (CMV) mismatch, CMV by polymerase chain reaction was checked weekly to evaluate for early CMV reactivation; Mrs. G.S. had very high glucose levels and remained on an insulin drip, and was also started on insulin glargine (Lantus).

One week postoperatively, the patient underwent a bronchoscopy and transbronchial biopsy. During the bronchoscopy, the anastomosis was found to be intact and the patient had minimal secretions. The bronchoalveolar lavage (BAL) showed negative growth and the transbronchial biopsy pathology result showed no evidence of acute cellular rejection (A0B0). Once the patient's transplant discharge teaching and medication teaching had been completed, the patient was discharged to home. Prior to discharge, the patient was started on low dose mycophenolate mofetil (CellCept) 500 mg twice a day. Her immunosuppression regimen consisted of CellCept 500 mg twice a day, prednisone 10 mg daily, and tacrolimus 1.5 mg twice a day with a lower goal level of 6 to 8 ng/mL.

1. What is the goal of the selection process when evaluating a patient for transplant candidacy?
2. Mrs. G.S. had induction therapy, and 24 hours later tacrolimus was initiated. What are the advantages of induction therapy?
3. What are the four types of rejection? Briefly describe each type.

## WANT TO KNOW MORE?

A wide variety of resources to enhance your learning and understanding of this chapter are available on thePoint.

You will find:

- References
- Selected readings
- NCLEX-style review questions
- Internet resources
- And more!

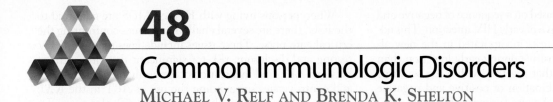

# 48

# Common Immunologic Disorders

Michael V. Relf and Brenda K. Shelton

## LEARNING OBJECTIVES

*Based on the content in this chapter, the reader should be able to:*

1. Use epidemiologic evidence to describe the current human immunodeficiency virus (HIV) and acquired immunodeficiency syndrome (AIDS) epidemics in the United States.

2. Describe the immunopathogenesis and natural history of HIV infection and AIDS.

3. Explain standard precautions and transmission-based precautions and their implementation in the intensive care unit.

4. Discuss the use of diagnostic testing and antiretroviral therapy in the management of HIV infection and AIDS.

5. Describe the pathophysiologic processes of the oncologic emergencies.

6. Discuss appropriate assessment data for each oncologic emergency derived from patient history and physical examination, clinical manifestations, and diagnostic studies.

7. Explain the anticipated medical management and rationale for the treatment of selected oncologic emergencies.

8. Describe relevant aspects of nursing management for each of the oncologic emergencies.

An intact immune system helps protect the body from a variety of antigens including bacteria, viruses, toxins, cancer cells, and foreign blood or tissues from another person or species.[1] When one or more components of this system are weakened or adversely altered, a person becomes susceptible to a variety of diseases including opportunistic infections and some cancers.

Primary immunodeficiency disorders (PIDs) are rare group of disorders resulting in poor or absent immune function with over 130 disorders identified.[2] Most PIDs are inherited; however, acquired forms have been identified. Examples of PIDs include agammaglobulinemia (a failure of B-lymphocyte precursors to mature into B lymphocytes and ultimately plasma cells), X-linked agammaglobulinemia or Bruton disease, Wiskott–Aldrich syndrome (involving both T and B lymphocytes and platelets), and severe combined immunodeficiency in which there is an absence of both T-lymphocyte and B-lymphocyte function.

An immunodeficiency is known as secondary if it is acquired later in life. Secondary immunodeficiencies have a variety of etiologies including malignancies (chronic lymphocytic leukemia, myeloma), drugs (cytotoxic agents, immunosuppressants used in organ transplantation, and steroids), viruses, nutritional deficits, metabolic disorders, and severe protein loss.[1]

This chapter is divided into two parts. The first part focuses on secondary immunodeficiency associated with HIV infection. The second part focuses on emergent situations precipitated by commonly occurring neoplastic disorders. The reader is encouraged to review Chapter 45, especially the material relating to the immune mechanisms (humoral and cell-mediated immunity, complement system, and phagocytosis/chemotaxis/opsonization). This review will help the reader appreciate the pathophysiologic changes occurring in the conditions discussed in this chapter.

## HUMAN IMMUNODEFICIENCY VIRUS INFECTION

Impaired cellular immunity is the underlying pathophysiologic consequence of AIDS, which is caused by HIV. In 1981, the first case reports of the illness known today as AIDS were reported to the Centers for Disease Control and Prevention (CDC).[3] Since early in the HIV/AIDS epidemics, case surveillance definitions have been used by public health professionals to stage HIV infection. In 2014, the HIV classification system and surveillance case definitions were further revised. In this most recent surveillance staging system, "a confirmed case that meets the criteria for diagnosis of HIV infection can be classified in one of five HIV infection stages (0, 1, 2, 3, or unknown). Stage 0 indicates early HIV infection, inferred from a negative or indeterminate HIV test result within 6 months of a confirmed positive result, and these criteria supersede and are independent of the criteria used for later stages. Stages 1, 2, and 3 are based on the CD4$^+$ T-lymphocyte count. If the CD4$^+$ count is missing or unknown, the CD4$^+$ T-lymphocyte percentage of total lymphocytes can be used to assign the stage. Cases with no information on CD4$^+$ T-lymphocyte count or percentage are classified as stage unknown. If a stage-3–defining opportunistic illness has been diagnosed, then the stage is 3 regardless of CD4 T-lymphocyte test results, unless the criteria described below for stage 0 are met."[4]

The 2014 surveillance definition added "specific criteria for defining a case of HIV-2 infection," classified "stages 1 to 3 of HIV infection on the basis of the CD4$^+$ T-lymphocyte count unless persons have had a stage-3–defining opportunistic illness," and combined "the adult and pediatric criteria for a confirmed case of HIV infection and specifies different criteria for staging HIV infection among three age groups (<1 year, 1 to 5 years, and ≥6 years). . . . Another important change is the addition of 'stage 0' based on a sequence of negative and positive test results indicative of early HIV infection. This addition takes advantage of tests incorporated in the new algorithms that are more sensitive during early infection than previously used tests, and that together with a less sensitive antibody test, yield a combination of positive and negative results enabling diagnosis of acute (primary) HIV infection, which occurs before the antibody response has fully developed. The addition of stage 0 allows for routine monitoring of the number of cases diagnosed within several months after infection, which includes the most highly infectious period when viral loads are extremely high and intervention might be most effective in preventing further transmission. The definition of stage 0 also will reduce confusion between acute HIV infection (part of stage 0), when CD4+ T-lymphocyte counts can be transiently depressed, and stage 3 (AIDS), an advanced stage of HIV infection when CD4+ T-lymphocyte values are usually persistently depressed."[4]

Since the 1980s, HIV infection has transformed from a life-limiting illness to a chronic illness manageable with strict adherence to antiretroviral therapy (ART) and other therapeutic interventions, including the prophylaxis and treatment of opportunistic infections. Despite significant treatment advances, it remains an incurable disease that is highly stigmatized in the United States and around the world.[5] Approximately one in eight HIV-infected individuals in the United States is unaware of his or her HIV status[6]; only 40% are engaged in care, only 37% are on ART, and only 30% have achieved viral suppression.[7] Thus, only three out of ten HIV-infected individuals in the United States are achieving the desired treatment outcome. Without treatment, a person infected with HIV will progress to AIDS and ultimately death in about 11 to 15 years. However, with early diagnosis, engagement in care, and strict adherence to ART and other therapies as needed, life expectancy can be extended into the early 70s, although differences by sex, race, HIV transmission risk group, and CD4 count do influence life expectancy.[8] To achieve this outcome, a cascade of events must occur.[9] The HIV treatment cascade focuses on identifying those infected, ensuring they are linked to and retained in care and treated with ART with the viral load suppressed.

Caring for persons with HIV or AIDS requires collaborative, interdisciplinary care throughout the course of the illness.[3] Early in the AIDS epidemic, many believed it to be futile and a waste of resources to admit persons living with AIDS to an intensive care unit (ICU).[10] Today, however, as persons living with HIV and AIDS are living longer, they are being admitted to the ICU for management of AIDS-related opportunistic infections, complications associated with ART, and medical problems unrelated to HIV infection.[11] The most common indication for admission to an ICU among persons infected with HIV is respiratory infection or respiratory failure and sepsis.[11,12] Other physiologic problems experienced by persons living with HIV or AIDS potentially requiring ICU care include immune reconstitution syndrome; atherogenic metabolic complications associated with ART; end-stage liver disease secondary to viral hepatitis; lactic acidosis associated with nucleoside reverse transcriptase inhibitors (NRTIs); end-stage renal disease secondary to HIV-associated nephropathy; hepatitis B or C; diabetes; and hypertension.[11] Similar to the general population, the leading cause of death among persons infected with HIV is cardiovascular disease.[13]

When persons living with HIV or AIDS are admitted to the ICU, there are several challenging issues confronting the critical care nurse. These issues include laws related to HIV testing and disclosure; risk for significant drug interactions between ART and medications commonly used in the ICU; and controversies surrounding the use of ART in the ICU. Therefore, to ensure quality, safe care, critical care nurses need to be familiar with ART for the following reasons[14]:

- to recognize life-threatening toxicities associated with ART
- to avoid drug interactions between ART and other classes of drugs that are common and potentially life-threatening
- to avoid promoting ART drug resistance, a situation that could have profound negative consequences for the person living with HIV or AIDS after discharge from the ICU.

For some persons, HIV or AIDS may be diagnosed during a hospitalization or critical illness. In 2006, the CDC issued *Revised Recommendations for HIV testing of adults, adolescents, and pregnant women in health-care* settings, which advocated the routine testing of all people who visit any health care setting.[15] The purpose of this report was to increase the rate of HIV testing in health care settings, foster earlier detection of HIV infection, identify and counsel persons with unrecognized HIV infection while linking them to clinical and prevention services, and further reduce the rate of perinatal or vertical (mother-to-child) transmission. Knowledge of an individual's HIV serostatus affects differential diagnosis and may influence the diagnostic and treatment options, including patient outcomes. Therefore, it is essential for critical care nurses to understand how HIV infection, as well as its sequelae and treatment, serves as a comorbid condition of the critically ill person or the primary admission diagnosis in the ICU.

## Epidemiology

The CDC estimates that more than 1.2 million people are living with HIV in the United States.[16] One in eight of those people living with HIV are unaware of their infection. As a consequence of increased survival, the prevalence of HIV and AIDS is increasing in the United States; in addition, the number of new infections remains high, with an estimated 50,000 Americans becoming newly infected with HIV annually. The majority of AIDS cases continue to occur in gay, bisexual, and other men who have sex with men (MSM). Half of new HIV infections annually and nearly half of the people living with HIV/AIDS are among MSM. However, heterosexuals and injection-drug users also continue to be diagnosed with HIV and AIDS. Like MSM, African Americans/Blacks are disproportionately affected by HIV and AIDS. Although African Americans/Blacks account for approximately 12% of the US population, they account for nearly half of all new HIV infections each year and half of the people living with HIV in the United States. While the epidemic continues in the historical urban epicenters of Washington, DC, New York City, and San Francisco, it has reached every US state, with the Southeastern United States having the highest rates of new HIV infections.[17] Of the 10 US states accounting for 65% of all new HIV infections in 2011, 7 are in the Southeastern United States.[17]

## Immunopathogenesis of HIV

The immunodeficiency associated with AIDS is caused by the viral agent HIV.[18,19] HIV is a single-stranded RNA virus that is part of the Retroviridae family in the genus *Lentivirus*. Two species of human primate lentiviruses are known to exist: HIV-1 and HIV-2. Their genetic cousins, simian immunodeficiency virus 1 and 2 (SIV-1 and SIV-2), are nonhuman primate lentiviruses. Recent evidence documents that there was extensive diversity of HIV-1 in the human primate population by 1960 and that the common ancestor to HIV-1 was spreading among humans 60 to 80 years before AIDS was first recognized in the 1980s.[20,21]

HIV is transmitted from person to person by blood and bodily fluids (semen, vaginal secretions, breast milk).[19] A variety of cells are susceptible to HIV infection including cells of the hematopoietic system, central nervous system (CNS), skin, gastrointestinal tract, and myocardium as well as the dendritic cells, renal tubular cells, hepatocytes, Kupffer cells, pulmonary fibroblasts, cells of the cervix, prostate, and testes, and dental pulp fibroblasts.[19] The biologic properties of the virus, its concentration in the bodily fluids, and the nature of the host's susceptibility at the cellular and immunologic levels influence transmission of HIV. Sexually transmitted infections (STIs) increase both the amount of infectious virus and the number of infected cells in the genitals and enhance HIV transmission. The lack of circumcision in males has been associated with an increased risk of infection related to the large number of dendritic cells in the foreskin and also with increased rates of transmission among uncircumcised men to their sexual partners.[19]

## Viral Replication

HIV is composed of nine genes responsible for invading host cells and replicating. HIV is composed of a small outer envelope, an inner core of genetic material (RNA), and three enzymes necessary for reproduction: reverse transcriptase, integrase, and protease (controlled by the pol—or polymerase—gene). Like all RNA viruses, HIV cannot reproduce on its own: it must attach to and invade other cells to reproduce. Figure 48-1 illustrates the process of viral replication.

After HIV enters the bloodstream, infection occurs with transmission of HIV across a mucosal barrier attaching itself to dendritic cells or Langerhans cells.[18] Propagation of HIV occurs initially in partially activated CD4$^+$ T cells, followed by massive propagation in activated CD4$^+$ T cells of the gut-associated lymphoid tissue. Then, dissemination of HIV to other secondary lymphoid tissues ensues, with establishment of stable HIV viral reservoirs following.

Having an affinity for CD4$^+$ receptors, HIV attaches to the CD4$^+$ receptors on the T lymphocytes, fusing with the host cell, shedding its outer envelope, and then integrating its viral core into the DNA of the host's cell. The viral RNA is incorporated into the DNA of the T-lymphocyte host with help from the enzyme integrase. After integration, viral RNA is transcribed into the host's DNA by way of the enzyme reverse transcriptase. After incorporation into the cell's DNA structure, the enzyme protease breaks the components down into functional pieces, which are then assembled into structurally intact, new infectious units called virions. This

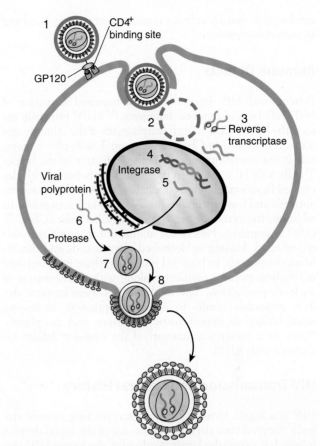

**FIGURE 48-1** Process of human immunodeficiency virus (HIV) replication. (1) Attachment of HIV to a CD4$^+$ receptor. (2) Internalization and uncoating of the virus with viral RNA and reverse transcriptase. (3) Reverse transcription, which produces a mirror image of the viral RNA and double-stranded DNA molecule. (4) Integration of viral DNA into host DNA using the integrase enzyme. (5) Transcription of the inserted viral DNA to produce viral messenger RNA. (6) Translation of viral messenger RNA to create viral polyprotein. (7) Cleavage of viral polyprotein into individual viral proteins that make up the new virus. (8) Assembly and release of the new virus from the host cell.

(Adapted from Porth C: Pathophysiology: Concepts of Altered Health States, 8th ed. Philadelphia, PA: Lippincott Williams & Wilkins, 2009.)

process tricks the host's cells into making components for more virions.

Eventually, the new virions undergo a process of coating and are then expelled from the host cell by budding. During budding, the parent cell releases a daughter cell with its cytoplasmic material, which begins existence as a separate cell. These daughter cells disseminate through the bloodstream and infect other cells. Approximately 30% of the viral burden in a person who is HIV positive is regenerated daily. This budding process weakens the cell wall of the original CD4$^+$ T cells, leading to cellular instability. This cellular instability—in combination with the direct cytopathic effects of HIV on CD4$^+$ cells and progenitor cells; the effect of HIV on cell membrane permeability; induction of apoptosis (programmed cell death) associated with immune activation; destruction of the bone marrow and lymphoid tissues; cytokine dysregulation; anti-CD4$^+$ cell cytotoxic activity; and anti-CD4$^+$ autoantibodies—results in a decline in the number of circulating CD4$^+$ T-cell lymphocytes. Ultimately, these complex mechanisms destroy cellular immune functioning, resulting in immunosuppression.[19]

## Immune Defects

Patients with HIV infection exhibit impaired activation of both cellular and humoral immunity.[18,19] HIV primarily infects the helper CD4+ T-cell lymphocytes of the immune system. As discussed in Chapter 45, these T cells play a major role in the overall immune response. Infection of the helper T cells with HIV results in profound lymphopenia with decreased functional abilities, including decreased response to antigens and loss of stimulus for T- and B-cell activation. In addition, the cytotoxic activity of the killer cells (CD8+ T cells) is impaired. Functional abilities of macrophages also are affected, leading to decreased phagocytosis and diminished chemotaxis. In humoral immunity, there is diminished antibody response to antigens, along with dysregulation of antibody production. The total effect of these immune defects ultimately results in immunosuppression, increasing susceptibility to opportunistic infections and neoplasms. Figure 48-2 presents a summary of the immune defects associated with AIDS.

## HIV Transmission and Natural History

HIV is a fragile virus and cannot survive long outside the body. Survival time depends on the size of the liquid droplet in which it exists: the larger the droplet, the longer HIV can remain alive. As the droplet dries, HIV dies. HIV has been isolated from all types of body fluids and tissues. However, not all body fluids have been implicated in the transmission of HIV. The four fluids from which large amounts of virus have been isolated and have been implicated in transmission are blood, semen, vaginal fluid, and breast milk.

The infectiousness of a fluid depends on the amount of virus present (viral load) in the fluid and the ability of that fluid to reach the target cell. For HIV to cause infection, it must leave the body of the infected host, successfully enter the new host's bloodstream, and attach itself to a CD4+ receptor site. The likelihood that this series of events will occur is low, especially because a certain amount of virus is required to cause an infection. The notion that HIV does not transmit easily is based on evidence suggesting that the probability of transmission ranges from 0.0001 to 0.0040 per sexual contact.[18] Small tears in the anus or vagina provide a portal of entry for virus present in blood, semen, and vaginal fluid. The virus in breast milk can enter through cuts or irritation in the gastrointestinal tract of the infant.

There are three known modes of HIV transmission[19]:
- Unprotected vaginal or anal sexual contact with an infected person, with unprotected receptive anal intercourse being the riskiest sexual behavior
- Inoculation with infected blood or blood products, which includes accidental needlestick injuries and risk for transmission with needle sharing by injection-drug users
- Vertical transmission from mother to child during delivery or through breast-feeding

After infection with HIV, a person does not immediately test positive for HIV; first, seroconversion must occur. Seroconversion is the development of antibodies that can be detected in the blood as a consequence of antigenic stimulation from HIV associated with exposure. In other words, seroconversion is the change from an HIV-negative result to an HIV-positive result. During the seroconversion process, the body recognizes HIV as an invader and develops antibodies, which are then detectable by enzyme-linked immunosorbent assay (ELISA). In most people, seroconversion occurs 2 to 8 weeks after exposure to HIV (average is 25 days).[22] During this time, a person can unknowingly transmit the virus, and an ELISA screening test may yield a false-negative result. In 97% of persons, seroconversion occurs within 3 months, but in extremely rare cases it can take up to 6 months for antibodies to develop.[22]

After a person is infected with HIV, manifestations of acute or primary HIV infection, also known as acute antiretroviral syndrome, occur 2 to 4 weeks later. The manifestations of acute HIV infection can present like other infectious viral disease such as mononucleosis and influenza. The most frequent manifestations associated with acute HIV infection include fever (96%), adenopathy (74%), pharyngitis (70%), rash (70%), myalgias (54%), and, less frequently, diarrhea (32%), headache (32%), nausea/vomiting (27%), hepatosplenomegaly (14%), weight loss (13%), thrush (12%), and neurologic symptoms (12%).[23]

During the acute HIV infection phase, there is usually a high viral load. It is not uncommon for an individual to be

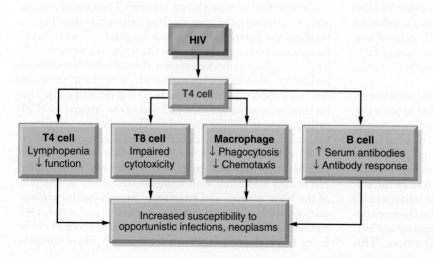

FIGURE 48-2 Summary of immune defects in AIDS.

unaware of his or her HIV serostatus and to test negative or indeterminate for HIV during this phase. Several studies suggest that as many as 40% of lifetime transmissions occur during this acute HIV infection phase. As previously stated, over 20% of all HIV-infected persons in the United States are not aware of their current serostatus and therefore have the potential to transmit the virus to another person. Although ELISA plays a valuable role in screening, it is not a confirmatory test for the diagnosis of HIV. Later in this chapter, other diagnostic tests used in HIV testing are discussed.

The risk of HIV transmission to health care workers is low if standard precautions are followed (Box 48-1).[24] Occupational exposure can occur through a percutaneous injury (needlestick), contact with mucous membrane, or contact with nonintact skin (chapped, abraded, or affected by dermatitis).[25] The estimated average risk for HIV transmission after a percutaneous injury is 0.3%. The estimated average risk for HIV transmission after a mucous membrane exposure is 0.09%.[25] To provide a mechanism for comparison, if a health care worker were to receive a percutaneous needlestick from a host who was antigen-positive for hepatitis B virus (HBV), hepatitis C virus (HCV), and HIV, the health care worker would have a 37% to 62% risk for acquiring HBV if previously not vaccinated and a 1.8% risk for acquiring HCV, in comparison to only a 0.3% risk for acquiring HIV. Factors that can influence HIV transmission in a health care setting include contact with a device that is visually contaminated with blood, exposure to a large quantity of blood, participating in a procedure in which a needle is placed in an artery or vein, and deep injuries.[25]

For many years, occupational and nonoccupational postexposure prophylaxis (PEP) has been offered to health care workers and persons with exposure to HIV. PEP should be started as soon as possible after exposure to HIV, preferably within hours but no later than within 72 hours.[25] After 72 hours, PEP is not recommended. The decision about when to initiate PEP is based on the type of exposure, risk assessment of the incident, and risk assessment for HIV. Combination therapy using two or three medications is recommended in PEP; the number of medications depends on the type of exposure and the risk status of the source. Whether an occupational or nonoccupational exposure, PEP is prescribed for 28 days and requires the person to maintain strict adherence, which may be difficult if toxicities or side effects develop. Laboratory tests for toxicity should occur at the time of exposure and 2 weeks later, and consist of a complete blood count (CBC) and renal and hepatic function tests. At the time of the exposure, persons exposed should have serologic testing followed by repeat testing at 6 weeks, 12 weeks, and 6 months after exposure.[25] The National HIV/AIDS Clinicians' Consultation Center is a 24-hours-a-day, 7-days-a-week resource to all healthcare professionals and includes a PEP hotline to help manage exposure not only to HIV but also to HBV and HCV (see http://nccc.ucsf.edu/ for more information).

Since there has not been a decline in the number of new infections in the United States, scientists, clinicians, public health specialists, and advocacy groups have debated the value of preexposure prophylaxis with ART as a mechanism to prevent HIV infection. In a large, multisite clinical trial, scientists identified that use of oral ART provided protection against the acquisition of HIV infection among MSM study participants.[26] Currently, the CDC recommends PrEP be considered for people who are HIV-negative and at substantial risk for HIV (http://www.cdc.gov/hiv/basics/prep.html). This includes uninfected individuals who have sex with a partner in serodiscordant relationships (an ongoing relationship with an HIV-infected partner); men who have sex with men who have had anal sex without a condom or who have been diagnosed with a sexually transmitted infection in the past 6 months; heterosexual men and women who do not regularly use a condom during sex whose partners' HIV status is unknown or at substantial risk for HIV (people who inject drugs, bisexual male partner); and people who have injected drugs in the past 6 months and have shared injection equipment.[27]

Regardless of the etiology of HIV infection, once infected with HIV, individuals will progress from the acute primary HIV infection phase to an asymptomatic phase. During this period, HIV viral replication continues, resulting in a decline of immune functioning. As the number of CD4$^+$ T cells declines, a number of infectious and noninfectious diseases begin to present. Table 48-1 describes the complications common at various CD4$^+$ T-cell counts. If not treated, the cellular immune system will continue to decline and the person living with HIV will continue to be at risk for or experience an increased number of infectious and noninfectious diseases. Once the CD4$^+$ T-cell count reaches 200 cells/mm$^3$, the infected person is considered immunosuppressed and at very high risk for a number of opportunistic infections and other problems. Box 48-2 on page 958 provides a list of AIDS-defining conditions.

## Assessment

### History and Physical Examination

The spectrum of clinical findings associated with acute HIV infection, clinical latency, and AIDS ranges from flulike symptoms, to a period of no symptoms, to a variety of infections and symptoms associated with immunosuppression, to unquestionable AIDS. Patients with HIV infection may become seriously ill, requiring frequent hospitalizations and care in the ICU. In the past, critical care nurses frequently encountered patients with AIDS experiencing life-threatening opportunistic infections. Today, as patients with HIV are living longer, critical care nurses are more frequently caring for this population as they experience other critical illnesses associated with aging, including cardiovascular disease, renal problems, trauma, or consequences of ART in addition to the complications of AIDS.

*Pneumocystis* pneumonia (PCP), which is caused by *Pneumocystis jiroveci* (formerly known as *Pneumocystis carinii*), is the most common opportunistic infection requiring admission to the ICU.[28] (Even though the name has changed, the abbreviation PCP is still used to describe the pathogen.) The *P. jiroveci* organism is considered a fungus based on its genetic makeup. The most common presenting symptoms of PCP include fever, exertional dyspnea, nonproductive cough, and a normal chest radiograph progressing to severe hypoxemia and respiratory failure.

The major indication for critical care of patients with PCP is impending or actual respiratory failure. Symptoms of respiratory compromise often are more severe than diagnostic

| BOX 48-1 | Summary of Isolation Precautions |
|---|---|

Standard Precautions: "Based on the principle that all blood, bodily fluids, secretions, excretions except sweat, non-intact skin and mucous membranes may contain transmissible infectious agents"

| Common Organisms | Key Elements |
|---|---|
| Hepatitis A virus<br>Hepatitis B/D virus<br>Hepatitis C virus<br>Human immunodeficiency virus (HIV)<br>*Pneumocystis jiroveci* | **Hand Hygiene**<br>• Before direct care contact<br>• Wash hands after touching blood, body fluids, secretions, excretions, and contaminated items, regardless of whether gloves are worn.<br>• Wash hands immediately after gloves are removed, between patient contacts, and whenever indicated to prevent transfer of microorganisms to other patients or environments. Use plain soap for routine handwashing and an antimicrobial or waterless antiseptic agent for specific circumstances.<br>• Wear clean, nonsterile gloves when touching blood, body fluids, excretions or secretions, contaminated items, mucous membranes, and nonintact skin. Change gloves between tasks on the same patient as necessary, and remove gloves promptly after use.<br>• Restrict use of artificial nails and nail polish.<br><br>**Use of Personal Protective Equipment**<br>• Wear mask, eye protection, or face shield during procedures and care activities that are likely to generate splashes or sprays of blood or body fluids. Use gown to protect skin and prevent soiling of clothing.<br><br>**Health Care Delivery System**<br>• Ensure that used patient care equipment that is soiled with blood or identified body fluids, secretions, and excretions is handled carefully to prevent transfer of microorganisms or cleaned and appropriately reprocessed if used for another patient.<br>• Use adequate environmental controls to ensure that routine care, cleaning, and disinfection procedures are followed.<br>• Handle, transport, and process linen soiled with blood and body fluids, excretions, and secretions in a manner that prevents skin and mucous membrane exposures, contamination of clothing, and transfer of microorganisms.<br><br>**Safe Injection Practices**<br>• Use previously identified techniques and equipment to prevent injuries when using needles, sharps, and scalpels and place these items in appropriate puncture-resistant containers after use. |

Airborne Precautions: Used in addition to standard precautions for "patients known or suspected with organisms transmitted by airborne droplets that remain suspended in the air and can be widely dispersed by air current"

| Common Organisms | Key Elements |
|---|---|
| *Mycobacterium tuberculosis*<br>Varicella<br>Measles<br>SARS | • Place the patient in private room with an isolation sign on the door that has monitored negative air pressure in relation to surrounding areas, 6–12 air changes per hour, and appropriate discharge of air outside or monitored filtration if air is recirculated.<br>• Keep the door closed to the patient room at all times and the patient in the room whenever possible.<br>• Use respiratory protection when entering room of patient with known or suspected TB. If patient has known or suspected rubeola (measles) or varicella (chickenpox), respiratory protection should be worn unless person entering room is immune to these diseases.<br>• Transport the patient out of the room only when necessary, and place a surgical mask on the patient if possible.<br>• Consult Centers for Disease Control and Prevention Guidelines for additional prevention strategies for TB. |

Droplet Precautions: Used in addition to standard precautions for "patients known or suspected to be infected with microorganisms transmitted by droplets generated during coughing, sneezing, talking, or during cough producing procedures"

| Common Organisms | Key Elements |
|---|---|
| Meningitis<br>Pertussis<br>Influenza (A, B, C, Avian, H1N1)<br>Mumps<br>Rubella<br>*Mycoplasma* | • Place the patient in private room with an isolation sign on the door, if available, or cohort patients if necessary. Door closed at all times.<br>• Spatial separation of at least 3 ft from other patients/visitors. Health care providers should wear a mask when working within 3 ft of the patient.<br>• Transport the patient out of the room only when necessary, and place a surgical mask on the patient if possible. |

## BOX 48-1  Summary of Isolation Precautions (*continued*)

Contact Isolation: Used in addition to standard precautions for "patients known or suspected to be infected or colonized with epidemiologically important microorganisms that can be transmitted by direct contact with the patient when performing care activities or indirect contact (touching) with environmental surfaces or patient care items"

| Common Organisms | Key Elements |
|---|---|
| *Clostridium difficile*<br>Respiratory syncytial virus<br>Pediculosis<br>Scabies<br>Multidrug resistant Staphylococcus aureus (MRSA)<br>Vancomycin resistant enterococcus (VRE)<br>Gram-negative bacteria | • Place the patient in private room with an isolation sign on the door, if available, or cohort patients if necessary. Door closed at all times.<br>• Change gloves after having contact with infective material. Remove gloves before leaving the patient environment, and wash hands with an antimicrobial or waterless antiseptic agent.<br>• Wear a gown if contact with infectious agent is likely or patient has diarrhea, ileostomy, colostomy, or wound drainage not contained by a dressing.<br>• Limit movement of the patient out of the room.<br>• When possible, dedicate the use of noncritical patient care equipment to a single patient to avoid sharing equipment. |

Adapted from Siegel JD, Rhinehart E, Jackson M, et al: The Healthcare Infection Control Practices Advisory Committee: 2007 Guideline for Isolation Precautions: Preventing Transmission of Infectious Agents in Healthcare Settings, June 2007. Retrieved from http://www.cdc.gov/ncidod/dhqp/pdf/isolation2007.pdf

## TABLE 48-1  Correlation Between CD4⁺ T-Cell Count and HIV Complications

| CD4$^+$ T-cell count*<br>(as cells/mm$^3$) | Infectious Complications | Noninfectious† Complications |
|---|---|---|
| >500 | Acute retroviral syndrome<br>Candidal vaginitis | Persistent generalized lymphadenopathy<br>Guillain-Barré syndrome<br>Myopathy<br>Aseptic meningitis |
| 200–500 | Pneumococcal and other bacterial pneumonia<br>Pulmonary tuberculosis (TB)<br>Herpes zoster<br>Oropharyngeal candidiasis (thrush)<br>Cryptosporidiosis, self-limited<br>Kaposi's sarcoma<br>Oral hairy leukoplakia | Cervical intraepithelial neoplasia<br>Cervical cancer<br>B-cell lymphoma<br>Anemia<br>Mononeuronal multiplex<br>Idiopathic thrombocytopenic purpura<br>Hodgkin's lymphoma<br>Lymphocytic interstitial pneumonitis |
| <200 | *Pneumocystis jiroveci* pneumonia<br>Disseminated histoplasmosis and coccidioidomycosis<br>Miliary/extrapulmonary TB<br>Progressive multifocal leukoencephalopathy | Wasting<br>Peripheral neuropathy<br>HIV-associated dementia<br>Cardiomyopathy<br>Vacuolar myelopathy<br>Progressive polyradiculopathy<br>Non-Hodgkin's lymphoma |
| <100 | Disseminated herpes simplex<br>Toxoplasmosis<br>Cryptococcosis<br>Cryptosporidiosis, chronic<br>Microsporidiosis<br>Candidal esophagitis | |
| <50 | Disseminated cytomegalovirus<br>Disseminated *Mycobacterium avium* complex | Primary central nervous system (CNS) lymphoma |

*Most complications occur with increasing frequency at lower CD4$^+$ T-cell counts.
†Some conditions categorized as noninfectious are often microbially mediated, such as lymphoma (Epstein-Barr virus), and cervical carcinoma (human papillomavirus).
From Bartlett JG, Gallant JE, Pham P: The Management of HIV Infection. Durham, NC: Knowledge Source Solutions, LLC, 2009, p 3.

studies, such as chest radiographs and blood gas values, indicate. Therefore, early aggressive therapy for PCP using intravenous (IV) trimethoprim and sulfamethoxazole (Bactrim, Septra) and corticosteroids is the treatment of choice. Corticosteroids are given to reduce the inflammation caused by the death of *P. jiroveci* in the lungs. Even with urgent, aggressive treatment, many patients require mechanical ventilation for progressive alveolar hypoventilation. Adverse reactions to trimethoprim and sulfamethoxazole, including nausea and vomiting, maculopapular rash, bone marrow suppression, anorexia, headache, crystalluria, and fever, reportedly occur in more than 50% of patients.

Patients with AIDS may also experience complex neurologic conditions including cryptococcal meningitis, toxoplasmosis, histoplasmosis, Creutzfeldt–Jakob disease (CJD) leading to progressive multifocal leukoencephalopathy, and CNS lymphomas. As with PCP, a priority is to reduce immunosuppression by initiating ART so that these opportunistic

Case Definition of AIDS for Surveillance

### Purposes: Indicator Conditions

- Candidiasis of bronchi, trachea, or lungs
- Candidiasis, esophageal
- Cervical cancer, invasive
- Coccidioidomycosis, disseminated or extrapulmonary
- Cryptococcosis, extrapulmonary
- Cryptosporidiosis, chronic intestinal (>1 month duration)
- Cytomegalovirus (CMV) disease (other than liver, spleen, or nodes)
- CMV retinitis (with loss of vision)
- Encephalopathy, HIV-related
- Herpes simplex: chronic ulcer(s) (>1 month duration); or bronchitis, pneumonitis, or esophagitis
- Histoplasmosis, disseminated or extrapulmonary
- Isosporiasis, chronic intestinal (>1 month duration)
- Kaposi's sarcoma
- Lymphoma, Burkitt's (or equivalent)
- Lymphoma, immunoblastic (or equivalent)
- Lymphoma, of brain, primary
- *Mycobacterium avium* complex or *Mycobacterium kansasii*, disseminated or extrapulmonary
- *Mycobacterium tuberculosis*, any site (pulmonary or extrapulmonary)
- *Mycobacterium*, other species or unidentified species, disseminated or extrapulmonary
- *Pneumocystis jiroveci* pneumonia
- Pneumonia, recurrent bacterial
- Progressive multifocal leukoencephalopathy (PML)
- *Salmonella* septicemia, recurrent
- Toxoplasmosis of brain
- Wasting syndrome due to HIV
- CD4$^+$ count 200 cells/mL or less

From Centers for Disease Control and Prevention. Revised surveillance case definitions for HIV infection among adults, adolescents, and children <18 months and for HIV infection and AIDS among children aged 18 months to less than 13 years—United States, 2008. Morb Mortal Wkly Rep 57(RR10): 1–8, 2008.

infections can be avoided. For the critical care nurse, treatment is usually associated with managing the neurologic compromise that includes increased intracranial pressure, seizures, and hemiparesis.

Although the early research related to HIV and AIDS was originally conducted in men, the body of knowledge about HIV and AIDS in women is significant, partially as a result of the natural history study of HIV in women also known as the Women's Interagency HIV Study.[29] Many recent studies, which have included women, suggest that men and women do not differ in terms of the general characteristics of HIV disease, except for the HIV-infected woman's increased risk for cervical dysplasia. The clinical course of infection—including time from HIV infection to AIDS, risk factors for HIV seroconversion, number and type of opportunistic illnesses, protection against infections, and the effectiveness of potent antiretroviral agents—appears similar in both men and women.

No organ system escapes involvement in HIV infection. Single infections may develop in critically ill patients with AIDS, but patients often have multiple infections simultaneously that require a variety of treatment strategies. The decrease in immune system functioning causes the multisystem manifestations to develop, resulting in an increase in opportunistic infections. Figure 48-3 presents manifestations of HIV infection and AIDS.

## Laboratory and Diagnostic Studies

### Tests Used to Detect HIV

Several serologic tests are used to determine whether a person has been exposed to HIV. The most widely used test for screening is the ELISA, which determines the presence of antibodies for HIV. The results of this rapid and inexpensive test are usually available in less than 1 hour. ELISA screening tests can be performed on either blood/plasma/serum or oral fluid.[23] Results are reported as either reactive (positive) or nonreactive (negative) and have a sensitivity (true positive) rate of 99.5% and specificity (true negative) rate of 99.994%.[23] Unfortunately, the presence of other antibodies may lead to a false-positive result—in other words, the test result may be HIV positive but the person is actually HIV negative. With ELISA, a positive/reactive ELISA is always repeated, and if the second ELISA is positive, confirmatory testing with Western blot is required.

Because of the "window period" associated with seroconversion, during the acute HIV infection phase, low production of antibodies at the time the test is performed or recency of infection may lead to a false-negative result. A false-negative result means that the test result was HIV negative but the person is actually HIV positive; therefore, persons should not be considered HIV negative until there are repeated negative results in a 6-month period. During this "window period," if a person engages in high-risk behaviors associated with HIV, another 6-month window is required to determine the individual's HIV status.

Rapid HIV testing is based on ELISA technology. Instead of sending the specimen to the laboratory and then obtaining results days later, as was standard procedure in the past, rapid HIV testing with ELISA yields results within 20 minutes. Frequently, this type of testing is done in emergency departments (EDs), labor and delivery units, and primary healthcare environments including ambulatory/outpatient clinics. Rapid HIV tests can be performed with either serum or saliva samples. Any positive ELISA, regardless of specimen type, still requires confirmatory testing with Western blot. In June 2010, the Food and Drug Administration (FDA) approved a fourth-generation HIV test. This contemporary HIV test incorporates p24 antigen testing with standard antibody testing and enables earlier and more accurate HIV detection, particularly during the window period.

All positive ELISAs are confirmed by a Western blot. The Western blot analysis is the most widely used confirmatory test and is highly sensitive and specific. The Western blot identifies the presence of antibodies to HIV-1 and/or HIV-2 proteins (depending on the specific assay). The Western blot screens for the following proteins: core (p17, p24, p55), polymerase (p31, p51, p66), and envelope (gp41, gp120, gp160).[23] In analyzing test results from a Western blot, the test is considered to be negative if no bands are present. To be positive, the Western blot results must include gp120/160 and either gp41 or p24. An indeterminate Western blot is the presence of any band not meeting positive criteria.

Several alternate FDA-approved HIV detection methods are available, but usually are not routinely used in screening adults. The polymerase chain reaction (PCR) test is frequently used in newborns and children to screen for HIV infection. Because it tests for genetic material of HIV rather than antibodies to the virus, it can identify HIV infection

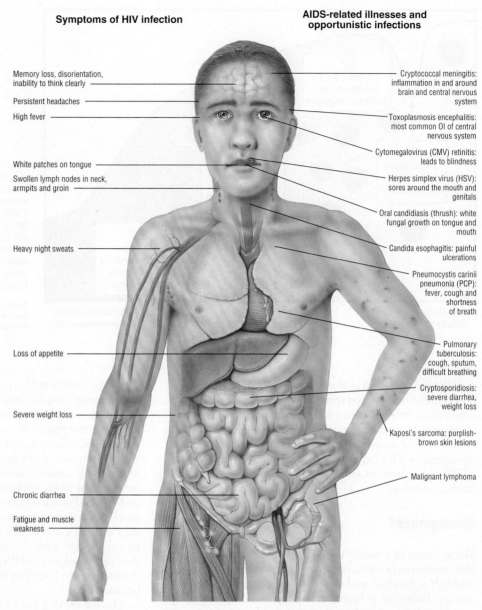

**Symptoms of HIV infection**

Memory loss, disorientation, inability to think clearly

Persistent headaches

High fever

White patches on tongue

Swollen lymph nodes in neck, armpits and groin

Heavy night sweats

Loss of appetite

Severe weight loss

Chronic diarrhea

Fatigue and muscle weakness

**AIDS-related illnesses and opportunistic infections**

Cryptococcal meningitis: inflammation in and around brain and central nervous system

Toxoplasmosis encephalitis: most common OI of central nervous system

Cytomegalovirus (CMV) retinitis: leads to blindness

Herpes simplex virus (HSV): sores around the mouth and genitals

Oral candidiasis (thrush): white fungal growth on tongue and mouth

Candida esophagitis: painful ulcerations

Pneumocystis carinii pneumonia (PCP): fever, cough and shortness of breath

Pulmonary tuberculosis: cough, sputum, difficult breathing

Cryptosporidiosis: severe diarrhea, weight loss

Kaposi's sarcoma: purplish-brown skin lesions

Malignant lymphoma

**FIGURE 48-3**   Manifestations of HIV infection and AIDS.

(From Anatomical Chart Company: Atlas of Pathophysiology, 3rd ed. Springhouse, PA: Springhouse, 2010, p 267.)

at a much earlier stage. Therefore, in adults, this test is frequently done when there has been a high-risk occupational or nonoccupational exposure.

As a consequence of the 2006 CDC recommendations, screening for HIV should be routinely performed in all healthcare settings for persons between the ages of 13 and 64. Furthermore, all patients initiating treatment for tuberculosis (TB) or seeking treatment for STIs should be routinely screened. All persons likely to be at high risk for HIV should be tested annually. According the CDC, "persons likely to be at high risk include injection-drug users and their sex partners, persons who exchange sex for money or drugs, sex partners of HIV-infected persons, and MSM or heterosexual persons who themselves or whose sex partners have had more than one sex partner since their most recent HIV test."[15]

### Tests Used to Evaluate Progression of HIV Infection

HIV nucleic acid testing, also called viral load testing, in combination with the CD4$^+$ T-cell lymphocyte count is currently

the best method available to determine progression on the HIV disease continuum. The viral load measures the amount of viral particles in a cubic mm (mm$^3$) of blood. The higher the viral load, the more HIV present to cause immune destruction and the more rapid the progression to AIDS.[23] Three methods can be used to determine the viral load: HIV RNA PCR, branched-chain DNA (bDNA), and nucleic acid sequence–based amplification. PCR is the most common method. The test results are used to determine the best time to begin ART and when a change in therapy may be indicated.

The CD4$^+$ T-cell count and percentage is another important evaluation tool used to stage HIV disease and to make decisions concerning the initiation of ART and prophylactic treatment for opportunistic organisms.[30] The normal CD4$^+$ T-cell count is around 1,000 cells/mm$^3$ in adults, and the count declines over time in the person with HIV not on treatment (Fig. 48-4). There is an inverse relationship between the viral load and CD4$^+$ T-cell count (Fig. 48-5). As HIV/AIDS progresses, the number of CD4$^+$ T cells declines, and the amount of HIV in the blood increases.

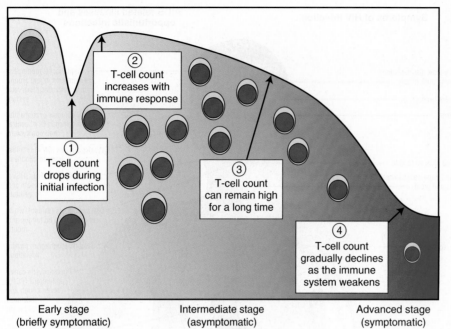

**FIGURE 48-4** Use of T-cell count (CD4) to stage HIV infection. (1) The T-cell count drops during initial infection because the virus is destroying the T cells. (2) Once the immune system starts to fight back, the T-cell count increases. T-cell counts can go up and down at different times during HIV disease, but they do not return to where they were before infection. (3) T-cell counts can remain fairly high for a long time—sometimes for years—but steadily lose ground.

(Redrawn from Glaxo Wellcome: HIV: Understanding the Disease. Research Triangle Park, NC: Author, 1995.)

Within figure:

② T-cell count increases with immune response

① T-cell count drops during initial infection

③ T-cell count can remain high for a long time

④ T-cell count gradually declines as the immune system weakens

Early stage (briefly symptomatic)

Intermediate stage (asymptomatic)

Advanced stage (symptomatic)

Other tests used to evaluate HIV infection include CBC, rapid plasma reagin (to screen for syphilis), chest radiograph, serum chemistries, Papanicolaou (Pap) tests to screen for cervical cancer in women and to screen for anal carcinoma in both men and women, purified protein derivative skin test (to screen for TB), hepatitis serology (to screen for HBV and HCV), toxoplasmosis serology, and cytomegalovirus (CMV) antibody serology.

## Management

Management of patients with HIV disease involves a complex, multisystem assessment, including diagnostic tests that establish a baseline and determine the appropriateness of therapy. Prognosis is based on the type and number of opportunistic infections that occur and the degree of immunosuppression. Patients with multiple opportunistic infections tend to be more seriously immunosuppressed and have a poorer prognosis.

## Control of Opportunistic Infection

The primary goal of management in critically ill HIV-infected patients is the prevention or resolution of infections, whether opportunistic, community-acquired, or health care associated. Opportunistic infections are the leading cause of death in patients with HIV infection; therefore, prevention is the cornerstone of treatment. Treatment of opportunistic infections is aimed at support of the involved system or systems. Treatment guidelines have been developed for prophylaxis against several organisms associated with HIV and AIDS. In April 2009, the *Guidelines for Prevention and Treatment of Opportunistic Infections in HIV-Infected Adults and Adolescents* were published.[30] The current organisms for which prophylaxis is strongly recommended include *P. jiroveci*, *Mycobacterium tuberculosis*, and *Toxoplasma gondii*. Organisms that

should be considered for prophylaxis include CMV, *Mycobacterium avium* complex, and varicella-zoster virus. In addition, vaccination guidelines should be implemented to prevent vaccine-preventable diseases including hepatitis A, hepatitis B, seasonal influenza, and *S. pneumoniae*.

Maintenance of safe infection control measures to prevent unnecessary contamination and complications in the ICU are essential when working with patients with HIV infection and AIDS. For current treatment guidelines associated with prophylaxis against common opportunistic infections associated with HIV and AIDS, critical care nurses are encouraged to collaborate with the interdisciplinary team and review data published on the HIV/AIDS pages of the CDC Web site (please refer to http://www.cdc.gov/hiv/default.htm for more information).

The use of ART has had a significant impact on the treatment of opportunistic infections. The number of opportunistic infections has significantly decreased because of advances in ART.[29,30] Prophylactic or suppressive treatment for PCP, toxoplasmosis, CMV infection, *M. avium* complex infection, leishmaniasis, cryptococcosis, and candidal thrush may be discontinued if the patient's CD4+ T-cell count increases sufficiently and is sustained, usually above 200 cells/mm³.[3,30] Administration of ART also can rapidly reduce viral load, thereby decreasing the incidence of complications.

## Antiretroviral Therapy

Persons living with HIV or AIDS who receive ART and maintain strict adherence can survive for many years after being infected with the virus.[6] The classes of antiretrovirals used to treat HIV include the nucleoside/nucleotide reverse transcriptase inhibitors (NRTIs), nonnucleoside reverse transcriptase inhibitors (NNRTIs), protease inhibitors (PIs), fusion inhibitors (FIs), integrase strand transfer inhibitors (INSTIs), and CCR5 antagonists (CCR5s).[31] These drug groups act by

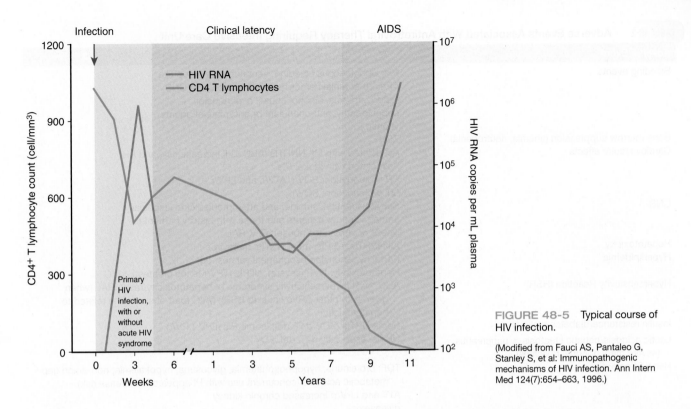

**FIGURE 48-5**  Typical course of HIV infection.

(Modified from Fauci AS, Pantaleo G, Stanley S, et al: Immunopathogenic mechanisms of HIV infection. Ann Intern Med 124(7):654–663, 1996.)

blocking the fusion of HIV with CD4$^+$ receptors (FIs) or work at different points along the replication cycle (INSTIs, NRTIs, NNRTIs) or inhibit the development of new virions (PIs).

The decision to initiate or change a person's therapy is determined by the presence or absence of symptoms along with the degree of immunosuppression that the patient is experiencing and the viral burden. The guidelines are based on the virologic, immunologic, and clinical status of the patient.[31] In the critical care environment, there is considerable debate about the appropriateness of initiating ART as well as using ART because of the potential for significant adverse effects (Table 48-2) and drug interactions. Therefore, it is important for critical care nurses to collaborate with the interdisciplinary team, especially the infectious diseases specialist, to obtain parameters for initiating and withholding ART medications when caring for critically ill persons living with HIV or AIDS. In regard to ART, either therapy needs to be fully administered or entirely withheld, because otherwise there is significant potential for viral resistance to develop.

For some persons with advanced AIDS, initiation of ART can lead to immune reconstitution inflammatory syndrome (IRIS). In this syndrome, an increase of symptoms consistent with an acute inflammatory or infectious process are present but not explained by a new infectious diagnosis. Clinically, a paradoxical worsening or new onset of infectious manifestations usually occurs as a result of improved immune functions and renewed inflammatory responses, an increase in the production of memory and naïve T cells, enhanced lymphoproliferation, increased interleukin-2 responses, and reduced production of some cytokines. The most frequent infectious processes associated with IRIS are TB, *Mycobacterium avium* complex, cryptococcosis, CMV, herpes zoster, HBV/HCV, and CJD. During IRIS, supportive therapy is indicated and aggressive treatment of the infectious diseases is indicated until the patient is clinically stabilized.

## Potent Combination Antiretroviral Therapy

Potent combination ART, also known as highly active ART, became the standard of practice in 1996. According to guidelines published by CDC in April 2015,[31] ART should be initiated in all patients, regardless of CD4$^+$ T-cell count or HIV viral load, to reduce the risk of disease progression and to prevent transmission of HIV. Contemporary evidence indicates that monotherapy with single NRTI, dual-NRTI, and triple-NRTI regimens is not recommended.[31] The three preferred ART regimens for treatment-naïve patients (those who have not previously taken ART) recommended by CDC in April 2015 include two nucleoside reverse transcriptase inhibitors and:

- Nonnucleoside reverse transcriptase inhibitor
- Protease inhibitor with a pharmacokinetic enhancer (cobicistat or ritonavir)
- Integrase strand transfer inhibitor

Regardless of the combination selected, ART has numerous treatment goals.[31] First, it is essential to maximally and durably suppress the HIV viral load to undetectable levels for as long as possible. Second, with viral suppression, it is then possible to restore and preserve immunologic function. Third, with the suppression of the viral load, it is also possible to reduce HIV disease transmission by HIV-positive persons. Fourth, with viral suppression and immune reconstitution, it is possible to reduce HIV-associated morbidity and mortality, ultimately improving survival. Finally, and equally important, ART can help to improve the quality of life of the person living with HIV or AIDS.

The decision to initiate ART or modify the regimen is complex and based on many factors. It is these issues, as well the significant risk for drug interactions and low trough

| TABLE 48-2 | Adverse Events Associated With Antiretroviral Therapy Requiring Intensive Care Unit |
| --- | --- |
| **Adverse Event** | **Associated ART** |
| Bleeding events | PIs: Spontaneous bleeding, hematuria in hemophilia<br>TPV: Intracranial hemorrhage associated with CNS lesions, trauma, alcohol abuse, hypertension, coagulopathy, anti-coagulant or anti-platelet agents, vitamin E |
| Bone marrow suppression (anemia, neutropenia) | ZDV |
| Cardiovascular effects | Associated with MI: NNRTIs (ABC, ddI increase risk) and PIs;<br>Associated with stoke: PIs<br>PR prolongation: SQV/r, ATV/r, and LPV/r<br>QT prolongation: SQV/r |
| CNS | Suicidal ideation, suicide, and attempted suicide (especially among younger patients and those with history of mental illness or substance abuse): EFV, RAL |
| Hepatotoxicity | All NNRTIs; all PIs; most NRTIs; maraviroc |
| Hyperlipidemia | Portal hypertension/esophageal varices: ddI<br>Hepatotoxicity: NVP (severe), all PIs (TPV/r is the greatest), MVC |
| Hypersensitivity Reaction (HSR) | ABC, NVP (hypersensitivity syndrome of hepatotoxicity/rash), RAL (when given with other ARVs causing HSR); MVC (part of syndrome related to hepatotoxicity) |
| Insulin resistance/diabetes mellitus | Some NRTIs (ZDV, d4T, ddI); some PIs (LPV, LPV/r) |
| Lactic acidosis/hepatic steatosis ± pancreatitis (severe mitochondrial toxicities) | NRTIs, especially d4T, ddI, ZDV |
| Renal Effects | TDF: proteinuria, hypophosphatemia, glycosuria, hypokalemia, non-anion gap metabolic acidosis (concurrent use with PI appears to increase risk)<br>ATV and LPV/r: Increased chronic kidney disease risk<br>IDV: pyuria, renal atrophy or hydronephrosis<br>IDV, ATV: Stone, crystal formation |
| Stevens-Johnson syndrome (SJS)/toxic epidermal necrosis (TEN) | NNRTs (NVP more than DLV, EFV, ETR, RPV); also reported with NRTIs (ddi, ZDV), PIs (FPV, DRV, IDV, LPV/r), INSTIs (RAL) ATV: |

From: Panel on Antiretroviral Guidelines for Adults and Adolescents: Guidelines for the use of antiretroviral agents in HIV-1-infected adults and adolescents. Department of Health and Human Services. Table 14, Antiretroviral Therapy-Associated Common and/or Severe Adverse Effects. Available at http://www.aidsinfo.nih.gov/ContentFiles/AdultandAdolescentGL.pdf

levels associated with poor absorption, that the ART regimen is carefully considered in the critical care environment. According to the CDC,[31] decisions about ART regimen selection should also be individualized in collaboration with the patient partner and should critically consider a number of factors, including:

- Comorbid conditions (eg, cardiovascular disease, chemical dependency, liver disease, psychiatric disease, renal diseases, or TB)
- Potential adverse drug effects
- Potential drug interactions with other medications
- Pregnancy or pregnancy potential
- Results of genotypic drug resistance testing
- Gender and pretreatment CD4 T-cell count if considering nevirapine
- HLA-B*5701 testing if considering abacavir
- Coreceptor tropism assay if considering maraviroc
- Patient adherence potential
- Convenience (eg, pill burden, dosing frequency, and food and fluid considerations)

HIV viral load levels are used to evaluate the effectiveness of ART. Once therapy has begun, a decrease in HIV viral load should occur within 2 to 8 weeks. According to the Department of Health and Human Services Panel on Antiretroviral Guides for Adults and Adolescents (p. C-5), "the minimal change in viral load considered to be statistically significant (2 standard deviations) is a threefold change (equivalent to a 0.5 $\log_{10}$ copies/mL change."[31] One key goal of therapy is suppression of viral load to below the limits of detection (below 40 to 75 copies/mL by most commercially available assays). For most individuals who are adherent to their antiretroviral regimens and who do not harbor resistance mutations to the prescribed drugs, viral suppression is generally achieved in 12 to 24 weeks.[31] Viral load assessment should be repeated every 3 to 4 months to monitor effectiveness.

There are times when the treatment does not achieve the desired effect; this is termed antiretroviral treatment failure. There are three types of treatment failure: virologic failure, immunologic failure, and clinical progression. *Virologic failure* is defined as a viral load that fails to decrease to nondetectable levels. *Immunologic failure* is defined as a lack of the immune system to increase the CD4$^+$ T-cell count by 25 to 50 cells/mm$^3$ over the patient's baseline within the first year of treatment or a drop in the CD4$^+$ T-cell count to below the patient's baseline. *Clinical progression* is defined as the occurrence or recurrence of an opportunistic illness after 3 months of receiving treatment with antiretroviral agents.[31] When failure occurs, virologic failure is most commonly the first to develop. Virologic failure is typically followed by immunologic failure and then clinical progression. The time interval between each is extremely varied and may be several years.

## Drug Resistance Testing

Genotypic and phenotypic resistance assays are frequently used in the provision of HIV care to assess viral strains and inform treatment decisions.[31] Genotypic assays assess mutations in relevant sections of the viral genome while phenotypic assays determine the ability of HIV to grow in the presence of different drug concentrations. Genotypic resistance testing is the most commonly used resistance assay in clinical practice. Genotypic assay results can be obtained within a few days after obtaining a blood sample, are more affordable, and have an increased sensitivity for detecting mixtures of wild-type virus and resistant virus.[31] A genotype assay should not be obtained if the viral load is less than 1,000 copies/mm.[31] Genotypic resistance testing helps to reduce the chance that antiretroviral treatment failure will occur, since ART is based on identified mutations and individual drug/class resistance profiles. Current guidelines recommend HIV drug-resistance testing in persons with HIV infection at entry into care regardless of whether ART will be initiated immediately or deferred.

## ART in the ICU Setting

As persons with HIV infection are admitted to the ICU, there are several issues that that the critical care nurse must consider in relation to ART.[14] First, for patients newly diagnosed with HIV infection while in the ICU, the multidisciplinary team will consider a variety of factors when deciding to either initiate or defer ART therapy in the ICU setting. Figure 48-6 provides an algorithm for decision making related to ART initiation in the ICU setting. Second, critical care nurses must also be aware of the numerous drug–drug interactions that exist between ART and other classes of drug.

## Summary

Critical care nursing practice will include an increasing number of people infected with HIV, as this population is living longer and as the number of people infected increases in the United States. Through collaborative, interdisciplinary practice, critical care nurses can optimize early identification of

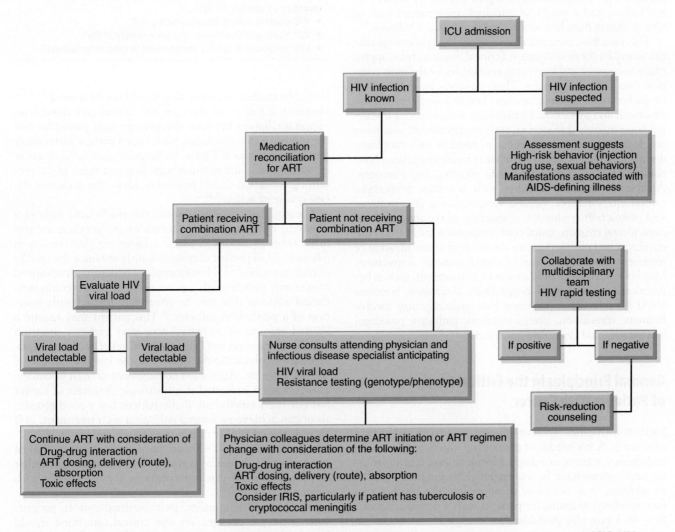

**FIGURE 48-6** Algorithm for making clinical decisions about initiating antiretroviral therapy (ART) in the intensive care unit (ICU). HIV, human immunodeficiency virus; IRIS, immune reconstitution inflammatory syndrome.

(From DeFreitas AA, D'Douza TL, Lazaro GJ, et al: Pharmacological considerations in human immunodeficiency virus–infected adults in the intensive care unit. Crit Care Nurse 33(2):46–57, 2013. Retrieved from http://ccn.aacnjournals.org/content/33/2/46.full.pdf)

those infected; provide compassionate, holistic care addressing complex physiologic, psychosocial and sometimes legal and ethical issues when working with those infected; and collaboratively management complex issues associated with ART in the critical care and acute care settings.

## ONCOLOGIC COMPLICATIONS AND EMERGENCIES

Oncologic emergencies are potentially life-threatening complications that occur as a result of malignancy or its treatment.[1,2] As many as 20% of people diagnosed with cancer have at least one oncologic emergency during the course of their disease.[2-4] The incidence of these emergencies increases as patients with cancer live longer and develop complications that relate to progressive or advanced disease.[3-7] The nature of emergencies requiring critical care management has also evolved as the natural history of common oncologic complications are better understood and managed on oncology units. Critical care is currently most often provided for patients with complications of sepsis, respiratory failure, organ failure, and acute onset oncologic emergencies such as airway obstruction, leukostasis, and tumor lysis syndrome.[6,7]

The nurse must recognize disease-related and patient-specific risk factors for the development of critical illness and plan appropriate assessment and intervention strategies for the most common oncologic emergencies. These emergencies are classified by pathophysiologic mechanisms: hematologic, anatomical–structural, and metabolic. Hematologic complications involving bone marrow dysfunction, such as engraftment syndrome and leukostasis, commonly occur in patients with neoplastic disorders. Disorders related to tumor or treatment-related bone marrow suppression include anemia, bleeding, and infections. Anatomical–structural disorders, such as cardiac tamponade, carotid artery rupture, hepatic veno-occlusive disease (sinusoid obstruction syndrome), obstruction of the superior vena cava, pleural effusion, spinal cord compression (SCC), and tracheobronchial obstruction, are the result of tumor invasion or treatment-related destruction of normal anatomical structures. Metabolic disruptions from cancer or its treatment, such as hypercalcemia, syndrome of inappropriate antidiuretic hormone (SIADH) secretion, and tumor lysis syndrome, may involve hormone stimulation, altered metabolic pathways, procoagulant activity, and electrolyte imbalances.[2,3,8–10]

## General Principles in the Critical Care of Patients With Cancer

Patients with cancer present unique concerns for the critical care nurse. A knowledge of preexisting illness, nature of the malignancy, treatment-related considerations, and prognostic implications must be incorporated into patient care.[1–11] In addition, it is necessary to appreciate the psychosocial factors related to caring for patients with a chronic disease.[1] Box 48-3 provides guidelines for evaluating an oncologic emergency.[1–3,12]

Ideally, before any acute event, the oncologist or primary care physician has discussed end-of-life care with the patient and family members, including the oncologic crises that

---

---

should be treated and those that should not be treated.[4–7,11,12] However, if this is not the case, the critical care nurse is an important liaison between the primary care physician and the intensive care physician. Each time a patient with cancer presents with critical illness, malignancy-associated prognostic variables and information regarding treatment of the presenting condition should be used to advise the patient of the best course of action.[1,10,11]

Clearly, there are times when the risk/benefit ratio of a lifesaving measure does not warrant its use, yet there are also many other situations in which a lifesaving intervention in a hopelessly ill patient may significantly enhance the quality of remaining life.[1,10–13] For example, a patient with advanced cancer may present with a potentially life-threatening pericardial effusion that can be effectively treated with insertion of a pericardial catheter.[14] This patient may require a limited amount of intensive care after catheter insertion and fluid drainage, but the symptom relief may be advantageous in enhancing the quality of the last few months of the patient's life. Aggressive management of most oncologic emergencies is indicated if a histologic diagnosis of cancer has not been established, if the patient has a good prognosis or can achieve prolonged palliation with treatment, or if there is the possibility of restoring functional status.[1,4–7,12–18] The guidelines in Box 48-3 are presented as a list of clinical questions that should be considered when deciding whether to provide critical care interventions for the patient with cancer.[1,4–7,12–15,17,19,20]

To provide high-quality, individualized care to patients with oncologic emergencies, the critical care nurse should know a few facts regarding critical illness and the patient with cancer. Box 48-4 presents important conclusions drawn from multiple studies of critical illness in patients with cancer.[1,3–8,13,18,21]

## BOX 48-4 — Critical Care of Cancer Patients: Conclusions From the Literature

### Incidence of Critical Illness
- Affects about 10% to 15% of patients
- Most common in patients with hematologic malignancy; lung cancer is most common diagnosis among patients with solid tumors
- Most common critical illnesses include respiratory failure requiring high oxygen concentration or mechanical ventilator support, renal replacement therapy, and septic shock with cardiovascular failure and requiring vasopressors. Other reasons include: adverse reactions to blood and antineoplastic therapies. hemoptysis, neurologic impairment, and postoperative observation

### Prognostics of Critical Illness
- Survival is better in the newly diagnosed patient who has not yet received antineoplastic therapy
- Survival often based upon candidate selection for critical care services; patients with severe and metastatic disease likely to have less successful outcomes from critical illness than patients in remission from disease
- Consistent trend toward ICU mortality rates close to those observed in the general population of critically ill patients (35% to 60%).
- Most important predictors of survival: status of the underlying malignant disease, and nature and number of organ failures
- Other poor prognostic variables: age extremes, concomitant health problems, severity of cancer, aggressiveness/potency of treatment, and reversibility of the specific crisis

# Hematologic Complications

## Bone Marrow Suppression

Cancer and its treatment often cause suppression of hematopoietic cell production or differentiation. Causes of bone marrow suppression are commonly associated with cancerous invasion of the bone, chemotherapy and some radiation treatments, or hematopoietic stem cell transplantation. The clinical consequences are symptoms related to decreased red blood cell production (anemia), decreased platelet production (thrombocytopenia), and decreased white blood cell (WBC) production (leukopenia).[22–24] Table 48-3 is a summary of the key clinical features of these three types of bone marrow suppression.[1,22–25] These disorders are not uniquely oncologic, but they are common in patients with cancer and influence the patient's response to other critical illnesses.

Other causes of bone marrow suppression must be considered if cancer-related etiologic factors are not present.[22] When serum tests are unclear in elucidating the etiology of bone marrow suppression, a bone marrow aspirate or biopsy may be performed to confirm whether the pathophysiologic process arises in the cell production phase. This test may require sedation and a local anesthetic before a large coring needle is used to remove the liquid red bone marrow from either the hip or sternum. Bone marrow biopsy determines whether the bone marrow defect is present during the

### TABLE 48-3 — Key Clinical Features of Bone Marrow Suppression

| Anemia | Thrombocytopenia | Leukopenia |
|---|---|---|
| **Definition** | | |
| *General criteria* <br> • Hemoglobin <12 mg% <br> • RBC count <3.0 × 10$^6$/mm$^3$ <br> • Hematocrit <32% <br> *Specific to types of anemia* <br> • Aplastic anemia <br> • Nutritional anemia <br> • Hemolytic anemia | Classified according to severity of thrombocytopenia and risk of bleeding: <br> • Mild: <100,000/mm$^3$ <br> • Mild: <1,000/mm$^3$ <br> • Moderate: <50,000/mm$^3$ <br> • Severe: <20,000/mm$^3$ | Classified according to severity of leukopenia and risk for infection <br> Decreased granulocytes (granulocytopenia) classified by severity of ANC <br> • Moderate: <500/mm$^3$ <br> • Severe: <100/mm$^3$ <br> Decreased lymphocytes (lymphocytopenia) classified by severity of absolute lymphocyte count <br> • Mild: <250 cells/mm$^3$ <br> • Moderate: <100 cells/mm$^3$ <br> • Severe: <50 cells/mm$^3$ |
| **Pathophysiology/Etiology/Contributing Factors** | | |
| *General* <br> • Bone marrow suppression (eg, chemotherapy, radiation to axial skeleton) <br> • Nutritional deficits—iron, protein, B vitamins <br> • Medications (estrogens, allopurinol [Zyloprim]) <br> *Aplastic anemia* <br> • Congenital disorders (eg, Fanconi's syndrome, maternal ingestion of thiazides) <br> • Viral infection <br> • Medications <br> *Nutritional anemia* <br> • Iron deficiency <br> • B-vitamin deficiency <br> *Hemolytic anemia* <br> • Immune hemolysis (viral illness, autoimmune disease) <br> • Sickle cell anemia <br> • PNH | • Bone marrow suppression (eg, chemotherapy, radiation to axial skeleton) <br> • Medications (nonsteroidal anti-inflammatory drugs) <br> • Large-bore intravenous lines (eg, IABP) <br> • High metabolic rate (eg, fevers) | • Bone marrow suppression (eg, chemotherapy, radiation to axial skeleton) <br> • Nutritional deficits <br> • Medications |

*(continued)*

**TABLE 48-3    Key Clinical Features of Bone Marrow Suppression (*continued*)**

| Anemia | Thrombocytopenia | Leukopenia |
|---|---|---|
| **Clinical manifestations** | | |
| • Due to decreased oxygen carrying and tissue delivery: fatigue, oliguria, chest pain, decreased bowel sounds, and constipation<br>• Due to decreased body insulation and vascular volume: hypothermia, hypotension, orthostasis<br>• Due to compensation for inadequate oxygen delivery to the tissue: tachycardia, tachypnea, cool extremities | • Due to decreased platelet plugging for normal vascular wear and tear: gum oozing, petechiae, occult blood in urine and stool<br>• Related to inadequate platelet response to injury: ecchymoses, hematomas, bleeding around procedure sites, frank hematuria, or gastrointestinal bleeding | *Granulocytopenia*<br>• Due to decreased phagocytic properties and recognition of invading microbes: fever, pain at site of potential infection, bacterial and fungal infecting organisms (after 7–10 d of granulocytopenia)<br>• Related to diminished inflammatory response: lack of localized erythema, swelling, or exudates<br>*Lymphocytopenia*<br>• Due to decreased cellular immune responses and recognition of foreign tissue or proteins: tissue anergy to pathogens, (opportunistic and viral infections more common) |
| **Diagnostic tests** | | |
| *General*<br>• RBC count<br>• Hematocrit and hemoglobin<br>• RBC morphology<br>*Aplastic anemia*<br>• Bone marrow aspirate and biopsy<br>*Nutritional anemia*<br>• Ferritin level<br>• Transferrin level<br>• Total iron-binding capacity<br>• Folate level<br>• Vitamin $B_{12}$ level<br>*Hemolytic anemia*<br>• Total and direct bilirubin<br>• Erythrocyte sedimentation rate<br>• RBC morphology<br>• Hemoglobin electrophoresis (sickle cell, PNH)<br>• Indium-tagged RBC survival studies | • Platelet count<br>• Bleeding time tests platelet quality to identify whether symptoms may be partly related to platelet function rather than number | • White blood cell count is initial screening tool, but analysis of actual cell count may be helpful<br>• ANC demonstrates the true number of granulocytes available for phagocytic activity<br>• Absolute lymphocyte count demonstrates the true number of lymphocytes available for recognition of foreign tissue and proteins |
| **Common nursing problems** | | |
| • Fatigue<br>• Activity intolerance<br>• Hypoxemia<br>• Digestion disorders | • Bleeding<br>• Altered body image | • Infection<br>• Risk for hemodynamic instability |
| **Medical management** | | |
| • Erythropoietin injections<br>• RBC transfusions<br>• Energy conservation | • Interleukin-11 (Oprelvekin) injections<br>• Platelet transfusions<br>• Bleeding precautions<br>• Thrombopoietin (Nplate) | • Granulocyte colony-stimulating factor (G-CSF) or granulocyte–macrophage colony-stimulating factor (GM-CSF) injections<br>• Broad-spectrum antimicrobial therapy |

ANC, absolute neutrophil count; PNH, paroxysmal nocturnal hemoglobinuria; IABP, intra-aortic balloon pump; RBC, red blood cell.

cellular production phase, and it may be a basis for clinical management.[1,23] Management of bone marrow suppression as a cluster involves determining whether the cause is time-limited and ascertaining the amount of supportive therapy required. Treatment may include administration of bone marrow growth factors specific to the deficient cellular component,[22,23] infusion of blood components or prophylactic clotting enhancement,[25] and broad-spectrum antimicrobial therapy to prevent life-threatening bleeding or infectious complications.[22–24,26]

## Engraftment Syndrome

Engraftment syndrome (also known as peri-engraftment syndrome, cytokine release syndrome, cytokine storm, hemophagocytic syndrome, and macrophage activation syndrome) is a recently identified disorder that occurs infrequently prior to or in association with the return of bone marrow growth after treatment of hematologic malignancies and hematopoietic stem-cell transplantation.[22,27–30] Patients most at risk for engraftment syndrome are women, those with acute leukemia (especially lymphocytic subtype), those who have just had haploidentical or fully myeloablative allogeneic hematopoietic stem cell transplantation (especially with human leukocyte antigen [HLA]-mismatched donors, umbilical cord stem cells), patient who previously received immunomodulatory agents (eg, bortezomib, lenalidomide) or syngeneic transplant, and those who have had transplantation for autoimmune disorders or solid tumors.[28-35] Patients who have had early engraftment after high-dose marrow-ablative treatment are also at risk for engraftment syndrome.[30]

### Pathophysiology

Regrowth of bone marrow cells, particularly myelocytes, results in release of inflammatory cytokines that produce vasodilation and capillary leaking similar to sepsis.[29-31] Lymphocytes and myelocytic precursors engraft the bone marrow earliest, and patients often still appear leukopenic at the onset of symptoms. Patients with engraftment syndrome often present with signs and symptoms similar to infection at a time when their blood counts are still low, and they are equally at risk for engraftment syndrome and severe infection. Therefore, it is extremely difficult to distinguish the two disorders.[28,30]

### Assessment

**HISTORY.** Engraftment syndrome often begins with fever, total-body erythema or rash, fluid retention, and symptoms of respiratory distress,[28-35] and these symptoms may be the only manifestations. However, many patients exhibit additional signs or symptoms of cytokine effects, such as oliguria or hematuria with elevated creatinine, abdominal discomfort with elevated aminotransferases, and gastrointestinal bleeding.[36] The Spitzer criteria for diagnosis includes these symptoms and the presence of the inflammatory marker of increased C-reactive protein.[29,31,37] The onset of symptoms is rapid, usually occurring over 24 to 48 hours, and symptoms dissipate after the neutrophils engraft and the WBC count reaches about 2,500 to 3,000/mm.[4,27,29,37] Newer literature describes this peri-transplantation syndrome as occurring as early as 4 days after transplant or as late as 14 days, and it may precede or coincide with engraftment.[30,36,38,39] Box 48-5 outlines key clinical manifestations that distinguish sepsis and engraftment syndrome.

**DIAGNOSTIC STUDIES.** There is no clearly definitive diagnostic test that can differentiate engraftment syndrome from sepsis, which it closely resembles. Even elevations of C-reactive protein are more reflective of inflammation than a true diagnostic test of differentiation.[29] The cornerstones of diagnosis are the constellation of clinical symptoms, subsequent increase in WBC count in patients with previous leukopenia, and absence of a positive microbial culture.[29,38,40]

### Management

Engraftment syndrome is managed supportively and conservatively. Patients are presumed septic and treated with broad-spectrum antimicrobial agents. Acetaminophen and diphenhydramine are administered as needed for erythema and pruritus. Hepatic dysfunction requires cautious monitoring and adjustment of fluids and medication doses as appropriate. IV fluids are used to prevent vasodilatory hypotension,

---

**BOX 48-5** | **Distinguishing Between Sepsis and Engraftment Syndrome**

**Sepsis**
- Fever, variable clinical features
- Variable symptom onset
- Variable skin manifestations
- Dyspnea, often with distinct infiltrates on chest radiography
- Thrombocytopenia; occasional mucous membrane bleeding
- Hypotension-related oliguria and elevated creatinine
- Hypotension-related hepatomegaly, elevated aminotransferases

**Engraftment Syndrome**
- Fever, sudden onset, often high and continuous
- Sudden symptom onset over 24 to 48 hour near engraftment period
- Erythema with or without pruritic total-body rash
- Dyspnea; bilateral diffuse alveolar infiltrates on chest radiography
- Gastrointestinal bleeding
- Unprecipitated oliguria, elevated creatinine, hematuria
- Unprecipitated hepatomegaly, elevated aminotransferases

---

but, occasionally, vasoconstricting agents such as phenylephrine or norepinephrine are necessary.[23] Rapid-acting IV corticosteroids have been used effectively when clinical symptoms are strongly suggestive of this disorder[36,38]; methylprednisolone dosed initially at 1 mg/kg/day is the usual treatment.[38] Post-transplantation cyclophosphamide has been used with perceived success at reducing the incidence of engraftment syndrome.[39] Small studies using thrombomodulin to counteract capillary permeability have also shown promise to reduce symptoms in engraftment syndrome.[40] Mechanical ventilation and renal replacement therapy are initiated as indicated, with the understanding and presumption that the syndrome is usually very short-lived.[36]

### Complications

The long-term outcome for most patients with engraftment syndrome is excellent, and there are no significant clinical sequelae.[27,28,30,33] Rarely do patients die or have long-term ischemic organ damage, although the incidence of acute graft-versus-host disease is more prevalent in these patients.[38,41] In situations in which negative sequelae have occurred, it has been difficult to determine whether engraftment syndrome or sepsis was the primary pathophysiologic process. For example, patients with a rapid onset and progression of respiratory distress syndrome may die of refractory hypoxemia, yet whether this has been caused by undiagnosed and untreated infection or engraftment syndrome cannot be determined.

## Leukostasis

Leukostasis is a disorder of excess circulating immature WBCs, resulting in hyperviscosity and microvascular occlusions.[42-46] Cancers such as acute leukemias are the primary cause of leukostasis, although the similar proliferative lymphomas, such as Burkitt and lymphoblastic lymphoma, have also been reported as triggering malignancies.[43,44] The incidence of symptomatic leukostasis in acute leukemia is estimated to be 5% to 30%,[2,46,47] and its association with high circulating immature WBCs confers a poor prognosis.[43,47,48] Initial mortality in patients with this syndrome is estimated to be approximately 40%.[45,49]

## Pathophysiology

Excess numbers of circulating WBCs, such as commonly occur in patients with acute leukemia, can cause a hyperviscosity syndrome that may lead to microcirculatory occlusion with ischemia and vessel rupture.[22,43,44] Several types of leukemia can cause elevated WBC counts, with greatest risk with acute monocytic leukemias of the M3v, M4, M5 subtypes, or acute lymphoblastic leukemia with 11q23 chromosome abnormality.[22,42,45,46] The immature myelocytes (blasts) found in acute nonlymphocytic leukemia have the greatest propensity for "stickiness" due to adhesion molecules and their interaction with endothelial vessel linings, and are most likely to cause leukostasis.[22,42,43,47] Risk for leukostasis is considered greatest when the WBC count is greater than 100,000/mm$^3$, although significant clinical symptoms may be present even when counts are in the 50,000/mm$^3$ range, especially if the WBC count is increasing rapidly or the cells are immature.[42,47,48] Vascular occlusion of the lungs and brain is most common, although coronary artery occlusion, renal failure, and splenic or bowel infarctions have been reported.[49,50] Hypoxic vasodilation is thought to worsen the clinical effects of vascular occlusions in the brain.[42,51]

## Assessment

**HISTORY.** Patients with leukostasis usually first present with respiratory or neurologic symptoms.[22,42,49–51] Onset of symptoms is acute (several hours to 1 day). Severe respiratory distress with hypoxemia and inflammatory alveolar infiltrates are the hallmarks of pulmonary involvement. It is difficult to determine the severity of hypoxemia because the immature WBC blasts consume the oxygen in the arterial blood gas (ABG) specimen, making the arterial blood oxygen level appear even lower than suspected based on clinical evidence. Oxygen saturation may be low (eg, 82% to 90%), but ABG oxygen levels may be only 30 mm Hg.[52,53] It is believed that immediate icing and rapid transit may reduce but not eliminate this testing problem. Neurologic leukostasis presents as mental status changes with clear focal deficits; vascular occlusions cause thrombotic or embolic strokes.[42,47,51,54,55] A recently defined and validated hyperleukocytosis-related retinopathy syndrome occurs owing to retinal artery occlusion with field cut blindness or tunnel vision.[54,56] Other clinical findings also associated with a poorer outcome in these patients include older age, monocytic cell line, bilirubin greater than 1.5 mg/dL, serum creatinine greater than 1.2 mg/dL, lactic dehydrogenase more than 2,000 IU, and thrombocytopenia less than 50,000/mm$^3$.[54]

**DIAGNOSTIC STUDIES.** Leukostasis may be suspected in high-risk groups, but the diagnosis is primarily made on the basis of clinical manifestations. In many instances, the existence of pathophysiologic complications such as infarction or stroke may validate the presumed diagnosis. Patients have specific diagnostic tests performed to assess their presenting symptoms. Chest radiography is often sufficient to diagnose pulmonary leukostasis.[49,50] A head computed tomography (CT) scan may reveal neurologic leukostasis.[42,51] Ultrasonography and magnetic resonance imaging (MRI) may also be performed. In pulmonary leukostasis, ABG results are used with a clear understanding of their diagnostic limitations.[42]

## Management

In leukostasis, the preferred management is to identify high-risk or early symptomatic patients and perform rapid cytoreduction, such as leukapheresis or high-dose chemotherapy, before the cells cause organ damage.[22,42–44,48,57,58] Some clinicians have noted that although leukapheresis does not have an impact on mortality, it does notably affect the number of WBCs and their influence on end-organ damage.[48,59] Therapeutic leukapheresis removes 20,000 to 40,000 WBCs per treatment, and once- or twice-daily treatments are often required until the WBC count is less than 30,000 to 40,000/mm.[43,47,57,60] If leukapheresis cannot be performed immediately, large amounts of IV fluids should be administered to dilute the blood and enhance renal excretion of metabolic toxins.[42,61] If leukapheresis is still not possible within a 12- to 24-hour period, and the patient's symptoms continue to worsen, exchange transfusions may be necessary.[22]

Many patients also receive immediate concomitant chemotherapy to prevent rapid cell regrowth or spontaneous tumor lysis syndrome with renal failure.[22,42] If possible, it is preferred that the necessary leukapheresis cycles be completed before starting chemotherapy; however, many patients are too sick for such treatment. In this situation, the critical care nurse must administer antimicrobial agents or chemotherapy between leukapheresis treatments. Despite some early controversies, chemotherapy may be administered concomitantly with continuous renal replacement therapy (CRRT), as the clearance rate with this dialysis therapy is less than normal kidney clearance, so there are no worries that the chemotherapy is being removed by the dialysis treatment.[45,62] This is not the case with hemodialysis, which does remove many chemotherapy agents. Low-dose cranial radiation (100 to 300 Gy) was once believed to stabilize cell membranes and destroy malignant cells, but this practice is now not recommended.[42,63] Patients with leukostasis receive supportive drug therapy with agents such as antimicrobials, diuretics, bronchodilators, phosphate-binding agents, rasburicase, and allopurinol, which are aimed at stabilizing their symptoms.[42,43,57]

It is important to recognize interventions that worsen the hyperviscosity of leukostasis and avoid these actions. Patients with acute leukemia are often anemic, but blood products should be administered with extreme caution and in combination with crystalloid fluids to avoid increased blood viscosity.[42,43] Diuretics may be given to enhance renal excretion of uric acid associated with tumor cells lysis, but also only in combination with crystalloid fluids to maintain normal vascular osmolarity.[61] Supportive interventions to reduce intracranial hemorrhage may include elevating the head of the bed and administering corticosteroids. Definitive treatment requires administration of chemotherapy directed against the leukemia. Box 48-6 lists nursing interventions aimed at reducing the risk for leukostasis-related complications.

**COMPLICATIONS.** Even in the face of appropriate, definitive treatment, patients with leukostasis may experience stroke, respiratory failure, bowel infarction, renal failure, or myocardial infarction. In many patients, some degree of

- Recognize patients at risk for leukostasis—acute myelocytic leukemia (with circulating blasts), white blood cell count more than 100,000/mm$^3$, renal dysfunction, dehydration.
- Administer large volumes of intravenous fluids to dilute cells and aid excretion of lysis components.
- Perform cytoreduction with leukapheresis or rapid-acting chemotherapy (eg, cyclophosphamide) as soon as possible.
- Treat organ system–specific leukostatic symptoms (eg, elevation of head of bed, bronchodilators).
- Administer drugs to reduce effects of tumor lysis: phosphate-binding drugs, allopurinol, rasburicase.
- Administer blood components cautiously early in the disease when hyperviscosity is problematic.
- Plan assessment interventions aimed at monitoring for ischemia or infarction of the body organs.

reversible organ ischemia develops, requiring supportive treatment.[22,42,58]

## Typhlitis/Necrotizing Enterocolitis

### Pathophysiology

Patients with severe or prolonged neutropenia are at risk for acute gastrointestinal symptoms related to the presence and activity of microbes within the gastrointestinal tract.[64–67] Resident Gram-negative organisms can produce serious clinical disease in patients without granulocytes.[26,68] Microbial infiltration of less perfused areas of the bowel, such as the cecum and appendix, produces an acute inflammation of the bowel wall, edema, and paralytic ileus,[64,65] a condition termed neutropenic enterocolitis (also known as typhlitis and ileocecal syndrome).[64] Gases produced by these bacteria can also lead to air in the bowel wall, ischemia, and possible infarction, which is termed necrotizing enterocolitis or pneumatosis intestinalis.[66,69] While reported more frequently in children, high-dose marrow suppressing therapy in any individual can lead to typhlitis.[64,70,71] Although older studies describe incidence rates of 20% to 40% of patients treated for leukemia or undergoing hematopoietic stem cell transplantation, recent reports suggest the incidence may vary from less than 1% to approximately 6% of such cases.[72–77] Despite a serious clinical presentation of acute abdominal infection, more than half of patients had negative blood cultures.[26,64]

### Assessment

**HISTORY.** Patients with prolonged or severe neutropenia are at risk for developing typhlitis, although other specific risks include presence of an appendix,[70] prior bowel surgery, and *Clostridium difficile* ("C. diff") infection.[68,69,78] Medications that have been linked to increased incidence of typhlitis include carboplatin, cyclophosphamide, cytosine arabinoside, daunomycin, docetaxel, doxorubicin, idarubicin, methotrexate, paclitaxel, pegylated asparaginase, pemetrexed, rituximab, topotecan, and vincristine.[64,69,78–82] Consistent administration of oral antimicrobials to sterilize the gut reduces the risk of bacterial translocation and subsequent sepsis. Nonadherence to this medication regimen has been associated with development of this disorder. Patients present with diffuse abdominal pain that is semi-localized in the right upper or middle quadrant of the abdomen.[66,68,71,76] Guarding, abdominal distention, diarrhea, and reduced bowel sounds are common, and rebound tenderness or gastrointestinal bleeding signals a more severe disease that has progressed to bowel ischemia and infarction.[64,66,68,71,74] Most patients demonstrate symptoms of acute abdominal sepsis such as fever, fluid shifting with oliguria, weight gain, and hypotension, although in antibiotic-controlled disease, these septic symptoms may be intermittent.[64,70,73,83]

**DIAGNOSTIC STUDIES.** Initial screening tests include an abdominal flat plate x-ray to detect possible air under the diaphragm, and a CT scan with contrast, while also evaluating lactic acid and amylase levels for signs of bowel ischemia.[64,72,84–86] An enlarged and edematous cecum is considered diagnostic, although other tests are better at predicting the severity of bowel wall injury or ischemia.[85,86]

### Management

Since recognition of this complication and its pathophysiologic origin, many clinicians have undertaken two primary preventive measures. First, high-risk patients are administered oral antimicrobial antibiotics (usually in liquid form) that destroy intestinal bacteria, producing sterile conditions within the bowel.[64–66] Second, patients with anticipated severe neutropenia are administered prophylactic hematopoietic growth factors, unless acute myeloid leukemia where there is concern the growth factors may enhance tumor growth.[65,69] These patients may perhaps then have reduced neutropenia. In patients who develop less severe typhlitis, potent broad-spectrum antimicrobials aimed to destroy a variety of both gram-positive and gram-negative bacteria, gut rest, and observation may be warranted and adequate until the patient's own WBCs repopulate their bone marrow and can destroy an existing infection.[72,83,86] Throughout the continuum of this complication, lactic acid levels are followed and IV fluids are administered to maintain gut perfusion.[69,70,86] Vasopressor agents are avoided if at all possible. In more serious cases, granulocyte transfusions have been administered in an attempt to boost the patient's immune activity.[64,87] In severe, sepsis-related disease or pneumatosis, emergent surgical resection may be necessary.[71,86,88,89]

### Complications

This continuum of bowel wall abnormalities may lead to acute bowel perforation, bowel infarction or gastrointestinal bleeding.[64,65,70] These serious consequence often herald poor outcomes as the patients are also too high of risk to consider surgical resection of the bowel, even though this intervention may be the only potentially effective measure to arrest the sepsis.

## Anatomical–Structural Complications

### Cardiac Tamponade

Cardiac tamponade is the result of accumulation of excess pericardial fluid or the presence of a tumor that compresses the heart, preventing return of venous blood and resulting in inability to create synchronized cardiac contraction and impaired blood ejection.[89–91] Direct involvement of the pericardium with cancer is rare, but effusions with malignant cell infiltration or therapy-induced capillary permeability has been reported more frequently.[90–92]

Progressive pericardial effusion is the most common etiology for tamponade in patients with cancer.[92] Malignancy can infiltrate the pericardium through local extension, hematogenous or lymphatic dissemination, or capillary permeability from cancer therapies causing excess fluid accumulation in the pericardial sac.[89,91] At autopsy, as many as 20% of people with cancer are found to have cardiac or pericardial metastases,[91] although established incidence has been considerably less frequent.[90]

### Pathophysiology

The pericardium is a double-walled sac that surrounds the heart and great vessels. A visceral layer lines the surface of the heart, and the parietal layer (or outer layer) moves freely. The pericardium supports the heart in a stable position and provides a frictionless sac for cardiac contractions. The pericardial cavity lies between the two layers and contains 10 to 50 mL of serous fluid.

Neoplastic cardiac tamponade results from the formation and accumulation of excessive amounts of fluid in the pericardial sac. This emergent condition may also be caused by encasement of the heart by tumor or postradiation pericarditis.[90,93] The severity of the tamponade is in direct proportion to the rate of fluid formation and the volume of fluid accumulated.[89] Slow accumulation may stretch the pericardium so that cardiac contractility is not adversely affected for months.[89,92] Normal diastolic filling is impaired by elevated pericardial pressures, and stroke volume is reduced. As stroke volume continues to fall, hypotension, compensatory tachycardia, and equalization and elevation of the mean left atrial, pulmonary arterial and venous, right atrial, and vena caval pressures occur. In an attempt to maintain arterial pressure, increase blood volume, and improve venous return, tachycardia worsens and peripheral vasoconstriction develop.[89,91] If the tamponade goes undiagnosed or untreated, circulatory collapse ensues.

Cancers of the esophagus or lung grow by direct extension into the pericardium, whereas distant primary cancers (eg, renal cell) metastasize to the pericardium through the bloodstream. Large chest tumors may also cause pericardial effusion due to lymphatic obstruction of pericardial fluid recirculation.[92] The primary tumors most commonly associated with pericardial effusion are tumors of the breast, lung, and esophagus; lymphoma; gastrointestinal carcinomas; melanoma; sarcoma; and leukemia.[91,92] Radiation pericarditis may be a causative factor, especially if the patient's heart was in the treatment field and if the total dose of radiation to this field exceeded 4,000 rad (40 Gy).[90,93] Biotherapeutic agents such as interleukin-2 (Aldesleukin), ipilimumab, and interferon-alpha cause increased capillary permeability and clinically significant pericardial effusions.[94] Pericardial effusion has also been reported in patients receiving arsenic trioxide, azacitidine, belinostat, cyclophosphamide, cytosine arabinoside, dasatinib, daunorubicin, doxorubicin, and paclitaxel.[92,94]

### Assessment

**HISTORY.** Signs and symptoms reflect the rapidity with which the fluid accumulates in the pericardial sac and, in the patient with cancer, are mainly those of right-sided heart failure due to slow accumulation.[92] Signs of effusion and tamponade include rapid, weak pulse; distant heart sounds; distended neck veins during inspiration (Kussmaul sign); pulsus paradoxus (inspiratory decrease in arterial blood pressure of greater than 10 mm Hg from baseline); ankle or sacral edema; edema; ascites; hepatosplenomegaly; hepatojugular reflex; lethargy; and altered level of consciousness.[89,90,92] Hypotension most likely signals progression to tamponade.[91] The patient may complain of dyspnea, cough, and retrosternal pain that is relieved by leaning forward. On occasion, a patient with a large effusion experiences epigastric pain, hiccups, hoarseness, nausea, and vomiting.[92,95]

**DIAGNOSTIC STUDIES.** A variety of studies are used to determine the presence and severity of cardiac tamponade. A chest film is used to determine the presence of cardiac enlargement, mediastinal widening, or hilar adenopathy.[89,90,92] The electrocardiogram (ECG) may show nonspecific abnormalities, including low QRS complex voltage in limb leads, electrical alternans, sinus tachycardia, precordial ST-segment elevations, and T-wave changes.[89,91,92,96–99] Echocardiography is the most sensitive and most specific noninvasive test for the presence of tamponade and is used routinely in most settings.[89,91,96–98] Two distinct echoes may be identified, one from effusion and the other from the posterior heart border. Spaces between these echoes indicate the size of the effusion or the thickness of the pericardium. Catheterization of the right side of the heart reveals pericardial tamponade or constriction but is performed infrequently because echocardiograms are routinely available.[96–98] Clarification of specific pathologic features and tumor involvement of the pericardium itself cannot be determined by echocardiogram and may require CT or MRI imaging.[96] Pericardiocentesis gives a positive cytologic result in the patient with metastatic cancer about 80% to 90% of the time.[91,97,98]

### Management

First, volume expansion is necessary because it increases venous pressure so that it is greater than the pericardial pressure, allowing increased venous return and improved cardiac output.[89,91,95] Oxygen administration is required, although assisted or mechanical ventilation may increase thoracic pressures, further impeding venous return and acutely worsening the tamponade.

The definitive treatment for pericardial effusion is fluid drainage.[96–98,100] Acute or life-threatening symptoms are indications for emergent pericardial drainage by needle or catheter pericardiocentesis. Without definitive treatment to alleviate the fluid in the pericardium, cardiac arrest occurs. Tamponade is likely to recur in 24 to 48 hours if treatment to prevent pericardial fluid reaccumulation is not initiated quickly.[96,98]

Factors that clinicians should consider when selecting a therapeutic option include the sensitivity of the primary tumor to specific treatment modalities, previous treatment, and the patient's life expectancy.[90–92] If effective drugs are available, systemic chemotherapy may be initiated after the patient is clinically stable.[90–92] This treatment have been most effective in patients with leukemia, lymphoma, and breast cancer who have pericardial effusion. In radiosensitive tumors such as lymphoma, radiation therapy may be the treatment of choice.[90–92] Research has shown that radiation therapy may control more than 50% of malignant pericardial effusions.[98] Insertion of a pericardial catheter guided by fluoroscopy or echocardiography to permit rapid fluid drainage is often the preferred immediate treatment.[89,90,98,100–102] The catheter may remain in place while anticancer therapy begins. Pericardial sclerosis through the pericardial catheter, which is rarely used, can control tamponade by causing adherence of the two pericardial layers and inhibiting fluid accumulation.[89,102] Intrapericardial chemotherapy with agents such as cisplatin and bleomycin has also been infrequently reported.[91,92,98,102] Intraoperative fluid drainage or shunting has been used with moderate success in extensive malignant disease.[89,91,96–98,100,101] In patients with a longer life expectancy and adequate performance status, an inferior pericardiotomy may be performed thoracoscopically. In this procedure, a pleural–pericardial window is created, which provides immediate relief of cardiac compression and tissue specimens for histologic diagnosis.[101] Fewer than 5% of patients have recurrence of symptoms after this procedure.[100,101] Pericardectomy is necessary if radiation-induced pericardial disease is not responsive to conservative medical management. This procedure should not take place if an extensive pericardial tumor is present because surgical morbidity and mortality rates are high.[91]

## Carotid Artery Rupture

Causes of a carotid artery rupture (or "blowout") are tumor erosion and rupture of the carotid artery. As nasopharyngeal cancers have become more prevalent with the advent of known human papilloma virus (HPV) involvement or the oropharynx, other great vessel erosions of the neck and superior mediastinum such as the innominate artery, internal jugular vein, and thyroid arteries have been reported and produce similar clinical consequences.[103,104] Such rupture results in the loss of large amounts of blood that, without rapid intervention, becomes life-threatening hemorrhage. Patients at risk for this oncologic emergency are primarily those with cancer of the head and neck, especially the squamous cell subtype, particularly after surgery or radiation, or with a wound infection. The incidence rate is this population is 2.6% to 4.5% of patient undergoing non-palliative treatment for the disease.[105,106] Affected patients occasionally have thyroid cancer, lymphoma, or melanoma.[107] Patients with a palpable pulse on top of a tumor, or in close proximity to it, have a greater risk for carotid vessel erosion.[102] In one systematic review, accelerated hyperfractionation of radiotherapy posed a greater risk than conventional or hyperfractionated schedules.[106]

### Pathophysiology

Rupture of a carotid artery is likely to occur when that vessel is weakened by invasion of tumor or by surgical manipulation.[103] Other causes of vessel weakness include simultaneous infection or skin flap necrosis. Late-onset vessel rupture has also been associated with radiation exposure with vascular aneurysm formation.[102]

### Assessment

The rupture of the artery may occur suddenly with forceful expulsion of large volumes of blood from the damaged vessel; however, the first sign of erosion or rupture usually is a small trickle of blood from the neck area or unexplained oral bleeding.[103] If the skin over the artery is intact, the patient

---

**QSEN BOX 48-7** | *PATIENT SAFETY*

**Cardinal Signs and Symptoms of Carotid Artery Rupture**
- Oozing blood from neck wound
- Unexplained oral bleeding
- Ecchymoses over neck region
- Sudden neck edema
- Retrosternal or epigastric chest pain
- Sense of impending doom, anxiety, or restlessness

---

may have darkened or ecchymotic skin changes, swelling, difficulty swallowing or breathing, retrosternal or high epigastric chest pain, and mental status changes. A unilateral headache or visual disturbance may also signal carotid artery bleeding. Box 48-7 lists the cardinal signs and symptoms of carotid artery rupture.

### Management

Patients identified at high risk for carotid artery rupture may have vascular stents placed during surgery as a preventive measure.[104] No diagnostic tests are performed at the time of bleed, as patients have been identified as at-risk in advance, and there is no time for diagnostic evaluation when an acute bleed occurs. If the bleeding begins subtly and evaluation is possible, angiography with interventional radiologic vessel ligation may be performed to minimize the blood flow to the tumor bed or oozing section of vessel. In addition, IV access should be in place, and blood should be typed and available for immediate transfusion.[105] Gauze, irrigation saline solution, and vascular clamps should be readily available at all times. The first emergency intervention in cases of suspected carotid artery rupture is constant digital pressure with saline-soaked cotton dressing wrapped around the two middle fingers and applied directly to the area over the artery. The nurse must not lessen pressure to see whether the bleeding has stopped or attempt to apply a hemostat; either of these steps increases the likelihood of further blood loss. Maintenance of the airway is essential. Only after the patient is in the operative suite and the operative area has been prepared should the pressure be released. The surgical treatment of choice is ligation of the damaged artery.[105] Embolization or stent placement may be alternatives.[108] Chapter 22 contains a detailed discussion of carotid artery surgery with assessment and nursing care.

### Complications

The overall mortality rate of carotid artery rupture is 40% to 60%.[108] This primarily results from inability to re-establish essential blood flow to the brain and massive blood loss. About 60% of patients who survive this complication have long-term neurologic deficits, the most common of which is hemiparesis.[106] The risk for hemiparesis is reduced by the prevention of shock and replacement of fluid for adequate perfusion of the brain through the opposite internal carotid artery.

## Sinusoidal Obstruction Syndrome

Sinusoidal obstruction syndrome (SOS), also known as hepatic veno-occlusive disease (HVOD), is occlusion of the venous vessels of the liver with inflammatory and fibrotic tissue.[109] The disease is a complication of high-dose radiation therapy and chemotherapy.[109–111] Its incidence is as low as 5% to 10% in patients receiving less myeloablative therapy and monoclonal antibody regimens but cumulatively 13.7% in one meta-analysis.[111,112] Earlier studies in hematopoietic stem cell transplantation, when total body irradiation was commonly used and busulfan was dosed without the benefits of dosing by serum blood levels, reported incidence was as high as 60% of post-transplant patients.[109,112,113]

Although SOS is most likely to develop in patients receiving high-dose alkylating agents (eg, cyclophosphamide, busulfan, thiotepa) or abdominal radiation, it also occurs in patients receiving the leukemic monoclonal antibody gemtuzumab, azathioprine, cisplatin, thioguanine, and oxaliplatin.[109,114, 115] Calcineurin inhibitors such as sirolimus and tacrolimus have been associated with the syndrome, as have azole antifungal agents.[114] Although not prevalent in the United States, worldwide SOS has been strongly linked to herbal remedies such as *Gynura segetum*, Tusangi, and teas containing pyrrolizidine alkaloids.[109,116–118] Dacarbazine and methotrexate may produce a clinical syndrome similar to sinusoid obstruction syndrome, but with more hypersensitivity features and infiltrative eosinophilia not seen with typical SOS.[114] Other risk factors in patients with cancer are baseline lower performance status/activity level, extensive pretreatment, unique disease genotypes, specific preparative regimen, older age, previous history of hepatitis, and baseline elevations of bilirubin or ferritin.[111,119]

## Pathophysiology

Through uncertain mechanisms, etiologic agents cause fibrotic changes in the endothelial layer that lines the walls of the veins and sinusoids in the liver, resulting in narrowed and stiff-walled venules that cause portal hypertensions and have a tendency for thrombosis. Venous flow through the liver is reduced and poral venous flow is reversed, with resulting congestion and eventual pressure-related hepatic damage.[109,120–122]

## Assessment

**HISTORY.** The earliest manifestations of SOS are fluid retention, elevated serum bilirubin, and nonspecific abdominal pain.[109] The onset of these symptoms occurs an average of 8 to 20 days after the therapy-triggering exposure; the time varies with the causative agent.[109,111,120] The clinical course begins primarily as one of weight gain, portal hypertension with ascites, painful hepatomegaly, and right-sided heart failure; it progresses over 1 to 3 weeks to include hepatic destruction with coagulopathies, thrombocytopenia, hyperammonemia, metabolic alkalosis, increased vagal tone, and hepatorenal failure.[109,111,119] Box 48-8 lists early and late clinical findings in SOS. Most patients with SOS have mild, reversible disease, and only 10% to 20% have severe, life-threatening manifestations.[109,111,119]

**DIAGNOSTIC STUDIES.** The first and most specific diagnostic test is the elevation of total and indirect bilirubin.[111,119] Aspartate transaminase (previously known as serum glutamic oxaloacetic transaminase) and alkaline phosphatase also increase early, and when progressive liver failure

**QSEN BOX 48-8** **PATIENT SAFETY**

### Signs and Symptoms of Sinusoidal Obstruction Syndrome (SOS)

**Early Findings**
- Weight gain
- Fluid retention, edema
- Painful hepatomegaly
- Increased total and direct bilirubin
- Increased aspartate aminotransferase and alkaline phosphatase

**Late Findings**
- Coagulopathies, thrombocytopenia
- Hyperammonemia
- Metabolic alkalosis
- Hepatorenal syndrome
- Right-sided heart failure
- Elevated aminotransferases
- Increased vagal tone

develops, hepatic aminotransferases also increase. Abdominal ultrasonography confirms hepatic enlargement and is used to rule out causal conditions, such as cholestasis and hepatic abscess.[119] The recent addition of ultrasonographic Doppler technology provides more conclusive evidence of hepatic veno-occlusive disease with validation of venous wall turgidity, estimated portal pressures, and the classic finding of portal venous blood flow.[111,119,122] Magnetic resonance angiography or computed tomography may be necessary to rule out Budd Chiari syndrome or hepatic parenchymal disease when other clinical and diagnostic parameters are inconclusive.[117,119] Several clinical classification systems have been developed to define the presence of SOS; severity grading systems have also been proposed and are being validated.[111,121]

In late or severe disease, the platelet count decreases, and coagulation studies such as prothrombin time or partial thromboplastin time are prolonged. A definitive diagnosis may be made only on the basis of liver biopsy. When it is necessary to differentiate hepatic veno-occlusive disease from other clinically similar processes, such as graft-versus-host disease, liver biopsy shows venule fibrosis.[111,119,120]

## Management

Because exact pathologic mechanisms of SOS are uncertain and the incidence of the disorder is declining, therapy is still presumptive and not clearly effective. Once SOS is suspected, supportive therapies, such as balancing fluid administration and diuresis, are implemented.[109,110,123] Transjugular intrahepatic portosystemic shunt and liver transplant procedures have been used in an attempt to enhance portal blood outflow with limited success.[123] Patients may require platelet and fresh frozen plasma transfusions, vasopressors, and ammonia-lowering therapies, such as lactulose.[109,111,122,123] Researchers have noted modest reports of successful symptom resolution with high-dose methylprednisolone, low-dose heparin, glutamine with high-dose vitamin E, ursodiol, and activated factor VII.[111,112,121–123] Agents not recommended for consideration owing to lack of efficacy include tissue plasminogen activator and N-acetylcysteine.[122,123] Defibrotide, an oligonucleotide derived from porcine intestinal mucosa that demonstrates simultaneous antithrombotic properties with microvascular protective features, producing minimal hemorrhagic risk, has been well-studied and recently licensed for treatment of SOS.[109,111,112,121–124] Renal replacement therapy is often required; continuous venovenous hemofiltration is often the preferred method of therapy because these patients exhibit increased vagal tone and a tendency for vasodilatory hypotension. Some experts advocate early implementation to preserve renal function and reduce the need for respiratory support.[123,124] Before the advent of CRRT, mechanical ventilation to control fluid imbalance–induced respiratory distress was often necessary.

No methods to prevent SOS have yet proved successful. Results of studies of low-dose heparin (subcutaneously or intravenously), prostaglandin E[1], and defibrotide as potential preventive agents have so far been inconclusive.[121–123]

### Complications

Patients with mild-to-moderate SOS experience complete reversal of the pathologic process.[109,111] It is uncertain whether supportive therapies have any influence on this outcome. Well-controlled studies clearly show that mortality is high in patients with total bilirubin levels greater than 15 to 18 mg/dL, renal dysfunction, high fibrinogen D-dimers, or a hepatic pressure gradient of greater than 20 mm Hg with an overall mortality rate averaging 21%.[111,121]

## Superior Vena Cava Syndrome

Superior vena cava syndrome (SVCS)—obstruction of the superior vena cava—results in venous blockage that produces pleural effusion and facial, chest, arm, and neck edema.[125–127] While known to be highly symptomatic, death due to SVCS is rare.[128]

### Pathophysiology

The superior vena cava is a thin-walled, low-pressure blood vessel in the mediastinal cavity that collects blood from the venous vessels that drain the head and neck and the upper thoracic cavity. The mediastinum is a rigid anatomical structure that contains the trachea, the vertebral column, the sternum and ribs, and the lymph nodes.

Most cases of SVCS result from mediastinal malignancies or involved lymph nodes that cause extrinsic compression or invade the vessel and impair return of venous blood.[125–128] More than 75% of cases are secondary to small cell or squamous cell lung cancers, and 10% to 15% are secondary to mediastinal lymphomas.[125,127–130] Other tumors that have been associated with SVCS include metastatic malignant melanoma, renal cell cancer, and thymic cancer.[125–128] Obstruction of the vessel lumen by a thrombus may also occur; it is most commonly caused by a central venous catheter or a hypercoagulability syndrome due to cancer.[125,127,128,131] Nonmalignant causes are less common but may include tuberculosis, syphilis, or granulomatous disease.[125,127] Box 48-9 summarizes the risk factors for SVCS.

### Assessment

**HISTORY.** Signs and symptoms of SVCS depend on the rapidity of compression of the superior vena cava. If it is compressed gradually and collateral circulation develops,

indications of SVCS may be more subtle.[125,127] Initial symptoms are most prominent in the early morning and include periorbital and conjunctival edema, facial swelling, and Stokes sign (tightness of the shirt collar).[125–127,132] These signs may disappear after the patient has been upright for a few hours. The patient may also complain of visual disturbances and headache. Altered consciousness and focal neurologic signs may result from brain edema and impaired cardiac filling. Late signs and symptoms include distention of the veins of the thorax and upper extremities, dysphagia, dyspnea, cough, hoarseness, and tachypnea. All patients, including children, most commonly visit health care providers because of dyspnea.[125–127] Pleural or pericardial effusions are present in some cases, compounding respiratory symptoms and providing a complex dimension for treatment planning.[125] Most pleural effusions are transudative and related to obstruction of pleural and lymphatic outflow.

**DIAGNOSTIC STUDIES.** Until recently, diagnostic evaluation of SVCS required multiple tests to validate the location, size, and vena caval involvement of tumors or thrombus. Conventional chest CT with IV contrast, venography, angiography, and radionuclide scans were necessary.[127] Currently, the spiral CT scan with contrast, which provides accurate information about tumor location and involvement of the vena cava, may be the only diagnostic test performed.[125,127,133,134] However, biopsy or cytologic tests may be required to establish a diagnosis in many patients because this syndrome is the presenting symptom at the time of diagnosis of cancer.[127]

### Management

Treatment is determined by the severity and rapidity of symptom onset. As many as 31% of patients experienced symptoms less than 2 weeks prior to presentation for evaluation and hence require emergent antineoplastic therapy as well as urgent diversive procedures[125]; the mean time to presentation in one study was 34 days.[135] The primary treatment of choice for SVCS caused by a tumor is radiation therapy, provided there is expected radiosensitivity.[125–127,136] Radiation therapy is initially given in high daily fractions (total dose of 300 to 500 cGy) for 2 to 4 days followed by 100 to 200 cGy for an additional 14 to 21 days.[125,136] Symptom relief occurs in 7 to 14 days.[127] Radiation therapy is given with palliative intent for SVCS in advanced cancer with little hope of total resolution.[127,136] Radiation of the mediastinal, hilar, and supraclavicular lymph nodes and any adjacent parenchymal lesions is appropriate in patients with locally advanced non–small cell lung cancer.

Patients who receive radiation therapy experience increased cough within 3 days of the start of therapy. During the initial 7 to 10 days, secretions are increased because of inflammation, but a dry irritation then develops, resulting in a dry, hacking cough with few secretions but possible bleeding.[125] Chemotherapy may be the treatment of choice for SVCS in patients with disseminated disease, such as small cell anaplastic carcinoma or lymphoma.[125–127,136] The agents used most often include high-dose regimens containing cyclophosphamide, cisplatin or carboplatin, bleomycin, etoposide, and doxorubicin.[127,136] The most common adverse effects of these agents include bone marrow suppression, cardiac toxicity, pneumonitis, and renal dysfunction.

Treatment of SVCS caused by a thrombus around a central venous catheter may include intravenous or catheter-directed antifibrinolytics or anticoagulants and possibly surgical removal of the catheter.[125,128,135–137] In any case, chest and neck central venous catheter placements should be avoided until effective treatment has been delivered.[125]

In some circumstances, the placement of stents or vascular grafts in the superior vena cava provides immediate symptomatic relief while patients receive definitive therapy.[125,127,135,136,138,139] It is unclear whether long-term anticoagulation is required. Caution must be taken and intensive observations are made to enhance early detection of bleeding as the tumor shrinks.[138] Supportive care is essential. Maintenance of a patent airway is of the highest priority.[125] Because many patients have severe dyspnea, they are unable to lie flat for their radiation therapy, and short-term airway intubation may be necessary. Clinicians may prescribe oxygen therapy, diuretics, steroids, and heparin, and their administration requires careful observation of patient response. If necessary, administration of corticosteroids for 3 to 7 days to decrease the edema associated with the disease and treatment is warranted.[128,136] The nurse teaches the patient not to bend over and to avoid Valsalva maneuvers. When the patient is in bed, the head should be at least in a semi-Fowler position. Elevation of the arms on pillows helps alleviate swelling; however, elevation of the legs is not helpful because this increases fluid volume in the torso.[125]

### Complications

Several complications may occur in patients with SVCS. Right-sided heart failure is the most common.[125] Such heart failure is usually self-limiting and is treated symptomatically with fluid restrictions, diuretics, and digoxin. Vessel rupture in SVCS when a tumor invades the vena cava is a great risk because the tumor shrinks with treatment. The incidence of vessel rupture is highest in patients with esophageal and lung cancer; peak incidence is 3 to 4 weeks after initiation of therapy.[127] Warning signs of vessel rupture are acute and sudden dyspnea, hypoxia, cough, and vascular collapse. Radiation pneumonitis, an inflammatory response in the radiation field that correlates with breath sound and radiographic changes reflective of alveolar capillary permeability, may occur 2 to 8 weeks after start of therapy in patients who receive chest radiation for SVCS.[125,127] Treatment of radiation pneumonitis involves corticosteroids and supportive therapy. SVCS recurs in 10% to 30% of patients.[127]

Severe obstruction results in impaired cardiac filling, and the venous congestion has also been associated with tracheal obstruction and cerebral edema.[140] Long-term obstruction has also been associated with portal hypertension and esophageal varices.[141]

## Pleural Effusion

### Pathophysiology

There is normally 30 to 150 mL of fluid between the visceral and parietal pleura that helps maintain a negative pleural pressure to facilitate lung expansion with minimum work of breathing. A pleural effusion is excess accumulation of fluid in the pleural space with subsequent impaired lung expansion and hypoxemia. When lymphatic obstruction (particularly of the thoracic duct), venous congestion, pleural inflammation, or excess capillary permeability occurs, the amount of fluid increases or does not drain properly.[142,143]

Although many nonmalignant conditions (eg, congestive heart failure, hypothyroidism) may cause pleural effusion, malignant conditions involving lymphatic obstruction or infiltration with malignant cells may also be the cause. Pleural effusions that result from volume overload, capillary permeability, or lymphatic obstruction produce a transudate characterized by the presence of albumin and the absence of cell fragments or enzymes in the pleural fluid.[142,144] Malignant cell infiltration or pleuritic infection causes pleural inflammation and exudates characterized by the release of red blood cells, WBCs, and lactate dehydrogenase into the pleural fluid.[144] As many as 50% of patients with cancer experience pleural effusions during the course of their disease, particularly in cancers of the lung or breast.[142,143] Other tumors commonly associated with pleural effusion include cancers of the kidney, ovary, or pancreas, sarcoma, and lymphoma.[142–144] Unilateral pleural effusions occur when the tumor is located in a single lung, but bilateral effusions are more common with abdominal cancers (eg, ovarian, pancreatic), hematologic malignancies, or when accompanied by ascites.[144,145] Pleural effusions are also associated with certain antineoplastic agents, the most common being all-trans-retinoic acid, cytarabine, dasatinib, docetaxel, fludarabine, imatinib, nilotinib, and pemetrexed.[94] Primary effusion lymphoma and mesothelioma are uncommon, but often present initially and in relapse with pleural and pericardial effusions.[146,147] The presence of pleural effusion is associated with a shorter life expectancy, averaging 3 to 12 months after diagnosis.[142] Predictors of better outcome include specific types of cancer and patients with higher performance status at diagnosis of effusion.[143,148]

Accumulation of pleural fluid leads to increased (more positive) pleural pressure. Higher pleural pressures increase the work of breathing, and collapsed alveoli cause decreased gas exchange and hypoxemia.[142]

### Assessment

**HISTORY.** The clinical findings in pleural effusion are related to the two major physiologic mechanisms: increased work of breathing and alveolar collapse. Excess pleural pressures decrease lung compliance ("stiff lungs"). Patients feel short of breath and must use their accessory muscles to breathe, and chest excursion on the affected side is reduced. When patients are in an upright position, the force of gravity pulls down the fluid, and breath sounds are diminished to the level of fluid. The pleural fluid takes up space in the chest, impeding lung expansion with consequent alveolar collapse. Symptoms that relate to this pathologic process are persistent cough and dyspnea, diminished breath sounds, unequal chest excursion, tracheal shift away from the effusion, and signs of hypoxemia (eg, dyspnea, anxiety, confusion, oliguria, decreased bowel sounds).[142-144]

**DIAGNOSTIC STUDIES.** The first diagnostic test performed to confirm the presence of pleural effusion is an upright chest radiograph or CT.[143] Lateral x-rays may be more sensitive that upright x-rays in small effusions.[149] The fluid accumulates in the lower lung, causing a blunted diaphragmatic dome and decreased radiolucence in the lower lung. Fluid accumulation often produces a meniscus of decreased radiolucence and a thickened lateral pleural lining, indicating fluid tracking up the side.[143] When alternative diagnoses such as hemothorax, infection, or tumor infiltrates are possible, the CT scan may be more accurate. After a pleural effusion is confirmed, a cytologic evaluation, which involves extraction of a sample of fluid and sending it for fluid chemistry and cytology, is necessary. Pleural fluid is categorized as transudative or exudative, which provides clues to the cause of the effusion.[149,150] The visual appearance of the effusion may also provide clues to the etiology: lymph produces chyle,[151] lung cancer has been associated with black fluid,[152] thick jelly-like exudate has also been associated with malignant cell infiltration,[153] and purulent or malodorous exudate is usually infectious.[150] Cytologic studies require at least 75 mL fluid to confirm the presence or absence of malignant cells; the results influence treatment decisions.[154] Multiple specimens may be necessary to confirm malignancy; it is estimated that cytology may be positive only half of the time when malignant cells are present.[149] When fluid cytology is inconclusive, pleural biopsy may be helpful in diagnosis of malignant infiltration.[150]

### Management

The treatment of pleural effusion depends on the etiologic mechanism, rapidity of symptom onset, degree of respiratory compromise, and overall goals of care.[142,149] Because many patients with malignant pleural effusion have limited survival, the selection of treatment that enhances quality of life with minimal time required for recovery is optimal.[149] When pleural effusions are small or have a nonmalignant cause, observation without definitive treatment may be indicated.[144,149] Aggressive antineoplastic therapy may be indicated when a large tumor causes lymphatic obstruction, heart failure, or pneumonitis that in turn causes pleural effusion.[143]

When malignant cells are present in the pleural fluid, management may be determined by overall treatment goals. Repeated therapeutic thoracenteses are often the preferred initial choice; this assumes that the ultimate cause of the pleural effusion is being treated or that the patient's life expectancy does not warrant more interventional measures.[142,143] When the patient's life expectancy is longer, and pleural effusions do not resolve with anticancer therapy and intermittent thoracenteses, treatment includes long-term chest catheter drainage or pleurodesis.[144,149] Long-term

pleural drainage via a soft tunneled catheter allows patients to have a means of draining excess fluid while remaining at home.[155,156] When drainage slows and patients become a good candidate for pleurodesis, they are admitted to the hospital for this procedure, although spontaneous pleural adherence has occurred. Alternatively, patients may be admitted for placement of a traditional chest catheter, and once drainage slows, pleurodesis may be performed. Pleurodesis, also called pleural sclerosing, involves intrapleural administration of a chemical (eg, doxycycline, bleomycin) or a mechanical agent (eg, talc slurry) to alter the pH of the pleural fluid and cause inflammatory adherence of the visceral and parietal pleura to each other.[157,158] Sclerosed pleura do not have the normal lubricating pleural fluid, and restrictive lung disease is the long-term consequence. Pleurodesis is successful only about 67% of the time, necessitating the availability of additional treatment options.[157] With the availability of tunneled pleural catheters and minimally invasive surgery, chest catheter pleurodesis is employed far less often.[143,144,158]

Pleurectomy is a thoracic surgical procedure that removes the entire pleura. Pleurectomy is effective but can be difficult to perform when long-term inflammation and pleurodesis attempts cause a friable pleura that is not easily separated. Chronic, long-term pleuroperitoneal shunts or implanted access devices have been used, but development of fibrin sheaths on the catheters often causes occlusion.[143] In cases where catheter drainage is unsuccessful, intracavitary chemotherapy with cisplatin, interferon, or pemetrexed have been used with moderate success.[143,159]

### Complications

Untreated pleural effusions that continue to accumulate lead to clinically significant alveolar collapse and respiratory failure, which may be caused by loss of gas-exchanging airways or mediastinal shifting with major airway obstruction. Progressive hypoxemia leads to profound respiratory acidosis and ischemic organ failure. Evacuation of an extensive and long-standing pleural effusion may result in re-expansion pulmonary edema or hypotension from fluid shifts.[142]

## Spinal Cord Compression

Spinal cord compression (SCC) occurs when tumor cells or collapsed vertebrae in the epidural space exert pressure on the spinal cord, which may result in permanent dysfunction (including paralysis) if not diagnosed and treated promptly.[160] The most common cause of SCC is compression fracture and vertebral collapse.[161] Epidural tumors are found in about 5% to 14% of patients with metastatic disease.[160,161] The tumors most often associated with spinal cord compression are breast, lung, kidney, and prostate, although other metastatic cancers have been occasionally seen.[160-164] Despite known risk factors, as many as 20% of patients may have SCC as their presenting symptomatology for cancer diagnosis.[164] Factors associated with effective local control and long-term survival after SCC include favorable histologic diagnosis, no visceral metastases, and a long-course radiation therapy schedule.[162]

### Pathophysiology

Two major pathophysiologic mechanisms are likely to result in SCC: (1) tumors arising within the epidural space through

**TABLE 48-4** Spinal Cord Compression: Etiology and Clinical Presentation

| Location of Lesion | Common Malignant Etiologies | Physical Symptoms | Autonomic Symptoms |
|---|---|---|---|
| Cervical spine | • Head and neck cancers<br>• Melanoma | • Radicular pain in the neck, occipital region, and shoulders (pain is often provoked by neck movement)<br>• Quadriplegia<br>• Upper extremity weakness (may be spastic or atrophic)<br>• Sensory loss in area of weakness<br>• Weakness or paralysis of the diaphragm may occur with lesion at or above C4 (may be unilateral or bilateral) | • Hypotension<br>• Bradycardia<br>• Loss of temperature autoregulation<br>• Autonomic hyperreflexia<br>• Gastric hypersecretion and paralytic ileus<br>• Reflex bowel, bladder, and penile erection<br>• Hoffman's sign (flicking of the middle finger induces flexion of the ipsilateral thumb or index finger) |
| Thoracic spine | • Breast cancer<br>• Gastric cancer<br>• Lung cancer<br>• Lymphoma<br>• Pancreatic cancer | • Pain (may be local, radicular, or both)<br>• Paraplegia<br>• Sensory loss below the level of the lesion<br>• Reflex abnormalities distal to the lesion | • Venous stasis and associated complications<br>• Reflex bowel, bladder, and penile erection |
| Lumbar spine | • Ovarian cancer<br>• Renal cell cancer<br>• Prostate cancer | • Bowel and bladder dysfunction<br>• Extensor plantar response | • Venous stasis and associated complications<br>• Reflex bowel, bladder, and penile erection |
| Cauda equina | • Bladder cancer<br>• Prostate cancer | • Pain (may be local, referred, or radicular)<br>• Sphincter disturbances<br>• Loss of buttock and leg sensation<br>• Lower extremity weakness/paralysis | • Areflexic bowel, bladder, and penile erection |

vertebral or lymphatic spread and (2) bony metastasis causing vertebral collapse with spinal cord and nerve root compression.[160–162] Permanent neurologic damage from proximal tumors may also occur if spinal circulation is compromised, such as in prolonged ischemia or hemorrhage.[160,165] Other disorders producing signs and symptoms of cord compression are paraneoplastic syndromes, radiation myelopathy, herpes zoster, pain from a pelvic or long bone metastasis, or cytotoxic drug effects.[160,162,165] Table 48-4 presents the tumors most likely to cause cord compression and the location of compression.

### Assessment

**HISTORY.** When a primary tumor presses on the spinal cord, signs and symptoms usually develop slowly. Problems develop more rapidly with metastatic disease. Most patients with SCC complain of progressive central or radicular back pain that often is aggravated by weight bearing, lying down, coughing, sneezing, or performing the Valsalva maneuver. Sitting relieves the pain.[160,163,165]

The earliest neurologic symptoms are sensory changes, such as numbness, paresthesia, and coldness.[160,163] Compression occurs most often in the thoracic section of the spinal cord, causing neurogenic bladder with urinary retention and incontinence. Patients may also lose the urge to defecate and are unable to bear down. Men on occasion lose the ability to have or maintain an erection. Metastases to the cauda equina frequently produce impaired urethral, vaginal, and rectal sensations; bladder dysfunction; decreased sensation in the lumbosacral dermatomes; and saddle anesthesia.[160,163,165] Box 48-10 describes spinal cord considerations in the older adult.

It is possible to determine the level of cord compression by the patient's report of pain during straight leg raising, neck flexion, or vertebral percussion. The upper limit of the

**BOX 48-10** CONSIDERATIONS for the Older Patient

**Spinal Cord Compression**

Signs and symptoms of SCC often begin as subtle and nonspecific back pain and sensory changes. The older patient may have concomitant diabetes mellitus or osteoarthritis that produces overlapping symptoms, delaying diagnosis of the oncologic complication. In addition, older persons often have bowel and bladder changes causing constipation or urinary incontinence, mimicking the more serious autonomic changes that occur in later SCC. People at high risk for SCC, such as those with known bone metastases, should be taught the importance of reporting and having evaluated all back pain and sensory changes, especially in the lower extremities. In SCC, palpable vertebral tenderness is more often present than with other nononcologic disorders.

sensory level is usually one or two vertebral bodies below the site of compression.[163,165] Lessened rectal tone and perineal sensation are observed with autonomic dysfunction. Deep tendon reflexes can be brisk with cord compression and diminished with nerve root compression.

Once patients experience pain, motor weakness and ataxia often follow.[160,161,163] Patients may complain that their arms or legs feel heavy. Some patients lose the ability to sense light touch, pain, and temperature. Over time, weakness may progress to spasm, paralysis, and muscle atrophy; sensations of deep pressure and position may disappear.[165]

**DIAGNOSTIC STUDIES.** A screening spinal radiograph will detect up to 80% of vertebral fractures and high risk for SCC, and may be used for initial, rapid evaluation in high-risk patients, particularly when an MRI is not readily available.[161,163,165] MRI is the diagnostic test of choice owing to its high sensitivity for neurologic tissues. MRI examinations can clearly demonstrate all epidural deposits as well as complete or partial block of the spinal cord.[160,163,165] A myelogram or CT scan may reveal spinal tumors, but these studies are less sensitive for diagnosing the presence and extent of cord compression. Lumbar puncture, which is used to obtain cerebrospinal fluid, reveals malignant cells in the presence of epidural disease.[160,165]

## Management

Factors considered in the selection of the best therapeutic option are the level of cord compression, the rate of neurologic deterioration, and previous use of radiation therapy.[166] The degree of spinal instability is used to determine the most immediate therapy, as an unstable spine has increased risk for permanent disability and less likelihood of responding to supportive or slower acting anticancer treatments.[166,167] Corticosteroids decrease peritumoral edema and neurologic dysfunction; however controversy exists as to whether the traditional high dose regimen remains preferable to a newer but less evidence-supported low-dose strategy.[162,167] High-dose dexamethasone, 10 mg as an initial dose, is administered to patients with neurologic symptoms before emergency diagnostic procedures are performed, and is continued during radiation therapy (4 to 20 mg every 6 hours) and then tapered.[162,167] It is not clear whether such steroid therapy affects final patient outcome.

Radiation therapy is appropriate when the tumor is determined to be radiosensitive, and should be initiated as soon as the diagnosis of cord compression has been confirmed.[168] Radiation portals include the entire area of blockage and two vertebral bodies above and below this area. More than 50% of patients with rapid neurologic deterioration improve with radiation therapy; however, patients with autonomic dysfunction or paraplegia have a poor prognosis with any therapy.[166-168]

Laminectomy, with or without placement of stabilization rods in the nearby vertebral bodies, may result in immediate decompression of the spinal cord and nerve roots.[167,168] The posterior approach is preferred but is often difficult because most metastases arise in the vertebral bodies anterior to the spinal cord.[167-169] The anterior approach is warranted for people with tumors that are believed to be resectable, making the clinical risks worth the aggressive surgical intervention.[169] Postoperative radiation therapy is used to shrink residual tumor, relieve pain, and improve the patient's functional status. If there is no previous histologic diagnosis of cancer, or if infection or epidural hematoma must be ruled out, then laminectomy can be used for both diagnosis and treatment. If high cervical cord compression precludes surgery, a neurologist should stabilize the patient's neck in halo traction to prevent respiratory paralysis.[166,167] If the patient continues to deteriorate neurologically despite high doses of steroids and radiation therapy, emergency decompression may be necessary.[169]

In some people, stabilization of the spine with vertebroplasty with or without kyphoplasty represents a less invasive and equally effective short-term resolution for acute cord compression and its associated pain.[166-170] Injection of physiologic cement (kyphoplasty) to reexpand collapsed vertebrae has been used to successfully prevent progression to SCC, but is contraindicated with an unstable spine.[170] If the tumor is

chemosensitive, chemotherapy concurrently with or soon after completion of radiation therapy or surgery may be appropriate. Chemotherapy may also be effective in patients with multiple myeloma who have had previous radiation therapy.[166,167] Systemic chemotherapy or hormonal therapy may be useful in certain types of tumors, such as lymphoma or prostatic cancer.

Pain management includes the administration of appropriate analgesics, bed rest, and patient support during position changes and transfer. Range-of-motion exercises are useful in patients with motor and sensory deficits. Bowel retraining and intermittent urinary catheterization may be necessary. Deep vein thrombosis prevention and frequent skin care is essential. Surgical wounds are particularly susceptible to skin breakdown (with possible wound dehiscence) because of limited mobility and the effects of concomitant corticosteroid therapy.[160]

## Tracheobronchial Obstruction

### Pathophysiology

Obstruction of the trachea or major branches of the bronchi with tumor results in respiratory distress and hypoxemia. The severity of symptoms depends on the rapidity of obstruction and degree of closure.[171] Tumors most likely to cause airway obstruction are lung cancer and lymphoma, although other metastatic tumors (eg, head and neck cancer, melanoma, thyroid, renal or breast cancer) and nonmalignant disorders (eg, amyloidosis, bronchomalacia) may also cause airway obstruction.[171] Left mainstem bronchus obstruction, poor performance status, and high anesthesia risk category are poor prognostic factors in outcomes for patients with central airway obstruction.[172,173]

### Assessment

**HISTORY.** Patients with tracheobronchial obstruction present with varying degrees of dyspnea depending on the amount and location of the obstruction and the rapidity of onset. Some patients with slowly developing tumors have compensated respiratory acidosis and minimal symptoms even with nearly complete obstruction. Other patients, especially those with lymphoma or small cell lung carcinoma, have rapidly growing tumors and severe symptoms even when the airway is less than 75% obstructed. Stridor is present in tracheal obstruction, and wheezing with unequal chest excursion is seen with bronchial obstruction.[171,174] Some patients presenting with severe respiratory distress actually have only partial airway obstruction, but the resultant narrowed airway leads to concomitant atelectasis or trapped secretions with pneumonia that may be mistaken as more severe tumor obstruction.[174]

**DIAGNOSTIC STUDIES.** Bronchoscopy makes it easy to detect tracheal or bronchial obstruction and grade its severity. However, bronchoscopy does not always reveal whether the airways are compressed extrinsically or invaded with tumor.[170] Bronchoscopy is used with spiral CT scans to provide a comprehensive description of the obstructive process that is used to guide therapy.[171]

### Management

Clinically significant obstruction of the major airways always necessitates immediate treatment, although the therapeutic plan varies according to tumor-specific factors and therapeutic goals. Emergent treatment of airway occlusion–induced hypoxemia or hypercapnia may require nasal inhalation or heliox-based nebulizer treatments. A combination of oxygen and helium that is lighter than pure oxygen, heliox enhances movement of the air beyond the area of obstruction and provides palliative relief until more aggressive operative measures are possible.[171] If air movement is adequate, bronchodilators and corticosteroids are administered to enhance ventilation, and if simultaneous pneumonia is suspected, antimicrobial therapy is instituted.[171]

Effective treatment for endobronchial tumors includes laser, cautery, photodynamic therapy, and endobronchial brachytherapy.[171,175,176] These therapies for tumors invading the major airways are highly successful for prolonging life as well as improving its quality. Most procedures entail use of a rigid bronchoscope under anesthesia, and patients usually experience a rapid recovery with little more than a sore throat and annoying cough for a few days afterward.[171,176] Endobronchial brachytherapy involves endotracheal intubation with precisely directed radiation therapy through an endobronchial catheter.[171,175,176] In laser therapy, electrocautery, photodynamic therapy, and endobronchial brachytherapy, close observation for airway bleeding is necessary, and clinicians may prescribe cough suppressants or low-dose corticosteroids to reduce the incidence of bleeding.[175]

Airway opening with tracheal or bronchial stents may provide temporary symptomatic relief while definitive anticancer treatment is implemented for palliative relief of symptoms.[171,175,176] For insertion of an airway stent, a rigid bronchoscope and light anesthesia are necessary, and multiple bronchoscopic procedures to assess or adjust placement are required. The most common problem with stents, especially if placed before shrinking the tumor, is displacement, because the airway naturally opens with the reduction of tumor. Displaced stents usually cause severe and sudden respiratory distress and require immediate interventional adjustment. Chronic lung infections after stent placement may occur, and are associated with high risk of occlusion and long-term stenosis.[176,177] In rare circumstances, or when stenting is not possible, patient positioning to shift the chest tumor off the major airway (eg, prone positioning) may provide temporary symptomatic relief while cancer therapy is used to shrink the tumor.

### Complications

Two severe complications that may occur are total airway occlusion and hemorrhage caused by tumor erosion into the nearby pulmonary vessels.[171,176] Treatment of total obstruction is the same as that of partial obstruction when an improvement in symptoms can be reasonably expected as a result of therapy. Emergent extracorporeal membrane oxygenation (ECMO) has also been used to bridge until the tumor shrinks. Treatment of hemorrhage, when recognized before massive bleeding occurs, may involve embolization. If severe hemorrhage occurs, it is necessary to insert a dual-lumen endotracheal tube or single-sided intubation and occlude the bleeding lung while ventilating the good lung until surgical repair can be performed. Airway obstruction may also lead to erosion through the airway and accompanying pneumothorax. In these circumstances, supportive therapy, such as chest tube insertion, may be used but is rarely helpful.

## Metabolic Complications

### Hypercalcemia

Hypercalcemia exists when the corrected serum calcium level is above 11 mg/dL (normal range, 8.5 to 10.5 mg/dL). This is the most common metabolic oncologic emergency that develops when the bones release more calcium into the extracellular fluid than can be filtered by the kidneys and excreted in the urine.[178] In the advent of effective prevention of bone demineralization using bisphosphonates, this complication has greatly reduced in incidence, and now most commonly a manifestation of refractory and end-stage malignancy.[178]

#### Pathophysiology

Ninety-nine percent of the calcium in the body is in an insoluble form in the bones. The remaining 1% is freely exchangeable calcium. The calcium of importance is the ionized calcium, which must be maintained within a precise range. Free total calcium levels may be affected by albumin, other serum proteins, or vascular volume status, and are most likely to be underestimated, even with standardized correction formulas.[179] Serum calcium levels are regulated by parathyroid hormone and calcitonin.[178] The release of parathyroid hormone from the parathyroid glands stimulates an increase in serum calcium levels, whereas the release of calcitonin produces a decrease in serum calcium levels.[178]

The three primary etiologies of hypercalcemia are (1) excessive quantities of intact parathyroid hormone (parathyroid origin) or humoral-mediated (malignant production) parathyroid-related hormone; (2) osteolysis with bone demineralization; and (3) excessive vitamin D activation.[180] Instances of nonbone hypercalcemia are often viewed as a hallmark of the presence of tumor. The incidence and severity of hypercalcemia may dramatically decrease when the patient's tumor is quiescent, and may become severe or difficult to manage when the tumor is active.[178]

Ectopic parathyroid hormone (PTH) may occur with primary parathyroidism (incidence less than 20% of cases), or with PTH or PTH-like substance production by tumor cells (44% to 60% of cases).[181] Differentiation of the precise mechanism of PTH activity may be unnecessary unless malignancy has not been previously identified.[178]

Destruction of the bone by metastatic invasion was once believed to be the most common cause of malignant hypercalcemia; however, reduction of skeletal events with prophylactic bisphosphonates has reduced the incidence of this etiology.[178] In patients with multiple myeloma, the abnormal plasma cells produce osteoclast-activating factor (OAF); however, hypercalcemia rarely develops in these patients unless they have inadequate renal function.[178] Patients with T-cell lymphoma have severe hypercalcemia related to the ectopic production of OAF, colony-stimulating factor, interferon-γ, and an active vitamin D metabolite.[170] Additional causes of hypercalcemia in the presence of malignancy include immobilization, renal insufficiency, thiazide diuretics, high dietary calcium or vitamin D intake, and low phosphate levels.[182,183] Table 48-5 lists causes of hypercalcemia in malignancy, proposed mechanisms, differential diagnosis, and preferred management.

| TABLE 48-5 | Evaluation and Management of Hypercalcemia | | |
|---|---|---|---|
| **Etiology** | **Pathogenesis** | **Diagnosis** | **Specific Treatment*** |
| Intact parathyroid hormone (PTH) elevation | Hormone from parathyroid excreted in large quantities such as with primary para-thyroidism or parathyroid adenoma<br>PTH Can be excreted directly from some tumors | ↑ serum total and ionized calcium, par-ticularly if malignancy in origin where value may be excessively high<br>↑ Intact PTH<br>Normal Phosphorous<br>Hypochloremic acidosis (↓Cl, ↓bicarbon-ate) present in milk-alkali syndrome<br>Urine calcium/creatinine ratio to differen-tiate acquired or familial parathyroid dysfunction | Parathyroidectomy<br>Treatment of malignancy |
| Parathyroid hormone (PTHrP)–related peptide elevation | | ↑ serum total and ionized calcium<br>↓ or normal Intact PTH<br>Normal Phosphorous | Bisphosphonates<br>Treatment of malignancy |
| Osteoclastic/osteoblastic activation | Calcium resorption (removal) from the bone increased | ↑ serum total and ionized calcium | Corticosteroids<br>Treatment of malignancy |
| High vitamin D (1,25-(OH)$_2$ vitamin D) | High vitamin D activation production leading to in-creased calcium absorption<br>Examples of causes: Granu-lomatous lung conditions, sarcoidosis, lymphoma | ↑ serum total and ionized calcium | |

*General treatment for hypercalcemia regardless of etiology includes administration of fluid boluses with or without diuretics.

Data from Crowley R, Gittoes N: How to approach hypercalcemia. Clin Med 13(3):287–290, 2013; Endres DB: Investigation of hypercalcemia. Clin Biochem 45(12):954–963, 2012; and Rosner MH, Dalkin AC: Electrolyte disorders associated with cancer. Adv Chronic Kidney Dis 21(1):7–17, 2014

## Assessment

**HISTORY.** The severity of signs and symptoms of hyper-calcemia often correlates with the serum calcium level. Mild calcium elevations may be asymptomatic or present as an-orexia, constipation, fatigue, or malaise. Moderate hyper-calcemia has presenting symptoms such as abdominal pain, nausea, bone pain, polyuria, and mental status changes. Most patients presenting with severe calcium elevations demon-strate dysrhythmias or neurologic symptoms such as somno-lence, combativeness, confusion, or coma.[180,184]

**DIAGNOSTIC STUDIES.** Elevated serum calcium and elevated ionized calcium are the hallmark diagnostic findings in hypercalcemia. The serum calcium measurement is often reported as an absolute number without considering that only the calcium bound to albumin is counted. A standard calcu-lation for correction of the serum calcium for a low albumin is performed by subtracting the patient's albumin from low normal, multiplying this number by a correction factor of 0.8, and adding this number to the reported calcium. Serum ion-ized calcium levels are more accurate, but because the normal value is 1.0 mEq/L (±0.02), its value may be underestimated in importance.[178]

After initial assessment of increased calcium levels, the specific etiology should be determined. Intact PTH is analyzed; when elevated, it is indicative of primary or sec-ondary parathyroidism. A normal intact PTH or elevated immunofluorescence PTH-related peptide may indicate humoral-mediated PTH elevations. Bone demineralization is characterized by normal PTH levels with low phosphorous and elevations in alkaline phosphatase.[185] Hyperphosphate-mia in the presence of hypercalcemia, especially in the ab-sence of kidney dysfunction, suggests vitamin-D mediated

disease.[180,185] Symptomatic patients usually have ECGs that show a bradycardia and prolonged PR, QRS, and QT intervals.

## Management

Medical management of hypercalcemia involves the use of IV fluids and drug therapy to enhance renal excretion of cal-cium and to decrease bone resorption. Acute hypercalcemia is initially treated with IV normal saline (0.9% NaCl) so-lution to dilute calcium levels and increase urinary calcium excretion.[165,175] When hypercalcemia is life-threatening, ag-gressive hydration (250 to 300 mL/h) and IV loop diuret-ics such as furosemide are necessary.[175] Hemodialysis with calcium-free dialysate has been used successfully for emer-gency management of life-threatening hypercalcemia.[176]

In most patients, treatment with hydration, diuretics, ap-propriate antitumor therapy, and mobilization is effective. Patients who do not respond to these therapies require hy-pocalcemic therapy indefinitely. Bisphosphonates are most frequently used. Currently, the most potent bisphospho-nate available is zoledronic acid. It is administered as an 8-mg 15-minute IV infusion daily for 3 days unless serum calcium levels decrease before that time.[178] Alternatively, bisphosphonate therapy with pamidronate may be given as a 90 mg infusion over 90 to 120 minutes. Denosumab, an FDA-licensed monoclonal antibody targeting rank ligand for prevention of bone breakdown, is also available to prevent skeletal related events, but its use in hypercalcemia has been limited.[180,185] In cases unresponsive to bisphosphonates, cal-citonin, corticosteroids, or strontium-98 may be useful.[178,186]

If possible, patients should ambulate to prevent osteoly-sis. It is necessary to eliminate constipation, which is usually caused by an increased level of calcium in the blood. Reduced oral intake of calcium or increased salt intake may be of some help. Patients should not take medications, such as thiazide diuretics and vitamins A and D, because they elevate the calcium level.[178] Close monitoring of fluid status is essential. Patients may receive up to 10 L of IV fluids daily, and the nurse should carefully measure intake and output. In addition, careful observation for overhydration is important. Potassium supplements may be necessary.

Hypercalcemia is a common oncologic emergency that can be prevented or diminished in a large number of patients with the appropriate prophylactic bisphosphonates, education, and precautions. Box 48-11 presents a teaching guide for patients with hypercalcemia.

### Complications

Permanent renal tubular abnormalities may develop in patients with prolonged hypercalcemia.[184] Sudden death from cardiac dysrhythmias may result from an acute increase in serum calcium. Long-term bisphosphonate use has been associated with severe osteonecrosis of the jaw. Specific risk factors for this complication are not yet clear.[181]

## Syndrome of Inappropriate Antidiuretic Hormone Secretion

SIADH secretion is a clinical disorder characterized by excess stimulation of pituitary excretion of antidiuretic hormone (ADH). Under normal circumstances, the posterior pituitary gland releases ADH in response to changes in plasma osmolality (concentration of solutes) and circulating blood volume. ADH release causes decreased urine production, oliguria, and increased water resorption. SIADH has several specific causes related to cancer and its treatment.[187] The clinical consequences of SIADH and its management strategies are discussed in Chapter 44.

### Pathophysiology

When thoracic or mediastinal tumors press on major cardiac vessels, the obstruction may impede cardiac output. The posterior pituitary gland perceives this to be a fall in circulatory volume and compensates by inappropriately secreting ADH, which in turn suppresses urinary output. The resulting volume expansion improves cardiac output but leaves the patient with a relative sodium deficiency (dilutional hyponatremia).[187]

In addition to the pressure of thoracic or mediastinal tumors on cardiac vessels, cancers and treatment-related factors can also precipitate SIADH. Small cell lung cancers or mixed cellularity lung cancers, pancreatic, renal, gastric, head and neck, thyroid cancer, neuroendocrine, and melanoma release an ADH-like substance.[180,187,188] Certain chemotherapeutic agents, such as cyclophosphamide, iphosphamide, imatinib, vincristine, vinorelbine and alemtuzumab, as well as morphine, may stimulate ADH release or potentiate its effects on the kidneys.[94,187] Ongoing evidence of SIADH after antineoplastic treatment is considered a poor prognostic sign, often a subtle indicator of persistent tumor.[187,188] Complicating this confusing clinical picture may be that brain injury, pulmonary infection, and HIV disease also cause SIADH.[189]

### Management

Treatment of the underlying malignancy is of primary importance in cancer-related SIADH.[190] Clinical evidence of excess ADH is present until the primary tumor stops compressing the major cardiac vessels or producing ADH-like substances. Antineoplastic therapy may include chemotherapy, radiation therapy, or corticosteroids. Fluid intake limited to 500 to 1,000 mL/d should result in a corrected fluid balance in 7 to 10 days.[187] Demeclocycline, an antibiotic that inhibits ADH secretion, may be effective; patients with chronic SIADH may receive demeclocycline, 900 to 1,200 mg/d.[187,189,190] Adverse effects include diarrhea, nausea, dysphagia, and photosensitivity. New specific vasopressin-receptor antagonists, called "vaptans," enhance water diuresis without sodium and potassium loss and show promise in the treatment of this disorder.[190] Oral agents such as tolvaptan inhibit only the V2 receptor, whereas the intravenous medication conivaptan blocks both V2 and V1a.[190] These agents should not be used in patients with liver disease and are not recommended for chronic treatment beyond 30 days.[190]

Diuretics are not used except in severe circumstances because they may produce additional electrolyte imbalances. However, the patient who is comatose or convulsing should receive 3% IV hypertonic saline solution and a potent loop diuretic, such as furosemide.[189,190] Fluid imbalances and hyponatremia may be severe enough to warrant initiation of mechanical ventilation; the need for this aggressive respiratory support is the most predictive of a mortality rate of 22% to 40%.[180,190]

---

**BOX 48-11**  *TEACHING GUIDE*  **Malignancy-Associated Hypercalcemia**

Patients at high risk for malignancy-associated hypercalcemia include those with:
- Bone metastases (most common in breast, lung, and colon cancer)
- Lung cancer
- Gastrointestinal cancers (gastric, pancreatic, colon)
- Hematologic cancers (leukemia, lymphoma, multiple myeloma)
- Renal (kidney) cancer
- Thyroid cancer

Patients with the risk factors below need to be instructed that additional factors increase their risk for developing hypercalcemia. These factors include:
- Lack of physical activity

- Low fluid status
- Poor kidney function

Critical care nurses can teach patients methods for preventing hypercalcemia as follows:
- Drink at least six to eight glasses of water every day.
- Eat salty foods.
- Remain physically active.
- Limit dairy products and vitamin D–enriched foods, such as milk, cheese, and yogurt.

# Tumor Lysis Syndrome

Tumor lysis syndrome is a metabolic imbalance caused by rapid cancer cell death occurring with clinical significance in 2% to 4% of high-risk patients.[191,192] Most patients with chemosensitive or radiosensitive tumors experience this complication 1 to 5 days after initiation of therapy.[191–193] However, there are documented instances of tumor lysis syndrome in rapidly proliferating disease such as acute leukemia or high-grade lymphoma even before treatment initiation.[192]

Patients at greatest risk for tumor lysis syndrome are those with bulky tumors that have a high growth rate (eg, acute leukemia or Burkitt lymphoma) and those with highly radiosensitive or chemosensitive tumors, such as small cell lung cancer and most malignant lymphomas.[191–193] Patients with preexisting renal dysfunction may be at greatest risk owing to their difficulty in clearing the metabolic waste products fast enough to prevent clinical complications.[193] Other patients at high risk are those with Merkel tumor, testicular cancer, hepatoblastoma, and medulloblastoma.[191]

## Pathophysiology

Rapid cell death causes the release of intracellular contents (potassium, phosphorus, and nucleic acids) into the circulating serum. The normal filtration mechanisms in the kidneys should immediately detect the levels of metabolic waste products and attempt to excrete them. If production is more rapid than excretion or renal insufficiency is present, accumulation of electrolytes and uric acid occurs in the serum. The most common abnormalities include hyperkalemia, hyperphosphatemia, and hyperuricemia.[191–193] High phosphorus causes the kidneys to excrete calcium, causing hypocalcemia. Hyperuricemia causes deposition of uric acid crystals in the urinary tract and may lead to renal failure.[191–193]

## Assessment

**HISTORY.** Signs and symptoms of tumor lysis syndrome are related to the specific electrolyte imbalances involved and renal dysfunction. Hyperkalemia, hyperphosphatemia, hypocalcemia, hyperuricemia, and acidosis may occur. Box 48-12 lists the typical clinical signs and symptoms associated with the metabolic abnormalities of tumor lysis syndrome.[180,191]

**DIAGNOSTIC STUDIES.** The electrolyte panel analysis is used to identify key abnormalities in patients at risk for tumor lysis syndrome. Elevated serum potassium, phosphate, uric acid, blood urea nitrogen, and creatinine, with low calcium, are reported. Acidosis may be present in patients with severely compromised renal function. The urinary uric acid/creatinine ratio is greater than 1. Renal ultrasonography is used to exclude ureteral obstruction.[194]

## Management

Treatment involves recognition of high-risk patients and promoting prevention through aggressive hydration, as well as administration of phosphate-binding agents and allopurinol for at least 48 hours before beginning chemotherapy. It is necessary to avoid agents that block tubular reabsorption of uric acid

---

**QSEN BOX 48-12** *PATIENT SAFETY*

### Signs and Symptoms of Tumor Lysis Syndrome

**Hyperkalemia**
- Peaked T waves on electrocardiogram (ECG)
- Dysrhythmias (tachycardia, ventricular ectopy/torsade de pointes [especially when potassium levels are >6.8 mEq/L])
- Muscle flaccidity, weakness
- Hyperactive bowel sounds, abdominal cramping, and diarrhea

**Hyperphosphatemia**
- Muscle weakness
- Bone marrow suppression (thrombocytopenia, leukopenia)
- Bone demineralization with tendency for pathologic fractures
- Renal dysfunction

**Hypocalcemia**
- Muscle tetany
- Seizures
- Short PR and QT intervals on ECG
- Dysrhythmias (tachycardia, ventricular ectopy/torsade de pointes)
- Hyperactive bowel sounds, abdominal cramping, and diarrhea

**Hyperuricemia**
- Uric acid crystals in urine
- Hematuria
- Oliguria, anuria
- Flank pain
- Renal failure

**Acidosis**
- Tachypnea
- Hypotension

---

(eg, aspirin, radiographic contrast, probenecid, thiazide diuretics). The goal is to keep the serum uric acid level within normal limits. Electrolyte disturbances are specifically treated as needed.[193–195]

IV fluids are given to ensure a urine volume of more than 3 L/d. In the past, IV sodium bicarbonate (4 g initially, then 1 to 2 g every 4 hours) has been administered to alkalinize the urine and reduce uric acid crystallization in the kidney tubules. Clinicians are now less likely to initiate alkalinization if the phosphate is high because calcium phosphate precipitation is equally likely to cause renal failure.[194–196] To measure urine output more accurately, insertion of a Foley catheter into the bladder is usually necessary. If oliguria or anuria develops, ureteral obstruction must be excluded. Phosphate-binding agents such as aluminum hydroxide are given every 2 to 4 hours in an effort to keep phosphate levels below 4 mg/dL.[191–194]

Concomitant diuresis or medications such as Kayexalate that enhance gastrointestinal excretion of potassium may effectively manage elevated serum potassium levels not prevented with hydration. Allopurinol, a xanthine oxidase inhibitor that blocks uric acid production, is administered in doses ranging from 300 to 900 mg/d. Because allopurinol is now available in an IV form given as 200 to 400 mg/m$^2$/d, rapid normalization of uric acid levels is an achievable objective.[191,192] Its greatest limitation is that it cannot assist in breakdown or clearance of already existing uric acid.[192] Rasburicase (Elitek) acts like the natural enzyme urate oxidase to oxidize uric acid to allantoin for excretion.[191,192,194] Rasburicase is used cautiously in patients at risk for glycoprotein deficiency (GPD) because of increased risk for hemolytic anemia. Severe hypersensitivity reactions have also been reported with rasburicase; therefore, careful observation of patients during infusion is warranted. The uric acid serum blood levels drawn on patients receiving rasburicase must be placed in an iced blood tube and transported to the laboratory on ice to ensure accurate levels.[191,192]

If diuresis does not occur within a few hours after the initiation of treatment, renal replacement therapy is needed. An initial hemodialysis treatment usually reduces the patient's uric acid levels by 50%, but most patients then receive several additional days of continuous renal replacement therapy

(CRRT) until electrolyte abnormalities and hyperuricemia resolve.[194] A low-calcium dialysate is used to prevent calcium phosphate precipitation. If peritoneal dialysis is used, albumin is added to the dialysate to increase uric acid protein binding and removal.

The focus of nursing care is on careful monitoring of fluid therapy, intake and output, and electrolyte balance. The use of prophylactic allopurinol, aggressive hydration, and early intervention with CRRT has reduced the incidence and severity of tumor lysis syndrome.[195]

## Clinical Applicability Challenges

---

### CASE STUDY

K.B. is a 45-year-old man with acute myelogenous leukemia diagnosed a month ago. He received cytosine arabinoside and idarubicin chemotherapy 16 days ago. He presented to the emergency department 4 hours ago with a fever of 102.2°F (39°C), chills, myalgias, somnolence, and right-sided abdominal pain. He has a past medical history of cholecystis with gallbladder removal 3 years ago. He has no other medical conditions. He is a nonsmoker, has light alcohol intake, and uses no other drugs, medications, or supplements.

When K.B. presented and was diagnosed with leukemia, he had a sinus infection and oral thrush. Despite negative cultures, he cleared infectious symptoms after antibiotics and chemotherapy. Most recently in clinic he experienced mild to moderate right-sided abdominal pain over the past 5 days, but no fever or constitutional symptoms until today. He was told that his blood count (CBC) was low owing to chemotherapy and that he should come immediately to the emergency department with any fever.

Physical examination revealed the following:

*Neurologic assessment:* K.B. was anxious but oriented to person, place, and time and had equal limb sensation and movement. He also reported diffuse right-sided abdominal pain rating 6 on a 1 to 10 scale (with 10 the greatest pain), but stated it was colicky in nature.

*Respiratory assessment:* Unlabored tachypnea with respirations at 28/min, normal chest excursion and breath sounds.

*Cardiovascular assessment:* Audible normal heart sounds, with normal point of maximal impulse. Radial pulses were full and bounding. There was an absence of jugular venous distention, trace peripheral edema, and slowed capillary refill. Mottling was noted on the lower legs, where pedal pulses were less than the upper extremity pulses. Pulse is 132 beats/min and regular, and K.B.'s blood pressure was 90/42 mm Hg.

*Gastrointestinal/genitourinary assessment:* Abdomen was firm, diffusely tender on palpation with rebound tenderness in right upper quadrant. K.B. reported moderate nausea and anorexia that had become more pronounced within the past week. Bowel sounds were diminished throughout but faint in the right upper quadrant. He reported he had not urinated in the past 8 hours and that his last urine was dark but not foul-smelling.

*Chest x-ray:* Normal.

*Electrocardiogram:* Normal sinus tachycardia.

*Arterial blood gas values on 3L nasal cannula:* pH 7.25, pCO$_2$ 32, pO$_2$ 66, and HCO$_3$ 13.

A peripheral IV was initiated for K.B., and the indwelling Hickman catheter was accessed and a cardiac monitor applied; blood was drawn for CBC and chemistry with phosphate, magnesium, lactic acid, amylase, and lipase. An indwelling catheter was placed for 60 mL dark urine, and Ringers lactate 2 L was administered wide open. Because of the fever, specimens for culture were obtained, followed by administration of acetaminophen (Tylenol) and piperacillin–tazobactam (Zosyn).

Upon arrival in the ICU, the nurse confirms these findings and verifies the CBC laboratory abnormalities are white blood cell count 0.002, Hgb 9.0, and platelets 32,000, thought to be related to his recent chemotherapy. Chemistry values of concern include Na 147, Cl 102, K 5.4, Mg 0.9, Phos 2.5, creatinine 2.2, and BUN 56. Additionally, K.B.'s serum lactic acid is 7.3, and amylase is 160.

An abdominal ultrasound is in order, as well as an abdominal CT scan with oral and IV contrast. The patient's heart rate and blood pressure initially respond to fluids with a heart rate reduction to 120/min and blood pressure increase to 106/50, but his temperature remains 101.8°F (38.8°C) despite acetaminophen and antimicrobial therapy. Staff contemplate using the Hickman catheter but are concerned that K.B. could have bacteremia, although the primary suspected source of infection is his abdomen. Given rebound tenderness, taut abdomen, diminished bowel sounds, and an elevated lactic acid, a surgery consult is requested.

Discussion of best management of K.B.'s possible infection and sources lead to concern for a line-related infection or a gram-negative infection, given his abdominal pain. A decision is made to broaden his antimicrobials to meropenem and vancomycin to cover a possible line-related bacteremia or abdominal infection. A central venous pressure from his Hickman catheter is obtained and shows good dynamics, and is recorded as a pressure of 3 mm Hg. (Soft catheters such as the Hickman do not always transmit pressures well, but can be trusted when there are good waveform dynamics. Other patients with chest masses may also have contraindications to central venous pressures owing to confounding factors that will falsely raise the values, but K.B. does not have these conditions.) Other aspects of the sepsis bundle interventions are considered, and K.B. is placed on a proton pump inhibitor, but deep vein thrombosis prophylaxis is deferred at this time owing to his thrombocytopenia. Given his renal impairment, a contrast prophylaxis fluid bolus of 1 L D5.5NS with 100 mEq NaHCO$^3$ is administered. The surgeon provides consultation and is most suspicious of typhlitis since K.B.'s gallbladder has already been removed. This diagnosis is confirmed by cecal wall thickening on CT scan; since K.B. has an intact appendix and is experiencing prolonged neutropenia, he is at risk for this complication. The oncologists state that they expect K.B.'s blood counts to return to normal within the upcoming 7 days, so there is a plan to attempt to avoid surgery if possible. K.B. is likely to be experiencing septic shock but is at high risk for poor operative outcomes,

so surgery is deferred for a short time to determine if IV antimicrobials, gut rest, and supportive care can resolve symptoms. The decision was made to follow serial amylase, lactic acid, and vital signs and reconsider treatment options if these values rise, or if vasopressors are required. Urgent treatment may include addition of an aminoglycoside antimicrobial, transfusion with allogeneic granulocytes, or reconsideration of the surgical risks.

1. In a patient with known severe myelosuppression with neutropenia, anemia, and thrombocytopenia, several oncologic emergencies may occur. Describe the emergent conditions K.B. is experiencing, as well as the physiologic basis of these emergencies.
2. Patients and families often are surprised by the sudden occurrence of an oncologic emergency. Develop a teaching plan for K.B. and his family.
3. Explore the psychosocial challenges of treating a young and previously healthy patient with recently diagnosed cancer.

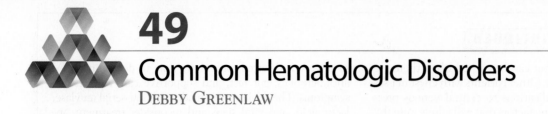

# 49

# Common Hematologic Disorders

DEBBY GREENLAW

## LEARNING OBJECTIVES

*Based on the content in this chapter, the reader should be able to:*

1. Describe the pathophysiology, assessment, and management of patients with disorders of red blood cells.

2. Discuss the pathophysiology, assessment, and management of patients with disorders of white blood cells.

3. Explain the pathophysiology, assessment, and management of patients with disorders of hemostasis.

Critically ill patients are at high risk for developing complications from a variety of hematologic disorders including red blood cell (RBC), white blood cell (WBC), platelet, and coagulation disorders. This chapter presents an overview of the pathophysiology, assessment, and management of these hematologic disorders.

## Disorders of Red Blood Cells

### Polycythemia

#### Polycythemia Vera

Polycythemia vera is a myeloproliferative disorder of increased RBC production resulting in a high hematocrit and an increased RBC mass. Increased RBC production causes decreased tissue oxygenation, increased blood viscosity, vascular insufficiency, and risk for thrombosis. As the disease progresses, some patients may develop bone marrow fibrosis, splenomegaly, and pancytopenia. See Spotlight on Genetics 49-1.

#### Secondary Polycythemia

Secondary polycythemia is a disorder of increased RBC production that can develop as a normal response to chronic hypoxia. Conditions causing chronic hypoxia include living at high altitudes, cardiopulmonary disease, sleep apnea, obesity hypoventilation syndrome, and exposure to carbon monoxide. Secondary polycythemia may also result from an inappropriate increase in erythropoietin production as a result of renal disease or, in rare cases, hepatic disease.

#### Assessment

Arterial and venous thrombosis resulting from the blood's hyperviscosity is the major concern. The patient with polycythemia is at increased risk for thromboembolic events such as myocardial and cerebral infarction, deep venous thrombosis, and pulmonary embolism.

It is important to review the patient's medical history for cardiac or pulmonary disease. Also, any history of arterial or venous thrombosis or smoking history is relevant. Table 49-1 lists additional clinical findings in polycythemia vera.

### SPOTLIGHT ON GENETICS 49-1

**HEMATOLOGIC SYSTEM—POLYCYTHEMIA VERA**

- Polycythemia vera is a condition characterized by an increased number of RBCs within the bloodstream and approximately 1 in 200,000 individuals are diagnosed each year.

- Mutations in the *JAK2* and *TET2* genes are associated with polycythemia vera. The function of the *TET2* gene is unknown. The *JAK2* gene provides instructions for making a protein that promotes the growth and division (proliferation) of cells.

- Polycythemia vera begins with one or more mutations in the DNA of a single hematopoietic stem cell, although it remains unclear exactly what initiates the disorder. A mutation in the *JAK2* gene seems to be particularly important for the development of polycythemia vera, as nearly all affected individuals have a mutation in this gene. *JAK2* gene mutations result in the production of a *JAK2* protein that is constantly turned on (constitutively activated), which improves the cell's ability to survive and increases production of blood cells

- Genetic and lab testing is available to diagnose polycythemia vera

Genetic Home Reference. Retrieved August 10, 2015, from http://ghr.nlm.nih.gov.

Pieri L, Pancrazzi A, Pacilli A, et al: JAK2V617F complete molecular remission in polycythemia vera/essential thrombocythemia patients treated with ruxolitinib. Blood 125(21):3352–3353, 2015.

#### Management

Serial phlebotomy is the first-line treatment for polycythemia vera. Generally 500 mL of blood is removed weekly until a hematocrit of less than 45% is achieved. Most patients managed by serial phlebotomy develop iron deficiency, which limits their ability to make RBCs and thus decreases the frequency of phlebotomy. The disadvantage of phlebotomy is that it stimulates bone marrow production, which leads to increased numbers of defective, sticky platelets. Antiplatelet aggregating agents, such as aspirin and dipyridamole, do not reduce thrombotic events and may increase the risk for bleeding.

| TABLE 49-1 | Clinical Findings and Related Causes in Polycythemia Vera |
|---|---|
| **Clinical Finding** | **Cause** |
| Dizziness, headache | Increased blood viscosity |
| Thrombosis | Increased blood viscosity, thrombocytosis, platelet defects |
| Pruritus | Elevated blood levels of histamine and/or increased skin mast cells |
| Bleeding tendency | Increased RBC/fibrin ratio; engorged capillaries and venules due to increased blood volume |
| Epigastric distress | Engorgement of gastric mucosa; increased blood histamine levels |
| Numbness and burning of toes | Peripheral vascular insufficiency |
| Cardiovascular insufficiency | Impaired tissue oxygenation due to increased blood viscosity |

Older patients with vascular disease are at high risk for thrombosis and require bone marrow suppression in addition to phlebotomy. Hydroxyurea is the medication of choice. Long-term therapy with bone marrow–suppressing agents has been associated with an increased risk for acute leukemia, so the potential benefits must be weighed against the anticipated duration of therapy. Measures to prevent thromboembolic complications should be instituted.

Treatment of secondary polycythemia focuses on correcting the underlying cause with long-term oxygen therapy, smoking cessation, weight loss, or surgical intervention as indicated. If these measures are ineffective, serial phlebotomy is required.

## Anemia

Anemia may be seen in the intensive care unit (ICU) as an incidental condition in a patient admitted to the unit for another acute illness, or as an acute condition requiring intensive monitoring and intervention. Typically, anemias are classified as blood loss, hemolytic (increased destruction of RBCs), or hypoproliferative (decreased production of RBCs). In addition, anemias can be classified by RBC size as microcytic, normocytic, or macrocytic.

Anemia is prevalent in critically ill patients. Acute blood loss, especially from intraoperative and gastrointestinal hemorrhage, is a frequent cause in the ICU setting. Phlebotomy for diagnostic tests has also been implicated: it is estimated that for every 100 mL of blood drawn, there is an associated decrease in hemoglobin of 0.7 g/dL and in hematocrit of 1.9%. Even with a conservative measurement of blood loss of 100 mL/d from phlebotomy, the impact is significant, especially in the patient who is hospitalized for several weeks in the ICU.

In addition to blood loss, disseminated intravascular coagulation (DIC) and a variety of hemolytic disorders can decrease the survival of RBCs, causing anemia in the critically ill. Nutritional deficiencies, inflammation, and sepsis contribute to anemia as well.

A brief review of the different types of anemia follows. Because the workup and treatment of many of these anemias does not take place in the critical care setting, the discussion is limited and specific to anemia in the critically ill.

### Blood Loss Anemia

Blood loss anemia is probably the most common anemia requiring admission of the patient to the ICU. Blood loss should always be ruled out in any acute anemia. The primary focus of patient management is to identify and treat the underlying source of blood loss.

Stress gastritis can be the source of significant blood loss. This complication is easier to prevent than it is to treat. All critically ill patients should be considered at risk, and prophylactic therapy with $H_2$-blockers or proton-pump inhibitors should be initiated; sucralfate is a secondary option. Endoscopy may be performed to evaluate for a gastrointestinal source of blood loss.

### Hemolytic Anemias

Hemolytic anemias result from the destruction of RBCs. They may be congenital or acquired, and can vary greatly in severity.

**CONGENITAL HEMOLYTIC ANEMIA.** The most common types of congenital hemolytic anemias are caused by enzyme defects or RBC membrane defects (Table 49-2). Most congenital RBC enzymatic deficiencies are glucose-6-phosphate dehydrogenase (G6PD) and pyruvate kinase deficiencies. Enzyme defects cause the RBCs to lyse when exposed to certain stressful conditions, such as drugs, chemicals, infections, surgery, or pregnancy. Substances to which people with G6PD deficiency may be susceptible are listed in Box 49-1.

**ACQUIRED HEMOLYTIC ANEMIA.** Acquired hemolytic anemias can have a number of causes (Table 49-3). In microangiopathic hemolytic anemia, RBCs are fragmented by vasculitis, collagen vascular disease, abnormal cardiac valves, arteriovenous (AV) malformations, thrombotic

| TABLE 49-2 | Congenital Hemolytic Anemias and Primary Interventions |
|---|---|
| **Type of Defect** | **Primary Interventions** |
| **Enzyme Defects** | |
| G6PD | Avoidance of agents that trigger hemolysis; hydration |
| Pyruvate kinase deficiency | Transfusion; splenectomy |
| **Red Blood Cell Membrane Defects** | |
| Hereditary spherocytosis | Splenectomy; folic acid supplements |
| Hereditary elliptocytosis | Usually no treatment required; folic acid supplements |
| Paroxysmal nocturnal hemoglobinuria | Corticosteroids, androgens, recombinant erythropoietin, iron therapy; transfusion as needed; anticoagulation therapy if thrombotic events; possible bone marrow transplantation |

## BOX 49-1 Substances That May Cause Hemolytic Anemia in Susceptible Individuals

**Congenital Hemolytic Anemia***

Norfloxacin
Methylene blue
Chloramphenicol
Nitrofurantoin
Sulfa drugs
Mothballs
Fava beans (Mediterranean variant of G6PD deficiency)

**Acquired Hemolytic Anemia**

Wasp and bee stings
Spider and snake bites
Copper and lead
Antineoplastic drugs, including mitomycin and cisplatin
Antimalarial drugs, primaquine and quinine
Quinidine
Methyldopa
Procainamide
NSAIDs
Penicillins
Cephalosporins

*G6PD deficiency.

### TABLE 49-3 Acquired Hemolytic Anemias and Potential Interventions

| Acquired Hemolytic Anemia | Interventions |
| --- | --- |
| **Microangiopathic** | Removal of causative factor; iron and folate supplements; transfusion |
| **Infectious agents** | Treatment of underlying infection; transfusion |
| **Liver disease** | Splenectomy; transfusion |
| **Autoimmune** | |
| *Warm antibody* | Glucocorticoids; splenectomy; immunosuppressive agents; transfusion |
| *Cold-reactive* | Avoidance of exposure to cold; transfusion; plasma exchange |
| *Drug-induced* | Discontinuation of drug; transfusion |

thrombocytopenic purpura (TTP), or DIC. Patients who experience hypothermia or cold cardioplegia with cardiac surgery may have RBCs with shortened life spans owing to membrane damage. Patients with RBCs recovered from the "cell saver" also experience significant membrane damage and hemolysis. Treatment focuses on removing the causative factor, such as replacing the abnormal heart valve or repairing the AV shunt. If this is not possible, the patient may be maintained on iron and folate supplements and periodic transfusions of RBCs.

Infectious agents may cause hemolytic anemia indirectly by causing splenomegaly or directly by invading the RBC and destroying its membrane. Malaria is an example of the latter. Patients are treated with transfusion support and anti-infective agents to address the underlying cause.

Abnormally shaped RBCs are frequently noticed in patients with liver disease. These patients may also have congestive splenomegaly, which causes sequestration and destruction of RBCs. In severe hemolysis, splenectomy and supportive RBC transfusions may be required.

Some patients can experience autoimmune hemolytic anemias. Warm autoimmune hemolytic anemia is the most common of these types. Approximately one half of all cases are idiopathic; known causative factors include collagen diseases, lymphoproliferative disorders, and drug reactions (see Box 49-1). Primary therapy is oral glucocorticoids to suppress the immune system. Additional treatments for patients who do not respond to glucocorticoids may include splenectomy, immunosuppressive agents, and intravenous immunoglobulin (IVIG).

Cold-reactive autoimmune hemolytic anemia is a disorder in which exposure to cold triggers complement-fixing immunoglobulin M antibodies to attach to RBCs in susceptible people, causing agglutination (clumping) and hemolysis (destruction). Often, these patients have an underlying lymphoproliferative disorder; others may have *Mycoplasma pneumoniae* infection, infectious mononucleosis, or hepatitis. If these patients require blood transfusion, use of a blood warmer and measures to keep the patient warm are recommended. Steroids and splenectomy are ineffective; intervention focuses on avoiding exposure to cold.

### Deficiency Anemias

Deficiency anemias include iron deficiency anemia, megaloblastic anemia, anemia of chronic disease, and aplastic anemia. Table 49-4 lists common interventions for these anemias.

**IRON DEFICIENCY ANEMIA.** Iron deficiency is the most common cause of anemia in adults. It is usually caused by chronic blood loss, but it may be due to inadequate iron intake or absorption. It is imperative in chronic blood loss to search for the underlying cause and correct it.

**MEGALOBLASTIC ANEMIAS.** Megaloblastic anemias are a group of anemias, most of which are caused by a deficiency of vitamin $B_{12}$ (cobalamin), folate, or both. Treatment entails correcting the deficiency.

Vitamin $B_{12}$ is poorly absorbed from the gut; therefore, intramuscular or subcutaneous injection is required. Most patients require maintenance injections monthly for the remainder of their lives. Body stores of folate can be restored with an oral folate supplement given daily for approximately 4 weeks. Once the deficiency is corrected, maintenance therapy is rarely necessary unless underlying factors, such as chronic alcoholism, are present.

### TABLE 49-4 Common Deficiency Anemias and Primary Interventions

| Type of Anemia | Primary Interventions |
| --- | --- |
| Iron deficiency anemia | Iron supplements; correction of underlying stressor |
| Megaloblastic anemia | Vitamin $B_{12}$ replacement; folic acid supplement |
| Anemia of chronic disease | Transfusion; recombinant erythropoietin; correction of underlying disorder |
| Aplastic anemia | Transfusion; immunosuppression; bone marrow transplantation |

**ANEMIA OF CHRONIC DISEASE.** Finally, anemia is seen with a number of chronic disorders, such as renal failure, infections, malignancies, and connective tissue diseases including rheumatoid arthritis. Anemia of chronic renal failure generally occurs when the creatinine clearance is less than 45 mL/min, and continues to worsen with increasing renal failure. Several mechanisms cause anemia of chronic disease, including suppression of RBC production, decreased RBC survival time, and low serum erythropoietin levels. Aspects of anemia in older patients are presented in Box 49-2. Treatment involves correcting the underlying cause, if possible. Transfusion may be of temporary benefit, although the survival of the transfused RBCs is reduced. Erythropoiesis-stimulating agents (ESAs) may be the treatment of choice for many people. ESAs are typically given intravenously or subcutaneously one to three times a week, with adjustments based on response.

**APLASTIC ANEMIA.** In aplastic anemia, there is deficiency of RBCs as well as WBCs and platelets; in other words, aplastic anemia is a condition of pancytopenia. In many cases, the cause of aplastic anemia is unknown. Possible factors include drugs, chemicals, viruses, and immunologic and congenital disorders (Box 49-3). In some patients, aplastic anemia is thought to result from replacement of normal cells by clones of cells that are incapable of normal hematopoiesis. Clinical features of aplastic anemia are related to the underlying pancytopenia and include anemia, infections, and bleeding.

Severe aplastic anemia is treated with transfusion support, immunosuppressive agents, and bone marrow transplantation. Drugs that stimulate bone marrow function are of no benefit in this condition. Bone marrow transplantation should be considered for patients younger than age 60. These patients should be considered for immediate transplantation and should not receive any transfusions or drug therapy before transplantation, if possible. Immunosuppressive therapy may be of benefit for older patients or those without a compatible donor for bone marrow transplantation.

## Assessment

The history of the patient with anemia includes assessment of blood loss as well as a thorough diet history. General symptoms of anemia include weakness, depressed mood, impaired cognitive function, and easy fatigability. Signs and symptoms indicative of decreased perfusion secondary to anemia are tachycardia, chest pain, dyspnea, and dizziness. Clinical consequences of anemia are impaired tissue oxygenation, impaired organ function, impaired susceptibility to thrombocytopenic bleeding, increased risk of postoperative mortality, increased probability of transfusion, and decreased survival.[1] Anemia in critically ill patients is similar in clinical presentation to the anemia of chronic disease, both of which lead to underproduction of RBCs.

Physical examination findings of anemia include pallor, tachycardia, hypotension, and signs of high-output heart failure. Patients with hemolytic anemia may have splenomegaly, jaundice, and dark urine owing to the excretion of bilirubin. It is necessary to review the intake and output records for fluid balance because hemodilution is common, particularly in the postoperative patient, due to aggressive intravenous hydration. All patients should have a stool guaiac test performed to look for occult gastrointestinal blood loss.

Typically, critically ill patients have low serum iron and total iron-binding capacity with elevated serum ferritin. While serum erythropoietin levels are mildly elevated, the concentration is inappropriately low for the severity of the anemia. The inflammatory response complicates the interpretation of iron studies in critical illness. Further laboratory assessment to evaluate anemia is discussed in Chapter 46.

## Management

The treatment of anemia starts with identifying the underlying cause. Iron supplementation may be indicated if there is clear evidence of iron deficiency. Iron sulfate, 325 mg by mouth two to three times per day, may be indicated. Parenteral iron may be administered when the patient is unable to take oral medications, or in the case of malabsorption or severe renal failure. Intramuscular iron injection may be painful and stain the patient's skin. Instead, intravenous injection is recommended. Close patient observation is necessary because severe anaphylactic reactions may occur with iron dextran (Box 49-4). Parenteral iron sucrose also has potential for anaphylactic reactions, but does not carry the same black box warning.

**BLOOD TRANSFUSION.** Critically ill patients differ in their age, diagnosis, comorbidities, and severity of illness.

---

**BOX 49-2** *CONSIDERATIONS for the Older Patient*

**Anemia**

Anemia is common in the elderly, and its prevalence increases with age. As with other cells, the body's capacity for red cell replacement decreases with aging, typically with a greater decline seen in men than women. Although most elderly people are able to maintain their hemoglobin and hematocrit levels within a normal range, they are unable to replace their red cells as promptly in situations such as bleeding.

In the elderly, anemia is usually the result of bleeding, infection, malignancy, or chronic disease. Combined deficiencies are common in older adults. Undiagnosed and untreated anemia is associated with decreased functional and self-care abilities and depression. It can also cause neurologic and cognitive disorders, cardiovascular complications, and increased risk for mortality. Orally administered iron is poorly used in older adults.

---

**BOX 49-3** **Causative Factors in Aplastic Anemia**

**Congenital (20% of Cases)**
Fanconi anemia
Familial aplastic anemia

**Acquired (80% of Cases)**
Idiopathic
Irradiation
Drugs: chloramphenicol, carbamazepine, sulfonamides, cimetidine, gold salts, acetazolamide
Chemicals: benzene and benzene derivatives, insecticides, cleaning solvents
Infections: non-A, non-B hepatitis, Epstein–Barr virus, HIV, mycobacteria
Immunologic: graft-versus-host disease, systemic lupus erythematosus
Pregnancy

**QSEN** **BOX 49-4**   *PATIENT SAFETY*

### Parenteral Administration of Iron Dextran

- Anaphylactic reactions, including fatalities, have followed the parenteral administration of iron dextran injection
- Have resuscitation equipment and personnel trained in the detection and treatment of anaphylactic reactions readily available
- Administer a test dose prior to the first therapeutic dose. Fatal reactions have followed the test dose and in situations where the test dose was tolerated

From U.S. Food and Drug Administration, U.S. Department of Health & Human Services: Dexferrum (Iron dextran injection)—Labeling Change. 2013. Retrieved January 5, 2015, from http://www.fda.gov/Safety/MedWatch /SafetyInformation/SafetyAlertsforHumanMedicalProducts/ucm186899.htm.

The risk versus benefit of blood transfusion in the critically ill patient is influenced by these factors and the patient's tolerance of anemia. In the past, hemoglobin transfusion triggers varied between 7 and 10 g/dL, most often between 8 and 9 g/dL. However, this practice has changed because of a number of factors associated with worse clinical outcomes occurring in patients receiving blood transfusions.[1]

**Therapeutic Considerations.** Currently, it is believed that transfusion of packed RBCs should be reserved for management of severe, active bleeding and for the patient who is experiencing serious symptoms from anemia. In other words, the practice should be to transfuse when the risks of decreased oxygen-carrying capacity outweigh the risks of transfusion, rather than relying on a specific hemoglobin or hematocrit trigger. The American College of Physicians has developed clinical guideline for the treatment of anemia in patients with heart disease, including transfusion decisions in specific critical care populations; see http://annals.org /article.aspx?articleid=1784292.

The normal compensatory mechanisms in response to the decreased oxygen supply in anemia (increased heart rate, increased cardiac output and index, decreased systemic vascular resistance) may not work efficiently or at all in critically ill patients. This deficit in compensatory mechanisms is particularly relevant in patients with cardiac disease and in those at high risk for myocardial infarction. For example, a patient with coronary stenosis may not have the normal response of vasodilation as a compensatory mechanism to the anemia. Likewise, increased cardiac output may not be achievable in patients with cardiomyopathy or pulmonary edema. In patients with sepsis, there is a general move toward less frequent use of RBC transfusions, with guidelines recommending transfusions only for a hemoglobin level of less than 7 g/dL in adults.[2,3]

**Complications.** Complications of blood transfusion may be noninfectious, infectious, or immunologic. Unfortunately, preventable fatal hemolytic reactions result from transfusion of ABO-incompatible blood. Signs and symptoms of acute transfusion reactions are listed in Box 49-5.

In critically ill patients, transfusion-related acute lung injury (TRALI) and transfusion-associated circulatory overload (TACO) are relevant complications. Both TRALI and TACO resemble acute respiratory distress syndrome (ARDS) with dyspnea, hypoxia, tachycardia, and noncardiogenic pulmonary edema; however, with TACO there is also evidence

**BOX 49-5**   **Signs and Symptoms of Acute Transfusion Reactions**

- Fever, chills/rigors, myalgia
- Urticaria (hives), rash, pruritus
- Angioedema (may be preceded by tingling)
- Dyspnea, stridor, wheeze, hypoxia
- Hypotension
- Severe anxiety or "feeling of impending doom"

of volume overload. Medical comorbidities that increase the risk of TACO include heart failure and renal impairment.

Viral screening of blood products and careful selection of donors have certainly decreased the risk for transfusion transmission of viruses, such as human immunodeficiency virus (HIV) and hepatitis C. However, there is still a risk posed by donors who donate during the infectious period before seroconversion occurs. In addition, blood screening methods do not exclude infectious agents such as hepatitis A virus, human parvovirus B19, cytomegalovirus (CMV), malaria, and disease-causing bacteria.

Exposure to the donor's leukocytes in transfusion may trigger an immune system response. Potential adverse outcomes include exacerbation of infections, earlier recurrence of malignancy, impaired wound healing and other postoperative complications, and increased likelihood of mortality.

To avoid some of these complications, consideration may be given to leukoreduced blood transfusion for critically ill patients. Leukoreduction is the process of removing WBCs from the blood product by filtration. Leukoreduced blood is less likely to cause antibodies to develop against specific blood types and less likely to cause febrile transfusion reactions. Also, leukoreduced blood greatly reduces the chance of CMV transmission.

**ERYTHROPOIESIS-STIMULATING AGENTS.** Administration of ESAs, such as epoetin and darbepoetin, in anemic critically ill patients is not recommended until clinical trials can demonstrate safety and efficacy data. These therapies can increase the risk of deep vein thrombosis.

### Nursing Care of the Patient With Anemia

Nursing interventions in all anemias support treatment protocols and measures to identify the underlying cause. Other important actions include assessing for adverse effects of replacement therapy and for signs and symptoms indicative of decreased perfusion. If transfusion therapy is prescribed, vigilance in identifying the correct patient and ensuring ABO compatibility is of utmost importance to prevent adverse and potentially fatal outcomes. Attention to the rate of infusion, administration of diuretics, and careful monitoring of fluid balance can reduce the risk of volume overload. In addition, measures to decrease metabolic needs and reduce oxygen demand should be instituted, including promotion of a restful environment, adequate pain control, and minimization of agitation. Supplemental oxygen may be needed to assist in maintaining adequate oxygen supply to the tissues.

Critical care nurses are in an ideal position to identify when phlebotomy appears excessive or unnecessary and to question the clinical justification for testing. Strategies to reduce phlebotomy blood loss should be instituted. These include eliminating standing orders for laboratory tests, organizing blood draws to eliminate duplicate testing, consolidating multiple collections, using smaller collection tubes, and using devices that return waste blood to the patient. The frequency of arterial blood gas collection can often be decreased by using noninvasive monitoring techniques, such as pulse oximetry and capnography.

## Sickle Cell Disease

### Pathophysiology

Sickle cell disease (SCD) is a chronic hereditary hemolytic anemia that occurs almost exclusively in people of African or African-Caribbean origin; however, a variety of other ethnic groups can be affected. The sickle cell gene results in abnormal hemoglobin, usually hemoglobin S (HbS). When oxygen and pH levels fall, HbS RBCs become elongated, sickle or crescent shaped, and rigid. These sickled cells are unable to pass through small blood vessels, causing inflammation, obstruction of the vessels, and decreased delivery of oxygen that perpetuates the cycle with more sickling. The cells are hemolyzed or destroyed when the body recognizes their abnormal structure.

### Clinical Presentation

The most common clinical picture in SCD is painful vaso-occlusive crisis. The crisis begins suddenly, sometimes as a consequence of infection or a change in temperature or for no identifiable reason. Severe deep pain is present in the long bones of the extremities. Sometimes the abdomen is affected by severe pain resembling an acute abdomen. The pain may be accompanied by fever, malaise, and leukocytosis.

SCD also results in organ damage with microinfarctions of the heart, skeleton, spleen, and central nervous system (CNS). Repeated splenic infarctions result in splenic failure, predisposing the patient to overwhelming infection, especially Gram-negative sepsis. Other manifestations of SCD that may be seen in the critical care patient are stroke, cardiac chamber enlargement, pulmonary hypertension, renal failure, and chronic leg ulcers.

Acute chest syndrome is caused by pulmonary infarction from fat embolism; bacterial infections likely contribute to its development as well. Symptoms include chest pain, fever, tachypnea, leukocytosis, and pulmonary infiltrates. Acute chest syndrome is a medical emergency, and if not treated properly, complications such as ARDS may develop.

### Management

Treatment of sickle cell crisis includes aggressive intravenous fluid hydration to decrease blood viscosity and maintain renal perfusion. The patient must be evaluated for infection, and if this is suspected, prompt treatment with broad-spectrum antibiotics is instituted until the causative organism is identified and the therapy can be tailored to the patient's needs. Oxygen administration may be needed to maintain adequate tissue perfusion. RBC transfusions are not usually required. Patients with SCD take folic acid supplementation and may take hydroxyurea, which helps prevent sickling.

The pain experienced by patients in sickle cell crisis is intense. Patients typically require around-the-clock dosing with a strong narcotic. Time-release narcotics and patient-controlled analgesia are two methods of delivering steady doses of pain medication. In addition to an opioid, nonsteroidal anti-inflammatory drugs (NSAIDs) may be given if not contraindicated. Patients with sickle cell crisis may not display overt signs of pain; this is typical for patients who experience chronic pain. The patient's report of pain, as well as clinical indicators, should be used in assessing pain.

Nursing care of the patient with sickle cell crisis includes close monitoring for response to interventions to promote tissue perfusion, treat infection, and effectively manage pain. A multidisciplinary approach may include input from pain management experts, social workers, psychiatrists, physical and occupational therapists, and infectious disease specialists.

## Disorders of White Blood Cells

### Leukopenia

Leukopenia refers to an abnormally low number of WBCs. The most common type of WBC deficiency is neutropenia, defined as a neutrophil count of less than 1,500 cells/mm³. Severe neutropenia, in which the neutrophil count is less than 200 cells/mm³, is referred to as agranulocytosis. Neutropenia can be seen as a result of a wide variety of conditions (Table 49-5). Leukopenia is most commonly drug related.

### Clinical Presentation

Because the neutrophil is essential to defense against bacterial and fungal infections, patients with neutropenia are susceptible to overwhelming infection and life-threatening sepsis. The risk of infection is related to the severity of the neutropenia. Untreated infections can be rapidly fatal, particularly if the neutrophil count is less than 250/mm³. In severe neutropenia, the usual signs of the inflammatory response to infection may be absent.

Neutrophils provide the first line of defense against organisms that inhabit the skin and gastrointestinal tract. Thus, skin infections and ulcerative lesions of the mouth are common infections in the neutropenic patient. The most frequent site of serious infection is the respiratory tract, a result of bacteria or fungi that frequently colonize the airways.

### Assessment

The history should include presence of viral infection or autoimmune disease. A thorough medication history, including over-the-counter preparations, should be obtained. Patients with neutropenia may present with mouth ulcers, fever, shaking chills, and systemic infection. Physical examination may reveal splenomegaly.

The presence of abnormal RBCs or WBCs suggests a primary bone marrow process. Laboratory studies should include viral serology for hepatitis and HIV as well as antinuclear antibody (ANA). Bone marrow aspiration and biopsy may be needed if the neutropenia is severe or the cause is not apparent.

### Management

Neutropenia is treated by removing or managing the underlying cause if known. If the patient is febrile, appropriate cultures and a chest radiograph should be obtained, followed

**TABLE 49-5  Causes of Neutropenia**

| Cause | Mechanism |
|---|---|
| Accelerated removal (eg, inflammation and infection) Drug-induced granulocytopenia | Removal of neutrophils from the circulation exceeds production |
| • Cytotoxic drugs used in cancer therapy | Depressed bone marrow function with decreased production of all blood cells |
| • Phenothiazines, propylthiouracil, and others | Toxic effect on bone marrow precursors |
| • Aminopyrine, certain sulfonamides, phenylbutazone, and others | Immune-mediated destruction |
| Periodic or cyclic neutropenia (occurs during infancy and later) | Unknown |
| Neoplasms involving bone marrow (eg, leukemias and lymphomas) | Overgrowth of neoplastic cells, which crowd out granulopoietic precursors |
| Idiopathic neutropenia that occurs in the absence of other disease or provoking influence | Autoimmune reaction |
| Felty syndrome | Intrasplenic destruction of neutrophils |

From Porth CM: Essentials of Pathophysiology, 2nd ed. Philadelphia, PA: Lippincott Williams & Wilkins, 2007, p 183.

by immediate broad-spectrum intravenous antibiotic therapy to prevent progression to septic shock and death. Signs and symptoms of infection without fever should also prompt administration of antibiotics in patients with neutropenia. If evidence of infection persists despite adequate antibiotic therapy, antifungal agents may be added to provide coverage for potential *Candida* or *Aspergillus* infections.

If the neutropenia is severe, treatment may include a hematopoietic growth factor (filgrastim, pegfilgrastim, or sargramostim) that stimulates bone marrow production of new neutrophils and enhances the activity of already circulating neutrophils. Additionally, patients with severe neutropenia or those with recurrent or serious infections may benefit from steroids. IVIG may improve the neutrophil count. Transfusions are used cautiously in patients who may require bone marrow transplantation.

## Neoplastic Disorders

Neoplastic disorders are characterized by new and abnormal growth of cells that may be benign or malignant. The clinical features of neoplastic disorders are determined largely by their site of origin. Lymphoproliferative disorders (disorders in which lymphoid tissue increases by reproducing) may originate in the bone marrow or in the lymph nodes and thymus. Leukemias and multiple myeloma are lymphoproliferative disorders of the bone marrow; lymphomas are lymphoproliferative disorders of the lymph nodes. Because blood cells circulate throughout the body, these neoplasms are systemically disseminated from the onset.

### Lymphoma

**HODGKIN LYMPHOMA.** Hodgkin lymphoma is a cancer of the lymphatic system, beginning as a malignancy in a single lymph node and then spreading to surrounding lymph nodes. A diagnosis of Hodgkin disease is confirmed by the presence of abnormal Reed–Sternberg cells in biopsied tissue.

**NON-HODGKIN LYMPHOMA.** Non-Hodgkin lymphoma (NHL) is a diverse group of malignancies that originate in the lymphoid cells. NHL can occur as a discrete mass, such as in a single lymph node, or as a widespread disease that affects multiple organ systems, including the bone marrow.

**CLINICAL PRESENTATION.** Symptoms of both types of lymphoma are related to the body area affected by the abnormal lymphoid cells. Constitutional symptoms include fever, fatigue, and weight loss. In the advanced stages, patients may have extensive chest disease and experience increasingly severe dyspnea. Bulky chest disease can cause superior vena cava syndrome. Abdominal disease can cause obstruction of the bowel or the ureters. Bone marrow involvement can lead to decreased production of RBCs, WBCs, and platelets. Extensive involvement of the lymphatic system can lead to impaired immune function and frequent, severe infections. Lymphoma of the CNS can cause headaches, visual disturbances, motor dysfunction, and increased intracranial pressure.

**MANAGEMENT.** The diagnosis, staging, and treatment of lymphomas are typically performed entirely on an outpatient basis. However, the critical care nurse may encounter the patient with lymphoma when complications arise from the disease or its treatment. Oncologic complications and their management are discussed in detail in Chapters 47 and 48.

### Leukemia

The leukemias are hematologic malignancies that affect the bone marrow and the lymph tissues. They are characterized by proliferation of hematopoietic stem cells, resulting in the accumulation of abnormal (leukemic) cells in the bone marrow and a decreased production of normal blood cells. These abnormal leukemic cells circulate in the bloodstream and infiltrate many body organs. Leukemias are commonly classified according to their predominant cell type (lymphoblastic or myelogenous) and whether the condition is acute or chronic. The chronic leukemias are not discussed in this chapter.

**ACUTE LYMPHOBLASTIC LEUKEMIA.** Acute lymphoblastic leukemia (ALL) is a disorder in which a clone of immature lymphocytes proliferates and replaces the normal cells of the bone marrow. The leukemic clones proliferate and infiltrate other normal tissues, such as the liver, spleen, and lymph nodes. Anemia, thrombocytopenia, and granulocytopenia are common. The spleen, liver, thymus, and lymph nodes are usually enlarged.

**ACUTE MYELOGENOUS LEUKEMIA.** A malignant disorder of hematopoietic stem cells, acute myelogenous leukemia (AML) causes abnormal production of the myeloid cell lines (erythrocyte, neutrophil, megakaryocyte, and macrophage). The malignant clones proliferate but do not differentiate into mature, functional cells. The blood, bone marrow, or both contain more than 30% immature blast cells. The proliferation of immature cells and bone marrow infiltration results in anemia, neutropenia, and thrombocytopenia. The patient's symptoms are related to these conditions. Splenomegaly is present in approximately one third of patients. Patients may require immediate interventions at the time of diagnosis for infections or anemia, or to achieve hemostasis.

**CLINICAL PRESENTATION.** Although ALL and AML are distinct disorders, they typically present with similar clinical features. These manifestations and their pathologic basis are summarized in Table 49-6.

Patients with leukocyte counts greater than 100,000 cells/mm$^3$ are at risk for leukostasis, a condition in which the high number of blasts increase blood viscosity, develop leukoblastic emboli, and aggregate in the capillaries. Manifestations include headache, confusion, CNS infarctions, acute respiratory insufficiency, and pulmonary infiltrates.

**MANAGEMENT.** Leukostasis requires immediate treatment to lower the blast count rapidly. Treatment involves emergent leukapheresis (removal of WBCs from the circulation) along with hydroxyurea. Chemotherapy should be initiated to stop leukemic cell production in the bone marrow.

A comprehensive discussion of diagnosis and treatment of leukemia is beyond the scope of this text. As in the patient with lymphoma, the patient with leukemia will typically be seen in the critical care unit as a result of complications of the disorder or its treatment. Refer to discussions of anemia, granulocytopenia, and thrombocytopenia in this chapter, as well as Chapters 47 and 48, for coverage of bone marrow or stem cell transplantation and oncologic emergencies.

## Nursing Care of the Patient With a White Blood Cell Disorder

The goals of nursing care of the patient with a WBC disorder are vigilant assessment for and prevention of infection, delivery of therapy, and management of disease and treatment-associated complications. Nursing interventions are guided by the treatment modality (eg, chemotherapy, radiation, bone marrow transplantation).

Meticulous attention to infection control procedures and vigilant surveillance of invasive therapeutic lines and equipment are mainstays of care. Attention must be paid during daily oral care to ensure that superinfection with *Candida* or herpesvirus has not developed. Antibacterial mouthwashes decrease the risk of infection. Severe mucositis may require opiates for pain control. Assessment for early indications of infection (eg, fever, chills, tachycardia, and tachypnea) may allow for prompt and aggressive initiation of pharmacologic therapies to reduce morbidity and mortality associated with infection in patients with WBC disorders.

Diarrhea may be a side effect of chemotherapy, neutropenia, or secondary causes. *Clostridium difficile* infection must be considered and treated if present. Digital rectal examinations should not be performed on neutropenic patients.

## Disorders of Hemostasis

Hemostasis is a finely balanced network of procoagulants (plasma coagulation factors and platelets) and anticoagulants. Hemostasis may be impaired by disruption of numerous interactions in the coagulation pathways or deficiencies or dysfunction in the required components for coagulation. Disorders of hemostasis include hypercoagulable states and bleeding disorders, whether from platelet defects (thrombocytopenia) or coagulation defects. Disorders of hemostasis are often seen in critically ill patients.[3]

## Platelet Disorders

Normally, approximately two thirds of platelets are circulating in the blood, and one third are sequestered or stored in the spleen. The life span of circulating platelets is 7 to 10 days. Thrombocytopenia occurs when there is decreased production or increased destruction of platelets or increased sequestration of platelets in the spleen. Common causes of thrombocytopenia are listed in Box 49-6. The most common causes seen in critical care patients are discussed here.

---

**TABLE 49-6** Clinical Manifestations of Acute Leukemia and Their Pathologic Basis

| Clinical Manifestations* | Pathologic Basis |
|---|---|
| Bone marrow depression | |
| Malaise, easy fatigability | Anemia |
| Fever | Infection or increased metabolism by neoplastic cells |
| Bleeding (petechiae, ecchymosis, gingival bleeding, epistaxis) | Decreased thrombocytes |
| Bone pain and tenderness upon palpation | Subperiosteal bone infiltration, bone marrow expansion, and bone resorption |
| Headache, nausea, vomiting, papilledema, cranial nerve palsies, seizures, coma | Leukemic infiltration of CNS |
| Abdominal discomfort | Generalized lymphadenopathy, hepatomegaly, splenomegaly due to leukemic cell infiltration |
| Increased vulnerability to infections | Immaturity of the white cells and ineffective immune function |
| Hematologic abnormalities: anemia, thrombocytopenia | Physical and metabolic encroachment of leukemia cells on RBC and thrombocyte precursors |
| Hyperuricemia and other metabolic disorders | Abnormal proliferation and metabolism of leukemic cells |

*Manifestations vary with the type of leukemia.
From Porth CM: Essentials of Pathophysiology, 2nd ed. Philadelphia, PA: Lippincott Williams & Wilkins, 2007, p 189.

| BOX 49-6 | Causes of Thrombocytopenia |
|---|---|
| **Decreased Platelet Production** | |
| Malignancy | Severe iron deficiency |
| Myelofibrosis | Infection (HIV, Hepatitis C, TB) |
| Chemotherapy | Alcohol use |
| Aplastic anemia | Folate, vitamin $B_{12}$ deficiency |
| **Splenic Sequestration of Platelets** | |
| Splenic enlargement | Splenic congestion |
| Tumor infiltration | Portal hypertension or liver disease |
| Infection | |
| **Increased Destruction of Platelets** | |
| Vascular prostheses, cardiopulmonary bypass | Autoimmune (antiphospholipid syndrome, systemic lupus erythematous) |
| Disseminated intravascular coagulation (DIC) | Immunodeficiencies |
| Sepsis | Drug-associated* |
| Vasculitis | Posttransfusion |
| Thrombotic thrombocytopenic purpura (TTP) | |
| Primary immune thrombocytopenia | |

*One of the most common causes of thrombocytopenia.

## Drug-Induced Thrombocytopenia

Thrombocytopenia in hospitalized patients is most commonly drug induced. The confirmation of this diagnosis occurs when the thrombocytopenia resolves after withdrawal of the causal medication. Medications commonly associated with thrombocytopenia include antineoplastic agents, heparin, histamine$_2$-blockers, trimethoprim-sulfamethoxazole, rifampin, vancomycin, amiodarone, and valproic acid.

### HEPARIN-INDUCED THROMBOCYTOPENIA.

After antineoplastic agents, heparin is the next most common drug associated with thrombocytopenia. Heparin-induced thrombocytopenia (HIT) is interesting in that thrombosis, rather than bleeding, may accompany the low platelet count. HIT places patients at risk for deep venous thrombosis, arterial occlusion, ischemic stroke, limb gangrene, myocardial infarction, and pulmonary embolism.

It is important to be aware that subcutaneous unfractionated heparin (UFH) or low-molecular-weight heparin (LMWH) delivered at treatment or prophylaxis dosing, by arterial or venous line flushes, through heparin-coated catheters, and intermittent heparin administered during dialysis may lead to HIT. Although HIT typically occurs 4 to 14 days after initiation of heparin therapy, it can occur as early as 10 hours after administration if the patient has been exposed to heparin within the previous 100 days. For patients who are starting heparin therapy, whether UFH or LMWH, the recommendation is to obtain a baseline platelet count and then repeat a platelet count within 24 hours of starting heparin. Clinical guidelines also suggest platelet count monitoring at least every 2 or 3 days up to 14 days, or until heparin therapy is stopped (whichever comes first).[4]

The hallmark of HIT is a decrease in platelet count to less than 50% of baseline or to fewer than 150,000/mm$^3$, or the occurrence of an unexplained thromboembolic event. Blood testing should be done for HIT antibodies.

For patients with confirmed or strongly suspected HIT, whether or not complicated by thrombosis, national guidelines recommend stopping heparin and using a non-heparin anticoagulant (eg, lepirudin, argatroban, fondaparinux, or bivalirudin).[4] Even if there is no clinical evidence of deep vein thrombosis, ultrasonography of the leg veins should be performed. Warfarin therapy should not be started until after the platelet count has substantially recovered, usually to at least 100,000/mm$^3$. Non-heparin anticoagulant should be continued until the platelet count has reached a stable plateau. Platelets are generally not transfused unless the patient is actively bleeding.

## Thrombotic Thrombocytopenic Purpura

TTP is an acute disorder with a mortality rate of 30% to 40%. Patients with TTP have absent or decreased levels of platelet-aggregating factor inhibitor, which is normally present in plasma. As a result, platelets become sensitized and clump in blood vessels, causing occlusion.

Five classic findings suggest TTP. Not every patient exhibits all five findings; however, the first two of the following must be present for the diagnosis to be considered:

- Thrombocytopenia and bleeding from increased consumption of platelets
- Microangiopathic hemolytic anemia from rupture of RBCs as they try to pass through partially occluded blood vessels
- Fever, possibly from hemolysis or vascular infarction of the hypothalamus
- Neurologic abnormalities, including fluctuating neurologic abnormalities, transient ischemic attacks, strokes, seizures, and coma from interrupted blood flow to the brain
- Renal dysfunction caused by obstruction of intraglomerular capillaries and infarction of the renal cortex.

Clinical features of TTP are described further in Table 49-7. Initiation of the disease process may be related to endothelial damage, autoimmune disorders, viral and bacterial infections, toxic agents, and genetic predisposition.

## Immune Thrombocytopenic Purpura

Immune thrombocytopenic purpura (ITP) is an immune-mediated disorder of platelet destruction. There are two

**TABLE 49-7   Clinical Manifestations of Thrombotic Thrombocytopenic Purpura**

| Abnormality | Findings |
|---|---|
| Thrombocytopenia | Epistaxis, gingival bleeding, ecchymosis, purpura, hematuria |
| Hemolytic anemia | Schistocytes, reticulocytosis, elevated serum lactate dehydrogenase and bilirubin, jaundice, pallor, weakness |
| Neurologic abnormalities | Headache, mental changes, confusion, visual problems, seizures, coma, aphasia, dysphasia, paresthesias |
| Renal dysfunction | Proteinuria, microscopic hematuria, elevated blood urea nitrogen and creatinine, renal failure |
| Fever | Persistent elevation of temperature during acute phase |
| Other | Abdominal pain, malaise, nausea, vomiting, weakness, chest pain |

distinct forms of ITP. Acute ITP typically occurs in childhood and may resolve spontaneously in several weeks. Autoimmune platelet destruction appears to be stimulated after a viral illness, even mild infections. Chronic ITP usually occurs in adults, more often in women than men. The platelet membrane is coated with an autoantibody (usually IgG), and the sensitized platelets are destroyed in the spleen and liver; therefore, platelet survival in the circulation is decreased. In at least 50% of patients with ITP, no known causative agent is identified; other patients may have underlying autoimmune, rheumatic, or lymphoproliferative diseases or HIV infection. A bone marrow examination is not necessary irrespective of age in patients presenting with typical ITP.[5]

### Assessment

The history, physical examination, and initial laboratory data help differentiate between the mechanisms of thrombocytopenia.

The patient history includes assessment of symptoms associated with any of the risk factors or associated disorders (see Table 49-7). A patient or family history of bleeding may help differentiate acquired and congenital disorders. Critical to the assessment is a medication and alcohol history. Fatigue, fever, weight loss, or night sweats may be associated with infection or malignancy. It is important to note a history of platelet transfusion.

The physical examination includes a thorough inspection of the skin for petechiae and bruising. It is important to also include the oropharynx as well as checking the stool for guaiac. Hypotension, tachycardia, and fever are suggestive of sepsis. A fever is also frequently present in TTP. An enlarged spleen suggests splenic sequestration of trapped blood from portal hypertension. In this setting, patients are likely to exhibit signs of liver disease, including jaundice, ascites, and extremity muscle wasting.

Laboratory examination is also significant. Signs and symptoms of low platelets vary depending on the platelet count. Platelet counts greater than 100,000/mm³ should result in normal hemostasis. Platelet counts less than 50,000/mm³ may lead to prolonged bleeding after procedures, easy bruising, and bleeding from the oral or gastrointestinal mucosa. Platelet counts less than 20,000/mm³ are associated with an exponential increase in the risk for bleeding. The nurse carefully assesses the patient for petechial rash or spontaneous bleeding such as epistaxis or bleeding gums. Platelet counts of less than 10,000/mm³ are associated with possible intracranial hemorrhage.

The complete blood count with differential is the most important first step in identifying the etiology of thrombocytopenia. It is important to check for accompanying anemia and leukopenia. If pancytopenia is present, bone marrow failure may be the cause of the problem; if this is suspected, a bone marrow biopsy may be performed. The presence of schistocytes on the differential may indicate TTP or DIC.

It is important to rule out artifactual thrombocytopenia caused by clumping of the platelets in a test tube containing ethylenediamine tetraacetic acid (lavender top). A report of platelet clumping should raise this suspicion. If the platelets are clumped, the automatic counter may inaccurately measure the number of platelets, resulting in a falsely low count; in this case, the sample should be redrawn in a citrate tube (blue top) or heparinized tube (green top).

Bleeding time is a test of platelet function. When the platelet count drops below 50,000/mm³, the bleeding time is significantly prolonged and is not useful. The bleeding time is a helpful test when a patient has mucosal bleeding but a normal platelet count. Evaluating prothrombin time (PT), partial thromboplastin time (PTT), and fibrin degradation products (FDPs) may help identify DIC and distinguish a hemolytic anemia from TTP. Additional studies that may be ordered to assist in determining the underlying etiology include HIV, HCV, and ANA screening as well as liver function tests.

### Management

The initial step in management of thrombocytopenia is to review the patient's medication list, placing on hold any drugs that may be suspected to induce thrombocytopenia. In addition, medications that inhibit platelet function should be avoided, including aspirin, antiplatelet agents, and NSAIDs. Avoidance of trauma is essential, and may even preclude the placement of central venous catheters and other invasive procedures. Evaluation of continued blood loss and assessment of daily laboratory data for adequacy of the platelet count and other parameters of hemostasis are important measures.

Patients with mild to moderate thrombocytopenia without bleeding require no treatment. Platelet transfusions are indicated when the platelet count is below 20,000 to 30,000/mm³ or in the case of spontaneous bleeding. A single donor unit of platelets is equivalent to six random donor platelets and should increase the platelet count by 30,000/mm³. The patient must be monitored for allergic reactions, anaphylaxis, and volume overload.

In sequestration or destruction-mediated thrombocytopenia, the response to platelet transfusion is typically very poor. Transfused platelets are destroyed very quickly by the same mechanism that causes the disease. Platelet transfusion should be used only for major life-threatening bleeding. In these patients, because the platelets may not last long, platelets need to be administered shortly before performing any invasive procedures.

TTP is an emergency because of its extremely high mortality rate. Early recognition and prompt initiation of treatment are imperative to improve patient survival. Acutely ill patients require plasma exchange in which plasmapheresis is used to remove 2 to 3 L of the patient's plasma, with an equal amount of fresh plasma given as replacement. Plasmapheresis is initiated as quickly as possible and repeated daily until the platelet count is greater than 150,000/mm³; this may take 5 to 10 days or more. Plasma exchange is superior to simple plasma infusion. However, because some patients do respond to simple plasma infusions, all patients should be infused immediately with fresh frozen plasma until plasma exchange can be arranged. Steroids are widely used in combination with plasmapheresis. Platelet transfusion is contraindicated even in severe thrombocytopenia because the transfused platelets may aggregate, resulting in myocardial infarction, stroke, coma, or death. Patients with TTP may be "cured," may relapse years later, or may have a chronic relapsing course.

Immunosuppression with corticosteroids is the initial therapy for ITP. With prednisone therapy it usually takes a few days before the count begins to rise. When the platelet count is critically low (5,000/mm³ or less) or the patient shows signs of serious bleeding, prednisone alone may not raise the platelet count rapidly enough. When a rapid increase in the platelet count is needed, IVIG, in addition to steroids, is highly successful. A typical treatment regimen is IVIG at 1 g/kg/d and prednisone 1 mg/kg/d. Patients with chronic ITP who fail to respond to steroids or are steroid dependent may require splenectomy. These patients should receive pneumococcal, meningococcal, and *Haemophilus influenzae* type B vaccines.

## Coagulation Disorders

Coagulation disorders can result from deficiencies or impairment of one or more of the clotting factors. These disorders of coagulation may be congenital or acquired. The most common congenital bleeding disorders are von Willebrand disease and hemophilia A. These disorders are caused by a deficiency in a specific factor. Numerous complications can occur as a result of these bleeding disorders (Table 49-8).

Management involves correcting the coagulation factor deficiency and treating sequelae that occur as a result of abnormal bleeding. Patients with mild hemophilia A and mild von Willebrand factor deficiency may respond to intravenous or nasal spray administration of desmopressin acetate, a hormone that temporarily stimulates the release of factor VIII to control bleeding. More severe cases of hemophilia A or active bleeding require intravenous infusion of factor VIII concentrate. More severe bleeding in von Willebrand

**TABLE 49-8** Complications in Coagulation Disorders

| Bleeding Site | Complication |
| --- | --- |
| Abdomen | Hypotension, hypovolemic shock |
| Muscle | Compartment syndrome |
| Joint | Hemarthrosis with destruction of bone and cartilage in joint capsule |
| Intracranial | Increased intracranial pressure |
| Retropharyngeal | Airway obstruction |
| Gastrointestinal | Anemia, melena |
| Urinary tract | Clots in ureters (especially after factor administration) |

disease requires factor VIII concentrate that contains von Willebrand factor. Von Willebrand factor is also found in cryoprecipitate, and factors VIII and IX are in fresh frozen plasma.

## Disseminated Intravascular Coagulation

### Pathophysiology

DIC is defined as the inappropriate triggering of the coagulation cascade and a breakdown in the normal feedback mechanisms in the body that allow for the dissolution of clots. Instead of a localized response to tissue damage or vascular injury, there is systemic coagulation activity, resulting in diffuse intravascular fibrin formation and widespread intravascular clotting. Eventually, coagulation factors become depleted as the body attempts to dissolve the newly formed clots. Because of the rapidity of intravascular thrombin formation, clotting factors are used up at a rate exceeding factor replenishment. In essence, there is an imbalance between the natural procoagulant and anticoagulant systems in the body. The result is unregulated thrombin activity, microvasculature thrombi, platelet consumption, and microangiopathic hemolytic anemia.

Activation of coagulation mechanisms also activates the fibrinolytic system. The breakdown of fibrin and fibrinogen results in FDPs and d-dimers; these products interfere with platelet function and the formation of the fibrin clot. In addition, plasmin can activate the complement and kinin systems, leading to increased vascular permeability, hypotension, and shock. Thus, the patient has a simultaneous, self-perpetuating combination of diffuse clotting and simultaneous hemorrhage occurring in response to the precipitating event as well as the potential for hemodynamic instability (Fig. 49-1).

### Etiology

DIC is a secondary complication of an underlying condition that serves as the initial triggering event for the inappropriate stimulation of clotting. It involves the activation of any of the coagulation pathways. The extrinsic pathway (tissue factor pathway) is activated by damage to the endothelial lining of blood vessels. Common causes include surgery, burns, heat stroke, a bacterial endotoxin, and malignant tumors. The intrinsic pathway (contact activation pathway) is activated when subendothelial tissue is exposed to the bloodstream and circulating factor XII comes in contact with the exposed tissue. The exposure may follow vascular injury or damage from immune complexes or bacterial endotoxins. The result is clot formation and activation of the coagulation cascade. Endotoxins released by Gram-negative bacteria and the resulting sepsis are significant triggers of DIC, accounting for approximately 20% of cases.

Shock or low-flow states can result in metabolic acidosis, tissue ischemia, and necrosis, which may also lead to clot formation. In cancer, a common etiology of DIC, the condition is caused by tumors eroding tissue, with subsequent release of thromboplastin or stimulation of factor XII from vascular injury, as well as by the autolysis of tumor cells in rapidly proliferating tumors. In cancers that are able to autolyse (eg, acute leukemia, Burkitt lymphoma, small cell lung cancer), the

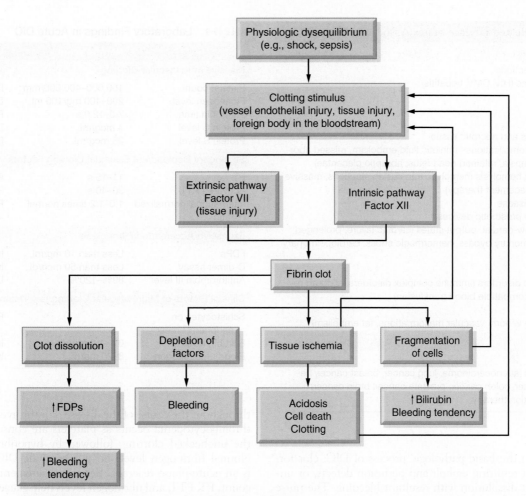

**FIGURE 49-1** Self-perpetuating cycle of thrombosis and bleeding in DIC.

cell fragments that result from the lysis are seen as "foreign bodies" and stimulate clotting. Still other cancers release procoagulants that enhance clotting (eg, mucin-producing adenocarcinomas, prostate and renal cancer, promyelocytic leukemias, and brain tumors).[4] Box 49-7 outlines some malignant and nonmalignant states of physiologic disequilibrium that can be precipitating factors for DIC.

### Clinical Presentation

Clinical consequences include systemic ischemia from the thrombi formation, as well as minor or major hemorrhage from ongoing fibrinolysis and depletion of clotting factors. A patient with DIC is vulnerable to a wide variety of complications resulting from the thrombotic or hemorrhagic disease processes. Thrombosis may result in ischemia or infarction in any organ, with concomitant loss of function. With depletion of clotting factors and platelets, bleeding into subcutaneous tissues, skin, and mucous membranes, or more serious hemorrhage, may result.

### Assessment

All critically ill patients are at risk for developing DIC because many are in the state of physiologic disequilibrium characterized by hypovolemia, hypotension, hypoxia, and acidosis, all of which have procoagulant effects. In addition,

the patient's critical illness may have been triggered by an injury that itself could result in the development of DIC. Increased awareness of DIC as a potentially catastrophic complication in the critically ill patient has resulted in earlier recognition and intervention. The critical care nurse who is armed with knowledge of physiologic norms and who uses a systemic approach to assessment may be the first person to identify the early signs of coagulation dysfunction and its probable trigger.

**HISTORY AND PHYSICAL EXAMINATION.** DIC may be acute in presentation, evidenced by severe clinical deterioration, or chronic in presentation, evidenced by mildly abnormal laboratory values and minimal, varied clinical symptoms. In chronic DIC, thrombosis is the prevalent disorder, and the degree of symptomatology is related to the ability of the liver and bone marrow to compensate for the disorder. Affected patients may have low-grade bleeding if factors become depleted, unexpected thrombotic events (including large vessel thrombi), or both. Chronic DIC must be ruled out in patients with multiple thrombotic sites developing simultaneously, serial thromboses, superficial venous thromboses, or arterial thromboses, especially in the presence of malignancy.

Most critical care nurses care for patients with acute DIC. It is important to realize that the assessment varies as the disease state evolves. Clinical assessment is organized

BOX 49-7 **Selected Disease States Associated With DIC**

**Nonmalignant**

Bacterial infections
Viral infections (HIV, CMV, hepatitis)
Burns
Heat stroke
Brain injury
Crush injuries and necrotic tissue
Obstetrical complications (amniotic fluid embolism, missed abortion, eclampsia, retained dead fetus, abruptio placentae)
Intravascular hemolysis (hemolytic transfusion reactions, massive blood replacement therapy)
Acute liver disease
Intravascular prosthetic devices
Prolonged low-cardiac output states (cardiac failure, prolonged cardiopulmonary bypass, hemorrhagic shock, cardiopulmonary arrest)
Vasculitis
Immunologic disorders (immune complex disorders, allograft reaction, incompatible blood transfusion)
Surgery
Other (snake venom, vascular malformations, fat embolism)

**Malignant**

Leukemias
Solid tumors (adenocarcinoma, lung cancer, breast cancer, hepatic cancer, colon cancer, prostate cancer, brain cancer)
Chemoradiation therapy

**TABLE 49-9** Laboratory Findings in Acute DIC

| Test | Normal Value | Value in DIC |
|---|---|---|
| **Massive Intravascular Clotting** | | |
| Platelet count | 150,000–400,000/mm³ | Decreased |
| Fibrinogen level | 200–400 mg/100 mL | Decreased |
| Thrombin time | 7.0–12.0 s | Prolonged |
| Protein C level | 4 mcg/mL | Decreased |
| Protein S level | 23 mcg/mL | Decreased |
| **Secondary Depletion of Essential Clotting Factors** | | |
| PT | 11–15 s | Prolonged |
| Activated PTT | 30–40 s | Prolonged |
| International normalized ratio | 1.0–1.2 times normal | Prolonged |
| **Excessive/Accelerated Fibrinolysis** | | |
| FDPs | Less than 10 mg/mL | Increased |
| D-dimer assay | Less than 50 mcg/dL | Increased |
| Antithrombin III level | 89%–120% | Decreased |
| **Clinical Effects of Microvascular Clotting/Cell Destruction** | | |
| Schistocytes on peripheral smear | | Present |
| Bilirubin level | 0.1–1.2 mg/dL | Increased |
| Blood urea nitrogen | 8–20 mg/dL | Increased |

according to the basic pathologic process of DIC: clot formation with resulting emboli and perfusion defects, or unchecked clot dissolution with resultant bleeding. The nurse evaluates the patient for signs and symptoms of inappropriate clotting: cyanosis, gangrene, mental status changes, altered level of consciousness, cerebrovascular accident, pulmonary embolus, bowel ischemia and infarction, and renal insufficiency or failure. Thrombosis may involve both arteries and veins. In addition, the nurse evaluates the patient for signs of bleeding from the nose, gums, lungs, gastrointestinal tract, surgical sites, injection sites, and intravascular access sites; hematuria; petechial rashes; and purpura fulminans. Bleeding is a manifestation of later disease because it is evidence of depletion of clotting factors.

Care of the patient with possible DIC requires constant reassessment and interpretation of findings. For example, the patient with a dull headache is likely to have a thrombotic defect, whereas a sudden and acute headache is more likely to be hemorrhagic. Dyspnea can be from a thrombotic disorder (pulmonary embolism) or from a hemorrhagic disorder (bleeding in the lungs). Either condition may present with hemoptysis and blood with suctioning. Hypotension may result from myocardial infarction (a thrombotic disorder) or cardiac tamponade (a hemorrhagic disorder). Ischemic bowel is characterized by decreased bowel sounds and a crampy and painful abdomen, with potential gastrointestinal bleeding, whereas gastrointestinal bleeding presents with heme-positive to melanotic stool and hyperactive bowel sounds.

**LABORATORY STUDIES.** Table 49-9 outlines studies that are commonly used to assess DIC. These studies, unfortunately, are neither specific nor sensitive, and results vary

throughout the course of the disease. For the average patient, thrombocytopenia occurs as platelets are consumed during the unchecked clotting, followed by hypofibrinogenemia. Normal fibrinogen levels do not preclude DIC because it is an acute-phase reactant. Serial measurements of platelet count, PT, PTT, and fibrinogen levels help gauge disease progression. Peripheral smears may reveal the presence of schistocytes, reflecting fragmentation of RBCs moving through clots or partially occluded vessels.

### Management

The backbone of therapy for DIC is eliminating the causative agent. The culprit that activates the clotting factors must be eliminated, whether through antibiotic or antifungal therapy for sepsis, antineoplastic therapy, rehydration, increasing oxygenation, or resolution of low-flow states. Unfortunately, some causes (such as burns, crush injury, and brain injury) cannot be as easily eliminated. General treatment principles include maintaining adequate fluid volume status and screening for and eliminating all medications that may enhance bleeding. Attention is also directed to correcting hypotension, hypoxia, and acidosis, all of which have procoagulant effects (Box 49-8).

Heparin therapy may be initiated to minimize further clotting. However, the risk of increased bleeding is always a major concern. In acute DIC, few clinical studies have shown heparin to be effective in slowing the coagulation cascade.

Replacement therapy and repletion of clotting factors are the focus of the treatment for significant hemorrhage. Fresh frozen plasma contains components of both the coagulation and fibrinolytic systems and can be given to normalize the international normalized ratio; the recommended dose is 10 to 20 mL/kg. Platelet transfusions are usually used only for patients with active bleeding or a platelet count of less than 20,000/mm³. Cryoprecipitate may be used for patients

**QSEN  BOX 49-8**  *COLLABORATIVE CARE GUIDE for the Patient With DIC*

| Outcomes | Interventions |
| --- | --- |
| **Impaired Gas Exchange** | |
| Arterial blood gases are within normal limits<br>Breath sounds are clear bilaterally | • Monitor pulse oximetry and/or arterial blood gases<br>• Maintain oxygen delivery whether noninvasive or mechanical ventilation<br>• Suction oropharynx and trachea carefully when necessary (see Chapter 25, Box 25-7)<br>• Turn, cough, deep-breathe, and use incentive spirometer every 2 hours |
| **Decreased Tissue Perfusion** | |
| Patient will achieve/maintain tissue perfusion | • Monitor tissue perfusion: color, temperature, pulses, level of consciousness, urinary output, and $SaO_2$/$PaO_2$<br>• Monitor vital signs every 1 to 4 hours based on clinical condition<br>• Monitor cardiac output, systemic vascular resistance, and pulmonary artery pressure every 4 hours if pulmonary artery catheter in place<br>• Administer blood products, positive inotropic agents, intravenous (IV) infusions as ordered |
| **Risk for Bleeding** | |
| Patient will not experience bleeding related to coagulopathies | • Monitor PT, PTT, and complete blood count daily; more frequently if monitoring for acute changes or response to therapy<br>• Assess every 2 to 4 hours for thrombotic and hemorrhagic manifestations<br>• Quantify degree of bleeding (count dressing changes, measure bodily drainage; test stool, urine, and emesis for heme)<br>• Assess organ systems for signs and symptoms: change in mental status with cerebral hemorrhage or thrombotic event; decreased $SaO_2$ and hemoptysis with pulmonary bleeding; visual changes (diplopia, blurred vision, visual field deficit) with retinal thrombosis/hemorrhage; back pain, flank pain, abdominal pain consistent with visceral organ bleeding<br>• Administer blood products and coagulation factors as indicated<br>• Maintain strict adherence to bleeding precautions<br>• Minimize invasive procedures and treatments<br>• Review and avoid medications that inhibit coagulation or promote thrombosis |
| **Electrolyte Imbalance** | |
| Patient is euvolemic<br><br>Mineral and electrolyte levels are within normal limits | • Trend daily weight<br>• Monitor intake and output; replace/diurese as required<br>• Maintain IV access and fluid replacement therapy<br>• Monitor and replace electrolytes daily and PRN |
| **Risk for Bleeding; Risk for Injury; Impaired Oral Mucous Membrane; Risk for Vascular Trauma** | |
| There is no evidence of bleeding due to preventable injury | • Institute bleeding precautions (soft toothbrush, electric razor, no rectal temperatures)<br>• Provide safe physical environment<br>• Apply pressure to puncture sites for 3 to 5 minutes, and then use pressure dressing |
| **Impaired Tissue Integrity** | |
| Skin will remain intact | • Turn patient every 2 hours and assess skin each time patient is repositioned for pressure areas, petechiae, and ecchymosis<br>• Assess injection sites and incisions for bleeding<br>• Consider pressure relief/reduction mattress, avoid shearing forces<br>• Use Braden scale to assess risk for skin breakdown |
| **Imbalanced Nutrition** | |
| Caloric and nutrient intake meets metabolic requirements per calculation (eg, basal energy expenditure) | • Provide enteral feeding or parenteral feeding if patient is NPO<br>• Assess for gastrointestinal bleeding and report<br>• Consult dietitian or nutritional support service |
| **Impaired Comfort** | |
| Patient will be as comfortable as possible as evidenced by stable vital signs or cooperation with treatments or procedures | • Objectively assess comfort/pain using a pain scale<br>• Correlate pain ratings with sites of potential ischemia or hemorrhage<br>• Provide analgesia and sedation as indicated by assessment<br>• Reassess patient for response to analgesia |
| **Ineffective Coping** | |
| Patient demonstrates decreased anxiety | • Provide areas of control to patient and family as possible (eg, performance of activities of daily living, visitors)<br>• Provide explanations and reassurance before procedures<br>• Consult palliative care and pastoral care as appropriate<br>• Provide for adequate rest and sleep<br>• Provide anxiolytics as indicated by assessment |
| **Teaching/Discharge Planning** | |
| Patient/significant others understand procedures and tests needed for treatment | • Educate patient and family regarding disease process, need for intensive monitoring, and actions taken to correct disorder<br>• Educate the patient and family regarding clinical parameters and patient presentation required for safe discharge from unit/hospital |

with plasma fibrinogen levels below 100 mg/dL. A single unit provides 200 mg of fibrinogen, as well as factor VIII, factor XII, and von Willebrand factor. The usual adult dose is 5 to 10 units, with each unit raising the fibrinogen level by 5 to 10 mg/dL. Depleted antithrombin III (necessary to balance clot production) can be replaced. RBC transfusions may be given to increase hemoglobin and oxygen-carrying capacity.

Localized bleeding should be minimized when possible. With venipuncture or removal of vascular access from compressible sites, pressure is applied for a minimum of 15 to 30 minutes or until bleeding has stopped. Sites are reassessed frequently for rebleeding because the initial clot may dissolve if the patient lacks the factors required to maintain hemostasis. Topical hemostatics may be used to provide superficial hemostasis.

## Clinical Applicability Challenges

### CASE STUDY

Mrs. G is a 45-year-old Hispanic woman who presents to the emergency department (ED) with complaints of malaise, fatigue, and severe headache. Two weeks ago, she was prescribed antibiotics by her primary care physician for an upper respiratory infection. In taking her history, she reports her urine has been bloody and her gums have been bleeding when she brushes her teeth. Findings on her physical examination include petechiae on her inner thighs and upper extremities; pale, jaundiced skin; and a mild temperature elevation. Laboratory tests are ordered by the ED nurse practitioner. Abnormal results include a markedly low platelet count of 10,000/mm$^3$, low hemoglobin at 9.5 mg/dL, mildly elevated total bilirubin at 2.6 mg/dL, and an elevated LDH of 713 U/L. Coagulation studies were essentially normal.

The patient was admitted to the ICU. Admission orders included a hematology consult and transfusion of fresh frozen plasma. The hematologist diagnosed TTP based on the patient's clinical presentation, laboratory data, and a review of the blood smear showing schistocytes (fragmented RBCs).

Mrs. G's clinical condition deteriorated rapidly. She became dyspneic and obtunded, and was intubated and placed on mechanical ventilation. High-dose corticosteroids were started, and she was scheduled for daily plasma exchanges. By day 7, her neurologic status improved, she was able to be extubated, and her platelet count had risen to 140,000/mm$^3$.

1. What hallmark findings of TTP did Mrs. G exhibit?
2. Why was not platelet transfusion part of the treatment of TTP?
3. What are some additional important nursing interventions for this patient?

### WANT TO KNOW MORE?

A wide variety of resources to enhance your learning and understanding of this chapter are available on thePoint.

You will find:

- References
- Selected readings
- NCLEX-style review questions
- Internet resources
- And more!

# PART 12

# Integumentary System

## 50

# Anatomy and Physiology of the Integumentary System

JOAN M. DAVENPORT

### LEARNING OBJECTIVES

*Based on the content in this chapter, the reader should be able to:*

1. Describe the features of the epidermis, dermis, and hypodermis.
2. Identify the appendages of the skin and state the purpose of each.
3. Discuss the homeostatic functions of the skin.
4. Explain the mechanism of infection resistance afforded by the integument.

The skin is described as protective, sensitive, reparative, and capable of maintaining a person's homeostasis. These physiologic features are explored in this chapter as functions of the anatomy of the skin and its appendages. The skin, which covers 1.2 to 2.3 m² of area, is the largest organ of the body and is supplied with one third of the circulating blood volume.[1] The three layers of the skin are the outer epidermis, the middle dermis, and the underlying hypodermis, or subcutaneous tissue. The appendages include the hair, nail, eccrine and apocrine sweat glands, and sebaceous glands. Figure 50-1 pictures the structures and layers of the skin. The functions of the skin include protection, sensation, water balance, temperature regulation, and vitamin production.

## Epidermis

This outer layer of the skin serves to protect underlying structures from invasion by microbes and other foreign substances. The cornified, external layer of the epidermis helps in the body's regulation of water loss. The innermost sublayer bends into the dermis and serves as the basis for the glands, nails, and hair roots. The epidermis does not have vascular supply; it depends on the dermal level for its nourishment.

Melanin and keratin are formed in the inner cellular layer of the epidermis. Melanocytes provide melanin, a pigment for both the skin and hair. This pigment provides the color for the skin and, more important, protects the underlying structures from ultraviolet light exposure by absorbing and scattering the radiation.[2]

Keratin is a tough protein that makes up hair, nails, and the tough, outer epidermal surface. These flattened scales of the skin slough continually and are replaced every 2 to 4 weeks.[2] The epidermis is actually made up of five distinct layers; the keratinocytes move from inner to outer sublayers as they mature. At the top, outermost layer, the keratinocytes are dead and are arranged in various thicknesses depending on the area of the body. In parts of the face, there is a thin stratum made up of a layer 15 cells deep. This contrasts with the thicker soles of the feet and palms of the hands, with at least 100 layers of keratinized cells.[2] It is these tough protein cells that serve to protect the underlying structures of the body.

## Dermis

The middle layer of the skin, the dermis, provides support for the outer epidermal layer. It is a very vascular connective tissue, and the blood vessels are integral to regulation of body temperature and blood pressure. The arteriovenous anastomoses, under control of the sympathetic nervous system and found in the dermal layer, are able to dilate or constrict in response to environmental conditions of heat and cold and to internal stimulation from anxiety or blood volume loss. The sensory function of the skin includes receptors for heat, cold, touch, pressure, and pain; these are located in the dermal layer. There is a great variety in the function of the nerve endings. Multiple stimuli are mediated centrally and result in patterned responses.[2]

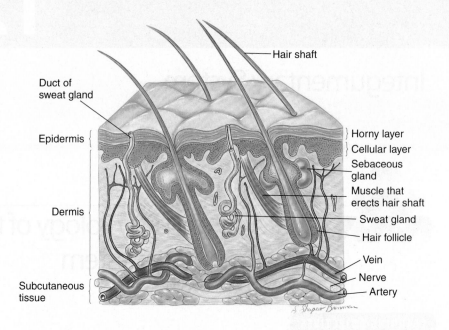

Duct of sweat gland
Hair shaft
Epidermis
Horny layer
Cellular layer
Sebaceous gland
Muscle that erects hair shaft
Dermis
Sweat gland
Hair follicle
Vein
Nerve
Subcutaneous tissue
Artery

**FIGURE 50-1**   Layers of the skin. (From Bickley LS, Szilagyi PG: Bates Guide to Physical Examination and History Taking, 11th ed. Philadelphia, PA: Lippincott Williams & Wilkins, 2013, p 171.)

The dermis is composed of two distinct layers. The papillary dermis is the more superficial of the two layers, lying just beneath the epidermis. This layer provides the attachment for the epidermis as the epidermal basal cells project into the papillary dermis.[3] The thicker underlayer of the dermis is the reticular dermis. Collagen is organized in a three-dimensional mesh pattern in this portion of the dermis. It is this mesh arrangement that allows the dermis to stretch with movement. Immune system components of the skin are found in the dermal layer and include macrophages, mast cells, T cells, and fibroblasts.[2]

## Hypodermis

The hypodermis or subcutaneous skin layer consists of connective tissue interspersed with fat. The fat of the hypodermis has the protective functions of heat retention and cushioning the underlying structures. In addition, the fat of the subcutaneous skin layer serves as storage for calories.[2]

## Skin Appendages

The hair, nails, and sebaceous and sweat glands are considered a part of the skin. These structures arise from or extrude through the epidermal or dermal skin layers.

## Sweat Glands

Eccrine sweat glands are distributed throughout the surface of the skin. These glands arise from the dermis and open at the skin surface. These specialized glands secrete sweat for the purpose of internal body temperature regulation. Apocrine sweat glands are not as widespread as the eccrine glands, are larger than eccrine glands, and open through a hair follicle of the axillae, nipples, areolae, groin, eyelids, and external ears.[2] Another difference between the two types of sweat glands is that the larger, less abundant apocrine glands secrete an oily substance with a particular odor. This odor is

used by animals to recognize the presence of other animals. In humans, the odor, known as body odor, is produced when the secretions come in contact with bacteria and when the fluid begins to decompose.[2]

## Sebaceous Glands

The sebaceous glands secrete sebum, a combination of triglycerides, cholesterol, and wax, through the hair follicle. These glands are situated over the entire surface of the skin except for the palms and soles of the feet. Sebaceous glands are inactive until puberty. At this time, they enlarge and are stimulated to secrete sebum by a rise in sex hormones. The sebum serves to keep the skin and hair from drying out.[2] By protecting the outer layer of the epidermis from undue drying, the sebum helps to conserve body heat. Table 50-1 summarizes the location and function of the eccrine, apocrine, and sebaceous glands.[4]

**TABLE 50-1**   Sweat and Sebaceous Glands

| Type of Gland | Location | Function |
|---|---|---|
| Eccrine sweat glands | All over body  Numerous in thick skin  Extended from dermis to epidermis | Regulate body temperature  Respond to emotional distress  Respond to physiologic stimuli |
| Apocrine sweat glands | Axillae  Nipples, breasts  Anogenital region  External ear canal  Eyelids | Respond to hormonal influences  Respond to emotional distress |
| Sebaceous glands | All over body except palms of hands, dorsum, and soles of feet | Produce sebum to lubricate hair and skin |

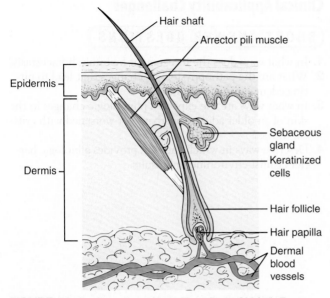

**FIGURE 50-2** Structures of hair. (From Porth CM (ed): Essentials of Pathophysiology, 4th ed. Philadelphia, PA: Wolters Kluwer, 2015, p 1147.)

## Hair

Epidermal cells in the dermis form the hair. Under the sebaceous gland, adjacent to the hair follicle, are the arrector pili muscles. Contraction of the arrector pili causes gooseflesh, a reduction of skin surface area, and reduced surface area for heat loss. Figure 50-2 shows the structures of the hair.

## Nails

Hardened plates of epidermal keratin cells grow from a curved groove over the distal dorsal fingertips. These nails serve to protect the fingers and toes and increase physical dexterity. The angle between the proximal nail fold and the nail plate is expected to be less than 180 degrees. Figure 50-3 illustrates the normal nail.

## Functions of the Skin

The epidermal layer of the integument provides protection against microbes, ultraviolet light exposure, and countless other threats. This tough, hardened outer layer also restricts water loss and thus helps to maintain organism homeostasis. The vascular dermis, with its rich supply of blood vessels, provides blood pressure and temperature-regulatory features. Nerve endings here supply receptors for heat, cold, touch, pressure, and pain.

Within this vascular dermal area, a potential space exists. This space, with its extracellular and extravascular fluid, may serve as a fluid reservoir to replace intravascular or intracellular fluid loss. This is also the place for fluid to migrate toward when intravascular hydrostatic pressure increases above the hydrostatic pressure with the dermal layer. This process produces the edema seen in patients.

The skin's ability to stretch with movement is also provided by the dermal collagen's mesh formation. The underlying hypodermal layers of connective tissue and fat serve to retain heat and to cushion the underlying structures. The appendages of the skin, the hair, nails, and glands contribute to the homeostatic function primarily by controlling heat loss with the hair's arrector pili muscles and secretions by the sebaceous and sweat glands. The integument is vital to an individual's survival.

The immune function of the skin is not to be overlooked. The most abundant of the immune cells within the dermal layer of the skin are the macrophages. Macrophages promote wound closure and tissue repair. Recent research has identified the macrophages as being a heterogenous group of cells responsive to the diverse functions as leukocyte extravasation, iron metabolism, and lymphangiogenesis.[5] Langerhans cells from the epidermis and dermal dendritic cells from the dermis provide a capacity for a response to antigens and to skin pathogens and are accountable for T-cell responses to these pathogens. Skin mast cells found close to the dermal blood vessels seem also linked to a response to environmental allergens and are implicated in autoimmune disease progression.

During critical care hospitalizations, there are many insults to the skin. Surgical wounds, vascular catheter insertions, opportunistic infections of the skin, nutritional compromise, and persistent pressure that leads to reduced blood flow are only a few of the challenges faced by the patient's integument. In older patients, age-related changes (Box 50-1; see also Chapters 12 and 51) leading to increased fragility of the skin and slower healing magnify the effects of these insults. Attention to the skin and appendages by the nurse maximizes this organ's functioning and results in protection of the patient.

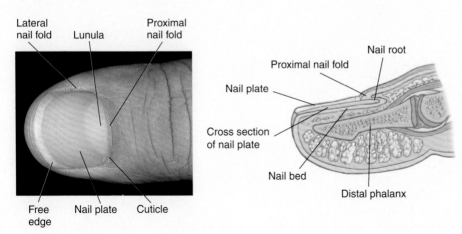

**FIGURE 50-3** The normal nail. (From Bickley LS, Szilagyi PG: Bates Guide to Physical Examination and History Taking, 11th ed. Philadelphia, PA: Lippincott Williams & Wilkins, 2013, p 172.)

<table>
<tr><td>BOX 50-1</td><td>**Anatomical and Physiological Changes in the Integumentary System That Occur With Aging**</td></tr>
</table>

- The skin becomes thinner, and there is a decrease in skin flexibility, placing the person at risk for epidermal tearing.
- The skin loses dermal elasticity, collagen, and mass, resulting in fine wrinkling, looseness, and sagging.
- The number of dermal blood vessels decreases; the vessels become thinner and more fragile, thus increasing the risk for bruising and hemorrhage.
- There is decreased density and activity of the eccrine and apocrine glands and decreased sebum production, resulting in dryness, itching, and decreased perspiration.
- Decreased peripheral circulation leads to slowed nail growth and brittle nails that split easily.
- Reduced hormone levels lead to thinning of the hair and transition from terminal to vellus hair.
- Decreased melanin leads to graying of the hair.
- Sun exposure over a long period of time leads to yellowing and thickening of the skin and the development of old age spots (solar lentigo).

## Clinical Applicability Challenges

### SHORT ANSWER QUESTIONS

1. In what ways does the integument maintain homeostasis?
2. What are the pathophysiologic changes that lead to pitting edema of the extremities?
3. In what ways are the expected physiologic changes in the skin of an older adult exacerbated or worsened with critical illness?
4. Describe ways in which the skin provides a biologic barrier against environmental insults.

### WANT TO KNOW MORE

A wide variety of resources to enhance your learning and understanding of this chapter are available on thePoint.

You will find:

- References
- Selected readings
- NCLEX-style review questions
- Internet resources
- And more!

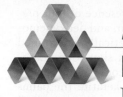

# 51

# Patient Assessment: Integumentary System

JOAN M. DAVENPORT AND JANET A. WULF

## LEARNING OBJECTIVES

*Based on the content in this chapter, the reader should be able to:*

1. Discuss the health history and physical assessment when evaluating a patient's skin.
2. Explain expected differences in skin color related to racial or skin tone characteristics.
3. Describe and recognize abnormal changes in skin color.
4. Explain and identify skin lesions resulting from increased vascularity.
5. Describe the significance of rashes related to infection or to allergic reaction.
6. Compare and contrast pitting and nonpitting edema.
7. Explain the cause of pressure ulcers and the Braden scale used to assess a patient for pressure ulcer development.
8. Discuss the features of malignant skin diseases.

The skin of a critically ill person is exposed to insults ranging from diminished blood flow and the resultant risk for pressure ulceration to rashes from hypersensitivity drug reactions and opportunistic infections. There is often ample opportunity for the critical care nurse to assess the skin—the intimacy involved in providing care to someone who is critically ill, the relative level of undress of the patient, and the attention to detail implicit in critical care nursing make integument assessment an ongoing and vital process.

## History

When caring for patients with skin disorders, it is important to obtain information from the health history (Box 51-1). The information is useful in guiding the physical examination and in determining appropriate interventions.

## Physical Examination

The assessment techniques necessary for an evaluation of the integument involve inspection and palpation.

### Inspection

Inspection of the general appearance of the skin includes assessment of color; determination of the presence of lesions, rashes, or increased vascularity; and assessment of the condition of the nails and hair.

### Color

Skin color is expected to be uniform over the body, except for the areas with greater degrees of vascularity. The genitalia, upper chest, and cheeks may appear pink or have a reddish tone in people with light skin. These same areas may appear darker in people with dark skin. Additional normal variations in skin color include those listed in Table 51-1.

---

**BOX 51-1** | **Health History for Integumentary Assessment**

**Chief Complaint**
- Patient's description of the problem

**History of the Present Illness**
- Complete analysis of the following signs and symptoms (using the NOPQRST format; see Box 17-1)
- Changes in skin color, pigmentation, temperature, or texture
- Changes in a mole
- Excess dryness or moisture
- Skin itching
- Excess bruising
- Delay in healing
- Skin rash or lesions
- Hair loss or increased growth
- Changes in hair texture
- Changes in nails

**Past Health History**
- Relevant childhood illnesses and immunizations: impetigo, scabies or lice exposure, measles, chickenpox, scarlet fever
- Past acute and chronic medical problems including treatments and hospitalizations: diabetes, peripheral vascular disease, Lyme disease, Parkinson disease, immobility, malnutrition, trauma, skin cancers, radiation treatments, HIV/AIDS
- Risk factors: age, ultraviolet sun exposure, tanning beds, exposure to dyes, toxic chemicals, insect bites, contact with some poisonous plants, autoimmune disease, exposure to extremes of temperature
- Past surgeries: skin biopsy
- Past diagnostic tests and interventions: allergy testing
- Medications: aspirin, antibiotics, barbiturates, sulfonamides, thiazide diuretics, oral hypoglycemic agents, tetracycline, antimalarials, antineoplastic agents, hormones, metals, topical steroids
- Allergies and reactions: foods, medications, contrast dyes, latex, soaps
- Transfusions

*(continued)*

**BOX 51-1** **Health History for Integumentary Assessment** (*continued*)

**Family History**
- Health status or cause of death of parents and siblings: skin cancer, autoimmune diseases

**Personal and Social History**
- Tobacco, alcohol, and substance use
- Family composition
- Occupation and work environment: farmers, roofers, creosote or coal workers, furniture repair and refinishing, gardeners
- Living environment: ability for self-care and hygiene, exposure to insects and pests, availability of indoor sleeping in environmental temperature extremes
- Diet
- Sleep patterns
- Exercise
- Cultural beliefs
- Spiritual/religious beliefs
- Coping patterns and social support systems
- Leisure activities
- Sexual activity
- Recent travel

**Review of Other Systems**
- Psychiatric/emotional: increased anxiety, nervousness, sleeplessness
- Neurologic: loss or decrease in sensation, numbness, pain or neuropathy, stroke
- Cardiovascular: swelling of extremities, cold extremities, varicose veins
- Gastrointestinal: change in diet, recent weight loss or gain, loss of appetite
- Musculoskeletal: immobility, weakness
- Metabolic: altered glucose level

**TABLE 51-1**    **Normal Variations in Skin Color**

| Normal Variation | Description |
|---|---|
| Moles (pigmented nevi) | Tan to dark brown; may be flat or raised |
| Stretch marks (striae) | Silver or pink; may be caused by weight gain or pregnancy |
| Freckles | Flat macules anywhere on the body |
| Vitiligo | Unpigmented skin area; more prevalent in people with dark skin |
| Birthmarks | Generally flat marks anywhere on the body; may be tan, red, or brown |

Skin color is determined by the presence of four pigments: melanin, carotene, hemoglobin, and deoxyhemoglobin. The amount of melanin is genetically determined and produces varying degrees of dark skin tone. Carotene, a yellow pigment, is in subcutaneous fat and is most evident in those areas with the most keratin: the palms and soles of the feet. Skin color abnormalities, such as pallor, cyanosis, jaundice, and erythema, manifest differently depending on the person's normal skin tone (Table 51-2).

The degree of oxygenation affects skin color. Hemoglobin, attached to red blood cells, transports oxygen to the tissues. A diminished flow of oxyhemoglobin through the cutaneous circulation results in pallor. In people with light skin, the skin appears very pale, without the usual pink undertones. In people with darker skin, pallor manifests as a yellowish-brown or ashen appearance (again, because the usual pink undertones are lost).

As hemoglobin gives up its oxygen to the tissues, the hemoglobin changes to deoxyhemoglobin. When deoxyhemoglobin is present in the cutaneous circulation, the skin takes on a blue cast, and the person is said to be cyanotic.[1] In light-skinned people, cyanosis may be seen as a grayish-blue color, especially in the palms and soles of the feet, the nail beds, the earlobes, the lips, and the mucous membranes. In those with darker skin, cyanosis appears as an ashen-gray color seen in the same areas.[2]

The yellowish hue of jaundice is indicative of liver disease or of hemolysis of red blood cells. In dark-skinned people, jaundice is seen as a yellowish-green color in the sclera, palms of the hands, and soles of the feet. In light-skinned people, jaundice is seen as a yellow coloration of the skin, sclera, lips, hard palate, and underside of the tongue. Bickley and Szilagyi[1] recommend using a transparent slide pressed against the lips to "blanch out the red color," making the yellow of jaundice more easily seen.

Another skin color abnormality is erythema. Erythema manifests as a reddish tone in light-skinned people and a deeper brown or purple tone in dark-skinned people. It is indicative of increased skin temperature caused by inflammation. The process of inflammation increases vascularity of the tissues, which produces the color alteration seen with erythema. Erythema may be expected with a surgical wound, due to the inflammatory process inherent in any tissue trauma. It is also seen in disease processes affecting the skin, such as cellulitis. In either case, the erythema is indicative of inflammation.

**TABLE 51-2**    **Skin Color Abnormalities**

| Skin Color Abnormality | Underlying Cause | Manifestation in Light-Skinned People | Manifestation in Dark-Skinned People |
|---|---|---|---|
| Pallor | Decreased blood flow (decreased oxyhemoglobin flow to tissues) | Excessively pale skin | Yellowish-brown or ashen color to the skin |
| Cyanosis | Increased deoxyhemoglobin in the cutaneous circulation | Grayish-blue color of the palms and soles of the feet, the nail beds, the lips, the earlobes, and the mucous membranes | Ashen-gray color of the conjunctiva, oral mucous membranes, and nail beds |
| Jaundice | Increased red blood cell hemolysis, liver disease | Yellow color of the sclera, lips, and hard palate | Yellow-green color of the sclera and palms and soles of the feet |
| Erythema | Inflammation | Reddish tone | Deeper brown or purple tone |

## Lesions

Skin lesions are variously described by their color, shape, cause, or general appearance (Tables 51-3 and 51-4). They are considered abnormal conditions and arise from many factors In general, it is important to note the anatomical location, distribution, color, size, and pattern of any abnormal skin lesion. In addition, details about the lesion's borders or edges, as well as whether the lesion is flat, raised, or sunken, should be noted. The length of time the lesion has been present and any environmental or medication exposure that may be considered contributory should also be noted.[3]

| TABLE 51-3 | Primary Skin Lesions | | |
|---|---|---|---|
| **Type** | **Description** | **Examples** | **Illustration** |
| Macule | Less than 1 cm in diameter, flat, nonpalpable, circumscribed, discolored | Brown: freckle, junctional nevus, lentigo, melasma<br>Blue: Mongolian spot, ochronosis<br>Red: drug eruption, viral exanthema, secondary syphilis<br>Hypopigmented: vitiligo, idiopathic guttate hypomelanosis | Macule |
| Patch | Greater than 1 cm in diameter, flat, nonpalpable, irregular shape, discolored | Brown: larger freckle, junctional nevus, lentigo, melasma<br>Blue: Mongolian spot, ochronosis<br>Red: drug eruption viral exanthema, secondary syphilis<br>Hypopigmented: vitiligo, idiopathic guttate hypomelanosis | Patch |
| Papule | Less than 1 cm in diameter, raised, palpable, firm | Flesh, white or yellow: flat wart, milium, sebaceous hyperplasia, skin tag<br>Blue or violaceous: venous lake, lichen planus, melanoma<br>Brown: seborrheic keratosis, melanoma, dermatofibroma, nevi<br>Red: acne, cherry angioma, early folliculitis, psoriasis, urticaria, and eczema | Papule |
| Nodule | Greater than 1 cm, raised, solid | Wart, xanthoma, prurigo nodularis, neurofibromatosis | Nodule |
| Plaque | Greater than 1 cm, raised, superficial, flat-topped, rough | Psoriasis, discoid lupus, tinea corporis, eczema, seborrheic dermatitis | Plaque |

(continued)

| TABLE 51-3 | Primary Skin Lesions (*continued*) | | |
|---|---|---|---|
| **Type** | **Description** | **Examples** | **Illustration** |
| Tumor | Large nodule | Metastatic carcinoma, sporotrichosis |  Tumor |
| Vesicle | Less than 1 cm, superficially raised, filled with serous fluid | Herpes simplex, herpes zoster, erythema multiforme, impetigo |  Vesicle |
| Bulla | Greater than 1-cm vesicle | Pemphigus, herpes gestationis, fixed drug eruption |  Bulla |
| Pustule | Raised, superficial, filled with cloudy, purulent fluid | Acne, candidiasis, rosacea, impetigo, folliculitis |  Pustule |
| Wheal | Raised, irregular area of edema, solid, transient, variable size | Hives, cholinergic urticaria, angioedema, dermatographism |  Wheal |
| Cyst | Raised, circumscribed, encapsulated with a wall and lumen, filled with liquid or semisolid | Digital mucus, epidermal inclusion, pilar |  Cyst |

From Rhoads J, Petersen SW: Advanced Health Assessment and Diagnostic Reasoning, 2nd ed. Philadelphia, PA: Lippincott Williams & Wilkins, 2013, pp 81–83.

**TABLE 51-4    Secondary Skin Lesions**

| Type | Description |
|------|-------------|
| Crust | Dried exudates over a damaged epithelium; may be associated with vesicles, bullae, or pustules. Large adherent crust is a scab. |
| Erosion | Loss of superficial epidermis; does not extend to the dermis; may be associated with vesicles, bullae, or pustules |
| Fissure | Crack in the epidermis usually extending into the dermis |
| Keloid | Hypertrophied scar tissue; secondary to collagen formation during healing; elevated irregular and red; more common in African Americans |
| Lichenification | Thickening and roughening of the skin; accentuated skin markings; may be secondary to repeated rubbing irritation and scratching |
| Scale | Skin debris on the surface of the epidermis secondary to desquamated, dead epithelium. Color and texture vary. |
| Scar | Skin mark left after healing of wound or lesion that represents replacement by connective tissue of the injured tissue. Young scars are red or purple. Mature scars are white or glistening. |
| Ulceration | Loss of epidermis, extending into dermis or deeper. Bleeding and scarring are possible. |

Adapted from Weber J, Kelley J: Health Assessment in Nursing, 4th ed. Philadelphia, PA: Wolters Kluwer Health/Lippincott Williams & Wilkins, 2010, p 199.

**TABLE 51-5    Vascular Lesions: Normal Variations**

| Normal Variation | Description |
|------------------|-------------|
| Nevus flammeus (port-wine stain), immature hemangioma (strawberry mark) | Range from dark red to pale pink and are considered birthmarks |
| Cherry angioma | Small, slightly raised, bright red lesions on the face, neck, and trunk; increase in size and number with advancing age |
| Capillary hemangioma | Red, irregular patch caused by capillary dilation in the dermis of the skin |
| Telangiectasis | Irregular, fine red lines caused by permanent dilation of a group of superficial vessels |

Vascular lesions can be either a normal variation or an abnormal finding. Vascular changes considered to be normal variants include nevus flammeus (port-wine stain), immature hemangioma (strawberry mark), telangiectasis, cherry angioma, and capillary hemangioma (Table 51-5). Abnormal vascular findings include petechiae, purpura, ecchymoses, spider angiomas, and urticaria (hives). These findings may indicate disease or injury and warrant further investigation by the critical care nurse.

*Petechiae* are purple or red, small (1 to 3 mm) lesions that are easily seen on light-skinned people and more difficult to see on those with dark skin (Fig. 51-1A). These tiny hemorrhages in the dermal or submucosal layers may appear anywhere on the body including oral mucosa and conjunctiva. They are caused by extravasated blood and do not disappear when pressure is applied to them.[3] Purpura are very similar to petechiae, only larger. Purpura may appear brownish-red.

*Ecchymoses* are bruises. They may appear as purple to yellowish-green rounded or irregular lesions and are more easily seen in people with light skin (see Fig. 51-1B). Ecchymoses occur as a result of trauma, when blood leaks from damaged blood vessels into the surrounding tissue.

*Spider angiomas* are fiery red lesions that are most often located on the face, neck, arms, or upper trunk (see Fig. 51-1C). Spider angiomas are seldom seen below the waist. They have a central body that is sometimes "raised and surrounded by erythema and radiating legs."[1] These lesions are most often associated with liver disease and vitamin B deficiency but also occur normally in some people.[1]

*Urticaria* is a reddened or white, raised, nonpitting plaque that often occurs as a result of an allergic reaction. The lesion often changes shape and size during the course of the reaction. The edema associated with urticaria is a result of local vasodilation and inflammation, which is followed by transudation of serous vascular fluid into the surrounding tissue.

### Rashes

Rashes identified during inspection may indicate infection or a reaction to drug therapy. Some of these rashes are identified by the names listed in Table 51-3. Identifying the type of lesion may help in identifying the cause of the rash. Attention

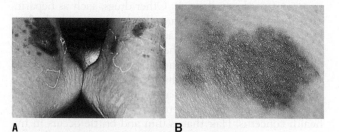

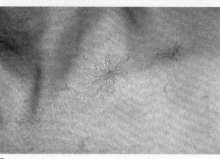

**FIGURE 51-1** Abnormal vascular lesions. **A:** Petechiae. **B:** Ecchymoses (bruises). **C:** Spider angiomas. (**A**, from Smeltzer SC, Bare BG: Textbook of Medical-Surgical Nursing, 9th ed. Philadelphia, PA: Wolters Kluwer Health/Lippincott Williams & Wilkins, 2000. **B**, from Bickley LS: Bates' Guide to Physical Examination and History Taking, 10th ed. Philadelphia, PA: Wolters Kluwer Health/Lippincott Williams & Wilkins, 2009, p 184. **C**, from Goodheart HP: Goodheart's Photoguide to Common Skin Disorders, 2nd ed. Philadelphia, PA: Lippincott Williams & Wilkins, 2003.)

to the development of a rash in association with a change in pharmacotherapy is essential to help identify the occurrence of an allergic hypersensitivity reaction.[4] The development of urticaria is often associated with food or drug reactions. Urticaria usually resolves completely over days to several weeks as the excess local fluid is reabsorbed. These lesions are often pruritic, and patient scratching may precipitate secondary skin abrasions, which can place the patient at risk for localized skin infections.

Skin infections are most often caused by fungi or yeasts and may range from superficial tinea pedis (athlete's foot) to intermediate yeast infections (eg, moniliasis resulting from *Candida albicans* infection) to deep fungal infections (eg, aspergillosis) that invade the underlying tissues. In the critical care setting, fungal and yeast infections are most often of the intermediate type and are the result of an opportunistic infection by normal flora. Antibiotics, corticosteroids, poor nutrition, and diabetes mellitus place the patient at risk for these infections. Candidiasis presents in the groin and under the breasts of female patients with erythema, a whitish pseudomembrane, and maculopapular satellite lesions.[5] Oral candidiasis, also known as thrush, manifests as a whitish coating of the oral mucosa, especially the tongue. This painful condition may produce fissures on the tongue and often restricts a patient's oral intake, further compromising the patient from a nutritional perspective.

### Condition of the Hair

The patient's terminal hair is inspected daily; the nurse notes the hair's quantity, distribution, and texture. Scalp hair should be resilient and evenly distributed.

Alopecia refers to hair loss and can be diffuse, patchy, or complete. Hair loss in the critical care setting can be associated with pharmacotherapy. Chemotherapy used in oncology treatment produces alopecia. Other drugs, such as heparin, used for a prolonged time may also be responsible for hair loss.[6] Hirsutism or increased facial, body, or pubic hair growth is an abnormal finding in the examination of women and children. Hirsutism has a familial pattern and is associated with menopause, endocrine disorders, and certain pharmacotherapies (eg, corticosteroids and androgenic medications).[2]

A change in the hair's texture may indicate ongoing health concerns. Hair that is thin and brittle occurs in hypothyroidism. In those with severe protein malnutrition, the hair color may appear reddish or bleached, and the hair texture is described as brittle and dry.[7]

Also not to be overlooked is the presence of infection or infestation of the scalp and hair. The patient's scalp and body hair are inspected regularly for evidence of flaking, sores, lice, louse eggs, scabies, and ringworm. During the inspection, the hair is parted in several areas to reveal the underlying scalp.

### Condition of the Nails

Nails, like hair, can be overlooked in the rush of critical care nursing; however, a careful inspection as part of the routine assessment can reveal information about the patient's general state of health. The nail bed is very vascular and is an excellent location for assessing the adequacy of the patient's peripheral circulation. The capillary refill test, done by blanching the nail beds and then releasing the pressure, should indicate a return of the pink tones in less than

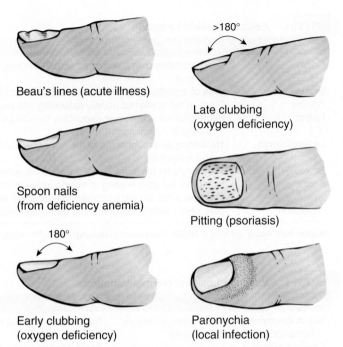

**FIGURE 51-2** Common nail disorders. (From Weber J, Kelley J: Health Assessment in Nursing, 4th ed. Philadelphia, PA: Wolters Kluwer Health/Lippincott Williams & Wilkins, 2010, p 203.)

3 seconds. Nail beds that are tinted bluish or purplish may indicate cyanosis; nail beds that are pale may indicate reduced arterial blood flow.

When the angle of the nail is 180 degrees or greater, clubbing is said to be present (see Chapter 24, Fig. 24-2). Clubbing is attributed to chronic hypoxemia. Other shapes that the nail takes on may provide clues to deficient nutritional states of the patient (Fig. 51-2). A spoon-shaped nail, called koilonychias, is associated with iron deficiency anemia.

Chronic disease states, such as cirrhosis, heart failure, and type II diabetes mellitus, may affect the nails by producing Terry nails.[1] These nails are whitish with a distal band of dark reddish-brown color, and the lunulae may not be visible (Fig. 51-3). Bands across the nails, especially in the older adult, may indicate protein deficiency. However, in dark-skinned individuals, lengthwise, linear dark stripes or diffuse

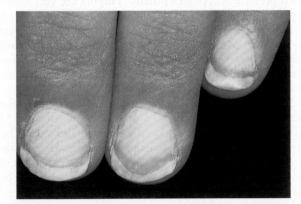

**FIGURE 51-3** Terry nails, seen in people with chronic diseases such as cirrhosis, congestive heart failure, and type II diabetes mellitus. (From Bickley LS: Bates' Guide to Physical Examination and History Taking, 10th ed. Philadelphia, PA: Lippincott Williams & Wilkins, 2009, p 193.)

brown, blue, or black pigmentation may be a normal finding.[5] Hyperkeratotic, dull, discolored, and distorted nails may indicate onychomycosis, a fungal infection of the nails seen frequently in critically ill patients; this condition is more common in toenails than fingernails. Risk factors include diabetes, poor venous and lymphatic drainage, poorly fitting shoes, history of athlete's foot, and increasing age.[8]

## Palpation

The skin is palpated for texture, moisture, temperature, mobility and turgor, and edema. Any evidence of discomfort arising from the areas palpated is noteworthy.

### Texture

Texture refers to the smoothness of the skin surface. It requires gentle palpation to assess. Rough skin occurs in patients with hypothyroidism.

### Moisture

The skin may be described as dry, oily, diaphoretic, or clammy. Dry skin may be seen in the patient with hypothyroidism. Skin is oily with acne and with increased activity of the sebaceous glands, as in Parkinson disease. Diaphoresis may be a response to increased temperature or increased metabolic rate. Hyperhidrosis is the term given to excessive perspiration. Bromhidrosis refers to foul-smelling perspiration. Low cardiac output states may produce skin that is referred to as clammy.

### Temperature

Temperature is usually assessed with the dorsal surface of the hand to identify the general skin temperature as warm or cool. The skin's temperature can also be used to assess the possibility of reduced blood flow from an arterial insufficiency, in which case the skin may be noticeably cooler distal to an occluding lesion.

### Mobility and Turgor

Mobility and turgor provide information about the health of the skin and may yield information about the patient's fluid volume balance. When assessed centrally, over the clavicles, the skin is expected to lift up easily and quickly return into place. Skin mobility may be decreased in scleroderma or in a patient with increased edema. Skin turgor is decreased in the patient with dehydration.[1]

### Edema

Edema is classified as either nonpitting or pitting. Nonpitting edema is that which does not depress with palpation. Nonpitting edema is seen in patients with a local inflammatory response and is caused by capillary endothelial damage. In addition to the edema, the skin is usually red, tender, and warm. Pitting edema is usually seen in the skin of the extremities and in dependent body parts. Pitting edema is identified as edema that retains the depression made when palpated. This type of edema can be further classified by the depth of the depression and, occasionally, by the amount of time it takes the pit to rebound (Table 51-6).

**TABLE 51-6** Pitting Edema Scale

| Scale | Depth of Indentation (mm) | Time to Return to Baseline | Descriptors |
|---|---|---|---|
| 1+ | 2 | Disappears rapidly | Trace |
| 2+ | 4 | 10–15 s | Mild |
| 3+ | 6 | 1–2 min | Moderate |
| 4+ | 8 | 2–5 min | Severe |

## Assessment of Pressure Ulcers

The development of pressure ulcers in the critically ill patient is a preventable complication. The patient with multiple-system dysfunction with concomitant fluid, electrolyte, and nutritional deficiencies is at high risk for pressure ulcers. Common pressure ulcer points include the occiput, scapula, sacrum, buttocks, ischium, heels, and toes. Pressure applied by the weight of the body causes a reduction in arterial and capillary blood flow, leading to these ischemic events. Therefore, frequent position changes are required to prevent the development of pressure ulcers.

Pressure ulceration on the toes occurs as a result of the pressure of the bed linen on the feet. Dressing devices and wound appliances can place pressure on underlying skin, resulting in reduced blood flow. The back of the neck of the patient with a tracheostomy tube must be assessed because the tube holder may be applied too tightly. The tape securing a nasogastric tube must be regularly removed and the condition of the tip of the nose, upper lip, and nares assessed for changes resulting from pressure from the tube.

Assisting the patient with frequent position changes is crucial in preventing pressure ulcers from developing. In addition, keeping the skin clean and dry is requisite in preventing pressure ulceration. Moisture increases the risk for maceration of the skin and promotes its breakdown. Infectious matter in wound drainage or feces increases the risk that an ulcer will progress and become a major source of sepsis.

Patients with decreased sensation or awareness (eg, from brain or spinal cord injury or from a peripheral neuropathy, such as that caused by diabetes) are at greater risk for ulceration because they do not recognize the discomfort from being in one position for extended periods. Similarly, patients with sedation or frequent analgesic dosing are at increased risk for problems related to their immobility. Patients with poor circulation, such as that caused by hypotension, heart failure, or peripheral vascular insufficiency, are also at higher risk because of the underlying possibility of tissue hypoxia. Lack of movement then serves only to accelerate the process of pressure ulcer development.

Identifying those people most at risk for pressure ulcer development is a focus of assessment. The National Pressure Ulcer Advisory Panel[9] recommends assessment on admission, change of status, prior to discharge, and as indicated by the patient's degree of risk and clinical setting. Recognizing that there are certain features that increase a patient's risk of developing pressure ulcers allows the critical care nurse to increase surveillance and implement preventive treatment modalities. Problems with sensory perception, moisture, incontinence, activity, mobility, nutrition, advanced age, and friction and shearing forces increase the patient's risk of developing pressure ulcers, which are debilitating and expensive

Braden Scale
# FOR PREDICTING PRESSURE SORE RISK

Patient's Name_____ Evaluator's Name_____

Date of Assessment [ ]

| SENSORY PERCEPTION<br>Ability to respond meaningfully to pressure-related discomfort | 1. Completely Limited:<br>Unresponsive (does not moan, flinch, or grasp) to painful stimuli, due to diminished level of consciousness or sedation.<br>OR<br>limited ability to feel pain over most of body surface. | 2. Very Limited:<br>Responds only to painful stimuli. Cannot communicate discomfort except by moaning or restlessness.<br>OR<br>has a sensory impairment which limits the ability to feel pain or discomfort over 1/2 of body | 3. Slightly Limited:<br>Responds to verbal commands, but cannot always communicate discomfort or need to be turned.<br>OR<br>has some sensory impairment which limits ability to feel pain or discomfort in 1 or 2 extremities. | 4. No Impairment:<br>Responds to verbal commands. Has no sensory deficit which would limit ability to feel or voice pain or discomfort. | |
|---|---|---|---|---|---|
| MOISTURE<br>Degree to which skin is exposed to moisture | 1. Constantly Moist:<br>Skin is kept moist almost constantly by perspiration, urine, etc. Dampness is detected every time patient is moved or turned. | 2. Very Moist:<br>Skin is often, but not always, moist. Linen must be changed at least once a shift. | 3. Occasionally Moist:<br>Skin is occasionally moist, requiring an extra linen change approximately once a day. | 4. Rarely Moist:<br>Skin is usually dry, linen only requires changing at routine intervals. | |
| ACTIVITY<br>Degree of physical activity | 1. Bedfast:<br>Confined to bed | 2. Chairfast:<br>Ability to walk severely limited or nonexistent. Cannot bear own weight and/or must be assisted into chair or wheelchair. | 3. Walks Occasionally:<br>Walks occasionally during day, but for very short distances, with or without assistance. Spends majority of each shift in bed or chair. | 4. Walks Frequently:<br>Walks outside the room at least twice a day and inside room at least once every 2 hours during waking hours. | |
| MOBILITY<br>Ability to change and control body position | 1. Completely Immobile:<br>Does not make even slight changes in body or extremity position without assistance. | 2. Very Limited:<br>Makes occasional slight changes in body or extremity position but unable to make frequent or significant changes independently. | 3. Slightly Limited:<br>Makes frequent though slight changes in body or extremity position independently. | 4. No Limitations:<br>Makes major and frequent changes in position without assistance. | |
| NUTRITION<br>Usual food intake pattern | 1. Very Poor:<br>Never eats a complete meal. Rarely eats more than 1/3 of any food offered. Eats 2 servings or less of protein (meat or dairy products) per day. Takes fluids poorly. Does not take a liquid dietary supplement.<br>OR<br>is NPO and/or maintained on clear liquids or IVs for more than 5 days. | 2. Probably Inadequate:<br>Rarely eats a complete meal and generally eats only about 1/2 of any food offered. Protein intake includes only 3 servings of meat or dairy products per day. Occasionally will take a dietary supplement.<br>OR<br>receives less than optimum amount of liquid diet or tube feeding. | 3. Adequate:<br>Eats over half of most meals. Eats a total of 4 servings of protein (meat, dairy products) each day. Occasionally will refuse a meal, but will usually take a supplement if offered.<br>OR<br>is on a tube feeding or TPN regimen which probably meets most of nutritional needs. | 4. Excellent:<br>Eats most of every meal. Never refuses a meal. Usually eats a total of 4 or more servings of meat and dairy products. Occasionally eats between meals. Does not require supplementation. | |
| FRICTION AND SHEAR | 1. Problem:<br>Requires moderate to maximum assistance in moving. Complete lifting without sliding against sheets is impossible. Frequently slides down in bed or chair, requiring frequent repositioning with maximum assistance. Spasticity, contractures or agitation leads to almost constant friction. | 2. Potential Problem:<br>Moves feebly or requires minimum assistance. During a move skin probably slides to some extent against sheets, chair, restraints, or other devices. Maintains relatively good position in chair or bed most of the time but occasionally slides down. | 3. No Apparent Problem:<br>Moves in bed and in chair independently and has sufficient muscle strength to lift up completely during move. Maintains good position in bed or chair at all times. | | |

**Braden Scale Scores**
1 = Highly Impaired
3 or 4 = Moderate to Low Impairment
Total Points Possible: 23
Risk Predicting Score: 16 or Less

NPO: Nothing by Mouth

IV: Intravenously
TPN: Total parenteral nutrition

Total Score [ ]

**FIGURE 51-4** The Braden Scale is a widely used screening tool to identify people at risk for pressure ulcers. (Courtesy of Barbara Braden and Nancy Bergstrom. Copyright, 1988. Reprinted with permission.)

to treat. Critically ill patients are among those with the most significant limitations of these parameters, and therefore are at very high risk for the development of pressure ulcers.

Many tools for assessing pressure ulcer risk use a point system.[9,10] The Braden Scale for Predicting Pressure Sore Risk, recommended in the guidelines set forth by the U.S. Agency for Health Care Policy and Research and widely used in hospital settings, requires the daily assessment of six parameters and provides a numerical score ranging from a very high risk score of 6 to a very limited risk or minimal risk score of 23 (Fig. 51-4).[10] Adults with a score below 16 (18 for older adults) are considered at risk, and specific interventions to prevent the development of ulceration are recommended.

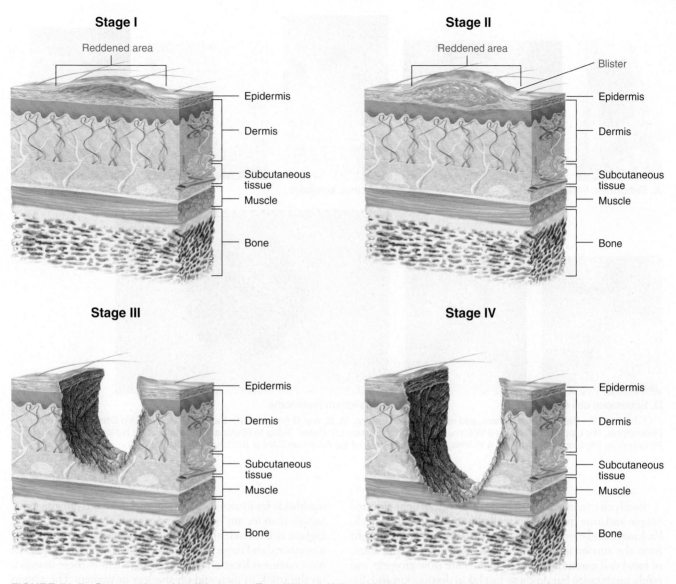

FIGURE 51-5    Pressure ulcers: identifying stage. (From Weber J, Kelley J: Health Assessment in Nursing, 4th ed. Philadelphia, PA: Wolters Kluwer Health/Lippincott Williams & Wilkins, 2010, pp 194–195.)

Studies suggest that stage 1 pressure ulcers are less likely to be identified in dark-skinned people, leading to higher incidence of pressure ulcers discovered at stage 2. Because erythema, the hallmark of stage 1 pressure ulcers, is not always easily detected in patients with darker skin tones, the National Pressure Ulcer Advisory Panel recommends assessing heat, edema, induration, or change in consistency in relation to surrounding skin as indicators of early tissue damage.[9]

During assessment of the skin, the nurse must be vigilant for signs of skin breakdown. The formation of pressure ulcers is illustrated in Figure 51-5. See Chapter 52 for the management of skin integrity.

## Assessment of Skin Tumors

Benign nevi and seborrheic keratoses are common, benign skin lesions. The benign nevus or mole appears in the first two to three decades, and its appearance remains unchanged over time. These lesions have clearly defined borders, are uniform in color, and are round or oval. The nevus is periodically assessed for changes because a change may indicate dysplasia of the tissue and the risk of melanoma. Seborrheic keratoses are common yellow to brown lesions that are described as velvety when touched (Fig. 51-6A). These lesions are often multiple and often symmetrically distributed on the trunk and face. Precancerous lesions (actinic keratoses) are thick, rough patches that develop on sun-exposed areas of the skin, especially in fair-skinned people (see Fig. 51-6B). They are described as dry, scaly, and rough textured; however, not all actinic keratoses look alike.[11] The color may vary from brown to red to yellowish-black, or they may appear as red bumps or scaly patches. They are often described as feeling like sandpaper. These lesions require attention because a few will develop into squamous cell carcinoma.[11,12]

Skin cancer is the most common type of cancer in the United States. In 2014, there were more than 3 million squamous or basal cell cancer diagnoses and more than 76,000 diagnoses of melanoma.[12] Basal cell and squamous cell cancers are often grouped as nonmelanoma skin cancers.

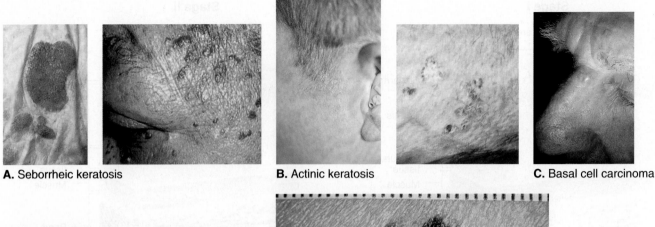

**A.** Seborrheic keratosis  **B.** Actinic keratosis  **C.** Basal cell carcinoma

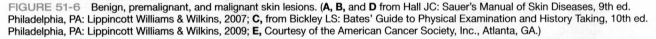

**D.** Squamous cell carcinoma  **E.** Malignant melanoma

**FIGURE 51-6**  Benign, premalignant, and malignant skin lesions. (**A, B,** and **D** from Hall JC: Sauer's Manual of Skin Diseases, 9th ed. Philadelphia, PA: Lippincott Williams & Wilkins, 2007; **C,** from Bickley LS: Bates' Guide to Physical Examination and History Taking, 10th ed. Philadelphia, PA: Lippincott Williams & Wilkins, 2009; **E,** Courtesy of the American Cancer Society, Inc., Atlanta, GA.)

Basal cell carcinomas are found exclusively in light-skinned people and arise from the hair follicles on the head and neck. Prolonged and cumulative exposure to ultraviolet (UV) light from the sun or indoor tanning is recognized as the cause of basal cell carcinoma. These tumors are slow growing and rarely metastasize but do cause local skin destruction and disfigurement. Basal cell carcinomas appear with pearly, raised borders and depressed centers (see Fig. 51-6C).[1]

Squamous cell carcinomas affect the skin and the mucous membranes. Like basal cell cancers, the primary cause is exposure to UV light. Radiation and tissue damage from scars, ulcers, and fistulas may give rise to squamous cell carcinomas. These cancers can be invasive and are more malignant than basal cell cancers if not treated promptly. As it develops, the carcinoma takes on a hyperkeratotic appearance and may ulcerate and bleed (see Fig. 51-6D).[12]

Malignant melanomas are highly metastatic lesions that come from the melanin-producing cells of the body. The worldwide frequency of malignant melanomas is growing more rapidly than for any other cancer except lung cancer. Those at highest risk include those with fair complexions, those prone to sunburn, and those with a family history of melanoma.[12] The most common location for the development of these lesions is on the trunk in men and on the legs in women. The tumors have irregular borders, are dark brown or black, and are usually larger than 6 mm (see Fig. 51-6E). The American Cancer Society[12] recommends a monthly self-assessment for melanoma using the "ABCDs": A is for asymmetry; B is for borders (are they irregular, ragged, notched, or blurred?); C is for color (dark brown or black, red, white, or blue?); and D is for diameter.

It is possible for the nurse in the critical care setting to perform a thorough assessment of a patient for suspect skin lesions that may be cancerous; the nurse may then refer the patient with a suspicious lesion to a dermatologist or oncologist, prompting the initiation of treatment much sooner than would otherwise be the case.

# Clinical Applicability Challenges

## CASE STUDY

Ms. Q. is a 49-year-old woman who was admitted to the intensive care unit 3 weeks ago with sepsis from a gangrenous foot. She has severe peripheral vascular disease, peripheral neuropathy, and chronic pain from a back injury since a motor vehicle accident 15 years ago for which she required a walker before this admission. Ms. Q. has diabetes mellitus, obesity, and impaired renal function. She has fluid volume overload and is undergoing diuresis, but she has moderate to severe edema in all extremities. Her right foot was amputated 1 week ago.

On day 2 of intravenous antibiotic therapy with Zosyn (piperacillin and tazobactam) through her left arm peripherally inserted central catheter, Ms. Q. develops a generalized petechial rash over her trunk and legs and complains of itching.

1. What factors increase Ms. Q.'s risk of a hypersensitivity reaction?
2. What orders does the nurse anticipate from the provider based upon this recent assessment?
3. What two factors related to Ms. Q.'s comorbid condition of diabetes mellitus increase her risk of gangrenous foot ulcer?

## WANT TO KNOW MORE?

A wide variety of resources to enhance your learning and understanding of this chapter are available on thePoint.

You will find:

- References
- Selected readings
- NCLEX-style review questions
- Internet resources
- And more!

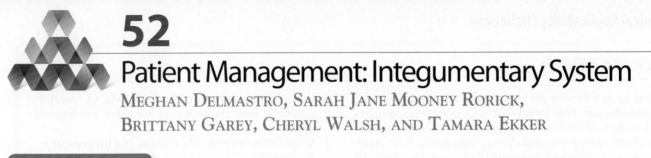

# 52

# Patient Management: Integumentary System

Meghan Delmastro, Sarah Jane Mooney Rorick,
Brittany Garey, Cheryl Walsh, and Tamara Ekker

## LEARNING OBJECTIVES

**Based on the content in this chapter, the reader should be able to:**

1. Explain the difference between pressure ulcers, leg ulcers, and skin tears.
2. Define specific terms related to wounds, including *acute wound, chronic wound, partial thickness, full thickness,* and *stages of wound healing.*
3. Explain the normal wound healing process.
4. Describe the different aspects of wound assessment and documentation.
5. Describe what is meant by *primary intention, secondary intention,* and *tertiary intention.*
6. Describe nursing care for patients with different types of wounds, including cleansing, debridement, wound dressings, pain management, and patient education.
7. Discuss the influence of nutrition and pharmacotherapy on wound healing.

Nursing management of wounds is both challenging and rewarding. Effective wound care requires a sound knowledge base and meticulous method. This chapter discusses types of wounds, including pressure ulcers, leg ulcers, and skin tears; the wound healing process; and nursing assessment, management, and patient teaching related to serious wounds that need ongoing care.

## Types of Wounds

A wound is a break in skin integrity. Wounds may be acute or chronic. An acute wound is a wound that follows an orderly, sequential healing process, resulting in an area that has anatomical and functional integrity.[1,2] Acute wounds are caused by surgery or trauma. Conversely, a chronic wound fails to yield an area that has anatomical and functional integrity. Chronic wounds fail to follow an orderly, sequential process because of precipitating factors such as diabetes, pressure, malnutrition, peripheral vascular disease, immune deficiencies, and infection.[1,2] An acute wound may become a chronic wound at any time.

Acute and chronic wounds may be defined as partial- or full-thickness wounds. Partial-thickness wounds involve the epidermis and may involve the dermis. A partial-thickness wound is a shallow wound that is usually moist and painful. The loss of the epidermis exposes nerve endings in the wound bed, creating the pain sensation in these superficial wounds. Full-thickness wounds involve the loss of the epidermis, dermis, and subcutaneous tissue, and they may involve muscle, tendons, ligaments, and bone. A full-thickness wound involves a large amount of tissue loss and appears as a crater or crevice. Pain sensation in full thickness wounds varies significantly.[1]

Pressure ulcers and leg ulcers are two specific types of wounds that may be seen in the critical care setting. Critically ill patients are at risk for developing pressure ulcers related to hemodynamic factors, disease processes, immobility, and nutritional deficits. Leg ulcers are due to specific disease processes. Both pressure ulcers and leg ulcers may complicate the critically ill patient's overall recovery.

The distinction between pressure ulcers and other types of wounds is essential. Current literature suggests that not all pressure ulcers are preventable; however, many health insurance providers, including Medicare and Medicaid, do not reimburse acute care facilities for Stage III and Stage IV pressure ulcer management if the wound developed during the current patient hospitalization.[3] This is an additional reason why accurate initial skin assessment is necessary.

### Pressure Ulcers

Pressure ulcers are wounds caused by pressure, shearing, and friction. Pressure ulcers start as acute wounds but become chronic in patients who have other risk factors. Risk factors for the development of pressure ulcers include prolonged and impaired mobility, incontinence, malnutrition, diabetes, spinal cord injuries, metastatic cancers, decreased level of consciousness, impaired mental status, and peripheral vascular disease.[1,2,4,5] A teaching guide for pressure ulcers is shown in Box 52-1.

A pressure ulcer is the only type of wound that is staged. Staging occurs when the wound is assessed and documented.

- **Stage I** is defined as nonblanchable erythema of intact skin. In patients with darker skin, the stage I pressure ulcer may be red, blue, or purple. It may be accompanied by hardness, induration, and edema.
- **Stage II** involves partial-thickness tissue loss and presents as a fluid-filled blistered or denuded area (a shallow open wound).
- **Stage III** is a full-thickness wound involving the subcutaneous tissue and presents as a crater.
- **Stage IV** is also a full-thickness wound involving a large amount of tissue loss. A Stage IV wound extends through the subcutaneous tissue and deep into the fascia, involving muscle, bone, ligament, or tendon.

- A pressure ulcer designated **unstageable** is covered by eschar (black, brown, tan) or slough (yellow, brown, gray, green, or tan), which prevents assessment of the wound bed. The wound must be débrided prior to staging.
- **Suspected deep tissue injury** is evidenced by a localized maroon or purple discolored area of intact skin or a blood-filled blister. The area is usually tender, mushy, or boggy.[4,5]

Reverse staging is inappropriate for pressure ulcers, because the tissue that fills in the wound bed is not the same as the tissue that has been lost. Lost muscle or subcutaneous tissue cannot be replaced. Therefore, it is appropriate to document "healing stage IV wound," but it is not appropriate to document "stage IV wound now stage III."

Pressure ulcers covered by eschar or slough are documented as "unstageable, wound covered by eschar/slough." If the wound is débrided, it may then be staged.

## Leg Ulcers

Leg ulcers are chronic wounds seen frequently in critically ill patients who have underlying health problems; they include venous stasis ulcers, arterial ulcers, and diabetic foot ulcers. Although patients with leg ulcers may be at high risk for pressure ulcers, leg ulcers are not pressure ulcers and are not staged.

### Venous Stasis Ulcers

Venous stasis ulcers are usually found on the medial aspect of the lower leg, superior to the medial malleolus.[1,2] The wound margins are irregular and present as shallow craters, and the wound margins and lower leg may have a ruddy appearance or hemosiderin staining.[1,2] The drainage from venous stasis ulcers may vary from mild to heavy. The primary treatment is compression therapy using an Unna boot or a multiple-wrap dressing.[1,2] Multiple-wrap dressings have the advantage of continuous compression, which may not be achieved with the Unna boot. The affected leg is elevated above heart level to decrease edema (edema impedes the healing process).

### Arterial Ulcers

Arterial ulcers (ischemic ulcers) are usually found on the distal leg, medial malleoli, or dorsal aspect of the foot and toes.[1,2]

The wound margins of arterial ulcers are round, smooth, well defined (*not* irregular), and frequently described as having a "punched-out" appearance.[1,2] Arterial ulcers have pale wound beds and may be shallow or deep. The affected leg may be cool to the touch, cyanotic, and pale with minimal hair distribution. The patient experiences increased pain to the affected area if the leg is elevated.[1,2] The primary dressing for arterial leg ulcers is an occlusive dressing. Healing does not occur unless the vascular deficit is addressed surgically and arterial circulation is restored.

### Diabetic Foot Ulcers

Diabetic foot ulcers are found in patients who have diabetes; they are frequently not initially recognized by the patient, owing to the patient's accompanying neuropathy. The primary locations for diabetic foot ulcers are the plantar aspect of the foot, the heels, and the metatarsals.[1,2] To promote wound healing, a dressing that provides a moist environment is most often used. The ulcer area usually needs débridement and must be assessed carefully for infection. Other treatment modalities include off-loading the patient's weight using special shoes. Osteomyelitis is always a concern in patients with diabetic foot ulcers. Healing is prolonged because of the diabetes. Therefore, it is important to aggressively manage the diabetes to promote an optimal healing environment.

## Skin Tears

Skin tears (partial-thickness wounds) are acute wounds secondary to the removal of tape or transparent occlusive dressings. Skin tears occur when the skin is thin and so fragile that it tears as tape or plastic film dressings are removed. Fragile skin may be due to age, disease process, nutritional status, drug therapy (ie, steroids), or a combination of these factors.

It is a common misconception that plastic film dressings, wound closure strips (Steri-Strips), or wound adhesives should be applied to skin tears. However, it is important to minimize the use of adhesives in all forms for patients prone to skin tears. Plastic film dressings and Steri-Strips potentiate more skin tears as they are removed or become dislodged. Because it is difficult to approximate the wound margins in a skin tear, wound adhesive frequently drips into the wound bed, prolonging healing and promoting infection.

Skin tears should be cleansed gently with normal saline solution or another institution-approved cleanser. Care is taken not to create a larger skin tear. After the wound area is cleansed, a hydrogel is applied to the wound and covered with a nonadherent dressing. The wound is wrapped with a self-adherent wrap, such as Kling or Coban, to hold the dressing in place without using tape on the skin.

## Wound Healing

Optimal wound healing occurs in a moist (not extremely wet or dry) environment.

### Phases of Wound Healing

The wound-healing process consists of three phases (Fig. 52-1). The first phase is the *inflammatory phase*, which occurs immediately after the wound occurs. At the time of injury, there is immediate vasoconstriction; this is the body's way of controlling bleeding. Once vasoconstriction occurs, platelets collect at the site and deposit fibrin to form a clot. The vasoconstriction

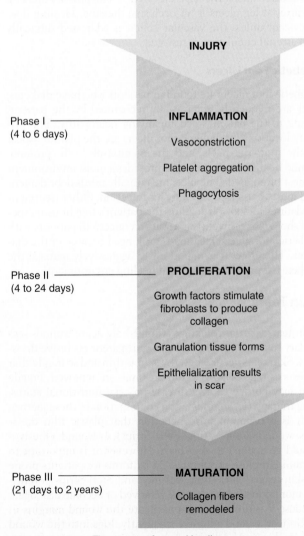

FIGURE 52-1  The stages of wound healing.

**Phase I** (4 to 6 days) — **INFLAMMATION**

Vasoconstriction

Platelet aggregation

Phagocytosis

**Phase II** (4 to 24 days) — **PROLIFERATION**

Growth factors stimulate fibroblasts to produce collagen

Granulation tissue forms

Epithelialization results in scar

**Phase III** (21 days to 2 years) — **MATURATION**

Collagen fibers remodeled

**INJURY**

---

**BOX 52-2**   *CONSIDERATIONS for the Older Patient*

**Factors That Affect Wound Healing**
- Less subcutaneous tissue
- More fragile skin secondary to age and drug therapy
- Increased number of precipitating risk factors for pressure ulcers
- Increased number of precipitating risk factors for chronic wounds
- Nutrition: Less than or more than body requirements
- Decreased ability to care for self with age
- Decreased immune system function
- Decreased pulmonary and cardiovascular function
- Increased potential for incontinence (urine and stool)

---

holds the wound together, and the platelets, with their fibrin clot formation, essentially "plug the hole." Phagocytosis also occurs during the inflammatory phase. Phagocytosis is the release of macrophages at the site of injury to destroy any bacteria that may be present and to remove the wound's cellular debris. This is the body's way of providing the optimal environment for wound healing (ie, a clean wound bed). It is at this time that growth factors are also present at the site of the injury. Overall, the inflammatory phase is estimated to last between 4 and 6 days. Visual assessment of the wound during the inflammatory phase reveals a wound with erythema and edema, and the patient experiences pain.

The second phase of wound healing is the *proliferation phase*. Growth factors stimulate the fibroblast to produce collagen. Collagen, along with new blood vessels and connective tissue, creates granulation tissue. Visual assessment of the wound at this point reveals a wound that is beefy red and shiny with a grainy or bumpy appearance. The appearance of granulation tissue prompts the wound margins to contract. Pulling together of the wound edges decreases the overall size of the wound. The last step of the proliferation phase is *epithelialization* or *reepithelialization*. Epithelialization results in a scar. The estimated overall duration of the proliferation phase is anywhere from 4 to 24 days.

The third and final phase of wound healing is the *maturation phase*, during which the collagen fibers are remodeled; this increases the tensile strength of the scar tissue. It has been estimated that only 70% to 80% of the skin's original strength is attained when the wound is healed. The maturation phase can extend from 21 days to 2 years. The outcome is always an area of tissue that is at greater risk for breakdown and more fragile than undamaged tissue.

If the wound becomes extremely wet or dry, the phases of wound healing occur at a slower rate. This may affect the final quality of the scar tissue with respect to anatomical and functional integrity as well as tensile strength. The patient's age and physical status also have an impact on the healing process (Box 52-2). Other factors that affect wound healing are listed in Table 52-1.

### Methods of Wound Healing

Wounds can heal through primary intention, secondary intention, or tertiary intention (Fig. 52-2).

Acute or surgical wounds typically heal by *primary intention*. The edges of the wound are drawn together (approximated);

| TABLE 52-1 | Factors Affecting Wound Healing | |
|---|---|---|
| **Factors** | **Rationale** | **Nursing Interventions** |
| Age of patient | The older the patient, the less resilient the tissues. | Handle all tissues gently. |
| Handling of tissues | Rough handling causes injury and delayed healing. | Handle tissues carefully and evenly. |
| Hemorrhage | Accumulation of blood creates dead spaces as well as dead cells that must be removed. The area becomes a growth medium for organisms. | Monitor vital signs. Observe incision site for evidence of bleeding and infection. |
| Hypovolemia | Insufficient blood volume leads to vasoconstriction and reduced oxygen and nutrients available for wound healing. | Monitor for volume deficit (circulatory impairment). Correct by fluid replacement as prescribed. |
| **Local Factors** | | |
| Edema | Reduces blood supply by exerting increased interstitial pressure on vessels | Elevate edematous part; apply cool compresses. |
| Inadequate dressing technique<br>  Too small<br>  Too tight | Permits bacterial invasion and contamination<br>Reduces blood supply carrying nutrients and oxygen | Follow guidelines for proper dressing technique. |
| Nutritional deficits | Protein–calorie depletion may occur.<br>Insulin secretion may be inhibited, causing blood glucose level to rise. | Correct deficits; this may require parenteral nutritional therapy.<br>Monitor blood glucose levels.<br>Administer vitamin supplements as prescribed. |
| Foreign bodies | Foreign bodies retard healing. | Keep wounds free of dressing threads and talcum and powder from gloves. |
| Oxygen deficit (tissue oxygenation insufficient) | Insufficient oxygen may be due to inadequate lung and cardiovascular function as well as localized vasoconstriction. | Encourage deep breathing, turning, controlled coughing. |
| Drainage accumulation | Accumulated secretions hamper healing process. | Monitor closed drainage systems for proper functioning.<br>Institute measures to remove accumulated secretions. |
| **Medications** | | |
| Corticosteroids | May mask presence of infection by impairing normal inflammatory response | Be aware of action and effect of medications patient is receiving. |
| Anticoagulants | May cause hemorrhage | |
| Broad-spectrum and specific antibiotics | Effective if administered immediately before surgery for specific pathology or bacterial contamination. If administered after wound is closed, ineffective because of intravascular coagulation. | |
| Patient overactivity | Prevents approximation of wound edges. Resting favors healing. | Use measures to keep wound edges approximated: taping, bandaging, splints.<br>Encourage rest. |
| Systemic disorders<br>  Hemorrhagic shock<br>  Acidosis<br>  Hypoxia<br>  Renal failure<br>  Hepatic disease<br>  Sepsis | These depress cell functions that directly affect wound healing. | Be familiar with the nature of the specific disorder. Administer prescribed treatment. Cultures may be indicated to determine appropriate antibiotic. |
| Immunosuppressed state | Patient is more vulnerable to bacterial and viral invasion; defense mechanisms are impaired. | Provide maximum protection to prevent infection. Restrict visitors with colds; institute mandatory hand hygiene by all staff. |
| Wound stressors<br>  Vomiting<br>  Valsalva maneuver<br>  Heavy coughing<br>  Straining | Produce tension on wounds, particularly of the torso. | Encourage frequent turning and ambulation and administer antiemetic medications as prescribed. Assist patient in splinting incision. |

From Smeltzer SC, Bare BG, Hinkle JL, et al: Brunner & Suddarth's Textbook of Medical–Surgical Nursing, 13th ed. Philadelphia, PA: Lippincott Williams & Wilkins, 2014.

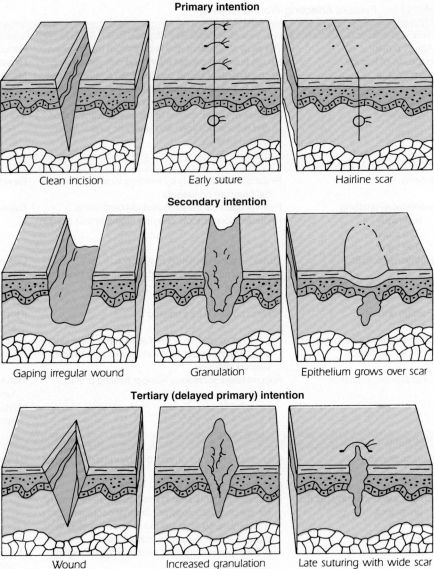

**Primary intention**

Clean incision    Early suture    Hairline scar

**Secondary intention**

Gaping irregular wound    Granulation    Epithelium grows over scar

**Tertiary (delayed primary) intention**

Wound    Increased granulation    Late suturing with wide scar

**FIGURE 52-2** Types of wound healing: primary intention healing, secondary intention healing, and tertiary intention healing.

(Adapted from Smeltzer SC, Bare BG, Hinkle JL, et al: Brunner & Suddarth's Textbook of Medical–Surgical Nursing, 13th ed. Philadelphia, PA: Lippincott Williams & Wilkins, 2014.)

this shortens the time required for the wound to heal to about 4 to 14 days overall. Primary intention is associated with a decreased risk of infection, minimal scarring, and decreased tissue loss.

Healing by *secondary intention* is seen most frequently in chronic wounds but can occur in acute wounds, when the wound edges cannot be approximated to each other because of a significant tissue loss. Examples of wounds that heal by secondary intention are pressure ulcers and venous stasis ulcers. The potential for infection is increased because of the inability to approximate the edges, thus leaving the area open to bacteria. Scarring may also be significant, depending on the amount of tissue loss.

The last form of wound repair is *tertiary intention*, which may also be called *delayed primary intention*. Tertiary (delayed primary) intention should not be confused with primary intention. With this type of wound healing, the wound is not closed for a period (usually 3 to 5 days) to allow infection, edema, or both, to resolve. During this time, the wound is packed or irrigated to remove exudate and cellular debris. When the edema and risk for infection have decreased, the

wound edges are approximated, and the wound is closed as it is in primary intention. Scarring is usually greater than that seen with primary intention but less than that seen with secondary intention.

## Wound Assessment

Wound assessment is performed in an orderly, sequential manner (Box 52-3). The location of the wound is defined as precisely as possible using anatomical terminology (eg, "medial aspect of the left lower leg, 10 cm distal to the knee"); this allows other healthcare professionals to visualize the location of the wound. Correct location is especially important if the patient has more than one wound. If photography is used to document the location and progression of the wound, room lighting and distance from the wound must be as identical as possible from one photograph to another to portray the wound accurately and consistently. Photography is used more frequently for chronic wounds than acute wounds.

BOX 52-3 Wound Assessment

**Location:** Document the location, using anatomical positions.

**Size:** Document the size, in centimeters or millimeters. Measure the length (by clock positions) from the 12- to 6-o'clock position. Measure the width from the 9- to 3-o'clock position.

**Depth:** Use a sterile swab to determine the depth of the wound (see Fig. 52-4).

**Undermining or tunneling:** Document the presence or absence of undermining or tunneling (see Fig. 52-5).

**Tissue type:** Describe the wound bed. If the wound bed is not visible, document the presence and condition of the eschar (scab), sutures, staples, or other wound closure.

**Drainage:** Note the presence or absence of drainage. If drainage is present, describe its odor, color, amount, and consistency.

**Wound margins:** Describe the wound margins (approximation, condition, and appearance of surrounding tissue).

**Drains and tubes:** Note the type of drain or tubing and its location (using anatomical or clock positions).

**Condition of dressing:** Describe the amount and type of drainage on the dressing, as well as the ease with which the dressing was removed.

**Pain:** Evaluate on a 0 to 10 scale (or other institution-approved assessment scale). Provide pain relief as needed before, during, and after wound assessment or dressing change.

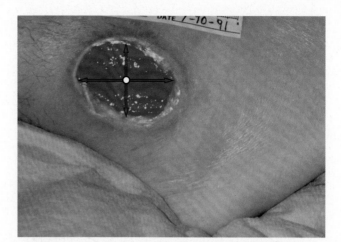

**FIGURE 52-3** Wound measurement. Linear measurements of a wound should be taken at the greatest length and width perpendicular to each other, as shown.

(From Baranoski S, Ayello EA: Wound Care and Essentials Practice Principles, 3rd ed. Philadelphia, PA: Lippincott Williams & Wilkins, 2012.)

**MEASURING THE WOUND.** The size of the wound should always be measured in centimeters, millimeters, or both.[2,4] Terminology such as "the size of a half dollar" should be avoided because it leads to inconsistent and inaccurate documentation. Linear measurements of a wound are taken at the greatest length and width, perpendicular to each other (Fig. 52-3).

Depth of the wound is measured by placing a sterile swab in the deepest area of the wound and marking the location of the wound's margin on the swab.[2] The sterile swab is dipped in normal saline solution before inserting it into the wound to minimize the potential of leaving cotton fibers in the wound. After removing the swab, measure from the distal tip of the swab to the area that was marked (Fig. 52-4). Documentation includes the depth in centimeters and also the location where the assessment was made (eg, "depth 5.8 cm in the distal wound bed in the 9-o'clock position"). Clear, concise documentation allows other healthcare professionals

to reassess the wound depth in the same area with each reevaluation.

**UNDERMINING AND TUNNELING.** Undermining and tunneling do not occur in acute wounds but can begin in acute wounds, so the nurse always assesses the wound for their presence. Undermining occurs when there is the loss of tissue along the wound margins, the "lip of tissue."[2] Tunneling is exactly what it implies: a tunnel opening somewhere in the wound bed. Tunneling can begin in acute wounds in which there are drains. (Note that if tunneling occurs, the wound is no longer considered an acute wound but has become a chronic wound.) A sinus tract is an opening somewhere in the wound bed that extends into the tissue, ending with a small pocket of open area. The process for assessing the direction and depth of tunneling is shown in Figure 52-5.

**WOUND MARGINS.** The wound margins are also assessed when performing a wound assessment. Are the edges well approximated? Is the surrounding tissue clean, dry, reddened, edematous, pale, intact, or blistered? Again, it is important

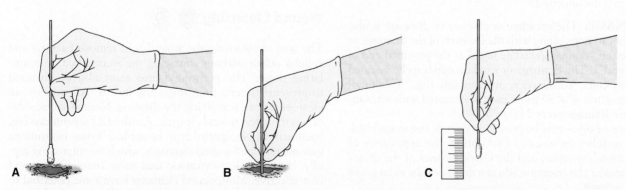

**FIGURE 52-4** Procedure for measuring wound depth. **A:** Put on gloves. Gently insert the swab into the deepest portion of the wound that you can see. **B:** Grasp the swab with your thumb and forefinger at the point corresponding to the wound margin. **C:** Carefully withdraw the swab while maintaining the position of your thumb and forefinger. Measure from the tip of the swab to that position.

(From Hess CT: Clinical Guide to Skin and Wound Care, 7th ed. Philadelphia, PA: Lippincott Williams & Wilkins, 2013.)

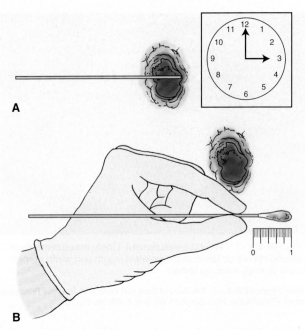

**A**

**B**

**FIGURE 52-5** Procedure for determining the direction and depth of tunneling. **A:** To assess the direction of tunneling, put on gloves and insert the swab into the sites where tunneling occurs. Progressing in a clockwise direction, document the deepest sites where the wound tunnels. (Twelve o'clock points in the direction of the patient's head, so in this example, tunneling occurs at three o'clock.) **B:** To assess the depth of tunneling, insert the swab into the tunneling areas, and grasp the swab where it meets the wound margin. Remove the swab, place it next to a measuring guide, and document the measurement centimeters.

(From Hess CT: Clinical Guide to Skin and Wound Care, 7th ed. Philadelphia, PA: Lippincott Williams & Wilkins, 2013.)

to be as exact as possible to paint an accurate picture of the wound margins for the next healthcare professional.

**TISSUE TYPE.** Determining the tissue type entails visual assessment of the wound bed. The tissue in the wound bed should be beefy red (as opposed to pale). The presence or absence of granulation tissue (shiny red, grainy, or bumpy tissue) is noted. The nurse assesses for necrotic tissue, which presents as black or brown tissue. Slough may also be present in the wound bed. Slough is yellow and stringy. If the wound bed is not visible, the presence or absence of eschar, sutures, staples, Steri-Strips, wound adhesives, or negative pressure dressings is documented.

**DRAINAGE.** The presence or absence of drainage is also important to note, along with the location of the drainage or exudate (eg, "drainage/exudate noted at the proximal end of the wound"). The drainage or exudate needs to be assessed for odor, color, consistency, and amount (eg, "abdominal dressing of ten 4″ × 4″ gauze pads is saturated with serosanguineous drainage every 2 hours").

Drains or tubes may be present in or near the wound bed. Drains or tubes are assessed for location, the appearance of the surrounding tissue, and the characteristics of the drainage. Consider the insertion site of a drain or tube as an acute wound in itself.

**DRESSING.** The dressing is assessed after it is removed. The soiled dressing's condition (eg, "saturated"), the ease with which the dressing was removed (eg, "sticking"), and

the location and type of drainage on the dressing are described. If the dressing came off without being removed by the nurse, this is noted as well (eg, "dressing found lying in bed—wound uncovered").

**PAIN.** Pain is assessed using an institution-approved standardized scale, such as the 0 to 10 scale. The patient should never be in pain while a wound is being assessed. If the patient experiences pain during wound assessment, the assessment should be stopped, and the patient should be medicated before continuing. Management of pain as it relates to wound assessment and care is discussed in more detail later in this chapter.

**DOCUMENTATION.** Wound documentation includes all descriptions and measurements, the presence and absence of pain during the procedure, and the type of dressing applied.[1,2,4,5] Many institutions use special wound measurement tools, wound assessment tools, and documentation tools (eg, flow sheets or computerized documentation) for wound documentation. Per Medicare guidelines, the presence or absence of wounds must be documented upon admission by both the physician and the nurse.

## Wound Care

### Wound Care Standards

The standards of wound care are established by the Agency for Healthcare Research and Quality (AHRQ), the Wound Ostomy and Continence Nurses (WOCN), the National Pressure Ulcer Advisory Panel (NPUAP), and the European Pressure Ulcer Advisory Panel (EPUAP). The most recent standards of care were set by the NPUAP and the EPUAP in 2014 and are considered the "gold standard." These standards, which are supported by evidence-based practice, guide institution policy and procedure. The Wound Ostomy and Continence Nurses Society (WOCN) issues clinical practice guidelines that apply evidence-based practice, new research and drugs, and the AHRQ standards.[6] The most current guidelines from these organizations are available through the organizations' websites. A free resource for practice guidelines is the National Guideline Clearinghouse, maintained by the Agency for Healthcare Research and Quality, a division of the US Department of Health and Human Services.[7]

### Wound Cleansing

The goal of cleansing the wound is to remove bacteria and cellular debris without damaging the wound bed or granulating tissue. The periwound area must also be cleansed to prevent bacteria from migrating into it. All wounds are cleansed before reapplying the dressing. Normal saline solution is the safest wound cleanser. Antibiotic preparations (eg, bacitracin or Neosporin) may be applied. Some institutions may use prepared wound cleansers, which are improving rapidly, becoming less cytotoxic and more time-efficient and cost-effective. Most wound cleansers have some potential to destroy granulating tissue (compared with normal saline solution) but are less toxic to granulating tissue than hydrogen peroxide or Betadine, which should be avoided. Other solutions to avoid when cleansing wounds are povidone–iodine, acetic acid, and sodium hypochlorite (Dakin solution). These solutions are toxic to epithelial cells and thus impede granulation and wound healing.

Open wounds are cleansed starting in the middle and moving outward in a circular motion to include the peri-wound area. Incisions are cleansed from top to bottom, again starting in the middle and moving outward to include the periwound area.

Impregnated gauzes for packing and various solutions (eg, Betadine and Dakin solution) may be used in the event that the wound is infected; however, they should not be used as a routine wound treatment for a prolonged time because they destroy granulating tissue and inhibit the normal healing process. Remember that the use of these products signals that the wound is not an acute wound but has become a chronic wound.

## Wound Débridement

At times, both acute wounds (ie, grafts) and chronic wounds need to be débrided. Débridement is the removal of necrotic (dead) or devitalized tissue. Necrotic or devitalized tissue presents as dark brown, black, yellow, pale, cyanotic, or crusty eschar and can result in a longer inflammatory process, decreased blood circulation, and increased bacterial growth.[1] To promote optimal wound healing, this tissue needs to be removed from the wound. The débridement process creates an "acute wound," and initiates the three phases of wound healing.

There are several methods of débridement: autolytic, chemical, mechanical, and laser. Occasionally, a combination of débridement methods may be used during different phases of the healing process. Combination therapy depends on the type of wound and its location, the patient's status, and physician preference.

### Autolytic Débridement

In autolytic débridement, the body breaks down necrotic or devitalized tissue through the use of endogenous enzymes.[1] This type of débridement is not the optimal choice for wounds that have large amounts of necrotic tissue. Autolytic débridement takes time: the body must use its own ability to lyse and dissolve necrotic tissue. Hydrocolloid dressings are frequently used to promote autolytic débridement.

### Chemical Débridement

Chemical débridement is accomplished using enzyme-based drugs that are applied topically to the wound. These agents dissolve nonviable tissue found within the wound bed.[1] Collagenase-based products such as Collagenase Santyl are the most commonly used enzymes for chemical debridement.

### Mechanical Débridement

Mechanical débridement can be accomplished by wet-to-dry dressings, whirlpool procedures, or ultrasound treatment. When using mechanical débridement, it is important to maintain awareness of the potential damage that can occur to the healthy tissue. Although wet-to-dry dressings are an effective method of débridement, they are not the primary treatment recommendation; care must be taken to change

to another method of wound care once the wound bed is dé-brided.

Hydrotherapy (whirlpool) can be effective for the treatment of larger wounds; however, the potential for infection is increased with multiple patients using the whirlpools.[1] There is also increased risk of wound maceration, which increases tissue loss and impedes wound closure. Ultrasound therapy is more often used for chronic wounds. However, studies have found it to be more effective for wound healing rather than débridement.[8]

### Sharps or Surgical Débridement

Surgical débridement can be performed using various techniques. Most commonly, a scalpel or scissors is used to clear the wound of all necrotic and devitalized tissue. Hydrosurgery is a relatively new technique that allows a surgeon to target the necrotic or devitalized tissue through the use of a high-velocity waterjet.[8] These surgical procedures may require anesthesia, intravenous conscious sedation, a local anesthetic, or a combination of the three.

### Laser Débridement

Laser débridement may also be used to provide a clean wound bed. Currently, laser débridement is not performed as frequently as autolytic, chemical, and mechanical débridement. Initial studies have shown this technique to be effective in the treatment of chronic wounds.[8]

### Biosurgical Débridement

Biosurgical débridement is the instillation of sterile larvae (maggots) into a wound. These sterile larvae selectively digest necrotic or devitalized tissue. However, this treatment may not be accepted well by the patient.[1]

## Wound Closure

The goal of all wound care is ultimately the closure of the wound and restoration of skin integrity. Wound closure is usually promoted by various types of treatments and dressings.

### Sutures, Staples, and Wound Adhesives

Sutures or staples must be cleaned with sterile normal saline solution or a wound cleanser. Immediately after surgery, the wound needs to be covered with a dry sterile dressing. Frequently after the initial postoperative period, the staples or sutures are left open to air.

Wound adhesives may be used on surgical or traumatic wounds to approximate the wound margins: sutures are used to close the underlying tissue, and the wound adhesive is applied topically to the wound margins as they are drawn together. Wound adhesives are not placed in the wound bed (only on the margins) because this may lead to delayed wound healing or infection. The wound adhesive appears as a shiny, clear coating over the incision.

Caution is needed when applying wound adhesives because of their liquid status. Wound adhesives may inadvertently spread to other areas. Extreme caution must be exercised when using wound adhesives near the eyes. Incisions in which wound adhesives are used must not be rubbed or soaked with any wound cleaner. They may be gently rinsed. Steri-Strips should not be used in conjunction with wound adhesives. Wounds in which a wound adhesive has been used are left uncovered.

### Percutaneous Drains

A drain may be inserted in the wound to prevent the pooling of exudate in the wound bed, which decreases healing and increases the potential of infection or tunneling. The most common types of drains are Hemovac drains, Penrose drains, Jackson–Pratt drains, and chest tubes. Basic care of all drains and chest tubes includes cleansing with sterile normal saline solution and applying a dressing. The dressing stabilizes the drain and prevents the drain insertion site from coming in contact with drainage and other potentially infectious surfaces.

Drain and tube insertion sites are never left open to air because of the risk of infection. If drainage from another source may potentially saturate the dressing (over the drain site), the dressing also needs to be occlusive. Drain tubing is stabilized with tape to decrease the potential for inadvertent dislodgment, removal, and pain. Inadvertent removal of a drain potentiates pain and infection, and increases the risk that an acute wound may become chronic.

### Vacuum-Assisted Wound Closure (Negative Pressure Therapy)

Vacuum-assisted wound closure (VAC) is a system that assists wound closure by providing localized negative pressure to the wound bed and wound margins (Fig. 52-6). VAC therapy can be used on numerous types of acute and chronic wounds. VAC therapy promotes wound healing by reducing edema and removing excess fluid in the wound bed, which facilitates angiogenesis and increased wound perfusion. This therapy stimulates wound bed contraction and draws wound edges together.[9,10]

Tubing, similar to that of suction tubing, is placed into a special foam dressing. The foam dressing is shaped in wedges that are cut to fit the wound. The sponge wedge and tubing are then covered with an occlusive transparent dressing. The tube is then connected to the vacuum unit at low suction levels (as directed by the manufacturer). If the dressing is not collapsed, there is a leak in the system, and the dressing must be replaced with attention given to the transparent occlusive dressing application. The transparent occlusive dressing must be securely in place to maintain negative pressure in the wound. Dressings have the appearance of being "vacuum packed" when the dressing is secure and occlusive.

With the VAC system, granulation tissue is stimulated, infection and bacterial colonization are decreased, and wound closure occurs in a moist "vacuum" environment. In addition, the VAC system decreases the frequency of dressing changes, thus decreasing patient discomfort and nursing time.[9,10]

The VAC system should be used with extreme caution in patients with active bleeding, those who are on anticoagulant therapy, and patients with a history of uncontrolled bleeding.[9,10] The VAC system is contraindicated for any patient with untreated osteomyelitis, necrotic tissue with eschar, malignancies of the wound, or nonenteric and unexplored fistulas. The foam wedge dressing is not to be placed in direct contact with exposed blood vessels, organs, or nerves. VAC sponges must be positioned on viable tissue; therefore, if necrotic tissue or devitalized tissue is present, the wound needs to be débrided before the VAC sponges can be placed. The VAC system may be used in an infected wound but only with appropriate antibiotic therapy.[9,10]

The use of the VAC system continues to increase as clinical case studies show positive patient outcomes in grafts, flaps, and orthopedic surgeries. The use of wound irrigations or instillations (antibiotics or anesthetic agents) in conjunction with this type of wound therapy is also promising.

VAC therapy has had an economic impact. It decreases the length of time for wound healing, as well as nursing labor, supplies, length of stay, complications, and hospital readmission, and it promotes the salvage of limbs.[9,10] In addition, this therapy has an emotional impact that can be directly related to the nursing diagnosis of Disturbed Body Image related to dysfunctional open wounds, scarring, or amputation.[11]

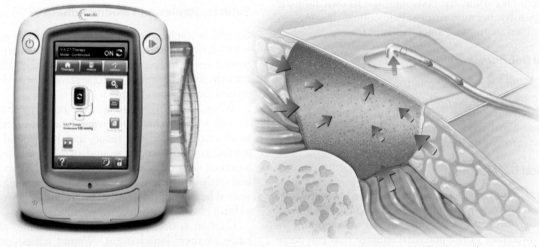

**FIGURE 52-6** A vacuum-assisted wound closure device (VAC) assists wound closure by providing localized negative pressure to the wound bed and wound margins.

It is the nurse's responsibility to be familiar with the operation and maintenance of the VAC system. Nursing responsibilities include wound assessment and documentation, along with placing the patient on the VAC system, changing the canister, and maintaining suction of the system. The wound should demonstrate progressive healing. If documentation fails to demonstrate progressive wound healing within 30 days, alternative therapies must be considered.

## Wound Dressings

The goal of wound dressings is to protect the wound from infection and promote a moist environment. There are hundreds of dressing products available. The dressing of choice depends on the wound characteristics, including tissue appearance, amount of exudate, and the patient's risk of infection.[1,12]

### Wet-to-Dry Dressings

A wound healing by secondary or tertiary intention is frequently packed with wet-to-dry dressings. The use of wet-to-dry dressings, or even simply dry dressings, is losing favor in the medical community owing to new studies that indicate that wounds heal faster with advanced wound dressings, such as those discussed below.[13] Wet-to-dry dressings have been shown to be detrimental to a healthy wound bed. Wounds need a moist environment to heal without impediment. Changing a wet-to-dry dressing every 8 or 12 hours leads to the dressing becoming exceptionally dry. Thus, when it is removed, indiscriminate débridement of both necrotic and granulating tissue occurs. This constant débriding of the wound (caused by frequent dressing changes) increases the patient's discomfort, promotes infection, slows the healing process, and may enlarge the wound. Wet-to-dry dressings affect not only wound healing but also healthcare costs by prolonging the healing time and increasing nursing labor and supply expenses.

### Hydrogels

Hydrogels are most often used for dry or necrotic wounds, such as arterial wounds, "dried out" venous stasis wounds, and vasculitic or rheumatologic ulcerations. They help maintain a moist wound environment, which promotes granulation, epithelialization, and autolytic débridement. Hydrogels have a water or glycerin base; they are available in sheets or gels that can be added to gauze packing to maintain moisture in the wound bed for longer periods of time.[1,12,14]

### Hydrocolloids

Hydrocolloids are most frequently used for minimally exudating wounds, such as in the care and treatment of stages I and II pressure ulcers and in the protection of hard-to-cover areas subject to friction. Hydrocolloids are occlusive, self-adhesive, and minimally absorptive. Hydrocolloids are advantageous because they are waterproof and only need to be changed every 3 to 5 days or if they are inadvertently removed. It is important to note that there is often a malodorous, yellow-brown drainage after removal of the dressing; this is normal in the absence of other signs of infection.[1] The manufacturer's recommendations should be consulted for

contraindications, which often include an actively infected wound bed.[1,12,13]

### Foam Dressings

Foam dressings are most frequently used for moderately draining wounds, such as stage II and III pressure ulcers, second-degree burns, and venous stasis ulcers. They are available in various shapes and sizes; some are self-adhesive while others may require a secondary dressing. When it is time to remove the foam dressing, it is simply lifted off the wound. Minimal trauma occurs to the wound bed and surrounding tissue. Foam dressings provide a moist wound environment that stimulates angiogenesis and autolysis.[1,12,14]

Contraindications to foam dressings vary according to the manufacturer. Caution should always be used if the wound is infected.

### Calcium Alginates and Hydrofiber Dressings

Wound healing by secondary or tertiary intention may also be promoted with calcium alginates or hydrofiber dressings. Calcium alginates are made from brown seaweed and are highly absorptive. They come in ropelike or flat pieces that must be "fluffed" and packed into the wound bed. Calcium alginates can hold up to 20 times their weight in wound drainage.[12,14]

Similar to calcium alginate, hydrofiber dressings are also for high exudating wounds. Made of carboxymethyl cellulose fibers, these dressings can hold up to three times as much drainage as the calcium alginates. They are available in sheets or ropes and can be used for wounds of various sizes. The dressing traps drainage and wound debris in its fibers, cleaning the wound and wicking away excess moisture.[12,14]

As the calcium alginate or hydrofiber dressing absorbs the wound drainage, its appearance changes from dry, fluffed strands to that of a gel that is easily removed from the wound. These dressings often need a secondary dressing and may be covered with foam, hydrocolloid, or a transparent dressing.[12,14]

Contraindications to calcium alginate and hydrofiber dressings vary and include dry nonexudating wounds; the manufacturers' information should be consulted for other contraindications.[12,13]

### Silver (Ag) Dressings

Silver dressings are dressings that have been impregnated with nanoparticles of the ion silver. Silver-impregnated dressings come in a variety of mediums, including foams, gels, creams, calcium alginates, and hydrofibers. These dressings have been shown to have anti-inflammatory and antimicrobial properties (they impede bacterial cell multiplication and migration). Many silver-impregnated dressings may be left in place for prolonged periods, which is advantageous for nursing care and patient self-care. Silver dressings work well in conjunction with other medical and pharmacotherapeutic treatments.[12,15]

### Honey Dressings

Medical Leptospermum honey, which is produced through a specific process, has been shown to have antibacterial effects and can help speed up wound healing. Leptospermum honey can be used as a gel or paste in dry wounds; a variety of dressing types impregnated with Leptospermum honey are also available for use in wounds with varying degrees of exudate.[16]

## Bilayered Dressings

Bilayered dressings are engineered dressings that are applied as "grafts" to wounds that fail to progress with other treatment modalities. These graft materials may be composed of fibroblast, collagen, and growth factors, depending on the type and brand. They act by giving the (noninfective) chronic wound a "jump start." Examples of these dressings are Apligraf, Integra, and Oasis. They are frequently used on venous stasis ulcers and diabetic foot ulcers or on exposed bone, tendon, or joints. The cost of these graft materials is much higher than conventional treatments; however, by "jump-starting" the process of wound healing, they may actually be more cost-effective in difficult cases.

## High-Volume Draining Wounds

Wound drainage, referred to as exudate, is composed of neutrophils, macrophages, cellular debris, proteins, and toxins. Exudate is the response of the body to the inflammatory phase. Some wounds may have copious to high volumes of exudate. High-volume-draining wounds generate more drainage than traditional gauze pad dressings and even advanced wound dressings can manage; for these wounds a composite dressing may be used. Composite dressings combine the physical attributes of two or more dressings to enhance absorptive capability. In some instances a vacuum-assisted wound device may be applied as well.

The goal of wound care is to contain the drainage and protect the surrounding tissue from breakdown. If the exudate cannot be controlled with a composite dressings and a vacuum-assisted device, alternatives must be considered. Frequently, the wound maybe "pouched" or "bagged." The same supplies used for ostomy pouching may be used for pouching a wound, or a product designed specifically for pouching high-volume draining wounds may be used (ie, an exudate management device). Pouching the high-volume draining wound allows for accurate measurement of output from the wound and protects the surrounding wound margins.

To pouch a wound, the skin is first cleaned with saline solution or an antibacterial soap and water, and then dried. The skin may then be prepared with a skin barrier wipe, which protects the skin and enhances the adherence of the wafer. The wound is measured or traced, and a wafer is cut to fit. Stoma paste is applied around the cutout area to prevent leakage of the drainage onto the skin.

A one- or two-piece pouching system may be used. With a one-piece pouching system, the wafer with pouch is applied to the wound. With a two-piece system, the wafer is applied first, and then the pouch is attached. Both systems use a closure device at the end of the pouch. A benefit of a two-piece system is that it allows for pouch removal so that the wound can be assessed without disturbing the wafer. The wound margins need to be assessed for skin breakdown when the system is changed and may be protected by a variety of skin wipes or protective ointments.

## Wound Cultures

All wounds are considered contaminated and have the potential to become infected. However, routine wound cultures are not recommended unless there are signs and symptoms of infection, such as fever, erythema, edema, induration, foul odor, purulent exudates, increased amount of exudate, abscess, cellulitis, discoloration of granulation tissue, friable granulation tissue (bleeds easily), increased or unexpected pain or tenderness, or an elevated white blood cell count.

Several methods may be used to culture a wound, including fluid biopsy, wound (tissue) biopsy, and surface culture (culture swab). A surface culture is usually done first. The wound is cleansed or irrigated with sterile normal saline solution before it is swabbed. Exudate and necrotic tissue are not cultured, because doing so provides invalid results. After the wound is cleansed, the swab is gently rolled or rotated, starting at the 12-o'clock position and moving in a zigzag pattern from side to side down the wound to the 6-o'clock position (Fig. 52-7).[2] Optimally, there should be 10 points of contact.[2]

A colony count of 100,000 organisms/mL indicates an infection that needs to be treated with the appropriate antibiotic.[17] At colony counts of greater than 100,000 organisms/mL, normal wound healing is inhibited, and the wound becomes a chronic wound.[2] Wounds that do not respond to antibiotic treatment need to be recultured. The most appropriate form of culture in this scenario is a wound biopsy. Wounds that contain necrotic tissue or tunneling need both aerobic and anaerobic cultures.

## Caring for and Preventing Pressure Ulcers

Pressure ulcer treatment, including the type of dressing used, depends on the stage of the wound, the amount and nature of drainage, the location of the wound, the condition of the ulcer bed and surrounding skin, and signs of infection. Stage I and II pressure ulcers are usually treated with hydrocolloid dressings. Stage III and IV pressure ulcers may be dressed using a filler in the wound bed and then covered with a hydrocolloid or occlusive transparent dressing. Another option for stage III and IV pressure ulcers is negative pressure wound therapy (the VAC system) as long as the wound meets criteria.

Treatment of any staged pressure ulcer includes cleansing and assessment of the wound to evaluate the effectiveness of the treatment plan. Manufacturer recommendations should be followed, especially in determining dressing change frequency. Dressings should be removed gently from the patient's skin to avoid injuring the peri-ulcer skin. Frequent

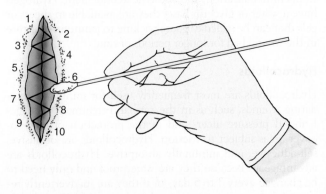

**FIGURE 52-7** Procedure for collecting a wound culture. The wound edges are swabbed using 10-point coverage.

(From Hess CT: Clinical Guide to Skin and Wound Care, 7th ed. Philadelphia, PA: Lippincott Williams & Wilkins, 2013.)

repositioning of any patient at risk of or with a pressure ulcer is important to promote perfusion and wound healing.[5]

### USE OF PRESSURE-RELIEVING DEVICES.
Pressure relief is a major component of wound care and of pressure ulcer prevention. A variety of methods may be used, ranging from low to high technology.[1,2,4,5] The easiest method of preventing pressure ulcers on the heels is to keep the heels off the bed by placing a pillow under the lower legs (a low-technology, cost-effective treatment). The pillow must be positioned to support the entire calf and avoid pressure on the Achilles tendon.[5] In general, ring- or donut-shaped devices should not be used because they create areas of high pressure around the edges that can lead to tissue damage.

A schedule for turning and positioning the patient is also an effective, easily implemented, and cost-effective intervention for relief of pressure. Recommended positioning for patients on bed rest include maintaining the head of bed no higher than 30 degrees and rotating the patient between left-, right-, back-lying, and prone positions as tolerated. Some critically ill patients will not tolerate these position changes; for these patients, specialty beds that incorporate reactive support surfaces should be used.[5] Many specialty beds inflate, deflate, alternate pressures, and laterally rotate. To prevent the occurrence of additional pressure ulcers, it is necessary to follow manufacturers' recommendations when positioning patients on specialty beds. Although these beds do relieve some pressure, they do not eliminate all pressure in the way that turning the patient from side to side does. Patients in a prone position are particularly at risk of facial and anterior body pressure ulcers and should be monitored closely with every position change.[5]

## Pain Management

In all areas of wound care (assessment, cleansing, dressing changes, and positioning), the nurse needs to focus on pain assessment and control. No procedure should occur without assessing for pain and then medicating the patient as needed. Once the pain is controlled, the nurse may proceed with the wound care. The choice of pain medication and the delivery method used (eg, continuous drip, epidural, patient-controlled analgesia pump, local anesthesia, medication-impregnated wound dressings) depends on the patient's status. Increased wound pain can indicate deterioration of the wound or infection; therefore, the nurse must reassess the wound if the patient reports increased pain.[5]

## Pharmacotherapy

Pharmacotherapy in wound care entails the use of pain medications and, in some cases, topical medications to improve wound healing. Pain medications are used to control pain during wound assessment, cleansing, and dressing changes. Growth hormones such as becaplermin (Regranex Gel 0.01%) may be used to stimulate wound healing. Topical steroid creams, such as clocortolone pivalate (Cloderm) and doxepin hydrochloride (Prudoxin), may be prescribed for wound care to relieve surface inflammation and pruritus of the wound margins. Topical phenytoin, a seizure medication that is known to cause gingival hyperplasia when taken orally, has been shown to increase collagen production and

deposition and increased wound strength in various types of wounds.[18] Topical atorvastatin has been studied minimally, but it has been shown to decrease wound healing times in stage I and II pressure ulcers in at least one clinical trial.[19]

Although silver-impregnated dressings are referred to as antimicrobials, they are considered a dressing and not a pharmacotherapeutic agent. Silver gels such as Silvasorb can be used instead of a silver-impregnated dressing. Silvasorb gel is a combination of silver and a hydrogel applied into the wound and is a controlled-release formula.

Xenaderm is a protective ointment composed of balsam of Peru, castor oil, and trypsin. This ointment increases blood flow to partial-thickness wounds while acting as a barrier in incontinent patients.

## Nutrition and Wound Healing

In critical care, monitoring nutritional status is as important as monitoring hemodynamics. Nutrition needs to be addressed early in the patient's admission to promote the optimal opportunity and environment for healing. Current guidelines recommend screening nutritional status in patients with or at risk for pressure ulcers upon admission to the hospital, with any significant changes in condition, and if progress is not made in wound closure. Guidelines also recommend evaluating intake, weight changes, hydration, and ability to eat independently, and assessing whether the patient needs further evaluation by an interprofessional nutrition team.[5]

Nutrition is paramount in critically ill patients or patients with wounds, whether the wounds are acute or chronic, because malnutrition extends the inflammatory phase and decreases immune function. To heal properly, the body needs adequate carbohydrates, fats, proteins, minerals, calories, vitamins, and hydration (Table 52-2).[1,2,20,21]

Protein is a basic and key component of all cellular activity. It is essential in the synthesis of enzymes involved in wound healing, the formation of cells, collagen, and connective tissues. Inadequate protein results in decreased skin and fascial wound strength, a decrease in immune system function, and a higher risk of infection. Proteins also affect oncotic pressure, which predisposes the patient to edema. Wound edema decreases the diffusion of oxygen and nutrients, impeding the healing process even more.

The recommendation for normal adult protein intake is 0.8g/kg/d, and the recommendation for older adults is 1g/kg/d. For optimal wound healing and for patients with or at risk for pressure ulcers, protein recommendations are even higher: 1.25 to 1.5g/kg/d.[20] Some patients with multiple deep wounds may require 1.5 to 2g/kg/d to maintain positive nitrogen balance. However, high doses of protein (2g/kg/d or greater) can cause dehydration in older adults and in patients with renal insufficiency, so these patients should be carefully monitored.[5,20]

Many studies have looked at nutritional supplementation with amino acids for improved wound healing. Arginine is involved in protein synthesis, cell growth, and collagen and is one of the best studied amino acids. However, arginine supplementation in critically ill patients is not recommended because it can increase nitric oxide production, which can cause greater hemodynamic instability. Other amino acids such as glutamine, methionine, cysteine, and lysine have not been studied sufficiently to be recommended at this time.[20]

**TABLE 52-2**    **Necessary Nutrients for Wound Healing**

| Nutrient | Function | Results of Deficiency |
|---|---|---|
| Proteins | Wound repair | Poor wound healing |
| | Clotting factor production | Hypoalbuminemia and generalized edema, which slows oxygen diffusion and metabolic transport mechanisms from the capillaries and cell membranes |
| | White blood cell production and migration | |
| | Cell-mediated phagocytosis | Lymphopenia |
| | Fibroblast proliferation | Impaired cellular immunity |
| | Neovascularization | |
| | Collagen synthesis | |
| | Epithelial cell proliferation | |
| | Wound remodeling | |
| Carbohydrates | Supply cellular energy | Body uses visceral and muscle proteins for energy |
| | Spare protein | |
| Fats | Supply cellular energy | Inhibited tissue repair |
| | Supply essential fatty acids | Use of visceral and muscle proteins for energy |
| | Cell membrane structure | |
| | Prostaglandin production | |
| Vitamin A | Collagen synthesis | Poor wound healing |
| | Epithelialization | Impaired immunity |
| Vitamin C | Membrane integrity | Impaired immunity |
| | Antioxidant | Poor wound healing |
| | | Capillary fragility |
| Vitamin K | Normal blood clotting | Increased risk for hemorrhage and hematoma formation |
| Iron | Collagen synthesis | Anemia, leading to increased risk for local tissue ischemia |
| | Enhances leukocytic bacterial activity | Impaired tensile strength |
| | Hemoglobin synthesis | |
| Zinc | Cell proliferation | Impaired collagen cross-linkage |
| | Cofactor for enzymes | Slow healing |
| | Vitamin A utilization | Alteration in taste |
| | | Anorexia |
| | | Impaired immunity |
| Copper | Collagen cross-linkage | Decreased collagen synthesis |
| | Red blood cell synthesis | Anemia |
| Pyridoxine, riboflavin, and thiamine | Energy production | Decreased resistance to infection |
| | Cellular immunity | Impaired wound healing |
| | Red blood cell synthesis | |
| Arginine | Increases local wound immune system | Decreased local wound immune system |
| | Nitrogen-rich (32% nitrogen, whereas the average amino acid is 16% nitrogen) | |
| | Precursor to proline, which is converted to hydroxyproline and then to collagen | |
| Glutamine | Primary fuel for fibroblasts | Less fuel for fibroblasts |
| | Preservation of lean body mass | |

From Hess CT: Clinical Guide: Wound Care, 7th ed. Ambler, PA: Lippincott Williams & Wilkins, 2012.

Although protein is a key component in the healing process, other nutrients play a role as well. Carbohydrates are the body's fuel source; they spare the proteins for use in cellular construction. Fats maintain cell membrane function and assist with the movement of minerals and fat-soluble vitamins in and out of the cell, although more research needs to be done to understand the role of fats in wound healing.[20] Vitamins act as catalysts in the body's chemical reactions and are also needed for protein and cellular replication. Minerals are needed in the body's biochemical reactions and control the movement of fluids into and out of the cell, through the process of osmosis.

In general, almost all patients with wounds are supplemented with a standard multivitamin with minerals. Studies have looked at additional, high dose supplementation of vitamin C, vitamin A, and minerals such as zinc, magnesium, and copper, since these micronutrients are important in wound healing[20]; however, reviews of these studies do not show improved wound healing in most patients. Current guidelines recommend supplementation of vitamins and minerals only if deficiencies are demonstrated or reasonably suspected.[20,21]

An adequate caloric intake is required for a wound to heal. Normal adult caloric intake varies greatly with factors such as activity level, but it is estimated between 25 and 40 kcal/kg/d. For optimal wound healing of chronic wounds and for patient with or at risk for pressure ulcers, caloric intake requirements are 30 to 35 kcal/kg/d.[2] Obese patients and older adults with wounds require nutritional care that is closely monitored and individualized. Ultimately, optimal nutritional care is achieved by consulting a dietitian, frequently evaluating the patient, and monitoring laboratory test results, such as indirect calorimetry and urine urea nitrogen levels, to maintain a positive nitrogen balance, along with the patient's basic intake, output, daily weights, anthropometrics, calorie count, and social history.

Evidence indicates that serum albumin and prealbumin levels should not be used to monitor acutely ill patients' nutritional status. Albumin and prealbumin levels are altered by inflammation, burns, cancer, hydration status, liver or renal disease, major surgery, and infection.[22,23]

Adequate hydration is paramount to ensure perfusion of the tissues. If the patient is hypovolemic, oxygen transport to the peripheral tissues is impaired. The optimal goal is to maintain hemodynamic stability. (For a thorough discussion of hemodynamic assessment, see Chapter 17.) Recommended daily fluid intake is 30 mL/kg, or 1 to 1.5 mL/kcal consumed. Fluid intake must be adjusted in patients with increased fluid demands—for example, those with high volume draining wounds, high protein intake, frequent emesis or diarrhea, or significant fluid shifts.

In critically ill patients, it is also important to account for the volume and nutritional content of their IV fluids and other medications. Fluids containing dextrose and medications such as propofol can greatly increase the patient's sugar and fat intake, respectively, on top of the enteral or parenteral nutrition they are receiving. Adjustments may have to be made to account for these other nutritional sources.

Patients who are experiencing frequent interruptions in their enteral or parenteral feedings due to NPO status for procedures or surgery should be closely monitored for adequate intake. Patients who are on nothing by mouth (NPO) status for longer than 24 to 48 hours are at risk for slowed healing owing to the lack of an adequate supply of protein, carbohydrates, and other nutrients.

## Patient Teaching and Discharge Planning

Patient teaching and discharge planning are ongoing processes that occur throughout the patient's hospital stay. Discharge planning for patients with wounds is a multidisciplinary challenge. An important part of discharge planning is ensuring that the patient or a family member knows how to care for the wound after the patient leaves the hospital.

One specific patient teaching point that nurses should help reinforce is the benefits of tobacco cessation. The effects of tobacco toxins are well documented and include vasoconstriction and thrombogenesis; this leads to inappropriate connective tissue formation and delayed wound healing.[24] While patients may not have the option of using tobacco while critically ill, it is important to reinforce this teaching point throughout the hospital stay so that patients are well informed long before discharge back to the home environment.

## Clinical Applicability Challenges

### CASE STUDY

Mrs. O. is a 60-year-old woman who is morbidly obese (204 kg) and has a history of type 2 diabetes, hypertension, and abdominal hernias. She presented to the emergency department 2 days ago, confused and complaining of severe abdominal pain. Her temperature was 102.9°F (39.4°C), blood pressure 83/46 (52), heart rate 122, and respiratory rate 34. Preliminary labs showed an elevated white blood cell count (17.5).

Mrs. O. was taken directly to the operating room for suspected small bowel perforation secondary to an obstruction. She was found to have several areas of strangulation and anastomotic leaks. Following surgery, Mrs. O. was admitted directly to the intensive care unit (ICU) for continued treatment of sepsis. She is intubated and sedated, and is dependent upon a norepinephrine drip. She is on broad-spectrum antibiotics and is receiving her nutrition via total parenteral nutrition.

Upon admission to the ICU, you complete a thorough skin assessment. Mrs. O. has a large surgical incision on the midline of her abdomen covered with a wound VAC. You also find an open area over her sacrum with a yellow/pink wound bed and small to moderate drainage. Mrs. O. is edematous and appears to have skin tears to her right hand where she previously had a peripheral IV (PIV). Her peripheral pulses are difficult to palpate; skin temperature is cool and capillary refill time is 4 seconds. Several hours later, while bathing Mrs. O., you find a large area with purple discoloration on a skin fold on her left posterior flank/back area.

1. Name and categorize each wound and recommend appropriate dressings.
2. What nursing interventions are important in preventing further skin breakdown?
3. What elements of Mrs. O.'s history still needs to be addressed in order to aid her wound healing?

### WANT TO KNOW MORE?

A wide variety of resources to enhance your learning and understanding of this chapter are available on thePoint.

You will find:

- References
- Selected readings
- NCLEX-style review questions
- Internet resources
- And more!

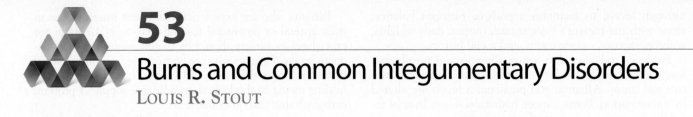

# 53

# Burns and Common Integumentary Disorders

Louis R. Stout

## LEARNING OBJECTIVES

### Based on the content in this chapter, the reader should be able to:

1. Discuss the classification of burn injuries.
2. Describe the pathophysiology of a burn injury.
3. Review the physiologic changes associated with each organ system in relation to a burn injury.
4. Discuss the initial priorities of caring for a patient with a burn injury.
5. Formulate a plan of care for a patient who has sustained a burn injury.
6. Discuss other types of injured patients who are cared for in the burn unit.

The number of burn injuries, hospitalizations, and deaths in the United States has been in a steady decline. Total burn injuries numbered over 2 million per year in the late 1950s and early 1960s. In comparison, in 2016, an estimated 486,000 burn injuries in the United States required medical treatment, with approximately 40,000 patients requiring hospitalization.[1] In 2016, an estimated 486,000 patients received medical treatment for burns[1]; about 40,000 of these patients were hospitalized related to burn injury, with 60% of them being admitted to hospital burn centers.

Great strides have been made in the technological and pharmacologic care of the burned patient. Today, a patient with over a 70% total body-surface area (TBSA) burn has a 50% chance of survival.[2] The trend toward outpatient management has contributed to the decreased number of hospitalized patients. From 1995 to 2005, the average length of stay for inpatient hospitalization declined from 13 to 8 days, and the mortality rate decreased from 6.2% to 4.7%.[1,2] Most recent data from 2012 for hospitalization remains at 8 days while mortality rates have declined further to 3.4%.[1]

Nearly 70% of burn patients are men; 72% of the injuries originate in the home; 43% are caused by fire or flame, closely followed by 34% from scald.[2] While 75% of burns affect less than 10% of the TBSA (90% of burns are less than 20% TBSA), these injuries are resource-intensive and often result in lifelong debilitation.[2] Of the patients with burns who are hospitalized, over 60% are treated at one of 127 specialized burn centers in the United States.[2] The American Burn Association (ABA) has established guidelines for transfer and referral of patients to burn centers.[3] Burn treatment centers are staffed by nurses, physicians, physical therapists, occupational therapists, recreational therapists, nutritionists, psychologists, social workers, and spiritual support staff.

Despite the dramatic reductions in incidence, an acute burn injury remains a leading cause of death with children 4 years and under and adults 65 and older particularly at risk. The advocacy of several national organizations has helped introduce more fire-resistant products, fire prevention programs, and legislation related to fire injury prevention (eg, flame-retardant children's sleepwear, smoke alarms, fire suppression systems).[1,2,4] Measures for safely preventing burns are given in Box 53-1.

---

**BOX 53-1** **TEACHING GUIDE** *Preventing Burns*

**Prevent Accidents in the Home**

- Install a smoke detector on each floor of your house; change the batteries twice a year.
- Plan an exit route in your house in the event of a fire and have routine fire drills once a month.
- Exercise caution with cooking. Avoid wearing clothes with sleeves that may dangle and accidentally ignite clothing.
- Exercise caution with foods that are cooked in a microwave.
- Keep pot and skillet handles turned inward on the stove.
- Never allow children to stand on an open oven door, as this may cause the entire stove to collapse.
- Never leave children unattended in a bathtub.
- Set your hot water heater no higher than 120°F.
- Never leave candles unattended and always be sure candles are fully extinguished.
- Have your furnace serviced once a year.
- Install a carbon monoxide detector.
- Never use the oven or barbeque grill as a heating source.

**Prevent Accidents Outside the Home**

- Only a responsible adult should handle fireworks. Never leave fireworks out where children can have access.
- Exercise caution with campfires and grills.
- Do not pour accelerant (gasoline, lighter fluid) on a lighted fire.
- If an electrical wire is found in contact with a tree, do not touch! Call the local electric company and police/fire company as soon as possible.
- Use sunscreens! Choose a sunscreen with ultraviolet A and ultraviolet B protection and a sun protection factor of 30. Apply every 2 to 3 hours.

**Should a Burn Occur**

- Stop the burning process by removing the source (refer to Box 53-2 for immediate treatment based on burn depth and size).

## Classification of Burn Injuries

Burn injuries are described in terms of causative agent, depth, and severity.

### Causative Agent

A burn injury usually results from energy transfer from a heat source to the body. The heat source may be thermal, chemical, electrical, or radiation-producing. Skin is an effective resistor; injury occurs when the agent exceeds the skin's threshold for resistance.

#### Thermal Burns

Thermal burns account for 86% of all burn injuries.[2] They may be caused by a flame source such as a house fire, a cooking accident, or a fiery explosion. Scald burns from steam or contact with a hot object, such as a cooking pan or hot steel, may also cause thermal injury.

#### Chemical Burns

Chemical injuries commonly occur after exposure to acids and alkali, including hydrofluoric acid, formic acid, anhydrous ammonia, and organic compounds. Other specific chemical agents that cause chemical burns include white phosphorus, certain elemental metals, nitrates, and hydrocarbons; these agents account for 3% of the number of burn cases admitted to reporting hospitals.[2]

Contact time has a critical effect on the severity of injury. Removal of contaminated clothing and water irrigation are crucial steps to limit the effects of the chemical. Regardless of the causative agent, the irrigation must continue once the patient arrives at the emergency department (ED). It is not useful to identify a specific agent to neutralize the acid or alkali agent responsible for the burn, because a neutralizing agent will also cause a chemical reaction in the neutralizing process, thereby risking further burn injury. For all chemical burns, hydrotherapy treatment should continue until the pain resolves; this could take 1 to 3 hours or longer. Chemicals in the eyes should be flushed continuously until a full evaluation can be completed by an ophthalmologist. Some agents, such as hydrofluoric acid, require specific treatments (eg, calcium chloride topical gels or dermal injections) to stop tissue destruction.[5,6]

#### Electrical Burns

Electrical burns are responsible for almost 4% of hospitalized burn patients each year.[2] The effects of electricity on the body are determined by the type of current (alternating or direct), the pathway of the current, the duration of contact, the resistance of the body tissue, and the amount of voltage. Because of their highly developed nervous system, humans are sensitive to very small electric currents. Electricity travels the path of least resistance; therefore, tissue, nerves, and muscle are easily damaged, whereas bone is not.

Low-voltage injuries are caused by 1,000 volts or less. They tend to occur at home and to involve the hands and oral cavities. The most common cause of low-voltage electric burns of the hand is contact with an extension cord in which the insulating material has worn off, either from overuse or

misuse. A low-voltage burn of the hand usually consists of a small, deep burn that may involve vessels, tendons, and nerves. Although these burns involve a small area of the hand, they may be severe enough to require amputation of a finger. Low-voltage electricity can also damage the oral cavity, leaving a permanent scar. These oral injuries occur most frequently in children between the ages of 1 and 2 years.[6] Most are caused by sucking on or biting an extension cord socket.

Whereas low-voltage current usually follows the path of least resistance (ie, nerves, blood vessels), high-voltage current takes a direct path between entrance and ground. Current is concentrated at the entrance to the body, then diverges centrally, and finally converges before exiting. The most severe damage to tissue occurs at the sites of contact, which are commonly referred to as entrance and exit wounds. High-voltage electric entry wounds are charred, centrally depressed, and leathery in appearance, often with resulting local muscle flexion; for example, contact with the hand is likely to present with the hand and forearm in a fixed, almost fully flexed position, often described as "claw-like." Exit wounds are more likely to "explode" as the charge exits.

### Depth

Many factors alter the response of body tissues to heat. The degree or depth of burn depends on (1) the temperature of the injuring agent, (2) the duration of exposure to the injuring agent, and (3) the areas of the body that are exposed to the injuring agent. Whereas the body can sustain prolonged exposure to moderate temperatures such as a hot tub of water (110°F or 43°C), significant damage can occur in as little as 1 second when the temperature exceeds 150°F (68°C). Hot water heaters are often installed with the setting at 140°F (60°C).[1,5,6] A safer setting would be 120°F (49°C), especially in homes with children or elderly family members.

Damage to the skin is frequently described according to the depth of injury and is defined in terms of superficial, partial-thickness, and full-thickness injuries, which correspond to the various layers of the skin (Fig. 53-1).

#### Superficial Burns

Superficial burn injuries are commonly known as first-degree burns. Superficial burns affect the epidermal layer and heal with minimal intervention. The skin is dry, red, blanches, and typically does not blister. Sunburn is a familiar example of a first-degree superficial burn injury; other examples include burns from very brief exposure to hot liquid, flash flame, or chemical agent. The burned skin is painful at first and later itches because of the stimulation of sensory receptors. Because of the continuous replacement of epidermal epithelial cells, this type of injury heals spontaneously without scarring in 3 to 5 days. Care of superficial burns is minimally supportive and is summarized in Box 53-2.

#### Partial-Thickness Burns

Partial-thickness burns (second-degree burns) are further differentiated into superficial and deep partial-thickness burns.

Superficial partial-thickness burns affect the epidermal and superficial dermal layers and usually heal with minimal intervention in 2 to 3 weeks (see Box 53-2). They result from

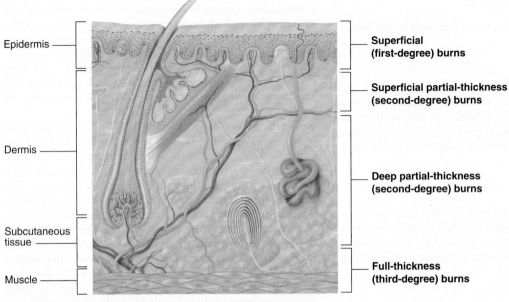

Epidermis — 

Dermis — 

Subcutaneous tissue — 

Muscle — 

Superficial (first-degree) burns

Superficial partial-thickness (second-degree) burns

Deep partial-thickness (second-degree) burns

Full-thickness (third-degree) burns

**FIGURE 53-1** Classification of burns by depth of injury. (Adapted from Anatomical Chart Company: Atlas of Pathophysiology, 3rd ed. Springhouse, PA: Springhouse, 2010, p 385.)

---

**BOX 53-2** | **Care of Superficial (First-Degree) Burns and Superficial Partial-Thickness (Second-Degree) Burns**

**Superficial (First-Degree) Burns**
- Apply ice packs or cold compresses.
- No dressing is required.
- Aloe gel with lidocaine can be applied topically as necessary for localized relief.
- Acetaminophen, aspirin, or ibuprofen can be taken as necessary for generalized discomfort.

**Superficial Partial-Thickness (Second-Degree) Burns**
- If the skin or blister is broken, wash the area with water and mild antiseptic soap.
- Apply a layer of silver sulfadiazine or bacitracin.
- Apply a layer of nonadherent gauze and secure with a gauze roll.
- Dressings should be changed twice a day.
- Wrap fingers and toes individually to prevent "webbing" of healing granulation tissue.
- The patient may continue his or her usual activity depending on the burned site.
- Dependent extremities should be elevated above the level of the heart to prevent excessive edema and promote venous return.
- The patient should be aware of signs and symptoms of infection, including fever, marked tenderness and erythema surrounding the burn wound, purulent drainage of pus, red streaks radiating from the wound, or pain that cannot be controlled with analgesics.
- The patient should follow up in 2 days with a primary care provider.

---

flash burns or scalds; the skin is characterized as moist and reddened, with blanching and blisters. The skin is hypersensitive and painful, and when healed show minimal scarring.

Deep partial-thickness burns affect the entire epidermal layer and deeper dermal layers, resulting in discomfort to pressure. They are caused by exposure to hot solids, flames, intense radiant energy, or chemicals. The skin is slightly moist-to-dry, mottled, and slow to blanch or does not blanch. Fluid resuscitation, nutritional status, and premorbid conditions may affect the healing potential of a deep partial-thickness burn injury. Deep partial-thickness burn injuries may have some spontaneous healing in 3 to 4 weeks but require surgical intervention (excision and skin grafting) if the burn is of any significant size. Delayed healing may result in scarring, contracture, and loss of function.

**Full-Thickness Burns**

Prolonged exposure to flame, a hot object, or a chemical agent or contact with high-voltage electricity can result in full-thickness burns (third-degree burns). These burns extend into the poorly vascularized adipose tissue and even into connective tissue, muscle or bones. All epidermal and dermal elements, including sweat glands and hair follicles, are destroyed. These burns may appear white, red, brown, or black. Reddened areas do not blanch in response to pressure because the underlying blood supply has been interrupted. Thrombosed blood vessels and capillaries may be visualized.[6,7] Full-thickness burns are insensate because the sensory receptors have been completely destroyed, and the patient may feel deep pressure only. In addition, the burns may appear sunken because of the destruction of underlying fat and muscle.

The loss of the hair follicle eliminates the ability of the skin to regenerate. A small wound (less than 4 cm) may be allowed to heal by granulation and migration of healthy epithelium from the wound margins. However, extensive, open full-thickness wounds leave the patient highly susceptible to overwhelming infection and malnutrition. Wound closure by skin grafting restores the integrity of the skin.

**Severity**

Burn severity is determined by the extent and depth of the burn and the causative agent, time, and circumstances surrounding the burn injury. To assess the severity of the burn, several factors must be considered:

- The percentage of body surface area burned
- The depth of the burn
- The anatomical location of the burn
- The person's age (Box 53-3)
- The person's medical history
- The presence of concomitant injury
- The presence of inhalation injury

Several methods using percentages of TBSA may be used to estimate the extent of a burn. The "rule of nines" or "rule of palms" allows for quick estimation until a detailed Lund and Browder assessment can be done. The "rule of nines" divides the body into parts in multiples of 9% (Fig. 53-2). Burns may involve only one surface of a body part or they may be circumferential. If only the anterior surface of the arm is burned, then the TBSA is estimated to be 4.5%. However, if the burn encircles the entire arm (from axilla to fingertips), then the value is 9%. The rule of palms can be used for estimating small scattered burns (eg, scald or grease burns). The patient's palmar surface (including the fingers) equals 1% of the patient's TBSA.

The Lund and Browder method (see Fig. 53-2) is highly recommended because it is more detailed and corrects for the large head-to-body ratio of infants and children. Surface measurements are assigned to each body part in terms of the age of the patient. However, because this method of measuring burn size is time consuming, it should be done after resuscitation efforts are well established.

A burn injury may range from a small blister to a massive full-thickness burn. Recognizing the need for a clear description of terms, the ABA developed the Injury Severity Grading System, which is used to determine the magnitude of the burn injury and to provide optimal criteria for hospital resources for patient care. The severity of burn injury is categorized into minor, moderate, and major, as outlined in Box 53-4. Minor burn injuries can be treated in the ED with outpatient follow-up every 48 hours, until the risk for infection is reduced and wound healing is underway. Patients with

moderate, uncomplicated burn injuries and those with major burn injuries should be referred to a regional burn center and, if appropriate, transferred for specialized care.

## Pathophysiology of Burn Injuries

### Localized Tissue Response

Cellular injury starts when tissues are exposed to an energy source (thermal, chemical, electrical, or radiation). The depth of the thermal injury is demonstrated by the extent of injury down through the layers of skin. Figure 53-3 depicts the concentric zones of a burn injury.[6] The zone of coagulation is the area where the most damage has been sustained; temperatures have exceeded 113°F (45°C). The necrotic tissue is black, gray, khaki, or white and has undergone protein coagulation and cell death. This area has lost the ability to recover and requires surgical intervention. The zone of stasis immediately surrounds the zone of coagulation. This area contains cells that are at the most risk during burn resuscitation. They can recover or become necrotic in the initial 24 to 72 hours, depending on the conditions and course of resuscitation. The zone of hyperemia is the area of increased blood flow that brings the needed nutrients to the tissue for recovery (*active hyperemia*) and removes the metabolic waste products (*reactive hyperemia*). This area heals rapidly and has no cell death.

### Systemic Response

Major changes at the cellular level are responsible for the tremendous systemic response noted in a patient with burns. The localized response causes a coagulation of cellular proteins, leading to irreversible cell injury with local production of complement, histamine, and oxygen free radicals (ie, by-products of oxidative processes). Oxygen free radicals alter cell lipids and proteins, affecting the integrity of the cell membrane. This is particularly problematic in the endothelium of the microvascular circulation, because disruption of the cell membrane leads to increased vascular permeability.[8,9] Increased vascular permeability leads to loss of plasma proteins into the interstitium and results in a marked decrease in circulating volume. The release of histamine, prostaglandins, and other vasoactive substances into the circulation contribute to the increased vascular permeability by increasing production of oxygen free radicals.[8–11] Increased vascular permeability leads to the formation of interstitial edema, which usually peaks within 24 to 48 hours of injury. It is hypothesized that the microvasculature takes weeks to restore itself completely to its premorbid state. The pulmonary vasculature is not spared: pulmonary interstitial edema forms, with intraalveolar hemorrhages. This initial pulmonary insult is thought to be a precursor to the development of acute respiratory distress syndrome (ARDS).[9]

Systemically, a burn injury causes a release of vasoactive substances, such as histamine, prostaglandins, interleukins (ILs), and arachidonic acid metabolites. These substances initiate the systemic inflammatory response syndrome (SIRS). The potent mediators and cytokines—nitric oxide, platelet-activating factor (PAF), serotonin, thromboxane $A_2$, and tumor necrosis factor (TNF)—deplete the intravascular

---

**BOX 53-3** *CONSIDERATIONS for the Older Patient*

**Burns**

Older patients respond differently to burn injuries because of age-related changes and diminished physiologic reserve. Preexisting medical conditions and complications as a result of injury are significant factors leading to mortality of the older burn patient. The adverse effects of trauma, including burns, can persist for an extended period after injury. Once injured, elderly patients may never regain their preinjury level of health. Postdischarge destination and care are challenging obstacles in discharge planning. Family interest in assuming caregiver responsibility, ability of the patient to render self-care, insurance, and financial limitations must be considered in planning for discharge. Many independent elderly patients will no longer be able to return home alone after a burn injury. Rehabilitation and long-term care facilities can create an emotional and financial burden on the family. In addition, acute rehabilitation requires the patient to participate in 3 hours of therapy each day. Many elderly patients are unable to meet this requirement, and thus may not be eligible for acute rehabilitation.

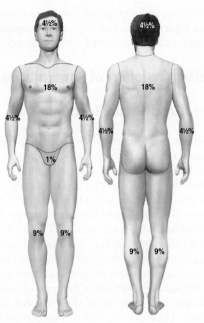

**A.** Rule of Nines

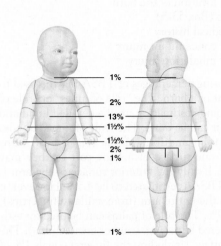

| AREA | PERCENT OF BURN | | | | | SEVERITY OF BURN | | TOTAL PERCENT |
|------|------|------|------|------|------|------|------|------|
| | 0–1 Year | 1–4 Years | 5–9 Years | 10–15 Years | Adult | 2° | 3° | |
| Head | 19 | 17 | 13 | 10 | 7 | | | |
| Neck | 2 | 2 | 2 | 2 | 2 | | | |
| Ant. Trunk | 13 | 13 | 13 | 13 | 13 | | | |
| Post. Trunk | 13 | 13 | 13 | 13 | 13 | | | |
| R. Buttock | 2½ | 2½ | 2½ | 2½ | 2½ | | | |
| L. Buttock | 2½ | 2½ | 2½ | 2½ | 2½ | | | |
| Genitalia | 1 | 1 | 1 | 1 | 1 | | | |
| R. U. Arm | 4 | 4 | 4 | 4 | 4 | | | |
| L. U. Arm | 4 | 4 | 4 | 4 | 4 | | | |
| R. L. Arm | 3 | 3 | 3 | 3 | 3 | | | |
| L. L. Arm | 3 | 3 | 3 | 3 | 3 | | | |
| R. Hand | 2½ | 2½ | 2½ | 2½ | 2½ | | | |
| L. Hand | 2½ | 2½ | 2½ | 2½ | 2½ | | | |
| R. Thigh | 5½ | 6½ | 8½ | 8½ | 9½ | | | |
| L. Thigh | 5½ | 6½ | 8½ | 8½ | 9½ | | | |
| R. Leg | 5 | 5 | 5½ | 6 | 7 | | | |
| L. Leg | 5 | 5 | 5½ | 6 | 7 | | | |
| R. Foot | 3½ | 3½ | 3½ | 3½ | 3½ | | | |
| L. Foot | 3½ | 3½ | 3½ | 3½ | 3½ | | | |
| **Total** | **Blue areas indicate 2°** **Red areas indicate 3°** | | | **Total** | | | | |

**B.** Lund and Browder chart

**FIGURE 53-2** **A:** The "rule of nines" method for determining percentage of body area with burn injury. **B:** Lund and Browder method for determining percentage of body area with burn injury. (**A:** Adapted from Anatomical Chart Company: Atlas of Pathophysiology, 3rd ed. Springhouse, PA: Springhouse, 2010, p 385.)

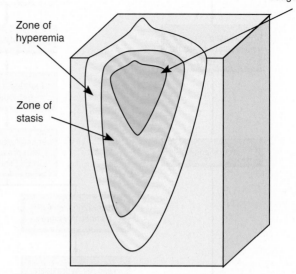

FIGURE 53-3 The concentric zones of a burn injury.

volume, decreasing blood flow to the kidneys and the gastrointestinal (GI) tract. If left uncorrected, hypovolemic shock, metabolic acidosis, and hyperkalemia may occur. Intestinal mucosal permeability also markedly increases and can become the primary source of bacterial infection. Early enteral feeding is one step to help prevent the translocation of bacteria.[12,13]

Nitric oxide relaxes smooth muscle and produces vasodilation and hypotension. It may also depress myocardial function and block platelet aggregation and adhesion. PAF initiates neutrophil and white blood cell (WBC) activation and produces tissue inflammation. PAF increases permeability of vessels, thereby decreasing myocardial contractility, causing vasodilation and hypotension. Some prostaglandins, and their activation, cause vasoconstriction, increased blood flow, and fever. Serotonin causes vasodilation, hypotension, and increased vessel permeability. TNF is responsible for numerous cellular responses, including increased formation of oxygen free radicals, which leads to injury of the lungs, GI tract, and kidneys; increased cytokine production; initial hyperglycemia followed by hypoglycemia; hypotension; metabolic acidosis; coagulopathy; and activation of the coagulation cascade.[9]

The end results of the local and systemic responses are dramatic if the burn covers more than 20% of the TBSA. The person with a major burn injury experiences a form of hypovolemic shock known as burn shock (Fig. 53-4); the severity and length is influenced by the depth and extent of burn, preexisting illness, and presence of inhalation injury.[8] Within minutes of thermal injury, a marked increase in capillary hydrostatic pressure occurs in the injured tissue, accompanied by an increase in capillary permeability. This results in a rapid shift of plasma fluid from the intravascular compartment across heat-damaged capillaries, into interstitial areas (resulting in edema), and to the burn wound itself. The loss of plasma fluid and proteins results in a decreased colloid osmotic pressure in the vascular compartment. As a result, fluid and electrolytes continue to leak from the vascular compartment, resulting in additional edema formation in the burned tissue and throughout the body. This "leak," which consists of sodium, water, and plasma proteins, is followed by a decrease in cardiac output, hemoconcentration of red blood cells, diminished perfusion to major organs, and generalized body edema.

The pathophysiologic response after burn injury is biphasic. In the early postinjury (ebb) phase, generalized organ hypofunction develops as a consequence of decreased cardiac output. Peripheral vascular resistance increases as a result of the neurohumoral stress response after trauma; this increases cardiac afterload, resulting in a further decrease in cardiac output. The increase in peripheral vascular resistance (selective vasoconstriction) and the hemoconcentration resulting from plasma fluid loss may cause the blood pressure to appear normal at first. However, if fluid replacement is inadequate, and plasma protein loss continues, hypovolemic shock soon occurs.

In patients receiving adequate fluid resuscitation, the cardiac output usually returns to normal in the latter part of the first 24 hours after burn injury. As plasma volume is replenished during the second 24 hours, the cardiac output increases to hypermetabolic levels (hyperfunction phase) and slowly returns to more normal levels as the burn wounds are closed.[9,12,14] In some instances, with burns exceeding 60% of the TBSA, depressed cardiac output does not respond to aggressive volume resuscitation. A myocardial depressant factor capable of depressing ventricular contractility by 60% has been identified. Myocardial depression in the early postburn period may also be the result of reduced coronary blood flow.[9,12]

The response of the pulmonary vasculature is similar to that of the peripheral circulation. However, pulmonary

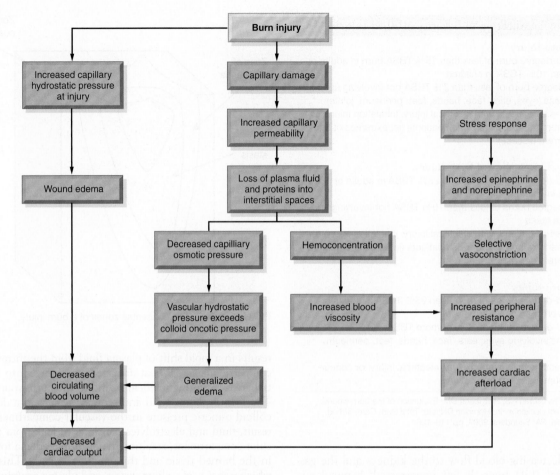

**FIGURE 53-4**    Fluid shifts in burn shock.

vascular resistance is greater and lasts longer. Immediately after burn injury, the patient may experience a mild, transient pulmonary hypertension. A decrease in oxygen tension and lung compliance may also be evident.

The loss of fluid throughout the body's intravascular space results in a thickened, sluggish flow of the remaining circulatory blood volume. The effects reach all body systems. This slowing of circulation permits bacteria and cellular material to settle in the lower portions of blood vessels, especially in the capillaries, which results in sludging.

The antigen–antibody reaction to burned tissue adds to circulatory congestion by the clumping or agglutination of cells. Coagulation problems occur as a result of the release of thromboplastin by the injury itself and the release of fibrinogen from injured platelets. If thrombi occur, they may cause ischemia of the affected part and lead to necrosis. Although of limited incidence in patients with burns, the increased coagulation process may develop into disseminated intravascular coagulation.

## Concomitant Problems

The actual burn is unlikely to cause the death of a patient; rather, it is complications resulting from other factors that are of concern. In the acute phase, the loss or impedance of a patent airway is the major issue.[15] After the first 5 to 7 days, the primary concern is that of infection.

## Pulmonary Injury

Pulmonary damage usually occurs within 24 to 48 hours of the injury and is secondary to the inhalation of combustible products, or may be the result of inhaled superheated air. In an incident involving large amounts of steam, the risk of injury is far greater because water has a heat-carrying capacity 4,000 times greater than air and has the ability to be inhaled deeply in the pulmonary system.[1,6] Pulmonary injury may also be the result of a systemic process related to SIRS.

Fiberoptic bronchoscopy permits direct visualization of the airways (facilitating evaluation of erythema, edema, ulceration, and enlarged vessels) as well as the removal of debris by lavage. Fiberoptic bronchoscopy should be completed when feasible and repeated as indicated during the acute phase to document the extent of the pulmonary injury and complete direct lavage when necessary.

### Carbon Monoxide Toxicity

Carbon monoxide is a nonirritating, odorless, colorless gas that is formed as a result of the incomplete combustion of any carbon fuel. Sources of carbon monoxide include hot water heaters, furnaces, tobacco smoke, and exhaust from vehicles. Carbon monoxide poisoning produces its effect on the body by competing with oxygen for uptake of hemoglobin, thereby acting as an asphyxiant. Because carbon monoxide affinity for hemoglobin is 200 to 300 times higher than oxygen, carbon monoxide readily displaces the oxygen, leading to the formation of carboxyhemoglobin and a reduction in systemic arterial oxygen content.[15–17] Carboxyhemoglobin shifts the oxyhemoglobin dissociation curve to the left, further decreasing the ability of the red blood cells to release oxygen to body tissues.[17] This may lead to severe anoxia and related brain injury.

The patient with a clear history of exposure to carbon monoxide is usually found in a closed environment in the presence of combusted gases, such as smoke, automobile exhaust, or fumes from a faulty furnace.[6] The signs of carbon monoxide poisoning depend on the carboxyhemoglobin level present in the patient's blood (Table 53-1).[16]

When carbon monoxide poisoning is suspected, 100% high-flow oxygen is administered. Carbon monoxide has a half-life of 4 hours if the patient breathes room air, but this is dramatically reduced to 45 minutes if the patient is breathing 100% oxygen. The patient should be maintained on 100% oxygen until the carboxyhemoglobin level is less than 10% and neurologic symptoms resolve.[6,15,16] Serial carboxyhemoglobin level measurements are the most accurate way to assess responsiveness to oxygen therapy.[16] Pulse oximetry is inaccurate when the carboxyhemoglobin level is elevated, because pulse oximetry cannot distinguish between oxygen and carbon monoxide on the hemoglobin. The analysis and trending of arterial blood gas (ABG) levels for acid–base balance, lactate levels, and bicarbonate are helpful to manage carbon monoxide poisoning with lactic or metabolic acidosis.[16]

### Inhalation Injury

Aside from carbon monoxide poisoning, thermal injury to the airway can result from smoke inhalation. Pulmonary damage from inhalation injury has historically been seen in less than 10% of the total burn cases but accounts for 20% to 84% of burn mortality and is a significant factor in increasing the hospital length of stay.[15,18] Three stages of injury have been described:

1. Acute pulmonary insufficiency may occur during the first 36 hours.
2. Pulmonary edema occurs in 5% to 30% of patients with burns between 6 and 72 hours after injury.
3. Bronchopneumonia appears in 15% to 60% of patients with burns 3 to 10 days after injury.

Upper airway injury is the result of inhalation of superheated air, which may cause blisters and edema in the supraglottic area around the vocal cords. This situation may cause airway obstruction and edema. Hoarseness, stridor, dyspnea, carbonaceous sputum, and tachypnea indicate airway compromise, which must be addressed immediately. Early intubation may thwart such disastrous occurrences.

Tracheobronchial and parenchymal lung injuries are usually a result of incomplete combustion of chemicals (eg, aldehyde, acrolein) or noxious gases, which results in a chemical pneumonitis. Pathophysiologic changes associated with lower lung injuries include impaired ciliary activity, hypersecretion, edema, inflammation, and bronchospasm.[6,15,18] Inflammatory changes in the trachea and alveoli occur within 24 hours of injury. The pulmonary tree becomes irritated and edematous. The alveoli may collapse, causing a decreased compliance, which leads to atelectasis. ARDS may develop rapidly. However, changes may not become apparent until the second 24 hours. Pulmonary edema is a possibility any time from the first few hours to 7 days after the injury. Subtle changes in the patient's sensorium may indicate hypoxia.

History and physical assessment findings that should alert the nurse to the potential for inhalation injury are given in Box 53-5. Serial ABG evaluations show a decreasing arterial oxygen tension ($PaO_2$). Usually, the admission chest film appears normal because changes are not reflected until 24 to 48 hours after the burn. A sputum specimen is obtained for culture and sensitivity studies. Laryngoscopy and bronchoscopy may be of value in determining the presence of extramucosal carbonaceous material (the most reliable sign of inhalation injury) and the state of the mucosa (blistering, edema, erythema). More specific confirmation of inhalation injury is achieved with the use of fiberoptic bronchoscopy, which permits direct examination of the proximal airway, and xenon-133 scintigraphy (ventilation–perfusion scanning).[6,15] Xenon-133 scintigraphy is helpful in establishing a diagnosis of injury to small airways and lung parenchyma.[15]

## Infection

There is no greater problem for the patient with burns than infection. Infection is the most common cause of death in patients with burns after the first 7 days.[19,20] Loss of the mechanical barrier between the human body and the environment is the first step in the weakening of defenses. All aspects of the immune system, including phagocytosis, soluble mediators of innate immunity such as complement, antibody production, and cellular (T-cell) defense systems, are compromised by severe burn injury.

Actions of the health care team can compromise patient survival. All catheters invading the body, including endotracheal tubes, central venous catheters, and bladder catheters,

---

**TABLE 53-1  Signs and Symptoms of Carbon Monoxide Poisoning**

| Carboxyhemoglobin Saturation (%) | Clinical Presentation |
|---|---|
| 10 | No symptoms |
| 20 | Headache, nausea/vomiting, dyspnea on exertion |
| 30 | Confusion, lethargy, tachypnea |
| 40–60 | Seizure, coma, changes on electrocardiogram |
| More than 60 | Death |

---

**QSEN BOX 53-5  *PATIENT SAFETY***

**History and Physical Examination Findings Suggestive of Inhalation Injury**

- History of incident occurring in a confined area
- Singed nasal or facial hairs
- Burns of the oral or pharyngeal mucous membranes
- Burns in the perioral area or neck
- Carbonaceous sputum
- Change in voice
- Change in level of consciousness

must be handled with as clean a technique as possible. Although the skin and gut are the source of endogenous bacteria, a greater threat to the patient is colonization with antibiotic-resistant pathogens carried by the burn team from other patients. The hands must be washed without fail before and after handling the patient, the patient's bed, or equipment. When dressings are removed and wounds exposed, sterile gloves must be worn. Frequent and meticulous hand washing alone probably prevents infection more than any other single action. Infection control policies vary from burn center to burn center, but the philosophy remains the same: Make *every* effort to minimize the transmission of bacteria from patient to patient.

Diagnosis of invasive infection in the patients with burns is unusually difficult. Most patients with burns meet two or more of the SIRS criteria because they are constantly and chronically exposed to the environment, and thus release inflammatory mediators. The ABA Consensus developed triggers that should prompt the healthcare team to look for an infection in the burn patient (Table 53-2). Manifestations of multisystem organ dysfunction, such as hypotension, hypoxia, decreased pulmonary compliance, renal failure, or hepatic dysfunction, are almost certain signs of septic shock.

Qualitative wound cultures done by swabbing the wound yield no new information other than the nature of the bacterial species colonizing the surface of the wound. A biopsy of the burn wound permits a quantitative assay of the number of colony-forming units (CFUs) of bacteria per gram of tissue. Burn wound sepsis is likely if the colony count is greater than 105 CFU/g, and the quantitative culture also allows isolation and identification of the invading organism.

## Trauma

Concomitant injuries such as fractures and head trauma pose significant risk for the patient with burns. The presentation of the burn patient can be horrific, but ensuring adequate airway, breathing, and circulation takes precedence over caring for specific injuries.[21] Cervical spine injuries should be stabilized and cleared. If head trauma is suspected, a computed tomography scan is obtained. The history of the burn injury is critical to assisting with the evaluation of the patient. The burn wounds may mask some of the classical signs of underlying injuries, such as ecchymosis or swelling. The burn incident may include an event such as an explosion, the patient being thrown or falling, or a motor vehicle crash. Patients with electrical injuries must be evaluated for fractures secondary to the violent muscular contraction after exposure, with special focus on the cervical spinous process and long bones.

# Assessment and Management of Burn Injuries

The initial assessment of the patient with burns is like that of any trauma patient. The ABA has identified criteria for referral to a burn center (Box 53-6). Whether the patient will say at the initial hospital or will be transferred to a burn center facility, the resuscitation phase begins immediately in the ED after the burn insult has occurred. The primary and secondary surveys are completed before transfer. Proper stabilization of the patient is crucial for successful transfer. As with any major trauma, the first hour is crucial, and the next 24 to 36 hours are also important. The management of fluid balance, the respiratory system, and nutrition is vital, and all systems have a major impact on the patient's survival.

## Resuscitative Phase

### Primary Survey

The following "A-B-C-D-E" parameters are assessed in the primary survey:

- **A**irway maintenance with cervical spine protection
- **B**reathing and ventilation
- **C**irculation with hemorrhage control
- **D**isability (assess neurologic deficit)
- **E**xposure (completely undress the patient, but maintain temperature)

---

**TABLE 53-2** American Burn Association (ABA) Consensus: Sepsis and Infections in Burns Versus Systemic Inflammatory Response Syndrome (SIRS)

| ABA Consensus | SIRS |
|---|---|
| Temperature greater than 39°C or less than 36.5°C | Temperature greater than 38°C or less than 36°C |
| Heart rate greater than 110 beats per minute | Heart rate greater than 90 bpm |
| Respiratory rate greater than 25 breaths per minute or minute ventilation greater than 12 L/min ventilated | Respiratory rate greater than 20 bpm or $PaCO_2$ less than 32 mm Hg |
| Thrombocytopenia less than 100,000/mcL | WBC greater than 12,000/mm³ or less than 4,000/mm³ or left shift greater than 10% bands |
| Hyperglycemia (no preexisting diabetes) or insulin resistance | |
| Enteral feeding intolerance | |

Concern for infection in case of at least three of the above conditions. bpm, breaths per minute.

From Greenhalgh DG, Saffle JR, Holmes JH, et al: American Burn Association consensus conference to define sepsis and infection in burns. J Burn Care Res 28(6):776–790, 2007.

---

**BOX 53-6** Criteria for Referral to a Burn Center

- Partial-thickness burns more than 10% of TBSA
- Burns that involve the face, hands, feet, genitalia, perineum, or major joints
- Third-degree burns in any age group
- Electrical burns, including lightning injury
- Chemical burns
- Inhalation injury
- Burn injury in patients with preexisting medical disorders that could complicate management, prolong recovery, or affect mortality
- Concomitant trauma, in which the burn injury poses the greatest risk for morbidity or mortality
- Children with burns in hospitals without qualified personnel or equipment for the care of children
- Patients with burns who will require special social, emotional, or long-term rehabilitative intervention

Data from the American Burn Association Burn Center Referral Criteria.

**AIRWAY.** On initial assessment of the patient with burns, the airway must be assessed immediately. The compromised airway may be controlled by a chin lift, jaw thrust, insertion of an oropharyngeal airway in an unconscious patient, or endotracheal intubation. It is crucial not to hyperextend the neck in patients with suspected cervical spine injuries. Partial to complete occlusion of the patent airway can occur rapidly in the burn patient throughout the acute phase, particularly in the presence of inhalation injury.

**BREATHING AND VENTILATION.** Ventilation requires adequate functioning of the lungs, chest wall, and diaphragm. To assess for breathing and ventilation, listen to the chest and verify breath sounds in each lung; assess adequacy of rate and depth of respiration; administer high-flow oxygen at 15 L/min using a nonrebreathing mask; and assess for circumferential full-thickness burns of the chest that may impair ventilation.

**CIRCULATION.** Assessment of the circulation includes a measurement of blood pressure and heart rate. Special attention should be paid to the distal pulses of any extremity with circumferential burns. Intravenous (IV) cannulation is performed by inserting two large-bore catheters into the skin that is unburned, if possible. A central venous catheter should be inserted when indicated. Doppler ultrasonography can be used to assess for pulses, specifically when diminishing or nonpalpable. Box 53-7 lists risk factors for impaired circulation.

**DISABILITY.** In the presence of burns alone, the patient will be alert and oriented. If this is not the case, associated injuries, such as inhalation injury, head trauma, substance abuse, or preexisting medical conditions, should be considered. The assessment is initiated by determining the patient's level of consciousness using the AVPU (**A**lert, responds to **V**erbal stimuli, responds to **P**ainful stimuli, **U**nresponsive) method.

**EXPOSURE.** All the patient's clothing and jewelry are removed to complete the primary and secondary survey. The environment should be warmed, because the burn patient has lost significant capacity to maintain body temperature. After examination, the patient is covered with a clean, dry sheet and warm blankets to prevent evaporative cooling. If possible, IV fluids are warmed at 98.6°F (37°C) to 104°F (40°C).

### Secondary Survey

The secondary survey, which is completed after resuscitative efforts are well established, consists of a detailed history and physical examination of the patient as well as a complete history of the event. Every attempt is made to determine exactly what happened (Box 53-8). A detailed neurologic examination is completed, and initial radiographic and laboratory studies are done. Resuscitative measures are ongoing and constantly evaluated.

A complete history and physical examination are the hallmarks of the secondary survey. It is not uncommon for patients to have comorbid diseases. Preexisting diseases, such as diabetes, hypertension, asthma, cancer, and stroke, should be documented. A medication list is obtained from the patient if possible, or a family member is asked to provide the information. In addition, any allergies, the person's tetanus immunization history, and the time of the person's last meal should be documented. Burn depth and burn size are assessed.

Burn injuries require a global assessment. The following laboratory and diagnostic studies are indicated for patients with burns:

- Complete blood count (CBC)
- Comprehensive chemistry panel, including blood urea nitrogen
- Creatinine level
- Urinalysis

---

**BOX 53-8** **Questions to Ask During a Secondary Survey**

**Thermal Burns**
- How did the burn occur?
- Did the burn occur inside or outside?
- Did the clothes catch fire?
- How long did it take to extinguish the fire?
- Were there any explosions?
- Was the patient found in a smoke-filled room?
- How did the patient escape?
- Did the patient jump out of a window?
- Were there other people injured or killed at the scene?
- Was the patient unconscious at the scene?
- Was there a motor vehicle crash?
- Was the car severely damaged?
- Was there a car fire?
- Are the purported circumstances of the injury consistent with the burn characteristics (is there possibility of abuse)?

**Scald Injuries**
- How did the burn occur?
- What was the temperature of the liquid?
- What was the liquid; how much liquid was involved?
- What was the burn cooled with?
- Who was present when the burn took place?
- Where did the burn take place? Is there possibility of abuse?

**Chemical Burns**
- What was the agent?
- How did the exposure occur?
- What was the duration of contact?
- Did contamination take place?

**Electrical Burns**
- What kind of electricity was involved?
- Did the patient lose consciousness?
- Did the patient fall?
- What was the estimated voltage?
- Was cardiopulmonary resuscitation administered at the scene?

---

**QSEN BOX 53-7** *PATIENT SAFETY*

**Risk Factors for Impaired Circulation**
- Progressive diminution of pulses despite adequate resuscitation
- Decreased capillary refill
- Decreased sensation
- Progressive worsening of pain
- Paresthesias
- Pallor of extremity

- ABG values to include carboxyhemoglobin determination
- Electrocardiogram
- Chest radiograph

After the primary and secondary surveys are complete, the burned area is usually covered with a dry sheet. This reduces the risk for infection and helps to maintain the patient's warmth. A cool compress can be applied to small superficial burns. If the patient has a high-voltage electrical burn or if cardiac changes are noted, continuous cardiac monitoring is indicated. If the patient has a chemical burn, the area is immediately flushed with large amounts of water to remove the chemical, and all contaminated clothing is removed and bagged. The caregiver should be cautious to avoid secondary exposure to chemical products.

If the patient will be transferred to a burn center, initiation of fluid resuscitation, insertion of a nasogastric tube (NGT), and insertion of an indwelling urinary catheter may be carried out during the secondary assessment.

### Providing Hemodynamic Support

Therapy for burn shock is aimed at supporting the patient through the period of hypovolemic shock until capillary integrity is restored. Fluid resuscitation is the primary intervention in the resuscitative phase in the intensive care unit (ICU) to maintain tissue perfusion and end organ function. Goals of fluid resuscitation are as follows:

- Correct fluid, electrolyte, and protein deficits.
- Replace continuing losses and maintain fluid balance.
- Prevent excessive edema formation.
- Maintain an hourly urinary output in adults of 30 to 50 mL/h (approximately 0.5 mL/kg/h).[6,8]

**FORMULAS FOR FLUID ADMINISTRATION.** Numerous formulas have been developed for fluid resuscitation (Box 53-9). Each has advantages and disadvantages. They differ primarily in terms of recommended volume administration and salt content. In general, lost crystalloid and colloid must be replaced rigorously. Free water, given as dextrose 5% in water ($D_5W$) with or without added electrolytes, is regulated so that insensible fluid loss is covered. Lactated Ringer solution is the crystalloid of choice because it is a balanced salt solution that closely approximates the composition of extracellular fluid.

The ABA recommends the use of the ABA consensus formula for the resuscitation of patients with burns. The formula is a combination of the modified Brooke formula and the Baxter (commonly called Parkland) formula. The ABA consensus formula prescribes 2 to 4 mL of lactated Ringer solution per kilogram of body weight per percentage TBSA burn:

$$\text{2–4 mL LR} \times \text{body weight in kg} \times \text{\% TBSA burn}$$

The total amount calculated is administered in the first 24 hours after injury. One-half is given in the first 8 hours *from the time of the burn,* one-fourth is given during the next 8 hours, and the remaining one-fourth is given over the next 8 hours.[6] The ABA consensus formula and the other fluid resuscitation formulas are guidelines; individual patients may require more or less fluid during the first 24 hours. Patients with electrical injuries, inhalation injuries, delayed

---

**BOX 53-9** | **Fluid Resuscitation Formulas**

**Baxter (Parkland) Formula**
- First 24 hours: Lactated Ringer solution (4 mL/kg/% TBSA); half given over first 8 hours, remaining half given over next 16 hours
- Second 24 hours: Dextrose in water, plus potassium- and colloid-containing fluid (0.3 to 0.5 mL/kg/% TBSA)

**Brooke Formula**
- First 24 hours: Lactated Ringer solution (1.5 mL/kg/% TBSA), plus colloid solution (0.5 mL/kg/% TBSA); half given over first 8 hours, remaining half given over next 16 hours
- Second 24 hours: Lactated Ringer solution (0.5 to 0.75 mL/kg/% TBSA), plus 5% dextrose in water ($D_5W$) (2 L)

**Modified Brooke Formula**
- First 24 hours: Lactated Ringer solution (2 mL/kg/% TBSA); half given over first 8 hours, remaining half given over next 16 hours
- Second 24 hours: Colloid solution (0.3 to 0.5 mL/kg/% TBSA), plus $D_5W$ to maintain adequate urine output

**Consensus Formula**
- First 24 hours: Lactated Ringer solution (2 to 4 mL/kg/% TBSA in adults; 3 to 4 mL/kg/% TBSA in children); half given over first 8 hours, remaining half given over next 16 hours
- Second 24 hours: Colloid-containing fluid (0.3 to 0.5 mL/kg/% TBSA), plus electrolyte-free fluid (in adults) or half-normal saline solution (in children) to maintain adequate urine output

**Dextran Formula**
- First 8 hours: Dextran 40 in saline (2 mL/kg/h), plus lactated Ringer solution infused to maintain urine output at 30 mL/h
- Second 8 hours: Fresh-frozen plasma (0.5 mL/kg/h) for 18 hours, plus additional crystalloid to maintain adequate urine output

**Evans Formula**
- First 24 hours: 0.9% normal saline solution (1 mL/kg/% TBSA), plus colloid solution (1 mL/kg/% TBSA); half given over first 8 hours, remaining half given over next 16 hours
- Second 24 hours: 0.9% normal saline solution (0.5 mL/kg/% TBSA), plus $D_5W$ (2 L)

---

resuscitation, prior dehydration at time of injury, and concomitant trauma often require more fluid than the formula predicted.

Other formulas contain various amounts of hypertonic saline or colloid. Hypertonic saline resuscitation lowers the amount of fluid that needs to be given to selected patients; however, it can cause severe hypernatremia and must be used cautiously. The argument against colloid administration within 12 hours of injury is that during this time, the diffuse postburn capillary leak allows colloids to extravasate through endothelial junctions. Therefore, colloid administration does not produce any demonstrable oncotic benefit over administration of a crystalloid while the capillary leak is present. The time at which capillary integrity is restored varies among people but usually is between 12 and 14 hours postinjury. Many physicians administer colloids at this point to restore albumin levels to 2.0 to 3.0 mg/dL. Controversy exists over the type of colloid to be administered, with some centers using salt-poor albumin, and others using fresh frozen plasma.

The challenge is to balance resuscitation since under- or over-resuscitation have significant consequences. Care must be taken to avoid fluid overload and pulmonary edema. This is often difficult because large amounts of fluids are given over a short period during fluid resuscitation immediately after the burn. For example, using the high range of the ABA consensus formula, a man weighing 75 kg who received burns over 50% of his body would require up to 15,000 mL of fluid (4 mL × 75 kg × 50% TBSA = 15,000 mL). Of this, 7,500 mL is to be administered during the first 8 hours, and 3,750 mL is to be administered in each of the second and third 8-hour periods. It is extremely difficult to avoid fluid overload and pulmonary edema when it is necessary to infuse large amounts of fluids so rapidly.

After the first 24 hours after injury, replacing the massive evaporative water loss is a major consideration in fluid management. The primary solution given at this time is $D_5W$, with the goal of keeping the patient's sodium concentration at 140 mEq/L. The fluid volume depends on the severity of injury, the age of the patient, the physiologic status of the patient, and any associated injuries. Consequently, the volume recommended by a resuscitation formula must be modified according to the person's response to therapy (Fig. 53-5).

Urine output is the single best indicator of fluid resuscitation in patients with previously normal renal function. The onset of spontaneous diuresis is a hallmark indicating the end of the resuscitative phase. Infusion rates can be decreased by 20% to 30% for 1 hour if the urine output is satisfactory and can be maintained for 2 hours; the reduction may then be repeated. It is essential that urinary outputs be maintained within normal limits of 30 to 50 mL/h (0.5 mL/kg/h) in the adult.[8] Other indications of adequate fluid replacement are listed in Box 53-10.

Patients are usually weighed daily. A gain of 15% of admission weight may be expected with large fluid resuscitation. Intake and output must be monitored meticulously. Patients who sustain deep muscle injury (ie, second- or third-degree burns or electrical injuries) are at risk for development of acute renal insufficiency. This renal dysfunction may be the result of inadequate fluid resuscitation, or it may be the consequence of the liberation of the myoglobin and hemoglobin from damaged cells. These compounds, sometimes called hemochromogens, may precipitate in renal tubules, resulting in acute tubular necrosis. Hemochromogens produce a clear reddish-brown color in the urine. Should hemochromogens appear in the urine, acidosis should be corrected promptly and IV fluids increased to maintain a brisk urine output

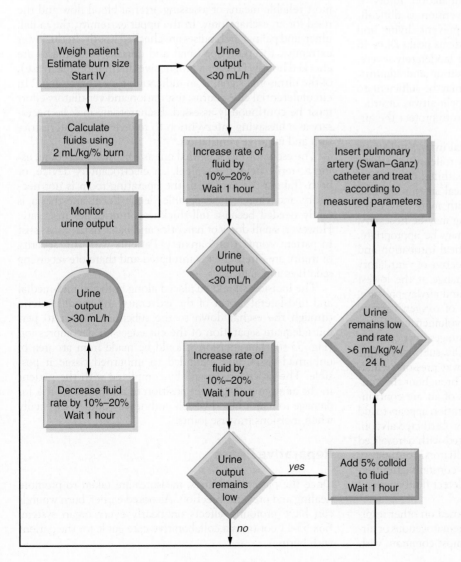

FIGURE 53-5  Initial 24-hour fluid management. (From Rue LW, Cioffi WG: Resuscitation of thermally injured patients. Crit Care Nurs Clin North Am 3(2):186, 1991.)

**Urinary output:** 30 to 70 mL/h (0.5 mL/kg/h)
**Pulse rate:** 100 to 120 bpm
**Central venous pressure (CVP):** less than 12 cm $H_2O$
**Pulmonary artery occlusion pressure (PAOP):** less than 18 mm Hg
**Lungs:** Clear
**Sensorium:** Clear
**Gastrointestinal tract:** Absence of nausea and adynamic ileus
**Arterial base deficit and lactate:** Normalizing values

*Central lines and Swan–Ganz catheters are not inserted routinely because of the danger of sepsis; however, they are used in selected instances.

(75 to 100 mL urine/h) until the urine returns to its normal clear yellow and there is no urinary myoglobin.

### Providing Pulmonary Support

Inhalation injury is the leading cause of death in the first 24 hours after burn injury. It increases the mortality rate by 20% alone and by as much as 60% when combined with pneumonia.[18,22,23] Goals for the successful treatment of inhalation injury include improving oxygenation and decreasing interstitial edema and airway occlusion.

The conventional treatment for inhalation injury is largely supportive because direct intervention is difficult. Humidified oxygen is administered to prevent drying and sloughing of the mucosa. Upper airway edema peaks 24 to 48 hours after injury. If the injury is mild or moderately severe, placing the patient in a high Fowler position and administering aerosolized racemic epinephrine may be sufficient to limit further edema formation. Severe upper airway obstruction may require endotracheal intubation to protect the airway until the edema subsides.[23]

In patients with mild tracheobronchial injury, atelectasis may be prevented by frequent pulmonary toilet, using a high Fowler position, coughing and deep breathing, chest physiotherapy, repositioning, frequent tracheal suctioning, and incentive spirometry.[15,16] In patients with more severe inhalation injury, more frequent suctioning may be necessary, and bronchoscopic removal of debris may be appropriate. These patients usually require endotracheal intubation and mechanical ventilatory support. The objective of ventilatory support is to provide adequate gas exchange at the lowest possible inspired oxygen concentration and airway pressure, in an attempt to reduce the incidence of oxygen toxicity and pulmonary barotrauma. The use of volumetric diffusive respiration (VDR) appears to offer advantages over conventional mechanical ventilation.[15,23] In VDR, subtidal volume breaths accumulate and build to a set airway pressure, which is then followed by passive exhalation. Throughout the ventilatory cycle, high-frequency pulsations of air are continuously administered. This method of inspiration appears to aid in ventilation and recruitment of partially obstructed alveoli.

Patients with bronchospasm are treated with aerosolized or intravenously administered bronchodilators. Respiratory parameters are monitored closely, with constant attention paid to breath sounds and vital signs to detect fluid overload as early as possible.

Bronchopneumonia may be superimposed on other respiratory problems at any time and may be hematogenous or airborne. Airborne bronchopneumonia is most common, with onset occurring soon after injury. It is often associated with a lower airway injury or aspiration. Hematogenous, or miliary, pneumonia begins as a bacterial abscess secondary to another septic source, usually the burn wound. The time of onset is usually 2 weeks after injury.

Prophylactic antibiotics and steroids have not been demonstrated to prevent the common complications of infection encountered in patients with inhalation injury. Researchers continue to look for new methods to decrease the incidence of nosocomial pneumonia in critically ill patients.

### Escharotomy

Any circumferential burn to an arm or leg may mimic compartment syndrome. Edema formation in the tissues under the tight, unyielding eschar of a circumferential burn of a deep partial-thickness or full-thickness injury produces significant vascular compromise in the affected limb.

To minimize the risk of circulatory compromise, the patient's rings, watch, and other jewelry are removed during the initial examination. Elevation and range of motion of the injured extremity may alleviate minimal degrees of circulatory distress. Skin color, sensation, capillary refill, and peripheral pulses are assessed and documented hourly in an extremity with a circumferential burn. Doppler ultrasonography is the most reliable means of assessing arterial blood flow and the need for an escharotomy. In the upper extremity, the radial, ulnar, and palmar arch pulses are checked hourly. In the lower extremity, the posterior tibial and dorsalis pedis pulses are checked hourly. Loss, or a progressive diminution (decrease), of the ultrasonic signal is an indication for escharotomy.[24] In circumferential chest burns, respiration and ventilatory effort must be continuously assessed. Escharotomy may be necessary as a lifesaving intervention to relieve chest wall restriction and improve ventilation.[21,24,25]

The escharotomy is carried out as a bedside procedure, using a sterile field and scalpel, an electrocautery device, or both. Taking the patient to the operating room is not necessary and causes unacceptable delay. Local anesthesia is rarely needed because full-thickness injuries are insensate. However, small doses of narcotics and benzodiazepines assist in patient comfort and anxiety. Patients with this severity of injury are often already intubated and therefore receiving sedatives and analgesics.

The incision should be placed along both the mid-medial and mid-lateral aspect of the extremity and should extend through the eschar down to the subcutaneous fat to permit adequate separation of the cut edges for decompression (Fig. 53-6). The incisions should be made from an area of unburned tissue and extended to unburned tissue if possible. The procedure should be completed with the patient in the anatomically correct position to minimize the risk for damage to major blood vessels and nerve bundles, especially when incisions traverse joints.

### Reparative Phase

Once the patient stabilizes, measures are taken to promote healing and prevent infection. As noted earlier, burn wounds can have profound effects on nearly every organ system. Box 53-11 contains a collaborative care guide for the patient with burns.

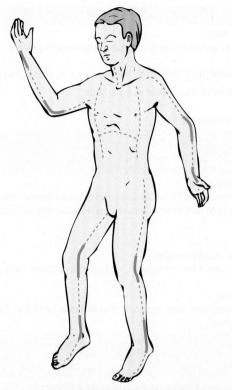

FIGURE 53-6 Preferred sites of escharotomy incisions.

## Ensuring Optimal Nutrition

Before the unique nutritional needs of patients with burns were fully recognized in the late 1970s, those who had severe burn injuries, and who survived, languished in a hospital ward with minimal oral intake until they became severely cachectic. It is now clear that appropriate nutrition plays a significant role in improving outcome for patients with severe burn injuries.

Although early parenteral feeding has been associated with increased mortality because of an increase in the risk for infection, early enteral feeding has been proposed because it may reduce the translocation of bacteria from the intestinal lumen even at low rates.[12,13] Passage of bacteria from the gut into the intestinal lymphatics or portal venous system probably occurs in all healthy people. However, the intestinal edema that accompanies the burn resuscitation period and the immunosuppression that follows make it difficult for the body to clear these microorganisms effectively. Microbial products—either live organisms or cell wall fragments—disseminate through the body, prompting the release of cytokines such as TNF, interleukin-1 (IL-1), and interleukin-6 (IL-6). These cytokines exacerbate the hypermetabolic response and may initiate SIRS.

The rationale for enteral feeding within the first 24 hours of injury is that the presence of food in the gut lumen reduces the rate of microbial translocation. Although

| **BOX 53-11** COLLABORATIVE CARE GUIDE for the Patient With a Burn | |
|---|---|
| **Outcomes** | **Interventions** |
| **Ineffective Airway Clearance**<br>**Impaired Gas Exchange**<br>**Ineffective Breathing Pattern** | |
| Patent airway is maintained. | • Auscultate breath sounds every 2 to 4 hours and as needed (PRN). |
| Lung is clear on auscultation. | • Assess for inhalation injury, and anticipate intubation.<br>• Assess quantity and color of tracheal secretions.<br>• Suction endotracheal airway when appropriate (see Chapter 25, Box 25-16).<br>• Hyperoxygenate and hyperventilate before and after each suction pass. |
| Peak, mean, and plateau pressures are within normal limits for a patient on a ventilator. | • Monitor airway pressures every 1 to 2 hours.<br>• Monitor lung compliance every 8 hours (see Chapter 24).<br>• Administer bronchodilators and mucolytics.<br>• Perform chest physiotherapy every 4 hours.<br>• Monitor airway pressures and lung compliance for improvement after interventions.<br>• Calculate $PaO_2/FiO_2$ ratio and oxygen index, monitoring trends. |
| There is no evidence of atelectasis or infiltrates. | • Turn side-to-side every 2 hours.<br>• Consider kinetic therapy or prone positioning.<br>• Daily chest x-ray. |
| Arterial blood gases (ABGs) are within normal limits. | • Initial and serial carboxyhemoglobin (carbon monoxide) levels until less than 10%.<br>• Monitor ABGs, monitor acid–base balance, lactate and bicarbonate levels. (Pulse oximeter and calculated $SaO_2$ are inaccurate measures in the presence of carbon monoxide.)<br>• Provide humidified oxygen.<br>• Consider hyperbaric therapy. |
| **Impaired Peripheral Tissue Perfusion**<br>**Risk for Imbalanced Body Temperature**<br>**Decreased Cardiac Perfusion** | |
| Blood pressure, heart rate, CVP, and pulmonary artery (PA) pressures are within normal limits. | • Assess vital signs every 1 hour.<br>• Assess hemodynamic pressures every 1 hour if patient has PA catheter.<br>• Administer intravascular volume as ordered to maintain preload (see below). |

| Outcomes | Interventions |
|---|---|
| Temperature is within normal limits. | • Monitor temperature every 1 hour.<br>• Maintain a warm environment, and use warming lights or blankets to prevent hypothermia.<br>• Treat fever by cooling the environment, and using antipyretics and cooling blankets. |
| Perfusion to extremities is maintained; pulses are intact. | • Monitor perfusion using Doppler and palpation every 1 hour.<br>• Elevate burned extremities.<br>• Prepare for escharotomy or fasciotomy. |

**Deficient Fluid Volume**
**Fluid Volume Excess**
**Electrolyte Imbalance**

| | |
|---|---|
| Restore and maintain fluid balance:<br>• Urine output 30 to 70 mL/h or 0.5 mL/kg/h.<br>• CVP 8 to 12 mm Hg; PAOP 12 to 18 mm Hg; blood pressure, within normal limits; heart rate 100 to 120 bpm. | • Assess intake and output every 1 hour.<br>• Give lactated Ringer's 2 to 4 mL/kg/% TBSA, divided into first 24-hours postburn.<br>• Monitor for spontaneous diuresis, and reduce intravenous infusion rate as indicated.<br>• Take daily weight. |
| Electrolytes, mineral, and renal function values are within normal limits. | • Monitor and replace minerals and electrolytes.<br>• Monitor blood urea nitrogen, creatinine, myoglobin, and urine electrolytes and glucose.<br>• Monitor neurologic status.<br>• Monitor and treat dysrhythmias.<br>• Monitor and limit water consumption; burn patients have extreme thirst and if allowed drastically decrease sodium level. |

**Risk for Activity Intolerance**
**Impaired Physical Mobility**
**Risk for Infection**

| | |
|---|---|
| Patient is free of joint contractures. | • Provide passive and active range-of-motion exercises every 1 to 2 hours.<br>• Apply positioning splints as needed. |
| There is no evidence of complications related to immobility. | • Turn and reposition every 2 hours.<br>• Consider kinetic therapy.<br>• Consider deep venous thrombosis prophylaxis. |
| There is no evidence of infection. | • Maintain strict sterile technique, and monitor technique of others.<br>• Maintain sterility of invasive catheters and tubes.<br>• Per hospital protocol, change dressings and invasive catheters. Culture wounds, blood, urine, as necessary.<br>• Monitor for changes in sputum or wounds.<br>• Monitor SIRS/sepsis using burn criteria: temperature, tachycardia, tachypnea or ↑minute ventilation, feeding intolerance, elevated glucose/insulin resistance. |

**Impaired Skin Integrity**

| | |
|---|---|
| Unburned skin will remain intact. | • Assess skin every 4 hours and each time patient is repositioned.<br>• Turn every 2 hours.<br>• Consider pressure relief/reduction mattress and devices. |
| Burns begin healing without complications. | • Treat burns per hospital protocol; apply topical medications and débride as indicated.<br>• Monitor skin graft viability.<br>• Protect grafted areas (eg, bed cradle, dressings).<br>• Consider air fluidized bed to enhance healing and relieve pressure from burned surface. |

**Imbalanced Nutrition: Less than Body Requirements**

| | |
|---|---|
| Caloric and nutrient intake meets metabolic requirements per calculation (eg, Basal Energy Expenditure). | • Provide enteral or parenteral nutrition within 24 hours of injury.<br>• Consult dietitian or nutritional support service to assess nutritional requirements with team.<br>• Monitor protein and calorie intake.<br>• Monitor albumin, prealbumin, transferrin, cholesterol, triglycerides, glucose, nitrogen balance. |

**Impaired Comfort**
**Acute Pain**

| | |
|---|---|
| Patient will have minimal pain (less than 5 on pain scale) and discomfort. | • Assess pain and discomfort using objective pain scale every 4 hours, PRN, and following administration of pain medication.<br>• Administer analgesics before procedures and monitor patient response.<br>• Use nonpharmacologic pain management techniques (eg, music, distraction, touch). |

| QSEN BOX 53-11 | *COLLABORATIVE CARE GUIDE for the Patient With a Burn (continued)* |
|---|---|
| **Outcomes** | **Interventions** |

**Ineffective Coping**
**Anxiety**

| | |
|---|---|
| Patient demonstrates decreased anxiety. | • Assess vital signs during treatments, discussions, and so forth. |
| | • Administer anxiolytics before treatments/procedures. |
| | • Consult social services, clergy, and so forth as appropriate. |
| | • Provide for adequate rest and sleep. |
| | • Encourage discussion regarding long-term effects of burns, available resources, and coping strategies. |

**Teaching/Discharge Planning**

| | |
|---|---|
| Patient/significant others understand procedures and tests needed for treatment. | • Prepare patient/significant others for procedures, such as débridement, escharotomy, fasciotomy, intubation, and mechanical ventilation. |
| Significant others understand the severity of the illness, ask appropriate questions, and anticipate potential complications. | • Explain the potential effects of burns and the potential for complications, such as infection, and respiratory or renal failure. |
| | • Encourage significant others to ask questions related to the management of burns, disfigurement, coping, and so forth. |

not proven definitively in the clinical setting of patients with burns, safety and simplicity of early feeding have been demonstrated. One approach is to slowly infuse tube feedings through the NGT at a rate of 10 to 20 mL/h. Although this clearly does not meet the nutritional needs of adult patients, it is enough to protect the gut mucosa. Long feeding tubes can be placed into the small bowel using endoscopy, fluoroscopy, or external magnetic guidance, and the rate steadily increased to meet the estimated calculated caloric requirements. The advantages of such tubes are higher and earlier rates of infusion and continuous feeding of patients during surgical procedures requiring general anesthesia. Patients with minor burns may be able to satisfy their caloric needs and fluid resuscitation through oral intake only.

Despite the theoretical advantages and need for the calories provided by enteral feeding, difficulties exist, and the technique cannot be used in all patients. Patients receive, on average, only 80% of the goal rate for enteral feedings because of frequent interruptions for patient care, including radiologic procedures and surgery. This deficit increases when patients develop intestinal ileus, as typically occurs with major infection. Osmotic diarrhea is troublesome, particularly when the patient's feces soil the burn dressings. A variety of techniques can be used to combat diarrhea, including the use of bulk-forming nutrients, retardation of bowel motility, and placement of a bowel management system.

The estimated caloric and protein needs of a patient may be met more reliably with parenteral than enteral feeding. The central venous catheter, which predisposes the patient to invasive infections (particularly infections with *Candida* species), is a disadvantage. Reports suggest that the rate of bacterial translocation is increased with the use of parenteral nutrition compared with enteral nutrition, and that infection rates are higher.[12,26] Long-term use of parenteral nutrition alone is associated with hepatobiliary dysfunction, including cholestatic hepatitis and acalculous cholecystitis. Nevertheless, parenteral nutrition can be used for patients who do not tolerate enteral feedings because of paralytic ileus of the intestine or prolonged diarrhea.

Burn injury results in an increase in the metabolic expenditure. Initial investigative work performed in the 1970s demonstrated that some patients with burns needed as many as 7,000 or 8,000 kcal/d to maintain weight. Although patients with burns still become hypercatabolic after injury, they do not become so to the same degree as in the past. Because of the effect of earlier enteral feeding and the introduction of procedures that promote early wound closure (early and aggressive excision and grafting and the use of biologic dressings), the increase in metabolic rate has diminished. Healing does not fully begin until the wounds are closed. Indirect calorimetry has shown that the most severe injuries require no more calories than twice the resting energy expenditure (REE) as described in the Harrison–Benedict formula. The REE calculated by the Harrison–Benedict formula is multiplied by a stress factor in direct proportion to the size of the burn (Box 53-12). The stress factor is judged conservatively to avoid overfeeding, which is associated with increased susceptibility to infection. Although indirect calorimetry prevents gross underestimation or overestimation of the patient's caloric needs, in most patients it is probably not superior to estimating their needs from a formula (such as the Harrison–Benedict formula) alone.[27,28]

| BOX 53-12 | **Stress Factors for Energy Expenditure Related to Burn Size (Harrison–Benedict Equations)** |
|---|---|

**Women:** $REE = 655 + [4.3 \times Wt\ (lb)] + [4.3 \times Ht\ (in)] - [4.7 \times Age]$

**Men:** $REE = 65 + [6.2 \times Wt\ (lb)] + [12.7 \times Ht\ (in)] - [6.8 \times age]$

| TBSA (%) | Stress Factor |
|---|---|
| 0 to 10 | 1.4 |
| 11 to 20 | 1.5 |
| 21 to 30 | 1.6 |
| 31 to 40 | 1.7 |
| 41 to 50 | 1.8 |
| 51 to 60 | 1.9 |
| Greater than 60 | 2.0 |

REE, resting energy expenditure.

Wound repair depends on amino acids, which are the building blocks of proteins. The type of amino acids used in enteral feedings varies. The amino acids arginine and glutamine have immune-enhancing properties, improve nitrogen retention, and maintain lean body mass. Formulas containing arginine supplements have been reported to reduce infections in trauma patients and to reduce length of stay of critically ill patients.

Judging the amount of protein necessary for recovery from burn injuries is difficult. Massive and unquantified loss of protein from the burn wound exudates precludes nitrogen balance studies based on urine excretion alone. Sequential measurements of serum proteins, such as transferrin and prealbumin, are a better index of the body's response to the amount and type of dietary protein given; however, few clinical studies show a correlation between an increase in serum proteins and improved clinical outcome. It is important to avoid overfeeding of protein because it predisposes patients to sepsis. Amounts of protein greater than 3 g/kg/d in adults are usually not tolerated because of azotemia. Dietary protein should be started at an administration rate of 1.2 g/kg/d and should be increased if there is not a subsequent increase in serum protein markers. A patient's diet can also be supplemented with vitamins A and C, and with the trace element zinc, all of which improve wound healing.[27]

Successful weaning of patients from nutritional supplements sometimes occurs earlier than expected. A regular diet with liquid supplements is offered within 24 hours of extubation. The increased thirst of patients with burns is used to encourage the intake of protein-containing solutions, either soy- or milk-based supplements, or protein-containing fruit drinks. Using supplements, patients can take up to 2,000 kcal each day. It is preferable to feed patients or allow them to feed themselves because of the inherent risks of feeding tubes and central lines.[28]

### Providing Musculoskeletal Support

Physical and occupational therapy begins on day 1 of a burn injury. Independent of the patient's general condition, injured upper and lower extremities can be elevated to allow adequate venous drainage and reduce edema. Passive exercises are initiated and, if alert and cooperative, the patient should participate in these exercises. Active and passive exercises to maintain joint range of motion are continued throughout hospitalization and the outpatient rehabilitation period.

Two important axioms influence rehabilitation. First, the burn wound will shorten by contraction until it meets an opposing force. Across a flexor surface, this may result in a contracture. Second, the position of comfort is the position of contracture. Range-of-motion exercises prevent tendon shortening and restriction of joint motion by burn scar contractures. As patients begin to recover and participate actively in therapy, exercises are designed to increase muscle strength and endurance. A return to activities of daily living frequently takes months.

An unfortunate consequence of contractures and immobility is heterotopic ossification. Heterotopic ossification develops when there is an abnormal deposition of calcium phosphate crystals in joint spaces or along tendons. Heterotopic ossification restricts the motion of joints, particularly in elbows and knees. Unlike the heterotopic ossification seen in patients with spinal cord injuries, the heterotopic ossification seen in patients with burns does not respond to treatment with etidronate disodium, and early surgical removal is not indicated. Resolution occurs with time in most patients, and few need surgical removal of the ossified crystals in the joints.

### Managing Pain

The pain associated with burns is managed aggressively. All narcotics are given intravenously because absorption of the drug is unpredictable when given intramuscularly or subcutaneously secondary to the hypermetabolic response and the fluid shifts.[6,24,29] Patients are given anxiolytics for anxiety related to appearance, procedures, and fear.[30] Patient-controlled analgesia (PCA) is ideal for patients who are awake, sufficiently oriented, and physically able to use the pump. PCA pumps can provide a continuous pain medication, with a "dose" available every 6 to 8 minutes for intermittent pain. The nurse can give the patient a "bolus" dose before procedures, such as dressing changes and physical therapy. Recommended narcotics include morphine, fentanyl, and hydromorphone.[21,29–31]

### Caring for the Wound

**CLEANSING.** The wound protocols of all burn centers and hospitals vary, but the most common wound cleansing involves water and chlorhexidine or saline solution and povidone–iodine (Betadine). Wounds are cleansed at each dressing change and are observed for signs of infection and rate of healing.

Hydrotherapy is the preferred approach of most burn centers because the warm, flowing water is beneficial to help loosen exudates, clean and assess the wound, and provide an opportunity for range-of-motion exercise. The solutions used vary and may contain salt, povidone–iodine, and bleach. Because the procedure is usually painful, patients should receive an analgesic 20 to 30 minutes before beginning and small, frequent doses throughout as needed. In addition, the patient should receive a complete explanation of, and assistance with, pain-controlling techniques (eg, imagery, music therapy). Additional support should be offered by providing ongoing explanations of what is to be done and why, and by permitting the patient to participate in care as much as possible. Patient participation encourages active range of motion and individual control of the procedure. Limiting the time the procedure takes is important to the patient's pain tolerance and temperature control. Hydrotherapy should be limited to 20 minutes to prevent extreme chilling, which increases metabolic demand.

Care must be taken to avoid cross-contamination of wounds during bathing procedures. For this reason, many centers no longer immerse patients in Hubbard tanks. Portable shower trolleys with disposable liners can provide hydrotherapy without the risk for contamination. These may be used in a central shower room or in facilities so equipped, or used directly in the patient's room, reducing the risk inherent in transporting the critically ill. Clean or healing wounds should be cleansed separately from contaminated wounds.

**APPLICATION OF TOPICAL ANTIMICROBIAL MEDICATIONS.** The choice of topical antimicrobial medications depends on the wound depth, location, and condition and on the presence of specific organisms. Common antimicrobial drugs used from time of admission to a burn unit include silver sulfadiazine (Silvadene), mafenide acetate (Sulfamylon), 0.5% silver nitrate, nitrofurazone, povidone–iodine, bacitracin, gentamicin, and nystatin (Table 53-3). No single drug is totally effective against all burn wound infections. Treatment is guided by in vitro testing or in vivo results. Eschar and granulating wound surfaces may be cultured three times weekly to identify contaminating organisms and determine antibiotic sensitivity.

Silver sulfadiazine is the primary topical drug of choice on admission. The most common adverse reaction is transient leukopenia; therefore, serial CBCs must be monitored. If the WBC count falls below 3,000 cells/mm$^3$, the physician will probably prescribe another topical agent. When the leukocyte count returns to normal (4,000 to 5,000 cells/mm$^3$), silver sulfadiazine therapy may be reinstituted.[32]

If the colony counts increase, the topical agent of choice is usually mafenide acetate cream, an effective broad-spectrum bacteriostatic agent. Mafenide acetate diffuses through third-degree eschar to the burn wound margin within 3 hours of application. Patient discomfort is common because mafenide acetate may cause a burning sensation as it penetrates the eschar tissue, lasting 20 to 30 minutes after application. This agent inhibits carbonic anhydrase, resulting in metabolic acidosis that is initially compensated for by hyperventilation. Oral administration of sodium citrate dihydrate (Bicitra) or IV sodium bicarbonate usually corrects this acid–base imbalance.

The application of topical antimicrobial drugs inhibits the rate of wound epithelialization and may increase the metabolic rate. Electrolyte imbalances (eg, sodium leaching by silver nitrate) and acid–base abnormalities may occur. The best topical drugs are water soluble because they do not hold in heat and macerate the wound. With the application of any topical drug, it is important to use sterile technique. Antimicrobial creams should be applied to a thickness recommended by the manufacturer and reapplied at the necessary frequency to maintain consistent coverage.

**DEBRIDEMENT.** Eschar covers the burn wound until it is excised or has separated spontaneously. Small burn wounds may be allowed to separate on their own if the wound shows no signs or symptoms of infection, the patient is hemodynamically stable, or the situation does not allow for excision. In theory, burn wound management is simple: it calls for debridement of the eschar and skin graft closure before the eschar becomes infected. However, the sometimes-serious systemic complications of burn injury, such as hypovolemia and sepsis, may delay this course of action significantly.

**Mechanical Debridement.** Mechanical debridement may be accomplished using forceps and scissors to gently lift and trim loose necrotic tissue. Another form of mechanical debridement is dressing the wound with coarse gauze in the form of wet-to-dry or wet-to-wet dressings. Wet-to-dry dressings consist of layers of moistened coarse mesh gauze. As the inner layer dries, it adheres to the wound, entrapping exudate and wound debris. The dressing should be removed at a 90-degree angle, and every effort should be made to avoid damaging fragile, newly granulating tissue. As the wound forms increasing amounts of granulation tissue, wet-to-wet dressings may be used to prevent desiccation and trauma; these dressings remain moist until the next dressing change. The dressing should be removed by first gently lifting from the edges toward the center of the wound and then removing the dressing at a 180-degree angle. This procedure prevents detachment of newly formed epithelial tissue.

**Enzymatic Debridement.** Enzymatic debridement involves the application of a proteolytic substance to burn wounds to shorten the time of eschar separation. Travase and Elase are commonly used agents. The wound is first cleaned and debrided of any loose necrotic material. The agent is then applied directly to the wound bed and covered with a layer of fine-mesh gauze. A topical antimicrobial agent is applied next, and the entire area is covered with saline-soaked gauze. The dressing is changed two to four times per day.

Enzymatic debridement has the advantage of eliminating the need for surgical excision; however, certain complications must be considered. Hypovolemia may occur as a result of excessive fluid loss through the wound; hence, no more than 20% TBSA should be treated in this manner. Cellulitis

**TABLE 53-3    Medications for Burn Wound Management**

| Agent | Advantages | Disadvantages | Nursing Considerations |
|---|---|---|---|
| **Mafenide acetate** | Broad-spectrum, penetrates eschar | Painful application, acid–base imbalances | Apply twice a day, leave open to air |
| **Silver nitrate** | Painless application, broad-spectrum, rare sensitivity | No eschar penetration, discolors wound and environmental surfaces, must be kept moist | Wet-to-wet dressing with nonadhering layer, followed by a gauze layer every 24 h |
| **Silver sulfadiazine** | Painless application, broad-spectrum, easy application | May cause transient leukopenia, minimal eschar penetration | Apply a moderate layer and wrap in a gauze dressing every 12 h |
| **Bacitracin** | Painless application, nonirritating | No eschar penetration, antimicrobial spectrum not as wide as above medications | Apply a thin layer and nonadhering dressing; if used on face, leave open to air |
| **Mupirocin** | Antimicrobial spectrum broader than bacitracin | Expensive | Apply a thin layer and nonadhering dressing; if used on face, leave open to air |
| **Neomycin** | Painless application | Antimicrobial spectrum not as wide as above medications | Apply a thin layer and nonadhering dressing; if used on face, leave open to air |

and maceration of normal skin may occur around the wound periphery, and patients often complain of a burning sensation lasting 30 to 60 minutes after enzyme application.

**Surgical Debridement.** In surgical excision, the wound is excised to viable bleeding points while minimizing the loss of viable tissue. Early excision has contributed significantly to the survival of people with major burns. The open burn causes hypermetabolism and a stress response that is not corrected until wound closure occurs. Surgical excision should be done as soon as the patient is hemodynamically stable, usually within 72 hours.[21,33,34]

After excision is complete, hemostasis must be achieved. This may be accomplished by topical thrombin sprayed on the wound or application sponges soaked in a 1:10,000 epinephrine solution.[21,33,34] After removal of necrotic tissue, the exposed underlying structures must be dressed with a temporary or permanent covering to provide protection and prevent infection.

**GRAFTS.** The ideal substitute for lost skin is an autograft of similar color, texture, and thickness from a close location on the body. Sheets of the patient's epidermis and a partial layer of the dermis are harvested from unburned locations using a dermatome. These grafts, referred to as split-thickness skin grafts, can be applied to the wound as a sheet graft or mesh grafts.

In a sheet graft, the harvested skin is applied to the surgically excised area. It is usually covered with a petrolatum-based gauze dressing. Over exposed areas such as the face and hands, a sheet graft gives a more natural appearance than a mesh graft.

Grafts must be inspected frequently to ensure that fluid is not collecting underneath them. Fluid accumulation is prevented by rolling a cotton-tipped applicator over the graft to express any trapped fluid. The sheet graft should be "pie-crusted" to allow for the expression of fluid through the closest opening; this avoids rolling the fluid to the edge of the graft, increasing the risk for dislodging the grafted tissue. After adherence has begun, usually after 24 hours, the fluid may be removed with a very small-gauge needle (26-gauge) to avoid disrupting the adherence of graft.

In a mesh graft, the harvested skin is slit, and the graft is then placed on the burn site. The slits (or interstices) allow the skin to expand, providing for greater coverage and drainage and facilitating draping over uneven surfaces. Mesh grafts frequently have to be expanded to obtain maximal coverage from each piece of autograft. An expansion ratio of 1:2 or 1:4 is often practical. Ratios such as 1:6 or 1:7 are used to cover large burns when donor tissue is limited. With these larger ratios, the expanded autograft is covered with either cadaver skin allografts, synthetic skin (Biobrane, Winthrop Pharmaceuticals), or negative pressure dressings.[21,35] In addition to physically stabilizing the fragile mesh, the cover decreases evaporation, heat loss, and bacterial contamination.

Dressings are used after surgery to immobilize the grafted area and prevent shearing and dislodging of the graft. Postoperative dressings also provide a degree of compression to minimize hematoma and seroma formation, but they may be a source of vascular compression in the extremities. Pulse checks distal to the dressings are documented every 4 hours for 24 hours after surgery. The dressings are usually left in place until the third postoperative day. Until that time, the dressings are moistened every 6 hours with a solution containing normal saline and polymyxin. The antibiotic solution keeps the fragile meshed grafts moist and protects against infection. On postoperative day 3, the dressings are removed and evaluated by the physician, who determines the success of the grafting, which is expressed in terms of percentages. The grafted area is then covered with a nonadherent dressing and a gauze layer, which are secured with a gauze roll. All components of the dressing are moistened with the antibiotic solution.

A variety of products are used at burn centers for donor site care, and burn surgeons vary in their preference as well. The donor site is covered during surgery with a single layer of fine-mesh gauze (eg, Biobrane, Acticoat).[35] Most products are kept in place until separation from the donor site begins. Positioning to prevent pressure on the site and to allow for drying is important. Daily inspection of the donor site is essential to detect early signs of infection or cellulitis.

The growth and subsequent graft placement of cultured epithelial autografts has become an important adjunct to permanent coverage of extensive burn wounds. Biopsies are taken from unburned skin, and cells are cultured in the laboratory. Sheets of cultured epithelial cells are attached to petrolatum-impregnated gauze and applied to the wound. The cultured cells are highly fragile, and the surgeon may elect to place the patient in traction for increased protection of the grafted tissue. After 7 to 10 days, the gauze application is removed, and a nonadherent dressing is applied to prevent mechanical trauma.

## Providing Psychological and Familial Support

Providing psychological support for the newly admitted patient with burns and the family is not the least of the many tasks facing the critical care nurse. The patient is often awake and alert, although anxious and overwhelmed by the suddenness and magnitude of injuries. With high anxiety levels and lack of knowledge pertaining to burns, the family approaches the burn unit with fear, hesitancy, and sometimes hysteria. The physical appearance of the patient and the high-technology atmosphere of the burn unit are frightening. Preparing the family for the initial visit by explaining what to expect and escorting them to the bedside is extremely important. Visitors are often overwhelmed on the first visit and stand silently with increasing feelings of anxiety and hopelessness. Burn injuries are dramatic and are psychologically traumatic for the patient and for those who witnessed the accident.

Counseling for the patient and the family begins on the day of admission. Families require constant support, and the burn team should plan weekly family meetings to discuss the patient's care plan and progress. This is often the all-important basis for establishing a trusting relationship for the long months of rehabilitation ahead. Critically ill patients with burns are likely to experience a series of small gains combined with intermittent setbacks, and this pattern does not stop until the burn wounds are closed, which can be 2 to 3 months after injury. The family needs to be informed and provided with the means to care for their own physical and psychological needs. Since burn centers tend to be regional, families of patients who were transferred from a great distance and who lack nearby support systems find the entire situation particularly stressful. The need to provide support for families cannot be overemphasized.

Patients with burns often become depressed and withdrawn, asking to be left alone and not to be made uncomfortable. The nurse should respond by making certain expectations of the patient clear. That is, the nurse should make it clear to the patient that, while the staff is there for them, the patient is to feed himself or herself, go to the bathroom unassisted, or do as much as his or her physical condition permits. At the same time, the nurse must communicate to the patient that the situation is not hopeless and that recovery is expected.

Hallucinations, confusion, and combativeness are also common in severely burned patients. Exhaustion, pain, and medications may distort reality and produce psychotic-like behavior.

The best way to handle regression in a patient with burns is to acknowledge it. First, the nurse must accept the fact that the patient may be unable to cope on an adult level with an injury of such magnitude and that the patient may be unstable emotionally and physically. Second, the nurse must devise ways to help the patient cope on an appropriate level. Interventions that usually help include following a regular schedule so that the patient knows what is expected, rewarding the patient for adult behavior, and permitting the patient as much control and choice as possible.

It is not uncommon for severely burned patients, and sometimes family members, to transfer their fears to a specific caregiver (physician, nurse, or therapist) and to complain that they are being treated unjustly or unkindly. Working with a psychiatric liaison nurse may help the burn survivor recognize and deal with his or her fears more effectively and help the caregiver support the patient by responding therapeutically. The recovery process is physically and emotionally burdensome on the entire staff as well; some burn centers employ behavioral health support to focus on staff.

Although the patient tends to concentrate on the present, the family members look to the future and want to know what to expect. Information about the patient's condition and treatments should be shared with them using an honest and open approach.

## Rehabilitative Phase

Patients with extensive burns require many months for recovery and rehabilitation. Physical and psychological rehabilitation measures are begun in the ICU and continue throughout the recovery period.

### Changes in Diet

The diet of the patient with burns should remain high in protein until all wounds have healed. As healing takes place, the diet should be tapered to meet normal caloric requirements. The patient with burns may become accustomed to eating frequently and in large amounts. After healing is complete, metabolism returns to normal, and weight will be gained if eating habits are not controlled properly.

### Prevention of Scarring and Contractures

Once regarded as inevitable, hypertrophic scarring and joint contractures are now largely preventable. Preventive measures start when the person is admitted to the hospital and continue for at least 12 months or until the scar is fully mature. Positioning the body with the extremities extended is extremely important. Although tightly flexed positions are preferred by patients for comfort, they result in severe contractures. Range-of-motion exercises should be carried out with each dressing change or more often if indicated. Special splints are used to maintain arm, legs, and hands in extended, yet functional, positions. Later, when the wounds have healed sufficiently, the person is custom-fitted for special pressure garments. The garment prevents hypertrophic scarring by applying continuous uniform pressure over the entire area of the burn. The garment must be worn almost 24 hours a day for approximately 1 year. The smooth elastic garment forms a shield that permits the person to wear normal clothing and resume ordinary activities much sooner.

Healed and grafted skin is dry and tight. Itching is a major patient complaint as healing occurs. Massaging a mild, nonirritating lotion into the healed skin provides lubrication, aids in range of motion, and promotes circulation.

### Psychological Rehabilitation

The burn survivor may have many psychological issues once discharge is nearing. The patient may be experiencing post-traumatic stress, anxiety, depression, or a combination of these. To ensure that these issues are effectively managed, the multidisciplinary team caring for the patient with burns must include mental health professionals.

## Other Injuries Treated in Burn Centers

Burn center referrals are not limited to traditional burn injuries (thermal, chemical, electrical, or radiation). Patients with disease processes that primarily involve the integumentary system have had better outcomes in burn centers because the unit is structured with the high levels of necessary resources for the required level of patient care. Patients who are referred to burn centers may have such conditions as toxic epidermal necrolysis syndrome (TENS), erythema multiforme minor, and extensive Stevens–Johnson syndrome (see Spotlight on Genetics 53-1), as well as diseases that may result in the loss of large amounts of tissue, such as necrotizing fasciitis, staphylococcal scalded skin syndrome, bullous pemphigoid, or pemphigus vulgaris. Patients with significant cold injuries may also be routinely referred to regional burn centers.

### Toxic Epidermal Necrolysis Syndrome

TENS is a superficial exfoliative dermatitis that has been linked to multiple sources, the most common being an adverse reaction to medications, the staphylococcal toxin, or viral infections.[36] The source may be undetermined. TENS can involve the entire mucosal surface of the body, including the oral mucosa and conjunctiva as well as the vaginal or urethral linings. The immediate concern is the oral lesions and possible occlusion of the respiratory system; intubation may be indicated as a supportive measure. The definitive diagnosis is made by sending a biopsy from

┌─────────────────────────────────────────┐
⬡ **SPOTLIGHT ON GENETICS 53-1**

**INTEGUMENTARY SYSTEM—STEVENS–JOHNSON SYNDROME/TOXIC EPIDERMAL NECROLYSIS**

- Stevens–Johnson syndrome/toxic epidermal necrolysis (SJS/TEN) is a rare but severe skin reaction most often triggered by particular medications. SJS/TEN often begins with a fever and flu-like symptoms. Within a few days, the skin begins to blister and peel, forming very painful raw areas that resemble a severe hot-water burn.
- Several genetic changes have been found to increase the risk of SJS/TEN in response to triggering factors such as medications. Most of these changes occur in genes that are involved in the normal function of the immune system.
- The genetic variations most strongly associated with SJS/TEN occur in the *HLA-B* gene. This gene is part of a family of genes called the human leukocyte antigen (HLA) complex. The HLA complex helps the immune system distinguish the body's own proteins from proteins made by foreign invaders. The *HLA-B* gene has many different normal variations, allowing each person's immune system to react to a wide range of foreign proteins. Certain variations in this gene occur much more often in people with SJS/TEN than in people without the condition.
- Genetic testing for *HLA-B* gene variant is available.

Genetic Home Reference. Retrieved August 10, 2015, from http://ghr.nlm.nih.gov; and Chung WH, Hung SI: Recent advances in the genetics and immunology of Stevens–Johnson syndrome and toxic epidermal necrosis. J Dermatol Sci 66(3):190–196, 2012.
└─────────────────────────────────────────┘

the involved tissue for microscopic examination where an epidermal split is observed at the junction of the epidermis and dermis.

Patients with TENS are often described by the percentage of their body surface area that is currently open, requiring fluid and electrolyte replacement for evaporative water loss through the open wounds. This disease is similar in its effects to a partial-thickness injury seen with a thermal burn. The lesions, with the nerve endings exposed to the environment, tend to be hypersensitive and extremely painful. If the soles of the feet are involved, ambulation is extremely painful and may lead to debilitation if physical activity is not maintained. Nutritional support is important to assist with the healing process; the insertion of a small-bore feeding tube may be indicated if caloric intake cannot be maintained, usually owing to oral lesions.

To increase survival, patients with TENS should be admitted to a burn center because of the complexity of wound care and the need for meticulous infection control standards. Historically, these patients have been treated with silver nitrate dressings, but more recently a variety of products, such as Acticoat and biologic dressings, have been used. The primary concern of wound care is that the dressings remain moist, not wet, at all times to decrease the desiccation of the dermal layer. Steroids are not indicated, and antibiotics are used only for specific infections.

## Necrotizing Fasciitis

Necrotizing fasciitis is a rapid and progressive inflammatory infection of the soft tissue that presents a diagnostic and therapeutic challenge. The pathogens enter the tissue through an open wound and spread rapidly in the extracellular space between the subcutaneous tissue and the fascia. It is classified into two types based on the culture findings. Type I is polymicrobial and accounts for 90% of the cases. Risk factors include postoperative status, obesity, diabetes, and older adulthood.[36] Type II accounts for the remaining 10% of cases and typically affects the upper and lower extremities. The infecting agent is Group A β-hemolytic streptococcus, with or without *Staphylococcus aureus*.[36] Diagnosis may be difficult initially because the external cutaneous damage may not be readily appreciated and the signs and symptoms may be diffuse. Early diagnosis is paramount, with timely and radical surgery being the definitive intervention. Necrotic tissue must be completely excised and explored to clean tissue borders. Broad-spectrum antibiotics are started preoperatively, and culture and Gram stain are used to provide guidance for the antibiotic regimen. Local and systemic infection must be completely controlled before wound closure is addressed.[13]

As in burn injuries, infection control is the primary component of wound management in necrotizing fasciitis. The need for extensive excision of tissue to the depth of the fascial compartments can result in extreme contractures and the loss of the protective mechanisms of the subcutaneous tissue (eg, protection from shearing and blunt forces, fat storage, temperature regulation).[36]

## Cold Injuries

Environmental exposure without appropriate protection may result in a cold injury. Although these injuries are more common in temperatures below freezing, their onset may also occur at relatively moderate temperatures depending on the length of the exposure and the person's condition at the time. Injuries may range from a localized frostbite to systemic lowering of the body's core temperature with hypothermia.

Frostbite is most often seen on the fingers, toes, and nose because they tend to be the most exposed to the environment with outdoor activity, and circulation is the most difficult to maintain in the microvasculature. With prolonged exposure, the intracellular and extracellular fluids of the body tissue become chilled and may eventually form ice crystals, impeding the blood flow to the area and leading to tissue destruction.[6] Mild cases involve only the skin and subcutaneous tissues, whereas the more severe cases involve deeper structures. The symptoms range from numbness and itching to paresthesia and decreased motion.[6]

Tissue should not be rewarmed until the patient is in an environment where the warming can be controlled and the temperature can be maintained. Rewarming the tissue involves risks because it may release a shower of microemboli. In addition, it is also extremely painful. Purplish or bluish blisters are left intact, whereas clear or white blisters are debrided, similar to burn blisters. To preserve as much length as possible for functionality, amputation is discouraged until definitive demarcation occurs, which can take weeks to months.[6,11]

# Clinical Applicability Challenges

## CASE STUDY

Mr. R., age 62, arrives in the emergency department via ambulance after sustaining burns from a house fire; he was found in his front yard with significant injuries. He is receiving oxygen at 4 L/min per nasal cannula and has one IV catheter infusing normal saline.

The ED staff conducts a primary and secondary survey in a warmed trauma room and places 100% humidified oxygen by nonrebreather mask on the patient. Since the accident, Mr. R. has complained of severe pain to the skin of his face and arms. His face is covered with carbon, and it is noted that he is becoming hoarse and has burnt facial hair.

The ED staff exposes Mr. R. and documents burns to the chest, abdomen, bilateral circumferential arms, face, neck, and upper back. Using the Rule of Nines, they estimate 55% TBSA burned. His preburn weight was 154 lb (70 kg).

A second IV is placed in Mr. R.'s other upper extremity. Based on his examination (facial burns, singed facial hair) and airway protection, Mr. R. is intubated and an indwelling urinary catheter is inserted. Fluid resuscitation is started, and analgesics are given per IV in frequent small doses for pain. The regional burn center is contacted, and Mr. R. is directly admitted to the burn ICU 3 hours after the burn injury.

Mr. R.'s vital signs are heart rate 138 bpm, blood pressure 105/56 mm Hg, respirations (assisted by ventilator) 12 breaths/min, and temperature 96.8°F (36.0°C). Breath sounds are auscultated, and coarse rhonchi are heard. Heart sounds are normal and rapid. The monitor displays sinus tachycardia without ectopy. Distal pulses on extremities with circumferential burns are assessed at least every hour. The upper extremities are checked more frequently because the pulses are diminished, and these are confirmed with Doppler ultrasound when not palpable. Bronchoscopy is performed, revealing erythema to the bilateral upper airways and no carbonaceous material; the bilateral lower airways appear to be uninjured. A fentanyl infusion and scheduled doses of lorazepam (Ativan) are given for analgesic relief and sedation, with additional dosing ordered for wound care and breakthrough pain. A nasogastric tube is inserted and arterial lines and central lines are placed.

When resuscitation is well underway, the Lund–Browder chart is completed, and a burn size of 44% TBSA

is calculated. Full-thickness burns (third-degree) account for 29% of the injuries; the burn area texture is leathery, and the surface is dry with thrombosed vessels. Prior to intubation, Mr. R. denied pain in these areas when touched or exposed to the air. The remaining partial-thickness burns are reddened, moist, and weeping serous fluid where thin-walled blisters have ruptured; when these are touched, Mr. R. has facial grimacing and his blood pressure rises. To determine estimated fluid requirements in the first 24 hours from the time of the burn, the burn resuscitation formula is calculated:

$$(2 \text{ mL}) \times (70 \text{ kg}) \times (44\% \text{ TBSA}) = 6{,}160 \text{ mL}$$

1st 8 Hours (from the time of the burn) = 3,080 mL

2nd 8 Hours = 1,540 mL

3rd 8 Hours = 1,540 mL

Mr. R. received 1,650 mL fluid at the transferring facility and 590 mL fluid while in transport and arrival to the burn center, which means that he needs an additional 1,960 mL of fluid in the first 8 hours from the time of the burn. It is now 4 hours since the time of the burn, so the fluid is divided for the remaining 4 hours, or 490 mL/h. Since the placement of the urinary catheter at the transferring facility, urine output has been 180 mL, or an average of 45 mL/h. Although this is currently adequate, it will be closely monitored because it has been trending down.

Urine outputs for hours 6 and 7 from the time of the burn are 23 and 17 mL, respectively, and the IV rate of fluid administration is increased by 20% to 588 mL/h. Urine output for hour 8 is 25 mL and the IV rate of fluid infusion is increased by 20% to 706 mL/h.

1. Discuss why fluid boluses are contraindicated and therefore not used during the resuscitation phase to treat marginally low hourly urine outputs. If the hourly urine output is exceeding the 0.5 mL/kg/h, how would you adjust the resuscitation infusion?
2. Discuss how you would secure Mr. R.'s medical devices: endotracheal tube, NGT, and peripheral IVs inserted through partial-thickness burns.
3. Discuss the signs and symptoms of ventilator compromise that would indicate the need for a chest escharotomy.

---

## WANT TO KNOW MORE?

A wide variety of resources to enhance your learning and understanding of this chapter are available on thePoint.

You will find:

- References
- Selected readings
- NCLEX-style review questions
- Internet resources
- And more!

# PART 13

# Multisystem Dysfunction

## 54

# Shock, Systemic Inflammatory Response Syndrome, and Multiple Organ Dysfunction Syndrome

Sarah R. Rosenberger, Kathryn T. Von Rueden, and Emily Smith Des Champs

### LEARNING OBJECTIVES

*Based on the content in this chapter, the reader should be able to:*

1. Describe common pathophysiologic processes involved in the generalized shock response.
2. Compare and contrast the etiology and clinical manifestations of the major types of shock.
3. Explain the anticipated management and rationale for treatment of the various shock states.
4. Describe patients at risk for development of shock and complications associated with the various shock states.
5. Discuss nursing management principles for patients with shock, systemic inflammatory response syndrome, and multiple organ dysfunction syndrome.

Under normal conditions, oxygen delivery ($DaO_2$) to the cells is sufficient to meet metabolic needs. Under stress, oxygen requirements of cells, tissues, and organs increase. Oxygen is consumed more rapidly, and compensatory mechanisms are initiated to meet the increased oxygen demands and restore perfusion to cells. The compensatory mechanisms are the same, regardless of the clinical condition causing cellular hypoperfusion. Clinical conditions that result in cellular hypoperfusion are often referred to as shock states.

## Pathophysiology of Shock

Although shock states have different causes and different clinical presentations, some features, such as hypoperfusion, hypercoagulability, and activation of the inflammatory response, are common to all shock states. Once a shock state develops, the subsequent course of illness is less dependent on the initial cause and more significantly influenced by the physiologic response to shock, including activation of the sympathetic nervous system, the inflammatory response, and the immune system. Thus, shock can be considered as a derangement of compensatory mechanisms that results in further circulatory and respiratory dysfunction with subsequent multiple organ damage.

## Tissue Oxygenation and Perfusion

Oxygenation of all organs and tissues is directly related to the cellular oxygen demands, adequacy of oxygen supply to meet demand, cellular extraction of oxygen from the blood, and the ability of the cells to use oxygen. The pulmonary system allows for the diffusion of oxygen into the blood. Oxygen binds with hemoglobin in the pulmonary capillaries to form oxyhemoglobin and carries oxygen to tissues; this is measured as arterial oxygen saturation ($SaO_2$). The cardiovascular system transports oxygenated blood to the cells for metabolism. $DaO_2$ is the amount of oxygen transported to the cells every minute. Typically, cells consume about 25% of the oxygen delivered; this utilization of oxygen is referred to as oxygen consumption ($VO_2$). Chapter 17 reviews how these oxygen parameters are calculated.

Under normal conditions, $VO_2$ is independent of $DaO_2$. When cells need to consume additional oxygen to produce energy in the form of adenosine triphosphate (ATP), they can extract the necessary amount required. However, during times of physiologic stress, $VO_2$ increases so significantly that it becomes dependent on $DaO_2$.[1,2]

Initial compensatory mechanisms by the respiratory, endocrine, and circulatory systems respond to the cells' need for oxygen by increasing $DaO_2$. These mechanisms include increasing respiratory rate, cardiac output (CO), antidiuretic hormone (ADH) release, and renin–angiotensin–aldosterone activity. If additional oxygen is required and the cells cannot extract the oxygen, they resort to anaerobic metabolism to produce ATP. Anaerobic metabolism is an inefficient method of energy production, and the amount of ATP produced is insufficient to meet cellular demands. Moreover, anaerobic metabolism produces lactate as a by-product; this can result in systemic metabolic acidosis. If oxygen availability continues to be insufficient to meet cellular demands for energy, cell death ensues. As more cells die, tissues and organs become progressively dysfunctional.[2,3]

During shock states, oxygen is consumed at a much greater rate than it is delivered. Oxygen supply is insufficient to meet oxygen demand, resulting in cellular hypoxia and dysfunction. To meet the increased need for cellular $VO_2$, the $DaO_2$ must be increased. Although it is not possible to manipulate cellular $VO_2$ directly, many interventions can be implemented to manipulate and increase $DaO_2$. In shock states, the primary goal is to maximize $DaO_2$ to meet cellular oxygen requirements in an effort to prevent tissue and cell death and maintain end-organ perfusion.

## Compensatory Mechanisms

Cellular perfusion depends on the synergy of multiple physiologic processes. The pulmonary, endocrine, and circulatory systems maintain an intricate balance to ensure oxygenation of arterial blood and delivery of oxygen to the cells by maintaining an adequate oxygenated blood supply and CO (Fig. 54-1). The autonomic nervous system assists in the orchestration of these coordinated efforts.

Compensatory mechanisms support $DaO_2$ to cells during states of hypoxia and hypoperfusion. Hypoxic states activate respiratory compensatory mechanisms that increase the depth and rate of respirations. The cardiovascular system increases CO to increase $DaO_2$ to the cells. During states of low perfusion (low blood pressure), compensatory mechanisms are initiated that result in increases in heart rate, systemic vascular resistance (SVR), preload, and cardiac contractility in an effort to restore appropriate circulatory volume. (See Chapters 16 and 17 for a discussion of these terms.) The fall in systemic blood pressure activates a series of neurohormonal responses to reestablish sufficient CO and perfusion to vital organs. These responses include decreased stimulation of baroreceptors, activation of the renin–angiotensin–aldosterone system (RAAS), and an increase in sympathetic response.

Continued sympathetic stimulation causes an increased heart rate and contractile force, increasing the CO. Arteriolar vasoconstriction increases SVR and blood pressure, and also shunts blood from less vital organs such as the stomach and intestines to vital organs, such as the heart, lungs, and brain. Preload and, subsequently, stroke volume and CO are increased by venoconstriction. The kidneys respond to sympathetic stimulation and local hypoperfusion by activating the RAAS. This increases vasoconstriction of the arterioles and veins, increasing SVR and blood pressure. Activation of the RAAS also stimulates the adrenal cortex to release aldosterone, which acts on the kidney to conserve sodium and water,

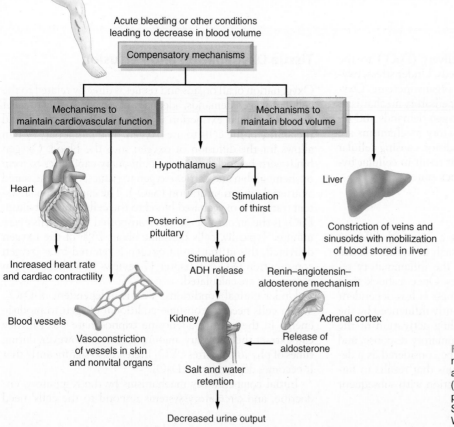

FIGURE 54-1 Compensatory mechanisms used to maintain circulatory function and blood volume in hypovolemic shock. (From Porth CM: Essentials of Pathophysiology: Concepts of Altered Health States, 3rd ed. Philadelphia, PA: Lippincott Williams & Wilkins, 2011, p 503.)

increasing circulating volume. A drop in blood pressure also causes the pituitary gland to release ADH. ADH stimulates water and sodium retention by the kidney, further increasing intravascular volume and thus preload. An increase of preload (from multiple sources) increases stroke volume, thereby increasing CO and blood pressure. Collectively, compensatory responses increase the circulating volume, blood pressure, and CO to provide perfusion and oxygen to the cells (Fig. 54-2).[2]

The goal in treating patients in shock states is to reestablish perfusion to provide adequate oxygen to meet the needs to the cells as quickly as possible. Early recognition of signs of shock and ongoing assessments guide therapeutic interventions. The nurse plays a key role in the ongoing assessment of shock. The patient's clinical presentation depends on the cause of the shock state and degree of compensation, as discussed later in this chapter. Clinical assessment parameters should be evaluated frequently to monitor the progression of shock and the effectiveness of interventions. Assessment parameters commonly found in all states of hypoperfusion include altered level of consciousness, tachypnea, arterial blood gases ($PaO_2$, $PaCO_2$, $SaO_2$), tachycardia, hypotension, decreased urine output, and metabolic acidosis (base deficit and serum lactate levels), and decreased central mixed venous oxygen saturation ($ScvO_2$) (refer to Chapter 17).

## Systemic Inflammatory Response Syndrome

The progression of shock states involves systemic activation of the inflammatory response. In addition to protective effects, the inflammatory response also has potentially detrimental effects that result in damage to tissues and organs.

The term *systemic inflammatory response syndrome* (SIRS) is used to describe patients in whom the inflammatory response is fully and systemically activated. Efforts have been made to identify patients in whom this systemic reaction is occurring, with the thought that prompt, effective intervention may prevent progression of the shock to an irreversible stage. SIRS is manifested by two or more conditions listed in Box 54-1.[4] The SIRS criteria are sometimes used as the triggers for initiating rapid response teams (see Chapter 14).

### Etiology

SIRS may be caused by any type of shock or by other insults such as massive blood transfusion, traumatic injury, brain injury, surgery, burns, and pancreatitis and infection.[5] Thus, SIRS criteria should be evaluated in any patient with shock or any condition that might lead to shock. Normally, the inflammatory response is an essential, tightly regulated and controlled protective mechanism of local response to invasion by microorganisms or to local tissue damage. However, in SIRS, this inflammatory response becomes an unregulated systemic response. Systemic inflammation results in the activation of endothelial cells, an immune response, and the coagulation cascade.

### Pathophysiology

Activation of the inflammatory response causes the release of various inflammatory mediators. Macrophages release inflammatory cytokines such as tumor necrosis factor alpha (TNFα) and interleukin-1 (IL-1).

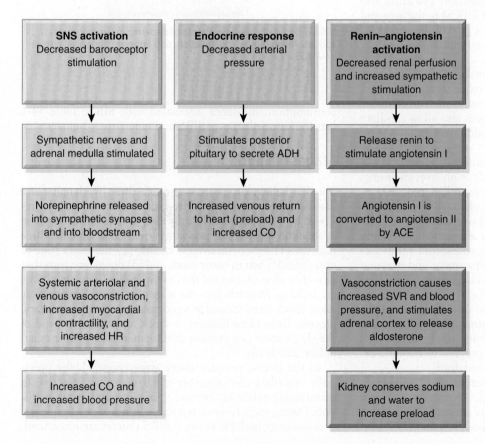

FIGURE 54-2 Compensatory mechanisms in shock. HR, heart rate; SNS, sympathetic nervous system.

### Identifying SIRS Criteria

- *Temperature*: Less than 36°C or greater than 38°C (100.4°F)
- *Heart Rate*: Greater than 90 bpm
- *Respiratory Rate*: Greater than 20 breaths/min
- *PaCO$_2$*: Less than 32 mm Hg (less than 4.3 kPa)
- *WBC Count*: Less than or equal to 4,000 cell/mm$^3$, greater than or equal to 12,000 cell/mm$^3$, or greater than 10% immature (band) forms

Endothelial cells that line blood vessels are central to the development of a local inflammatory response. In the absence of inflammation, endothelial cells provide an anticoagulant surface and controlling permeability of vessels.[6] In a localized inflammatory response, endothelial cells near the site of inflammation become activated as a result of mediators released by injured tissue cells. Under normal circumstances there are tight junctions between the endothelial cells that line blood vessels. During proinflammatory states, cytokines cause these tight junctions to separate, which increases capillary permeability and allows plasma to leak into the interstitial spaces. Activated endothelial cells express cell-surface proteins that attract platelets and neutrophils. A procoagulant endothelial surface is formed in the area. Platelets are activated, aggregate, and adhere to endothelial cells to form platelet plugs. The coagulation cascade is also activated. Fibrin, the end product of the coagulation cascade, forms strands around the clot to give it stability and strength. Microthrombi form in the capillaries and obstruct blood flow to repair injury.[6] Proinflammatory cytokines also attract phagocytic white blood cells (WBCs) to the area and activate the complement cascade. The goal of the combined activity of WBCs and complement proteins is the elimination of the invading microorganism.[2]

WBCs, platelets, and activated endothelial cells release vasodilating substances such as nitric oxide (NO), histamine, and bradykinin to enhance blood flow to the site of injury and promote healing. These substances also allow capillary leak from blood vessels, resulting in additional extravasation of plasma and coagulation factors.

In SIRS, the inflammatory response is systemic: it occurs throughout the body. The result is an overwhelming, unregulated inflammation with uncontrolled coagulation, disruption of capillaries and intravascular volume loss, maldistribution of circulating volume, and oxygen supply and demand imbalance.[2,7] Endothelial cells are activated in many vessels throughout the body, causing widespread extravasation of fluid into the interstitial compartment and systemic activation of the immune system and coagulation cascade (Fig. 54-3). A substantial amount of extravascular fluid accumulates, and microthrombi form in capillaries and in the interstitium. The combination of intravascular coagulation and decreased circulating blood volume results in reduced perfusion of vital organs, which can progress to multiple organ dysfunction syndrome (MODS) and death.

Events surrounding the complex interactions of the multiple inflammatory mediators of SIRS remain an active area of clinical research. Several mediators are believed to play a key role in the maldistribution of blood flow and DaO$_2$ and

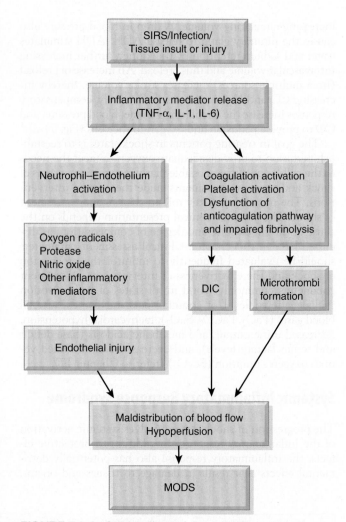

**FIGURE 54-3** Cellular effects of systemic inflammatory response. Inflammation, coagulation, and impaired fibrinolysis result in MODS.

consumption imbalance associated with SIRS. Table 54-1 lists the key mediators of SIRS and summarizes their activity.

## Stages of Shock

Shock is believed to progress through three overlapping and increasingly severe phases, the last of which cannot be reversed by known means. It is difficult to determine the phase of shock in a particular person at a particular time for three reasons: (1) shock has diverse causes, (2) the exact time of onset is unknown in many cases, and (3) diagnostic tests that provide a clear measure of the extent of shock at a given time are lacking. Nevertheless, the stages are useful because they allow shock to be viewed as a progressive rather than a static process. Early identification of shock and timely reversal of the shock state can prevent development of multiple organ failure and death.[2,8,9]

In the initial, nonprogressive stage (stage 1), the previously described compensatory mechanisms are effective in maintaining relatively normal vital signs and tissue perfusion. During stage 1, shock is poorly diagnosed and frequently goes unrecognized. However, if SIRS criteria are recognized,

**TABLE 54-1  Mediators of the Inflammatory/Immune Responses**

| Mediator | Description of Activity | Clinical Response |
|---|---|---|
| Endotoxin | • Produced by certain bacterial cells<br>• Activates complement system and coagulation cascades<br>• Activates macrophages, which release TNF and IL-1 | • Increased microvascular permeability, vasodilation, third spacing, microthrombi formation<br>• Inflammatory response |
| TNF | • Released by monocyte–macrophages<br>• Multiple effects locally and systemically<br>• Stimulates other mediator activity | • Hypotension, tachycardia, myocardial depression, tachypnea, hyperglycemia, metabolic acidosis, third spacing, fever, microvascular vasoconstriction |
| IL-1 | • Released by monocyte–macrophages<br>• Stimulates leukocytosis<br>• Triggers production of acute-phase proteins and release of amino acids from skeletal muscle<br>• Activates procoagulant activity<br>• Decreases vascular responsiveness to catecholamines | • Increased WBCs<br>• High urinary nitrogen excretion and muscle wasting<br>• Elevated coagulation laboratory values<br>• Decreased SVR with impaired response to low dosages of vasopressor or synthetic catecholamine agents |
| IL-6 | • Released by monocytes, helper T cells, and macrophages<br>• Increases inflammatory response<br>• B-cell stimulation and differentiation<br>• Synergistic with IL-1 | • Fever<br>• Antibody secretion |
| Complement cascade | • Activated in response to pathogen surface, lectin, or antigen–antibody complex<br>• Identifies, invades, and lyses foreign particles and cells<br>• Stimulates neutrophils (and oxygen radicals) and IL-1<br>• Degranulates mast cells and basophils | • Edema formation: fluid leakage into interstitial space as a result of vasodilation and increased vascular permeability<br>• All effects of IL-1 |
| Platelet aggregating factor | • Released by mast cells, basophils, macrophages, neutrophils, platelets, and damaged endothelium<br>• Increases platelet aggregation<br>• Increases neutrophil adhesion<br>• Increases vascular permeability and bronchoconstriction<br>• Negative inotropic effects on the heart | • Formation of microthrombi, thus impaired perfusion<br>• Bronchoconstriction, rhonchi and wheezes, increased pulmonary airway pressures<br>• Decreased heart contractility, with impaired response to low dosages of vasopressor and inotropic agents |
| Arachidonic acid metabolites | • Stimulation of the release of metabolites prostaglandins (PG), thromboxanes (TX), and leukotrienes (LT)<br>• PGF and TXA2 cause pulmonary hypertension, vasoconstriction, and platelet activation and aggregation<br>• PGE, PGD, and prostacyclin cause vasodilation and decreased platelet aggregation<br>• Leukotrienes increase neutrophil chemotaxis, vascular constriction, and vascular permeability<br>• Increases gastric permeability to Gram-negative bacteria<br>• Inhibits leukocyte adhesion and platelets | • Oxygenation and ventilation difficulties, increased airway resistance, wheezing<br>• Fluid leakage from intravascular into interstitial space, edema formation<br>• Vasodilation, increased capillary permeability, and hypotension |
| Oxygen radicals | • Generate metabolites ($O_2$, $H_2O_2$, OH-) during the respiratory burst of the neutrophils<br>• Damage cell structure and interfere with cell activities<br>• Damage endothelial cells, which stimulate the coagulation system<br>• Increases vascular permeability | • Inflammatory response, fever<br>• Microthrombi formation<br>• Fluid leakage from intravascular into interstitial space, edema formation |

early shock may be successfully recognized and treated and the patient may make a full recovery.

In the intermediate, progressive phase (stage 2), compensatory mechanisms that maintain normal perfusion begin to fail, metabolic and circulatory derangements become more pronounced, and activation of the inflammatory and immune responses may fully develop. Signs of failure in one or more organs may become apparent. In stage 2 of shock, interventions that target both the cause of the shock and the resultant metabolic, circulatory, and inflammatory responses may result in salvage of the patient.

In the final, irreversible stage (stage 3), cellular and tissue injury is so severe that correction of metabolic, circulatory, and inflammatory derangements is difficult or impossible, and cellular hypoxia and death ensue. MODS develops, often resulting in the demise of the patient, as discussed later in this chapter.

As previously mentioned, any shock state can trigger a SIRS response and, if left unrecognized and untreated, can cause MODS. Understanding the classification, etiology, and clinical presentation of shock enables clinicians to more rapidly identify and manage shock, thus improving the likelihood of patient survival.

## Classification of Shock

Shock can be classified as *hypovolemic, cardiogenic,* or *distributive.* Hypovolemic and distributive shock occur because of inadequate venous return to the heart. Inadequate venous return may result from hypovolemia (dehydration, hemorrhage) or widespread vasodilation (sepsis, anaphylaxis, or loss of sympathetic tone with a spinal cord injury), which cause a relative hypovolemia. Cardiogenic shock is caused by the failure of the heart to pump effectively. Pump failure may result from myocardial infarction, abnormal heart rate or rhythm, or impaired diastolic filling.[10,11]

## Hypovolemic Shock

### Etiology

Hypovolemic shock is a result of inadequate circulating volume. Most commonly, hypovolemic shock is caused by sudden blood loss or severe dehydration. Some injuries, such as burns, cause significant fluid shifts from the intravascular space to the interstitial space, resulting in hypovolemia. (Chapter 53 discusses the care of patients with burns.) Hypovolemia in critically ill patients involves both intracellular and extracellular

compartments. Acute fluid volume loss does not allow the normal compensatory mechanisms to restore an appropriate circulating volume rapidly enough. If left untreated, hypovolemia may lead to a variety of secondary complications, such as hypotension, electrolyte and acid–base disturbances, and organ dysfunction resulting from hypoperfusion (Fig. 54-4).

## Pathophysiology

A sudden loss of intravascular volume decreases venous return to the heart and results in reduced CO. Compensatory mechanisms are initiated to increase the circulating volume through the activation of the sympathetic nervous system and neurohormonal responses (see Fig. 54-1). Existing blood volume is shunted to the vital organs (heart, lungs, and brain), causing hypoperfusion to other organs such as the liver, stomach, and kidneys. If volume is not replaced, compensatory mechanisms eventually become ineffective. The failure of the compensatory mechanisms to restore adequate circulating volume causes cellular hypoperfusion and the inability to meet cellular oxygen requirements for metabolism. Cells commit to anaerobic metabolism in an effort to meet their ATP requirements; this results in lactic acid production and metabolic acidosis.

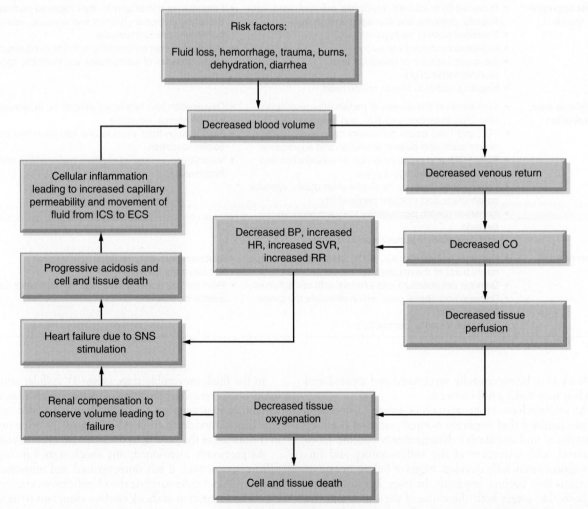

**FIGURE 54-4** Hypovolemic shock. BP, blood pressure; ECS, extracellular space; HR, heart rate; ICS, intracellular space; RR, respiratory rate; SNS, sympathetic nervous system.

Failed compensatory mechanisms, which were initiated to restore CO, eventually cause the myocardium to fatigue. Sympathetic stimulation to increase heart rate, contractility, and SVR escalates the workload of the heart. Ejection of a higher volume of blood against a higher SVR requires utilization of more oxygen and energy. Such stress on the heart causes an increase in myocardial metabolism and myocardial oxygen consumption ($MvO_2$). The continued lack of circulating volume prevents appropriate $DaO_2$ to the heart, creating a vicious cycle. End-organ perfusion, or adequate oxygenation to essential organs such as the brain, heart, lungs, and kidneys, is impaired. The inability of the circulatory system to provide end-organ perfusion forces conversion to anaerobic metabolism. Anaerobic metabolism cannot provide enough ATP to meet energy demands. Inadequate ATP production causes ischemic damage, which may progress to end-organ failure (see Fig. 54-4).

## Assessment

Clinical findings are directly related to the severity and acuity of volume loss (Table 54-2). Some patients, especially older patients or those who have chronic diseases, have more subtle compensatory responses, which may be overlooked. Box 54-2 lists considerations for older patients in shock. Serial assessments of physical and laboratory data may uncover trends that guide treatment and prevent cardiovascular collapse.

### History

A thorough history of the patient's presenting problem may reveal risk factors for hypovolemic shock. Patients experiencing significant blood loss because of gastric hemorrhage or liver or splenic rupture from trauma require rapid replacement of circulating volume to prevent the consequences of hypovolemia.

### Physical Findings

Patients with hypovolemic shock have the following signs and symptoms caused by poor organ perfusion:

- Altered mentation, ranging from lethargy to unresponsiveness
- Rapid and deep respirations, which gradually become labored and more shallow as the patient's condition deteriorates
- Cool and clammy skin, with weak and thready pulses
- Tachycardia from activation of the sympathetic nervous system
- Hypotension
- Decreased urine output; urine is darker and more concentrated because the kidneys are conserving fluid.

### Laboratory Studies

Useful laboratory studies include serum lactate, arterial pH, and base deficit to assess the presence of anaerobic metabolism as a marker of inadequate $DaO_2$. Test results can be used to measure the effectiveness of resuscitation. A serum lactate level that remains elevated after initial resuscitation is a poor prognostic indicator.[12,13] Metabolic laboratory studies and serum electrolyte measures assist with adjustment of fluid and electrolytes. Serial hemoglobin and hematocrit and coagulation panels may be drawn to assess the need for blood or blood product replacement. However, the hemoglobin and hematocrit may not directly reflect the severity of blood loss from either hemoconcentration caused by dehydration or hemodilution caused by the infusion of large volumes of intravenous (IV) fluid.

## Management

Management of hypovolemic shock focuses on restoring circulating volume and resolving the cause of volume loss. Composition of volume replacement therapy depends on

**TABLE 54-2    Clinical Findings Associated With Blood Volume Loss (Estimated) in Hypovolemic Shock**

| Less than 500 mL Blood Loss | 500–1,000 mL Blood Loss | 1,000–2,000 mL Blood Loss | 2,000–3,000 mL Blood Loss |
|---|---|---|---|
| None | • Tachycardia (↑HR greater than 20% of patient's baseline)<br>• Hypotension (↓SBP greater than 10% of patient's baseline)<br>• Pulses weaker<br>• Skin and extremities cool to touch<br>• ↓Urine output<br>• Hemodynamics: within normal limits CO, ↑SVR<br>• Mild acidosis (↑base deficit, ↑lactic acid) | • Tachycardia (↑HR greater than 20%–30% of patient's baseline)<br>• Hypotension (↓SBP greater than 10%–20% of patient's baseline)<br>• Cool, diaphoretic skin<br>• Poor peripheral pulses<br>• ↓Urine output (less than 30 mL/h)<br>• Hemodynamics: ↓CO, ↑SVR<br>• Progressive acidosis (↑base deficit, ↑lactic acid)<br>• Tachypnea (↑RR greater than 10% of patient's baseline)<br>• $SvO_2$ less than 60%, $ScVO_2$ less than 70%<br>• Altered level of consciousness: restlessness, agitation, confusion, or obtunded | • Tachycardia (↑HR greater than 20%–30% of patient's baseline)<br>• Hypotension (↓SBP greater than 10%–20% of patient's baseline)<br>• Marked peripheral vasoconstriction: cold extremities, poor peripheral pulses, pallor<br>• Oliguria → anuria<br>• Hemodynamics: ↓CO, ↑SVR<br>• Severe acidosis (↑base deficit, ↑lactic acid)<br>• Tachypnea (↑RR greater than 10%–20% of patient's baseline)<br>• $SvO_2$ less than 55%–60%<br>• Mental stupor |

RR, respirations; HR, heart rate.

what was lost. First-line therapy for volume resuscitation is typically crystalloid solution. Isotonic solutions, such as lactated Ringer's solution or 0.9% normal saline solution, are preferred over hypotonic solutions (5% dextrose solution). Blood and blood products are administered to replace red blood cells, platelets, and clotting factors lost with severe bleeding. Other colloid solutions (albumin and synthetic volume expanders) may be used to assist in the resuscitation process, especially if blood loss is the primary cause.

The use of colloids in the early phase of fluid replacement is controversial. Because colloids normally remain within the intravascular space more so than crystalloids, patients generally require smaller volumes of colloids for resuscitation. However, because capillary membrane permeability is increased in shock, the large colloid molecules leak from the blood vessels into the extravascular space, shifting more fluid from the intravascular space to interstitial tissues and thereby worsening the hypovolemia. Current research suggests that colloids are not superior to crystalloids in treating hypovolemia in critically ill patients.[14–16] Box 54-3 summarizes some of the known complications of fluid resuscitation.

### Nursing Management

Nursing management of hypovolemic shock focuses on the restoration of circulating volume through volume administration. Obtaining and maintaining adequate IV access is essential. Ideally, large-bore (16-gauge or larger) IV catheters are inserted into large veins or central veins to facilitate with the rapid infusion of fluids. Care must be taken to administer fluids rapidly but without compromising the pulmonary system. Large volumes of fluids given too quickly may cause pulmonary congestion and inhibit adequate ventilation, further compromising $DaO_2$ to the tissues. Fluids should also be warmed during infusion to limit the negative

effects of hypothermia. Frequent monitoring and documentation of blood pressure, heart rate, respiratory rate and depth, oxygen saturation, urine output, and mentation, as well as laboratory results and interventions, are essential.

## Cardiogenic Shock

### Etiology

Cardiogenic shock results from loss of contractile function of the heart. Cardiogenic shock is usually diagnosed by the presence of systemic and pulmonary hemodynamic alterations, which result from inadequate CO and tissue perfusion. Typically, this occurs when more than 40% of ventricular mass is damaged. The most common cause of cardiogenic shock is an extensive left ventricular myocardial infarction. Acute cardiogenic shock following a myocardial infarction is associated with in-hospital mortality rates of more than 50%.[11] Other causes of cardiogenic shock include papillary muscle rupture, ventricular septal rupture, cardiomyopathy, acute myocarditis, cardiac valve disease, and dysrhythmias. A thorough history provides the information necessary to predict whether a patient is at risk for developing cardiogenic shock.

Box 54-4 shows independent predictors for development of cardiogenic shock. Patients with several risk factors have a greater than 50% chance of developing cardiogenic shock.[11] Identifying patients at risk for development of cardiogenic shock and formulating strategies for prevention is extremely important. It is important to explore all causes of decreased CO before initiating therapy. Patients with acute myocardial infarction may require rapid revascularization with thrombolytics (see Chapter 21), percutaneous coronary intervention (see Chapter 18), or cardiac surgery (see Chapter 22).

**BOX 54-3** | **Complications of Volume Resuscitation by Fluid Type**

| Crystalloid and Colloid | Packed Red Blood Cells |
|---|---|
| Dilutional coagulopathy | Acidosis (banked blood has pH 6.9–7.1) |
| Dilutional thrombocytopenia | Left shift on the oxyhemoglobin dissociation curve (banked blood is deficient in 2,3-DPG) |
| Hypothermia | |
| Increased hemorrhage | Hyperkalemia |
| Pulmonary edema | Immunologic and infectious complications |
| Intracranial hypertension (patients with traumatic brain injury) | Dilutional coagulopathy |
| | Dilutional thrombocytopenia |
| | Hypothermia |

**Risk Factors for Inpatient Development of Cardiogenic Shock**
- Increased age (elderly)
- Left ventricular ejection fraction less than 35% on hospital admission
- Large myocardial infarction
- Previous myocardial infarction
- Presence of chronic comorbidities (diabetes mellitus, hypertension)
- Altered mental status
- Hemodynamic instability

## Pathophysiology

Cardiogenic shock is caused by loss of ventricular contractile force, which results in decreased stroke volume and decreased CO (Fig. 54-5). Similar to hypovolemic shock, neuroendocrine compensatory mechanisms are activated to improve perfusion by increasing preload and afterload. Stimulation of the RAAS and the sympathetic nervous system causes vasoconstriction and increases afterload (see Fig. 54-1). Although vasoconstriction increases blood pressure, the increase in afterload causes increased myocardial workload, intraventricular filling pressures, and myocardial oxygen requirements. Elevated afterload therefore reduces effective contraction and inhibits ejection. Ventricular filling pressures increase because of the increased preload, but lack of contractility prevents complete ejection. The ventricle becomes distended, further impairing effective contraction, and CO continues to decrease. Compensatory mechanisms continue the vicious cycle of elevated ventricular filling pressures and SVR, in combination with an inability of the heart to eject an adequate volume of blood into circulation. Pulmonary vascular pressures rise as left ventricular function declines, resulting in pulmonary congestion. Pulmonary congestion and increased pressure in the pulmonary capillaries cause fluid to leak into the interstitium and alveoli, impairing the diffusion of oxygen from alveoli into the pulmonary capillaries. A vicious cycle ensues related to decompensation: myocardial contraction is further impaired, pulmonary congestion worsens, and $DaO_2$ to the heart and other organs is inadequate to support aerobic metabolism.

Inadequate oxygenation of myocardial tissue exacerbates the anaerobic metabolism and further decreases contractility. These stressors placed on the failing heart may result in cardiac arrest.

## Assessment

Patients who are at high risk for cardiogenic shock require close monitoring. Assessment parameters are similar to those for congestive heart failure but the signs and symptoms are more severe. The nurse should follow assessment findings over time in order to identify subtle changes that signal the beginning of cardiogenic shock.

### Physical Findings

Clinical manifestations associated with cardiogenic shock are outlined in Box 54-5. In addition to the signs and symptoms listed in the box, patients with cardiogenic shock often experience recurrent chest pain, which may indicate extension of the infarcted tissue. Other clinical findings are directly related to the decrease in CO.

### Laboratory Studies

Presence of elevated myocardial tissue markers, accompanied by progressive hemodynamic compromise and clinical deterioration, are hallmarks of acute myocardial infarction and extensive myocardial necrosis, which may precede cardiogenic shock. Laboratory studies such as creatine phosphokinase

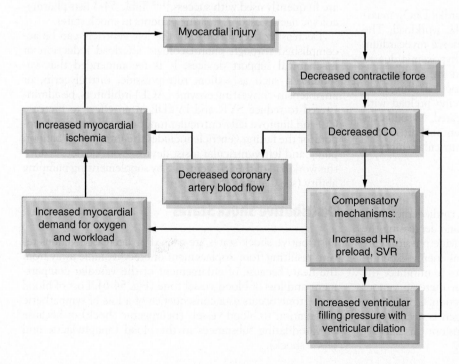

FIGURE 54-5 Cardiogenic shock. HR, heart rate.

> **BOX 54-5**   **Clinical Manifestations of Cardiogenic Shock**
>
> **Hemodynamic Findings**
> SBP less than 90 mm Hg
> MAP less than 70 mm Hg
> Cardiac index less than 2.2 L/min/m$^2$
> Pulmonary artery occlusion pressure (also known as pulmonary artery wedge pressure) greater than 18 mm Hg
> SVR greater than 1,400 dynes/s/cm$^5$
>
> **Noninvasive Findings**
> Thready, rapid pulse
> Narrow pulse pressure
> Distended neck veins
> Dysrhythmias
> Chest pain
> Cool, pale, moist skin
> Oliguria
> Decreased mentation
>
> **Pulmonary Findings**
> Dyspnea
> Increased respiratory rate
> Inspiratory crackles, possible wheezing
> Arterial blood gas measures show a decrease in PaO$_2$
> Respiratory alkalosis
>
> **Radiographic Findings**
> Enlarged heart
> Pulmonary congestion

and cardiac troponin I are released in the bloodstream by dying cardiac cells. Brain natriuretic peptide and N-terminal pro-brain natriuretic peptide are produced and released by the ventricle when it is stretched owing to increased intraventricular pressure. These markers can be used to help determine both the presence and severity of heart failure.[17]

## Management

Management is aimed at increasing myocardial DaO$_2$, maximizing CO, and decreasing left ventricular workload. The goals of treatment are to protect and preserve myocardium and improve tissue perfusion. Reversing hypoxemia due to pulmonary congestion and metabolic acidosis can improve the response to other therapies. Left ventricular filling pressures are often elevated; therefore, reducing preload with diuretics or nitrate infusion may be indicated. Vasodilators and intra-aortic balloon pumps are interventions directed at reducing afterload, thus improving left ventricular emptying and reducing myocardial workload.

### Nursing Management

Nursing management for the patient with cardiogenic shock centers on conserving myocardial energy and decreasing the workload of the heart. Nurses need to provide physical care and periods of rest to minimize myocardial energy expenditure. Use of opioid analgesics and sedatives to minimize the sympathetic nervous system response can increase venous capacitance and decrease resistance to ejection. Opioids also relieve ischemic pain. Supplemental oxygen is necessary to optimize arterial oxygen content and diffusion; this may require initiation of mechanical ventilation.

Dysrhythmias often occur with acute myocardial infarction, ischemia, or acid–base imbalances and can further decrease CO. Use of antiarrhythmic agents, cardioversion, or pacing can help restore a stable heart rhythm and enhance CO.

Electrolytes, specifically potassium, calcium, and magnesium, are essential to maintaining the action potential to drive myocardial contraction, and may need to be replaced to provide optimal conditions for the damaged myocardial muscle.

The critical care nurse must obtain, follow, and carefully interpret the patient's hemodynamic parameters to achieve the goal of optimizing CO. Optimal filling pressures assist in restoring CO but must be attained cautiously. As mentioned, left ventricular filling pressures, pulmonary artery pressures, and pulmonary artery occlusion pressures may be elevated, and diuresis should be used to reduce these pressures. If the left ventricular filling pressure is too low, fluids may be used, but they must be stopped when filling pressures increase without a subsequent increase in CO. In general, a preload (left ventricular end-diastolic pressure [LVEDP]) of 14 to 18 mm Hg should be maintained. Achieving an "optimal filling pressure" by administering fluids and diuretics is not always an easy task. Slow fluid administration or diuresis requires diligent assessment of the effectiveness of the interventions.

Pharmacologic agents can be used to augment CO, but they too must be used cautiously. Many agents can increase MvO$_2$ without having an appreciable effect on CO. Decisions to use some pharmacologic agents are based on overall risk–benefit considerations. The sympathomimetic drugs norepinephrine and epinephrine may enhance CO by increasing contractility, heart rate, or SVR but simultaneously increase cardiac work. In addition, stimulation of β-2 receptors by epinephrine may produce dilation in peripheral vascular beds that robs vital organs of blood. Agents with positive inotropic effects that have less activity on vascular tone, such as low-dose dopamine, dobutamine, amrinone, and milrinone, are frequently used with success.[11,18] Table 54-3 lists pharmacologic agents used in treating patients in shock states.

Decreasing the workload of the left ventricle can be accomplished through pharmacologic afterload reduction or mechanical support devices. It is recommended that vasodilators, such as sodium nitroprusside, nitroglycerin, or angiotensin-converting enzyme (ACE) inhibitors, be administered to reduce SVR and LVEDP in an effort to increase CO and improve left ventricular function.[18] Mechanical support for the failing ventricle includes the intra-aortic balloon pump and left ventricular assist device. Both devices reduce the workload of the left ventricle by supplementing pumping ability (see Chapter 18).

## Distributive Shock States

Distributive shock states are caused by decreased venous return resulting from displacement of blood volume away from the heart because of enlargement of the vascular compartment and loss of blood vessel tone (Fig. 54-6). Loss of blood vessel tone occurs as a consequence of a loss of sympathetic innervation to blood vessels (neurogenic shock) or because of vasodilating substances in the blood (anaphylactic and septic shock).

**TABLE 54-3** Pharmacologic Drugs Used in the Treatment of Shock*

| Drug | Heart Rate | Effects on Contractility | Systemic Venous Resistance | Nursing Considerations |
|---|---|---|---|---|
| Dopamine (Intropin) | ↑ | ↑↑ | ↑ | Hemodynamic effects are dose dependent<br>May increase MO₂ demands |
| Epinephrine (Adrenaline) | ↑↑ | ↑↑ | ↑ | May induce ventricular dysrhythmias<br>May increase MO₂ demands<br>β₂ Activity may dilate peripheral beds |
| Norepinephrine (also known as levarterenol [Levophed]) | ↑ | ↑ | ↑↑↑ | Monitor peripheral circulation closely; may increase MO₂ |
| Phenylephrine (Neo-Synephrine) | | | ↑↑ | May induce dysrhythmias |
| Vasopressin (Pitressin) | | ↑ | ↑↑ | Monitor peripheral circulation closely; may increase MO₂ |
| Sodium nitroprusside (Nipride) | ↑ | | ↓↓ | Hemodynamic effects are dose dependent; adjust dosage slowly |
| Nitroglycerine (Tridil) | ↑ | | ↓ | Hemodynamic effects are dose dependent; adjust dosage slowly; tolerance may develop |
| Amrinone (Inocor) | ↑ | ↑ | ↓ | May increase MO₂ demands |
| Milrinone (Primacor) | ↑ | ↑↑ | ↓ | May increase MO₂ demands<br>Monitor for tachyarrhythmias |
| Dobutamine (Dobutrex) | ↑ | ↑↑ | ↓ | May increase MO₂ demands<br>Monitor for tachyarrhythmias |

MO₂, myocardial oxygen consumption. ↑ small effect; ↑↑ moderate effect; ↑↑↑ large effect.

*All agents should be administered through a central venous catheter and using a volumetric pump.

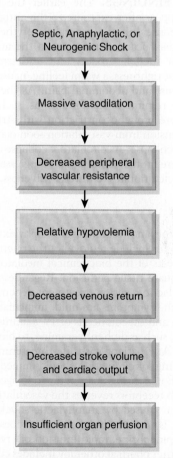

**FIGURE 54-6** Distributive shock states are caused by decreased venous return as a result of displacement of blood volume away from the heart due to enlargement of the vascular compartment and loss of blood vessel tone.

## Neurogenic Shock

### Etiology

Neurogenic shock results from loss or disruption of sympathetic tone, which causes peripheral vasodilation and subsequent decreased tissue perfusion. The disturbance of sympathetic tone may be caused by any event that disrupts the sympathetic nervous system. The most common cause of neurogenic shock is a spinal cord injury above the level of T6, because sympathetic innervation occurs above this level. Other causes include spinal analgesia, drugs, or other central nervous system problems.

### Pathophysiology

Neurogenic shock is characterized by hypotension, bradycardia, and hypothermia. When sympathetic tone is lost, unopposed parasympathetic response results in uncontrolled arterial vasodilation and a decrease in SVR. Simultaneous venous vasodilation results in blood pooling and decreases preload. Unopposed parasympathetic stimulation leads to bradycardia, even in the presence of falling blood pressure. Unlike other shock states in which falling blood pressure would cause an increased heart rate, in neurogenic shock, disruption of the sympathetic nervous system inhibits the stimulation of baroreceptors in the aortic arch and carotid sinus. Vasodilation causes decreased preload and thus stroke volume. The decrease in both stroke volume (from decreased preload) and heart rate leads to decreased CO, resulting in inadequate tissue perfusion. Hypothermia results from uncontrolled heat loss from excessive vasodilation.[19,20]

### Assessment

Physical findings in the patient with neurogenic shock are largely related to excessive vasodilation and the impaired response to this process. Patients demonstrate decreased central venous pressure (CVP), CO, and SVR combined with bradycardia. Unlike many shock states in which the patient may feel cold and clammy, often the skin is warm owing to massive vasodilation.

## Management

Prevention and treatment of hypotension through careful fluid resuscitation is a high priority. The patient's effective circulating volume may be dramatically decreased because of venous pooling. In general, the systolic blood pressure (SBP) should be kept over 90 mm Hg. If fluid administration alone is not adequate to restore the blood pressure, vasopressors may be added. The goal of pharmacology in neurogenic shock is to mimic the sympathetic nervous system. The use of agents with α-adrenergic activity, such as norepinephrine, promotes vasoconstriction, while β-adrenergic agonists, such as dopamine, increase heart rate and contractility.[19] (Refer to Chapter 37 for detailed information on spinal cord injury and associated complications such as neurogenic shock.)

## Anaphylactic Shock

Anaphylaxis results from an allergic reaction to a specific allergen that evokes a life-threatening hypersensitivity response. The three most common causes of anaphylaxis in adults are foods, insect stings, and medications.[21] If left untreated, vascular collapse can occur, resulting in greatly decreased tissue perfusion and death. Prompt intervention is critical.

### Etiology

Antigens, the substances that elicit the allergic response, can be introduced through injection or ingestion, or through the skin or respiratory tract. A number of substances are capable of evoking anaphylaxis in humans, including drugs, blood products, diagnostic agents, hormones, enzymes, and venom from insects, spiders, snakes, and jellyfish.

Anaphylaxis may be either immunoglobulin E (IgE) mediated or non–IgE mediated. IgE-mediated anaphylaxis occurs as a result of the immune response to a specific antigen. The first time the immune system is exposed to the antigen, a very specific IgE antibody is formed and circulates in the blood. When a second exposure to this antigen occurs, the antigen binds to this circulating IgE, which then activates mast cells and basophils, triggering release of histamine, prostaglandins, leukotrienes, and other biochemical mediators that initiate anaphylaxis.

Anaphylactoid or non–IgE-mediated reactions occur without the presence of IgE antibodies. It is thought that direct activation of mediators causes this response. One common anaphylactoid reaction is associated with nonsteroidal anti-inflammatory drugs (NSAIDs), including aspirin.[22] If there has been an anaphylactoid reaction to one agent, restrictions should include all NSAIDs, because any of them could elicit a second reaction.

### Pathophysiology

The antibody–antigen reaction causes antibody-specific mast cells and basophils to secrete substances such as histamine, leukotrienes, eosinophil chemotactic substance, heparin, prostaglandins, neutrophil chemotactic substance, and platelet-activating factor 2 (Fig. 54-7). These substances, particularly histamine, prostaglandins, and leukotrienes, cause systemic vasodilation, increased capillary permeability, bronchoconstriction, coronary vasoconstriction, and urticaria (hives). Some of the other substances precipitate a continued downward spiral by causing myocardial depression, inflammation, excessive secretion of mucus, and peripheral vasodilation.[23] The diffuse arterial vasodilation creates a maldistribution of blood volume to tissues, and venous dilation decreases preload, decreasing CO. Increased capillary permeability leads to loss of vascular volume, further decreasing CO and subsequently impairing tissue perfusion. Initial symptoms include itching, urticaria, and some difficulty breathing due to bronchoconstriction. Death from circulatory collapse or extreme bronchoconstriction may occur within minutes or hours.

### Assessment

Anaphylactic shock may have no predisposing factors. Therefore, avoiding known allergens is usually the best way to prevent anaphylactic shock. It is necessary to obtain a thorough history of allergies and responses to drugs, foods, blood products, or anesthetic agents. Moreover, it is important to recognize the various clinical presentations.

**PHYSICAL FINDINGS.** The earlier the symptoms of anaphylaxis appear after exposure to the antigen, the more severe the response. Initially, generalized erythema, urticaria, and pruritus may occur in response to the antigen. Other symptoms may include anxiety and restlessness, dyspnea, wheezing, chest tightness, a warm feeling, nausea and vomiting, angioedema, and abdominal pain. As the episode progresses, severe respiratory manifestations, such as laryngeal edema or severe bronchoconstriction with stridor, may develop. Hypotension from vasodilation soon occurs and leads to circulatory collapse. As circulatory collapse or hypoxemia related to severe bronchoconstriction progresses, the level of consciousness deteriorates to unresponsiveness.

### Management

Early recognition and treatment of anaphylaxis is essential. Therapeutic goals include removal of the offending antigen, reversal of effects of the biochemical mediators, and restoration of adequate tissue perfusion. Regardless of the cause of the anaphylactic reaction, treatment depends on clinical symptoms. If the symptoms are mild, immediate therapy includes oxygen and subcutaneous or IV administration of an antihistamine, such as diphenhydramine, to block the effects of histamine. Any patient with life-threatening changes in airway, breathing, or circulation should immediately receive epinephrine. Epinephrine is an adrenergic agonist; stimulation of α and β receptors reverses the vasodilation and bronchoconstriction caused by anaphylactic shock (Box 54-6). If the patient is severely hypotensive or does not respond promptly to epinephrine, rapid infusion of crystalloid fluids is essential. Other pharmacotherapy includes corticosteroids, bronchodilators, and, if absolutely necessary, vasoconstrictors and positive inotropic agents to combat circulatory collapse.[23,24]

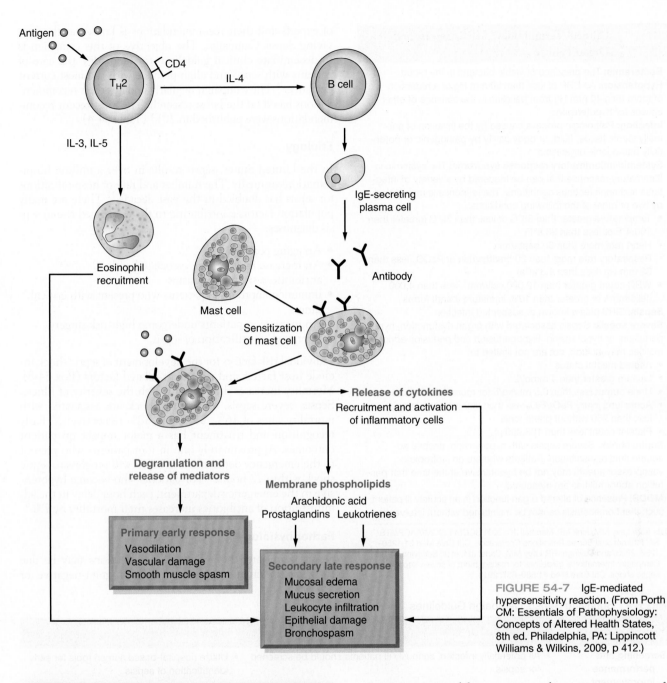

FIGURE 54-7 IgE-mediated hypersensitivity reaction. (From Porth CM: Essentials of Pathophysiology: Concepts of Altered Health States, 8th ed. Philadelphia, PA: Lippincott Williams & Wilkins, 2009, p 412.)

**BOX 54-6** **Epinephrine Dosage in Anaphylaxis: Adults**

Epinephrine 1:1,000 dilution (1 mg/mL), 0.2 to 0.5 mL intramuscularly or subcutaneously every 5 minutes, as necessary, should be used to control symptoms and increase blood pressure in patients experiencing anaphylaxis.

Data from Lieberman P, Nicklas RA, Randolph C, et al: Anaphylaxis: A practice parameter update 2015. Ann Allergy Asthma Immunol 115(5):341–384, 2015.

**NURSING MANAGEMENT.** Nursing care involves maintaining an adequate airway and monitoring patient response to the antigen. The nurse also monitors respirations, heart rate, blood pressure, and level of anxiety, and institutes comfort measures related to the dermatologic manifestations. If the agent causing the anaphylaxis is unknown, evaluation for allergies and future risk for anaphylaxis should be completed. Patient education regarding prevention and treatment is critical for any person who experiences a significant anaphylactic or anaphylactoid reaction.

## Septic Shock

Septic shock is a complex and generalized process that involves all organ systems. Sepsis, severe sepsis, and septic shock represent progressive stages of the same illness in response to infection. In 1991, the Society of Critical Care Medicine and the American College of Chest Physicians established universal definitions for the term sepsis and other associated clinical conditions[4] to promote earlier detection of and intervention for these states, improve outcomes, and standardize the terminology used in research protocols. Several consensus conferences have subsequently modified the existing definitions for accuracy, reliability, and clinical utility of the diagnosis of sepsis (Box 54-7).[25] The current international committee

**BOX 54-7** Clinical Terminology: SIRS, Sepsis, and Organ Failure

**Bacteremia:** The presence of viable bacteria in the blood
**Hypotension:** An SBP of less than 90 mm Hg or a reduction of more than 40 mm Hg from baseline in the absence of other causes for hypotension
**Infection:** Pathologic process caused by the invasion of normally sterile tissue, fluid, or body cavity by pathogenic or potentially pathogenic organisms
**Systemic inflammatory response syndrome:** The systemic inflammatory response that can be triggered by a variety of infectious and noninfectious conditions. The response is manifested by two or more of the following conditions:

- Temperature greater than 38°C or less than 36°C (greater than 100.4°F or less than 96.8°F)
- Heart rate more than 90 beats/min
- Respiratory rate more than 20 breaths/min or $PaCO_2$ less than 32 mm Hg (less than 4.3 kPa)
- WBC count greater than 12,000 cell/$mm^3$, less than 4,000 cells/$mm^3$, or greater than 10% immature (band) forms

**Sepsis:** SIRS plus a known or suspected infection
**Severe sepsis:** Sepsis associated with organ dysfunction, hypoperfusion, or hypotension. Hypoperfusion and perfusion abnormalities may include, but are not limited to:

- Altered mental status
- Lactate greater than 4 mmol/L
- Urine output less than 0.5 mL/kg/h for more than 2 hours
- Acute lung injury $PaO_2/FiO_2$ less than 200 with pneumonia; less than 250 without pneumonia
- Platelet count less than 100,000 μL

**Septic shock:** Severe sepsis with hypotension, despite adequate fluid resuscitation. Patients who are on inotropic or vasopressor agents may not be hypotensive at the time that perfusion abnormalities are measured.

**MODS:** Presence of altered organ function in an acutely ill patient such that homeostasis cannot be maintained without intervention.

Data from Levy MM, Fink MP, Marshall JC: 2001 SCCM/ESICM/AACP/ATS/SIS International Sepsis Definitions Conference. Crit Care Med 31:1250–1256, 2003; and Dellinger RP, Levy MM, Carlet JM, et al: Surviving Sepsis Campaign: International guidelines for management of severe sepsis and septic shock. Crit Care Med 41:580–637, 2013.

of experts and their recommendations is known as the Surviving Sepsis Campaign. The objective of this campaign is to disseminate clinical guidelines to standardize the care of patients with sepsis and align practice with the most current evidence.[26] The campaign regularly updates their recommendations based on the latest research. The most recent recommendations were published in 2013 (Table 54-4).

## Etiology

In the United States, sepsis results in over a million hospitalizations annually. The number and rate of hospitalizations for sepsis has doubled in the past decade.[27] There are many population factors contributing to the continued rise in sepsis diagnoses:

- An aging population
- An increase in infections associated with antibiotic-resistant organisms
- Immunocompromised patients who present with critical illness
- An increase in patients undergoing high-risk surgery
- Improved identification of sepsis.

Individual risk factors for the development of septic shock include host factors and treatment-related factors (Box 54-8). Mortality increases dramatically with the severity of illness. Sepsis, severe sepsis, and septic shock are associated with mortality rates of 16%, 25%, and 50% respectively.[28] Early recognition and treatment has a major impact on patient outcomes. Approximately one in four patients who present to the emergency department in sepsis will progress to septic shock within 72 hours.[26] For patients who become hypotensive in the emergency department, each hour delay in the administration of antibiotics increases their mortality by 7%.[8]

## Pathophysiology

Sepsis is initiated by an infection. Infections may be due to a variety of microorganisms such as gram-negative or

**TABLE 54-4** Surviving Sepsis Campaign Guidelines

| Collaborative Care Focus | Surviving Sepsis Guidelines | Interventions and Patient Care Considerations |
| --- | --- | --- |
| Screening and performance improvement | • All potentially infected, seriously ill patients should be screened for sepsis | • Utilize hospital-based screen tools for early identification of sepsis |
| Oxygenation, ventilation | **Mechanical ventilation**<br>• For patients requiring mechanical ventilation, a tidal volume (Vt) of 6 mL/kg should be used, with an upper limit plateau pressure of 30 cm $H_2O$ or less<br>• Permissive hypercapnia may be tolerated in patients with elevated plateau pressures and tidal volumes<br>• Positive end-expiratory pressure should be applied to prevent lung collapse at end expiration<br>• The head of bed should be raised to at least 30 degrees unless contraindicated to prevent ventilator-associated pneumonia<br>• A weaning protocol with spontaneous breathing trial should be in place to promote ventilator weaning even in patients who are arousable, hemodynamically stable, have no new life-threatening conditions, and are not requiring high levels of $FiO_2$ or ventilatory support<br>• Prone position may be considered in patients with ARDS requiring high levels of $FiO_2$ or plateau pressure<br>• The use of recruitment maneuvers may be considered for patients with severe and refractory hypoxemia | • Maintain a patent airway<br>• Auscultate breath sounds every 2–4 h and PRN<br>• Suction endotracheal airway when appropriate (see Chapter 25)<br>• Hyperoxygenate and hyperventilate before and after each suction pass<br>• Monitor pulse oximetry and end-tidal $CO_2$<br>• Monitor arterial blood gases as indicated by changes in noninvasive parameters<br>• Monitor intrapulmonary shunt (Qs/Qt and $PaO_2/FiO_2$)<br>• Monitor airway pressures every 1–2 h<br>• Consider kinetic therapy<br>• Consider a daily chest x-ray (see Chapter 27) |

| Collaborative Care Focus | Surviving Sepsis Guidelines | Interventions and Patient Care Considerations |
|---|---|---|
| Circulation, perfusion | **Initial resuscitation**<br>• Resuscitation should begin as soon as sepsis is identified<br>• Fluid resuscitation should initially begin with crystalloid boluses<br>• In the initial 6-h period after identifying sepsis:<br>  • Use vasopressors for hypotension that does not respond to initial fluid resuscitation to maintain a MAP of 65 mm Hg or higher<br>  • In the event of persistent hypotension after initial fluid administration (MAP less than 65 mm Hg), or if initial lactate was 4 mmol/L or more, reassess volume status and tissue perfusion and document findings as noted in the Intervention and Patient Care Consideration column | • Administer intravascular fluids and vasopressors per protocol<br>• Lactate level may confirm hypoperfusion in patients who are not hypotensive. Monitor serum lactate level on admission and then at least once daily<br>• Assess vital signs, including adequacy of urine output hourly<br>• Document reassessment of volume status and tissue perfusion as follows:<br>  • Have a licensed independent practitioner repeat focused exam (after initial fluid resuscitation), including vital signs, cardiopulmonary, capillary refill, pulse, and skin findings<br>OR<br>  • Do two of the following:<br>   • Measure CVP<br>   • Measure ScvO$_2$<br>   • Perform bedside cardiovascular ultrasound<br>   • Perform dynamic assessment of fluid responsiveness with passive leg raise or fluid challenge |
| | **Ongoing hemodynamic management**<br>• Continue to use fluid challenge techniques as long as associated with clinical improvement; albumin may also be considered for patients requiring substantial amounts of crystalloids<br>• Vasopressors should be considered for patients unresponsive to fluid challenges (inadequate blood pressure and organ perfusion)<br>• Norepinephrine is recommended as the first-choice vasopressor<br>• Low-dose dopamine should not be used for renal protection as a part of the treatment for severe sepsis<br>• Epinephrine may be added to or considered as an alternative agent in septic shock that responds poorly to norepinephrine<br>• Low-dose vasopressin (less than 0.03 units/min) is not recommended; higher does vasopressin (0.03–0.04 units/min) are reserved for salvage therapy | • Assess hemodynamic pressures hourly if patient has an arterial, CVP, or pulmonary artery catheter in place<br>• If available, monitor SvO$_2$ via a specialty pulmonary artery catheter or ScvO$_2$ via central venous catheter<br>• Monitor for response to fluid challenge with increases in blood pressure or urine output<br>• Monitor for evidence of intravascular volume overload<br>• Vasopressors should be administered through central venous access whenever possible<br>• For patients on vasopressors, an arterial catheter should be placed as soon as possible for accurate monitoring of blood pressures |
| | • Inotropic therapy may be initiated for patients with low CO despite adequate fluid resuscitation<br>• Dobutamine may be used to increase CO/index to normal levels; it is not recommended to target supranormal levels<br>• Patients with hypotension should also receive a vasopressor to maintain MAP | • Monitor CO and cardiac index per hospital protocol<br>• Monitor hemoglobin and hematocrit |
| | • Blood products: After the initial resuscitation is complete, administer red blood cells only when the hemoglobin is less than 7 g/dL<br>  • The target hemoglobin is 7–9 g/dL for patients without significant coronary artery disease, acute hemorrhage, or lactic acidosis | • During transfusion, observe for signs of transfusion reaction<br>• Monitor coagulation parameters |
| Sedation, analgesia, and neuromuscular blockade | • A sedation protocol should be used in conjunction with a standardized sedation scale for patient evaluation<br>• Sedation should be minimized by using discrete end points and administered with either intermittent boluses or continuous infusion<br>• Neuromuscular blocking agents (NMBAs) should be avoided whenever possible. NMBAs may be considered for a short course (less than 48 h) in patients with early sepsis-induced ARDS | • Monitor sedation level per sedation scale<br>• Continuous infusion of sedative agents should be interrupted daily for assessment of patient status while awake, with subsequent re-titration as indicated by sedation protocol and assessment |

*(continued)*

**TABLE 54-4** Surviving Sepsis Campaign Guidelines (*continued*)

| Collaborative Care Focus | Surviving Sepsis Guidelines | Interventions and Patient Care Considerations |
|---|---|---|
| **Fluids, electrolytes, and glycemic control** | • Blood glucose: After initial stabilization, blood glucose level should target less than 180 mg/dL<br>• A blood glucose protocol should be used to identify hyperglycemia and initiate timely glucose regulation with insulin infusion | • Monitor intake and output every 1 h<br>• Monitor blood glucose every 1–2 h until stabilized, then every 4 h<br>• Initiate insulin protocol for blood glucose greater than 180 mg/dL<br>• Monitor electrolytes daily and PRN<br>• Replace electrolytes as ordered<br>• Monitor blood urea nitrogen, creatinine, serum osmolality, and serum electrolyte values daily |
| | • Renal replacement therapy with intermittent hemodialysis and continuous renal replacement therapy (CRRT) are considered equivalent. CRRT may be preferable in the hemodynamically unstable patient | • Monitor fluid balance and hemodynamic stability of patients receiving renal replacement therapy |
| **Identifying and treating the cause of sepsis** | • The patient should be formally evaluated for a focus of infection. Any known or suspected source of infection should be removed or treated within 12 h of diagnosis, if feasible<br>• Cultures should be obtained before antimicrobial therapy is initiated if possible but should not delay the administration of antimicrobial therapy more than 45 min<br>• At least two sets of aerobic and anaerobic blood cultures should be obtained with at least one culture specimen drawn percutaneously<br>• At least one culture specimen from each vascular access device inserted more than 48 h prior should be obtained to rule out lines as the source of infection<br>• Other sources of infection should be considered and cultured as clinically indicated (ie, urine, wounds, respiratory secretions) | • Obtain urine, sputum, and blood cultures as ordered |
| | • IV antibiotics should be started as early as possible and always within the first hour of recognizing severe sepsis or septic shock<br>• Initial therapy should include medications with activity against the likely pathogen, with consideration of patterns of resistance in the hospital and community | • Obtain wound and central vascular line tip culture specimens as ordered<br>• Administer antibiotics as ordered<br>• Monitor serum antibiotic levels as ordered<br>• Consider infectious disease consult<br>• Monitor SIRS criteria listed in Box 54-1 |
| **Preventing new infection** | • The antimicrobial regimen should be reassessed daily to optimize activity and prevent development of resistance<br>• Chlorhexidine gluconate, an oral decontamination agent, should be used to reduce the risk of ventilator-associated pneumonia in patients with severe sepsis | • Adjust antibiotics based on culture results<br>• Use strict aseptic technique during procedure, and monitor technique of others<br>• Maintain sterility of invasive catheters and tubes<br>• Perform daily mouth care to reduce risk of ventilator-associated pneumonia |
| **Deep venous thrombosis (DVT) prophylaxis** | • Patients with sepsis should receive prophylaxis against DVT<br>  • For patients with severe sepsis both pharmacologic and mechanical prophylaxis should be considered<br>  • Unless contraindicated, pharmacologic prophylaxis is preferred over mechanical prophylaxis | • Monitor for signs and symptoms of DVT (redness, swelling, tenderness, or pain in calf) |
| **Stress ulcer prophylaxis** | • Patients with severe sepsis or bleeding risk factors should receive stress ulcer prophylaxis<br>• Patients without risk factors should not receive stress ulcer prophylaxis.<br>  • The preferred agents are $H_2$ blockers or proton-pump inhibitors | • Monitor for signs and symptoms of peptic ulcer disease (abdominal pain, gastrointestinal bleeding) |
| **Setting goals of care** | • Communicate likely outcomes and realistic goals of treatment to patients and family<br>• Address goals of care within 72 h of ICU admission<br>• Incorporate goals of care into treatment decisions<br>• Consider less aggressive support or withdrawal of support if in the best interest of the patient | • Consult social services, clergy, and palliative care team as appropriate<br>• Provide for adequate rest and sleep |

Data from Dellinger RP, Levy MM, Carlet JM, et al: Surviving Sepsis Campaign: International guidelines for management of severe sepsis and septic shock. Crit Care Med 41:580–637, 2013; and Surviving Sepsis Campaign: Updated Bundles in Response to New Evidence. Retrieved April 2015, from http://www.survivingsepsis.org/SiteCollectionDocuments/SSC_Bundle.pdf.

## Risk Factors for the Development of Septic Shock

**Host Factors**
- Extremes of age
- Malnutrition
- General debilitation
- Chronic debilitation
- Chronic illness
- Drug or alcohol abuse
- Neutropenia
- Splenectomy
- Multiple organ failure

**Treatment-Related Factors**
- Use of invasive catheters
- Surgical procedures
- Traumatic or thermal wounds
- Invasive diagnostic procedures
- Mechanical ventilation
- Drugs (antibiotics, cytotoxic agents, steroids)

gram-positive bacteria, fungi, and viruses. In some patients, multiple causative organisms are identified, but in many patients the causative organism is never identified. Microorganisms may be introduced through the pulmonary system, urinary tract, or gastrointestinal system; through wounds; or through invasive devices.

Septic shock results from complex interactions among invading microorganisms and immune, inflammatory, and coagulation systems, which result in a proinflammatory and hypercoagulable state (Fig. 54-8). Both gram-negative and gram-positive organisms may directly stimulate the inflammatory response and other aspects of the immune system that activate cytokines, complement, and coagulation systems. In response to the presence of microorganisms, macrophages and helper T cells secrete the proinflammatory cytokines, such as TNFα and IL-1β. As previously discussed, these cytokines induce endothelial dysfunction and result in increased capillary permeability. Normally, anti-inflammatory cytokines are also released to balance the proinflammatory response. Type 2 helper T cells secrete the anti-inflammatory cytokines IL-4 and IL-10. But in some patients, anti-inflammatory cytokines fail to balance the proinflammatory cytokines, and the excessive proinflammatory response activates the coagulation cascade.[7]

Another important aspect of sepsis is the imbalance between procoagulant and anticoagulant factors. Endotoxins, substances embedded in the cell walls of invading microorganisms, stimulate endothelial cells to release tissue factor. The release of tissue factor activates the coagulation cascade, causing the conversion of fibrinogen to fibrin. Fibrin binds to platelet plugs that have adhered to damaged endothelial cells, forming a stable fibrin clot. These clots, known as microthrombi, form throughout the microvasculature and cause obstruction of vessels, leading to additional injury and ischemia to distal tissues. Normally, anticoagulant factors (protein C, protein S, antithrombin III, tissue factor pathway inhibitor) modulate coagulation, preventing

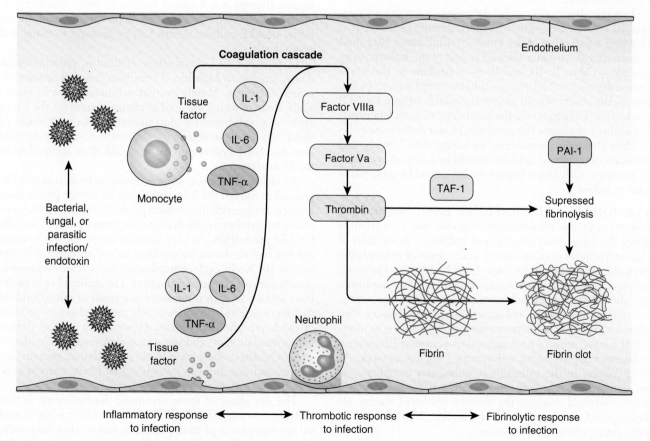

**FIGURE 54-8** Inflammatory/immune response in septic shock. TAFi, thrombin-activated fibrinolysis inhibitor; PAI-1, plasminogen-activator inhibitor-1. (Copyright © 2001, Eli Lilly and Company. All rights reserved.)

widespread microthrombi formation. Thrombin binds with thrombomodulin on endothelial cells, "activating" protein C. Activated protein C then inactivates factors V and VIII and inhibits the synthesis of plasminogen-activator inhibitor, which then allows plasmin to break down the fibrin–platelet clots.[29] In sepsis, the levels of these anticoagulant factors is decreased, resulting in a procoagulant state that increases microthrombi formation and contributes to further inflammation.[7] Recognition that the proinflammatory and procoagulant responses result in a loss of homeostasis of almost every organ system is key to understanding sepsis.

**CARDIOVASCULAR ALTERATIONS.** In general, septic shock is associated with three major pathophysiologic effects on the cardiovascular system: vasodilation, maldistribution of blood flow, and myocardial depression.

Proinflammatory cytokines stimulate the release of NO from endothelial cells. NO is a potent vasodilator and causes widespread vasodilation. Because of this vasodilation, there is decreased SVR, decreased venous return to the heart, and thus decreased CO. Other inflammatory mediators, including endothelin, are released from endothelial cells and cause vasoconstriction in other vascular beds.[30] The combination of vasodilation and vasoconstriction produces maldistribution of blood flow in all microcirculation.[31]

Early in septic shock, activation of the sympathetic nervous system and release of vasodilatory substances such as NO promote development of a hyperdynamic state, with high CO and low SVR. Later, as circulating cardiac depressants increase, the heart becomes hypodynamic, with low CO and increased SVR.

In septic shock, myocardial depression is evident in a decreased ventricular ejection fraction, dilation of the ventricles, and a flattening of the Frank–Starling curve after fluid resuscitation. Cytokines released as part of the inflammatory cascade—TN-α, IL-1β, and IL-6—contribute to this myocardial depression. NO also contributes to dysfunction by impairing the ability of cells to utilize available oxygen for ATP production. Consequently, the heart demonstrates functional impairment of contractility and ventricular performance.[11,32]

Hemodynamic parameters, including $ScvO_2/SvO_2$ and measures of metabolic acidosis, should be followed over time to recognize early tissue hypoperfusion caused by progressive cardiac failure.

**PULMONARY ALTERATIONS.** Events initiated by activation of the inflammatory response and its mediators affect the lungs both directly and indirectly. Activation of the sympathetic nervous system and release of epinephrine from the adrenal medulla cause bronchodilation. However, inflammatory cytokines override the effect of epinephrine, and the net result is bronchoconstriction. More importantly, inflammatory mediators and activated neutrophils cause capillary leak into the pulmonary interstitium, resulting in interstitial edema, areas of poor pulmonary perfusion (shunting), pulmonary hypertension, and increased respiratory work. As fluid collects in the interstitium, pulmonary compliance is reduced, gas exchange is impaired, and hypoxemia occurs. Interstitial fluid damages the alveolar epithelial barrier, allowing fluid to accumulate in the alveoli. This further impairs oxygenation and ventilation.

The pulmonary alterations described previously may culminate in acute respiratory distress syndrome (ARDS),

which is frequently associated with septic shock.[33,34] Mechanical ventilation, which is common in patients with ARDS, may provide an avenue of entry for microorganisms into the lungs. Alveolar infiltrates are fertile areas for bacterial growth; therefore, a secondary pneumonia may develop, possibly caused by a different organism than that which produced the sepsis. See Chapter 27 for more information about ARDS.

**HEMATOLOGIC ALTERATIONS.** Platelet abnormalities also occur in septic shock, because endotoxin indirectly causes platelet aggregation and subsequent release of more vasoactive substances such as serotonin and thromboxane $A_2$. Platelets aggregate in the microvasculature of septic patients. Overactivation of the coagulation cascade without the counterbalance of adequate fibrinolysis compromises tissue perfusion by obstructing blood flow both regionally and globally, as described above. Over time, clotting factors are depleted and a coagulopathy occurs, with the potential of progressing to disseminated intravascular coagulation (DIC).[29]

**METABOLIC ALTERATIONS.** Septic shock induces a hypermetabolic state characterized by an increase in resting energy consumption, extensive protein and fat catabolism, negative nitrogen balance, hyperglycemia, and hepatic gluconeogenesis. Excessive catecholamine release stimulates gluconeogenesis and insulin resistance. This compromises cellular metabolism, causing hyperglycemia in critically ill patients who do not have diabetes. Owing to insulin resistance, cells are progressively unable to use glucose, protein, and fat as energy sources. Hyperglycemia that is resistant to insulin therapy is a frequent finding in early shock. Eventually, glycogen energy stores are depleted and, without an influx of ATP, cellular pumps fail, progressing to tissue and organ death.

In response to lack of effect of insulin, proteins break down, leading to high blood urea nitrogen and urinary nitrogen excretion. Muscle protein is broken down to amino acids, some of which are used as energy sources for the Krebs cycle or as substrates for gluconeogenesis. In later stages of shock, the liver is unable to use the amino acids because of its own metabolic dysfunction. Amino acids then accumulate in the bloodstream.

As shock progresses, adipose tissue is broken down (lipolysis) to furnish the liver with lipids for energy production. Hepatic triglyceride metabolism produces ketones, which circulate to peripheral cells that can use them in the Krebs cycle for ATP production. As liver function decreases, triglycerides are not broken down; they collect in the mitochondria and inhibit the Krebs cycle, contributing to increased anaerobic metabolism and lactate production. The ability of cells to extract and use oxygen is impaired as a result of mitochondrial dysfunction. Oxidants are normally produced as a by-product of oxidative phosphorylation. However, in critical illness, an accumulation of oxidants occurs that results in oxidative stress. Oxidative stress causes lipid peroxidation, protein oxidation, and mutations in mitochondrial DNA, thereby contributing to cell death.

The net effect of these metabolic derangements is that cells become energy starved. This energy deficit is implicated in the emergence of multiple organ failure that frequently develops regardless of interventions designed to support the circulatory and organ systems.[3]

## Assessment

A thorough understanding of the mediator responses that occur during sepsis aids in assessing and evaluating the response to treatment.

**PHYSICAL FINDINGS.** The earliest signs of septic shock—tachycardia, increased respiratory rate, abnormal WBC count, and either fever or hypothermia—reflect the SIRS. Because of the exaggerated inflammatory response with release of vasoactive mediators, the clinical presentation of the patient is complex. The patient may become edematous yet intravascularly depleted, and areas of microthrombi and vasoconstriction obstruct perfusion. As fluid replacement occurs, the leaking capillary beds shift the fluid interstitially, requiring more fluid resuscitation, which may further exacerbate interstitial edema. Perfusion imbalances cause ischemia in some vascular beds, such as the splanchnic circulation, skin, and extremities; this may lead to necrosis. Inappropriate systemic activation of the coagulation system depletes the body's stores of clotting factors, and spontaneous bleeding may occur. Consistent with the hyperdynamic state, CO may initially be high; however, it is insufficient to maintain adequate perfusion because of the inappropriately low SVR.

**LABORATORY STUDIES.** The rapid progression of illness and severity-related mortality associated with sepsis make early identification paramount. Early diagnosis of sepsis is often made by assessment of patient risk factors and clinical findings (see Box 54-8) but may also be enhanced by laboratory and diagnostic studies. Specific laboratory studies including WBC count with differential, platelet count, lactate, $SvO_2$ or $ScvO_2$, creatinine, glucose, and bilirubin help to quantify the severity of the patient's presentation.[26] Laboratory and diagnostic studies that may help to identify and direct the management of sepsis are summarized in Box 54-9.

---

**BOX 54-9** **Physiologic Data Helpful in Diagnosing Sepsis**

- **Cultures:** blood, sputum, urine, surgical or nonsurgical wounds, sinuses, and invasive catheters; positive results are not necessary for diagnosis.
- **CBC:** WBCs usually will be elevated and may decrease with progression of shock.
- **Chemistry panel:** hyperglycemia may be evident, followed by hypoglycemia in later stages.
- **Arterial blood gases:** metabolic acidosis with mild hypoxemia ($PaO_2$ less than 80 mm Hg) and possibly compensatory respiratory alkalosis ($PaCO_2$ less than 35 mm Hg).
- **CT scan:** may be needed to identify sites of potential abscesses.
- **Chest and abdominal radiographs:** may reveal infectious processes.
- **SvO_2 or ScvO_2:** can assist in the assessment of adequacy of oxygen delivery and consumption.
- **Lactate level:** decreasing levels of serum lactate indicate aerobic metabolism is able to meet cellular energy requirements. Elevated levels indicate inadequate perfusion and utilization of anaerobic metabolism to meet cellular energy requirements.
- **Base deficit:** elevated levels indicate inadequate perfusion and anaerobic metabolism.
- **EtCO_2:** decreasing $EtCO_2$ is an early indicator of inadequate regional and global tissue perfusion.

---

## Management

Septic shock requires a prompt, aggressive, multidisciplinary team approach with monitoring and treatment facilities found in an intensive care unit. The primary treatment goals are to maximize $DaO_2$ to meet cellular oxygen demand requirements and to halt the exaggerated inflammatory response. Initiating early treatment within the first 3 hours of identification has been shown to slow the decompensation of patients in a septic state and decrease the risk for multiorgan failure.[13,35] Initial interventions include large-volume fluid resuscitation, obtaining serum lactate level and blood cultures, and antibiotic administration. Subsequent interventions include continuing resuscitation and assuring adequate perfusion—for example, invasive hemodynamic monitoring, blood administration, and the use of vasoactive medications. A systematic protocol to drive these interventions is described in the Surviving Sepsis Guidelines.[26] The use of a sepsis protocol or sepsis 3-hour and 6-hour bundles improves timely interdisciplinary management of severe sepsis and septic shock, and is associated with improved survival.[9,35-37] The Surviving Sepsis Guidelines have been adopted by many hospitals. Several recent large randomized controlled trials have demonstrated that strict adherence to the 6-hour bundle to reach targeted endpoints did not improve survival as compared to usual care directed by emergency and critical care clinicians.[38-40] However, these studies did demonstrate that critical elements improving survival are rapid identification of sepsis, early acquisition of blood cultures followed by initiation of antibiotics, and volume administration. The interventions discussed below outline the evidence-based strategies that drive care of patients with sepsis. The use of a sepsis protocol or sepsis bundle improves timely interdisciplinary management of septic shock and is associated with improved survival.[9,35-37]

**PREVENTION.** Because morbidity and mortality from septic shock are so high, it is imperative that preventive infection control measures are in place. In critically ill patients, the body's natural defense mechanisms are often impaired, and protection from hospital-acquired (nosocomial) infections is essential. Nosocomial infections increase length of hospital stay and are associated with substantial costs, ranging from $5,800 to $12,700 for a case of sepsis and $11,100 to $22,300 for a case of pneumonia.[41] Therefore, a critical aspect of nursing care involves meticulous adherence to aseptic technique, thorough hand washing, and a continuing awareness of potential sites and causes of infection.[42]

**IDENTIFICATION AND TREATMENT OF INFECTION.** Source identification and control of infection is of paramount importance. A thorough assessment during nursing activities may identify new areas of erythema or drainage that lead to the early identification of infection or sepsis.[42] Blood and other relevant fluids such as sputum and urine samples should be collected for culture immediately upon diagnosis. Empiric broad-spectrum antibiotic therapy with coverage against gram-negative and gram-positive bacteria and anaerobes must be initiated as soon as possible.[8,43] Once the infectious organism has been isolated, antibiotic therapy should be narrowed to antibiotics effective against that specific organism to try to minimize development of antibiotic resistance. If a source is identified, definitive measures to alleviate the cause of sepsis may include resection, drainage of purulent tissues or secretions, or removal of contaminated intravascular devices.[26,42]

However, antimicrobial treatment of sepsis and source control are not sufficient to treat the generalized inflammatory reactions seen with septic shock. Supportive measures establish and maintain adequate tissue perfusion, and other therapies aim to block or interfere with the action of the various mediators implicated in shock. Aspects of supportive care include the following:

- Restoring intravascular volume
- Maintaining an adequate CO
- Ensuring adequate ventilation and oxygenation
- Restoring balance between coagulation and anticoagulation
- Providing an appropriate metabolic environment.

**Restoration of Intravascular Volume.** Adequate volume replacement is important for reversing hypotension. Patients may require several liters or more of fluid because of mediator-induced vasodilation and capillary leak, as discussed above. Fluid replacement should be guided by hemodynamic parameters, urine output, and indicators of metabolic acidosis (end-tidal carbon dioxide, base deficit, lactic acid levels). The Surviving Sepsis Campaign Guidelines recommend an initial fluid resuscitation challenge of at least 30 mL/kg of crystalloids in the first 3 hours of treatment. Fluid resuscitation may be guided by multiple assessment parameters.[26] Invasive monitoring devices, such as arterial catheters, some of which can provide CO and stroke volume variation, and central venous catheters that can monitor CVP and venous oxygen saturation (ScvO$_2$ or SvO$_2$), may be helpful in guiding fluid resuscitation.[44] A downward trend in the indicators of anaerobic metabolism, such as serum lactate, and reversal of metabolic acidosis are indicators of improved tissue perfusion. In addition to crystalloid fluids, colloid fluids such as blood products may be administered even in the absence of bleeding. Colloid fluid products enhance the delivery of oxygen to cells and maintain intravascular volume. Blood administered to reach specific levels of hemoglobin, however, has not demonstrated clear superiority in patient outcomes.[16,38–40] Administering the fluid and closely monitoring the response to fluid therapy are important nursing responsibilities (see Table 54-4).

**Maintenance of Adequate Cardiac Output.** In the early phase of septic shock, CO may be normal or elevated. However, the CO is not adequate to maintain tissue oxygenation and perfusion because of decreased SVR and peripheral vasodilation. As septic shock progresses, CO begins to decrease because of cardiac dysfunction. Because DaO$_2$ is dependent on CO, maintenance of CO is a primary therapeutic goal.

If adequate volume replacement does not improve tissue perfusion, vasoconstricting drugs can be administered to support circulation. The Surviving Sepsis Campaign Guidelines recommend vasoactive drugs be administered to target a mean arterial pressure (MAP) of 65 mm Hg. Norepinephrine is the first-line vasopressor for patients in septic shock.[26,45,46] Vasopressin, epinephrine, or dopamine may be used as second-line agents.[26,32] For patients with persistently low CO despite adequate fluid resuscitation and goal MAP, dobutamine is the recommended first-line inotropic agent to improve cardiac contractility.[26] It is recommended that dobutamine be titrated to normal but not elevated CO (see Table 54-4).

**Maintenance of Adequate Ventilation and Oxygenation.** Maintaining a patent airway, augmenting ventilation, and ensuring adequate oxygenation in the patient with septic shock usually require endotracheal intubation and mechanical ventilation. As previously discussed, these patients are at high risk for the development of ARDS. Low tidal volume (lung-protective) ventilation strategies limit further lung injury related to mechanical ventilation. The Surviving Sepsis Campaign Guidelines recommend a tidal volume of 6 mL/kg predicted body weight and plateau pressures no greater than 30 cm H$_2$O. Other strategies to improve oxygenation in sepsis include the use of higher levels of PEEP, recruitment maneuvers, and prone positioning where available.[26] Assessment of circulatory support, ventilation, and oxygenation is essential. (For nursing management of patients on mechanical ventilation, see Chapter 25.) The patient's DaO$_2$ and VO$_2$ needs are evaluated frequently. The goal is to maximize DaO$_2$ to ensure that VO$_2$ remains independent of DaO$_2$. Aerobic metabolism is maintained, and tissue energy needs are satisfied through the delivery of adequate oxygen to the cells.

**Restoration of Balance Between Coagulation and Anticoagulation.** The systemic release and depletion of coagulation factors is well known in sepsis; however, the management of this complication remains a challenge. Pharmacologic interventions to replete individual clotting factors, such as protein C, have failed to produce improvement in clinical outcomes.[47,48] Similarly, the use of fresh frozen plasma has been suggested to replete all clotting factors; this too has failed to improve outcomes and is not recommended.[26] Expert opinion from the Surviving Sepsis Campaign Guidelines suggests some patients may benefit from repletion of platelets in the setting of thrombocytopenia; however, additional research is needed to show definitive benefit.[26] Currently there is no proven intervention to restore the balance between coagulation and anticoagulation in patients with sepsis.

**Maintenance of Metabolic Environment.** The many and varied metabolic derangements associated with septic shock necessitate frequent monitoring of hematologic, renal, and hepatic function. Nutritional stores are depleted, and the patient requires supplemental nutrition to prevent malnutrition and to optimize cellular function. Despite increased metabolic needs, many patients with sepsis are unable to tolerate full caloric feeding; higher feeding is associated with increased enteral complications, infectious complications, and mortality. Trophic feeding, or underfeeding, to a maximum of 500 kcal per day is recommended in the early treatment of sepsis.[26] Enteral nutrition is the preferred route of nutritional support because it maintains the integrity of the gastrointestinal tract, decreases infection, and decreases mortality in patients with sepsis or a hypotensive event.[49]

Intolerance of enteral feeding may necessitate the use of total parenteral nutrition, but ideally, a small amount of enteral nutrition can still be delivered. Immune-modulated diets were once thought to replenish depleted nutrients, but more recent studies have identified complications related to the immune-modulated diets, and recent research has shown no difference in mortality.[26]

## Multiple Organ Dysfunction Syndrome

MODS is defined as a progressive physiologic failure of several organ systems in acutely ill patients. The physiologic threat is so disruptive to systemic homeostasis that homeostasis cannot be maintained without intervention.[4] The inability to maintain end-organ perfusion and oxygenation because of SIRS or any type of shock may result in MODS.

### Etiology

The exact cause of MODS is unknown. Release of systemic inflammatory mediators found in SIRS (see Table 54-1) may play a role in the etiology of MODS.[2,7] The inflammatory and procoagulant effects on systemic vasculature cause tissue hypoxia and necrosis at end organs.[6] In addition, inflammatory mediators disrupt cell junctions, not only in the endothelium but in the in gut mucosa as well. A loss of integrity of the gut mucosal barrier liberates bacterial toxins from the gut by a process called translocation. Gastrointestinal toxins circulate systemically, causing further damage to multiple organs.

### Pathophysiology

Several mechanisms may contribute to the pathophysiology of MODS; it appears to result from a cascade of bacterial factors, endothelial injury, inflammatory mediator release, disturbed hemostasis, and microcirculatory failure (see Fig. 54-3). Mitochondrial dysfunction and reduced ATP production are implicated in organ failure.[3] It is suggested that MODS may even be an adaptive state, allowing organs time to recover from injury and insult.[3]

Damage to organs may be primary or secondary and cause organ failure. A primary insult refers to a direct injury to an organ that results in organ dysfunction. For example, severe blunt chest trauma injures the lungs and may cause ARDS. Secondary insult is due to mechanisms operable in shock states. For example, a wound infection may cause sepsis, but the resultant SIRS and septic shock may cause ARDS. (ARDS is discussed in Chapter 27.)

In MODS, dysfunction and the inflammatory response in one organ may trigger dysfunction in another.[3,50,51] Therefore, failure of a particular organ makes the failure of a second or third organ more likely. Usually, the first organs to manifest signs of dysfunction are the lungs, heart, and kidneys. Liver failure tends to occur later because the liver has a considerable compensatory capacity. If hypoperfusion persists, all vital organs may fail. It is paramount that interventions increase end-organ perfusion and oxygenation and lessen the inflammatory response during the clinical management of shock states to prevent or limit MODS.

The lungs are particularly vulnerable to failure because the capillary beds act as a filter that is exposed to cytokines, mediators, and activated neutrophils. Capillary leakage causes interstitial edema, which impairs pulmonary gas exchange. The epithelial cells lining the alveoli are affected by inflammatory mediators. The disruption of the epithelium allows fluid, mediators, and coagulation factors to flood the alveoli, further impairing pulmonary gas exchange.[33] Respiratory failure associated with MODS is akin to ARDS and is discussed in detail in Chapter 27.

The cardiovascular system dysfunction includes reduced CO secondary to dysrhythmias and myocardial depression, as well as abnormalities in the peripheral vascular system, including vasodilation and hypotension that is unresponsive to fluid administration, increased capillary permeability, and maldistribution of blood flow.[3,51] The most common hematologic dysfunction is thrombocytopenia, which occurs because of increased consumption of platelets due to microthrombi formation and sequestration of platelets in the spleen, as well as impaired thrombopoiesis as a result of bone marrow suppression. This increases the risk for DIC in MODS.[7] (See Chapter 49 for a discussion of DIC.)

Neurologic dysfunction can be manifested by altered levels of consciousness, confusion, and delirium. The dysfunction may be secondary to poor cerebral perfusion or an increase in metabolic substances that are neurotoxic (ammonia), or it can be due to electrolyte imbalances. Renal dysfunction can occur secondary to poor renal perfusion and prolonged ischemia to renal tubular cells, or intrarenal causes such as nephrotoxic drugs. Renal failure may also be a direct result of mechanical ventilation from altered cardiovascular function, or to ventilator-induced lung injury and resultant cytokine release.[50,51] Progressive liver dysfunction results in hepatic failure. Hepatic failure affects multiple body systems, because the liver has so many functions, including synthesis of albumin, clotting factors, and drug metabolism. And, as previously discussed, hepatic failure can lead to impaired mitochondrial function and the ability of cells to use oxygen.[3]

### Assessment

Early recognition and management of MODS is essential to improve the likelihood of survival.[52]

Assessment of vital signs for signs of SIRS, including hypotension, tachycardia, tachypnea, hypothermia, and hyperthermia, is crucial in all hospitalized patients, particularly those at risk for developing shock and MODS. Close surveillance of laboratory values for changes in coagulation parameters, platelet count, WBCs, lactate, renal function, and other studies discussed in this chapter provides early indicators that a patient may be developing organ dysfunction. Several scoring systems exist to determine the extent of MODS, but to date there has not been uniform acceptance of one tool over another.[53]

### Management

Nurses have a key role in preventing, recognizing, and managing patients with MODS. Prevention strategies include enforcement of measures to prevent nosocomial infections, such as proper positioning (head of bed elevated during mechanical ventilation), oral care, turning and skin care, invasive catheter care, and wound care.[42] Unfortunately, no specific medical treatment for MODS, other than supportive care, is available. Management focuses on treating hemodynamic and metabolic derangements as described in the management of sepsis described above (see Table 54-4). Treatment directed at specific organ systems, other than supportive measures such as continuous renal replacement therapy and low–tidal volume ventilation, has not been shown to result in improved survival in patients with MODS. This may reflect the interdependence of organ systems and the systemic character of MODS. However, evidence suggests that early identification of patients with a high likelihood of developing MODS and early normalization of ScvO$_2$, arterial lactate concentration, base deficit, and pH lead to a more benign hospital course with decreased inpatient mortality.[44]

## Clinical Applicability Challenges

---

### CASE STUDY

J. N. is a 65-year-old woman who is postop day 5 status post hip fracture with open reduction with internal fixation secondary to a fall at home. She is currently being treated on the medical-surgical unit. She has a history of type 2 diabetes, hypertension, coronary artery disease, and an ischemic stroke 5 years ago that left her with some residual right-sided weakness. Her medications include metoprolol, lisinopril, atorvastatin, aspirin, metformin, and a multivitamin. The oncoming nurse notices that Ms. N. is increasingly drowsy and lethargic as compared to the previous day. The previous day, she had been alert, oriented and communicative, and had begun working with physical therapy in preparation for rehabilitation

On physical examination, Ms. N is pale, diaphoretic, and lethargic. She arouses to voice but is able only to state her first name. Her vital signs are as follows: blood pressure, 78/49 mm Hg; heart rate, 130; respiratory rate, 26; and temperature, 36.9°C. Oxygen saturation by pulse oximetry is 99% on room air. Her indwelling urinary catheter has put out 120 mL of cloudy, concentrated urine in the past 12 hours. A second large-bore IV catheter is started, and specimens are sent immediately for laboratory analysis, including two sets of blood cultures and a urine culture. She is given a liter bolus of normal saline solution. Her laboratory results are as follows: sodium, 143 mmol/L; potassium, 3.9 mmol/L; blood urea nitrogen, 32 mg/dL; creatinine, 0.9 mg/dL; glucose, 104 mg/dL; lactate, 2.1 mmol/L; hemoglobin, 11.1 g/dL; hematocrit, 33.5%; and WBC count, 14.2 cell/mm$^3$. Her urinalysis reveals greater than 10,000 WBCs and is positive for nitrites and leukocyte esterase. Chest x-ray findings are normal.

After the first liter of fluid, her blood pressure is 84/52 mm Hg, and a second liter bolus of normal saline solution is given. She is also given ceftriaxone 1 g IV and ampicillin 2 g IV and is transferred to the medical intensive care unit. A central line is inserted for fluid and medication administration and monitoring of CVP and ScvO$_2$. An arterial line is inserted for continuous blood pressure, stroke volume, and CO monitoring. She receives an additional liter of normal saline solution to increase her CVP mm Hg, but her MAP hovers around 55 to 60 mm Hg, and urine output remains about 20 mL/h. Norepinephrine is started at 1 mcg/min and titrated to 8 mcg/min to achieve a goal MAP of 65 mm Hg or greater.

Six hours into her intensive care unit stay, Ms. N develops a fever at 38.7°C. At this time, her ScvO$_2$ is 64% and the lactate level has increased to 3.4 mmol/L. Dobutamine is started at 5 mcg/kg/min, her urine output begins to improve, and her ScvO$_2$ rises to 71%. Her heart rate decreases to 105 beats/min. She is started on subcutaneous heparin for venous thromboembolism prophylaxis as well as famotidine for stress ulcer prophylaxis, and antibiotic therapy is continued. Her glucose level has risen to 190 mg/dL, so an insulin drip is started to maintain glucose level less than 180 mg/dL. Overnight, she remains on norepinephrine and dobutamine, receives an additional liter of normal saline solution to maintain CVP at 8 to 12 mm Hg, and makes 30 to 60 mL/h of urine.

The next morning, Ms. N's lactate level has decreased to 1.8 mmol/L, and ScvO$_2$ remains 70% to 75%. Other laboratory results include hemoglobin 10.1 g/dL, hematocrit 30.2%, and WBC count 13.6 cell/mm$^3$. The nurse is able to decrease the norepinephrine incrementally without a drop in MAP. The laboratory reports growth of Gram-negative rods in the urine sent for culture, and antibiotic therapy is narrowed to a fluoroquinolone. On examination, J. N. is more alert and is oriented to place and person. Her heart rate is 85 to 90, respiratory rate is 16, and temperature is 36.5°C. In the afternoon, her lactate level is 1.4 mmol/L and ScvO$_2$ is 72%. The dobutamine is discontinued. Close monitoring of her MAP, CVP, and ScvO$_2$ is continued. She remains stable overnight and is transferred to the step-down unit for continuing care the following day.

1. Discuss the importance of, and barriers to, early antibiotic administration in sepsis.
2. Discuss the serum lactate level as a measure of tissue perfusion and prognostic indicator in shock states.
3. What nursing interventions can be implemented to avoid urinary tract infections?

---

### WANT TO KNOW MORE?

A wide variety of resources to enhance your learning and understanding of this chapter are available on thePoint.

You will find:

- References
- Selected readings
- NCLEX-style review questions
- Internet resources
- And more!

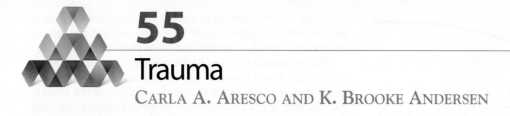

# 55

# Trauma

CARLA A. ARESCO AND K. BROOKE ANDERSEN

## LEARNING OBJECTIVES

*Based on the content in this chapter, the reader should be able to:*

1. Compare and contrast mechanisms of trauma injury.
2. Describe phases of initial assessment and related care of the trauma patient.
3. Discuss the assessment, management, and nursing care of patients with thoracic, abdominal, musculoskeletal, and maxillofacial trauma.
4. Describe early and late complications of trauma and the impact of these complications on mortality.

Trauma is defined by the *American Heritage Dictionary* as "Serious injury to the body, as from physical violence or an accident."[1] Injury is defined by the National Safety Council as "physical harm or damage to the body resulting from an exchange, usually acute, of mechanical, chemical, thermal, or other environmental energy that exceeds the body's tolerance."[2] Unintentional injuries include motor vehicle crashes (MVCs), poisonings, falls, choking, drowning, fires, and mechanical suffocation. Intentional injuries are divided into four subgroups; intentional self-harm (suicide), assault (homicide), legal intervention, and war operations.[2] This chapter specifically discusses mechanical injury.

Trauma is one of the leading causes of critical illness and death in the United States, with unintentional injury being the number one cause of death in age groups 1 through 44 years and the fifth leading cause of death overall.[2,3] In 1990, there were 5 million trauma deaths, and this number is expected to rise to 8 million by 2020.[4] Despite safety improvements, MVCs are still the number one cause of civilian trauma. Globally, the "war on terror" has increased the importance and incidence of military trauma.

## Mechanism of Injury

Awareness of the mechanism of injury can help the healthcare provider clarify the type of injury, predict the eventual outcome, and identify common injury combinations. An injury may exist in a trauma patient without the classical signs; knowing the mechanism of injury may prompt additional diagnostic workup and reassessment.

The mechanism of injury is related to the type of injuring force and the subsequent tissue response. Injury occurs when a force deforms tissues beyond their failure limits. Wounds vary depending on the injuring agent. The effect of injury also depends on personal and environmental factors, such as the person's age and sex, the presence or absence of underlying disease process, and the geographic region.

Force may or may not be penetrating. The injury delivered from force depends on the energy delivered and the area of contact. In penetrating injury, the concentration of force is to a small area. In blunt or nonpenetrating injury, the energy is distributed over a large area. The predominant feature affecting the impact is speed, or acceleration:

$$Force = mass \times acceleration$$

## Blunt Injury

Mechanisms of blunt injury include MVCs, falls, assaults, and contact sports. Multiple injuries are common with blunt trauma, and these injuries are often more life-threatening than penetrating injuries because the extent of the injury is less obvious and the diagnosis can be more difficult.

Blunt injury is caused by a combination of forces. These forces include acceleration, deceleration, shearing, crushing, and compressive resistance:

- *Acceleration* is an increase in the velocity (or speed) of a moving object.
- *Deceleration* is a decrease in the velocity of a moving object.
- *Shearing* occurs across a plane when structures slip relative to each other.
- *Crushing* occurs when continuous pressure is applied to a body part.
- *Compressive resistance* is the ability of an object or structure to resist squeezing forces or inward pressure.

In blunt trauma, injury occurs when there is direct contact between the body surface and the injuring agent. It is the direct impact that causes the greatest injury. Indirect forces are transmitted internally with dissipation of energy to the internal structure. The extent of injury from an indirect force depends on transference of energy from an object to the body. Injury occurs as a result of energy released and the tendency for the tissues to be displaced on impact.

Acceleration–deceleration injuries are the most common causes of blunt trauma. Before an MVC, the occupant and the car are traveling at the same speed. During the crash, both the occupant and the car decelerate to zero, but not necessarily at the same rate. There are actually three collisions involved in one crash: the first is the car with another object; the second is the occupant's body with the interior

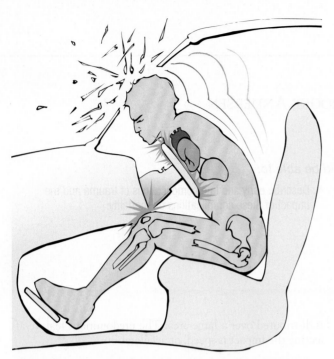

**FIGURE 55-1** In a motor vehicle crash, if the driver is not wearing a seat belt and an airbag is not deployed, damage may occur in various sections of the body. Without the use of restraints, injuries would occur to the skull, scalp, face, sternum, ribs, heart, liver, or spleen. Bones of the pelvis and lower extremities also may be damaged.

of the car; and the third is the internal tissues with the rigid body surface structure. For example, rapid deceleration in an MVC can cause direct injury to tissue. Subsequently, injury occurs as internal organs impinge on bony internal structures and cause major vessels to undergo stretching and bowing.

Although there may be bruising and/or burns to the face and chest from an airbag being deployed, airbags, along with wearing shoulder and lap restraints, reduce the incidence and severity of injury. Without a seatbelt, there is also a high risk of ejection from the vehicle resulting in further injuries.

These types of restraints reduce the force with which a person strikes a surface. Figure 55-1 demonstrates the type of injuries that could occur without these restraints.

The occupant's position in the vehicle also makes a difference in the blunt injury received. When a vehicle strikes a pedestrian, it is important to visualize the size of the vehicle and the size of the pedestrian. The area of impact can vary depending on these factors (Fig. 55-2).

## Penetrating Injury

Penetrating trauma refers to an injury produced by foreign objects penetrating the tissue. The severity of the injury is related to the structures damaged. The mechanism of injury is caused by the energy created and dissipated by the penetrating object into the surrounding areas. The amount of tissue damaged by a bullet is determined by the amount of energy that transfers into the tissue along with the amount of time it takes for the transfer to occur. It is important to note that the external appearance of the wound does not reflect the extent of internal injury.

Velocity determines the extent of cavitation and tissue damage. Low-velocity missiles localize the injury to a small radius from the center of the tract and have little disruptive effect. They cause little cavitation and blast effect, essentially only pushing the tissue aside. High-velocity missiles can cause more serious injury because of the amount of energy and cavitation produced. The damage depends on three factors: the density and compressibility of the tissue injured, the missile's velocity, and the fragmentation of the primary missile. High-velocity bullets compress and accelerate tissue away from the bullet, causing a cavity to form around the bullet and its entire tract. Shotguns are short-range, low-velocity weapons that use multiple lead pellets encased in a larger shell for ammunition. Each pellet is a missile. Figure 55-3 illustrates damage caused by shotguns at close and medium range.

It is important to obtain a brief description of the mechanism of gunshot injuries, including the weapon, the ammunition, and ballistics. This essential information is used to

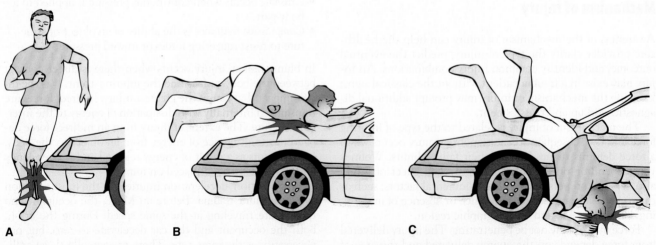

**A**   **B**   **C**

**FIGURE 55-2** Pedestrians may be hurt critically when hit by a moving vehicle. **A:** A common injury is the fracture of the tibia and fibula at the time of impact. **B:** Impact when the pedestrian strikes the hood of the car may cause fractured ribs and a ruptured spleen. **C:** Injuries to the head and additional fractures of the extremities may occur as the pedestrian rolls off the braking car or is thrown by the impact.

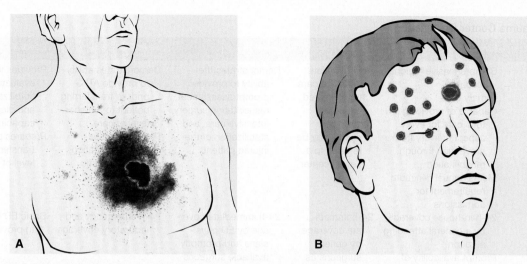

**FIGURE 55-3**   Damage is caused by shotguns at two different distances. **A:** At close range, the opening is extensive and is surrounded by blood splatters and powder burns. **B:** At medium range (8 to 10 ft), the larger entry wound is surrounded by individual pellet wounds.

guide the assessment of patients who sustain injuries from these weapons. All trauma patients must be undressed and inspected for entrance and exit wounds during the assessment process.

A stab wound or impalement is a low-velocity injury. The main injury determinants are length, width, and trajectory of the penetrating object and the presence of vital organs in the area of the wound. Although the injuries tend to be localized, deep organs and multiple body cavities can be penetrated.

## Initial Assessment and Management

When a trauma patient is brought to the emergency department or the trauma resuscitation unit, it is imperative to obtain a thorough history of the preceding events. This initial evaluation aids in assessment and treatment and can decrease morbidity and mortality. During this initial assessment, it is important to obtain as much detail as possible about the circumstances surrounding the injury, including the mechanism of injury. To facilitate initial assessment, intervention, and triage of the trauma victim, the American College of Surgeons (ACS) has developed the Advanced Trauma Life Support course. This course presents guidelines that provide an organized, standardized approach to the initial assessment of trauma patients, increasing the speed of the primary assessment and minimizing the risk that injuries will be overlooked.

## Prehospital Management

Prehospital management begins immediately after the patient is injured. The primary goal is to move the patient to the location that will provide definitive management as quickly as possible.[5] Care begins in the prehospital arena and is continued throughout the hospital stay. The principal factor influencing prehospital care is the transport time to the trauma center. Delivering the right care to the right patient in the right time is the purpose of trauma systems.[6] The Centers for Disease Control (CDC) and the Committee on Trauma (COT) have developed a National Trauma Triage

Protocol to assist prehospital providers in triaging patients to a trauma center.[5,6,7]

The advanced trauma life support guidelines state that the emphasis for assessment and management in the prehospital phase should be placed on maintaining the airway, ensuring adequate ventilation, controlling external bleeding and preventing shock, maintaining spine immobilization, and transporting the patient immediately to the closest appropriate facility.[5] The prehospital priority of maintaining adequate airway, breathing, and circulation (ABC) may be difficult because of the mechanism of injury. It is imperative that cervical spine immobilization be maintained at all times during airway management and transport to definitive care. After assessing and managing the ABCs, the trauma patient's neurologic status is assessed, including level of consciousness and pupil size and reaction. Once this primary assessment is complete, a secondary assessment is performed to determine any other injuries.

The prehospital providers must consider the facility that will receive the patient. Trauma systems have been designed to get the "right patient to the right resources in the right time frame." Table 55-1 details the various requirements for Level I through Level IV trauma centers. Transporting the patient to a Level I facility allows definitive care to be initiated earlier in the process, thereby reducing patient mortality. The creation of trauma centers and trauma programs has had a positive effect on outcomes in severely injured patients.[6]

Research has shown that injury-related mortality is significantly reduced with organized systems of trauma care, including prehospital care, acute care, and rehabilitation. Inclusive trauma systems have been designed to care for all injured patients and involve all acute care facilities to the extent that their resources allow.[8]

## In-Hospital Management

In-hospital patient management entails a rapid primary evaluation and resuscitation of vital functions, a more detailed secondary survey, a tertiary survey to identify specific injuries, and initiation of definitive care. Table 55-2 outlines the initial

**TABLE 55-1** Trauma Center Designation

| | Level I | Level II | Level III | Level IV | Level V |
|---|---|---|---|---|---|
| **Definition** | Comprehensive regional resource<br>Tertiary care<br>Capable of providing total care for every aspect of injury from prevention through rehabilitation<br>Meets annual minimum requirement for admissions | Able to initiate definitive care for all injured patients<br>Tertiary care needs may be referred to a Level I center | Demonstrates the ability to provide prompt assessment, resuscitation surgery, intensive care, and stabilization of the injured patient | Demonstrates ability to provide ATLS prior to transferring patient to a higher level of care<br>Provides evaluation, stabilization, and diagnostic capabilities | Provides initial evaluation, stabilization, and diagnostic capabilities<br>Prepares patient for transfer to higher level of care |
| **Surgeon availability** | 24-h in-house coverage by a general attending surgeon<br>Prompt availability of specialties (orthopedic, neuro, oral and maxillofacial, etc.) | 24-h immediate coverage by general surgeons as well as coverage by other specialties | 24-h immediate coverage by ED physicians and promptly available surgeons | 24-h emergency and laboratory coverage | Basic ED facilities to provide ATLS |
| **Research center** | Required | Not required | Not required | Not required | Not required |
| **Education, prevention, and outreach** | Required | Required | Required (continuing education for the RN, allied health personnel and/or trauma team) | Required (involved with prevention efforts and active community outreach) | Has developed transfer agreements to higher level of care |

Data from American Trauma Society: Trauma center levels explained. Retrieved January 27, 2016, from http://www.amtrauma.org/?page=TraumaLevels

assessment and management of the patient with trauma, commonly referred to as the "ABCDEs" of trauma care. According to the ACS, adhering to this sequence allows for the efficient identification of life-threatening conditions.[3,5] Optimal care of the trauma patient includes a preplanned emergency phase involving a predetermined response team with defined roles and expectations. This is necessary so that multiple procedures can be performed simultaneously. The team leader is a

physician. It is the leader's responsibility to assess the patient, order and interpret the diagnostic studies, and prioritize the diagnostics and therapeutic concerns.

### Primary Survey

During the primary survey, each priority of care is dealt with in order. The patient's assessment does not continue to the

**TABLE 55-2** Initial Assessment and Management of the Patient With Trauma

| Parameter | Assessment | Interventions |
|---|---|---|
| **Airway** | Air exchange<br>Airway patency | Jaw thrust, chin lift<br>Removal of foreign bodies<br>Suctioning<br>Oropharyngeal or nasopharyngeal airway<br>Endotracheal intubation (orally or nasally)<br>Cricothyrotomy |
| **Breathing** | Respirations (rate, depth, effort)<br>Color<br>Breath sounds<br>Chest wall movement and integrity<br>Position of trachea | Supplemental oxygen<br>Ventilation with bag–valve device<br>Treatment of life-threatening conditions (eg, tension pneumothorax) |
| **Circulation** | Pulse, blood pressure<br>Capillary refill<br>Obvious external bleeding<br>Electrocardiogram | Hemorrhage control: direct pressure, elevate extremity, pneumatic antishock garment<br>Intravenous therapy: crystalloids, blood transfusion<br>Treatment of life-threatening conditions (eg, cardiac tamponade)<br>Cardiopulmonary resuscitation |
| **Disability** | Level of consciousness<br>Pupils | — |
| **Exposure** | Inspection of body for injuries | — |

next phase until each preceding priority is effectively managed. For example, if a patient does not have a patent airway, breathing and ventilation cannot be established. Therefore, it is during this initial phase that life-threatening injuries are identified and managed. So, if the patient does not have a patent airway, endotracheal intubation, chest tube insertion, and central vascular line access may be initiated and intravenous (IV) fluid and blood products may be administered to maintain life-sustaining vital signs before moving on to the next phase of the evaluation. Initial radiographs and procedures are dependent on the findings in the primary survey. However, chest, abdomen, and pelvis imaging is generally completed at this time.

Assessing the patient for evidence of hypovolemia is essential. Blood loss can result from an external injury, associated with obvious bleeding, or from an internal injury, where bleeding may not be obvious. Any of these injuries can lead to inadequate tissue perfusion, which equals traumatic shock. It is necessary to first stop the bleeding with compression or surgery and then replace the lost intravascular volume. Some signs of hypovolemia include pallor, poor skin integrity, diaphoresis, tachycardia, and hypotension. Usually, trauma patients arrive at the trauma center with a large-bore IV line already in place, with IV fluid running in rapidly.

During the resuscitation period, electrocardiography (ECG) is performed. The patient is placed on a monitor with pulse oximetry and end-tidal carbon dioxide monitoring. A Foley catheter and a nasogastric or orogastric tube are placed, and blood specimens are sent to the laboratory for evaluation. Blood work includes evaluation of electrolytes, hemoglobin and hematocrit, blood type and crossmatch, and arterial blood gases (ABGs), if the patient is believed to have a high level of injury.

The nurse also assesses the patient for hypothermia. The trauma patient is often subjected to environmental factors, which, along with his or her altered physiologic state and possibly wet clothing, predispose the patient to hypothermia. Some measures, such as the infusion of room-temperature IV fluids or exposure of the patient's body to inspect for injuries, can exacerbate hypothermia. Warm fluids and blankets are used whenever possible to increase body temperature or maintain normothermia.

## Secondary Survey

Once the primary survey is completed, a more detailed secondary survey is initiated. This survey begins at the head and works down to the patient's feet. Non–life-threatening injuries are revealed during this survey. During this time, a plan is developed and the appropriate diagnostic tests (eg, radiographs, ultrasound studies, computed tomography [CT] scans, angiographic studies) are ordered. This is also the time when a more detailed patient history can be obtained, as well as important information regarding the mechanism of injury. The nurse asks the field providers for information regarding the incident because the patient may not be able to speak or may not remember the event. Family and friends might be helpful in providing additional information about the patient.

Questions the nurse asks before or during the trauma patient's arrival to the hospital include the following:

- Was the person involved in an MVC? Was the person wearing a restraining device? If the person was hit by a vehicle, was the person on foot or on a bike? What kind of vehicle was involved? Where was the person at the time of impact? What was the speed, point of impact, type of impact? Was there a fatality at the scene?
- Is blunt or penetrating trauma the main concern?
- Did the patient fall? How far? Was the fall off a ladder or down a flight of stairs?

Based on the information obtained from field providers or family members of the patient, other injuries may be suspected, and further investigation may be warranted. This is especially true in intubated, comatose, or paralyzed patients who are unable to verbalize their complaints. It is also important to remember that the elderly and the very young are patient populations that are more likely to have life-threatening injuries without obvious signs and symptoms.[3] The nurse continuously reassesses the trauma patient because injuries often go undetected.

## Tertiary Survey

The tertiary survey is completed on all trauma patients admitted to the intensive care unit (ICU). It is necessary to identify all of the patient's injuries completely. To do this, another head-to-toe examination is completed, an assessment of the patient's response to resuscitation is made, films are reviewed with the radiologist, laboratory values are reviewed, and every effort is made to obtain or complete a preinjury medical history. Delays in injury identification are common. However, if the injury is found within 24 hours of admission, it is not considered a missed injury.

## Fluid Resuscitation

Most trauma patients have a fluid volume deficit that must be corrected. The goal of fluid resuscitation is to maintain perfusion to the vital organs, especially the heart and the brain, by restoring circulating volume. A recent study examines the phenomenon of hypotensive resuscitation, in which "overresuscitation before management of bleeding could potentially increase the rate of blood loss."[5] Another study suggests that "initial liberal fluid resuscitation strategies may be associated with higher mortality in injured patients."[4]

Fluid administration is one of the most basic concepts in resuscitation and is also a part of the daily routine of medically managed patients in the hospital. To guide fluid resuscitation, the nurse uses physical assessment and hemodynamic parameters. Two factors affect the choice of fluid: how the volume loss occurred and which solutes need to be replaced.

Mechanism of injury is thought to affect *acute coagulopathy of trauma* (ACOT).[9] ACOT, which increases mortality, occurs in the early postinjury phase of trauma, and requires increased transfusions.[9] In the last decade, it has been recognized that with increased transfusions it is necessary to supply coagulation factors (plasma) and platelets in 1:1 ratio with red cells.[3,10] With this in mind, it is important to address the underlying problem causing the loss of fluids, electrolytes, or both. With aggressive fluid resuscitation, many patients have total-body edema and ascites. The two main complications of aggressive fluid resuscitation are hypothermia and coagulopathy.

## Crystalloids

Typically, crystalloids are administered to the trauma patient. Crystalloids are an aqueous solution that contains

| TABLE 55-3 | Intravenous Fluid |
|---|---|
| **Isotonic** | • *Example:* 0.9 normal saline solution<br>• Equivalent to the tonicity of the human body<br>• Causes minimal shifts between intracellular and extracellular fluid |
| **Hypotonic** | • *Example:* 5% dextrose in water (D5W), 0.45% sodium chloride<br>• Tonicity is less than that of human body<br>• May cause swelling, pulls into intracellular and interstitial space |
| **Hypertonic** | • *Example:* 3% saline solution<br>• Tonicity is more than that of human body<br>• Pulls fluid into the extracellular space to increase volume |

Data from Crawford A, Harris H: I.V. fluids: What nurses need to know. Nursing 41(5): 30–38, 2011

electrolytes and nonelectrolytes that will diffuse into all body fluid compartments; they are used to expand the patient's volume status. The volume of crystalloid replacement needed by the patient tends to be greater than the amount of blood lost. Crystalloids can be further classified by their tonicity (ie, the amount of sodium in the solution) as isotonic, hypotonic, and hypertonic (Table 55-3).

Hypertonic saline has been shown to enable a more rapid restoration of cardiac function with a smaller volume of fluid. It is supplied either in a 3%, 7.5%, or 23.4% sodium chloride (NaCl) solution. As little as 4 mL/kg, if given rapidly, may have the same hemodynamic effect as several liters of isotonic crystalloid. Hypertonic saline solution has the effect of shifting water into the plasma; this water comes from the red blood cells, interstitial space, and tissue. The result is a rapid increase in blood volume, which supports and improves hemodynamics. Hypertonic saline solution increases the mean arterial pressure and cardiac output, which then leads to peripheral vasodilation.[10] However, some studies have indicated that no change in survival rates were demonstrated in patients given hypertonic saline solution versus lactated Ringer solution.

The initial management of trauma patients often requires the infusion of 2 L of isotonic crystalloid as rapidly as possible, while trying to achieve a normal heart rate and blood pressure.[3,4,9] However, research has shown that the infusion of crystalloids in patients with hypotension can cause more harm by displacing a hemostatic clot, causing more bleeding.[3,9] The infusion of crystalloid also further dilutes the patient's hemoglobin and can increase intraperitoneal blood loss. It is now recommended that after 2 L of crystalloid infusion, consideration be given for blood transfusion.[3]

## Colloids

Colloids can also be given to resuscitate a trauma patient. Colloids, such as albumin, dextran, and hetastarch, create oncotic pressure, which encourages fluid retention and movement of fluid into the intravascular space. Colloids have a longer duration of action because they are larger molecules and stay in the intravascular compartment longer. They are also more efficient in expanding plasma volume, use a smaller volume, and increase colloid osmotic pressure.

Proponents of colloid use have argued that a lesser volume of fluid is necessary to achieve hemodynamic stability, and that the fluid is retained in the intravascular space longer. Despite possible advantages, there is no clear evidence that colloids are superior to crystalloids for resuscitation of the trauma patient. Potential complications, such as anaphylaxis and coagulopathy, have been reported with certain colloids. These potential adverse effects, together with higher costs, make colloids less desirable than crystalloids for use in resuscitation of trauma patients.

## Blood Products

Blood products are considered an excellent resuscitation fluid. Red blood cells increase oxygen-carrying capacity and allow for volume expansion. It is well known that the maintenance of adequate oxygen delivery is critical in the bleeding trauma patient; therefore, packed red blood cells are the mainstay of treatment. Blood also stays in the intravascular space for longer periods of time compared with the other resuscitation fluids. Although there is some concern about bloodborne pathogens and transfusion reactions, it is essential to understand the advantages offered by blood transfusion.

Blood should be transfused when patients are hemodynamically unstable or are showing signs of tissue hypoxia despite crystalloid infusion. Crossmatched blood is preferred but may not be available if emergent transfusion prohibits type and crossmatching of the patient's blood. O-negative blood is the preferred type of uncrossmatched blood, especially in women of childbearing age. O-positive blood may be used in male and postmenopausal female patients. If the patient requires large amounts of blood, transfusion of fresh frozen plasma and platelets is initiated. It is important to replace coagulation factors and platelets not contained in blood. In the event of massive blood transfusions, the risk of acute respiratory distress syndrome (ARDS) and disseminated intravascular coagulation (DIC) is heightened. An extended period of hypotension increases the possibility of renal failure.

Autotransfusion is another modality commonly used in the hemorrhaging trauma patient. Obviously, the nature of trauma prevents patients from donating their own blood, as they may for an elective surgery. However, sometimes blood can be salvaged. Most often, blood is saved from a chest tube underwater seal device. A cell saver is connected into the system, and the blood from the wound collects there. Once full, the cell saver is disconnected from the underwater seal device, and this blood is then transfused into the patient using a macroaggregate filter.

## Blood Substitutes

Blood substitutes do not require crossmatching and do not carry the risk of bloodborne pathogen transmission. Blood substitutes have a long shelf life and are not immunosuppressive. Blood substitutes have oxygen-carrying capacity and oxygen dissociation capability of natural hemoglobin; in addition, they have the ability to maintain hemodynamic stability and intravascular perseverance. Some examples of blood substitutes are hemoglobin-based oxygen carriers and perfluorocarbons.[10]

## Damage Control

For unstable patients, abbreviated surgery may be used to stabilize potentially fatal problems, followed by more extensive surgeries after initial resuscitation.[5] This approach is referred to as damage control. Uncontrolled bleeding and iatrogenic interventions ultimately result in hypothermia, coagulopathy, and acidosis; each of these exacerbates the other, causing a spiraling cycle with death as the ultimate result.[5] Damage-control surgery is designed to avoid or correct this lethal triad until definitive management can occur.

Damage control involves using a staged approach to patients with multiple injuries. The stages are as follows:

- *Stage 1*: Stop hemorrhage, control contamination, and perform closure methods to close wounds temporarily.
- *Stage 2*: Correct physiologic abnormalities in the ICU by warming and ensuring adequate resuscitation as well as correcting coagulopathy.
- *Stage 3 (final stage)*: Definitive operative management.

The philosophy of damage control is to use abbreviated surgical interventions before the development of irreversible physiologic end points.[5] Traditionally, damage control was used for abdominal trauma, but it is now used for all types of trauma that require immediate surgery.

### Definitive Care

Increasingly, trauma care consists of nonoperative management of stable patients. Traditionally, solid organ injuries, both blunt and penetrating, were treated with surgery. Today, many trauma surgeons are choosing nonoperative management for their patients whenever possible. Ever more sophisticated techniques for visualization of internal structures, such as CT, ultrasonography, and angiography, have reduced the need for immediate surgical exploration in many cases. Without question, CT offers improved accuracy and high sensitivity and specificity.[11,12] It provides more information to aid in diagnosing injuries that may have been missed without it. Using CT to discharge a patient earlier, or to clear the patient for an earlier surgery with another service, makes sense from a patient care and economic perspective. Many of these visualization techniques can be used for management as well as diagnosis. For example, angiographic interventions may be used to embolize a hemorrhaging internal vessel, obviating the need for invasive surgical intervention.

Patients who are treated nonoperatively require frequent assessment and are admitted to the ICU for that purpose. To observe the patient effectively, the nurse must be aware of potential injuries and associated signs and symptoms. Attention is also given to the management of preexisting medical conditions and the identification of injuries missed during treatment of life-threatening problems. Once again, knowledge regarding the mechanism of injury is necessary. Finally, the patient is monitored for the development of complications. The critical care nurse must be aware of potential complications and related risk factors associated with various injuries. Certain situations, such as prolonged extrication, prolonged hypothermia, respiratory or cardiac arrest, massive fluid resuscitation, and massive blood transfusions, suggest an increased likelihood of severe injuries and a greater chance of complications and death after trauma. A collaborative care guide for the patient with multisystem trauma is given in Box 55-1.

---

**QSEN BOX 55-1**    *COLLABORATIVE CARE GUIDE for the Patient With Multisystem Trauma*

| Outcomes | Interventions |
| --- | --- |
| **Impaired Gas Exchange: Ineffective Breathing Pattern** | |
| The patient will maintain a patent airway. | • Auscultate breath sounds.<br>• Perform frequent assessments.<br>• Intubate if needed.<br>• Provide supplemental oxygen PRN. |
| The patient will maintain an SaO₂ of 95% or more and have adequate ABG values. | • Provide pulmonary toilet (chest physiotherapy and incentive spirometry).<br>• Intubate.<br>• Monitor ABGs. |
| The patient will be able to take deep breaths and will be free of anxiety. | • Use mechanical ventilation if necessary to support adequate ventilation.<br>• Provide adequate pain medication to promote deep breathing (patient-controlled analgesia [PCA], epidural, round-the-clock medications)<br>• Medicate before pain increases.<br>• Use antianxiety drugs as necessary. |
| **Risk for Shock: Decreased Cardiac and Peripheral Tissue Perfusion** | |
| The patient will maintain an adequate blood pressure, heart rate, and respiratory rate. | • Monitor respiratory rate and depth.<br>• Use ECG monitor.<br>• Administer intravenous (IV) fluids and packed red blood cells to ensure adequate intravascular volume and oxygen-carrying capacity.<br>• Administer medications, such as vasoactive and inotropic agents, after intravascular volume is restored.<br>• Install pulmonary artery catheter/A-line.<br>• Assess skin color and capillary refill time. |
| The patient will not experience deep venous thrombosis. | • Use prophylactic anticoagulants unless contraindicated.<br>• Apply antiembolic stockings.<br>• Use pneumatic compression devices. |

*(continued)*

**QSEN BOX 55-1** | *COLLABORATIVE CARE GUIDE for the Patient With Multisystem Trauma (continued)*

| Outcomes | Interventions |
|---|---|
| **Electrolyte Imbalance: Risk for Imbalanced Fluid Volume** | |
| The patient will maintain an adequate intake and output. | • Monitor blood pressure, heart rate, central venous pressure, pulmonary capillary wedge pressure, IV fluid.<br>• Use Foley catheter to monitor urine output.<br>• Consider insensible fluid loss in output.<br>• Monitor laboratory values. |
| The patient will maintain electrolyte balance. | • Replace electrolytes PRN.<br>• Monitor ECG. |
| **Risk for Activity Intolerance: Impaired Physical Mobility** | |
| The patient's range of motion will be maintained. | • Consult physical/occupational therapist.<br>• Use splints PRN.<br>• Do range-of-motion exercises every 8 hours.<br>• Out of bed as tolerated. |
| **Impaired Tissue Integrity** | |
| The patient will not experience skin breakdown. | • Monitor skin every 4 hours.<br>• Turn patient every 2 hours and PRN.<br>• Use pressure-relieving devices.<br>• Remove splints to monitor skin.<br>• Provide prescribed wound care.<br>• Monitor wound for evidence of infection. |
| **Imbalanced Nutrition** | |
| The patient will maintain an adequate calorie intake to meet metabolic needs. | • Arrange dietary/nutrition consult.<br>• Use total parenteral nutrition/lipids if enteral nutrition contraindicated.<br>• Tube feeds: Encourage enteral nutrition when possible.<br>• Check prealbumin and electrolytes.<br>• Monitor for weight loss. |
| **Impaired Comfort** | |
| The patient will maintain a pain score of <5. | • Administer adequate pain medication.<br>• Use PCA/epidural PRN.<br>• Arrange pain consult if needed.<br>• Use sedation as needed.<br>• Monitor vital signs. |
| **Ineffective Coping: Disturbed Body Image: Impaired Individual Resilience** | |
| The patient will maintain as much control as possible. | • Inform patient of procedures.<br>• Establish a schedule with the patient if possible.<br>• Provide an alternate means of communication if necessary, such as lip reading, writing, and a communication board. |
| The patient and family will cope effectively with the traumatic event. | • Provide repeated information.<br>• Encourage use of appropriate coping.<br>• Encourage use of support systems.<br>• Arrange social work consult. |
| **Teaching/Discharge Planning** | |
| The patient will be involved in discharge planning. | • Discuss discharge with patient.<br>• Allow patient to make decisions if possible. |
| The patient will understand injuries and complications of injuries. | • Provide discharge instructions accordingly with injury.<br>• Provide patient with list of injuries. |

## Assessment and Management of Specific Injuries

Although this section discusses traumatic injuries related to specific areas of the body, the nurse must keep in mind that head-to-toe assessment is required for each trauma patient. Physical assessment of each organ system is indicated, as described in previous chapters throughout this text.

## Thoracic Trauma

Thoracic injuries range from simple abrasions and contusions to life-threatening insults to the thoracic viscera. Although these injuries are associated with a high mortality rate, most can be managed with simple chest tube insertion, mechanical ventilation, aggressive pain control, and other supportive care. Great vessel injuries or disruption to the heart usually result in immediate death. Early deaths (30 minutes to 3 hours after injury) are related to cardiac tamponade, tension pneumothorax, aspiration, or airway obstruction.[13,14]

Immediate life-threatening injuries require evaluation and treatment during the primary survey. Examples of these include airway obstruction, tension pneumothorax, cardiac tamponade, open pneumothorax, massive hemothorax, and flail chest (Fig. 55-4). Potentially life-threatening injuries,

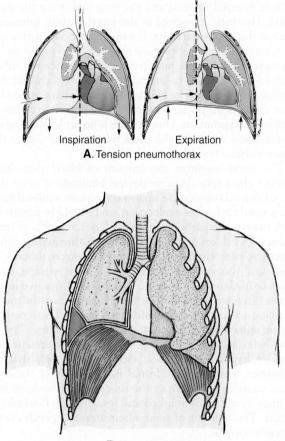

**A.** Tension pneumothorax

**B.** Hemothorax

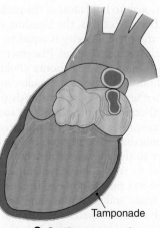

Tamponade

**C.** Cardiac tamponade

**FIGURE 55-4** **A:** Tension pneumothorax. **B:** Hemothorax. **C:** Cardiac tamponade.(**B,** Courtesy of Neil O. Hardy, Westpoint, Conn. **C,** Courtesy of LifeART image © 2007 Lippincott Williams & Wilkins. All rights reserved.)

such as thoracic aortic disruption, tracheobronchial disruption, myocardial contusion, traumatic diaphragm tear, esophageal disruption, and pulmonary contusion, should be addressed during the secondary survey.[15]

In thoracic injury, the first priority is always airway management. This includes immediate airway control as well as adequate oxygenation and protection from aspiration. Airway obstruction may be the result of another injury or the primary problem. The most common causes of airway obstruction are the tongue, avulsed teeth, dentures, secretions, and blood. Other causes of airway obstruction include injuries to the trachea, thyroid cartilage, or cricoid process.

## Tracheobronchial Trauma

Injuries to the trachea or bronchi can be caused by blunt or penetrating trauma and frequently are accompanied by esophageal and vascular damage. Ruptured bronchi often are present in association with upper rib fractures and pneumothorax. Severe tracheobronchial injury is associated with a high mortality rate; however, with continued improvements in prehospital care and transport, more of these patients are surviving.

Airway injuries often are subtle. Presenting signs include dyspnea (occasionally the only sign), hemoptysis, cough, subcutaneous emphysema, anxiety, hoarseness, stridor, air hunger, hypoventilation, use of accessory muscles, sternal and subscapular retractions, diaphragm breathing, apnea, and cyanosis. Cyanosis may be a late sign. A chest radiograph can alert the physician to a possible injury; however, diagnosis usually is made with bronchoscopy or during surgery. Tracheobronchial injury is considered whenever a persistent air leak accompanies a pneumothorax.

Small lung lacerations or pleural tears can be managed conservatively with mechanical ventilation delivered through an endotracheal tube or tracheostomy. Larger injuries may require surgical repair. Simultaneous independent lung ventilation, in which each lung is ventilated separately (each with a dedicated ventilator), may also be used.

Nursing care involves the assessment of oxygenation and gas exchange, along with appropriate pulmonary care. During the first few days, the physician may perform a bronchoscopy to visualize the repair site and provide more effective secretion removal. Pneumonia is a potential short-term complication, whereas tracheal stenosis may occur later.

## Bony Thorax Fractures

Rib fractures, sternal fractures, and flail chest are thoracic fractures commonly seen in trauma patients. They occur when the applied force exceeds the strength of the thoracic cage. Rib fractures are common injuries. They are clinically significant as markers of serious intrathoracic and abdominal injuries, sources of significant pain, and predictors of pulmonary deterioration. With rib fractures, the most common associated thoracic injuries are pneumothorax, hemothorax, and pulmonary contusion, and the most frequently injured abdominal organs are the liver and the spleen.[16] The greatest concerns for nurses caring for patients with such injuries are pain, ineffective ventilation, and secretion control. Ribs 1 and 2 are usually protected by the clavicle, scapula, humerus, and surrounding muscles. If these ribs are fractured, it often signifies that high-impact trauma and other injuries—for example, to the aorta, the thorax, and the spine—are very likely, and this should be investigated. Ribs 4 through 10 are most commonly fractured in blunt trauma. If these ribs are fractured, there are often associated underlying lung injuries. Fractures of the lower ribs (8 through 12) can also be associated with injury to the liver or other abdominal structures. Sternal fractures are associated with blunt trauma.

Flail chest is an injury that involves multiple rib fractures. These fractures can be anterior, posterior, or lateral, and usually a sternal fracture is present as well. The stability of the thorax is disrupted, and the rib cage no longer moves in unison. The diagnosis of flail chest is made on the basis of a fracture of two or more ribs, in two or more separate locations, causing an unstable segment. This creates a free-floating segment of rib or sternum.[16] The injured area does not respond to the action of the respiratory muscles; rather, it moves in accordance with the changes in intrapleural pressure. The flail segment movement is paradoxical, hence the term paradoxical breathing. The flail segment causes a decrease in the normal negative pressure of the chest, thereby decreasing ventilation and causing some degree of hypoxia. The flail segment follows pleural pressure instead of respiratory muscle activity. As the patient's pulmonary status worsens, the paradoxical movement of the flail segment increases. Initially, muscular splinting may mask the injury until the patient becomes fatigued. This patient may require intubation and mechanical ventilation.[16]

Initial management of patients with bony thorax fractures includes airway management, pain management, and oxygen therapy to maintain adequate saturation. The nurse must consider the underlying structures and the possible injury to them. Treatment of flail chest includes turning the patient with the injured side down to improve oxygenation. This is often difficult because of the need to maintain cervical spine immobilization. Other treatment modalities include internal splinting, accomplished by placing the intubated patient on positive-pressure ventilation. Sometimes surgical repair is performed, especially if a thoracotomy is necessary for other reasons. Surgical repair may help decrease the need for prolonged mechanical ventilation.

## Pleural Space Injuries

For the purpose of this chapter, the term *pleural space injury* is used in reference to pneumothorax (intrapleural air collection), hemothorax (intrapleural blood collection), and hemopneumothorax (interpleural air and blood collections). Pleural space injuries are caused by disruption of an intrathoracic structure, which allows air or blood to build up in the pleural layers, thereby leading to a decrease in negative intrathoracic pressure. Sometimes, air and blood continue to build up in the pleural cavity, causing increased tension, which leads to a tension pneumothorax or a tension hemothorax. Either blunt or penetrating trauma may result in a pleural space injury.

The mechanism of injury may lead the nurse to suspect a pleural space injury. For example, an unrestrained driver whose chest hits the steering wheel has a great potential for this injury. When assessing the patient, respiratory distress may be evident along with altered ventilation, which leads to impaired gas exchange. Impaired gas exchange may be evidenced by restlessness, anxiety, tachypnea, decreased oxygenation, poor color, and diaphoresis. The nurse continuously reassesses the patient, because even if the original injury is small, it can expand, causing a life-threatening emergency.

Chest radiography is usually used to diagnose pleural space injuries. Sometimes, if the pneumothorax is less than 20% of the chest cavity, it may not be seen initially on chest film. A chest CT scan often shows the smaller pleural space injuries.

Treatment of pleural space injuries includes appropriate management of the patient's airway, ventilation, and oxygenation. A large-bore chest tube, such as a 40-French tube, is often inserted to reexpand the lung and drain the air or blood. This tube is inserted in the fourth or fifth intercostal space at the midaxillary line. For trauma patients with a simple pneumothorax, a chest tube may be placed in the second intercostal space at the midclavicular line. Once the tube is inserted, it is attached to an underwater seal system and then attached to suction. The effects of treatment are assessed by chest radiograph, physical examination, and observation for improved oxygenation. Often, there is an air leak in the underwater seal system of the chest tube drainage device that ceases within a few days.

The nurse monitors the amount of blood that drains into the chest tube drainage device. Drainage of more than 250 mL/h for 2 consecutive hours may indicate a missed injury or the need for further exploration, and should be reported.[16]

A massive hemothorax is defined as 1.5 to 4 L of intrathoracic blood loss and constitutes a life-threatening injury. A massive hemothorax is often caused by severe thoracic injuries, and the source of bleeding is a large systemic blood vessel or mediastinal structure. Patients with massive hemothorax often arrive at the emergency department or trauma resuscitation unit in cardiopulmonary arrest. These patients require immediate thoracotomy to control bleeding. The patients who are not in cardiopulmonary arrest present with signs of hypovolemic shock (see Chapter 54), dyspnea, tachypnea, and cyanosis. Initial management of these patients includes treatment of the shock state. Two large-bore IV lines should be established and resuscitation fluid administered. The amount of fluid administered depends on the patient's response.

A left massive hemothorax is more common than a right one and is often associated with aortic rupture. The chest cavity is large enough to hold most of the patient's circulating blood volume. Because of this, the bleeding stops only when the pressure in the pleural cavity is equal to or greater than the pressure in the damaged vessel. Placement of a chest tube in a patient with massive hemothorax could lead to exsanguination by eliminating the tamponade caused by a closed chest injury. If a chest tube is inadvertently placed, it should be clamped until exploratory thoracotomy can be performed.

Tension pneumothorax is a life-threatening condition that requires immediate recognition. It may be the result of a primary injury to the thorax, or it may be a delayed complication related to tracheobronchial injury or mechanical ventilation. Tension pneumothorax is caused by air entering the pleural space and becoming trapped without an exit. A one-way valve closed system is formed. This causes a compression of one or more of the intrathoracic structures (trachea, heart, lungs, and great vessels) and prohibits them from functioning adequately. The outcome is ventilation failure, compromised venous return, and insufficient cardiac output.[14]

Tension pneumothorax is often difficult to diagnose in the trauma patient because of other injuries the patient may have, as well as the presence of a shock state. It may not be diagnosed until the patient has decompensated. The nurse may notice that it is difficult to ventilate the patient, despite an open airway. There is often a drop in the patient's oxygenation. Other signs of tension pneumothorax include chest asymmetry, tracheal shift, neck vein distention (unless the patient is hypovolemic), decreased breath sounds on the affected side, and evidence of decreased cardiac output (eg, decreased blood pressure and poor tissue perfusion).[14]

Treatment of tension pneumothorax requires immediate decompression of the trapped air. This is done initially by placing a 14- or 16-gauge needle into the pleural space, usually between the second to fourth anterior intercostal space. An immediate rush of air should escape, and the patient's ventilation should improve. Supplemental oxygen is provided to the patient before decompression. After emergent decompression, the needles are changed to chest tubes. This is done to allow the lungs to expand as well as to prevent a reoccurrence. Lastly, additional assessment is necessary to determine the cause of tension pneumothorax. The nurse must continue to assess and reassess the patient.

## Pulmonary Contusion

A pulmonary contusion is a bruising of the lung parenchyma, often caused by blunt trauma. It is the most common lung injury. It is often apparent on the chest radiograph and CT as ill-defined, patchy, ground-glass density regions of opacification in mild contusion to widespread areas of consolidation in more severe injury. CT is more sensitive in diagnosing pulmonary contusions, because it may take up to 24 hours for the pulmonary contusion to show up on chest radiograph.[13] However, the presence of a scapular fracture, rib fractures, or a flail chest should lead to the suspicion of a possible underlying pulmonary contusion. In fact, pulmonary contusion should be anticipated in any patient who sustains significant high-energy blunt chest trauma. The most common mechanism for pulmonary contusion is MVCs.

Pulmonary contusion occurs when rapid deceleration ruptures capillary cell walls, causing hemorrhage and extravasation of plasma and protein into alveolar and interstitial spaces. This results in atelectasis and consolidation, leading to intrapulmonary shunting and hypoxemia. Presenting signs and symptoms include dyspnea, rales, hemoptysis, and tachypnea. Severe contusions also result in increasing peak airway pressures, hypoxemia, and respiratory acidosis. Pulmonary contusion may mimic ARDS; both are poorly responsive to high fractions of inspired oxygen ($FiO_2$). ARDS is discussed in detail in Chapter 27. The greater the degree of pulmonary contusion, the greater the degree of ventilatory impairment.

Treatment of pulmonary contusion is supportive. Patients with a mild contusion require close observation with frequent ABG measurements or pulse oximetry monitoring. Additional nursing interventions include frequent respiratory assessment, pulmonary care, and pain control. Chest physiotherapy and continuous epidural analgesia also may be beneficial. An oximetric pulmonary artery catheter and arterial line usually are placed to facilitate monitoring of ABGs, hemodynamics, and respiratory parameters (oxygen delivery, oxygen consumption, intrapulmonary shunt).

Severe pulmonary contusion may require ventilatory support with positive end-expiratory pressure (PEEP). Although alveolar ventilation improves as PEEP is added, blood flow to alveoli may diminish, leading to an increased intrapulmonary shunt. To optimize tissue perfusion and oxygenation, each change in PEEP requires assessment of the status of the shunt, oxygen delivery, and other indicators of tissue perfusion (cardiac output, blood pressure, and urine output). For adequate pain control, epidural or intrapleural infusions of analgesics or an intracostal nerve block may be necessary. In severe cases of respiratory compromise, increased sedation or paralysis may be indicated to decrease energy expenditure and oxygen requirements. A rotation bed also may be considered to promote pulmonary toilet and respiratory gas exchange. Positioning the patient with the injured side up is beneficial in the case of a severe unilateral contusion. In rare instances, when the patient does not respond to traditional mechanical ventilation, prone positioning and high-frequency jet ventilation may be used. Another mode of ventilation commonly used is airway pressure-release ventilation.

Fluid management also is important. Intake and output, daily weights, central venous pressure, and pulmonary artery and capillary wedge pressures are monitored to guide fluid administration. Medications may need to be more concentrated to compensate for excess fluid intake, and diuretics may be required periodically. Severe fluid restriction is not indicated; instead, fluid balance should be maintained at a normal level (euvolemia) to support optimal cardiac output and oxygen delivery. The contused lung should show radiographic signs of improvement within 72 hours. The presence of persistent infiltrates may indicate complications, such as pneumonia or superimposed ARDS. Long-term sequelae include prolonged reduced functional residual capacity, dyspnea, and fibrosis.

## Blunt Cardiac Injuries

Blunt cardiac injuries encompass a wide spectrum of clinical manifestations ranging from asymptomatic myocardial bruise to cardiac rupture and death.[13] These injuries include cardiac wall rupture, valvular disruption, coronary artery dissection, and cardiac contusions. Table 55-4 describes the blunt cardiac injury (BCI) classification according to the sequelae of the injury. There are few clinical signs and symptoms of BCI. Chest pain is usually the most common, and others secondary to thoracic injuries often occur (eg, dyspnea, chest wall ecchymosis, flail chest). It is thought to be overdiagnosed because of the lack of a gold standard test.[13]

**TABLE 55-4  Blunt Cardiac Injury (BCI) Classification According to the Sequelae of the Injury**

| Classification | Description |
| --- | --- |
| 1 | BCI with cardiac free wall rupture |
| 2 | BCI with septal rupture |
| 3 | BCI with coronary artery injury |
| 4 | BCI with cardiac failure |
| 5 | BCI with complex dysrhythmias |
| 6 | BCI with minor electrocardiographic or cardiac enzymes abnormalities |

From Schultz JM, Trunkey DD: Blunt cardiac injury. Crit Care Clin 20:57–70, 2004.

Cardiac contusions, the most common form of blunt cardiac injuries, are usually caused by blunt trauma as the heart hits the sternum during rapid deceleration. A contusion can also develop if the heart is compressed between the sternum and the spine. Symptoms vary from none (common) to severe congestive heart failure and cardiogenic shock. Complaints of chest pain must be evaluated carefully after trauma. Nonspecific ECG changes, which can include any type of dysrhythmia, are frequently seen. A dysrhythmia always indicates a cardiac contusion until proven otherwise. Atrial dysrhythmias and conduction disturbances may be seen with right-sided cardiac injuries; ventricular disturbances are more likely after left-sided cardiac injuries.

A cardiac contusion is suspected when there is a history of severe anterior blunt trauma and the patient has chest wall bruising and fractures of the ribs or sternum. A 12-lead ECG is performed to detect any electrical abnormalities. Most patients with cardiac contusions have ECG abnormalities on admission.[13] However, there is no correlation between the complexity of the dysrhythmia and the degree of the cardiac contusion. These patients are placed on continuous cardiac monitoring, and blood is drawn for cardiac isoenzyme and troponin studies. Although cardiac enzymes lack specificity in terms of diagnosis, they are used to guide therapy.[13]

Controversy exists over the standard of care for patients with cardiac contusion. Because there is no standard in diagnosing this injury, there is also no standard in treatment. Continuous monitoring must be done to evaluate for symptomatic dysrhythmias, especially ventricular irritability and conduction defects. Echocardiography or multigated angiography may be helpful in determining any muscle defect or damage. In general, patients are treated to relieve their symptoms.

### Penetrating Cardiac Injury

In most cases, a penetrating injury to the heart results in prehospital death.[13] Those who survive do so because of cardiac tamponade. Cardiac tamponade and hypovolemic shock are the common presenting signs.[13] The right ventricle is injured most often because of its anterior location.[13] Occasionally, small stab wounds to the ventricles seal themselves because of the thick ventricular musculature. Treatment of hemodynamically stable patients remains controversial. In some instances, monitoring with serial CT scanning or with pericardial and pleural ultrasonography is acceptable. In other cases, surgery to create a thoracoscopic pericardial window may be necessary to aid in the diagnosis of ongoing hemorrhage and to drain pericardial fluid collections. In the presence of ongoing hemorrhage and shock, lost blood volume is replaced, and the patient is immediately transported to the operating room for a median sternotomy and exploration. In severe cases, a thoracotomy in the emergency department may be required as a lifesaving measure.

After surgical repair, appropriate central lines and arterial line are placed to facilitate careful hemodynamic monitoring. Vasopressors or inotropic agents may be necessary to maintain adequate blood pressure and cardiac output. Fluid and electrolyte balance, along with cardiac rhythm, must be monitored closely. Heart sounds are assessed to detect murmurs, indicating valvular or septal defects, and for signs of congestive heart failure. Chest and mediastinal tube drainage

are recorded frequently. Fresh frozen plasma and platelets are administered, as indicated, to correct coagulopathies. Complications include continued hemorrhage and postcardiotomy syndrome.

### Cardiac Tamponade

Cardiac tamponade, known as both a symptom and injury, can result from both penetrating and blunt trauma. It is a life-threatening injury that needs to be immediately assessed and treated. Cardiac tamponade is caused by blood filling the pericardium and compressing the heart, causing decreased cardiac filling, which leads to reduced cardiac output and eventually shock. Bleeding into the pericardial sac (hemopericardium) or a small pericardial rupture may or may not cause cardiac tamponade, depending on the amount of pressure in the pericardium.

The pericardial sac normally holds about 25 mL of fluid, which serves to cushion and protect the heart. Only a small amount of pericardial blood (50 to 100 mL) is necessary to increase intrapericardial pressure.[13] Continued bleeding increases the pressure rapidly, and the patient presents with signs and symptoms of cardiac tamponade.

Classical symptoms include decreased blood pressure, muffled heart sounds, and increased central venous pressure manifested by distended neck veins (Beck triad). Another key sign to cardiac tamponade is pulsus paradoxus, a drop in systemic blood pressure during inspiration caused by a fall in cardiac output. Because these signs may be obscured in the hypovolemic trauma victim, patients with a history of precordial trauma must be treated with a high index of suspicion. Diagnosis of cardiac tamponade is not easy. An echocardiogram is most useful in the diagnosis and is readily available, but cardiac tamponade is a clinical diagnosis.[13]

Treatment of cardiac tamponade includes airway control, oxygenation, hemodynamic support, and rapid transport to a definitive care center. The rapid transfusion of IV fluids increases venous pressure and ultimately improves cardiac output as well as provides the needed time to prepare for interventions. Ultimately, the treatment of cardiac tamponade is drainage of blood from the pericardial sac (pericardiocentesis)[13]; this is the only life-sustaining intervention. Nursing management of a patient with cardiac tamponade includes airway protection and ventilatory support, hemodynamic support, and assistance with interventions provided to the patient.

### Aortic Injuries

Sudden shearing forces caused by rapid deceleration are usually the cause of blunt aortic injuries.[13] These injuries remain associated with significant early mortality and are thought to be the second leading cause of traumatic death following head injuries[17]; 80% to 90% of patients die before reaching the hospital.[13,16,17] The location and size of the disruption determine its significance. MVCs are the primary causes of this injury.[16,17] Of the patients who make it to the hospital alive, 75% are hemodynamically unstable and 50% die before repair. Many of these patients have other significant injuries. Angiography was previously the gold standard for diagnosis of aortic injuries; however, with the advances in CT scanning, this modality is now the gold standard, with a sensitivity of 100% and specificity of 80% to 85%.[16] This new standard is beneficial for smaller centers that may not have the ability to perform angiography and previously would have had to transfer patients to a higher level of care.

Because the thoracic aorta is very mobile, the tears occur at points of fixation. There are three common locations of vessel rupture. The most common is at the aortic isthmus, just distal to the left subclavian artery, where the vessel is attached to the chest wall by the ligamentum arteriosum. The two other sites of rupture are in the ascending aorta, where the aorta leaves the pericardial sac, and at the entry to the diaphragm. The inner layers of the vessel tear on impact from deceleration. The outer layers remain intact and balloon out into a pseudoaneurysm. A partial circumferential hematoma may also be tamponaded by surrounding tissues. Both of these mechanisms may prolong survival, but only for a limited time.

Penetrating mediastinal injuries or thoracic injuries caused by blunt trauma should raise suspicion of aortic injury. Other injuries that may raise suspicion include first or second rib fractures, high sternal fractures, clavicular fractures at the sternal margin, and massive left-sided hemothorax.

Loss of effective blood transport because of major vessel rupture is the main physiologic problem associated with aortic rupture. The goal of assessment is to identify evidence of poor perfusion beyond the aortic lesion. Many patients are asymptomatic on presentation. Findings associated with aortic injuries are listed in the Patient Safety box (Box 55-2).

A supine chest radiograph is obtained to aid in diagnosis of an aortic injury. After spinal injury has been ruled out, an upright chest radiograph may be obtained as well. If a widened mediastinum is detected on radiograph, additional evaluation is necessary for definitive management. A positive CT scan may indicate the need for surgical repair. The torn aorta may require end-to-end anastomosis or, more commonly, the placement of a synthetic graft. Thoracic endovascular repair (TEVAR) has rapidly gained popularity because it is minimally invasive and has positive short term outcomes; it is the preferred mode of therapy.[18] Cardiopulmonary bypass may be necessary for repair of the ascending aorta or the aortic arch. However, repair of the descending thoracic aorta is usually accomplished during aortic cross-clamping. Because this maneuver occludes distal blood flow, it is imperative that the cross-clamp time be as brief as possible (preferably less than 30 minutes). To prevent leakage from the repair site, vasodilators may be administered after surgery to reduce afterload. After replacement of intravascular volume, a vasopressor may be added to support adequate blood pressure. Nursing care focuses on hemodynamic monitoring with a pulmonary artery catheter and titrating medications to maintain optimal blood pressure. Autotransfusion may also be necessary.

Complications are related to the level of the tear and the extent of altered perfusion. Hypoperfusion and resulting damage to organs below the level of the laceration can result from the injury itself or from prolonged cross-clamping during repair. Serious complications resulting from prolonged cross-clamp time include renal failure, bowel ischemia, lower extremity weakness, or permanent paralysis of the lower extremities. Other sequelae, such as ARDS or DIC, can be a consequence of hemorrhagic shock and multiple blood transfusions.

## Abdominal Trauma

Abdominal trauma can be caused by both blunt and penetrating injuries. Abdominal injuries can rapidly lead to death secondary to hemorrhage, shock, and sepsis. Missed abdominal injuries are a frequent cause of trauma deaths. Compared with penetrating trauma, blunt abdominal trauma is associated with more fatalities because many of the injuries are "hidden," and often, more obvious but less severe injuries lead to a delay in diagnosis. Deaths that occur more than 48 hours after abdominal injury are due to sepsis and its complications. In intra-abdominal trauma, rarely does single-organ or single-system injury occur.

The abdomen contains both solid and hollow organs. The solid organs include the liver, spleen, pancreas, and kidneys. The hollow organs include the intestines, stomach, gallbladder, and urinary bladder. Clinicians divide the abdomen into three main regions to facilitate description of the location of the injury. The three areas are the following:

1. The peritoneal area, which includes the diaphragm, liver, spleen, stomach, transverse colon, and the portion covered by the bony thorax.
2. The retroperitoneal area, which includes the aorta, vena cava, pancreas, kidney, ureters, and parts of the duodenum and colon.
3. The pelvis, which includes the rectum, bladder, uterus, and the iliac vessels.

MVCs are the most common cause of blunt abdominal trauma, although assaults, falls, pedestrian–motor vehicle collisions, and industrial accidents also contribute to blunt abdominal injuries. These injuries occur as the result of compressive, crushing, shearing, and deceleration forces. Diagnosis of blunt abdominal trauma can be difficult, especially if there are multisystem injuries. If the patient has abdominal tenderness or guarding, hemodynamic instability, lumbar spine injury, pelvic fracture, retroperitoneal or intraperitoneal air, or unilateral loss of the psoas shadow on radiograph, visceral damage should be suspected.

Blunt trauma is likely to cause serious damage to solid organs, and penetrating trauma most often damages the hollow organs. The compression and deceleration of blunt trauma leads to fractures of solid organ capsules and parenchyma,

---

**QSEN BOX 55-2 PATIENT SAFETY**

**Signs and Symptoms of Aortic Injuries**
- Pulse deficit in any area, particularly lower extremities or left arm
- Hypotension unexplained by other injuries
- Upper extremity hypertension relative to lower extremities
- Interscapular pain or sternal pain
- Precordial or interscapular systolic murmur caused by turbulence across the disrupted area
- Hoarseness caused by hematoma pressure around the aortic arch
- Respiratory distress or dyspnea
- Lower extremity neuromuscular or sensory deficit

Data from Frawley PM: Thoracic trauma. In: McQuillan KA, Flynn Makic MB, Whalen E, et al (eds): Trauma Nursing, 4th ed. Philadelphia, PA: WB Saunders, 2009, pp 614–677.

whereas hollow organs can collapse and absorb the force. However, the bowel, which occupies most of the abdominal cavity, is prone to injury by penetrating trauma. In general, solid organs respond to trauma with bleeding. Hollow organs rupture and release their contents into the peritoneal cavity, causing inflammation and infection.

Stab wounds, impalements, and gunshot wounds can cause penetrating trauma. Injury patterns differ depending on the mechanism. If the mechanism of penetrating trauma is a stab wound, knowledge of the size, shape, and length of the instrument used is helpful in determining the extent of intra-abdominal damage. There is a decreased likelihood of finding an injury requiring operative repair as compared to gunshot injuries.[11] Impalement is considered a "dirty" wound. "Dirty" wounds can result in high mortality secondary to the infection that is caused by bacterial contamination and subsequent multisystem organ failure. Gunshot wounds (missile injuries) are difficult to evaluate. The amount of major vessel disruption and multiple organ involvement are predictors of mortality. The velocity and amount of energy dispersed by the bullet often determine the extent of injury. A bullet can rebound off organs or bones, changing its trajectory and causing massive internal damage to organs and vessels. The blast effect from bullets can also cause significant intra-abdominal injury.[19]

Abdominal trauma requires continual assessment. Frequently, unrecognized abdominal trauma is a cause of preventable death. The nurse must be organized and methodical in the approach to patient assessment. The nurse needs to understand the mechanism of injury as well as the patient's complaints to perform an adequate assessment and identify potentially life-threatening abdominal injuries. It is important to remember that in blunt trauma, the validity of the physical examination alone is questionable. It is often unreliable if alcohol, illicit drugs, analgesics, or narcotics were involved or if the patient has a reduced level of consciousness. In penetrating trauma, the physical examination tends to be more reliable. Usually, a primary survey is completed, and the patient is resuscitated before the abdomen is assessed. During the secondary survey, the abdomen is assessed and reassessed, and laboratory and diagnostic tests are performed. An orogastric or nasogastric tube and a Foley catheter are placed during the secondary survey phase.

Often, diagnosis of penetrating trauma requires local wound exploration. However, it is important to note the site of the injury because wound exploration depends on mechanism and location. If the injury is in the anterior abdominal region (anterior costal margins to the inguinal creases between the anterior axillary lines), the likelihood that the peritoneum has been penetrated is low. If the injury is in the thoracoabdominal region (fourth intercostal space anteriorly and seventh intercostal space posteriorly to inferior costal margins), exploration is not recommended because there is an increased risk for tension pneumothorax. The patient requires a laparoscopy, thoracoscopy, or exploratory laparotomy. Exploration tends to be difficult in flank or back wounds. The patient usually requires a triple-contrast CT.

Diagnostic testing may include focused abdominal sonography for trauma (FAST), diagnostic peritoneal lavage (DPL), a chest radiograph (to determine gross abnormalities as well as any organ displacement), and an abdominal CT scan. Many trauma centers are performing FAST on all

trauma patients. This is an ideal diagnostic study because it is portable, fast, and reproducible.[5] It is performed by placing an ultrasound probe over various areas on the abdomen to determine whether free fluid is located in those areas. The areas evaluated are Morison's pouch in the right upper quadrant, the pericardial sac, the splenorenal region in the left upper quadrant, and the pelvis (suprapubic region). If the results of FAST are positive and the patient is hemodynamically unstable, an exploratory laparotomy is performed. The FAST allows the practitioner to forego other diagnostic tests and proceed to immediate operation.[12]

A DPL is a quick diagnostic procedure that is used during the resuscitation phase of care in hemodynamically unstable trauma patients to diagnose intra-abdominal bleeding (Box 55-3). DPL is not performed as regularly now because the FAST has proved to be very effective and efficient in diagnosing the immediate need for surgical intervention. Other indications for use may include the following:

- Unexplained hypotension, decreased hematocrit, or shock
- Equivocal results of abdominal examination
- Altered mental status caused by brain injury or alcohol or drug intoxication
- Spinal cord injury
- Distracting injuries, such as major orthopedic fractures or chest trauma

If the results of DPL are positive and the patient is hemodynamically unstable, an exploratory laparotomy is performed.

There are several contraindications to performing a DPL. These include morbid obesity, third-trimester pregnancy,

---

**BOX 55-3** | **Diagnostic Peritoneal Lavage**

**Indications**
- Blunt abdominal injury with:
  - Altered mental status
  - Unexplained hypotension, decreased hematocrit, shock
  - Equivocal results of abdominal examination
  - Spinal cord injury
  - Distracting injuries (eg, orthopedic fractures, chest trauma)
- Penetrating abdominal trauma (if exploration is not indicated)

**Possible Contraindications**
- History of multiple abdominal operations
- Third-trimester pregnancy
- Advanced cirrhosis of the liver
- Morbid obesity
- Known history of coagulopathy

**Technique**
1. Insert lavage catheter into peritoneal cavity through 1- to 2-cm incision.
2. Attempt to aspirate peritoneal fluid.
3. Infuse normal saline or Ringer lactate by gravity.
4. Turn patient from side to side (unless contraindicated).
5. Allow fluid to run back into bag by gravity.
6. Send specimens to laboratory.

**Positive Results**
- 10 to 20 mL gross blood on initial aspirate
- Greater than 100,000 red blood cells/mm$^3$
- Greater than 500 white blood cells/mm$^3$
- Elevated amylase level
- Presence of bile, bacteria, or fecal matter

advanced cirrhosis, a history of coagulopathy, and a history of multiple abdominal surgeries.[12] There is an increased risk for omental laceration and visceral or vascular perforation if DPL is performed in patients with these findings.

When performing DPL, it is important to first ensure that the patient has a Foley catheter and an orogastric or nasogastric tube in place to decompress the stomach and the bladder. Decompression of the stomach and bladder guards against accidental perforation when the lavage catheter is placed. Once the Foley catheter and an orogastric or nasogastric tube are placed, the lavage catheter is inserted into the peritoneal space. If less than 10 mL of frank blood is returned, a 1-liter bag of warm crystalloid (lactated Ringer solution or 0.9% normal saline solution) is infused into the peritoneum. After the infusion is complete, the IV bag is placed in a dependent position to allow the fluid to exit the abdomen by gravity. A sample of the fluid is then sent to the laboratory for evaluation.

CT scans are now being used more often in trauma patients. In blunt trauma, the CT scan has become the mainstay of diagnosis for abdominal injury, with a 92% to 97% sensitivity and 98% specificity. Often, the CT scan is performed with both IV and oral contrast agents to visualize the organs and note any disruption. The CT scan allows visualization of the peritoneal, retroperitoneal, and pelvic areas and permits estimation of the amount of fluid in these areas. CT scans are also used to grade solid organ injuries. Limitations to the use of CT include penetrating trauma, the amount of time required to perform the study, the need to transport the patient out of the resuscitation area, and the requirement that the patient must be hemodynamically stable and have limited movement during the study.

## Trauma to the Esophagus and Diaphragm

Esophageal injury is rare and very difficult to diagnose because of the lack of clinical signs initially and the severity of other injuries. Esophageal injuries often go unrecognized until sepsis develops. Esophageal injuries have a high death rate. Penetrating trauma is the most likely cause of esophageal injury; usually the cervical esophagus is where the injury occurs. The clinical symptoms are subtle. Presenting symptoms that should lead to a suspicion of esophageal injury include a hemothorax or pneumothorax without rib fractures.

Diagnosis includes CT scan of the chest, abdomen, and pelvis with and without contrast. Esophagoscopy, flexible endoscopy, and swallow studies are also performed. Treatment for esophageal injury is surgical repair. The patient is kept without anything by mouth (NPO) with a nasogastric tube to continuous suction, and antibiotic therapy is initiated. Nursing considerations include paying close attention to the airway of the patient, ventilation, oxygenation, and hemodynamic support.

Diaphragm rupture is more common in blunt injury (MVC and falls from height) than in penetrating injury.[20] Such rupture occurs more frequently on the left side because there the diaphragm is not protected by the liver. Injury is often secondary to the rising and falling associated with respiration. If a diaphragm rupture is suspected, it is necessary to look for both thoracic and abdominal injury. It is not uncommon to see abdominal contents in the thorax, which subsequently causes bowel strangulation in approximately 30% of patients. Respiratory compromise may also be seen because of impairment of lung capacity and displacement of normal lung tissue.

The clinical picture of diaphragm rupture depends on the size and site of injury. This injury is often difficult to diagnose because there is minimal bleeding and the patient is often asymptomatic. Clinical findings may include marked respiratory distress, dyspnea, decreased breath sounds on the affected side, positive bowel sounds in the thorax, palpation of abdominal contents when inserting a chest tube, and paradoxical movement of the abdomen when breathing.

Chest radiography is the initial modality used to diagnose diaphragm rupture; however, findings are often normal or nonspecific. The presence of abdominal contents in the chest denotes an injury. If an injury is suspected, ultrasound and a CT scan should be performed. DPL may be falsely negative. The only definitive treatment for diaphragm rupture is surgical repair.

## Trauma to the Stomach and Small Bowel

Significant gastric injury is rare. Small bowel injuries are much more common. Although frequently damaged by penetrating trauma, the small bowel can also burst when subjected to blunt trauma.[21] The multiple convolutions occasionally form a closed loop, which can rupture when subjected to increased pressure caused by impact with a steering wheel or seat belt. The bowel's mobility around fixed points (such as the ligament of Treitz) predisposes it to shearing injuries with deceleration.

Blunt small bowel or gastric injury can present with blood in the nasogastric aspirate or hematemesis. Physical signs often are absent, and CT findings may be subtle and nonspecific. Close observation is required; often, the diagnosis is not made until peritonitis develops. Penetrating injuries usually cause positive results on DPL. Although a mild bowel contusion can be managed conservatively (gastric decompression and withholding oral intake), surgery usually is necessary to repair penetrating wounds or bowel rupture.

Postoperative decompression with a gastric tube is maintained until bowel function returns. In most cases, a feeding jejunostomy tube is placed distal to the repair site, and tube feedings can be initiated early in the postoperative course. As the concentration and rate of feedings are advanced slowly, frequent assessment for signs of intolerance (distention, vomiting) is essential.

Because the stomach and small bowel contain an insignificant amount of bacteria, the risk for sepsis is small after rupture of these organs. If the injury goes unrecognized, there is a risk for sepsis. On the other hand, the acidic gastric juice is irritating to the peritoneum and may cause peritonitis. Potential complications related to stomach and small bowel trauma are listed in the accompanying Patient Safety box (Box 55-4). Some of these conditions may necessitate additional surgical procedures.

---

**QSEN BOX 55-4** *PATIENT SAFETY*

### Complications Related to Stomach and Small Bowel Trauma
- Intolerance to tube feedings
- Peritonitis
- Postoperative bleeding
- Hypovolemia caused by third spacing
- Development of a fistula or obstruction

## Trauma to the Duodenum and Pancreas

The pancreas and duodenum are discussed together because these retroperitoneal organs are closely related anatomically and physiologically. A great deal of force is necessary to injure these organs because they are well protected deep in the abdomen. Most injuries are related to penetrating trauma.[5] Injuries to adjacent organs almost always are present. The retroperitoneal location makes these injuries difficult to diagnose with DPL. An abdominal CT scan is very useful in this instance. Signs and symptoms may include an acute abdomen, increased serum amylase levels, epigastric pain radiating to the back, nausea, and vomiting.

Small lacerations or contusions may require only the placement of drains, whereas larger wounds need surgical repair. Most pancreatic injuries require postoperative closed-suction drainage to prevent fistula formation. Distal pancreatectomy and Roux-en-Y anastomosis are two procedures commonly performed for injuries to the body and tail of the pancreas. Occasionally, the spleen also must be removed because of its multiple vascular attachments to the pancreas. Damage to the head of the pancreas is associated with duodenal injury and severe hemorrhage because of the close proximity of vascular structures. Surgical procedures used in these cases include pancreaticoduodenectomy, Roux-en-Y anastomosis, and, on rare occasions, total pancreatectomy.

Postoperative nursing assessment and care are similar for the various procedures. Patency of drains must be maintained, and the patient must be monitored for the development of fistulas, the most common complication. Skin protection is important if a cutaneous fistula does develop because of the high enzyme content of pancreatic fluid. Assessment of fluid and electrolyte balance is also important because a pancreatic fistula results in fluid loss, along with loss of potassium and bicarbonate. Pancreatic stimulation can be decreased by administering parenteral hyperalimentation or jejunal feedings instead of an oral diet. The onset of diabetes mellitus is rare unless a total pancreatectomy is performed.

Primary repair or resection with reanastomosis is sufficient to manage most penetrating duodenal injuries. A duodenostomy tube may be placed for decompression and a jejunostomy tube for feeding. Blunt trauma to the duodenum can cause an intramural hematoma, which may lead to duodenal obstruction. The diagnosis is made with a diatrizoate (Gastrografin) upper gastrointestinal study. A complete obstruction usually requires surgical drainage of the hematoma.

## Trauma to the Colon

Usually, injury to the colon results from penetrating trauma. The nature of the injury most often dictates surgical exploration (exploratory laparotomy). Primary repair may be considered if the patient is hemodynamically stable and the injury is small and without fecal contamination. In some situations, such as injury to the left colon or when there is massive blood loss, an exteriorized repair or colostomy is required. A cecostomy tube may be placed for colon decompression. Subcutaneous tissue and skin of the incision site are often left open to decrease the chance of wound infection. The colon has a high bacteria count; spillage of the contents predisposes the patient to intra-abdominal sepsis and abscess formation.

Postoperative nursing care focuses on prevention of infection. Dressing changes are necessary for open incisions, and prophylactic antibiotics may be used. In the case of an exteriorized colon repair, resection and end-to-end anastomosis is performed, and the repair site is exteriorized to facilitate identification of a leak. The exteriorized colon must be kept moist and covered with a nonadherent dressing or bag to protect the integrity of the sutures. Because sepsis is a major complication of colon injuries, a series of radiographic and surgical procedures may be required to locate and drain abscesses.

A teaching guide for patients who have undergone a laparotomy can be found in Box 55-5.

---

**BOX 55-5** **TEACHING GUIDE**  *After a Laparotomy*

**Patient Activity**
- No tub baths or showers while the staples/stitches are in place.
- If you are tired, rest.
- Only lift what you can easily lift with one hand.
- You may eat your normal diet.
- Take your temperature once a day at the same time and write it down.
- Maintain a normal schedule with your bowel movements.
- If you become constipated, drink more fruit juices.
- Do not drive until you have your doctor's permission.

**Wound Care**
- It is important to keep the staple/stitch line clean.
- Monitor your wound closely.
- Cleanse the area once a day. To do this, you will need 4" × 4" gauze pads and a solution of half peroxide/half saline solution.
- Wash your hands.
- Open the gauze pad and leave the pad on the paper.
- Pour a small amount of the peroxide/saline solution on the center of the pad while it is lying on the paper.

- Pick up the pad, pulling all four corners together without touching the center.
- Wipe over the stitches/staples from top to bottom, covering them well with the solution. It is normal to see bubbles when cleaning with this solution. Wipe the area only once with a single gauze pad.
- Repeat.
- Allow the area to air dry.
- Tape a gauze pad over the stitch or staple line to prevent rubbing or irritation caused by a belt or waistband.

**Signs of Infection**
- Swelling around the site
- Increased redness
- Increased tenderness
- Warmth around the site
- Wound edges separating
- Increased drainage
- Foul-smelling drainage
- Change in color of drainage
- Temperature of 101°F or higher
- Vomiting, diarrhea, or constipation

## Trauma to the Liver

Along with the spleen, the liver is the most commonly injured abdominal organ.[5] Both blunt and penetrating trauma can cause hepatic injuries. Fractures of the right lower ribs increase suspicion for a liver injury. Presenting signs and symptoms may include right upper quadrant pain, rebound tenderness, hypoactive or absent bowel sounds, or signs of hypovolemic shock. Box 55-6 presents the liver injury scale.

Because the liver has been shown to heal itself, hemodynamically stable patients with liver injuries are now managed nonoperatively. Manipulation during surgery tends to cause more bleeding; thus, observation is now considered the standard treatment unless the patient is hemodynamically unstable or has frank peritonitis.[22] CT scans are performed to verify bleeding cessation. Hepatic trauma can cause a large blood loss into the peritoneum, but bleeding may stop spontaneously. In some instances, bleeding vessels may be ligated or embolized. Small lacerations are repaired, whereas larger injuries may require segmental resection or débridement. In the case of uncontrollable hemorrhage, the liver is packed. After packing, the abdomen may be closed or simply covered and left open; an additional surgical procedure is required within the next few days to remove the packing and repair the laceration. Large liver injuries also need postoperative drainage of bile and blood with closed-suction drains.

After surgery, coagulopathies may be present. Incomplete hemostasis also is a possibility and must be differentiated from coagulopathy-induced bleeding. Severe bleeding resulting from incomplete hemostasis requires clot removal, packing, and additional repair. With a coagulopathy, bleeding arises from numerous sites, whereas with incomplete hemostasis, the bleeding is mainly from the surgical site.

Nursing care of patients with liver injuries includes the replacement of blood products while monitoring the hematocrit and coagulation studies. Assessment of the character and amount of tube drainage, along with fluid balance, also is essential. Potential complications of liver injury include hepatic or perihepatic abscess, biliary obstruction or leak, sepsis, ARDS, and DIC. In 6 to 8 weeks, physical examination findings should be improved. To prevent rebleeding, patients should not participate in contact sports until a repeated CT scan shows healing of the injury.

## Trauma to the Spleen

Along with the liver, the spleen is the most commonly injured abdominal organ, usually as a result of blunt trauma. In 60% of patients sustaining blunt trauma, the spleen is the only organ injured. Because of its vascularity, the spleen has a tendency to lose blood rapidly.[5] Presence of left lower rib fractures increases suspicion for a splenic injury. Presenting signs and symptoms include left upper quadrant pain radiating to the left shoulder (Kehr sign), hypovolemic shock, and the nonspecific finding of an increased white blood cell count. FAST, DPL or abdominal CT is usually necessary for diagnosis. Box 55-7 provides the splenic injury scale.

Management for splenic injuries includes observation, embolization, or surgery, depending on the hemodynamic stability of the patient, preexisting conditions, and the grade of splenic injury. Hemodynamically unstable patients with a positive FAST or DPL require immediate surgery to determine the source of bleeding. Hemodynamically stable patients with low-grade injury (grades I to III) without any evidence of bleeding on CT scan or FAST can be observed closely. Patients with contrast extravasation on CT or with abdominal blush on CT may have a higher rate of failure and may require embolization. Also, patients with neurologic compromise, who are unreliable to observe, may require surgery.

Approximately 50% to 70% of hemodynamically stable patients—usually adults with lower-grade injuries and most children—are treated nonoperatively with observation and embolization. An observation period of 5 days is the standard. The

---

### BOX 55-6  Liver Injury Scale

**Hematomas**
- **Grade I hematomas:** subcapsular; involving less than 10% of surface area
- **Grade II hematomas:** subcapsular, intraparenchymal hematoma; involving 10% to 50% of surface area, <10 cm in diameter
- **Grade III hematomas:** subcapsular, involving more than 50% of surface area, or ruptured and actively bleeding; intraparenchymal hematoma greater than or equal to 10 cm or expanding

**Lacerations**
- **Grade I lacerations:** capsular tear less than 1 cm deep
- **Grade II lacerations:** capsular tear 1 to 3 cm deep, <10 cm long
- **Grade III lacerations:** more than 3 cm deep
- **Grade IV lacerations:** parenchymal disruption involving 25% to 75% hepatic lobe or 1–3 Couinaud segments within a single lobe
- **Grade V lacerations:** involving more than 75% hepatic lobe parenchymal disruption; or >3 Couinaud segments within a single lobe; vascular injury includes retrohepatic vena cava and juxtahepatic venous injuries
- **Grade VI lacerations:** vascular hepatic avulsion

Data from Kokabi N, Shuaib W, Xing M, et al: Intra-abdominal solid organ injuries: An enhanced management algorithm. Can Assoc Radiol J 65:301–309, 2014

---

### BOX 55-7  Splenic Injury Scale

**Hematomas**
- **Grade I hematomas:** subcapsular <1 cm thick
- **Grade II hematomas:** subcapsular 1 to 3 cm thick
- **Grade III hematomas:** splenic capsular disruption, subcapsular hematoma >3 cm thick, parenchymal hematoma >3 cm in diameter
- **Grade IVa hematomas:** involving ruptured parenchyma with active bleeding

**Lacerations**
- **Grade I lacerations:** less than 1 cm deep
- **Grade II lacerations:** 1 to 3 cm deep
- **Grade III lacerations:** more than 3 cm deep
- **Grade IVa lacerations:** splenic vascular injury (AV fistula or pseudoaneurysm); shattered spleen
- **Grade IVb lacerations:** Active intraperitoneal bleeding

Data from Olthof D, van der Viles CH, Scheerder MJ et al: Reliability of injury grading systems for patients with blunt splenic trauma. Injury 45(1): 146–150, 2014

patient is admitted to a monitored bed and watched carefully for hypotension and signs of bleeding. Hemoglobin and hematocrit (H&H) analyses are performed every 6 hours until stable. The patient is initially placed on bed rest, although there is no clinical evidence to support this practice. The patient is kept NPO until his or her H&H is stable, and then begins a diet. Patients with a higher-grade injury require longer observation.

Early complications of splenic trauma include recurrent bleeding, subphrenic abscess, and pancreatitis resulting from surgical trauma. Rupture of an expanding subscapular hematoma or pseudoaneurysm may present days or weeks after an initial normal examination. Late complications consist of thrombocytosis and overwhelming postsplenectomy sepsis (OPSS). Because the spleen plays an important role in the body's response to infection, a splenectomy predisposes the patient to an increased risk for infection. Pneumococcus, an encapsulated microorganism resistant to phagocytosis, is the organism that most often infects patients after splenectomy. OPSS frequently begins with the onset of pneumococcal pneumonia, which progresses to a fulminant sepsis. Postsplenectomy patients increase their immunity toward pneumococcal infections by receiving a polyvalent pneumococcal vaccine (Pneumovax). Complications of OPSS include adrenal insufficiency and DIC. OPSS has a high incidence and mortality rate, especially within 1 year of surgery. Patient and family teaching should focus on information about signs and symptoms of infection.

### Trauma to the Kidneys

Injury to the kidney may lead to a "free" hemorrhage, contained hematoma, or the development of an intravascular thrombus. Sudden deceleration injury can cause the kidney to move, avulsing smaller renal vessels or tearing the renal artery intima, which also may lead to vessel thrombosis. Blunt and penetrating trauma can also cause a laceration or contusion of the renal parenchyma or rupture of the collecting system. Lower rib or lumbar vertebral fractures, along with liver and spleen injuries, should raise suspicion of an associated renal injury. Signs and symptoms, when present, consist of hematuria, pain, a flank hematoma, or ecchymosis over the flank. Because the bleeding is retroperitoneal, it can be difficult to detect. A helical CT scan, ultrasound, or an IV pyelogram (less commonly used) usually provides the diagnosis.

Renal injuries are graded based on their severity; increased grade correlates with decreased function. Many renal injuries can be managed conservatively with observation and bed rest until gross hematuria resolves. Some studies suggest that bed rest can be avoided unless hematuria increases or resumes after ambulation.[23] However, in some instances (mainly for vascular injury), surgical repair or nephrectomy is necessary.

Postoperative assessment and support of renal function are imperative. Optimal fluid balance must be maintained. Low-dose dopamine may be ordered to promote renal perfusion. Major complications consist of arterial or venous thrombosis and acute renal failure. Other complications include bleeding, perinephric abscess, the development of a urinary fistula, and late onset of hypertension.

### Trauma to the Bladder

The bladder can be lacerated, ruptured, or contused, most often as the consequence of blunt trauma (usually because of a full bladder at the time of injury). Bladder injuries frequently are associated with pelvic fractures. Gross hematuria is typically noted with bladder rupture.[24] Presence of blood at the urethral meatus, a scrotal hematoma, or a displaced prostate gland requires examination for urethral injuries with a CT scan or conventional cystography before the insertion of a urinary catheter. CT cystogram is the gold standard for diagnosing this injury.[24]

A bladder injury can cause intraperitoneal or extraperitoneal urine extravasation. Extraperitoneal extravasation, usually associated with pelvic fractures, can often be managed with urinary catheter drainage. However, intraperitoneal extravasation (associated with a high-force injury) requires surgery. This injury has a high mortality rate because of associated injuries that occur secondary to the force involved. A suprapubic cystostomy tube may be placed. Complications are infrequent, but infection resulting from the urinary catheter or sepsis from extravasation of infected urine can occur. Patients may complain of an inability to void or of shoulder pain (caused by extravasation of urine into the peritoneal space).

## Musculoskeletal Injuries

Although musculoskeletal injuries take a long time to heal and can often result in lifelong disability, they are usually not considered life threatening unless there is a traumatic amputation or pelvic fracture. Routinely, the musculoskeletal assessment is done in the secondary survey after hemodynamic stabilization. These injuries do require prompt recognition and stabilization to promote optimal recovery and function.

There are a variety of causes of trauma-related musculoskeletal injuries; the major causes include MVCs, falls, assaults, and industrial, farming, and home accidents. Musculoskeletal injuries are often associated with other injuries to the body. It is important to understand the circumstances surrounding, and the mechanism involved in, musculoskeletal trauma. Force might be applied to one area, but the transferred energy and distribution of force may cause injury somewhere else. For example, in a person who falls off a two-story building and lands on his or her feet, one would expect to find calcaneus or ankle fractures, but the transference of energy may also cause a pelvic or lumbar spine fracture. Obviously, if the patient is conscious, he or she can verbalize his or her pain. However, fractures and sprains often go unrecognized because the patient is not able to verbalize and communicate the location of his or her pain.

### Types of musculoskeletal injuries

There are many types of musculoskeletal injuries, including fractures, fracture dislocations, amputations, and trauma to the soft tissue (ie, skin, muscle, tendons, ligaments, and cartilage).

**FRACTURE.** Fracture classification is based on type, cause, and anatomical location. Several fracture types are shown in Figure 55-5. If the skin is broken at the fracture site, the injury is considered to be an "open" fracture. If the skin is intact, the injury is said to be a "closed" fracture. An open fracture is further classified as grade I, II, or III, depending on the tissue damage involved.

**DISLOCATION.** Dislocation occurs when the articulating surfaces of a joint are no longer in contact because of

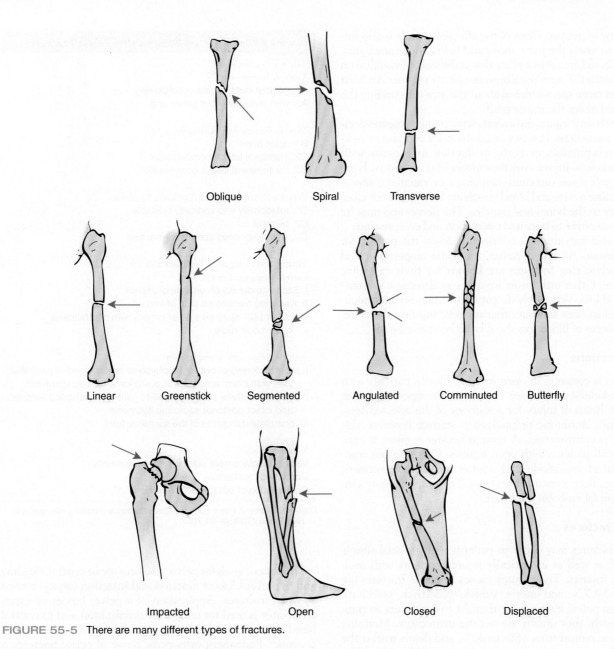

Oblique  Spiral  Transverse

Linear  Greenstick  Segmented  Angulated  Comminuted  Butterfly

Impacted  Open  Closed  Displaced

FIGURE 55-5  There are many different types of fractures.

joint disruption. Joint mobility may be restricted. There may also be associated vascular or nerve injury with dislocations. Ligamentous injury usually accompanies dislocations because ligaments stretch or tear at the time of dislocation.

**AMPUTATION.** Amputations are classified according to the amount of tissue, nerve, and vascular damage. A cut or guillotine amputation has clean lines and well-defined edges, whereas a crush amputation has more soft tissue damage and the edges are not as well defined. An avulsion amputation occurs when a force stretches and tears away tissues, causing nerves and vessels to be torn in different areas than the bone.

### Assessment

As in all trauma patients, initial assessment begins with the primary survey. Once this is complete and the patient is hemodynamically stable, the secondary assessment is conducted. When trauma patients are admitted to the

resuscitation unit, cervical spine, chest, and pelvis films are obtained first. Sometimes, thoracic and lumbar spine films are obtained, depending on the mechanism of injury. The initial pelvic film tells the nurse whether the patient has a life-threatening pelvic fracture. If this is the case, immobilization of the pelvis should be maintained to prevent exsanguination. Immobilization of the pelvis is achieved with a C-clamp, external fixator, pelvic binder, or sheets wrapped tightly around the patient to attempt to stop the bleeding.

During the secondary survey, if limb swelling, ecchymosis, or deformity is noted, that extremity should be immobilized. Proper imaging is ordered to determine the extent of the injury. The nurse tests the extremities for capillary refill (less than 2 seconds is normal), pulses, crepitus, muscle spasm, movement, sensation, and pain.

The most common studies used to diagnose musculoskeletal injuries are plain radiographs, CT, and magnetic resonance imaging (MRI). When obtaining radiographs, it is important to get two views of the affected area. It is also important to assess the joint above and below the injured area. If the affected area is in a place that is difficult to visualize on plain films, a CT scan usually gives a better picture. An MRI also gives more specific detail about the area surrounding the injury and about the injury itself.

As with any injury, musculoskeletal trauma requires continuous assessment. It is not uncommon for vascular or neurologic compromise, or both, to develop in patients with musculoskeletal injury. Any musculoskeletal injury involving bone or soft tissue can cause neurologic or vascular compromise because nerves and blood vessels are located in such close proximity to the bones and muscles. The nerves and muscles are very sensitive to impaired circulation and compression.

It is also important to continually assess the patient for hypovolemia. As stated earlier, traumatic amputation and major pelvic ring fractures are known for their extensive blood loss. Other orthopedic injuries can also cause substantial blood loss. Very rarely do patients sustain severe musculoskeletal injuries without other systemic injuries; therefore, other sources of blood loss should also be investigated.

## Complications

Infection is common in open injuries. Ideally, patients with musculoskeletal trauma are brought to the operating room within 6 hours of injury for a washout of the affected area. Sometimes, antibiotic prophylaxis is started; however, this practice is controversial. A tetanus booster is given if indicated to all patients with open injuries. Other serious complications of musculoskeletal injuries include compartment syndrome, deep venous thrombosis (DVT), pulmonary embolus, and fat embolus syndrome.

## Pelvic Fractures

Pelvic fractures may occur in patients with isolated simple fractures as well as in critically injured patients with multisystem injuries. The primary causes of pelvic fractures are MVCs, MCCs, and motor vehicle–pedestrian collisions. Although pelvic fractures are thought to contribute to traumatic death, they usually are not the main cause. Mortality rates have ranged from 18% to 40%, and death within the first 24 hours was most often a result of acute blood loss. The risk for death is increased in patients who have open pelvic fractures or who have been hit by a motor vehicle. Pelvic ring fractures are associated with high-energy mechanisms, and patients often have soft tissue injury. In hemodynamically unstable patients, it is imperative to find the site of bleeding and control it. Bleeding can occur from three major sources: arterial, venous, and cancellous bone.

Physical examination for pelvic fractures begins with inspection for abrasions, lacerations, contusions, and symmetry of the lower extremities. Palpation to assess for rotational and vertical instability is then necessary. Rectal and vaginal examinations should be performed to assess for a urethral tear in males and an open fracture in females.

Radiographic evaluation of pelvic injuries includes an anteroposterior view. This film can detect up to 90% of pelvic fractures. Other radiographs include pelvic inlet and outlet views and lateral sacral views. CT scan is also used to evaluate the sacroiliac joints as well as the extent of the injury. See Box 55-8 for classification of pelvic fractures.

---

**BOX 55-8** **Classification Schemes for Pelvic Fractures**

**Tile's Classification**
Type A, Stable
A1, without involvement of pelvic ring
A2, with involvement of pelvic ring

Type B, Rotationally Unstable
B1, open book
B2, ipsilateral lateral compression
B3, contralateral lateral compression

Type C, Rotationally and Vertically Unstable
C1, rotationally and vertically unstable
C2, bilateral
C3, with associated acetabular fracture

**Young and Burgess Classification**
Lateral Compression (LC)
I, Sacral compression on side of impact
II, Iliac wing fracture on side of impact
III, LCI or LCII injury on side of impact with contralateral open-book injury

Anterior–Posterior Compression
I, slight widening of pubis symphysis or anterior part of sacroiliac joint with intact anterior and posterior sacroiliac ligaments
II, widened anterior part of sacroiliac joint with disrupted anterior and intact posterior sacroiliac ligaments
III, complete disruption of the sacroiliac joint

Vertical Shear
Vertical displacement anteriorly and posteriorly
Combined mechanism
Combination of other injury patterns

Data from Walker J: Pelvic fractures: Classification and nursing management. Nurs Stand 26(10):49–58, 2011

---

Treatment goals for pelvic fractures are to control bleeding and to prevent loss of function and infection (sepsis) caused by open fractures. Application of a pelvic binder or external fixator is used for temporary stabilization and to control bleeding. Embolization is also indicated for hemorrhage control.[25] Permanent orthopedic repair of pelvic fractures is usually performed within 24 to 72 hours after injury when the patient is adequately resuscitated and hemodynamically stable. This can be accomplished with either internal or external fixation.

## Compartment Syndrome

Compartment syndrome occurs when the pressure within the fascia-enclosed muscle compartment is increased, causing blood flow to the muscles and nerves in the compartment to become compromised. The final result is cellular anoxia; it is suspected based on mechanism of injury. This ischemia then leads to tissue damage, which compromises nerve and muscle function. A prolonged elevation of compartmental pressure leads to death of the muscles and nerves involved. Normal compartment pressure is between 0 and 8 mm Hg. Capillary blood flow is believed to become compromised at 20 mm Hg, pain develops at a pressure between 20 and 30 mm Hg, and ischemia occurs at pressures greater than 30 mm Hg. Patients with higher diastolic pressures are able to tolerate higher tissue pressures without ischemic damage. Fasciotomy is recommended when the compartment pressure approaches 20 mm Hg below the diastolic pressure. Hypotensive trauma patients may experience significant muscle ischemia at lower compartment pressures.

Patients with compartment syndrome complain of increased pain in the affected area. Compartment syndrome occurs most often with long bone fractures in the lower leg or forearm. The pain is described as being "out of proportion" to the injury. The most reliable early sign of compartment syndrome is decreased sensation. The compartment involved is firm, and the patient eventually has paresthesia. Pallor and pulselessness are late signs of compartment syndrome. When the compartment syndrome has progressed to the point that the patient is showing late signs, loss of the affected extremity is threatened. The nurse must constantly monitor the affected extremity and compare it with the unaffected extremity. If any of the signs or symptoms of compartment syndrome are present, the orthopedic or general surgeon should be notified immediately so that compartment pressures can be measured. If it is deemed that the compartment pressures are high, a fasciotomy is performed to release the pressure and save the extremity. The extremity should never be elevated when compartment syndrome is suspected because this will decrease arterial inflow and exacerbate ischemia.

### Deep Venous Thrombosis

DVT is a significant risk for all trauma patients, especially those with musculoskeletal injuries. It is known as a common, life-threatening complication of major trauma. The danger of DVT is that it may progress to pulmonary embolus. The administration of low-dose heparin or low–molecular-weight heparin and the use of intermittent pneumatic compression devices are recommended to prevent DVT.[26] The pathophysiology of DVT, and later pulmonary embolus, is related to Virchow triad:

1. Venous stasis from decreased blood flow, decreased muscular activity, and external pressure on the deep veins
2. Vascular damage or concomitant pathologic state
3. Hypercoagulability

The nurse assesses for signs and symptoms of DVT on a regular basis. These include swelling of the affected area, tachycardia, fever, and distal skin color and temperature changes. If these signs or symptoms are found, they should be reported immediately. Sometimes, an acute pulmonary embolus is the first indication of DVT.

### Pulmonary Embolus

A pulmonary embolus occurs when a blood clot dislodges from the vein, travels through the heart, and lodges in the pulmonary artery, obstructing blood flow. Sudden onset of dyspnea is the classical sign of a pulmonary embolus, but signs and symptoms vary, depending on the size of the clot and the number of vessels occluded. Signs and symptoms may include a decline in oxygenation, substernal chest pain, hypovolemic relative shock, tachypnea, shortness of breath, anxiety, a feeling of impending doom, a low-grade fever, an altered level of consciousness, and a pale, dusky, or cyanotic skin color. Often, a patient with a pulmonary embolus also has a DVT.[26]

### Fat Embolism Syndrome

Fat emboli are fat globules in the lung tissue and peripheral circulation after a long bone fracture or major trauma. Fat emboli may or may not cause systemic symptoms. Fat embolism syndrome is a serious (but rare) manifestation of fat emboli that involves a classical triad of symptoms: hypoxemia, neurologic decline, and petechial rash. It usually occurs within 24 to 72 hours of injury. Clinical indications include tachypnea, dyspnea, and hypoxemia. Many patients develop neurologic changes after respiratory distress, which are usually completely reversible. Petechial rash often occurs on the head, neck, anterior thorax, axilla, and subconjunctivals; it typically lasts 5 to 7 days. Nurses should be aware of the potential for fat embolism syndrome and monitor the patient for hypoxemia with pulse oximetry.

## Maxillofacial Trauma

Despite laws that mandate lower speed limits and the use of air bags and seat belts, the incidence of maxillofacial trauma remains high because the face is unprotected during rapid deceleration. The degree of maxillofacial injury is directly related to the force at impact when the face makes contact with a stationary object. As the force increases, the amount of energy that is dispersed increases, causing an increase in injury. Penetrating injury is less common than blunt injury in patients with maxillofacial trauma.

As with any trauma patient, initial management priorities remain ABC.[27] The trauma team cannot be distracted from these priorities by obvious deformities that may be associated with maxillofacial injuries. Maxillofacial trauma can cause airway obstruction and death if airway and breathing are not adequately and urgently established. When the primary survey is completed, an adequate assessment of the maxillofacial injuries is performed. Figure 55-6 shows maxillae fractures according to Le Fort classification.

When assessing for maxillofacial injuries, the nurse assesses soft tissues as well as bony structures. The nurse inspects the face for symmetry and then palpates systematically to observe for any movement of bony structures. Cranial nerves are assessed. Often, maxillofacial injuries coincide with head injuries, reinforcing the importance of a thorough

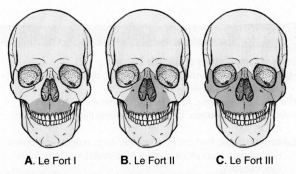

| **A.** Le Fort I | **B.** Le Fort II | **C.** Le Fort III |

**FIGURE 55-6**  Le Fort fractures. **A:** Le Fort I: Transverse disarticulation of the maxillary dentoalveolar process from the remaining basal bone of maxilla and midface. **B:** Le Fort II: Pyramidal fracture involving entire maxilla and nasal complex. **C:** Le Fort III: Complete craniofacial–midface disassociation.

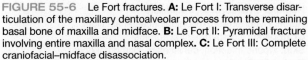

(Courtesy of Neil O. Hardy, Westpoint, CT.)

neurologic examination (see Chapter 33). Any midface fractures that communicate through the orbit require a thorough ocular assessment and frequent reassessment.

Most maxillofacial injuries involve the soft tissue. In any soft tissue injury, there is potential for contamination; therefore, each patient's immunization to tetanus is assessed and, if needed, a tetanus booster is given. All wounds are assessed for dirt, grease, particles, and other contaminants. Many wounds require an operation for washout to débride the tissue and clean the area.[27] These injuries are usually not life threatening and are treated in the appropriate order. However, even a small abrasion to a person's face can lead to a lifetime of disfigurement; therefore, all injuries must be attended to appropriately.

As stated earlier, in any type of trauma, but especially in maxillofacial trauma when the patient's airway may be compromised, it is imperative to assess and maintain an adequate airway for the patient continuously. Loss of an artificial airway (eg, inadvertent removal of the endotracheal tube) can be life threatening because of soft tissue swelling. It is also essential to assess for and treat hypovolemia secondary to hemorrhage from facial arteries. Epistaxis may also occur with any fracture that communicates with the nose. The nurse continuously assesses the patient's neurologic status and reports any abnormalities. The patient's pain and anxiety must be assessed and treated. Many patients with maxillofacial injuries are robbed of their senses: they may be unable to see, smell, taste, or speak secondary to their injury. This is an anxiety-provoking situation; patients require continuous reassurance and medication as necessary. Many maxillofacial injuries require multiple surgeries before the patient is definitively treated.

## Complications of Multiple Trauma

Complications associated with multiple trauma are numerous (Box 55-9). Because most trauma patients are in the ICU when these complications develop, the nurse plays an essential role in detecting, preventing, and treating them.

The unexpected nature of trauma tends to amplify fear and anxiety. Therefore, nursing care must also provide psychosocial support for the seriously injured patient and his or her family. A multidisciplinary approach that recognizes concerns and offers frequent explanations is recommended. Special considerations for older trauma patients can be found in Box 55-10.

---

**QSEN** **BOX 55-9** *PATIENT SAFETY*

**Delayed Complications of Multiple Trauma**

**Hematologic:** Hemorrhage, coagulopathy, disseminated intravascular coagulation
**Cardiac:** Dysrhythmia, heart failure, ventricular aneurysm
**Pulmonary:** Atelectasis, pneumonia, emboli (fat or thrombotic), ARDS
**Gastrointestinal:** Peritonitis, adynamic ileus, mechanical bowel obstruction, acalculous cholecystitis, anastomotic leak, fistula, bleeding
**Hepatic:** Liver abscess, liver failure
**Renal:** Hypertension, myoglobinuria, renal failure
**Orthopedic:** Compartment syndrome
**Skin:** Wound infection, dehiscence, skin breakdown
**Systemic:** Sepsis

---

Death after multiple traumatic injuries, when it occurs, may occur immediately, or it may occur as a result of early or late complications. Immediate deaths occur at the scene and within minutes of the injury. Most common causes of immediate deaths are brainstem or high spinal cord injury, cardiac rupture, transection of the great vessels, and airway obstruction.

## Early Complications

Severe head injuries and hemorrhage are the early complications of multiple trauma most often responsible for causing death within hours of the injury, usually in the emergency department or operating room. Often, death at this stage can be prevented with quick assessment, resuscitation, and management of injuries.

Management of head injuries is discussed in Chapter 36. To prevent exsanguination, hemorrhage must be controlled and volume resuscitation begun with the infusion of crystalloids and blood. Patients may require emergent surgical ligation or packing, or embolization by angiography. Massive hemorrhage complicated by hypothermia, metabolic acidosis, and coagulopathy is highly lethal.

## Late Complications

Late complications of multiple trauma include hypovolemic shock, infection and septic shock, ARDS, and multiple organ dysfunction syndrome (MODS).

### Hypovolemic Shock

Massive hemorrhage or continued bleeding because of incomplete hemostasis or an undiagnosed injury can lead to

---

**BOX 55-10** *CONSIDERATIONS for the Older Patient*

**Trauma**

- Unintentional Injury is the ninth most frequent cause of death among the elderly.
- The older person is injured less frequently than the younger person; however, when an older person does sustain injuries, the injuries are more likely to be life threatening.
- The injuries occurring in the elderly population tend to be less severe but are associated with a greater risk of death.
- Falls are the most prominent cause of trauma in the older person followed by MVC, pedestrian versus a vehicle, and burns.
- Financial burden of trauma care related to the elderly is close to $9 billion annually
- Constant monitoring is essential with the older trauma patient.
- Providers should have a decreased threshold for invasive monitoring with an elderly patient, secondary to predisposing conditions and past medical history.
- Management considerations are as follows:
  - Consider cervical osteoarthritis when intubation is necessary.
  - Pain management should be more local if possible (eg, epidural catheter, nerve block).
  - Fluid management should be done cautiously. Older adults require adequate rapid fluid replacement without excess. Consider a pulmonary artery or central venous pressure line for guidance in fluid replacement.
  - Older adults tend to become hypothermic more quickly than younger people. Use warm fluid and warming devices as indicated.

Data from Holleran RS: Elderly trauma. Crit Care Nurs Q 38(3):298–311, 2015

hypovolemic shock and eventually to decreased organ perfusion. The various organs respond differently to the decrease in perfusion caused by hypovolemia. Multiple blood transfusions are often necessary, further increasing the likelihood of ARDS and MODS.

## Infection and Septic Shock

Another frequent and potentially serious complication of multiple trauma is infection. The risk of infection is increased after close-range shotgun blasts, high-velocity penetrating injuries, penetrating wounds to the colon, prolonged surgery, multiple blood transfusions, and injury to multiple organs. Other risk factors include advanced age, underlying immunosuppression, and a history of diabetes mellitus.

Infections can range from a minor wound infection to fulminant sepsis syndrome and septic shock. In septic shock, the release of toxins causes dilation of vessels, leading to venous pooling that results in a decreased venous return. Initially, cardiac output increases to compensate for decreased systemic vascular resistance. Eventually, the compensatory mechanisms fail, and cardiac output falls along with blood pressure and organ perfusion (ie, septic shock).

To treat sepsis effectively, the source of infection must be found and eradicated. The nurse must watch for the sometimes subtle indicators of sepsis. Hyperthermia or hypothermia and altered mental status are often present early in the septic process, as well as tachycardia, tachypnea, and an increase in the white blood cell count. These findings should prompt further assessment to detect a possible infectious source.

When sepsis is suspected, cultures are obtained, antibiotics are prescribed, radiologic studies are done, and exploratory surgery frequently is performed. Intra-abdominal abscess is a frequent cause of sepsis. Some abscesses can be drained percutaneously, whereas others require surgery. After the surgical drainage of an abdominal abscess, the incision is left open with drains in place to allow healing and prevent recurrence. Other sources of infection are invasive lines, the urinary tract, and the lungs. Pneumonia is a common cause of sepsis in trauma patients. Risk factors for pneumonia include advanced age, aspiration, underlying pulmonary disease, thoracic or abdominal surgery, and prolonged intubation.

Hemodynamics are altered and metabolic demands are increased during sepsis. The typical patient exhibits elevated cardiac output, decreased systemic vascular resistance, and increased oxygen consumption. Hemodynamics must be supported and a balance between oxygen delivery and oxygen consumption maintained. Research suggests that early nutritional support decreases the development of sepsis and MODS. Enteral feeding should be used whenever possible because it is associated with a lower incidence of sepsis than total parenteral nutrition.

## Acute Respiratory Distress Syndrome

ARDS is the most frequent manifestation of multiple organ failure (MOF) after trauma.[28] It occurs in 12% to 25% of injured patients and has a mortality rate of 50% to 80%.[28] Patients with MOF and ARDS have longer hospital stays, increased cost, and worse long-term quality of life.[28]

ARDS is a constellation of the following symptoms: shortness of breath, reduced lung compliance, and severe hypoxemia refractory to oxygen and bilateral pulmonary infiltrates. ARDS can be caused by direct injury (eg, pneumonia, aspiration of gastric contents, inhalation injury, fat emboli) or indirect injury (insult anywhere in the body, eg, sepsis, multiple blood transfusions, shock, burns). In a recent study, predictors of ARDS consisted of an ISS greater than 25, age over 65 years, hemorrhagic shock (SBP less than 90 on admission), pulmonary contusion, and massive transfusion (more than 10 units of RBCs within the first 24 hours of admission).[28] Another study linked gender to ARDS, stating that females are more likely than males to develop it.[29]

Sepsis may predispose the patient to ARDS (see Chapter 27). In addition to sepsis, specific injuries (eg, head trauma, pulmonary contusion, multiple major fractures), massive blood transfusions, aspiration, and pneumonia can also increase the likelihood of ARDS. With a mortality rate between 50% and 80%, ARDS is characterized by hypoxemia with shunting, decreased lung compliance, tachypnea, dyspnea, and the appearance of diffuse bilateral pulmonary infiltrates.

Treatment of ARDS is multifaceted. Initially, therapy is aimed at treatment of the primary cause. Fluid and hemodynamic management, management of infection, adequate nutrition, mechanical ventilation, and supportive oxygen delivery are incorporated in the therapeutic regimen. The main goal of ARDS treatment is to increase oxygen in the body.

## Systemic Inflammatory Response Syndrome

Systemic inflammatory response syndrome (SIRS) describes a pathophysiologic response to a cascade of events precipitated by shock, which usually occurs after trauma. A controlled inflammatory response takes place, designed to heal wounds and ward off infection. Continuous stimulation or severe infection may result in sustained inflammation—SIRS. The result is an imbalance of cellular oxygen supply and demand, causing an oxygen extraction deficit.

## Multiple Organ Dysfunction Syndrome

Sixty percent of trauma patients have clinical signs of sepsis without an apparent bacterial source. Many factors have been associated with the development of MODS, including hemorrhage, massive blood transfusion, hypovolemic shock, and sepsis. Characterized by the failure of two or more organs, MODS accounts for many late deaths in trauma patients. Usually, the lungs are the first organs to fail (heralded by the onset of ARDS), followed by the liver, gastrointestinal tract, and kidneys.

Liver failure can result from initial damage, vascular compromise, shock, or sepsis. Jaundice is a common indicator of deteriorating liver function, although other causes, such as posttraumatic biliary obstruction, must be ruled out. Liver function tests are diagnostic. Liver failure can lead to a decreased level of consciousness, abnormal clotting study results, and hypoglycemia (see Chapter 41).

Gastrointestinal failure, which manifests with hemorrhage from stress ulcers, requires blood transfusion. Prophylactic neutralization of gastric acid can minimize the risk of bleeding (see Chapter 41).

Renal failure can be precipitated by a renal injury, ischemia, radiographic contrast material, rhabdomyolysis, hypovolemia (due to hemorrhage, third spacing), or sepsis. Initial signs include increasing blood urea nitrogen and serum creatinine levels. Renal failure may be polyuric or oliguric. Dialysis may be necessary (see Chapter 30).

Cardiovascular failure, DIC, metabolic changes (eg, hyperglycemia, metabolic acidosis), and central nervous system changes, ranging from confusion to obtundation, also may be evident in MODS. See Chapter 49 for a discussion of DIC.

### Psychosocial Considerations

Today's elderly are more active and mobile than ever before; however, this leads to an increased risk of injury. As medical advances extend life expectancy, the elderly population (65 years and older) are expected to be more than 21% of the US population by the year 2050.[30] Currently, the elderly represent 13% of the US population.[30] Elderly trauma patients are the fastest growing segment of patients admitted to trauma centers, and are expected to account for 39% of trauma admissions by 2050.[30] It is important to remember that there is a progressive functional decline that occurs with normal aging that affects each body system. This makes the elderly more physiologically frail and unable to tolerate the stresses of injury as compared to the younger population.[30]

Obesity is becoming another issue in trauma care. Although there are many studies that state obese patients have an increase in mortality and morbidity, the current literature is inconclusive. The difference is thought to be attributed to a decrease in mobility, longer hospitalizations, higher incidence of respiratory complications, higher VTE, and higher nosocomial infection rates.[31] The obese patient requires an increase in hospital resources, such as special equipment to get him or her out of bed and mobile.

Patients' families are another important issue complicating trauma care: you are caring not only for the patient but also for the family. Trauma is an unexpected event that disrupts the lives of family members as well as the patient. Both patient and family members experience grief and denial. Many ICUs and resuscitation areas offer 24-hour visiting and presence during resuscitation to support the patient and the family.

## Clinical Applicability Challenges

---

### CASE STUDY

Ms. A., a 30-year-old woman, was crossing the street when she was struck by a vehicle. There was a witness to the accident who called 911. First responders arrived in the ER with the patient. Her initial vitals were temperature 94.1°F, heart rate 147, blood pressure 82/41, respiratory rate 24, and oxygen saturation 90%.

After the primary survey and initial resuscitation, the patient was found on chest radiography to have several broken ribs and a hemothorax. The physician placed a large-bore chest tube in order to drain the blood, and 1000 cc of blood was evacuated into the pleural vac. The patient's respiratory status improved after chest tube placement, and the patient was sent to radiology for a CT scan. CT revealed that the patient had a grade 3 spleen injury and a grade 2 liver injury. When she returned from radiology, she was hypotensive and tachycardic, with a heart rate of 155 and a blood pressure of 78/36. You also noticed that there were 300 cc additional blood in the chest tube pleural vac. You notified the physician, and Ms. A. was taken emergently to the operating room for a thoracotomy. In the operating room, she received 6 units of packed red blood cells and 3 units of fresh frozen plasma.

After the operation, Ms. A. was admitted to the ICU on a ventilator with stable vital signs. The chest tube output had now slowed down and was only 25 to 50 cc per hour. The patient had stabilized and seemed to be recovering from her traumatic injuries. Two days later, on hospital day 3, she was extubated and began participating in physical therapy. On hospital day 5, when you did your A.M. assessment, Ms. A. seemed slightly confused, and you noticed that she was tachycardic with a heart rate or 123 and tachypneic with a respiratory rate of 20. You notified the physician, who came to the bedside to evaluate the patient. Ms. A. was much better the next day, and after 2 weeks in the hospital she was transferred to rehab.

1. After reviewing Ms. A.'s case, what additional information would be important to gather from the first responders?
2. Based on Ms. A.'s initial set of vitals, you suspect that she is suffering from hypovolemia. What type of fluid and what amount would you initially administer?
3. What amount of chest tube output indicates continued bleeding and should cause concern for a missed injury? What amount of blood is considered a massive hemothorax?
4. On hospital day 5, your patient has become slightly confused, tachypneic, and tachycardic. What is your main concern for this patient, and what other data must you gather?

---

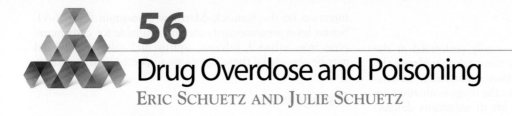

# 56

# Drug Overdose and Poisoning

ERIC SCHUETZ AND JULIE SCHUETZ

**LEARNING OBJECTIVES**

*Based on the content in this chapter, the reader should be able to:*

1. Explain the initial assessment and management of acutely poisoned or overdosed patients.

2. Describe the groups of symptoms that may help identify the drugs or toxins to which a patient may have been exposed.

3. Compare and contrast methods used to prevent absorption and enhance elimination of a drug or toxin.

4. Formulate a plan of care for the poisoned patient.

In 2013, more than 2.2 million exposures to various drugs and toxins were reported to the American Association of Poison Control Centers. Of these exposures, 2,937 resulted in death.[1] The types of toxic exposure reported to poison control centers are diverse: herbal remedies purchased at health food stores, snake and arthropod envenomations, alcohol or drugs, fumes emitted by faulty furnaces, poisonous plants, and industrial hazardous material spills or releases.

Therapy for toxic exposure changes rapidly, based on clinical experience and new research information. Health care professionals may find it challenging to keep abreast of the most advanced therapy. Fortunately, phone consultation with poison control centers offers rapid access to this information. A local poison control center can be reached nationwide by calling 1-800-222-1222. The services of a local poison control center are a useful resource for both health care professionals and the public. Nurses, pharmacists, and physicians with specialized training in clinical toxicology staff such centers.

This chapter presents general guidelines for the assessment and management of the acutely poisoned or overdosed patient. It lists commonly observed poisonings and contains a collaborative care guide for the patient with cocaine toxicity. The chapter ends with a section discussing prevention through patient teaching.

## The Poisoned or Overdosed Patient

Poisonings and drug overdoses can cause quick physical and mental changes in a person. Bystanders are usually the ones who must initiate care and call a poison control center or emergency number.

### Poisoning

The most common routes of exposure in poisoning are inhalation, ingestion, and injection. Toxic chemical reactions can compromise cardiovascular, respiratory, central nervous, hepatic, gastrointestinal (GI), and renal systems.

Most exposures to toxic fumes occur in the home. Poisoning may result from the improper mixing of household cleaning products or malfunctioning household appliances that release carbon monoxide. Burning wood, gas, oil, coal, or kerosene also produces carbon monoxide. Carbon monoxide gas is colorless, odorless, tasteless, and nonirritating, which makes it especially dangerous.

The ingestion of poisons and toxins occurs in various settings and in different age groups. Poisoning in the home usually occurs when children ingest household cleaners or medicines. Improper storage of these items contributes to such accidents. Plants, pesticides, and paint products are also potential household poisons. Because of mental or visual impairment, illiteracy, or a language barrier, older adults may ingest incorrect amounts of medications. In addition, poisoning may occur in the health care environment when medications are administered improperly.

Similarly, poisoning can also occur in the health care environment when a medication normally given only by the subcutaneous or intramuscular route is given intravenously, or when the incorrect medication is injected. Poisoning by injection can also occur in the setting of substance abuse, as when an addict inadvertently injects bleach or too much heroin.

### Substance Abuse and Overdose

Most poisoned patients are admitted to a critical care unit for an intentional or suspected suicidal overdose. These patients frequently have histories of mental illness, substance abuse problems, or both. Often, withdrawal symptoms complicate the assessment of potential toxidromes. A toxidrome is a syndrome (group of signs and symptoms) associated with overdose or exposure to a particular category of drugs and toxins.

Commonly abused substances are nicotine, alcohol, heroin, marijuana, narcotic analgesics, amphetamines, benzodiazepines, and cocaine. Some children and adolescents turn to common household substances because they are readily available. People who attempt to manage stress through substance abuse require a comprehensive treatment program to address their coping and adaptation problems.

### Assessment

A health care facility's systematic approach to the assessment of the poisoned or overdosed patient includes performing triage, obtaining the patient's history, performing a physical examination, and conducting laboratory studies.

## Triage

Although some type of triage is usually performed at the scene or by an emergency response team, triage is always the first step performed in the emergency department. Two essential questions to be considered in the triage evaluation are the following: (1) Is the patient's life in immediate danger? (2) Is the patient's life in potential danger? If the patient's life is in immediate danger, the goals of immediate treatment are patient stabilization and evaluation and management of airway, breathing, and circulation (ABC).

## History

A history of the patient's exposure provides a framework for managing the poisoning or overdose. Key points include identifying the drugs or toxins, the time and duration of the exposure, first-aid treatment given before arrival at the hospital, allergies, and any underlying disease processes or related injuries. This information may be obtained from the patient, family members, friends, rescuers, or bystanders.

## Physical Examination

A quick but thorough physical examination is essential. Preliminary examination results lead to the in-depth evaluation and serial assessment of affected systems (actual or anticipated). As noted previously, a toxidrome is a group of signs and symptoms associated with overdose or exposure to a particular category of drugs and toxins. Recognizing the presence of a toxidrome may help identify the toxins or drugs to which the patent was exposed, and the crucial body systems that may be involved. Table 56-1 lists four common toxidromes with their signs and symptoms and common causes.

## Laboratory Studies

Relevant clinical laboratory data are vital to the assessment of the poisoned or overdosed patient. Tests that provide clues to the agents taken by the patient include electrolytes, hepatic function, urinalysis, electrocardiography, and serum osmolality tests. A serum level measurement of acetaminophen is obtained in all patients who have overdosed because acetaminophen is a component of many prescription and over-the-counter preparations. In the event of an acetaminophen overdose, the level is plotted against the time since

ingestion on the Rumack–Matthew nomogram (Fig. 56-1). Serum level measurements are also available for carbamazepine, iron, ethanol, lithium, aspirin, and valproic acid and may be obtained if these agents are suspected in an overdose.

## Management

Management of the poisoned or overdosed patient is aimed at preventing absorption of and further exposure to the agent. After triage to determine the status of the patient's ABC, the patient must be stabilized. Treatment begins with first aid at the scene and continues in the emergency department and often in the critical care unit. Advanced general management involves further steps to prevent absorption and enhance elimination of the agent. Antidotes, antivenins, or antitoxins, when available, may be administered. The health care team must further support vital functions and monitor and treat multisystem effects. Patient and family teaching to prevent future exposures is another part of the nurse's management strategy.

## Stabilization

Stabilization of patients includes performing the steps summarized in Box 56-1, which are also discussed in the following list:

- *Airway patency.* Nasotracheal or endotracheal intubation may be necessary to adequately maintain and protect the patient's airway.
- *Breathing.* Mechanical ventilation may be necessary to support the patient. Many drugs and toxins depress the respiratory drive. Patients therefore may require ventilator assistance until the drugs or toxins are eliminated from the body.
- *Circulation.* Complications range from shock caused by fluid loss to fluid overload. These are often related to the patient's hydration status and the ability of the cardiovascular system to adjust to drug- or toxin-induced changes. For example, rattlesnake envenomations often cause third spacing of fluid into the area of the bite, leading to intravascular hypovolemia. As a consequence, the patient develops hypotension, which usually responds to aggressive intravenous (IV) fluid therapy. Some toxic drug ingestions impair myocardial contractility, and fluid overload may result because of the heart's inability to pump

### TABLE 56-1 Toxidromes

| Toxidrome | Signs/Symptoms | Common Causes |
|---|---|---|
| **Anticholinergic agents** | Delirium; dry, flushed skin; dilated pupils; elevated temperature; decreased bowel sounds; urinary retention; tachycardia | Antihistamines, atropine, jimson weed |
| **Cholinergic agents** | Excessive salivation, lacrimation, urination, diarrhea, and emesis; diaphoresis, bronchorrhea, bradycardia, fasciculations, central nervous system (CNS) depression, constricted pupils | Organophosphate insecticides (eg, malathion, diazinon); carbamate insecticide (eg, carbaryl, propoxur) |
| **Opioid agents** | CNS depression, respiratory depression, constricted pupils, hypotension, hypothermia | Opiates (eg, codeine, morphine, propoxyphene, heroin), diphenoxylate (eg, diphenoxylate/atropine sulfate [Lomotil]) |
| **Sympathomimetic agents** | Agitation, tachycardia, hypertension, seizures, metabolic acidosis | Amphetamines, cocaine, theophylline, caffeine |

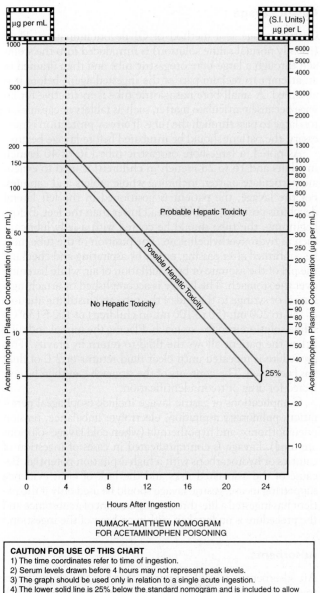

RUMACK–MATTHEW NOMOGRAM
FOR ACETAMINOPHEN POISONING

**CAUTION FOR USE OF THIS CHART**
1) The time coordinates refer to time of ingestion.
2) Serum levels drawn before 4 hours may not represent peak levels.
3) The graph should be used only in relation to a single acute ingestion.
4) The lower solid line is 25% below the standard nomogram and is included to allow for possible errors in acetaminophen plasma assays and estimated time from ingestion of an overdose.

**FIGURE 56-1** Semilogarithmic plot of plasma acetaminophen levels versus time. (From Rumack BH, Matthew HJ: Acetaminophen poisoning and toxicity. Pediatrics 55:871–876, 1975.)

**BOX 56-1** | **Nursing Interventions**

For the Stabilization of the Poisoned or Overdosed Patient
- Assess, establish, and maintain the airway.
- Evaluate respiratory effort.
- Maintain adequate circulation.
- Monitor cardiac function.
- Maintain or correct acid–base balance and electrolyte homeostasis.
- Assess mentation.
- Protect individual from injury during period of acute confusion or unresponsiveness.
- Identify injuries and disease processes that increase risk.
- Measure vital signs and temperature frequently to track changes.

effectively. In these cases, fluid balance needs to be carefully controlled. Invasive monitoring (eg, central venous pressure, pulmonary artery catheter, Foley catheter with urometer) and drug therapy may be necessary to prevent or minimize complications such as pulmonary edema.

- *Cardiac function.* Many drugs and toxins cause cardiac conduction delays and dysrhythmias. The history of the drugs or toxins involved may not be reliable or even known, especially when patients are found unconscious or have attempted suicide. In these cases, continuous cardiac monitoring and 12-lead electrocardiograms (ECGs) help detect cardiotoxic effects.
- *Acid–base balance and electrolyte homeostasis.* Electrolyte abnormalities and metabolic acidosis frequently occur, which may require serial measurements of electrolytes and arterial blood gases (ABGs), as well as other specific laboratory tests. For example, serial measurements of electrolytes, ABGs, and salicylate levels are the means of evaluating aspirin toxicity.
- *Mentation.* Many factors can affect the patient's mental status. Hypoglycemia and hypoxemia are two that can be life threatening but easily addressed by administering oxygen and IV dextrose until laboratory results are available. Naloxone (Narcan) is a narcotic antagonist that reverses narcotic-induced central nervous system and respiratory depression. It is often initially given to comatose patients. However, it must be given cautiously because it can precipitate withdrawal in narcotic-dependent individuals, which may present as violent, agitated behavior, thus placing nurses and other health care providers in danger. In the critical care unit, it may be necessary to continue to administer boluses of naloxone to a patient because of its short duration of action compared with the duration of action of most opioids. In such circumstances, it may be necessary to give naloxone by continuous infusion.[2]
- *Injuries associated with toxic exposure and underlying disease processes.* Any injuries associated with toxic exposure and other underlying disease processes identified during the initial physical examination are treated or monitored, or both. For example, the street drug phencyclidine may provoke violent, agitated, bizarre behavior, leading to trauma during the acute toxic phase. Also, for instance, the patient with preexisting ischemic heart disease may not be able to tolerate the hypoxemia associated with carbon monoxide poisoning as well as a young, healthy patient.
- *Vital signs and temperature.* The critical or potentially critical patient's vital signs and temperature are measured frequently to track changes indicating additional problems.

## Initial Decontamination

First aid may be given by a bystander, health care provider, or emergency response team or in the emergency department. The physicochemical properties of the agent and the amount, route, and exposure time help determine the type and extent of management required. Decontamination methods for ocular, dermal, inhalation, and ingestion exposures follow.

### Ocular Exposure

Many substances can accidentally splash into the eyes. When this happens, the eyes must be flushed to remove the agent.

Immediate irrigation with lukewarm water or normal saline solution is recommended. Continuous flooding of the eyes with a large glass of water or low-pressure shower should be done for 15 minutes. The patient should blink the eyes open and closed during the irrigation. An ophthalmologic examination is needed if ocular irritation or visual disturbance persists after irrigation.

### Dermal Exposure

When dermal exposure occurs, the patient should flood the skin with lukewarm water for 15 to 30 minutes. Most companies that produce or use chemical agents have showers for this purpose. The patient should remove any clothing that may have been contaminated. After standing under running water for the allotted time, the patient should then wash the area gently with soap and water and rinse thoroughly.

Some toxins may require further decontamination. For example, three separate soap-and-water washings or showers are recommended to decontaminate a person who has been exposed to organophosphate pesticides (eg, malathion or diazinon). Protective clothing should be worn to reduce the risk for toxicity while handling contaminated clothing or assisting with skin decontamination.

Although it may seem logical to apply an acid to neutralize a base exposure and a base to neutralize an acid exposure, this can be quite dangerous. Neutralization is the reaction between an acid and a base in which the $H^+$ of the acid and the $OH^-$ of the base react to produce $H_2O$ (water) and heat. The heat produced by this reaction is significant enough to cause burns. Therefore, neutralizing the skin after a dermal exposure is not recommended.

### Inhalation Exposure

A person who has experienced an inhalation exposure should be moved to fresh air as quickly as possible. The responder must also protect himself or herself from the airborne toxin. Further evaluation is needed if the patient experiences respiratory irritation or shortness of breath. Large-scale exposures or those that occur at the workplace may require consultation with a HazMat team, a group of individuals specially trained to manage exposures to hazardous materials.

### Ingestion Exposure

Milk or water dilutes ingested irritants, such as bleach, or caustics, such as drain cleaner. After such an ingestion, adults should drink 8 oz of milk or water, and children should drink 2 to 8 oz (based on their size). Further evaluation is necessary after dilution if there is mucosal irritation or burns. Because of the risk for aspiration, ingestions should not be diluted when they are accompanied by seizures, depressed mental status, or loss of the gag reflex. Again, neutralization is not used because of the risk for thermal burn.

## Gastrointestinal Decontamination

Gastric lavage, adsorbents, cathartics, and whole-bowel irrigation are used to prevent absorption of, and forestall toxicity from, almost all drugs and a variety of toxins. The American Academy of Pediatrics no longer recommends the use of emetics (such as of ipecac syrup) for GI decontamination.

### Gastric Lavage

Gastric lavage is a method of GI decontamination. Fluid (usually normal saline solution) is introduced into the stomach through a large-bore orogastric tube and then drained in an attempt to reclaim part of the ingested agent before it is absorbed. A small-bore nasogastric tube is ineffective for lavage because particulate matter, such as tablets or capsules, is too large to pass through the tube. If airway protection is necessary, the patient should be intubated before lavage begins.

As noted, a large-bore orogastric tube (36 to 40 French in adults and 16 to 28 French in children) is used to evacuate particulate matter, including whole tablets and capsules. For the lavage, the patient is positioned in the left lateral decubitus position, with the head lower than the feet. Before beginning, the tube should be coated with a jelly lubricant such as hydroxyethylcellulose. The position of the tube must be confirmed after passing, either by aspirating and checking the pH of the aspirate or by insufflation of air, while listening over the stomach. The lavage is accomplished by attaching a funnel or syringe to the end of the tube and instilling aliquots of 150 to 200 mL (50 to 100 mL in children) of 100 F (38°C) saline solution into the stomach. Placing the funnel and tube below the patient allows the fluid to return by gravity. This procedure is repeated until clear fluid returns or 2 L of fluid has been used. The contents of the stomach can then be collected for drug or toxin identification.

Complications of gastric lavage include esophageal perforation, pulmonary aspiration, electrolyte imbalance, tension pneumothorax, and hypothermia (when cold lavage solutions are used). Lavage is contraindicated in cases of ingestion of caustics or hydrocarbons with a high aspiration potential. Because of the associated risks and the lack of clear evidence supporting its use, gastric lavage should be used only if the patient has ingested a life-threatening amount of a substance and the procedure is undertaken within an hour of the ingestion.[2]

### Adsorbents

An adsorbent is a solid substance that has the ability to attract and hold another substance to its surface ("to adsorb"). Activated charcoal is an effective nonspecific adsorbent of many drugs and toxins. Activated charcoal adsorbs, or traps, the drug or toxin to its large surface area and prevents absorption from the GI tract. Box 56-2 identifies both drugs and toxins that are adsorbed effectively by activated charcoal and those not adsorbed effectively.

Activated charcoal is a fine black powder that is given as a slurry with water, either orally or by nasogastric or orogastric tube, as soon as possible after the ingestion. Commercially available activated charcoal products may be mixed with 70% sorbitol to decrease grittiness, increase palatability, and serve as a cathartic. The usual dose that is given is one 50 g bottle. Administration of more than one dose is controversial and is usually limited to overdoses of large quantities of aspirin, valproic acid, and theophylline. Activated charcoal is used cautiously in patients with diminished bowel sounds and is contraindicated in patients with bowel obstruction.[2]

### Cathartics

A cathartic is a substance that causes or promotes bowel movements. The use of cathartics alone in the management of poisoning is not an acceptable means of GI decontamination. In

---

| BOX 56-2 | Adsorption of Drugs and Toxins by Activated Charcoal |
|---|---|

**Drugs and Toxins Well Adsorbed by Activated Charcoal**
- Acetaminophen
- Amphetamines
- Antihistamines
- Aspirin
- Barbiturates
- Benzodiazepines
- β-Blockers
- Calcium-channel blockers
- Cocaine
- Opioids
- Phenytoin
- Theophylline
- Valproic acid

**Drugs and Toxins Not Well Adsorbed by Activated Charcoal**
- Acids
- Alkalis
- Alcohols
- Iron
- Lithium
- Metals

---

theory, cathartics decrease the absorption of drugs and toxins by speeding their passage through the GI tract, thereby limiting their contact with mucosal surfaces. Magnesium citrate or 70% sorbitol is often used. Currently, however, there is no clinical evidence that shows that a cathartic can reduce the bioavailability of drugs or improve the outcome of poisoned patients. Data regarding the effectiveness of mixing cathartics with activated charcoal are not yet available. Clearly, more research needs to be done in this area of clinical practice.[2]

### Whole-Bowel Irrigation

The goal of whole-bowel irrigation is to give large volumes of a polyethylene glycol with electrolytes solution rapidly (1 to 2 L/h) to flush the patient's bowel mechanically without creating electrolyte disturbances. Used as a bowel preparation for colonoscopy, this solution is also used as a GI decontamination procedure for patients who have ingested bags or vials of narcotics to avoid arrest, for drug smugglers who pack their GI tracts with narcotics (either orally or rectally), and for patients who have overdosed on modified-release pharmaceuticals.

Commercial products used in whole-bowel irrigation include GoLYTELY and Colyte. Both products are dispensed as powders and are given after adding water. Whole-bowel irrigation is contraindicated in the patient with bowel obstruction or perforation.[2]

## Enhanced Elimination of the Drug or Toxin

The pharmacologic and kinetic characteristics of a drug or toxin greatly influence the severity and length of the clinical course in the acutely poisoned or overdosed patient. The absorption rate, body distribution, metabolism, and elimination must be considered when choosing methods to eliminate the drug or toxin from the body.

### Multiple-Dose Activated Charcoal

Administering multiple doses of activated charcoal can result in greater adsorption of certain drugs such as aspirin, valproic acid, and theophylline. Multiple-dose activated charcoal is given orally, by nasogastric tube, or by orogastric tube every 2 to 6 hours. Complications of multiple-dose activated charcoal include aspiration and bowel obstruction.[2]

### Alteration of Urine pH

Alkalinizing the patient's urine enhances excretion of drugs that are weak acids by increasing the amount of ionized drug in the urine. This form of enhanced elimination is also termed ion trapping. The urine is alkalinized by administering a continuous IV infusion of 1 to 3 ampules of sodium bicarbonate per 1 L of fluid. Urine alkalinization is frequently used in patients experiencing a salicylate overdose. Complications of alkalinization include cerebral or pulmonary edema and electrolyte imbalances. Urine acidification is no longer recommended because it results in low drug clearance and has a risk of complications such as rhabdomyolysis.

### Hemodialysis

Hemodialysis is the process of altering the solute composition of blood by removing it from an artery, diffusing it across a semipermeable membrane (between the blood and a salt solution), then returning it into a vein. It is used in moderate to severe intoxications to remove a drug or toxin rapidly when more conservative methods (eg, gastric lavage, activated charcoal, antidotes) have failed or in patients with decreased renal function. Hemodialysis requires consultation with a nephrologist and specially trained nurses to perform the procedure and monitor the patient. Low molecular weight, low protein binding, and water solubility are factors that make a drug or toxin suitable for hemodialysis. Drugs and toxins that may be removed by hemodialysis include ethylene glycol (commonly found in antifreeze), methanol, lithium, salicylates, and theophylline.[2]

### Hemoperfusion

Hemoperfusion removes drugs and toxins from the patient's blood by pumping the blood through a cartridge of adsorbent material, such as activated charcoal. An advantage of hemoperfusion over hemodialysis is that the total surface area of the dialyzing membrane is much greater with the hemoperfusion cartridges. As in hemodialysis, drugs that have high tissue-binding characteristics and a large volume distributed outside the circulation are not good candidates for hemoperfusion because little drug is found in the blood. Although rarely used in the poisoned and overdosed population, hemoperfusion has been used successfully in patients experiencing a theophylline overdose.[2]

### Chelation

Chelation involves the use of binding agents to remove toxic levels of metals from the body, such as mercury, lead, iron, and arsenic. Examples of chelating agents are dimercaprol (BAL in oil), calcium disodium edetate (EDTA), succimer (DMSA), and deferoxamine. Concerns about the toxicity of the chelators; their tissue distribution characteristics; and the stability, distribution, and elimination of the chelator–metal complex make chelation a complicated procedure.

## Hyperbaric Oxygenation Therapy

In hyperbaric oxygenation therapy (HBO) therapy, oxygen is administered to a patient in an enclosed chamber at a pressure greater than the pressure at sea level (eg, 1 atm). This therapy is sometimes used in carbon monoxide poisoning. In room air, the half-life of carbon monoxide is 5 to 6 hours, whereas in 100% oxygen it is 90 minutes, and in an HBO chamber it is 20 minutes. Complications of HBO therapy include pressure-related otalgia, sinus pain, tooth pain, and tympanic membrane rupture. Confinement anxiety, convulsions, and tension pneumothorax also have been observed in patients receiving HBO therapy.[3]

## Antagonists, Antitoxins, and Antivenins

In pharmacology, an antagonist is a substance that counteracts the action of another drug. Although the general public often believes there is an antidote for every drug or toxin, the opposite is closer to the truth. There are, in fact, very few antidotes. Antidotes for specific intoxications are listed in Table 56-2.

Antitoxins neutralize a toxin. For instance, botulism antitoxin trivalent (equine) is available through the Centers for Disease Control and Prevention to counteract the effects of botulism.

Antivenins are antitoxins that neutralize the venom of the offending snake or spider. There are several antivenins; each is active against a specific venom. Crotalidae polyvalent immune Fab (CroFab), for example, is approved by the US Food and Drug Administration (FDA) for the treatment of a snakebite by a North American pit viper, and CroFab is produced using a purification process that removes the Fc fragment and leaves only the Fab fragments of the immunoglobulins; typically, this results in a product that causes fewer reactions in humans. Antivenins are available for black widow spider bites (*Latrodectus mactans*; equine) as well as for envenomations by the eastern and Texas coral snake (*Micrurus fulvius*; equine). However, there are many venomous snakes and spiders for which no antivenin exists. Envenomation from one of these species is treated with symptomatic and supportive care.[5,6]

## Continuous Patient Monitoring

Seriously poisoned or overdosed patients may require continued monitoring for hours or days after exposure. Physical examination, the use of diagnostic tools, and careful assessment of clinical signs and symptoms provide information about the patient's progress and guide medical and nursing management. Diagnostic tools include the following:

- *Electrocardiography.* Electrocardiography can provide evidence of drugs causing dysrhythmias or conduction delays (eg, tricyclic antidepressants).
- *Radiology.* Many substances are radiopaque or can be visualized using a contrast-enhanced computed tomography scan (eg, heavy metals, button batteries, some modified-release tablets or capsules, aspirin concretions, cocaine or heroin containers). Chest radiographs provide evidence of aspiration and pulmonary edema.
- *Electrolytes, ABGs, and other laboratory tests.* Acute poisoning can cause an imbalance in a patient's electrolyte levels, including sodium, potassium, chloride, carbon dioxide content, magnesium, and calcium. Signs of inadequate ventilation or oxygenation include cyanosis, tachycardia, hypoventilation, intercostal muscle retractions, and altered mental status. Such signs should be evaluated by pulse oximetry and ABG measurements. Seriously poisoned patients require routine screening of electrolytes, ABGs, creatinine, and glucose; complete blood count; and urinalysis.
- *Anion gap.* The anion gap is a simple, cost-effective tool that uses common serum measurements, such as sodium, chloride, and bicarbonate, to help evaluate the poisoned patient for certain drugs or toxins. The anion gap represents the difference between unmeasured anions and cations in the blood. Using measured anions and a cation, the anion gap is calculated using the following formula:

$$[Na] - ([Cl] + [HCO_3]) = \text{anion gap}$$

The normal value for the anion gap is approximately 8 to 16 mEq/L. An anion gap that exceeds the upper normal value can indicate metabolic acidosis caused by an accumulation of acids in the blood. Drugs, toxins, or medical conditions that

---

**TABLE 56-2**  **Antidotes for Specific Drugs and Toxins**

| Drug/Toxin | Antidote |
|---|---|
| Acetaminophen | *N*-acetylcysteine (NAC) (Mucomyst [PO], Acetadote [IV]) |
| Anticholinergics | Physostigmine (Antilirium) |
| Benzodiazepines | Flumazenil (Romazicon) |
| β-Blocking agents | Glucagon |
| Calcium-channel blockers | Glucagon, calcium chloride, hyperinsulinemia-euglycemia |
| Carbon monoxide | Oxygen |
| Cyanide | Lilly Cyanide Antidote Kit: amyl nitrite, sodium nitrite, and sodium thiosulfate, Cyanokit (hydroxocobalamin) |
| Digoxin | Digoxin-specific fab fragments (Digibind or DigiFab) |
| Ethylene glycol | Fomepizole (Antizol)*, ethanol |
| Methanol | Fomepizole (Antizol)†, ethanol |
| Nitrites | Methylene blue |
| Opioids | Naloxone (Narcan) |
| Organophosphate insecticides | Atropine, pralidoxime |

*Bennen DP, Bohra RB, Cook MD, et al: Antidote use in the critically Ill poisoned patient. J Intensive Care Med 21:255–277, 2006.
†Haddad L, Shannon M, Winchester J: Clinical Management of Poisoning and Drug Overdose, 4th ed. Philadelphia, PA: WB Saunders.

can produce an elevated anion gap include iron, isoniazid (INH), lithium, lactate, carbon monoxide, cyanide, toluene, methanol, metformin, ethanol, ethylene glycol, salicylates, hydrogen sulfide, strychnine, diabetic ketoacidosis, uremia, seizures, and starvation. Although these substances and processes can cause an elevated anion gap, a normal anion gap alone does not preclude a toxic exposure.

- *Osmolal gap.* The osmolal gap is the difference between the measured osmolality (using the freezing point depression method) and the calculated osmolality. The calculated osmolality is derived using laboratory values for the major osmotically active substances in the serum, such as sodium, glucose, and blood urea nitrogen (BUN). Like the anion gap, it is a simple, cost-effective tool for evaluating the poisoned patient for certain drugs or toxins. The calculated osmolality (using serum electrolyte values) is defined as follows:

$$2(Na^+) + \frac{glucose}{18} + \frac{BUN}{2.8}$$
$$= \text{calculated osmolality}$$

The osmolal gap is then calculated as follows:

Measured osmolality − calculated osmolality = osmolal gap

An osmolal gap that exceeds 10 mOsm is abnormal. Toxins that can cause an elevated osmolal gap include ethanol, ethylene glycol, and methanol. If an ethanol level is known, it can be factored into the following equation:

$$2(Na^+) + \frac{glucose}{18} + \frac{BUN}{2.8} + \frac{BAL}{4.6}$$
$$= \text{calculated osmolality}$$

where BAL is the blood alcohol level measured in milligrams per deciliter.

- *Toxicology screens.* A toxicology screen is a laboratory analysis of a body fluid or tissue to identify drugs or toxins. Although saliva, spinal fluid, and hair may be analyzed, blood or urine samples are used more frequently. The number and type of drugs assessed by toxicology screens vary. Each screen tests for specific drugs or agents. For example, drug abuse screens usually identify several common street or prescription drugs, whereas a coma panel detects common drugs that cause CNS depression. Comprehensive screens include many drugs (ranging from antidepressants to cardiac drugs to alcohols) and are more expensive. A number of factors limit the role of toxicology screens in managing poisonings or overdoses. The test sample must be collected while the drug or toxin is in the body fluid or tissue used for testing. For example, cocaine is a rapidly metabolized drug; however, its metabolite, benzoylecgonine, can be detected in the urine for several hours after cocaine use. Also, a toxicology screen with a negative result does not necessarily mean that no drug or toxin is present, but rather that none of the drugs or toxins for which a patient has been screened is present. For example, γ-hydroxybutyrate is not included in toxicology screens because it is rapidly metabolized to small, unmeasurable molecules.

Patient care in some of the more common poisonings and overdoses is summarized in Table 56-3. Clinical manifestations

**TABLE 56-3  Common Patient Care in Poisonings and Overdoses**

| Drug/Substance | Clinical Presentation and Assessment | Intervention |
|---|---|---|
| **Acetaminophen (APAP)** | | |
| Common OTC antipyretic and analgesic<br>Often sold as a component of combination drugs for pain, cough, cold, and sleep<br>Examples: OTC remedies such as Tylenol, Tylenol Extended Relief, Tempra, Liquiprin, Panadol, Excedrin PM (diphenhydramine-APAP) and in controlled-substance combination drugs such as oxycodone-APAP (Percocet), codeine-APAP (Tylenol #3), hydrocodone-APAP (Vicodin)<br>Acetaminophen toxicity: hepatotoxicity and occasionally renal dysfunction, 1–3 d postingestion | • *Phase 1 (up to 24 h postingestion)*: anorexia, nausea, malaise<br>• *Phase 2 (24–48 h postingestion)*: clinical picture improves, increase in AST, ALT, and total bilirubin, prolongation of prothrombin time<br>• *Phase 3 (72–96 h postingestion)*: peak hepatotoxicity usually observed<br>• Coagulopathies<br>• Jaundice<br>• AST and ALT may rise into the 10,000–20,000 IU/L range and return to normal without the patient experiencing long-term sequelae.<br>• Chronic toxicity well described in the medical literature | *Prevention of absorption:*<br>• Activated charcoal<br><br>*Laboratory:*<br>• Draw acetaminophen level at 4 h (or later if patient presents late to the health care facility), plot level on the Rumack–Matthew nomogram (see Fig. 56-1) to determine whether antidote is indicated.<br>• Monitor daily AST, ALT, total bilirubin, blood urea nitrogen, creatinine, and prothrombin time in patients with a toxic acetaminophen level.<br><br>*Treatment:*<br>Antidote: NAC<br>• Oral: NAC, Mucomyst<br>  • Loading dose: 140 mg/kg orally<br>  • Maintenance doses: 70 mg/kg orally every 4 h for a total of 17 maintenance doses<br>  • Dilute NAC (20% solution) 3:1 with a soft drink or juice<br>  • Repeat any dose not retained 1 h, may need antiemetics to control vomiting*<br>• IV: Acetadote<br>  • Loading dose: 150 mg/kg in 200 mL of D5W IV over 60 min<br>  • First maintenance dose: 50 mg/kg in 500 mL of D5W IV over 4 h<br>  • Second maintenance dose: 100 mg/kg in 1,000 mL of D5W IV over 16 h<br>• Supportive care |

*(continued)*

**TABLE 56-3** Common Patient Care in Poisonings and Overdoses (*continued*)

| Drug/Substance | Clinical Presentation and Assessment | Intervention |
|---|---|---|
| **Amphetamines** | | |
| Group of drugs used therapeutically for narcolepsy, short-term treatment of obesity, and attention-deficit disorder<br><br>As drugs of abuse, used for ability to stimulate CNS to combat fatigue or produce a "high"<br><br>Prescription amphetamines and related agents: methylphenidate (Ritalin), dextroamphetamine (Dexedrine), mixed salts of amphetamine (Adderall)<br><br>Street names: speed, uppers, crank, E, X, ecstasy, ice, crystal | • Flushing<br>• Diaphoresis<br>• Restlessness<br>• Talkativeness<br>• Irritability<br>• Confusion<br>• Panic<br>• Seizures<br>• Intracranial hemorrhage<br>• Hypertension<br>• Tachycardia<br>• Chest pain<br>• Myocardial infarction<br>• Cardiac dysrhythmias<br>• Palpitations<br>• Peripheral vasoconstriction<br>• Nausea<br>• Vomiting<br>• Chronic amphetamine toxicity may lead to the development of paranoia or hallucinations.<br>• IV abusers may also have complications such as hepatitis, sepsis, abscesses, and HIV infection. | *Prevention of absorption:*<br>• Activated charcoal<br><br>*Laboratory:*<br>• Monitor electrolytes and acid–base status<br>• Urine drug screen may detect amphetamines<br><br>*Treatment:*<br>• External cooling measures for hyperthermia<br>• Benzodiazepines to control agitation<br>• Severe hypertension controlled with IV nitroprusside (Nipride), other drugs suggested<br>• Supportive care |
| **Benzodiazepines** | | |
| Antianxiety agents, anticonvulsants, muscle relaxants, and sedatives<br><br>Examples: alprazolam (Xanax), clonazepam (Klonopin), diazepam (Valium), lorazepam (Ativan), midazolam (Versed)<br><br>Primarily cause CNS and respiratory depression. Due to their low order of toxicity, fatalities unlikely unless ingested with other CNS depressants | • Respiratory depression<br>• Airway protection/gag reflex<br>• Lethargy<br>• Coma<br>• Confusion<br>• Slurred speech<br>• Ataxia | *Prevention of absorption:*<br>• Activated charcoal<br><br>*Laboratory:*<br>• Urine drug screen may detect benzodiazepines.<br><br>*Treatment:*<br>• Flumazenil reverses CNS and respiratory depression; due to risk in unmasking controlled seizures, flumazenil is contraindicated in the face of simultaneous potential seizure causing overdose.<br>• Supportive care |
| **Carbon Monoxide** | | |
| Colorless, odorless gas that is a component of automobile exhaust, natural gas or propane furnace emissions, cigarette smoke, wood stove emissions, and pollution<br><br>Methylene chloride, a component found in some paint strippers, is metabolized in the body to carbon monoxide after inhaled or ingested<br><br>It displaces oxygen from the hemoglobin, leading to hypoxia<br><br>It is absorbed rapidly by inhalation and combines readily with hemoglobin due to a greater affinity than oxygen<br><br>Fetal carboxyhemoglobin levels are possibly 10%–15% greater than the maternal carboxyhemoglobin level | • Flu-like symptoms<br>• Headache<br>• Nausea<br>• Vomiting<br>• Syncope<br>• Fatigue<br>• Weakness<br>• Lack of concentration<br>• Irritability<br>• Chest pain, especially in people with underlying cardiovascular disease<br>• Occasionally, irreversible changes in memory and personality<br>• Fetotoxicity<br>• People usually report feeling better when not in the area of the carbon monoxide; for example, if the exposure is occurring in the home because of a faulty furnace, the person will often report a decrease or resolution of symptoms when away from the home. | *Prevention of absorption:*<br>• Fresh air<br><br>*Laboratory:*<br>• Carboxyhemoglobin levels<br><br>*Treatment:*<br>• 100% oxygen until all signs and symptoms resolve<br>• Thorough neurologic examination<br>• Hyperbaric oxygenation therapy (HBO) to decrease half-life; however, due to lack of available HBO chambers, use is limited and efficacy not well documented by research<br>• Supportive care |

| Drug/Substance | Clinical Presentation and Assessment | Intervention |
|---|---|---|
| **Cocaine** | | |
| Common street drug that produces a temporary feeling of well-being for the user<br>Routes of exposure: IV, snorting, smoking<br>Street names: crack, rock, coke, snow, blow<br>Toxic effects related to the rapid onset of CNS and cardiac stimulation | • Tachycardia<br>• Hypertension<br>• Cardiac dysrhythmias<br>• Chest pain<br>• Myocardial infarction<br>• Aortic dissection<br>• Bowel infarction<br>• Hyperthermia<br>• Anxiety<br>• Seizures<br>• Tactile hallucinations ("cocaine bugs")<br>• Cerebral hemorrhage<br>• Cerebral infarction<br>• Rhabdomyolysis<br>• Rapid onset of toxic effects<br>• In pregnant women, abruptio placentae or abortion possible<br>• Chronic snorting, nasal septal perforation<br>• If clinical presentation is inconsistent with cocaine alone, possibly adulterants, substitutes, co-ingestants, or withdrawal | *Prevention of absorption (for ingested packets):*<br>• Activated charcoal<br>• Whole-bowel irrigation<br><br>*Laboratory:*<br>• Urine drug screen to detect metabolite of cocaine: benzoylecgonine<br>• Cardiac enzymes as indicated to rule out myocardial infarction<br><br>*Treatment:*<br>• Benzodiazepines such as diazepam (Valium) usually control hyperactivity, hypertension, tachycardia, anxiety, hyperthermia, and seizures.<br>• Phenobarbital may be necessary if seizures not controlled with benzodiazepines.<br>• Life-threatening hyperthermia may be reduced by external cooling measures.<br>• Cardiac monitoring and serial 12-lead ECG are used to evaluate dysrhythmias and myocardial ischemia.[†]<br>• Monitor for other organ ischemia or infarction.<br>• Provide supportive care. |
| **Halogenated Hydrocarbons** | | |
| Agents used as propellants and refrigerants<br>Freon, dichlorodifluoromethane (Freon 12) and trichloromonofluoromethane (Freon 11) included in this category<br>Exposures to leaking household air conditioners are usually minor, causing transient eye, nose, and throat irritation; dizziness; and palpitations<br>More concentrated exposures such as in industrial spills or deliberate abuse ("huffing") associated with possible fatal ventricular dysrhythmias (due to myocardial sensitization to catecholamines) and pulmonary edema | • Eye, nose, and throat irritation<br>• Cough<br>• Dizziness<br>• Disorientation<br>• Palpitations<br>• Bronchial constriction<br>• Pulmonary edema<br>• Ventricular dysrhythmias<br>• Frostbite possible with dermal exposures | *Prevention of absorption:*<br>• Fresh air<br><br>*Laboratory:*<br>• No specific laboratory tests<br><br>*Treatment:*<br>• Quiet environment<br>• Cardiac monitoring<br>• Frostbite: complete rewarming<br>• Supportive care |
| **Heroin** | | |
| Common street drug that produces a temporary euphoria in the user<br>Routes of exposure: IV, snorting<br>Street names: dope, smack, junk | • Miosis<br>• Decreased respiratory drive<br>• Decreased level of consciousness<br>• "Nodding" | *Prevention of absorption:*<br>• Not applicable<br><br>*Laboratory:*<br>• As clinically indicated<br>• Serum toxicology screen<br><br>*Treatment:*<br>• Careful administration of naloxone<br>• Referral to substance abuse counselor |
| **Lysergic Acid Diethylamide (LSD)** | | |
| Common name for psychedelic drug LSD<br>Common drug of abuse since its rise in popularity in the 1960s<br>Street drug: available in tablet, capsule, sugar cubes, or as a substance on blotting paper known as "blotter acid" | • Anxiety<br>• Impaired color perception<br>• Impaired judgment<br>• Paranoia or ideas of persecution<br>• Time distortions<br>• Blood pressure normal<br>• Tachycardia<br>• Tachypnea | *Prevention of absorption:*<br>• Activated charcoal<br>• Cathartic<br><br>*Laboratory:*<br>• Urine drug screen<br><br>*Treatment:*<br>• Acute anxiety may be managed with IV or oral diazepam (Valium). |

*(continued)*

**TABLE 56-3**   **Common Patient Care in Poisonings and Overdoses** (*continued*)

| Drug/Substance | Clinical Presentation and Assessment | Intervention |
|---|---|---|
| One source of LSD is ingestion of morning glory seeds<br>In addition to the psychedelic experience, may result in physical effects and behavior-related trauma during the acute toxic phase | • Slight temperature elevation<br>• Flashbacks (transient recurrences of a psychedelic experience) possible after a period of abstinence, may recur for years<br>• Trauma due to behavioral changes associated with LSD use | • A quiet, nonstimulating environment may be useful while trying to help the patient who is experiencing a bad reaction.<br>• Evaluate for evidence of trauma.<br>• Provide supportive care. |

**Methanol**

| | | |
|---|---|---|
| Highly toxic antifreeze and solvent<br>Available forms: most windshield washer fluids, Sterno canned heat, and components of some paints, gasoline additives, and shellacs<br>Toxic effects: life-threatening acidosis and irreversible blindness, caused by the toxic metabolite, not the methanol itself | • Blurred vision<br>• Decreased visual acuity<br>• Subjective description of vision as if walking in a snowstorm<br>• Retinal edema<br>• Hyperemia of the optic disk<br>• Headache<br>• Vertigo<br>• Lethargy<br>• Confusion<br>• Coma<br>• Nausea<br>• Vomiting<br>• Abdominal pain<br>• Metabolic acidosis | *Prevention of absorption:*<br>• Syrup of ipecac<br>• Gastric lavage<br>• Activated charcoal and cathartic are of little value<br><br>*Laboratory:*<br>• Methanol level drawn 1 h postingestion<br>• Serial electrolytes<br>• If using ethanol therapy, serial glucose and blood ethanol level monitored every hour initially<br><br>*Treatment:*<br>• Treatment is aimed at preventing the formation of toxic metabolites with either Antizol (4-methylpyrazole: 4-MP) or ethanol.<br>• Hemodialysis usually indicated for methanol levels more than 50 mg/dL, visual changes, renal failure, or refractory acidosis.<br>• Folic acid administration to assist with oxidation of the toxic metabolite formic acid to carbon dioxide<br>• Supportive care |

**Salicylates**

| | | |
|---|---|---|
| Group of drugs used primarily for anti-inflammatory, antipyretic, and analgesic properties<br>Common sources: aspirin, some formulations of Alka-Seltzer, Aspergum, Pepto-Bismol, sunscreens, liniments such as Icy Hot, and oil of wintergreen (methylsalicylate)<br>Life-threatening metabolic acidosis, cerebral edema, and pulmonary edema from salicylism<br>Aspirin ingestions difficult to manage due to the formation of a mass of aspirin in the gastrointestinal (GI) tract called a concretion<br>Concretion formation leads to delayed absorption and therefore delayed toxicity<br>Chronic salicylism more common in older adults and easily missed due to lack of careful history taking<br>Higher salicylate levels tolerated with acute overdose as opposed to chronic toxicity | • Tinnitus<br>• Tachypnea<br>• Pulmonary edema<br>• Confusion<br>• Lethargy<br>• Seizures<br>• Cerebral edema<br>• Respiratory alkalosis coupled with metabolic acidosis (initially)<br>• Hypokalemia<br>• Platelet dysfunction<br>• Hypothrombinemia<br>• GI hemorrhage<br>• Nausea<br>• Vomiting<br>• Hyperthermia<br>• Dehydration | *Prevention of absorption:*<br>• Syrup of ipecac<br>• Gastric lavage<br>• Multiple-dose activated charcoal<br>• Single-dose cathartic<br><br>*Laboratory:*<br>• Serial salicylate levels<br>• Serial electrolytes<br>• Arterial blood gas (ABG) as indicated<br>• Hematologic and coagulation studies<br><br>*Treatment:*<br>• IV hydration<br>• Urinary excretion is enhanced by urine alkalinization (urine pH = 7.5–8.0); IV fluid is usually $D_5W$ with 20–40 mEq KCl and 2–3 ampules of sodium bicarbonate/L to infuse at a rate of 2–3 mL/kg/h to achieve equal urine output (Note: It is difficult to alkalinize the urine without a normal serum potassium level.)<br>• Potassium is replaced IV as needed.<br>• Monitor onset of cerebral or pulmonary edema; chest radiograph is taken as needed.<br>• Hemodialysis is indicated for renal failure, cerebral edema, pulmonary edema, refractory acidosis, chronic salicylate level more than 50 mg/dL, or acute salicylate level more than 100 mg/dL postingestion.<br>• Provide supportive care<br>• Note: Treatment is based on serial salicylate levels and clinical presentation; each case is individually assessed and managed. |

| Drug/Substance | Clinical Presentation and Assessment | Intervention |
|---|---|---|
| **Tricyclic Antidepressants (TCA)** | | |
| Class of drugs prescribed for depression and chronic pain<br>Examples: amitriptyline (Elavil), clomipramine (Anafranil), desipramine (Norpramin), doxepin (Adapin, Sinequan), imipramine (Tofranil), nortriptyline (Pamelor, Aventyl), protriptyline (Vivactil), and trimipramine (Surmontil) | • Tachycardia<br>• Ventricular dysrhythmias (including ventricular tachycardia and ventricular fibrillation)<br>• Cardiac conduction delays (eg, QRS > 100 ms)<br>• Hypotension<br>• Agitation<br>• Sedation<br>• Seizures<br>• Coma<br>• Dry, flushed skin<br>• Decreased GI motility<br>• Urinary retention<br>• Metabolic acidosis | *Prevention of absorption:*<br>• Syrup of ipecac contraindicated because of the rapid onset of sedation or seizures<br>• Gastric lavage<br>• Activated charcoal<br>• Cathartic<br><br>*Laboratory:*<br>• Serum TCA levels not clinically useful in managing overdoses<br>• Urine drug screen for TCAs<br>• Serial electrolytes and ABGs as indicated<br><br>*Treatment:*<br>• Prepare for rapid onset of cardiovascular collapse<br>• Seizures may be treated initially with IV benzodiazepines (diazepam, lorazepam) and, if necessary, phenobarbital.<br>• Ventricular dysrhythmias may initially be controlled with systemic alkalinization (keeping blood pH +7.45–7.55 using IV boluses of sodium bicarbonate or intubation and hyperventilation); ventricular dysrhythmias not controlled with systemic alkalinization may be controlled with lidocaine or bretylium (Bretylol); do not use procainamide (Pronestyl) or quinidine due to effects on cardiac conduction similar to those of TCAs.<br>• Cardiac conduction delays (eg, QRS > 100 ms) also are treated with systemic alkalinization as outlined in previous point; conduction delays not responsive to systemic alkalinization may be treated with phenytoin<br>• Hypotension may be addressed initially with Trendelenburg position and IV fluids; if necessary, follow with dopamine infusion; norepinephrine (Levophed) may be necessary.<br>• Provide supportive care. |

ALT, alanine aminotransferase; AST, aspartate aminotransferase; OTC, over the counter.

*Wright RO, Anderson AC, Lesko SL, et al: Effect of metoclopramide dose on preventing emesis after oral administration of *N*-acetylcysteine for acetaminophen overdose. J Toxicol Clin Toxicol 37:35–42, 1999.

†McCord J, Jneid H, Hollander J, et al: Management of cocaine-associated chest pain and myocardial infarction: A scientific statement from the American Heart Association Acute Cardiac Care Committee of the Council on Clinical Cardiology. Circulation 117:1897–1907, 2007.

are included in the table. Management of the patient who is toxic with cocaine is summarized in Box 56-3.[7,8]

## Patient Teaching

One of the interventions the nurse can perform in the emergency department or intensive care unit is preventive teaching. All patients (and parents of pediatric patients) who have survived a toxic encounter should be taught how to prevent such an incident from recurring. Parents of young children need information on child-proofing their home. Family teaching guidelines for lead poisoning are included in Box 56-4. Finally, a summary of poison prevention for the older patient can be found in Box 56-5.

In addition, carbon monoxide detectors alert families to problems in their homes. Utility companies and local health and fire authorities can help identify and remove sources of fumes.

---

**QSEN  BOX 56-3**   *COLLABORATIVE CARE GUIDE for the Patient With Cocaine Toxicity*

| Outcomes | Interventions |
|---|---|
| **Impaired Gas Exchange due to Medication Overdose** | |
| ABGs are within normal limits | • Monitor pulse oximetry and ABGs<br>• Validate significant changes in pulse oximetry with co-oximetry arterial saturation measurement |
| Respiratory rate and depth are within normal limits | • Monitor every 15 minutes, then every 1 hour<br>• Prepare for intubation and mechanical ventilation (see Collaborative Care Guide for the Patient on Mechanical Ventilation, p 538) |

*(continued)*

**QSEN BOX 56-3**   *COLLABORATIVE CARE GUIDE for the Patient With Cocaine Toxicity (continued)*

| Outcomes | Interventions |
|---|---|
| **Decreased Cardiac Tissue Perfusion**<br>**Ineffective Thermoregulation: Risk for Imbalanced Body Temperature** | |
| Blood pressure and heart rate are within normal limits<br>Patient is free of dysrhythmias<br>There is no evidence of myocardial dysfunction, such as altered ECG or cardiac enzymes | • Monitor vital signs every 15 minutes then hourly<br>• Provide continuous ECG monitoring<br>• Monitor 12-lead ECG daily and PRN<br>• Monitor cardiac enzymes, magnesium, phosphorus, calcium, and potassium as ordered<br>• Assess for chest pain<br>• Monitor ECG for dysrhythmias and changes consistent with evolving myocardial infarction |
| • Patient is euthermic | • Assess temperature every 15 to 30 minutes, then hourly<br>• Provide a cool environment, and institute cooling strategies (eg, hypothermia blanket, tepid sponge bath), as indicated |
| **Electrolyte Imbalance**<br>**Risk for Imbalanced Fluid Volume** | |
| Patient's urine output >30 mL/h (or >0.5 mL/kg/h) | • Take intake and output hourly<br>• Administer fluids and diuretics to maintain intravascular volume and renal function per order |
| There is no evidence of electrolyte imbalance or renal dysfunction | • Monitor electrolytes daily and PRN<br>• Replace electrolytes as ordered<br>• Monitor BUN, creatinine, serum osmolality, and urine electrolytes daily |
| **Risk for Injury** | |
| There is no evidence of seizure activity | • Monitor for seizure activity<br>• Administer anticonvulsants<br>• Assess anticonvulsant levels daily if indicated<br>• Maintain calm, quiet environment |
| Patient does not harm self | • Institute seizure precautions<br>• Institute fall precautions<br>• Assess need for physical or chemical restraint to protect from self-injury<br>• Monitor agitation and administer sedation when appropriate<br>• Evaluate risk for suicide and take measures to protect patient |
| **Impaired Skin Integrity** | |
| There is no evidence of skin breakdown | • Document skin integrity every 8 hour<br>• Turn and reposition every 2 hour<br>• Use Braden Scale to assess risk for skin breakdown |
| **Imbalanced Nutrition** | |
| • Caloric and nutrient intake meets metabolic requirements per calculation (eg, basal energy expenditure) | • Provide parenteral or enteral nutrition if patient is NPO<br>• Consult dietitian or nutritional support service<br>• Monitor protein and calorie intake<br>• Monitor albumin, prealbumin, transferrin, cholesterol, triglycerides, and glucose |
| **Impaired Comfort** | |
| Patient will have minimal discomfort related to withdrawal from cocaine and other substances | • Obtain toxicology screen to identify other substances used by the patient<br>• Treat drug withdrawal and overdose symptoms promptly and with appropriate intervention (eg, remove from circulation, administer antidote, administer methadone) |
| **Ineffective Coping**<br>**Ineffective Health Maintenance**<br>**Risk-prone Health Behavior** | |
| Patient and family acknowledge substance abuse | • Assess patient and family response to overdose<br>• Support healthy coping behaviors<br>• Consult substance abuse counselor and social worker<br>• Encourage patient discussion regarding use of illegal drugs, support system, financial concerns, and readiness for substance abuse treatment |
| **Teaching/Discharge Planning** | |
| • Patient and family have information about treatment and self-help resources | • Assess patient and family knowledge and understanding of substance abuse<br>• Provide literature and explanations to patient and family regarding substance abuse, treatment, relapse, legal issues, and self-help groups |
| Patient and family each have a plan for follow-up care | • Refer family to self-help resources<br>• If patient agrees, initiate referral for substance abuse rehabilitation<br>• Coordinate referral with patient, family, and social worker to address other possible issues (eg, housing, financial issues, long-term care planning) |

Lead is commonly found in old homes, in paint, plumbing, and dinnerware.

- Lead is excreted more slowly than it is absorbed, leading to a buildup of lead in the body.
- Accumulation of lead in high levels is frequently missed through lack of blood lead level screening, and not detected until effects such as learning disabilities are diagnosed.
- Children can be tested for lead by their health care providers.
- The local health department can provide lead poisoning treatment and information about lead abatement programs.

**Accidental Poisoning**

- Poison control centers receive many calls from or related to older adults regarding accidental poisonings.
- Telephone numbers for the health care provider and the poison control center should be in a readily accessible place.
- The older population uses more medicine than any other age group.
- Older people may be more susceptible to the effects of drugs.
- When questions arise concerning drugs, a responsible adult should not hesitate to call a health care provider.
- The patient should not change the dose or discontinue taking prescription drugs without first consulting the physician or nurse.
- Avoid doubling medication when a pill is forgotten. The patient should seek the advice of his or her physician, nurse, or pharmacist.
- Medications and alcohol should not be mixed without first checking with the pharmacist for possible interactions.
- The pharmacist can provide large-print labels.
- A medication calendar or diary will help the older person keep track of the dosing schedule.
- Pill dispensers are helpful for the patient who has to take a variety of pills or who has trouble remembering the prescribed schedule.
- Individual pharmacies may be willing to place patient's medications into daily dose blister packs.
- When a medication is discontinued, the remaining medication should be discarded with regard for the environment; for example, it may be returned to a pharmacy for responsible disposal.

## Clinical Applicability Challenges

**CASE STUDY**

D.C. is a 41-year-old woman who just presented to the emergency department, claiming that 15 minutes ago she took 25 of bupropion (Wellbutrin XL, 150 mg), as a suicide gesture. D.C. appears alert and slightly anxious, and has the following vitals: heart rate, 110; blood pressure, 144/88; respiratory rate (RR) 16, temperature 36.8°C (98.2°F), oxygen saturation 100% on room air, finger stick (FS) glucose level = 98. Her skin appears warm and moist; her pupils are 3 to 4 mm and reactive. She denies using alcohol or other drugs, and says she has been taking the Wellbutrin for depression for several months.

The triage nurse called the poison center, who recommended giving D.C. 50 g of activated charcoal and beginning IV fluid administration and cardiac monitoring; observing for 24 hours for seizures, with benzodiazepines as needed; checking levels of acetaminophen (APAP), aspirin (ASA), and alcohol (ETOH); performing a urine toxicology screen for drugs of abuse; and scheduling a psychiatric evaluation. Activated charcoal was given with no vomiting; IV fluids were started and cardiac monitoring was begun. Within an hour, D.C. had a 30-second seizure; 2 mg of IV lorazepam was given and the seizure resolved.

An ICU bed was available, and D.C. was admitted for observation. While D.C. was in the ICU, the lab results and the levels of APAP, ASA, and ETOH were all below detection. No drugs of abuse were detected in the urine. D.C. continued to be observed in the ICU for 24 hours, and she was then transferred to the psychiatric unit for help with her suicidal ideations.

1. Explain why it was helpful for the triage nurse to call the poison center.
2. Why was it necessary to check the levels of APAP, ASA, and ETOH?
3. Why was a urine toxicology screen necessary?

**WANT TO KNOW MORE?**

A wide variety of resources to enhance your learning and understanding of this chapter are available on thePoint.

You will find:

- References
- Selected readings
- NCLEX-style review questions
- Internet resources
- And more!

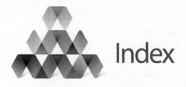

# Index

Note: Page numbers followed by *f* indicate figures; those followed by *t* indicate tables; and those followed by *b* indicate box.

## A

AAA (abdominal aortic aneurysm), 347
AACN. *See* American Association of Critical-Care Nurses (AACN)
Abacavir, 960
Abciximab, 279*b*
Abdomen
  assessment of, 769–773
    auscultation in, 770, 771*f*
    inspection in, 770
    palpation in, 771–773, 772*f*
    percussion, 770–771, 772*f*
  counter of, abnormal, 770*t*
Abdominal aortic aneurysm (AAA), 347
Abdominal aortic pulsations, 770*t*
Abdominal contour, 770*t*
Abdominal distention, in pediatric patients, 101
Abdominal films, 778*t*
Abdominal sounds, abnormal, 771*t*
Abdominal trauma, 1083–1088, 1084*b*
  to bladder, 1088
  colonic, 1086, 1086*b*
  diaphragmatic, 1085
  duodenal and pancreatic, 1086
  esophageal, 1085
  hepatic, 1087, 1087*b*
  renal, 1088
  splenic, 1087–1088, 1087*b*
Abdominal twitching, cardiac pacing and, 318
Abducens nerve (cranial nerve VI), 623*t*
  assessment of, 647–649, 648*f*
ABGs. *See* Arterial blood gases (ABGs)
Abruption placentae, 113
Abscesses, pancreatic, 815
Absorptive dressings, 1021
Abuse, of older patients, 133–134
A/C (assist-control) ventilator mode, 469
Acalculia, 643*t*
Acapella valve, 450
ACC/AHA (American College of Cardiology/American Heart Association Guidelines), 351–352
Accelerated idioventricular rhythm (AIVR), on electrocardiography, 228
Acceleration-deceleration injuries, 711
Acceleration injuries, 711
Access problems, with continuous renal replacement therapy, 570
ACE (angiotensin-converting enzyme) inhibitors, 269, 366, 408
Acebutolol, 265*t*
Acetaminophen
  intoxication by, 1100*t*, 1101*t*
    antidote for, 1100*t*
  for pain management, 51, 51*t*
Acetylcholine, as neurotransmitter, 612, 628*f*, 630
Achromatopsia, 643*t*
Acid-base balance, 544–555*t*, 554
  alterations of, 442
    in renal failure, 599–600
  anion gap and, 554–555, 556*t*

evaluating, 444
  management of
    in drug overdose/poisoning, 1096
    in renal failure, 599–600
Acid-suppressive therapy, for gastrointestinal bleeding, 801–802
Acidosis
  diabetic ketoacidosis and. *See* Diabetic ketoacidosis (DKA)
  metabolic, 443, 540*f*, 554–555*t*
  renal system, 538, 540, 540*f*
  respiratory, 442–443, 554*t*
Acid(s), 442. *See also* PH
ACLS guideline, 267, 325, 331, 407
Acoustic nerve (cranial nerve VIII), 624*t*, 649
Acoustic neuromas, 676*t*
Acquired immunodeficiency syndrome (AIDS). *See* Human immunodeficiency virus (HIV)
ACS (acute coronary syndrome), 373
ACTH (adrenocorticotropic hormone), 837, 846, 850, 860*t*
  neuroendocrine response to stress and, 863*t*
Actinic keratosis, 1010*f*
Action, nursing excellence and, 95–96
Action potentials, 612–613
Activated charcoal, for drug overdose/poisoning, 1098
Activated clotting time, normal values for, 196*t*
Activated partial thromboplastin time (aPTT), 911
  normal values for, 196*t*
Active fixation lead, for cardiac pacing, 310*b*
Active transport, renal tubular reabsorption and, 538
Activities of daily living (ADLs), dysfunction in, evaluation of, 650
Acute coagulopathy of trauma (ACOT), 1075
Acute coronary syndrome (ACS), 373
Acute Kidney Injury Network (AKIN) criteria, 584, 585*t*
Acute lymphocytic leukemia (ALL), 988
Acute myelogenous leukemia (AML), 988–989
Acute myocardial infarction (AMI), 372–487
  acute coronary syndrome, 373
  angina pectoris, 375–377. *See also* Angina pectoris
  assessment in, 379–385
    diagnostic tests in, 380
    history in, 379–380
    physical examination in, 380
  atherosclerosis and, 374–375
    pathophysiology of, 374–375
    risk factors for, 375
  cardiac rehabilitation, 391
  complications, 389–391
    acute kidney injury, 390–391
    dysrhythmia, 390
    hemodynamic, 391, 391*b*
    hyperglycemia, 391
    left ventricular free wall rupture, 389–390

    myocardial, 391*b*
    pericardial, 391*b*
    thromboembolic, 390
    ventricular septal wall rupture, 389
  infarction location and, 378
  infarction size in, 378
  infarction type and, 379
  management of, 385–389
    early, 385–386
    fibrinolytic therapy for, 386
    hemodynamic monitoring, 387
    intensive and intermediate care management, 386–389
    percutaneous coronary intervention, 385–386
    pharmacological, 387
  pathophysiology, 373–374
Acute pancreatitis (AP)
  assessment, 813–815, 815*b*
  complications
    cardiovascular, 815*b*, 816
    local, 815, 815*b*
    metabolic, 815*b*, 816
    pulmonary, 815–816, 815*b*
    renal, 815*b*, 816
  etiology, 812–813, 813*b*
  management
    fluid and electrolyte replacement, 816
    medical, 816
    nutritional support, 817
    pain management, 816–817
    surgical, 817
  pathophysiology, 813
  severity of, predicting, 814–815, 815*b*
Acute respiratory distress syndrome (ARDS)
  assessment of, 523–525
    diagnostic studies in, 525
    history in, 523–524
    physical examination in, 524–525, 524*t*
  case study of, 532
  complications, prevention of, 531, 531*b*
  diagnostic criteria for, 519–520
  etiology of, 519–520
  incidence of, 519–520, 520*b*
  management of, 525–530, 526*b*, 528*b*, 529–530*b*
    collaborative care guide for, 529–530*b*
    mechanical ventilation for, 526–527
    nutritional support for, 528–529, 529–530*b*
    oxygen delivery for, 526
    pharmacological, 527–528
    positioning and, 527, 528*b*
    sedation, 528
  outcomes and conclusion of, 531–532
  pathophysiology of, 520–523
    pathological changes and, 520–522, 520*t*, 521*f*, 522*f*
    stages of, 523, 523*t*